General Dilution Chart (m...

D1298674

Amount of Drug Required in Grams	Amount of Diluent						
	1,000 mL	500 mL	250 mL				
	mcg/mL	mcg/mL	mcg/mL	mcg/mL	mcg/mL	mcg/mL	mcg/mL
20 mg	20	40	80	160	200	400	800
19 mg						0	760
18 mg						0	720
17 mg						0	680
16 mg						0	640
15 mg						0	600
14 mg						0	560
13 mg						0	520
12 mg						0	480
11 mg						0	440
10 mg						0	400
9 mg						0	360
8 mg	8					0	320
7 mg	7	14				0	280
6 mg	6	12	24			0	240
5 mg	5	10	20	40	50	00	200
4.5 mg	4.5	9	18	36	45	90	180
4 mg	4	8	16	32	40	80	160
3.5 mg	3.5	7	14	28	35	70	140
3 mg	3	6	12	24	30	60	120
2.5 mg	2.5	5	10	20	25	50	100
2 mg	2	4	8	16	20	40	80
1.5 mg	1.5	3	6	12	15	30	60
1 mg	1	2	4	8	10	20	40
0.5 mg	0.5	1	2	4	5	10	20
0.25 mg	0.25	0.5	1	2	2.5	5	10

To use chart:
1. Find mcg/mL desired, track to amount of diluent desired and amount of drug in mg required.
2. Find amount of drug in mg required, track to diluent desired and/or mcg/mL desired.
3. Find amount of diluent required, track to amount of drug in mg and/or mcg/mL desired.

Formula: Substitute any number for X

X mg diluted in 1,000 mL = X mcg/mL (1 mg in 1,000 mL = 1 mcg/mL)
X mg diluted in 500 mL = 2 X mcg/mL (1 mg in 500 mL = 2 mcg/mL)
X mg diluted in 250 mL = 4 X mcg/mL (1 mg in 250 mL = 4 mcg/mL)
X mg diluted in 125 mL = 8 X mcg/mL (1 mg in 125 ml = 8 mcg/mL)
X mg diluted in 100 mL = 10 X mcg/mL (1 mg in 100 mL = 10 mcg/mL)
X mg diluted in 50 mL = 20 X mcg/mL (1 mg in 50 mL = 20 mcg/mL)
X mg diluted in 25 mL = 40 X mcg/mL (1 mg in 25 mL = 40 mcg/mL)

Some variation occurs from manufacturer's overfill or if the drug is in liquid form. If absolute accuracy is required, these variations can be avoided by withdrawing an amount in mL from the diluent equal to manufacturer's overfill and/or an amount equal to the amount in mL of the drug. Consult the pharmacist for specific information on manufacturer's overfill of infusion fluids used in your facility.

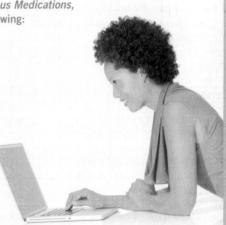

HOW TO USE THIS BOOK

STEP 1

Refer to the index at the back of the book. You can find any drug by any name in less than 5 seconds. All drugs are cross-indexed by generic and all known trade names. The index is easily distinguished by a printed blue bar at the edge of the pages. Drugs are also indexed by pharmacologic action. With one turn of the page, all drugs included in the text with similar pharmacologic actions and their page numbers are available to you. Everything is strictly alphabetized; you will never be required to refer to additional pages to locate a drug.

STEP 2

Turn to the single page number given after the name of the drug. All information about the drug is included as continuous reading. You will rarely be required to turn to another section of the book to be completely informed. Specific breakdowns of each drug (Usual Dose, Pediatric Dose, Dose Adjustments, Dilution, Compatibility, Rate of Administration, Actions, Indications and Uses, Precautions, Contraindications, Drug/Lab Interactions, Side Effects, and Antidote) are consistent in format and printed in boldface type. Subheadings under these categories are in boldface. Scan quickly for a Usual Dose check, Dose Adjustment, Drug/Lab Interaction, Side Effect, or Antidote or carefully read all included information. The choice is yours. A quick scan will take 5 to 10 seconds. Even the most complicated drugs will take less than 2 minutes to read completely. Read each monograph carefully and completely before administering a drug to a specific patient for the first time and review it any time a new drug is added to the patient's drug profile.

That's it! A fast, complete, and accurate reference for anyone administering intravenous medications. The spiral binding is specifically designed to lie flat, leaving your hands free to secure needed supplies, prepare your medication, or even ventilate a patient while you read the needed information.

Develop the "look it up" habit. Clear, concise language and simplicity of form contribute to quick, easy use of this handbook. Before your first use, read the preface; it contains lots of helpful information.

Check out the *Intravenous Medications* website for monographs no longer included in this text and for other useful IV medication information:

http://evolve.elsevier.com/IVMeds

INTRAVENOUS MEDICATIONS

A Handbook for Nurses and Health Professionals

BETTY L. GAHART, RN
Nurse Consultant in Education
Napa, California
Former Director, Education and Training
Queen of the Valley Medical Center
Napa, California

ADRIENNE R. NAZARENO, PharmD
Clinical Manager, Department of Pharmacy
Queen of the Valley Medical Center
Napa, California

MEGHAN Q. ORTEGA, RN, BSN
Staff Nurse/Home Care
Formerly of Continuum Pediatric Nursing
Chicago, Illinois

THIRTY-THIRD EDITION

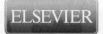

ELSEVIER

3251 Riverport Lane
St. Louis, Missouri 63043

INTRAVENOUS MEDICATIONS

ISBN: 978-0-323-29739-4

Notices

Knowledge and best practice in this field are constantly changing. As new research and experience broaden our understanding, changes in research methods, professional practices, or medical treatment may become necessary.

Practitioners and researchers must always rely on their own experience and knowledge in evaluating and using any information, methods, compounds, or experiments described herein. In using such information or methods they should be mindful of their own safety and the safety of others, including parties for whom they have a professional responsibility.

With respect to any drug or pharmaceutical products identified, readers are advised to check the most current information provided (i) on procedures featured or (ii) by the manufacturer of each product to be administered, to verify the recommended dose or formula, the method and duration of administration, and contraindications. It is the responsibility of the practitioners, relying on their own experience and knowledge of their patients, to make diagnoses, to determine dosages and the best treatment for each individual patient, and to take all appropriate safety precautions.

To the fullest extent of the law, neither the Publisher nor the authors, contributors, or editors, assume any liability for any injury and/or damage to persons or property as a matter of products liability, negligence or otherwise, or from any use or operation of any methods, products, instructions, or ideas contained in the material herein.

Previous editions copyrighted 1973, 1977, 1981, 1984, 1988, 1989, 1990, 1991, 1993, 1994, 1995, 1996, 1997, 1998, 1999, 2000, 2001, 2002, 2003, 2004, 2005, 2006, 2007, 2008, 2009, 2010, 2011, 2012, 2013, 2014, 2015, 2016

ISBN: 978-0-323-29739-4
ISSN: 1556-7443

Executive Content Strategist: Sonya Seigafuse
Senior Content Development Specialist: Billie C. Sharp
Publishing Services Manager: Jeff Patterson
Senior Project Manager: Jodi M. Willard
Design Direction: Ryan Cook

Printed in the United States of America

Last digit is the print number: 9   8   7   6   5   4   3   2   1

NURSING AND PHARMACOLOGY CONSULTANTS

KIM HUBER, PharmD
Clinical Pharmacist
Memorial Medical Center
Modesto, California

GREGORY D. NAZARENO, PharmD
Staff Pharmacist
John Muir Medical Center
Walnut Creek, California

MERRILEE NEWTON, RN, MSN
Administrative Director of Quality and
    Infection Prevention—Retired
Alta Bates Summit Medical Center
Berkeley, California;
Co-Regional Quality Director
Sutter Health East Bay

REVIEWERS

DANA H. HAMAMURA, PharmD, RPh
Clinical Pharmacist
Emergency Department
University of Colorado Hospital
Aurora, Colorado

JOSHUA J. NEUMILLER, PharmD, CDE, FASCP
Assistant Professor of Pharmacotherapy
College of Pharmacy
Washington State University
Spokane, Washington

CHRISTOPHER T. OWENS, PharmD, MPH
Associate Professor and Chair
Department of Pharmacy Practice and
    Administrative Sciences
Idaho State University College of Pharmacy
Pocatello, Idaho

RANDOLPH E. REGAL, BS, PharmD
Clinical Associate Professor
Adult Internal Medicine
University of Michigan Hospital and
    College of Pharmacy
Ann Arbor, Michigan

TRAVIS E. SONNETT, PharmD, FASCP
Clinical Pharmacy Specialist
Mann-Grandstaff VA Medical Center;
Clinical Assistant Professor
College of Pharmacy
Washington State University
Spokane, Washington

This Year 2017 edition marks the forty-fourth year of publication of *Intravenous Medications*.

In this thirty-third edition, a total of 25 new drugs approved by the FDA for intravenous use have been incorporated. They include **brivaracetam (Briviact)**, an anticonvulsant used as adjunctive therapy in the treatment of partial-onset seizures in patients 16 years of age and older with epilepsy; **cangrelor (Kengreal)**, an antiplatelet agent and adjunct to PCI; **coagulation factor X (Coagedex)**, indicated for the treatment of factor X deficiency in adult and pediatric patients; **crotalidae immune F(ab^9)$_2$ (Anavip)**, an equine-derived antivenin for the management of adult and pediatric patients with North American rattlesnake envenomation; **daratumumab (Darzalex)** and **elotuzumab (Empliciti)**, both indicated for the treatment of multiple myeloma; **defibrotide sodium (Defitelio)**, indicated for the treatment of veno-occlusive disease; **idarucizumab (Praxbind)**, indicated for the reversal of Pradaxa; **necitumumab (Portrazza)**, indicated for the treatment of metastatic squamous non–small-cell lung cancer (SNSCLC) in combination with gemcitabine and cisplatin; **obiltoxaximab (Anthim)**, indicated for the treatment of anthrax in combination with appropriate antibiotics; **reslizumab (Cinquair)**, indicated for the treatment of severe asthma; **sebelipase alfa (Kanuma)**, a treatment for lysosomal acid deficiency; **sugammadex injection (Bridion)**, indicated for the reversal of neuromuscular blockade induced by rocuronium or vecuronium; **trabectedin (Yondelis)**, indicated for the treatment of unresectable or metastatic liposarcoma or leiomyosarcoma; and, lastly, **von Willebrand factor (recombinant [Vonvendi])**, used for on-demand treatment of bleeding episodes in adults with von Willebrand disease. Eleven of these new drugs are presented in individual monographs alphabetically within the text. **Brivaracetam (Briviact)**, **crotalidae immune F(ab^9)$_2$ (Anavip)**, and **defibrotide sodium (Defitelio)** are found in Appendix E. **Sebelipase alfa (Kanuma)** is posted on the Evolve website.

Four new antihemophilic factors have been approved—**antihemophilic factor (recombinant) (Nuwiq, Kovaltry, and Kovaltry Bio-Set)**, and **antihemophilic factor (recombinant), PEGylated (Adynovate)** for the treatment of hemophilia A. These four drugs have been incorporated into the antihemophilic factor monograph. **Asparaginase *Erwinia chrysanthemi* (Erwinase)**, an antineoplastic agent, has been incorporated into the pegaspargase monograph. Two new **factor IX products (Ixinity [recombinant]** and **Idelvion [recombinant] albumin fusion protein)**, indicated for control and prevention of bleeding episodes with hemophilia B (**Ixinity** in patients 12 years of age and older, and **Idelvion** in adult and pediatric patients), have been incorporated in the factor IX monograph. **Infliximab-dyyb (Inflectra)**, a biosimilar preparation of infliximab, has been incorporated into the infliximab monograph. A new **liposomal form of irinotecan (Onivyde)** for the treatment of pancreatic cancer has been incorporated in the irinotecan monograph, and an encapsulated form of **melphalan (Evomela)** for the treatment of multiple myeloma has been incorporated into the melphalan monograph.

Many new uses have been approved for established drugs, and numerous safety issues have been identified by the FDA. All of these changes are incorporated so our readers have the most current information available.

We continually strive to make information in this handbook informative and easier to access. We continue to identify drugs with a Black Box Warning **BBW** in the main heading of the monograph. In addition, Black Box Warning statements are shaded in light gray and a different typeface is used for instant identification wherever they appear in the text. *Blue-screened text* emphasizes a special circumstance not covered by a Black Box Warning. The FDA is now identifying **Limitations of Use** of drugs under Indications. Previously this information has been placed in Precautions.

In the past, we have incorporated the Common Toxicity Criteria (CTC) provided by the U.S. Department of Health and Human Services, the National Institutes of Health, and the National Cancer Institute. This listing has been expanded and updated by these organizations and is too expansive to be included in an appendix. Web access to this material is available at **www.cancer.gov**. Search for CTCAE (Common Terminology Criteria for Adverse Events Version 4.0). Printed copies are available free of charge; call 1-800-4-CANCER (1-800-422-6237).

We are all aware that **The Joint Commission** and the **Institute for Safe Medication Practices (ISMP)** have strongly emphasized various ways to reduce errors in drug ordering and administration. One of their suggestions is to refer to a drug by both its generic and its trade name. *Intravenous Medications* is the only reference that has consistently used both names since its first publication. They also recommend that symbols (e.g., $<$, $>$, $\leq$, $\geq$,) be spelled out. **Although we have always spelled out most of them, they are now all spelled out. The only exception is in charts when there isn't room for the spelled-out version.** The symbols are included in the Key to Abbreviations (p. xviii) if you need a refresher. **Some of the other ways in which we assist with safe administration** is to spell out the word *units*, use Gm instead of gm so it is not confused with mg, use mcg instead of μg, and drop all trailing 0s (as in 1.0) to prevent overdoses. **The Joint Commission, the ISMP, the American Pharmaceutical Association, and several other organizations have identified "High-Alert Medications" (a list of medications with the highest risk of injury when misused).** The websites of these organizations contain considerable information and identify common risk factors and suggested strategies. From the authors' viewpoint, **all drugs given by the IV route should be considered high-alert medications.** They have an immediate effect, are irretrievable, and can cause life-threatening side effects with incorrect usage.

We join The Joint Commission in urging you to pay special attention to **how tubes and catheters are connected to patients.** The Joint Commission challenges the manufacturers of these devices to redesign them in ways that will make dangerous misconnection much less possible. Look up The Joint Commission suggestions. A preventive measure not mentioned by The Joint Commission is the **simple practice of labeling every line at the point of entry into the patient.** This should be done whenever more than a single piece of tubing (IV or other) is connected to a patient. Multiple-lumen catheters, 3-way stopcocks, chest tubes, nasogastric tubes, and any other tubing entering the patient should be labeled with its contents or use at the connection closest to the patient. In today's health care settings, patients frequently have multiple tubes inserted into their bodies. Correct labeling takes only a few seconds at the time of insertion and saves many moments of precious time every time the line needs to be accessed. Misconnection errors may be fatal; establish all of these suggestions as a standard of practice, and misconnection errors will be avoided.

IV solutions prepared in flexible plastic containers have generated Safety Alerts by the FDA. As a reminder: Do not hang IV infusions in flexible plastic containers **in series connection, do not pressurize** IV infusions in flexible plastic containers **to increase flow rates without first fully evacuating residual air from the container, and do not use vented IV administration sets** with IV infusions in flexible plastic containers. **All may result in air embolism.**

Elsevier offers electronic versions of *Intravenous Medications* for handheld devices, tablets, laptops, and desktop computers. These electronic versions are convenient and portable alternatives or supplements to the printed book. In addition, all drugs currently on the Evolve IV Meds website (http://evolve.elsevier.com/IVMeds) for *Intravenous Medications* (because of space limitations for the print version) are either incorporated in these electronic versions or have a direct link to them. Although the electronic versions are accessible wherever you have an electronic device, keep in mind that on some devices the entire monograph may not be visible at the same time. It is the user's responsibility to be familiar with the complete monograph and *all* aspects of each drug before administration.

Health care today is an intense environment. The speed of change is overwhelming, but the authors and publisher of *Intravenous Medications* have a commitment to provide all health care professionals who have the responsibility to administer IV medications with annual editions that incorporate complete, accurate, and current information in a clear, concise, accessible, and reliable tool. FDA websites are monitored throughout the year and provide many important updates, such as dose changes, new pediatric doses, additional disease-specific doses, refinements in dosing applications, new indications, new drug interactions, additional precautions, updates on post-marketing side effects, and new information on antidotes. Most drugs currently approved for intravenous use are included. Exceptions are opaque dyes and some radioactive therapeutic agents used in radiology, some general anesthetics used only in the OR, and a few rarely used drugs. To stay within the confines of the spiral binding, selected diagnostic agents, muscle relaxants intended for use only in the OR, and several other rarely used drugs have been moved to the Evolve IV Meds website: http://evolve.elsevier.com/IVMeds. (See p. xiii for a listing.) Helpful charts for dilution and/or rate of administration are incorporated in selected monographs. A General Dilution Chart to simplify calculations is found on the inside front cover. Front matter material provides a Key to Abbreviations and Important IV Therapy Facts.

Intravenous Medications is designed for use in critical care areas, at the nursing station, in the office, in public health and home care settings, and by students and the armed services. Pertinent information can be found in a few seconds. Take advantage of its availability and quickly review every intravenous medication before administration.

The nurse is frequently placed in a variety of difficult situations. While the physician verbally requests or writes an order, the nurse must evaluate it for appropriateness and may need to prepare it, administer it, and observe the effects. Intravenous drugs are instantly absorbed into the bloodstream, leading, it is hoped, to a prompt therapeutic action, but the risk of an inappropriate reaction is a constant threat that can easily become a frightening reality. It will be the nurse who must initiate emergency measures should adverse effects occur. This is an awesome responsibility.

If, after reviewing the information in *Intravenous Medications,* you have any questions about any order you are given, clarify it with the physician, consult the pharmacist, or consult your supervisor. The circumstances will determine whom you will approach first. If the physician thinks it is imperative to carry out an order even though you have unanswered questions, never hesitate to request that the physician administer the drug, drug combination, or dose himself or herself. In this era of constant change, the physician should be very willing to supply you, your supervisor, and/or the pharmacist with current studies documenting the validity and appropriateness of orders.

All information presented in this handbook is pertinent only to the intravenous use of the drug and not necessarily to intramuscular, subcutaneous, oral, or other means of administration.

Our sincere appreciation is extended to Gregory Nazareno, Kim Huber, and Merrilee Newton for their ongoing participation in our efforts to bring you current, accurate, and relevant information; and to Sonya Seigafuse, Billie Sharp, Charlene Ketchum, Jeff Patterson, Jodi M. Willard, and Amy Buxton at Elsevier and Joe Rekart at Graphic World, who are the editors, production staff, and design staff that make the publishing of *Intravenous Medications* happen each year.

We also wish to thank you, the users of this reference. By seeking out this information, you serve your patients' needs and contribute to the safe administration of IV meds. We will continue to strive to earn your trust and confidence as we look forward together to an exciting future for health care.

Betty L. Gahart   Adrienne R. Nazareno

Myла L. Ortega

CONTENTS

Selected Agents Not Included in the Book, *Evolve website*

Designed to facilitate quick reference, each entry begins with the generic name of the drug in boldface type. **Drugs with a Black Box Warning are identified with a symbol BBW in the main heading.** Phonetic pronunciations appear just below the generic name. Drug categories follow. The primary category may be followed by additional ones representing the multiple uses of a drug. Associated trade names are under the generic name. Boldface type and alphabetical order enable the reader to verify correct drug names easily. The use of a Canadian maple leaf symbol (🍁) after a trade name indicates availability in Canada only. The pH is listed in the lower right-hand corner of the title section. While this information is not consistently available, it is provided whenever possible. It represents the pH of the undiluted drug, the drug after reconstitution, or the drug after dilution for administration.

Headings within drug monographs are as follows:

Usual Dose: Doses recommended are the usual range for adults unless specifically stated otherwise. This information is presented first to enable the nurse to verify that the physician order is within acceptable parameters while checking the order and before preparation. If there are any questions, much time can be saved in clarifying them. If premedication is indicated, it will be noted here.

Pediatric Dose: Pediatric doses are specifically stated if they vary from mg/kg of body weight or M^2 dose recommended for adults. Not all drugs are recommended for use in children. See Maternal/Child for information on safety and effectiveness for use in pediatric patients. To prevent unintentional overdose, a premixed solution such as DUPLEX or Galaxy containers available in a specific dose (e.g., 1 Gm, 2 Gm) should be used in pediatric patients <u>only when</u> the individual dose is the entire contents of the container and not any fraction thereof.

Infant and/or Neonatal Dose: Included if available and distinct from Pediatric Dose. See Maternal/Child for information on safety and effectiveness for use in pediatric patients, including infants and neonates.

Dose Adjustments: Any situation that requires increasing or decreasing a dose is mentioned here. The range covers adjustments needed for elderly, debilitated, or hepatic or renal impairment patients; adjustments required by race or gender; or adjustments required in the presence of other medications or as physical conditions are monitored.

Dilution: Specific directions for dilution are given for all drugs if dilution is necessary or permissible. Drugs, diluents, and solutions must be appropriate for IV use. Certain medications may be available in more than one form (e.g., Advantage, Duplex); follow manufacturer's directions for reconstitution and stability. The manufacturing and approval of generics seems to be accelerating. They are usually similar to the trade version but may differ slightly, so be sure to double-check the dose and dilution requirements. Appropriate diluents are listed. The Solution Compatibility Chart on the inside back cover has been expanded and updated. Diluents that are not identified in Dilution will be listed in this chart. This is the only reference that provides calculation examples to simplify dilution and accurate dose measurement. Charts are available in selected monographs. If recommendations for pediatric dilutions are available, they are listed. In some situations mcg or mg/mL dilutions partially account for this variation. To prevent unintentional overdose, a premixed solution such as DUPLEX or Galaxy containers available in a specific dose (e.g., 1 Gm, 2 Gm) should be used in pediatric patients <u>only when</u> the individual dose is the entire contents of the container and not any fraction thereof. If there are any doubts, consult with the pharmacist and/or pediatric specialist. Generic dilution charts for grams to milligrams and milligrams to micrograms are featured on the inside front cover and facing page.

Filters: A subheading. Content here includes information included in prescribing information and information we have requested from manufacturers. Many drugs are filtered during the manufacturing process. There are numerous variations in recommendations for filtration after the manufacturing process. Filters are single-use one-way streets and are most effective when used at the last stage of mixing or dilution or in-line as administered to the patient. Most manufacturers expect that a drug distributed in an ampule will be filtered to eliminate the possibility of glass being drawn into a syringe on withdrawal of the drug. This is always a two-needle process. One process uses a standard needle to withdraw from the ampule; that needle is then replaced with a needle filter to inject the drug into the diluent. If it will not be added to a diluent, use the needle filter to withdraw from the ampule and replace it with a new standard needle to administer. When questioned, many manufacturers suggest following a specific hospital's standard, which may recommend that a drug distributed as a powder be filtered either with a needle filter on withdrawal from the vial, after reconstitution as added to the diluent, or with an in-line filter on delivery to the patient. Some acknowledge that in selected situations (e.g., open heart surgery) everything is filtered at some point before delivery to the patient. Although these responses are helpful, none of them clarify specific information about a drug. For questions, the manufacturer's pharmacist is available.

Storage: A subheading. Content here includes such items as stability, refrigeration versus room temperature, predilution versus postdilution. Newly approved generics may have slight differences; check the manufacturer's recommendations.

COMPATIBILITIES

The focus of this section is **compatibility. Any drug not listed as compatible should be considered incompatible. *Incompatibilities are listed only when specifically identified by the manufacturer. No third-party incompatibilities are listed.***

Some monographs include only general information because that is all that is available. It may include the manufacturer's recommendation to administer separately from other drugs or the potential for reaction with some plastic infusion bags or tubing. Other monographs include manufacturers' statements regarding the potential inactivation or inhibition of one drug on another.

Compatibilities listed by the manufacturer are listed first, followed by **compatibilities** listed by another source, which may be divided into **additive and Y-site. *Any drug not listed as compatible should be considered incompatible.*** Drugs are alphabetized by generic name for ease in locating the drugs with which you are working. To make identification easier, common trade names accompany generic names, or examples are presented for drug categories. No other reference consistently provides this helpful information.

Because compatibilities may be influenced by many factors (e.g., temperature, pH, concentration, time together in solution, a specific order of mixing), **it is imperative that you verify compatibilities with your pharmacist.** Knowledge is growing daily in this field, and your pharmacist should have current information on the pharmacy computer or access to extensive references. Many compatibility studies have been done by other parties for both additive and Y-site compatibilities. Almost all are based on specific concentrations, which may or may not relate to usual doses or recommended concentrations.

Occasionally sources disagree on compatibility. If there is conflicting information about a compatibility, you will be told that this is not recommended by the manufacturer, or *the individual drugs that may have a conflict will be underlined.*

What steps should you consider before administering any drug?

- If the drug you wish to administer is not listed in the **Compatibility** section, ***consider it to be incompatible.*** To administer, you must turn off the infusing IV (at the stopcock or with a clamp close to the Y-site), flush the line with a solution compatible to both drugs (and/or solutions), administer the required drug, and flush the line again before turning the previously infusing IV back on. If you are unable to discontinue the infusion IV, you must have another IV access (e.g., a multi-lumen catheter, a second IV line, or a heparin lock). Some drugs actually require separate tubing.

- If compatibilities are included in the package insert from the manufacturer, it will be so stated. If the manufacturer lists drugs as compatible by additive or Y-site and doesn't list concentrations, this is a good assurance of compatibility. If concentrations are listed, review the concentrations of both drugs to make sure they are within the defined parameters.

- If the drug you wish to administer is listed in the **Compatibility** section of the access you wish to use (e.g., **additive or Y-site**), *you must consult with the pharmacist to confirm any specific conditions that may apply.* After your consultation, write the results of your consultation regarding the specific directions for coadministering drugs on the patient's medication record or nursing care plan so others will not need to retrace your research steps when the medication is to be given again.
- When combining drugs in a solution (additives), always consider the required rate adjustments of each drug. Can each drug produce the desired effect at the suggested rate, or is continuous adjustment necessary for one drug, making the combination impractical?
- Y-site means that the specific drug in a specific monograph is compatible at its Y-site with an injection or an infusion containing one of the drugs listed under Y-site. The reverse Y-site compatibility may not be true.
- Although some drugs may be listed as compatible at the Y-site, some drugs can be administered at the Y-site only if they are further diluted in compatible solutions and given as an infusion (e.g., potassium concentrates [e.g., acetates, chlorides, phosphates], saline solution in concentrations greater than 0.9% or NS, amino acids, and dextrose solutions greater than 10% [unless in small amounts such as 50 mL dextrose 50% in insulin-induced hypoglycemia]).
- Because today's hospital units are very specialized (e.g., cancer care, emergency room, intensive coronary care, various intensive care units, transplant units, and orthopedic units to name just a few), nursing staff in each of these areas most likely administer similar combinations of drugs to their patients. *Take the initiative and research the drug combinations that are most frequently used on your unit. Then consult with the pharmacist and make your own compatibility chart for additives and Y-site (if applicable).* By creating a chart specific to your unit, you will limit the number of consults required with the pharmacist to combinations that fall outside the parameters you have researched. This approach will save time for every nurse on your unit and will give each of you the necessary compatibility information to administer the IV drug combinations specific to your unit.
- The Solution Compatibility Chart on the inside back cover has been expanded and updated. Diluents that are not identified in Dilution will be listed in this chart.

Rate of Administration: Accepted rates of administration are clearly stated. As a general rule, a slow rate is preferred. 25-gauge needles aid in giving a small amount of medication over time. Problems with rapid or slow injection rates are indicated here. Adjusted rates for infants, children, or the elderly are listed when available. Charts are available in selected monographs.

Actions: Clear, concise statements outline the origin of each drug, how it affects body systems, its length of action, and methods of excretion. If a drug crosses the placental barrier or is secreted in breast milk, it will be mentioned here if that information is available.

Indications and Uses: Uses recommended by the manufacturer are listed. **Limitations of Use** are now being identified by the manufacturer or FDA for some drugs. Unlabeled uses are stated as such.

Contraindications: Contraindications are those specifically listed by the manufacturer. Consult with the physician if an ordered drug is contraindicated for the patient. The physician may have additional historical information that alters the situation or may decide that use of the drug is indicated in a critical situation.

Precautions: The section on precautions covers many areas of information needed before injecting any drug, including Black Box warnings from the prescribing information. Most Black Box Warnings appear in this Precautions section; however, **all actual Black Box Warning statements are shaded** in light gray **and a different typeface is used** for instant identification wherever they appear in the text. The range of information in this category covers all facets not covered under specific headings. Each listing is as important as the next. To make it easier for spot checks (after reading the entire monograph), additional subdivisions are included.

Monitor: A subheading that includes information such as required prerequisites for drug administration, parameters for evaluation, and patient assessments.

Patient Education: A subheading that addresses only specific, important issues required for short-term IV use. It is expected that the health professional will always review the major points in the drug profile with any conscious patient, side effects to expect, how to cope with them, when to report them, special requirements such as the intake of extra fluids, and an overall review of what the drug does, why it is needed, and how long the patient can anticipate receiving it. Patient Medication Guides approved by the FDA are available for most drugs, and it is recommended that the patient review the Medication Guide whenever possible before beginning treatment and repeat the review as indicated.

Maternal/Child: A subheading that addresses FDA pregnancy categories (see Appendix B for a complete explanation), any known specifics affecting patients capable of conception, safety for use during lactation, safety for use in pediatric patients, and any special impact on infants and neonates.

Elderly: A subheading that is included whenever specific information impacting this patient group is available. Always consider age-related organ impairment (e.g., cardiac, hepatic, renal, insufficient bone marrow reserve), history of previous or concomitant disease or drug therapy, and route of excretion when determining dose and evaluating side effects.

Drug/Lab Interactions: Drug/drug or drug/lab interactions are listed here. To help identify these interactions more easily, **single drugs, drug categories when there are multiple drugs, and specific tests are in boldface type.** If a conflict with the patient's drug profile is noted, consult a pharmacist immediately. Increasing or decreasing the effectiveness of a drug can be a potentially life-threatening situation. Check with the lab first on drug/lab interactions; acceptable alternatives are usually available. After this consultation, notify the physician if appropriate. To facilitate recognition, common trade names accompany generic names or examples are presented for drug categories. No other reference consistently provides this helpful information.

Side Effects: In some monographs, the most common side effects may be listed first, followed by the most serious side effects. In all monographs, alphabetical order simplifies confirmation that a patient's symptom could be associated with specific drug use. Specific symptoms of overdose are listed where available or distinct from usual doses.

Post-Marketing: Post-marketing side effects reported that have not been previously recorded in the prescribing information are listed.

Antidote: Specific antidotes are listed in this section if available. In addition, specific nursing actions to reverse undesirable side effects are clearly stated—an instant refresher course for critical situations.

Within a heading there may be references to other sections within an individual monograph (e.g., see Precautions, see Monitor, see Dose Adjustments, see Maternal/Child). These references indicate additional requirements and should be consulted before administering the drug.

KEY TO ABBREVIATIONS

<	less than	CVA	cerebrovascular accident
>	more than	CVP	central venous pressure
1/4NS	one-fourth normal saline (0.2%)	D10NS	10% dextrose in normal saline
1/3NS	one-third normal saline (0.33%)	D10W	10% dextrose in water
1/2NS	one-half normal saline (0.45%)	D5/1/4NS	5% dextrose in one-quarter normal
ABGs	arterial blood gases		saline (0.2%)
ACE	angiotensin converting enzyme	D5/1/3NS	5% dextrose in one-third normal
ACT	activated coagulation time		saline (0.33%)
AF	atrial fibrillation	D5/1/2NS	5% dextrose in one-half normal saline
A/G	albumin-to-globulin ratio		(0.45%)
AIDS	acquired immunodeficiency syndrome	D5LR	5% dextrose in lactated Ringer's
ALT	(SGPT) alanine aminotransferase		solution
AMI	acute myocardial infarction	D5NS	5% dextrose in normal saline
ANC	absolute neutrophil count	D5R	5% dextrose in Ringer's solution
aPTT	activated partial thromboplastin time	D5W	5% dextrose in water
ARDS	adult respiratory distress syndrome/	DC	discontinued
	acute respiratory distress syndrome	DEHP	Diethylhexylphthalate
AST	(SGOT) aspartate aminotransferase	DIC	disseminated intravascular
AUC	area under the curve		coagulation
AV	atrioventricular	dL	deciliter(s) (100 mL)
BMD	bone mass density	DNA	deoxyribonucleic acid
BP	blood pressure	ECG	electrocardiogram
BSA	body surface area	EEG	electroencephalogram
BUN	blood urea nitrogen	ESRD	end-stage renal disease
BWFI	bacteriostatic water for injection	F	Fahrenheit
C	Celsius	GI	gastrointestinal
Ca	calcium	GFR	glomerular filtration rate
CABG	coronary artery bypass graft	Gm	gram(s)
CAD	coronary artery disease	gr	grain(s)
CAPD	continuous ambulatory peritoneal	gtt	drop(s)
	dialysis	GU	genitourinary
CBC	complete blood cell count	Hb	hemoglobin
CDAD	Clostridium difficile–associated	Hct	hematocrit
	diarrhea	HCV	hepatitis C virus
CHF	congestive heart failure	Hg	mercury
Cl	chloride	HIV	human immunodeficiency virus
CMV	cytomegalovirus	hr	hour
CNS	central nervous system	HR	heart rate
CO2	carbon dioxide	HSCT	hematopoietic stem cell transplant
COPD	chronic obstructive pulmonary disease	IBW	ideal body weight
CPK	creatine-kinase	ICU	intensive care unit
CrCl	creatinine clearance	IgA	immune globulin A
CRF	chronic renal failure	IGIV	immune globulin intravenous
CRT	controlled room temperature (20° to	ÍL	microliters, μL, mm³
	25° C [68° to 77° F])	IM	intramuscular
CSF	cerebrospinal fluid	INR	International Normalized Ratio
C/S	culture and sensitivity	IP	intrapleural
CTCAE	Common Terminology Criteria for	IU	international unit(s)
	Adverse Events	IV	intravenous

IVIG	intravenous immune globulin	**PRCA**	pure red cell aplasia
K	potassium	**PRES**	posterior reversible encephalopathy
KCl	potassium chloride		syndrome
kg	kilogram(s)	**PSVT**	paroxysmal supraventricular
L	liter(s)		tachycardia
lb	pound(s)	**PT**	prothrombin time
LDH	lactic dehydrogenase	**PTT**	partial thromboplastin time
LFT	liver function test	**PVC**	polyvinyl chloride; premature
LR	lactated Ringer's injection or solution		ventricular contraction
M	molar	**R**	Ringer's injection or solution
M²	meter squared	**RBC**	red blood cell
MAO	monoamine oxidase	**refrigerate**	temperature at 2° to 8° C (36° to
MAP	mean arterial pressure		46° F)
mcg	microgram(s)	**RNA**	ribonucleic acid
mCi	millicurie(s)	**RT**	room temperature
mEq	milliequivalent	**RTS**	room-temperature stable
Mg	magnesium	**SA**	sinoatrial
mg	milligram(s)	**SC**	subcutaneous
MI	myocardial infarction	**SIADH**	syndrome of inappropriate antidiuretic
min	minute		hormone
mL	milliliter	**SOB**	shortness of breath
mmol	millimole(s)	**SCr**	serum creatinine
mm³	cubic millimeters, μL, ÍL	**S/S**	signs and symptoms
MDRSP	multidrug-resistant *Streptococcus*	**SW or SWI**	sterile water for injection
	pneumoniae	**TEN**	toxic epidermal necrolysis
MRI	magnetic resonance imaging	**TIA**	transient ischemic attacks
Na	sodium	**TLS**	tumor lysis syndrome
NaCl	sodium chloride	**TNA**	3-in-1 combination of amino acids,
NCI	National Cancer Institute; see CTCAE		glucose, and fat emulsion
ng	nanogram (millimicrogram)	**TPN**	2-in-1 combination of amino acids and
NS	normal saline (0.9%)		glucose; total parenteral nutrition
NSAID	nonsteroidal anti-inflammatory drug	**TRALI**	transfusion-related acute lung injury
NSCLC	non–small-cell lung cancer	**TT**	thrombin time
NSR	normal sinus rhythm	μ**L**	microliters, mm³, ÍL
N/V	nausea and vomiting	**ULN**	upper limits of normal
OTC	over-the-counter	**URI**	upper respiratory infection
PAC	premature atrial contraction	**UTI**	urinary tract infection
Pao₂	arterial oxygen pressure	**VF**	ventricular fibrillation
PCA	patient-controlled analgesia	**VS**	vital signs
PCP	*Pneumocystis jiroveci* pneumonia	**VT**	ventricular tachycardia
pg	picogram	**v/v**	volume-to-volume ratio
pH	hydrogen ion concentration	**WBC**	white blood cell
PML	progressive multifocal	**WBCT**	whole blood clotting time
	leukoencephalopathy	**w/v**	weight-to-volume ratio
PO	by mouth/orally	**w/w**	weight-to-weight ratio

IMPORTANT IV THERAPY FACTS

- Read the Preface and Format and Contents sections at least once. They'll answer many of your questions and save time.

USUAL DOSE

- Doses calculated on body weight are usually based on pretreatment weight and not on edematous weight.
- Normal renal or hepatic function is usually required for drugs metabolized by these routes.
- Formula to calculate creatinine clearance (CrCl) from serum creatinine value (Cockcroft-Gault equation):

$$\text{Males: } \frac{\text{Weight in kg} \times (140 - \text{Age in years})}{72 \times \text{Serum creatinine (mg/dL)}} = \text{CrCl}$$

Females: $0.85 \times$ Male CrCl value calculated from above formula.

- Children: $\text{K} \times \dfrac{\text{Linear length or height (cm)}}{\text{SCr (mg/100 mL)}}$

  K for children >1 year of age $= 0.55$
  K for infants $= 0.45$
- Lean Body Weight (LBW)
  Males $= 50$ kg $+ 2.3$ kg for each inch over 5 feet.
  Females $= 45.5$ kg $+ 2.3$ kg for each inch over 5 feet.
  Children weighing 15 kg or less—Use actual body weight in kg.
- Formula to calculate body surface area (BSA):

$$\text{BSA (M}^2) = \sqrt{\frac{\text{Height (cm)} \times \text{Weight (kg)}}{3600}}$$

- To prevent unintentional overdose, a premixed solution such as DUPLEX or Galaxy containers available in a specific dose (e.g., 1 Gm, 2 Gm) should be used in pediatric patients <u>only when</u> the individual dose is the entire contents of the container and not any fraction thereof.

DILUTION

- Check all labels (drugs, diluents, and solutions) to confirm appropriateness for IV use.
- Sterile technique is imperative in all phases of preparation.
- Use a filter needle when withdrawing IV meds from ampules to eliminate possible pieces of glass.
- Pearls: 1 Gm in 1 Liter yields 1 mg/mL
  1 mg in 1 Liter yields 1 mcg/mL
  % of a solution equals the number of grams/100 mL
  (5% = 5 Gm/100 mL)
- Pediatric dilution: If you dilute 6.0 mg/kg in 100 mL, 1 mL/hr
  equals 1.0 mcg/kg/min
  If you dilute 0.6 mg/kg in 100 mL, 1 mL/hr
  equals 0.1 mcg/kg/min
- To prevent unintentional overdose, a premixed solution such as DUPLEX or Galaxy containers available in a specific dose (e.g., 1 Gm, 2 Gm) should be used in pediatric patients <u>only when</u> the individual dose is the entire contents of the container and not any fraction thereof.
- See charts on inside front cover.

- Do not use bacteriostatic diluents containing benzyl alcohol for neonates. May cause a fatal toxic syndrome. S/S include CNS depression, hypotension, intracranial hemorrhage, metabolic acidosis, renal failure, respiratory problems, seizures.
- Ensure adequate mixing of all drugs added to a solution.
- When combining drugs in a solution (additives), always consider the required rate adjustment of each drug.
- Examine solutions for clarity and any possible leakage.
- Frozen infusion solutions should be thawed at room temperature (25° C [77° F]) or under refrigeration. Do not force by immersion in water baths or in the microwave. All ice crystals must be melted before administration. Do not refreeze.
- Syringe prepackaging for use in specific pumps is now available for many drugs. Concentrations are often the strongest permissible, but length of delivery is accurate.
- Controlled room temperature (CRT) is considered to be 25° C (77° F). Most medications tolerate variations in temperature from 15° to 30° C (59° to 86° F).

INCOMPATIBILITIES
- Some manufacturers routinely suggest discontinuing the primary IV for intermittent infusion; usually done to avoid any possibility of incompatibility. Flushing the line before and after administration may be indicated and/or appropriate for some drugs.
- The brand of intravenous fluids or additives, concentrations, containers, rate and order of mixing, pH, and temperature all affect solubility and compatibility. Consult your pharmacist with any question, and document appropriate instructions on care plan.

TECHNIQUES
- **Do not hang** IV infusions in flexible plastic containers **in series connection, do not pressurize** IV infusions in flexible plastic containers **to increase flow rates without first fully evacuating residual air from the container, and do not use vented IV administration sets** with IV infusions in flexible plastic containers. **All may result in air embolism.**
- Confirm patency of peripheral and/or central sites. Avoid extravasation.
- Avoid accidental arterial injection; can cause gangrene.

RATE OF ADMINISTRATION
- Life-threatening reactions (time-related overdose or allergy) are frequently precipitated by a too-rapid rate of injection.
- If a common IV line is used to administer other drugs through the same IV line, flush the IV line before and after each infusion with a compatible solution (e.g., NS, D5W). When flushing before administration, be sure to flush with an amount adequate to clear the previous drug (e.g., mL of drug or mL of lumen of catheter). When flushing after administration, be sure to flush with an amount at least equal to that of the drug administered (e.g., mL of drug or mL of lumen of catheter).

PATIENT EDUCATION
- A well-informed patient is a great asset; review all appropriate drug information with every conscious patient.

SIDE EFFECTS
- Reactions may be caused by a side effect of the drug itself, allergic response, overdose, or the underlying disease process.

RESOURCES

PUBLICATIONS

The following publications have been used as a resource to assemble the information found in *Intravenous Medications*. Additional and more detailed information on drugs may be found in these publications:

American Heart Association: *Handbook of Emergency Cardiovascular Care for Health Care Providers, 2015.*

American Hospital Formulary Service Drug Information 2016, Bethesda, Md, American Society of Health-System Pharmacists (updated via website).

ASHP Publications: *Handbook on Injectable Drugs,* ed 18, 2015, American Society of Health-System Pharmacists, Inc.

Drug Facts and Comparisons, St Louis, 2016, Facts and Comparisons Division, Wolters Kluwer Health.

Lexi-Comp's Drug Information Handbook, ed 22, 2013-2014, Hudson, Ohio, American Pharmacists Association.

Elsevier Guide to Oncology Drugs and Regimens, Huntington, NY, 2006, Elsevier.

The Johns Hopkins Hospital: *The Harriet Lane Handbook,* ed 20, St Louis, 2014, Mosby.

Manufacturers' literature.

WEBSITE RESOURCES

http://www.accessdata.fda.gov/scripts/cder/drugsatfda—Drug Approvals and Updates

http://www.fda.gov/safety/medwatch/default.htm—Safety Information

http://evolve.elsevier.com/IVMeds

http://www.cancer.gov—Common Terminology Criteria for Adverse Events (CTCAE)

http://www.blackboxrx.com—A listing of all drugs with a black box warning

ABATACEPT

(a-**BAY**-ta-sept)

Antirheumatic agent

Orencia

pH 7.2 to 7.8

USUAL DOSE

Dose is based on body weight in kilograms as shown in the following chart. After the initial dose, repeat administration at 2 and 4 weeks. Administer every 4 weeks thereafter. May be used as monotherapy or concomitantly with disease-modifying antirheumatic drugs (DMARDs) other than TNF antagonists; see Contraindications and Drug Interactions. May be given by SC injection or as an IV infusion in adults; formulation and dose are different; see Indications and prescribing information.

Abatacept Adult Dosing Guidelines		
Body Weight (kg)	Dose (mg)	Number of Vials
<60 kg	500 mg	2 vials
60 to 100 kg	750 mg	3 vials
>100 kg	1,000 mg	4 vials

Patients transitioning from IV therapy to subcutaneous administration should administer the first subcutaneous dose instead of the next scheduled IV dose. Abatacept is dosed weekly in the subcutaneous regimen and may be initiated with or without an IV loading dose. If the subcutaneous regimen is initiated with an IV loading dose, determine loading dose as outlined in the previous chart. The first subcutaneous injection should be administered within a day of the IV loading dose.

PEDIATRIC DOSE

Pediatric patients 6 to 17 years of age who weigh less than 75 kg: 10 mg/kg/dose based on patient's body weight at each administration. After the initial dose, repeat administration at 2 and 4 weeks. Administer every 4 weeks thereafter.

Pediatric patients 6 to 17 years of age who weigh more than 75 kg: See Usual Dose and the Abatacept Adult Dosing Guidelines chart. Do not exceed a maximum dose of 1,000 mg.

DOSE ADJUSTMENTS

There is a trend toward a higher clearance with increasing body weight; see Usual Dose. No specific dose adjustments are required based on age or gender when corrected for body weight. ▪ Withhold therapy in patients with severe infections. ▪ The effects of renal or hepatic impairment have not been studied.

DILUTION

Using **ONLY the silicone-free disposable syringe provided** with each vial and an 18- to 21-gauge needle, reconstitute each 250-mg vial with 10 mL SWFI; final concentration is 25 mg/mL. (If reconstituted with a siliconized syringe, the solution must be discarded.) Direct stream of SWFI toward side of vial. Do not use vial if vacuum is not present. Rotate or swirl vial gently until contents have dissolved. Do not shake. After dissolution, vent vial with a needle to dissipate any foam that may be present. Solution should be clear and colorless to pale yellow. Reconstituted solution must be further diluted to 100 mL as follows: From a 100-mL infusion bag or bottle, withdraw a volume of NS equal to the volume of reconstituted abatacept solution required for the patient's dose (for 2 vials, remove 20 mL; for 3 vials, remove 30 mL; for 4 vials, remove 40 mL). Using the **same silicone-free disposable syringe provided,** slowly add the reconstituted abatacept into the infusion bag or bottle. Mix gently.

Filter: Administration through a 0.2- to 1.2-micron, nonpyrogenic, low–protein binding filter is required.

Storage: Refrigerate unopened vials at 2° to 8° C (36° to 46° F). Do not use beyond expiration date. Protect from light. Before administration, the diluted solution may be stored at RT or refrigerated; however, infusion of the diluted solution should be completed within 24 hours of reconstitution. Discard diluted solution if not administered within 24 hours. Any unused portion in a vial must be discarded.

COMPATIBILITY

Manufacturer states, "Should not be infused concomitantly in the same intravenous line with other agents." **Compatibility** studies have not been performed.

RATE OF ADMINISTRATION

Administration through a 0.2- to 1.2-micron, nonpyrogenic, low–protein binding filter is required.

A single dose equally distributed over 30 minutes.

ACTIONS

A soluble fusion protein that consists of the extracellular domain of human cytotoxic, T-lymphocyte–associated antigen 4 linked to the modified Fc portion of human immunoglobulin G1 (IgG1). Produced by recombinant DNA technology. Acts as a selective biologic response modulator by inhibiting T-lymphocyte activation, which is implicated in the pathogenesis of rheumatoid arthritis. Reduces pain and joint inflammation and slows the progression of structural damage to bone and cartilage. Mean half-life is 13.1 days (range 8 to 25 days).

INDICATIONS AND USES

Reduce the S/S, induce a major clinical response, inhibit the progression of structural damage, and improve the physical function in adult patients with moderately to severely active rheumatoid arthritis. May be used as monotherapy or concomitantly with DMARDs other than TNF antagonists. SC injection may be used in adult patients unable to receive an infusion, and/or adult infusion patients may transition to SC injection; see prescribing information. ▪ Reduce the S/S in pediatric patients 6 years of age and older with moderately to severely active polyarticular juvenile idiopathic arthritis. May be used as monotherapy or concomitantly with methotrexate.

Limitations of Use: Should not be administered concomitantly with TNF antagonists (e.g., adalimumab [Humira], etanercept [Enbrel]) or other biologic rheumatoid arthritis therapy, such as anakinra (Kineret).

CONTRAINDICATIONS

Known hypersensitivity to abatacept or any of its components (maltose, monobasic sodium phosphate). See Limitations of Use and Drug/Lab Interactions.

PRECAUTIONS

Concurrent use with a TNF antagonist (e.g., adalimumab [Humira], etanercept [Enbrel]) is associated with an increased risk of infections with no associated increased efficacy when compared with use of the TNF antagonist alone. Concurrent use is not recommended; see Contraindications and Drug/Lab Interactions. ▪ Hypersensitivity reactions, including anaphylaxis, have been reported and can occur after the first infusion. Emergency medical equipment and medications for treating these reactions must be readily available. ▪ Serious infections, including sepsis and pneumonia, have been reported; some have been fatal. Patients receiving concomitant immunosuppressive therapy may be at increased risk. ▪ Use caution in patients with a history of recurrent infections, underlying conditions that may predispose them to infections, or chronic, latent, or localized infections; see Monitor. ▪ Antirheumatic therapies have been associated with hepatitis B reactivation. Screening for viral hepatitis should be done before starting therapy with abatacept. Patients who screened positive for hepatitis were excluded from clinical studies. ▪ Use with caution in patients with COPD. May be at increased risk for developing respiratory adverse events (e.g., COPD exacerbation, cough, dyspnea, rhonchi). ▪ A small number of patients have developed binding antibodies to abatacept. No correlation of antibody development to clinical response or adverse events has been observed. ▪ T-cells mediate cellular immune responses. Therefore drugs that inhibit T-cell activation, including abatacept, may affect patient defenses against infection and malignancies. The impact of abatacept on the development and course of malignancies is not fully understood. ▪ See Maternal/Child.

Monitor: Evaluate patients for latent tuberculosis (TB) with a TB skin test. Patients testing positive in TB screening should be treated with a standard TB regimen before initiating therapy with abatacept. ▪ Screening for viral hepatitis is recommended before initiating therapy with abatacept; virus may reactivate with abatacept treatment. ▪ Monitor for S/S of infection, especially if transitioning patient from TNF antagonist therapy to therapy with abatacept. Discontinue therapy if a serious infection develops. ▪ Monitor COPD patients for worsening of respiratory status. ▪ Monitor for S/S of hypersensitivity or infusion-related reactions; see Side Effects. ▪ Do not administer live virus vaccines during or within 3 months of use. ▪ See Precautions and Drug/Lab Interactions.

Patient Education: Read manufacturer's patient information sheet before each infusion. ▪ Review medication list and vaccination status with physician; see Precautions. ▪ Report S/S of allergic reaction (e.g., rash, itching, wheezing), infusion reaction (e.g., dizziness, headache), or infection promptly. Discuss previous infections, current infections, or exposure to TB.

Maternal/Child: Category C: safety for use in pregnancy has not been established. Has been shown to cross the placenta in animal studies. Use caution. ▪ Discontinue breast-feeding. ▪ A pregnancy registry has been established; contact manufacturer. ▪ Safety and effectiveness for use in pediatric patients under 6 years of age not established. ▪ Safety and effectiveness for uses other than juvenile idiopathic arthritis in pediatric patients have not been established. ▪ Safety and effectiveness of subcutaneous injection is not known in patients under 18 years of age. ▪ Patients with juvenile idiopathic arthritis should be brought up-to-date with all immunizations before initiating therapy with abatacept.

Elderly: Specific differences in safety and efficacy not noted. Incidence of infection and malignancy is higher in the elderly. Use caution; see Precautions.

DRUG/LAB INTERACTIONS
Formal drug interaction studies have not been conducted. ▪ Has been used with methotrexate, NSAIDs (e.g., naproxen [Naprosyn, Aleve], ibuprofen [Motrin, Advil]), corticosteroids (e.g., prednisone), azathioprine, chloroquine (Aralen), gold (Myochrysine), hydroxychloroquine (Plaquenil), leflunomide (Arava), and sulfasalazine (Azulfidine). ▪ Methotrexate, NSAIDs, corticosteroids, and TNF antagonists do not appear to influence abatacept clearance. ▪ Concurrent use with a **TNF antagonist** (e.g., adalimumab [Humira], etanercept [Enbrel], infliximab [Remicade]) is associated with an increased risk of serious infections and no significant additional efficacy over use of the TNF antagonist alone. Concurrent use is not recommended. ▪ With the IV formulation, falsely elevated blood glucose readings may occur on the day of the infusion with **specific blood glucose monitoring systems** that react to drug products containing maltose. IV formulation contains maltose; SC formulation does not contain maltose; see prescribing information. ▪ Safety and efficacy of concurrent use with **anakinra** (Kineret) has not been established. Concurrent use is not recommended. ▪ **Live virus vaccines** should not be given concurrently with or within 3 months of abatacept. ▪ May blunt the effectiveness of some **vaccinations.**

SIDE EFFECTS
In adult and pediatric patients, side effects are similar in type and frequency. The most commonly reported side effects are headache, nasopharyngitis, nausea, and upper respiratory tract infections. The most serious adverse effects are infections and malignancies. Infections are the most likely adverse event to cause interruption or discontinuation of therapy. Acute infusion-related reactions (cough, dyspnea, dizziness, flushing, headache, hypertension, hypotension, nausea, pruritus, rash, urticaria, wheezing) have been reported and usually occur within 1 hour of the infusion. Hypersensitivity reactions (anaphylaxis [rare], dyspnea, hypotension, urticaria) have been reported, usually within

24 hours of infusion. Other reactions include back or extremity pain, COPD exacerbation, dyspepsia, immunogenicity (antibody formation), and rhonchi.

Post-Marketing: Vasculitis (including cutaneous vasculitis and leukocytoclastic vasculitis).

ANTIDOTE

Notify physician of any side effects; most will be treated symptomatically. During clinical studies, most infusion-related reactions were mild to moderate, and therapy was discontinued in very few patients. Discontinue abatacept for any serious reaction or infection. Therapy may need to be interrupted in patients who develop infections. Treat infusion and hypersensitivity reactions as indicated (e.g., oxygen, diphenhydramine, epinephrine, corticosteroids, vasopressors, and/or fluids). Resuscitate as necessary.

ABCIXIMAB	Antiplatelet agent
(ab-**SIX**-ih-mab)	Antithrombotic
	Monoclonal antibody
ReoPro	**pH 7.2**

USUAL DOSE

Administered concomitantly with heparin and aspirin as described in Clinical Studies; see prescribing information.

Percutaneous coronary intervention: 0.25 mg/kg as an IV bolus administered 10 to 60 minutes before percutaneous coronary intervention (PCI). Follow with a continuous infusion of 0.125 mcg/kg/min (weight adjusted) to a maximum of 10 mcg/min (non–weight adjusted) for 12 hours.

Unstable angina not responding to conventional medical therapy with planned PCI within 24 hours: 0.25 mg/kg as an IV bolus followed by an 18- to 24-hour continuous infusion of 10 mcg/min. Discontinue abciximab 1 hour after the PCI.

Based on an integrated analysis of data from all studies, the following guidelines may be used to minimize the risk for bleeding:

- When abciximab is initiated 18 to 24 hours before PCI, the aPPT should be maintained between 60 and 85 seconds during the abciximab and heparin infusion period.
- During PCI, the ACT should be maintained between 200 and 300 seconds.
- If anticoagulation is continued in these patients following PCI, the aPTT should be maintained between 55 and 75 seconds.

DILUTION

Available in 5-mL vials (2 mg/mL). Solution must be clear. Must be filtered with a nonpyrogenic, low–protein binding, 0.2- or 5-micron filter before administering the bolus and a 0.2- or 0.22-micron filter before administering the infusion; see Filters. Filtering of the infusion may be done during preparation or at administration, using the appropriate in-line filter. Do not shake.

IV injection: Bolus injection may be given undiluted.

Infusion: Withdraw desired dose and further dilute with NS or D5W (5 mL [10 mg] diluted with 250 mL NS or D5W equals 40 mcg/mL).

Filters: Must be filtered before administering the bolus and the infusion. Bolus may be given using a sterile, nonpyrogenic, low–protein binding, 0.2- or 5-micron syringe filter. Filtering of the infusion may be done during preparation using a sterile, nonpyrogenic, low–protein binding, 0.2- or 5-micron syringe filter or at administration using an in-line, sterile, nonpyrogenic, low–protein binding, 0.2- or 0.22-micron filter; see Dilution.

Storage: Refrigerate before use. Do not freeze. Check expiration date on vial. Contains no preservative; discard any unused portion.

COMPATIBILITY

Consider any drug NOT listed as compatible to be INCOMPATIBLE until consulting a pharmacist; specific conditions may apply.

According to the manufacturer, no **incompatibilities** have been shown with IV fluids or commonly used cardiovascular drugs; however, administration through a separate IV line and not mixing with other medications is recommended. No **incompatibilities** observed with glass bottles or polyvinyl chloride bags and administration sets.

One source suggests the following **compatibilities:**

Y-site: Adenosine (Adenocard), argatroban, atropine, bivalirudin (Angiomax), diphenhydramine (Benadryl), fentanyl, metoprolol (Lopressor), midazolam (Versed).

RATE OF ADMINISTRATION

IV injection: An initial dose as a bolus injection; filtration required.

Infusion: See Usual Dose. Must be administered through an in-line, nonpyrogenic, low-protein binding filter (0.2 or 0.22 microns), if not done during preparation, and controlled by a continuous infusion pump. A 40-mcg/mL solution (10 mg in 250 mL) at a rate of 10.5 mL/hr will deliver 7 mcg/min, and 15 mL/hr will deliver 10 mcg/min. Discard unused portion at the end of the infusion.

ACTIONS

The fab fragment of the chimeric human-murine monoclonal antibody, abciximab binds to the glycoprotein GPIIb/IIIa receptor of human platelets and produces rapid dose-dependent inhibition of platelet function. It inhibits platelet aggregation by preventing the binding of fibrinogen, von Willebrand factor, and other adhesive molecules to GPIIb/IIIa receptor sites on activated platelets. Also binds to the vitronectin receptor found on platelets and on the endothelial and smooth muscle cells of the vessel wall. The vitronectin receptor mediates the procoagulant properties of platelets and the proliferative properties of vascular endothelial and smooth muscle cells. Onset of action is rapid, reducing platelet aggregation to less than 20% of baseline within 10 minutes. Inhibition of platelet function is temporary following a bolus dose, but can be sustained at greater than 80% by continuous IV infusion. Has prevented acute thrombosis and resulted in lower rates of thrombosis as compared to aspirin and/or heparin. Initial half-life is 10 minutes. Second phase half-life is 30 minutes. After the infusion is ended, platelet function generally recovers gradually over 48 hours. In most patients, bleeding time returns to less than 12 minutes within 12 to 24 hours. Some abciximab remains in the circulation for 15 days or more.

INDICATIONS AND USES

An adjunct to PCI for the prevention of cardiac ischemic complications in patients undergoing PCI and in patients with unstable angina not responding to conventional medical therapy when PCI is planned within 24 hours. Safety and effectiveness of abciximab use in patients not undergoing PCI have not been established. Used concurrently with aspirin and heparin.

CONTRAINDICATIONS

Active internal bleeding, administration of oral anticoagulants (e.g., warfarin [Coumadin]) within 7 days unless PT is at or less than 1.2 times control, aneurysm, arteriovenous malformation, bleeding diathesis, clinically significant GI or GU bleeding within 6 weeks, history of CVA within 2 years, history of CVA with significant residual neurologic deficit, history of vasculitis (presumed or documented), hypertension (severe and uncontrolled), intracranial neoplasm, known hypersensitivity to any component of abciximab or to murine proteins, major surgery or trauma within 6 weeks, thrombocytopenia (less than 100,000/mm^3), or the use of IV dextran before PCI or intent to use it during PCI.

PRECAUTIONS

Administered only in the hospital under the direction of a physician knowledgeable in its use and with appropriate diagnostic, laboratory, and surgical facilities available. ▪ May cause major bleeding complications (e.g., retroperitoneal bleeding, spontaneous GI and GU bleeding, bleeding at the arterial access site). Fatalities have occurred. ▪ Risk of bleeding may be minimized by using weight-adjusted dosing of abciximab and low-dose weight-adjusted doses of heparin, with adherence to stricter anticoagulation guidelines, careful vascular access site management, discontinuation of heparin after the procedure, and early sheath removal. ■ Incidence of major bleeding is increased in patients receiving heparin, other anticoagulants, or thrombolytics (e.g., alteplase [tPA], reteplase [r-PA], streptokinase). Consider if benefits will outweigh risks, and proceed with extreme caution if use is considered necessary. ■ Incidence of major bleeding is also increased if PCI occurs within 12 hours of the onset of symptoms of an acute MI, if the PCI procedure is prolonged (lasting more than 70 minutes), or if PCI procedure fails. ■ Extreme care must be taken in accessing the femoral artery for femoral sheath placement. Only the anterior wall of the femoral artery should be punctured (avoid a Seldinger [through and through technique] for obtaining sheath access). ■ Avoid femoral vein sheath placement if possible. ■ Hypersensitivity reactions, including anaphylaxis, can occur at any time (a protein solution). Emergency drugs and equipment must always be available. ■ Thrombocytopenia, including severe thrombocytopenia, has been reported. Usually seen within the first 24 hours of abciximab administration. ■ Administration may result in the formation of human antichimeric antibody (HACA). Can cause hypersensitivity reactions including anaphylaxis, thrombocytopenia, or diminished benefit if abciximab is readministered at another time or other monoclonal antibodies are administered. Incidence and severity of thrombocytopenia may be increased with readministration. ■ See Drug/Lab Interactions.

Monitor: Before initiating, obtain results of baseline CBC, platelet count, PT, ACT, and aPTT. Type and cross-match would also be appropriate. ■ Monitor heparin anticoagulation (ACT or aPTT) and PT closely. ■ While a femoral sheath is in place, the patient must be on strict bed rest, head of the bed should be less than 30 degrees, and the appropriate limb(s) restrained in a straight position. Monitor sheath insertion site(s) and distal pulses of affected leg(s) frequently while sheath is in place and for 6 hours after removal. Measure any hematoma and monitor for enlargement. ■ Monitor platelet count 2 to 4 hours following the bolus dose and at 24 hours or before discharge, whichever is first. More frequent monitoring may be indicated. ■ Monitor patient carefully and frequently for signs of bleeding; take vital signs (avoiding automatic BP cuffs); observe any invaded sites at least every 15 minutes (e.g., sheaths, IV sites, cutdowns, punctures, Foleys, NGs); watch for hematuria, hematemesis, hemoptysis, bloody stool, petechiae, hematoma, flank pain, muscle weakness; and do neuro checks every hour. Continue until clotting functions move toward normal. ■ Use care in handling patient; avoid arterial puncture, venipuncture, and IM injection. Use extreme precautionary methods and only compressible sites if these procedures are absolutely necessary. Apply pressure for 30 minutes to any invaded site and then apply pressure dressings. Saline or heparin locks are suggested to facilitate blood draws. ■ Minimize use of urinary catheters, nasotracheal intubation, nasogastric tubes, and automatic blood pressure cuffs. Discontinue heparin after PCI and remove sheath no sooner than 2 hours and no later than 6 hours after heparin is discontinued (aPTT must be at or less than 50 seconds or ACT at or less than 175 seconds). After removal, apply pressure to the femoral artery for at least 30 minutes. When hemostasis is confirmed, apply a pressure dressing. Maintain strict bed rest for at least 6 to 8 hours after sheath removal and/or abciximab is discontinued or 4 hours after heparin is discontinued, whichever is later. ■ Throughout process medicate as needed for back or groin pain and nausea or vomiting. ■ Remove pressure dressing before ambulation. ■ In the event of serious, uncontrolled bleeding or the need for emergency surgery, discontinue abciximab. Platelet function may be partly restored with platelet transfusions. ■ See Precautions, Drug/Lab Interactions, and Antidote.

Patient Education: Compliance with all measures to minimize bleeding (e.g., strict bed rest, positioning) is imperative. ■ Avoid use of razors, toothbrushes, and other sharp items. ■ Use caution while moving to avoid excessive bumping. ■ Report all episodes of bleeding and apply local pressure if indicated. ■ Expect oozing from IV sites.

Maternal/Child: Category C: use only if clearly needed and with extreme caution. ▪ Safety for use during breast-feeding not established. Not known if it is secreted in breast milk; use extreme caution; probably best to postpone breast-feeding until bleeding time approaches normal. ▪ Safety and effectiveness for use in pediatric patients not established. **Elderly:** No overall difference in safety or efficacy observed in patients between 65 and 75 years of age as compared with younger patients. Insufficient data to determine whether patients age 75 or older respond differently. ▪ Increased risk of major bleeding complications if weight less than 75 kg; see Precautions. ▪ Consider age-related organ impairment, concomitant disease, or drug therapy; may also increase risk of bleeding.

DRUG/LAB INTERACTIONS

Formal drug interaction studies have not been conducted. ▪ Use with extreme caution with other drugs that affect hemostasis (e.g., **thrombolytics** [e.g., alteplase (tPA), streptokinase], **anticoagulants** [e.g., heparin, warfarin (Coumadin)], **NSAIDs** [e.g., ibuprofen (Advil, Motrin), naproxen (Aleve, Naprosyn)], **platelet aggregation inhibitors** [e.g., clopidogrel (Plavix), dipyridamole (Persantine), ticlopidine (Ticlid)] and **other glycoprotein GPIIb/IIIa receptor antagonists** [e.g., eptifibatide (Integrilin), tirofiban (Aggrastat)], **and selected antibiotics** [e.g., cefotetan]). ▪ **Dextran solutions** increased the risk of major bleeding events when used concurrently with abciximab; see Contraindications. ▪ **HACA titer** may precipitate an acute hypersensitivity reaction with other **diagnostic or therapeutic monoclonal antibodies** (e.g., muromonab-CD3). ▪ Has been administered to patients with ischemic heart disease treated concomitantly with heparin, warfarin, beta-adrenergic receptor blockers (e.g., metoprolol [Lopressor]), calcium channel antagonists (e.g., diltiazem [Cardizem]), angiotensin-converting enzyme inhibitors (e.g., enalapril [Vasotec]), nitrates, ticlopidine (Ticlid), and aspirin.

SIDE EFFECTS

May cause major bleeding incidents (e.g., femoral artery or other access site, intracranial hemorrhage, spontaneous gross hematuria and other GU bleeds, spontaneous hematemesis and other GI bleeds, pulmonary alveolar hemorrhage, retroperitoneal bleeding). Decreases in hemoglobin greater than 5 Gm/dL or intracranial hemorrhage were defined as major during trials. Thrombocytopenia is common and may require platelet transfusion. Abdominal pain, back pain, bradycardia, chest pain, headache, hypotension, nausea, peripheral edema, positive HACA response, hypersensitivity reactions (including anaphylaxis), puncture site pain, and vomiting may occur. Other side effects that may occur are anemia, arrhythmias (e.g., atrial fibrillation/flutter, bradycardia, complete AV block, supraventricular tachycardia, ventricular PVCs, tachycardia, or fibrillation), confusion, hyperesthesia, intermittent claudication, leukocytosis, limb embolism, pericardial effusion, pleural effusion or pleurisy, pneumonia, pulmonary edema, pulmonary embolism, and visual disturbances.

ANTIDOTE

Stop the infusions of abciximab and heparin if any serious bleeding not controllable with pressure occurs. Stop infusion in patients with failed PCI. Stop infusion if a hypersensitivity reaction occurs. Treat hypersensitivity reactions as indicated; may require epinephrine, airway management, oxygen, IV fluids, antihistamines (e.g., diphenhydramine [Benadryl]), corticosteroids (e.g., hydrocortisone sodium succinate [Solu-Cortef]), and pressor amines (e.g., dopamine). Keep physician informed. If an acute platelet decrease occurs (less than 100,000/mm^3 or a decrease of at least 25% from pretreatment value), obtain additional platelet counts in separate tubes containing ethylenediaminetetraacetic acid (EDTA), citrate, and heparin. This is to exclude pseudothrombocytopenia due to anticoagulant interaction. If true thrombocytopenia is verified, discontinue abciximab immediately. Platelet transfusions may be required. Heparin and aspirin should also be avoided if the platelet count drops below 60,000/mm^3.

ACETAMINOPHEN BBW

(ah-**SEAT**-ah-**MIN**-oh-fen)

Ofirmev

Antipyretic
Analgesic

pH 5.5

USUAL DOSE

May be given as a single or repeated dose. Minimum dosing interval is 4 hours. No dose adjustment is necessary when converting from oral to IV dosing.

Care must be taken to avoid dosing errors, which could result in accidental overdose and death. In particular, be careful to ensure that:

- Dose in milligrams and milliliters is not confused
- Dosing is based on weight for patients under 50 kg
- Infusion pump is programmed properly
- Maximum single dose and the maximum total daily dose of acetaminophen from all sources (i.e., IV, oral, and rectal) and all products containing acetaminophen do not exceed maximum limits.

Summary of Acetaminophen Dosing in Adults and Adolescents				
Age-Group	Dose Given q 4 hr	Dose Given q 6 hr	Maximum Single Dose	Maximum Total Daily Dose of Acetaminophen (By All Routes)
Adults and adolescents (13 years and older) weighing ≥50 kg	650 mg	1,000 mg	1,000 mg	4,000 mg in 24 hr
Adults and adolescents (13 years and older) weighing <50 kg	12.5 mg/kg	15 mg/kg	15 mg/kg	75 mg/kg in 24 hr (up to 3,750 mg)

PEDIATRIC DOSE

Pediatric patients 2 to 12 years of age: 15 mg/kg every 6 hours or 12.5 mg/kg every 4 hours. Do not exceed a maximum single dose of 15 mg/kg or a maximum daily dose of 75 mg/kg/day. See comments under Usual Dose.

DOSE ADJUSTMENTS

A reduced total daily dose of acetaminophen may be appropriate in patients with hepatic impairment or active liver disease. ■ A reduced total daily dose and longer dosing intervals may be appropriate in patients with a CrCl less than or equal to 30 mL/min.

DILUTION

Available in a single-use vial containing 1,000 mg/100 mL (10 mg/mL) of acetaminophen. For adults and adolescent patients weighing 50 kg or more requiring a 1,000-mg dose, administer the dose by inserting a vented intravenous set through the septum of the 100-mL vial. Doses less than 1,000 mg should be withdrawn from the vial and placed into a separate empty container before administration to avoid inadvertent administration of an overdose. Withdraw appropriate dose (650 mg or weight-based) from 100-mL vial and place in an empty container (e.g., syringe, glass bottle, plastic intravenous container) for intravenous infusion.

Filter: Information not available.

Storage: Store unopened vial at CRT. Do not refrigerate or freeze. Discard 6 hours after entry into vial or transfer into an empty container. Single-use vial. Discard any unused solution.

COMPATIBILITY

Manufacturer states, "Do not add other medications to solution. **Incompatible** with diazepam and chlorpromazine. Do not administer simultaneously."

One source suggests the following **compatibilities.**

Solutions: D5W, NS.

Y-site: Buprenorphine (Buprenex), butorphanol (Stadol), cefoxitin (Mefoxin), ceftriaxone (Rocephin), clindamycin (Cleocin), D5LR, D5NS, D10W, dexamethasone (Decadron), diphenhydramine (Benadryl), dolasetron (Anzemet), droperidol (Inapsine), fentanyl, granisetron (Kytril), heparin, hydrocortisone sodium succinate (Solu-Cortef), hydromorphone (Dilaudid), ketorolac (Toradol), lidocaine, lorazepam (Ativan), LR, mannitol (Osmitrol), meperidine (Demerol), methylprednisolone sodium succinate (Solu-Medrol), metoclopramide (Reglan), midazolam (Versed), morphine, nalbuphine, ondansetron (Zofran), piperacillin/tazobactam (Zosyn), potassium chloride, prochlorperazine (Compazine), ranitidine (Zantac), sufentanil (Sufenta), vancomycin.

RATE OF ADMINISTRATION

Administer as an infusion, equally distributed over 15 minutes. Pediatric doses up to 600 mg may be drawn up into a syringe and delivered via a syringe pump.

ACTIONS

A nonsalicylate antipyretic and a nonopioid analgesic agent. Exact mechanism of action is unknown but is thought to act through central actions. Widely distributed into most tissues except fat. Low protein binding (10% to 25%). Half-life is approximately 2 to 3 hours. Metabolized in the liver via three different pathways. Metabolites excreted in the urine.

INDICATIONS AND USES

Management of mild to moderate pain. ▪ Management of moderate to severe pain with adjunctive opioid analgesics. ▪ Reduction of fever.

CONTRAINDICATIONS

Known hypersensitivity to acetaminophen or to any components of the IV formulation. ▪ Patients with severe hepatic impairment or severe active liver disease.

PRECAUTIONS

Acetaminophen has been associated with cases of acute liver failure, at times resulting in liver transplant and death. Most cases of liver injury are associated with the use of acetaminophen at doses that exceed the maximum daily limits and often involve more than one acetaminophen-containing product. Do not exceed the maximum recommended daily dose. ▪ Use with caution in patients with hepatic impairment or active hepatic disease, alcoholism, chronic malnutrition, severe hypovolemia (e.g., due to dehydration or blood loss), or severe renal impairment (CrCl less than or equal to 30 mL/min). ▪ Serious skin reactions such as acute generalized exanthematous pustulosis, Stevens-Johnson syndrome, and toxic epidermal necrolysis have been reported rarely. ▪ Hypersensitivity and anaphylactic reactions have been reported. ▪ Care must be taken when prescribing, preparing, or administering acetaminophen to avoid dosing errors, which could result in accidental overdose and death; see Usual Dose. ▪ Antipyretic effects may mask fever in patients treated for postsurgical pain.

Monitor: Monitor for S/S of hypersensitivity reaction (e.g., respiratory distress; pruritus; rash; swelling of the face, mouth, and throat; urticaria). ▪ Monitor for S/S of serious skin reactions. ▪ Baseline SCr and liver function tests may be indicated.

Maternal/Child: Category C: epidemiologic data on oral acetaminophen use in pregnant women show no increased risk of major congenital malformations. Safety of IV formulation for use in pregnancy not established. Use only if clearly needed. ▪ Assess benefit versus risk before use during labor and delivery. ▪ Safety for use in breast-feeding not established. Acetaminophen is secreted in human milk in small quantities after oral administration. Use caution. ▪ Safety and effectiveness for treatment of acute pain or fever has not been studied in pediatric patients less than 2 years of age.

Elderly: No overall differences in safety and efficacy were observed between older and younger patients, but greater sensitivity of some older individuals cannot be ruled out.

DRUG/LAB INTERACTIONS

Substances that induce or regulate hepatic cytochrome enzyme CYP2E1 (e.g., ethanol, isoniazid) may alter the metabolism of acetaminophen and increase its hepatotoxic potential. Effects have not been studied. ▪ Ethanol may induce hepatic cytochromes and may act as a competitive inhibitor of the metabolism of acetaminophen. ▪ Chronic acetaminophen doses of 4,000 mg/day may cause an increase in INR in patients stabilized on **warfarin**. Effect of short-term use on INR has not been studied. Monitoring of INR recommended. ▪ **Many available analgesics contain acetaminophen in combination with another analgesic** (e.g., hydrocodone/acetaminophen [Vicodin, Norco], oxycodone/acetaminophen [Percocet]). **Over-the-counter cold and allergy preparations** may also contain acetaminophen in combination with other active ingredients. Monitor total daily dose of acetaminophen coming from all possible sources.

SIDE EFFECTS

Adult patients: The most common adverse reactions were headache, insomnia, nausea, and vomiting. Less frequently reported side effects included anxiety, dyspnea, fatigue, hypersensitivity reaction, hypertension, hypokalemia, hypotension, increased aspartate aminotransferase, infusion site pain, muscle spasms, peripheral edema, and trismus.

Pediatric patients: The most common adverse reactions were agitation, atelectasis, constipation, nausea, pruritus, and vomiting. Less commonly reported side effects included abdominal pain, anemia, diarrhea, fever, headache, hypersensitivity reaction, hypertension, hypervolemia, hypoalbuminemia, hypokalemia, hypomagnesemia, hypophosphatemia, hypotension, hypoxia, increased hepatic enzymes, injection site pain, insomnia, muscle spasm, oliguria, pain in extremities, periorbital edema, peripheral edema, pleural effusion, pulmonary edema, rash, stridor, tachycardia, and wheezing.

Overdose: Hepatic necrosis, renal tubular necrosis, hypoglycemic coma, and thrombocytopenia.

Post-Marketing: Hypersensitivity and anaphylaxis (e.g., respiratory distress; pruritus; rash; swelling of the face, mouth, and throat; urticaria).

ANTIDOTE

Notify the physician of significant side effects. Discontinue immediately at the first appearance of skin rash or any other sign of hypersensitivity. Treat as indicated (e.g., diphenhydramine, epinephrine, albuterol). Resuscitate as necessary. If an acetaminophen overdose is suspected, obtain a serum acetaminophen level and baseline liver function studies. *N*-acetylcysteine antidote may be indicated. See acetylcysteine monograph. Contact a regional poison control center for additional information.

ACETAZOLAMIDE SODIUM
(ah-set-ah-**ZOE**-la-myd **SO**-dee-um)

Antiglaucoma
Anticonvulsant
Diuretic
Urinary alkalinizer

Diamox   pH 9.2

USUAL DOSE
Antiglaucoma agent: 250 mg to 1 Gm/24 hr. May be given as 250-mg doses at 4- to 6-hour intervals. In the treatment of secondary glaucoma and in the preoperative treatment of some cases of acute congestive (closed-angle) glaucoma, the preferred dose is 250 mg every 4 hours. In acute cases, to rapidly lower intraocular pressure, an initial single dose of 500 mg followed by 125 to 250 mg at 4-hour intervals may be given.

Edema of congestive heart failure or drug therapy: 250 to 375 mg or 5 mg/kg of body weight as a single dose daily; when loss of edematous fluid stops, reduce to every other day or give for 2 days followed by a day of rest.

Anticonvulsant: *Adults and pediatric patients:* Dose in epilepsy may range from 8 to 30 mg/kg/24 hr in divided doses every 6 to 12 hours (2 to 7.5 mg/kg every 6 hours or 4 to 15 mg/kg every 12 hours). Reduce initial daily dose when given with other anticonvulsants.

Urinary alkalinization: *Adults and pediatric patients:* 5 mg/kg/dose every 8 to 12 hours.

PEDIATRIC DOSE
See Maternal/Child.

Acute antiglaucoma agent: 5 to 10 mg/kg every 6 hours. Do not exceed 1,000 mg/24 hr.

Edema of congestive heart failure or drug therapy: 5 mg/kg as a single dose daily or every other day; see comment under Usual Dose. Do not exceed 1,000 mg/24 hr.

Slowly progressive hydrocephalus in infants 2 weeks to 10 months (unlabeled): 20 mg/kg/24 hr in equally divided doses every 8 hours (8.3 mg/kg every 8 hours). Up to 100 mg/kg/24 hr or a maximum dose of 2 Gm/24 hr has been used.

DOSE ADJUSTMENTS
Reduced dose required when introducing acetazolamide into a treatment regimen with other anticonvulsants. ■ Administer every 12 hours in patients with a CrCl from 10 to 50 mL/min. Avoid use in patients with a CrCl less than 10 mL/min (ineffective).

DILUTION
Each 500 mg should be diluted in 5 mL SWFI. May then be given by IV injection or added to standard IV fluids. IM administration not recommended.

Storage: Reconstituted solution stable for 12 hours at RT or 3 days refrigerated.

COMPATIBILITY   (Underline Indicates Conflicting Compatibility Information)
Consider any drug NOT listed as compatible to be INCOMPATIBLE until consulting a pharmacist; specific conditions may apply.
One source suggests the following **compatibilities:**

Additive: Ranitidine (Zantac).

Y-site: Diltiazem (Cardizem).

RATE OF ADMINISTRATION
500 mg or fraction thereof over at least 1 minute or added to IV fluids to be given over 4 to 8 hours.

ACTIONS
A potent carbonic anhydrase inhibitor and nonbacteriostatic sulfonamide, acetazolamide depresses the tubular reabsorption of sodium, potassium, and bicarbonate. Excreted unchanged in the urine, producing diuresis, alkalinization of the urine, and a mild degree of metabolic acidosis.

INDICATIONS AND USES

Adjunctive treatment of edema due to congestive heart failure, drug-induced edema, centrencephalic epilepsies (petit mal, unlocalized seizures), chronic simple (open-angle) glaucoma, and secondary glaucoma, and preoperatively in acute angle-closure glaucoma when delay of surgery is desired to lower intraocular pressure. ▪ Used orally for acute mountain sickness.

Unlabeled uses: Metabolic alkalosis, urine alkalinization, respiratory stimulant in COPD.

CONTRAINDICATIONS

Depressed sodium and potassium levels, hyperchloremic acidosis, marked kidney or liver disease, adrenocortical insufficiency, hypersensitivity to acetazolamide or any of its components. Long-term use contraindicated in some glaucomas.

PRECAUTIONS

Chemically related to sulfonamides; may cause serious reactions in sensitive patients. ▪ May be alternated with other diuretics to achieve maximum effect. ▪ Greater diuretic action is achieved by skipping a day of treatment rather than increasing dose; failure in therapy may be due to overdose or too-frequent dosage. ▪ IM administration not recommended. Administration by IV injection is preferred. ▪ Use with caution in impaired respiratory function (e.g., pulmonary disease, edema, infection, obstruction); may cause severe respiratory acidosis. ▪ Potassium excretion is proportional to diuresis. Hypokalemia may result from diuresis or with severe cirrhosis. ▪ Introduce or withdraw gradually when used as an anticonvulsant.

Monitor: Obtain baseline CBC and platelet count before use and monitor during therapy. ▪ Periodic monitoring of electrolytes is recommended.

Patient Education: Consider birth control options.

Maternal/Child: Category C: has been shown to be teratogenic in animal studies. Use during pregnancy only if potential benefit justifies potential risks to the fetus. ▪ Discontinue breast-feeding or discontinue acetazolamide. ▪ Safety for use in pediatric patients not established, but no problems are documented.

Elderly: Use caution; no documented problems, but age-related renal impairment may be a factor.

DRUG/LAB INTERACTIONS

May cause hypokalemia with concurrent use of **steroids.** ▪ Hypokalemia may cause toxicity and fatal cardiac arrhythmias with **digoxin** or interfere with **insulin or oral antidiabetic agent** response, thus causing hyperglycemia. ▪ Alkalinization of urine potentiates **amphetamines, ephedrine, flecainide** (Tambocor), **methenamine, procainamide, pseudoephedrine** (Sudafed), **quinidine, and tricyclic antidepressants** (e.g., amitriptyline [Elavil]) by decreasing rate of excretion. ▪ May decrease response to **lithium, methotrexate, some antidepressants, phenobarbital, salicylates, and urinary anti-infectives** by increasing rate of excretion. ▪ Metabolic acidosis induced by acetazolamide may potentiate **salicylate** toxicity (anorexia, tachypnea, lethargy, coma, and death can occur with high-dose aspirin). ▪ Alkalinity may cause **false-positive urinary protein** and possibly **urinary steroid tests.** ▪ May depress **iodine uptake** by the thyroid.

SIDE EFFECTS

Minimal with short-term therapy. Respond to symptomatic treatment or withdrawal of drug: acidosis, anorexia, bone marrow suppression, confusion, crystalluria, drowsiness, fever, hemolytic anemia, hypokalemia (ECG changes, fatigue, muscle weakness, vomiting), paresthesias, photosensitivity, polyuria, rash, renal calculus, thrombocytopenic purpura.

ANTIDOTE

Notify physician of any adverse effects and discontinue drug if necessary. Treat hypersensitivity reactions as indicated; may require epinephrine, airway management, oxygen, IV fluids, antihistamines (e.g., diphenhydramine [Benadryl]), corticosteroids (e.g., hydrocortisone sodium succinate [Solu-Cortef]), and pressor amines (e.g., dopamine). Moderately dialyzable (20% to 40%).

ACETYLCYSTEINE INJECTION BBW*

(ah-see-till-**SIS**-tay-een in-**JEK**-shun)

Antidote

Acetadote

pH 6 to 7.5

*This drug is on the Black Box Warning list; however, a BBW is not provided in the parenteral prescribing information.

USUAL DOSE (Adult and Pediatric)

Assess the potential risk of hepatotoxicity by determining plasma or serum acetaminophen concentrations as early as possible but no sooner than 4 hours following an acute overdose. Acetylcysteine may be withheld until acetaminophen assay results are available as long as initiation of treatment is not delayed beyond 8 hours postingestion; see Precautions and Monitor. Total dose equals 300 mg/kg given as three separate doses and administered over 21 hours. Total volume administered for patients less than 40 kg and for those requiring fluid restriction can be adjusted as clinically needed; see Dosing chart for patients who weigh from 5 to 20 kg and from 21 to 40 kg. Consider osmolarity; see Dilution and Precautions.

Distribute doses as indicated in the following guidelines:

Dosing for patients who weigh 5 to 20 kg:
Loading dose: 150 mg/kg diluted in 3 mL/kg of diluent administered over 1 hour.
Second dose: 50 mg/kg diluted in 7 mL/kg of diluent administered over 4 hours.
Third dose: 100 mg/kg diluted in 14 mL/kg of diluent administered over 16 hours.

	Acetylcysteine Dosage Guide by Weight in Patients 5 to 20 kg					
Body Weight (kg)	Loading Dose: 150 mg/kg diluted in 3 mL/kg of diluent administered over 1 hour		Second Dose: 50 mg/kg diluted in 7 mL/kg of diluent administered over 4 hours		Third Dose: 100 mg/kg diluted in 14 mL/kg of diluent administered over 16 hours	
	Total Acetylcysteine Dose (mg)	Diluent Volume (mL)	Total Acetylcysteine Dose (mg)	Diluent Volume (mL)	Total Acetylcysteine Dose (mg)	Diluent Volume (mL)
5 kg	750 mg	15 mL	250 mg	35 mL	500 mg	70 mL
10 kg	1,500 mg	30 mL	500 mg	70 mL	1,000 mg	140 mL
15 kg	2,250 mg	45 mL	750 mg	105 mL	1,500 mg	210 mL
20 kg	3,000 mg	60 mL	1,000 mg	140 mL	2,000 mg	280 mL

Dosing for patients who weigh 21 to 40 kg:
Loading dose: 150 mg/kg diluted in 100 mL of diluent administered over 1 hour.
Second dose: 50 mg/kg diluted in 250 mL of diluent administered over 4 hours.
Third dose: 100 mg/kg diluted in 500 mL of diluent administered over 16 hours.

	Acetylcysteine Dosage Guide by Weight in Patients 21 to 40 kg		
Body Weight (kg)	Loading Dose: 150 mg/kg in 100 mL of diluent administered over 1 hour	Second Dose: 50 mg/kg in 250 mL of diluent administered over 4 hours	Third Dose: 100 mg/kg in 500 mL of diluent administered over 16 hours
	Total Acetylcysteine Dose (mg)	Total Acetylcysteine Dose (mg)	Total Acetylcysteine Dose (mg)
21 kg	3,150 mg	1,050 mg	2,100 mg
30 kg	4,500 mg	1,500 mg	3,000 mg
40 kg	6,000 mg	2,000 mg	4,000 mg

Continued

Dosing for patients who weigh 41 to 100 kg:
Loading dose: 150 mg/kg diluted in 200 mL of diluent administered over 1 hour.
Second dose: 50 mg/kg diluted in 500 mL of diluent administered over 4 hours.
Third dose: 100 mg/kg diluted in 1,000 mL of diluent administered over 16 hours.

Acetylcysteine Dosage Guide by Weight in Patients 41 to 100 kg			
Body Weight (kg)	Loading Dose: 150 mg/kg in 200 mL of diluent administered over 1 hour	Second Dose: 50 mg/kg in 500 mL of diluent administered over 4 hours	Third Dose: 100 mg/kg in 1,000 mL of diluent administered over 16 hours
	Total Acetylcysteine Dose (mg)	Total Acetylcysteine Dose (mg)	Total Acetylcysteine Dose (mg)
41 kg	6,150 mg	2,050 mg	4,100 mg
50 kg	7,500 mg	2,500 mg	5,000 mg
60 kg	9,000 mg	3,000 mg	6,000 mg
70 kg	10,500 mg	3,500 mg	7,000 mg
80 kg	12,000 mg	4,000 mg	8,000 mg
90 kg	13,500 mg	4,500 mg	9,000 mg
100 kg	15,000 mg	5,000 mg	10,000 mg

Dosing for patients who weigh more than 100 kg:
Limited data available. Manufacturer recommends:
Loading dose: 15,000 mg diluted in 200 mL administered over 1 hour.
Second dose: 5,000 mg diluted in 500 mL of diluent administered over 4 hours.
Third dose: 10,000 mg diluted in 1,000 mL of diluent administered over 16 hours.

DOSE ADJUSTMENTS
Therapy extending beyond 21 hours may be considered in rare cases such as suspected massive overdose, concomitant ingestion of other substances, or in patients with pre-existing liver disease. In these cases, absorption and/or half-life of acetaminophen may be prolonged. Obtain acetaminophen levels and ALT/AST and INR before the end of the 21-hour infusion. If acetaminophen levels are still detectable, or in cases in which ALT/AST is still increasing or INR remains elevated, continue the infusion and contact a regional poison control center. ▪ Specific information and/or recommendations are not available for patients with impaired hepatic or renal function.

DILUTION
May be diluted in D5W, ½NS, or SWFI. See Usual Dose for dilution guidelines based on weight. Total volume administered should be adjusted for patients less than 40 kg or for those requiring fluid restriction. Hyponatremia and seizures may result from large volumes in small children. ▪ A hyperosmolar solution. Caution is advised when the diluent volume is decreased; hyperosmolarity of the solution is increased as shown in the following chart.

Acetylcysteine Concentration and Osmolarity			
Acetylcysteine Concentration (mg/mL)	Osmolarity in ½NS (mOsmol/L)	Osmolarity in D5W (mOsmol/L)	Osmolarity in SWFI (mOsmol/L)
7 mg/mL	245 mOsmol/L	343 mOsmol/L	91 mOsmol/L*
24 mg/mL	466 mOsmol/L	564 mOsmol/L	312 mOsmol/L

*Osmolarity should be adjusted to a physiologically safe level (generally not less than 150 mOsmol/L in children).

Color of acetylcysteine may change from colorless to a slight pink or purple once the stopper is punctured; quality is not affected.
Filters: Data not available and use is not required by manufacturer. Studies on the use of filters are planned.

Storage: Store unopened vials at CRT. Diluted solution is stable for 24 hours at CRT. Do not use previously opened vials for IV administration. Discard unused portions.

COMPATIBILITY
Manufacturer states, "**Compatible** with D5W, ½NS, and SWFI."

RATE OF ADMINISTRATION
Usual total infusion time of all 3 doses is 21 hours. Rate reduction may be required to manage S/S of infusion reactions; see Monitor and Antidote.

Loading dose: An infusion evenly distributed over 60 minutes.

Second dose: An infusion evenly distributed over 4 hours.

Third dose: An infusion evenly distributed over 16 hours.

ACTIONS
Protects the liver by maintaining or restoring the glutathione levels (metabolites formed after an overdose of acetaminophen may deplete the hepatic stores of glutathione and cause binding of the metabolite to protein molecules within the hepatocyte, resulting in cellular necrosis). It may also act by forming an alternate compound and detoxifying the reactive metabolite. Half-life is approximately 5.6 hours. Metabolizes to various compounds. Crosses the placental barrier. Some excretion in urine.

INDICATIONS AND USES
To prevent or lessen hepatic injury after ingestion of a potentially hepatotoxic quantity of acetaminophen. Overdose incidences are divided into two types: (1) acute ingestion, or (2) repeated supratherapeutic ingestion (RSI).

CONTRAINDICATIONS
Known hypersensitivity to acetylcysteine or any of its components.

PRECAUTIONS
Should be administered in a facility equipped to monitor the patient and respond to any medical emergency. ▪ Most effective against severe hepatic injury when administered within 8 hours of ingestion. Administration before 4 hours does not allow enough time to determine an actual need for treatment with acetylcysteine; serum levels drawn before 4 hours have passed may be misleading. Effectiveness diminishes gradually after 8 hours. Should be administered if 24 hours or less has passed since ingestion, because the reported time of ingestion may not be correct and it does not appear to worsen the patient's condition. ▪ Total volume administered should be adjusted for patients less than 40 kg and for patients requiring fluid restriction. If volume is not adjusted, fluid overload can occur, potentially resulting in hyponatremia, seizure, and death; see Usual Dose. ▪ Anaphylactoid reactions have been reported and usually occur soon after initiation of the infusion. Use caution in patients with asthma or a history of bronchospasm. Death occurred in a patient with asthma. ▪ Acute flushing and erythema of the skin may occur. These reactions usually occur within 30 to 60 minutes of beginning the infusion and often resolve spontaneously despite continued infusion. ▪ Clearance decreased and half-life prolonged in patients with various stages of liver damage (Child-Pugh scores of 5 to 13). ▪ The Rumack-Matthew nomogram does not apply to patients with repeated supratherapeutic ingestion (RSI), which is defined as ingestion of acetaminophen at doses higher than those recommended for extended periods of time. For treatment information, see prescribing information for a professional assistance line for acetaminophen overdose, or contact a regional poison control center. ▪ The Rumack-Matthew nomogram may underestimate the risk for hepatotoxicity in some patients with risk factors such as chronic alcoholism, malnutrition, or CYP2E1 enzyme-inducing drugs (e.g., isoniazid [INH]). ▪ Vial stopper does not contain natural rubber latex. ▪ See Monitor and Antidote.

Monitor: Acute ingestion of 150 mg/kg or more of acetaminophen may result in hepatic toxicity. Obtain baseline hepatic function studies and monitor throughout detoxification process.

Preferred method of treatment: Estimate time of acetaminophen ingestion. If less than 24 hours since overdose, draw serum for an acetaminophen level at 4 hours postingestion or as soon as possible thereafter to clarify the need for intervention with acetylcysteine. The serum acetaminophen level should be evaluated on the Rumack-Matthew nomogram to determine the probability of toxicity (see package insert for copy of nomogram). ▪ If serum acetaminophen level is below the treatment line on the nomogram, discontinue the acetylcysteine if initiated as a precaution. If the plasma level is above the treatment line on the nomogram, initiate or continue treatment.

Secondary options for treatment: If serum acetaminophen levels are not available within 8 hours, initiate treatment. Do not delay treatment more than 8 hours postingestion. ▪ If time of ingestion is unknown or if the patient is unreliable, consider empiric initiation of acetylcysteine treatment. ▪ If a serum acetaminophen level is not available or cannot be interpreted and less than 24 hours has elapsed since ingestion, administer acetylcysteine regardless of the quantity reported to have been ingested.

All treatment options: Obtain serum acetaminophen level and baseline ALT, AST, bilirubin, blood glucose, BUN, electrolytes, PT, and SCr. Monitor as indicated by results. ▪ Monitor BP and HR before, during, and after the infusion. ▪ Evaluate serum acetaminophen level on the Rumack-Matthew nomogram. ▪ Infusion reactions may begin with acute flushing and erythema of the skin. May resolve spontaneously despite continued infusion of acetylcysteine or may progress to an acute hypersensitivity reaction and/or anaphylaxis. Observe continuously for initial S/S of a hypersensitivity reaction (e.g., hypotension, rash, shortness of breath, wheezing). ▪ In suspected toxicity resulting from the extended-release acetaminophen preparation, an acetaminophen level drawn fewer than 8 hours postingestion may be misleading. Draw a second level at 4 to 6 hours after the initial level. If either acetaminophen level falls above the toxicity line, acetylcysteine treatment should be initiated. ▪ See Precautions and Antidote.

Patient Education: Report S/S of hypersensitivity promptly (e.g., flushing, itching, shortness of breath, feeling of faintness).

Maternal/Child: Category B: use during pregnancy only if clearly needed. ▪ Use caution; safety for use during breast-feeding not established; effects unknown. After 30 hours, acetylcysteine should be cleared from maternal blood, and breast-feeding can be resumed. ▪ No adequate or well-controlled studies in pediatric patients, but it has been used. Efficacy appears to be similar to that seen in adults; see Side Effects. ▪ Administered to a small number of preterm infants during clinical studies (a mean rate of 4.2 mg/kg/hr for 24 hours); half-life prolonged to approximately 11 hours in these newborns. ▪ Acetylcysteine was measurable in the circulation and cord blood of three newborns whose mothers were treated for acetaminophen overdose. No adverse side effects were noted, and none of the infants had evidence of acetaminophen poisoning.

Elderly: Differences in response compared with younger adults not known.

DRUG/LAB INTERACTIONS
Drug-drug interaction studies have not been done.

SIDE EFFECTS
Adult and pediatric patients: Pruritus, rash, and urticaria have been reported most frequently and most commonly occur during the initial loading dose. Other reported side effects include anaphylactoid reactions, angioedema, dyspepsia, dysphoria (abnormal thinking or confusion), dyspnea, edema, erythema of the skin, eye pain, facial flushing, gait disturbances, hypotension, nausea and vomiting, palmar erythema, respiratory symptoms (e.g., bronchospasm, chest tightness, cough, respiratory distress, shortness of breath, stridor, wheezing), sweating, syncope, tachycardia, vasodilation.

Overdose: S/S of acute toxicity in animals included ataxia, convulsions, cyanosis, hypoactivity, labored respiration, and loss of righting reflex.

ANTIDOTE
Keep physician informed of all side effects. Flushing and erythema of the skin are expected. If other symptoms of a hypersensitivity reaction occur (e.g., bronchospasm, dyspnea, hypotension, wheezing), discontinue acetylcysteine and treat with diphenhydramine (Benadryl) or epinephrine as indicated. After symptoms subside, the infusion may be carefully resumed. If S/S of hypersensitivity recur, discontinue infusion permanently and consider alternate treatments. Contact a regional poison control center for possible treatment alternatives.

ACYCLOVIR

(ay-**SYE**-kloh-veer)

Zovirax

Antiviral

pH 10.5 to 11.6

USUAL DOSE

In all situations for adults, adolescents, children, and neonates, do not exceed a maximum dose of 20 mg/kg every 8 hours.

Adults and adolescents (12 years of age and older):

Herpes simplex infections; mucosal and cutaneous HSV infections in immunocompromised patients: 5 mg/kg of body weight every 8 hours for 7 days.

Severe initial clinical episodes of herpes genitalis: 5 mg/kg every 8 hours for 5 days.

Herpes simplex encephalitis: 10 mg/kg every 8 hours for 10 days.

Herpes zoster infections (shingles) in immunocompromised patients: 10 mg/kg every 8 hours for 7 days.

PEDIATRIC DOSE

Pediatric patients under 12 years of age:

Herpes simplex infections; mucosal and cutaneous HSV infections in immunocompromised patients: 10 mg/kg every 8 hours for 7 days.

Herpes simplex encephalitis: *Pediatric patients over 3 months of age:* 20 mg/kg every 8 hours for 10 days.

Herpes zoster infections (shingles) in immunocompromised patients: 20 mg/kg every 8 hours for 7 days.

NEONATAL DOSE

Neonatal herpes simplex virus infections: *Birth to 3 months:* 10 mg/kg every 8 hours for 10 days. Doses of 15 mg/kg to 20 mg/kg every 8 hours have been used for up to 14 to 21 days; safety and efficacy have not been established.

DOSE ADJUSTMENTS

Calculate dose by ideal body weight in obese individuals. ▪ Reduced dose may be indicated in the elderly based on the potential for decreased renal function and concomitant disease or drug therapy. ▪ In adults and pediatric patients with impaired renal function, reduce dose and/or adjust dosing interval based on CrCl as indicated in the following chart.

Acyclovir Dosage Adjustments for Adults and Pediatric Patients with Renal Impairment		
Creatinine Clearance (mL/min per 1.73 M^2)	Percent of Recommended Dose	Dosing Interval (hours)
>50 mL/min	100%	Every 8 hr
25-50 mL/min	100%	Every 12 hr
10-25 mL/min	100%	Every 24 hr
0-10 mL/min	50%	Every 24 hr

Plasma concentrations decrease with hemodialysis; adjustment of the dosing schedule is recommended so that an additional dose is administered after each dialysis. No supplemental dose is indicated in peritoneal dialysis after adjustment of the dosing interval.

DILUTION

Initially dissolve each 500 mg with 10 mL SWFI (1,000 mg with 20 mL). Concentration equals 50 mg/mL. Do not use bacteriostatic water for injection (BWFI); will cause precipitation. Shake well to dissolve completely. Also available in liquid vials. Withdraw the desired dose and further dilute in an amount of solution to provide a concentration less than 7 mg/mL (70-kg adult at 5 mg/kg equals 350 mg dissolved in a total of 100 mL of solution equals 3.5 mg/mL). **Compatible** with most standard electrolyte and glucose infusion solutions.

Filters: No data available from manufacturer.

Storage: Store unopened vials at CRT. Use reconstituted solution within 12 hours; high pH may result in etching of glass vial surface after 12 hours. Use solution fully diluted for administration within 24 hours. Manufacturer will supply data showing stability for longer periods under specific conditions.

COMPATIBILITY   (Underline Indicates Conflicting Compatibility Information)
Consider any drug NOT listed as compatible to be INCOMPATIBLE until consulting a pharmacist; specific conditions may apply.
Manufacturer lists bacteriostatic water for injection (BWFI) as **incompatible**. Dilution in biologic or colloidal fluids (e.g., blood products, protein solutions) is not recommended.

One source suggests the following **compatibilities:**
Additive: Fluconazole (Diflucan), meropenem (Merrem IV).
Y-site: Allopurinol (Aloprim), amikacin, amphotericin B cholesteryl (Amphotec), ampicillin, anidulafungin (Eraxis), caspofungin (Cancidas), cefazolin (Ancef), cefotaxime (Claforan), cefoxitin (Mefoxin), ceftaroline (Teflaro), ceftazidime (Fortaz), ceftriaxone (Rocephin), cefuroxime (Zinacef), chloramphenicol (Chloromycetin), cisatracurium (Nimbex), clindamycin (Cleocin), dexamethasone (Decadron), diltiazem (Cardizem), dimenhydrinate, diphenhydramine (Benadryl), docetaxel (Taxotere), doripenem (Doribax), doxorubicin liposomal (Doxil), doxycycline, droperidol (Inapsine), erythromycin (Erythrocin), etoposide phosphate (Etopophos), famotidine (Pepcid IV), fentanyl, filgrastim (Neupogen), fluconazole (Diflucan), gallium nitrate (Ganite), gentamicin, granisetron (Kytril), heparin, hydrocortisone sodium succinate (Solu-Cortef), hydromorphone (Dilaudid), imipenem-cilastatin (Primaxin), linezolid (Zyvox), lorazepam (Ativan), magnesium sulfate, melphalan (Alkeran), meperidine (Demerol), meropenem (Merrem IV), methylprednisolone (Solu-Medrol), metoclopramide (Reglan), metronidazole (Flagyl IV), milrinone (Primacor), morphine, multivitamins (M.V.I.), nafcillin (Nallpen), nalbufine, oxacillin (Bactocill), paclitaxel (Taxol), pemetrexed (Alimta), penicillin G potassium, pentobarbital (Nembutal), potassium chloride (KCl), propofol (Diprivan), ranitidine (Zantac), remifentanil (Ultiva), sodium bicarbonate, sulfamethoxazole/trimethoprim, teniposide (Vumon), theophylline, thiotepa, tobramycin, vancomycin, zidovudine (AZT, Retrovir).

RATE OF ADMINISTRATION
A single dose must be administered at a constant rate over 1 hour as an infusion. Renal tubular damage will occur with too-rapid rate of injection. Acyclovir crystals will occlude renal tubules. Use of an infusion pump or microdrip (60 gtt/mL) recommended.

ACTIONS
An antiviral agent with activity against herpes simplex virus types 1 (HSV-1) and 2 (HSV-2) and varicella-zoster virus (VZV). Inhibits replication of viral DNA. Widely distributed in tissues and body fluids. Metabolized to a small extent in the liver. Half-life is approximately 2.5 hours. Excreted mainly as unchanged drug in the urine. Crosses the placental and blood-brain barriers. Secreted in breast milk.

INDICATIONS AND USES
Treatment of initial and recurrent mucosal and cutaneous herpes simplex (HSV-1 and HSV-2) infections in immunosuppressed patients. ■ Severe initial clinical episodes of herpes genitalis in immunocompetent patients. ■ Herpes simplex encephalitis. ■ Neonatal herpes simplex virus infections. ■ Herpes zoster infections (shingles) in immunocompromised patients. ■ Oral acyclovir is used to treat varicella zoster (chickenpox).
Unlabeled uses: Prevention of HSV reactivation in HSCT, treatment of disseminated HSV or VZV, or empiric treatment of suspected encephalitis in immunocompromised patients with cancer.

CONTRAINDICATIONS
Hypersensitivity to acyclovir or valacyclovir (Valtrex). The ganciclovir monograph indicates a contraindication for ganciclovir with acyclovir.

PRECAUTIONS

Confirm diagnosis of herpes simplex virus (HSV-1 or HSV-2) through laboratory culture. Initiate therapy as quickly as possible after symptoms are identified. ▪ For IV use only; avoid IM or SC injection. ▪ Use caution in patients with underlying neurologic abnormalities, those with serious renal, hepatic, or electrolyte abnormalities, or significant hypoxia. ▪ Use caution in patients receiving interferon or intrathecal methotrexate, or with patients who have had previous neurologic reactions to cytotoxic drugs. ▪ Incidence of CNS adverse events may be more common in the elderly or in patients with decreased renal function. ▪ Isolates of herpes simplex viruses (HSV-1, HSV-2) and varicella-zoster virus (VZV) with reduced susceptibility to acyclovir have been identified. Consider the possibility of viral resistance to acyclovir in patients who show poor clinical response. ▪ Thrombotic thrombocytopenic purpura/hemolytic uremic syndrome (TTP/HUS) has been reported in immunocompromised patients receiving acyclovir. Deaths have occurred. ▪ See Contraindications.

Monitor: Maintain adequate hydration and urine flow before and during infusion. Encourage fluid intake of 2 to 3 L/day. ▪ Monitor CBC, liver function tests, and renal function; abnormal renal function (decreased CrCl can occur), concomitant use of other nephrotoxic drugs, pre-existing renal disease, and dehydration make further renal impairment with acyclovir more likely. ▪ Confirm patency of vein; will cause thrombophlebitis. Rotate site of infusion.

Patient Education: Maintain adequate hydration. Virus remains dormant and can still spread to others. ▪ Avoid sexual intercourse when visible herpes lesions are present. Use condoms routinely.

Maternal/Child: Category B: use during pregnancy only if benefits outweigh risk to fetus. ▪ Breast milk concentrations can be higher than maternal serum concentrations. Discontinue breast-feeding or evaluate very carefully. ▪ 10 mg/kg and 20 mg/kg doses in pediatric patients from 3 months to 16 years achieved concentrations similar to those in adults receiving 5 mg/kg to 10 mg/kg. ▪ Use with caution in neonates; they have an age-related decrease in clearance and an increase in half-life (3.8 hours).

Elderly: Effectiveness is similar to younger adults. ▪ Plasma concentrations are higher in the elderly compared to younger adults; may be due to age-related changes in renal function. ▪ Duration of pain after healing was longer in patients 65 years or older. ▪ Incidence of side effects (e.g., CNS adverse events [coma, confusion, hallucinations, somnolence], dizziness, nausea, renal adverse events, vomiting) was increased. ▪ See Dose Adjustments and Precautions.

DRUG/LAB INTERACTIONS

See Precautions. May cause neurotoxicity (e.g., severe drowsiness and lethargy) with **zidovudine.** ▪ Concurrent use with other **nephrotoxic agents** (e.g., aminoglycosides [gentamicin, tobramycin], cisplatin) may increase risk of nephrotoxicity, especially in patients with pre-existing renal impairment. ▪ Potentiated by **probenecid.** ▪ Synergistic effects with **ketoconazole and interferon** have been noted. Clinical importance not established. ▪ In one case report, a patient stabilized on **phenytoin and valproic acid** experienced seizures and a reduction in antiepileptic drug serum concentrations when acyclovir was added to the regimen.

SIDE EFFECTS

Acute renal failure, aggressive behavior, agitation, angioedema, ataxia, coma, confusion, delirium, diaphoresis, disseminated intravascular coagulation (DIC), dizziness, dysarthria (difficulty articulating words), elevated transaminase levels, encephalopathy, hallucinations, headache, hematuria, hemolysis, hives, hyperbilirubinemia, hypersensitivity reactions (e.g., anaphylaxis), hypotension, inflammation at injection site, lethargy, nausea, obtundation, phlebitis, rash, seizures, transient increased BUN or SCr levels, tremors, vomiting. Some patients (fewer than 1%) may have abdominal pain, anemia, anorexia, anuria, chest pain, diarrhea, edema, fatigue, fever, hemoglobinemia, hepatitis, hypokalemia, ischemia of digits, jaundice, leukocytosis, light-headedness, myalgia, neutropenia, neutrophilia, paresthesia, psychosis, pulmonary edema with cardiac tamponade, rigors, skin reactions (e.g., erythema multiforme, Stevens-Johnson syndrome, toxic epidermal necrolysis), thirst, thrombocytosis, thrombocytopenia, visual abnormalities.

ANTIDOTE

Notify physician of all side effects. Discontinue drug with onset of CNS side effects. Treatment will be symptomatic and supportive. Adequate hydration is indicated to prevent precipitation of acyclovir in the renal tubules. A 6-hour session of hemodialysis will reduce plasma acyclovir concentration by approximately 60%. Hemodialysis may be indicated in patients with acute renal failure and anuria. Treat anaphylaxis and resuscitate as necessary.

ADENOSINE
(ah-**DEN**-oh-seen)

Adenocard, Adenoscan

Antiarrhythmic
Diagnostic agent

pH 4.5 to 7.5

USUAL DOSE

Adenocard: Conversion of acute paroxysmal supraventricular tachycardia (PSVT): 6 mg initially as a rapid bolus by the peripheral IV route. If supraventricular tachycardia not eliminated in 1 to 2 minutes, give 12 mg. May repeat 12-mg dose in 1 to 2 minutes if needed. Do not exceed 12 mg in any single dose. Give undiluted directly into a vein. If given into an IV line, use the port closest to the insertion site and follow with a rapid NS flush to be certain the solution reaches the systemic circulation.

Do not administer a repeat dose to patients who develop a high-level block on one dose of adenosine.

Adenoscan: Noninvasive diagnosis of coronary artery disease with thallium tomography: 140 mcg/kg/min (0.14 mg/kg/min) as a 6-minute continuous peripheral infusion (total dose of 0.84 mg/kg). Injection should be as close to the venous access as possible. Inject thallium at 3 minutes. May be injected directly into adenosine infusion set. Dose should be based on total body weight. There are no data on the safety or efficacy of alternative Adenoscan infusion protocols. Safety and efficacy of Adenoscan administered by the intracoronary route have not been established. ▪ See Drug/Lab Interactions.

PEDIATRIC DOSE

See Maternal/Child.

Adenocard: Conversion of acute paroxysmal supraventricular tachycardia (PSVT) in pediatric patients weighing less than 50 kg: 0.05 to 0.1 mg/kg. May increase dose by 0.05 to 0.1 mg/kg increments every 2 minutes until PSVT is terminated or maximum dose is reached (0.3 mg/kg or 12 mg). AHA guidelines recommend 0.1 mg/kg rapid IV push. Follow each dose with a 5- to 10-mL NS flush. Double to 0.2 mg/kg if a second dose is required. Maximum first dose 6 mg. Maximum second dose and maximum single dose is 12 mg. ▪ See comments in Usual Dose.

Pediatric patients weighing more than 50 kg: Same as Usual Dose.

DOSE ADJUSTMENTS

Metabolism of adenosine is independent of hepatic or renal function. No dose adjustment indicated. ▪ See Drug/Lab Interactions; alternative therapy (e.g., calcium channel blockers) may be indicated.

DILUTION

Solution must be clear; do not use if discolored or particulate matter present. Give undiluted for both indications.

Storage: Store at CRT 15° to 30° C (59° to 86° F); refrigeration will cause crystallization. If crystals do form, dissolve by warming to room temperature. Discard unused portion.

COMPATIBILITY

Consider any drug NOT listed as compatible to be INCOMPATIBLE until consulting a pharmacist; specific conditions may apply.

Manufacturer states that thallium-201 is **compatible** with Adenoscan and may be injected directly into the Adenoscan infusion set.

One source suggests the following **compatibilities:**

Y-site: Abciximab (ReoPro).

RATE OF ADMINISTRATION

Adenocard: *Conversion of acute PSVT:* Must be given as a rapid bolus IV injection over 1 to 2 seconds. Follow each dose with NS flush; see Usual Dose.

Adenoscan: *Pharmacologic stress testing:* See Usual Dose.

ACTIONS

A naturally occurring nucleoside present in all cells of the body. Has many functions. When given as a rapid IV bolus of 6 or 12 mg, adenosine usually has no systemic hemodynamic effects. As a rapid IV bolus, it has antiarrhythmic properties, slowing cardiac conduction (particularly at the AV node), interrupting re-entry pathways through the AV node, and restoring sinus rhythm in patients with PSVT, including PSVT associated with Wolff-Parkinson-White syndrome. When used as a diagnostic aid and given as a continuous infusion, adenosine acts as a vasodilator. Dilates normal coronary vessels, increasing blood flow. Has little effect on stenotic arteries. When administered with thallium-201, helps differentiate between areas of heart supplied by normal blood flow and areas supplied by stenotic coronary arteries. When larger doses are given by infusion, adenosine decreases BP and produces a reflexive increase in HR. Adenocard and Adenoscan have the same molecular structure, same solvent, diluent, and concentration. The difference in their actions is in the rate of administration; however, the FDA has approved Adenocard for converting PSVT and Adenoscan for pharmacologic stress testing. When used for treatment of PSVT, it is effective within 1 minute. When used for diagnostic purposes, maximum effect is reached within 2 to 3 minutes of starting the infusion. Coronary blood flow velocity returns to basal levels within 1 to 2 minutes after the infusion is discontinued. Half-life is estimated to be less than 10 seconds. Adenosine is salvaged immediately by erythrocytes and blood vessel endothelial cells and metabolized for natural uses throughout the body (regulation of coronary and systemic vascular tone, platelet function, lipolysis in fat cells, intracardiac conduction).

INDICATIONS AND USES

Adenocard: To convert acute paroxysmal supraventricular tachycardia (PSVT) to normal sinus rhythm; a first-line agent according to AHA. Includes PSVT associated with accessory bypass tracts (Wolff-Parkinson-White syndrome). Does not convert atrial flutter, atrial fibrillation, or ventricular tachycardia to normal sinus rhythm (NSR).

Adenoscan: Adjunct to thallium-201 myocardial perfusion scintigraphy in patients unable to exercise adequately. (Results are similar to exercise stress testing.)

CONTRAINDICATIONS

Known hypersensitivity to adenosine. ▪ Sinus node disease, such as symptomatic bradycardia or sick sinus syndrome, and second- or third-degree AV block unless a functioning artificial pacemaker is in place. ▪ Known or suspected bronchoconstrictive or bronchospastic lung disease (e.g., asthma).

PRECAUTIONS

Both preparations: Emergency resuscitation drugs and equipment must always be available. ▪ May produce short-lasting first-, second-, or third-degree heart block or sinus bradycardia. Usually self-limiting due to short half-life. Patients who develop high-level block should not be given additional doses of adenosine. ▪ May cause dyspnea, bronchoconstriction, and respiratory compromise. Use with caution in patients with obstructive lung disease not associated with bronchoconstriction (e.g., emphysema, bronchitis). Avoid use in patients with bronchoconstrictive or bronchospastic disease (e.g., asthma); see Contraindications.

Adenocard: Valsalva maneuver may be used before use of adenosine in PSVTs if clinically appropriate. ▪ Transient or prolonged episodes of asystole and ventricular fibrillation have been reported. Deaths have occurred. In most instances, these cases were associated with the concomitant use of digoxin (Lanoxin) and, less frequently, with digoxin and verapamil. ▪ Some slowing of ventricular response may occur if atrial flutter or fibrillation is also present.

Adenoscan: Use with caution in patients with pre-existing first-degree AV block or bundle branch block. ▪ Fatal and nonfatal cardiac arrest, sustained ventricular tachycardia (requiring resuscitation), and MI have been reported. Avoid use in patients with S/S of myocardial ischemia (e.g., unstable angina) or cardiovascular instability; may be at increased risk for adverse cardiac events. ▪ Can cause significant hypotension. Use with caution in patients with autonomic dysfunction, stenotic valvular heart disease, pericarditis or pericardial effusion, stenotic carotid artery disease with cerebrovascular insufficiency, or uncorrected hypovolemia; may be at increased risk for hypotensive complications. ▪ Hemorrhagic and ischemic cerebrovascular accidents have occurred. ▪ New onset or recurrence of convulsive seizures has occurred following administration of Adenoscan. Some seizures are prolonged and require emergent anticonvulsive management. Aminophylline may increase the risk of seizures associated with Adenoscan; see Antidote. ▪ Hypersensitivity reactions (e.g., chest discomfort, dyspnea, erythema, flushing, throat tightness, and rash) have occurred. ▪ Hypertension has been reported; usually resolves spontaneously within several minutes but, in some cases, has lasted for several hours. ▪ Atrial fibrillation has been reported. In reported cases, it began 1.5 to 3 minutes into the infusion, lasted for 15 seconds to 6 hours, and spontaneously converted to NSR.

Monitor: *Adenocard: Conversion of acute PSVT:* Must reach systemic circulation; see Usual Dose. ▪ ECG monitoring during administration recommended. Monitor BP. At the time of conversion to normal sinus rhythm, PVCs, PACs, atrial fibrillation, sinus bradycardia, sinus tachycardia, skipped beats, and varying degrees of AV nodal block are seen on the ECG in many patients. Usually last only a few seconds and resolve without intervention. ▪ Less likely to precipitate hypotension if arrhythmia does not terminate.

Adenoscan: Pharmacologic stress testing: ECG monitoring during administration recommended. Monitor HR and BP at regular intervals during infusion. ▪ Obtain images when infusion complete and redistribution images 3 to 4 hours later. ▪ Monitor for S/S of hypersensitivity reactions.

Patient Education: Avoid consumption of any products containing methylxanthines, including caffeinated coffee, tea, or other caffeinated beverages; caffeine-containing drug products; aminophylline; and theophylline before the myocardial perfusion imaging study. ▪ Review medical history (e.g., history of seizures or respiratory compromise). ▪ Promptly report any potential side effects.

Maternal/Child: Category C: use in pregnancy only if clearly needed. Some references recommend avoiding early pregnancy. ▪ Safety for use in pediatric patients not established, but has been used for conversion of PSVT in neonates, infants, children, and adolescents. Safety for use in pharmacologic stress testing in patients under 18 years not established. ▪ Interrupt nursing after administration of Adenoscan.

Elderly: Response similar to that seen in younger patients; however, greater sensitivity of some older patients cannot be ruled out. May have diminished cardiac function, nodal dysfunction, concomitant disease, or drug therapy that may alter hemodynamic function and produce severe bradycardia or AV block.

DRUG/LAB INTERACTIONS

Both preparations: Effects antagonized by **methylxanthines** (e.g., caffeine, theophylline); larger doses may be required or adenosine may not be effective. ▪ Potentiated by **dipyridamole** (Persantine); smaller doses of adenosine may be indicated. Safety and efficacy of adenosine in the presence of dipyridamole have not been systematically evaluated. ▪ Cardiovascular effects increased by **nicotine;** rapid injection may induce anginal pain. ▪ May produce a higher degree of heart block with **carbamazepine** (Tegretol). ▪ Concomitant use with **digoxin alone or digoxin in combination with verapamil** associated with rare cases of ventricular fibrillation; see Precautions. ■ See Usual Dose. ■ **Adenoscan:** Before using Adenoscan for pharmacologic stress testing, avoid (or withhold for at least 5 half-lives) **adenosine antagonists** (e.g., methylxanthines) **and/or potentiators** (e.g., dipyridamole). ■ Has been used with other cardioactive agents such as **beta-adrenergic blockers** (e.g., metoprolol [Lopressor], atenolol [Tenormin]), **angiotensin-converting enzyme inhibitors** (e.g., lisinopril [Prinivil, Zestril], enalapril [Vasotec]), **and calcium channel blockers** (e.g., diltiazem [Cardizem], verapamil [Calan]) without apparent adverse interactions, but its effectiveness with these agents has not been fully evaluated.

SIDE EFFECTS

Both preparations: Generally predictable, short lived, and easily tolerated. Most will appear immediately and last less than 1 minute. Atrial fibrillation, bronchospasm, chest pressure or discomfort, dizziness, dyspnea and/or shortness of breath, facial flushing, GI discomfort, headache, hypertension, light-headedness, nausea, numbness, PACs, PVCs, sinus bradycardia, sinus tachycardia, skipped beats, varying degrees of AV nodal block. Less than 1% of patients complain of apprehension; blurred vision; burning; chest pain; head pressure; heavy arms; hyperventilation; hypotension; metallic taste; neck and back pain; palpitations; pressure in groin; seizures; sweating; throat, neck, or jaw discomfort; tight throat; and tingling in arms. Serious side effects may include arrhythmias (persistent), including VT, VF, atrial fibrillation, and torsades de pointes; bronchospasm (severe); myocardial infarction; pulmonary edema; third-degree AV block. Asystole with fatal outcome has been reported.

Post-Marketing: *Both preparations:* Seizure activity, including tonic-clonic (grand mal) seizures, and loss of consciousness. *Adenoscan:* Cardiac failure, cerebrovascular accident (including intracranial hemorrhage), fatal and nonfatal cardiac arrest, hypersensitivity reactions, injection site reactions, myocardial infarction, respiratory arrest, throat tightness, ventricular arrhythmia, vomiting. *Adenocard:* Atrial fibrillation, bradycardia, prolonged asystole, torsades de pointes, transient increase in blood pressure, VF, VT.

ANTIDOTE

Notify physician of any side effect that lasts more than 1 minute. If a side effect persists, decrease rate of infusion (Adenoscan [pharmacologic stress testing]). Discontinue in any patient who develops severe respiratory difficulties or in any patient who develops persistent or symptomatic high-grade AV block or hypotension. Treat side effects symptomatically if indicated. Bradycardia may be refractory to atropine. Short half-life generally precludes overdose problems, but aminophylline 50 to 125 mg as a slow infusion is a competitive antagonist. Methylxanthine use (e.g., aminophylline) is not recommended in patients who experience seizures in association with Adenoscan. Resuscitate as necessary.

ADO-TRASTUZUMAB EMTANSINE BBW

(a-do-tras-**TU**-zoo-mab em-**TAN**-seen)

Monoclonal antibody
Antineoplastic

Kadcyla

pH 5

USUAL DOSE

3.6 mg/kg as an infusion every 3 weeks (21-day cycle) until disease progression or unacceptable toxicity. *Do not administer doses greater than 3.6 mg/kg. Do not substitute adotrastuzumab (Kadcyla) for or with trastuzumab.*

DOSE ADJUSTMENTS

No dose adjustment is indicated in patients with mild or moderate renal impairment. In patients with severe renal impairment (CrCl less than 30 mL/min), no dose adjustments can be recommended because of the limited data available. ▪ If a planned dose is delayed or missed, *do not wait until the next planned cycle;* administer as soon as possible, and adjust the schedule to maintain a 3-week interval between doses. ▪ The recommended dose reduction schedule for adverse events and dose modification guidelines for various adverse events are listed in the following charts.

Recommended Ado-Trastuzumab Dose Reduction Schedule for Adverse Events*	
Dose Reduction Schedule	Dose Level to Administer
Starting dose	3.6 mg/kg
First dose reduction	3 mg/kg
Second dose reduction	2.4 mg/kg
Requirement for further dose reduction	Discontinue treatment

*Ado-trastuzumab dose should not be re-escalated after a dose reduction is made.

Ado-Trastuzumab Dose Modification Guidelines for Increased Serum Transaminases (AST/ALT)		
Grade 2 (>2.5 to ≤5 × ULN)	Grade 3 (>5 to ≤20 × ULN)	Grade 4 (>20 × ULN)
Treat at same dose level.	Do not administer until AST/ALT recovers to Grade ≤2, and then reduce one dose level.	Permanently discontinue adotrastuzumab.

ALT, Alanine transaminase; *AST,* aspartate transaminase; *ULN,* upper limit of normal.

Ado-Trastuzumab Dose Modification Guidelines for Hyperbilirubinemia		
Grade 2 (>1.5 to ≤3 × ULN)	Grade 3 (>3 to ≤10 × ULN)	Grade 4 (>10 × ULN)
Do not administer until total bilirubin recovers to Grade ≤1, and then treat at same dose level.	Do not administer until total bilirubin recovers to Grade ≤1, and then reduce one dose level.	Permanently discontinue ado-trastuzumab.

Ado-Trastuzumab Dose Modification Guidelines for Left Ventricular Dysfunction				
Symptomatic CHF	LVEF <40%	LVEF 40% to ≤45% and Decrease Is ≥10% Points from Baseline	LVEF 40% to ≤45% and Decrease Is <10% Points from Baseline	LVEF >45%
Discontinue ado-trastuzumab.	Do not administer ado-trastuzumab. Repeat LVEF assessment within 3 weeks. If LVEF <40% is confirmed, discontinue ado-trastuzumab.	Do not administer ado-trastuzumab. Repeat LVEF assessment within 3 weeks. If LVEF has not recovered to within 10% points from baseline, discontinue ado-trastuzumab.	Continue treatment with ado-trastuzumab. Repeat LVEF assessment within 3 weeks	Continue treatment with ado-trastuzumab.

CHF, Congestive heart failure; LVEF, left ventricular ejection fraction.

Ado-Trastuzumab Dose Modification Guidelines for Thrombocytopenia	
Grade 3	Grade 4
Platelets 25,000/mm³ to <50,000/mm³	Platelets <25,000/mm³
Do not administer ado-trastuzumab until platelet count recovers to ≤Grade 1 (≥75,000/mm³), and then treat at same dose level.	Do not administer ado-trastuzumab until platelet count recovers to ≤Grade 1 (≥75,000/mm³), and then reduce one dose level.

Ado-Trastuzumab Dose Modification Guidelines for Other Adverse Events	
Adverse Event	Action
Serum transaminases >3 × ULN and concomitant total bilirubin >2 × ULN	Permanently discontinue ado-trastuzumab.
Diagnosed with nodular regenerative hyperplasia (NRH)	Permanently discontinue ado-trastuzumab.
Diagnosed with interstitial lung disease (ILD) or pneumonitis	Permanently discontinue ado-trastuzumab.
Grade 3 or 4 peripheral neuropathy	Temporarily discontinue ado-trastuzumab until resolution to ≤Grade 2.

DILUTION
Specific techniques required; see Precautions. Check vial label to avoid medication errors; should read Kadcyla (ado-trastuzumab emtansine), **NOT** trastuzumab. Trade name (Kadcyla) should be clearly recorded (or stated) in the patient file to improve traceability of biological medicinal products.

Available in single-dose vials of 100 mg/vial and 160 mg/vial. Slowly inject 5 mL of SWFI into the 100-mg vial or 8 mL of SWFI into the 160-mg vial to yield a solution containing 20 mg/mL. Swirl vial gently; ***do not shake***. Solution should be clear to slightly opalescent and colorless to light brown. Withdraw the calculated dose and transfer to an infusion bag of 250 mL of NS. *Do not use D5W.* Avoid foaming by gently inverting bag to mix. ***Do not shake.*** Immediate use preferred.

Filters: Use of a 0.2- or 0.22-micron, in-line, polyethersulfone (PES) filter required for administration.

Storage: Store vials until time of reconstitution in refrigerator at 2° to 8° C (36° to 46° F). *Do not freeze or shake original vials or reconstituted or diluted solutions.* Reconstituted vials should be used immediately but may be stored for up to 24 hours in a refrigerator at 2° to 8° C (36° to 46° F). Diluted solutions should also be used immediately but can be refrigerated for up to 24 hours. The storage time of the diluted solution is in addition to the time allowed for the reconstituted vials. Discard unused reconstituted or diluted drug after 24 hours.

COMPATIBILITY

Manufacturer states, "Do not mix Kadcyla (ado-trastuzumab emtansine), or administer as an infusion, with other medicinal products." **Incompatible** with D5W.

RATE OF ADMINISTRATION

For IV infusion only. Do not administer as an IV push or bolus. Use of a 0.2- or 0.22-micron, in-line, polyethersulfone (PES) filter required. Slow or interrupt the infusion if patient develops an infusion-related reaction; see Dose Adjustments, Precautions, and Antidote.

First infusion: Administer over 90 minutes.

Subsequent infusions: If initial and/or prior infusions are well tolerated, subsequent infusions may be administered over 30 minutes.

Delayed or missed infusions: Administer at the dose and rate tolerated in the most recent infusion.

ACTIONS

A HER2-targeted antibody-drug conjugate (ADC) that contains the humanized anti-HER2 IgG1, trastuzumab, covalently linked to the microtubule inhibitory drug DM1 (a maytansine derivative). Specific processes result in the intracellular release of DM1-containing cytotoxic catabolites. Binding of DM1 to tubulin disrupts microtubule networks in the cell, which results in cell-cycle arrest and apoptotic cell death. Ado-trastuzumab emtansine also inhibits HER2 receptor signaling, mediates antibody-dependent cell-mediated cytotoxicity, and inhibits shedding of the HER2 extracellular domain in human breast cancer cells that overexpress HER2. Maximum concentrations have been observed close to the end of an infusion. DM1 is metabolized in the liver by CYP3A4/5. Elimination half-life is approximately 4 days.

INDICATIONS AND USES

Used as a single agent in the treatment of patients with HER2-positive, metastatic breast cancer who previously received trastuzumab and a taxane separately or in combination. Patients should have either received prior therapy for metastatic disease or developed a recurrence of disease during or within 6 months of completing other chemotherapy.

CONTRAINDICATIONS

Manufacturer states, "None."

PRECAUTIONS

Follow guidelines for handling cytotoxic agents. See Appendix A, p. 1331. ▪ *Do not administer doses greater than 3.6 mg/kg.* ▪ *Do not substitute ado-trastuzumab (Kadcyla) for or with trastuzumab.* ▪ Serious hypersensitivity and/or infusion reactions have occurred. Ado-trastuzumab has not been studied in patients who had trastuzumab permanently discontinued because of infusion-related reactions and/or hypersensitivity; treatment with ado-trastuzumab is not recommended for these patients. ▪ Administer under the direction of a physician knowledgeable in its use in a facility with adequate diagnostic and treatment facilities to monitor the patient and respond to any medical emergency. ▪ Exposure to ado-trastuzumab can result in embryo-fetal death or birth defects; see Patient Education and Maternal/Child. ▪ Hepatotoxicity, predominantly increases in serum transaminases, has been observed. Serious hepatotoxicity has been reported, including liver failure and death. ▪ Cases of nodular regenerative hyperplasia (NRH) of the liver have been identified from liver biopsies; one case was fatal. NRH may lead to noncirrhotic portal hypertension. ▪ Cardiac toxicity has been reported. Treatment with ado-trastuzumab may lead to reductions in left ventricular ejection fraction (LVEF). ▪ Interstitial lung disease (ILD), including pneumonitis, has been reported. Some have resulted in acute respiratory distress syndrome or fatal outcome. Patients with dyspnea at rest due to complications of advanced malignancy and comorbidities may be at increased risk for pulmonary toxicity. ▪ Hemorrhagic events, including CNS, respiratory, and GI hemorrhage, have been reported. Some resulted in fatal outcomes. Hemorrhagic events were observed in patients with no known risk factors, as well as in patients with thrombocytopenia and in patients receiving anticoagulation or antiplatelet therapy; see Drug Interactions. ▪ Peripheral neuropathy (predominantly sensory) has been reported. ▪ Effects on patients with severe renal impairment and/or hepatic impairment have not been studied. ▪ A protein substance; has potential for immunogenicity. ▪ See Dose Adjustments, Monitor, and Antidote.

Monitor: Verify nonpregnancy status before beginning ado-trastuzumab therapy. ▪ Assess HER2 status before beginning ado-trastuzumab therapy. Testing should be done by a laboratory with demonstrated proficiency in the testing process. ▪ Obtain baseline CBC and differential with platelets before treatment and before each scheduled dose. ▪ Obtain baseline AST, ALT, and bilirubin before treatment and before each scheduled dose (every 3 weeks). ▪ Obtain baseline LVEF before treatment and at regular intervals (e.g., every 3 months) to confirm it remains within the prescribed parameters. ▪ Avoid extravasation; monitor infusion site closely. ▪ Monitor for S/S of a hypersensitivity or infusion reaction (e.g., bronchospasm, chills, dyspnea, fever, flushing, hypotension, pruritus, rash, tachycardia, urticaria, and wheezing). Observe closely during and for 90 minutes after the first infusion and during and for at least 30 minutes after subsequent infusions. ▪ Consider a possible diagnosis of NRH in patients with clinical symptoms of portal hypertension and/or with cirrhosis-like patterns seen on the computed tomography (CT) scan of the liver but with normal transaminases and no other manifestations of cirrhosis. Diagnosis can be confirmed only by histopathology. ▪ Monitor for S/S of ILD (e.g., cough, dyspnea, fatigue, and pulmonary infiltrates). May or may not occur as sequelae of infusion reactions. ▪ Monitor for thrombocytopenia (platelet count less than 50,000/mm^3). Nadir occurs by Day 8 and generally improves to Grade 0 or 1 (equal to or greater than 75,000/mm^3) by the next scheduled dose. Initiate precautions to prevent excessive bleeding (e.g., inspect IV sites, skin, and mucous membranes; use extreme care during invasive procedures; test urine, emesis, stool, and secretions for occult blood). ▪ Monitor for S/S of peripheral neuropathy (e.g., paresthesias, tingling, weakness).

Patient Education: Avoid pregnancy; potential serious risk to fetus. Effective contraception required while receiving therapy and for 7 months following the last dose. ▪ If ado-trastuzumab is administered during pregnancy or if the patient becomes pregnant while receiving ado-trastuzumab within 7 months following the last dose of ado-trastuzumab, report exposure immediately to the Genentech Adverse Event Line. ▪ During infusion, promptly report S/S of an infusion or hypersensitivity reaction (e.g., asthenia, bronchospasm, chills, dizziness, dyspnea, fatigue, fever, flushing, hypotension, nausea, pruritus, rash, urticaria, vomiting, wheezing). ▪ Promptly report S/S of acute hepatitis (e.g., abdominal pain, anorexia, dark urine, generalized pruritus, jaundice, nausea, vomiting). ▪ Report new-onset or worsening SOB, cough, swelling of ankles/legs, weight gain. ▪ See Appendix D, p. 1333.

Maternal/Child: Category D: avoid pregnancy; may cause fetal harm. Exposure can result in embryo-fetal death and birth defects. Oligohydramnios, fatal pulmonary hypoplasia, skeletal abnormalities, and embryo-fetal death have been reported in post-marketing reports for trastuzumab; see Patient Education. ▪ Encourage patients who are exposed during pregnancy or within 7 months before conception to enroll in the MotHER Pregnancy Registry. ▪ Discontinue breast-feeding during treatment with ado-trastuzumab and for 7 months after completion of therapy. ▪ Safety and effectiveness for use in pediatric patients not established.

Elderly: Age does not affect the pharmacokinetics of ado-trastuzumab.

DRUG/LAB INTERACTIONS

No formal drug interaction studies have been done. ▪ DM1, the cytotoxic component of ado-trastuzumab, is metabolized mainly by CYP3A4 and to a lesser extent by CYP3A5. **Avoid concomitant use of strong CYP3A4 inhibitors** (e.g., atazanavir [Reyataz], clarithromycin [Biaxin], indinavir [Crixivan], itraconazole [Sporanox], ketoconazole [Nizoral], nefazodone, nelfinavir [Viracept], ritonavir [Norvir], saquinavir [Invirase], telithromycin

[Ketek], voriconazole [VFEND]). Consideration of an alternate medication with no or minimal potential to inhibit CYP3A4 is recommended, or delay ado-trastuzumab treatment until the strong CYP3A4 inhibitors have cleared from the circulation (approximately 3 elimination half-lives of the inhibitors). If coadministration cannot be delayed, closely monitor patients for adverse reactions. ▪ Possible increased risk of hemorrhage when administered concomitantly with **anticoagulants** (e.g., warfarin [Coumadin]) and/or **antiplatelet agents** (e.g., clopidogrel [Plavix]). Consider additional monitoring when concomitant use is medically necessary.

SIDE EFFECTS

Constipation, epistaxis, fatigue, headache, hemorrhage, increased transaminases, musculoskeletal pain, nausea, and thrombocytopenia were most common. Serious side effects include embryo-fetal toxicity, hepatotoxicity (including hepatic failure), hypersensitivity and/or infusion-related reactions, left ventricular dysfunction, neurotoxicity, nodular regenerative hyperplasia, portal hypertension, pulmonary toxicity, and thrombocytopenia. Abdominal pain, anemia, arthralgia, asthenia, blurred vision, chills, conjunctivitis, cough, diarrhea, dizziness, dry eyes, dry mouth, dysgeusia, dyspepsia, dyspnea, epistaxis, fever, hypertension, hypokalemia, increased blood alkaline phosphatase, increased lacrimation, insomnia, myalgia, neutropenia, peripheral edema, pneumonitis, pruritus, rash, stomatitis, urinary tract infections, and vomiting have also been reported.

ANTIDOTE

Notify physician of all side effects. Most will be treated symptomatically. If signs of an infusion reaction occur, slow or interrupt the infusion and treat appropriately. Monitor patients carefully until symptoms resolve. Discontinue immediately for a serious hypersensitivity or infusion-related reaction. Treat hypersensitivity reactions with epinephrine, antihistamines, corticosteroids, bronchodilators, and oxygen. See Dose Adjustments for recommendations to reduce dose of, delay, or permanently discontinue ado-trastuzumab in cases of serious side effects (e.g., hyperbilirubinemia, increased serum transaminases, reduction in LVEF, nodular regenerative hyperplasia [NRH], peripheral neuropathy, pulmonary toxicity [ILD or pneumonitis], thrombocytopenia). Resuscitate as indicated.

ALBUMIN (HUMAN)
(al-**BYOO**-min **HU**-man)

**Plasma volume expander
(plasma protein fraction)**

Albumin (Human Preservative Free) 5%, 20%, & 25%, Albuminar 5% & 25%, AlbuRx 5% & 25%, Albutein 5% & 25%, Buminate 5% & 25%, Flexbumin 25%, Human Albumin Grifols 25%, Normal Serum Albumin, Plasbumin 5%, 20%, & 25%

pH 6.4 to 7.4

USUAL DOSE
Variable, depending on patient condition (e.g., presence of hemorrhage, hypovolemia, or shock, pulse, BP, hemoglobin and hematocrit, and amount of pulmonary or venous congestion present). Fluid and protein requirements and underlying condition determine the concentration of albumin used. 5% is usually indicated in hypovolemic or intravascularly depleted patients, and 20% or 25% is appropriate when fluid and sodium intake should be minimized (e.g., cerebral edema, hypoproteinemia, pediatric patients). The initial dose is usually 12.5 to 25 Gm. Amount of 5% given may be increased to 0.5 Gm/lb of body weight (10 mL/lb) with careful monitoring of the patient. Available as 5% solution (5 Gm/100 mL), 20% solution (20 Gm/100 mL), or 25% solution (25 Gm/100 mL). The maximum dose is 6 Gm/kg/24 hr or 250 Gm in 48 hours (250 Gm is equal to 5 liters of 5% or 1 liter of 25%). In the absence of active hemorrhage, the total dose usually does not exceed the normal circulating mass of albumin (e.g., 2 Gm/kg of body weight).

Hypoproteinemia (hypoalbuminemia): 50 to 75 Gm as a 5% or 25% solution. Repeat doses may be required in patients who continue to lose albumin.

Hypovolemia: 12 to 25 Gm as a 5%, 20%, or 25% solution. May be repeated in 15 to 30 minutes if response inadequate. If 25% solution is used, additional fluids may be needed.

Burns: Electrolyte replacement and crystalloids (e.g., IV fluids) to maintain plasma volume are required in the first 24 hours. Then begin with 25 Gm and adjust as necessary to maintain albumin level from 2 to 3 Gm/dL.

Acute nephrosis or acute nephrotic syndrome: 20 to 25 Gm of a 25% solution with a loop diuretic (e.g., furosemide [Lasix], torsemide [Demadex]) daily for 7 to 10 days.

Hemodialysis: 100 mL of a 20% or 25% solution.

Red blood cell resuspension: 20 to 25 Gm of a 20% or 25% solution/liter of RBCs.

Cardiopulmonary bypass: Achieve a plasma albumin of 2.5 Gm/dL and hematocrit concentration of 20% with either a 5% or 25% solution. Use crystalloids (IV fluids) as a pump prime.

PEDIATRIC DOSE
0.5 to 1 Gm/kg/dose. 25% solution is usually used in infants and other pediatric patients; *do not use in preterm infants.* Monitor hemodynamic response closely. Maximum dose 6 Gm/kg/24 hr or 250 Gm/48 hr.

Hypoproteinemia (hypoalbuminemia): 0.5 to 1 Gm/kg/dose. Repeat every 1 to 2 days as needed.

Hypovolemia: 0.5 to 1 Gm/kg/dose. May be repeated in 15 to 30 minutes if response inadequate.

Hemolytic disease of the newborn: 1 Gm/kg (4 mL/kg) of 25% albumin. One source recommends giving 1 hour before exchange transfusion. Another recommends 1 to 2 hours before blood transfusion or with transfusion (exchange 50 mL of albumin 25% for 50 mL plasma). *Do not use in preterm infants.*

Burns: See Usual Dose.

DILUTION

May be given undiluted or further diluted with NS or D5W for infusion. NS is the preferred diluent. When sodium restriction is required, D5W may be substituted. The use of SWFI as a diluent is not recommended. Life-threatening hemolysis and acute renal failure can result if a sufficient volume of SWFI is used as a diluent. The 5% product is isotonic and osmotically approximates human plasma. One volume of 25% to four volumes of diluent is isotonic. Use only clear solutions.

Storage: Store at CRT. Use within 4 hours after opening. Discard unused portions.

COMPATIBILITY

Consider any drug NOT listed as compatible to be INCOMPATIBLE until consulting a pharmacist; specific conditions may apply.

Do not use SWFI as a diluent; see Dilution. Manufacturers state, "Do not mix with protein hydrolysates, amino acid mixtures, or solutions containing alcohol." Manufacturers also state, "May be administered in conjunction with or combined with other parenterals such as whole blood, plasma, glucose, saline, or sodium lactate."

One source suggests the following **compatibilities:**

Y-site: Diltiazem (Cardizem), lorazepam (Ativan).

RATE OF ADMINISTRATION

Variable, depending on indication, present blood volume, patient response, and concentration of solution. A too-rapid rate, especially in the presence of normal blood volume, may cause circulatory overload and pulmonary edema. Averages are:

Normal blood volume: 1 to 2 mL/min.

Deficient blood volume (hypovolemia): A single dose as rapidly as tolerated. Repeat dose as rapidly as tolerated if indicated. As volume approaches normal, slow 5% to 1 to 2 mL/min and 25% to 1 mL/min to prevent circulatory overload and pulmonary edema.

Hypoproteinemia: 2 to 3 mL/min in adults; a single dose over 30 to 120 minutes in pediatric patients.

Infants and other pediatric patients: For uses other than hypovolemia and hypoproteinemia, the rate of administration should be about one fourth to one half the adult rate.

ACTIONS

A sterile natural plasma protein substance prepared by a specific process, which makes it free from the danger of serum hepatitis. A blood volume expander that accounts for 70% to 80% of the colloid oncotic pressure of plasma. Expands blood volume proportionately to amount of circulating blood, improves cardiac output, prevents marked hemoconcentration, aids in reduction of edema, and raises serum protein levels. Low sodium content helps to maintain electrolyte balance and should promote diuresis in presence of edema (contains 130 to 160 mEq sodium/L). Also acts as a transport protein that binds both endogenous and exogenous substances, including bilirubin and certain drugs.

INDICATIONS AND USES

Hypovolemia (with or without shock [actual or impending], with or without hemorrhage); 5% if hypovolemic, 25% if adequate hydration or edema is present. ■ Hypoalbuminemia from inadequate production (e.g., burns, congenital analbuminemia, endocrine disorders, infection, liver disease, major injury, malignancy, malnutrition). ■ Hypoalbuminemia from excessive catabolism (e.g., burns, major injury, nephrosis, pancreatitis, pemphigus [chronic relapsing skin disease], peritonitis, thyrotoxicosis). ■ Hypoalbuminemia from loss from the body (e.g., hemorrhage, burn exudates, excessive renal excretion, exfoliative dermatoses, exudative enteropathy [e.g., inflammatory bowel disease]). ■ Hypoalbuminemia from redistribution within the body (e.g., cirrhosis with ascites, inflammatory conditions, major surgery). ■ Hypoalbuminemia secondary to pulmonary edema in adult respiratory distress syndrome (ARDS). ■ Raising plasma oncotic pressure to treat edema of nephrosis. ■ Cardiopulmonary bypass surgery. ■ Hemolytic disease of the newborn (bilirubin binding activity) as adjunct to exchange transfusion. ■ Provide adequate volume and prevent hypoproteinemia as an adjunct to RBC resuspension.

Unlabeled uses: Large-volume paracentesis, spontaneous bacterial peritonitis in patients with cirrhosis.

CONTRAINDICATIONS

Anemia (severe) or cardiac failure in the presence of normal or increased intravascular volume, hypersensitivity to albumin, pulmonary edema. ▪ Buminate 25% should not be used in patients with chronic renal impairment; contains aluminum.

PRECAUTIONS

Whole blood or packed cells probably indicated if more than 1,000 mL 5% albumin required in hemorrhage; are adjunctive to use of large amounts of serum albumin to prevent anemia. Is not a substitute for whole blood in situations in which both the oxygen-carrying capacity and plasma volume expansion provided by whole blood are required. ▪ May be given regardless of patient blood group. ▪ Use caution in hypertension, low cardiac reserve, hepatic or renal failure, or lack of albumin deficiency. ▪ Use caution in patients with normal or increased intravascular volume; however, patients with hypoproteinemia may have normal blood volume. ▪ Use caution in patients with burns, hypoproteinemia, or hypovolemia; an FDA-issued Dear Doctor letter identified concerns of an excess mortality rate when albumin administration was compared to NS administration in these critically ill patients. Trauma patients with concomitant traumatic brain injuries may also be at risk for increased mortality. ▪ Made from human plasma and may contain infectious agents (e.g., HIV, Creutzfeldt-Jakob disease, hepatitis B, hepatitis C). Numerous steps in the manufacturing process are used to make the potential for infection extremely remote. ▪ 25 Gm of albumin is the osmotic equivalent of 2 units of fresh-frozen plasma. 25 Gm of albumin provides as much plasma protein as 500 mL of plasma or 2 units of whole blood. ▪ Albumin is not a source of nutrition.

Monitor: Monitor BP. ▪ Monitor for S/S of a hypersensitivity reaction (e.g., chest pain, dizziness, dyspnea, fever, flushing, hypotension, nausea, pruritus, rash, rigors, urticaria). ▪ Hemoglobin, hematocrit, electrolyte, and serum protein evaluations are mandatory during therapy. Alkaline phosphatase may be elevated. ▪ Hyponatremia may result from administration of large volumes of albumin diluted in D5W; additional monitoring of electrolytes may be required. ▪ Observe patient carefully for increased bleeding resulting from more normal BP, circulatory embarrassment, pulmonary edema, or lack of diuresis. Central venous and/or pulmonary wedge pressure readings are most helpful. ▪ Maintain hydration with additional fluids, especially in dehydrated patients. ▪ Normal plasma albumin is 3.5 to 6 Gm/dL.

Maternal/Child: Category C: safety for use during pregnancy not established. ▪ Do not use 25% solution in preterm infants.

Elderly: Monitor fluid intake carefully; more susceptible to circulatory overload and pulmonary edema. ▪ Plasma albumin levels may be more volatile.

DRUG/LAB INTERACTIONS

Specific information not available.

SIDE EFFECTS

Chills, fever, headache, hypotension, nausea, salivation, skin rash or hives, tachycardia, vomiting.

Major: Congestive heart failure, decreased myocardial contractility, hypersensitivity reactions including anaphylaxis (rare), precipitous hypotension, pulmonary edema, salt and water retention.

ANTIDOTE

Notify the physician of all side effects. Minor side effects are generally tolerated and treated symptomatically. For major side effects, discontinue albumin and treat symptomatically. Resuscitate as necessary.

ALDESLEUKIN BBW
(al-des-**LOO**-kin)

Antineoplastic
Immunomodulator
Biologic response modifier
Recombinant interleukin-2

Interleukin-2 Recombinant, Proleukin

pH 7.2 to 7.8

USUAL DOSE
(International units [IU])
Patient selection restricted. Prescreening and baseline studies required; see Precautions/ Monitor.

Standard high-dose regimen: _Intermittent IV:_ 600,000 international units (IU)/kg (0.037 mg/kg) every 8 hours for 14 doses. After 9 days of rest, repeat for up to 14 more doses; this constitutes one course (two 5-day [14 or fewer doses] treatment cycles separated by a rest period of 9 days). Treat with 28 doses or until dose-limiting toxicity requiring ICU-level support occurs. Dose is based on actual patient weight.

Retreatment: Evaluate for response 4 weeks after course completion and again before scheduling start of the next course. Additional courses are considered if there is some tumor shrinkage following the previous course and retreatment is not contraindicated. At least 7 weeks from hospital discharge should elapse before a subsequent course is administered.

Sometimes given in combination with other agents.

DOSE ADJUSTMENTS
Information on dosing in obese and underweight patients is not available; base dose on actual patient weight. ▪ Doses are frequently withheld for toxicity. Doses are actually withheld, not reduced in amount. Median number of doses actually administered in a first course is 20 for metastatic renal cell carcinoma patients and 18 for metastatic melanoma patients. Continuous infusions can be interrupted as indicated by patient symptoms. ▪ Hold doses and restart based on the following chart:

Guidelines for Holding Doses of Aldesleukin	
Hold Dose for	May Give Next Dose if
CARDIOVASCULAR	
Atrial fibrillation, supraventricular tachycardia, bradycardia that requires treatment or is recurrent or persistent.	Patient is asymptomatic with full recovery to normal sinus rhythm.
Systolic BP <90 mm Hg with increasing requirements for pressors.	Systolic BP ≥90 mm Hg and stable or improving requirements for pressors.
Any ECG change consistent with MI or ischemia with or without chest pain; suspicion of cardiac ischemia or myocarditis.	Patient is asymptomatic; MI and myocarditis have been ruled out; clinical suspicion of angina is low; there is no incidence of ventricular hypokinesia.

Guidelines for Holding Doses of Aldesleukin—cont'd	
Hold Dose for	**May Give Next Dose if**
PULMONARY	
O_2 saturation <90%.	O_2 saturation >90%.
CENTRAL NERVOUS SYSTEM	
Mental status changes (e.g., agitation, confusion, lethargy, somnolence). May result in coma.	Mental status changes completely resolved.
BODY AS A WHOLE	
Sepsis syndrome; patient is clinically unstable.	Sepsis syndrome has resolved; patient is clinically stable; infection is under treatment.
UROGENITAL	
SCr >4.5 mg/dL or a SCr of ≥4 mg/dL in presence of severe volume overload, acidosis, or hyperkalemia.	SCr <4 mg/dL, and fluid and electrolyte status is stable.
Persistent oliguria, urine output of <10 mL/hr for 16 to 24 hr with rising SCr.	Urine output >10 mL/hr with a decrease of SCr >1.5 mg/dL or normalization of SCr.
DIGESTIVE	
Signs of hepatic failure, including encephalopathy, increasing ascites, liver pain, hypoglycemia.	Discontinue for remainder of current course. May consider a new course of treatment in 7 weeks if all signs of hepatic failure have resolved.
Stool guaiac repeatedly >3 to 4$^+$.	Stool guaiac negative.
SKIN	
Bullous dermatitis or marked worsening of pre-existing skin condition (avoid topical steroid therapy).	Resolution of all signs of bullous dermatitis.

- After withholding a dose, no dose should be given until patient is globally assessed and specific criteria for restarting aldesleukin are met.

DILUTION (International units [IU])

Each 22,000,000 IU vial (1.3 mg) must be reconstituted with 1.2 mL of preservative-free SWFI (18,000,000 IU/mL [1.1 mg (1,100 mcg)/mL]). Sterile technique imperative. Direct diluent to side of vial and gently swirl to avoid excess foaming. Do not shake. Further dilute the calculated dose in 50 mL D5W. Desired final infusion concentration is 30 to 70 mcg/mL. If the total dose is 1.5 mg or less (patient weighs less than 40 kg), the dose of aldesleukin should be diluted in a smaller volume of D5W so the final concentration remains in the acceptable range. Plastic infusion containers are preferred over glass. Do not use any filters for dilution or administration. Do not use any other diluent or infusion solution; may cause increased aggregation. Bring to room temperature before administration.

Filters: Do not use any filters for dilution or administration.

Storage: Store in refrigerator before and after reconstitution and dilution. Do not freeze. Protect from light. No stability problems will occur at CRT for 48 hours after dilution but has no preservatives. Do not use beyond expiration date on vial.

COMPATIBILITY (Underline Indicates Conflicting Compatibility Information)

Consider any drug NOT listed as compatible to be INCOMPATIBLE until consulting a pharmacist; specific conditions may apply.

Manufacturer recommends not mixing with other drugs in the same container. Bacteriostatic water for injection (BWFI) or NS will increase aggregation.

One source suggests the following **compatibilities:**

Y-site: Amphotericin B (conventional), calcium gluconate, diphenhydramine (Benadryl), dopamine, fluconazole (Diflucan), foscarnet (Foscavir), heparin, magnesium sulfate, metoclopramide (Reglan), ondansetron (Zofran), potassium chloride (KCl), ranitidine (Zantac), sulfamethoxazole/trimethoprim, vancomycin.

RATE OF ADMINISTRATION

Intermittent IV: A single dose as an intermittent infusion over 15 minutes. Flush main line IV with D5W before and after each use. Manufacturer recommends that any keep-open IV in place for intermittent administration be D5W.

ACTIONS

A genetically engineered recombinant protein that possesses the biologic activity of naturally occurring interleukin-2. Exact mechanism of action is unknown. Immunoregulatory properties include enhancement of lymphocyte mitogenesis and stimulation of long-term growth of human interleukin-2 dependent cell lines, enhancement of lymphocyte cytotoxicity, induction of killer cell (lymphokine-activated [LAK] and natural [NK]) activity, and induction of interferon-gamma production. Immunologic effects occur in a dose-dependent manner and include activation of cellular immunity with profound lymphocytosis, eosinophilia, and thrombocytopenia, as well as the production of cytokines, including tumor necrosis factor, IL-1, and gamma interferon. In vivo experiments in murine tumor models have shown inhibition of tumor growth. Following a short infusion, aldesleukin distributes rapidly into the kidneys, liver, lungs, and spleen. Half-life is approximately 85 minutes. Eliminated by metabolism in the kidney with little or no bioactive protein excreted in urine.

INDICATIONS AND USES

Prescreening mandatory. Eligibility requirements for treatment are specific; see Precautions and Contraindications. ▪ Treatment of metastatic renal cell carcinoma in adults. Patient selection should include assessment of performance status. See prescribing information for details. ▪ Treatment of adults with metastatic melanoma.

Unlabeled uses: Acute myelogenous leukemia after autologous BMT.

CONTRAINDICATIONS

Abnormal thallium stress test or pulmonary function tests. ▪ Known hypersensitivity to interleukin-2 or any component of aldesleukin. ▪ Patients with organ allografts. ▪ Exclude from treatment any patient with significant cardiac, pulmonary, renal, hepatic, or CNS impairment; any patient requiring treatment with steroidal agents; and any patient at higher risk for cardiovascular adverse events during periods of hypotension and fluid shifts.

Retreatment is permanently contraindicated in patients who experienced specific toxicities in a previous course of therapy (see the following chart).

Contraindications for Retreatment with Aldesleukin	
Organ System	**Symptom**
Cardiovascular	Sustained ventricular tachycardia ≥5 beats. Cardiac rhythm disturbances not controlled or unresponsive to management. Chest pain with ECG changes consistent with angina or myocardial infarction. Cardiac tamponade.
Pulmonary	Intubation required more than 72 hours.
Renal	Renal failure requiring dialysis for more than 72 hours.
Central nervous system	Coma or toxic psychosis lasting more than 48 hours. Repetitive or difficult-to-control seizures.
Gastrointestinal	Bowel ischemia or perforation. Bleeding requiring surgery.

PRECAUTIONS

Administered in the hospital under the supervision of a qualified physician (usually a medical oncologist and/or immunologist). Intensive care facilities and specialists in cardiopulmonary and/or intensive care medicine must be available. ▪ Capillary leak syndrome (CLS [extravasation of plasma proteins and fluid into the extravascular space and loss of vascular tone]) can begin immediately after aldesleukin treatment starts and results in hypotension and reduced organ perfusion that can be severe enough to result in death. CLS may be associated with angina, arrhythmias (supraventricular and ventricular), edema, GI bleed or infarction, mental status changes, myocardial infarction, renal insufficiency, and respiratory insufficiency requiring intubation. Extravasation of protein and fluid into the extravascular space will lead to edema and the creation of new effusions. ▪ Therapy should be restricted to patients with normal cardiac and pulmonary functions as defined by appropriate tests. ▪ Use extreme caution in patients with normal thallium stress tests and pulmonary function tests who have a history of prior cardiac or pulmonary disease. ▪ Patients who have had a nephrectomy are eligible for treatment if SCr is less than 1.5 mg/dL (85% of patients in one study). ▪ Mental status changes (e.g., irritability, confusion, depression) may be indicators of bacteremia or early bacterial sepsis, hypoperfusion, occult CNS malignancy, or direct aldesleukin-induced CNS toxicity. Mental status changes due solely to aldesleukin may progress for several days before recovery begins. Permanent neurologic deficits have been reported. ▪ Withhold administration in patients who develop moderate to severe lethargy or somnolence; continued administration may result in coma. ▪ May exacerbate disease symptoms in clinically unrecognized or untreated CNS metastases. Thoroughly evaluate and treat CNS metastases before aldesleukin therapy. Should be neurologically stable and have a negative CT scan. New neurologic signs, symptoms, and anatomic lesions following aldesleukin therapy have been reported in patients without evidence of CNS metastases. Clinical manifestations include agitation, ataxia, change in mental status, hallucinations, obtundation, speech difficulties, and coma. Cortical lesions and demyelination have been seen using MRI studies. Neurologic S/S usually resolve following discontinuation of therapy; however, there have been reports of permanent damage. ▪ Use extreme caution in patients with a history of seizures (may cause seizures), patients with fixed requirements for large volumes of fluid (e.g., hypercalcemia), those with autoimmune disorders (e.g., Crohn's disease, ulcerative colitis, psoriasis), previous cytotoxic drug therapy or radiation therapy, and patients sensitive to *Escherichia coli*–derived proteins. ▪ May cause autoimmune disease and inflammatory disorders or exacerbate pre-existing conditions (e.g., Crohn's disease, diabetes mellitus, scleroderma, inflammatory arthritis, oculobulbar myasthenia gravis, glomerulonephritis, cholecystitis, cerebral vasculitis, thyroiditis, Stevens-Johnson syndrome, bullous pemphigoid). ▪ Serious manifestations of eosinophilia involving eosinophilic infiltration of cardiac and pulmonary tissues can occur following aldesleukin administration. ▪ Associated with impaired neutrophil function and an increased risk of disseminated infection, including sepsis and bacterial endocarditis. Pre-existing bacterial infections should be adequately treated before beginning therapy. Patients with indwelling central lines are at increased risk for infection with gram-positive organisms. Antibiotic prophylaxis with ciprofloxacin, nafcillin, oxacillin, or vancomycin has been associated with a reduced incidence of staphylococcal infections. ▪ Induces significant hypotension; discontinue antihypertensives during treatment. ▪ Kidney and liver function are impaired during aldesleukin therapy. ▪ May impair thyroid function; changes may suggest autoimmunity; thyroid replacement therapy has been required in a few patients. ▪ May cause hyperglycemia and/or diabetes mellitus. ▪ Anti-aldesleukin antibodies have been detected in some patients. Impact of antibody formation on efficacy and safety of aldesleukin is unknown. ▪ See Drug/Lab Interactions.

Monitor: A central venous catheter (double or triple lumen) is frequently ordered on admission (required for continuous infusion). A minimum of two IV lines is usually required (one for the aldesleukin and its keep-open IV and one for other needed fluids and medications). One line could suffice if absolutely necessary since aldesleukin would be discontinued when colloids are administered. Flushing of line with D5W before and after aldesleukin is imperative. Ability to record CVP and draw blood samples should be available. ▪ Admission chest x-ray, ECG, CBC with differential and platelet count, blood chemistries including electrolytes and renal and liver function tests, T_3, T_4, PT, PTT, urinalysis, and body weight should be obtained. Adequate pulmonary function, normal arterial blood gases, and normal ejection fraction and unimpaired wall motion (confirmed by thallium stress test and/or a stress echocardiogram) should be documented. ▪ During drug administration obtain daily CBC with differential and platelet count, blood chemistries including electrolytes, renal and hepatic function tests, and chest x-rays. ▪ Continuous cardiac monitoring is indicated (required with BP below 90 mm Hg or any cardiac irregularity). ▪ Monitoring and flexibility in management of fluid balance and organ perfusion status are imperative. Requires constant management and balancing of effects of fluid shifts to prevent the consequences of hypovolemia (e.g., impaired organ perfusion) or fluid accumulation (e.g., edema, pulmonary edema, ascites, pulmonary effusion), which may exceed the patient's tolerance. ▪ Assess hypovolemia by central venous catheterization and frequent central venous pressure monitoring. Administer colloids (albumin, plasmanate) or crystalloids (IV fluids) as indicated for a BP drop of 20 mm Hg or greater or a systolic BP less than 90. ▪ Frequent neuro checks required (note agitation, blurred vision, confusion, depression, irritability, and persistent somnolence). ▪ Vital signs and strict I&O are required every 2 to 4 hours (much more frequently as side effects develop). ▪ Weigh daily. ▪ Assess thyroid function periodically. ▪ An ECG and cardiac enzymes are indicated for any S/S of chest pain, murmurs, gallops, irregular rhythm, or palpitations. A repeat thallium study is indicated for evidence of cardiac ischemia or CHF; may indicate ventricular hypokinesia due to MI or myocarditis. ▪ Obtain a urinalysis as indicated. ▪ Assess pulmonary function through examination, vital signs, and pulse oximetry. Arterial blood gases are indicated for any dyspnea or respiratory impairment. ▪ Some routine medications are indicated prophylactically to reduce the incidence of side effects and to promote patient comfort. The morning of the first treatment, begin standard antipyretic therapy (e.g., acetaminophen 650 mg PO q 4 hr) and NSAIDs (e.g., naprosyn 500 mg q 12 hr PO) for fever and arthralgia. Use an H_2 antagonist (e.g., ranitidine 150 mg PO q 12 hr) to prevent GI bleeding. Continue administration of these drugs until 12 hours after last dose of aldesleukin. Low-dose dopamine 1 to 5 mcg/kg/min can help maintain organ perfusion and urine output if given at initial onset of CLS before hypotension occurs. Antiemetics, antidiarrheals, antichill/rigors (meperidine), antihistamines, and moisturizing skin lotions will also be used throughout treatment; see Antidote for specifics. ▪ If fever occurs several days into treatment or recurs after subsiding, assume infection first, then drug. Confusion, depression, or irritability may also suggest infection. Draw cultures; administer appropriate antibiotics. ▪ Patients who have had nephrectomies may be more at risk for increases in serum BUN or creatinine, electrolyte shifts, and reduced urine output. Evaluate fluid, electrolyte, and acid-base status promptly if any of the above occur. Gradual increases without other complications (marked fluid overload, hyperkalemia, acidosis) are frequently tolerated (SCr must not exceed 4.5 mg/dL). ▪ Maintain pulmonary status as needed with O_2 and diuretics (furosemide). Assess pulmonary status with chest x-rays. ▪ Monitor central and peripheral IV sites to reduce potential for infection. ▪ No restrictions on activity; use caution ambulating (orthostatic hypotension). ▪ No restrictions on diet. Encouragement may be required (anorexia and/or mouth sores). ▪ Monitor for thrombocytopenia (platelet count less than 50,000/mm^3). Initiate precautions to prevent excessive bleeding (e.g., inspect IV sites, skin, and mucous membranes; use extreme care during invasive procedures; test urine, emesis, stool, and secretions for occult blood). ▪ Specific preparation required for discharge; refer to literature. ▪ Manufacturer supplies excellent brochures for nurses and physicians with detailed guidelines in chart form on all aspects of monitoring, toxicity, and treatment. ▪ Complete review and adequate preparation of all aspects of this therapy with the patient and family are imperative. Can reduce psychologic stress of toxicity. ▪ Tumor regression has continued for up to 12 months after one or more courses of therapy. ▪ See Dose Adjustments, Contraindications, and Antidote.

Patient Education: Many side effects will occur; report any changes you perceive so they can be evaluated and treated if needed (e.g., changes in breathing, chest or other pain, temperature, mood, light-headedness, fatigue). ▪ Request assistance for ambulation and always sit on the side of the bed first. ▪ Take only prescribed medications. ▪ Avoid alcohol. ▪ Use of effective contraceptive measures recommended for fertile men and women. ▪ Use 15 SPF sunscreen in sunlight to protect against photosensitivity. ▪ See Appendix D, p. 1333, for additional information. ▪ Manufacturer supplies a patient education booklet; review thoroughly and discuss with your physician and nurse.

Maternal/Child: Category C: benefits must outweigh risks. Contraceptive measures required before initial administration and throughout treatment. ▪ Discontinue breastfeeding. ▪ Safety for use in pediatric patients under 18 years of age not established; studies show responsiveness and toxicity similar.

Elderly: Response rates and toxicity similar to that seen in younger adults; however, some increased incidence of severe urogenital toxicities and dyspnea was noted in the elderly. ▪ Use caution; consider age-related organ impairment.

DRUG/LAB INTERACTIONS

May cause interactions with **psychotropic drugs** (e.g., analgesics, antiemetics, narcotics, sedatives, tranquilizers) because aldesleukin also affects central nervous function. ▪ Concomitant use with **cardiotoxic agents** (e.g., doxorubicin [Adriamycin]), **hepatotoxic agents** (e.g., methotrexate, asparaginase), **myelotoxic agents** (e.g., cytotoxic chemotherapy, radiation therapy), **and nephrotoxic agents** (e.g., aminoglycosides, indomethacin) may increase toxicity in these organ systems and/or delay excretion of these agents, increasing their toxicity. ▪ Acute, atypical adverse reactions have been reported in patients treated with aldesleukin and subsequently administered **radiographic iodinated contrast media.** Reactions have included chills, diarrhea, edema, fever, hypotension, nausea, oliguria, pruritus, rash, and vomiting. Most reactions were reported when contrast media were given within 4 weeks after the last dose of aldesleukin. ▪ **Glucocorticoids** (e.g., dexamethasone [Decadron]) reduce aldesleukin-induced side effects but also reduce its antitumor effectiveness. ▪ Aldesleukin-induced hypotension may be potentiated by **beta-blockers** (e.g., metoprolol, atenolol) **and other antihypertensive agents** (e.g., ACE inhibitors [e.g., enalapril (Vasotec), lisinopril (Zestril)], calcium channel blockers [e.g., diltiazem (Cardizem), verapamil]). ▪ Concurrent use with **interferon-alfa** may increase incidence of MI, myocarditis, ventricular hypokinesia, and severe rhabdomyolysis. ▪ May cause hypersensitivity reactions in patients receiving combination regimens (**high-dose aldesleukin and antineoplastics** [e.g., dacarbazine, cisplatin, tamoxifen, interferon-alfa]). ▪ Aldesleukin may decrease clearance and increase plasma levels of **indinavir** (Crixivan). ▪ Capable of altering numerous lab values; see literature.

SIDE EFFECTS

Frequent, predictable, often severe; are usually clinically manageable and frequently require intensive care management. Begin to occur shortly after therapy begins (chills, fatigue, fever, hypotension, nausea, vomiting). Frequency and severity are dose-related and schedule-dependent. Most are reversible within 2 or 3 days of discontinuation of therapy. Even with intensive management, side effects can progress to death.

Initially anorexia, arthralgia, chills, fatigue, fever, nausea, and vomiting occur. Initial symptoms of capillary leak syndrome are edema, electrolyte abnormalities, hypotension, oliguria, respiratory distress, significant weight gain, tachycardia. Effects of CLS **successively** result in *hypovolemia,* which in turn leads to hypotension → hypoperfusion → sinus tachycardia → angina → myocardial ischemia and infarction → arrhythmias (supraventricular and ventricular) → decreased renal perfusion → prerenal azotemia → oliguria → anuria; *fluid retention/weight gain,* which in turn leads to rales → dyspnea → cough → tachypnea → hypoxia → pleural effusion → respiratory insufficiency requiring intubation → diarrhea → edema of the bowel → refractory acidosis → edema → ascites; and *breakdown of blood-brain barrier* (neuropsychiatric toxicity [e.g., agitation, combativeness, confusion, hallucinations, lethargy, psychosis, somnolence]). Abdominal pain and GI bleeding may be related to diarrhea, vomiting, stomatitis, duodenal ulcer formation, bowel ischemia, infarction, or perforation. Cerebral edema and concomitant medications may impact many side effects. Lethargy and/or somnolence may lead to coma. Anemia and thrombocytopenia may occur; coagulation abnormalities (PT, PTT) reflect liver dysfunction. Hemodynamic effects similar to septic shock may be caused by tumor necrosis factor. Erythematous rash and pruritus (can progress to dry desquamation) can occur in almost all patients and are extremely uncomfortable. See Precautions and Drug/Lab Interactions.

Post-Marketing: Anaphylaxis, angioedema, cardiac tamponade, cardiomyopathy, cellulitis, cerebral hemorrhage, cerebral lesions, cholecystitis, colitis, demyelinating neuropathy, encephalopathy, eosinophilia, extrapyramidal syndrome, fatal endocarditis, fatal subdural and subarachnoid hemorrhage, febrile neutropenia, gastritis, hepatitis, hepatosplenomegaly, hypertension, hyperthyroidism, injection site necrosis, insomnia, intestinal obstruction, lymphocytopenia, myopathy, myositis, neuralgia, neuritis, neutropenia, pneumonia (bacterial, fungal, viral), retroperitoneal hemorrhage, rhabdomyolysis, urticaria.

ANTIDOTE

Temporarily discontinue aldesleukin and notify physician immediately of arrhythmias or rhythm changes, chest pain, marked changes in HR, positive neuropsychiatric check (agitation, blurred vision, persistent extreme somnolence), systolic BP below 90 mm Hg, apical HR over 120, temperature over 38° C (100.4° F), respirations over 25/min, complaints of dyspnea, decreased breath sounds, increased sputum production, severe diarrhea associated with refractory acidosis, vomiting refractory to treatment, acute changes in GI status. May be restarted based on patient response. Hold any subsequent dose for failure to maintain organ perfusion; see Dose Adjustments. Fever is routinely treated with acetaminophen and indomethacin or naprosyn; increased doses may be needed. Suggested treatments include slow IV meperidine (Demerol) 25 to 50 mg for chills and rigidity; diphenoxylate (Lomotil) or loperamide (Imodium) PO for diarrhea (these meds may not help and diarrhea may be dose-limiting); diphenhydramine (Benadryl) 25 mg PO q 6 hr, a soothing skin cream (Eucerin), and oatmeal baths for urticaria and pruritus; temazepam (Restoril) for insomnia; ondansetron (Zofran) or prochlorperazine (Compazine) for nausea. Treat edema with furosemide (Lasix) once BP has normalized. IV fluids, albumin or plasmanate, and Trendelenburg positioning are used to maintain fluid balance and BP. If organ perfusion and BP are not sustained by dopamine 1 to 5 mcg/kg/min as a continuous infusion, increase to 6 to 10 mcg/kg/min or add phenylephrine (1 to 5 mcg/kg/min). Prolonged use of pressors at relatively high doses may cause cardiac arrhythmias. Treat arrhythmias as indicated (usually sinus or supraventricular tachycardia [adenosine, verapamil]). Use O_2 for decreased PaO_2. Use packed RBCs for anemia and to ensure maximum oxygen-carrying capacity. Platelet transfusions are indicated for thrombocytopenia or to reduce risk of GI bleeding. Use of blood modifiers to treat bone marrow toxicity may be indicated (e.g., darbepoetin alfa [Aranesp], epoetin alfa [Epogen], filgrastim [Neupogen, Zarxio], pegfilgrastim [Neulasta], sargramostim [Leukine]). Special precautions may be required (e.g., avoid IM injections; test urine, emesis, stool, secretions for occult blood). All treatment is supportive; recovery should begin within a few hours of cessation of aldesleukin. With normalized BP, diuretics (furosemide [Lasix]) can hasten recovery. Low-dose haloperidol (Haldol) may help severe mental status changes.

More rapid onset of dose-limiting toxicities will occur with overdose. **Dexamethasone (Decadron)** is indicated to counteract life-threatening toxicities. May result in loss of therapeutic effect.

ALEMTUZUMAB BBW
(**ah**-lem-**TOOZ**-uh-mab)

Monoclonal Antibody
Antineoplastic
Immunomodulator

Campath ▪ Lemtrada

pH 6.8 to 7.4

USUAL DOSE

CAMPATH

Premedication, dose escalation to the recommended maintenance dose, and anti-infective prophylaxis are required.

Premedication: Oral diphenhydramine (Benadryl) 50 mg and acetaminophen (Tylenol) 500 to 1,000 mg should be administered 30 minutes before the first dose, at dose escalations, and as clinically indicated. For cases in which severe infusion-related reactions have occurred, corticosteroids may be administered to help prevent or minimize subsequent reactions.

Dose escalation: Dose escalation is required at initiation of dosing or if dosing is held for 7 or more days during treatment. Initiate at a dose of 3 mg daily. When this dose is tolerated (infusion-related toxicities are Grade 2 or less), the daily dose should be increased to 10 mg. When the 10-mg dose is tolerated, the maintenance dose of 30 mg may be initiated. In most cases, dose escalation to the maintenance dose of 30 mg can be achieved in 3 to 7 days.

Maintenance dose: 30 mg/day administered three times a week on alternate days (i.e., Monday, Wednesday, Friday). Total duration of therapy, including dose escalation, is 12 weeks. Single doses greater than 30 mg or cumulative weekly doses greater than 90 mg have been associated with an increased incidence of pancytopenia and should **not** be administered.

Anti-infective prophylaxis: Administer sulfamethoxazole/trimethoprim DS twice daily three times a week (or equivalent) as *Pneumocystis jiroveci* pneumonia (PCP) prophylaxis and famciclovir (Famvir) 250 mg twice daily or equivalent as herpetic prophylaxis at the start of alemtuzumab therapy. Continue PCP and herpes viral prophylaxis for a minimum of 2 months after completion of therapy or until the CD4+ count is equal to or greater than 200 cells/mm³, whichever occurs later.

LEMTRADA

Pretreatment: Complete any necessary immunizations at least 6 weeks before treatment with Lemtrada. Determine whether the patient has a history of varicella or has been vaccinated for varicella zoster virus (VZV). If not, test the patient for antibodies to VZV and consider vaccination if antibody-negative. Postpone treatment until 6 weeks after VZV vaccination.

Premedication: *Corticosteroids:* Administer high-dose corticosteroids (1,000 mg methylprednisolone [Solu-Medrol] or equivalent) immediately before Lemtrada infusion for the first 3 days of each treatment course. Also consider pretreatment with antihistamines and/or antipyretics.

Herpes prophylaxis: Administer antiviral prophylaxis for herpetic viral infections starting on the first day of each treatment course and continue for a minimum of 2 months following treatment with Lemtrada or until the CD4+ lymphocyte count is ≥200 cells/μL, whichever occurs later.

Lemtrada: Recommended dose is 12 mg/day administered by IV infusion for 2 treatment courses.

First treatment course: 12 mg/day as an infusion on 5 consecutive days (60 mg total dose).

Second treatment course: 12 mg/day as an infusion on 3 consecutive days (36 mg total dose) administered 12 months after the first treatment course.

DOSE ADJUSTMENTS

CAMPATH AND LEMTRADA

Withhold alemtuzumab during serious infections or other serious adverse reactions until resolution. *Continued*

CAMPATH

There are no dose modifications recommended for lymphopenia. ▪ Discontinue alemtuzumab for autoimmune anemia or autoimmune thrombocytopenia. ▪ Recommendations for dose modification for severe neutropenia or thrombocytopenia are listed in the following chart.

Alemtuzumab Dose Modification for Neutropenia or Thrombocytopenia	
Hematologic Values	**Dose Modification***
ANC less than 250/mm³ and/or platelet count equal to or less than 25,000/mm³	
First occurrence	Withhold alemtuzumab therapy. Resume alemtuzumab at 30 mg when ANC is equal to or greater than 500/mm³ and platelet count is equal to or greater than 50,000/mm³.
Second occurrence	Withhold alemtuzumab therapy. Resume alemtuzumab at 10 mg when ANC is equal to or greater than 500/mm³ and platelet count is equal to or greater than 50,000/mm³.
Third occurrence	Discontinue alemtuzumab therapy.
Equal to or greater than 50% decrease from baseline in patients initiating therapy with a baseline ANC equal to or less than 250/mm³ and/or a baseline platelet count equal to or less than 25,000/mm³	
First occurrence	Withhold alemtuzumab therapy. Resume alemtuzumab at 30 mg upon return to baseline value(s).
Second occurrence	Withhold alemtuzumab therapy. Resume alemtuzumab at 10 mg upon return to baseline value(s).
Third occurrence	Discontinue alemtuzumab therapy.

*If the delay between dosing is equal to or more than 7 days, resume alemtuzumab therapy at 3 mg and escalate to 10 mg and then to 30 mg as tolerated; see Usual Dose and Rate of Administration.

DILUTION
CAMPATH

Available as a 30 mg/1 mL single-use vial. **Do not shake** vial before use. Contains no preservatives; sterile technique is imperative. Withdraw the necessary amount of Campath from the vial into a syringe:

- To prepare the 3-mg dose, withdraw 0.1 mL into a 1-mL syringe calibrated in increments of 0.01 mL.
- To prepare the 10-mg dose, withdraw 0.33 mL into a 1-mL syringe calibrated in increments of 0.01 mL.
- To prepare the 30-mg dose, withdraw 1 mL in either a 1-mL or 3-mL syringe calibrated in 0.1-mL increments.

Inject the appropriate dose into 100 mL of NS or D5W. Gently invert the bag to mix solution. Discard any unused drug.

LEMTRADA

Available as a 12 mg/1.2 mL single-use vial. **Do not freeze or shake** vial before use. Contains no preservatives; sterile technique is imperative. Withdraw 1.2 mL of Lemtrada from the vial into a syringe and inject into 100 mL of NS or D5W. Gently invert the bag to mix solution.

Filters: Filtering no longer recommended by the manufacturer.

Storage: Campath: Store vials in refrigerator at 2° to 8° C (36° to 46° F). **Do not freeze or shake**. If accidentally frozen, thaw at 2° to 8° C before administration. Protect from direct sunlight.

Lemtrada: Store vials in refrigerator at 2° to 8° C (36° to 46° F) in original carton to protect from light. **Do not freeze or shake.**

Campath and Lemtrada: Prepared solution may be stored at RT (15° to 30° C) or refrigerated. Protect from light and use within 8 hours of dilution.

COMPATIBILITY

Campath and Lemtrada: Manufacturer states, "Do not add or simultaneously infuse other drug substances through the same intravenous line."

Campath: Compatible with PVC bags and PVC or polyethylene-lined PVC administration sets.

RATE OF ADMINISTRATION

Campath and Lemtrada: *Do not administer* as an IV push or bolus.

Campath: A single dose as an infusion over 2 hours. Subcutaneous administration is unlabeled but has been used.

Lemtrada: A single dose as an infusion over 4 hours starting within 8 hours of dilution. Extend duration of infusion if clinically indicated.

ACTIONS

A recombinant, DNA-derived, humanized monoclonal antibody (Campath-1H) that binds to the 21-28 kD cell surface glycoprotein, CD52. CD52 is expressed on the surface of both normal and malignant B- and T-lymphocytes, natural killer (NK) cells, most monocytes, macrophages, and a subpopulation of granulocytes. Alemtuzumab binding has been observed in lymphoid tissues, the mononuclear phagocyte system, and the male reproductive tract. A proportion of bone marrow cells, including some CD34+ cells, also express variable levels of CD52. The proposed mechanism of action for **Campath** is antibody-dependent cellular-mediated lysis following cell surface binding of Campath to the leukemic cells. The precise mechanism of action by which **Lemtrada** exerts its therapeutic effects in multiple sclerosis is unknown but is presumed to involve binding to CD52. Following cell surface binding to T- and B-lymphocytes, **Lemtrada** results in antibody-dependent cellular cytolysis and complement-mediated lysis. Circulating T- and B-lymphocytes are depleted after each treatment course. Lymphocyte counts then increase slowly over time, with B-cell counts recovering within 6 months and T-cell counts recovering after 12 months. Alemtuzumab exhibits nonlinear kinetics. **Campath** AUC and half-life increase with repeated dosing. Mean half-life was 11 hours (range 2 to 32 hours) after the first 30-mg dose and was 6 days (range 1 to 14 days) after the last 30-mg dose. The half-life of **Lemtrada** was approximately 2 weeks and was comparable between courses.

INDICATIONS AND USES

Cᴀᴍᴘᴀᴛʜ

Treatment of B-cell chronic lymphocytic leukemia (B-CLL).

Lᴇᴍᴛʀᴀᴅᴀ

Treatment of patients with relapsing forms of multiple sclerosis (MS). Because of its safety profile, use is generally reserved for patients who have had an inadequate response to two or more drugs indicated for the treatment of MS.

CONTRAINDICATIONS

Cᴀᴍᴘᴀᴛʜ

Manufacturer states, "None."

Lᴇᴍᴛʀᴀᴅᴀ

Contraindicated in patients who are infected with human immunodeficiency virus (HIV) because it causes prolonged reductions of CD4+ lymphocyte counts.

PRECAUTIONS

Cᴀᴍᴘᴀᴛʜ ᴀɴᴅ Lᴇᴍᴛʀᴀᴅᴀ

Administered by or under the direction of a physician specialist in a facility with adequate diagnostic and treatment facilities to monitor patient and respond to any medical emergency.

Cᴀᴍᴘᴀᴛʜ

Serious and, in rare instances, fatal pancytopenia/marrow hypoplasia, autoimmune idiopathic thrombocytopenia, and autoimmune hemolytic anemia have been reported. Have occurred at recommended dose. Do not exceed maximum daily or weekly recommended dose. See Usual Dose, Dose Adjustments, and Antidote. ▪ Serious and sometimes fatal bacterial, viral, fungal, and protozoan infections have been reported. Prophylaxis directed against *Pneumocystis jiroveci* pneumonia and herpes virus infections has been shown to decrease but not eliminate the occurrence of these infections. See Usual

Dose, Dose Adjustments, Monitor, and Antidote. ▪ Serious and sometimes fatal infusion reactions can occur; see Monitor. ▪ Use caution in patients who have had previous cytotoxic agents or radiation therapy or who have received agents that may cause blood dyscrasias; see Drug/ Lab Interactions. ▪ Administer only irradiated blood products to avoid transfusion-associated graft-versus-host disease (TAGVHD) unless immediate transfusion is required. ▪ A small percentage of patients have developed antibodies to alemtuzumab.

LEMTRADA

Available only through the Lemtrada REMS program because of the risks of autoimmunity, infusion reactions, and malignancies; see prescribing information. ▪ May cause serious, sometimes fatal, autoimmune conditions such as immune thrombocytopenia and antiglomerular basement membrane disease. ▪ Immune thrombocytopenia (ITP) has occurred and has been diagnosed more than 3 years after the last Lemtrada dose. Antiplatelet antibodies did not precede ITP onset. ▪ Glomerular nephropathies (e.g., antiglomerular basement membrane [anti-GBM] disease) have occurred, and some resulted in ESRD requiring renal transplantation. May occur up to 40 months after the last dose of Lemtrada. ▪ Newly diagnosed autoimmune thyroid disorders (e.g., Graves' disease, hyperthyroidism, hypothyroidism) have been reported and have occurred more than 7 years after the first Lemtrada dose. ▪ Autoimmune cytopenias (e.g., neutropenia, hemolytic anemia, pancytopenia) have occurred. ▪ *Causes cytokine release syndrome, which may result in serious and life-threatening infusion reactions.* ▪ *May cause an increased risk of malignancies, including thyroid cancer, melanoma, and lymphoproliferative disorders.* ▪ Cases of lymphoproliferative disorders and lymphoma have occurred in Lemtrada-treated patients with MS, including a MALT lymphoma, Castleman's disease, and a fatality following treatment of non–Epstein Barr virus-associated Burkitt's lymphoma. ▪ Because Lemtrada is an immunomodulatory therapy, caution should be exercised in initiating it in patients with pre-existing or ongoing malignancies. ▪ Serious infections, including appendicitis, gastroenteritis, herpes viral infections (genital herpes, herpes simplex, herpes zoster, oral herpes), human papillomavirus (HPV), pneumonia, tooth infection, and tuberculosis, have occurred. Fungal infections (e.g., oral and vaginal candidiasis), listeria infections (e.g., listeria meningitis) have also been reported. ▪ Serious and sometimes fatal bacterial, fungal, protozoan, and viral infections, including those due to reactivation of latent infections reported with Campath, may occur. ▪ No data are available on reactivation of hepatitis B virus (HBV) or hepatitis C virus (HCV) because these patients were excluded from trials. Consider screening patients at high risk for HBV or HCV infections; may be at risk for irreversible liver damage. ▪ Hypersensitivity pneumonitis and pneumonitis with fibrosis have occurred. ▪ Potential for immunogenicity; patients have developed antibodies to alemtuzumab. ▪ Lymphopenia is common; total lymphocyte counts increased to reach the lower limit of normal 6 to 12 months after each course of Lemtrada. ▪ See Monitor and Drug/Lab Interactions.

Monitor: *Campath:* Obtain a baseline CBC, including differential and platelet count. Monitor weekly or more frequently if worsening anemia, neutropenia, or thrombocytopenia develops. ▪ Infusion reactions, including angioedema, anaphylactoid shock, ARDS, bronchospasm, cardiac arrhythmias and/or arrest, chills, fever, hypotension, MI, N/V, pulmonary infiltrates, rash, respiratory arrest, rigors, shortness of breath, syncope, and/or urticaria may occur. Reactions may be severe. Acute infusion-related reactions were most common during the first week of therapy in clinical studies. Premedicate patient and monitor carefully during infusion. Gradual escalation to the recommended maintenance dose is required at the initiation of therapy and after interruption of therapy for 7 or more days. See Usual Dose. ▪ Monitor for CMV infection during and for at least 2 months after completion of therapy. Treat confirmed infection or viremia as indicated with ganciclovir (Cytovene) or equivalent. ▪ Monitor blood pressure and hypotensive symptoms carefully in patients with ischemic heart disease and in patients taking antihypertensive medications; see Drug/Lab Interactions. ▪ Monitor for thrombocytopenia (platelet count less than 50,000/mm³). Initiate precautions to prevent excessive bleeding (e.g., inspect IV sites, skin, and mucous membranes; use extreme care during invasive procedures; test urine, emesis, stool, and secretions for occult blood). ▪ CD4+ counts should be followed after therapy until recovery to equal to or greater than 200 cells/mm³. See Usual Dose.

Lemtrada: Obtain baseline CBC with differential, serum creatinine levels, urinalysis with urine cell counts, and a test of thyroid function (e.g., thyroid-stimulating hormone [TSH] level). Repeat CBC, SCr, and urinalysis at monthly intervals and repeat TSH every 3 months. Continue for 48 months after the last dose. After 48 months, perform testing based on clinical findings that suggest autoimmunity (e.g., ITP, anti-GBM disease, thyroid disorders, cytopenias). ▪ TB screening recommended before initiating therapy with Lemtrada. Treat appropriately if screening is positive. ▪ Monitor vital signs before the infusion and periodically during the infusion. ▪ Monitor for S/S of an infusion reaction (e.g., anaphylaxis, angioedema, bradycardia, bronchospasm, chest pain, fever, headache, hypertension, hypotension, rash, tachycardia [including atrial fibrillation], transient neurologic symptoms) during and for a minimum of 2 hours after each infusion. Serious infusion reactions have been reported more than 24 hours after an infusion. ▪ Additional monitoring may be indicated in patients predisposed to cardiovascular or pulmonary compromise. ▪ Monitor for symptoms of thyroid cancer (e.g., new lump or swelling in the neck, pain in the front of the neck, persistent hoarseness or other voice changes, trouble swallowing or breathing, a constant cough). ▪ Perform baseline and yearly skin examinations to monitor for melanoma. ▪ Monitor for thrombocytopenia (platelet count less than 50,000/mm³). Initiate precautions to prevent excessive bleeding (e.g., inspect IV sites, skin, and mucous membranes; use extreme care during invasive procedures; test urine, emesis, stool, and secretions for occult blood). ▪ Monitor for S/S of anti-GBM disease (e.g., elevated SCr levels, hematuria or proteinuria, hemoptysis [from alveolar hemorrhage]) during treatment and after treatment is completed. ▪ Monitor for S/S of infection and consider delaying administration in patients with active infection until the infection is fully controlled. ▪ Annual HPV screening is recommended for female patients. ▪ See Drug/Lab Interactions.

Patient Education: *Campath and Lemtrada:* Promptly report any unusual side effects or signs of bleeding or bruising, infection (e.g., fever), or infusion reaction (e.g., difficulty breathing, rash). ▪ See Appendix D, p. 1333.

Campath: Women of childbearing potential and men of reproductive potential should use effective contraceptive methods during treatment and for a minimum of 6 months following therapy. ▪ Irradiation of blood products is required.

Lemtrada: Review Medication Guide before each treatment course. ▪ To avoid in utero exposure to Lemtrada, women of childbearing potential should use effective contraceptive measures during treatment and for 4 months following therapy. ▪ Serious infusion reactions may occur after the infusion is complete. ▪ Seek immediate medical help for bruising, petechiae, spontaneous mucocutaneous bleeding (e.g., epistaxis, hemoptysis), or heavier than normal or irregular menstrual bleeding. ▪ Promptly report chest pain or tightness, cough, dark urine, hemoptysis, jaundice, shortness of breath, tachycardia, wheezing. ▪ May cause thyroid disorders. Promptly report symptoms (e.g., weight loss or gain, fast heartbeat or palpitations, eye swelling, constipation, or feeling cold). ▪ May increase the risk of suicidal thoughts and behavior. Promptly report emergence or worsening of S/S of depression, any unusual changes in mood or behavior, or thoughts about self-harm. ▪ Avoid or adequately heat foods that are potential sources of *Listeria monocytogenes*. ▪ Periodic laboratory monitoring required for prolonged period of time (48 months or longer).

Maternal/Child: *Campath and Lemtrada:* Category C: may cause fetal harm. Should be used during pregnancy only if the potential benefit justifies the potential risk to the fetus.

Campath: Discontinue breast-feeding during treatment. ▪ Safety and effectiveness for use in pediatric patients not established.

Lemtrada: Placental transfer of antithyroid antibodies resulting in neonatal Graves' disease has been reported. Use during pregnancy only if the potential benefit justifies the potential risk to the fetus. ▪ May induce persistent thyroid disorders. Untreated hypothyroidism in pregnant women increases the risk of miscarriage and may have effects on the fetus, including cognitive impairment and dwarfism. ▪ Discontinue breast-feeding. ▪ Safety and effectiveness for use in pediatric patients less than 17 years of age not established.

Elderly: *Campath:* Differences in safety and efficacy related to age have not been observed to date, but study numbers have been small.

Lemtrada: Clinical studies did not include sufficient numbers of patients age 65 and over. Differences in response compared with younger adults not known.

DRUG/LAB INTERACTIONS

CAMPATH AND LEMTRADA

Do not administer **chloroquine or live virus vaccines** to patients receiving alemtuzumab. ▪ Campath and Lemtrada both contain the same active ingredient, **alemtuzumab.** Before use in a patient who has received **either Campath or Lemtrada** previously, consider the potential for additive and long-lasting effects on the immune system.

CAMPATH

No formal drug interaction studies have been performed. ▪ May cause additive effects with **bone marrow–suppressing agents, radiation therapy, or agents that cause blood dyscrasias** (e.g., amphotericin B, antithyroid agents [Methimazole (Tapazole)], azathioprine, chloramphenicol, ganciclovir [Cytovene], interferon, plicamycin [Mithracin], zidovudine [AZT, Retrovir]). ▪ May intensify effects of **antihypertensive medications;** see Monitor.

LEMTRADA

Concomitant use with antineoplastic or immunosuppressive therapies could increase the risk of immunosuppression.

SIDE EFFECTS

CAMPATH

The most common serious side effects are cytopenias (anemia, lymphopenia, neutropenia, thrombocytopenia), immunosuppression/infections (CMV viremia, CMV infection, other infections), and infusion reactions (chills, dyspnea, fever, hypotension, nausea, rash, tachycardia, urticaria). GI symptoms (abdominal pain, N/V) and neurologic symptoms (insomnia, anxiety) are also reported commonly. Hypersensitivity reactions (including anaphylaxis), anorexia, arrhythmias, asthenia, autoimmune hemolytic anemia or autoimmune idiopathic thrombocytopenia, constipation, cough, depression, dizziness, dyspepsia, edema, epistaxis, febrile neutropenia, Goodpasture's syndrome, Graves' disease, Guillain-Barré syndrome, headache, hypertension, infections (e.g., pneumonia, Epstein-Barr virus [EBV], progressive multifocal leukoencephalopathy [PML], and several other opportunistic infections), malaise, mucositis, myalgias, optic neuropathy, pain, purpura, rhinitis, serum sickness, somnolence, tremor, tumor lysis syndrome, and many others have been reported.

LEMTRADA

The most common serious side effects include autoimmunity, glomerular nephropathies, immune thrombocytopenia, infections, infusion reactions, malignancies, other autoimmune cytopenias, pneumonitis, and thyroid disorders. The most common side effects reported include abdominal pain, arthralgia, back pain, diarrhea, dizziness, fatigue, fever, flushing, fungal infections, headache, herpes viral infection, insomnia, nasopharyngitis, nausea and vomiting, oropharyngeal pain, pain in extremities, paresthesia, pruritus, rash, sinusitis, thyroid gland disorders, upper respiratory tract infection, urinary tract infection, urticaria. Immunogenicity and suicidal behavior have also been reported. All side effects listed under Campath may occur.

Post-Marketing: *Campath:* Aplastic anemia, cardiotoxicity (e.g., cardiomyopathy, CHF, and decreased ejection fraction [some patients had been previously treated with cardiotoxic agents]), chronic inflammatory demyelinating polyradiculoneuropathy, EBV-associated lymphoproliferative disorder, fatal infusion reactions, fatal transfusion-associated graft-versus-host disease, reactivation of latent viruses, serum sickness.

Lemtrada: Post-marketing symptoms under Campath may occur.

ANTIDOTE

CAMPATH AND LEMTRADA

Notify physician of all side effects. Treatment of most reactions will be supportive. Therapy should be temporarily discontinued during serious infection, serious hematologic toxicity (except lymphopenia), or other serious toxicity until the infection or adverse event resolves. Discontinue medication for severe reactions. Infusion reactions may be treated with acetaminophen, antihistamines (e.g., diphenhydramine), corticosteroids (e.g., hydrocortisone), and meperidine as indicated. Treat hypersensitivity reactions with epinephrine, antihistamines, and corticosteroids as needed. Resuscitate as indicated.

CAMPATH

Discontinue medication permanently for severe reactions, including autoimmune anemia or thrombocytopenia. Administration of irradiated blood products and/or blood modifiers (e.g., darbepoetin [Aranesp], epoetin alfa [Epogen], filgrastim [Neupogen, Zarxio], pegfilgrastim [Neulasta], sargramostim [Leukine]) may be indicated to treat bone marrow toxicity. Median durations of neutropenia were 28 to 37 days, and median durations of thrombocytopenia were 9 to 21 days. Median time to recovery of CD4+ counts to equal to or greater than 200/mm^3 is 2 to 6 months; however, full recovery of CD4+ and CD8+ counts may take more than 12 months. Discontinue alemtuzumab and provide supportive therapy in overdose.

LEMTRADA

Consider pretreatment with antihistamines and/or antipyretics. If ITP is suspected, obtain a CBC. If ITP is confirmed, treat appropriately. If anti-GBM disease is suspected, urgent evaluation and treatment are required. Anti-GBM disease can lead to renal failure requiring dialysis or transplantation and can be life threatening if left untreated.

ALFENTANIL HYDROCHLORIDE
(al-**FEN**-tah-nil hy-droh-**KLOR**-eyed)

General anesthetic
Opioid analgesic agonist
Anesthesia adjunct

pH 4 to 6

USUAL DOSE

Adults and pediatric patients 12 years of age and older: Dose must be individualized and titrated to the desired effect in each patient according to body weight, physical status, underlying pathologic condition, use of other drugs, and type and duration of surgical procedure and anesthesia. Usually used in conjunction with short-acting barbiturates (e.g., thiopental [Pentothal]), neuromuscular blocking agents (e.g., pancuronium, succinylcholine), and an inhalation anesthetic (e.g., nitrous oxide) to maintain balanced anesthesia. Use reduced doses of a neuromuscular blocking agent prophylactically to prevent muscle rigidity or to induce muscle relaxation after rigidity occurs. Full paralyzing doses may be used after loss of consciousness. Use of a benzodiazepine (e.g., diazepam [Valium], midazolam [Versed]) may reduce induction dose requirements, decrease time to loss of consciousness, and diminish patient recall; see Drug/Lab Interactions. See Dose Adjustments.

Alfentanil Dosing Guidelines for Use During General Anesthesia	
SPONTANEOUSLY BREATHING/ASSISTED VENTILATION	
	Induction of analgesia: 8-20 mcg/kg Maintenance of analgesia: 3-5 mcg/kg q 5-20 min or 0.5-1 mcg/kg/min Total dose: 8-40 mcg/kg
ASSISTED OR CONTROLLED VENTILATION	
Incremental injection (To attenuate response to laryngoscopy and intubation)	Induction of analgesia: 20-50 mcg/kg Maintenance of analgesia: 5-15 mcg/kg q 5-20 min Total dose: Up to 75 mcg/kg
CONTINUOUS INFUSION	
(To provide attenuation of response to intubation and incision)	Infusion rates are variable and should be titrated to the desired clinical effect. SEE INFUSION DOSAGE GUIDELINES (BELOW) Induction of analgesia: 50-75 mcg/kg Maintenance of analgesia: 0.5-3 mcg/kg/min (average rate 1-1.5 mcg/kg/min) Total dose: Dependent on duration of procedure
ANESTHETIC INDUCTION	
	Induction of anesthesia: 130-245 mcg/kg Maintenance of analgesia: 0.5-1.5 mcg/kg/min or general anesthetic Total dose: Dependent on duration of procedure At these doses, truncal rigidity should be expected and a muscle relaxant should be utilized Administer slowly (over 3 minutes) Concentration of inhalation agents reduced by 30%-50% for initial hour
MONITORED ANESTHESIA CARE (MAC)	
For sedated and responsive, spontaneously breathing patients	Induction of MAC: 3-8 mcg/kg Maintenance of MAC: 3-5 mcg/kg q 5-20 min or 0.25-1 mcg/kg/min Total dose: 3-40 mcg/kg

Alfentanil Dosing Guidelines for Use During General Anesthesia—cont'd
SPONTANEOUSLY BREATHING/ASSISTED VENTILATION
INFUSION DOSAGE
Continuous infusion: 0.5-3 mcg/kg/min administered with nitrous oxide/oxygen in patients undergoing general surgery. Following an anesthetic induction dose of alfentanil, infusion rate requirements are reduced by 30%-50% for the first hour of maintenance. Changes in vital signs that indicate a response to surgical stress or lightening of anesthesia may be controlled by increasing the alfentanil to a maximum of 4 mcg/kg/min and/or administration of bolus doses of 7 mcg/kg. If changes are not controlled after three bolus doses given over a 5-minute period, a barbiturate, vasodilator, and/or inhalation agent should be used. Infusion rates should always be adjusted downward in the absence of these signs until there is some response to surgical stimulation. Rather than an increase in infusion rate, 7 mcg/kg bolus doses of alfentanil or a potent inhalation agent should be administered in response to signs of lightening of anesthesia within the last 15 minutes of surgery. Alfentanil infusion should be discontinued at least 10 to 15 minutes before the end of surgery. Discontinue 10 to 15 minutes before end of procedures in general anesthesia. Continue infusion to end of procedure during MAC, then discontinue.

PEDIATRIC DOSE
Safety for use in pediatric patients under 12 years of age not established; not recommended. Half-life and duration of action is decreased in pediatric patients; more frequent supplemental doses may be required; see Maternal/Child.

DOSE ADJUSTMENTS
Reduce dose of one or both agents when given in combination with other CNS depressants (e.g., barbiturates, inhalation anesthetics, narcotic analgesics, tranquilizers). ▪ Calculate dose based on lean body weight in obese patients (more than 20% above ideal body weight). ▪ Reduced initial dose required in elderly or debilitated patients (a 40% reduction was required in one study); reduced supplemental doses, a slower infusion rate, or longer intervals between doses may be required based on effects of initial dose. ▪ Doses appropriate for general population may cause serious respiratory depression in vulnerable patients. ▪ Reduced dose may be required in hypothyroidism and in impaired hepatic function. ▪ See Drug/Lab Interactions.

DILUTION
IV injection: Small volumes may be given undiluted (usually by the anesthesiologist). Use of tuberculin syringe recommended (1 mL equals 500 mcg). Further dilution with 5 mL of SWFI or NS to facilitate titration is appropriate.

Infusion: Dilute 20 mL alfentanil with 230 mL NS, D5NS, D5W, or LR to achieve a concentration of 40 mcg/mL. Desired concentration range is 25 to 80 mcg/mL.

Storage: Store ampules at CRT; protect from light and freezing.

COMPATIBILITY
Consider any drug NOT listed as compatible to be INCOMPATIBLE until consulting a pharmacist; specific conditions may apply.
One source suggests the following **compatibilities:**
Y-site: Bivalirudin (Angiomax), cisatracurium (Nimbex), dexmedetomidine (Precedex), etomidate (Amidate), fenoldopam (Corlopam), hetastarch in electrolytes (Hextend), linezolid (Zyvox), propofol (Diprivan), remifentanil (Ultiva).

RATE OF ADMINISTRATION
IV injection: Administer over a minimum of 3 minutes. Rapid administration of lower doses or administration of full anesthetic doses will result in muscle rigidity, apnea, respiratory paralysis, loss of vascular tone, and hypotension. Titrate rate to desired patient response.
Infusion: See Usual Dose.

ACTIONS

An opioid derivative, narcotic analgesic, and descending CNS depressant. Less potent than fentanyl milligram for milligram, but achieves higher plasma concentrations. Produces hypnosis and respiratory depressant actions that outlast its analgesic effect. Onset of action is immediate. Produces analgesic effects in 1 minute. Peak effect (respiratory depression and analgesia) occurs within 1½ to 2 minutes. With induction doses, loss of consciousness occurs within 1 to 2 minutes. Provides dose-related protection against hemodynamic responses to surgical stress. Histamine release rarely occurs. May cause rigidity of chest, pharynx, and abdominal muscles, inhibiting ventilation; see Precautions/Monitor, Side Effects, Antidote. Duration of action is 5 to 10 minutes. Has a terminal half-life of 90 to 111 minutes. Cumulative effects are somewhat less than with fentanyl or sufentanil, but with repeat doses recovery may be prolonged. Recovery should occur within 10 to 15 minutes of end of procedure or 25 to 30 minutes after last incremental dose or discontinuing the infusion. Metabolized in the liver. Excreted as metabolites in urine. Crosses the placental barrier. Secreted in breast milk.

INDICATIONS AND USES

Analgesic adjunct given in incremental doses in the maintenance of anesthesia with barbiturate/nitrous oxide/oxygen. ■ Analgesic administered by continuous infusion with nitrous oxide/oxygen in the maintenance of general anesthesia. ■ Primary anesthetic agent for the induction of anesthesia in patients undergoing general surgery requiring endotracheal intubation and mechanical ventilation. ■ Analgesic component for monitored anesthesia care (MAC) during surgical or diagnostic procedures.

CONTRAINDICATIONS

Known hypersensitivity to alfentanil or known intolerance to other opioid agonists (e.g., fentanyl, sufentanil). Use during labor and delivery not recommended.

PRECAUTIONS

For IV use only. ■ Administered by or under the direct observations of the anesthesiologist. Must have responsibility only for anesthesia and continuous observation of the patient during surgery and/or procedure. ■ Oxygen, controlled ventilation equipment, opioid antagonists (e.g., naloxone), neuromuscular blocking agents (e.g., pancuronium, succinylcholine [Anectine]), and all emergency drugs and equipment must be immediately available. ■ Staff must be skilled in medical management of critically ill patients, cardiovascular resuscitation, and airway management. ■ Use caution; plasma clearance reduced and recovery time prolonged in the elderly and in patients with impaired liver function (half-life prolonged [up to 5.8 hours]); reduced dose may be indicated. ■ Use caution in patients with pulmonary disease, decreased respiratory reserve, or potentially compromised respiration. May cause rigidity of chest and abdominal muscles, decrease respiratory drive, and increase airway resistance; may require assisted or controlled ventilation. ■ Use caution in patients with head injury or increased intracranial pressure; risk of respiratory depression is increased. ■ Respiratory depression may cause an increased Pco_2, cerebral vasodilation, and increased intracranial pressure. Clinical course of head injury may be obscured. ■ Use caution in patients with bradyarrhythmias. ■ In general, narcotic analgesics are contraindicated in acute or severe bronchial asthma and when an upper airway obstruction or significant respiratory depression is present. ■ Use caution in patients with hypothyroidism; risk of respiratory depression and prolonged CNS depression is increased. Reduced doses may be indicated. ■ See Drug/Lab Interactions.

Monitor: Can cause rigidity of respiratory muscles; concurrent use of a neuromuscular blocking agent can prevent or reverse muscle rigidity to permit controlled ventilation. ■ Adequate preoperative hydration is recommended to reduce incidence of hypotension. ■ Observe for hypotension, apnea, upper airway obstruction, and/or oxygen desaturation. Monitor vital signs and oxygen saturation continuously. If not unconscious, patient will appear to be asleep and forget to breathe unless commanded to do so. ■ Additional doses of alfentanil can be used to control tachycardia and hypertension during surgery. ▪ Prolonged postoperative monitoring may be indicated; respiratory depression, respiratory arrest, bradycardia, asystole, arrhythmias, and hypotension may occur after initial recovery. ▪ Keep patient supine; orthostatic hypotension and fainting may occur. ▪ Has a short duration of action; pain medication may be required soon after initial recovery. ▪ See Precautions and Drug/Lab Interactions.

Patient Education: Avoid alcohol or other CNS depressants (e.g., antihistamines, benzodiazepines [e.g., diazepam (Valium)]). ▪ Blurred vision, dizziness, drowsiness, or lightheadedness may occur; request assistance with ambulation. ▪ Review all medications for interactions.

Maternal/Child: Category C: safety for use in pregnancy not established; has embryocidal effects in rats and rabbits. ▪ Not recommended for use during labor and delivery. ▪ Postpone breast-feeding for at least 24 hours after use of alfentanil. ▪ Muscle rigidity is more common in neonates than in older children or adults.

Elderly: See Dose Adjustments and Precautions. ▪ May markedly decrease pulmonary ventilation. ▪ Decreased protein binding, decreased clearance, and possible increased brain sensitivity may make the elderly more sensitive to effects (e.g., respiratory depression, extended recovery time, urinary retention, constipation). ▪ Lower doses may provide effective analgesia. ▪ Consider age-related organ impairment; elimination half-life is extended, and postoperative recovery may be delayed.

DRUG/LAB INTERACTIONS

Use of **benzodiazepines** (e.g., diazepam [Valium], midazolam [Versed]) may decrease dose of alfentanil required and decrease patient recall, but when given immediately before or in conjunction with high doses of alfentanil, benzodiazepines may produce vasodilation, severe hypotension, and result in delayed recovery. ▪ After an anesthetic induction dose of alfentanil, requirements for **volatile inhalation anesthetics** (e.g., nitrous oxide) **and/or alfentanil infusion** are reduced by 30% to 50% for the first hour of maintenance. ▪ **Beta-adrenergic blocking agents** (e.g., metoprolol, timolol) may be used preoperatively to decrease hypertensive episodes during surgical procedures, but chronic use (including ophthalmic preparations) may also increase the risk of initial bradycardia. ▪ Respiratory depression, CNS depression, hypotensive effects, and duration of action increased with concomitant administration of other **CNS depressants** (e.g., antidepressants, antihistamines, barbiturates, benzodiazepines, haloperidol, inhalation anesthetics, narcotic analgesics, phenothiazines). Reduced doses of one or both agents usually required. ▪ Clearance decreased by **cimetidine** (Tagamet) **and erythromycin;** risk of prolonged or delayed respiratory depression may be increased. ▪ Respiratory depressant effects are additive with **neuromuscular blocking agents** (e.g., pancuronium, succinylcholine). ▪ Other opioids have caused severe hypertension with **MAO inhibitors** (e.g., selegiline [Eldepryl]). Use extreme caution; beta-blockers (e.g., propranolol) and vasodilators (e.g., nitroglycerin) should be available. ▪ Duration of action may be prolonged with other **agents that inhibit hepatic enzymes** (e.g., azole antifungals [e.g., itraconazole (Sporanox)], beta-blockers [e.g., metoprolol (Lopressor), propranolol, timolol (Novo-Timol)], calcium channel blockers [e.g., diltiazem (Cardizem), verapamil], fluoroquinolones [e.g., ciprofloxacin (Cipro), levofloxacin (Levaquin)], MAO inhibitors). ▪ Monitor closely for S/S of respiratory depression and CNS depression with concurrent use of **protease inhibitors** (e.g., saquinavir [Invirase], ritonavir [Norvir]). ▪ Use of **naltrexone** (ReVia) would require increased doses of alfentanil; may cause prolonged respiratory depression and/or circulatory collapse. Discontinue naltrexone several days before elective surgery if use of an opioid is necessary. ▪ Analgesic effects may be antagonized by **opioid agonist/antagonist analgesics;** may also cause additive CNS and respiratory depressant effects. ▪ May delay **gastric emptying** and invalidate diagnostic tests. ▪ May interfere with some **hepatobiliary imaging.** ▪ Delay **plasma amylase and lipase measurements** for at least 24 hours.

SIDE EFFECTS

Average dose: Bradycardia and hypotension may occur shortly after administration. Respiratory depression caused by alfentanil and/or muscle rigidity may progress to apnea. Agitation, arrhythmias (e.g., bradycardia, tachycardia), blurred vision, bradypnea, chest wall rigidity, dizziness, euphoria, headache, hypercapnia (increased CO_2), hypersensitivity reactions (e.g., anaphylaxis, bronchospasm, itching, laryngospasm, urticaria), hypertension, hypotension, muscle rigidity (skeletal muscles including abdomen, chest, pharynx, neck, and extremities), myoclonic movements, nausea, postoperative confusion, respiratory sedation, shivering, skeletal muscle movements, sleepiness, vomiting.

Overdose: Bradycardia; circulatory depression; cold, clammy skin; dizziness (severe); drowsiness (severe); hypotension; nervousness or restlessness (severe); pinpoint pupils of eyes; respiratory depression; weakness (severe).

ANTIDOTE

Many side effects are medical emergencies. Manage respiratory depression during surgery via endotracheal intubation and assisted or controlled ventilation; prolonged mechanical ventilation may be required. Treat postoperative respiratory depression with naloxone; titrate dose carefully to improve respirations without reversing analgesic effects or causing other adverse effects (hypertension and tachycardia may result in left ventricular failure and pulmonary edema, especially in cardiac patients). Treat bradycardia with atropine, or alfentanil-induced bradycardia can be antagonized with the use of a neuromuscular blocking agent with vagolytic activity (e.g., pancuronium). Treat hypotension by placing the patient in a Trendelenburg position, if possible; administer IV fluids and a vasopressor (e.g., norepinephrine [Levophed], dopamine) if indicated. Naloxone may reverse hypotension postoperatively. Muscle rigidity during anesthesia induction or surgery must be controlled with neuromuscular blocking agents and controlled ventilation with oxygen. Use a neuromuscular blocking agent prophylactically to prevent muscle rigidity or to induce muscle relaxation after rigidity occurs. Neuromuscular blocking agents with vagolytic activity (e.g., pancuronium) may decrease risk of alfentanil-induced bradycardia and hypotension, but may increase the risk of hypertension or tachycardia in some patients. In patients with compromised cardiac function and/or those receiving a beta-adrenergic blocking agent preoperatively, a nonvagolytic neuromuscular blocking agent (e.g., succinylcholine) may increase the incidence and severity of bradycardia and hypotension. Respiratory depressant effects of neuromuscular blocking agents are additive with alfentanil. Postoperatively, naloxone may be used in small incremental doses to reverse skeletal muscle rigidity. Resuscitate as necessary.

ALLOPURINOL SODIUM
(al-oh-**PYOUR**-ih-nohl **SO**-dee-um)

Antigout
Antihyperuricemic
Antineoplastic adjunct

Aloprim

pH 11.1 to 11.8

USUAL DOSE
IV and oral doses are therapeutically equivalent. Oral dose can replace an IV dose at any time. See Monitor.

200 to 400 mg/M^2/day as a single infusion or in equally divided doses at 6-, 8-, or 12-hour intervals (50 to 100 mg/M^2 every 6 hours, 67 to 133 mg/M^2 every 8 hours, or 100 to 200 mg/M^2 every 12 hours). Total dose should not exceed 600 mg/day.

PEDIATRIC DOSE
Recommended starting dose is 200 mg/M^2/day. Usually given in equally divided doses at 6- to 8-hour intervals (50 mg/M^2 every 6 hours or 67 mg/M^2 every 8 hours). Another source says the daily dose may be given at 6-, 8-, or 12-hour intervals or as a single daily infusion. Studies found no significant difference in dose response in pediatric patients. See comments in Usual Dose.

DOSE ADJUSTMENTS
In patients with impaired renal function not on dialysis, reduce dose based on CrCl according to the following chart.

Allopurinol Dosing in Impaired Renal Function	
CrCl (mL/min)	Dose
10-20 mL/min	200 mg daily
3-10 mL/min	100 mg daily
<3 mL/min	100 mg daily at extended intervals (more than 24 hr if necessary)

Treat with the lowest effective dose to minimize side effects. ▪ Dose with normal renal function may be increased or decreased based on electrolytes and serum uric acid levels. ▪ Lower doses and/or extended intervals may be required in the elderly; consider potential for decreased organ function, concomitant disease, or other drug therapy. ▪ See Drug/Lab Interactions.

DILUTION
Available as a single-dose vial containing 500 mg of allopurinol. Reconstitute with 25 mL of SWFI (yields 20 mg/mL). Swirl until completely dissolved. Must be further diluted with NS or D5W. Maximum concentration for administration is 6 mg/mL. 19 mL of additional diluent per 20 mg (1 mL) yields 1 mg/mL, 9 mL of additional diluent yields 2 mg/mL, and 2.3 mL of additional diluent yields 6 mg/mL.

Storage: Store unopened vials at CRT. Do not refrigerate the reconstituted and/or diluted product; begin infusion within 10 hours of reconstitution.

COMPATIBILITY
Consider any drug NOT listed as compatible to be INCOMPATIBLE until consulting a pharmacist; specific conditions may apply.

Manufacturer recommends administering sequentially and flushing before and after administration. Manufacturer lists the following drugs as **incompatible:** amikacin, amphotericin B (conventional), carmustine (BiCNU), cefotaxime (Claforan), chlorpromazine (Thorazine), clindamycin (Cleocin), cytarabine (ARA-C), dacarbazine (DTIC), daunorubicin (Cerubidine), diphenhydramine (Benadryl), doxorubicin (Adriamycin), doxycy-cline, droperidol (Inapsine), floxuridine (FUDR), gentamicin, idarubicin (Idamycin), imipenem-cilastatin (Primaxin), mechlorethamine (nitrogen mustard) (Mustargen), me-peridine (Demerol), methylprednisolone (Solu-Medrol), metoclopramide (Reglan), mi-nocycline (Minocin), nalbuphine, ondansetron (Zofran), prochlorperazine (Compazine), promethazine (Phenergan), sodium bicarbonate, streptozocin (Zanosar), tobramycin, vinorelbine (Navelbine). *Do not use solutions containing sodium bicarbonate.*

One source suggests the following **compatibilities:**

Y-site: Acyclovir (Zovirax), aminophylline, aztreonam (Azactam), bleomycin (Blenox-ane), bumetanide, buprenorphine (Buprenex), butorphanol (Stadol), calcium gluconate, carboplatin (Paraplatin), cefazolin (Ancef), cefotetan, ceftazidime (Fortaz), ceftriaxone (Rocephin), cefuroxime (Zinacef), cisplatin, cyclophosphamide (Cytoxan), dactinomy-cin (Cosmegen), dexamethasone (Decadron), doxorubicin liposomal (Doxil), enalaprilat (Vasotec IV), etoposide (VePesid), famotidine (Pepcid IV), filgrastim (Neupogen), fluco-nazole (Diflucan), fludarabine (Fludara), fluorouracil (5-FU), furosemide (Lasix), gal-lium nitrate (Ganite), ganciclovir (Cytovene IV), granisetron (Kytril), heparin, hydrocor-tisone sodium succinate (Solu-Cortef), hydromorphone (Dilaudid), ifosfamide (Ifex), lorazepam (Ativan), mannitol, mesna (Mesnex), methotrexate, metronidazole (Flagyl IV), mitoxantrone (Novantrone), morphine, potassium chloride (KCl), ranitidine (Zantac), sulfamethoxazole/trimethoprim, teniposide (Vumon), thiotepa, ticarcillin/clavulanate (Timentin), vancomycin, vinblastine, vincristine, zidovudine (AZT, Retrovir).

RATE OF ADMINISTRATION

Manufacturer's recommendation not available. A maximum dose should take at least $^{1}/_{2}$ to 1 hour or more based on volume with diluent and patient comfort and/or requirements. Include in hydration fluids. See Compatibility.

ACTIONS

A xanthine oxidase inhibitor. Metabolized to oxypurinol. Acts on purine catabolism without disrupting the biosynthesis of purines. Reduces the production of uric acid by inhibiting the biochemical reactions immediately preceding its formation. Decreases uric acid concentrations in both serum and urine. Prevents or decreases urate deposition, de-creasing the occurrence or progression of gout or urate nephropathy. Reduction of serum uric acid concentration occurs in 2 to 3 days. Peak concentrations are related to dose. Pharmacokinetic and plasma profiles of allopurinol and oxypurinol, as well as half-lives and systemic clearance, are similar with IV or oral administration. Systemic exposure to oxypurinol is also similar by both routes at each dose level. Cleared by glomerular filtra-tion; some oxypurinol is reabsorbed in the kidney tubules. Secreted in breast milk.

INDICATIONS AND USES

Management of patients with leukemia, lymphoma, and solid tumor malignancies who are receiving cancer therapy that causes elevations of serum and urinary uric acid levels and who cannot tolerate oral therapy. Consider prophylactic use before initiation of and during chemotherapy in patients who are NPO, are nauseated and vomiting, or have malabsorption problems, dysphagia, or GI tract dysfunctions. Used prophylactically be-fore the initiation of and during chemotherapy to prevent hyperuricemia caused by tumor lysis syndrome (TLS) and its sequela, acute uric acid nephropathy (AUAN).

Unlabeled uses: Preservation of cadaveric kidneys for transplantation.

CONTRAINDICATIONS

Any patient who has had a severe reaction to allopurinol (usually a hypersensitivity reaction).

PRECAUTIONS

For IV infusion only. ▪ A skin rash or other beginning signs of hypersensitivity may be followed by exfoliative, urticarial, and purpuric lesions; Stevens-Johnson syndrome; generalized vasculitis; irreversible hepatotoxicity; and/or rarely death. ▪ Incidence of hypersensitivity reactions may be increased in patients with decreased renal function who are receiving concurrent thiazides (e.g., chlorothiazide [Diuril]); use with cau-tion. ▪ See Drug/Lab Interactions.

Monitor: Whenever possible, begin allopurinol therapy 24 to 48 hours before the start of chemotherapy known to cause tumor cell lysis (including adrenocorticosteroids). ▪ Monitor serum uric acid levels and electrolytes before and during therapy. Monitor serum uric acid levels to determine dose and frequency required to maintain uric acid levels within the normal range. ▪ Hydration with 3,000 mL/M^2/day (twice the level of maintenance fluid replacement) is recommended to promote a high volume of urine output (more than 2 L/day in adults) with low urate concentration. ▪ Maintain urine at neutral or slightly alkaline pH. To increase solubility of uric acid, alkalinity of urine may be increased with sodium bicarbonate. ▪ Monitor renal and hepatic systems before and during therapy. ▪ Monitoring of liver function suggested in patients with pre-existing liver disease, in patients with increases in liver function tests, and in patients who develop anorexia, pruritus, or weight loss. ▪ Observe for symptoms of TLS (e.g., hyperuricemia, hyperkalemia, hyperphosphatemia, and hypocalcemia). If untreated, may develop AUAN leading to renal failure requiring hemodialysis. ▪ Bone marrow suppression has been reported; monitor CBC periodically.

Patient Education: Maintain adequate hydration, avoid alcoholic drinks, and report nausea and vomiting and decreased urine production. ▪ Report promptly blood in the urine, painful urination, irritation of the eyes, skin rash, or swelling of the lips or mouth. ▪ Major acute toxicities may be allergic or renal. ▪ May cause drowsiness; use caution in activities that require alertness. Request assistance for ambulation.

Maternal/Child: Category C: potential benefits must justify potential risks to fetus. ▪ Use caution if required during breast-feeding.

Elderly: Lower-end initial doses or extended intervals may be appropriate in the elderly; see Dose Adjustments.

DRUG/LAB INTERACTIONS

May increase toxicity of **didanosine** (Videx); concurrent use not recommended. ▪ Inhibits metabolism and increases effects and toxicity of **thiopurines** (e.g., azathioprine, mercaptopurine [Purinethol]). Reduce dose of thiopurine to one third to one fourth. ▪ **Uricosuric agents** (e.g., sulfinpyrazone [Anturane], probenecid, colchicine) may increase elimination of active metabolites of allopurinol; may increase urinary excretions of uric acid. ▪ Prolongs half-life of **dicumarol;** monitor PT or PTT and adjust anticoagulant dose as indicated. ▪ Frequency of skin rash increased with **ampicillin/amoxicillin.** ▪ Bone marrow suppression may be increased when given concurrently with **cytotoxic agents** (e.g., cyclophosphamide [Cytoxan]); risk of bleeding or infection may be increased. ▪ May prolong half-life of **chlorpropamide** (Diabinese). ▪ Hypersensitivity reactions may be increased with **ACE inhibitors** (e.g., enalapril) **or thiazide diuretics** (e.g., chlorothiazide [Diuril]). ▪ Concurrent use with **cyclosporine** (Sandimmune) may increase cyclosporine serum levels. A reduced dose of cyclosporine may be indicated; monitoring of cyclosporine serum levels suggested. ▪ May decrease clearance and increase toxicity of **theophyllines** (e.g., Aminophylline).

SIDE EFFECTS

Fewer than 1% of patients have had side effects directly attributable to allopurinol. Most were hypersensitivity reactions (e.g., nausea and vomiting, rash, and renal failure/insufficiency) and of mild to moderate severity. Xanthine crystalluria has been rarely reported in long-term therapy with oral allopurinol.

ANTIDOTE

Discontinue allopurinol at the first sign of skin rash or any other allergic reaction. Do not restart. Keep physician informed of all side effects. Symptoms of TLS require immediate intervention and correction of electrolyte abnormalities to avoid kidney damage. Treat hypersensitivity reactions as indicated; may require epinephrine (Adrenalin), diphenhydramine (Benadryl), corticosteroids (hydrocortisone), and/or oxygen. Allopurinol is dialyzable, but effectiveness of hemodialysis or peritoneal dialysis in an overdose is not known.

ALPHA₁-PROTEINASE INHIBITOR (HUMAN)

(**AL**-fah **PRO**-teen-ayse in-**HIB**-ih-ter [**HU**-man])

Alpha₁-antitrypsin
replenisher

Alpha₁-antitrypsin, Alpha₁-PI, Aralast NP, Glassia, Prolastin-C, Zemaira

pH 7.2 to 7.8 (Aralast NP) ■
pH 6.6 to 7.4 (Prolastin-C)

USUAL DOSE

60 mg/kg once a week as an infusion.

Manufacturers of Prolastin-C recommend immunizing every patient against hepatitis B before administration. If immediate treatment is required, give a single dose of hepatitis B immune globulin (human) 0.06 mL/kg IM at the same time as the initial dose of hepatitis B vaccine.

DILUTION

All preparations: Bring components to room temperature (diluent [SWFI], lyophilized preparation of alpha₁-PI, or ready-to-use solution). Must be used within 3 hours of reconstitution or entry into vial. Must be filtered before or during administration.

Aralast NP and Prolastin-C: Insert one end of the double-ended transfer needle (shortest end for Prolastin-C) into the diluent. Invert the bottle of diluent and insert the other end of the transfer needle at a 45-degree angle into the alpha₁-PI; diluent will be drawn into the alpha₁-PI by a vacuum. Remove the diluent bottle and transfer device.

Aralast NP—Allow the reconstituted solution to stand until contents appear to be in solution, then swirl gently to completely dissolve. May take 5 to 10 minutes. **Do not shake or invert vial until ready to withdraw contents.** Solution should be colorless to slightly yellow to yellowish-green. A few small visible particles may occasionally remain and will be removed by the microaggregate filter. Reconstituted product from several vials may be pooled into an empty, sterile IV solution container. Use the sterile 20-micron filter provided for transfer.

Prolastin-C—Swirl vigorously for 10 to 15 seconds immediately after adding diluent to thoroughly break up cake, then swirl continuously until the powder is completely dissolved. Some foaming will occur. Reconstituted product from several vials may be pooled into an empty, sterile IV solution container. If particles are visible, remove by passing through a sterile filter (e.g., 15-micron filter [not supplied]) used for administering blood products.

Glassia: Available as a single-use vial containing 1 Gm of functional alpha₁-PI in 50 mL of ready-to-use solution. Solution should be clear and colorless to yellow-green. Do not use if product is cloudy. Infusion can be made directly from the vial, or vials may be pooled in an empty, sterile IV container. When infusing directly from the vial, use a vented spike adapter and a 5-micron in-line filter (neither is supplied). When infusing from a sterile IV container, use a vent filter (not supplied) to withdraw Glassia from the vial, and then use the supplied 5-micron filter needle to transfer Glassia into the infusion container. Attach an IV administration set and administer through an additional 5-micron in-line filter (not supplied).

Zemaira: Insert the white end of the double-ended transfer needle into the center of the upright diluent vial. Invert the diluent vial and insert the green end of the double-ended transfer needle into the center of the product vial. Use minimum force. Diluent will be drawn into the alpha₁-PI by a vacuum. Wet the lyophilized cake completely by gently tilting the product vial. Do not allow the air inlet filter to face downward, and use care not to lose the vacuum. Remove the diluent bottle and transfer device. Gently swirl until the powder is completely dissolved. May take 5 to 10 minutes. **Do not shake or invert vial until ready to withdraw contents.** Reconstituted product from several vials may be pooled into an empty, sterile IV solution container. Administer through an infusion set with a 5-micron in-line filter (not supplied).

Aralast NP will yield a 0.5 Gm/25 mL vial or a 1 Gm/50 mL vial (20 mg/mL).

Glassia will yield a 1 Gm/50 mL vial (20 mg/mL).

Prolastin-C will yield a 1 Gm/20 mL vial (50 mg/mL).

Zemaira will yield a 1 Gm/20 mL vial (50 mg/mL).

Filters: All products must be filtered before or during administration. Manufacturers supply either a filter needle to withdraw alpha₁-PI from the vial or may supply an in-line filter (to be used in the IV line or for pooling); see Dilution for other filter requirements.

Storage: Refrigerate **Glassia** in carton until use. Contains no preservatives and no latex. **Aralast NP and Prolastin-C** should be stored at temperatures not to exceed 25° C (77° F). **Zemaira** may be refrigerated before reconstitution or stored at temperatures up to 25° C (77° F). **All Preparations:** Avoid freezing. Do not use after expiration date on vials. Must be used within 3 hours of reconstitution or entry into vial.

COMPATIBILITY

Manufacturers state, "Should be given alone, without mixing with other agents or diluting solutions."

RATE OF ADMINISTRATION

Aralast NP: Do not exceed 0.08 mL/kg/min.

Prolastin-C, Zemaira: 0.08 mL/kg/min is recommended.

Glassia: Do not exceed 0.04 mL/kg/min.

If an infusion reaction or other adverse effects occur, a reduced rate or interruption of the infusion may be indicated until symptoms subside; see Side Effects and Antidote.

ACTIONS

Aralast NP, Prolastin-C, Zemaira are sterile, stable, lyophilized preparations. **Glassia** is a ready-to-use solution. All are obtained from human plasma. Increases and maintains functional levels of alpha₁-PI in the epithelial lining of the lower respiratory tract. Provides adequate antineutrophil elastase activity in the lungs of individuals with alpha₁-antitrypsin deficiency. Weekly infusions of alpha₁-PI usually maintain serum levels above a target threshold of 11 micromoles. Numerous processes employed during manufacture to eliminate potential for viral transmission from human plasma; see Precautions.

INDICATIONS AND USES

Treatment of congenital alpha₁-antitrypsin deficiency, a potentially fatal deficiency; used for chronic replacement (augmentation and maintenance therapy) only in individuals with alpha₁-antitrypsin deficiency and selected types of clinically demonstrated emphysema.

CONTRAINDICATIONS

Individuals with selective IgA deficiencies (IgA level less than 15 mg/dL for **Aralast NP**) who have known antibodies against IgA (anti-IgA antibodies). IgA may be present and severe reactions, including anaphylaxis, can occur. ▪ Known hypersensitivity to any alpha₁-PI product or any product components.

PRECAUTIONS

For IV use only. Confirm diagnosis of congenital alpha₁-antitrypsin deficiency with selected clinically demonstrated emphysema. ▪ May contain trace amounts of IgA. Patients with selective or severe IgA deficiency and with known antibodies to IgA have a greater risk for developing severe hypersensitivity and anaphylactic reactions; see Contraindications. ▪ Each unit of plasma is tested and found nonreactive to HIV antibody, Creutzfeldt-Jakob disease, hepatitis B surface antigen, and hepatitis C. Transmission of these viruses is still possible. ▪ Will increase plasma volume; use caution in patients at risk for circulatory overload. ▪ Long-term effects from continued use are not known. ▪ Individuals severely deficient in endogenous alpha₁-PI are unable to maintain an adequate antiprotease defense and are subject to more rapid proteolysis of the alveolar walls leading to chronic lung disease. Pulmonary infections, including pneumonia and acute bronchitis, are common in these individuals.

Monitor: Monitor V/S and observe patient continuously throughout infusion. ▪ Blood levels of alpha₁-PI have been maintained above the functional level of 80 mg/dL with this replacement therapy. Serum levels determined by commercial immunologic assays may not reflect actual functional alpha₁-PI levels. ▪ Assess lung sounds and rate and quality of respirations before each infusion. ▪ Monitor for S/S of a hypersensitivity reaction (e.g., dyspnea, flushing, hypotension, rash, tachycardia); emergency equipment, medications, and supplies must be available.

Patient Education: Inform of risks and of safety precautions taken during manufacturing process. ▪ Note changes in breathing pattern or sputum production; avoid smoking. ▪ Report S/S of a hypersensitivity reaction promptly (e.g., dyspnea, faintness, hypotension, hives, tightness of the chest). ▪ Report S/S of parvovirus B19 (e.g., chills, drowsiness, fever, and runny nose, followed 2 weeks later by a rash and joint pain). Parvovirus B19 may be more serious in pregnant women and immune-compromised individuals.

Maternal/Child: Category C: use in pregnancy only when clearly needed. May present risk to fetus; benefits must justify risks. ▪ Safety for use during breast-feeding not established; effects unknown. ▪ Safety for use in pediatric patients not established.

Elderly: Differences in response compared to younger adults not known. As for all patients, dosing for elderly patients should be appropriate to their overall situation.

DRUG/LAB INTERACTIONS

No specific information available; see Compatibility.

SIDE EFFECTS

All formulations: Consider risk potential for contracting AIDS, Creutzfeldt-Jakob disease, hepatitis B, or hepatitis C. Hypersensitivity reactions, including anaphylaxis, chills, dyspnea, hypotension, rash, and tachycardia, have been reported; see Contraindications.

Aralast NP: Cough, headache, musculoskeletal discomfort, and pharyngitis are most common. Asthma, back pain, bloating, bronchitis, dizziness, pain, peripheral edema, rash, rhinitis, sinusitis, somnolence, and viral infection may occur.

Glassia: Dizziness and headache are most common. Chest discomfort, cough, increased hepatic enzymes, sinusitis, and URI have been reported. Cholangitis, exacerbation of COPD, and severe headache may occur.

Prolastin-C: Chills, headache, hot flush, pruritus, and rash were most common. A severe abdominal and extremity rash occurred in one patient and recurred in two patients on rechallenge.

Zemaira: Asthenia, bronchitis, chest pain, cough, dizziness, fever, headache, injection site pain and/or hemorrhage, paresthesia, pruritus, rhinitis, sinusitis, sore throat, and upper respiratory infections may occur.

ANTIDOTE

All side effects except potential transmission of viral diseases usually subside spontaneously. Keep the physician informed. If side effects occur, interrupt or discontinue infusion until symptoms subside, then resume at a tolerated rate. Discontinue alpha₁-PI and treat anaphylaxis (antihistamines, epinephrine, corticosteroids) as indicated. Resuscitate as necessary.

ALPROSTADIL BBW

(al-**PROSS**-tah-dill)

Prostaglandin E₁, Prostin VR Pediatric

Prostaglandin
(ductus arteriosus
patency adjunct)

USUAL DOSE
Pediatric patients: Begin with 0.05 to 0.1 mcg/kg of body weight/min. When therapeutic response is achieved, reduce infusion rate in increments to the lowest dose that maintains the response (e.g., reduce from 0.1 to 0.05 or from 0.025 to 0.01 mcg/kg/min). If necessary, dose may be increased gradually to a maximum of 0.4 mcg/kg/min. Generally these higher rates do not produce greater effects. May be given through infusion in a large vein or, if necessary, through an umbilical artery catheter placed at the ductal opening.

DILUTION
Each 500 mcg (1 mL) must be further diluted with NS or D5W. When using a volumetric infusion chamber, the appropriate amount of IV infusion solution should be added to the chamber first. The undiluted alprostadil should then be added to the IV infusion solution, avoiding direct contact of the undiluted solution with the wall of the volumetric infusion chamber; see Compatibility. Various volumes of infusion solution may be used depending on infusion pump capabilities and desired infusion rate.

Guidelines for Dilution of 500 mcg (1 mL) of Alprostadil and Rate of Infusion for Desired Dose of Alprostadil			
Diluent (mL)	Concentration (mcg/mL)	Desired Dose (mcg/kg/min)	Rate of Infusion (mL/min/kg)
250 mL	2 mcg/mL	0.1 mcg/kg/min	0.05 mL/min/kg
100 mL	5 mcg/mL	0.1 mcg/kg/min	0.02 mL/min/kg
50 mL	10 mcg/mL	0.1 mcg/kg/min	0.01 mL/min/kg
25 mL	20 mcg/mL	0.1 mcg/kg/min	0.005 mL/min/kg

Storage: Refrigerate until dilution. Prepare fresh solution for administration every 24 hours.

COMPATIBILITY
Consider any drug NOT listed as compatible to be INCOMPATIBLE until consulting a pharmacist; specific conditions may apply.
Manufacturer states that undiluted alprostadil may interact with the plastic sidewalls of the volumetric infusion chamber, causing a change in the appearance of the chamber and creating a hazy solution. Should this occur, the solution and the volumetric infusion chamber should be replaced; see Dilution.

One source suggests the following **compatibilities:**
Y-site: Ampicillin, cefazolin (Ancef), cefotaxime (Claforan), chlorothiazide (Diuril), dobutamine, dopamine, fentanyl, gentamicin, methylprednisolone (Solu-Medrol), nitroprusside sodium, tobramycin, vancomycin, vecuronium.

RATE OF ADMINISTRATION
See Usual Dose. Infusion pump capable of delivering 0.005, 0.01, 0.02, or 0.05 mL/min/kg required. Use for the shortest time possible at the lowest rate therapeutically effective. Decrease rate of infusion *stat* if a significant fall in arterial pressure occurs.

ACTIONS
A naturally occurring acidic lipid. A prostaglandin. Has various pharmacologic effects, including vasodilation, inhibition of platelet aggregation, and stimulation of the intestinal and uterine smooth muscle. Lowers blood pressure by decreasing peripheral resistance. A reflex increase in cardiac output and heart rate accompany the reduction in blood pressure. Smooth muscle of the ductus arteriosus is susceptible to alprostadil's relaxing ef-

fect. Infants with congenital defects that restrict the pulmonary or systemic blood flow may benefit from alprostadil infusion. In some infants with restricted pulmonary blood flow, an increase in blood pO_2 was observed. In some infants with restricted systemic blood flow, an increase in pH in those who were acidotic, an increase in SBP, and a decrease in the ratio of pulmonary artery pressure to aortic pressure were seen. Rapid metabolism by oxidation (80% in one pass through the lungs) necessitates administration by continuous infusion. Remainder excreted as metabolites in the urine.

INDICATIONS AND USES
Temporarily maintain the patency of the ductus arteriosus until corrective or palliative surgery can be performed on neonates who have congenital heart defects and who depend on the patent ductus for survival. Such congenital heart defects include pulmonary atresia, pulmonary stenosis, tricuspid atresia, tetralogy of Fallot, interruption of the aortic arch, coarctation of the aorta, or transposition of the great vessels. ▪ Used by intercavernosal injection to treat impotence.

CONTRAINDICATIONS
None known.

PRECAUTIONS
Usually administered by trained personnel in pediatric intensive care facilities. ▪ Establish a diagnosis of cyanotic heart disease (restricted pulmonary blood flow). Not indicated for infant respiratory distress syndrome (hyaline membrane disease). ▪ Response is poor in infants with Po_2 values of 40 torr or more or those more than 4 days old. More effective with lower Po_2. ▪ Apnea has been experienced in 10% to 12% of treated neonates; see Monitor. ▪ Use caution in neonates with bleeding tendencies; inhibits platelet aggregation. ▪ Administration of alprostadil to neonates may result in gastric outlet obstruction secondary to antral hyperplasia. Appears to be related to duration of therapy and cumulative dose. Risk of long-term infusion should be weighed against the possible benefits in a critically ill neonate; see Monitor. ▪ Cortical proliferation of the long bones has been observed in infants during long-term infusions. May regress after withdrawal of drug.

Monitor: Monitor respiratory status continuously. Ventilatory assistance must be immediately available. May cause apnea, especially in infants under 2 kg. Apnea usually appears during the first hour of infusion. ▪ Monitor arterial pressure intermittently by umbilical artery catheter, auscultation, or Doppler transducer. Decrease rate of infusion *stat* if a significant fall in arterial pressure occurs. ▪ Decrease or stop infusion if infant develops increased respiratory distress; bleeding, bruising, or hematoma formation; or sudden changes in cardiac status (e.g., decreased BP, bradycardia, cardiac arrest, cyanosis). ▪ Measure effectiveness with increase of Po_2 in infants with restricted pulmonary blood flow and increase of BP and blood pH in infants with restricted systemic blood flow. ▪ Monitor for evidence of antral hyperplasia and gastric outlet obstruction in neonates receiving more than 120 hours of therapy at recommended doses.

DRUG/LAB INTERACTIONS
No drug interactions have been reported between alprostadil and the therapy that is standard in neonates with restricted pulmonary or systemic blood flow. Standard therapy includes **antibiotics** such as penicillin or gentamicin; **vasopressors** such as dopamine and isoproterenol; **cardiac glycosides**; and **diuretics** such as furosemide. ▪ Inhibits **platelet aggregation.**

SIDE EFFECTS
Apnea, bradycardia, cardiac arrest, cerebral bleeding, cortical proliferation of long bones, diarrhea, DIC, edema, fever, flushing, hyperextension of the neck, hyperirritability, hypokalemia, hypotension, hypothermia, seizures, sepsis, tachycardia. Many other side effects have occurred in 1% or less of infants receiving alprostadil.

Overdose: Apnea, bradycardia, fever, flushing, hypotension.

ANTIDOTE

Notify physician of all side effects. Discontinue immediately if apnea occurs. Institute emergency measures. If infusion is restarted, use extreme caution. Decrease or stop infusion if infant develops increased respiratory distress; bleeding, bruising, or hematoma formation; or sudden changes in cardiac status (e.g., decreased BP, bradycardia, cardiac arrest, cyanosis). Decrease rate if pyrexia, hypotension, or fall in arterial pressure occurs.

ALTEPLASE
(**AL**-teh-playz)

Thrombolytic agent

Activase, rt-PA❋, Tissue Plasminogen Activator, tPA ▪ Cathflo Activase

pH 7.3

USUAL DOSE

Selected indications (e.g., acute ischemic stroke, acute myocardial infarction [AMI] in patients weighing less than 65 or 67 kg) require exact weight-adjusted dosing. To deliver an accurate dose without possibility of overdose, calculate desired dose and withdraw any amount **NOT** needed from a 50- or 100-mg vial and discard. In all situations follow total dose with at least 30 mL of NS or D5W through the IV tubing to ensure administration of total dose.

ACUTE MYOCARDIAL INFARCTION

Administer as soon as possible after onset of symptoms. Total dose is based on patient weight and should not exceed 100 mg regardless of selected administration regimen (accelerated infusion and 3-hour infusion are outlined in the following sections).

Accelerated infusion: Recommended accelerated infusion dose consists of an IV bolus over 1 to 2 minutes followed by an IV infusion as shown in the following chart.

Accelerated Infusion Weight-Based Doses for Patients with AMI			
Patient Weight (kg)	IV Bolus	First 30 Minutes	Next 60 Minutes
>67 kg	15 mg	50 mg	35 mg
≤67 kg	15 mg	0.75 mg/kg	0.5 mg/kg

The safety and efficacy of accelerated infusion of alteplase have been investigated only with concomitant administration of heparin and aspirin. See comments under Usual Dose.

3-hour infusion: For patients weighing 65 kg or more, administer a total dose of 100 mg titrated over 3 hours as an IV infusion. Initially, administer 60 mg over the first hour (with 6 to 10 mg of this administered as a bolus over 1 to 2 minutes). Follow with 20 mg/hr for 2 hours. For smaller patients (less than 65 kg), calculate total dose using 1.25 mg/kg of body weight administered over 3 hours (with 0.075 mg/kg administered as a bolus over 1 to 2 minutes). Follow with 0.675 mg/kg over the first hour and 0.25 mg/kg for 2 hours. Weight-based doses are shown in the following chart. See comments under Usual Dose.

3-Hour Infusion Weight-Based Doses for Patients with AMI			
Patient Weight (kg)	Bolus	Rest of 1st Hour	2nd Hour	3rd Hour
≥65 kg	6 to 10 mg	50 to 54 mg	20 mg	20 mg
<65 kg	0.075 mg/kg	0.675 mg/kg	0.25 mg/kg	0.25 mg/kg

Continued

ACUTE ISCHEMIC STROKE

Administer as soon as possible but within 3 hours after onset of symptoms. Perform non–contrast-enhanced CT or MRI before administration to rule out intracranial bleed. Recommended dose is 0.9 mg/kg. Do not exceed the maximum dose of 90 mg. See comments in Usual Dose. Give a bolus of 10% of the calculated dose over 1 minute followed by balance of calculated dose (90%) as an infusion evenly distributed over 60 minutes. Do not give aspirin, heparin, or warfarin for 24 hours; see Precautions.

PULMONARY EMBOLISM

100 mg administered over 2 hours as an IV infusion. Begin parenteral anticoagulation near the end of or immediately following the alteplase infusion when the partial thromboplastin time (PTT) or thrombin time (TT) returns to twice normal or less.

CENTRAL VENOUS ACCESS DEVICE (CVAD) OCCLUSIONS, CATHFLO ACTIVASE

See Rate of Administration, Precautions, Monitor, and Maternal/Child.

Patient weight 30 kg or greater: Instill 2 mg in 2 mL into the occluded catheter.

Patient weight less than 30 kg: Instill 110% of the internal lumen volume of the occluded catheter into the occluded catheter. Do not exceed 2 mg in 2 mL.

Attempt to aspirate blood from the catheter after 30 minutes of dwell time. If catheter function has been restored, aspirate 4 to 5 mL of blood in patients equal to or greater than 10 kg or 3 mL of blood in patients less than 10 kg to remove Cathflo Activase and residual clot, then gently irrigate the catheter with NS.

If catheter function has not been restored (unable to aspirate blood), allow the first dose to remain in the catheter for 90 additional minutes of dwell time and then attempt to aspirate again (total elapsed time is 120 minutes). If catheter function has been restored, aspirate and irrigate as above. If function has not been restored, a second dose may be instilled and the dwell time and aspiration process repeated.

DILUTION

Myocardial infarction, stroke, and pulmonary embolism: Must be reconstituted with SWFI without preservatives (provided by manufacturer). Available in 50- and 100-mg vials. May be administered as reconstituted solution at 1 mg/mL or further diluted immediately before administration in an equal volume of NS or D5W to yield a concentration of 0.5 mg/mL using either polyvinyl chloride bags or glass vials. Slight foaming is expected; let stand for several minutes to dissipate large bubbles. Do not shake. Mix by swirling or slow inversion; avoid agitation during dilution.

50-mg vial: Use a large-bore (18-gauge) needle and syringe to direct the stream of provided diluent (SWFI) into the lyophilized cake. A vacuum must be present when the diluent is added to the powder for injection. Do not use if vacuum is not present.

Bolus dose can be given when indicated by IV injection through a med port or by IV pump. To obtain bolus dose, **do not** prime syringe used with air; insert needle into the alteplase vial stopper to withdraw dose. Administer balance of dose using either a polyvinyl chloride bag or glass vial and infusion set. Adjust pump rate of delivery as required. Complete by flushing tubing with IV solution.

100-mg vial: Does not contain a vacuum. Diluent and transfer device provided. Insert one end of transfer device into upright vial of diluent (do not invert diluent vial yet). Hold alteplase vial upside down and push center of vial down onto piercing pin. Now invert vials and allow diluent to flow into alteplase. Small amount (0.5 mL) of diluent will not transfer. Swirl gently to dissolve. Do not shake. Process takes several minutes. Remove any quantity of drug in excess of that specified for patient treatment; see Usual Dose.

Bolus dose can be given when indicated by IV injection through a med port or by IV pump. When withdrawing the bolus dose from a 100-mg vial, the needle should be inserted away from the puncture mark made by the transfer device. Administer the balance of dose by inserting an infusion set into puncture site created by piercing pin. Hang by plastic capping on bottom of vial. Prime tubing with alteplase and administer. Adjust pump rate of delivery as required. Complete by flushing tubing with IV solution.

Cathflo Activase for CVAD occlusion: Supplied as a sterile lyophilized powder in 2-mg vials. Must be reconstituted with 2.2 mL of SWFI without preservatives. Direct diluent stream into the powder. Allow to stand undisturbed until large bubbles dissipate; may foam slightly. Mix by swirling gently; do not shake. Should be completely dissolved within 3 minutes. Final concentration is 1 mg/mL. If the 2-mg vials are not available, some pharmacies dilute 50 mg of alteplase with 50 mL of SWFI without preservatives (1 mg/mL). Withdraw 2.2 mL (2.2 mg) to 2- or 5-mL sterile disposable syringes. In studies these were transferred to sterile glass vials and frozen. Defrost and use as needed (22 prepared doses).

Filters: Specific information not available.

Storage: *Systemic alteplase:* Protect from light in cartons. May be stored at CRT or refrigerated before and/or after reconstitution. Manufacturer recommends reconstitution immediately before use. Must be used within 8 hours of reconstitution. Discard unused solution. Stable as a 0.5 mg/mL solution in NS or D5W for 8 hours at CRT.

Cathflo Activase: Refrigerate unopened vials; protect from light during extended storage. Reconstitution immediately before use is recommended, but solution may be used up to 8 hours after reconstitution if refrigerated at 2° to 30° C (36° to 46° F). Do not use beyond expiration date on vial. Discard unused solution.

COMPATIBILITY

Consider any drug NOT listed as compatible to be INCOMPATIBLE until consulting a pharmacist; specific conditions may apply.

Manufacturer states, "No other medication should be added to infusion solutions containing alteplase; see Dilution.

One source suggests the following **compatibilities:**

Y-site: Lidocaine, metoprolol (Lopressor), and propranolol through **Y-site** of free-flowing alteplase infusion.

RATE OF ADMINISTRATION

Systemic alteplase: See specific rates for each diagnosis under Usual Dose. In all situations use an infusion pump (preferred) or a metriset with microdrip (60 gtt/mL) and IV tubing to facilitate accurate administration. Flushing of IV line required. NS preferred for flushing of IV line.

Cathflo Activase: Avoid excessive pressure or force while attempting to clear catheters; see Usual Dose, Precautions, and Monitor.

ACTIONS

A tissue plasminogen activator and enzyme produced by recombinant DNA. It binds to fibrin in a thrombus and converts plasminogen to plasmin. Plasmin digests fibrin and dissolves the clot. With therapeutic doses, a decrease in circulating fibrinogen makes the patient susceptible to bleeding. Onset of action is prompt, effecting patency of the vessel within 1 to 2 hours in most patients. Prompt opening of arteries increases probability of improved function. Cleared from the plasma by the liver within 5 (50%) to 10 (80%) minutes after the infusion is discontinued. Some effects may linger for 45 minutes to several hours.

INDICATIONS AND USES

Systemic alteplase: Use in acute myocardial infarction (AMI) for the reduction of the incidence of congestive heart failure and the reduction of mortality associated with AMI. ▪ Treatment of acute ischemic stroke. Exclude intracranial hemorrhage as the primary cause of stroke S/S before initiation of treatment. ▪ Lysis of acute massive pulmonary embolism defined as (1) acute pulmonary emboli obstructing blood flow to a lobe or to multiple lung segments, or (2) acute pulmonary emboli accompanied by unstable hemodynamics (e.g., failure to maintain BP without supportive measures).

Limitation of use: In patients with AMI, the risk of stroke may outweigh the benefit produced by thrombolytic therapy in patients whose AMI puts them at low risk for death or heart failure.

Cathflo Activase: Restoration of function to CVADs as assessed by the ability to withdraw blood.

Unlabeled uses: *Systemic alteplase:* Treatment of acute ischemic stroke 3 to 4.5 hours after symptom onset. Has been shown to restore blood flow to frostbitten limbs. Has been used in peripheral arterial occlusion, prosthetic valve thrombosis, and submassive pulmonary embolism.

CONTRAINDICATIONS

All indications: Known hypersensitivity to alteplase or its components.

Acute myocardial infarction/pulmonary embolism: Do not administer for the treatment of AMI or pulmonary embolism in the following situations in which the risk of bleeding is greater than the potential benefit: active internal bleeding, bleeding diathesis, history of recent cerebrovascular accident, recent (within 3 months) intracranial or intraspinal surgery or serious head trauma, current severe uncontrolled hypertension, presence of intracranial conditions that may increase the risk of bleeding (e.g., some neoplasms, arteriovenous malformation, or aneurysm).

Acute ischemic stroke: Do not administer to treat acute ischemic stroke in the following situations in which the risk of bleeding is greater than the potential benefit: current intracranial hemorrhage (on pretreatment evaluation), subarachnoid hemorrhage, active internal bleeding, presence of intracranial conditions that may increase the risk of bleeding (e.g., some neoplasms, arteriovenous malformation, or aneurysm), recent (within 3 months) intracranial or intraspinal surgery or serious head trauma, bleeding diathesis, or current severe uncontrolled hypertension.

PRECAUTIONS

All systemic indications: Administered under the direction of a physician knowledgeable in its use and with appropriate emergency drugs and diagnostic and laboratory facilities available. ▪ Bleeding is the most common complication. May be internal bleeding (involving intracranial or retroperitoneal sites or the GI, GU, or respiratory tracts) or external bleeding, especially at arterial and venous puncture sites. Use extreme care with the patient; avoid IM injections and any trauma to the patient who is taking alteplase. Avoid invasive procedures (e.g., arterial puncture and venipuncture). If these procedures are absolutely necessary, use extreme precautionary methods. To minimize bleeding from noncompressible sites, avoid internal jugular and subclavian venous punctures. If an arterial puncture is necessary, use an upper extremity vessel that is accessible to manual compression, apply pressure for at least 30 minutes, and monitor the puncture site closely. ▪ Fatal cases of hemorrhage associated with traumatic intubation in patients receiving alteplase have been reported. ▪ Aspirin and heparin have been administered concomitantly with and following infusions of alteplase in the management of AMI and PE. However, the administration of heparin and aspirin concomitantly with and following infusions of alteplase for the treatment of acute ischemic stroke during the first 24 hours after symptom onset has not been investigated. Because heparin, aspirin, or alteplase may cause bleeding complications, carefully monitor for bleeding. Hemorrhage can occur 1 or more days after administration of alteplase while patients are still receiving anticoagulant therapy. ▪ The risk of bleeding with alteplase therapy for all systemic indications is increased and should be weighed against the anticipated benefit in any of the following conditions: recent major surgery or procedure (e.g., CABG, obstetric delivery, organ biopsy, previous puncture of noncompressible vessels), recent intracranial hemorrhage, recent GI or GU bleeding, cerebrovascular disease, hypertension (systolic above 175 mm Hg or diastolic above 110 mm Hg), recent trauma, high likelihood of left heart thrombus (e.g., mitral stenosis with atrial fibrillation), acute pericarditis, subacute bacterial endocarditis, hemostatic defects (including those secondary to severe hepatic or renal disease), significant liver dysfunction, pregnancy, hemorrhagic ophthalmic conditions (e.g., diabetic hemorrhagic retinopathy), septic thrombophlebitis or occluded AV cannula at seriously infected site, patients taking anticoagulants, advanced age, or any situation in which bleeding might be hazardous or difficult to manage because of location. ▪ Cholesterol embolism has been reported rarely; see Side Effects. ▪ Orolingual angioedema has been reported in patients with acute MI and acute ischemic stroke. Onset may occur during or up to 2 hours after infusion. May be associated with concomitant use of angiotensin-converting enzyme inhibitors. Most resolved with prompt treatment; see Drug/Lab Interactions and Antidote.

Myocardial infarction: Reperfusion arrhythmias can occur (e.g., sinus bradycardia, accelerated idioventricular rhythm, PVCs, ventricular tachycardia); have antiarrhythmic medications available.

Acute ischemic stroke: Because of the higher risk of intracranial hemorrhage in patients treated for acute ischemic stroke, treatment facility must be able to provide evaluation and management of intracranial hemorrhage. ▪ Risk of intracranial hemorrhage may be increased in patients with severe neurologic deficit at presentation. ▪ Treatment may begin before coagulation study results are known in patients without recent use of oral anticoagulants or heparin. Discontinue infusion if pretreatment INR is greater than 1.7 or if an elevated aPTT is identified. ▪ Use caution in patients with blood glucose values less than 50 mg/dL or greater than 400 mg/dL; risk of misdiagnosis of acute ischemic stroke is increased. ▪ Safety and efficacy in patients with minor neurologic deficit or rapidly improving symptoms before treatment is begun have not been studied; use is not recommended.

Pulmonary emboli: Treatment with alteplase does not constitute adequate treatment of underlying deep venous thrombosis. ▪ Risk of re-embolization due to lysis of underlying DVT should be considered.

Cathflo Activase: Consider causes of catheter dysfunction other than thrombus formation (e.g., catheter malposition, mechanical failure, constriction by a suture, lipid deposits or drug precipitates within the catheter lumen). ▪ Do not apply vigorous suction during attempts to determine catheter occlusion; may risk damage to the vascular wall or collapse of soft-walled catheters. Avoid excessive pressure during instillation of Cathflo Activase into the catheter; may cause rupture of the catheter or expulsion of the clot into the circulation. ▪ Use caution with patients who have active internal bleeding, thrombocytopenia, or other hemostatic defects (including those secondary to hepatic or renal disease). ▪ Use caution in patients who have conditions for which bleeding constitutes a significant hazard, who would be difficult to manage because of location of the bleeding, who are at high risk for embolic complications (e.g., venous thrombosis in the region of the catheter), or who have had any of the following within 48 hours: surgery, obstetric delivery, percutaneous biopsy of viscera or deep tissues, or puncture of noncompressible vessels. ▪ Use caution in the presence of known or suspected infection in the catheter; may release a localized infection into the systemic circulation. ▪ See Monitor. ▪ Safety and effectiveness of doses greater than 2 mg have not been established.

Monitor: *All systemic indications:* Establish a separate IV line for alteplase. ▪ Obtain appropriate laboratory studies (e.g., PT, TT, PTT, INR, aPTT, CBC, fibrinogen levels, platelets). ▪ Diagnosis-specific baseline studies (e.g., ECG, troponin in myocardial infarction, noncontrast CT brain scan, neurologic assessment in acute ischemic stroke, and lung scan or pulmonary angiography in pulmonary embolism) are indicated. ▪ Monitor the patient carefully and frequently for pain and signs of bleeding; observe catheter sites frequently and apply pressure dressings to any recently invaded site; watch for hematuria, hematemesis, bloody stool, petechiae, hematoma, flank pain, or muscle weakness; perform neuro checks. Continue until normal clotting function returns. ▪ Monitor BP and maintain within appropriate limits with antihypertensives or vasopressors as indicated. ▪ Monitor for signs of orolingual angioedema during and for several hours after infusion. ▪ Watch for extravasation; may cause ecchymosis and/or inflammation. Restart IV at another site. Moist compresses may be helpful. ▪ See Precautions and Drug/Lab Interactions.

Myocardial infarction: Monitor ECG.

Acute ischemic stroke: Before the initiation of therapy, determine actual time of onset of stroke. ▪ During and following alteplase administration, frequently monitor and control BP. The 2013 AHA/ASA guidelines for early management of acute ischemic stroke recommend monitoring BP and performing neurologic assessments every 15 minutes for 2 hours, every 30 minutes for 6 hours, then every 1 hour for 18 hours. ▪ Hemorrhage in the brain occurs frequently during treatment with alteplase; monitor carefully. Acute neurologic deterioration, new headache, acute hypertension, or nausea and vomiting may indicate the occurrence of intracranial hemorrhage. If intracranial hemorrhage is suspected, discontinue alteplase and obtain a CT scan.

Cathflo Activase: Aseptic technique imperative. ▪ Avoid force while attempting to clear catheters; may rupture catheter or dislodge clot into the circulation. ▪ To prevent air from entering the open catheter and the circulatory system, instruct the patient to exhale and hold his/her breath any time the catheter is not connected to the IV tubing or a syringe. ▪ See Precautions.

Patient Education: Compliance with all measures to minimize bleeding (e.g., strict bed rest) is very important. ▪ Avoid use of razors, toothbrushes, and other sharp items. Use caution while moving to avoid excessive bumping. ▪ Report all episodes of bleeding and apply local pressure if indicated. Expect oozing from IV sites.

Maternal/Child: *Systemic alteplase:* Category C: safety for use in pregnancy and breast-feeding not established. ▪ Safety and effectiveness for use in pediatric patients not established.

Cathflo Activase: Category C: use during pregnancy only if benefits justify potential risk to the fetus. ▪ Use caution during breast-feeding. ▪ Has been used in patients 2 weeks to 17 years of age. Rates of serious adverse events as well as restoration of catheter function similar to adults.

Elderly: *Systemic alteplase:* Possible increased risk of bleeding with advanced age (e.g., age greater than 77 years). In acute ischemic stroke, efficacy results suggest a reduced but still favorable clinical outcome for elderly patients treated with alteplase.

Cathflo Activase: No incidents of intracranial hemorrhage, embolic events, or major bleeding events were observed during studies. ▪ Use caution in the elderly with conditions known to increase the risk of bleeding; see Precautions.

DRUG/LAB INTERACTIONS

Risk of bleeding may be increased by any medicine that affects blood clotting, including **anticoagulants** (e.g., heparin, warfarin [Coumadin]); **any medication that may cause hypoprothrombinemia, thrombocytopenia, or GI ulceration or bleeding** (e.g., selected antibiotics [e.g., cefotetan], aspirin, NSAIDs [e.g., ibuprofen (Advil, Motrin), naproxen (Aleve, Naprosyn)]); **and/or any other medication that inhibits platelet aggregation** (e.g., clopidogrel [Plavix], dipyridamole [Persantine], glycoprotein GPIIb/IIIa receptor antagonists [e.g., abciximab (ReoPro), eptifibatide (Integrilin), tirofiban (Aggrastat)]). If concurrent or subsequent use is indicated, monitor patient closely. ▪ Orolingual angioedema has been reported. Many patients, including patients with acute ischemic stroke, were receiving **angiotensin-converting enzyme inhibitors** (e.g., enalapril [Vasotec], enalaprilat [Vasotec IV], lisinopril [Zestril]). ▪ **Coagulation tests and measures of fibrinolytic activity** may be unreliable; specific procedures can be used; notify the lab of alteplase use.

SIDE EFFECTS

Systemic alteplase: Bleeding is most common: internal (GI tract, GU tract, retroperitoneal, or intracranial sites) and superficial or external bleeding (ecchymosis, epistaxis, gingival bleeding, venous cutdowns, arterial punctures, sites of recent surgical intervention). Mild to serious hypersensitivity reactions (e.g., anaphylactoid reaction, laryngeal edema, orolingual angioedema, rash, urticaria) have occurred. Cholesterol embolization can occur with thrombolytics but has been reported rarely. It may present with acute renal failure, bowel infarction, cerebral infarction, gangrenous digits, hypertension, livedo reticularis, myocardial infarction, pancreatitis, purple toe syndrome, retinal artery occlusion, rhabdomyolysis, or spinal cord infarction. Fatalities have been reported.

Post-Marketing: The following events may be life threatening:

Acute ischemic stroke (AIS): Cerebral edema, cerebral herniation, new ischemic stroke, seizure.

Acute myocardial infarction (AMI): Arrhythmias, AV block, cardiac arrest, cardiac tamponade, cardiogenic shock, electromechanical dissociation, fever, heart failure, hypotension, mitral regurgitation, myocardial reinfarction, myocardial rupture, nausea and/or vomiting, pericardial effusion, pericarditis, pulmonary edema, recurrent ischemia, thromboembolism.

Pulmonary embolism (PE): Hypotension, pleural effusion, pulmonary edema, pulmonary re-embolization, thromboembolism.

Cathflo Activase: Gastrointestinal bleeding, sepsis, and venous thrombosis have occurred. There were no reports of intracranial hemorrhage or pulmonary emboli during clinical trials.

ANTIDOTE

Systemic alteplase: Notify physician of all side effects. Note even the most minute bleeding tendency. Oozing at IV sites is expected. Control minor bleeding by local pressure. For severe bleeding in a critical location or suspected intracranial bleeding, discontinue alteplase and any heparin therapy immediately. Obtain PT, aPTT, platelet count, and fibrinogen. Draw blood for type and cross-match. Transfuse as indicated. Consider protamine if heparin has been used. Treat reperfusion arrhythmias with appropriate antiarrhythmic; VT or VF may require cardioversion. If anaphylaxis occurs, discontinue infusion immediately and initiate appropriate treatment. Treat minor hypersensitivity reactions symptomatically. If angioedema occurs, treat promptly with antihistamines (e.g., diphenhydramine [Benadryl]), IV corticosteroids, or epinephrine and consider discontinuing the alteplase infusion; resuscitate as necessary.

Cathflo Activase: Discontinue Cathflo Activase and withdraw it from the catheter if serious bleeding in a critical location (e.g., intracranial, gastrointestinal, retroperitoneal, pericardial) occurs. Discontinue drug and treat anaphylaxis as indicated; resuscitate as necessary. In the event of accidental administration of a 2-mg dose directly into the systemic circulation, the concentration of circulating levels of alteplase would be expected to return to exogenous levels of 5 to 10 ng/mL within 30 minutes.

AMIFOSTINE
(am-ih-**FOS**-teen)

Ethyol

Antidote
Antineoplastic adjunct
Cytoprotective agent

USUAL DOSE
PROPHYLACTIC REDUCTION OF CISPLATIN-INDUCED NEPHROTOXICITY, PROPHYLACTIC REDUCTION OF CISPLATIN-INDUCED NEUROTOXICITY (UNLABELED), AND PROPHYLACTIC REDUCTION OF ANTINEOPLASTIC AGENT BONE MARROW TOXICITY (UNLABELED)

Must be administered in conjunction with cisplatin. Adequate hydration and premedication required before administration; see Premedication below, Monitor, and cisplatin monograph.

Premedication: Premedication to prevent severe nausea and vomiting is recommended before each dose. Usual regimen includes dexamethasone 20 mg IV and a serotonin $5HT_3$ receptor antagonist (e.g., ondansetron [Zofran], granisetron [Kytril]) given before and in conjunction with amifostine infusion. Additional antiemetics (e.g., aprepitant [EMEND]) may be required based on the chemotherapy drugs administered.

Amifostine: 910 mg/M^2. Cisplatin dose must be given within 30 minutes of starting the amifostine infusion, but only after the full dose of amifostine is administered.

REDUCTION OF MODERATE TO SEVERE XEROSTOMIA FROM RADIATION OF THE HEAD AND NECK

Premedication: Premedication to prevent nausea and vomiting is recommended before each dose. Oral $5HT_3$ receptor antagonists alone or in combination with other antiemetics are recommended. Adequate hydration required; see Monitor.

Amifostine: 200 mg/M^2 once daily as a 3-minute infusion, starting 15 to 30 minutes before standard fraction radiation therapy.

DOSE ADJUSTMENTS

Dosing should be cautious in the elderly. Consider potential for decreased organ function and concomitant disease or drug therapy.

Reduction of cumulative renal toxicity with chemotherapy: Temporarily discontinue the infusion if the systolic BP decreases significantly from the baseline value. See the following chart.

Guideline for Interrupting Amifostine Infusion Due to Decrease in Systolic Blood Pressure					
	Baseline Systolic Blood Pressure (mm Hg)				
	<100	100-119	120-139	140-179	≥180
Decrease in systolic blood pressure during infusion of amifostine (mm Hg)	20	25	30	40	50

Infusion may be restarted to deliver the full dose if the BP returns to normal within 5 minutes and the patient is asymptomatic. If the BP does not return to baseline within 5 minutes and/or the patient is symptomatic (e.g., bradycardia, fainting, unconscious), the full dose cannot be delivered and subsequent doses should be reduced to 740 mg/M^2.

DILUTION

Each 500-mg vial should be reconstituted with 9.7 mL of NS (50 mg/mL). May be further diluted with NS to concentrations from 5 to 40 mg/mL. An additional 2.5 mL of NS will yield 40 mg/mL; 90 mL NS will yield 5 mg/mL.

Filters: Not required by manufacturer. Additional data not available.

Storage: Store at CRT before reconstitution. Reconstituted or diluted solution prepared in PVC infusion bags is stable for 5 hours at room temperature or 24 hours if refrigerated.

COMPATIBILITY

Consider any drug NOT listed as compatible to be INCOMPATIBLE until consulting a pharmacist; specific conditions may apply.
Use of any additive, diluent, or solution other than NS is not recommended by manufacturer.

One source suggests the following **compatibilities:**
Y-site: Amikacin, aminophylline, ampicillin, ampicillin/sulbactam (Unasyn), aztreonam (Azactam), bleomycin (Blenoxane), bumetanide, buprenorphine (Buprenex), butorphanol (Stadol), calcium gluconate, carboplatin (Paraplatin), carmustine (BiCNU), cefazolin (Ancef), cefotaxime (Claforan), cefotetan, cefoxitin (Mefoxin), ceftazidime (Fortaz), ceftriaxone (Rocephin), cefuroxime (Zinacef), ciprofloxacin (Cipro IV), clindamycin (Cleocin), cyclophosphamide (Cytoxan), cytarabine (ARA-C), dacarbazine (DTIC), dactinomycin (Cosmegen), daunorubicin (Cerubidine), dexamethasone (Decadron), diphenhydramine (Benadryl), dobutamine, docetaxel (Taxotere), dopamine, doxorubicin (Adriamycin), doxycycline, droperidol (Inapsine), enalaprilat (Vasotec IV), etoposide (VePesid), famotidine (Pepcid IV), fluconazole (Diflucan), fludarabine (Fludara), fluorouracil (5-FU), furosemide (Lasix), gallium nitrate (Ganite), gemcitabine (Gemzar), gentamicin, granisetron (Kytril), heparin, hydrocortisone sodium succinate (Solu-Cortef), hydromorphone (Dilaudid), idarubicin (Idamycin), ifosfamide (Ifex), imipenem-cilastatin (Primaxin), leucovorin calcium, lorazepam (Ativan), magnesium sulfate, mannitol (Osmitrol), mechlorethamine (nitrogen mustard), meperidine (Demerol), mesna (Mesnex), methotrexate, methylprednisolone (Solu-Medrol), metoclopramide (Reglan), metronidazole (Flagyl IV), mitomycin (Mutamycin), mitoxantrone (Novantrone), morphine, nalbuphine, ondansetron (Zofran), pemetrexed (Alimta), potassium chloride (KCl), promethazine (Phenergan), ranitidine (Zantac), sodium bicarbonate, streptozocin (Zanosar), sulfamethoxazole/trimethoprim, teniposide (Vumon), thiotepa, ticarcillin/clavulanate (Timentin), tobramycin, vancomycin, vinblastine, vincristine, zidovudine (AZT, Retrovir).

RATE OF ADMINISTRATION

Reduction of cumulative renal toxicity with chemotherapy: A single dose evenly distributed over 15 minutes. Complete amifostine dose but begin cisplatin within 30 minutes after beginning amifostine. Amifostine must be given over 15 minutes; longer infusion times increase the risk of side effects, especially hypotension. Shorter infusion times have not been studied.
Reduction of moderate to severe xerostomia from radiation of the head and neck: A single dose evenly distributed over 3 minutes. Begin infusion 15 to 30 minutes before standard fraction radiation therapy.

ACTIONS

A cytoprotective agent. Rapidly metabolized by alkaline phosphatase in tissues to an active metabolite that can reduce the nephrotoxic effects of cisplatin and the toxic effects of radiation on normal oral tissues. This protective metabolite is generated in greater amounts in normal tissues versus tumor tissues and is available to bind to and detoxify reactive metabolites of cisplatin and/or radiation. It reduces the incidence of cisplatin toxicity including nephrotoxicity but does not cause other toxic reactions. Its protective metabolite can also scavenge reactive oxygen species generated by exposure to either cisplatin or radiation. May adversely affect antitumor effects of cisplatin. Rapidly cleared from plasma with an elimination half-life of 8 minutes. Pretreatment with antiemetics does not alter its actions. Measurable levels of the metabolite have been found in bone marrow; minimal excretion in urine.

INDICATIONS AND USES

Reduce the cumulative renal toxicity associated with repeated administration of cisplatin in patients with advanced ovarian cancer. May allow higher cumulative doses of cisplatin and cyclophosphamide. ▪ Reduce the incidence of moderate to severe xerostomia (dryness of the mouth from salivary gland dysfunction) in patients undergoing postoperative radiation treatment for head and neck cancer, where the "radiation port" includes a substantial portion of the parotid glands.

Unlabeled uses: Reduce acute and cumulative hematologic toxicity associated with various chemotherapy regimens (e.g., cisplatin, cyclophosphamide, carboplatin; see literature). ▪ Decrease frequency or severity of cisplatin-induced neurotoxicity. ▪ Prevention of radiation proctitis in rectal cancer.

CONTRAINDICATIONS

Known sensitivity to aminothiol compounds or mannitol. ▪ Not recommended for patients receiving chemotherapy for malignancies if chemotherapy can produce significant survival benefit or cure; may interfere with effectiveness of chemotherapy regimen and reduce incidence of cure. ▪ Not recommended for patients who are hypotensive, dehydrated, or for those receiving antihypertensive therapy that cannot be stopped for 24 hours before amifostine is administered. ▪ Not recommended for patients receiving definitive radiotherapy. Tumor-protective effect in this setting has not been ruled out.

PRECAUTIONS

Use caution in the elderly and in patients with pre-existing cardiovascular or cerebrovascular conditions (e.g., arrhythmias, congestive heart failure, history of stroke, history of ischemic heart disease). ▪ Hypotension and nausea and vomiting can be severe; use caution in any situation in which these side effects may have serious consequences. ▪ Discontinue antihypertensive therapy 24 hours before administering amifostine. ▪ Hypersensitivity reactions, including anaphylaxis and severe cutaneous reactions, have been reported; see Monitor and Side Effects. Deaths have occurred. ▪ Facilities for monitoring the patient and responding to any medical emergency must be available.

Monitor: *All indications:* Adequate hydration required before administration of amifostine. ▪ Monitor fluid balance carefully, especially in conjunction with highly emetogenic chemotherapy (e.g., cisplatin). ▪ See Usual Dose for premedication requirements. Additional antiemetics may be required to offset nausea and vomiting of chemotherapy drugs. ▪ Keep patient in supine position during and immediately after the infusion. ▪ Hypersensitivity and/or severe cutaneous reactions may occur during or after infusion; monitor closely before, during, and after administration. Serious cutaneous reactions may develop weeks after initiation of therapy. ▪ Monitor serum calcium. Risk of hypocalcemia increased in some patients (e.g., nephrotic syndrome or patients receiving multiple doses). Calcium supplements may be required. ▪ See Dose Adjustments, Rate of Administration, and Antidote.

Reduction of cumulative renal toxicity with chemotherapy: Discontinue antihypertensive therapy if indicated; see Contraindications, Precautions, Drug/Lab Interactions. ▪ Obtain baseline BP and monitor at least every 5 minutes during and immediately after the infusion. Continue monitoring BP as indicated. ▪ Hypertension may be exacerbated by several causes (e.g., interruption of antihypertensive therapy, IV hydration). Monitor BP closely. ▪ Hypotension can occur at any time but is more frequent toward the end of the infusion, and recovery usually begins within 5 to 6 minutes after infusion is discontinued.

Reduction of xerostomia from radiation: Monitor BP before and immediately after the infusion and as indicated by results.

Patient Education: Void before administration. ▪ May produce significant hypotension. Effects may be additive with medications currently being taken. Review all medications (prescription and nonprescription) with nurse and/or physician. ▪ Must remain in supine position until BP is stabilized, then request assistance for ambulation. ▪ Report feelings of faintness or nausea promptly. ▪ Promptly report development of any rash or skin condition.

Maternal/Child: Category C: use only if potential benefits justify risk to fetus; embryotoxic in rabbits at doses lower than required for humans. ▪ Discontinue breast-feeding. ▪ Safety for use in pediatric patients not established; experience is limited.

Elderly: Response similar to younger adults; however, dosing should be cautious; see Dose Adjustments. ▪ Monitor fluid balance closely; avoid dehydration. ▪ Hypotension may be sudden and severe; monitor closely. ▪ See Contraindications and Precautions.

DRUG/LAB INTERACTIONS

Antihypertensive therapy (e.g., ACE inhibitors [e.g., enalapril], **calcium channel blocking agents** [e.g., nicardipine, verapamil], **diuretics** [e.g., furosemide, torsemide], **nitroglycerin, nitroprusside sodium**) should be discontinued 24 hours before amifostine administration; see Contraindications. ▪ Use extreme caution in any patient receiving medications with **hypotensive effects** (**antidepressants, benzodiazepines, beta-adrenergic blocking agents** [e.g., atenolol, esmolol, metoprolol, propranolol], **lidocaine, magnesium, narcotics, nitrates, paclitaxel, procainamide**); will cause additive hypotension.

SIDE EFFECTS

Hypotension and severe nausea and vomiting occur frequently. Hypotension may be associated with apnea, arrhythmias (e.g., atrial fibrillation/flutter, bradycardia, extrasystoles, tachycardia), chest pain, dyspnea, hypoxia, myocardial ischemia, and rarely renal failure, respiratory and cardiac arrest, seizures, and unconsciousness. Dehydration, dizziness, feelings of cold or warmth, flushing, hiccups, hypocalcemia, loss of consciousness, somnolence, and/or transient hypertension or exacerbation of pre-existing hypertension may occur. Hypersensitivity reactions (e.g., anaphylaxis [rare], arrhythmias, chest tightness, chills, cutaneous eruptions, dyspnea, fever, hypoxia, laryngeal edema, pruritus, sneezing, urticaria) have occurred. Most cutaneous eruptions, pruritus, and urticaria were mild; however, serious skin reactions such as erythema multiforme, exfoliative dermatitis, rash, Stevens-Johnson syndrome (rare), toxic epidermal necrolysis, and urticaria have been reported. Serious skin reactions have been reported more frequently when amifostine is used as a radioprotectant.

Overdose: Hypotension is the most likely symptom. Anxiety and reversible urinary retention have occurred at higher doses. Up to 3 doses have been given within 24 hours without unexpected side effects.

ANTIDOTE

Keep physician informed of side effects. Treatment of nausea and vomiting is imperative to encourage patients to continue treatment with full doses of chemotherapeutic agents. Hypotension may be dose-limiting. If the systolic BP decreases significantly (see Dose Adjustments chart), temporarily discontinue the amifostine still infusing, place the patient in Trendelenburg position, and administer an infusion of NS at a separate site. Vasopressors (e.g., dopamine, norepinephrine [Levophed]) may be required. If indicated, restart infusion if BP returns to baseline within 5 minutes and patient is asymptomatic. Discontinue amifostine immediately and permanently if an acute hypersensitivity or cutaneous reaction occurs. Dermatologic consult may be required. Treat anaphylaxis and resuscitate as necessary.

AMIKACIN SULFATE BBW
(am-ih-**KAY**-sin **SUL**-fayt)

Antibacterial
(aminoglycoside)

pH 3.5 to 5.5

USUAL DOSE
Up to 15 mg/kg of body weight/24 hr equally divided into 2 or 3 doses at equally divided intervals (5 mg/kg every 8 hours or 7.5 mg/kg every 12 hours). Dosage based on ideal weight of lean body mass. Do not exceed a total adult dose of 15 mg/kg/24 hr in an average weight patient or 1.5 Gm in heavier patients by all routes in 24 hours.

Studies suggest that in certain populations a single daily dose of 15 to 20 mg/kg (instead of divided into 2 or 3 doses) may provide higher peak levels and enhance drug effectiveness while actually reducing or having no adverse effects on risk of toxicity. Various procedures for monitoring blood levels are in use. Some health facilities are monitoring with trough levels; others may draw levels at predetermined times and plot the concentration on nomograms. Depending on the protocol in place, doses or intervals may be adjusted. See Dose Adjustments and Precautions.

PEDIATRIC DOSE
15 to 22.5 mg/kg/24 hr equally divided into 2 or 3 doses and given every 8 to 12 hours (5 to 7.5 mg/kg every 8 hours or 7.5 to 11.25 mg/kg every 12 hours). Do not exceed 1.5 Gm/24 hr. A single daily dose is also being used in pediatric patients. See comments under Usual Dose.

NEWBORN DOSE
See Maternal/Child.
10 mg/kg of body weight as a loading dose, then 7.5 mg/kg/dose. Intervals of 7.5 mg/kg dose adjusted based on age as follows:
Under 28 weeks' gestation and less than 7 days of age: Give every 24 hours.
Under 28 weeks' gestation and over 7 days or 28 to 34 weeks' gestation and under 7 days of age: Give every 18 hours.
28 to 34 weeks' gestation and over 7 days of age or over 34 weeks' gestation and under 7 days of age: Give every 12 hours.
Over 34 weeks' gestation and over 7 days of age: Give every 8 hours.

DOSE ADJUSTMENTS
Reduce daily dose commensurate with amount of renal impairment and/or increase intervals between injections. ▪ Once-daily dosing is not usually used in patients with ascites, burns covering more than 20% of the total body surface area, CrCl less than 40 mL/min (including patients requiring dialysis), CrCl greater than 120 mL/min, cystic fibrosis, endocarditis, mycobacterium infections, or in infants or pregnancy. ▪ Reduced dose or extended intervals may be required in the elderly. ▪ See Drug/Lab Interactions.

DILUTION
Each 500 mg or fraction thereof is diluted with 100 to 200 mL D5W, D5NS, or NS. Amount of diluent may be decreased proportionately with dosage for infants and other pediatric patients. Available for pediatric injection as 50 mg/mL.
Storage: Stable for 24 hours at RT at concentrations of 0.25 and 5 mg/mL when diluted in specific solutions; see prescribing information.

COMPATIBILITY
(Underline Indicates Conflicting Compatibility Information)
Consider any drug NOT listed as compatible to be INCOMPATIBLE until consulting a pharmacist; specific conditions may apply.
Do not physically premix with other drugs; administer separately as recommended by manufacturer. Inactivated in solution with beta-lactam antibiotics (e.g., cephalosporins, penicillins) and vancomycin. Do not mix in the same solution. Appropriate spacing required because of physical **incompatibilities**. See Drug/Lab Interactions.

One source suggests the following **compatibilities:**

Solution: Manufacturer lists D5W, D5/¹/₄NS, D5/¹/₂NS, NS, LR, D5 in Normosol M (Plasma-Lyte 56 in D5W), D5 in Normosol R (Plasma-Lyte 148 in D5W). Other sources list additional solutions.

Y-site: Acyclovir (Zovirax), amifostine (Ethyol), amiodarone (Nexterone), <u>anidulafungin (Eraxis)</u>, aztreonam (Azactam), bivalirudin (Angiomax), <u>caspofungin (Cancidas)</u>, cefepime (Maxipime), ceftaroline (Teflaro), ceftazidime (Fortaz), cisatracurium (Nimbex), cyclophosphamide (Cytoxan), dexamethasone (Decadron), dexmedetomidine (Precedex), diltiazem (Cardizem), docetaxel (Taxotere), doripenem (Doribax), enalaprilat (Vasotec IV), esmolol (Brevibloc), etoposide phosphate (Etopophos), fenoldopam (Corlopam), filgrastim (Neupogen), fluconazole (Diflucan), fludarabine (Fludara), foscarnet (Foscavir), furosemide (Lasix), gemcitabine (Gemzar), granisetron (Kytril), hetastarch in electrolytes (Hextend), hydromorphone (Dilaudid), idarubicin (Idamycin), labetalol, levofloxacin (Levaquin), linezolid (Zyvox), lorazepam (Ativan), magnesium sulfate, melphalan (Alkeran), meperidine (Demerol), midazolam (Versed), milrinone (Primacor), morphine, nicardipine (Cardene IV), ondansetron (Zofran), paclitaxel (Taxol), pemetrexed (Alimta), remifentanil (Ultiva), sargramostim (Leukine), teniposide (Vumon), thiotepa, tigecycline (Tygacil), vinorelbine (Navelbine), warfarin (Coumadin), zidovudine (AZT, Retrovir).

RATE OF ADMINISTRATION

A single dose over at least 30 to 60 minutes. Infants should receive a 1- to 2-hour infusion.

ACTIONS

An aminoglycoside antibiotic with neuromuscular blocking action. Bactericidal against many gram-negative organisms resistant to other antibiotics including other aminoglycosides such as gentamicin, kanamycin, and tobramycin. Well distributed through all body fluids. Usual half-life is 2 to 3 hours. Crosses the placental barrier. Excreted in the kidneys. Cross-allergenicity does occur between aminoglycosides.

INDICATIONS AND USES

Short-term treatment of serious infections caused by susceptible organisms (e.g., gram-negative bacteria) generally resistant to alternate drugs that have less potential toxicity. ▪ Effective in infections of the respiratory and urinary tracts, CNS (including meningitis), skin and soft tissue, intra-abdominal (including peritonitis), bacterial septicemia (including neonatal sepsis), burns, and postoperative infections. ▪ Considered initial therapy in suspected gram-negative infections after culture and sensitivity is drawn. ▪ In certain severe infections (e.g., neonatal sepsis), empiric concomitant treatment with an antibiotic effective against gram-positive organisms (e.g., penicillin) may be required until the results of C/S are obtained.

Unlabeled uses: Treatment of *Mycobacterium avium* complex, a common infection in AIDS (part of a multiple [3 to 5] drug regimen), tuberculosis.

CONTRAINDICATIONS

Known amikacin or aminoglycoside sensitivity. Sulfite sensitivity may be a contraindication.

PRECAUTIONS

Sensitivity studies indicated to determine susceptibility of causative organism to amikacin. ▪ Response should occur in 24 to 48 hours. Safety for use longer than 14 days not established. ▪ Superinfection may occur from overgrowth of nonsusceptible organisms. ▪ May contain sulfites; use caution in patients with asthma. ▪ Single daily dosing has been used effectively in abdominal, pelvic inflammatory, and GU infections in patients with normal renal function. Not recommended in bacteremia caused by *Pseudomonas aeruginosa,* endocarditis, meningitis, during pregnancy or in patients less than 6 weeks postpartum. Limited data available for use in all other situations (e.g., burns, cystic fibrosis, elderly, pediatrics, renal impairment). ▪ Potentially nephrotoxic, ototoxic, and neurotoxic. Risk of nephrotoxicity and neurotoxicity (e.g., auditory and vestibular ototoxicity) increased in patients with pre-existing renal damage or in normal renal function with prolonged use. Partial or total irreversible deafness may continue to develop after amikacin is discontinued. ▪ Use with caution in patients with muscular disorders (e.g., myasthenia gravis, parkinsonism) because these drugs may aggravate muscle weakness. ▪ *Clostridium difficile*–associated diarrhea (CDAD) has been reported. May range from mild diarrhea to fatal colitis. Consider in patients who present with diarrhea during or after treatment with amikacin. ▪ See Monitor and Drug/Lab Interactions.

Monitor: Maintain good hydration. ▪ Narrow range between toxic and therapeutic levels. Periodically monitor peak and trough concentrations. Manufacturer recommends avoiding peak serum concentrations greater than 35 mcg/mL and trough serum concentrations above 10 mcg/mL. ▪ Monitor urine protein, presence of cells and casts, and decreased specific gravity. Watch for decreased urine output, rising BUN and SCr, and declining CrCl levels. Dose adjustment may be necessary. ▪ Closely monitor patients with impaired renal function for nephrotoxicity and neurotoxicity (e.g., auditory and vestibular ototoxicity); nephrotoxicity may be reversible. ▪ In extended treatment, monitor serum levels, electrolytes, and renal, auditory, and vestibular functions frequently. ▪ See Drug/Lab Interactions.

Patient Education: Report promptly any changes in balance, hearing loss, weakness, or dizziness. ▪ Consider birth control options. ▪ Promptly report diarrhea or bloody stools that occur during treatment or up to several months after an antibiotic has been discontinued; may indicate CDAD and require treatment.

Maternal/Child: Category D: avoid pregnancy. Potential hazard to fetus. ▪ Safety for use during breast-feeding not established; use extreme caution. ▪ Peak concentrations are generally lower in infants and young children. ▪ Use extreme caution in premature infants and neonates; immature kidney function will result in prolonged half-life.

Elderly: Consider less toxic alternatives. ▪ Longer intervals between doses may be more important than smaller doses. ▪ Monitor renal function and drug levels carefully. Measurement of CrCl more useful than BUN or SCr to assess renal function. ▪ Half-life prolonged.

DRUG/LAB INTERACTIONS

Synergistic when used in combination with **beta-lactam antibiotics** (e.g., cephalosporins, penicillins) **and vancomycin.** Synergism may be inconsistent; see Compatibility. ▪ Concurrent use topically or systemically with any other **ototoxic or nephrotoxic agents** should be avoided. May have dangerous additive effects with **anesthetics** (e.g., enflurane), **other neuromuscular blocking antibiotics** (e.g., kanamycin), **diuretics** (e.g., furosemide [Lasix]), **beta-lactam antibiotics** (e.g., cephalosporins), **vancomycin, and many others.** ▪ Neuromuscular blocking muscle relaxants (e.g., atracurium [Tracrium], succinylcholine) are potentiated by aminoglycosides. *Apnea can occur.* ▪ Aminoglycosides are potentiated by **anticholinesterases** (e.g., edrophonium), **antineoplastics** (e.g., nitrogen mustard, cisplatin).

SIDE EFFECTS

Occur more frequently with impaired renal function, higher doses, prolonged administration, in dehydrated or elderly patients, and in patients receiving other ototoxic or nephrotoxic drugs. Fever, headache, hypotension, nausea, paresthesias, seizures, skin rash, tremor, vomiting.

Major: Albuminuria, anemia, arthralgia, azotemia, CDAD, eosinophilia, loss of balance, neuromuscular blockade, oliguria, ototoxicity, RBCs and WBCs or casts in urine, respiratory depression or arrest, rising SCr.

ANTIDOTE

Notify physician of all side effects. If minor side effects persist or any major symptom appears, discontinue drug and notify physician. Treatment is symptomatic, or a reduction in dose may be required. In overdose hemodialysis may be indicated. Monitor fluid balance, CrCl, and plasma levels carefully. Complexation with ticarcillin may be as effective as hemodialysis. Consider exchange transfusion in the newborn. Calcium salts or neostigmine may reverse neuromuscular blockade. Treat CDAD with fluids, electrolytes, protein supplements, and oral vancomycin (Vancocin) or metronidazole (Flagyl) as indicated. In severe cases, surgical evaluation may be indicated. Resuscitate as necessary.

AMINOCAPROIC ACID
(a-mee-noh-ka-**PROH**-ick **AS**-id)

Antifibrinolytic
Antihemorrhagic

Amicar

pH 6 to 7.6

USUAL DOSE
4 to 5 Gm initially over 1 hour. Follow with 1 Gm/hr for 8 hours or until bleeding is controlled. In acute bleeding syndromes, the 4- to 5-Gm dose may be given as a continuous infusion over the first hour, followed by a continuous infusion of 1 Gm/hr for 8 hours or until bleeding is controlled. Maximum dose is 30 Gm/24 hr.

Prevent recurrence of subarachnoid hemorrhage (unlabeled): 36 Gm/24 hr. One source suggests administering 18 Gm in 400 mL D5W every 12 hours for 10 days. Follow with oral therapy.

Prevention of perioperative bleeding during cardiac surgery (unlabeled): 10 Gm as an infusion over 20 to 30 minutes before skin incision. Follow with 1 to 2.5 Gm/hr (usually 2 Gm/hr) until the end of the operation. Infusion may be continued for 4 hours after protamine reversal of heparin. In addition, 10 Gm may be added to the cardiopulmonary bypass circuit priming solution. An alternate regimen is 10 Gm over 20 to 30 minutes before skin incision, followed by 10 Gm after heparin administration, then 10 Gm when cardiopulmonary bypass is discontinued and before protamine reversal of heparin. Another source suggests a loading dose of 80 mg/kg over 20 minutes followed by 30 mg/kg/hr, or a loading dose of 60 mg/kg over 20 minutes followed by 30 mg/kg/hr plus a 10-mg/kg dose in the priming solution of the cardiopulmonary bypass pump.

PEDIATRIC DOSE
Acute bleeding syndromes (unlabeled): See Maternal/Child. *Loading dose:* 100 to 200 mg/kg. Follow with a maintenance dose of 100 mg/kg/dose every 4 to 6 hours. Maximum dose is 30 Gm/24 hr.

DOSE ADJUSTMENTS
May accumulate in patients with renal impairment, and reduced doses are suggested; however, specific recommendations are not available from the manufacturer. Another source suggests decreasing dose to 15% to 25% of the normal dose in patients with renal impairment.

DILUTION
1 Gm equals 4 mL of prepared solution. Further dilute with **compatible** infusion solutions (NS, D5W, SWFI, or Ringer's solution). Up to 50 mL of diluent may be used for each 1 Gm.

Storage: Before use store at CRT. Do not freeze.

COMPATIBILITY
Compatible in D5W, Ringer's solution, and NS. One source suggests **compatibility** at the **Y-site** with fenoldopam (Corlopam).

RATE OF ADMINISTRATION
5 Gm or fraction thereof over first hour in 250 mL of solution; then administer each succeeding 1 Gm over 1 hour in 50 to 100 mL of solution. Use of an infusion pump for accurate dose recommended. Rapid administration or insufficient dilution may cause hypotension, bradycardia, and/or arrhythmia.

ACTIONS
A 6-aminohexanoic acid that acts as an inhibitor of fibrinolysis. Inhibits plasminogen activator substances; to a lesser degree inhibits plasmin activity. Increases fibrinogen activity in clot formation by inhibiting the enzyme required for destruction of formed fibrin. Onset of action is prompt, but will last less than 3 hours. Partially metabolized. Half-life is 2 hours. Excreted in urine. Easily penetrates RBCs and tissue cells after prolonged administration.

INDICATIONS AND USES

Useful in enhancing hemostasis when fibrinolysis contributes to bleeding. ▪ Treatment of fibrinolytic bleeding, which may be associated with surgical complications following heart surgery (with or without cardiac bypass procedures) and portacaval shunt, hematologic disorders such as aplastic anemia, acute and life-threatening abruptio placentae, hepatic cirrhosis, and neoplastic disease such as carcinoma of the prostate, lung, stomach, and cervix. ▪ Urinary fibrinolysis (normal physiologic phenomenon), which may result from severe trauma, anoxia, shock, surgical hematuria complications following prostatectomy and nephrectomy, or nonsurgical hematuria resulting from polycystic or neoplastic disease of the GU system.

Unlabeled uses: Prevent recurrence of subarachnoid hemorrhage. ▪ Control of bleeding in thrombocytopenia. ▪ Prevention of perioperative bleeding during cardiac surgery. ▪ Prophylaxis and treatment during dental surgical procedures (hemophilia and/or hemorrhage).

CONTRAINDICATIONS

Evidence of an active intravascular clotting process. ▪ Uncertainty as to whether the cause of bleeding is primary fibrinolysis (PF) or disseminated intravascular coagulation (DIC). This distinction must be made before administration; see Precautions. ▪ Do not use aminocaproic acid in the presence of DIC without concomitant heparin.

PRECAUTIONS

Should not be administered without a definite diagnosis and/or lab findings indicative of hyperfibrinolysis. ▪ The following tests are used to differentiate primary fibrinolysis (PF) from disseminated intravascular coagulation (DIC). Platelet count should be normal in PF but is usually decreased in DIC; protamine paracoagulation test is negative in PF and positive in DIC (a precipitate forms when protamine sulfate is dropped into citrated plasma); euglobulin clot lysis test is abnormal in PF but normal in DIC. ▪ In life-threatening situations, transfusion and other appropriate emergency measures may be required. ▪ Avoid use in patients with hematuria of upper urinary tract origin. Has caused glomerular capillary thrombosis in the renal pelvis and ureters, leading to intrarenal obstruction. ▪ Use with caution in patients with cardiac disease. May cause hypotension and bradycardia. Endocardial hemorrhage and fatty degeneration of the myocardium have been reported in animals. ▪ Use with caution in patients with hepatic disease. Etiology of bleeding may be multifactorial and difficult to diagnose. ▪ Use with caution in patients with renal impairment; see Dose Adjustments. Kidney stones have been reported in animal studies. ▪ Skeletal muscle weakness with necrosis of muscle fibers has been reported after prolonged use; see Monitor. ▪ An increased incidence of certain neurologic deficits (e.g., cerebral ischemia, cerebral vasospasm, hydrocephalus) associated with the use of antifibrinolytic agents in the treatment of subarachnoid hemorrhage has been reported. Relationship to drug therapy versus natural disease process or diagnostic procedures (e.g., angiography) is unclear.

Monitor: See Precautions and Contraindications. ▪ Use only in conjunction with general and specific tests to determine the amount of fibrinolysis present (e.g., fibrinogen, PT, aPTT). ▪ Monitor lab evaluations as appropriate for diagnosis (e.g., platelet count, clotting factors, CPK, AST). ▪ Vital signs, intake and output, any signs of bleeding, and neurologic assessment should be monitored based on patient condition. ▪ Observe for thromboembolic complications (e.g., chest pain, dyspnea, edema, hemoptysis, leg pain, or positive Homans' sign). ▪ Monitor for S/S of skeletal muscle damage. May range from mild myalgias with weakness to severe proximal myopathy with rhabdomyolysis, myoglobinuria, and acute renal failure. ▪ Monitor lab evaluations as appropriate for diagnosis (e.g., platelet count, clotting factors, CPK, AST).

Patient Education: Move slowly with help to avoid orthostatic hypotension.

Maternal/Child: Category C: safety for use in pregnancy and breast-feeding not established. ▪ Safety for use in pediatric patients not established but is used. ▪ Contains benzyl alcohol, which has been associated with "gasping syndrome" in neonates (sudden onset of gasping respirations, hypotension, bradycardia, and cardiovascular collapse).

Elderly: Consider age-related impaired organ function; reduced dose may be indicated.

DRUG/LAB INTERACTIONS

Potential for thrombus formation increased with concurrent use of **estrogens.** ▪ Frequently used with **clotting factor complexes** (e.g., factor IX complex, anti-inhibitor coagulant complex), but risk of thrombus formation may be increased. Delay administration for 8 or more hours after clotting factor complexes. ▪ Prolongation of template **bleeding time** has been reported during continuous infusions exceeding 24 Gm/day.

SIDE EFFECTS

Generally well tolerated. Abdominal pain, agranulocytosis, bradycardia, coagulation disorder, confusion, cramps, decreased vision, diarrhea, dizziness, dyspnea, edema, grand mal seizure, hallucinations, headache, hypersensitivity reactions (including anaphylaxis), hypotension, increased BUN and CPK, injection site reactions, intracranial hypertension, leukopenia, malaise, muscle weakness, myalgia, myopathy, myositis, nausea, peripheral ischemia, pruritus, pulmonary embolism, renal failure, rhabdomyolysis, rash, stuffy nose, stroke, syncope, tearing, thrombocytopenia, thrombophlebitis, thrombosis, tinnitus, vomiting.

Overdose: Acute renal failure, convulsions, death.

ANTIDOTE

Treat side effects symptomatically. Discontinue use of drug with any suspicion of thrombophlebitis, thromboembolic complications, or if CPK is elevated (myopathy). In life-threatening situations, fresh whole blood transfusions, fibrinogen infusions, and other emergency measures may be required. May be removed by hemodialysis or peritoneal dialysis.

AMINOPHYLLINE
(am-ih-**NOFF**-ih-lin)

Bronchodilator
Respiratory stimulant

(79% Theophylline), Theophylline Ethylenediamine

pH 8.6 to 9

USUAL DOSE
To obtain maximum benefit with minimal risk of adverse effects, dosing must be individualized based on serum theophylline concentration and patient response. Monitor frequently to avoid toxicity. Only aminophylline premixed in solution or aminophylline containing 20 mg of theophylline for each 25 mg of aminophylline is intended for IV use (approximately 79% theophylline). *All doses are based on lean body weight;* theophylline does not distribute into fatty tissue. *All doses listed are milligrams of aminophylline to be administered.*

BRONCHODILATION IN ACUTE ASTHMA OR BRONCHOSPASM
With an average mean volume of distribution of 0.5 L/kg (range is 0.3 to 0.7 L/kg), each mg/kg of theophylline given over 30 minutes should result in an average 2 mcg/mL increase in serum theophylline concentration.

Adults, children, infants and neonates who *have not* received a theophylline preparation in the previous 24 hours: An *initial loading dose* of 5 to 6 mg/kg of lean body weight (5.7 mg of aminophylline is equal to 4.6 mg/kg of theophylline) should produce a serum concentration of 10 mcg/mL (range 6 to 16 mcg/mL). Measure serum theophylline concentration in 30 minutes to determine if additional loading doses are indicated. Once a serum concentration of 10 to 15 mcg/mL is obtained with loading dose(s), it should be maintained with a continuous infusion. Rate of infusion is based on the pharmacokinetic parameters (e.g., volume of distribution, clearance, concomitant disease states) of the specific patient population and should achieve a target serum concentration of 10 mcg/mL. See Dose Adjustments and Monitor for recommendations of serum theophylline testing after an infusion is started.

Adults, children, infants and neonates who *have* received a theophylline preparation in the previous 24 hours: *A serum theophylline concentration must be obtained before considering any loading dose.* Calculate the appropriate loading dose with the following formula.

$$D = (\text{Desired C} - \text{Measured C}) \times (V)$$

D is the loading dose, C is the serum theophylline concentration, and V is the volume of distribution (0.5 L/kg). Desired serum concentration in this situation should be conservative (e.g., 10 mcg/mL) to allow for variability in the volume of distribution; carefully evaluate the patient condition and risk versus benefit. It is not recommended by the manufacturer, but another source suggests that a smaller loading dose may be considered if it is not immediately possible to obtain a theophylline serum concentration. Carefully evaluate the patient's condition and risk versus benefit. The potential for theophylline toxicity must be ruled out. For example, if significant respiratory distress is present, a smaller loading dose of 2.5 mg/kg should increase the theophylline level by approximately 5 mcg/mL. In the absence of toxicity, this increase is unlikely to cause significant side effects and may improve the clinical picture. In all situations, measure serum theophylline concentration in 30 minutes to determine if additional loading doses are indicated. Once a serum concentration of 10 to 15 mcg/mL is obtained with or without loading dose(s), it should be maintained with a continuous infusion. Rate of infusion is based on the pharmacokinetic parameters (e.g., volume of distribution, clearance, concomitant disease states) of the specific patient population and should achieve a target serum concentration of 10 mcg/mL. See Dose Adjustments and Monitor for recommendations of serum theophylline testing after an infusion is started.

Maintenance infusion: Desired theophylline serum concentration is 10 mcg/mL. Most maintenance doses can be reduced within the first 12 hours based on serum theophylline levels and depending on patient condition and response; see Dose Adjustments. Because of a large interpatient variability in theophylline clearance, each patient may differ from the mean value used to calculate these infusion rates. Another serum concentration is recommended one expected half-life after starting the continuous infusion; see Dose Adjustments.

Aminophylline Infusion Rates Following an Appropriate Loading Dose	
Patient Population	Aminophylline Infusion Rate in mg/kg/hr[a] (Actual theophylline administered in mg/kg/hr is in parentheses)
Neonates up to 24 days of age	1.27 mg/kg *every 12 hours* (1 mg/kg *every 12 hours*)[b]
Neonates over 24 days of age	1.9 mg/kg *every 12 hours* (1.5 mg/kg *every 12 hours*)[b]
Infants 6 to 52 weeks of age	mg/kg/hr = [(0.008 × Age in weeks) + 0.21[c]] ÷ 0.79
Children 1 to 9 years	1 mg/kg/hr (0.8 mg/kg/hr)
Children 9 to 12 years	0.875 mg/kg/hr (0.7 mg/kg/hr)
Adolescent smokers 12 to 16 years	0.875 mg/kg/hr (0.7 mg/kg/hr)
Adolescent nonsmokers 12 to 16 years	0.625 mg/kg/hr (0.5 mg/kg/hr)[d]
Adults (healthy nonsmokers 16 to 60 years)	0.5 mg/kg/hr (0.4 mg/kg/hr)[d]
Elderly over 60 years	0.375 mg/kg/hr (0.3 mg/kg/hr)[e]
Cardiac decompensation, cor pulmonale, liver dysfunction, sepsis with multiorgan failure, or shock	0.25 mg/kg/hr (0.2 mg/kg/hr)[e]

[a]Lower initial dose may be required for patients receiving other drugs that decrease theophylline clearance (e.g., cimetidine [Tagamet]).
[b]To achieve a target concentration of 7.5 mcg/mL for neonatal apnea.
[c]The 0.21 factor was not adjusted from the theophylline formula because it may not have the same proportional value. See package insert or contact Abbott if additional information desired.
[d]Not to exceed 900 mg/day unless serum levels indicate need for a larger dose.
[e]Not to exceed 400 mg/day or 21 mg/hr (17 mg/hr as theophylline) unless serum levels indicate need for a larger dose.

REVERSE ADENOSINE-MEDIATED EFFECTS OF DIPYRIDAMOLE IN ADULTS (UNLABELED)
50 to 100 mg over 30 to 60 seconds. Do not exceed a rate of 50 mg/30 sec. Maximum dose is 250 mg.
NEONATAL DOSE
Apnea and bradycardia of prematurity (unlabeled): *Loading dose:* 5 to 6 mg/kg given over 20 to 30 minutes. See all criteria under Usual Dose.
Maintenance dose: See Maintenance Infusion under Usual Dose. Manufacturer recommends keeping serum theophylline level at 7.5 mcg/mL. Another source recommends 1 to 2 mg/kg/dose every 6 to 8 hours.
DOSE ADJUSTMENTS
To determine if the concentration is accumulating or declining from the post–loading dose level, a serum concentration is recommended one expected half-life after starting the continuous infusion; see the following chart or see literature for a complete summary. If the level is declining (higher than average clearance), consider an additional loading dose or increasing the infusion rate. If the level is increasing, assume accumulation and decrease the infusion rate before the level exceeds 20 mcg/mL.

Continued

Theophylline Half-Life (Approximate)	
Age	Half-Life Mean (Range) in Hours
Premature neonates, see Maternal/Child	
3 to 15 days	30 (17 to 43) hours
25 to 57 days	20 (9.4 to 30.6) hours
Term infants, see Maternal/Child	
1 to 2 days	25.7 (25 to 26.5) hours
3 to 30 weeks	11 (6 to 29) hours
Children	
1 to 4 years	3.4 (1.2 to 5.6) hours
4 to 12 years	Not reported in studies
13 to 15 years	Not reported in studies
16 to 17 years	3.7 (1.5 to 5.9) hours
Adults (16 to 60 years) and healthy nonsmoking asthmatics	8.7 (6.1 to 12.8) hours
Elderly (over 60 years); nonsmokers with normal cardiac, liver, and renal function	9.8 (1.6 to 18) hours

There are huge variances in patients with concurrent illness or altered physiologic states (e.g., acute pulmonary edema, COPD, cystic fibrosis, fever with acute viral respiratory illness in pediatric patients [9 to 15 years], liver disease, pregnancy, sepsis with multi-organ failure, thyroid disease); see package insert. ▪ In patients with cor pulmonale, cardiac decompensation, liver dysfunction, or in those taking drugs that markedly reduce theophylline clearance (e.g., cimetidine [Tagamet]), the initial aminophylline infusion rate should not exceed 21 mg/hr (17 mg/hr as theophylline) unless serum concentrations can be monitored every 24 hours. Up to 5 days may be required before steady state is reached in these patients; see Drug Interactions. ▪ To decrease the risk of side effects associated with unexpected large increases in serum theophylline concentration, dose adjustment recommendations should be considered as the upper limit.

Final Dose Adjustment Guided by Serum Theophylline Concentration*	
Peak Serum Concentration	Dose Adjustment
Less than 9.9 mcg/mL	If symptoms are not controlled and current dose is tolerated, increase infusion rate about 25%. Recheck serum concentration after 12 hours in pediatric patients and 24 hours in adults for further dose adjustment.
10 to 14.9 mcg/mL	If symptoms are controlled and current dose is tolerated, maintain infusion rate and recheck serum concentration at 24-hour intervals. If symptoms are not controlled and current dose is tolerated, consider adding additional medication(s) to treatment regimen.
15 to 19.9 mcg/mL	Consider 10% decrease in infusion rate to provide greater margin of safety, even if current dose is tolerated.†
20 to 24.9 mcg/mL	Decrease infusion rate by 25%, even if no side effects are present. Recheck serum concentration after 12 hours in pediatric patients and 24 hours in adults to guide further dose adjustment.

Continued

Final Dose Adjustment Guided by Serum Theophylline Concentration*—cont'd	
Peak Serum Concentration	**Dose Adjustment**
25 to 30 mcg/mL	Stop infusion for 12 hours in pediatric patients and 24 hours in adults and decrease subsequent infusion rate at least 25% even if no side effects are present. Recheck serum concentration after 12 hours in pediatric patients and 24 hours in adults to guide further dose adjustment. If symptomatic, stop infusion and consider need for overdose treatment; see Antidote.
Over 30 mcg/mL	Stop the infusion and treat overdose as indicated; see Antidote. If aminophylline is subsequently resumed, decrease infusion rate by at least 50% and recheck serum concentration after 12 hours in pediatric patients and 24 hours in adults to guide further dose adjustment.

*Dose increases should not be made in patients with an acute exacerbation of symptoms unless the steady-state serum theophylline concentration is less than 10 mcg/mL.

†Dose reduction and/or serum theophylline concentration measurement is indicated whenever side effects are present, physiologic abnormalities that can reduce theophylline clearance occur (e.g., sustained fever), or a drug that interacts with theophylline is added or discontinued; see Precautions and Drug/Lab Interactions.

DILUTION
Check vial carefully; must state, "For IV use." Warm to room temperature. Only the 25 mg/mL solution may be given by IV injection undiluted, but further dilution for infusion in at least 100 to 200 mL of D5W is preferred. NS or dextrose in saline solutions may be used. Available prediluted. Crystals will form if solution pH falls below 8.

Storage: Usually stored between 15° and 30° C (59° and 86° F). Protect from light and freezing.

COMPATIBILITY   (Underline Indicates Conflicting Compatibility Information)
Consider any drug NOT listed as compatible to be INCOMPATIBLE until consulting a pharmacist; specific conditions may apply.

Manufacturer states, "Should not be mixed in a syringe with other drugs but should be added separately to the IV solution," and recommends discontinuing other solutions infusing at the same site if there is a potential problem with admixture **incompatibility.** Manufacturer recommends avoiding admixtures with alkali labile drugs (e.g., epinephrine, norepinephrine [Levophed], isoproterenol [Isuprel], penicillin G potassium). Precipitation in acidic media may occur with the undiluted solution but not to dilute solutions in IV infusions.

One source suggests the following **compatibilities:**

Additive: Amikacin, ascorbic acid, calcium gluconate, chloramphenicol (Chloromycetin), dexamethasone (Decadron), dimenhydrinate, diphenhydramine (Benadryl), dopamine, erythromycin (Erythrocin), esmolol (Brevibloc), fat emulsion IV, flumazenil (Romazicon), furosemide (Lasix), heparin, hydrocortisone sodium succinate (Solu-Cortef), lidocaine, meropenem (Merrem IV), methyldopate, methylprednisolone (Solu-Medrol), midazolam (Versed), nafcillin (Nallpen), nitroglycerin IV, pentobarbital (Nembutal), phenobarbital (Luminal), potassium chloride (KCl), ranitidine (Zantac), sodium bicarbonate, vancomycin.

Y-site: Allopurinol (Aloprim), amifostine (Ethyol), amphotericin B cholesteryl (Amphotec), anidulafungin (Eraxis), aztreonam (Azactam), bivalirudin (Angiomax), ceftaroline (Teflaro), ceftazidime (Fortaz), cisatracurium (Nimbex), cladribine (Leustatin), dexmedetomidine (Precedex), diltiazem (Cardizem), docetaxel (Taxotere), doripenem (Doribax), doxorubicin liposomal (Doxil), enalaprilat (Vasotec IV), esmolol (Brevibloc), etoposide phosphate (Etopophos), famotidine (Pepcid IV), filgrastim (Neupogen), fluconazole (Diflucan), fludarabine (Fludara), foscarnet (Foscavir), gallium nitrate (Ganite), gemcitabine (Gemzar), granisetron (Kytril), heparin, hetastarch in electrolytes (Hextend), hydrocortisone sodium succinate (Solu-Cortef), labetalol, levofloxacin (Levaquin), linezolid (Zyvox), melphalan (Alkeran), meropenem (Merrem IV), micafungin (Mycamine), morphine, nicardipine (Cardene IV), paclitaxel (Taxol), pancuronium, pemetrexed (Alimta), piperacillin/tazobactam (Zosyn), potassium chloride (KCl), propofol (Diprivan), ranitidine (Zantac), remifentanil (Ultiva), sargramostim (Leukine), tacrolimus (Prograf), teniposide (Vumon), thiotepa, vecuronium.

RATE OF ADMINISTRATION

A single dose over a minimum of 20 to 30 minutes. Most references suggest a minimum of 30 minutes. Do not exceed an average rate of 1 mL or 25 mg/min when giving by IV injection or as an infusion. Rapid administration may cause cardiac arrhythmias. Discontinue primary infusion if theophylline administered by piggyback or additive tubing and a possible **incompatibility** problem exists.

Reverse adenosine-mediated effects of dipyridamole: See Usual Dose.

ACTIONS

An alkaloid xanthine derivative. It relaxes smooth muscle in the airways (bronchodilation) and suppresses the response of the airways to stimuli (nonbronchodilator prophylactic effects). Cardiac output, urinary output, and sodium excretion are increased. Skeletal and cardiac muscles are stimulated, as is the CNS to a lesser degree. There is peripheral vasodilation. It decreases pulmonary artery pressure and lowers the threshold of the respiratory center to CO_2. Well distributed throughout the body. In adults and pediatric patients over 1 year of age, 90% of a dose is metabolized in the liver. Because of a large interpatient variability in theophylline clearance, half-life varies extensively based on age, concurrent illness, or altered physiologic state; see Dose Adjustments, Precautions, Maternal/Child, and Elderly. Excreted in a changed form in the urine. Crosses the placental barrier. Secreted in breast milk.

INDICATIONS AND USES

Adjunct to inhaled beta-2 selective agonists (e.g., albuterol) and systemic corticosteroids for the treatment of acute exacerbations of the symptoms and reversible airflow obstruction associated with asthma and other chronic lung diseases (e.g., emphysema, chronic bronchitis).

Unlabeled uses: Apnea and bradycardia of prematurity. ▪ Reduce bronchospasm in cystic fibrosis and acute descending respiratory infections. ▪ Relieve periodic apnea and increase arterial blood pH in patients with Cheyne-Stokes respirations. ▪ Reverse adenosine-mediated effects of dipyridamole- (Persantine), adenosine- (Adenoscan), or regadenoson- (Lexiscan) induced adverse reactions (e.g., angina pectoris, bronchospasm, severe hypotension, ventricular arrhythmias).

CONTRAINDICATIONS

Known hypersensitivity to theophylline or ethylenediamine.

PRECAUTIONS

There is an increase in the volume of distribution of theophylline (primarily due to reduction in plasma protein binding) in premature neonates, patients with hepatic cirrhosis, uncorrected acidemia, the elderly, and women during the third trimester of pregnancy. Toxicity may occur in the therapeutic range. ▪ Theophylline clearance may be reduced in neonates (term and premature); children less than 1 year; elderly (over 60 years); infants less than 3 months of age with reduced renal function; patients with acute pulmonary edema, congestive heart failure, cor pulmonale, hypothyroidism, liver disease (e.g., cirrhosis, acute hepatitis), sepsis with multiorgan failure, shock; or in patients with a fever of 102° F or more for 24 hours or more, or lesser temperature elevations for longer periods. Risk of severe toxicity increased in these patient populations; dose reduction and more frequent monitoring may be required. ▪ Use with extreme caution in patients with active peptic ulcer disease, cardiac arrhythmias (not including bradyarrhythmias), or seizures; may exacerbate these conditions. ▪ Initiate oral therapy as soon as symptoms are adequately improved. ▪ See Maternal/Child and Drug/Lab Interactions.

Monitor: Monitor serum levels as directed in Usual Dose and Dose Adjustments to achieve maximum benefit with minimum risk. Each 0.5 mg/kg will increase serum theophylline by 1 mcg/mL. 10 mcg/mL to less than 20 mcg/mL is considered therapeutic. Peak serum level is best measured 20 to 30 minutes after initial loading dose, a half-life after the initial infusion, or 12 to 14 hours into continuous infusion. ▪ Monitor vital signs, including lung sounds. ▪ Monitor for all signs of toxicity; see Side Effects. Serious toxicity may not be preceded by less severe side effects. ▪ Serum theophylline measurements are indicated before making a dose increase; whenever signs or symptoms of toxicity are present; whenever a new illness presents, an existing illness worsens, or a change in treatment regimen is initiated that may alter theophylline clearance (e.g., sustained fever, hepatitis [see Precautions], or drugs that may interact [see Drug/Lab Interactions]); and every 24 hours throughout the infusion. ▪ Stop the IV infusion and obtain a serum theophylline concentration immediately in any patient on aminophylline who develops nausea or vomiting (particularly repetitive vomiting) or if any other signs of toxicity occur, even if another cause is suspected. ▪ Dose increases should not be made in patients with an acute exacerbation of symptoms unless the steady-state serum theophylline concentration is less than 10 mcg/mL. ▪ Patients with a very high initial clearance rate (low steady-state serum theophylline concentrations at above-average doses) are likely to experience large changes in serum concentration in response to dose changes. ▪ Maintain hydration. ▪ See Precautions, Maternal/Child, Elderly, and Drug/Lab Interactions.

Patient Education: Do not take or discontinue any prescription or over-the-counter medication, including herbal products, without physician's approval. ▪ Promptly report S/S of toxicity (e.g., nausea and vomiting).

Maternal/Child: Category C: use in pregnancy only if clearly indicated. ▪ Neonates may have therapeutic blood levels and may develop apnea from theophylline withdrawal. ▪ Elimination of drug is prolonged in premature infants, neonates, and children up to 1 year. Use with extreme caution in pediatric patients. Has caused fatal reactions. Elimination reaches maximum values by 1 year of age, remains fairly constant to 9 years of age, and slowly decreases by approximately 50% to adult values at 16 years of age. ▪ Pediatric patients under the age of 1 year, as well as neonates with decreased renal function, require careful attention to dosing and frequent monitoring of serum theophylline concentrations. ▪ Secreted in breast milk; some sources recommend discontinuing breastfeeding. If the decision is made to breast-feed, monitor infant for evidence of side effects.

Elderly: Compared to healthy young adults, clearance of theophylline is decreased an average of 30% in healthy elderly. Monitor dosing carefully; frequent serum theophylline concentrations are recommended. See Dose Adjustments, Precautions, and Monitor.

DRUG/LAB INTERACTIONS

Review of patient drug profile by pharmacist is imperative at time of initiation of aminophylline and with any change in medication regimen. ▪ Do not use one **xanthine derivative** concurrently with another **xanthine derivative, ephedrine, or other sympathomimetic drugs.** ▪ Xanthines antagonize or potentiate or are themselves antagonized or potentiated by many drug groups. Monitor serum levels as indicated. **Theophylline clearance increased and serum levels decreased by aminoglutenide, barbiturates, carbamazepine** (Tegretol), **ethmozine** (Moricizine), **isoproterenol** (Isuprel), **hydantoins** (e.g., phenytoin [Dilantin]), **rifampin** (Rifadin), **smoking, sulfinpyrazone** (Anturane). **Theophylline clearance decreased and serum levels increased by alcohol, allopurinol, beta-adrenergic blockers** (e.g., propranolol), **cimetidine** (Tagamet), **ciprofloxacin** (Cipro IV), **clarithromycin, disulfiram** (Antabuse), **enoxacin** (Penetrex), **erythromycin, estrogen-containing oral contraceptives, fluvoxamine** (Luvox), **interferon alfa-A, methotrexate, mexiletine, pentoxifylline** (Trental), **propafenone** (Rythmol), **tacrine** (Cognex), **thiabendazole** (Mintezol), **ticlopidine** (Ticlid), **troleandomycin** (TAO), **verapamil.** ▪ Inhibits **pancuronium;** increased doses of pancuronium may be required to achieve neuromuscular blockade. ▪ **Carbamazepine** (Tegretol) **and loop diuretics** (e.g., furosemide [Lasix]) may increase or decrease serum levels. ▪ Reduces sedative effect of **benzodiazepines** (e.g., diazepam [Valium], midazolam [Versed]) **and of propofol** (Diprivan); increased doses of sedatives may be required. To avoid respiratory depression, reduce sedative dose if aminophylline is discontinued or if dose is significantly reduced. ▪ May decrease **lithium** levels. Dose adjustment and monitoring of lithium levels may be indicated. ▪ Concurrent use with **halothane** may induce cardiac arrhythmias. ▪ Concurrent use with **ketamine** may lower aminophylline seizure level. ▪ Concurrent use with **ephedrine** may increase nausea, nervousness, and insomnia. ▪ May increase **lab values** for free fatty acids, glucose, HDL, LDL, total cholesterol, uric acid, and urinary free cortisol excretion. ▪ Caffeine and xanthine metabolites in neonates or patients with renal dysfunction may cause readings from some **immunoassay techniques** to be higher than the actual serum theophylline concentration. ▪ Interferes with **dipyridamole-assisted MI perfusion studies.**

SIDE EFFECTS

Headache, insomnia, nausea, vomiting most common when peak serum concentrations are less than 20 mcg/mL. Rarely a severe hypersensitivity reaction of the skin (e.g., exfoliative dermatitis) may occur. Toxicity resulting in death may occur suddenly at levels less than 20 mcg/mL, especially in certain populations (see Precautions); may occur more frequently with serum levels above 20 mcg/mL. Anxiety, cardiac arrest, arrhythmias (e.g., atrial fibrillation, ventricular fibrillation), convulsions, delirium, dizziness, flushing, hyperpyrexia, intractable seizures, nausea, peripheral vascular collapse, persistent vomiting, restlessness, temporary hypotension.

Overdose: *Acute:* Acid/base disturbances, arrhythmias (e.g., sinus tachycardia), hyperglycemia, hypokalemia, seizures (usually with serum concentrations over 100 mcg/mL), vomiting, and death have occurred.

Chronic: All of the above plus various arrhythmias, seizures (with serum concentration greater than 30 mcg/mL), and death.

ANTIDOTE

With onset of any side effect, discontinue drug and notify physician. ▪ Stop the IV infusion and obtain a serum theophylline concentration immediately in any patient on aminophylline who develops nausea or vomiting (particularly repetitive vomiting) or if any other signs of toxicity occur, even if another cause is suspected. ▪ For mild symptoms the physician may choose to continue the drug at a decreased dose and rate of administration. All side effects will be treated symptomatically. Maintain adequate ventilation and adequate hydration. Grand mal seizures may not respond to anticonvulsants. Diazepam (Valium) may be most effective. Treat atrial arrhythmias with verapamil, ventricular arrhythmias with lidocaine or procainamide. Use dopamine for hypotension. Do not use stimulants. Resuscitate as necessary.

MANUFACTURER'S SPECIFIC RECOMMENDATIONS FOR ACUTE AND CHRONIC OVERDOSE
Acute overdose (e.g., excessive loading dose or excessive infusion rate for less than 24 hours) or chronic overdose (e.g., excessive infusion rate for more than 24 hours): Serum concentration 20 to 30 mcg/mL: Stop the infusion, monitor the patient, and obtain a serum theophylline concentration in 2 to 4 hours to ensure that the concentration is decreasing.
Acute overdose with a serum concentration of 30 to 100 mcg/mL or chronic overdose with serum concentrations greater than 30 mcg/mL in patients less than 60 years of age: Stop the infusion. Administer multiple-dose, oral-activated charcoal and measures to control emesis. Monitor the patient and obtain serial theophylline concentrations every 2 to 4 hours to determine the effectiveness of therapy and to determine further treatment decisions. Institute extracorporeal removal if emesis, seizures, or cardiac arrhythmias cannot be adequately controlled.
Acute overdose with a serum concentration greater than 100 mcg/mL or chronic overdose with serum concentrations greater than 30 mcg/mL in patients 60 years or older: Stop the infusion. Consider prophylactic anticonvulsant therapy. Administer multiple-dose oral-activated charcoal and measures to control emesis. Consider extracorporeal removal, even if the patient has not experienced a seizure. Monitor the patient and obtain serial theophylline concentrations every 2 to 4 hours to determine the effectiveness of therapy and to determine further treatment decisions.
Extracorporeal removal: Weigh risk versus benefits. Charcoal hemoperfusion is the most effective and increases theophylline clearance up to sixfold, but hypotension, hypocalcemia, and platelet consumption and bleeding diatheses may occur. Hemodialysis is about as efficient as multiple-dose oral-activated charcoal and has a lower risk of serious complications. Consider hemodialysis when charcoal hemoperfusion is not feasible and multiple-dose oral-activated charcoal is ineffective because of intractable emesis. Serum theophylline concentrations may rebound 5 to 10 mcg/mL after either treatment is discontinued due to redistribution of theophylline from the tissue compartment. Peritoneal dialysis is ineffective, and exchange transfusions in neonates have been minimally effective.

AMIODARONE HYDROCHLORIDE

Antiarrhythmic

(am-ee-**OH**-dah-rohn hy-droh-**KLOR**-eyed)

Nexterone

pH 4.08

USUAL DOSE

TREATMENT AND PROPHYLAXIS OF VENTRICULAR TACHYCARDIA (VT) AND VENTRICULAR FIBRILLATION (VF)

1,000 mg over the first 24 hours in 3 distinct segments; two loading infusions and a maintenance infusion. Use of a dedicated central venous catheter preferred.

Rapid loading infusion: 150 mg specifically diluted solution (1.5 mg/mL) over 10 minutes (15 mg/min). Follow immediately with the slow loading infusion.

Slow loading infusion: 360 mg specifically diluted solution (1.8 mg/mL) at 1 mg/min over the next 6 hours.

Maintenance infusion: 540 mg of 1.8 mg/mL solution at 0.5 mg/min over 18 hours. Maintenance infusion is usually continued at 0.5 mg/min for 48 to 96 hours or until ventricular arrhythmias are stabilized. May be continued with caution for up to 2 to 3 weeks. Transfer to oral therapy as soon as feasible (guidelines are in package insert).

TREATMENT OF BREAKTHROUGH VENTRICULAR FIBRILLATION (VF) OR HEMODYNAMICALLY UNSTABLE VENTRICULAR TACHYCARDIA (VT)

At any time that breakthrough VF or hemodynamically unstable VT occurs during administration, a supplemental rapid loading infusion (150 mg over 10 minutes) may be repeated. May be specifically diluted 1.5 mg/mL solution or rate of the maintenance infusion (1.8 mg/mL) may be temporarily increased to equal 150 mg (83.33 mL) over 10 minutes. During trials total doses above 1,800 to 2,100 mg (including added doses for breakthrough VF/VT) increased the risk of hypotension. In life-threatening arrhythmias, AHA guidelines state that this rapid loading infusion (150 mg over 10 minutes) may be repeated every 10 minutes as needed and recommend a maximum cumulative dose of 2.2 Gm/24 hr.

CARDIAC ARREST (UNLABELED)

300 mg (6 mL) or 5 mg/kg as a bolus injection. Flush with 10 mL D5W or NS. Should be given through a separate IV line immediately after the first dose of epinephrine (1 mg) and before the fourth electrical countershock. Supplemental doses of 150 mg (3 mL) may be given for recurrent bouts of VT/VF. AHA guidelines recommend a first dose of 300 mg IV push and a second dose, if needed, of 150 mg IV push. After return of spontaneous circulation (ROSC), initiate the slow loading infusion and maintenance infusion as above. If effective, discontinue amiodarone and reassess arrhythmia management within 6 to 24 hours.

SUPRAVENTRICULAR ARRHYTHMIAS (UNLABELED)

150 mg over 10 minutes as a loading dose (15 mg/min). Follow with an infusion of 360 mg over 6 hours (1 mg/min) followed by a maintenance infusion of 0.5 mg/min for 18 hours. Other regimens used during studies to convert atrial fibrillation and atrial flutter to sinus rhythm include 5 mg/kg over 3 to 5 minutes; 5 to 7 mg/kg as a 30- to 60-minute infusion followed by a continuous infusion of 1.2 to 1.8 Gm/24 hr followed with oral dosing until a 10-Gm total dose is reached; or an infusion of 2 mg/kg/hr continued for up to 2 hours after conversion to a stable sinus rhythm or a maximum dose of 2,400 mg/24 hr.

INTRAVENOUS TO ORAL TRANSITION

Guidelines for IV to oral transition are located in manufacturer's literature. See Prescribing Information or consult pharmacist.

PEDIATRIC DOSE

Safety for use in pediatric patients (particularly infants and neonates) not established and not recommended; see Contraindications and Maternal/Child.

Continued

Treatment of refractory pulseless VT, VF (unlabeled): AHA guidelines recommend 5 mg/kg by IV bolus (maximum single dose is 300 mg). May repeat to a maximum of 15 mg/kg/24 hr. Total dose in adolescents is 2.2 Gm/24 hr.

Treatment of perfusing supraventricular and ventricular arrhythmias (unlabeled): AHA guidelines recommend 5 mg/kg as an infusion over 20 to 60 minutes (maximum single dose 300 mg). May repeat to a maximum of 15 mg/kg/24 hr. Total dose in adolescents is 2.2 Gm/24 hr.

DOSE ADJUSTMENTS
Rate of maintenance infusion may be increased to achieve effective arrhythmia suppression. ▪ Not required in renal or hepatic disease. Another source suggests a reduced dose in hepatic failure. ▪ Dose selection should be cautious in the elderly. Reduced initial doses may be indicated based on the potential for decreased organ function and concomitant disease or drug therapy.

DILUTION
Available as a premixed solution in 1.5 mg/mL and 1.8 mg/mL concentrations or as a vial that must be further diluted. To further dilute vials, do not use evacuated glass intravenous bottles. Use only commercially available D5W (D5W or NS may be used for Nexterone) solutions in polyolefin or glass containers in any prepared solution that will be given over more than 2 hours. PVC containers are suitable only for dilution of the rapid loading dose; see Compatibility and Precautions.

Rapid-loading infusion: Dilute 150 mg (3 mL) in 100 mL D5W; concentration is 1.5 mg/mL (D5W or NS may be used for Nexterone).

Slow-loading infusion and maintenance infusion: Dilute 900 mg (18 mL) in 500 mL D5W; concentration is 1.8 mg/mL (D5W or NS may be used for Nexterone). Dilutions from 1 to 6 mg/mL have been used for maintenance solutions after the first 24 hours. Use of a central venous catheter is recommended; however, concentrations over 2 mg/mL for longer than 1 hour must be administered through a central venous catheter. Higher concentrations (3 to 6 mg/mL) have caused peripheral vein phlebitis and hepatocellular necrosis; see Precautions.

Cardiac arrest (unlabeled): Loading dose (300 mg or 5 mg/kg) or supplemental boluses (150 mg) may be given undiluted. Has also been diluted in up to 20 mL D5W (D5W or NS may be used for Nexterone).

Filters: Use of a 0.2-micron in-line filter recommended by manufacturer. States "filtering does not affect potency." Another source suggests no significant loss of drug potency with the use of a 0.22-micron cellulose ester membrane filter.

Storage: Store ampules and premixed solutions in their carton at CRT. Use solutions diluted in PVC containers within 2 hours; use those diluted in glass or polyolefin containers within 24 hours. Protect from light and freezing.

COMPATIBILITY   (Underline Indicates Conflicting Compatibility Information)
Consider any drug NOT listed as compatible to be INCOMPATIBLE until consulting a pharmacist; specific conditions may apply.

Manufacturer recommendations include: Do not use evacuated glass intravenous bottles. Administer through a dedicated IV line (central venous catheter preferred). Absorbs to PVC tubing but loss accounted for in specified dose; follow infusion regimen closely. Leaches out plasticizers, including DEHP, from IV tubing. The degree of leaching increases when the solution is infused at a higher concentration or a slower infusion rate than recommended. Manufacturer lists aminophylline, argatroban, bivalirudin (Angiomax), cefazolin (Ancef), ceftazidime (Fortaz), digoxin (Lanoxin), furosemide (Lasix), heparin, imipenem-cilastatin (Primaxin), magnesium sulfate, mezlocillin (Mezlin), nitroprusside sodium (Nitropress), piperacillin/tazobactam (Zosyn), potassium phosphates, sodium bicarbonate, and sodium phosphates as **incompatible** at the **Y-site** with amiodarone in D5W. Aminophylline, ampicillin/sulbactam (Unasyn), and micafungin (Mycamine) in NS are also listed as **incompatible** at the **Y-site**.

One source suggests the following **compatibilities:**

Additive: Dobutamine, furosemide (Lasix), lidocaine, potassium chloride (KCl), procainamide (Pronestyl), quinidine, verapamil.

Y-site: Amikacin, amphotericin B (conventional), atracurium (Tracium), atropine, calcium chloride, calcium gluconate, caspofungin (Cancidas), cefazolin (Ancef), ceftaroline (Teflaro), ceftriaxone (Rocephin), cefuroxime (Zinacef), ciprofloxacin (Cipro IV), clindamycin (Cleocin), dexmedetomidine (Precedex), dobutamine, dopamine, doripenem (Doribax), doxycycline, epinephrine (Adrenalin), eptifibatide (Integrilin), erythromycin (Erythrocin), esmolol (Brevibloc), famotidine (Pepcid IV), fenoldopam (Corlopam), fentanyl, fluconazole (Diflucan), furosemide (Lasix), gentamicin, hetastarch in electrolytes (Hextend), insulin (regular), isoproterenol (Isuprel), labetalol, lidocaine, lorazepam (Ativan), magnesium sulfate, methylprednisolone (Solu-Medrol), metoprolol (Lopressor), midazolam (Versed), milrinone (Primacor), morphine, nesiritide (Natrecor), nitroglycerin IV, nitroprusside sodium, norepinephrine (Levophed), penicillin G potassium, phentolamine (Regitine), phenylephrine (Neo-Synephrine), potassium chloride (KCl), procainamide (Pronestyl), tirofiban (Aggrastat), tobramycin, vancomycin, vasopressin, vecuronium.

RATE OF ADMINISTRATION

Volumetric pump required for administration. Surface properties of diluted solution reduce drop size; use of a drop counter infusion set causes underdosing. Use of a 0.2-micron in-line filter is also recommended. A central venous catheter is recommended for all concentrations and is required for concentrations greater than 2 mg/mL. Adhere to prescribed rates; risk of hypotension is increased in the first hours of treatment and with increased rates; may cause secondary renal or hepatic failure; see Precautions. Avoid IV bolus doses in patients with marked cardiomegaly; a continuous infusion is preferred. Do not use plastic containers in a series; could result in air embolism.

Rapid loading infusion or breakthrough treatment of VF/VT: 150 mg over 10 minutes (15 mg/min). Do not exceed a rate of 30 mg/min.

Slow loading infusion: 1 mg/min or 33.3 mL/hr (0.556 mL/min) of 1.8 mg/mL solution for 6 hours.

Maintenance infusion: 0.5 mg/min or 16.6 mL/hr (0.278 mL/min) of 1.8 mg/mL solution for 18 hours. A continuing maintenance solution should deliver 720 mg/24 hr at 0.5 mg/min whether the concentration is 1.8 mg/mL or 6 mg/mL. May be continued at this rate for up to 2 to 3 weeks as described in Usual Dose.

Cardiac arrest (unlabeled): Loading or supplemental doses by IV bolus injection. Follow with 10 mL flush of D5W or NS through Y-tube or three-way stopcock. May be given through a free-flowing infusion of D5W (D5W or NS may be used for Nexterone). After return of spontaneous circulation (ROSC), initiate the slow loading and maintenance infusions as above.

ACTIONS

An antiarrhythmic agent. Generally considered a Class III antiarrhythmic drug, but possesses characteristics of all four antiarrhythmic classes. Decreases number of VT/VF events. It prolongs the duration of action potentials in cardiac fibers, depresses conduction velocity, slows conduction and prolongs refractoriness at the AV node, and exhibits some alpha and beta blockade activity. Raises the threshold for VF and may prevent its recurrence. Also has vasodilatory effects that decrease cardiac workload and myocardial oxygen consumption. Uptake by the myocardium is rapid; antiarrhythmic effect is prompt (clinically relevant within hours); however, full effect may take days. Has an exceptionally long half-life. Metabolized in the liver by cytochrome P_{450} enzymes (specifically CYP3A4 and CYP2C8). Primarily excreted in bile. Crosses placental barrier. Secreted in breast milk.

INDICATIONS AND USES

Initiation of treatment and prophylaxis of frequently recurring VF and hemodynamically unstable VT in patients refractory to other therapy. Used until ventricular arrhythmias are stabilized; usually 48 to 96 hours, but may be given for longer periods. ▪ Treatment of patients taking oral amiodarone who are unable to take oral medication.

Unlabeled uses: Conversion of atrial fibrillation to a normal sinus rhythm and maintenance of a normal sinus rhythm. ■ Cardiac arrest with persistent VT or VF if defibrillation, CPR, and vasopressor administration have failed. ■ Control of hemodynamically stable monomorphic VT, polymorphic VT with a normal baseline QT interval, or wide-complex tachycardia of uncertain origin. ■ Control of rapid ventricular rate due to accessory pathway conduction in pre-excited atrial arrhythmias. ■ Heart rate control in patients with atrial fibrillation and heart failure with no accessory pathway. ■ Pharmacologic adjunct to ICD (implantable cardioverter defibrillator) therapy to suppress symptomatic ventricular tachyarrhythmias in otherwise optimally treated patients with heart failure.

CONTRAINDICATIONS

Cardiogenic shock; corneal refractive laser surgery; known hypersensitivity to amiodarone or any of its components, including iodine; marked sinus bradycardia; second- or third-degree AV block unless a functioning pacemaker is available; sinus node dysfunction. See Drug/Lab Interactions. ■ Not recommended for use in neonates or infants. ■ Contraindicated with nelfinavir (Viracept) and ritonavir (Norvir).

PRECAUTIONS

Usually administered by or under the direction of the physician specialist with facilities for monitoring the patient and responding to any medical emergency. ■ Because of the long half-life of amiodarone and its metabolite, the potential for adverse reactions or interactions, as well as observed adverse effects, can persist following amiodarone withdrawal. ■ Correct hypokalemia and hypomagnesemia before use; may exaggerate a prolonged QTc and cause arrhythmias (e.g., torsades de pointes). ■ May cause increases in liver enzymes and bilirubin levels, but abnormal baseline hepatic enzymes are not a contraindication to use. ■ Use of higher than recommended loading dose concentrations and increased rates of administration have been associated with hepatocellular necrosis, hepatic coma, acute renal failure, and death. ■ May worsen existing arrhythmias or precipitate new ones, primarily torsades de pointes or new-onset VF. Deaths have occurred. ■ Combination of amiodarone with other antiarrhythmics that can prolong the QTc interval should be reserved for patients with life-threatening ventricular arrhythmias who do not respond to single agent therapy; see Drug/Lab Interactions. ■ Risk of QTc prolongation is increased (with or without torsades de pointes) with other medications that can prolong the QTc (e.g., fluoroquinolones [e.g., levofloxacin (Levaquin)], macrolide antibiotics [e.g., erythromycin (Erythrocin)], azoles [e.g., fluconazole (Diflucan)]); see Drug/Lab Interactions. ■ Hypotension is the most common side effect. Usually occurs within the first several hours of therapy and appears to be rate-related. Do not exceed initial rates recommended by manufacturer. In some cases, hypotension has been refractory to treatment. Deaths have occurred. See Monitor and Antidote. ■ May cause visual impairment (e.g., optic neuropathy or optic neuritis); has progressed to permanent blindness. ■ May cause pulmonary toxicity (e.g., ARDS, bronchospasm, cough, dyspnea, hemoptysis, hypoxemia, pulmonary fibrosis, wheezing). Usually seen with long-term use, but acute pulmonary hypersensitivity has been reported after short-term IV use and with or without IV use. Has progressed to respiratory failure and death. The elderly and patients with pre-existing lung disease may be at increased risk and have a poorer prognosis if pulmonary toxicity develops; see Side Effects. ■ Monitor patients undergoing general anesthesia closely; may increase sensitivity to myocardial depressant and conduction defects of halogenated inhalation anesthetics (hypotension and atropine-resistant bradycardia). ■ Use caution in patients with cardiomyopathy, hepatic failure, left ventricular dysfunction, or thyroid dysfunction. ■ May cause hypothyroidism or hyperthyroidism. Amiodarone-induced hyperthyroidism may result in thyrotoxicosis and/or the possibility of arrhythmia breakthrough or aggravation. Deaths have occurred. Severe hypothyroidism and myxedema coma, sometimes fatal, have been reported. ■ Thyroid nodules and/or thyroid cancer have been reported in patients treated with amiodarone. ■ Anaphylactic/anaphylactoid reactions, some fatal, have been reported. ■ See Compatibility and Drug/Lab Interactions.

Monitor: Continuous ECG and HR monitoring is mandatory to observe for arrhythmias. Watch for QTc prolongation; may cause proarrhythmia (torsades de pointes). ■ Monitor for bradycardia and AV block. A temporary pacemaker should be available. Consider the possibility of hyperthyroidism if new signs of arrhythmia appear. ■ Monitor BP closely to minimize hypotension (occurs frequently with initial rates); see Rate of Administration, Precautions, and Antidote. ■ Confirm patency of vein. Reduce rate or concentration for pain or redness at injection site. Incidence of phlebitis markedly increased with concentrations above 2.5 mg/mL. For infusions longer than 1 hour, do not exceed a concentration of 2 mg/mL unless a central venous line is used. ■ Monitor serum electrolytes and acid-base balance, especially in patients with prolonged diarrhea and those receiving diuretics. ■ Monitor liver enzymes (AST, ALT, GGT) and bilirubin for elevations indicating progressive injury. ■ Monitor pulmonary status (e.g., Fio_2, Sao_2, Pao_2, chest x-ray); baseline pulmonary function tests recommended; repeat as indicated. ■ Monitor thyroid function tests before treatment and periodically thereafter. Patients with a history of thyroid nodules, goiter, or other thyroid dysfunction and the elderly should be monitored closely. Amiodarone is eliminated slowly, and abnormal function tests may persist for weeks or months after it is discontinued. ■ Regular ophthalmic exams, including funduscopy and slit lamp exams, are recommended. Prompt ophthalmic exams recommended at first sign of visual impairment. May require discontinuation of amiodarone therapy. ■ Serum amiodarone levels greater than 2.5 mcg/mL have been associated with a higher incidence of side effects. ■ Monitor for S/S of anaphylaxis/anaphylactoid reactions (e.g., cardiac arrest, cold sweat, cyanosis, flushing, hyperhidrosis, hypotension, hypoxia, rash, shock, tachycardia). ■ See Precautions and Drug/Lab Interactions.

Patient Education: Most manufacturers of corneal refractive laser surgery devices contraindicate this procedure in patients receiving amiodarone. ■ Report promptly any feelings of faintness, difficulty breathing, or pain or stinging along injection site. Review side effect profile, including S/S of hypothyroidism or hyperthyroidism. ■ Nonhormonal birth control recommended. ■ Numerous drug interactions. Review all medications, including OTC medications, with physician or pharmacist. ■ Avoid grapefruit juice if transitioned to oral amiodarone.

Maternal/Child: Category D: can cause fetal harm; avoid pregnancy or use only if benefit to mother justifies risk to fetus. Fetal exposure may increase potential for adverse experiences, including cardiac, thyroid, neurodevelopmental, neurologic, and growth effects in neonates. ■ Discontinue breast-feeding. ■ Safety for use during labor and delivery not established. ■ Safety and effectiveness for use in pediatric patients not established. ■ A manufacturer's warning letter has been issued citing potentially fatal or developmental side effects in infants and neonates; see Contraindications. Another source suggests amiodarone may adversely affect male reproductive tract development in infants, neonates, and toddlers. ■ Vials contain benzyl alcohol, which has been associated with "gasping syndrome" in neonates (sudden onset of gasping respirations, hypotension, bradycardia, and cardiovascular collapse).

Elderly: Differences in response between the elderly and younger patients have not been identified; however, clearance is slower and half-life may be doubled (up to 47 days). See Dose Adjustments.

DRUG/LAB INTERACTIONS

Amiodarone has a long half-life; drug interactions may persist long after it is discontinued. *Contraindicated with nelfinavir (Viracept) and ritonavir (Norvir).* Should not be given concurrently with **ibutilide** (Corvert). ■ Concurrent use with other **antiarrhythmic agents** (e.g., flecainide [Tambocor], procainamide [Pronestyl], quinidine) increases their serum concentrations and may result in additive increases in QT prolongation and serious arrhythmias. Manufacturer recommends reducing the dose of previously given antiarrhythmic agents by 30% to 50% several days after starting amiodarone and then evaluating the need for continued therapy with the other antiarrhythmic agent after the effects of amiodarone have been established. Monitor serum levels if possible. ■ QT prolongation has been reported with concomitant administration of amiodarone and **fluoroquinolones** (e.g., levofloxacin [Levaquin]), **halogenated inhalation anesthetic agents** (e.g., desflurane [Suprane], sevoflurane [Ultane]), **macrolide antibiotics** (e.g., erythromycin [Erythrocin]), **azoles** (e.g., fluconazole [Diflucan]), **lithium, loratadine** (Claritin), **phenothiazines** (e.g., prochlorperazine [Compazine], promethazine [Phenergan]), **trazodone** (Desyrel), **tricyclic antidepressants** (e.g., amitriptyline [Elavil], desipramine [Norpramin]), **and grapefruit juice (oral therapy);** see Precautions. ▪ May decrease metabolism and increase serum levels of **digoxin.** Reduce digoxin dose by 50% or withdraw completely when amiodarone therapy is initiated. ▪ Use with **potassium-depleting diuretics** (e.g., chlorothiazide [Diuril], furosemide [Lasix], indapamide [Lozol]) may lead to increased risk of arrhythmias due to hypokalemia. ▪ Inhibits metabolism and increases anticoagulant effect (e.g., increased PT and INR) of **warfarin** (Coumadin). Dose reduction of the anticoagulant and careful monitoring of PT or INR recommended. Effects may persist long after amiodarone is discontinued. ▪ Coadministration with dabigatran (Pradaxa) may result in an elevated serum concentration of dabigatran. ▪ May decrease metabolism and increase serum levels of **cyclosporine** (Sandimmune), **flecainide** (Tambocor), **hydantoins** (e.g., phenytoin [Dilantin]), **lidocaine, methotrexate, procainamide** (Pronestyl), **quinidine, and theophyllines** (Aminophylline). May cause toxicity; monitor serum levels. Reduced doses indicated. ▪ Concomitant use with **HMG-CoA reductase inhibitors** that are CYP3A4 substrates (e.g., lovastatin [Mevacor], simvastatin [Zocor]) has been associated with myopathy/rhabdomyolysis. In patients taking amiodarone, limit the dose of lovastatin to 40 mg daily and limit the dose of simvastatin to 20 mg daily. Lower starting and maintenance doses of other CYP3A4 substrates (e.g., atorvastatin [Lipitor]) may also be required. ▪ May cause bradycardia, decreased cardiac output, and hypotension with **fentanyl** (Sublimaze). ▪ Amiodarone clearance increased and plasma levels decreased with **cholestyramine** (Questran), **phenytoin** (Dilantin), **rifampin** (Rifadin), **and St. John's wort.** ▪ **Cimetidine** (Tagamet) **and protease inhibitors** (e.g., indinavir [Crixivan]) may decrease clearance and increase plasma levels of amiodarone. ▪ Concomitant use of **drugs with depressant effects on the sinus and AV node** (e.g., beta-blockers [e.g., propranolol], calcium channel blockers [e.g., diltiazem (Cardizem), verapamil], clonidine, digoxin) can potentiate the electrophysiologic and hemodynamic effects of amiodarone, resulting in bradycardia, sinus arrest, and AV block. Monitoring of heart rate required. ▪ May inhibit conversion of **clopidogrel** (Plavix) to its active metabolite, resulting in ineffective inhibition of platelet aggregation. ▪ May inhibit conversion of the prodrug **cyclophosphamide** (Cytoxan) to its active metabolite. ▪ Monitor patients undergoing **general anesthesia** closely. May increase sensitivity to myocardial depressant and conduction defects of **halogenated inhalation anesthetics** (hypotension and atropine-resistant bradycardia). ▪ PO use for longer than 2 weeks may decrease metabolism and increase serum levels of **dextromethorphan** (Robitussin DM), **methotrexate, and phenytoin.** ▪ See Precautions.

SIDE EFFECTS

Hypotension or pain at the IV site are the most common side effects. Agranulocytosis, anaphylaxis, anemia (aplastic and/or hemolytic), angioedema, anorexia, arrhythmias (e.g., AV block, bradycardia, new onset VT/VF, sinus arrest, torsades de pointes), adult respiratory distress syndrome (ARDS), ataxia, cardiac arrest, cardiogenic shock, confusion, congestive heart failure, delirium, disorientation, dizziness, dry eyes, hallucinations, hepatotoxicity (liver function test abnormalities), impotence, muscle weakness, myopathy, nausea, nephrotoxicity, neutropenia, pancreatitis, pancytopenia, paresthesias, peripheral neuropathy, photosensitivity, pleuritis, pruritus, pseudotumor cerebri (swelling that resembles a tumor), pulmonary toxicity (including bronchiolitis obliterans organizing pneumonia [may be fatal]), renal impairment, respiratory disorders (including cough, dyspnea, hemoptysis, hypoxia, pulmonary infiltrates and/or mass on chest x-ray, respiratory failure), rhabdomyolysis, skin disorders (e.g., epididymitis, erythema multiforme, exfoliative dermatitis, Stevens-Johnson syndrome, toxic epidermal necrolysis [may be fatal]), syndrome of inappropriate antidiuretic hormone secretion (SIADH), thrombocytopenia, thyroid dysfunction, and visual impairment/loss of vision may occur. In addition to these side effects, overdose or extended use may cause hepatic and/or renal failure secondary to hypotension.

Overdose: AV block, bradycardia, cardiogenic shock, death, hepatotoxicity, hypotension.

ANTIDOTE

Keep physician informed of all side effects and treat promptly as appropriate; many are life threatening. Reduce rate and/or concentration for pain at IV site. Monitor hepatic enzymes closely. Reduce rate or discontinue for progressive hepatic injury. Treat hypotension and cardiogenic shock by slowing the infusion rate. Vasopressors (e.g., dopamine, norepinephrine [Levophed]), inotropic agents (e.g., digoxin), and volume expansion may be indicated. Slow infusion rate or discontinue if bradycardia and/or AV block occur; may require a temporary pacemaker. If torsades de pointes occurs, stop all cardioactive drugs (e.g., antiarrhythmics, digoxin, antidepressants, phenothiazines) and normalize electrolytes (e.g., potassium, magnesium). Atrial overdrive pacing may be required to stabilize cardiac rhythm. Dose reduction or discontinuation of amiodarone may be required if thyroid abnormalities develop. Thyroid hormone supplementation may be required in hypothyroidism. Initiation of antithyroid drugs (e.g., propylthiouracil [PTU]), beta-blockers (e.g., propranolol), and/or temporary corticosteroid therapy may be necessary for treatment of hyperthyroidism. In severe thyrotoxicosis where amiodarone cannot be discontinued, thyroidectomy may be used as treatment. Experience with surgical intervention is limited; could induce thyroid storm. Amiodarone is not dialyzable. Resuscitate as necessary.

AMPHOTERICIN B BBW* ■
AMPHOTERICIN B LIPID-BASED PRODUCTS
(am-foe-**TER**-ih-sin)

Antifungal
Antiprotozoal (AmBisome)

Abelcet, AmBisome, Amphotec   pH 5.7 to 8 ■ 5 to 6

---

*The Black Box Warning applies only to the generic formulation.

USUAL DOSE

Each product has different biochemical, pharmacokinetic, and pharmacodynamic properties. They are not interchangeable from dose to dose, in a given patient, between each other or conventional amphotericin.

ABELCET (AMPHOTERICIN B LIPID COMPLEX INJECTION)

Adults and pediatric patients: 5 mg/kg/24 hr as an infusion. Repeat daily until clinical response or mycologic cure.

AMPHOTEC (AMPHOTERICIN B CHOLESTERYL SULFATE COMPLEX FOR INJECTION)

Adults and pediatric patients: 3 to 4 mg/kg/24 hr as an infusion. Pretreatment with antipyretics, antihistamines, or corticosteroids may be indicated; see Precautions and Antidote. On the first day of treatment, begin with a test dose of 10 mL of the final diluted preparation and infuse over 15 to 30 minutes. Observe the patient for the next 30 minutes. If there is no adverse reaction, continue with the calculated dose. May be increased to 6 mg/kg/24 hr if there is no improvement or if the fungal infection progresses. See Indications.

AMBISOME (AMPHOTERICIN B LIPOSOME FOR INJECTION)

Adults, children, and infants over 1 month of age: All doses are by infusion.

Empirical therapy in febrile, neutropenic patients: 3 mg/kg/24 hr.

Continued

Systemic fungal infections (e.g., *Aspergillus, Candida, Cryptococcus*): 3 to 5 mg/kg/24 hr.
Treatment of cryptococcal meningitis in HIV-infected patients: 6 mg/kg/24 hr.
Visceral leishmaniasis in immunocompetent patients: 3 mg/kg/24 hr on Days 1 through 5. Repeat 3 mg/kg on Day 14 and on Day 21. A repeat course of therapy may be useful if parasitic clearance is not achieved.
Visceral leishmaniasis in immunocompromised patients: 4 mg/kg/24 hr on Days 1 through 5. Repeat 4 mg/kg on Days 10, 17, 24, 31, and 38. During clinical studies parasitic clearance was not achieved or relapse within 6 months occurred in 88.2% of patients. Usefulness of repeat courses not determined.

GENERIC (CONVENTIONAL AMPHOTERICIN B)

Adults and pediatric patients: Begin with a test dose of 0.1 mg/kg up to 1 mg maximum dose in 20 mL D5W. Infuse over 20 to 30 minutes. Determine size of therapeutic dose by intensity of reaction over a 2- to 4-hour period. Usual starting dose is 0.25 mg/kg of body weight/24 hr. Gradually increase dose by 5 to 10 mg/day (0.125 to 0.25 mg/kg in pediatric patients) to a final dose of 0.5 to 0.7 mg/kg. Total daily dose may range up to 1 mg/kg/day, or up to 1.5 mg/kg/24 hr may be given on alternate-day therapy. Several months of therapy are usually required and recommended for cure. Dosage must be adjusted to each specific patient. In some instances, higher doses can be used. Do not exceed a total daily dose of 1.5 mg/kg under any circumstances.

DOSE ADJUSTMENTS

ABELCET: Full dose usually required; base on SCr and overall patient condition.
AMPHOTEC/AMBISOME: No dose adjustments suggested.
GENERIC (CONVENTIONAL): In all situations, gradual dose increases are essential. Whenever medicine is not given for 7 days or longer, restart treatment at lowest dosage level.
Patients with impaired cardio-renal function or a severe reaction to the test dose: Initiate with smaller daily doses (i.e., 5 to 10 mg).
Patients who experience amphotericin-induced nephrotoxicity: One source recommends reducing the total daily dose by 50% or administering the dose every other day.
Severe and rapidly progressive fungal infection: Initiate treatment with a daily dose of 0.3 mg/kg.

DILUTION

ABELCET: Available in 100-mg (20-mL) vials. Shake vial until all yellow sediment is dissolved. Maintain aseptic technique. Withdraw an exact total daily dose from one or more vials using one or more syringes and 18-gauge needles. Replace needle(s) on syringe(s) with the 5-micron filter(s) supplied with each vial. A new filter must be used for each 400 mg (80 mL) of Abelcet. Empty syringe contents through filter into an infusion of D5W. 4 mL of diluent (D5W) is required for each 1 mL (5 mg) of Abelcet to achieve a final concentration of 1 mg/mL. For *pediatric* and/or fluid-restricted patients (e.g., patients with cardiovascular disease) reduce diluent by half (approximate concentration of 2 mg/mL).

AMPHOTEC: Available in 50-mg or 100-mg vials. Reconstitute by rapidly adding 10 mL of SWFI for each 50 mg of Amphotec (5 mg/mL). Use of a 20-gauge needle is recommended. Shake gently, rotating the vial until all solids have dissolved. May be opalescent or clear. Must be further diluted for infusion with D5W (see the following chart). Final desired concentration is approximately 0.6 mg/mL (range with recommended amounts of diluent is 0.16 mg/mL to 0.83 mg/mL). Do not filter or use an in-line filter. See Compatibility and Rate of Administration.

Guidelines for Dilution of Amphotec		
Dose of Amphotec (mg)	Volume of Reconstituted Amphotec (mL)	Infusion Bag Size for D5W for Injection (mL)
10-35 mg	2-7 mL	50 mL
35-70 mg	7-14 mL	100 mL
70-175 mg	14-35 mL	250 mL
175-350 mg	35-70 mL	500 mL
350-1,000 mg	70-200 mL	1,000 mL

AMBISOME: Reconstitute each 50-mg vial with 12 mL SWFI (without a bacteriostatic agent) to yield 4 mg/mL. Shake vial vigorously for 30 seconds; forms a yellow translucent suspension. Withdraw an exact total daily dose from one or more vials using one or more 20-mL syringes and needles. Replace needle(s) with the 5-micron filter(s) supplied with each vial. A new filter must be used for each 50-mg vial. Empty syringe contents through filter into an infusion of D5W. Use sufficient diluent to achieve a final concentration of 1 to 2 mg/mL, pH 5 to 6. For **pediatric patients:** may be further diluted to concentrations of 0.2 to 0.5 mg/mL for infants and small children to provide adequate volume for infusion.

GENERIC (CONVENTIONAL): A 50-mg vial is initially diluted with 10 mL of SWFI (without a bacteriostatic agent); 5 mg equals 1 mL. Shake well until solution is clear. Further dilute each 1 mg in at least 10 mL of D5W. Dextrose must have a pH above 4.2. Concentration of solution must not be greater than 0.1 mg/mL. Do not use any other diluent. Use a sterile 20-gauge or larger needle at each step of the dilution. Maintain aseptic technique. Larger pore 1-micron filters may be used. Use only fresh solutions without evidence of precipitate or foreign matter. Light sensitive; protect from light during administration.

Filters: Abelcet: 5-micron filter(s) supplied with each vial. A new filter must be used for each 400 mg (80 mL) of Abelcet. Empty syringe contents through filter into an infusion solution. Do not use an in-line filter.

Amphotec: Do not filter or use an in-line filter.

AmBisome: 5-micron filter(s) supplied with each vial. A new filter must be used for each 50-mg vial. Empty syringe contents through filter into an infusion solution. Do not use an in-line filter smaller than 1 micron.

Generic (Conventional): Larger pore 1-micron filters may be used; see Dilution.

Storage: Abelcet: Before reconstitution, refrigerate in carton until time of use and protect from light. Do not freeze. Diluted solution is stable 48 hours if refrigerated and an additional 6 hours at room temperature. Discard unused drug.

Amphotec: Store unopened vials in carton at CRT. Refrigerate reconstituted or diluted solutions; must be used within 24 hours. Do not freeze. Discard unused drug.

AmBisome: Unopened vials may be stored at temperatures up to 25° C (77° F). Vials reconstituted with SWFI may be refrigerated for up to 24 hours. Do not freeze. Infusion of fully diluted solution must begin within 6 hours. Discard unused drug.

Generic (Conventional): Before reconstitution, refrigerate vials and protect from light. Do not freeze. Preserve concentrate in refrigerator up to 7 days or 24 hours at room temperature. Use diluted solution promptly.

COMPATIBILITY   (Underline Indicates Conflicting Compatibility Information)

Consider any drug NOT listed as compatible to be INCOMPATIBLE until consulting a pharmacist; specific conditions may apply.

ALL FORMULATIONS

In all situations, use a separate infusion line or flush an existing line with D5W before and after administration.

ABELCET

Do not mix with any other diluent, drug, or solution. Use only D5W. Manufacturer states that **compatibility** with any other diluent has not been established. Another source lists **compatibility** at the **Y-site** with anidulafungin (Eraxis), doripenem (Doribax), telavancin (Vibativ).

AMBISOME/AMPHOTEC/GENERIC

Do not mix with any other diluent, drug, or solution. Use only SWFI for reconstitution and D5W for dilution for infusion. Use of any other solution or the presence of a bacteriostatic agent (e.g., benzyl alcohol) may cause precipitation. Another source lists AmBisome as **compatible** at the **Y-site** with anidulafungin (Eraxis), doripenem (Doribax).

AMPHOTEC

One source suggests the following **compatibilities:**

Y-site: Acyclovir (Zovirax), aminophylline, cefoxitin (Mefoxin), clindamycin (Cleocin), cytarabine (ARA-C), dexamethasone (Decadron), doripenem (Doribax), fentanyl, furosemide (Lasix), ganciclovir (Cytovene IV), granisetron (Kytril), hydrocortisone sodium succinate (Solu-Cortef), ifosfamide (Ifex), lorazepam (Ativan), mannitol, methotrexate, methylprednisolone (Solu-Medrol), nitroglycerin IV, sulfamethoxazole/trimethoprim, sufentanil (Sufenta), vinblastine, vincristine, zidovudine (AZT, Retrovir).

GENERIC (CONVENTIONAL)

One source suggests the following **compatibilities:**

Additive: *Not recommended by manufacturer.* Fluconazole (Diflucan), heparin, hydrocortisone sodium succinate (Solu-Cortef), sodium bicarbonate.

Y-site: Aldesleukin (Proleukin, Interleukin-2), amiodarone (Nexterone), cisatracurium (Nimbex), diltiazem (Cardizem), doripenem (Doribax), remifentanil (Ultiva), sargramostim (Leukine), tacrolimus (Prograf), teniposide (Vumon), thiotepa, zidovudine (AZT, Retrovir).

RATE OF ADMINISTRATION

ALL AMPHOTERICINS: Rapid infusion may cause hypotension, hypokalemia, arrhythmia, and shock. Infusion reactions can occur with all amphotericin B formulations. See Precautions, Side Effects, and Antidote. With all formulations, flush existing line with D5W before and after administration or use a separate IV line.

ABELCET: Total daily dose as an infusion at 2.5 mg/kg/hr. Contents of diluted solution must be mixed by shaking at least every 2 hours. Do not use an in-line filter.

AMPHOTEC: See rate for test dose in Usual Dose. Give total daily dose as an infusion at 1 mg/kg/hr. Infusion time may be shortened to a minimum of 2 hours for patients who show no evidence of intolerance or infusion-related reactions. May be extended for acute reactions or if infusion volume is not tolerated. Do not use filters.

AMBISOME: Total daily dose as an infusion over 2 hours. Use of a controlled infusion device is recommended. Infusion time may be shortened to a minimum of 1 hour for patients who show no evidence of intolerance or infusion-related reactions. Infusion time may be extended for patient discomfort or acute reactions or if infusion volume is not tolerated. Do not use any in-line filter less than 1 micron.

GENERIC (CONVENTIONAL): Daily dose over 2 to 6 hours by slow IV infusion. Expected reactions usually less severe with slower rate. A minimum 1-micron filter may be used.

ACTIONS

Antifungal antibiotic agents that bind to the sterol component of fungal cell membranes resulting in leakage of cellular contents. May be fungistatic or fungicidal according to body fluid concentration and susceptibility of the fungus. Abelcet is amphotericin B complexed with two phospholipids in a 1:1 drug-to-lipid ratio. Amphotec is amphotericin B complexed with cholesteryl sulfate in a colloidal dispersion in a 1:1 drug-to-lipid ratio. AmBisome is amphotericin B intercalated into a liposomal membrane with several components. Assay tests cannot distinguish lipid-based amphotericin from conventional amphotericin B. Modification of amphotericin to the various lipid-based products alters the drug's functional properties. It allows for increased levels of drug at the site of action (usually areas where the fungi are). Overall effect is increased effectiveness with less toxicity. Not effective against bacteria, rickettsiae, or viruses. Long terminal half-life probably reflects a slow redistribution from tissues. Actual distribution to organs is somewhat selective and may help to decide which product is best to use in a given situation. Route of metabolism not known. Excreted very slowly in the urine.

INDICATIONS AND USES

ABELCET: Treatment of invasive fungal infections in patients who are refractory to or intolerant of conventional amphotericin B therapy.

AMPHOTEC: Treatment of invasive aspergillosis in patients refractory to or intolerant of conventional amphotericin B or in patients in whom conventional amphotericin treatment has failed.

AMBISOME: Empirical therapy for presumed fungal infection in febrile, neutropenic patients. ▪ Treatment of patients with aspergillosis, candida, and/or cryptococcus infections refractory to conventional amphotericin B or in patients in whom renal impairment or unacceptable toxicity precludes the use of conventional amphotericin B. ▪ Treatment of visceral leishmaniasis. ▪ Treatment of cryptococcal meningitis in HIV-infected patients.

GENERIC (CONVENTIONAL): Treatment of fungal infections that are progressive and potentially fatal, such as aspergillosis, cryptococcosis, blastomycosis, and disseminated forms of candidiasis, coccidioidomycosis, and histoplasmosis, mucormycosis, and sporotrichosis. These infections must be caused by specific organisms. Not recommended for treatment of noninvasive forms of fungal disease in patients with normal neutrophil counts.

Unlabeled uses: AmBisome has been used to prevent fungal infections in bone marrow transplant patients.

CONTRAINDICATIONS

All amphotericin formulations: Known sensitivity to amphotericin B or any components of its formulations unless a life-threatening situation is present.

PRECAUTIONS

ALL AMPHOTERICIN FORMULATIONS: Diagnosis should be positively established by culture or histologic study. ▪ Close clinical observation is imperative. Anaphylaxis has occurred; emergency equipment and supplies must be available. ▪ Infusion reactions are common and usually occur 1 to 3 hours after the start of the infusion. Frequency and severity of reactions generally diminish with subsequent doses. Pretreatment with antipyretics, antihistamines (e.g., diphenhydramine [Benadryl]), and/or selective use of corticosteroids may be indicated. ▪ Use caution in patients receiving leukocyte transfusions; may cause acute pulmonary toxicity. Separate times of administration as much as possible. ▪ Nephrotoxicity is the usual dose-limiting factor for use of conventional amphotericin B. Impairment may improve with dose reduction or alternate-day therapy, but some residual dysfunction is possible. Lipid-based formulations are associated with less nephrotoxicity. Most studies show equivalent or superior effectiveness compared with conventional amphotericin. Introduction of lipid-based products to patients with increased CrCl and BUN from conventional amphotericin has decreased the CrCl and BUN.

ABELCET: Renal toxicity is dose dependent but has been consistently less nephrotoxic than conventional amphotericin B.

AMPHOTEC/AMBISOME: Incidence of renal toxicity significantly lower than with conventional amphotericin B.

GENERIC (CONVENTIONAL): Should be used primarily for treatment of patients with progressive and potentially life-threatening fungal infections. It should not be used to treat noninvasive forms of fungal disease such as oral thrush, vaginal candidiasis, and esophageal candidiasis in patients with normal neutrophil counts. ▪ To prevent overdose, verify product name and dose, especially if dose exceeds 1.5 mg/kg. ▪ Therapy is often initiated in infusion centers. ▪ A small amount of heparin added to the infusion may reduce the incidence of thrombophlebitis. ▪ Meperidine (Demerol), nonsteroidal anti-inflammatory agents (e.g., ibuprofen), or hydrocortisone before administration may prevent febrile reactions, including chills; corticosteroids not recommended for concomitant use in other situations because they exaggerate hypokalemia. ▪ Prophylactic antiemetics and antihistamines are also appropriate.

Monitor: *All amphotericin formulations:* Obtain baseline CBC, PT, serum electrolytes, renal (e.g., creatine kinase, BUN, SCr) and liver function (e.g., ALT, AST) tests. Repeat frequently during therapy; recommended weekly. Monitor PT as indicated during therapy. ▪ Discontinue or reduce dose until renal function improves if increase in BUN or SCr is clinically significant. Side effects (e.g., hypokalemia, hypomagnesemia, impaired renal function) may be life threatening. ▪ Monitor vital signs and I&O. Record every 30 minutes for up to 4 hours after infusion is complete. ▪ Monitor for S/S of hypersensitivity or infusion reactions (e.g., chest pain, dizziness, dyspnea, fever, flushing, hypotension, nausea, pruritus, rash, rigors, urticaria). ▪ Encourage fluids to maintain hydration.

Patient Education: *All amphotericin formulations:* Review all medical conditions and medications before beginning treatment. ▪ Discomfort associated with infusion. ▪ Promptly report S/S of an acute reaction (e.g., anorexia, chills, fever, headache, hypotension, nausea or vomiting, shortness of breath). ▪ Long-term therapy required to effect a cure. ▪ Report diarrhea, fever, increased or decreased urination, loss of appetite, sore throat, stomach pain, and any unusual bleeding or bruising, tiredness, or weakness. ▪ Maintain adequate hydration.

Maternal/Child: *All amphotericin formulations:* Category B: has been used successfully during pregnancy but adequate studies not available. Use only if clearly needed. ▪ Safety for use in breast-feeding and pediatric patients not established. Discontinue nursing. ▪ Conventional amphotericin B has been used in pediatric patients. Lipid-based preparations have been used in pediatric patients without any unexpected side effects. Safety of use of AmBisome in infants under 1 month of age not established.

Elderly: Consider age-related impaired body functions. Lipid-based preparations have been used without unexpected side effects.

DRUG/LAB INTERACTIONS

Drug interaction studies have not been done for lipid-based preparations, but interactions similar to conventional amphotericin B are expected. ▪ **Corticosteroids** will increase hypokalemia and may cause arrhythmias. Use with caution only if indicated to control drug reactions or, if necessary, monitor serum electrolytes and cardiac function closely. ▪ Hypokalemic effect may be increased with **thiazides,** may potentiate **digoxin** toxicity, and/or may enhance the curariform effect of **neuromuscular blocking agents** (e.g., rocuronium [Zemuron], succinylcholine); monitor serum potassium levels. ▪ Avoid use or use extreme caution with other **nephrotoxic drugs** (e.g., **aminoglycosides** [e.g., gentamicin, tobramycin], **selected antibiotics** [e.g., vancomycin], **anesthetics** [e.g., methoxyflurane]), **antituberculars** [e.g., capreomycin (Capestat)], **diuretics** [e.g., furosemide (Lasix), torsemide (Demadex)], **pentamidine).** Nephrotoxic effects are additive. Frequent monitoring of renal function indicated if any other nephrotoxic drug must be used. ▪ Nephrotoxicity and myelotoxicity are both increased when given concurrently with **zidovudine** (AZT, Retrovir). ▪ Potentiates nephrotoxicity of **cyclosporine;** alternate immunosuppressive therapy recommended. ▪ Concurrent use with **antineoplastic agents** (e.g., cisplatin, methotrexate) **or radiation therapy** may increase renal toxicity and incidence of bronchospasm and hypotension. ▪ Enhances antifungal effects of **flucytosine** (Ancobon) **and other anti-infectives.** May increase toxicity. ▪ Antagonism between amphotericin B and **imidazole antifungals** (e.g., ketoconazole, miconazole, fluconazole) has been reported. ▪ Acute pulmonary toxicity occurred in patients receiving **leukocyte transfusion;** separate administration times as much as possible. ▪ **False elevations of serum phosphate** may occur if patient samples are analyzed using the PHOSm assay.

SIDE EFFECTS

Lipid-Based Preparations: Most side effects similar to conventional amphotericin B but occur with less frequency and intensity. Acute reactions, including fever and chills, may occur within 1 to 3 hours of starting the infusion. Infusion-related cardiorespiratory reactions may include dyspnea, hypertension, hyperventilation, hypotension, hypoxia, tachycardia, and vasodilation. Arrhythmia, bronchospasm, and shock can occur. Anaphylaxis and cardiac arrest from overdose have been reported.

GENERIC (CONVENTIONAL): Common even at doses below therapeutic; may begin to occur within 15 to 20 minutes: anorexia, chills, convulsions, diarrhea, fever, headache, phlebitis, vomiting. Anaphylactoid reactions, anemia, cardiac disturbances (including fibrillation and arrest), coagulation defects, hypertension, hypokalemia, hypotension, and numerous other side effects occur fairly frequently. Renal function impaired in 80% of patients. May reverse after treatment ends, but some permanent damage likely.

Post-Marketing: *AmBisome:* Agranulocytosis, angioedema, bronchospasm, cyanosis/hypoventilation, edema, erythema, hemorrhagic cystitis, pulmonary edema, rhabdomyolysis.

ANTIDOTE

ALL AMPHOTERICIN FORMULATIONS: Notify the physician of all side effects. Many are reversible if the drug is discontinued. Some will respond to symptomatic treatment. Acute reactions (e.g., fever, chills, hypotension, nausea, and vomiting) usually lessen with subsequent doses. These acute infusion-related reactions can be managed by pretreatment with antipyretics, antihistamines, and/or corticosteroids or reduction of the rate of infusion and prompt treatment with antihistamines and/or corticosteroids and meperidine (Demerol) for chills. If anaphylaxis or serious respiratory distress occurs, discontinue amphotericin and treat as necessary. Give no further infusions. Hemodialysis not effective in overdose. Discontinue if BUN and alkaline phosphatase are abnormal. Dantrolene has been used to prevent (50 mg PO) or treat (50 mg IV) severe, shaking chills.

GENERIC (CONVENTIONAL): Administration of conventional amphotericin B on alternate days may decrease the incidence of some side effects. Urinary alkalinizers may minimize renal tubular acidosis.

ABELCET/AMPHOTEC: Overdose has caused cardiac arrest. Discontinue drug and treat symptomatically.

AMPICILLIN SODIUM
(am-pih-**SILL**-in **SO**-dee-um)

Antibacterial
(penicillin)

pH 8 to 10

USUAL DOSE

Range is from 1 to 12 Gm/24 hr for adults and pediatric patients weighing 20 kg or more. Larger doses may be indicated based on the seriousness of the infection. Some clinicians suggest a weight of 40 kg to receive adult dose range.

Respiratory tract or skin and skin structure infections: 250 to 500 mg every 6 hours.

GI or GU infections: 500 mg every 6 hours.

Septicemia or bacterial meningitis: 8 to 14 Gm or 150 to 200 mg/kg/24 hr in equally divided doses every 3 to 4 hours (18.75 to 25 mg/kg every 3 hours or 25 to 33.3 mg/kg every 4 hours). Administer IV a minimum of 3 days; then may be given IV or IM.

Treatment of gonorrhea: 500 mg. Repeat in 8 to 12 hours. May repeat 2-dose regimen IV or IM if indicated. Ceftriaxone (Rocephin) IV or IM is most commonly used.

Listeriosis: 50 mg/kg every 6 hours.

Prevention of bacterial endocarditis in dental or respiratory tract surgery or instrumentation: 2 Gm of ampicillin 30 minutes before procedure.

Prevention of bacterial endocarditis in GI, GU, or biliary tract surgery or instrumentation: *Low to moderate risk:* A single dose of 2 Gm of ampicillin 30 minutes before procedure. *Moderate to high risk:* 2 Gm of ampicillin in conjunction with gentamicin 1.5 mg/kg (up to 80 mg) 30 minutes before procedure. Repeat 1 Gm of ampicillin or give oral amoxicillin 1 Gm in 6 hours.

Continued

Prophylaxis in high-risk cesarean section patients: 1 to 2 Gm immediately after clamping cord.

Prophylaxis of neonatal group B *Streptococcal* disease: 2 Gm to the mother during labor. Should be given at least 4 hours before delivery to ensure amniotic fluid concentrations and placental transfer of ampicillin. May repeat 1 to 2 Gm every 4 to 6 hours until delivery. Continue treatment postpartum if active signs of maternal infection develop. Routine use of prophylaxis in neonates born to these mothers is not recommended; risk must be assessed on an individual basis for each infant.

Leptospirosis (unlabeled): 500 mg to 1 Gm every 6 hours.

Typhoid fever (unlabeled): 25 mg/kg every 6 hours.

PEDIATRIC DOSE

Range is from 25 to 400 mg/kg of body weight/24 hr for pediatric patients weighing less than 20 kg. Some clinicians suggest a weight up to 40 kg is appropriate for pediatric use. Do not exceed adult dose or 12 Gm.

Respiratory tract or skin and skin structure infections: 25 to 50 mg/kg/24 hr in equally divided doses every 4 to 6 hours (4.16 to 8.3 mg/kg every 4 hours or 6.25 to 12.5 mg/kg every 6 hours).

GI or GU infections: 50 to 100 mg/kg/24 hr in equally divided doses every 6 hours (12.5 to 25 mg/kg every 6 hours).

Septicemia or bacterial meningitis: 100 to 200 mg/kg/24 hr in equally divided doses every 3 to 4 hours (12.5 to 25 mg/kg every 3 hours or 16.6 to 33.3 mg/kg every 4 hours).

Empiric treatment of bacterial meningitis in infants and children 2 months to 12 years of age: Some clinicians recommend 200 to 400 mg/kg/24 hr in equally divided doses every 4 to 6 hours (33.3 to 66.6 mg/kg every 4 hours to 50 to 100 mg/kg every 6 hours). Given in conjunction with chloramphenicol. Satisfactory response should occur within 48 hours or initiate alternate therapy. Administer any regimen IV a minimum of 3 days, then may be given IV or IM.

Prevention of bacterial endocarditis in dental or respiratory tract surgery or instrumentation: 50 mg/kg of ampicillin 30 minutes before procedure.

Prevention of bacterial endocarditis in GI, GU, or biliary tract surgery or instrumentation: *Low to moderate risk:* A single dose of 50 mg/kg 30 minutes before procedure. *Moderate to high risk:* 50 mg/kg of ampicillin in conjunction with gentamicin 1.5 mg/kg (up to 80 mg) 30 minutes before procedure. Repeat 25 mg/kg of ampicillin or oral amoxicillin in 6 hours.

NEONATAL DOSE

Age up to 7 days: *Weight less than 2,000 Gm:* 25 mg/kg every 12 hours. *2,000 Gm or more:* 25 mg/kg every 8 hours.

Over 7 days of age: *Weight less than 1,200 Gm:* 25 mg/kg every 12 hours. *1,200 to 2,000 Gm:* 25 mg/kg every 8 hours. *More than 2,000 Gm:* 25 mg/kg every 6 hours.

Empiric treatment of bacterial meningitis in neonates and infants less than 2 months of age: 100 to 300 mg/kg/24 hr in equally divided doses (e.g., 33.3 to 100 mg/kg every 8 hours) in conjunction with IM gentamicin. Administer any regimen IV a minimum of 3 days, then may be given IV or IM.

Bacterial meningitis in neonates and infants less than 2 months of age:

Age up to 7 days: *Weight less than 2,000 Gm:* 50 to 75 mg/kg every 12 hours.

2,000 Gm or more: 50 to 75 mg/kg every 8 hours.

Over 7 days of age: *Weight less than 2,000 Gm:* 50 mg/kg every 8 hours.

2,000 Gm or more: 50 mg/kg every 6 hours.

DOSE ADJUSTMENTS

Patients with a CrCl of 10 to 50 mL/min may require the usual dose every 6 to 12 hours. Reduce dose by increasing interval to 12 to 24 hours in severe renal impairment (CrCl less than 10 mL/min). Another source suggests no dose adjustment with a CrCl of 30 mL/min or greater and dosing every 8 hours for a CrCl of 10 mL/min or less. Administer 250 mg every 12 hours to peritoneal dialysis patients. Hemodialysis patients should receive 1 to 2 Gm after dialysis on dialysis days.

DILUTION

Each 500 mg or fraction thereof must be reconstituted with at least 5 mL of SWFI. Use within 1 hour of reconstitution. May be further diluted in 50 mL or more of selected IV solutions. Stable for 8 hours at concentrations up to 30 mg/mL in NS, LR, sodium lactate, or SWFI. Stable in D5/^{1}/$_2$NS or 10% invert sugar in water for 4 hours at concentrations up to 2 mg/mL. Stable in D5W for 4 hours at concentrations up to 2 mg/mL but only for 2 hours at concentrations up to 20 mg/mL. Must be administered before stability expires.

COMPATIBILITY   (Underline Indicates Conflicting Compatibility Information)

Consider any drug NOT listed as compatible to be INCOMPATIBLE until consulting a pharmacist; specific conditions may apply.

Inactivated in solution with aminoglycosides (e.g., amikacin, gentamicin). Do not mix in the same solution. Appropriate spacing and/or separate sites required. See Drug/Lab Interactions.

One source suggests the following **compatibilities:**

Additive: Aztreonam (Azactam), cefepime (Maxipime), clindamycin (Cleocin), erythromycin (Erythrocin), furosemide (Lasix), heparin, hydrocortisone sodium succinate (Solu-Cortef), lincomycin (Lincocin), metronidazole (Flagyl IV), ranitidine (Zantac), verapamil.

Y-site: Acyclovir (Zovirax), alprostadil, amifostine (Ethyol), anidulafungin (Eraxis), aztreonam (Azactam), bivalirudin (Angiomax), calcium gluconate, cisatracurium (Nimbex), cyclophosphamide (Cytoxan), dexmedetomidine (Precedex), diltiazem (Cardizem), docetaxel (Taxotere), doxapram (Dopram), doxorubicin liposomal (Doxil), enalaprilat (Vasotec IV), esmolol (Brevibloc), etoposide phosphate (Etopophos), famotidine (Pepcid IV), filgrastim (Neupogen), fludarabine (Fludara), foscarnet (Foscavir), gemcitabine (Gemzar), granisetron (Kytril), heparin, hetastarch in electrolytes (Hextend), hetastarch in NS (Hespan), hydrocortisone sodium succinate (Solu-Cortef), hydromorphone (Dilaudid), 6% hydroxyethyl starch (Voluven), insulin (regular), labetalol, levofloxacin (Levaquin), linezolid (Zyvox), magnesium sulfate, melphalan (Alkeran), meperidine (Demerol), milrinone (Primacor), morphine, multivitamins (M.V.I.), pantoprazole (Protonix IV), pemetrexed (Alimta), phytonadione (vitamin K$_1$), potassium chloride (KCl), propofol (Diprivan), remifentanil (Ultiva), tacrolimus (Prograf), teniposide (Vumon), theophylline, thiotepa, vancomycin.

RATE OF ADMINISTRATION

A single dose over 10 to 15 minutes when given by IV injection. In 100 mL or more of solution, administer at prescribed infusion rate but never exceed IV injection rate. Too-rapid injection may cause seizures.

ACTIONS

A semi-synthetic penicillin. Bactericidal against many gram-positive and some gram-negative organisms. Appears in all body fluids. Appears in cerebrospinal fluid only if inflammation is present. Crosses the placental barrier. Excreted in urine. Secreted in breast milk.

INDICATIONS AND USES

Highly effective against severe infections caused by gram-positive and some gram-negative organisms (e.g., respiratory tract, skin and skin structure, GI and GU, bacterial meningitis, endocarditis, listeriosis, septicemia). Not effective with penicillinase-producing staphylococci. ■ Prevention of bacterial endocarditis in dental and respiratory tract surgery or instrumentation. ■ Prevention of bacterial endocarditis in GI, GU, or biliary surgery or instrumentation. Used concurrently with gentamicin. ■ Drug of choice during labor for prevention of neonatal group B streptococcal infections.

Unlabeled uses: Prophylaxis in high-risk cesarean section patients. Treatment of leptospirosis. Treatment of typhoid fever.

CONTRAINDICATIONS

Known penicillin or cephalosporin sensitivity (not absolute); see Precautions. Infectious mononucleosis because of increased incidence of rash.

PRECAUTIONS

Hypersensitivity reactions, including fatalities, have been reported in patients undergoing penicillin therapy; most likely to occur in patients with a history of penicillin allergy or sensitivity to multiple allergens. There have been reports of individuals with a history of penicillin hypersensitivity experiencing severe reactions when treated with cephalosporins. Check history of previous hypersensitivity reactions to penicillins, cephalosporins, or other allergens. Actual incidence of cross-allergenicity not established but may be more common with first-generation cephalosporins. ▪ Sensitivity studies indicated to determine susceptibility of the causative organism to ampicillin. ▪ To reduce the development of drug-resistant bacteria and maintain its effectiveness, ampicillin should be used to treat or prevent only those infections proven or strongly suspected to be caused by bacteria. ▪ Avoid prolonged use of this drug; superinfection caused by overgrowth of nonsusceptible organisms may result. ▪ *Clostridium difficile*–associated diarrhea (CDAD) has been reported. May range from mild diarrhea to fatal colitis. Consider in patients who present with diarrhea during or after treatment with ampicillin. ▪ Side effects increased in some patients; see Side Effects.

Monitor: Watch for early symptoms of hypersensitivity reactions, especially in individuals with a history of allergic problems. ▪ AST may be increased. Renal, hepatic, and hematopoietic function should be checked during prolonged therapy. ▪ May cause thrombophlebitis; observe carefully and rotate infusion sites.

Patient Education: May require alternate birth control. ▪ Promptly report diarrhea or bloody stools that occur during treatment or up to several months after an antibiotic has been discontinued; may indicate CDAD and require treatment.

Maternal/Child: Category B: use only if clearly needed. ▪ May cause diarrhea, candidiasis, or allergic response in nursing infants. ▪ Elimination rate markedly reduced in neonates.

Elderly: Consider degree of age-related impaired renal function.

DRUG/LAB INTERACTIONS

Streptomycin potentiates bactericidal activity against enterococci. ▪ May be used concurrently with **aminoglycosides** (e.g., gentamicin), but these drugs must never be mixed in the same infusion (mutual inactivation). If given concurrently, administer at separate sites. ▪ May be antagonized by **bacteriostatic antibiotics** (e.g., chloramphenicol, erythromycin, and tetracyclines); may interfere with bactericidal action. ▪ Concomitant use with **beta-adrenergic blockers** (e.g., propranolol) may increase risk of anaphylaxis and inhibit treatment. ▪ Potentiated by **probenecid;** toxicity may result. ▪ Increased risk of bleeding with **heparin.** ▪ May decrease clearance and increase toxicity of **methotrexate.** ▪ Decreases effectiveness of **oral contraceptives;** breakthrough bleeding or pregnancy could result. ▪ Ampicillin-induced skin rash potentiated by **allopurinol** (Aloprim). ▪ False-positive glucose reaction with **Clinitest and Benedict's or Fehling's solution.** ▪ May cause **false values** in other lab tests; see literature.

SIDE EFFECTS

Primarily hypersensitivity reactions such as anaphylaxis, exfoliative dermatitis, rashes, and urticaria. May cause CDAD. Hypersensitivity myocarditis can occur (fever, eosinophilia, rash, sinus tachycardia, ST-T changes, and cardiomegaly). Anemia, leukopenia, and thrombocytopenia have been reported. Thrombophlebitis will occur with long-term use. Higher than normal doses may cause neurologic adverse reactions including convulsions, especially with impaired renal function. Incidence of side effects increased in patients with viral infections or those taking allopurinol (Aloprim).

ANTIDOTE

Notify the physician of any side effect. For severe symptoms, discontinue the drug, treat hypersensitivity reactions (antihistamines, epinephrine, corticosteroids), and resuscitate as necessary. Hemodialysis is effective in overdose. Treat CDAD with fluids, electrolytes, protein supplements, and oral vancomycin (Vancocin) or metronidazole (Flagyl) as indicated. In severe cases, surgical evaluation may be indicated.

AMPICILLIN SODIUM AND SULBACTAM SODIUM
(am-pih-**SILL**-in **SO**-dee-um and sull-**BACK**-tam **SO**-dee-um)

Antibacterial
(penicillin and beta-lactamase inhibitor)

Unasyn   pH 8 to 10

USUAL DOSE
Adults and pediatric patients weighing 40 kg or more: 1.5 to 3 Gm every 6 hours (1 Gm ampicillin with 0.5 Gm sulbactam to 2 Gm ampicillin with 1 Gm sulbactam). All commercial preparations in the United States have a 2:1 ratio of ampicillin to sulbactam (e.g., 1.5 Gm = 1 Gm ampicillin plus 0.5 Gm sulbactam). Do not exceed 4 Gm *sulbactam*/24 hr. *All doses in this monograph include ampicillin and sulbactam within the recommended dose.*

PEDIATRIC DOSE
IV use for more than 14 days is not recommended. See comments under Adult Dose.
Skin and skin structure infections in pediatric patients over 1 year of age and less than 40 kg: 300 mg/kg/day (200 mg/kg ampicillin and 100 mg/kg sulbactam) in equally divided doses as an infusion every 6 hours (75 mg/kg every 6 hours).
The American Academy of Pediatrics suggests use in pediatric patients over 1 month of age in the following doses.
Mild to moderate infections: 150 to 225 mg/kg/day (100 to 150 mg/kg of ampicillin and 50 to 75 mg/kg sulbactam) in equally divided doses as an infusion every 6 hours (37.5 to 56.5 mg/kg every 6 hours).
Severe infections: 300 to 450 mg/kg/day (200 to 300 mg/kg of ampicillin and 100 to 150 mg/kg of sulbactam) in equally divided doses as an infusion every 6 hours (75 mg/kg to 112.5 mg/kg every 6 hours).

DOSE ADJUSTMENTS
May be indicated in the elderly. ▪ Reduce total daily dose in impaired renal function according to the following chart.

Ampicillin/Sulbactam Dose Guidelines in Impaired Renal Function	
Creatinine Clearance (mL/min per 1.73 M²)	Dose/Frequency
30 mL/min or more	Usual recommended dose q 6 to 8 hr
15 to 29 mL/min	Usual recommended dose q 12 hr
5 to 14 mL/min	Usual recommended dose q 24 hr
Hemodialysis patients*	Usual recommended dose q 24 hr On day of dialysis, give immediately after dialysis

*One source recommends 1.5 to 3 Gm every 12 to 24 hours for hemodialysis patients, given after dialysis on dialysis days. A dose of 3 Gm/24 hr has been recommended for peritoneal dialysis patients.

DILUTION
Each 1.5 Gm or fraction thereof must be initially reconstituted with 4 mL of SWFI (375 mg/mL). Allow to stand to dissipate foaming. Solution should be clear. Must be further diluted to a final concentration of 3 to 45 mg/mL in one of the following solutions and given by slow IV injection or as an intermittent IV infusion: D5W, D5/^{1}/$_2$NS, 10% invert sugar in water, LR, ^{1}/$_6$ M sodium lactate solution, or NS. 3 Gm/L equals 3 mg/mL, 3 Gm/125 mL equals 24 mg/mL. Also available in piggyback vials and ADD-Vantage vials for use with ADD-Vantage infusion containers.
Storage: Store at CRT before dilution. Stable in all specifically listed solutions in any dilution for at least 2 hours. Stability in each solution varies (see literature).

COMPATIBILITY   (Underline Indicates Conflicting Compatibility Information)
Consider any drug NOT listed as compatible to be INCOMPATIBLE until consulting a pharmacist; specific conditions may apply.
May be inactivated in solution with aminoglycosides (e.g., amikacin, gentamicin). Do not mix in the same solution. Appropriate spacing and/or separate sites required. See Drug/Lab Interactions.

One source suggests the following **compatibilities:**
Additive: Aztreonam (Azactam).
Y-site: Amifostine (Ethyol), anidulafungin (Eraxis), aztreonam (Azactam), bivalirudin (Angiomax), cisatracurium (Nimbex), dexmedetomidine (Precedex), diltiazem (Cardizem), docetaxel (Taxotere), enalaprilat (Vasotec IV), etoposide phosphate (Etopophos), famotidine (Pepcid IV), fenoldopam (Corlopam), filgrastim (Neupogen), fluconazole (Diflucan), fludarabine (Fludara), gallium nitrate (Ganite), gemcitabine (Gemzar), granisetron (Kytril), heparin, hetastarch in electrolytes (Hextend), insulin (regular), linezolid (Zyvox), meperidine (Demerol), morphine, paclitaxel (Taxol), palonosetron (Aloxi), pemetrexed (Alimta), remifentanil (Ultiva), tacrolimus (Prograf), telavancin (Vibativ), teniposide (Vumon), theophylline, thiotepa, vancomycin.

RATE OF ADMINISTRATION
IV injection: A single dose over a minimum of 10 to 15 minutes.
Intermittent IV: A single dose over 15 to 30 minutes or longer, depending on amount of solution. Too-rapid injection may cause seizures.

ACTIONS
A semi-synthetic penicillin. The addition of sulbactam extends the antibacterial spectrum of ampicillin to include many bacteria normally resistant to it and to other beta-lactam antibacterials. A broad-spectrum antibiotic and beta-lactamase inhibitor effective against selected gram-positive, gram-negative, and anaerobic organisms (see literature). Inhibits bacterial cell wall synthesis. Peak serum levels achieved by end of infusion. Widely distributed into many body tissues and fluids. Half-life is 1 hour. Crosses the placental barrier. Excreted in the urine. Secreted in breast milk.

INDICATIONS AND USES
Treatment of skin and skin structure and intra-abdominal and gynecologic infections due to susceptible strains of specific organisms.

CONTRAINDICATIONS
History of serious hypersensitivity reactions (e.g., anaphylaxis or Stevens-Johnson syndrome) to ampicillin, sulbactam, or other beta-lactam antibacterial drugs (e.g., penicillins and cephalosporins). ▪ Patients with a previous history of cholestatic jaundice/hepatic dysfunction associated with ampicillin/sulbactam. ▪ Infectious mononucleosis because of increased incidence of rash.

PRECAUTIONS
Hypersensitivity reactions, including fatalities, have been reported in patients undergoing penicillin therapy; most likely to occur in patients with a history of penicillin allergy or sensitivity to multiple allergens. There have been reports of individuals with a history of penicillin hypersensitivity experiencing severe reactions when treated with cephalosporins. Check history of previous hypersensitivity reactions to penicillins, cephalosporins, or other allergens. Actual incidence of cross-allergenicity not established but may be more common with first-generation cephalosporins. ▪ Hepatic dysfunction, including hepatitis and cholestatic jaundice, has been associated with the use of ampicillin/sulbactam. Hepatic toxicity is usually reversible; however, deaths have been reported. ▪ Studies indicated to determine the causative organism and susceptibility to ampicillin/sulbactam. ▪ To reduce the development of drug-resistant bacteria and maintain its effectiveness, ampicillin and sulbactam should be used to treat or prevent only those infections proven or strongly suspected to be caused by bacteria. ▪ Avoid prolonged use of this drug; superinfection caused by overgrowth of nonsusceptible organisms may result. ▪ *Clostridium difficile*–associated diarrhea (CDAD) has been reported.

May range from mild diarrhea to fatal colitis. Consider in patients who present with diarrhea during or after treatment with ampicillin and sulbactam.

Monitor: Watch for early symptoms of hypersensitivity reactions, especially in individuals with a history of allergic problems. ▪ AST may be increased. Renal, hepatic, and hematopoietic function should be checked during prolonged therapy. Hepatic function should be monitored at regular intervals in patients with hepatic impairment. ▪ May cause thrombophlebitis. Observe carefully and rotate infusion sites.

Patient Education: Promptly report fever, rash, sore throat, unusual bleeding or bruising, severe stomach cramps and/or diarrhea, seizures. ▪ May require alternate birth control. ▪ Promptly report diarrhea or bloody stools that occur during treatment or up to several months after an antibiotic has been discontinued; may indicate CDAD and require treatment.

Maternal/Child: Category B: studies in rabbits have not shown adverse effects on fertility or in the fetus. Use only if clearly needed. ▪ May cause diarrhea, candidiasis, or allergic response in nursing infants. ▪ Safety for IV use in pediatric patients over 1 year of age has been established for skin and skin structure infections but not for other uses; however, it is in use. Elimination rate markedly reduced in neonates. ▪ Safety and effectiveness of IM use in pediatric patients not established.

Elderly: Consider degree of age-related impaired renal function. ▪ See Dose Adjustments.

DRUG/LAB INTERACTIONS

Concurrent use with probenecid may increase ampicillin and sulbactam blood levels. ▪ Frequently used concomitantly with **aminoglycosides** (e.g., gentamicin), but these drugs must never be mixed in the same infusion (mutual inactivation). If given concurrently, administer at separate sites. ▪ May be antagonized by **bacteriostatic antibiotics** (e.g., chloramphenicol, erythromycin, tetracyclines); may interfere with bactericidal action. ▪ May decrease clearance and increase toxicity of **methotrexate.** ▪ Ampicillin-induced skin rash potentiated by **allopurinol** (Aloprim). ▪ False-positive glucose reaction with **Clinitest and Benedict's or Fehling's solution.** ▪ May cause **false values** in other lab tests; see literature.

SIDE EFFECTS

Full scope of hypersensitivity reactions, including anaphylaxis, is possible. Diarrhea and rash occur most frequently. Abdominal distension; burning, discomfort, and pain at injection site; candidiasis; chest pain; chills; decreased hemoglobin, hematocrit, RBC, WBC, lymphocytes, neutrophils, and platelets; decreased serum albumin and total protein; dysuria; edema; epistaxis; erythema; facial swelling; fatigue; flatulence; glossitis; headache; increased alkaline phosphatase, BUN, creatinine, LDH, AST, ALT; increased basophils, eosinophils, lymphocytes, monocytes, and platelets; itching; malaise; mucosal bleeding; nausea and vomiting; RBCs and hyaline casts in urine; substernal pain; thrombophlebitis; tightness in throat; and urine retention can occur. May cause CDAD. Higher than normal doses may cause neurologic adverse reactions, including convulsions, especially with impaired renal function.

Post-Marketing: Acute generalized exanthematous pustulosis, agranulocytosis, black "hairy" tongue, cholestasis, cholestatic hepatitis, erythema multiforme, exfoliative dermatitis, gastritis, hemolytic anemia, hyperbilirubinemia, jaundice, positive direct Coombs' test, Stevens-Johnson syndrome, stomatitis, thrombocytopenic purpura, toxic epidermal necrolysis, tubulointerstitial nephritis, and urticaria.

ANTIDOTE

Notify the physician of any side effect. For severe symptoms, discontinue the drug, treat hypersensitivity reactions as indicated (e.g., antihistamines, epinephrine, corticosteroids) and resuscitate as necessary. Treat CDAD with fluids, electrolytes, protein supplements, and oral vancomycin (Vancocin) or metronidazole (Flagyl) as indicated. In severe cases, surgical evaluation may be indicated. Hemodialysis may be effective in overdose.

ANIDULAFUNGIN

(a-**nid**-yoo-luh-**FUN**-jin)

Antifungal
(echinocandin)

Eraxis

USUAL DOSE

Candidemia and other Candida infections (intra-abdominal abscess and peritonitis): Begin with a *loading dose* of 200 mg as an infusion on Day 1. Follow with a daily dose of 100 mg as an infusion beginning on Day 2. Base duration of treatment on patient's clinical response. In general, antifungal therapy should continue for at least 14 days after the last positive culture.

Esophageal candidiasis: Begin with a *loading dose* of 100 mg as an infusion on Day 1. Follow with a daily dose of 50 mg as an infusion beginning on Day 2. Treat for a minimum of 14 days and for at least 7 days following resolution of symptoms. Relapse of esophageal candidiasis has occurred in patients with HIV infections; suppressive antifungal therapy may be considered after a course of treatment.

DOSE ADJUSTMENTS

No dose adjustment is indicated based on age, gender, or race; in patients with any degree of renal or hepatic insufficiency; or in patients using concomitant medications that are known metabolic substrates, inhibitors, or inducers of cytochrome P_{450} (CYP450) isoenzymes; see Drug/Lab Interactions. ▪ No dose adjustment is required in patients with HIV who are receiving concomitant antiretroviral therapy (e.g., HIV protease inhibitors [e.g., amprenavir (Agenerase), indinavir (Crixivan), nelfinavir (Viracept), ritonavir (Norvir), saquinavir (Invirase)]).

DILUTION

Each 50-mg vial must be reconstituted with 15 mL of SWFI, and each 100-mg vial must be reconstituted with 30 mL of SWFI. The resulting concentration is 3.33 mg/mL. Aseptically transfer the reconstituted dose (50, 100, or 200 mg) into the appropriately sized IV container of D5W or NS for infusion as shown in the following chart. The final concentration of infusion solution is 0.77 mg/mL.

Dilution Requirements for Administration of Anidulafungin				
Dose (mg)	Number of Unit Packs Required	Total Reconstituted Volume (mL)	Volume of NS or D5W for Infusion	Total Infusion Volume (mL)
50 mg	1-50 mg	15 mL	50 mL	65 mL
100 mg	2-50 mg or 1-100 mg	30 mL	100 mL	130 mL
200 mg	4-50 mg or 2-100 mg	60 mL	200 mL	260 mL

Filters: No data available from manufacturer.

Storage: Store unopened vials at 2° to 8° C (36° to 46° F). Do not freeze. Excursions for 96 hours up to 25° C (77° F) are permitted, and the vial can be returned to storage at 2° to 8° C. Reconstituted solution can be stored at up to 25° C (77° F) for up to 24 hours. Infusion solution can be stored at temperatures up to 25° C for up to 48 hours or stored frozen for at least 72 hours.

COMPATIBILITY   (Underline Indicates Conflicting Compatibility Information)

Consider any drug NOT listed as compatible to be INCOMPATIBLE until consulting a pharmacist; specific conditions may apply.

Manufacturer states, "Do not mix or co-infuse with other medications or electrolytes. **Compatibility** of anidulafungin with intravenous substances, additives, or medications other than D5W or NS has not been established."

One source suggests the following **compatibilities:**

Y-site: Acyclovir (Zovirax), amikacin, aminophylline, amphotericin B lipid complex (Abelcet), amphotericin liposomal (AmBisome), ampicillin, ampicillin/sulbactam (Unasyn), carboplatin (Paraplatin), cefazolin (Ancef), cefepime (Maxipime), cefoxitin (Mefoxin), ceftazidime (Fortaz), ceftriaxone (Rocephin), cefuroxime (Zinacef), ciprofloxacin (Cipro IV), cisplatin, clindamycin (Cleocin), cyclophosphamide (Cytoxan), cyclosporine (Sandimmune), cytarabine (ARA-C), daunorubicin (Cerubidine), dexamethasone (Decadron), digoxin (Lanoxin), dobutamine, docetaxel (Taxotere), dopamine, doripenem (Doribax), doxorubicin (Adriamycin), epinephrine (Adrenalin), erythromycin (Erythrocin), etoposide phosphate (Etopophos), famotidine (Pepcid IV), fentanyl, fluconazole (Diflucan), fluorouracil (5-FU), furosemide (Lasix), ganciclovir (Cytovene IV), gemcitabine (Gemzar), gentamicin, heparin, hydrocortisone sodium succinate (Solu-Cortef), ifosfamide (Ifex), imipenem-cilastatin (Primaxin), leucovorin calcium, levofloxacin (Levaquin), linezolid (Zyvox), meperidine (Demerol), meropenem (Merrem IV), methylprednisolone (Solu-Medrol), metronidazole (Flagyl IV), midazolam (Versed), morphine, mycophenolate (CellCept IV), norepinephrine (Levophed), paclitaxel (Taxol), pantoprazole (Protonix IV), phenylephrine (Neo-Synephrine), piperacillin/tazobactam (Zosyn), potassium chloride, quinupristin/dalfopristin (Synercid), ranitidine (Zantac), sulfamethoxazole/trimethoprim, tacrolimus (Prograf), ticarcillin/clavulanate (Timentin), tobramycin, vancomycin, vincristine, voriconazole (VFEND IV), zidovudine (AZT, Retrovir).

RATE OF ADMINISTRATION
Flush IV line with D5W or NS before and after infusion. **Do not exceed an infusion rate of 1.1 mg/min** (equivalent to 1.4 mL/min or 84 mL/hr when diluted as directed). Infusion at a rate greater than 1.1 mg/min may cause histamine-mediated reactions (e.g., bronchospasm, dyspnea, flushing, hypotension, pruritus, rash, urticaria).

ACTIONS
A semi-synthetic lipopeptide, anidulafungin is an echinocandin, the newest class of antifungal agents. Acts by inhibiting the synthesis of 1,3-beta-D-glucan, an integral component of the fungal cell wall not present in mammalian cells. Extensively protein bound. Steady state is achieved after a loading dose. Not metabolized, it undergoes slow chemical degradation. Hepatic metabolism has not been observed. Anidulafungin is not a clinically relevant substrate, inducer, or inhibitor of cytochrome P_{450} (CYP450) isoenzymes. Terminal half-life ranges from 40 to 50 hours. Some excretion in feces, with minimal excretion in urine.

INDICATIONS AND USES
Treatment of the following fungal infections: candidemia and other forms of *Candida* infections (intra-abdominal abscess and peritonitis) and esophageal candidiasis. **Limitation of use:** Has not been studied in *Candida* infections associated with endocarditis, osteomyelitis, and meningitis. ■ Has not been studied in sufficient numbers of neutropenic patients to determine effectiveness.

CONTRAINDICATIONS
Hypersensitivity to anidulafungin or any of its components (e.g., fructose, mannitol, polysorbate 80, tartaric acid, sodium hydroxide, and/or hydrochloric acid) or to other echinocandins (e.g., micafungin [Mycamine]).

PRECAUTIONS
Do not give as an IV bolus; for IV infusion only. ■ Abnormal liver function tests have been reported. Isolated cases of significant hepatic dysfunction, hepatitis, or worsening hepatic failure have occurred. Incidence may be increased in patients with serious underlying conditions who are receiving additional concomitant medications. Evaluate risk versus benefit of continued anidulafungin therapy. ■ During studies, endoscopically documented relapse rates were higher in patients treated for esophageal candidiasis with anidulafungin than in patients treated with fluconazole (Diflucan). ■ *Candida* isolates with reduced susceptibility to anidulafungin have been reported, which suggests a poten-

tial for development of drug resistance. Clinical significance unknown. Cross-resistance with other echinocandins (e.g., micafungin [Mycamine]) has not been studied. ▪ Has been shown to be active against *Candida albicans* resistant to fluconazole (Diflucan). ▪ See Monitor and Antidote.

Monitor: Specimens for fungal culture, serologic testing, and histopathologic testing should be obtained before therapy to isolate and identify causative organisms. Therapy may begin as soon as all specimens are obtained and before results are known. Reassess after test results are known. ▪ Baseline CBC with differential and platelet count, BUN, and liver function tests (e.g., ALT, AST) may be indicated. ▪ Monitor for evidence of impaired hepatic function (e.g., increased ALT, AST, serum alkaline phosphatase). ▪ Monitor for S/S of infusion-related, possibly histamine-related, adverse reactions (e.g., bronchospasm, dyspnea, flushing, hypotension, pruritus, rash, urticaria). ▪ Anaphylaxis, including shock, has been reported. Monitor for S/S of a hypersensitivity reaction (e.g., bronchospasm, dyspnea, hives, hypotension, pruritus, rash, swelling of eyelids, lips, or face); discontinue infusion if a hypersensitivity reaction occurs.

Patient Education: Promptly report any hypersensitivity or infusion-related reactions (e.g., bronchospasm, dyspnea, dizziness, flushing, itching, rash, urticaria). Report S/S of liver dysfunction (anorexia, fatigue, jaundice, nausea and vomiting, dark urine, or pale stools).

Maternal/Child: Category B: use during pregnancy only if benefits justify risk to fetus. Some abnormalities, including skeletal changes, occurred in animal studies. ▪ Use caution if required during breast-feeding. Secreted in milk of drug-treated rats; not known if anidulafungin is secreted in human milk. ▪ Safety and effectiveness for use in pediatric patients 16 years of age or younger have not been established; however, some immunocompromised pediatric (2 through 11 years) and adolescent (12 through 17 years) patients with neutropenia were included in studies; see prescribing information.

Elderly: Differences in response compared to younger adults not identified.

DRUG/LAB INTERACTIONS

Anidulafungin is not a clinically relevant substrate, inducer, or inhibitor of cytochrome P_{450} (CYP450) isoenzymes. It is considered unlikely that it will have a clinically relevant effect on the metabolism of drugs metabolized by CYP450 isoenzymes and/or other drugs likely to be coadministered with it. ▪ No dose adjustment of either drug is indicated when coadministered with **cyclosporine** (Sandimmune), **tacrolimus** (Prograf), **or voriconazole** (VFEND IV). ▪ No dose adjustment of anidulafungin is indicated when it is coadministered with **liposomal amphotericin B** (AmBisome) **or rifampin** (Rifadin).

SIDE EFFECTS

Patients treated for candidemia and other *Candida* infections: Deep vein thrombosis; diarrhea; elevated ALT, AST, alkaline phosphatase; fever; hypokalemia; insomnia; nausea; vomiting.

Patients treated for esophageal candidiasis: Anemia; diarrhea; dyspepsia (aggravated); elevated ALT, AST, and gamma-glutamyl transferase; fever; headache; leukopenia; nausea; neutropenia; phlebitis; rash; and vomiting.

Histamine-mediated reactions (e.g., bronchospasm, dyspnea, flushing, hypotension, pruritus, rash, urticaria) or hypersensitivity reactions (including anaphylaxis) may occur. Significant hepatic dysfunction (e.g., hepatitis, hepatocellular damage, hyperbilirubinemia, or hepatic failure) has occurred. Many other side effects have been reported in small numbers of patients.

Post-Marketing: Anaphylactic reaction, anaphylactic shock, bronchospasm.

ANTIDOTE

Notify physician of all side effects; most will be treated symptomatically. Reduce rate of infusion if a histamine-mediated reaction occurs. If a hypersensitivity reaction occurs, discontinue anidulafungin and treat as indicated. Appropriate treatment may include oxygen, epinephrine, antihistamines (e.g., diphenhydramine [Benadryl]), vasopressors (e.g., dopamine), corticosteroids, IV fluids, and ventilation equipment. S/S indicative of hepatic side effects may require evaluation of benefits versus risk of continuing anidulafungin therapy. Not removed by hemodialysis. Resuscitate as indicated.

ANTIHEMOPHILIC FACTOR (HUMAN ▪ RECOMBINANT ▪ RECOMBINANT [Fc FUSION PROTEIN] ▪ RECOMBINANT [PEGYLATED] ▪ RECOMBINANT [PORCINE SEQUENCE]*)

Antihemophilic agent

(an-tie-hee-moe-**FIL**-ik **FAK**-tor)

AHF, Factor VIII ▪ **Hemofil M, Koate DVI, Monoclate-P**
▪ **Advate, Helixate FS, Kogenate FS, Kogenate FS Bio-Set, Kovaltry, Kovaltry Bio-Set, Novoeight, Nuwiq, Recombinate, Xyntha, Xyntha Solofuse** ▪ **Eloctate** ▪ **Adynovate** ▪ **Obizur***

*Recombinant (Porcine Sequence [Obizur]) is indicated for use only in acquired hemophilia. Not indicated for use in congenital hemophilia A.

Available factor VIII products and their origins include the following:

Hemofil M, Koate DVI, Monoclate-P (Human): Blood product derivatives. May contain trace amounts of mouse or hamster protein.

Advate, Helixate FS, Kogenate FS, Kogenate FS Bio-Set, Kovaltry, Kovaltry Bio-Set, Novoeight, Xyntha, Xyntha Solofuse (Recombinant): Stabilized without human albumin. No human or animal-derived proteins are used in the purification or formulation processes. May contain trace amounts of mouse or hamster protein.

Recombinate (Recombinant): Stabilized in human albumin. May contain bovine protein and trace amounts of mouse or hamster protein.

Eloctate (Recombinant): B-domain–deleted recombinant factor VIII Fc (BDD-rFVIIIFc) fusion protein is the active ingredient. No human or animal-derived proteins are used in the purification or formulation processes.

Nuwiq (Recombinant): B-domain–deleted recombinant factor VIII (BDD-rFVIII) is the active ingredient. No human or animal-derived proteins are used in the purification or formulation processes.

Adynovate (Recombinant) PEGylated: The cell culture, pegylation, purification process, and formulation do not use additives of human or animal origins. May contain trace amounts of hamster protein.

Obizur* (Recombinant): Porcine sequence. May contain trace amounts of hamster protein.

Alphanate and Humate P (see AHF and von Willebrand Factor Complex monograph): From human plasma; intermediate and high purity.

USUAL DOSE (International units [IU])

Adults and pediatric patients: Dosing is completely individualized. Dose, frequency, and duration of treatment are based on severity of the factor VIII deficiency, location and extent of bleeding, clinical condition of the patient, desired antihemophilic factor level, body weight, and presence of factor VIII inhibitors. Measure factor VIII level before administration. In general, a dose of 1 IU/kg will raise the plasma factor VIII activity by 2 IU/dL. On average, a plasma antihemophilic factor level of 20% to 40% of normal is required to control minor hemorrhage. A level of 30% to 60% of normal may be required to control moderate bleeding; greater percentages are required for major bleeding or surgical procedures.

All products except Obizur use a variation of the following formula.

To calculate the dose needed based on a desired factor VIII increase (%):

Dose (IU) = Body weight (kg) × Desired factor VIII increase (IU/dL or % of normal) × 0.5

Continued

To calculate the expected % factor VIII increase for a given dose:

Expected % factor VIII increase = (# Units administered × 2) ÷ Body weight (kg)

The following charts outline AHF dosing recommendations for the various AHF products. *Consult individual product labeling for more detailed information.*

Control and Prevention of Bleeding Episodes				
	AHF Product	**Required Peak Postinfusion Factor VIII Activity (as % of Normal or IU/dL)**	**Dose (IU/kg)**	**Frequency and Duration of Therapy**
Minor Early hemarthrosis, mild muscle bleed, or mild oral bleed Superficial muscle or soft tissue and oral bleeds	Advate	20 to 40	10 to 20 IU/kg	Repeat every 12 to 24 hr (8 to 24 hr in patients under 6 years of age) for 1 to 3 days until bleeding is resolved or healing is achieved.
	Adynovate	20 to 40	10 to 20 IU/kg	Repeat every 12 to 24 hr until bleeding is resolved.
	Eloctate	40 to 60	20 to 30 IU/kg	Repeat every 24 to 48 hr (12 to 24 hr in patients under 6 years of age) until bleeding is resolved or healing is achieved.
	Helixate FS Kogenate FS	20 to 40	10 to 20 IU/kg	Repeat dose if there is evidence of further bleeding until bleeding is resolved.
	Koate DVI	20	10 IU/kg	May respond to a single dose. Repeat if there is evidence of further bleeding.
	Kovaltry Kovaltry Bio-Set	20 to 40	See formula	Repeat every 12 to 24 hr for at least 1 day until bleeding episode as indicated by pain is resolved or healing is achieved.
	Monoclate P	30	See formula	May respond to a single dose. Repeat if there is evidence of further bleeding.
	Novoeight Recombinate Xyantha Hemofil M	20 to 40	See formula	Repeat every 12 to 24 hr for at least 1 day (usually 1 to 3 days) until bleeding is resolved or healing is achieved.
	Nuwiq	20 to 40	See formula	Repeat every 12 to 24 hr for at least 1 day, until bleeding is resolved.
Moderate Moderate bleeding into muscle, bleeding into oral cavity, definite hemarthroses, and known trauma	Advate	30 to 60	15 to 30 IU/kg	Repeat every 12 to 24 hr (8 to 24 hr in patients under 6 years of age) for 3 days or more until bleeding is resolved or healing is achieved.
	Adynovate	30 to 60	15 to 30 IU/kg	Repeat every 12 to 24 hr until bleeding is resolved.
	Eloctate	40 to 60	20 to 30 IU/kg	Repeat every 24 to 48 hr (12 to 24 hr in patients under 6 years of age) until bleeding is resolved or healing is achieved.

Continued

		Control and Prevention of Bleeding Episodes—cont'd		
	AHF Product	Required Peak Postinfusion Factor VIII Activity (as % of Normal or IU/dL)	Dose (IU/kg)	Frequency and Duration of Therapy
Moderate Moderate bleeding into muscle, bleeding into oral cavity, definite hemarthroses, and known trauma—cont'd	Helixate FS Kogenate FS	30 to 60	15 to 30 IU/kg	Repeat every 12 to 24 hr until bleeding is resolved.
	Koate DVI Monoclate P	30 to 50	Initial: 15 to 25 IU/kg Repeat: 10 to 15 IU/kg	Repeat with lower dose every 8 to 12 hr if needed until bleeding is resolved or healing is achieved.
	Kovaltry Kovaltry Bio-Set	30 to 60	See formula	Repeat every 12 to 24 hr for 3 to 4 days or more until pain and acute disability are resolved.
	Novoeight Recombinate Xyntha Hemofil M	30 to 60	See formula	Repeat every 12 to 24 hr until pain and acute disability are resolved and/or adequate local hemostasis is achieved (approximately 3 to 4 days).
	Nuwiq	30 to 60	See formula	Repeat every 12 to 24 hr for 3 to 4 days or more until bleeding is resolved.
Major Significant GI bleed; intracranial, intra-abdominal, or intrathoracic bleeding; CNS bleeding; bleeding into retropharyngeal or retroperitoneal spaces or iliopsoas sheath or into eyes/retina; fractures; head trauma	Advate	60 to 100	30 to 50 IU/kg	Repeat every 8 to 24 hr (6 to 12 hr in patients under 6 years of age) for 3 days or more until bleeding is resolved or healing is achieved.
	Adynovate	60 to 100	30 to 50 IU/kg	Repeat every 8 to 24 hr until bleeding is resolved.
	Eloctate	80 to 100	40 to 50 IU/kg	Repeat every 12 to 24 hr (8 to 24 hr in patients under 6 years of age) until bleeding is resolved or healing is achieved (approximately 7 to 10 days).
	Helixate FS Kogenate FS	80 to 100	Initial: 40 to 50 IU/kg Repeat: 20 to 25 IU/kg	Every 8 to 12 hr until bleeding is resolved.
	Koate DVI Monoclate P	80 to 100	Initial: 40 to 50 IU/kg Repeat: 20 to 25 IU/kg	Every 8 to 12 hr until bleeding is resolved.
	Kovaltry Kovaltry Bio-Set	60 to 100	See formula	Repeat every 8 to 24 hr until bleeding is resolved.
	Novoeight Recombinate Xyantha Hemofil M	60 to 100	See formula	Repeat every 8 to 24 hr until bleeding is resolved (approximately 7 to 10 days).
	Nuwiq	60 to 100	See formula	Repeat every 8 to 24 hr until bleeding is resolved.

Continued

Perioperative Management (Surgical Prophylaxis)			
Type of Surgery	AHF Product	Required Peak Postinfusion Factor VIII Activity (as % of Normal or IU/dL)	Dose, Frequency, and Duration of Therapy
Minor Including tooth extraction	Advate	60 to 100	A single bolus infusion (30 to 50 IU/kg) beginning within 1 hr of operation. Optional additional dosing every 12 to 24 hr as needed to control bleeding. For dental procedures, adjunctive therapy may be considered.
	Eloctate	50 to 80	25 to 40 IU/kg. Repeat every 24 hr (12 to 24 hr in patients under 6 years of age). Continue for at least 1 day until healing is achieved.
	Helixate FS Kogenate FS	30 to 60	15 to 30 IU/kg. Repeat every 12 to 24 hr until bleeding is resolved.
	Koate DVI	Not listed	See Major. Less intensive treatment schedules may provide adequate hemostasis.
	Kovaltry Kovaltry Bio-Set	30 to 60 Preoperative and postoperative	See formula. Repeat every 24 hr for at least 1 day until healing is achieved.
	Monoclate P	30 to 50	Initial dose of 15 to 25 IU/kg. Follow with repeat doses of 10 to 15 IU/kg every 8 to 12 hr if needed.
	Novoeight	30 to 60	See formula. Repeat every 24 hr for at least 1 day until healing is achieved.
	Nuwiq	30 to 60 Preoperative and postoperative	See formula. Repeat dose every 24 hr. Continue at least 1 day until healing is achieved.
	Recombinate Hemofil M	60 to 80	See formula. A single infusion plus oral antifibrinolytic therapy within 1 hr is sufficient in approximately 70% of cases.
	Xyantha	30 to 60	See formula. Repeat every 12 to 24 hr for 3 to 4 days until adequate local hemostasis is achieved. For tooth extraction, a single infusion plus oral antifibrinolytic therapy within 1 hr may be sufficient.
Major Examples include intracranial, intra-abdominal, or intrathoracic surgery, joint replacement surgery	Advate	80 to 120 Preoperative and postoperative	Preoperative: 40 to 60 IU/kg. Verify 100% activity has been achieved before surgery. Maintenance: 40 to 60 IU/kg every 8 to 24 hr (6 to 24 hr in patients under 6 years of age) depending on desired level of factor VIII and state of wound healing.
	Eloctate	80 to 120 Preoperative and postoperative	Preoperative: 40 to 60 IU/kg. Verify 100% activity has been achieved before surgery. Follow with a repeat dose of 40 to 50 IU/kg after 8 to 24 hr (6 to 24 hr in patients under 6 years of age) and then every 24 hr to maintain factor VIII activity within target range until adequate wound healing; then continue for at least 7 days to maintain factor VIII activity within target range.

Continued

Perioperative Management (Surgical Prophylaxis)—cont'd			
Type of Surgery	AHF Product	Required Peak Postinfusion Factor VIII Activity (as % of Normal or IU/dL)	Dose, Frequency, and Duration of Therapy
Major Examples include intracranial, intraabdominal, or intrathoracic surgery, joint replacement surgery— cont'd	Helixate FS Kogenate FS	100	50 IU/kg preoperatively to achieve 100% activity. Repeat every 6 to 12 hr to keep factor VIII activity in desired range. Continue until healing is achieved.
	Koate DVI	100	50 IU/kg. Verify 100% activity has been achieved before surgery. Repeat infusions every 6 to 12 hr initially and for a total of 10 to 14 days until healing is complete.
	Kovaltry Kovaltry Bio-Set	80 to 100 Preoperative and postoperative	See formula. Repeat every 8 to 24 hr until adequate wound healing is achieved, then continue for at least another 7 days to maintain factor VIII activity of 30% to 60% (IU/dL).
	Monoclate P	80 to 100	See formula. A second dose, $^1/_2$ the amount of the initial dose, should be given in 5 hours. Dose to achieve factor VIII levels of at least 30% (IU/dL) for 10 to 14 days.
	Novoeight	80 to 100 Preoperative and postoperative	See formula. Continue every 8 to 24 hr until adequate wound healing. Continue at reduced dose for at least 7 days to maintain a factor VIII activity at 30% to 60% (IU/dL).
	Nuwiq	80 to 100 Preoperative and postoperative	See formula. Repeat dose every 8 to 24 hr until adequate wound healing, then continue therapy for at least another 7 days to maintain a factor VIII activity of 30% to 60% (IU/dL).
	Recombinate Hemofil M	80 to 100 Preoperative and postoperative	See formula. Continue every 8 to 24 hr depending on the state of wound healing.
	Xyantha	60 to 100	See formula. Continue every 8 to 24 hr until threat is resolved or, in the case of surgery, until adequate local hemostasis and wound healing are achieved.

Obizur (porcine preparation): Obizur does not use a formula. **Indicated for use only in acquired hemophilia. Not indicated for use in congenital hemophilia A.** The recommended dose of Obizur for minor, moderate, and/or major bleeding is 200 units/kg as an initial dose. Subsequent doses may be given every 4 to 12 hours and should be titrated to individual clinical response and to maintain recommended factor VIII trough levels (50% to 100% of normal for minor or moderate bleeding and 100% to 200% of normal for an acute bleed, decreasing to 50% to 100% of normal after acute bleed is controlled, if required). Maintain the factor VIII activity within the target range. Plasma levels of factor VIII should not exceed 200% of normal or 200 units/dL.

Routine prophylaxis to prevent or reduce the frequency of bleeding (e.g., severe factor VIII deficiency with frequent hemorrhages):

Advate: 20 to 40 units/kg every other day (3 to 4 times per week). Alternately, an every-third-day dosing regimen targeted to maintain factor VIII trough levels greater than or equal to 1% may be used. Adjust dose based on patient response.

Adynovate: Administer 40 to 50 IU /kg 2 times per week. Adjust dose based on patient's clinical response.

Continued

Eloctate: Initiate therapy with a dose of 50 units/kg every 4 days. Adjust dose based on patient response (range 25 to 65 units/kg at 3- to 5-day intervals). More frequent or higher doses up to 80 units/kg may be required in pediatric patients less than 6 years of age.

Helixate FS and Kogenate FS: *Adults:* 25 units/kg 3 times a week. *Pediatric patients:* 25 units/kg every other day.

Kovaltry, Kovaltry Bio-Set: *Adults and adolescents:* 20 to 40 IU/kg 2 or 3 times a week. *Pediatric patients 12 years of age or younger:* 25 to 50 IU/kg twice weekly, 3 times weekly, or every other day according to individual requirements.

Novoeight: *Adults and adolescents (12 years of age or older):* 20 to 50 units/kg 3 times a week or 20 to 40 IU/kg every other day. *Pediatric patients (less than 12 years of age):* 25 to 60 IU/kg 3 times a week or 25 to 50 IU/kg every other day.

Nuwiq: *Adults and adolescents (12 to 17 years of age):* 30 to 40 IU/kg every other day. *Pediatric patients (2 to 11 years of age):* 30 to 50 IU/kg every other day or 3 times per week.

DOSE ADJUSTMENTS

Titrate the dose to the patient's clinical response. ▪ If factor VIII level fails to increase as expected or if bleeding is not controlled after administration of the calculated dose, factor VIII antibodies are probable; may respond to an increased dose, especially if titer is less than 10 Bethesda units/mL. Frequent determinations of circulating AHF levels indicated. ▪ Higher or more frequent dosing may be required in pediatric patients.

DILUTION

Products are available in multiple strengths. Actual number of AHF units is shown on each vial. Consult package insert of product to obtain product-specific information on dilution. All preparations provide diluent, and most provide administration equipment that may include transfer devices, needles (single- or double-ended), filters or filter needles, syringes, vial adapters, and/or administration sets for each vial. Use only the diluent provided, and maintain strict aseptic technique. Warm to room temperature (25° C) before dilution and maintain throughout administration to avoid precipitation of active ingredients. If more than one package is required to achieve the desired dose, multiple packages may be drawn into the same container (e.g., syringe). Follow manufacturer's instructions. Products do not contain a preservative, and all products must be used within 3 hours of reconstitution (4 hours for Novoeight).

Filters: Supplied by manufacturer if required.

Storage: Consult package insert of product to obtain product-specific information on storage requirements. Before reconstitution, store all formulations in original packages to protect from light at 2° to 8° C (35° to 46° F). (Recombinate may be stored at RT or under refrigeration.) Do not freeze. **All formulations except Adynovate and Obizur** can be stored at CRT for 2 months or longer before reconstitution. **Adynovate** can be stored at CRT for up to 1 month. Do not return to the refrigerator after storage at CRT. **Obizur** should be refrigerated until use. Do not use beyond expiration dates on bottles.

COMPATIBILITY

Administration through a separate line without mixing with other IV fluids or medications is recommended.

RATE OF ADMINISTRATION

Use administration set supplied by manufacturer, if provided. Rate of administration is based on patient comfort. Reduce rate of infusion or temporarily discontinue if there is a significant increase in heart rate or if S/S of hypersensitivity occur.

Advate, Adynovate: A single dose over 5 minutes or less. Do not exceed a rate of 10 mL/min.

Eloctate, Hemofil M: A single dose administered at a rate not to exceed 10 mL/min.

Helixate FS, Kogenate FS, Kogenate FS Bio-Set, Kovaltry, Kovaltry Bio-Set: A single dose over 1 to 15 minutes is usually well tolerated.

Koate-DVI: A single dose over 5 to 10 minutes.

Monoclate-P: A single dose at a rate of 2 mL/min.

Novoeight: A single dose over 2 to 5 minutes.

Nuwiq: A single dose at a maximum rate of 4 mL/min.

Obizur: A single dose at a rate of 1 to 2 mL/min.
Recombinate (reconstituted with 5 mL of SWFI): Do not exceed a rate of 5 mL/min.
Recombinate (reconstituted with 10 mL SWFI): Do not exceed a rate of 10 mL/min.
Xyntha, Xyntha Solofuse: A single dose over several minutes, based on patient comfort.

ACTIONS

AHF is one of nine major factors in the blood that must act in sequence to produce co-agulation, or clotting. It is the specific clotting factor deficient in patients with hemo-philia A (classic hemophilia). Administration of AHF can temporarily correct the coagu-lation defect in these patients. One international unit (IU) of AHF is approximately equal to the level of factor VIII activity in 1 mL of fresh pooled human plasma. **Adynovate** ex-hibits an extended terminal half-life through pegylation of the parent molecule, Advate, which reduces binding to the physiologic factor VIII clearance receptor (LRP1).
Recombinant porcine sequence AHF (Obizur): Patients with acquired hemophilia have nor-mal factor VIII genes but develop autoantibodies against their own factor VIII (i.e., in-hibitors). These autoantibodies neutralize circulating human factor VIII and create a functional deficiency of factor VIII. Obizur temporarily replaces the inhibited endoge-nous factor VIII that is needed for effective hemostasis in patients with acquired hemo-philia A.

INDICATIONS AND USES

On-demand treatment and control of bleeding episodes in adults and pediatric patients with hemophilia A (congenital factor VIII deficiency) **(all products *except* Adynovate and Obizur).** ▪ Perioperative management (surgical prophylaxis) in adults and pediatric pa-tients with hemophilia A **(all products *except* Obizur).** ▪ Routine prophylaxis to prevent or reduce the frequency of bleeding in adults and pediatric patients with hemophilia A **(Advate, Eloctate, Helixate FS, Kogenate FS, Kovaltry, Kovaltry Bio-Set, Novoeight, Nuwiq).** ▪ Routine prophylaxis to prevent bleeding episodes and risk of joint damage in pediatric patients without pre-existing joint damage **(Helixate FS, Kogenate FS).** ▪ Control and pre-vention of bleeding episodes in adolescent and adult patients (12 years and older) with hemophilia A and routine prophylaxis to reduce the frequency of bleeding episodes **(Adynovate).** ▪ Treatment of bleeding episodes in adults with *acquired hemophilia A* **(Obizur).**
Limitations of use: *All products:* Not indicated for treatment of von Willebrand disease. *Obizur:* Safety and efficacy of **Obizur** has not been established in patients with a baseline anti-porcine factor VIII inhibitor titer of greater than 20 Bethesda units. ▪ **Obizur is not indicated for treatment of congenital hemophilia A.**

CONTRAINDICATIONS

All products: Hypersensitivity to the specific product or to any component of a product (e.g., mouse, hamster, or bovine protein [monoclonal antibody–derived factor VIII, por-cine sequence]; various stabilizers; polysorbate 80).

PRECAUTIONS

Should be administered under the direction of a physician specialist. ▪ Hypersensitivity reactions (including anaphylaxis) are possible. ▪ Formation of neutralizing antibodies (inhibitors) to factor VIII can occur; see Monitor. ▪ Plasma-derived products may con-tain infectious agents that can cause disease (e.g., viruses and, theoretically, the Creutzfeldt-Jakob disease agent). The risk that these products will transmit an infectious agent has been reduced by screening plasma donors, testing for the presence of viruses, and inactivating and/or removing certain viruses during manufacturing. Hepatitis A and parvovirus 19 have been reported infrequently with plasma-based products, usually in immunocompromised patients or pregnant women. ▪ Intravascular hemolysis can occur when large volumes of plasma-derived products are given to individuals with blood groups A, B, or AB. Monitor for progressive anemia. ▪ Components of some products may contain latex; use caution to avoid a hypersensitivity reaction. ▪ Hemophilic pa-tients with cardiovascular risk factors or diseases may be at the same risk as nonhemo-philic patients for developing cardiovascular events when clotting has been normalized by treatment with factor VIII. ▪ Treatment of choice when volume or RBC replacement

is not needed; avoids hypervolemia and hyperproteinemia. ▪ Not useful to treat other coagulation factor deficiencies. ▪ Catheter-related infections may occur if antihemophilic factor is administered via central venous access devices (CVADs). These infections have not been associated with the actual AHF product. ▪ Desmopressin may be the preferred treatment for mild to moderate hemophilia A (AHF levels that are at least 5%).
Monitor: *All products:* Identification of factor VIII deficiency with determination of circulating AHF levels should be obtained before administration. Monitor plasma factor VIII activity by the one-stage clotting assay to confirm that adequate factor VIII levels have been achieved and maintained. Adjust dose as indicated. ▪ Monitor heart rate before and during treatment. ▪ Monitor for the development of factor VIII inhibitors. Should be suspected if factor VIII plasma levels are not obtained or if bleeding is not controlled with an appropriate dose. The Bethesda inhibitor assay determines if factor VIII inhibitors are present. Bethesda Units (BU) are used to report inhibitor levels. ▪ Monitor patients with a known or suspected inhibitor to factor VIII more frequently. ▪ Monitor for S/S of a hypersensitivity reaction (e.g., anaphylaxis, angioedema, chest tightness, dizziness, dyspnea, face swelling, fever, flushing, hypotension, laryngeal edema, nausea, paresthesia, pruritus, rash, tachycardia, urticaria, vomiting, wheezing). ▪ Monitor patients with CVADs for S/S of infection. ▪ See Precautions.
Obizur: Monitor factor VIII activity 30 minutes and 3 hours after initial dose and 30 minutes after subsequent doses. Use of the Nijmegen-Bethesda inhibitor assay is recommended.
Patient Education: *All products:* Read manufacturer-supplied patient product information. ▪ Instruction for self-administration and proper storage and preparation may be appropriate. ▪ Discontinue antihemophilic factor and immediately report S/S of a hypersensitivity reaction (e.g., hives, hypotension, itching, rash, tightness of the chest, wheezing). ▪ Review prescription and nonprescription medications with a health care provider. ▪ Contact provider for lack of clinical response. May indicate development of inhibitors. ▪ Consult with health care provider before travel. Bring an adequate supply of AHF based on current treatment regimen.
Plasma-derived products: Report S/S of hepatitis A (e.g., persistent poor appetite and tiredness, fever, dark urine, yellowing of the skin, nausea, vomiting, and abdominal pain). ▪ Report S/S of parvovirus B19 (e.g., chills, drowsiness, fever, and runny nose followed 2 weeks later by a rash and joint pain).
Maternal/Child: Category C: use during pregnancy only if clearly needed. ▪ Use caution during breast-feeding. ▪ Advate, Helixate FS, Kogenate FS, Kovaltry, Kovaltry Bio-Set, and Recombinate have been used in pediatric patients of all ages, including infants. Other formulations are indicated for use in pediatric patients but did not include newborns in clinical trials. ▪ *All products:* Clearance (based on kg body weight) is higher in the pediatric population. Half-life is shorter; see Dose Adjustments. ▪ *Adynovate:* Safety and effectiveness in pediatric patients less than 12 years of age not established. ▪ *Obizur:* Safety and efficacy for use in pediatric patients not established.
Elderly: Numbers in clinical studies insufficient to determine if the elderly respond differently from younger subjects.

DRUG/LAB INTERACTIONS
Specific information not available.

SIDE EFFECTS
May respond to reduced rate of administration. Serious adverse reactions include hypersensitivity reactions and factor VIII inhibitors.
Plasma-based AHF: Abdominal pain, blurred vision, bradycardia, chills, clouding or loss of consciousness, diarrhea, dizziness, dysgeusia, factor VIII inhibition, fever, flushing, headache, hemolytic anemia, hyperfibrinogenemia, hypersensitivity reactions (anaphylaxis, backache, chills, erythema, fever, hives, hypotension, nausea, pruritus, rash, tightness of chest, urticaria, wheezing), lethargy, paresthesias, somnolence, stinging at infusion site, tachycardia, tingling, or vomiting may occur.

Recombinant products: The most commonly reported side effects included arthralgia, back pain, central venous access device–associated infections, chills, cough, dry mouth, epistaxis, fever, flushing, headache, increased hepatic enzymes, infusion site reactions (e.g., inflammation, pain), inhibitor formation in previously untreated or minimally treated patients, limb injury, malaise, nasopharyngitis, nausea, nonneutralizing anti–factor VIII antibody formation, paresthesia, skin-associated hypersensitivity reactions (e.g., pruritus, rash, urticaria), vertigo, and generalized hypersensitivity reactions, including anaphylaxis.

Obizur: In clinical trials, development of inhibitors to porcine factor VIII occurred in more than 5% of patients.

ANTIDOTE

Most side effects usually subside spontaneously in 15 to 20 minutes and are generally related to the rate of infusion. Keep the physician informed. Slow or discontinue infusion temporarily if heart rate increases or beginning S/S of a hypersensitivity reaction occur. Discontinue immediately and treat hypersensitivity reactions (antihistamines, epinephrine, corticosteroids). Resuscitate as necessary.

114

ANTIHEMOPHILIC FACTOR ▪ VON WILLEBRAND FACTOR COMPLEX (HUMAN)

(an-tie-hee-moe-**FIL**-ik **FAK**-tor)

Alphanate, Humate-P

USUAL DOSE
(International units [IU])

Completely individualized. Based on degree of deficiency, desired antihemophilic factor level, body weight, severity of bleeding, and presence of factor VIII inhibitors. One international unit (IU) of factor VIII or 1 IU of von Willebrand factor:Ristocetin Cofactor (vWF:RCof) is approximately equal to the level of factor VIII activity or vWF:RCof found in 1 mL of fresh pooled human plasma.

ALPHANATE

Treatment of hemophilia A (adults): Dose requirements and frequency are calculated on the basis of an expected initial response of 2% of normal FVIII:C IU/kg of body weight administered. Assess adequacy of treatment by clinical effects and monitoring of factor VIII activity. See Precautions. The following general dosages are recommended for adult patients:

Alphanate Dose Guidelines for the Treatment of Adults with Hemophilia A	
Hemorrhagic Event	Dosage (AHF FVIII:C IU/kg body weight)
Minor hemorrhage: Bruises, cuts, or scrapes or uncomplicated joint hemorrhage	FVIII:C levels should be brought to 30% of normal (15 FVIII IU/kg twice daily) until hemorrhage stops and healing has been achieved (1 to 2 days).
Moderate hemorrhage: Nose, mouth, and gum bleeds; dental extractions; hematuria	FVIII:C levels should be brought to 50% (25 FVIII IU/kg twice daily). Continue until healing has been achieved (2 to 7 days on average).
Major hemorrhage: Joint or muscle hemorrhage, major trauma, hematuria, intracranial and/or intraperitoneal bleeding	FVIII:C levels should be brought to 80% to 100% of normal for at least 3 to 5 days (40 to 50 FVIII IU/kg twice daily). Then maintain at 50% (25 FVIII IU/kg twice daily) until healing has been achieved. May require treatment for up to 10 days.
Surgery	Before surgery, FVIII:C levels should be brought to 80% to 100% of normal (40 to 50 FVIII IU/kg twice daily). For the next 7 to 10 days or until healing has been achieved, patient should be maintained at 60% to 100% FVIII levels (25 to 50 FVIII IU/kg twice daily).

IU, International unit.

Alphanate Dose Guidelines for Prophylaxis During Surgery and Invasive Procedures of Adult and Pediatric Patients with von Willebrand Disease (Except Type 3 Patients Undergoing Surgery)	
Bleeding Prophylaxis for Surgical or Invasive Procedures	Dosage (AHF vWF:RCof IU/kg body weight)
Adult	Preoperative dose: 60 vWF:RCof IU/kg body weight. Subsequent infusions: 40 to 60 vWF:RCof IU/kg body weight at 8- to 12-hour intervals as clinically needed. Dosing may be reduced after the third postoperative day. Continue treatment until healing is complete.
Adult	**Minor procedure:** vWF activity of 40% to 50% for at least 1 to 3 days postoperatively.
Adult	**Major procedure:** vWF activity of 40% to 50% for at least 3 to 7 days postoperatively.
Pediatric	Initial dose: 75 vWF:RCof IU/kg body weight. Subsequent infusions: 50 to 75 vWF:RCof IU/kg body weight at 8- to 12-hour intervals as clinically needed. Dosing may be reduced after the third postoperative day. Continue treatment until healing is complete.

IU, International unit.

Humate-P

Treatment of hemophilia A (adults): As a general rule, 1 IU of factor VIII activity per kg body weight will increase the circulating factor VIII level by approximately 2 IU/dL. Assess adequacy of treatment by clinical effects and monitoring of factor VIII activity. See Precautions. The following general dosages are recommended for adult patients:

Humate-P Dose Recommendations for the Treatment of Hemophilia A*	
Hemorrhage Event	Dosage (IU† FVIII:C/kg body weight)
Minor • Early joint or muscle bleed • Severe epistaxis	Loading dose 15 IU FVIII:C/kg to achieve FVIII:C plasma level of approximately 30% of normal; one infusion may be sufficient If needed, half of the loading dose may be given once or twice daily for 1-2 days
Moderate • Advanced joint or muscle bleed • Neck, tongue, or pharyngeal hematoma without airway compromise • Tooth extraction • Severe abdominal pain	Loading dose 25 IU FVIII:C/kg to achieve FVIII:C plasma level of approximately 50% of normal Followed by 15 IU FVIII:C/kg every 8-12 hours for first 1-2 days to maintain FVIII:C plasma level at 30% of normal Then same dose once or twice a day for up to 7 days or until adequate wound healing
Life-threatening • Major operations • Gastrointestinal bleeding • Neck, tongue, or pharyngeal hematoma with potential for airway compromise • Intracranial, intra-abdominal, or intrathoracic bleeding • Fractures	Initially 40-50 IU FVIII:C/kg Followed by 20-25 IU FVIII:C/kg every 8 hours to maintain FVIII:C plasma level at 80%-100% of normal for 7 days Then continue the same dose once or twice a day for another 7 days to maintain the FVIII:C level at 30%-50% of normal

*In all cases, the dose should be adjusted individually by clinical judgment of the potential for compromise of a vital structure and by frequent monitoring of factor VIII activity in the patient's plasma.
†*IU*, International unit.

Continued

Treatment of von Willebrand Disease (vWD) (adults and pediatric patients): As a rule, 40-80 IU vWF:RCof (corresponding to 16 to 32 IU factor VIII in Humate-P) per kg body weight given every 8 to 12 hours. Repeat doses are administered as needed based on monitoring of appropriate clinical and laboratory measures. Expected levels of vWF:RCof are based on an expected in vivo recovery of 1.5 IU/dL rise per IU/kg vWF:RCof administered. The administration of 1 IU of factor VIII per kg body weight can be expected to lead to a rise in circulating vWF:RCof of approximately 3.5 to 4 IU/dL. The following general dosages are recommended for adult and pediatric patients:

Humate-P Dose Recommendations for Treatment of von Willebrand Disease in Adult and Pediatric Patients		
Classification	Hemorrhage	Dosage (IU* vWF:RCof/kg body weight)
TYPE 1		
Mild *(Where use of desmopressin is known or suspected to be inadequate)* Baseline vWF:RCof activity typically >30% of normal (i.e., >30 IU/dL)	**Major (examples)** • Severe or refractory epistaxis • GI bleeding • CNS trauma • Traumatic hemorrhage	Loading dose 40 to 60 IU/kg Then 40 to 50 IU/kg every 8 to 12 hours for 3 days to keep the nadir level of vWF:RCof >50% of normal (i.e., >50 IU/dL) Then 40 to 50 IU/kg daily for a total of up to 7 days of treatment
Moderate or Severe Baseline vWF:RCof activity typically <30% of normal (i.e., <30 IU/dL)	**Minor (examples)** • Epistaxis • Oral bleeding • Menorrhagia	40 to 50 IU/kg (1 or 2 doses)
	Major (examples) • Severe or refractory epistaxis • GI bleeding • CNS trauma • Hemarthrosis • Traumatic hemorrhage	Loading dose of 50 to 75 IU/kg Then 40 to 60 IU/kg every 8 to 12 hours for 3 days to keep the nadir level of vWF:RCof >50% of normal (i.e., >50 IU/dL) Then 40 to 60 IU/kg daily for a total of up to 7 days of treatment *Factor VIII:C levels should be monitored and maintained according to the guidelines for hemophilia A therapy†*
TYPE 2 (ALL VARIANTS) AND TYPE 3		
	Minor (clinical indications above)	40 to 50 IU/kg (1 or 2 doses)
	Major (clinical indications above)	Loading dose of 60 to 80 IU/kg Then 40 to 60 IU/kg every 8 to 12 hours for 3 days to keep the nadir level of vWF:RCof >50% of normal (i.e., >50 IU/dL) Then 40 to 60 IU/kg daily for a total of up to 7 days of treatment *Factor VIII:C levels should be monitored and maintained according to the guidelines for hemophilia A therapy†*

IU, International unit.
†In instances where both FVIII and vWF levels must be monitored.

Prevention of excessive bleeding during and after surgery in vWD: In the case of emergency surgery, administer a loading dose of 50 to 60 IU/kg Humate-P and closely monitor the patient's trough coagulation factor levels. Measurement of incremental in vivo recovery (IVR) and assessment of baseline plasma vWF:RCof and FVIII:C levels are recommended in all patients before surgery. Calculation of the loading dose requires four values: the target peak plasma vWF:RCof level, the baseline vWF:RCof level, body weight (BW) in kilograms, and IVR. If individual recovery values are not available, a standardized loading dose can be used based on an assumed vWF:RCof IVR of 2 IU/dL per IU/kg of vWF:RCof product administered.

vWF:RCof and FVIII:C Humate-P Loading Dose Recommendations for the Prevention of Excessive Bleeding During and After Surgery			
Type of Surgery	vWF:RCof Target Peak Plasma Level	FVIII:C Target Peak Plasma Level	Calculation of Loading Dose (to be administered 1 to 2 hours before surgery)
Major	100 IU/dL	80 to 100 IU/dL	Δ* vWF:RCof × BW (kg)/IVR† = IU vWF:RCof required If incremental IVR is not available, assume an IVR of 2 IU/dL per IU/kg and calculate the loading dose as follows: (100 − Baseline plasma vWF:RCof) × BW (kg)/2 In the case of emergency surgery, administer a dose of 50 to 60 IU/kg.
Minor/oral ‡	50 to 60 IU/dL	40 to 50 IU/dL	Δ* vWF:RCof × BW (kg)/IVR† = IU vWF:RCof required

*Δ = Target peak plasma vWF:RCof − Baseline plasma vWF:RCof.
†IVR = Incremental recovery as measured in the patient.
‡Oral surgery is defined as removal of fewer than three teeth, if the teeth are nonmolars and have no bony involvement. Removal of more than one impacted wisdom tooth is considered major surgery due to the expected difficulty of the surgery and the expected blood loss, particularly in subjects with type 2A or type 3 vWD. Removal of more than two teeth is considered major surgery in all patients.

vWF:RCof and FVIII:C Target Trough Plasma Level and Minimum Duration of Treatment Recommendations for Subsequent Maintenance Doses of Humate-P for the Prevention of Excessive Bleeding During and After Surgery					
	vWF:RCof Target Trough Plasma Levels*		FVIII:C Target Trough Plasma Levels*		Minimum Duration of Treatment
Type of Surgery	Up to 3 Days Following Surgery	After Day 3	Up to 3 Days Following Surgery	After Day 3	
Major	>50 IU/dL	>30 IU/dL	>50 IU/dL	>30 IU/dL	72 hours
Minor	≥30 IU/dL	—	—	>30 IU/dL	48 hours
Oral†	≥30 IU/dL	—	—	>30 IU/dL	8 to 12 hours‡

*Trough levels for either coagulation factor should not exceed 100 IU/dL.
†See note on oral surgery in previous chart.
‡At least one maintenance dose following surgery based on individual pharmacokinetic values.

PEDIATRIC DOSE
Treatment of hemophilia A (unlabeled): For immediate control of bleeding, follow the general recommendations for dosing and administration for adults. See Usual Dose and Maternal/Child.

DOSE ADJUSTMENTS
Adjust subsequent doses based on FVIII:C plasma level achieved or as outlined in specific charts.

DILUTION
Consult individual product instructions in the package insert; each product has a specific process for dilution. Information may be updated frequently. **Alphanate** provides diluent, a double-ended transfer needle, and a microaggregate filter for use in administration. **Humate-P** provides diluent and a filter transfer set.
Alphanate and Humate-P: Actual number of AHF units is shown on each vial. Use only the diluent provided and maintain strict aseptic technique. Use a plastic syringe to prevent binding to glass surfaces. Warm to room temperature (25° C) before dilution and maintain throughout administration to avoid precipitation of active ingredients.

Filters: Filters supplied by manufacturer; see Dilution.

Storage: *Alphanate:* Refrigerate before use. Avoid freezing. May be stored at CRT for up to 2 months. Label vial with date removed from refrigeration. *Humate-P:* Store up to 25° C (up to 77° F). Avoid freezing. *Alphanate and Humate-P:* Do not refrigerate after reconstitution. Confirm expiration date on vial. Administer within 3 hours of reconstitution to ensure sterility. Discard any unused solution.

COMPATIBILITY

Specific information not available. Administration through a separate line without mixing with other IV fluids or medications is generally recommended for these products.

RATE OF ADMINISTRATION

Inject solution slowly. Rapid administration may result in vasomotor reactions.

Humate-P recommends a maximum rate of 4 mL/min.

Alphanate recommends a maximum rate not to exceed 10 mL/min.

ACTIONS

A purified, sterile, lyophilized concentrate of antihemophilic factor (factor VIII) and von Willebrand Factor (vWF). Factor VIII is an essential cofactor in the activation of factor X, leading ultimately to the formation of thrombin and fibrin. It is the specific clotting factor deficient in patients with hemophilia A (classic hemophilia). vWF is important for correcting the coagulation defect in patients with von Willebrand disease (vWD). It promotes platelet aggregation and platelet adhesion on damaged vascular endothelium and acts as a stabilizing carrier protein for the procoagulant protein factor VIII. vWF activity is measured with an assay that uses an agglutinating cofactor called Ristocetin (RCof). The vWF:RCof assay provides a quantitative measurement of vWF function by determining how well vWF helps platelets adhere to one another. Reduced vWF:RCof activity indicates a deficiency of vWF. Following administration of FVIII/vWF, there is a rapid increase of plasma factor VIII activity, followed by a rapid decrease in activity and then a slower rate of decrease in activity. The mean initial half-life in hemophilic patients is 8.3 to 27.5 hours with Alphanate and 12.2 hours (range: 8.4 to 17.4 hours) with Humate-P. In patients with vWD, bleeding time decreases. Antihemophilic factor/von Willebrand Factor Complex is obtained from pooled human fresh-frozen plasma. Multiple methods of purification are used to inactivate infectious agents, including viruses.

INDICATIONS AND USES

ALPHANATE

Prevention and control of bleeding in patients with factor VIII deficiency due to hemophilia A or acquired factor VIII deficiency. ▪ Prophylaxis for surgical and/or invasive procedures in adult and pediatric patients with von Willebrand disease (vWD) (type 1 or 2) in which the use of desmopressin is either ineffective or contraindicated. ▪ Not indicated for patients with severe vWD (type 3).

HUMATE-P

Treatment and prevention of bleeding in adult patients with hemophilia A. ▪ Treatment of spontaneous and trauma-induced bleeding episodes and prevention of excessive bleeding during and after surgery in adult and pediatric patients with severe vWD or with mild or moderate vWD in which the use of desmopressin is known or suspected to be inadequate. ▪ Safety and efficacy of prophylactic dosing to prevent spontaneous bleeding and to prevent excessive bleeding related to surgery have not been established in patients with vWD.

CONTRAINDICATIONS

ALPHANATE: None known when used as indicated.

HUMATE-P: History of anaphylactic or severe systemic response to AHF-vWF preparations or known hypersensitivity to any of its components.

PRECAUTIONS

ALPHANATE AND HUMATE-P: For IV use only. ▪ Health care professionals should use caution during administration; may have risk of exposure to viral infection. ▪ Important to establish that coagulation disorder is caused by factor VIII or vWF deficiency. Not useful in treatment of other deficiencies. ▪ Manufactured from human plasma. Risk of transmitting infectious agents (e.g., HIV, hepatitis and, theoretically, Creutzfeldt-Jakob disease) has been greatly reduced by screening, testing, and manufacturing techniques. However, risk of transmission cannot be totally eliminated. ■ Hepatitis A and B vaccines are recommended for patients receiving plasma derivatives. ■ Thrombotic events have been reported. Use caution in patients with known risk factors for thrombosis. Incidence may be higher in females. ■ Inhibitors may develop with large or frequent doses; see Monitor.

Monitor: Complex contains blood group isoagglutinins (anti-A and anti-B). When very large or frequently repeated doses are needed, as when inhibitors are present or when presurgical and postsurgical care is involved, patients of blood groups A, B, and AB should be monitored for signs of intravascular hemolysis and decreasing hematocrit values; see Antidote. ■ Replacement therapy should be monitored by appropriate coagulation tests, especially in cases involving major surgery. Monitor factor VIII and vWF:RCof as indicated in dosing guidelines.

Patient Education: Prophylactic hepatitis A and hepatitis B vaccines recommended. ■ Report symptoms of possibly transmitted viral infections immediately. Symptoms may include anorexia, arthralgias, fatigue, jaundice, low-grade fever, nausea, or vomiting. ■ Report rash or any other sign of hypersensitivity reaction promptly.

Maternal/Child: Category C: use only if clearly needed. ■ Adequate and well-controlled studies with long-term evaluation of joint damage have not been done in pediatric patients. Joint damage may result from suboptimal treatment of hemarthroses. ■ Safety and effectiveness for use in neonates with vWD has not been established. Has been used safely in infants, children, and adolescents with vWD.

Elderly: Numbers insufficient to determine differences in response compared with younger adults. Consider overall status in dosing.

DRUG/LAB INTERACTIONS
Specific information not available.

SIDE EFFECTS
Alphanate and Humate-P: Usually well tolerated. Rare cases of hypersensitivity reactions, including anaphylaxis, have been reported (symptoms may include chest tightness, edema, fever, pruritus, rash, throat tightness). Other reported side effects include chills, headache, lethargy, nausea and vomiting, paresthesia, phlebitis, somnolence, and vasodilation. Inhibitors of factor VIII may occur.

Post-Marketing: *Alphanate:* In addition to the above, cardiac arrest, femoral venous thrombosis, flushing, itching, joint pain, pulmonary embolus, seizure, shortness of breath, swelling of the parotid gland, urticaria. *Humate-P:* Hypersensitivity reactions (including anaphylaxis), development of inhibitors to factor VIII, hemolysis, hypervolemia, thromboembolic complications.

ANTIDOTE
Keep physician informed of all side effects. If mild reactions occur (mild allergic reaction, chills, nausea, or stinging at the infusion site) and additional treatment is indicated, a product from a different lot should be considered. Discontinue immediately at first sign of a moderate to severe hypersensitivity reaction. Treat as necessary (antihistamines, epinephrine, corticosteroids). Development of acute hemolytic anemia, increased bleeding tendency, or hyperfibrinogenemia may require transfusion with Type O red blood cells. Discontinue administration of Alphanate/Humate-P and consider alternative therapy. Resuscitate as necessary.

ANTI-INHIBITOR COAGULANT COMPLEX BBW   Antihemorrhagic
(an-**TIE**-in-**HIH**-bih-tor coe-**AG**-you-lant **COM**-plex)

Feiba

USUAL DOSE

A unit of **Feiba (nanofiltered and vapor heated)** is expressed as factor VIII inhibitor bypassing activity. Identification of factor VIII inhibitor levels and PT mandatory before administration.

FEIBA

Range is 50 to 100 units/kg.

Specific suggested dosing regimens include:

Joint hemorrhage: 50 units/kg; repeat at 12-hour intervals if indicated. May be increased to 100 units/kg if indicated. Continue treatment until clinical improvement (e.g., mobilization of the joint, reduction of swelling, relief of pain). *Do not exceed 200 units/kg/24 hr.*

Mucous membrane bleeding: 50 units/kg; repeat at 6-hour intervals if indicated. Monitor visible bleeding sites and hematocrit closely. May be increased to 100 units/kg every 6 hours for up to 2 doses if bleeding does not stop. *Do not exceed 200 units/kg/24 hr.*

Serious soft tissue hemorrhage: 100 units/kg; repeat at 12-hour intervals if indicated.

Other severe hemorrhage (e.g., CNS bleeding): 100 units/kg; repeat at 12-hour intervals if indicated. Feiba may be indicated at 6-hour intervals until clear clinical improvement occurs.

DILUTION

Actual number of units shown on each vial. Use only the diluent provided and maintain strict aseptic technique. Bring to room temperature before reconstitution. Follow manufacturer's guidelines for reconstitution using the BAXJECT device. May stick to sides of glass syringes; use of plastic syringes recommended. Gently swirl. Do not shake. May be given through Y-tube or three-way stopcock of infusion set. To avoid hypotension from prekallikrein activator (PKA), give **Feiba** within 3 hours of reconstitution.

Filters: The manufacturer of *Feiba* uses a needleless transfer device and has no recommendation for use of an in-line filter.

Storage: Within the indicated shelf life, may be stored in original packaging to protect from light at RT (not to exceed 25° C [77° F]). Do not freeze.

COMPATIBILITY

Specific information not available. Administration through a separate line without mixing with other IV fluids or medications is generally recommended. If anti-inhibitor coagulant is given as a continuous IV, one source says heparin 5 to 10 units/mL of concentrate may be added to avoid thrombophlebitis.

RATE OF ADMINISTRATION

If symptoms of too-rapid infusion (headache, flushing, changes in BP or pulse rate) occur, discontinue until symptoms subside. Restart at a lower rate.

Feiba: Do not exceed 2 units/kg/min.

ACTIONS

An activated prothrombin complex prepared from pooled human plasma. Controls bleeding in patients with factor VIII inhibitors. Mechanism of action is not well understood. Onset of response is usually within 12 hours. Peak response is usually seen within 36 to 72 hours.

Feiba: 1 unit of activity is the amount of anti-inhibitor coagulant complex (AICC) that will shorten the aPTT of a high-titer factor VIII inhibitor reference plasma to 50% of the blank value.

INDICATIONS AND USES

Prophylaxis and treatment of hemorrhagic complications in hemophiliacs (hemophilia A or B) with factor VIII inhibitors who are bleeding or will undergo elective or emergency surgery. Anti-inhibitor coagulant complex (AICC) is most frequently indicated if presenting factor VIII inhibitor levels are above 5 to 10 Bethesda units (BU) or rise to that level following treatment with antihemophilic factor (AHF). Patients whose factor VIII inhibitor levels are between 5 and 10 BU and whose inhibitor levels remain at those levels may be treated with either AHF or AICC. Patients whose inhibitor levels are less than or equal to 5 BU and whose inhibitor levels remain at those levels may be treated with AHF.

Unlabeled uses: Feiba has been used in the prophylaxis and treatment of hemorrhagic complications in nonhemophiliacs with acquired inhibitors to factors VIII, XI, and XII.

CONTRAINDICATIONS

Patients with a normal coagulation mechanism; patients with significant signs of DIC; treatment of bleeding due to coagulation factor deficiencies in the absence of inhibitors to coagulation factors VIII or IX.

PRECAUTIONS

Anamnestic responses (development of antibodies, reducing effectiveness of the drug) with a rise in factor VIII inhibitor titers have been seen in up to 20% of cases. ▪ Thrombotic and thromboembolic events have been reported (e.g., DIC, venous thrombosis, pulmonary embolism, MI, and stroke). Risk of complications may be increased in surgical patients, in patients with thrombotic risk factors, and in patients receiving higher doses. Patients receiving more than 100 units/kg/dose or 200 mg/kg/day are at increased risk for DIC or acute coronary ischemia. Use high doses only as long as necessary to stop bleeding. ▪ Patients with DIC, advanced atherosclerotic disease, crush injury, septicemia, or concomitant treatment with recombinant factor VIIa (e.g., NovoSeven RT) have an increased risk of developing thrombotic events due to circulating tissue factor (TF) or predisposing coagulopathy. ▪ Use with caution and only if there are no therapeutic alternatives in patients at risk for DIC or arterial or venous thrombosis or in patients with existing thrombotic conditions (e.g., MI or venous thrombosis). ▪ Use with caution in patients with a history of coronary heart disease, liver disease, or postoperative immobilization, in the elderly, and in neonates; weigh benefits versus risk. ▪ Do not use Feiba for the treatment of bleeding episodes resulting from coagulation factor deficiencies. ▪ Made from human plasma and may contain infectious agents (e.g., HIV, Creutzfeldt-Jakob disease, hepatitis B, or hepatitis C). Numerous steps in the manufacturing process are used to reduce the potential for infection. ▪ See Drug/Lab Interactions.

Monitor: Monitor PT before and after treatment. Use only accurate means of treatment evaluation; see Drug/Lab Interactions. ▪ Monitor vital signs before, during, and after the infusion. ▪ Monitor for S/S of acute coronary ischemia, DIC, and other thrombotic or thromboembolic events (e.g., changes in BP and HR, chest pain, cough, respiratory distress); see Antidote. ▪ Laboratory indications of DIC may include decreased fibrinogen, decreased platelet count, and/or the presence of fibrin-fibrinogen degradation products (FDP) or significantly prolonged TT, PT, or PTT. ▪ Monitor for S/S of a hypersensitivity reaction (e.g., rash, shortness of breath).

Patient Education: Manufactured from pooled human plasma. Possibility of viral transmission exists. Promptly report S/S of viral infections (e.g., chills, drowsiness, fever, runny nose followed by joint pain, rash, and/or S/S of hepatitis A [e.g., days to weeks of poor appetite, low-grade fever, and tiredness followed by abdominal pain, dark urine, jaundice, nausea, vomiting]).

Maternal/Child: Category C: use only if clearly needed. ▪ Data not available for use in newborns. ▪ Safety for use in breast-feeding not established.

Elderly: May have increased risk for thromboembolic complications.

DRUG/LAB INTERACTIONS

Not recommended for use with **antifibrinolytic products** (aminocaproic acid, tranexamic acid). Feiba has been used with **antifibrinolytics;** however, they should be used with caution and not administered until at least 12 hours after Feiba. ▪ aPTT, WBCT, and other **clotting factor tests** do not correlate with clinical improvement. Attempts to normalize these values may lead to overdose and DIC.

SIDE EFFECTS

Anaphylaxis, bradycardia, chest pain, chills, cough, decreased fibrinogen concentration, decreased platelet count, DIC, fever, flushing, headache, hypertension, hypotension, myocardial infarction, prolonged PT, prolonged PTT, prolonged thrombin time, respiratory distress, tachycardia, thrombosis or thromboembolism, urticaria. Consider risk potential of contracting AIDS or hepatitis.

Overdose: Increased risk for DIC, MI, or thromboembolism.

Post-Marketing: Anaphylactic reaction, DIC, hypersensitivity, hypoaesthesia, facial hypoaesthesia, hypotension, injection site pain, thromboembolism, thrombosis.

ANTIDOTE

If side effects occur, discontinue the infusion and notify the physician. May be resumed at a slower rate or discontinued, or an alternate product may be used. Symptoms of DIC (BP and pulse rate changes, respiratory discomfort, chest pain, cough, prolonged clotting tests, cyanosis of hands and feet, persistent bleeding from puncture sites or mucous membranes) require discontinuation of the infusion and immediate treatment. Treat anaphylaxis or other hypersensitivity reactions (changes in BP or HR [may indicate prekallikrein activity]) with antihistamines, epinephrine, corticosteroids and resuscitate as necessary.

ANTITHROMBIN III (HUMAN)

(an-tie-**THROM**-bin)

AT-III, Thrombate III

Anticoagulant
Antithrombotic

pH 6.5 to 7.5

USUAL DOSE   (International units [IU])

Loading dose, maintenance dose, and dosing intervals are completely individualized based on confirmed diagnosis (see Precautions), patient weight, clinical condition, degree of deficiency, type of surgery or procedure involved, physician judgment, desired level of antithrombin III (AT-III), and actual plasma levels achieved as verified by appropriate lab tests. One unit/kg should raise the level of AT-III by 1.4%. The desired AT-III level after the first dose should be about 120% of normal (normal is 0.1 to 0.2 Gm/L). AT-III levels must be maintained at normal or at least above 80% of normal for 2 to 8 days depending on individual patient factors. Usually achieved by administration of a maintenance dose once daily. Concomitant administration of heparin usually indicated; see Drug/Lab Interactions.

Calculate the initial loading dose using the following formula (assumes a plasma volume of 40 mL/kg):

$$\text{Dosage units} = \frac{(\text{Desired AT-III level [\%]} - \text{Baseline AT-III [\%]}) \times \text{Body weight (kg)}}{\div 1.4\%}$$

For a 70-kg patient with a baseline AT-III level of 57% the initial dose of Thrombate III would be (120% − 57%) × 70 ÷ 1.4 = 3,150 international units (IU). Measurement of plasma levels is suggested preinfusion, 20 minutes postinfusion (peak), 12 hours postinfusion, and preceding next infusion (trough). If recovery differs from the anticipated rise of 1.4% for each IU/kg, modify the formula accordingly. If the above patient has a 20-minute AT-III level of 147%, the increase in AT-III measured for each 1 IU/kg administered is (147% − 57%) × 70 kg ÷ 3,150 IU = 2% rise for each IU/kg administered. This in vivo recovery would be used to calculate future doses. A maintenance dose of approximately 60% of the loading dose every 24 hours is the average required to maintain plasma levels between 80% and 120%. Dose and interval based on plasma levels.

DOSE ADJUSTMENTS
See Drug/Lab Interactions.

DILUTION
Diluent, double-ended needles for dilution, and filter needle for aspiration into a syringe are provided. Warm unopened diluent and concentrate to room temperature. Enter diluent bottle with double-ended transfer needle first. Enter vacuum concentrate bottle with double-ended transfer needle at a 45-degree angle. Direct diluent from above to sides of vial to gently moisten all contents. Remove diluent bottle and transfer needle; swirl continuously until completely dissolved. Draw into a syringe through the filter needle. Remove filter needle; replace with an administration set (not provided). For larger doses, several bottles may be drawn into one syringe. Use a separate filter needle for each bottle.

Filters: Filter needle supplied by manufacturer; see Dilution. For larger doses, several bottles may be drawn into one syringe. Use a separate filter needle for each bottle.

Storage: Store in refrigerator before dilution; avoid freezing. Do not refrigerate after reconstitution. Use within 3 hours of reconstitution.

COMPATIBILITY
Administration through a separate line without mixing with other IV fluids or medications is recommended.

RATE OF ADMINISTRATION
Too-rapid injection may cause dyspnea.
A single dose over 10 to 20 minutes.

ACTIONS
Manufactured from human plasma, purified and heat treated through specific processes, AT-III is a plasma-based protein produced by the body to inactivate specific clotting proteins and control clot formation. Identical to heparin cofactor I, a factor in plasma necessary for heparin to exert its anticoagulant effect. It inactivates thrombin and the activated forms of factors IX, X, XI, and XII (all coagulation enzymes except factors VIIa and XIIIa). Increases AT-III levels within 30 minutes and has a half-life of up to 3 days.

INDICATIONS AND USES
Treatment of patients with hereditary AT-III deficiency to prevent thrombosis during surgical or obstetric procedures (replacement therapy) or during acute thrombotic episodes.

CONTRAINDICATIONS
None when used as indicated.

PRECAUTIONS
For IV use only. ▪ Confirm diagnosis of hereditary AT-III deficiency based on a clear family history of venous thrombosis as well as decreased plasma AT-III levels and the exclusion of acquired deficiency. Present laboratory tests may not be able to identify all cases of congenital AT-III deficiency. ▪ Every unit of plasma used to manufacture AT-III is tested and found nonreactive for HBsAg and negative for antibody to HIV by FDA-approved tests, then heat-treated by a special process. Even with these precautions, individuals who receive multiple infusions may develop viral infection, particularly non-A, non-B hepatitis. HIV infection remains a remote possibility. ▪ May reverse heparin resistance.

Monitor: See varying methods for measuring AT-III levels under Usual Dose. Should be measured at least twice daily until the patient is stabilized and peak and trough levels established, then measured daily. All blood work should be drawn immediately before the next infusion of AT-III.

Patient Education: Inform of risks of thrombosis in connection with pregnancy and surgery and the fact that AT-III deficiency is hereditary.

Maternal/Child: Neonatal AT-III levels should be measured immediately after birth if parents are known to have AT-III deficiency (fatal neonatal thromboembolism [e.g., aortic thrombi] has occurred). Treatment of the neonate should be under the direction of a physician knowledgeable about coagulation disorders. Normal full-term and premature infants have lower than adult averages of AT-III plasma levels. ▪ Category B: use only if clearly indicated. Fetal abnormalities not noted when administered in the third trimester. ▪ Safety for use in pediatric patients not established.

DRUG/LAB INTERACTIONS

Half-life of AT-III decreases with concurrent **heparin** treatment. The anticoagulant effect of heparin is enhanced, and a reduced dose of heparin and low-molecular-weight heparins (LMWHs) is indicated to avoid bleeding.

SIDE EFFECTS

Bowel fullness, chest pain, chest tightness, chills, cramps, dizziness, fever, film over eye, foul taste in mouth, hives, light-headedness, oozing and hematoma formation, and shortness of breath have occurred with Thrombate III. Some patients with acquired AT-III deficiency diagnosed with disseminated intravascular coagulation (DIC) have had diuretic and vasodilatory effects. Rapid infusion may cause dyspnea.

ANTIDOTE

Levels of 150% to 210% found in a few patients have not caused any apparent complications. Observe for bleeding. Reduce rate of infusion immediately for dyspnea. Decrease rate or interrupt infusion as indicated until side effects subside. Keep physician informed of patient's lab values and condition.

ANTITHROMBIN RECOMBINANT

(an-tie-**THROM**-bin re-**KOM**-be-nant)

Atryn

Anticoagulant
Antithrombotic

pH 7

USUAL DOSE

(International units [IU])

Dose must be individualized for each patient and is based on the pretreatment level of functional antithrombin (AT) (expressed in percent of normal) and on body weight in kilograms according to the following chart. Treatment goal is to restore and maintain functional AT activity levels between 80% and 120% (0.8 to 1.2 IU/mL) of normal. Treatment should be initiated before delivery or approximately 24 hours before surgery to ensure AT level is in the target range. Different dosing formulas are used for the treatment of surgical and pregnant patients. Pregnant women being treated with antithrombin recombinant for any peripartum or perioperative event, including a cesarean section, should be treated according to the dosing formula for pregnant women.

Antithrombin Recombinant Dosing Formula for Surgical Patients and Pregnant Women	
Loading Dose (IU)	Maintenance Dose (IU/hr)
Surgical Patients	
$\dfrac{(100\text{-Baseline AT activity level})}{2.3} \times$ Body weight (kg)	$\dfrac{(100\text{-Baseline AT activity level})}{10.2} \times$ Body weight (kg)
Pregnant Women	
$\dfrac{(100\text{-Baseline AT activity level})}{1.3} \times$ Body weight (kg)	$\dfrac{(100\text{-Baseline AT activity level})}{5.4} \times$ Body weight (kg)

Check AT level just after surgery or delivery; AT activity may be rapidly decreased by surgery or delivery. If AT activity level is below 80%, administer an additional bolus dose to rapidly restore decreased AT activity level. Then restart the maintenance dose at the same rate of infusion as before the bolus. Monitor AT activity at least once or twice daily and adjust doses according to the chart in Dose Adjustments. Continue treatment until adequate follow-up anticoagulation is established.

DOSE ADJUSTMENTS

Antithrombin Recombinant AT Activity Monitoring and Dose Adjustment			
Initial Monitor Time	AT Level	Dose Adjustment	Recheck AT Level
2 hr after initiation of treatment	<80%	Increase by 30%	2 hr after each dose adjustment
	80% to 100%	None	6 hr after initiation of treatment or dose adjustment
	>120%	Decrease by 30%	2 hr after each dose adjustment

DILUTION

Bring vials to RT no more than 3 hours before reconstitution. Each vial contains approximately 1,750 IU; exact potency is stated on the carton and label. Immediately before use, each vial **must** be reconstituted with 10 mL SWFI. **Do not shake.** Draw the reconstituted solution from one or more vials into a sterile syringe. May administer reconstituted solution directly or may further dilute in an infusion bag containing NS (e.g., dilute to obtain a final concentration of 100 IU/mL). Administer using an infusion set with a 0.22-micron in-line filter.

Filters: Use of a 0.22-micron in-line filter required during infusion.

Storage: Before use, refrigerate vials between 2° and 8° C (36° and 46° F). Use reconstituted or diluted solution within 8 to 12 hours of preparation. Do not use beyond expiration date on vial. Discard unused product.

COMPATIBILITY

Specific information not available. Because of specific use and unique formulation, consider administering through a separate line without mixing with other IV fluids or medications.

RATE OF ADMINISTRATION

Loading dose: Administer as an infusion over 15 minutes. Follow immediately with the **maintenance dose** as a continuous infusion at the calculated IU/hr rate.

ACTIONS

A recombinant human antithrombin produced by DNA technology. A DNA coding sequence for human antithrombin and a mammary gland–specific DNA sequence are introduced into genetically engineered goats. The goats' milk contains the antithrombin. The amino acid sequence of antithrombin recombinant is identical to that of human plasma-derived antithrombin. Purified through numerous processes to eliminate potential viruses. AT is the principal inhibitor of thrombin and factor Xa. AT neutralizes the activity of thrombin and factor Xa by forming a complex that is rapidly removed from the circulation. When AT is bound to heparin, the ability of antithrombin to inhibit thrombin and factor Xa can be enhanced by greater than 300- to 1,000-fold. Half-life range based on IU/kg is 11.6 to 17.7 hours. This recombinant formulation has a shorter half-life and more rapid clearance compared with plasma-derived antithrombin (e.g., Thrombate III). Secreted in breast milk.

INDICATIONS AND USES

Prevention of perioperative and peripartum thromboembolic events in patients with hereditary antithrombin deficiency. ▪ **Not indicated for treatment** of thromboembolic events in patients with hereditary antithrombin deficiency.

CONTRAINDICATIONS

Known hypersensitivity to goat and goat milk proteins.

PRECAUTIONS

For IV use only. ▪ Confirm diagnosis of hereditary antithrombin deficiency. ▪ Hypersensitivity reactions may occur at any time during the infusion, thus requiring discontinuation of the infusion. ▪ The anticoagulant effect of drugs that use antithrombin to exert their anticoagulation (e.g., heparin, low-molecular-weight heparins such as enoxaparin [Lovenox]) may be altered when antithrombin recombinant is added or withdrawn. Avoid excessive or insufficient anticoagulation by monitoring coagulation tests suitable for the anticoagulant used (e.g., aPTT and anti-factor Xa activity). To avoid bleeding or thrombosis, perform these tests regularly and at close intervals, especially during the first hours after the start or withdrawal of antithrombin recombinant. ▪ See Drug/Lab Interactions.

Monitor: Specific coagulation tests are required before administration and throughout the infusion process; see Usual Dose and Precautions. ▪ Monitor throughout the infusion for S/S of a hypersensitivity reaction (e.g., hives, hypotension, generalized urticaria, tightness of the chest, wheezing, and/or anaphylaxis). ▪ Monitor for S/S of bleeding or thrombosis.

Patient Education: Inform physician of a past or present allergy to goats or goat milk. ▪ Promptly report S/S of a hypersensitivity reaction (e.g., rash, shortness of breath, wheezing). ▪ Risk of bleeding increased when used with other anticoagulants. Report bleeding from any source.

Maternal/Child: Category C: use during pregnancy only if clearly needed. Studies have not shown that antithrombin recombinant increases the risk of fetal abnormalities if administered during the third trimester of pregnancy. Adverse reactions have not been reported in neonates born to women treated with antithrombin recombinant during clinical trials. ▪ Indicated for prevention of thromboembolic events in women with hereditary antithrombin deficiency during labor and delivery. ▪ Levels that appear in breast milk are estimated to be the same as in normal lactating women; however, use only if clearly needed and with caution during breast-feeding. ▪ Safety and effectiveness for use in pediatric patients not established.

Elderly: Numbers in clinical studies insufficient to determine if elderly patients respond differently than younger subjects. Dosing should be cautious in the elderly. Reduced doses may be indicated based on the potential for decreased organ function and concomitant disease or drug therapy.

DRUG/LAB INTERACTIONS

The anticoagulant effect of **heparin and low-molecular-weight heparin** is enhanced by antithrombin. Concurrent use with these anticoagulants may alter the half-life of antithrombin. Concurrent use with **heparin, low-molecular-weight heparins** such as enoxaparin (Lovenox), **or other anticoagulants** that use antithrombin to exert their anticoagulant effect must be monitored clinically and biologically. To avoid excessive anticoagulation, perform regular coagulation tests (aPTT and, where appropriate, anti-factor Xa activity) at close intervals and adjust the dose of anticoagulant as indicated.

SIDE EFFECTS

Hemorrhage and infusion site reactions were most commonly reported. Hemorrhage may be serious (intra-abdominal, hemarthrosis, and postprocedural). Less common side effects include feeling hot, hematoma, hematuria, hepatic enzyme abnormalities, hypersensitivity reactions (including anaphylaxis), and noncardiac chest pain.

ANTIDOTE

Keep physician informed of patient's lab values and condition. Discontinue the infusion if a hypersensitivity reaction occurs. ▪ Treat anaphylaxis immediately with oxygen, epinephrine (Adrenalin), antihistamines (e.g., diphenhydramine [Benadryl]), vasopressors (e.g., dopamine), corticosteroids, albuterol, IV fluids, and ventilation equipment as indicated. Resuscitate as necessary.

ANTI-THYMOCYTE GLOBULIN (RABBIT) BBW

Immunosuppressant

(an-tie-**THI**-mo-cite **GLOB**-you-lin)

Thymoglobulin, Atgam (equine)*

pH 7 to 7.4

USUAL DOSE

Premedication: To reduce the incidence and intensity of side effects during the infusion of anti-thymocyte globulin; premedication 1 hour before the infusion with corticosteroids (e.g., dexamethasone [Decadron]), acetaminophen (e.g., Tylenol), and/or an antihistamine (e.g., diphenhydramine [Benadryl]) is recommended.

Anti-thymocyte globulin: 1.5 mg/kg of body weight daily for 7 to 14 days. Given as an infusion into a high-flow vein. Used in conjunction with maintenance immunosuppression (e.g., tacrolimus [Prograf], mycophenolate [Cell-Cept]); see Drug/Lab Interactions.

DOSE ADJUSTMENTS

Reduce dose by one-half if WBC count is between 2,000 and 3,000 cells/mm^3 or if platelet count is between 50,000 and 75,000 cells/mm^3. ▪ Consider withholding dose or stopping anti-thymocyte therapy if WBC count falls below 2,000 cells/mm^3 or platelets fall below 50,000 cells/mm^3.

DILUTION

Calculate the number of vials required (25 mg/vial); 5 mL of SWFI as diluent per vial is supplied. Drug and diluent must be warmed to room temperature before dilution. Absolute sterile technique required throughout dilution process. For each vial required use a new syringe and needle. Withdraw 5 mL of diluent and inject into lyophilized powder. Rotate vial gently until powder is completely dissolved. Do not shake. Each reconstituted vial contains 25 mg (5 mg/mL). Must be further diluted by transferring into 50 mL of infusion solution (saline or dextrose) for each 25 mg of anti-thymocyte globulin. Total volume is usually between 50 to 500 mL. Invert the infusion bag gently once or twice to mix the solution.

Filters: Use of a 0.22-micron in-line filter recommended.

Storage: Refrigerate and protect from light until removed to prepare for reconstitution. Do not freeze. Do not use after expiration date on vial. Use reconstituted vials within 4 hours. Use infusion solutions immediately. Discard unused drug.

COMPATIBILITY
(Underline Indicates Conflicting Compatibility Information)

Consider any drug NOT listed as compatible to be INCOMPATIBLE until consulting a pharmacist; specific conditions may apply.

Administration through a separate line without mixing with other IV fluids or medications is suggested because of specific use and potential for anaphylaxis.

One source suggests the following **compatibilities:**

Y-site: <u>Heparin</u>, hydrocortisone sodium succinate (Solu-Cortef).

RATE OF ADMINISTRATION

Use of a high-flow vein and a 0.22-micron filter recommended. Well-tolerated and less likely to produce side effects (e.g., chills and fever) when administered at the recommended rate and the patient is premedicated.

Initial dose: A total daily dose equally distributed over a minimum of 6 hours.

Subsequent doses: A total daily dose equally distributed over a minimum of 4 hours.

ACTIONS

A purified, pasteurized, gamma immune globulin, obtained by immunization of rabbits with human thymocytes. Mechanism of action not fully understood. May induce immu-

---

*See Index for monograph of Lymphocyte Immune Globulin, the equine product of Anti-Thymocyte Globulin.

nosuppression by T-cell depletion and immune modulation. Made up of a variety of antibodies that recognize key receptors on T-cells (those cells responsible for attacking and rejecting a foreign substance within the body). Anti-thymocyte globulin antibodies can inactivate and kill these T-cells, thus reversing the rejection process. May prevent organ loss and reduce the need for retransplantation. T-cell depletion is usually observed within a day of initiating thymoglobulin therapy. Half-life averages 2 to 3 days but the drug remains active, targeting the offending immune cells for days to weeks after treatment.

INDICATIONS AND USES
Treatment of kidney transplant acute rejection in conjunction with concomitant immunosuppression.

Unlabeled uses: Compassionate use in the treatment of acute rejection in bone marrow, heart, and liver transplants. Treatment of myelodysplastic syndrome (MDS).

CONTRAINDICATIONS
Patients with a known allergy to rabbit proteins, an acute viral illness, or a history of anaphylaxis during rabbit immunoglobulin administration.

PRECAUTIONS
Administered only under the direction of a physician experienced in immunosuppressive therapy and management of renal transplant patients in a facility with adequate laboratory and supportive medical resources. ▪ Not considered effective for treating antibody-mediated (humoral) rejections. ▪ Prolonged use or overdose in combination with other immunosuppressive agents may cause over-immunosuppression resulting in severe infections and may increase the incidence of lymphoma or posttransplant lymphoproliferative disease (PTLD) or other malignancies. Use of appropriate antiviral, antibacterial, antiprotozoal, and/or antifungal prophylaxis is recommended. In clinical trials, viral prophylaxis with ganciclovir infusion was used. ▪ In clinical trials, anti-rabbit antibodies developed in 68% of patients. Controlled studies on repeat use of anti-thymocyte globulin in patients with anti-rabbit antibodies have not been conducted. Use caution if repeat courses are indicated; monitoring of lymphocyte count is recommended to ensure that T-cell depletion is achieved. ▪ If anaphylaxis occurs during or after therapy, further administration of anti-thymocyte globulin is contraindicated.

Monitor: Close clinical observation is imperative. Monitor for side effects during and after infusion. Anaphylaxis has occurred; emergency equipment, medications, and supplies must be available. ▪ Obtain baseline and monitor WBC and platelet counts during therapy. Thrombocytopenia or neutropenia may occur and are reversible following dose adjustment; see Dose Adjustments. ▪ Monitoring of the lymphocyte count (i.e., total lymphocyte count and T-cell counts [absolute and/or subset]) may help assess the degree of T-cell depletion. ▪ Monitor carefully for signs of infection. ▪ Prophylactic antibiotics may be indicated pending results of C/S in a febrile neutropenic patient. ▪ See Precautions and Drug/Lab Interactions.

Patient Education: Imperative that all medications (especially immunosuppressants) be reviewed with physician. ▪ Report any previous hypersensitivity/anaphylactic reaction. ▪ Report acute viral infections immediately. ▪ Promptly report chest pain, irregular or rapid heartbeat, shortness of breath, swelling of the face or throat, or wheezing during infusion of medication. ▪ See Appendix D, p. 1333. ▪ May be associated with an increased risk of malignancy.

Maternal/Child: Category C: safety for use during pregnancy and breast-feeding not established. Safety and effectiveness for use in pediatric patients not established. Use only if clearly needed. ▪ Has been used in pediatric patients in limited European studies and in the United States for compassionate use. Response similar to adults.

Elderly: Specific information not available.

DRUG/LAB INTERACTIONS
Concurrent use with **immunosuppressants** (e.g., azathioprine, cyclosporine [Sandimmune], mycophenolate [Cell-Cept], tacrolimus [Prograf]) may potentiate the immunosuppressive action of these agents; many transplant centers decrease maintenance immunosuppression therapy during the period of antibody therapy. ▪ May **stimulate the**

production of antibodies, which cross-react with rabbit immune globulins. ▪ May interfere with **rabbit antibody-base immunoassays** and with **cross-match or panel-reactive antibody cytotoxicity assays.**

SIDE EFFECTS

Are dose-limiting. Abdominal pain, asthenia, diarrhea, dizziness, dyspnea, fever, headache, hyperkalemia, hypertension, infection, infusion reaction (e.g., chills and fever), leukopenia, malaise, nausea, pain, peripheral edema, tachycardia, and thrombocytopenia were reported frequently. Anaphylaxis has been reported.

Overdose: Leukopenia or thrombocytopenia.

ANTIDOTE

Notify physician of all side effects. Most can be managed symptomatically. Manage leukopenia or thrombocytopenia during therapy or in overdose with dose reduction. Infusion reactions are managed with premedication and reduction in the rate of infusion. Treat infections aggressively; see Precautions. May require discontinuation of therapy. Discontinue infusion and/or therapy immediately if anaphylaxis occurs. Treat anaphylaxis immediately with epinephrine (Adrenalin), diphenhydramine (Benadryl), oxygen, vasopressors (e.g., dopamine), corticosteroids, IV fluids, and ventilation equipment as indicated. Resuscitate as necessary.

ANTIVENIN CROTALIDAE POLYVALENT IMMUNE FAB (OVINE)

Antivenin

(an-tee-**VEN**-in kro-**TAL**-ih-day pol-ih-**VAY**-lent im-**MYOUN** fab)

CroFab

USUAL DOSE

Contact a regional poison control center for individual treatment advice.

Premedication: Premedication may be indicated for patients with allergies. Obtain blood work before administration; see Contraindications, Precautions, and Monitor. Initiate as soon as possible after crotalid snakebite in patients who develop signs of progressive envenomation (e.g., worsening local injury, coagulation abnormality, or systemic signs of envenomation); see Monitor. Has been effective when given within 6 hours of snakebite.

Initial dose: Skin testing for sensitivity to serum is not required. 4 to 6 vials is the recommended initial dose based on clinical experience. Adjust based on severity of envenomation when patient is initially assessed. Observe for up to 1 hour after initial dose administered. Desired outcome is complete control of the envenomation (i.e., complete arrest of local manifestations and return of coagulation tests and systemic signs to normal).

Repeat doses: If control of symptoms is not accomplished by the initial dose, give an additional dose of 4 to 6 vials. This dose may be repeated until initial control of the envenomation syndrome has been achieved. After initial control has been established, give additional 2-vial doses every 6 hours for up to 18 hours (3 doses). Optimal dosing following the 18-hour scheduled dose has not been determined. Additional 2-vial doses may be given as directed by the treating physician, based on the patient's clinical response. Up to 18 vials have been given without any observed direct toxic effect. Scheduled dosing rather than PRN dosing may provide better control of envenomation symptoms caused by the continued leaking of venom from depot sites.

PEDIATRIC DOSE

Absolute venom dose following snakebite is expected to be the same in pediatric patients and adults; no dose adjustment for age is required. See Maternal/Child.

DOSE ADJUSTMENTS

No dose adjustments recommended.

DILUTION

Reconstitute each vial with 18 mL NS. Mix by continuous gentle swirling. Do not shake. Further dilute the contents of the reconstituted vials in 250 mL NS and mix by gently swirling.

Storage: Refrigerate unopened vials; do not freeze. Reconstituted vials and diluted solution must be used within 4 hours.

COMPATIBILITY

Specific information not available. Administration through a separate line without mixing with other IV fluids or medications is suggested because of specific use and potential for anaphylaxis.

RATE OF ADMINISTRATION

Initiate infusion at a rate of 25 to 50 mL/hr for the first 10 minutes. Carefully observe for hypersensitivity reactions. If no adverse reaction occurs, increase rate to 250 mL/hr so that total dose is administered over 1 hour. Reduce rate of administration if infusion-related reactions occur (e.g., fever, low back pain, nausea, wheezing), and monitor closely.

ACTIONS

A venom-specific Fab fragment of immunoglobulin G (IgG) obtained from the blood of healthy sheep flocks immunized with one of four snake venoms; see Indications for specific venoms. To obtain the final product, the four different monospecific antivenins are mixed. Works by binding and neutralizing venom toxins, facilitating their redistribution away from target tissues and their elimination from the body. Half-life is estimated to be 12 to 23 hours.

INDICATIONS AND USES

Management of patients with North American Crotalid envenomation. The term *Crotalid* is used to describe the Crotalinae subfamily (formerly known as Crotalidae) of venomous snakes and includes rattlesnakes, copperheads, cottonmouths/water moccasins. Early use (within 6 hours) is advised to prevent clinical deterioration and the occurrence of systemic coagulation abnormalities.

CONTRAINDICATIONS

Known history of hypersensitivity to sheep, papaya, or papain unless benefits outweigh risks and appropriate management for anaphylactic reactions is readily available.

PRECAUTIONS

Usually administered in the hospital by or under the direction of the physician specialist with adequate diagnostic and treatment facilities readily available. ▪ Patients with allergies to dust mites, latex, papain, chymopapain, other papaya extracts, the pineapple enzyme bromelain, or sheep protein may be at risk for a hypersensitivity reaction to this antivenin; see Contraindications; use caution. ▪ Contains 0.03 mg of mercury per vial (ethyl mercury from thimerosal). Exposure from 18-vial dose is 0.6 mg of mercury. Definitive data not available; literature suggests that information related to methyl mercury toxicities may be applicable. ▪ Recurrent coagulation abnormalities (e.g., decreased fibrinogen, decreased platelets, and elevated PT), defined as the return of a coagulation abnormality after it has been successfully treated with antivenin, were observed in patients who experienced coagulation abnormalities during their initial hospitalization and occurred in approximately one half of patients studied. Crotalidae immune fab has a shorter persistence in the blood than crotalid venoms, which can leak from depot sites over a prolonged period of time; repeat dosing to prevent or treat such recurrence may be necessary. Optimal dosing to prevent recurrent coagulopathy has not been determined. ▪ Use caution if a repeat course of treatment is required for a subsequent envenomation episode; crotalidae immune fab is a foreign protein and antibodies may develop, producing sensitivity.

Monitor: Before antivenin is administered, draw adequate blood for baseline studies (e.g., type and cross-match, CBC, hematocrit, platelet count, PT, bleeding and coagulation times, BUN, electrolytes, and bilirubin). ▪ Severity of envenomation is based on six body categories: cardiovascular, gastrointestinal, hematologic, local wound (e.g., pain, swelling, and ecchymosis), nervous system, and pulmonary effects. Specific parameters of minimal, moderate, and severe envenomation are outlined in the following chart.

Definition of Minimal, Moderate, and Severe Envenomation Used in Clinical Studies of Crotalidae Polyvalent Immune Fab	
Envenomation Category	Definition
Minimal	*Swelling, pain, and ecchymosis* limited to the immediate bite site. *Systemic signs and symptoms* absent. *Coagulation parameters* normal with no clinical evidence of bleeding.
Moderate	*Swelling, pain, and ecchymosis* involving less than a full extremity or, if bite was sustained on the trunk, head, or neck, extending less than 50 cm. *Systemic signs and symptoms* may be present but not life-threatening, including but not limited to nausea, vomiting, oral paresthesia or unusual tastes, mild hypotension (systolic BP less than 90 mm Hg), mild tachycardia (HR less than 150), and tachypnea. *Coagulation parameters* may be abnormal, but no clinical evidence of bleeding present. Minor hematuria, gum bleeding, and nosebleeds are allowed if they are not considered severe in the investigator's judgment.
Severe	*Swelling, pain, and ecchymosis* involving more than an entire extremity or threatening the airway. *Systemic signs and symptoms* are markedly abnormal, including severe alteration of mental status, severe hypotension, severe tachycardia, tachypnea, or respiratory insufficiency. *Coagulation parameters* are abnormal, with serious bleeding or severe threat of bleeding.

- Anaphylactic and anaphylactoid reactions, delayed hypersensitivity reactions (late serum reaction or serum sickness), and a possible febrile response to immune complexes formed by animal antibodies and neutralized venom components may occur. Observe all patients continuously for signs and symptoms of an acute hypersensitivity reaction (e.g., angioedema, bronchospasm with wheezing or cough, erythema, hypotension, pruritus, stridor, tachycardia, urticaria). ■ Follow-up monitoring is required for S/S of delayed hypersensitivity reactions or serum sickness (e.g., arthralgia, fever, myalgia, rash). ■ Monitor all vital signs at frequent intervals. Observe for signs of shock; treat with IV fluids, blood products, plasma expanders, vasopressors (e.g., dopamine) as indicated. ■ Keep emergency equipment available at all times, including oxygen, epinephrine, antihistamines (e.g., IV diphenhydramine [Benadryl]), corticosteroids, albuterol, vasopressors (e.g., dopamine), and ventilation equipment. ■ Initiate two IV lines as soon as possible—one to be used for supportive therapy, the other for antivenin and electrolytes. ■ If coagulation abnormalities occur, consider other disease processes associated with coagulation disorders (e.g., cancer, collagen disease, CHF, diarrhea, elevated temperature, hepatic disorder, hyperthyroidism, poor nutritional state, steatorrhea, vitamin K deficiency). ■ Monitor patients who experience coagulopathy due to snakebite during hospitalization for initial treatment for several weeks after discharge. Recurrent coagulopathy may persist for 1 to 2 weeks or more. Assess the need for retreatment and/or use of anticoagulant or antiplatelet agents. ■ Supportive measures to treat other manifestations of the snakebite (e.g., hypotension, pain, swelling, wound infection) should be implemented.

Patient Education: Immediately report any S/S of delayed hypersensitivity reactions or serum sickness (e.g., pruritus, rash, or urticaria occurring after discharge). ■ Promptly report unusual bruising or bleeding (e.g., nosebleeds, excessive bleeding after toothbrushing or superficial injuries, blood in stools or urine, excessive menstrual bleeding, petechiae). May occur for up to 1 week or longer and indicate need for additional treatment.

Maternal/Child: Category C: use during pregnancy only if clearly needed. ▪ Use caution; safety for use during breast-feeding not established. ▪ Exposure to mercury has been associated with neurologic and renal toxicities. Developing fetuses and very young children are most susceptible and are at greater risk.

Elderly: No specific studies on elderly patients.

DRUG/LAB INTERACTIONS
Studies have not been conducted.

SIDE EFFECTS
Pruritus, rash, and urticaria are frequent side effects. Anorexia, back pain, cellulitis, chest pain, chills, circumoral paresthesia, cough, delayed hypersensitivity reactions (late serum reaction or serum sickness), ecchymosis, febrile response to immune complexes formed by animal antibodies and neutralized venom components, general paresthesia, hypersensitivity reactions including anaphylaxis, hypotension, increased sputum, myalgia, nausea, nervousness, recurrent coagulopathy, and wound infection have occurred.

Post-Marketing: Angioedema, bronchospasm, delayed hypersensitivity reactions (epigastric pressure, fever, hives, itching, rash), dizziness, dyspnea, erythema, failure to achieve initial control, headache, lip swelling, recurrent coagulopathy with medically significant bleeding, recurrent swelling (refractory to treatment), sweating, tachycardia, tachypnea, thrombocytopenia (refractory to treatment), tongue swelling, tracheal edema, treatment failure resulting in death, wheezing, worsening eyesight.

ANTIDOTE
Keep physician informed of all side effects and extent or progression of envenomation. Reduce the rate of administration if infusion-related reactions occur (e.g., fever, low back pain, nausea, wheezing). Monitor closely and discontinue antivenin if symptoms worsen or a hypersensitivity reaction occurs. Treat hypersensitivity reactions and/or anaphylaxis immediately with oxygen, epinephrine, antihistamines (e.g., IV diphenhydramine [Benadryl]), corticosteroids, albuterol, vasopressors (e.g., dopamine), and ventilation equipment as indicated. Recurrent coagulopathy may require rehospitalization and additional antivenin administration. Resuscitate as necessary.

ARGATROBAN
(ahr-**GAT**-troe-ban)

Anticoagulant
(direct thrombin inhibitor)

pH 3.2 to 8.8

USUAL DOSE
Discontinue all parenteral anticoagulants (e.g., heparin) and obtain baseline blood tests including an aPTT (prophylaxis or treatment) and ACT (PCI) before administration of argatroban; see Monitor.

Prophylaxis or treatment of thrombosis in patients with heparin-induced thrombocytopenia (HIT/HITTS): Begin *argatroban* with an initial dose of 2 mcg/kg/min as a continuous infusion. Steady-state levels usually obtained within 1 to 3 hours. Check the aPTT in 2 hours. Adjust the mcg/kg/min dose (not to exceed 10 mcg/kg/min) as clinically indicated until the steady-state aPTT is 1.5 to 3 times the initial baseline value (not to exceed 100 seconds).

Anticoagulant in patients with or at risk for HIT/HITTS undergoing percutaneous coronary interventions (PCI): *Aspirin* 325 mg 2 to 24 hours before planned PCI was administered in studies. After venous or arterial sheaths are in place, begin *argatroban* with an initial infusion of 25 mcg/kg/min via a large-bore IV line. Next, administer a bolus of 350 mcg/kg over 3 to 5 minutes. 5 to 10 minutes after completion of bolus dose, check the ACT. The PCI may proceed if the ACT is greater than 300 seconds but less than 450 seconds. If

ACT is less than 300 seconds, give an additional IV bolus of 150 mcg/kg, increase the infusion rate to 30 mcg/kg/min, and check the ACT in 5 to 10 minutes. If ACT is greater than 450 seconds, decrease the infusion rate to 15 mcg/kg/min and recheck the ACT in 5 to 10 minutes. When a therapeutic ACT has been achieved (between 300 and 450 seconds), the infusion dose in effect at the time the therapeutic ACT is achieved should be continued for the duration of the procedure. For situations outside these parameters, see Dose Adjustments. If anticoagulation is required after PCI, continue argatroban but lower infusion rate to 2 mcg/kg/min. Draw an aPTT in 2 hours and adjust the infusion rate as clinically indicated (not to exceed 10 mcg/kg/min) to reach an aPTT between 1.5 and 3 times baseline value (not to exceed 100 seconds); see All Situations in Monitor if transfer to oral anticoagulation is indicated.

DOSE ADJUSTMENTS
All situations: No dose adjustment indicated in patients with impaired renal function, or based on age or gender.

Prophylaxis or treatment of thrombosis in patients with heparin-induced thrombocytopenia (HIT/HITTS): Reduce initial dose to 0.5 mcg/kg/min in patients with moderate or severe hepatic impairment. There is a fourfold decrease in argatroban clearance in these patients; titrate dose carefully and monitor aPTT closely.

Anticoagulant in patients with or at risk for HIT/HITTS undergoing percutaneous coronary interventions (PCI): In case of dissection, impending abrupt closure, thrombus formation during the procedure, or inability to achieve or maintain an ACT over 300 seconds, additional bolus doses of 150 mcg/kg may be given and the infusion rate increased to 40 mcg/kg/min. Check the ACT after each additional bolus or change in rate of infusion. ▪ In patients with hepatic impairment undergoing PCI, carefully titrate argatroban until desired level of anticoagulation is achieved. See Precautions for patients with clinically significant liver disease.

DILUTION
Available premixed at a final concentration of 1 mg/mL or as a 250-mg vial that must be diluted in 250 mL of NS, D5W, or LR to a concentration of 1 mg/mL. Mix by repeated inversion of the diluent bag for a minimum of 1 minute. Solution may initially be briefly hazy. Do not expose prepared solutions to direct sunlight.

Storage: Store vials in carton at CRT, protected from light and freezing. Diluted solution stable in ambient indoor light for 24 hours at 20° to 25° C (68° to 77° F). Light-resistant measures such as foil protection for IV lines are not necessary. Stable for up to 96 hours protected from light and stored at CRT or refrigerated. Store premixed vials in original carton at 20° to 25° C (68° to 77° F). Do not refrigerate or freeze. Protect from light.

COMPATIBILITY
Consider any drug NOT listed as compatible to be INCOMPATIBLE until consulting a pharmacist; specific conditions may apply.

Manufacturer states, "Should not be mixed with other drugs prior to dilution in a suitable IV fluid." Consider specific use and dose adjustment requirements.

One source suggests the following **compatibilities:**

Y-site: Abciximab (ReoPro), atropine, diltiazem (Cardizem), diphenhydramine (Benadryl), dobutamine, dopamine, eptifibatide (Integrilin), fenoldopam (Corlopam), fentanyl, furosemide (Lasix), hydrocortisone sodium succinate (Solu-Cortef), lidocaine, metoprolol (Lopressor), midazolam (Versed), milrinone (Primacor), morphine, nesiritide (Natrecor), nitroglycerin IV, nitroprusside sodium, norepinephrine (Levophed), phenylephrine (Neo-Synephrine), tirofiban (Aggrastat), vasopressin, verapamil.

RATE OF ADMINISTRATION
Prophylaxis or treatment of thrombosis in patients with heparin-induced thrombocytopenia (HIT/HITTS):

Argatroban Infusion Rates for 2 mcg/kg/min Dose (1 mg/mL Final Concentration)	
Body Weight (kg)	Infusion Rate (mL/hr)
50 kg	6 mL/hr
60 kg	7 mL/hr
70 kg	8 mL/hr
80 kg	10 mL/hr
90 kg	11 mL/hr
100 kg	12 mL/hr
110 kg	13 mL/hr
120 kg	14 mL/hr
130 kg	16 mL/hr
140 kg	17 mL/hr

Anticoagulant in patients with or at risk for HIT/HITTS undergoing percutaneous coronary interventions (PCI): See Usual Dose and/or Dose Adjustments for specific rates and criteria.

ACTIONS
An anticoagulant that is a highly selective synthetic direct thrombin inhibitor. It reversibly binds to the thrombin active site and exerts its anticoagulant effects by inhibiting thrombin-catalyzed or induced reactions, including fibrin formation; activation of coagulation factors V, VIII, and XIII and protein C; and platelet aggregation. Highly selective for thrombin with little or no effect on related serine proteases (trypsin, factor Xa, plasmin, and kallikrein). Inhibits both free and clot-bound thrombin. Does not require the cofactor antithrombin III for antithrombic activity. Produces a dose-dependent increase in aPTT, ACT, INR, PT, and TT. Anticoagulant effects are immediate. Steady-state levels of both drug and anticoagulant effect are usually attained within 1 to 3 hours and are maintained until the infusion is discontinued or the dose adjusted. Distribution is primarily in the extracellular fluid. Metabolized in the liver. Half-life range is 39 to 51 minutes. Excreted primarily in feces with some excretion in urine.

INDICATIONS AND USES
An anticoagulant for prophylaxis or treatment of thrombosis in patients with heparin-induced thrombocytopenia (HIT). ▪ An anticoagulant in patients with or at risk for heparin-induced thrombocytopenia undergoing percutaneous coronary intervention (PCI). May be used in combination with aspirin.

CONTRAINDICATIONS
Hypersensitivity to argatroban or any of its components and patients with overt major bleeding.

PRECAUTIONS
All situations: Hemorrhage can occur at any site. Use with extreme caution in disease states and other circumstances in which there is an increased danger of hemorrhage, including severe hypertension; immediately following lumbar puncture; spinal anesthesia; major surgery, especially involving the brain, spinal cord, or eye; hematologic conditions associated with increased bleeding tendencies such as congenital or acquired bleeding disorders and gastrointestinal lesions such as ulcerations. ▪ Concomitant therapy with thrombolytic agents (e.g., alteplase [tPA], reteplase [Retavase], streptokinase), antiplatelet agents, or other anticoagulants may increase the risk of bleeding, including life-threatening intracranial bleeding; see Drug/Lab Interactions. ▪ Safety and effectiveness of argatroban for cardiac indications other than PCI in patients with HIT not established. ▪ Use caution in

patients with hepatic disease; argatroban clearance is decreased fourfold and elimination half-life is increased. Full reversal of anticoagulant effect may require longer than 4 hours. See Dose Adjustments.

PCI: Avoid use of argatroban in PCI patients with clinically significant hepatic disease or AST/ALT levels greater than 3 times the upper limit of normal. These patients were not included in clinical trials.

Monitor: *All situations:* Obtain baseline and monitor platelet count, hemoglobin, hematocrit, and occult blood in stool in addition to required aPTT or ACT; see Usual Dose and specific parameters as follows. ▪ Other coagulation tests (e.g., PT, INR, and TT) are affected by argatroban, but therapeutic ranges for these tests have not been identified. ▪ Observe carefully for symptoms of a hemorrhagic event (e.g., unexplained fall in hematocrit, fall in BP, or any other unexplained symptom). ▪ HIT is a serious, immune-mediated complication of heparin therapy that may result in subsequent venous and arterial thrombosis. Initial treatment of HIT is to discontinue all heparin, but patients still require anticoagulation for prevention and treatment of thromboembolic events. ▪ Initiate oral anticoagulation with warfarin (Coumadin) when appropriate. Do not use a loading dose of warfarin; use the expected daily dose. Monitor INR daily. Concurrent use with warfarin results in prolongation of the PT and INR beyond that produced by warfarin alone. With doses of argatroban up to 2 mcg/kg/min, argatroban can be discontinued when the INR is greater than 4 on combined therapy. After argatroban is discontinued, repeat the INR in 4 to 6 hours. If the INR is below the desired therapeutic range, resume the infusion of argatroban and repeat the procedure daily until the desired therapeutic range on warfarin alone is reached. See Drug/Lab Interactions. With doses of argatroban more than 2 mcg/kg/min the INR relationship is less predictable. Reduction of dose to 2 mcg/kg/min is recommended.

Prophylaxis or treatment of thrombosis: Obtain a baseline aPTT before treatment begins. Repeat aPTT in 2 hours, after any dose adjustment, and as indicated to achieve desired target aPTT of 1.5 to 3 times baseline. ▪ No enhancement of aPTT response was observed in subjects receiving repeated administration of argatroban. Repeated administration has been tolerated with no loss of anticoagulant activity and no evidence of neutralizing antibodies. No change in dose is required.

PCI: Obtain baseline ACT before dosing; repeat ACT 5 to 10 minutes after bolus dosing, after a change in infusion rate, and at the end of the PCI procedure. Draw additional ACTs every 20 to 30 minutes during a prolonged procedure. ▪ Follow standard procedures for maintenance and care of venous or arterial sheaths. Remove sheaths no sooner than 2 hours after discontinuing argatroban and when ACT has decreased to less than 160 seconds. ▪ See Dose Adjustments if anticoagulation is required after PCI.

Patient Education: Report all episodes of bleeding. ▪ Report tarry stools. ▪ Compliance with all measures to minimize bleeding is very important (e.g., avoid use of razors, toothbrushes, other sharp items). ▪ Use caution while moving to avoid excess bumping.

Maternal/Child: Category B: use during pregnancy only if clearly needed. ▪ Discontinue breast-feeding. ▪ Safety and effectiveness for use in pediatric patients under 18 years of age not established. ▪ Has been used in a small number of pediatric patients with HIT or HITTS who require an alternative to heparin therapy. See package insert for dosing recommendations and monitoring parameters. Clearance is decreased in seriously ill pediatric patients.

Elderly: Response similar to that in younger patients. See Dose Adjustments for the elderly with impaired liver function.

DRUG/LAB INTERACTIONS

If argatroban is to be initiated after cessation of **heparin** therapy, allow sufficient time for heparin's effect on the aPTT to decrease. ▪ Drug interactions have not been demonstrated between argatroban and concomitantly administered **aspirin or acetaminophen.** ▪ Risk of bleeding may be increased by any medicine that affects blood clotting, including **anticoagulants** (e.g., heparin, warfarin [Coumadin]); **any medication that may cause hypoprothrombinemia, thrombocytopenia, or GI ulceration or bleeding** (e.g., selected antibiotics [e.g., cefotetan], aspirin, NSAIDs [e.g., ibuprofen (Advil, Motrin), naproxen (Aleve, Naprosyn)]); **and/or any other medication that inhibits platelet aggregation** (e.g., clopidogrel [Plavix], dipyridamole [Persantine], glycoprotein GPIIb/IIIa receptor antagonists [e.g., abciximab (ReoPro), eptifibatide (Integrilin), tirofiban (Aggrastat)], plicamycin [Mithracin], sulfinpyrazone [Anturane], ticlopidine [Ticlid], valproic acid [Depacon]). If concurrent or subsequent use is indicated, monitor aPTT and PT closely. ▪ In clinical testing, was not found to interact with **digoxin or erythromycin** (a potent inhibitor of CYP3A4/5). ▪ Concurrent use with **warfarin** results in prolongation of the PT and INR beyond that produced by warfarin alone; see Monitor. The combination causes no further reduction in vitamin K dependent factor Xa than that seen with warfarin alone. Relationship between INR obtained on combined therapy and INR obtained on warfarin alone is dependent on both the dose of argatroban and the thromboplastin reagent used.

SIDE EFFECTS

All situations: Bleeding is the most frequent adverse event. Hypersensitivity reactions (e.g., coughing, dyspnea, hypotension, rash) have been reported, most frequently in patients who also received streptokinase or contrast media.

Prophylaxis or treatment of thrombosis: The most common side effects are cardiac arrest, diarrhea, dyspnea, fever, hypotension, and sepsis. Hemorrhagic events included a decreased hemoglobin and hematocrit, GI bleed, GU bleed, hematuria, hemoptysis, intracranial bleed, limb and below-knee amputation stump, and multisystem hemorrhage and DIC. Abdominal pain, abnormal renal function, arrhythmias (e.g., atrial fibrillation, ventricular tachycardia), cerebrovascular disorder, coughing, nausea, pain, pneumonia, UTI, and vomiting have occurred.

PCI: The most common side effects are back pain, chest pain, headache, hypotension, nausea, and vomiting. Retroperitoneal and GI bleeding occurred in a few patients. Other minor bleeding included coronary arteries; a decreased hemoglobin and hematocrit; GI bleeding; GU bleeding; hematuria; groin, hemoptysis, and access site (venous or arterial). Abdominal pain, bradycardia, fever, and MI and other serious coronary events have occurred.

Overdose: Symptoms of acute toxicity in animals included clonic convulsions, coma, loss of righting reflex, paralysis of hind limbs, and tremors.

ANTIDOTE

No specific antidote is available. Obtain aPTT, ACT, and/or other coagulation tests. Overdose with or without bleeding may be controlled by discontinuing argatroban or by decreasing the infusion dose; aPTT should return to baseline within 2 to 4 hours after discontinuation. Reversal may take longer in patients with hepatic impairment. If life-threatening bleeding develops and excessive plasma levels of argatroban are suspected, immediately stop argatroban infusion. Determine aPTT and hemoglobin, and prepare for blood transfusion as appropriate. Follow current guidelines for treatment of shock as indicated (fluid, vasopressors [e.g., dopamine], Trendelenburg position, plasma expanders [e.g., albumin, hetastarch]). Approximately 20% of argatroban may be cleared through dialysis.

ARSENIC TRIOXIDE BBW

(**AR**-sen-ik try-**OKS**-ide)

Antineoplastic

Trisenox

pH 7.5 to 8.5

USUAL DOSE

12-lead ECG, serum electrolytes (calcium, magnesium, and potassium), and serum creatinine required before beginning therapy; see Monitor.

Induction schedule: 0.15 mg/kg of body weight daily as an infusion until bone marrow remission. Total induction dose should not exceed 60 doses.

Consolidation schedule: Begin 3 to 6 weeks after completion of induction therapy. 0.15 mg/kg daily for 25 doses over a period of up to 5 weeks.

PEDIATRIC DOSE

Pediatric patients from 5 to 16 years of age: See Usual Dose. See Maternal/Child.

DOSE ADJUSTMENTS

Patients with severe renal impairment (CrCl less than 30 mL/min) or severe hepatic impairment (Child-Pugh Class C) should be closely monitored for toxicity. Dose reduction may be indicated. ▪ Use in dialysis has not been studied.

DILUTION

Specific techniques required; see Precautions. Ampule contains 10 mg/10 mL (1 mg/mL). Dilute each daily dose with 100 to 250 mL D5W or NS immediately after withdrawal from the ampule and give as an infusion.

Storage: Store ampules at CRT. Do not freeze. Do not use beyond expiration date. Discard unused portions of each ampule; contains no preservatives. Diluted solutions are stable for 24 hours at RT and 48 hours if refrigerated.

COMPATIBILITY

Manufacturer states, "Do not mix arsenic trioxide with other medications."

RATE OF ADMINISTRATION

A single daily dose as an infusion over 1 to 2 hours. May be extended up to 4 hours if acute vasomotor reactions are observed (e.g., flushing, hypertension, hypotension, pallor). May be given through a peripheral vein; a central venous catheter is not required.

ACTIONS

An antineoplastic agent. Mechanism of action not understood. May cause morphologic changes and DNA fragmentation in selected promyelocytic leukemia cells and damage or degrade selected fusion proteins. In clinical trials, median time to bone marrow remission was 44 days and to onset of complete remission (absence of visible leukemic cells in bone marrow and peripheral recovery of platelets and WBC with a confirmatory bone marrow about 30 days later) was 53 days. Responses were seen in all age-groups ranging from 6 to 72 years. Arsenious acid is the pharmacologically active species of arsenic trioxide. Metabolized in the liver (not by the cytochrome P_{450} family of isoenzymes). Elimination half-life is 10 to 14 hours. Arsenic is stored mainly in liver, kidney, heart, lung, hair, and nails. Excreted in urine. Crosses the placental barrier. Secreted in breast milk.

INDICATIONS AND USES

Induction of remission and consolidation in patients with acute promyelocytic leukemia (APL) who are refractory to, or have relapsed from, retinoid and anthracycline chemotherapy, and whose APL is characterized by the presence of the t(15;17) translocation or PML/RAR-alpha gene expression.

Unlabeled uses: Orphan drug status for treatment of chronic myeloid leukemia (CML), acute promyelocytic leukemia (APL), multiple myeloma (MM), malignant glioma, myelodysplastic syndrome, liver cancer, and chronic lymphocytic leukemia (CLL).

CONTRAINDICATIONS

Known hypersensitivity to arsenic.

PRECAUTIONS

Follow guidelines for handling cytotoxic agents. See Appendix A, p. 1331. ▪ Administered by or under the direction of a physician experienced in the management of patients with acute leukemia, with facilities for monitoring the patient and responding to any medical emergency. ▪ Symptoms similar to those associated with retinoic-acid–acute promyelocytic leukemia (RA-APL) or APL differentiation syndrome (dyspnea, fever, pleural or pericardial effusions, pulmonary infiltrates, and weight gain with or without leukocytosis) have been reported in some patients treated with arsenic trioxide and can be fatal. See Monitor and Antidote. ▪ May cause QT interval prolongation and complete atrioventricular block. QT prolongation can lead to torsades de pointes, which can be fatal. Risk of torsades de pointes is increased by extent of QT prolongation, concomitant administration of QT prolonging drugs, a history of torsades de pointes, pre-existing QT interval prolongation, congestive heart failure, administration of potassium-wasting diuretics, or other conditions that result in hypokalemia or hypomagnesemia; see Drug/Lab Interactions. QT prolongation was observed between 1 and 5 weeks after infusion and returned toward baseline by the end of 8 weeks after infusions were complete. ▪ Has been associated with the development of hyperleukocytosis. WBC counts during induction were higher than during consolidation. Treatment with additional chemotherapy was not required. ▪ Use caution in patients with impaired renal function; exposure may be increased. Monitor patients with severe renal impairment (CrCl less than 30 mL/min) closely for toxicity; dose reduction may be required. ▪ Use with caution in patients with impaired hepatic function. Data are limited. Monitor patients with severe hepatic impairment (Child-Pugh Class C) closely for toxicity.

Monitor: *Before initiating therapy:* Obtain baseline 12-lead ECG, CBC with differential, platelet count, coagulation profile (e.g., PT), serum electrolytes (e.g., calcium, magnesium, and potassium), and serum creatinine. Correct pre-existing electrolyte abnormalities and, if possible, discontinue drugs that are known to prolong the QT interval; see Drug/Lab Interactions. If the QT interval is greater than 500 msec, corrective measures should be completed and the QT interval reassessed with serial ECGs before starting arsenic trioxide. *During therapy:* Monitor electrolytes, CBC (including differential), platelet count, and coagulation profile (e.g., PT) at least twice weekly during induction and weekly during consolidation. May be indicated more frequently. Keep potassium concentrations above 4 mEq/dL and magnesium concentrations above 1.8 mg/dL. ▪ Monitor ECG weekly and more frequently in unstable patients. No data on the effect of arsenic trioxide on the QT interval during the infusion. If the QT interval is greater than 500 msec at any time during therapy, reassess the patient, correct concomitant risk factors, and consider risk/benefit of continuing versus suspending arsenic trioxide. If syncope or rapid or irregular heartbeat develops, the patient should be hospitalized for ECG monitoring and monitoring of serum electrolytes. Temporarily discontinue arsenic trioxide. Do not resume therapy until the QT interval is less than 460 msec, electrolyte abnormalities are corrected, and syncope and irregular heartbeat cease. ▪ Monitor for thrombocytopenia (platelet count less than 50,000/mm³). Initiate precautions to prevent excessive bleeding (e.g., inspect IV sites, skin, and mucous membranes; use extreme care during invasive procedures; test urine, emesis, stool, and secretions for occult blood). ▪ Monitor for signs of APL differentiation syndrome (e.g., abnormal chest auscultatory findings or radiographic abnormalities, dyspnea, weight gain, and unexplained fever). If symptoms occur, irrespective of the leukocyte count, begin immediate treatment with high-dose steroids (e.g., dexamethasone 10 mg IV twice daily); continue for at least 3 days or longer until S/S resolve. Termination of arsenic trioxide treatment is not usually required. ▪ See Precautions.

Patient Education: Avoid pregnancy; may cause fetal harm. Nonhormonal birth control recommended. Notify physician immediately if a pregnancy is suspected. ▪ Report dizziness, dyspnea, fainting, fever, rapid or irregular heartbeat, and weight gain immediately. ▪ Review all prescription and nonprescription drugs with your physician. ▪ See Appendix D, p. 1333.

Maternal/Child: Category D: avoid pregnancy. May cause fetal harm. Effective birth control required. ▪ Discontinue breast-feeding. ▪ Limited clinical data for pediatric use. In one study, five patients ranging in age from 5 to 16 years were included in clinical studies, and three achieved a complete response. In another study, the toxicity profile observed in 13 pediatric patients was similar to that seen in adults. ▪ Safety and effectiveness for pediatric patients under 4 years of age not established.

Elderly: Response similar to that in younger patients. ▪ Monitor renal function closely.

DRUG/LAB INTERACTIONS

Concurrent use with **other drugs that prolong the QT interval, including antiarrhythmics** (e.g., amiodarone [Nexterone], disopyramide [Norpace], ibutilide [Corvert], mexiletine, procainamide [Pronestyl], quinidine), **antihistamines, azole antifungals** (e.g., itraconazole [Sporanox]), **fluoroquinolones** (e.g., levofloxacin [Levaquin]), **phenothiazines** (e.g., thioridazine [Mellaril]), **and tricyclic antidepressants** (e.g., amitriptyline [Elavil], imipramine [Tofranil]) may cause torsades de pointes and could be fatal. ▪ Concurrent use with drugs that may cause hypokalemia or other electrolyte abnormalities (e.g., **amphotericin B, diuretics** [e.g., furosemide (Lasix)]) may increase the risk of hypokalemia and cardiac arrhythmias.

SIDE EFFECTS

Abdominal pain, anemia, chest pain, cough, diarrhea, dizziness, dyspnea, edema, fatigue, headache, hyperglycemia, hyperkalemia, hypertension, hypokalemia, hypomagnesemia, hypotension, hypoxia, itching, leukocytosis, nausea, neutropenia (may be febrile), palpitations, pleural effusion, rash, thrombocytopenia, URI, and vomiting. Numerous other side effects have been reported (see literature).

Major: Adverse events rated Grade 3 or 4 on the Common Terminology Criteria for Adverse Events (CTCAE) were common. APL differentiation syndrome, atrial arrhythmias, hyperglycemia, hyperleukocytosis, QT interval 500 msec or more (with or without torsades de pointes) also occurred.

Overdose: Acute arsenic toxicity (e.g., confusion, convulsions, and muscle weakness).

Post-Marketing: Pancytopenia, peripheral neuropathy, ventricular extrasystoles, and tachycardia associated with QT prolongation.

ANTIDOTE

Keep physician informed of all side effects. Those classified as average will usually be treated symptomatically. Major side effects may be fatal and require aggressive treatment as well as temporarily withholding or discontinuing arsenic trioxide. In all situations, monitor electrolytes; maintain potassium and magnesium within prescribed limits. Treat APL differentiation syndrome immediately with high-dose steroids (dexamethasone [Decadron] 10 mg IV twice daily) for at least 3 days or until signs and symptoms resolve (interruption of arsenic trioxide therapy not consistently required). Temporarily discontinue arsenic trioxide for QT prolongation 500 msec or more; see Monitor for recommendations, and promptly treat any serious or symptomatic arrhythmia (e.g., conduction abnormalities, VT, torsades de pointes). Discontinue therapy and treat acute arsenic intoxication with dimercaprol (BAL) 3 mg/kg IM every 4 hours until immediate life-threatening toxicity subsides. Then treat with penicillamine 250 mg PO up to four times a day (approximately 1 Gm/day). Hyperleukocytosis was not treated with additional chemotherapy during clinical trials.

ATROPINE SULFATE
(**AH**-troh-peen **SUL**-fayt)

Anticholinergic
Antiarrhythmic
Antidote

pH 3 to 6.5

USUAL DOSE
IV administration is usually preferred, but subcutaneous, intramuscular, and endotracheal administration are possible. For administration via an endotracheal tube, dilute 1 to 2 mg in no more than 10 mL of SWFI or NS.

Titrate dose based on HR, PR interval, BP, and symptoms. Manufacturer-recommended adult doses are outlined in the following chart.

Manufacturer-Recommended Adult Dosage		
Use	Dose	Repeat
Antisialagogue or other antivagal	0.5 to 1 mg	1 to 2 hours
Organophosphorus* or muscarinic mushroom poisoning	2 to 3 mg†	20 to 30 minutes
Bradyasystolic cardiac arrest	1 mg	3 to 5 minutes; 3 mg maximum total dose

*Atropine is given in conjunction with pralidoxime for organophosphate insecticide and nerve agent poisoning.
†Higher doses have been used in severe poisoning. Consult a regional poison control center.

Other sources recommend the following doses:

Inhibition of salivation and secretions (preanesthesia): 0.4 to 0.6 mg 30 to 60 minutes preoperatively and repeat every 4 to 6 hours as needed.

Bradycardia: 0.5 mg every 3 to 5 minutes, not to exceed a total dose of 3 mg or 0.04 mg/kg.

Reversal of neuromuscular blockade: 15 to 30 mcg/kg administered with neostigmine or 7 to 10 mcg/kg administered with edrophonium. Administer in a separate syringe either concurrently or a few minutes before administering the anticholinesterase agent. If bradycardia is present, administer atropine first.

Cardiac asystole or pulseless electrical activity: AHA guidelines state, "Routine use during pulseless electrical activity or asystole is unlikely to have a therapeutic benefit."

PEDIATRIC DOSE
Fatal dose of atropine in pediatric patients may be as low as 10 mg. See Maternal/Child.

Dosing in pediatric patients has not been well studied. The manufacturer lists a usual initial dose of 0.01 to 0.03 mg/kg. Doses less than 0.1 mg have been associated with a paradoxical bradycardia.

Other sources recommend the following doses:

Inhibition of salivation and secretions (preanesthesia): *Infants; weight less than 5 kg:* 0.02 mg/kg/dose. There is no documented minimum dose for patients in this age/weight range. *Infants and children; weight equal to or more than 5 kg:* 0.01 to 0.02 mg/kg/dose; maximum single dose should not exceed 0.4 mg. Minimum recommended dose is 0.1 mg. May repeat every 4 to 6 hours.

Bradycardia: *Infants; weight less than 5 kg:* 0.02 mg/kg/dose. There is no documented minimum dose for patients in this age/weight range. *Infants and children; weight equal to or more than 5 kg:* 0.02 mg/kg/dose; maximum single dose should not exceed 0.5 mg. May repeat one time in 3 to 5 minutes; maximum total dose should not exceed 1 mg. Minimum recommended dose is 0.1 mg.

Antidote for acute poisoning from exposure to anticholinesterase compounds (e.g., organophosphate compounds, nerve gases, mushroom poisoning): 0.05 to 0.1 mg/kg; repeat every

5 to 10 minutes until muscarinic signs and symptoms subside. Administer repeat doses as needed based on recurrence of symptoms.

Reversal of neuromuscular blockade: 0.01 to 0.02 mg/kg of atropine concomitantly with 0.04 mg/kg of neostigmine. See Usual Dose for additional information.

DOSE ADJUSTMENTS

Reduced dose may be indicated in the elderly based on decreased organ function and/or concomitant disease or other drug therapy. ▪ See Drug/Lab Interactions and Pediatric Dose.

DILUTION

May be given undiluted. Do not add to IV solutions. Inject through Y-tube or three-way stopcock of infusion set. Also available in combination with edrophonium (Enlon-Plus) to reverse nondepolarizing neuromuscular blocking agents.

Storage: Store at CRT.

COMPATIBILITY   (Underline Indicates Conflicting Compatibility Information)

Consider any drug NOT listed as compatible to be INCOMPATIBLE until consulting a pharmacist; specific conditions may apply.

One source suggests the following **compatibilities:**

Additive: Dobutamine, furosemide (Lasix), meropenem (Merrem IV), sodium bicarbonate, verapamil.

Y-site: Abciximab (ReoPro), amiodarone (Nexterone), argatroban, bivalirudin (Angiomax), dexmedetomidine (Precedex), doripenem (Doribax), etomidate (Amidate), famotidine (Pepcid IV), fenoldopam (Corlopam), fentanyl, heparin, hydrocortisone sodium succinate (Solu-Cortef), hydromorphone (Dilaudid), meropenem (Merrem IV), methadone (Dolophine), morphine, nafcillin (Nallpen), palonosetron (Aloxi), potassium chloride (KCl), propofol (Diprivan), tirofiban (Aggrastat).

RATE OF ADMINISTRATION

Administer undiluted by rapid IV injection. Slow injection may cause a paradoxical bradycardia.

ACTIONS

Atropine is an anticholinergic drug and a potent belladonna alkaloid. An antimuscarinic agent that competitively antagonizes the muscarine-like actions of acetylcholine and other choline esters. Produces local, central, and peripheral effects on the body. Main therapeutic uses are peripheral, affecting smooth muscle, cardiac muscle, and exocrine gland cells. Increases heart rate and cardiac output and dries secretions. Widely distributed, metabolized by the liver via enzymatic hydrolysis, and excreted in urine. Half-life in adults is approximately 3 hours. Half-life in pediatric patients and adults over 65 years of age may be more than doubled. Crosses placental barrier. Secreted in breast milk.

INDICATIONS AND USES

Temporary blockade of severe or life-threatening muscarinic effects (e.g., as an antisialagogue, an antivagal agent, an antidote for organophosphorus or muscarinic mushroom poisoning, and for treatment of bradyasystolic cardiac arrest).

CONTRAINDICATIONS

Manufacturer states, "None." Other sources list hypersensitivity to atropine. No contraindications exist in the treatment of life-threatening organophosphorus or carbamate insecticide or nerve agent poisoning.

PRECAUTIONS

Use with caution in patients with coronary artery disease. When recurrent use is essential, the total dose should be restricted to 2 to 3 mg (0.03 to 0.04 mg/kg) to avoid the detrimental effects of atropine-induced tachycardia on myocardial oxygen demand. ▪ May precipitate acute glaucoma. ▪ May convert partial organic pyloric stenosis into complete obstruction. ▪ May cause complete urinary retention in patients with prostatic hypertrophy. ▪ May cause thickening of bronchial secretions and the formation of viscid mucous plugs in patients with chronic lung disease. ▪ Use with caution in patients with cardiovascular disease, pulmonary disease, autonomic neuropathy, GI disease (e.g., paralytic ileus, intestinal atony, severe ulcerative colitis, toxic megacolon), hyperthyroidism, myasthenia gravis, and renal impairment.

Monitor: Vital signs and/or ECG based on specific situation. ▪ Monitor for resolution or return of symptoms in episodes of poisoning. ▪ Monitor for S/S of atropine toxicity (e.g., blurred vision, delirium, fever, muscle fasciculations, hot, dry skin).

Patient Education: Use caution if task requires alertness; may cause blurred vision, dizziness, or drowsiness. ▪ Report eye pain, flushing, or skin rash promptly. ▪ Report dry mouth, difficulty urinating, constipation, or increased light sensitivity.

Maternal/Child: Category C: safety for use in pregnancy, breast-feeding, and pediatric patients not established. ▪ Pediatric patients may be more sensitive to anticholinergic effects.

Elderly: May be more sensitive to adverse effects. ▪ Potential for constipation and urinary retention increased. ▪ See Dose Adjustments.

DRUG/LAB INTERACTIONS

May have additive effects when used in combination with **other agents with anticholinergic properties** (e.g., amantadine [Symmetrel], glycopyrrolate [Robinul], phenothiazines [e.g., prochlorperazine (Compazine)], tricyclic antidepressants [e.g., amitriptyline (Elavil), imipramine (Tofranil)]). ▪ May potentiate effects of many oral drugs by delaying gastric emptying and increasing absorption (e.g., **atenolol, digoxin, nitrofurantoin, thiazide diuretics**). ▪ Decreases the rate of **mexiletine** absorption without altering the relative oral bioavailability. ▪ Antagonizes **anticholinesterase inhibitors** (e.g., edrophonium [Tensilon], pyridostigmine [Regonol]).

SIDE EFFECTS

Most side effects of atropine are directly related to its antimuscarinic action. Blurred vision, dryness of the mouth, photophobia, and tachycardia commonly occur. Other possible reactions include anhidrosis (leading to heat intolerance), constipation, dilation of the pupils, flushing, gastroesophageal reflux, heat prostration from decreased sweating, hypersensitivity reactions (e.g., skin rashes that in some cases progressed to exfoliation), nausea, paralytic ileus, postural hypotension, tachycardia, urinary hesitancy and retention (especially in males), and vomiting.

Overdose: *Excessive doses* may cause ataxia; difficulty swallowing; dilated pupils; dizziness; fatigue; hot, dry skin; palpitations; restlessness; thirst; and tremor. *Toxic doses* may lead to restlessness and excitation, hallucinations, delirium, and coma. *Severe intoxication* may lead to depression and circulatory collapse, paralysis, coma, respiratory failure, and death.

ANTIDOTE

Discontinue if side effects increase or are severe. Notify physician. Use standard treatments to manage cardiac arrhythmias. Physostigmine salicylate (Antilirium) (1 to 4 mg [0.5 to 1 mg in pediatric patients]) reverses most cardiovascular and CNS effects. Repeat doses as needed. Diazepam (Valium) or a short-acting barbiturate may be administered as needed to control marked excitement and convulsions. Large doses should be avoided because central depressant action may coincide with the depression that occurs late in atropine poisoning. Central stimulants are not recommended. Artificial respiration with oxygen may be necessary. Ice bags and alcohol sponges help to reduce fever, especially in pediatric patients. Atropine is not removed by dialysis.

AZACITIDINE
(ay-za-**SYE**-ti-deen)

Antineoplastic

Vidaza

USUAL DOSE
Premedication: Prophylactic administration of antiemetics (e.g., granisetron [Kytril], ondansetron [Zofran]) is indicated before each dose.

First treatment cycle: An initial dose of 75 mg/M^2 as an IV infusion or as a SC injection once daily for 7 days is recommended for all patients regardless of baseline hematology.

Subsequent treatment cycles: Cycles should be repeated every 4 weeks. Dose may be increased to 100 mg/M^2 if no beneficial effect is seen after 2 treatment cycles and if no toxicity other than nausea and vomiting has occurred. Treatment is recommended for a minimum of 4 to 6 cycles; however, a complete or partial response may require additional treatment cycles. Repeat cycles may be administered as long as the patient continues to benefit. See Dose Adjustments for dose delay or reduction recommendations for hematologic response, renal toxicities, and/or electrolyte disturbances.

DOSE ADJUSTMENTS
After administration of the recommended dosage for the first cycle, adjust dosage for subsequent cycles based on nadir counts and hematologic response as outlined in the following chart.

Dose Adjustments of Azacitidine Based on Baseline Hematologic Responses	
In any given subsequent cycle for patients with a baseline (start of treatment) WBC equal to or greater than 3 × 10^9/L (3,000 cells/mm^3), ANC equal to or greater than 1.5 × 10^9/L (1,500 cells/mm^3), and platelets equal to or greater than 75 × 10^9/L (75,000 cells/mm^3): Adjust the dose based on nadir counts according to the following chart.	

Nadir Counts		% Dose in the Next Cycle
ANC (cells/mm^3)	Platelets (cells/mm^3)	
<500 cells/mm^3	<25,000 cells/mm^3	50%
500 to 1,500 cells/mm^3	25,000 to 50,000 cells/mm^3	67%
>1,500 cells/mm^3	>50,000 cells/mm^3	100%

In any given subsequent cycle for patients with a baseline (start of treatment) WBC less than 3 × 10^9/L (3,000 cells/mm^3), ANC less than 1.5 × 10^9/L (1,500 cells/mm^3), or platelets less than 75 × 10^9/L (75,000 cells/mm^3): Adjust the dose based on nadir counts and bone marrow biopsy cellularity at the time of the nadir according to the following chart. *The exception is the presence of clear improvement in differentiation (% of mature granulocytes is higher and ANC is higher than at the onset of that course) at the time of the next cycle. If this improvement occurs, the dose of the current treatment should be continued.*

WBC or Platelet Nadir (% Decrease in Counts from Baseline)	Bone Marrow Biopsy Cellularity at Time of Nadir (%)		
	30% to 60%	15% to 30%	<15%
	% Dose in the Next Course		
50% to 75%	100%	50%	33%
>75%	75%	50%	33%

Continued

If a nadir as defined in this chart has occurred, the next course of treatment should be given 28 days after the start of the preceding course, provided that both the WBC and the platelet count are greater than 25% above the nadir and are rising. If a greater than 25% increase above the nadir is not seen by day 28, counts should be reassessed every 7 days. If a 25% increase is not seen by Day 42, the patient should be treated with 50% of the scheduled dose.

Dose adjustments of azacitidine based on renal function and serum electrolytes: If unexplained reductions in serum bicarbonate levels to less than 20 mEq/L occur, reduce the dose by 50% on the next course. ▪ If unexplained elevations of BUN or SCr occur, delay the next cycle until values return to baseline and then reduce the dose by 50% on the next course. Severe renal impairment (CrCl less than 30 mL/min) has no major effect on exposure of azacitidine after multiple SC administrations. Therefore azacitidine can be administered to patients with renal impairment without Cycle 1 dose adjustment. (IV route was not studied.) ▪ Use care in dose selection for the elderly; reduced doses may be indicated based on overall renal function.

DILUTION

Specific techniques required; see Precautions. Available as a lyophilized powder in single-use vials containing 100 mg. More than one vial may be required for a single dose. Reconstitute each vial with 10 mL SWFI. Vigorously shake or roll each vial until all solids are dissolved. Solution equals 10 mg/mL. Withdraw the required amount of azacitidine to deliver the desired dose and inject into a 50- or 100-mL infusion bag of NS or LR. Administration must be complete within 1 hour of reconstitution. Discard unused portions appropriately.

Filters: Specific information not available.

Storage: Store in cartons at CRT. Reconstituted solutions may be held at 25° C (77° F), but administration must be complete within 1 hour of reconstitution.

COMPATIBILITY

Consider any drug NOT listed as compatible to be INCOMPATIBLE until consulting a pharmacist; specific conditions may apply.

Manufacturer lists azacitidine as **incompatible** with D5W, hetastarch, or any solution that contains bicarbonate. These solutions have the potential to increase the rate of degradation of azacitidine.

RATE OF ADMINISTRATION

A single dose equally distributed over 10 to 40 minutes. Administration must be complete within 1 hour of reconstitution.

ACTIONS

A pyrimidine nucleoside analog of cytidine. Azacitidine is believed to exert its antineoplastic effects by causing hypomethylation of DNA and direct cytotoxicity on abnormal hematopoietic cells in the bone marrow. Cytotoxic effects cause the death of rapidly dividing cells, including cancer cells that are no longer responsive to normal growth-control mechanisms. Nonproliferating cells are relatively insensitive to azacitidine. This hypomethylation may restore normal function to genes that are critical for cellular differentiation and proliferation and also allow the formation of normal bone marrow cells. May be metabolized by the liver. Half-life is 4 hours. Primarily excreted in urine with minimal excretion in feces.

INDICATIONS AND USES

Treatment of patients with the following French-American-British (FAB) myelodysplastic syndrome (MDS) subtypes such as refractory anemia (RA), refractory anemia with ringed sideroblasts (if accompanied by neutropenia or thrombocytopenia or requiring transfusions), refractory anemia with excess blasts (RAEB), refractory anemia with excess blasts in transformation (RAEB-T), and chronic myelomonocytic leukemia (CMMoL).

CONTRAINDICATIONS

Known hypersensitivity to azacitidine or mannitol; patients with advanced malignant hepatic tumors.

PRECAUTIONS

Follow guidelines for handling cytotoxic agents; see Appendix A, p. 1331. ▪ If azacitidine comes into contact with skin, immediately wash with soap and water. If it comes into contact with mucous membranes, flush thoroughly with water. ▪ Administer by or under the direction of a physician specialist in a facility with adequate diagnostic and treatment facilities to monitor the patient and respond to any medical emergency. ▪ Use caution in patients with liver disease; potentially hepatotoxic in patients with severe pre-existing hepatic impairment; see Contraindications. Cases of progressive hepatic coma and death have been reported in patients with extensive tumor burden due to metastatic disease, especially when baseline albumin is less than 3 Gm/dL. ▪ Rare reports of renal abnormalities (e.g., elevated serum creatinine, renal failure, and death) have occurred in patients treated with azacitidine in combination with other chemotherapeutic agents for non-MDS conditions. Patients with renal impairment may be at increased risk for renal toxicity. ▪ Renal tubular acidosis (a fall in serum bicarbonate to less than 20 mEq/L in association with an alkaline urine and hypokalemia [serum potassium less than 3 mEq/L]) developed in 5 patients with chronic myelogenous leukemia (CML) treated with azacitidine and etoposide. ▪ The effects of race or hepatic impairment on the pharmacokinetics of azacitidine have not been studied. ▪ Anemia, leukopenia, neutropenia, and thrombocytopenia may be dose-limiting toxicities. ▪ Patients with MDS produce poorly functioning and immature blood cells and experience anemia, bleeding, fatigue, infection, and weakness. High-risk MDS patients may experience bone marrow failure, which may lead to death from bleeding and infection. ▪ MDS can progress to acute leukemia.

Monitor: Obtain a baseline CBC with platelets, and monitor before each dosing cycle and as indicated to monitor response and toxicity between cycles. ▪ Obtain baseline renal and hepatic function (BUN, SCr, bilirubin) studies and electrolytes; monitor during treatment as indicated. Renal function should be monitored before each dosing cycle. ▪ Use prophylactic antiemetics to reduce nausea and vomiting and to increase patient comfort. ▪ Monitor for S/S of infection. Prophylactic antibiotics may be indicated pending results of C/S in a febrile neutropenic patient. ▪ Monitor for thrombocytopenia (platelet count less than 50,000/mm³). Initiate precautions to prevent excessive bleeding (e.g., inspect IV sites, skin, and mucous membranes; use extreme care during invasive procedures; test urine, emesis, stool, and secretions for occult blood). ▪ Avoid administration of live virus vaccine to immunocompromised patients. ▪ Observe for S/S of a hypersensitivity reaction; specific information not available. ▪ See Precautions and Antidote.

Patient Education: Avoid pregnancy; nonhormonal birth control recommended for both males and females. Women should report a suspected pregnancy immediately. Males should not father a child during treatment with azacitidine. ▪ Inform physician about any underlying liver or renal disease.

Maternal/Child: Category D: avoid pregnancy; may cause fetal harm. Males should not father a child while receiving treatment with azacitidine. ▪ Discontinue breast-feeding; has the potential for causing serious harm to nursing infants. ▪ Safety and effectiveness for use in pediatric patients not established.

Elderly: Safety and effectiveness similar to younger adults. ▪ Consider age-related renal impairment; dosing should be cautious; see Dose Adjustments. Monitor renal function.

DRUG/LAB INTERACTIONS

Formal drug interaction studies have not been completed. ▪ Effect on metabolism by some known microsomal enzyme inhibitors or inducers has been studied in vitro. Does not appear to inhibit CYP2B6 or CYP2C8. Potential to inhibit other P_{450} enzymes is not known. Does not appear to induce CYP1A2, CYP2C19, or CYP3A4/5. ▪ Do not administer **live virus vaccines** to patients receiving antineoplastic agents.

SIDE EFFECTS

Hypokalemia, petechiae, rigors, and weakness are the most common side effects. Other common side effects include anemia; constipation; diarrhea; ecchymosis; fatigue; fever; infection; injection site bruising, erythema, and pain; leukopenia; nausea; neutropenia;

thrombocytopenia; and vomiting. Febrile neutropenia, fever, leukopenia, neutropenia, pneumonia, and thrombocytopenia were the most frequent cause of dose reduction, delay, and discontinuation. Infusion site erythema or pain and catheter site reactions such as infection, erythema, or hemorrhage were reported with IV administration. Elevated SCr, hepatic coma, hypokalemia, renal failure, and renal tubular acidosis have also been reported. Numerous other side effects may be associated with azacitidine.

Post-Marketing: Injection site necrosis, interstitial lung disease, necrotizing fasciitis (including fatal cases), Sweet's syndrome (acute febrile neutrophilic dermatosis), tumor lysis syndrome.

ANTIDOTE
Notify physician of any side effects. Most will be treated symptomatically. Dose may be reduced or delayed for hematologic toxicity, renal toxicity, or electrolyte disturbances. See Dose Adjustments for specific criteria. Blood and blood products, antibiotics, and other adjunctive therapies must be available. No known antidote; monitor blood counts and provide supportive care in overdose. ▪ Resuscitate as necessary.

AZATHIOPRINE SODIUM BBW
(ay-zah-**THIGH**-oh-preen **SO**-dee-um)

Immunosuppressant

pH 9.6

USUAL DOSE
3 to 5 mg/kg of body weight/24 hr. Begin treatment within 24 hours of renal homotransplantation. In some cases, doses are given 1 to 3 days before transplantation. Maintenance dose is 1 to 3 mg/kg/24 hr. Individualized adjustment is imperative. Do not increase to toxic levels because of threatened rejection. Oral and IV doses are therapeutically equivalent; transfer to oral therapy as soon as practical.

DOSE ADJUSTMENTS
Dose reduction is recommended in patients with reduced thiopurine *S*-methyltransferase (TPMT) activity; see Precautions. ▪ Reduce dose in impaired kidney function (especially immediately after transplant or with cadaveric kidneys) and in persistent negative nitrogen balance. ▪ Dose reduction may be required if there is a rapid fall or a persistently low leukocyte count. ▪ Decrease dose to one third to one fourth of the usual dose when given concomitantly with allopurinol. Consider further dose reduction or alternative therapy in patients with low or absent TPMT activity who are receiving both drugs. ▪ To minimize risk of malignancy secondary to immunosuppression, immunosuppressive drug therapy should be maintained at the lowest effective levels. ▪ See Drug/Lab Interactions and Precautions/Monitor.

DILUTION
Specific techniques suggested; see Precautions. Each 100 mg should be initially reconstituted with 10 mL of SWFI. Swirl the vial gently until completely in solution. May be further diluted in a minimum of 50 mL of NS, D5W, or D5NS and given as an infusion. See Compatibility.

Storage: Store unopened vials at 20° to 25° C (68° to 77° F). Protect from light. Use diluted solution within 24 hours.

COMPATIBILITY
Specific information not available. Listed as **incompatible** with preservatives (e.g., methylparaben, phenol, propylparaben). Administer separately. Converts to 6-mercaptopurine in alkaline solutions and sulfhydryl compounds. Flush IV line with a **compatible** IV fluid before and after administration.

RATE OF ADMINISTRATION

A single dose properly diluted and infused over 30 to 60 minutes. Actual range may be 5 minutes to 8 hours.

ACTIONS

An immunosuppressive antimetabolite that aids in inhibition of renal homograft rejection. It is chemically cleaved to the antineoplastic compound 6-mercaptopurine. Exact method of action is unknown. It suppresses hypersensitivities of the cell-mediated type and causes variable alterations in antibody production. Action depends on the temporal relationship to antigenic stimulus or engraftment. Has little effect on established graft rejections or secondary responses. Also suppresses disease manifestations and underlying pathology of autoimmune disease (e.g., rheumatoid arthritis [RA]). Exact mechanism of action is unknown. Metabolized readily with small amounts excreted in the urine. Crosses placental barrier. Secreted in breast milk.

INDICATIONS AND USES

Adjunct to prevent rejection in renal homotransplantation. ▪ Used PO to treat rheumatoid arthritis; see package insert.

CONTRAINDICATIONS

Known hypersensitivity to azathioprine. ▪ Patients with rheumatoid arthritis who have been treated with alkylating agents (e.g., chlorambucil [Leukeran], cyclophosphamide [Cytoxan], melphalan [Alkeran]) may have a prohibitive risk of malignancy if treated with azathioprine.

PRECAUTIONS

Follow guidelines for handling cytotoxic agents; see Appendix A, p. 1331. ▪ Usually administered in the hospital by or under the direction of a physician experienced in immunosuppressive therapy and management of organ transplant patients. ▪ Adequate laboratory and supportive medical resources must be available. ▪ Chronic immunosuppression increases the risk of malignancy. Reports of malignancy include posttransplant lymphoma, increased risk of developing lymphoma and other malignancies (particularly of the skin), and hepatosplenic T-cell lymphoma (HSTCL) in patients with inflammatory bowel disease. Has mutogenic potential to both men and women. Patients with Crohn's disease or inflammatory bowel disease, particularly adolescents and young adults, may have a higher risk of malignancies, including hepatosplenic T-cell lymphoma (HSTCL), with azathioprine alone or in combination therapy with TNF blockers (e.g., infliximab [Remicade]). Safety and efficacy of azathioprine for treatment of Crohn's disease and ulcerative colitis have not been established. ▪ Severe leukopenia, thrombocytopenia, macrocytic anemia, and/or pancytopenia may occur. ▪ Serious infections (bacterial, fungal, protozoal, viral, and opportunistic infections, including reactivation of latent infections) may occur and can be fatal. ▪ Progressive multifocal leukoencephalopathy (PML), including fatal PML, has been reported in patients treated with immunosuppressants, including azathioprine. ▪ Rapid bone marrow suppression progressing to severe, life-threatening myelotoxicity may occur in patients with inherited intermediate, low, or absent TPMT. Genotyping or phenotyping may help identify these patients. Accurate phenotyping results are not possible in patients who have received recent blood transfusions. TPMT testing cannot substitute for required CBC and platelet monitoring. ▪ Hematologic toxicities are dose-related and may be more severe in renal transplant patients whose homograft is undergoing rejection. ▪ A GI hypersensitivity reaction (e.g., severe nausea and vomiting) has been reported. May also cause diarrhea, elevations of liver function tests, fever, hypotension, malaise, myalgias, and rash. Usually develops within the first several weeks of therapy and resolves when azathioprine is discontinued.

Monitor: Monitor CBC with platelets weekly for the first month, twice monthly for the second and third months, then monthly or more frequently if dose adjustments or other therapy changes are necessary. Drug should be withdrawn or dose reduced at first sign of abnormally large fall in the leukocyte count or other evidence of persistent bone marrow suppression. ▪ Observe constantly for signs of infection. Prophylactic antibiotics may be indicated pending results of C/S in a febrile neutropenic patient. ▪ Monitor for S/S of malignancies such as HSTCL (e.g., abdominal pain, hepatomegaly, night sweats, persistent fever, weight loss). ▪ Periodic assessment of liver function tests indicated for early detection of hepatotoxicity. ▪ Consider PML in patients with new-onset or changes to pre-existing neurologic manifestations; consider consultation with a neurologist as clinically indicated. Consider dose reduction; however, reduced immunosuppression may cause graft rejection.

Patient Education: Avoid pregnancy; nonhormonal birth control recommended. ▪ Promptly report abdominal pain, fever, unusual bruising or bleeding, and/or S/S of infection. ▪ Obtain all lab work as directed. ▪ Wear protective clothing and use sunscreen to limit exposure to sunlight and ultraviolet light. ▪ Risk of malignancy increased with chronic immunosuppression. ▪ See Appendix D, p. 1333.

Maternal/Child: Category D: avoid pregnancy. Can cause fetal harm. ▪ Discontinue breast-feeding. ▪ Safety and effectiveness for use in pediatric patients not established.

Elderly: Dose selection should be cautious; consider age-related renal impairment; see Dose Adjustments. Monitor renal function.

DRUG/LAB INTERACTIONS

Allopurinol (Aloprim) inhibits the metabolism of azathioprine, increasing its activity and toxicity. Reduce dose of azathioprine to one third or one fourth of usual; see Dose Adjustments. ▪ Inhibits anticoagulant effects of **warfarin** (Coumadin). ▪ Concurrent use with **bone marrow suppressants, radiation therapy, other immunosuppressants** (e.g., cyclosporine [Sandimmune]) **or other drugs that may cause blood dyscrasias** (e.g., sulfamethoxazole/trimethoprim [Bactrim]) may increase toxicity. ▪ Concurrent use with **ACE inhibitors** (e.g., captopril) may induce anemia and severe leukopenia. ▪ Plasma levels of the metabolite 6-MP may be increased by **methotrexate.** ▪ **Aminosalicylates** (e.g., sulfasalazine [Azulfidine], mesalamine [Asacol, Pentasa], olsalazine [Dipentum]) may inhibit TPMT, increasing the risk of toxicity. Use caution if concomitant therapy is required. ▪ **Ribavirin** (Rebetol, Vizoral) inhibits azathioprine metabolism. Concurrent use may induce severe pancytopenia. Dose adjustment and careful monitoring required if concurrent use necessary. ▪ Antibody response to **vaccines** may be suppressed. Do not use **live virus vaccines** in patients receiving azathioprine.

SIDE EFFECTS

Principal and potentially serious side effects are hematologic and gastrointestinal. Risk of infection and malignancy are also significant. Frequency and severity of side effects depend on dose, duration of therapy, and on patient's underlying condition and concomitant therapy. Leukopenia and/or thrombocytopenia are dose-dependent and dose limiting. Other side effects include alopecia; anemia; anorexia; arthralgia; bleeding; diarrhea; fever; hepatic veno-occlusive disease; hepatosplenic T-cell lymphoma; hepatotoxicity characterized by elevation of serum alkaline phosphatase, bilirubin, and serum transaminases (e.g., ALT, AST); hypotension; infection; jaundice; malaise; myalgias; nausea; neoplasia; oral lesions; pancreatitis; skin rash; Sweet's syndrome (acute febrile neutrophilic dermatosis); vomiting. A GI hypersensitivity reaction (e.g., severe nausea and vomiting) has been reported; see Precautions.

ANTIDOTE

Notify the physician of all side effects. Most can be treated symptomatically and may reverse when the drug is discontinued. The GI hypersensitivity reactions can occur within hours of a rechallenge. Drug may be decreased or discontinued or other immunosuppressive agents utilized. Hematopoietic depression may require temporary or permanent discontinuation of treatment and may be indicated even if rejection of graft may occur. Dialysis may be useful in overdose (partially dialyzable).

AZITHROMYCIN
(az-**zith**-roh-**MY**-sin)

Zithromax

Antibacterial
(azalide/macrolide)

pH 6.4 to 6.6

USUAL DOSE
Community-acquired pneumonia: 500 mg as a single daily dose for a minimum of 2 days. Follow with 500 mg of oral azithromycin as a single daily dose. Total course of therapy (IV + oral) should be 7 to 10 days.

Pelvic inflammatory disease: 500 mg as a single daily dose for 1 to 2 days. Follow with 250 mg of oral azithromycin as a single daily dose. Total course of therapy (IV + oral) should be 7 days. If anaerobic microorganisms are also suspected, concurrent administration of an antibacterial agent with anaerobic activity is recommended (e.g., metronidazole [Flagyl]).

DOSE ADJUSTMENTS
Reduced dose may be required in impaired liver or renal function; see Precautions. ▪ See Drug/Lab Interactions.

DILUTION
Each 500-mg vial must be reconstituted with 4.8 mL SWFI. Shake well to ensure dilution (100 mg/mL). Further dilute each 500 mg of reconstituted solution with 250 to 500 mL of one of the following solutions: D5W, NS, 1/2NS, D5/1/3NS, D5/1/2NS, D5/1/2NS with 20 mEq KCl, LR, D5LR, D5/Normosol M, D5/Normosol R. 500 mL diluent yields 1 mg/mL, 250 mL yields 2 mg/mL. Concentrations greater than 2 mg/mL have caused local IV site reactions and should be avoided.

Storage: Reconstituted or diluted solution stable at CRT for 24 hours. Diluted solution stable for up to 7 days if refrigerated.

COMPATIBILITY
(Underline Indicates Conflicting Compatibility Information)

Consider any drug NOT listed as compatible to be INCOMPATIBLE until consulting a pharmacist; specific conditions may apply.

Manufacturer states, "Other IV substances, additives, or medications should not be added to azithromycin, or infused simultaneously through the same IV line." Flush IV line with a **compatible** IV fluid before and after administration.

One source suggests the following **compatibilities:**

Y-site: Bivalirudin (Angiomax), caspofungin (Cancidas), ceftaroline (Teflaro), dexmedetomidine (Precedex), diphenhydramine (Benadryl), dolasetron (Anzemet), doripenem (Doribax), droperidol (Inapsine), hetastarch in electrolytes (Hextend), ondansetron (Zofran), telavancin (Vibativ), tigecycline (Tygacil).

RATE OF ADMINISTRATION
Do not give by IV bolus; must be infused over at least 1 hour.

1 mg/mL dilution: A single dose equally distributed over 3 hours.

2 mg/mL dilution: A single dose equally distributed over 1 hour.

ACTIONS
A macrolide/azalide antibiotic. Active against selected organisms, including aerobic gram-positive and gram-negative organisms and other organisms, including *Chlamydia* and *Mycoplasma pneumoniae.* Interferes with microbial protein synthesis by binding a ribosomal subunit of a susceptible microorganism. Terminal half-life of 68 hours allows for once-daily dosing. Prolonged half-life is thought to result from extensive uptake and subsequent release of drug from tissues. Studies to assess the metabolism of azithromycin have not been performed. Oral formulation is excreted primarily as unchanged drug in bile. Up to 14% excreted in urine within 24 hours. Excreted in breast milk in small amounts.

INDICATIONS AND USES

Treatment of community-acquired pneumonia and pelvic inflammatory disease caused by specific organisms (e.g., *Staphylococcus aureus, Streptococcus pneumoniae, Haemophilus influenzae, Neisseria gonorrhoeae, Chlamydia trachomatis*. See product insert for complete list in patients who require initial IV therapy). Many other indications for oral use.

CONTRAINDICATIONS

Hypersensitivity to azithromycin, erythromycin, or any macrolide antibiotic or ketolide antibiotic (e.g., telithromycin [Ketek]). ▪ Patients with a history of cholestatic jaundice/hepatic dysfunction associated with prior use of azithromycin.

PRECAUTIONS

For IV use only. ▪ Specific sensitivity studies are indicated to determine susceptibility of the causative organism to azithromycin. ▪ To reduce the development of drug-resistant bacteria and maintain its effectiveness, azithromycin should be used only to treat or prevent infections proven or strongly suspected to be caused by bacteria. ▪ Has demonstrated cross-resistance with erythromycin-resistant gram-positive organisms. Most strains of *Enterococcus faecalis* and methicillin-resistant staphylococci are resistant to azithromycin. ▪ Serious hypersensitivity reactions, including angioedema, anaphylaxis, and dermatologic reactions (e.g., Stevens-Johnson syndrome, toxic epidermal necrolysis) have been reported. Use extreme caution; hypersensitivity reactions have recurred even after azithromycin was discontinued and hypersensitivity reactions treated. ▪ Principally eliminated in the liver; use caution in patients with impaired hepatic function. Hepatotoxicity, including abnormal liver function, hepatitis, cholestatic jaundice, hepatic necrosis, and hepatic failure, have been reported; deaths have occurred. ▪ Use caution in patients with impaired renal function; no data available on effects of IV azithromycin. ▪ Macrolide antibiotics (including azithromycin) have caused ventricular arrhythmias, including ventricular tachycardia and torsades de pointes, which can be fatal. Consider risk/benefit of azithromycin use in at-risk patients, such as patients with known prolonged QT intervals, a history of torsades de pointes, congenital long QT syndrome, bradyarrhythmias, or uncompensated heart failure; patients taking drugs known to prolong the QT interval; patients with ongoing pro-arrhythmic conditions (e.g., uncorrected hypokalemia or hypomagnesemia) or clinically significant bradycardia; and patients receiving Class Ia (quinidine, procainamide) or Class III (amiodarone, dofetilide [Tikosyn], sotalol [Betapace AF]) antiarrhythmic agents. ▪ Timing of transfer to oral therapy should be based on clinical response. ▪ Avoid prolonged use; superinfection caused by overgrowth of nonsusceptible organisms may result. ▪ *Clostridium difficile*–associated diarrhea (CDAD) has been reported. May range from mild diarrhea to fatal colitis. Consider in patients who present with diarrhea during or after treatment with azithromycin. ▪ May cause exacerbations of symptoms of myasthenia gravis or new onset of myasthenia syndrome.

Monitor: Monitor vital signs. ▪ Observe closely for signs of a hypersensitivity reaction; see Antidote. ▪ Monitoring of liver function may be indicated; see Precautions. ▪ ECG monitoring for QT prolongation may be indicated; see Precautions. ▪ Monitor infusion site for inflammation and/or extravasation. ▪ Contains 4.96 mEq of sodium/vial. Observe for electrolyte imbalance and cardiac irregularities. May aggravate CHF. ▪ See Drug/Lab Interactions and Antidote.

Patient Education: Discontinue azithromycin and report any signs of an allergic reaction immediately (difficulty breathing, itching, rash, swelling). ▪ Discontinue azithromycin and report S/S of hepatitis (e.g., dark urine, jaundice, loss of appetite, malaise, nausea and vomiting). ▪ Promptly report diarrhea or bloody stools that occur during treatment or up to several months after an antibiotic has been discontinued; may indicate CDAD and require treatment. ▪ Review all prescription and nonprescription medications with your health care provider.

Maternal/Child: Category B: safety for use during pregnancy and breast-feeding not established; use with caution and only if clearly needed. ▪ Safety and effectiveness for use in pediatric patients under 16 years of age not established. ▪ Has been administered to pediatric patients age 6 months to 16 years by the oral route. The most common side effects in this age-group included abdominal pain, diarrhea, headache, nausea, rash, and vomiting.

Elderly: Response similar to that seen in younger adults. May be more susceptible to development of drug-associated effects on the QT interval than younger patients. ▪ Consider age-related organ impairment.

DRUG/LAB INTERACTIONS

May have a modest effect on the pharmacokinetics of **atorvastatin** (Lipitor), **carbamazepine** (Tegretol), **cetirizine** (Zyrtec), **didanosine** (Videx), **efavirenz** (Sustiva), **fluconazole** (Diflucan), **indinavir** (Crixivan), **midazolam** (Versed), **rifabutin** (Mycobutin), **sildenafil** (Viagra), **theophylline, sulfamethoxazole/trimethoprim** (Bactrim, Septra), or **zidovudine** (AZT, Retrovir). No dose adjustment required with coadministration of these drugs. ▪ **Efavirenz and fluconazole** may have a modest effect on the pharmacokinetics of azithromycin. No dose adjustment is necessary with coadministration of these drugs. ▪ May increase the anticoagulant effects of **warfarin** (Coumadin); monitoring of PT is indicated. ▪ Coadministration with nelfinavir (Viracept) results in increased azithromycin levels. Dose adjustment is not recommended, but close monitoring for known side effects (e.g., liver enzyme abnormalities, hearing impairment) is suggested. ▪ In healthy subjects, coadministration of azithromycin and chloroquine (known to prolong the QT interval) increased the QTc interval in a dose- and concentration-dependent manner; see Precautions. ▪ *Other macrolide antibiotics cause interactions when given concomitantly with the following drugs; azithromycin has not been studied.* ▪ May inhibit metabolism and increase serum levels and effects of **cyclosporine** (Sandimmune), **phenytoin** (Dilantin), **and terfenadine;** reduced doses of these drugs may be indicated. ▪ May increase **digoxin levels;** monitoring of digoxin levels is indicated. ▪ May cause acute ergot toxicity (severe peripheral vasospasm and dysesthesia) with **ergotamine or dihydroergotamine.**

SIDE EFFECTS

Usually mild to moderate in severity and reversible after azithromycin discontinued. The most commonly reported side effects are abdominal pain, diarrhea, nausea and vomiting. Less frequently reported side effects include anemia; anorexia; cough; dizziness; dyspnea; facial edema; fatigue; fungal infections; hypotension; increase in AST, ALT, and/or alkaline phosphatase levels; injection site pain or local inflammation; malaise; oral candidiasis; pancreatitis; pharyngitis; pleural effusion; pruritus; rashes; rhinitis; stomatitis; vaginitis.

Post-Marketing: Arrhythmias (e.g., ventricular tachycardia, QT prolongation, and torsades de pointes), CDAD, CNS toxicity (e.g., agitation, convulsions, headache, somnolence, syncope), constipation, hematologic abnormalities (e.g., decreased platelet count, leukopenia, neutropenia), hepatotoxicity (e.g., hepatitis and cholestatic jaundice, cases of hepatic necrosis, and hepatic failure [some resulting in death]), hypersensitivity reactions (e.g., anaphylaxis, angioedema, and dermatologic reactions [including Stevens-Johnson syndrome, toxic epidermal necrolysis, and urticaria]), interstitial nephritis, and acute renal failure.

ANTIDOTE

Notify physician of any side effects. Discontinue azithromycin for hypersensitivity reactions and S/S of hepatotoxicity. Treat hypersensitivity reactions as indicated and resuscitate as necessary. Additional hypersensitivity reactions have recurred after azithromycin has been discontinued and initial treatment completed. Prolonged observation is required. Mild cases of CDAD may respond to discontinuation of azithromycin. Treat CDAD with fluids, electrolytes, protein supplements, and oral vancomycin (Vancocin) or metronidazole (Flagyl) as indicated. In severe cases, surgical evaluation may be indicated.

AZTREONAM
(az-**TREE**-oh-nam)

Azactam

Antibacterial
(monobactam)

pH 4.5 to 7.5

USUAL DOSE
Dose determined by susceptibility of the causative organism(s), severity and site of infection, and condition of the patient.

Urinary tract infection: 500 mg to 1 Gm every 8 to 12 hours.

Moderately severe systemic infections: 1 or 2 Gm every 8 to 12 hours.

Severe systemic or life-threatening infections: 2 Gm every 6 or 8 hours. Use the full suggested dose. Do not exceed 8 Gm/24 hr.

Normal renal function required. Duration of therapy depends on the severity of the infection. Continue for at least 2 days after all symptoms of infection subside. Can produce therapeutic serum levels given intraperitoneally in dialysis fluid.

PEDIATRIC DOSE
See Maternal/Child.

Mild to moderate infections: 30 mg/kg every 8 hours.

Moderate to severe infections: 30 mg/kg every 6 or 8 hours. Maximum recommended dose is 120 mg/kg/24 hr.

Cystic fibrosis: 50 mg/kg every 6 to 8 hours. Maximum dose is 8 Gm/24 hr.

NEONATAL DOSE
Neonatal doses are **unlabeled;** see Maternal/Child.

30 mg/kg/dose. Interval between doses based on age and weight as follows:

Less than 1,200 Gm and 0 to 4 weeks of age: Give every 12 hours.

Less than 2,000 Gm and 0 to 7 days of age: Give every 12 hours.

1,200 to 2,000 Gm and over 7 days of age: Give every 8 hours.

More than 2,000 Gm and 0 to 7 days of age: Give every 8 hours.

More than 2,000 Gm and over 7 days of age: Give every 6 hours.

DOSE ADJUSTMENTS
Dosing in the elderly should be cautious and reduced based on CrCl; consider potential for decreased organ function and concomitant disease or drug therapy. ▪ Prolonged serum levels may occur in patients with renal insufficiency. After an initial loading dose of 1 or 2 Gm, reduce succeeding doses by 50% in patients with CrCl between 10 and 30 mL/min/1.73 M^2. ▪ After an initial loading dose of 500 mg, 1 Gm, or 2 Gm, reduce succeeding doses by 75% in patients with CrCl less than 10 mL/min/1.73 M^2 or in patients supported by dialysis. For serious or life-threatening infections, in addition to the maintenance doses, give 12.5% of the initial dose after each dialysis session.

DILUTION
Usually light yellow, may become slightly pink on standing; does not affect potency.

IV injection: Reconstitute a single dose with 6 to 10 mL of SWFI. Shake immediately and vigorously. Use immediately and discard any unused solution.

Intermittent IV: Initially reconstitute each single dose with a minimum of 3 mL of SWFI. Shake immediately and vigorously. Must be further diluted in at least 50 mL of D5W, NS, or other **compatible** infusion solutions for each 1 Gm of aztreonam (see chart on inside back cover or literature). Concentration should not exceed 20 mg/mL or 2% w/v. Available in vials and premixed Galaxy infusion bags.

Storage: Store vials at RT before use. Concentrations exceeding 2% should be used promptly unless prepared with SWFI or NS. Other reconstituted or diluted solutions are stable for 48 hours at CRT or up to 7 days if refrigerated. Vials are for single use only; discard unused amounts. Store aztreonam in Galaxy plastic containers at or below

−20° C (−4° F). Thaw frozen container at RT or in a refrigerator. **Do not** force thaw by immersion in a water bath or by microwave irradiation. Thawed solutions are stable for 14 days refrigerated or for 48 hours at RT. Do not refreeze.

COMPATIBILITY   (Underline Indicates Conflicting Compatibility Information)
Consider any drug NOT listed as compatible to be INCOMPATIBLE until consulting a pharmacist; specific conditions may apply.
Manufacturer lists as **incompatible** with metronidazole (Flagyl IV), nafcillin (Nallpen).

One source suggests the following **compatibilities:**
Solution: See chart on inside back cover. Others listed by manufacturer include D5/Ionosol B, Isolyte E, D5/Isolyte E, D5/Isolyte M, Normosol-R, D5/Normosol-R, D5/Normosol-M, Mannitol 5% and 10%, D5/Plasma-Lyte, Travert injection 10%, Travert injection 10% and Electrolytes (multiple).
Additive: Manufacturer lists ampicillin, cefazolin (Ancef), clindamycin (Cleocin), gentamicin, tobramycin, and vancomycin diluted in specific concentrations and in specific solutions and states, "Other admixtures are not recommended."

Other sources list ampicillin/sulbactam (Unasyn), cefoxitin (Mefoxin), ciprofloxacin (Cipro IV), linezolid (Zyvox), mannitol (Osmitrol), vancomycin.
Y-site: Allopurinol (Aloprim), amifostine (Ethyol), amikacin, aminophylline, ampicillin, ampicillin/sulbactam (Unasyn), bivalirudin (Angiomax), bleomycin (Blenoxane), bumetanide, buprenorphine (Buprenex), butorphanol (Stadol), calcium gluconate, carboplatin (Paraplatin), carmustine (BiCNU), caspofungin (Cancidas), cefazolin (Ancef), cefotaxime (Claforan), cefotetan, cefoxitin (Mefoxin), ceftazidime (Fortaz), ceftriaxone (Rocephin), cefuroxime (Zinacef), ciprofloxacin (Cipro IV), cisatracurium (Nimbex), cisplatin, clindamycin (Cleocin), cyclophosphamide (Cytoxan), cytarabine (ARA-C), dacarbazine (DTIC), dactinomycin (Cosmegen), daptomycin (Cubicin), dexamethasone (Decadron), dexmedetomidine (Precedex), diltiazem (Cardizem), diphenhydramine (Benadryl), dobutamine, docetaxel (Taxotere), dopamine, doxorubicin (Adriamycin), doxorubicin liposomal (Doxil), doxycycline, droperidol (Inapsine), enalaprilat (Vasotec IV), etoposide (VePesid), etoposide phosphate (Etopophos), famotidine (Pepcid IV), fenoldopam (Corlopam), filgrastim (Neupogen), fluconazole (Diflucan), fludarabine (Fludara), fluorouracil (5-FU), foscarnet (Foscavir), furosemide (Lasix), gallium nitrate (Ganite), gemcitabine (Gemzar), gentamicin, granisetron (Kytril), heparin, hetastarch in electrolytes (Hextend), hydrocortisone sodium succinate (Solu-Cortef), hydromorphone (Dilaudid), idarubicin (Idamycin), ifosfamide (Ifex), imipenem-cilastatin (Primaxin), insulin (regular), leucovorin calcium, linezolid (Zyvox), magnesium sulfate, mannitol, mechlorethamine (nitrogen mustard), melphalan (Alkeran), meperidine (Demerol), mesna (Mesnex), methotrexate, methylprednisolone (Solu-Medrol), metoclopramide (Reglan), morphine, nalbuphine, nicardipine (Cardene IV), ondansetron (Zofran), pemetrexed (Alimta), piperacillin/tazobactam (Zosyn), potassium chloride (KCl), promethazine (Phenergan), propofol (Diprivan), quinupristin/dalfopristin (Synercid 20 mg/mL), ranitidine (Zantac), remifentanil (Ultiva), sargramostim (Leukine), sodium bicarbonate, sulfamethoxazole/trimethoprim, teniposide (Vumon), theophylline, thiotepa, ticarcillin/clavulanate (Timentin), tigecycline (Tygacil), tobramycin, vancomycin, vinblastine, vincristine, vinorelbine (Navelbine), zidovudine (AZT, Retrovir).

RATE OF ADMINISTRATION
IV injection: A single dose equally distributed over 3 to 5 minutes.
Intermittent IV: A single dose over 20 to 60 minutes. May be given through Y-tube or three-way stopcock of infusion set. Do not infuse simultaneously with other drugs or solutions except in proven **compatibility.** Flush common IV tubing before and after administration.

ACTIONS

A synthetic monobactam antibiotic. Bactericidal through inhibition of bacterial cell wall synthesis to a wide spectrum of specific gram-negative aerobic organisms, including *Pseudomonas aeruginosa*. Has activity in the presence of some beta-lactamases (both penicillinases and cephalosporinases) of gram-negative and gram-positive bacteria. Therapeutic levels widely distributed into many body fluids and tissues. Serum half-life averages 1.7 hours; range is 1.5 to 2 hours. Primarily excreted in the urine with some excretion through feces. Crosses placental barrier. Secreted in breast milk.

INDICATIONS AND USES

Treatment of serious lower respiratory tract, urinary tract, skin and skin structure, gynecologic, and intra-abdominal infections and bacterial septicemia. Most effective against specific gram-negative organisms (see literature). ▪ Adjunctive therapy to surgery for the management of infections caused by susceptible organisms, including abscesses, infections complicating hollow viscus perforations, cutaneous infections, and infections of serous surfaces.

CONTRAINDICATIONS

Known hypersensitivity to aztreonam or its components.

PRECAUTIONS

Specific studies are indicated to identify the causative organism and susceptibility to aztreonam. ▪ To reduce the development of drug-resistant bacteria and maintain its effectiveness, aztreonam should be used to treat or prevent only those infections proven or strongly suspected to be caused by bacteria. ▪ Before C/S data are available, concurrent initial antimicrobial therapy with agents to cover gram-positive and/or anaerobic microorganisms may be indicated in seriously ill patients. ▪ Avoid prolonged use of drug; superinfection caused by overgrowth of nonsusceptible organisms may result. ▪ Cross-reactivity with other beta-lactam antibiotics (e.g., penicillins, cephalosporins, and/or carbapenems) is rare but can occur with or without prior exposure. Use with caution in patients with a history of hypersensitivity reactions to beta-lactam antibiotics. ▪ *Clostridium difficile*–associated diarrhea (CDAD) has been reported. May range from mild diarrhea to fatal colitis. Consider in patients who present with diarrhea during or after treatment with aztreonam. ▪ Epidermal necrolysis has been reported rarely in patients receiving aztreonam who have undergone BMT and have other risk factors (e.g., graft-versus-host disease, radiation therapy, sepsis).

Monitor: Watch for early symptoms of a hypersensitivity reaction. Use caution in patients with known sensitivity to penicillins, cephalosporins, or carbapenems. ▪ Monitor renal and hepatic function, especially in the elderly. ▪ Monitor renal function with concurrent administration of higher doses or prolonged administration of aminoglycosides (e.g., gentamicin). ▪ May cause thrombophlebitis. Use small needles and large veins and rotate infusion sites.

Patient Education: Report pain or burning at injection site or S/S of a hypersensitivity reaction (e.g., difficulty breathing, flushing, itching, rash). ▪ Promptly report diarrhea or bloody stools that occur during treatment or up to several months after an antibiotic has been discontinued; may indicate CDAD and require treatment.

Maternal/Child: Category B: use in pregnancy only if clearly needed. ▪ Consider discontinuing breast-feeding. ▪ Safety and effectiveness for use in infants under 9 months of age and for treatment of pediatric patients with septicemia and skin and skin-structure infections (where the skin infection is believed or known to result from *H. influenzae* type b) not established. ▪ Higher doses of aztreonam may be indicated in pediatric patients with cystic fibrosis. ▪ IV route is suggested for pediatric patients; data are limited for IM injection and impaired renal function.

Elderly: Reduced doses may be indicated. Monitor renal function; see Dose Adjustments. ▪ Response is similar to that seen in younger patients; however, clearance is decreased and half-life is prolonged.

DRUG/LAB INTERACTIONS

Antagonism may occur with **beta-lactamase–inducing antibiotics** (e.g., cefoxitin, imipenem); do not use concurrently. ■ Aztreonam and **aminoglycosides** have been shown to be synergistic against many gram-negative aerobic bacilli. May be used concomitantly in severe infections. Nephrotoxicity and ototoxicity can be markedly increased when both drugs are utilized. ■ **Probenecid and furosemide** do increase blood levels; not clinically significant. ■ Significant interactions between aztreonam and concomitantly administered **gentamicin, nafcillin** (Nallpen), **clindamycin** (Cleocin), **and metronidazole** (Flagyl) have not been seen in single-dose pharmacokinetic studies. ■ Bactericidal activity of aztreonam may be antagonized by **chloramphenicol** (Chloromycetin). ■ See Side Effects.

SIDE EFFECTS

Diarrhea, nausea and vomiting, phlebitis/thrombophlebitis, and rash occur most frequently. Less frequently reported reactions include abdominal cramps; allergic reactions (e.g., anaphylaxis, angioedema, bronchospasm); altered taste; CDAD; confusion; diaphoresis; diplopia; dizziness; dyspnea; elevated alkaline phosphatase, AST, ALT, and SCr; eosinophilia; erythema multiforme; exfoliative dermatitis; fever; halitosis; headache; hematologic changes (e.g., anemia, neutropenia); hepatitis; hypotension; insomnia; jaundice; mouth ulcer; nasal congestion; numb tongue; paresthesia; petechiae; positive Coombs' test; prolonged PT and PTT; pruritus; purpura; seizures; sneezing; tinnitus; toxic epidermal necrosis; transient ECG changes (ventricular bigeminy and PVCs); urticaria; vaginitis; vertigo.

ANTIDOTE

Notify physician of any side effects. Discontinue the drug if indicated. Treat hypersensitivity reactions as indicated and resuscitate as necessary. Mild cases of CDAD may respond to discontinuation of drug. Treat CDAD with fluids, electrolytes, protein supplements, and oral vancomycin (Vancocin) or metronidazole (Flagyl) as indicated. In severe cases, surgical evaluation may be indicated. Hemodialysis or peritoneal dialysis may be useful in overdose.

BASILIXIMAB BBW

(**bah**-zih-**LIX**-ih-mab)

Simulect

Recombinant monoclonal antibody
Immunosuppressant

USUAL DOSE

Basiliximab should only be administered once it has been determined that the patient will receive the graft and concomitant immunosuppression. Patients who have received a previous course of basiliximab should only be re-exposed to a subsequent course of therapy with extreme caution. Used concurrently with cyclosporine (Sandimmune) and corticosteroids.

Organ rejection prophylaxis in renal transplant: 2 doses of 20 mg each as an infusion. Administer the first dose within 2 hours before transplantation. Give the second dose 4 days after transplantation. Withhold the second dose if complications such as severe hypersensitivity reactions to basiliximab or graft loss occur.

PEDIATRIC DOSE

Less than 35 kg: 2 doses of 10 mg each (discard remaining product after each dose).
35 kg or more: 2 doses of 20 mg each.

In all pediatric patients, administer the first dose within 2 hours before transplantation. Give the second dose 4 days after transplantation. See Actions and Maternal/Child. Withhold second dose if complications occur (e.g., hypersensitivity reactions or graft loss).

DOSE ADJUSTMENTS

No dose adjustments indicated.

DILUTION

Reconstitute each single 20-mg vial with 5 mL of SWFI. Reconstitute each 10-mg vial with 2.5 mL SWFI. Shake gently to dissolve powder. After reconstitution, may be given as an IV injection or may be further diluted to 50 mL with NS or D5W. When mixing, gently invert to avoid foaming; do not shake.

Storage: Store unopened vials in the refrigerator (2° to 8° C [36° to 46° F]). Should be used within 4 hours of reconstitution. If necessary, may be refrigerated for up to 24 hours. Discard prepared solution after 24 hours.

COMPATIBILITY

Manufacturer states, "Other drug substances should not be added or infused simultaneously through the same IV line." No **incompatibilities** observed with polyvinyl chloride bags and administration sets.

RATE OF ADMINISTRATION

May be given through a peripheral or central vein.

IV injection: May be given as a bolus injection over 30 to 60 seconds. Incidence of N/V and local reaction including pain increased.

Infusion: A single dose properly diluted over 20 to 30 minutes.

ACTIONS

A chimeric (murine/human) monoclonal antibody produced by recombinant DNA technology. Functions as an immunosuppressant. Specifically binds to and blocks the interleukin-2 receptor alpha chain (IL-2Rα, also known as CD25 antigen), thereby inhibiting IL-2 driven proliferation of activated T-cells, which play a key role in organ rejection. Reduces/minimizes acute rejection. IL-2Rα is expressed selectively on activated, but not resting, T-cells. This selectivity prevents the profound generalized immunosuppression seen with other immunosuppressants used in organ transplantation and may decrease the risk of infection and development of lymphoproliferative disorders. Two 20-mg doses block the receptor for 4 to 6 weeks posttransplantation, the critical risk period for acute organ rejection. Has reduced the incidence of biopsy-confirmed acute rejections while minimizing side effects seen with other immunosuppressants. Clinical benefit demonstrated in a broad range of patients, regardless of age, gender, race, donor type, or history of diabetes mellitus as long as serum levels exceed 0.2 mg/mL (by ELISA). Mean half-life is 4 to 10.4 days. Half-life is increased (5.2 to 17.8 days) and distribution volume and clearance are decreased by about 50% in pediatric patients 2 to 11 years of age. Crosses the placental barrier. May be secreted in breast milk.

INDICATIONS AND USES
Prophylaxis of acute organ rejection in patients receiving renal transplants. Used as part of an immunosuppressive regimen that includes cyclosporine and corticosteroids. Dosing regimen may also include either azathioprine or mycophenolate (CellCept IV).

CONTRAINDICATIONS
Known hypersensitivity to basiliximab or any of its components (composite of human and murine antibodies).

PRECAUTIONS
Usually administered by or under the direction of a physician experienced in immunosuppressive therapy and management of organ transplant patients. Adequate laboratory and supportive medical resources must be available. ■ Severe acute (onset within 24 hours) hypersensitivity reactions including anaphylaxis have been reported both with initial exposure and/or following re-exposure after several months. Emergency equipment and drugs for the treatment of severe hypersensitivity reactions must be readily available. Withhold the second dose of basiliximab if a hypersensitivity reaction occurs. ■ Readministration after an initial course of therapy has not been studied in humans, but other monoclonal antibodies have precipitated anaphylactoid reactions. ■ Potential for causing lymphoproliferative disorders, cytomegalovirus (CMV), and other opportunistic infections is unknown. ■ Use with caution in patients with infections or malignancies. ■ It is not known whether basiliximab use will have a long-term effect on the ability of the immune system to respond to antigens first encountered during induced immunosuppression. ■ Low titers of anti-idiotype antibodies and human antimurine antibodies (HAMA) to basiliximab have been detected in some patients during treatment; no adverse effects have been noted.
Monitor: Obtain baseline CBC with differential and platelets and baseline renal and liver tests if not already completed for other immunosuppressant agents. ■ Monitor vital signs. ■ Observe closely for signs of infection (fever, sore throat, tiredness) or unusual bleeding or bruising. ■ Prophylactic antibiotics may be indicated pending results of C/S in a febrile immunosuppressed patient. ■ Symptoms of cytokine release syndrome (e.g., chills, fever, dyspnea, and malaise) have not been reported but may occur; observe carefully. ■ See Drug/Lab Interactions.
Patient Education: Report difficulty in breathing or swallowing, rapid heartbeat, rash, or itching immediately. ■ Report swelling of lower extremities and weakness. ■ Avoid pregnancy; nonhormonal birth control preferred. Women with childbearing potential should use effective contraception before beginning basiliximab therapy, during therapy, and for 2 months after completion. ■ See Appendix D, p. 1333.
Maternal/Child: Category B: use during pregnancy only if benefits justify the potential risk to the fetus. Avoid pregnancy; effective contraception required; see Patient Education. ■ Discontinue breast-feeding. ■ Has been used in pediatric patients from 2 to 15 years of age. No adequate or well-controlled studies completed. See differences in Actions. Most frequent side effects were fever and urinary infections.
Elderly: Age-related dosing not required. Adverse events similar to younger adults. Use caution when giving immunosuppressive drugs to the elderly.

DRUG/LAB INTERACTIONS
Has been administered concurrently with **antilymphocyte globulin** (ALG), **antithymocyte globulin** (ATG), **azathioprine, corticosteroids, cyclosporine** (Sandimmune), **muromonab CD3** (Orthoclone), **and mycophenolate** (CellCept); no additional adverse reactions noted. ■ **May increase or decrease numerous lab values,** including serum calcium and potassium and fasting blood glucose.

SIDE EFFECTS
Basiliximab did not appear to alter the pattern, frequency, or severity of known side effects associated with the use of immunosuppressive drugs. Abdominal pain, anemia,

constipation, diarrhea, edema, fever, headache, hyperkalemia, hypersensitivity reactions (including anaphylaxis, bronchospasm, capillary leak syndrome, cardiac failure, cytokine release syndrome, dyspnea, hypotension, pruritus, pulmonary edema, rash, respiratory failure, sneezing, tachycardia, urticaria, wheezing), hypertension, hypokalemia, insomnia, nausea, pain, peripheral edema, upper respiratory infections, urinary tract infections. Incidence of N/V and local reaction including pain increased with bolus injection. Severe hypersensitivity reactions (including anaphylaxis), capillary leak syndrome, and cytokine release syndrome have been reported. Incidence of infections, lymphomas, or other malignancies similar to placebo groups in studies.

ANTIDOTE

Notify physician of all side effects. Most will be treated symptomatically. Basiliximab may be discontinued or alternate immunosuppressive agents substituted. Discontinue immediately if anaphylaxis occurs, and treat with oxygen, epinephrine, corticosteroids, and/or antihistamines (e.g., diphenhydramine [Benadryl]). Resuscitate as necessary.

BELATACEPT BBW
(bel-**AT**-a-sept)

Nulojix

Immunosuppressant

pH 7.2 to 7.8

USUAL DOSE

Administration of higher-than-recommended doses or more frequent dosing of belatacept is not recommended because of an increased risk of posttransplant lymphoproliferative disorder (PTLD), progressive multifocal leukoencephalopathy (PML), and serious CNS infections.

Premedication is not required. Base the total infusion dose on actual body weight at the time of transplantation.

Dosing of Belatacept for Kidney Transplant Recipients*	
Dosing for Initial Phase	**Dose**
Day 1 (day of transplantation, before implantation) and Day 5 (approximately 96 hours after Day 1 dose)	10 mg/kg
End of Week 2 and Week 4 after transplantation	10 mg/kg
End of Week 8 and Week 12 after transplantation	10 mg/kg
Dosing for Maintenance Phase	**Dose**
End of Week 16 after transplantation and every 4 weeks (plus or minus 3 days) thereafter	5 mg/kg

*The dose prescribed must be evenly divisible by 12.5 mg (evenly divisible increments are 0, 12.5, 25, 37.5, 50, 62.5, 75, 87.5, and 100). For example: At 10 mg/kg/dose, a patient weighing 64 kg would receive 640 mg. The closest doses evenly divisible by 12.5 below and above 640 mg are 637.5 mg and 650 mg. The nearest dose is 637.5 mg, and this would be the actual prescribed dose.

Regimen includes basiliximab (Simulect) induction, mycophenolate mofetil (MMF, CellCept), and corticosteroids.

Basiliximab: 20 mg IV on the day of transplantation and 4 days later.

Mycophenolate mofetil: 1 Gm twice daily as an initial dose. Adjust dose based on clinical signs of adverse events or efficacy failure.

Corticosteroid doses should be consistent with those used in clinical trials. In clinical trials, the median corticosteroid doses were tapered to approximately 15 mg (10 to 20 mg) per day by the first 6 weeks and remained at approximately 10 mg (5 to 10 mg) per day for the first 6 months posttransplant; see Precautions. Actual corticosteroid dosing in clinical trials is summarized in the following chart.

Actual Corticosteroid[a] Dosing in Studies 1 and 2		
	Median (Q1-Q3) Daily Dose[b,c]	
Day of Dosing	Study 1	Study 2
Week 1	31.7 mg (26.7 to 50 mg)	30 mg (26.7 to 50 mg)
Week 2	25 mg (20 to 30 mg)	25 mg (20 to 30 mg)
Week 4	20 mg (15 to 20 mg)	20 mg (15 to 22.5 mg)
Week 6	15 mg (10 to 20 mg)	16.7 mg (12.5 to 20 mg)
Month 6	10 mg (5 to 10 mg)	10 mg (5 to 12.5 mg)

[a]Corticosteroid = Prednisone or prednisolone.
[b]Protocols allowed for flexibility in determining corticosteroid dose and rapidity of taper after Day 15. It is not possible to distinguish corticosteroid doses used to treat acute rejection versus doses used in a maintenance regimen.
[c]Q1 and Q3 are the 25th and 75th percentiles of daily corticosteroid doses, respectively.

DOSE ADJUSTMENTS

Do not modify the dose during the course of therapy unless there is a change in body weight of greater than 10%. ▪ Age, gender, race, renal function, hepatic function, diabetes, and concomitant dialysis do not affect the clearance of belatacept.

DILUTION

Belatacept is for IV infusion only. *Must be reconstituted/prepared using only the silicone-free disposable syringe provided with each vial. This syringe will be required for both reconstitution and the preparation of the final infusion. Maintain sterility. Any solution prepared with other than the provided silicone-free syringe must be discarded* (contact the manufacturer to obtain an additional supply of silicone-free disposable syringes).

Each vial contains 250 mg of belatacept lyophilized powder. Calculate the number of vials needed to provide the total infusion dose. Reconstitute the contents of each vial with 10.5 mL of SWFI, NS, or D5W using the silicone-free disposable syringe and an 18- to 21-gauge needle. Direct the stream of diluent to the glass wall of the vial. To avoid foaming, rotate the vial and swirl gently until contents are completely dissolved. *Avoid prolonged or vigorous agitation. Do not shake.* Reconstituted solution yields 25 mg/mL and should be clear to slightly opalescent and colorless to pale yellow. Calculate the total volume of reconstituted solution required to provide the prescribed dose:

Volume of 25 mg/mL belatacept solution (in mL) = Prescribed dose (in mg) ÷ 25 mg/mL

The reconstituted solution must be further diluted in infusion fluid. If reconstituted with SWFI, dilute with either NS or D5W. If reconstituted with NS, further dilute with NS. If reconstituted with D5W, further dilute with D5W. From the appropriate-size infusion bag or bottle (typically an infusion volume of 100 mL is appropriate, but volumes from 50 to 250 mL may be used), withdraw a volume of infusion fluid equal to the total volume of reconstituted belatacept required to provide the prescribed dose. Using the same silicone-free disposable syringe used for reconstitution, withdraw the required amount of belatacept and inject it into the infusion bag or bottle. Gently rotate to ensure mixing. Concentration should range from 2 mg/mL to 10 mg/mL.

Filters: Must be administered with a nonpyrogenic, low–protein binding, 0.2- to 1.2-micron filter.

Storage: Refrigerate vials of lyophilized powder at 2° to 8° C (36° to 46° F) in carton to protect from light. The reconstituted solution should be further diluted in infusion fluid immediately. The infusion must be completed within 24 hours. Infusion solution can be refrigerated protected from light for up to 24 hours. A maximum of 4 hours of those 24 hours can be at RT 20° to 25° C (68° to 77° F) and room light. Discard any unused solution remaining in vials.

COMPATIBILITY

Manufacturer states, "Must be reconstituted/prepared using only the silicone-free disposable syringe provided with each vial. Any solution prepared with other than the provided silicone-free syringe must be discarded" and "Infuse in a separate line; should not be infused concomitantly in the same IV line with other agents."

RATE OF ADMINISTRATION

A single dose evenly distributed over 30 minutes.

ACTIONS

A selective T-cell costimulation blocker. Produced by recombinant DNA technology. Binds to CD80 and CD86 on antigen-presenting cells, thereby blocking CD28-mediated costimulation of T-lymphocytes. Belatacept binds to CD80 and CD86 more readily than abatacept (the parent molecule from which it is derived). Belatacept-mediated costimulation blockade results in the inhibition of cytokine production by T-cells required for antigen-specific antibody production by B-cells and inhibits T-lymphocyte proliferation. Activated T-lymphocytes are the predominant mediators of immunologic rejection. Half-life ranges from 6.1 to 15.1 days. In clinical trials, trough concentrations were consistently maintained from 6 months up to 3 years posttransplant. Increasing body weight may result in a trend toward higher clearance.

INDICATIONS AND USES

Prophylaxis of organ rejection in adult patients receiving a kidney transplant. Used in combination with basiliximab (Simulect) induction, mycophenolate mofetil (CellCept), and corticosteroids.

Limitation of use: Use only in patients who are Epstein-Barr virus (EBV) seropositive. ▪ Use for prophylaxis of organ rejection in transplanted organs other than the kidney not established. Not recommended for use in liver transplant patients; risk of graft loss and death is increased.

CONTRAINDICATIONS

Transplant recipients who are Epstein-Barr virus (EBV) seronegative or who have unknown EBV serostatus because of risk of posttransplant lymphoproliferative disorder (PTLD) predominantly involving the CNS.

PRECAUTIONS

For IV use only. ▪ Usually administered by or under the direction of a physician experienced in immunosuppressive therapy and management of organ transplant patients. Adequate laboratory and supportive medical resources must be available. ▪ Increased risk for developing posttransplant lymphoproliferative disorder (PTLD), predominantly involving the CNS, compared with patients on a cyclosporine-based regimen. Recipients without immunity to Epstein-Barr virus (EBV) are at a particularly increased risk; therefore use in EBV-seropositive patients only. Do not use belatacept in transplant recipients who are EBV-seronegative or who have unknown EBV serostatus. ▪ Other known risk factors for PTLD include cytomegalovirus (CMV) infection and T-cell–depleting therapy. Use T-cell–depleting therapies to treat acute rejection with caution. CMV prophylaxis is recommended for at least 3 months after transplantation. Patients who are EBV seropositive and CMV seronegative may be at increased risk for PTLD compared with patients who are EBV seropositive and CMV seropositive. ▪ Minimization of the corticosteroid dose to 5 mg/day between Day 3 and Week 6 posttransplantation has been associated with an increased rate and grade of acute rejection, particularly Grade III rejection. Graft loss occurred in some patients. Corticosteroid use should be consistent with clinical trial experience; see Usual Dose. ▪ Increased susceptibility to infection and possible development of malignancies may result from immunosuppression. Increased risk of developing other malignancies, including malignancies of the skin, appears related to intensity and duration of use. Avoid prolonged exposure to UV light and sunlight. Risk of developing bacterial, viral (e.g., CMV and herpes), fungal, and protozoal infections, including opportunistic infections such as tuberculosis (TB) or polyoma virus–associated nephropathy (PVAN), is increased and may lead to serious (including fatal) outcomes. Prophylaxis for *Pneumocystis jiroveci* is recommended after transplantation. ▪ PML (a rapidly progressive and fatal opportunistic infection of the CNS that is caused by the JC virus) has been reported. ▪ Infusion-related reactions have occurred within 1 hour of infusion; however, no serious reactions or anaphylaxis have been reported. ▪ Use in liver transplant patients is not recommended; see Limitation of Use. ▪ Anti-belatacept antibody development was not associated with an altered clearance of belatacept. The clinical impact of anti-belatacept antibodies has not been determined. ▪ Do not administer live virus vaccines; see Drug/Lab Interactions.

Monitor: Ascertain EBV serology before starting therapy with belatacept. ▪ Monitor for new or worsening neurologic, cognitive, or behavioral signs and symptoms. May indicate PTLD or PML. ▪ Evaluate patients for latent tuberculosis (TB). Patients testing positive in TB screening should be treated with a standard TB regimen before initiating belatacept therapy. ▪ Monitor for S/S of infection; see Antidote. ▪ Monitor renal function closely and consider PVAN if renal function is deteriorating. ▪ New-onset diabetes, dyslipidemia, and hypertension may occur; monitor blood sugar, lipid panel, and BP. ▪ See Precautions.

Patient Education: Read manufacturer's patient information sheet before each infusion. ▪ Risk of other malignancies, especially skin cancer, is increased. Limit exposure to sunlight and UV light. Wear protective clothing and use a sunscreen with a high protection factor. ▪ Promptly report confusion, thinking problems, and loss of memory; decreased strength or weakness on one side of the body; and changes in mood or behavior, walking or talking, and vision. ▪ Promptly report S/S of infection (e.g., fever, malaise). Adherence to prescribed antimicrobial prophylaxis is imperative. ▪ May cause fetal harm. Pregnancy Registry available to monitor maternal-fetal outcomes.

Maternal/Child: Category C: may cause fetal harm. Use only if potential benefit to mother outweighs potential risk to fetus. ▪ Discontinue breast-feeding. ▪ Safety and effectiveness for use in pediatric patients less than 18 years of age not established.

Elderly: Safety or effectiveness similar to that seen in younger adults.

DRUG/LAB INTERACTIONS

A change of **mycophenolic acid (MPA)** exposure may occur with a crossover from **cyclosporine to belatacept** or from **belatacept to cyclosporine** in patients concomitantly receiving **MMF.** Cyclosporine decreases MPA exposure by preventing enterohepatic recirculation of MPA, whereas belatacept does not. A higher MMF dosage may be needed after switching from belatacept to cyclosporine because cyclosporine may result in lower MPA concentrations and increase the risk of graft rejection. A lower MMF dosage may be needed after switching from cyclosporine to belatacept because belatacept may result in higher MPA concentrations and increase the risk for adverse reactions related to MPA. ▪ No dosage adjustments are needed for **drugs metabolized via CYP1A2** (e.g., caffeine), **CYP2C9** (e.g., losartan [Cozaar]), **CYP2D6** (e.g., dextromethorphan), **CYP3A** (e.g., midazolam [Versed]), and **CYP2C19** (e.g., omeprazole [Prilosec]). ▪ Avoid the use of **live vaccines** during treatment with belatacept, including but not limited to intranasal influenza, measles, mumps, rubella, oral polio, BCG, yellow fever, varicella, and Ty21a typhoid vaccines.

SIDE EFFECTS

Anemia, constipation, cough, diarrhea, fever, graft dysfunction, headache, hyperkalemia, hypertension, hypokalemia, leukopenia, nausea, peripheral edema, urinary tract infection, and vomiting are most common. Posttransplant lymphoproliferative disorder (PTLD), predominantly CNS PTLD; other malignancies; and serious infections, including JC virus–associated progressive multifocal leukoencephalopathy (PML) and polyoma virus-associated nephropathy (PVAN), are the most serious potential side effects and may be life threatening. Abdominal pain, acne, anxiety, arthralgia, back pain, bronchitis, cytomegalovirus (CMV) and herpes infections, dyslipidemia, dysuria, hematuria, hypercholesterolemia, hyperglycemia, hyperuricemia, hypocalcemia, hypomagnesemia, hypophosphatemia, hypotension, influenza, insomnia, nasopharyngitis, proteinuria, renal tubular necrosis, tremor, tuberculosis, and upper respiratory infections may occur.

ANTIDOTE

Notify physician of all side effects. Most will be treated symptomatically. If PML is suspected, confirmation of the diagnosis by consultation with a neurologist, brain imaging, CSF testing for JC viral DNA, and/or brain biopsy is indicated. If PML is confirmed, consider reducing or discontinuing immunosuppression, taking into account the risk to the allograft. Therapy may need to be interrupted in patients who develop infections. Treat infusion reactions as indicated. Resuscitate as necessary.

BELIMUMAB
(be-**LIM**-ue-mab)

Monoclonal antibody

Benlysta

pH 6.5

USUAL DOSE

Premedication: Consider premedication (e.g., antihistamines [e.g., diphenhydramine (Benadryl)], H_2 antagonists [e.g., ranitidine (Zantac)], and/or corticosteroids [e.g., dexamethasone (Decadron)]) to help prevent or minimize hypersensitivity/infusion reactions. **Belimumab:** 10 mg/kg as an infusion at 2-week intervals for the first 3 doses. Administer at 4-week intervals thereafter.

DILUTION

Available in two strengths (120 mg or 400 mg). Allow vial to reach RT before reconstitution (approximately 10 to 15 minutes). Reconstitute the 120-mg vial with 1.5 mL SWFI and the 400-mg vial with 4.8 mL SWFI. Concentration for both will equal 80 mg/mL. Direct the SWFI toward the side of the vial to minimize foaming. Gently swirl for 60 seconds. Allow to sit at RT and gently swirl for 60 seconds every 5 minutes until completely dissolved. ***Do not shake.*** Reconstitution may take up to 30 minutes. Protect from sunlight. Solution should be opalescent and colorless to pale yellow. Small air bubbles are expected and are acceptable. If reconstituted with a mechanical swirler, do not exceed 500 rpm and/or a duration of 30 minutes. Desired dose of the reconstituted solution must be further diluted to 250 mL with NS by withdrawing and discarding a volume equal to the desired dose from a 250-mL infusion bag or bottle of NS. Add the desired dose of belimumab to the infusion bag or bottle and invert to mix the solution; see Storage.
Filters: No data available from manufacturer.
Storage: Before use, refrigerate vials (2° to 8° C [36° to 46° F]) in original carton, protected from light. Do not freeze. Avoid exposure to heat. Do not use beyond expiration date. Reconstituted solution, if not used immediately, should be refrigerated protected from direct sunlight. Solution diluted in NS may be refrigerated or kept at RT. Total time from reconstitution to completion of the infusion should not exceed 8 hours. Discard any unused product.

COMPATIBILITY

Manufacturer states, "**Incompatible** with dextrose solutions," "No **incompatibilities** with polyvinylchloride or polyolefin bags observed," and "Should not be infused concomitantly in the same IV line with other agents."

RATE OF ADMINISTRATION

A single dose, properly diluted, as an infusion equally distributed over 1 hour. Slow or interrupt infusion rate if an infusion reaction develops.

ACTIONS

A recombinant, DNA-derived, humanized monoclonal antibody. It is a B-lymphocyte stimulator (BLyS)–specific inhibitor that blocks the binding of soluble BLyS (a B-cell survival factor) to its receptors on B-cells. Does not bind with B-cells directly. However, by binding BLyS, it inhibits the survival of B-cells (including auto-reactive B-cells) and reduces the differentiation of B-cells into immunoglobulin-producing plasma cells. Significantly reduces circulating CD19+, CD20+, naïve, and activated B-cells, plasmacytoid cells, and the SLE B-cell subset. Reductions in IgG and anti-dsDNA and increases in complement (C3 and C4) were observed as early as Week 8 and sustained through Week 52. Terminal half-life is 19.4 days.

INDICATIONS AND USES

Treatment of adult patients with active, autoantibody-positive, systemic lupus erythematosus (SLE) who are receiving standard therapy.

Limitation of use: Not recommended in patients with severe active lupus nephritis or severe active central nervous system lupus; has not been studied in these situations.

CONTRAINDICATIONS

Patients who have experienced an anaphylactic hypersensitivity reaction with belimumab.

PRECAUTIONS

For IV infusion only. ▪ Administered under the direction of a physician knowledgeable in its use in a facility with adequate diagnostic and treatment facilities to monitor the patient and respond to any medical emergency. ▪ Serious hypersensitivity/infusion reactions, including anaphylaxis and death, have occurred. Acute hypersensitivity reactions usually occur within hours of the infusion. Nonacute reactions, including rash, nausea, fatigue, myalgia, headache, and facial edema, may occur up to a week following the infusion. Patients with a history of multiple drug allergies or significant hypersensitivity may be at increased risk. Administration of premedications (which can mask or mitigate a reaction) and the overlap in S/S may make it difficult to distinguish between a hypersensitivity reaction and an infusion reaction. ▪ Serious and sometimes fatal infections have been reported. Use with caution in patients with chronic infections. Therapy should not be started if a patient is receiving any therapy for a chronic infection. ▪ Cases of JC virus–associated progressive multifocal leukoencephalopathy (PML) resulting in neurologic deficits, including fatal cases, have been reported. Risk factors for PML include treatment with immunosuppressant therapies and impairment of immune function. ▪ Psychiatric events, including depression, insomnia, and anxiety, have been reported. Most patients had a history of depression or other serious psychiatric disorders and were receiving psychoactive medications. ▪ More deaths were reported with belimumab than with placebo during the controlled period of clinical trials. Etiologies included cardiovascular disease, infection, and suicide. No single cause of death predominated. ▪ The impact of treatment with belimumab on the development of malignancies is not known. ▪ Anti-belimumab antibodies developed in a small percentage of patients. Clinical relevance is unknown. ▪ Response rates were lower in black/African-American patients; use with caution. ▪ Use in patients with impaired renal or hepatic function has not been studied.

Monitor: Obtain a baseline CBC, including a differential and platelet count. Monitor as indicated. ▪ Monitor for hypersensitivity reactions carefully during and for an appropriate period of time after administration; delayed onset of severe hypersensitivity reactions has been reported. S/S reported include anaphylaxis, angioedema, dyspnea, hypotension, pruritus, rash, and urticaria. ▪ On the day of the infusion, monitor for S/S of an infusion reaction (e.g., bradycardia, headache, hypotension, myalgia, nausea, rash, urticaria). ▪ Monitor for S/S of PML, such as new-onset or deteriorating neurologic signs. Consultation with a neurologist is recommended. ▪ Consider interrupting therapy if a new infection develops during treatment with belimumab.

Patient Education: Women of childbearing potential should use effective contraceptive methods during treatment and for a minimum of 4 months after the final treatment. ▪ Manufacturer has established a pregnancy registry, and patients who are or who become pregnant are encouraged to register. ▪ Tell your health care provider if you are allergic to any medications. ▪ Promptly report difficulty breathing; dizziness or fainting; headache; itching; nausea; skin rash, redness, or swelling; swelling of the face, lips, mouth, tongue, or throat; may indicate a hypersensitivity/infusion reaction. ▪ Promptly report bloody diarrhea, chest discomfort or pain, chills, cold sweats, coughing up mucus, dizziness, fever, nausea, new or worsening depression or suicidal thoughts, pain or burning with urination, unusual changes in behavior or mood. ▪ Promptly report new or worsening neurologic symptoms (e.g., confusion, difficulty talking or walking, loss of balance, memory loss, or vision problems).

Maternal/Child: Category C: use during pregnancy only if the potential benefit justifies the potential risk to the fetus. ▪ Discontinue breast-feeding. ▪ Safety and effectiveness for use in pediatric patients not established.

Elderly: Numbers in clinical studies are insufficient to determine if the elderly respond differently than younger subjects; use with caution.

DRUG/LAB INTERACTIONS

Formal drug interaction studies have not been performed. ▪ Has not been studied in combination with other **biologics, including B-cell–targeted therapies or IV cyclophosphamide;** concurrent use is not recommended. ▪ Do not administer **live virus vaccines** for 30 days before or concurrently with belimumab. ▪ Has been administered concomitantly with corticosteroids, antimalarials, immunomodulatory and immunosuppressive agents (including azathioprine, methotrexate, and mycophenolate), angiotensin-pathway antihypertensives, HMG-CoA reductase inhibitors (statins), and NSAIDs without meaningful clinical effect on belimumab pharmacokinetics.

SIDE EFFECTS

Bronchitis, depression, diarrhea, fever, insomnia, nasopharyngitis, migraine, nausea, pain in extremities, and pharyngitis were most commonly reported. The most common serious infections included bronchitis, cellulitis, pneumonia, and urinary tract infections. Anxiety, cystitis, depression, hypersensitivity/infusion reactions, influenza, leukopenia, sinusitis, and viral gastroenteritis also were reported.

Post-Marketing: Fatal anaphylaxis.

ANTIDOTE

Notify physician of all side effects. Treatment of most side effects will be supportive. Consider interrupting therapy if a new infection develops during treatment with belimumab. If PML is confirmed, consider discontinuing immunosuppressant therapy, including belimumab. Slow or interrupt infusion rate if an infusion reaction develops. Infusion reactions may be treated with acetaminophen, antiemetics (e.g., ondansetron [Zofran]), antihistamines (e.g., diphenhydramine [Benadryl]), H$_2$ antagonists (e.g., ranitidine [Zantac]), or corticosteroids (e.g., hydrocortisone sodium succinate [Solu-Cortef]) as indicated. Discontinue if a serious hypersensitivity reaction occurs. Treat hypersensitivity reactions as indicated; may require epinephrine, airway management, oxygen, IV fluids, antihistamines (e.g., diphenhydramine [Benadryl]), corticosteroids (e.g., hydrocortisone sodium succinate [Solu-Cortef]), and pressor amines (e.g., dopamine).

BELINOSTAT
(be-**LIN**-oh-stat)

Antineoplastic

Beleodaq

USUAL DOSE
1,000 mg/M^2 administered over 30 minutes by IV infusion once each day on Days 1 through 5 of a 21-day cycle. Cycles can be repeated every 21 days until disease progression or unacceptable toxicity.

DOSE ADJUSTMENTS
Before the start of each cycle and before resuming treatment following toxicity, the absolute neutrophil count (ANC) should be greater than or equal to 1×10^9/L (1,000/mm^3), and the platelet count should be greater than or equal to 50×10^9/L (50,000/mm^3). ▪ Other toxicities must be NCI-CTCAE Grade 2 or less before retreatment. ▪ Reduce the starting dose of belinostat to 750 mg/M^2 in patients known to be homozygous for the UGT1A*28 allele. ▪ See the following chart for dose modifications for hematologic and nonhematologic toxicities. Base the dose adjustments for thrombocytopenia and neutropenia on platelet and absolute neutrophil nadir (lowest value) counts in the preceding cycle of therapy.

Dose Modifications for Hematologic and Nonhematologic Toxicities	
Hematologic Toxicities	**Dose Modification**
Platelet count $\geq 25 \times 10^9$/L and nadir ANC $\geq 0.5 \times 10^9$/L	No change
Nadir ANC $<0.5 \times 10^9$/L (any platelet count)	Decrease dose by 25% (750 mg/M^2)
Platelet count $<25 \times 10^9$/L (any nadir ANC)	Decrease dose by 25% (750 mg/M^2)
Nonhematologic Toxicities	**Dose Modification**
Any CTCAE Grade 3 or 4 adverse reaction*	Decrease dose by 25% (750 mg/M^2)
Recurrence of CTCAE Grade 3 or 4 adverse reaction after two dose reductions	Discontinue Beleodaq

*For nausea, vomiting, and diarrhea, dose modify only if the duration is greater than 7 days with supportive management.

DILUTION
Specific techniques required; see Precautions. Available in single-use vials containing lyophilized powder equivalent to 500 mg belinostat. Reconstitute each vial with 9 mL of SWI (concentration is 50 mg/mL). Swirl contents until no visible particles remain. Withdraw the required dose and transfer to an infusion bag containing 250 mL of NS. Do not use if cloudiness or particulates are observed.

Filters: Use of an infusion set with a 0.22-micron in-line filter is required for administration.

Storage: Store in original packaging at CRT until use. Reconstituted vials may be stored for up to 12 hours at (15° to 25° C (59° to 77° F). Fully diluted solution may be stored at 15° to 25° C (59° to 77° F) for up to 36 hours, including infusion time.

COMPATIBILITY
Specific information not available.

RATE OF ADMINISTRATION
A single dose as an IV infusion equally distributed over 30 minutes. Infusion time may be extended to 45 minutes for infusion site pain or other symptoms potentially attributable to the infusion.

ACTIONS
A histone deacetylase (HDAC) inhibitor. HDACs catalyze the removal of acetyl groups from the lysine residues of histones and some nonhistone proteins. In vitro, belinostat caused the accumulation of acetylated histones and other proteins, inducing cell-cycle

arrest and/or apoptosis of some transformed cells. It shows preferential cytotoxicity toward tumor cells compared with normal cells. Highly bound to protein. Primarily metabolized by UGT1A1. Also undergoes some metabolism by selected cytochrome P_{450} isoenzymes. Elimination half-life is 1.1 hours. Excreted in urine.

INDICATIONS AND USES

Treatment of patients with relapsed or refractory peripheral T-cell lymphoma. Approval is based on tumor response rate and duration of response. An improvement in survival or disease-related symptoms has not been established.

CONTRAINDICATIONS

Manufacturer states, "None."

PRECAUTIONS

Follow guidelines for handling cytotoxic agents. See Appendix A, p. 1331. ▪ Usually administered by or under the direction of a physician specialist with adequate diagnostic and treatment facilities to monitor the patient and respond to any medical emergency. ▪ Can cause thrombocytopenia, leukopenia (neutropenia and lymphopenia), and/or anemia. See Monitor and Dose Adjustments. ▪ Serious and sometimes fatal infections, including pneumonia and sepsis, have occurred. Do not administer belinostat to patients with an active infection. Patients with a history of extensive or intensive chemotherapy may be at higher risk for life-threatening infections. ▪ Can cause fatal hepatotoxicity and liver function test abnormalities. Interrupt or adjust dose until recovery, or permanently discontinue belinostat based on the severity of the hepatic toxicity. ▪ Tumor lysis syndrome (TLS) has occurred. May cause acute renal failure requiring dialysis and can be fatal. ▪ Gastrointestinal toxicity has been reported. ▪ Use caution in patients with hepatic impairment. Patients with moderate and severe hepatic impairment (total bilirubin greater than 1.5 × ULN) were excluded from clinical trials. ▪ See Monitor.

Monitor: Obtain baseline CBC, including platelets, and monitor weekly. ▪ Obtain baseline serum chemistry tests, including renal and hepatic function, before the start of the first dose of each cycle. ▪ Observe closely for signs of infection. Prophylactic antibiotics may be indicated pending results of C/S in a febrile neutropenic patient. ▪ Monitor for S/S of TLS; early signs are flank pain and hematuria. May further develop to a rapid reduction in tumor volume, renal insufficiency, hyperkalemia, hypocalcemia, hyperuricemia, or hyperphosphatemia. Monitoring of serum electrolytes, uric acid, and renal function indicated. ▪ Prevention and treatment of hyperuricemia due to TLS may be accomplished with adequate hydration and, if necessary, allopurinol (Aloprim) and alkalinization of urine. ▪ Monitor for thrombocytopenia (platelet count less than 50,000 mm³). Initiate precautions to prevent excessive bleeding (e.g., inspect IV sites, skin, and mucous membranes; use extreme care during invasive procedures; test urine, emesis, stool, and secretions for occult blood). ▪ Nausea, vomiting, and diarrhea may require the use of antiemetic and/or antidiarrheal medications. Use prophylactically to increase patient comfort.

Patient Education: Review manufacturer's patient information leaflet. ▪ Avoid pregnancy. Nonhormonal birth control recommended. ▪ Promptly report nausea, vomiting, and diarrhea; antiemetics and/or antidiarrheals may be indicated. ▪ Promptly report symptoms of infection (e.g., fever). ▪ Report bloody stools, bruising, fatigue. ▪ Monitoring of liver function is imperative. ▪ See Appendix D, p. 1333.

Maternal/Child: Category D: avoid pregnancy. A genotoxic drug that targets rapidly dividing cells; may cause teratogenicity and/or embryo-fetal death. May impair male fertility. ▪ Discontinue breast-feeding. ▪ Safety and effectiveness for use in pediatric patients not established.

Elderly: Patients 65 years of age and older had a higher response rate to belinostat than did younger adults. ▪ No clinically meaningful differences in serious side effects were observed in patients based on age.

DRUG/LAB INTERACTIONS

Avoid concomitant administration of belinostat with **strong inhibitors of UGT1A1** (e.g., atazanavir [Reyataz], indinavir [Crixivan], ketoconazole [Nizoral]). ▪ Belinostat did not increase the AUC or C_{max} of **warfarin** (Coumadin). Dose adjustment of warfarin is not required when coadministered with belinostat. ▪ Likely a glycoprotein (P-gp) substrate but not likely to inhibit P-gp.

SIDE EFFECTS

The most common side effects reported are anemia, fatigue, fever, nausea and vomiting. Serious side effects reported include hematologic toxicity (anemia, lymphopenia, neutropenia, thrombocytopenia), hepatotoxicity and liver function abnormalities, increased SCr, infections (pneumonia, sepsis), multiorgan failure, and tumor lysis syndrome. Anemia, fatigue, febrile neutropenia, and multiorgan failure were reported as the reason for discontinuation of treatment. Other side effects reported include abdominal pain, chills, constipation, cough, decreased appetite, diarrhea, dizziness, dyspnea, headache, hypokalemia, hypotension, increased blood lactate dehydrogenase, infusion site pain, peripheral edema, phlebitis, prolonged QT, pruritus, and rash. Treatment-related deaths have occurred.

ANTIDOTE

Notify physician of all side effects. Minor side effects may be treated symptomatically. Supportive therapy as indicated will help sustain the patient in toxicity. Interrupt or adjust dose until recovery, or permanently discontinue belinostat based on the severity of the hematologic or hepatic toxicity. Hematologic toxicity may require dose adjustment. Neutropenia may be treated with filgrastim (Neupogen, Zarxio). Severe thrombocytopenia or anemia may require transfusion. Should a hypersensitivity reaction occur, treat as indicated.

BENDAMUSTINE HYDROCHLORIDE

(ben-deh-**MUS**-teen)

Bendeka, Treanda

Antineoplastic
Alkylating agent

pH 2.5 to 3.5

USUAL DOSE

Premedication: Premedication with antihistamines (e.g., diphenhydramine [Benadryl]), antipyretics (e.g., acetaminophen [Tylenol]), and corticosteroids may be indicated; see Monitor and Antidote.

Chronic lymphocytic leukemia (CLL): 100 mg/M^2 as an IV infusion on Days 1 and 2 of a 28-day cycle. May be repeated for up to 6 cycles.

Non-Hodgkin's lymphoma (NHL): 120 mg/M^2 as an IV infusion on Days 1 and 2 of a 21-day cycle. May be repeated for up to 8 cycles.

DOSE ADJUSTMENTS

Chronic lymphocytic leukemia (CLL) and non-Hodgkin's lymphoma (NHL): Delay treatment for Grade 4 hematologic toxicity or clinically significant nonhematologic toxicity equal to or greater than Grade 2. In addition, dose reduction may be indicated; see specific indication. Reinitiate treatment, if indicated, when nonhematologic toxicity has recovered to equal to or less than Grade 1 and/or the ANC has recovered to equal to or greater than 1,000 cells/mm^3 and platelets have recovered to equal to or greater than 75,000 cells/mm^3. ▪ No dose adjustment indicated based on age or gender; see Precautions.

Chronic lymphocytic leukemia (CLL): Reduce dose to 50 mg/M^2 on Days 1 and 2 of each cycle for Grade 3 or greater hematologic toxicity. If Grade 3 or greater toxicity recurs, reduce dose to 25 mg/M^2 on Days 1 and 2 of each cycle. ▪ Reduce dose to 50 mg/M^2 on Days 1 and 2 of each cycle for clinically significant Grade 3 or greater nonhemato-

Continued

logic toxicity. ■ Dose re-escalation in subsequent cycles may be considered by the treating physician.

Non-Hodgkin's lymphoma (NHL): Reduce dose to 90 mg/M² on Days 1 and 2 of each cycle for Grade 4 hematologic toxicity. If Grade 4 toxicity recurs, reduce the dose to 60 mg/M² on Days 1 and 2 of each cycle. ■ Reduce dose to 90 mg/M² on Days 1 and 2 of each cycle for Grade 3 or greater nonhematologic toxicity. If Grade 3 or greater toxicity recurs, reduce the dose to 60 mg/M² on Days 1 and 2 of each cycle.

DILUTION

Specific techniques required; see Precautions. Treanda is available in **two formulations:** a solution **(Treanda Injection)** and a lyophilized powder **(Treanda for Injection).** Formulations have different concentrations. **Do not mix or combine the two formulations.**

Treanda Injection is available as a solution in 45 mg/0.5 mL and 180 mg/2 mL single-use vials. **Do not use with devices containing polycarbonate or acrylonitrile-butadiene-styrene (ABS), including closed-system transfer devices (CSTDs), adaptors, and syringes when preparing the infusion bag.** Must be diluted in a biosafety cabinet or a containment isolator. Aseptically withdraw the volume needed for the required dose and transfer to a 500-mL infusion bag of NS or D2.5/¹/₂NS using a polypropylene syringe with a metal needle and polypropylene hub. (Polypropylene syringes are translucent in appearance.) Final concentration of infusion solution should be 0.2 to 0.7 mg/mL. Mix thoroughly; solution should be clear and colorless to slightly yellow; see Compatibility. After dilution of **Treanda Injection** in the infusion bag, devices that contain ABS or polycarbonate, including infusion sets, may be used.

Treanda for Injection is available as a lyophilized powder in 25- and 100-mg single-use vials. **If a CSTD or adaptor that contains polycarbonate or ABS is to be used as supplemental protection during preparation, use only this formulation (Treanda for Injection).** Reconstitute each 25-mg vial with 5 mL SWFI and each 100-mg vial with 20 mL SWFI; concentration is 5 mg/mL. Shake well. Should completely dissolve in 5 minutes. Within 30 minutes of reconstitution, withdraw the desired dose from the vial(s) and further dilute in 500 mL of NS or D2.5/¹/₂NS. Final concentration should be 0.2 to 0.6 mg/mL. Mix thoroughly; solution should be clear and colorless to slightly yellow.

Bendeka is available as a ready-to-dilute solution in 100 mg/4 mL multiple-dose vials. Withdraw the volume needed for the required dose and immediately transfer into a 50-mL infusion bag of NS, D5W, or D2.5/¹/₂NS. The final concentration should be 1.85 to 5.6 mg/mL. The final admixture should be a clear and colorless to yellow solution.

Generic bendamustine hydrochloride as a lyophilized powder has recently been approved. Prescribing information was not available at the time of this printing. Read labeling carefully. Product formulation, dilution, storage, and precautions around administration may differ among the various products.

Filters: Specific information not available.

Storage: *All formulations:* Retain in original package to protect from light. **Bendeka** must be stored in the refrigerator at 2° to 8° C (36° to 46° F). Solution diluted in NS or D2.5/¹/₂NS is stable for 6 hours at RT (15° to 30° C [59° to 86° F]) and room light or for 24 hours refrigerated at 2° to 8° C (36° to 46° F). Solution diluted in D5W is stable for 3 hours at RT (15° to 30° C [59° to 86° F]) and room light or for 24 hours refrigerated at 2° to 8° C (36° to 46° F). Administration must be completed within these times (e.g., 3, 6, or 24 hours based on type of storage and solution used). **Bendeka** is supplied as a multiple-dose vial that is stable for up to 28 days when stored in its original carton under refrigeration. Manufacturer recommends no more than 6 dose withdrawals from each vial. **Treanda Injection** must be stored in the refrigerator at 2° to 8° C (36° to 46° F). Solution diluted in NS or D2.5/¹/₂NS is stable for 2 hours at RT (15° to 30° C [59° to 86° F]) and room light or for 24 hours refrigerated at 2° to 8° C (36° to 46° F). Administration must be completed within these times (e.g., 2 or 24 hours based on type of storage). **Treanda for Injection** may be stored at CRT. Solution diluted in NS or D2.5/¹/₂NS is stable for

3 hours at RT (15° to 30° C [59° to 86° F]) and room light or for 24 hours refrigerated at 2° to 8° C (36° to 46° F). Administration must be completed within these times. Discard any unused solution.

COMPATIBILITY

Manufacturer states, "Use SWFI for reconstitution (for **Treanda for Injection**) and then (for **both formulations**) either NS or D2.5/¹/₂NS for dilution. No other diluents have been shown to be **compatible**."

Treanda Injection: Contains N,N-dimethylacetamide (DMA), which is **incompatible** with devices that contain polycarbonate or ABS. Devices, including CSTDs, adaptors, and syringes that contain polycarbonate or ABS, have been shown to dissolve when they come into contact with DMA. This **incompatibility** leads to device failure (e.g., leaking, breaking, or operational failure of CSTD components), possible product contamination, and potential serious adverse health consequences to the practitioner or patient.

RATE OF ADMINISTRATION

Bendeka: *All indications:* Total daily dose as an infusion equally distributed over 10 minutes.

Treanda: *Chronic lymphocytic leukemia (CLL):* Total daily dose as an infusion equally distributed over 30 minutes.

Non-Hodgkin's lymphoma (NHL): Total daily dose as an infusion equally distributed over 60 minutes.

ACTIONS

A bifunctional mechlorethamine derivative. An alkylating agent. Active against both quiescent and dividing cells. Exact mode of action unknown. May lead to cell death by damaging the DNA in cancer cells as well as by disrupting normal cell division. Highly protein bound. Distributes freely in human red blood cells. Extensively metabolized via hydrolytic, oxidative, and conjugative pathways. Excreted in urine and feces.

INDICATIONS AND USES

Treatment of patients with chronic lymphocytic leukemia (CLL). Study demonstrated a higher rate of overall response and a longer progression-free survival for bendamustine compared with chlorambucil (Leukeran). Effectiveness compared with first-line therapies other than chlorambucil has not been studied. ▪ Treatment of patients with indolent B-cell non-Hodgkin's lymphoma that has progressed during or within 6 months of treatment with rituximab (Rituxan) or a rituximab-containing regimen.

CONTRAINDICATIONS

Bendeka: Known hypersensitivity to bendamustine, polyethylene glycol 400, propylene glycol, or monothioglycerol.

Treanda: Known hypersensitivity to bendamustine.

PRECAUTIONS

Follow guidelines for handling cytotoxic agents. See Appendix A, p. 1331. ▪ Administered by or under the direction of the physician specialist in a facility equipped to monitor the patient and respond to any medical emergency. ▪ Do not use in patients with a CrCl less than 40 mL/min. Use with caution in patients with mild or moderate renal impairment; no formal studies conducted. ▪ Use with caution in patients with mild hepatic impairment. Do not use in patients with moderate hepatic impairment (AST or ALT 2.5 to 10 times the ULN and total bilirubin 1.5 to 3 times the ULN) or severe hepatic impairment (total bilirubin greater than 3 times the ULN). No formal studies conducted. ▪ Myelosuppression may be severe and require dose delays and/or subsequent dose reductions. Deaths from myelosuppression-related adverse reactions have occurred; see Dose Adjustments. ▪ Infections, including hepatitis, pneumonia, and sepsis, have been reported. Has been associated with septic shock and death. ▪ Patients treated with bendamustine are at risk for reactivation of infections, including (but not limited to) hepatitis B, cytomegalovirus, *Mycobacterium tuberculosis,* and herpes zoster; see Monitor. ▪ Infusion reactions are common. In rare instances anaphylaxis or anaphylactoid reactions have occurred. Usually occur in the second and/or subsequent cycles of therapy.

- Tumor lysis syndrome (TLS) has been reported and may occur in the first treatment cycle. S/S are rapid reduction in tumor volume, renal insufficiency, hyperkalemia, hypocalcemia, hyperuricemia, or hyperphosphatemia. May lead to acute renal failure and death. ▪ Skin reactions, including rash, toxic skin reactions, and bullous exanthema, have been reported; see Drug/Lab Interactions and Antidote. ▪ Premalignant and malignant diseases, including myelodysplastic syndrome, myeloproliferative disorders, acute myeloid leukemia, and bronchial carcinoma have been reported. Causal relationship has not been determined.

Monitor: Patients should undergo appropriate measures (including clinical and laboratory monitoring, prophylaxis, and treatment) for infection and/or infection reactivation before treatment. ▪ Obtain baseline CBC with differential and platelet count. Monitor CBC with differential weekly, and monitor platelet count each cycle. Hematologic nadir usually occurs in the third week. If recovery to recommended values does not occur by the first day of the next scheduled cycle, delay dose until recovery occurs; see Dose Adjustments. ▪ Obtain baseline CrCl, AST, ALT, and total bilirubin; repeat as indicated. ▪ Monitor closely for S/S of infusion or hypersensitivity reactions (e.g., chills, fever, pruritus, rash). Discontinue bendamustine if a severe reaction occurs. Inquire about possible symptoms that suggest a minor reaction after the first infusion. Consider premedication with antihistamines (e.g., diphenhydramine [Benadryl]), antipyretics (e.g., acetaminophen [Tylenol]), and corticosteroids in patients who have experienced a Grade 1 or 2 infusion reaction; see Antidote. ▪ Monitor for S/S of TLS. In patients at risk for TLS, prevention and treatment of hyperuricemia may be accomplished with vigorous hydration. Allopurinol has been used during the beginning of bendamustine therapy; see Drug/Lab Interactions. Monitor uric acid levels. Monitor electrolytes, particularly potassium, and treat as indicated. ▪ Monitor patients with skin reactions closely. Withhold or discontinue bendamustine if skin reactions are severe or progressive. ▪ Use prophylactic antiemetics to reduce nausea and vomiting and increase patient comfort. ▪ Observe for S/S of infection (e.g., fever) or reactivation of infection. Prophylactic antibiotics may be indicated pending results of C/S in a febrile neutropenic patient. ▪ Monitor for thrombocytopenia (platelet count less than 50,000 cells/mm³). Initiate precautions to prevent excessive bleeding (e.g., inspect IV sites, skin, and mucous membranes; use extreme care during invasive procedures; test urine, emesis, stool, and secretions for occult blood). ▪ Monitor IV site for signs of extravasation during and after administration (e.g., infection, pain, redness, swelling, necrosis); extravasation has resulted in hospitalization.

Patient Education: Avoid pregnancy; nonhormonal birth control is recommended for both men and women throughout treatment and for 3 months after treatment is complete; report a suspected pregnancy immediately. May pose a risk to reproductive capacity in both males and females. ▪ Promptly report signs of infection (e.g., chills, fever) or allergic reaction (e.g., dyspnea, itching, rash) and severe or worsening skin reactions, including itching or rash. ▪ Frequent laboratory monitoring required. ▪ Promptly report IV site burning or stinging. ▪ Report other side effects such as nausea, vomiting, or diarrhea. Symptomatic treatment can be provided. ▪ May cause fatigue. Avoid driving or operating any dangerous tools or machinery if this side effect is experienced. ▪ See Appendix D, p. 1333.

Maternal/Child: Category D: avoid pregnancy; can cause fetal harm. May also cause impaired spermatogenesis, azoospermia, and total germinal aplasia in males. Males and females of childbearing age must use birth control. ▪ If the drug is used during pregnancy or if the patient becomes pregnant during therapy, inform the patient of the potential hazard to the fetus. ▪ Has the potential for serious side effects; discontinue breastfeeding. ▪ Effectiveness for use in pediatric patients not established. Evaluation of one small Phase 1/2 trial suggests that the safety profile in pediatric patients is similar to that seen in adults; see prescribing information.

Elderly: Side effect profile similar for all age-groups studied.

Chronic lymphocytic leukemia (CLL): Response to bendamustine was improved in all age-groups over the response to chlorambucil; however, response in the elderly was less than in younger adults. The progression-free survival time was somewhat longer for younger adults compared with those 65 years of age or older.

Non-Hodgkin's lymphoma (NHL): Effectiveness and duration of response similar for all age-groups.

DRUG/LAB INTERACTIONS

No formal drug interaction studies have been conducted. ▪ Active metabolites of benda-mustine are formed via cytochrome P_{450} CYP1A2. **Inhibitors of CYP1A2** (e.g., ciprofloxa-cin [Cipro], fluvoxamine [Luvox]) may increase plasma concentrations of bendamustine and decrease plasma concentrations of active metabolites. **Inducers of CYP1A2** (e.g., omeprazole [Prilosec], smoking) may decrease plasma concentrations of bendamustine and increase plasma concentrations of its active metabolites. Use caution or consider alternative treatments if concomitant treatment with CYP1A2 inhibitors or inducers is indicated. ▪ Not likely to inhibit metabolism via other selected CYP isoenzymes or to induce the metabolism of substrates of cytochrome P_{450} enzymes. ▪ Cases of Stevens-Johnson syndrome (SJS) and toxic epidermal necrolysis (TEN) have been reported with concomitant administration of **allopurinol and other medications known to cause these syndromes** (e.g., rituximab [Rituxan]). ▪ In vitro data suggest that P-glycoprotein breast cancer resistance protein (BCRP) and/or other efflux transporters may have a role in bendamustine transport.

SIDE EFFECTS

Anorexia, constipation, cough, diarrhea, dyspnea, fatigue, fever, headache, myelosup-pression (anemia, febrile neutropenia, leukopenia, lymphopenia, neutropenia, thrombo-cytopenia), nausea, rash, stomatitis, vomiting, and weight loss were most common. Other side effects reported include asthenia; chills; decreased CrCl; dry mouth; elevated AST, ALT, and bilirubin levels; herpes simplex; hypersensitivity and/or infusion reactions (e.g., anaphylaxis [rare], pruritus, rash); hypertension; hyperuricemia; infections; mal-aise; malignancies; mucosal inflammation; nasopharyngitis; pneumonia; sepsis; somno-lence; stomatitis; TLS; and weakness. Hypersensitivity reactions and fever required study withdrawal in some patients.

Post-Marketing: Anaphylaxis, cardiac disorders (atrial fibrillation, CHF [some fatal], MI [some fatal], palpitation), extravasation resulting in hospitalization, infusion site reac-tions (irritation, pain, phlebitis, pruritus, swelling), pancytopenia, *Pneumocystis jiroveci* pneumonia, pneumonitis, Stevens-Johnson syndrome, and toxic epidermal necrolysis.

Overdose: Ataxia, cardiac arrhythmias, convulsions, respiratory distress, sedation, tremor.

ANTIDOTE

Keep physician informed of all side effects and hematologic parameters. Side effects may decrease in severity with reduced dose. Bone marrow depression may require withhold-ing bendamustine until recovery occurs. Administration of whole blood products (e.g., packed RBCs, platelets, leukocytes) may be required. Selected blood modifiers (e.g., erythropoiesis-stimulating agents [ESAs (Aranesp, Epogen, Mircera)], filgrastim [Neupo-gen, Zarxio], pegfilgrastim [Neulasta], sargramostim [Leukine]) may be indicated to treat bone marrow toxicity. Discontinue the infusion immediately for any life-threatening side effect (e.g., clinically significant bronchospasm, cardiac arrhythmias, severe hypoten-sion). Consider premedication with antihistamines (e.g., diphenhydramine [Benadryl]), antipyretics (e.g., acetaminophen [Tylenol]), and corticosteroids in subsequent cycles in patients who have experienced a Grade 1 or 2 hypersensitivity and/or infusion reaction. Grade 3 or 4 reactions have not typically been rechallenged; consider discontinuing bendamustine. Withhold or discontinue bendamustine if skin reactions are severe or pro-gressive. There is no specific antidote. Supportive therapy as indicated will help sustain the patient in toxicity. ECG monitoring may be indicated to evaluate cardiac side effects.

BEVACIZUMAB `BBW`
(beh-vah-**SIZZ**-ih-mab)

Recombinant monoclonal antibody
Angiogenesis inhibitor
Antineoplastic

Avastin

pH 6.2

USUAL DOSE

Do not begin therapy until at least 28 days after major surgery. Surgical incisions should be fully healed. May be used in combination with other antineoplastic agents or as a single agent. See Dose Adjustments, Monitor, and Precautions. Continue treatment until disease progression or unacceptable toxicity occurs.

Metastatic carcinoma of the colon or rectum: Administered as an infusion. Recommended doses are either 5 mg/kg or 10 mg/kg every 2 weeks when used in combination with intravenous 5-FU–based chemotherapy. Administer 5 mg/kg when used in combination with bolus IFL (irinotecan [Camptosar], fluorouracil [5-FU], leucovorin calcium). Administer 10 mg/kg when used in combination with FOLFOX4 (fluorouracil [5-FU], leucovorin calcium, and oxaliplatin [Eloxatin]).

Administer 5 mg/kg every 2 weeks or 7.5 mg/kg every 3 weeks when used in combination with a fluoropyrimidine-irinotecan–based or a fluoropyrimidine-oxaliplatin–based chemotherapy regimen in patients who have progressed on a first-line bevacizumab-containing regimen.

Nonsquamous, non–small-cell lung cancer: 15 mg/kg as an infusion every 3 weeks in combination with carboplatin (Paraplatin) and paclitaxel (Taxol).

Glioblastoma: 10 mg/kg every 2 weeks.

Metastatic renal cell carcinoma: 10 mg/kg every 2 weeks in combination with interferon alfa.

Cervical cancer: 15 mg/kg as an infusion every 3 weeks administered in combination with one of the following chemotherapy regimens: paclitaxel (Taxol) and cisplatin, or paclitaxel and topotecan (Hycamtin).

Platinum-resistant recurrent epithelial ovarian, fallopian tube, or primary peritoneal cancer: 10 mg/kg every 2 weeks in combination with one of the following chemotherapy regimens: paclitaxel, pegylated liposomal doxorubicin, or topotecan (weekly); or 15 mg/kg every 3 weeks in combination with topotecan (every 3 weeks).

DOSE ADJUSTMENTS

No dose adjustments are recommended based on age, gender, or race. ▪ No dose adjustments are recommended for patients with impaired hepatic or renal function; bevacizumab was not studied in these patients. ▪ Permanently discontinue if GI perforation, fistula formation in the GI tract (e.g., enterocutaneous, esophageal, duodenal, rectal), intra-abdominal abscess, fistula formation involving an internal organ, wound dehiscence (parting of the sutured lips of a surgical wound) or wound healing complications requiring medical intervention, serious bleeding, severe arterial thromboembolic event, life-threatening (Grade 4) venous thromboembolic events (including pulmonary embolism), nephrotic syndrome, hypertensive crisis or hypertensive encephalopathy, or posterior reversible encephalopathy syndrome (PRES) develops; see Monitor and Precautions. ▪ Temporarily discontinue if moderate to severe proteinuria (equal to or greater than 2 Gm/24 hr), severe hypertension not controlled with medical management, and/or a severe infusion reaction occurs; see Monitor and Precautions. ▪ Withhold bevacizumab for at least 4 weeks before elective surgery (half-life is approximately 20 days but has a wide range). Incision must be fully healed before therapy is resumed.

DILUTION

Available in single-use vials containing 100 mg in 4 mL or 400 mg in 16 mL (25 mg/mL). Calculate desired dose and choose the appropriate vial or combination of vials. Withdraw the required volume of bevacizumab and dilute in a total volume of 100 mL of NS.

Filters: Not required by manufacturer; however, studies using a 0.2-micron in-line filter were done, and drug potency appeared to be maintained.

Storage: Store in original carton in refrigerator at 2° to 8° C (36° to 46° F). Protect from light. *Do not shake or freeze.* Diluted solutions may be refrigerated for up to 8 hours. Contains no preservatives; unused portions must be discarded.

COMPATIBILITY

Manufacturer states, "Should not be administered with or mixed with dextrose solutions." **Incompatibilities** with polyvinylchloride or polyolefin bags have not been observed.

RATE OF ADMINISTRATION

Do not administer as an IV push or bolus. Must be given as an infusion. Administer following concurrent chemotherapy. Infusion reactions are not common but may occur; see Monitor.

Initial infusion: A single dose equally distributed over 90 minutes.

Second infusion: If the initial infusion is well tolerated, the second infusion may be administered equally distributed over 60 minutes.

Subsequent infusions: If the 60-minute infusion is well tolerated, subsequent infusions may be administered equally distributed over 30 minutes.

ACTIONS

A humanized IgG_1 monoclonal antibody produced by recombinant DNA technology. Has antiangiogenesis properties; it binds to and inhibits the biologic activity of human vascular endothelial growth factor (VEGF). The interaction of VEGF with its receptors leads to endothelial cell proliferation and new blood vessel formation. By binding VEGF, bevacizumab prevents the interaction of VEGF with its receptors on the surface of endothelial cells, thus inhibiting the development of new blood vessels around tumors (a tumor-starving mechanism) and resulting in a reduction of microvascular growth and an inhibition of metastatic disease progression. Predicted time to steady-state was 100 days. Half-life is approximately 20 days (range is 11 to 50 days). IgG antibodies may cross the placental barrier and be secreted in breast milk.

INDICATIONS AND USES

First-line or second-line treatment of metastatic carcinoma of the colon or rectum. Used in combination with intravenous 5-fluorouracil–based chemotherapy (e.g., IFL, FOLFOX4). ■ Second-line treatment of metastatic colorectal cancer in patients who have progressed on a first-line bevacizumab-containing regimen. Used in combination with fluoropyrimidine-irinotecan–based or fluoropyrimidine-oxaliplatin–based chemotherapy. ■ First-line treatment of patients with unresectable, locally advanced, recurrent, or metastatic nonsquamous, non–small-cell lung cancer. Given in combination with carboplatin and paclitaxel. ■ Treatment of glioblastoma in adult patients as a single agent for patients with progressive disease following prior therapy. (Effectiveness is based on an improvement in objective response rate. There are no data showing an improvement in disease-related symptoms or increased survival with bevacizumab.) ■ Treatment of metastatic renal cell cancer. Given in combination with interferon alfa. ■ Treatment of persistent, recurrent, or metastatic carcinoma of the cervix. Given in combination with paclitaxel and cisplatin or paclitaxel and topotecan. ■ Treatment of patients with platinum-resistant recurrent epithelial ovarian, fallopian tube, or primary peritoneal cancer who received no more than 2 prior chemotherapy regimens. Given in combination with paclitaxel, pegylated liposomal doxorubicin, or topotecan.

Limitation of use: Bevacizumab is not indicated for adjuvant treatment of colon cancer.

CONTRAINDICATIONS

Manufacturer states, "No known contraindications." However, bevacizumab must be discontinued if GI perforation, wound dehiscence requiring medical intervention, serious bleeding, nephrotic syndrome, or hypertensive crisis develops; see Antidote. ■ Use with caution in patients with known hypersensitivity to murine proteins, bevacizumab, or any of its components. ■ Not recommended for use in patients with recent hemoptysis (greater than or equal to ¹/₂ teaspoon of red blood). ▪ Avoid use in patients with ovarian cancer who have evidence of rectosigmoid involvement by pelvic examination or bowel involvement on CT scan or clinical symptoms of bowel obstruction.

PRECAUTIONS

Do not administer as an IV push or bolus. Must be given as an infusion. ▪ Should be administered by or under the direction of a physician specialist in a facility equipped to monitor the patient and respond to any medical emergency. ▪ Has been shown to impair wound healing; withhold bevacizumab for a minimum of 28 days after major surgery; surgical incision must be fully healed. Withhold at least 28 days before elective surgery (half-life is approximately 20 days but has a wide range). Appropriate intervals between surgery and the beginning of bevacizumab therapy and/or the end of bevacizumab therapy and subsequent elective surgery have not been determined. ▪ GI perforation with or without fistula formation and/or intra-abdominal abscesses has occurred; deaths have been reported. The majority of cases occurred within the first 50 days of initiation of bevacizumab. Consider GI perforation in any patient with complaints of abdominal pain associated with constipation, fever, nausea, and vomiting. ▪ Nongastrointestinal fistula formation has been reported, in some cases with a fatal outcome. Fistula formations involving tracheoesophageal, bronchopleural, biliary, vaginal, renal, and bladder areas have been reported. Most events occurred within the first 6 months of bevacizumab therapy. ▪ Necrotizing fasciitis (including fatal cases) has been reported, usually secondary to wound healing complications, gastrointestinal perforation, or fistula formation. ▪ Severe or fatal hemorrhage, including CNS hemorrhage, epistaxis, GI bleed, hematemesis, hemoptysis, and vaginal bleeding occurred up to five times more frequently in patients receiving bevacizumab. Do not administer bevacizumab to patients with serious bleeding or hemoptysis. ▪ May cause severe hypertension that may be persistent. Treatment is required; see Monitor and Antidote. ▪ Posterior reversible encephalopathy syndrome (PRES) has been reported. Onset of symptoms occurred from 16 hours to 1 year after initiation of therapy. May present with blindness and other visual and neurologic disturbances, confusion, headache, lethargy, and seizures. Mild to severe hypertension may be present. MRI is required to confirm diagnosis. Symptoms usually resolve gradually with discontinuation of bevacizumab and treatment of hypertension. ▪ Severe neutropenia, febrile neutropenia, and infection with neutropenia have been reported in patients treated with myelosuppressive chemotherapy plus bevacizumab. ▪ Proteinuria occurred during studies and progressed to nephrotic syndrome in some patients. Findings consistent with thrombotic microangiopathy have been found on kidney biopsy in some patients. In other patients, proteinuria decreased within several months after therapy was discontinued. Increased serum creatinine levels have occurred and may not return to baseline. ▪ CHF has been reported. Incidence is higher in patients receiving chemotherapy plus bevacizumab compared with patients receiving chemotherapy alone. ▪ Infusion reactions are infrequent but have occurred. S/S may include chest pain, diaphoresis, Grade 3 hypersensitivity, headache, hypertension, hypertensive crisis associated with neurologic S/S, oxygen desaturation, rigors, and wheezing. ▪ Serious and sometimes fatal arterial thromboembolic events (e.g., CVA [stroke], MI, TIA, angina) have been reported. Incidence is greater with bevacizumab given in combination with chemotherapy as compared to those receiving chemotherapy alone. Risk increased in patients with a history of arterial thromboembolism or diabetes and in patients greater than 65 years of age. ▪ Venous thromboembolic events (e.g., deep vein thrombosis, intra-abdominal thrombosis, and pulmonary embolism) have been reported. Patients treated for persistent, recurrent, or metastatic cervical cancer with bevacizumab may be at increased risk for venous thromboembolic events; see Antidote. ▪ Avastin may cause fetal harm; see Maternal/Child. ▪ Bevacizumab increases the risk of ovarian failure (defined as amenorrhea lasting 3 or more months, FSH level equal to or greater than 30 mIU/mL, and a negative serum β-HCG pregnancy test). Recovery of ovarian function occurred in some but not all women following discontinuation of therapy. Long-term effects of bevacizumab exposure on fertility are unknown. ▪ A protein substance, it has the potential for producing an immune response. Neutralizing antibodies against bevacizumab have been found using a specific immunosorbent assay; clinical significance is not known. ▪ See Drug/Lab Interactions and Antidote.

Monitor: Obtain baseline BP, CBC with differential and platelets, electrolytes, and urinalysis. ▪ Monitor for S/S of an infusion reaction (e.g., chest pain, chills, diaphoresis, headache, hypertension, hypertensive crisis associated with neurologic S/S, oxygen desaturation, wheezing). ▪ Monitor V/S and BP at least every 2 to 3 weeks; monitor more frequently in patients with hypertension. ACE inhibitors, beta-blockers, calcium channel blockers, and diuretics may be used to manage hypertension. Continue to monitor BP at regular intervals after therapy is discontinued. ▪ Repeat CBC with differential and platelets and electrolytes as indicated. ▪ Use of prophylactic antibiotics may be indicated pending C/S in a febrile, neutropenic patient. ▪ Monitor for the development or worsening of proteinuria by serial dipstick urinalysis. Patients with a 2+ or greater urine dipstick reading should undergo further assessment with a 24-hour urine collection. Monitor patients with moderate to severe proteinuria until improvement and/or resolution is observed. Repeat urinalyses and/or 24-hour urine collections as indicated. ▪ Monitor for S/S of CHF (e.g., cyanosis, dyspnea on mild exertion, edema, fatigue on exertion, hypoxemia, intolerance to cold, jugular venous distension, orthopnea, pulmonary rales, tachycardia, third heart sound). ▪ Check surgical wounds for wound dehiscence. ▪ Monitor for S/S of any type of bleeding. ▪ Monitor for GI perforation or fistula formulation (e.g., abdominal pain, constipation, fever, hypotension, nausea and vomiting). ▪ Monitor for S/S of thromboembolic events. ▪ See Dose Adjustments, Rate of Administration, Precautions, and Antidote.

Patient Education: May cause fetal harm; avoid pregnancy. Use effective contraception during treatment with and for 6 months after the last dose of bevacizumab; see Maternal/Child. Women should report a suspected pregnancy immediately. ▪ Increases risk of ovarian failure and may impair fertility. ▪ Full disclosure of health history is imperative. ▪ Promptly report any unusual or unexpected symptoms or side effects (e.g., abdominal pain, bleeding from any source, constipation, dyspnea, fever, persistent cough, rigors, sudden onset of worsening neurologic function, vomiting, wound separation). ▪ Routine monitoring of BP required. ▪ See Appendix D, p. 1333.

Maternal/Child: May cause fetal harm based on findings from animal studies and the drug's mechanism of action. Females of reproductive potential are advised to use effective contraception during treatment with bevacizumab and for 6 months after the last dose of bevacizumab. Multiple congenital malformations have been observed in rabbits. Animal models link angiogenesis and VEFG and VEFG Receptor 2 to critical aspects of female reproduction, embryofetal development, and postnatal development. ▪ May cause ovarian failure in premenopausal women; long-term effects on fertility are unknown. ▪ Discontinue breast-feeding during treatment with bevacizumab and for a prolonged period following treatment (half-life 20 days [range 11 to 50 days]). ▪ Safety and effectiveness for use in pediatric patients (including glioblastoma) not established. Nonmandibular osteonecrosis has been reported in pediatric patients less than 18 years of age who have received bevacizumab. Bevacizumab is not approved for this patient population. ▪ Dose-related physeal dysplasia (variations in the growth plate) occurred in tested juvenile monkeys; partially reversible after therapy is discontinued.

Elderly: Overall survival was similar compared to younger adults; however, the incidence of some side effects was increased (e.g., anemia, anorexia, arterial thromboembolic events [e.g., CVA (stroke), MI, TIA, angina], asthenia, CHF, constipation, deep thrombophlebitis, dehydration, diarrhea, dyspepsia, edema, epistaxis, fatigue, GI hemorrhage, hypertension, hypokalemia, hyponatremia, hypotension, ileus, increased cough, leukopenia, nausea and vomiting, proteinuria, sepsis, venous thromboembolic events [e.g., deep vein thrombosis, intra-abdominal thrombosis, pulmonary embolism], voice alteration).

DRUG/LAB INTERACTIONS

Drug interaction studies have not been completed. ▪ Has been administered concurrently with a regimen of **irinotecan, 5-fluorouracil, and leucovorin.** Studies indicate no significant effect of bevacizumab on the pharmacokinetics of irinotecan or its active metabolite SN-38. ▪ Has been administered with **carboplatin, paclitaxel, and interferon alfa.** ▪ Several cases of microangiopathic hemolytic anemia (MAHA) have been reported in patients with solid tumors who are receiving concomitant therapy with bevacizumab and **sunitinib malate** (Sutent). This combination therapy is not approved and not recommended. ▪ **ACE inhibitors, beta-blockers, calcium channel blockers, and diuretics** have been coadministered to control hypertension.

SIDE EFFECTS

The most common side effects include back pain, dry skin, epistaxis, exfoliative dermatitis, headache, hypertension, lacrimation (excess), proteinuria, rectal hemorrhage, rhinitis, and taste alteration. Major, dose-limiting, and potentially life-threatening side effects include arterial thromboembolic events (e.g., angina, cerebral infarction, MI, TIA), bleeding episodes (e.g., CNS hemorrhage, epistaxis [severe], GI hemorrhage, hemoptysis, vaginal bleeding), GI perforations, hypertensive crises, infusion reactions, nongastric intestinal fistula formation, posterior reversible encephalopathy syndrome (PRES), proteinuria and/or nephrotic syndrome, surgery and wound healing complications, and venous thromboembolic events. Other reported side effects included abdominal pain, abnormal gait, alopecia, anorexia, anxiety, asthenia, bilirubinemia, CHF, colitis, confusion, constipation, cough, dehydration, diarrhea, dizziness, dry mouth, dysarthria, dyspepsia, dysphonia, dyspnea, edema, fatigue, flatulence, hematologic toxicity (e.g., anemia, leukopenia, neutropenia, thrombocytopenia), hyperglycemia, hypertension, hypoalbuminemia, hypokalemia, hypomagnesemia, hyponatremia, hypotension, ileus, increased serum creatinine, infection, myalgia, nail disorder, nausea, pain, palmar-plantar erythrodysesthesia syndrome, pneumonitis, renal thrombotic microangiopathy (manifested as severe proteinuria), sensory neuropathy, sepsis, skin discoloration, skin ulcer, stomatitis, syncope, urinary frequency and urgency, venous thromboembolic events (e.g., deep vein thrombosis, intra-abdominal thrombosis, pulmonary embolism), voice alteration, vomiting, weight loss.

Post-Marketing: Anastomotic ulceration, acute hypertensive episodes, gallbladder perforation, GI fistula formation (e.g., gastrointestinal, enterocutaneous, esophageal, duodenal, rectal), GI perforation, GI ulcer, hepatobiliary disorders, intestinal necrosis, intra-abdominal abscess, mesenteric venous occlusion, nasal septum perforation, necrotizing fasciitis, nonmandibular osteonecrosis, osteonecrosis of the jaw, ovarian failure, pancytopenia, polyserositis, pulmonary hypertension.

ANTIDOTE

Keep physician informed of all side effects. May constitute a medical emergency or will be treated symptomatically as indicated. Permanently discontinue if any of the following develop: GI perforation, fistula formation in the GI tract (e.g., enterocutaneous, esophageal, duodenal, rectal), intra-abdominal abscess, fistula formation involving an internal organ, formation of a tracheoesophageal fistula or any Grade 4 fistula, wound dehiscence or wound healing complications requiring medical intervention, necrotizing fasciitis, serious bleeding requiring medical intervention, nephrotic syndrome, a severe arterial thromboembolic event, life-threatening (Grade 4) venous thromboembolic events (including pulmonary embolism), PRES, hypertensive crisis, or hypertensive encephalopathy. Treat these side effects aggressively; see Precautions and Monitor. Discontinue bevacizumab for severe infusion reactions and treat as indicated (e.g., epinephrine, diphenhydramine [Benadryl], IV fluids, oxygen). Data on rechallenge not available. Temporarily discontinue if moderate to severe proteinuria (equal to or greater than 2 Gm/24 hr) occurs. Resume therapy when proteinuria is less than 2 Gm/24hr; see Monitor and Precautions. Temporarily discontinue if severe hypertension not controlled with medical management occurs; see Monitor and Precautions. Thromboembolic events (e.g., deep vein thrombosis, intra-abdominal thrombosis, pulmonary embolism) were treated with full-dose warfarin (Coumadin) during clinical trials. Monitor INR closely. Bleeding occurred in patients with elevated INRs; relationship to bevacizumab not determined. Withhold bevacizumab for at least 28 days before elective surgery (half-life is approximately 20 days but has a wide range). Incision must be fully healed before therapy is resumed.

BIVALIRUDIN
(**by**-val-ih-**ROO**-din)

Anticoagulant

Angiomax

pH 5 to 6

USUAL DOSE

Initiate just before percutaneous coronary intervention (PCI) or percutaneous transluminal coronary angioplasty (PTCA). Given in combination with aspirin.

Aspirin: 300 to 325 mg before PCI and daily thereafter.

FOR PATIENTS WHO **DO NOT HAVE** HEPARIN-INDUCED THROMBOCYTOPENIA (**HIT**) OR HEPARIN-INDUCED THROMBOCYTOPENIA AND THROMBOSIS SYNDROME (**HITTS**):

Bivalirudin: Begin with an IV bolus dose of 0.75 mg/kg. Follow immediately with an infusion at 1.75 mg/kg/hr for the duration of the PCI/PTCA procedure. Perform an ACT 5 minutes after the bolus dose has been administered. An additional bolus dose of 0.3 mg/kg should be given if needed (e.g., ACT less than 225 seconds). Administration with a glycoprotein IIb/IIIa inhibitor (e.g., abciximab [ReoPro], eptifibatide [Integrilin], tirofiban [Aggrastat]) should be considered in any of the following circumstances:

- Decreased TIMI (0 to 2) or slow reflow (Thrombolysis in Myocardial Infarction [TIMI])
- Dissection with decreased flow
- New or suspected thrombus
- Persistent residual stenosis
- Distal embolization
- Unplanned stent placement
- Suboptimal stenting
- Side branch closure
- Abrupt closure, clinical instability
- Prolonged ischemia

FOR PATIENTS WHO **DO HAVE** HIT/HITTS:

Bivalirudin: Begin with an IV bolus dose of 0.75 mg/kg. Follow with an infusion at a rate of 1.75 mg/kg/hr for the duration of the PCI procedure.

For ongoing treatment postprocedure: Infusion may be continued for 4 hours post PCI/PTCA at the discretion of the treating physician. In patients with ST-segment elevation myocardial infarction (STEMI), continuation of the bivalirudin infusion at a rate of 1.75 mg/kg/hr for up to 4 hours post PCI/PTCA should be considered to mitigate the risk of stent thrombosis. After 4 hours, a reduced infusion rate of 0.2 mg/kg/hr may be administered for up to 20 hours if indicated.

DOSE ADJUSTMENTS

Reduce infusion rate in impaired renal function as indicated in the following chart. No reduction in the bolus dose is needed.

Guidelines for Bivalirudin Dose Adjustments in Impaired Renal Function*	
Renal Function (GFR)	Infusion Rate (mg/kg/hr)
GFR >30 mL/min	1.75 mg/kg/hr
GFR ≤30 mL/min	1 mg/kg/hr
Patients on hemodialysis	0.25 mg/kg/hr

*The ACT should be monitored in renally impaired patients.

DILUTION

Bolus and initial infusion: Reconstitute each 250-mg vial with 5 mL SWFI. Gently swirl to dissolve. Reconstituted solution is clear to opalescent and colorless to slightly yellow.

Withdraw and discard 5 mL from a 50-mL infusion bag containing D5W or NS. Add the contents of the reconstituted vial to the infusion bag to yield a final concentration of 5 mg/mL. Each 250-mg vial must be further diluted to 50 mL of D5W or NS as described (e.g., 1 vial in 50 mL, 2 vials in 100 mL, and 5 vials in 250 mL).

Low-rate infusion: Withdraw 5 mL from a 500-mL infusion bag of D5W or NS. After reconstitution as above, the 250-mg vial should be further diluted in the infusion bag to yield a final concentration of 0.5 mg/mL.

Storage: Store unopened vials at CRT. Do not freeze reconstituted or diluted solution. Reconstituted solution stable for 24 hours refrigerated. Concentrations between 0.5 mg/mL and 5 mg/mL are stable at RT for up to 24 hours. Discard unused portion of reconstituted solution.

COMPATIBILITY   (Underline Indicates Conflicting Compatibility Information)
Consider any drug NOT listed as compatible to be INCOMPATIBLE until consulting a pharmacist; specific conditions may apply.

Manufacturer lists alteplase (Activase, tPA), amiodarone (Nexterone), amphotericin B (conventional), chlorpromazine (Thorazine), diazepam (Valium), prochlorperazine (Compazine), reteplase (Retavase, r-PA), streptokinase, and vancomycin as **incompatible** through the same IV line (**Y-site** or piggyback). Dobutamine is **compatible** at concentrations up to 4 mg/mL but **incompatible** at a concentration of 12.5 mg/mL. No **incompatibilities** observed with glass bottles or polyvinyl chloride bags and administration sets.

One source suggests the following **compatibilities:**

Y-site: Abciximab (ReoPro), alfentanil, amikacin, aminophylline, ampicillin, ampicillin/sulbactam (Unasyn), atropine, azithromycin (Zithromax), aztreonam (Azactam), bumetanide, butorphanol (Stadol), calcium gluconate, cefazolin (Ancef), cefepime (Maxipime), cefotaxime (Claforan), cefotetan, cefoxitin (Mefoxin), ceftazidime (Fortaz), ceftriaxone (Rocephin), cefuroxime (Zinacef), ciprofloxacin (Cipro IV), clindamycin (Cleocin), dexamethasone (Decadron), digoxin (Lanoxin), diltiazem (Cardizem), diphenhydramine (Benadryl), <u>dobutamine</u>, dopamine, doxycycline, droperidol (Inapsine), enalaprilat (Vasotec IV), ephedrine, epinephrine (Adrenalin), epoprostenol (Flolan), eptifibatide (Integrilin), erythromycin (Erythrocin), esmolol (Brevibloc), famotidine (Pepcid IV), fentanyl, fluconazole (Diflucan), furosemide (Lasix), gentamicin, heparin, hydrocortisone sodium succinate (Solu-Cortef), hydromorphone (Dilaudid), isoproterenol (Isuprel), labetalol, levofloxacin (Levaquin), lidocaine, lorazepam (Ativan), magnesium, mannitol (Osmitrol), meperidine (Demerol), methylprednisolone (Solu-Medrol), metoclopramide (Reglan), metoprolol (Lopressor), metronidazole (Flagyl IV), midazolam (Versed), milrinone (Primacor), morphine, nalbuphine, nitroglycerin IV, nitroprusside sodium, norepinephrine (Levophed), phenylephrine (Neo-Synephrine), piperacillin/tazobactam (Zosyn), potassium chloride, procainamide (Pronestyl), promethazine (Phenergan), ranitidine (Zantac), sodium bicarbonate, sufentanil (Sufenta), sulfamethoxazole/trimethoprim, theophylline, ticarcillin/clavulanate (Timentin), tirofiban (Aggrastat), tobramycin, verapamil, warfarin (Coumadin).

RATE OF ADMINISTRATION
The following chart details, by patient weight in kilograms, the amount of the bolus dose, the rate in mL/hr of the initial infusion, and the rate in mL/hr of the subsequent infusion.

Bivalirudin Dosing Guidelines		
Using 5 mg/mL Concentration		Using 0.5 mg/mL Concentration
Weight (kg)	Bolus (0.75 mg/kg) (mL)	Infusion (1.75 mg/kg/hr) (mL/hr)	Subsequent Low-rate Infusion (0.2 mg/kg/hr) (mL/hr)
43-47	7 mL	16 mL/hr	18 mL/hr
48-52	7.5 mL	17.5 mL/hr	20 mL/hr
53-57	8 mL	19 mL/hr	22 mL/hr
58-62	9 mL	21 mL/hr	24 mL/hr
63-67	10 mL	23 mL/hr	26 mL/hr
68-72	10.5 mL	24.5 mL/hr	28 mL/hr
73-77	11 mL	26 mL/hr	30 mL/hr
78-82	12 mL	28 mL/hr	32 mL/hr
83-87	13 mL	30 mL/hr	34 mL/hr
88-92	13.5 mL	31.5 mL/hr	36 mL/hr
93-97	14 mL	33 mL/hr	38 mL/hr
98-102	15 mL	35 mL/hr	40 mL/hr
103-107	16 mL	37 mL/hr	42 mL/hr
108-112	16.5 mL	38.5 mL/hr	44 mL/hr
113-117	17 mL	40 mL/hr	46 mL/hr
118-122	18 mL	42 mL/hr	48 mL/hr
123-127	19 mL	44 mL/hr	50 mL/hr
128-132	19.5 mL	45.5 mL/hr	52 mL/hr
133-137	20 mL	47 mL/hr	54 mL/hr
138-142	21 mL	49 mL/hr	56 mL/hr
143-147	22 mL	51 mL/hr	58 mL/hr
148-152	22.5 mL	52.5 mL/hr	60 mL/hr

ACTIONS

An anticoagulant that is a specific and reversible direct thrombin inhibitor. It directly inhibits thrombin by specifically binding both to the catalytic site and to the anion-binding exosite of circulating and clot-bound thrombin. It inhibits coagulant effects by preventing thrombin-mediated cleavage of fibrinogen to fibrin and activation of factors V, VIII, and XIII. Exhibits dose- and concentration-dependent anticoagulant activity as evidenced by prolongation of ACT, aPPT, PT and TT. Anticoagulant effect is immediate. Cleared from plasma by a combination of renal mechanisms and proteolytic cleavage. The binding of bivalirudin to thrombin is reversible, resulting in recovery of thrombin active site functions. Coagulation times return to baseline approximately 1 hour after completion of infusion. Half-life averages 25 minutes. 20% of unchanged drug excreted in urine.

INDICATIONS AND USES

An anticoagulant for use in patients with unstable angina undergoing percutaneous trans-luminal coronary angioplasty (PTCA). (Used in place of heparin.) Used concurrently with aspirin. ■ As an anticoagulant for use in patients undergoing percutaneous coronary intervention (PCI). Used in combination with aspirin and may be used in combination with glycoprotein IIb/IIIa inhibitor (e.g., abciximab [ReoPro], eptifibatide [Integrilin]) as medically indicated. ■ As an anticoagulant in patients with, or at risk for, heparin-induced thrombocytopenia (HIT) or heparin-induced thrombocytopenia and thrombosis syndrome (HITTS) undergoing PCI.

Limitation of use: Safety and effectiveness not established in patients with acute coronary syndrome who are not undergoing PTCA or PCI.

Unlabeled uses: Heparin-induced thrombocytopenia (HIT), ST-elevation myocardial infarction (STEMI) undergoing PCI. ▪ Used as a substitute for heparin in patients with acute HIT who require cardiac surgery (e.g., coronary artery bypass graft [CABG]).

CONTRAINDICATIONS

Hypersensitivity to bivalirudin or its components; active major bleeding.

PRECAUTIONS

For IV use only. ▪ Most bleeding associated with the use of bivalirudin in PCI/PTCA occurs at the site of arterial puncture; however, hemorrhage can occur at any site. Consider a hemorrhagic event if there is an unexplained fall in BP or hematocrit or other unexplained symptom and discontinue bivalirudin. ▪ Has been associated with an increased risk of thrombus formation when used in gamma brachytherapy (percutaneous intracoronary brachytherapy). Fatalities have occurred. Imperative to maintain meticulous catheter technique, with frequent aspiration and flushing to minimize conditions of stasis within the catheter and vessels. ▪ Acute stent thrombosis (fewer than 4 hours) has been observed at a greater frequency in bivalirudin-treated patients compared with heparin-treated patients with STEMI undergoing primary PCI. Patients should remain for at least 24 hours in a facility capable of managing ischemic complications and should be carefully monitored following primary PCI for S/S consistent with myocardial ischemia. ▪ Use with caution in disease states and other circumstances in which there is an increased risk of bleeding, including severe hypertension; immediately following lumbar puncture; spinal anesthesia; major surgery, especially involving the brain, spinal cord, or eye; hematologic conditions associated with increased bleeding tendencies such as congenital or acquired bleeding disorders and gastrointestinal lesions such as ulcerations. ▪ Half-life extended in patients with impaired renal function; see Dose Adjustments. ▪ Limited data regarding re-exposure to bivalirudin; positive antibodies developed in 2 patients, and neither developed clinical evidence of a hypersensitivity reaction. ▪ See Drug/Lab Interactions.

Monitor: Before therapy, obtain platelet count, hemoglobin and hematocrit, SCr, ACT, and aPTT. ▪ Dose is not titrated to ACT; however, the ACT was checked at 5 minutes and again in 45 minutes during original clinical studies. ▪ Monitor anticoagulation status in patients with impaired renal function receiving reduced doses. ▪ Observe carefully for symptoms of a hemorrhagic event (e.g., unexplained fall in hematocrit, fall in BP, or any other unexplained symptom). ▪ Monitor STEMI patients undergoing primary PCI for S/S consistent with myocardial ischemia for a minimum of 24 hours following the procedure.

Patient Education: Risk of bleeding may be increased; discuss medical history and list of all medications (prescription and over-the-counter) with your health care provider; see Drug Interactions. ▪ Report all episodes of bleeding. ▪ Report tarry stools. ▪ Compliance with all measures to minimize bleeding is very important (e.g., avoid use of razors, toothbrushes, other sharp items). ▪ Use caution while moving to avoid excess bumping.

Maternal/Child: Category B: safety for use during pregnancy not established. May have adverse effects on the fetus and the potential for maternal bleeding is increased, particularly during the third trimester. Use only if clearly needed. ▪ Not known if bivalirudin is secreted in human milk; use caution if required during breast-feeding. ▪ Safety and effectiveness for use in pediatric patients not established.

Elderly: Response similar to younger adults. ▪ See Dose Adjustments for the elderly with impaired renal function. ▪ Bleeding events are more common in the elderly.

DRUG/LAB INTERACTIONS

Coadministration with **heparin, warfarin, thrombolytics** (e.g., alteplase [Activase], reteplase [Retavase], tenecteplase [TNKase]), **or glycoprotein IIb/IIIa inhibitors** is associated with an increased risk of major bleeding events. ▪ Concomitant use with **other agents that alter** hemostasis such as **other anticoagulants** (e.g., enoxaparin [Lovenox], apixaban [Eliquis], rivaroxaban [Xarelto]), **nonsteroidal anti-inflammatory drugs** (e.g., ibuprofen [Advil, Motrin], naproxen [Aleve, Naprosyn]), **and platelet aggregation inhibitors** (e.g., clopidogrel [Plavix], prasugrel [Effient]) may increase the risk of bleeding. ▪ No experience with coadministration of bivalirudin and plasma expanders such as dextran. ▪ Bivalirudin affects INR; therefore INR measurements made in patients who have been treated with bivalirudin may not be useful for determining the appropriate dose of warfarin.

SIDE EFFECTS

Bleeding is the most frequent adverse event; incidence in clinical studies was less than with heparin. Fever, headache, and thrombocytopenia were also commonly reported. Abdominal pain, angina pectoris, anxiety, back pain, bradycardia, dyspepsia, hypertension, hypotension, injection site pain, insomnia, nausea, nervousness, pain, pelvic pain, urinary retention, and vomiting have occurred.

Post-Marketing: Cardiac tamponade, elevated INR, fatal hemorrhage, hypersensitivity reactions (including anaphylaxis), pulmonary hemorrhage, and thrombus formation during PCI with and without intracoronary brachytherapy, including reports of fatal outcomes.

Overdose: Death due to hemorrhage.

ANTIDOTE

No specific antidote is available. Overdose with or without bleeding may be controlled by discontinuing bivalirudin. Discontinuation leads to a gradual reduction in anticoagulant effects due to metabolism of the drug depending on dose/overdose and concentration achieved. ACT or aPTT should return to normal within 1 to 4 hours after discontinuation. Reversal may take longer in patients with renal impairment. If life-threatening bleeding develops and excessive plasma levels of bivalirudin are suspected, immediately stop infusion. Determine aPTT, ACT, and hemoglobin and prepare for blood transfusion as appropriate. Follow current guidelines for treatment of shock as indicated (fluid, vasopressors [e.g., dopamine], Trendelenburg position, plasma expanders [e.g., albumin, hetastarch]). Treat hypersensitivity reactions as indicated; may require epinephrine, airway management, oxygen, IV fluids, antihistamines (e.g., diphenhydramine [Benadryl]), corticosteroids (e.g., hydrocortisone sodium succinate [Solu-Cortef]), and pressor amines (e.g., dopamine). Bivalirudin is partially removed by hemodialysis.

BLEOMYCIN SULFATE BBW
(blee-oh-**MY**-sin **SUL**-fayt)

Antineoplastic
(antibiotic)

Blenoxane

pH 4.5 to 6

USUAL DOSE
Squamous cell carcinoma, non-Hodgkin's lymphoma, testicular carcinoma: 0.25 to 0.5 units/kg of body weight/dose (10 to 20 units/M^2), once or twice weekly (1 unit equals 1 mg). The first two doses in lymphoma patients should not exceed 2 units in order to rule out hypersensitivity.

Hodgkin's disease: Dosage as above. After a 50% response, a maintenance dose of 1 unit daily or 5 units weekly is recommended.

DOSE ADJUSTMENTS
Unit/kg dose based on average weight in presence of edema or ascites. ▪ Dose selection in the elderly should be cautious; consider decreased renal function and concomitant disease or drug therapy. ▪ Reduce dose in impaired renal function as indicated in the following chart.

CrCl (mL/min)	Bleomycin Dose
50 mL/min and above	100%
40-50 mL/min	70%
30-40 mL/min	60%
20-30 mL/min	55%
10-20 mL/min	45%
5-10 mL/min	40%

DILUTION
Specific techniques required; see Precautions. Each 15 units or fraction thereof must be reconstituted with 5 mL or more of NS. For IV injection, further dilution is not necessary, but has been further diluted in 50 to 100 mL NS and given as an intermittent infusion. May be given through Y-tube or three-way stopcock of a free-flowing IV.

Filters: No data available from manufacturer. Another source indicates no significant drug loss with the use of a 0.22-micron filter.

Storage: Refrigerate powder. Diluted solution stable at room temperature for 24 hours.

COMPATIBILITY
Consider any drug NOT listed as compatible to be INCOMPATIBLE until consulting a pharmacist; specific conditions may apply.

Manufacturer states, "Should not be reconstituted or diluted with D5W or other dextrose-containing diluents."

One source suggests the following **compatibilities:**

Additive: Amikacin, dexamethasone (Decadron), diphenhydramine (Benadryl), fluorouracil (5-FU), gentamicin, heparin, streptomycin, tobramycin, vinblastine, vincristine.

Y-site: Allopurinol (Aloprim), amifostine (Ethyol), aztreonam (Azactam), cisplatin, cyclophosphamide (Cytoxan), doxorubicin (Adriamycin), doxorubicin liposomal (Doxil), droperidol (Inapsine), etoposide phosphate (Etopophos), filgrastim (Neupogen), fludarabine (Fludara), fluorouracil (5-FU), furosemide (Lasix), gemcitabine (Gemzar), granisetron (Kytril), heparin, leucovorin calcium, melphalan (Alkeran), methotrexate, metoclopramide (Reglan), mitomycin (Mutamycin), ondansetron (Zofran), paclitaxel (Taxol), piperacillin/tazobactam (Zosyn), sargramostim (Leukine), teniposide (Vumon), thiotepa, vinblastine, vincristine, vinorelbine (Navelbine).

RATE OF ADMINISTRATION

IV injection: Each 15- to 30-unit dose over 10 minutes.
Intermittent infusion: A single dose over 15 to 30 minutes or 1 unit/minute.

ACTIONS

An antibiotic antineoplastic agent, cell cycle phase-specific, that seems to act by splitting and fragmentation of double-stranded DNA. Inhibits DNA synthesis and, to a lesser extent, RNA and protein synthesis. It localizes in tumors. Improvement usually noted within 2 to 3 weeks. Widely distributed throughout the body. Inactivated by an enzyme that is widely distributed in normal tissue with the exception of the skin and lungs. Half-life is approximately 2 hours. About 60% to 70% excreted in urine.

INDICATIONS AND USES

Testicular carcinoma; may induce complete remission with vinblastine and cisplatin. ■ Palliative treatment, adjunct to surgery or radiation, in patients not responsive to other chemotherapeutic agents or those with squamous cell carcinoma of the skin, head, esophagus, neck, or GU tract, including the cervix, vulva, scrotum, and penis; in Hodgkin's disease and other lymphomas. ■ Injected into pleural cavity to treat malignant pleural effusion.

CONTRAINDICATIONS

Patients who have demonstrated a hypersensitive or idiosyncratic reaction to it.

PRECAUTIONS

Follow guidelines for handling cytotoxic agents. See Appendix A, p. 1331. ■ May be given by the IM, IV, SC, or IP routes. ■ Administered by or under the direction of the physician specialist. ■ Administer in a facility with adequate diagnostic and treatment facilities to monitor the patient and respond to any medical emergency. ■ May be used with other antineoplastic drugs to achieve tumor remission. ■ Pulmonary toxicity may progress from nonspecific pneumonitis to pulmonary fibrosis and death. Pulmonary toxicity increases markedly with advancing age or with total doses greater than 400 units but has been seen in younger patients and in patients treated with lower doses. It may occur at lower doses when bleomycin is used in combination with other antineoplastic agents. Risk of developing pulmonary toxicity is greater when O_2 is administered in surgery. To prevent this side effect, it has been recommended that the FiO_2 be maintained at concentrations approximating that of room air during surgery and in the postoperative period. Additionally, fluid replacement should be closely monitored and focus more on colloid (e.g., albumin) administration rather than on crystalloid (e.g., NS, LR) administration. ■ A severe idiosyncratic reaction (similar to anaphylaxis) has been reported in approximately 1% of lymphoma patients. S/S include hypotension, mental confusion, fever, chills, and wheezing; may be immediate or delayed for several hours. More common after the first or second doses. ■ Use with extreme caution in patients with significant renal impairment or compromised pulmonary function.

Monitor: Obtain a baseline chest x-ray, and recheck every 1 to 2 weeks to detect pulmonary changes. ■ To identify subclinical pulmonary toxicity, monitor pulmonary diffusion capacity for carbon monoxide monthly. Should remain 30% to 35% above pretreatment value. Earliest signs of pulmonary toxicity are rales and dyspnea. ■ Monitor renal, hepatic, and central nervous systems and skin for symptoms of toxicity. ■ Determine patency of vein; avoid extravasation. ■ Maintain adequate hydration. ■ Prophylactic antiemetics may reduce nausea and vomiting and increase patient comfort. ■ Observe closely for all signs of infection. Prophylactic antibiotics may be indicated pending results of C/S in a febrile neutropenic patient. ■ Acetaminophen, diphenhydramine (Benadryl), and steroids (e.g., hydrocortisone) may be used prophylactically to reduce incidence of fever and anaphylaxis. ■ See Precautions.

Patient Education: Use nonhormonal contraception. ■ Report any possible side effects promptly. ■ Report stinging or burning at IV site promptly. ■ See Appendix D, p. 1333. ■ Pulmonary toxicity more likely in smokers.

Maternal/Child: Category D: avoid pregnancy. ■ Not recommended during breastfeeding. ■ Safety and effectiveness for use in pediatric patients not established. Volume of distribution and half-life is comparable to that in adults.

Elderly: Response similar to that seen in younger adults; however, pulmonary toxicity is more common in patients older than 70 years of age. ▪ See Dose Adjustments; monitoring of renal function suggested.

DRUG/LAB INTERACTIONS

See Precautions. ▪ Vascular toxicities (e.g., myocardial infarction, CVA, thrombotic microangiopathy, cerebral arteritis) or Raynaud's phenomenon have occurred rarely when bleomycin is used in combination with **other antineoplastic agents.** ▪ May decrease GI absorption of **digoxin and hydantoins** (e.g., phenytoin). ▪ Do not administer **live virus vaccines** to patients receiving antineoplastic drugs. ▪ Causes sensitization of lung tissue to O_2; increases risk of pulmonary toxicity with **O_2 and general anesthetics.** ▪ **Cisplatin** may inhibit renal elimination and increase toxicity.

SIDE EFFECTS

Alopecia, anorexia, chills, dyspnea, fever, hypotension, malaise, nausea, phlebitis (infrequent), rales, scleroderma-like skin changes, stomatitis, tenderness of the skin, tumor site pain, vomiting, weight loss.

Major: Severe idiosyncratic reaction similar to anaphylaxis (up to 6 hours after test dose), chest pain (acute with sudden onset suggestive of pleuropericarditis), pneumonitis, pulmonary fibrosis, skin toxicity (including nodules on hands, desquamation of skin, hyperpigmentation, and gangrene).

ANTIDOTE

Notify the physician of all side effects. Minor side effects will be treated symptomatically. Discontinue the drug immediately and notify the physician of any symptom of major side effects. Provide immediate treatment (epinephrine [Adrenalin] and diphenhydramine [Benadryl] for anaphylaxis, antibiotics and steroids for pneumonitis) or supportive therapy as indicated.

BLINATUMOMAB BBW

(**BLIN**-a-**TOOM**-oh-mab)

Blincyto

Antineoplastic
Monoclonal antibody

pH 7

USUAL DOSE

Hospitalization is recommended for the first 9 days of the first cycle and the first 2 days of the second cycle; see Precautions.

Premedication: Administer dexamethasone 20 mg IV 1 hour before the first dose of blinatumomab of each cycle, 1 hour before a step dose (such as Cycle 1, Day 8), or when restarting an infusion after an interruption of 4 or more hours.

Blinatumomab: A single cycle of treatment consists of 4 weeks of continuous intravenous infusion followed by a 2-week treatment-free interval.

Patients at least 45 kg in weight: *Cycle 1:* 9 mcg/day on Days 1 through 7, then increase to 28 mcg/day on Days 8 through 28.

Subsequent cycles: 28 mcg/day on Days 1 through 28. Allow for at least 2 treatment-free weeks between cycles. A treatment course consists of up to 2 cycles for induction followed by 3 additional cycles for consolidation treatment (up to a total of 5 cycles).

DOSE ADJUSTMENTS

For an interruption of no longer than 7 days, continue the same cycle to a total of 28 days of infusion, including the days before and after the interruption in that cycle. If an interruption due to an adverse event is longer than 7 days, start a new cycle. ▪ No dose adjustment is needed for patients with a baseline CrCl equal to or greater than 30 mL/min. No information is available for patients with a CrCl less than 30 mL/min or for patients on hemodialysis.

Dose Adjustment of Blinatumomab for Toxicity		
Toxicity	Grade*	Action
Cytokine release syndrome (CRS)	Grade 3	Withhold blinatumomab until resolved, then restart at 9 mcg/day. Escalate to 28 mcg/day after 7 days if the toxicity does not recur.
Cytokine release syndrome (CRS)	Grade 4	Discontinue blinatumomab permanently.
Neurologic toxicity	Seizure	Discontinue blinatumomab permanently if more than one seizure occurs.
Neurologic toxicity	Grade 3	Withhold blinatumomab until toxicity is no more than Grade 1 (mild) and for at least 3 more days, then restart at 9 mcg/day. Escalate to 28 mcg/day after 7 days if the toxicity does not recur. If the toxicity occurred at 9 mcg/day, or if the toxicity takes more than 7 days to resolve, discontinue blinatumomab permanently.
Neurologic toxicity	Grade 4	Discontinue blinatumomab permanently.
Other clinically relevant adverse reactions	Grade 3	Withhold blinatumomab until toxicity is no more than Grade 1 (mild), then restart at 9 mcg/day. Escalate to 28 mcg/day after 7 days if the toxicity does not recur. If the toxicity takes more than 14 days to resolve, discontinue blinatumomab permanently.
Other clinically relevant adverse reactions	Grade 4	Consider discontinuing blinatumomab permanently.

*Based on the Common Terminology Criteria for Adverse Events (CTCAE). Grade 3 is severe, and Grade 4 is life-threatening.

DILUTION

To minimize medication errors, including underdose and overdose, it is imperative that the instructions for preparation (including admixing) and administration be followed exactly. Contains no preservatives; aseptic technique must be strictly observed. Must be prepared in an ISO Class 5 or better laminar flow hood by appropriately trained personnel. Consult the prescribing information before preparation begins and again if questions arise during reconstitution, preparation, or administration. Contact manufacturer if needed. Available in a package that includes a 35-mcg vial of blinatumomab and a vial of IV solution stabilizer. Additional single-use syringes, 21- to 23-gauge needles, preservative-free SWFI, a 250-mL prefilled infusion bag of NS, and polyolefin, PVC non-DEHP, or EVA IV tubing with a sterile, nonpyrogenic, low–protein-binding, 0.2-micron in-line filter are required. Confirm compatibility with the infusion pump to be used. When preparing an IV bag, remove the air from the IV bag. This is particularly important for use with an ambulatory infusion pump.

Preparation of a 9 mcg/day dose to be infused over 24 hours at a rate of 10 mL/hr:

1. Use a prefilled 250-mL infusion bag of NS (the typical overfill to a total volume of 265 to 275 mL is required; adjust volume if indicated).
2. Using a 10-mL syringe, aseptically transfer **5.5 mL** of the IV solution stabilizer to the IV bag of NS. Gently mix to avoid foaming. Discard remaining IV solution stabilizer. The IV stabilizer is used to prevent adhesion of blinatumomab to IV bags and IV lines. *Do not reconstitute blinatumomab with the IV solution stabilizer.*
3. Using a 5-mL syringe, reconstitute one vial of blinatumomab using 3 mL of preservative-free SWFI. Direct SWFI toward the side of the vial. Gently swirl contents to avoid excess foaming. *Do not shake.* Final blinatumomab concentration is 12.5 mcg/mL. Solution should be clear to slightly opalescent and colorless to slightly yellow. *Do not use if solution is cloudy or has precipitated.*
4. Using a 1-mL syringe, aseptically transfer **0.83 mL** of the reconstituted solution of blinatumomab into the IV bag. Gently mix the contents of the bag to avoid foaming.
5. Attach the IV tubing to the IV bag with the sterile 0.2-micron in-line filter. *Remove air from the IV bag and prime the IV line only with the prepared solution for infusion. Do not prime with NS.*

Preparation of a 9 mcg/day dose to be infused over 48 hours at a rate of 5 mL/hr: Repeat Steps 1 through 5 above **EXCEPT** in Step 4, use a 3-mL syringe to aseptically transfer **1.7 mL** of the reconstituted solution of blinatumomab into the IV bag. Gently mix the contents of the bag to avoid foaming.

Preparation of a 28 mcg/day dose to be infused over 24 hours at a rate of 10 mL/hr: Repeat Steps 1 through 5 above **EXCEPT** in Step 2, transfer **5.6 mL** of the IV solution stabilizer to the IV bag of NS and, in Step 4, transfer **2.6 mL** of the reconstituted solution of blinatumomab into the IV bag.

Preparation of a 28 mcg/day dose to be infused over 48 hours at a rate of 5 mL/hr:

1. Use a prefilled 250-mL infusion bag of NS (the typical overfill to a total volume of 265 to 275 mL is required; adjust volume if indicated).
2. Using a 10-mL syringe, aseptically transfer **5.6 mL** of the IV solution stabilizer to the IV bag of NS. Gently mix to avoid foaming. Discard remaining IV solution stabilizer vials. The IV stabilizer is used to prevent adhesion of blinatumomab to IV bags and IV lines. *Do not reconstitute blinatumomab with the IV solution stabilizer.*
3. Use 2 vials of blinatumomab. Using a 5-mL syringe, reconstitute each vial of blinatumomab using 3 mL of preservative-free SWFI. Direct SWFI toward the side of the vial. Gently swirl contents to avoid excess foaming. *Do not shake.* Final blinatumomab concentration is 12.5 mcg/mL. Solution should be clear to slightly opalescent and colorless to slightly yellow. *Do not use if solution is cloudy or has precipitated.*
4. Using a 3-mL syringe, aseptically transfer **5.2 mL** of the reconstituted solution of blinatumomab into the IV bag (2.7 mL from one vial and the remaining 2.5 mL from the second vial). Gently mix the contents of the bag to avoid foaming.

5. Attach the IV tubing to the IV bag with the sterile 0.2-micron in-line filter. *Remove air from the IV bag and prime the IV line only with the prepared solution for infusion. Do not prime with NS.*

Filters: Must be administered using IV tubing that contains a sterile, nonpyrogenic, low–protein-binding, 0.2-micron in-line filter.

Storage: Refrigerate vials of blinatumomab and IV solution stabilizer at 2° to 8° C (36° to 46° F) in the original package and protect from light until time of use. Do not freeze. If not used immediately, the reconstituted vial may be refrigerated for up to 24 hours or kept at room temperature (23° to 27° C [73° to 81° F]) for up to 4 hours. Prepared solutions may be refrigerated for up to 8 days or kept at room temperature for up to 48 hours. Storage times **include** infusion time. Protect from light in all dilutions. Discard if not administered within the maximum time frames for storage. Do not return solution that has been stored at RT to the refrigerator.

COMPATIBILITY
Manufacturer states, "Blinatumomab should be infused through a dedicated lumen."

RATE OF ADMINISTRATION
Do not flush the blinatumomab infusion line, especially when changing infusion bags. Flushing when changing bags or at completion of the infusion can result in overdose. Administer as a continuous IV infusion over 24 to 48 hours at a constant flow rate using a programmable, lockable, nonelastomeric infusion pump with an alarm.

24-hour infusion: A complete dose delivered at 10 mL/hr.
48-hour infusion: A complete dose delivered at 5 mL/hr.

ACTIONS
Blinatumomab is produced by recombinant technology. It is a bispecific, CD19-directed, CD3T-cell engager that binds to CD19 expressed on cells of B-lineage origin and to CD3 expressed on T-cells. It activates endogenous T-cells by connecting CD3 in the T-cell receptor (TCR) complex with CD19 on benign and malignant B-cells. Through various processes it results in redirected lysis of CD19+ cells. During the continuous intravenous infusion (over 4 weeks), the pharmacodynamics response was characterized by T-cell activation and initial redistribution, reduction in peripheral B-cells, and transient cytokine elevation. The highest elevation of cytokines occurs during the first 2 days following the initiation of dosing and usually returns to baseline within 24 to 48 hours. In subsequent cycles, cytokine elevation is less intense. With a continuous infusion, steady-state serum concentration was achieved within a day and remained stable over time during studies. Metabolic pathway has not been characterized. Degradation into small peptides and amino acids via catabolic pathways is suspected. Half-life was 2.11 hours. Negligible amounts excreted in urine.

INDICATIONS AND USES
Treatment of Philadelphia chromosome-negative relapsed or refractory B-cell precursor acute lymphoblastic leukemia (ALL).

CONTRAINDICATIONS
Known hypersensitivity to blinatumomab or to any component of the product formulation.

PRECAUTIONS
Administered under the direction of a physician or health care professional knowledgeable in its use. Hospitalization is recommended for the first 9 days of the first cycle and the first 2 days of the second cycle. For all subsequent cycle starts and re-initiation (e.g., if treatment is interrupted for 4 or more hours), supervision by a health care professional or hospitalization is recommended. Adequate diagnostic and treatment facilities to monitor the patient and respond to any medical emergency should be available. ▪ Cytokine release syndrome (CRS), which may be life-threatening or fatal, has occurred. Interrupt or discontinue blinatumomab as recommended. ▪ Infusion reactions have occurred and may be clinically indistinguishable from manifestations of CRS. ▪ Disseminated intravascular coagulation (DIC), capillary leak syndrome (CLS), and hemophagocytic lymphohistiocytosis/macrophage activation syndrome (HLH/MAS) have been reported

with CRS. ▪ Neurologic toxicities that may be severe, life-threatening, or fatal have occurred. Interrupt or discontinue blinatumomab as recommended. ▪ Serious infections (e.g., bacteremia, catheter-site infections, opportunistic infections, pneumonia, sepsis) were observed in 25% of patients; some were life-threatening or fatal. ▪ Tumor lysis syndrome (TLS), which may be life-threatening or fatal, has been observed. ▪ Neutropenia and febrile neutropenia, including life-threatening cases, have been observed. ▪ Changes showing leukoencephalopathy have been identified by cranial MRI, especially in patients with prior treatment with cranial irradiation and antileukemic chemotherapy (including systemic high-dose methotrexate or intrathecal cytarabine). Clinical significance unknown. ▪ Preparation and administration errors have occurred; follow instructions carefully. ▪ No formal pharmacokinetic studies have been conducted in patients with hepatic or renal impairment. ▪ A therapeutic protein, there is a potential for immunogenicity. Notify manufacturer if anti-blinatumomab antibodies with a clinically significant effect are suspected.

Monitor: Obtain baseline CBC (including, but not limited to, WBC and ANC). Repeat during each cycle as indicated. ▪ Obtain baseline ALT, AST, GGT, and total bilirubin. Elevation in liver enzymes has been seen in isolation and in conjunction with CRS. Repeat during treatment as indicated. ▪ Monitor for S/S of CRS (e.g., asthenia; fever; headache; hypotension; increased ALT, AST, and total bilirubin; nausea); see Precautions. ▪ Monitor for S/S of neurologic toxicities (e.g., confusion and disorientation, convulsions, coordination and balance disorders, disturbances in consciousness, encephalopathy, speech disorders). Neurologic toxicities occurred in approximately 50% of patients, with Grade 3 or higher events occurring in 15% of patients. The median time to onset was 7 days. Most events resolved with treatment interruption, but some resulted in discontinuation of blinatumomab. ▪ Observe closely for S/S of infection (e.g., chills, cough, fever, pain with urination). Prophylactic antibiotics and surveillance testing during treatment may be indicated. Treat appropriately. ▪ Monitor for S/S of hypersensitivity (e.g., hypotension, rash, urticaria, tightness of the chest, wheezing) or S/S of an infusion reaction (e.g., breathing problems, chills, fever, or rash). ▪ Monitor for S/S of TLS (e.g., hyperkalemia, hyperphosphatemia, hyperuricemia, hypocalcemia, metabolic acidosis, urate crystalluria, and renal failure). Flank pain and hematuria are early signs. To prevent TLS, initiate appropriate prophylactic measures, including pretreatment nontoxic cytoreduction and on-treatment hydration. Management may require temporary interruption or discontinuation of blinatumomab.

Patient Education: Keep the area around the intravenous catheter clean to reduce the risk of infection. ▪ Do not adjust the setting on the infusion pump; may result in dosing errors. Notify the doctor or nurse immediately if there is a problem with the infusion pump or the pump alarms. ▪ There is a risk of seizures or a loss of consciousness. Refrain from driving and/or engaging in hazardous occupations or activities (e.g., operating heavy or potentially dangerous machinery). ▪ Promptly report S/S that may be associated with cytokine release syndrome and infusion reactions (e.g., chills, fatigue, fever, hypotension, nausea and vomiting, rash, wheezing). ▪ Promptly report S/S of neurologic toxicities (e.g., confusion, convulsions, speech disorders) and S/S of infection, including pneumonia.

Maternal/Child: Category C: use during pregnancy only if the potential benefit justifies the potential risk to the fetus. ▪ Discontinue breast-feeding. ▪ Limited experience in pediatric patients; see prescribing information for suggested doses. ▪ See Appendix D, p. 1333.

Elderly: Safety and effectiveness similar to that seen in younger adults. The elderly experienced a higher rate of neurologic toxicities, including cognitive disorder, confusion, encephalopathy, and serious infections.

DRUG/LAB INTERACTIONS

No formal drug interaction studies have been conducted. ■ Initiation of blinatumomab treatment causes transient release of cytokines that **may suppress CYP$_{450}$ enzymes**. Highest risk is during the first 9 days of the first cycle and the first 2 days of the second cycle in patients receiving concomitant CYP$_{450}$ substrates, particularly those with a narrow therapeutic index. Monitor these patients for toxicity (e.g., warfarin [Coumadin]) or drug concentrations (e.g., cyclosporine [Sandimmune]) and adjust the dose of the concomitant drug as needed.

SIDE EFFECTS

Constipation, febrile neutropenia, fever, headache, hypokalemia, nausea, peripheral edema, rash, and tremor are most common. Cytokine release syndrome, neurologic toxicities, infections, tumor lysis syndrome, elevated liver enzymes, febrile neutropenia, and leukencephalopathy are the most serious side effects. Other reported side effects include abdominal pain, anemia, arthralgia, back pain, bone pain, chest pain, chills, cough, decreased appetite, diarrhea, dizziness, dyspnea, fatigue, hyperglycemia, hypertension, hypomagnesemia, hypophosphatemia, hypotension, insomnia, neutropenia, pain in an extremity, thrombocytopenia, vomiting, and weight increase. Many other side effects occurred in lesser percentages of patients.

ANTIDOTE

Notify physician of all side effects. Minor side effects may be treated symptomatically. Supportive therapy as indicated will help sustain the patient in toxicity. Interrupt the infusion and/or discontinue blinatumomab for cytokine release syndrome, neurologic toxicities, and/or tumor lysis syndrome; see Dose Adjustments. Interrupt the infusion for CRS, neurologic toxicities, TLS, prolonged neutropenia, transaminases greater than 5 times the ULN, a bilirubin more than 3 times the ULN, or other clinically relevant adverse reactions. Discontinue blinatumomab as outlined in Dose Adjustments. In the event of overdose, interrupt the infusion, monitor the patient for signs of toxicity, and provide supportive care. Consider re-initiation of blinatumomab at the correct therapeutic dose when all toxicities have resolved and no earlier than 12 hours after interruption of the infusion. Treat an infusion reaction as indicated. Treat a hypersensitivity reaction immediately with oxygen, epinephrine (Adrenalin), antihistamines (e.g., diphenhydramine [Benadryl]), vasopressors (e.g., dopamine), corticosteroids, albuterol, IV fluids, and ventilation equipment as indicated. Resuscitate as necessary.

BORTEZOMIB

Antineoplastic

(bore-**TEH**-zo-mib)

Velcade

pH 2 to 6.5

USUAL DOSE

See Dose Adjustments for recommended starting dose modifications for patients with moderate to severe hepatic impairment.

Previously untreated multiple myeloma: 1.3 mg/M^2/dose as an IV bolus. Given in combination with oral melphalan (Alkeran) and oral prednisone for nine 6-week cycles as outlined in the following chart. For Cycles 1 to 4, administer twice weekly (Days 1, 4, 8, 11, 22, 25, 29, 32). For Cycles 5 to 9, administer once weekly (Days 1, 8, 22, 29). At least 72 hours should elapse between consecutive doses of bortezomib.

Dosage Regimen for Patients with Previously Untreated Multiple Myeloma Twice-Weekly Bortezomib (Cycles 1-4 When Used in Combination with Melphalan and Prednisone)											
Week	1				2	3		4		5		6
Bortezomib (1.3 mg/M^2)	Day 1	—	—	Day 4	Day 8	Day 11	Rest period	Day 22	Day 25	Day 29	Day 32	Rest period
Melphalan (9 mg/M^2) Prednisone (60 mg/M^2)	Day 1	Day 2	Day 3	Day 4	—	—	Rest period	—	—	—	—	Rest period

Once-Weekly Bortezomib (Cycles 5-9 When Used in Combination with Melphalan and Prednisone)											
Week	1				2	3		4		5		6
Bortezomib (1.3 mg/M^2)	Day 1	—	—	—	Day 8	—	Rest period	Day 22	—	Day 29	—	Rest period
Melphalan (9 mg/M^2) Prednisone (60 mg/M^2)	Day 1	Day 2	Day 3	Day 4	—	—	Rest period	—	—	—	—	Rest period

Previously untreated mantle cell lymphoma: 1.3 mg/M^2/dose as an IV bolus. Given in combination with intravenous rituximab, cyclophosphamide, doxorubicin, and oral prednisone (VcR-CAP) for six 3-week cycles as outlined in the following chart. Bortezomib is administered first, followed by rituximab. Bortezomib is administered twice weekly for 2 weeks (Days 1, 4, 8, 11), followed by a 10-day rest period on Days 12 to 21. For patients with a response first documented at Cycle 6, two additional VcR-CAP cycles are recommended. At least 72 hours should elapse between consecutive doses of bortezomib.

Dosage Regimen for Patients with Previously Untreated Mantle Cell Lymphoma							
Twice Weekly Bortezomib (Six 3-week Cycles)*							
Week	1					2		3
Bortezomib (1.3 mg/M^2)	Day 1	—	—	Day 4	—	Day 8	Day 11	Rest period
Rituximab (375 mg/M^2) Cyclophosphamide (750 mg/M^2) Doxorubicin (50 mg/M^2)	Day 1	—	—	—	—	—	—	Rest period
Prednisone (100 mg/M^2)	Day 1	Day 2	Day 3	Day 4	Day 5	—	—	Rest period

*Dosing may continue for 2 more cycles (for a total of 8 cycles) if response is first seen at Cycle 6.

Relapsed multiple myeloma and relapsed mantle cell lymphoma: 1.3 mg/M²/dose as an IV bolus 2 times a week for 2 weeks (Days 1, 4, 8, and 11). Follow with a 10-day rest period (Days 12 through 21). At least 72 hours should elapse between doses of bortezomib (e.g., Days 1, 4, 8, and 11). A treatment cycle is 21 days. See Dose Adjustments. For extended therapy of more than 8 cycles, bortezomib may be administered on the above standard schedule or, for relapsed multiple myeloma, on a maintenance schedule of once weekly for 4 weeks (Days 1, 8, 15, and 22), followed by a 13-day rest period (Days 23 to 35).

Patients with multiple myeloma who have previously responded to treatment with bortezomib (either alone or in combination) and who have relapsed at least 6 months after their prior therapy may be started on bortezomib at the last tolerated dose. Retreated patients are administered bortezomib twice weekly (Days 1, 4, 8, and 11) every 3 weeks for a maximum of 8 cycles. At least 72 hours should elapse between consecutive doses of bortezomib. Bortezomib may be administered either alone or in combination with dexamethasone.

Combination therapy in multiple myeloma (unlabeled in bortezomib prescribing information):
Bortezomib: Administer 1.3 mg/M² as an IV bolus on Days 1, 4, 8, and 11 every 3 weeks. **Doxil:** Administer 30 mg/M² on Day 4 following bortezomib. Continue for up to 8 cycles until disease progression or the occurrence of unacceptable toxicity.

DOSE ADJUSTMENTS
Dose adjustments are based on clinical toxicities. ▪ Dose adjustments are not required for patients with renal insufficiency, including those requiring dialysis. Bortezomib may be partially removed by dialysis. Administer after dialysis. ▪ Dose adjustments based on age, gender, or race have not been evaluated; see Precautions. ▪ See the following charts for recommended starting dose modifications for patients with moderate to severe hepatic impairment; dose adjustments in combination therapy with melphalan and prednisone; dose adjustments in combination therapy with rituximab, cyclophosphamide, doxorubicin, and prednisone; and bortezomib-related neuropathic pain and/or peripheral sensory or motor neuropathy in relapsed multiple myeloma and mantle cell lymphoma.

Recommended Starting Dose Modification for Bortezomib in Patients with Hepatic Impairment			
	Bilirubin Level	SGOT (AST) Levels	Modification of Starting Dose
Mild	≤1 × ULN	>ULN	None
Mild	>1 to 1.5 × ULN	Any	None
Moderate	>1.5 to 3 × ULN	Any	Reduce bortezomib to 0.7 mg/M² in the first cycle. Consider dose escalation to 1 mg/M² or further dose reduction to 0.5 mg/M² in subsequent cycles based on patient tolerance.
Severe	>3 × ULN	Any	

Combination therapy with melphalan and prednisone in previously untreated multiple myeloma: Before each treatment cycle, platelet count should be equal to or greater than 70 × 10⁹/L, and ANC should be equal to or greater than 1 × 10⁹/L. Nonhematologic toxicities should have resolved to Grade 1 or baseline. Dose modifications for subsequent cycles are outlined in the following chart.

Continued

| Dose Modifications During Cycles of Combination Bortezomib, Melphalan, and Prednisone Therapy* ||
Toxicity	Dose Modification or Delay
Hematologic toxicity during a cycle: If prolonged Grade 4 neutropenia or thrombocytopenia, or thrombocytopenia with bleeding, is observed in the previous cycle	Consider reducing the melphalan dose by 25% in the next cycle.
If platelet count is ≤30 × 10⁹/L or ANC is ≤0.75 × 10⁹/L on a bortezomib-dosing day (other than Day 1)	Withhold bortezomib dose.
If several bortezomib doses in consecutive cycles are withheld due to toxicity	Reduce bortezomib dose by 1 dose level (from 1.3 mg/M^2 to 1 mg/M^2, or from 1 mg/M^2 to 0.7 mg/M^2).
Grade ≥3 nonhematologic toxicities	Withhold bortezomib therapy until symptoms of the toxicity have resolved to Grade 1 or baseline. Bortezomib may then be reinitiated with 1 dose-level reduction (from 1.3 mg/M^2 to 1 mg/M^2, or from 1 mg/M^2 to 0.7 mg/M^2). For bortezomib-related neuropathic pain and/or peripheral neuropathy, hold or modify bortezomib as outlined in the chart for dose modification for bortezomib-related neuropathic pain and/or peripheral neuropathy.

*Graded according to Common Terminology Criteria for Adverse Events (CTCAE).

Combination therapy with IV rituximab, cyclophosphamide, doxorubicin, and oral prednisone in previously untreated mantle cell lymphoma: Before the first day of each cycle (other than Cycle 1), platelet count should be equal to or greater than $100 × 10^9$/L, and ANC should be equal to or greater than $1.5 × 10^9$/L. Hemoglobin should be equal to or greater than 8 g/dL, and nonhematologic toxicities should have resolved to Grade 1 or baseline. Dose modifications for Days 4, 8, and 11 are outlined in the following chart.

| Dose Modifications on Days 4, 8, and 11 During Cycles of Combination Bortezomib, Rituximab, Cyclophosphamide, Doxorubicin, and Prednisone Therapy ||
Toxicity	Dose Modification or Delay
Hematologic Toxicity	
Grade 3 or higher neutropenia or a platelet count below 25 × 10⁹/L	Withhold bortezomib therapy for up to 2 weeks until the patient has an ANC at or above 0.75 × 10⁹/L and a platelet count at or above 25 × 10⁹/L. • If the toxicity does not resolve after bortezomib has been withheld, discontinue bortezomib. • If toxicity resolves such that the patient has an ANC at or above 0.75 × 10⁹/L and a platelet count at or above 25 × 10⁹/L, bortezomib dose should be reduced by 1 dose level (from 1.3 mg/M^2 to 1 mg/M^2, or from 1 mg/M^2 to 0.7 mg/M^2).
Grade 3 or higher nonhematologic toxicities	Withhold bortezomib therapy until symptoms of the toxicity have resolved to Grade 2 or better. Bortezomib may then be re-initiated with 1 dose-level reduction (from 1.3 mg/M^2 to 1 mg/M^2, or from 1 mg/M^2 to 0.7 mg/M^2). For bortezomib-related neuropathic pain and/or peripheral neuropathy, hold or modify bortezomib as outlined in the chart for dose modification for bortezomib-related neuropathic pain and/or peripheral neuropathy.

For information concerning rituximab, cyclophosphamide, doxorubicin, and prednisone, see manufacturer's prescribing information.

Relapsed multiple myeloma and relapsed mantle cell lymphoma: Withhold dose if a Grade 3 nonhematologic toxicity (e.g., 6 to 10 emeses/24 hr, severe infection) or a Grade 4 hematologic toxicity (e.g., thrombocytopenia less than 25,000/mm^3) occurs. When symptoms have resolved, resume treatment with a dose reduced by 25% (1.3 mg/M^2/dose reduced to 1 mg/M^2/dose, 1 mg/M^2/dose reduced to 0.7 mg/M^2/dose). ▪ See doxorubicin monograph for additional dose adjustments required in Doxil and bortezomib combination therapy for treatment of multiple myeloma. ▪ Reduce dose in patients who develop bortezomib-related neuropathic pain and/or peripheral sensory or motor neuropathy according to the following chart.

Recommended Dose Modification for Bortezomib-Related Neuropathic Pain and/or Peripheral Sensory or Motor Neuropathy*	
Severity of Peripheral Neuropathy Signs and Symptoms	Modification of Dose and Regimen
Grade 1 (asymptomatic; loss of deep tendon reflexes or paresthesias) without pain or loss of function	No action.
Grade 1 with pain or Grade 2 (moderate symptoms; limiting instrumental Activities of Daily Living [ADL])†	Reduce dose to 1 mg/M^2.
Grade 2 with pain or Grade 3 (severe symptoms; limiting self-care ADL‡)	Withhold therapy until toxicity resolves. When toxicity resolves, re-initiate with a reduced dose of 0.7 mg/M^2 and change treatment schedule to once per week.
Grade 4 (life-threatening consequences; urgent intervention indicated)	Discontinue bortezomib.

*Graded according to Common Terminology Criteria for Adverse Events (CTCAE).
†Instrumental ADL (e.g., preparing meals, shopping for groceries or clothes, using telephone, managing money).
‡Self-care ADL (e.g., bathing, dressing and undressing, feeding self, using the toilet, taking medications, and not bedridden).

DILUTION
Specific techniques required; see Precautions. Reconstitute each 3.5-mg vial **only with 3.5 mL NS.** Concentration equals 1 mg/mL. *The SC route uses less diluent and results in a different concentration (2.5 mg/mL).* To prevent overdosage, use caution when diluting and calculating volume to administer. Manufacturer supplies a sticker that specifies indicated route of administration. Place sticker on syringe of prepared bortezomib.
Storage: Stable until expiration date when stored at CRT in original package and protected from light. Reconstituted solution stable at 25° C (77° F) for up to 8 hours in a syringe or in original vial when exposed to normal indoor lighting. Must be given within 8 hours.

COMPATIBILITY
Specific information not available. Consider specific use; consult pharmacist.

RATE OF ADMINISTRATION
A single dose as an IV bolus injection over 3 to 5 seconds. May be given into a peripheral vein. To ensure the full dose is administered, flush with NS after injection.

May also be given through an IV port if the primary IV is temporarily discontinued. Flush with NS before and after administration.

ACTIONS
A reversible inhibitor of the 26S proteasome, which is a large protein complex that degrades ubiquitinated proteins. The blocking of this proteasome disrupts numerous biologic pathways related to the growth and survival of cancer cells and can lead to cell death. Distributes widely to peripheral tissues. Over 80% is bound to plasma proteins.

Mean elimination half-life after multiple doses ranges from 76 to 108 hours after the 1.3 mg/M^2 dose. Metabolized in the liver via selected cytochrome P$_{450}$ enzymes. Pathways of elimination in humans have not been determined.

INDICATIONS

Treatment of patients with multiple myeloma. ▪ Treatment of patients with mantle cell lymphoma.

Unlabeled use: Treatment of multiple myeloma in combination with doxorubicin liposomal injection (Doxil) in patients who have received one prior therapy but have not previously received bortezomib. (Indication in Doxil prescribing information.)

CONTRAINDICATIONS

Hypersensitivity to bortezomib, boron, or mannitol (not including local reactions); intrathecal administration.

PRECAUTIONS

Follow guidelines for handling cytotoxic agents. See Appendix A, p. 1331. ▪ For IV or SC use only. ▪ Administered by or under the supervision of a physician experienced in the use of antineoplastic therapy in a facility equipped to monitor the patient and respond to any medical emergency. ▪ Bortezomib therapy causes peripheral neuropathy. Both sensory and motor peripheral neuropathy have been reported. Use caution in patients with pre-existing peripheral neuropathy; symptoms may worsen. Many have been treated previously with neurotoxic agents. Incidence of peripheral neuropathy may be less with SC administration. Use of the SC route may be considered for patients who have pre-existing or are at high risk for peripheral neuropathy. ▪ May cause orthostatic/postural hypotension. Use with caution in patients with a history of syncope, in patients receiving concomitant medications that may cause hypotension, and in patients who are dehydrated. ▪ Hypersensitivity reactions (including anaphylactic reactions) have been reported. ▪ Thrombocytopenia and neutropenia have been reported; see Monitor. ▪ Gastrointestinal and intracerebral hemorrhages have occurred during thrombocytopenia in association with bortezomib. ▪ Acute development or exacerbation of CHF and/or new onset of decreased left ventricular ejection fraction has been reported. ▪ Acute diffuse infiltrative pulmonary disorders of unknown etiology such as pneumonitis, interstitial pneumonia, lung infiltration, and acute respiratory distress syndrome (ARDS) have occurred. ▪ Pulmonary hypertension in the absence of left heart failure or significant pulmonary disease has been reported. ▪ Posterior reversible encephalopathy syndrome (PRES), formerly termed reversible posterior leukoencephalopathy syndrome (RPLS), has occurred. Patients may present with blindness, confusion, headache, hypertension, lethargy, seizure, or other visual or neurologic disturbances. MRI may be used to confirm diagnosis. ▪ Use caution in patients with moderate to severe liver impairment. Clearance decreased; see Monitor and Dose Adjustments. Use caution in patients who are receiving multiple concomitant medications and/or who have serious underlying medical conditions; asymptomatic increases in liver enzymes, hyperbilirubinemia, hepatitis, and rare cases of acute liver failure have been reported. May be reversible if bortezomib is discontinued. Information on rechallenging these patients is limited. ▪ Tumor lysis syndrome has been reported; patients with a high tumor burden are at increased risk. ▪ GI adverse events, including constipation, diarrhea, ileus, nausea, and vomiting, have been reported and may require treatment. ▪ Consider antiviral prophylaxis. Herpes simplex and herpes zoster reactivation have been reported.

Monitor: Obtain baseline CBC with differential and platelet count; repeat before each cycle and monitor as needed during treatment. Monitor platelet count before each dose. ▪ Obtain baseline electrolytes, including serum calcium and potassium and serum and urine M-protein. Monitor fluid and electrolyte balance and replace as indicated. Prevent dehydration. ▪ Obtain baseline bilirubin and AST and repeat as indicated; see Dose Adjustments. Monitor patients with impaired liver function closely for S/S of bortezomib toxicity. ▪ Monitor BP closely. Dehydration and/or concomitant medications may cause hypotension. Assist with ambulation. ▪ Monitor patients at risk for or with existing heart disease closely for S/S of CHF (e.g., exertional dyspnea, orthopnea, edema, tachycardia, pulmonary rales, a third heart sound, jugular venous distention) and/or for new onset of decreased left ventricular ejection fraction. ▪ Confirm patency of vein; however, tissue damage did not occur with extravasation during clinical studies. ▪ Use prophylactic antiemetics to reduce nausea and vomiting and increase patient comfort. ▪ Antidiarrheal medication (e.g., loperamide [Imodium]) may be indicated. ▪ Monitor for S/S of peripheral neuropathy (e.g., hyperesthesia [sensitivity of skin], hypoesthesia [impairment of any sense, especially touch], neuropathic pain or weakness, paresthesia [abnormal sensation such as burning, prickling]). Incidence may be increased in patients treated previously with neurotoxic agents (e.g., cisplatin, thalidomide [Thalomid], vinca alkaloids [e.g., vincristine]). See Dose Adjustments; may require change of dose or schedule. Improvement in or a resolution of peripheral neuropathy has been reported following dose adjustment or discontinuation of bortezomib. ▪ Monitor for neutropenia and thrombocytopenia (platelet count less than $50,000/mm^3$). Occurs in a cyclical pattern with nadirs occurring after the last dose of each cycle and typically recovering before initiation of the next cycle. Initiate precautions to prevent excessive bleeding (e.g., inspect IV sites, skin, and mucous membranes; use extreme care during invasive procedures; test urine, emesis, stool, and secretions for occult blood). ▪ Monitor uric acid levels before and during therapy. Allopurinol and/or alkalinization of the urine may be indicated for serious tumor lysis syndrome. ▪ Hypoglycemia and hyperglycemia have been reported in patients taking oral diabetic agents. Monitor blood glucose levels and adjust antidiabetic medications as indicated; see Drug/Lab Interactions. ▪ Monitor respiratory status closely. Any change in condition should be evaluated promptly and treated as indicated. ▪ Monitor for S/S associated with development of PRES (e.g., blindness, confusion, headache, hypertension, lethargy, seizures, and other visual and neurologic disturbances).

Patient Education: Avoid pregnancy; use effective contraceptive measures. Should pregnancy occur, notify physician immediately and discuss potential hazards. ▪ May cause dizziness, fatigue, hypotension, or syncope; use caution when driving or operating machinery. ▪ Review all medications with your physician and/or pharmacist; effects of medications for high blood pressure and other medications that may lower blood pressure may increase hypotension. Other agents may increase peripheral neuropathy. May interfere with medications for diabetes. ▪ Review of monitoring requirements and adverse events before therapy is imperative. ▪ Avoid dehydration; promptly report diarrhea, dizziness, fainting spells, light-headedness, and vomiting. ▪ Promptly report any signs of infection (e.g., chills, fever, night sweats) or signs of bleeding (e.g., bruising, tarry stools, blood in urine, pinpoint red spots on skin). ▪ Promptly report symptoms of peripheral neuropathy (e.g., burning sensation, skin sensitivity, impairment of any sense [especially touch]). If these symptoms pre-existed, report if they seem to be worse. ▪ Promptly report shortness of breath or swelling of the ankles, feet, or legs. ▪ Report any visual or neurologic disturbances. ▪ See Appendix D, p. 1333.

Maternal/Child: Category D: avoid pregnancy; may cause fetal harm. Use of effective contraception required. ▪ Discontinue breast-feeding. ▪ Safety and effectiveness for use in pediatric patients not established.

Elderly: Safety and effectiveness similar to other age-groups; however, greater sensitivity in the elderly cannot be ruled out. In clinical trials, patients over 65 years of age had a slightly increased incidence of Grade 3 or 4 toxicity.

DRUG/LAB INTERACTIONS

Drug interaction studies are limited. ▪ Coadministration with **prednisone and melphalan** (Alkeran) increases bortezomib exposure. Increase is unlikely to be significant. ▪ Has been administered with **omeprazole** (Prilosec) without effect. ▪ Coadministration of **dexamethasone** has no effect on bortezomib levels. ▪ Bortezomib is a substrate of CYP3A4, 2C19, and 1A2; concomitant administration of **inhibitors or inducers of selected cytochrome P$_{450}$ enzymes** may cause toxicity or reduce effectiveness of bortezomib. Consult pharmacist. **Inhibitors** may reduce metabolism and increase serum levels of bortezomib. ▪ Coadministration with **ketoconazole** (Nizoral), an inhibitor, increases bortezomib exposure. Monitor for toxicity. Other examples of **inhibitors** may include cimetidine (Tagamet), erythromycins, grapefruit juice, antifungal agents (e.g., itraconazole [Sporanox]), nefazodone, ritonavir (Norvir), verapamil. Patients receiving bortezomib in conjunction with a strong CYP3A4 inhibitor should be closely monitored. ▪ **Inducers** may increase metabolism and decrease serum levels and effectiveness of bortezomib. Examples of **inducers** may include carbamazepine (Tegretol), phenobarbital (Luminal), phenytoin (Dilantin), rifampin (Rifadin). Concomitant use of **strong CYP3A4 inducers** (e.g., rifampin [Rifadin]) is not recommended. ▪ **St. John's wort** may decrease levels of bortezomib unpredictably. Concurrent use should be avoided. ▪ Hypotension may be increased by **agents that induce hypotension** (e.g., alcohol, antihypertensives [e.g., ACE inhibitors (e.g., lisinopril)], beta-blockers [e.g., atenolol (Tenormin)], opioid narcotics, sildenafil [Viagra], tricyclic antidepressants [e.g., amitryptyline (Elavil), imipramine (Tofranil)]). ▪ Peripheral neuropathy may be increased by numerous agents. Some examples are **acyclovir** (Zovirax), **amiodarone** (Nexterone), **antineoplastics** (e.g., cisplatin, **vinca alkaloids** [e.g., vincristine]), **foscarnet** (Foscavir), **isoniazid** (INH), **nitrofurantoin** (Furadantin), **thalidomide** (Thalomid), **statins** (e.g., lovastatin [Mevacor], simvastatin [Zocor]). ▪ May increase or decrease the effects of **oral antidiabetic agents** (e.g., glyburide [DiaBeta], glipizide [Glucotrol]). Monitor blood glucose levels and adjust dose of antidiabetic medication as indicated.

SIDE EFFECTS

Diarrhea, fatigue, peripheral neuropathy, excessive vomiting, and thrombocytopenia may be dose limiting. Most common side effects reported include anemia, anorexia, constipation, diarrhea, fatigue, fever, leukopenia, lymphopenia, nausea and vomiting, neuralgia, neutropenia, peripheral neuropathy, rash, and thrombocytopenia. Abdominal pain, arthralgia, asthenia, bronchitis, cardiac failure, chills, cough, dehydration, dizziness, dysesthesia, edema, headache, hypertension, hypotension, malaise, nasopharyngitis, paresthesia, peripheral edema, pneumonia, psychotic disorders (e.g., anxiety, agitation, confusion, insomnia, mental status change, suicidal ideation), reactivation of herpesvirus infections (zoster and simplex), respiratory tract infections, upper abdominal pain, weakness, and weight loss have also been reported. Numerous other side effects have been reported that may or may not be related to bortezomib and may include hypersensitivity reactions (including anaphylaxis and immune complex–mediated hypersensitivity), ARDS and other pulmonary disorders, bleeding (e.g., GI, intracerebral), CVA, GI disorders (serious [e.g., acute pancreatitis, ischemic colitis, paralytic ileus]), hepatic disorders (e.g., cholestasis, liver failure, portal vein thrombosis), hyperbilirubinemia, hypernatremia, hyperuricemia, hypocalcemia, hypokalemia, hyponatremia, infections (e.g., aspergillosis, bacteremia, herpes, listeriosis, oral candidiasis, septic shock, toxoplasmosis, URI), MI, pleural effusion, PRES, pulmonary embolism, pulmonary hypertension, renal disorders (e.g., acute or chronic renal failure, calculus, hemorrhagic cystitis, hydronephrosis), respiratory distress, and tumor lysis syndrome.

Post-Marketing: Acute diffuse infiltrative pulmonary disease, acute febrile neutrophilic dermatosis (Sweet's syndrome), acute pancreatitis, blindness, cardiac arrhythmias (including complete AV block), cardiac tamponade, deafness (bilateral), DIC, dysautonomia, encephalopathy, hepatitis, herpes meningoencephalitis, ischemic colitis, ophthalmic herpes, optic neuropathy, progressive multifocal leukoencephalopathy (PML), and toxic epidermal necrolysis. 2% of patients died. Cause of death may have been related to bortezomib and included cardiac arrest, CHF, pneumonia, renal failure, respiratory failure, and sepsis.

Overdose: Profound progressive hypotension, tachycardia, and decreased cardiac contractility. Symptomatic hypotension and thrombocytopenia with fatal outcomes have been reported in patients who received more than twice the recommended dose.

ANTIDOTE

Keep physician informed of all side effects. Most will be treated symptomatically as indicated. Temporarily discontinue bortezomib if Grade 4 thrombocytopenia occurs (less than 25,000/mm^3); may be resumed at a reduced dose after thrombocytopenia is resolved. Severe thrombocytopenia may require platelet transfusions. Reduce dose, withhold dose, or discontinue based on S/S of peripheral neuropathy. Symptoms of peripheral neuropathy may improve or return to baseline if bortezomib is discontinued. Hypotension may respond to adjustment of antihypertensive medications, hydration, or administration of mineralocorticoids. Recovery from neutropenia may be spontaneous or may be treated with filgrastim (Neupogen, Zarxio) or pegfilgrastim (Neulasta). Treat anemia as indicated with whole blood products (e.g., packed RBCs) or blood modifiers (e.g., darbepoetin alfa [Aranesp], epoetin alfa [Epogen]). For new or worsening cardiopulmonary symptoms, consider interrupting bortezomib until a prompt and comprehensive diagnostic evaluation is conducted. For symptoms of serious liver dysfunction, interrupt bortezomib to assess reversibility. Discontinue bortezomib in patients who develop PRES. In overdose, monitor V/S continuously and provide supportive care. Maintain BP with dopamine, epinephrine, or norepinephrine (Levophed) as needed. Maintain body temperature. There is no specific antidote; supportive therapy will help sustain the patient in toxicity. Resuscitate as indicated.

BRENTUXIMAB VEDOTIN BBW

(bren-**TUX**-i-mab ve-**DOE**-tin)

Antineoplastic
(monoclonal antibody)

Adcetris

pH 6.6

USUAL DOSE

1.8 mg/kg as an IV infusion over 30 minutes every 3 weeks. For patients weighing more than 100 kg, base calculated dose on a weight of 100 kg (i.e., dose should not exceed 180 mg). Continue treatment until disease progression or unacceptable toxicity. For classical Hodgkin lymphoma (HL) post–autologous hematopoietic stem cell transplantation (post–auto-HSCT) consolidation treatment, initiate brentuximab treatment within 4 to 6 weeks post–auto-HSCT or upon recovery from auto-HSCT. Continue treatment until a maximum of 16 cycles, disease progression, or unacceptable toxicity.

DOSE ADJUSTMENTS

Dose Modification of Brentuximab in Renal Impairment	
Mild (CrCl >50-80 mL/min) or Moderate (CrCl 30-50 mL/min)	1.8 mg/kg up to 180 mg.
Severe (CrCl <30 mL/min)	Avoid use (see Precautions).

Dose Modification of Brentuximab in Hepatic Impairment	
Mild (Child-Pugh A)	1.2 mg/kg up to 120 mg.
Moderate (Child-Pugh B) or Severe (Child-Pugh C)	Avoid use (see Precautions).

Dose Modification of Brentuximab in Peripheral Neuropathy	
New or worsening Grade 2 or 3 neuropathy	Hold dosing until neuropathy improves to Grade 1 or baseline; then restart at 1.2 mg/kg.
Grade 4 peripheral neuropathy	Discontinue brentuximab.

Dose Modification of Brentuximab with Neutropenia	
Grade 3 or 4 neutropenia	Hold dosing until neutropenia resolves to baseline or Grade 2 or lower. Consider G-CSF prophylaxis (e.g., filgrastim [Neupogen]) for subsequent cycles in patients who experience Grade 3 or 4 neutropenia.
Recurrent Grade 4 neutropenia despite the use of G-CSF prophylaxis	Consider discontinuation or dose reduction of brentuximab to 1.2 mg/kg.

DILUTION

Specific techniques required; see Precautions. Each vial contains 50 mg of brentuximab. Calculate the number of vials required. For example, in a 70-kg patient:

1. 1.8 mg/kg × 70 kg =126 mg
2. 126 mg ÷ 50 mg/vial = 2.5+ vials; so 3 vials would be needed

Reconstitute each vial with 10.5 mL of SWFI to yield 5 mg/mL. Direct the stream of diluent toward the side of the vial. Gently swirl to aid dissolution. *Do not shake.* Solution should be clear to slightly opalescent and colorless. Withdraw the calculated dose from the vials (126 mg [from the previous example] ÷ 5 mg/mL = 25.2 mL). This calculated dose must be further diluted in a minimum of 100 mL of NS, D5W, or LR to achieve a final concentration of 0.4 to 1.8 mg/mL. Gently invert to mix the solution.

Filters: No specific recommendations stated.

Storage: Refrigerate vials in carton at 2° to 8° C (36° to 46° F) to protect from light. Immediate further dilution of reconstituted vials is preferred; however, they may be refrigerated for up to 24 hours. Do not freeze. Immediate use of fully diluted solution is preferred; however, it may be refrigerated but must be used within 24 hours of reconstitution. Do not freeze.

COMPATIBILITY

Manufacturer states, "Do not mix with, or administer as an infusion with, other medicinal products."

RATE OF ADMINISTRATION

A single dose as an IV infusion equally distributed over 30 minutes.

ACTIONS

A CD30-directed antibody-drug conjugate (ADC). Produced by recombinant DNA technology with three components: (1) the chimeric IgG1 antibody cAC10, specific for human CD30; (2) the microtubule-disrupting agent MMAE; and (3) a protease-cleavable linker that covalently attaches MMAE to cAC10. Anticancer activity is thought to result from the binding of the ADC to CD30-expressing cells, followed by internalization of the ADC-CD30 complex and the release of MMAE via proteolytic cleavage. Binding of MMAE to tubulin disrupts the microtubule network within the cell, inducing cell-cycle arrest and apoptotic death of the cells. Terminal half-life is approximately 4 to 6 days. Minimal to no accumulation noted with every-3-week dosing. Minimal metabolism of MMAE occurs via oxidation by CYP3A4/5. Moderate amounts excreted as mostly unchanged MMAE in feces and urine.

INDICATIONS AND USES

Treatment of patients with classical Hodgkin lymphoma (HL) after failure of autologous hematopoietic stem cell transplantation (auto-HSCT) or after failure of at least two prior multiagent chemotherapy regimens in patients who are not auto-HSCT candidates. ▪ Treatment of patients with classical HL who are at high risk for relapse or progression as post–auto-HSCT consolidation. ▪ Treatment of patients with systemic anaplastic large cell lymphoma (sALCL) after failure of at least one prior multiagent chemotherapy regimen. This indication is based on response rates. No data demonstrating improvement in patient outcomes or survival has been demonstrated.

CONTRAINDICATIONS

Concomitant use with bleomycin due to pulmonary toxicity; see Drug/Lab Interactions.

PRECAUTIONS

Follow guidelines for handling cytotoxic agents. See Appendix A, p. 1331. ▪ For IV infusion only; do not administer as an IV push or bolus. ▪ Usually administered in a setting with adequate diagnostic and treatment facilities to monitor the patient and respond to any medical emergency. ▪ JC virus infection resulting in progressive multifocal leukoencephalopathy (PML) and death can occur. ▪ Causes a peripheral neuropathy that is predominantly sensory and cumulative. Peripheral motor neuropathy has also been reported. ▪ Infusion-related reactions, including anaphylaxis, have occurred; see Monitor and Antidote. ▪ Prolonged (1 week or longer) severe neutropenia, febrile neutropenia, and Grade 3 or Grade 4 thrombocytopenia or anemia can occur. G-CSF prophylaxis may be indicated; see Dose Adjustments. ▪ Serious infections and opportunistic infections (e.g., bacteremia, pneumonia, sepsis/septic shock) have been reported. ▪ Risk of tumor lysis syndrome is increased in patients with rapidly proliferating tumor and high tumor burden. ▪ Frequency of Grade 3 or higher adverse reactions and deaths was greater in patients with severe renal impairment compared with patients with normal renal function; see Dose Adjustments. ▪ Frequency of Grade 3 or higher adverse reactions and deaths was greater in patients with moderate and severe hepatic impairment compared with patients with normal hepatic function; see Dose Adjustments. ▪ Serious cases of hepatotoxicity, including fatal outcomes, have been reported. May occur after the first dose or after rechallenge. Pre-existing liver disease, elevated baseline liver enzymes, and concomitant medications may increase the risk of hepatotoxicity. ▪ Noninfectious pulmonary toxicity (including acute respiratory distress syndrome [ARDS], interstitial lung disease, and pneumonitis), some with a fatal outcome, have been reported. ▪ Stevens-Johnson syndrome (SJS) and toxic epidermal necrolysis (TEN), including fatal outcomes, have been reported. ▪ Patients who develop persistently positive antibodies demonstrated a higher incidence of infusion-related reactions. ▪ Patients enrolled in the clinical trials for classical HL post–auto-HSCT consolidation received standard infection prophylaxis for herpes simplex virus (HSV), varicella-zoster virus (VZV), and *Pneumocystis jiroveci* pneumonia (PCP) after auto-HSCT. ▪ Influence of renal or hepatic impairment on the pharmacokinetics of brentuximab is not known.

Monitor: Obtain baseline CBC and monitor before each dose. Consider more frequent monitoring for patients with Grade 3 or 4 neutropenia. Dose delay, reduction, or discontinuation of therapy may be required; see Dose Adjustments. ▪ Obtain baseline and periodic SCr, liver enzymes, and bilirubin. ▪ Monitor for S/S of neuropathy (e.g., a burning sensation, discomfort, hyperesthesia, hypoesthesia, neuropathic pain, paresthesia, weakness). New or worsening neuropathy may require a delay of therapy, change in dose, or discontinuation of therapy; see Dose Adjustments. ▪ Monitor closely during infusion for S/S of hypersensitivity or infusion reactions (e.g., back pain, chills, cough, dyspnea, fever, headache, nausea, pruritus, rash, vomiting). Patients who have experienced a prior infusion-related reaction should be premedicated for subsequent infusions; may include acetaminophen, an antihistamine, and a corticosteroid. Immediately and permanently discontinue brentuximab if anaphylaxis occurs. ▪ Monitor for S/S of bacterial, fungal, or viral infections. Prophylactic antibiotics may be indicated pending results of C/S in a febrile neutropenic patient. ▪ Monitor for early signs of tumor lysis syndrome (e.g., flank pain and hematuria); monitoring of uric acid levels may be required; maintain hydration. Allopurinol and/or alkalinization of urine may be indicated. ▪ Monitor for S/S of PML (e.g., changes in mood or unusual behavior; confusion; thinking problems; loss of memory; changes in vision, speech, or walking; and decreased strength or weakness on one side of the body); see Antidote. ▪ Monitor for S/S of pulmonary toxicity, including cough and dyspnea. ▪ Monitor for serious dermatologic reactions. ▪ Monitor for thrombocytopenia (platelet count less than 50,000/mm^3). Initiate precautions to prevent excessive bleeding (e.g., inspect IV sites, skin, and mucous membranes; use extreme care during invasive procedures; test urine, emesis, stool, and secretions for occult blood).

Patient Education: Avoid pregnancy. Use effective birth control. Report a suspected pregnancy immediately. ▪ Promptly report S/S of infection (e.g., chills, cough, fever of 100.5° F or greater, pain with urination). ▪ Promptly report S/S of peripheral neuropathy (e.g., muscle weakness, numbness or tingling of the hands or feet). ▪ Promptly report S/S of an infusion reaction (e.g., breathing problems, chills, fever, or rash within 24 hours of an infusion). ▪ Promptly report changes in mood or unusual behavior; confusion; thinking problems; loss of memory; changes in vision, speech, or walking; and decreased strength or weakness on one side of the body. ▪ Promptly report symptoms of pancreatitis or hepatotoxicity (abdominal pain, anorexia, dark urine, fatigue, jaundice). ▪ Report symptoms of pulmonary toxicity (e.g., cough or shortness of breath). ▪ See Appendix D, p. 1333.

Maternal/Child: Category D: avoid pregnancy; can cause fetal harm. ▪ Discontinue breast-feeding. ▪ Safety and effectiveness for use in pediatric patients not established.

Elderly: Numbers in clinical studies insufficient to determine if elderly patients respond differently than younger subjects. Safety and effectiveness not established.

DRUG/LAB INTERACTIONS
Concomitant use with **bleomycin** is contraindicated; has resulted in an increased risk of pulmonary toxicity compared with other chemotherapy regimens; see Precautions and

Side Effects ▪ In vitro data indicate that monomethyl auristatin E (MMAE) is a substrate and an inhibtor of CYP3A4/5 and a substrate of the efflux transporter P-glycoprotein (P-gp). ▪ Coadministration with **ketoconazole** (Nizoral), a potent CYP3A4 inhibitor, increases exposure to MMAE; monitor patients receiving ketoconazole or other potent **CYP3A4 inhibitors** (e.g., clarithromycin [Biaxin], itraconazole [Sporanox], nefazodone, saquinavir [Invirase]) closely for adverse reactions. ▪ Coadministration with **rifampin** (Rifadin), a potent CYP3A4 inducer, reduces exposure to MMAE, reducing its effectiveness. ▪ Coadministration with **P-gp inhibitors** (e.g., amiodarone [Nexterone], clarithromycin [Biaxin], ritonavir [Norvir], verapamil) may increase exposure to MMAE. Monitor closely for adverse reactions. ▪ MMAE does not inhibit other CYP enzymes at relevant clinical concentrations and is not expected to alter the exposure to drugs that are metabolized by CYP3A4 enzymes, including midazolam (Versed).

SIDE EFFECTS
Anemia, cough, diarrhea, fatigue, fever, nausea, neutropenia, peripheral sensory neuropathy, rash, thrombocytopenia, upper respiratory tract infection, and vomiting are most common. Neutropenia and peripheral neuropathy can be severe and dose-limiting. Other severe side effects include anaphylaxis and infusion reactions, hepatotoxicity, PML, serious dermatologic reactions (e.g., SJS and TEN), serious infections (including opportunistic infections), and tumor lysis syndrome. Abdominal pain, alopecia, anorexia, anxiety, arthralgia, back pain, chills, constipation, dizziness, dry skin, dyspnea, headache, insomnia, lymphadenopathy, muscle spasms, myalgia, night sweats, oropharyngeal pain, peripheral edema, pain (including extremity pain), pruritus, and weight loss have also occurred.

Post-Marketing: Febrile neutropenia, hepatotoxicity, hyperglycemia, noninfectious pulmonary toxicity (including ARDS, interstitial lung disease, and pneumonitis), pancreatitis, PML, serious infections (including opportunistic infections), toxic epidermal necrolysis.

ANTIDOTE
Notify physician of all side effects. Treatment of most reactions will be supportive. No known antidote for overdose. Dose delay, dose modification, or discontinuation of therapy may be required in patients with severe or prolonged neutropenia, peripheral neuropathy, or hepatotoxicity. G-CSF prophylaxis may be considered in patients with Grade 3 or Grade 4 neutropenia. If PML is suspected, hold brentuximab. Confirmation of the diagnosis by consultation with a neurologist, brain imaging, CSF testing for JC viral DNA, and/or brain biopsy is indicated. If PML is confirmed, discontinue brentuximab. In the event of new or worsening pulmonary symptoms, hold therapy until evaluation is complete and symptoms have improved. Discontinue if severe dermatologic reaction occurs and treat as indicated. Interrupt the infusion for an infusion-related reaction and institute approriate medical management. Discontinue the infusion immediately and treat anaphylaxis with oxygen, epinephrine (Adrenalin), antihistamines (e.g., diphenhydramine [Benadryl]), vasopressors (e.g., dopamine), corticosteroids, albuterol, and IV fluids as indicated. Resuscitate as necessary.

BUMETANIDE BBW

(byou-**MET**-ah-nyd)

Diuretic (loop)

pH 6.8 to 7.8

USUAL DOSE

0.5 to 1 mg. May be repeated at 2- to 3-hour intervals. Do not exceed 10 mg/24 hr. Can be used for patients allergic to furosemide. 1:40 mg ratio (bumetanide to furosemide) is used to determine dose. Individualize dose and schedule; see Precautions/Monitor.

DOSE ADJUSTMENTS

Start at lower end of dosing range in the elderly. Consider decreased cardiac, hepatic, or renal function; concomitant disease; and other drug therapy.

DILUTION

May be given undiluted. Not usually added to IV solutions but **compatible** with D5W, NS, and LR. Usually given through Y-tube or three-way stopcock of infusion set. Use only freshly prepared solutions for infusion. Discard after 24 hours.

COMPATIBILITY   (Underline Indicates Conflicting Compatibility Information)

Consider any drug NOT listed as compatible to be INCOMPATIBLE until consulting a pharmacist; specific conditions may apply.

One source suggests the following **compatibilities:**

Additive: Furosemide (Lasix).

Y-site: Allopurinol (Aloprim), amifostine (Ethyol), aztreonam (Azactam), bivalirudin (Angiomax), caspofungin (Cancidas), ceftaroline (Teflaro), cisatracurium (Nimbex), cladribine (Leustatin), dexmedetomidine (Precedex), diltiazem (Cardizem), docetaxel (Taxotere), doripenem (Doribax), etoposide phosphate (Etopophos), filgrastim (Neupogen), gemcitabine (Gemzar), granisetron (Kytril), hetastarch in electrolytes (Hextend), lorazepam (Ativan), melphalan (Alkeran), meperidine (Demerol), micafungin (Mycamine), milrinone (Primacor), morphine, oxaliplatin (Eloxatin), pemetrexed (Alimta), piperacillin/tazobactam (Zosyn), propofol (Diprivan), remifentanil (Ultiva), teniposide (Vumon), thiotepa, vinorelbine (Navelbine).

RATE OF ADMINISTRATION

A single dose by IV injection over 1 to 2 minutes. Give infusion at prescribed rate.

ACTIONS

A sulfonamide diuretic, antihypertensive, and antihypercalcemic agent related to the thiazides. A loop diuretic agent. Extremely potent. Onset of action is within minutes and duration of action may last 4 to 6 hours. Apparently acts on the proximal and distal ends of the tubule and the ascending limb of the loop of Henle to excrete water, sodium, chloride, and potassium. Will produce diuresis in alkalosis or acidosis. Rapidly distributed, it is excreted primarily in the urine.

INDICATIONS AND USES

Edema associated with congestive heart failure, cirrhosis of the liver with ascites, renal diseases including nephrotic syndrome. ▪ Acute pulmonary edema. ▪ Edema unresponsive to other diuretic agents. ▪ Diuresis in patients allergic to furosemide. ▪ Adjunct in combination with other antihypertensive agents in the treatment of hypertensive crisis.

Unlabeled uses: Treatment of hypercalcemia.

CONTRAINDICATIONS

Anuria, known hypersensitivity to bumetanide. Use caution in patients with hepatic coma or in states of severe electrolyte depletion. Do not use until condition is improved or corrected. See Precautions.

PRECAUTIONS

May be used concurrently with aldosterone antagonists (e.g., spironolactone [Aldactone]) for more effective diuresis and to prevent excessive potassium loss. ▪ May increase blood glucose; has precipitated diabetes mellitus. ▪ May lower serum calcium level, causing tetany. ▪ In rare instances may precipitate an acute attack of gout. ▪ Risk of ototoxicity increased with higher doses, rapid injection, decreased renal function, or concurrent use with other ototoxic drugs; see Drug/Lab Interactions. ▪ Patients allergic to sulfonamides may have an allergic reaction to bumetanide. ▪ Excessive doses can lead to profound diuresis with water and electrolyte depletion.

Monitor: Monitor for excessive diuresis with water and electrolyte depletion. Routine checks on electrolyte panel, CO_2, serum glucose, uric acid, and BUN are necessary during therapy. Potassium chloride replacement may be required.

Patient Education: Hypotension may cause dizziness; move slowly, and request assistance to sit on edge of bed or ambulate. ▪ May decrease potassium levels and require a supplement.

Maternal/Child: Category C: use in pregnancy only if clearly needed. ▪ Consider discontinuing breast-feeding. ▪ Safety and effectiveness for use in pediatric patients not established. ▪ Has been used in infants age 4 days to 6 months at doses ranging from 0.005 mg/kg to 0.1 mg/kg. Maximal diuretic effect seen at doses of 0.035 to 0.04 mg/kg. Elimination half-life decreases during the first month of life from approximately 6 hours at birth to 2.4 hours at 1 month.

Elderly: Response similar to that seen in younger patients; however, dose selection should be cautious; see Dose Adjustments. Consider increased sensitivity to hypotensive and electrolyte effects and increased risk of circulatory collapse or thromboembolic episodes. ▪ Monitoring of renal function suggested.

DRUG/LAB INTERACTIONS

Causes excessive potassium depletion with **corticosteroids, thiazide diuretics** (e.g., hydrochlorothiazide), **amphotericin B** (all formulations). ▪ Potentiates **antihypertensive drugs** (e.g., nitroglycerin, nitroprusside sodium); reduced dose of the antihypertensive agent or both drugs may be indicated. ▪ May cause transient or permanent deafness with doses exceeding the usual or when given in conjunction with **other ototoxic drugs** (e.g., aminoglycosides [e.g., gentamicin], cisplatin). ▪ **Amphotericin B** (all formulations) may increase potential for ototoxicity and nephrotoxicity; avoid concurrent use. ▪ Nephrotoxicity increased by other **nephrotoxic agents** (e.g., acyclovir [Zovirax], aminoglycosides, ciprofloxacin [Cipro], cyclosporine [Sandimmune], vancomycin); avoid concurrent use. ▪ May increase serum levels of **lithium** (may cause toxicity). ▪ May cause cardiac arrhythmias with **amiodarone** (Nexterone) **or digoxin** (potassium depletion). ▪ Risk of cardiotoxicity increased with **pimozide** (Orap) **and sparfloxacin** (Zagam); concurrent use not recommended. ▪ May enhance or inhibit actions of **nondepolarizing muscle relaxants** (e.g., atracurium [Tracrium]) **or theophyllines.** ▪ May cause hyperglycemia with **insulin or sulfonylureas** (e.g., tolbutamide) by decreasing glucose tolerance. ▪ Effects may be inhibited by **ACE inhibitors** (e.g., captopril), **NSAIDs** (e.g., ibuprofen [Motrin]), **probenecid, or** in patients with cirrhosis and ascites who are taking **salicylates.** ▪ May cause profound diuresis and serious electrolyte abnormalities with **thiazide diuretics** (e.g., chlorothiazide [Diuril]) because of synergistic effects. ▪ Do not use concomitantly with **ethacrynic acid** (Edecrin); risk of ototoxicity markedly increased. ▪ Smoking may increase secretion of ADH-decreasing diuretic effects and cardiac output. ▪ See Precautions.

SIDE EFFECTS

Usually occur in prolonged therapy, seriously ill patients, or following large doses.

Abdominal pain, arthritic pain, azotemia, dizziness, ECG changes, elevated SCr, encephalopathy, headache, hyperglycemia, hyperuricemia, hypocalcemia, hypochloremia, hypomagnesemia, hyponatremia, hypotension, impaired hearing, muscle cramps, nausea, pruritus, rash.

Major: Anaphylactic shock, blood volume reduction, circulatory collapse, dehydration, excessive diuresis, hypokalemia, metabolic acidosis, thrombocytopenia, vascular thrombosis, and embolism.

ANTIDOTE

If minor side effects are noted, discontinue the drug and notify the physician, who may treat the side effects symptomatically and continue the drug. If side effects are progressive or any major side effect occurs, discontinue the drug immediately and notify the physician. Treatment of major side effects is symptomatic and aggressive and includes fluid and electrolyte replacement. Resuscitate as necessary.

BUPRENORPHINE HYDROCHLORIDE
(byou-pren-**OR**-feen hy-droh-**KLOR**-eyed)

Narcotic analgesic
(agonist-antagonist)
Anesthesia adjunct

Buprenex

pH 3.5 to 5.5

USUAL DOSE
Pain control: 0.3 mg (1 mL). Repeat every 6 hours as necessary. May be repeated in 30 to 60 minutes, if indicated. These dose recommendations have been lowered because of excessive respiratory depression with doses up to 0.6 mg. 25 to 250 mcg/hr has been given as a continuous infusion to manage postoperative pain.

Reverse fentanyl-induced anesthesia (unlabeled): 0.3 to 0.8 mg 1 to 4 hours after induction of anesthesia and 30 minutes before end of surgery.

PEDIATRIC DOSE
2 to 12 years of age: Pain control: 2 to 6 mcg/kg of body weight every 4 to 8 hours. A repeat dose in 30 to 60 minutes is not recommended. Longer intervals (6 to 8 hours) are suggested and should provide sufficient pain relief. Determine appropriate interval through clinical assessment. See Maternal/Child.

DOSE ADJUSTMENTS
Reduce dose by one half in high-risk patients (e.g., elderly or debilitated, respiratory disease), when other CNS depressants have been given, and in the immediate postoperative period; see Drug/Lab Interactions. ▪ Reduced dose may be required in impaired liver function.

DILUTION
IV injection: May be given undiluted.

Infusion: May be further diluted with NS, D5W, D5NS, or LR injection and given as an infusion. 1 mg in 250 mL = 4 mcg/mL; 3 mg in 250 mL = 12 mcg/mL.

Filters: Not required by manufacturer; however, 0.2-micron filters were used during manufacturing. No loss of drug potency expected.

Storage: Before use, store at CRT. Avoid freezing and/or prolonged exposure to light.

COMPATIBILITY
Consider any drug NOT listed as compatible to be INCOMPATIBLE until consulting a pharmacist; specific conditions may apply.

One source suggests the following **compatibilities:**

Y-site: Acetaminophen (Ofirmev), allopurinol (Aloprim), amifostine (Ethyol), aztreonam (Azactam), cisatracurium (Nimbex), cladribine (Leustatin), docetaxel (Taxotere), etoposide phosphate (Etopophos), filgrastim (Neupogen), gemcitabine (Gemzar), granisetron (Kytril), linezolid (Zyvox), melphalan (Alkeran), oxaliplatin (Eloxatin), pemetrexed (Alimta), piperacillin/tazobactam (Zosyn), propofol (Diprivan), remifentanil (Ultiva), teniposide (Vumon), thiotepa, vinorelbine (Navelbine).

RATE OF ADMINISTRATION
Titrate slowly according to symptom relief and respiratory rate.

IV injection: A single dose over 3 to 5 minutes.

Infusion: See Usual Dose. Use of a metriset (60 gtt/min) or a controlled infusion device recommended.

ACTIONS
A synthetic narcotic agonist-antagonist analgesic. Thirty times as potent as morphine in analgesic effect (0.3 mg equivalent to 10 mg morphine) and has the antagonist effect of naloxone in larger doses. Does produce respiratory depression. Pain relief is effected in 2 to 3 minutes and lasts up to 6 hours. Metabolized in the liver. Primarily excreted through feces. Crosses the placental barrier. Secreted in breast milk.

INDICATIONS AND USES
Relief of moderate to severe pain.
Unlabeled use: Reverse fentanyl-induced anesthesia.

CONTRAINDICATIONS
Hypersensitivity to buprenorphine.

PRECAUTIONS
Usually given IM. ▪ May precipitate withdrawal symptoms if stopped too quickly after prolonged use or if patient has been on opiates. ▪ Use caution in asthma, respiratory depression or difficulty from any source, impaired renal or hepatic function, the elderly or debilitated, myxedema or hypothyroidism, adrenocortical insufficiency, CNS depression or coma, toxic psychoses, prostatic hypertrophy or urethral stricture, acute alcoholism, delirium tremens, or kyphoscoliosis. ▪ May elevate cerebrospinal fluid pressure; use caution in head injury, intracranial lesions, and other situations with increased intracranial pressure.
Monitor: Naloxone, oxygen, and controlled respiratory equipment must be available. Naloxone is only partially effective in reversing respiratory depression. ▪ Observe patient frequently and monitor vital signs. ▪ Keep patient supine to minimize side effects; orthostatic hypotension and fainting may occur. Observe closely during ambulation. ▪ Pain control usually more effective with routinely administered doses. Determine appropriate interval through clinical assessment.
Patient Education: Avoid use of alcohol or other CNS depressants (e.g., antihistamines, diazepam [Valium]). ▪ Use caution performing any task requiring alertness; may cause dizziness, euphoria, and sedation. ▪ Request assistance for ambulation. ▪ May be habit forming.
Maternal/Child: Category C: safety for use during pregnancy, labor and delivery, or breastfeeding not established. Use only when clearly needed. ▪ Not recommended in pediatric patients under 2 years of age but has been used in pediatric patients as young as 9 months of age.
Elderly: See Dose Adjustments. ▪ May be more sensitive to effects (e.g., respiratory depression, urinary retention, constipation, dizziness). ▪ Analgesia should be effective with lower doses. ▪ Consider possibility of decreased organ function.

DRUG/LAB INTERACTIONS
Respiratory and CNS effects may be additive with **barbiturate anesthetics** (e.g., thiopental [Pentothal]); reduced doses of both drugs may be indicated. ▪ May cause respiratory depression and cardiovascular collapse with **diazepam** (Valium); reduced doses of both drugs may be indicated. ▪ May decrease analgesic effects of **other narcotics;** avoid concurrent use. ▪ Clearance decreased and serum levels increased by **cytochrome P$_{450}$ inhibitors** (e.g., azole antifungal agents [e.g., itraconazole (Sporanox)], macrolide antibiotics [e.g., erythromycin], protease inhibitors [e.g., ritonavir (Norvir)]). Monitor with concurrent use; dose adjustment may be indicated. ▪ Clearance increased and serum levels decreased by **cytochrome P$_{450}$ inducers** (e.g., carbamazepine [Tegretol], phenytoin [Dilantin], rifampin [Rifadin]). Use caution; dose adjustments may be indicated. ▪ Manufacturer suggests caution when used in combination with **MAO inhibitors** (e.g., selegiline [Eldepryl]).

SIDE EFFECTS
Excessive sedation is a major side effect. Has caused death from respiratory depression. Acute and chronic hypersensitivity reactions (e.g., anaphylaxis, angioneurotic edema, bronchospasm, hives, pruritus, rash), bradycardia, clammy skin, constipation, cyanosis, dizziness, dyspnea, headache, hypertension, hypotension, nausea, pruritus, tachycardia, vertigo, visual disturbances, vomiting.

ANTIDOTE
With increasing severity of any side effect or onset of symptoms of overdose, discontinue the drug and notify the physician. Naloxone hydrochloride will help to reverse respiratory depression, but is not as effective as it is with other narcotics. A patent airway, artificial ventilation, oxygen therapy, and other symptomatic treatment must be instituted promptly. Treat anaphylaxis and resuscitate as necessary.

BUSULFAN BBW

(byou-**SUL**-fan)

Busulfex

Antineoplastic
(alkylating agent)

pH 3.4 to 3.9

USUAL DOSE

Administered in combination with cyclophosphamide as a component of a conditioning regimen before bone marrow or peripheral blood progenitor cell replacement support.

Premedication: Premedicate patients with phenytoin (use of other anticonvulsants not recommended) and an antiemetic (e.g., $5HT_3$ antiemetics such as ondansetron [Zofran], granisetron [Kytril]). Continue antiemetic administration on a fixed schedule throughout busulfan therapy. See Monitor, Drug Interactions, and Side Effects.

Busulfan: 0.8 mg/kg of ideal body weight (IBW) or actual body weight, whichever is lower, administered through a central venous catheter every 6 hours for 4 days (16 doses). Six hours after the 16th busulfan dose (on BMT day minus 3 [3 days prior to BMT]), begin cyclophosphamide at a dose of 60 mg/kg/day for 2 days. Before and after each infusion, flush the catheter line with 5 mL NS or D5W.

PEDIATRIC DOSE

See Maternal/Child.

Initial doses are based on a small trial and are unlabeled. Therapeutic drug monitoring and dose adjustment based on AUC determination following the first dose are recommended. See manufacturer's literature for details.

Actual body weight equal to or less than 12 kg: 1.1 mg/kg.

Actual body weight greater than 12 kg: 0.8 mg/kg.

DOSE ADJUSTMENTS

In obese or severely obese patients, dose should be based on an adjusted ideal body weight (AIBW). Calculate as follows:

$$AIBW = IBW + 0.25 \times (\text{Actual weight [kg]} - IBW)$$

- Busulfan has not been studied in patients with renal or hepatic insufficiency. See Precautions.

DILUTION

Specific techniques required; see Precautions. Supplied in vials containing 60 mg/10 mL (6 mg/mL). Must be diluted before infusion with either NS or D5W. The diluent volume should be 10 times the busulfan volume to ensure a final concentration of approximately 0.5 mg/mL. Remove calculated dose of busulfan from vial. Inject the contents of the syringe into an intravenous bag or syringe that contains the calculated amount of diluent. Always add the busulfan to the diluent rather than the diluent to the busulfan. Mix thoroughly by inverting several times. The dose for a 70-kg patient would be prepared using the following steps:

1. 70 kg × 0.8 mg/kg = 56 mg.
2. 56 mg ÷ 6 mg/mL = 9.3 mL busulfan needed.
3. 9.3 × 10 = 93 mL.
4. Add 9.3 mL of busulfan to 93 mL of NS or D5W.

Filters: 5-micron nylon filter has been used; see Compatibility.

Storage: Refrigerate. Busulfan diluted with NS or D5W is stable for 8 hours at room temperature, but infusion must be completed within that time. When diluted with NS and refrigerated, it is stable for 12 hours, but infusion must be completed within that time.

COMPATIBILITY

Do not use polycarbonate syringes or polycarbonate filter needles. Manufacturer states, "Do not infuse concomitantly with another intravenous solution of unknown **compatibility.** Flush central venous catheter line before and after administration with at least 5 mL of NS or D5W."

RATE OF ADMINISTRATION

Before and after each infusion, flush the catheter line with 5 mL NS or D5W.

Busulfan: Infuse over 2 hours using an infusion pump.

Cyclophosphamide: Infuse over 1 hour.

ACTIONS

A bifunctional alkylating agent. Cell cycle phase–nonspecific. Interferes with DNA replication, leading to cytotoxicity and cell death. Distributes equally into plasma and CSF. Metabolized in the liver. Excreted partially in the urine, primarily as metabolites.

INDICATIONS AND USES

For use in combination with cyclophosphamide as a conditioning regimen prior to allogeneic hematopoietic progenitor cell transplantation for chronic myelogenous leukemia. **Unlabeled uses:** Component of pretransplant conditioning regimens in patients undergoing bone marrow transplant for acute myeloid leukemia and nonmalignant diseases (e.g., sickle cell disease). ▪ Patients 5 to 16 years of age undergoing allogeneic hematopoietic stem cell transplantation (HSCT).

CONTRAINDICATIONS

Previous hypersensitivity to busulfan or any of its components (polyethylene glycol and dimethylacetamide).

PRECAUTIONS

Follow guidelines for handling cytotoxic agents. See Appendix A, p. 1331.
▪ Administered by or under the direction of a physician who is experienced in allogeneic hematopoietic stem cell transplantation, the use of cancer chemotherapeutic drugs, and the management of patients with severe pancytopenia. ▪ Adequate diagnostic and treatment facilities must be readily available to manage therapy and any complications that arise. ▪ Profound myelosuppression, including granulocytopenia, thrombocytopenia, anemia, or any combination of these will occur. ▪ Seizures have been reported. Use caution when administering to patients with a history of seizures or head trauma or patients who are receiving other potentially epileptogenic drugs (e.g., imipenem-cilastatin [Primaxin], meperidine [Demerol]). ▪ Anticonvulsant prophylactic therapy should be initiated with phenytoin before busulfan treatment. ▪ High busulfan AUC values (greater than 1,500 μM·min) may be associated with an increased risk of developing hepatic veno-occlusive disease (HVOD). Patients who have received prior radiation therapy, three or more cycles of chemotherapy, or a prior progenitor cell transplant may be at an increased risk of developing hepatic HVOD with the recommended busulfan dose and regimen. ▪ Cardiac tamponade has been reported in pediatric patients with thalassemia who received high doses of oral busulfan and cyclophosphamide. No patients treated in the busulfan injection trials experienced cardiac tamponade. ▪ Bronchopulmonary dysplasia with pulmonary fibrosis is a rare but serious complication following chronic busulfan therapy. Average onset of symptoms is 4 years after therapy (range: 4 months to 10 years). ▪ May cause cellular dysplasia in many organs. Dysplasia may be severe enough to cause difficulty in interpretation of exfoliative cytologic examinations of the lungs, bladder, breast, and the uterine cervix. ▪ Secondary malignancies, including acute nonlymphocytic leukemia, myeloproliferation syndrome, and carcinoma have been reported in patients treated with alkylating agents.

Monitor: Obtain a baseline and a daily CBC, including differential and platelet count, during treatment and until engraftment is demonstrated. Absolute neutrophil count (ANC) dropped below $0.5 \times 10^9/L$ at a median of 4 days posttransplant and recovered at a median of 13 days when prophylactic G-CSF was used. Thrombocytopenia (platelets less than 25,000/mm³ or platelet transfusion required) occurred at a median of 5-6 days. ▪ Monitor for signs of local or systemic infection or bleeding. Antibiotic therapy and platelet and RBC support should be used when medically indicated. ▪ Monitor for thrombocytopenia (platelet count less than 50,000/mm³). Initiate precautions to prevent excessive bleeding (e.g., inspect IV sites, skin, and mucous membranes; use extreme care during invasive procedures; test urine, emesis, stool, and secretions for occult blood). ▪ Serum transaminases, alkaline phosphatase, and bilirubin should be obtained daily through transplant day 28 to monitor for signs of hepatotoxicity and the onset of hepatic VOD. Jones' criteria may be used to diagnose VOD (hyperbilirubinemia and two of the following three findings: painful hepatomegaly, weight gain more than 5%, or ascites). ▪ Obtain baseline and periodic uric acid concentrations. ▪ Use of anticonvulsants other than phenytoin may result in higher busulfan plasma AUCs and an increased risk of VOD or seizures. When other anticonvulsants are used, plasma busulfan AUC should be monitored; see Drug/Lab Interactions.

Patient Education: Nonhormonal birth control recommended. ▪ May be at increased risk of developing a secondary malignancy. ▪ See Appendix D, p. 1333.

Maternal/Child: Category D: avoid pregnancy. Can cause fetal harm. Has mutagenic potential. ▪ Discontinue breast-feeding. ▪ Safety and efficacy for use in pediatric patients not established. Clearance has been shown to be higher in pediatric patients than in adults, necessitating the development of alternative dosing regimens for oral busulfan in pediatric patients. A recent small pharmacokinetic study suggests an unlabeled dosing regimen; see Pediatric Dose and manufacturer's literature.

Elderly: Has been used in a small number of patients over 55 years of age. All achieved myeloablation and engraftment.

DRUG/LAB INTERACTIONS

Itraconazole (Sporanox), **metronidazole** (Flagyl), **and cyclophosphamide** (Cytoxan) decrease busulfan clearance, increasing the AUC and risk of toxicity. ▪ **Phenytoin** increases the clearance of busulfan. Because the pharmacokinetics of busulfan were studied in patients treated with phenytoin, the clearance of busulfan at the recommended dose may be lower and the AUC higher in patients not treated with phenytoin. ▪ **Acetaminophen** (Tylenol) may decrease clearance of busulfan. Avoid administration of acetaminophen 72 hours prior to or with busulfan therapy. ▪ Do not administer **live virus vaccines** to patients receiving antineoplastic drugs. ▪ Busulfan has been used with **fluconazole** (Diflucan), **ondansetron** (Zofran), **and granisetron** (Kytril). ▪ May cause additive effects with **bone marrow–suppressing agents or agents that cause blood dyscrasias** (e.g., amphotericin B, antithyroid agents, azathioprine, chloramphenicol, ganciclovir [Cytovene], interferon, plicamycin [Mithracin], zidovudine) **and radiation therapy.** Adjust busulfan dose based on blood cell counts. ▪ Risk of uric acid nephropathy increased with **sulfinpyrazone** (Anturan); allopurinol may be preferred to prevent or treat hyperuricemia. ▪ See Precautions.

SIDE EFFECTS

Profound myelosuppression, including granulocytopenia, thrombocytopenia, anemia, or a combination of these, will occur in 100% of patients. ▪ Other nonhematologic adverse events occurring in more than 20% of patients include abdominal pain or enlargement, ALT elevation, anorexia, anxiety, asthenia, back pain, chest pain, chills, constipation, cough, creatinine elevation, depression, diarrhea, dizziness, dry mouth, dyspepsia, dyspnea, edema, epistaxis, fever, headache, hyperbilirubinemia, hyperglycemia, hypersensitivity reactions, hypertension, hypervolemia, hypocalcemia, hypokalemia, hypomagnesemia, infection, inflammation or pain at injection site, insomnia, lung disorders, nausea, pain, pruritus, rash, rectal disorder, rhinitis, seizures, stomatitis (mucositis), tachycardia, third-degree heart block, thrombosis, vasodilation (flushing or hot flashes), vomiting, weight gain secondary to edema. ▪ Graft-versus-host disease, hepatic veno-occlusive disease and death have also been reported. ▪ Dimethylacetamide (DMA), the solvent used in busulfan formulation, has been associated with adverse reactions such as confusion, hallucinations, hepatotoxicity, lethargy, and somnolence. The relative contribution of DMA to neurologic and hepatic toxicities observed with busulfan is difficult to determine. ▪ Numerous other side effects have occurred.

Post-Marketing: Febrile neutropenia, thrombotic microangiopathy, tumor lysis syndrome, and severe bacterial, viral (e.g., CMV viremia), and fungal infections and sepsis.

ANTIDOTE

Treat minor side effects symptomatically. In the absence of hematopoietic progenitor cell transplantation, the normal dosage of busulfan injection constitutes an overdose. Monitor hematologic status closely, and institute supportive measures as indicated. Administration of whole blood products (e.g., packed RBCs, platelets, leukocytes) and/or blood modifiers (e.g., darbepoetin alfa [Aranesp], epoetin alfa [Epogen], filgrastim [Neupogen, Zarxio], pegfilgrastim [Neulasta], sargramostim [Leukine]) may be indicated to treat bone marrow toxicity. Dialysis and administration of glutathione may be considered in an overdose (busulfan is metabolized by conjugation with glutathione).

BUTORPHANOL TARTRATE

(byou-**TOR**-fah-nohl **TAHR**-trayt)

Narcotic analgesic
(agonist-antagonist)
Anesthesia adjunct

Butorphanol Tartrate PF, Stadol, Stadol PF   pH 3 to 5.5

USUAL DOSE

Pain control: 1 mg. Repeat every 3 to 4 hours as necessary. Range is 0.5 to 2 mg.

Preoperative or preanesthetic: 2 mg 60 to 90 minutes before surgery. Individualize dose. Usually given IM.

Labor: 1 to 2 mg at full term in early labor; may be repeated after 4 hours. Use alternate analgesia if delivery is expected to occur within 4 hours.

Adjunct to balanced anesthesia: 2 mg just before induction or 0.5 to 1 mg in increments during anesthesia. Increments may be up to 0.06 mg/kg and should be based on previous sedative, analgesic, and hypnotic drugs. Patients seldom require less than 4 mg or more than 12.5 mg. Administered only under the direction of the anesthesiologist.

DOSE ADJUSTMENTS

Reduce dose to one half of the recommended dose and increase the interval between doses to at least 6 hours for impaired liver or renal function and in the elderly; adjust as indicated by patient response. ■ Another source suggests that patients with a glomerular filtration rate (GFR) of 10 to 50 mL/min receive 75% of the usual dose given at the normal dosage interval and that patients with a GFR less than 10 mL/min receive 50% of the usual dose given at the normal dosage interval. No dose adjustment is necessary for patients with a GFR greater than 50 mL/min. ■ Reduce dose when other CNS depressants have been given and in the immediate postoperative period. Use the smallest effective dose and extend intervals between doses. ■ See Drug/Lab Interactions.

DILUTION

May be given undiluted. Avoid aerosol spray while preparing a syringe for use. Rinse with cool water following skin contact. Available preservative free.

Storage: Store at CRT. Protect from light and freezing.

COMPATIBILITY

Consider any drug NOT listed as compatible to be INCOMPATIBLE until consulting a pharmacist; specific conditions may apply.

One source suggests the following **compatibilities:**

Additive: Droperidol (Inapsine).

Y-site: Acetaminophen (Ofirmev), allopurinol (Aloprim), amifostine (Ethyol), aztreonam (Azactam), bivalirudin (Angiomax), cisatracurium (Nimbex), cladribine (Leustatin), dexmedetomidine (Precedex), docetaxel (Taxotere), doxorubicin liposomal (Doxil), enalaprilat (Vasotec IV), esmolol (Brevibloc), etoposide phosphate (Etopophos), fenoldopam (Corlopam), filgrastim (Neupogen), fludarabine (Fludara), gemcitabine (Gemzar), granisetron (Kytril), hetastarch in electrolytes (Hextend), labetalol, linezolid (Zyvox), melphalan (Alkeran), nicardipine (Cardine IV), oxaliplatin (Eloxatin), paclitaxel (Taxol), pemetrexed (Alimta), piperacillin/tazobactam (Zosyn), propofol (Diprivan), remifentanil (Ultiva), sargramostim (Leukine), teniposide (Vumon), thiotepa, vinorelbine (Navelbine).

RATE OF ADMINISTRATION
Each 2 mg or fraction thereof over 3 to 5 minutes. Frequently titrated according to symptom relief and respiratory rate.

ACTIONS
A potent narcotic analgesic with some narcotic agonist-antagonist effects. Exact mechanism of action is unknown. Analgesia similar to morphine is produced. Does produce respiratory depression, but this does not increase markedly with larger doses. Pain relief is effected almost immediately, peaks at 30 minutes, and lasts about 2 to 4 hours. Causes some hemodynamic changes that increase the workload of the heart. Metabolized in the liver. Excreted in urine and feces. Crosses the blood-brain barrier and placental barrier. Secreted in breast milk.

INDICATIONS AND USES
Relief of moderate to severe pain. ▪ Preoperative or preanesthetic medication, as a supplement to anesthesia. ▪ Relief of pain during early labor.

CONTRAINDICATIONS
Hypersensitivity to butorphanol or its components (some products contain benzethonium chloride).

PRECAUTIONS
Not used for narcotic-dependent patients because of antagonist activity. ▪ May increase cardiac workload; use in myocardial infarction, ventricular dysfunction, and coronary insufficiency only if benefits outweigh risks. ▪ Use caution in respiratory depression or difficulty from any source, obstructive respiratory conditions, head injury, and impaired liver or kidney function. ▪ May elevate cerebrospinal pressure. ▪ Prolonged continuous use may result in physical dependence or tolerance. ▪ In overdose situations, always consider the possibility of multiple drug ingestion.
Monitor: Naloxone, oxygen, and controlled respiratory equipment must be available. Duration of action of butorphanol usually exceeds that of naloxone; repeated dosing may be necessary. ▪ Observe patient frequently and monitor vital signs. ▪ Keep patient supine to minimize side effects; orthostatic hypotension and fainting may occur. Observe closely during ambulation. ▪ Pain control usually more effective with routinely administered doses. Determine appropriate interval through clinical assessment.
Patient Education: Avoid use of alcohol or other CNS depressants (e.g., antihistamines, diazepam [Valium]). ▪ Use caution performing any task requiring alertness; may cause dizziness, euphoria, and sedation. ▪ Request assistance for ambulation. ▪ May be habit forming.
Maternal/Child: Category C: safety for use in pregnant women before 37 weeks' gestation not established; use only if benefit justifies potential risk to fetus. ▪ Has been used safely during labor of term infants. Has been associated with transient (10 to 90 minutes) sinusoidal fetal heart rate patterns. Use caution if abnormal fetal heart rate is present; manufacturer states "was not associated with adverse outcomes." Alternative analgesia suggested if delivery is expected to occur within 4 hours. ▪ Use caution in breast-feeding; an estimated 4 mcg/L has been found in breast milk; may be clinically insignificant. ▪ Safety and effectiveness for use in pediatric patients under 18 years of age not established.
Elderly: Mean half-life may be extended by 25%, may be more sensitive to effects (e.g., respiratory depression, constipation, dizziness, urinary retention). ▪ Analgesia should be effective with lower doses; see Dose Adjustments. ▪ Consider decreased organ function, concomitant disease, or other drug therapy.

DRUG/LAB INTERACTIONS

Potentiated by **cimetidine** (Tagamet), **phenothiazines** (e.g., chlorpromazine [Thorazine]), **droperidol** (Inapsine), **and CNS depressants** such as narcotic analgesics, general anesthetics, alcohol, anticholinergics, antihistamines, barbiturates, benzodiazepines (e.g., diazepam [Valium]), hypnotics, MAO inhibitors, neuromuscular blocking agents (e.g., atracurium [Tracrium]), psychotropic agents, and sedatives. Reduced doses of both drugs may be indicated; use the smallest effective dose of butorphanol and/or extend intervals between doses. ■ Effects may be altered by other **medications that affect hepatic metabolism of drugs** (e.g., aminophylline, erythromycin). Reduced doses of butorphanol and/or longer intervals between doses may be indicated. ■ May decrease analgesic effects of **other narcotics;** avoid concurrent use. ■ Will cause an increase in conjunctival changes with **pancuronium.**

SIDE EFFECTS

Dizziness, nausea and/or vomiting, and somnolence occur most frequently. Abdominal pain, anorexia, anxiety, asthenia, bronchitis, clammy skin, confusion, constipation, cough, diplopia, dizziness, drug dependence, dry mouth, dyspnea, euphoria, floating feeling, flushing, hallucinations, headache, hypersensitivity reactions (e.g., pruritis), hypotension, insomnia, lethargy, nervousness, palpitations, paresthesia, respiratory depression, sweating, tremor, unusual dreams, vasodilation, vertigo, warmth. May cause increased pulmonary artery pressure, pulmonary wedge pressure, left ventricular end-diastolic pressure, systemic arterial pressure, pulmonary vascular resistance, and cardiac workload.

Overdose: Cardiovascular insufficiency, hypoventilation, coma, and death. May be associated with ingestion of multiple drugs.

ANTIDOTE

With increasing severity of any side effect or onset of symptoms of overdose, discontinue the drug and notify the physician. Most side effects will be treated symptomatically. Treat hypertension with antihypertensives (e.g., nitroglycerin, nitroprusside sodium). Naloxone hydrochloride will reverse respiratory depression. Duration of action of butorphanol usually exceeds that of naloxone; repeated dosing may be necessary. A patent airway, adequate ventilation, oxygen therapy, and other symptomatic treatment must be instituted promptly. Vasodilation may cause hypotension.

C1 ESTERASE INHIBITOR (HUMAN OR RECOMBINANT)

(C 1 **ES**-ter-ase in-**HIB**-it-or)

Berinert, Cinryze, Ruconest

Available C1 esterase inhibitor products include:
Berinert: Plasma-derived C1 esterase inhibitor (human) pH 4.5 to 8.5
Cinryze: Plasma-derived C1 esterase inhibitor (human) pH 6.6 to 7.4
Ruconest: (Recombinant) C1 esterase inhibitor pH 6.8

USUAL DOSE   (International units [IU])
BERINERT
Treatment of an acute attack: 20 international units/kg (IU/kg) as an IV injection. Doses lower than 20 international units/kg (IU/kg) should not be administered.

CINRYZE
Routine prophylaxis dosing: 1,000 units as an IV injection over 10 minutes (1 mL/min). May be repeated every 3 or 4 days as necessary for routine prophylaxis against angioedema attacks in patients with hereditary angioedema (HAE).

RUCONEST
Treatment of an acute attack: 50 international units/kg (IU/kg) with a maximum of 4,200 international units (IU) administered as a slow IV injection over approximately 5 minutes. If symptoms persist, a second dose may be administered. Do not exceed 4,200 international units/dose (IU/dose).

DILUTION
BERINERT
Available in a kit containing one 500–international unit (IU) vial of Berinert, one 10-mL vial of SWFI, one Mix2Vial filtered transfer set, and one alcohol swab. Bring components to room temperature. Berinert is a lyophilized concentrate and requires reconstitution. The Mix2Vial transfer set provided requires a specific technique to accomplish reconstitution; see manufacturer's literature for instructions. Alternately, for each vial of Berinert and provided diluent, place all components on a flat surface, remove the flip caps from the drug and diluent vials, swab the vials with alcohol, and allow them to dry. Insert one end of a double-ended transfer needle into the diluent. Invert the diluent bottle and insert the other end of the transfer needle into the drug vial. Diluent will be drawn into the drug vial by a vacuum. Remove the transfer device and diluent vial. Gently swirl the drug vial to fully dissolve. Solution should be colorless, clear, and free from visible particles. Do not use if solution is cloudy, discolored, or contains particulates. Concentration equals 50 units/mL. Calculate volume required to supply the calculated dose. Attach a vented filter spike to a 10-mL (or larger) syringe and withdraw the contents. Contents of multiple vials may be pooled in a single administration device (e.g., syringe). Use a new double-ended transfer needle and a new vented filter spike or a new unused Mix2Vial for each vial requiring reconstitution.

CINRYZE
If refrigerated, bring components to RT (two 500-unit vials of Cinryze and two 5-mL vials of SWFI [not supplied by manufacturer]). Use of a silicone-free syringe is recommended for reconstitution and administration. Access the diluent vial before the Cinryze vial to prevent loss of vacuum. For each 500-unit vial, insert one end of a double-ended transfer needle into the SWFI diluent. Invert the bottle of diluent and rapidly insert the other end of the transfer needle into the slightly angled Cinryze vial. Diluent will be drawn into the Cinryze vial by a vacuum. Do not use if there is no vacuum. Remove the transfer device and diluent vial. Gently swirl the Cinryze vial until the powder is completely dissolved. Do not use if solution is turbid or discolored (should be colorless to

slightly blue and clear). Attach a filter needle to a 10-mL syringe and withdraw 500 units (5 mL) from each vial (total dose 1,000 units in 10 mL [100 units/mL]).

Ruconest

Bring components to room temperature (vials of Ruconest and SWFI as diluent [not supplied by manufacturer]). Remove the flip caps from the drug and diluent vials, swab the vials with alcohol, and allow them to dry. Using the syringe/needle or syringe/vial adapter, withdraw 14 mL of SWFI from the diluent vial. Remove the syringe and transfer the diluent to the Ruconest vial. Add the diluent slowly to avoid forceful impact on the powder. Swirl the vial slowly to mix and avoid foaming. If indicated, repeat this procedure using another 14 mL of diluent using a new vial adapter and a second vial of Ruconest. Concentration equals 150 international units/mL (IU/mL). Calculate volume required to supply the calculated dose and draw up into a syringe. Contents of both vials may be pooled into a single administration syringe. Do not use if solution is cloudy, discolored, or contains particulates.

Filters: Berinert: A Mix2Vial filtered transfer set is provided for each single-use dose or, alternately, a double-ended needle and a vented filter spike are required.

Cinryze and Ruconest: Specific information not available.

Storage: All Formulations: Store in carton at 2° to 25° C (36° to 77° F) until ready for use. Do not freeze. Protect from light. Do not use beyond expiration date. For single use only. Discard unused drug.

Berinert: Reconstituted solution must be used within 8 hours; do not refrigerate or freeze.

Cinryze: Reconstituted solution must be administered at RT within 3 hours of preparation.

Ruconest: Use reconstituted solution immediately, or refrigerate and use within 8 hours. Do not freeze.

COMPATIBILITY

Berinert: Manufacturer states, "Do not mix Berinert with other medicinal products, and administer by a separate infusion line."

Cinryze: Manufacturer states, "Do not mix with other materials."

Ruconest: Manufacturer states, "Do not mix with other medicinal products or solutions. Administer by a separate infusion line."

RATE OF ADMINISTRATION

Berinert: A single dose at a rate of approximately 4 mL/min.

Cinryze: A single dose equally distributed over 10 minutes (1 mL/min).

Ruconest: A single dose equally distributed over approximately 5 minutes.

ACTIONS

C1 esterase inhibitor is a normal constituent of human blood and is a serine proteinase inhibitor. It has an important inhibiting potential on several of the major cascade systems, including the complement system, the intrinsic coagulation (contact) system, the fibrinolytic system, and the coagulation cascade. Hereditary angioedema (HAE) patients have low levels of endogenous or functional C1 esterase inhibitor. Although the events that induce attacks of angioedema in HAE patients are not well defined, it is thought that increased vascular permeability and the clinical manifestation of HAE attacks (e.g., local tissue swelling of hands, feet, limbs, face, intestinal tract, and airway [larynx or trachea]) are primarily mediated through contact system activation. Suppression of contact system activation by C1 esterase inhibitor through the inactivation of plasma kallikrein and factor XIIa is thought to modulate vascular permeability by preventing the generation of bradykinin. Supplying additional C1 esterase inhibitor activity by IV injection facilitates the normal process. Plasma levels of C1 inhibitor increase within 1 hour or less of IV administration of Cinryze. The mean half-life is 22 hours for **Berinert,** 56 hours for **Cinryze,** and 2.5 hours for **Ruconest.**

INDICATIONS AND USES

Berinert: Treatment of acute abdominal, facial, or laryngeal attacks of hereditary angioedema (HAE) in adult and adolescent patients. ▪ Safety and effectiveness for use as prophylactic therapy not established.

CINRYZE: Routine prophylaxis against angioedema attacks in adolescent and adult patients with HAE.

RUCONEST: Treatment of acute attacks in adult and adolescent patients with HAE.

Limitation of use: RUCONEST: Effectiveness not established in HAE patients with laryngeal attacks.

CONTRAINDICATIONS

ALL FORMULATIONS: Known life-threatening hypersensitivity reactions, including anaphylaxis to C1 esterase inhibitor preparations.

RUCONEST: Is contraindicated in patients with a history of allergy to rabbits or rabbit-derived products.

PRECAUTIONS

ALL FORMULATIONS: For intravenous use only. ▪ Initiate treatment under the supervision of a qualified health care professional experienced in the treatment of HAE. ▪ Severe hypersensitivity reactions, including anaphylaxis, may occur. Epinephrine should be immediately available. See Antidote. ▪ Serious arterial and venous thromboembolic (TE) events (e.g., basilar artery thrombosis, multiple pulmonary microemboli, and thrombosis) have been reported at recommended doses of C1 esterase inhibitor products, and other TE events (e.g., myocardial infarction, pulmonary embolism, arterial thrombosis, deep vein thrombosis) have been reported in patients receiving off-label high-dose C1 esterase inhibitor therapy. Risk factors may include the presence of an indwelling venous catheter/access device, prior history of thrombosis, underlying atherosclerosis, use of oral contraceptives or certain androgens, morbid obesity, and immobility. Weigh benefits of treatment versus risk.

BERINERT AND CINRYZE: Made from human plasma and may contain infectious agents (e.g., HIV, Creutzfeldt-Jakob disease, hepatitis B, or hepatitis C). Numerous steps in the manufacturing process are used to reduce the potential for infection.

Monitor: ALL FORMULATIONS: Observe for symptoms of a hypersensitivity reaction (e.g., anaphylaxis, generalized urticaria, hives, hypotension, tightness in the chest, wheezing). Reaction may occur during injection or after injection is complete. ▪ Symptoms of an HAE attack may be similar to S/S of hypersensitivity reactions. Evaluate carefully to initiate the correct treatment. There is usually no itching or hives with an HAE attack. ▪ Monitor patients with known risk factors for thrombotic events during and after administration; see Precautions.

Patient Education: ALL FORMULATIONS: Inform patients of the risks for infectious agent transmission and of safety precautions taken during the manufacturing process. ▪ Promptly report symptoms of a hypersensitivity reaction (e.g., difficulty breathing, feeling faint, hives, itching, tightness in the chest, wheezing). ▪ Promptly report symptoms of a possible thrombosis (e.g., altered consciousness or speech; loss of sensation or motor power; new-onset swelling and pain in the abdomen, chest, or limbs; shortness of breath). ▪ Appropriately trained patients may self-administer upon recognition of an HAE attack. However, given the potential for airway obstruction during an acute laryngeal HAE attack, patients experiencing such an attack should be advised to seek immediate medical attention after self-administration of **Berinert**. ▪ Discuss all medications used (e.g., prescription, nonprescription, over-the-counter, herbal, supplements) with the physician. ▪ Consult a health care professional before travel.

Maternal/Child: BERINERT AND CINRYZE: Category C: safety and effectiveness for use during pregnancy, labor, and delivery have not been established; use only if clearly needed.

RUCONEST: Category B: safety and effectiveness during pregnancy, labor, and delivery have not been established; use only if clearly needed.

ALL FORMULATIONS: Not known if C1 esterase inhibitor is secreted in human milk; use only if clearly needed during breast-feeding. ▪ **Berinert:** Safety and effectiveness for use in pediatric patients less than 12 years of age not established. ▪ **Cinryze:** Safety and effectiveness for use in neonates, infants, or other pediatric patients not established. Clinical studies included patients 9, 14, and 16 years of age. ▪ **Ruconest:** Safety and effectiveness were evaluated in 17 adolescent patients (13 to 17 years of age) treated for 52 HAE attacks with no serious adverse reactions. Abdominal pain, headache, and oropharyngeal pain did occur.

Elderly: ALL FORMULATIONS: Numbers in clinical studies insufficient to determine if the elderly respond differently than do younger subjects.

DRUG/LAB INTERACTIONS

ALL FORMULATIONS: No drug interaction studies have been conducted.

SIDE EFFECTS

BERINERT: The most common side effect observed was dysgeusia (an altered sense of taste). An increase in the severity of pain associated with HAE was the most serious side effect during clinical trials. Other reported side effects include abdominal pain, back pain, diarrhea, facial pain, headache, muscle spasm, nausea, and vomiting.

CINRYZE: The most common side effects reported include headache, nausea, rash, and vomiting. The most serious reaction observed in clinical studies was a cerebrovascular accident. Hypersensitivity reactions, including anaphylaxis, hives, hypotension, tightness of the chest, urticaria, and wheezing, have occurred.

RUCONEST: The most common side effects reported include diarrhea, headache, and nausea. Hypersensitivity with anaphylaxis was the most serious reaction reported.

Post-Marketing: BERINERT: Reported side effects from use outside the United States include hypersensitivity/anaphylactic reactions, viral transmission (e.g., acute hepatitis C), chills, fever, and injection site pain or redness.

CINRYZE: Local infusion site reactions (including inflammation or hematoma) and thromboembolic events (including catheter-related and deep venous thrombosis, transient ischemic attack, and stroke).

RUCONEST: Abdominal pain and rash.

ANTIDOTE

ALL FORMULATIONS: Keep the physician informed of side effects. Interrupt or discontinue injection if indicated (e.g., hypersensitivity reaction, thrombotic event). If appropriate and if symptoms subside, infusion may be resumed at a tolerated rate. ▪ Discontinue C1 esterase inhibitor and treat anaphylaxis immediately with oxygen, epinephrine (Adrenalin), antihistamines (e.g., diphenhydramine [Benadryl]), vasopressors (e.g., dopamine), corticosteroids, albuterol, IV fluids, and ventilation equipment as indicated. Resuscitate as necessary.

CABAZITAXEL BBW
(ka-**BAZ**-i-**TAX**-el)

Antineoplastic agent
(taxane)

Jevtana

USUAL DOSE
Premedication: Must be premedicated at least 30 minutes before each dose to reduce the risk and/or severity of hypersensitivity reactions. Usual regimen includes IV administration of an antihistamine (diphenhydramine [Benadryl] 25 mg or equivalent), a corticosteroid (dexamethasone [Decadron] 8 mg or equivalent steroid), and an H_2 antagonist (ranitidine [Zantac] 50 mg or equivalent H_2 antagonist).

Antiemetic prophylaxis is recommended and may be given orally or IV as needed.
Cabazitaxel: 25 mg/M^2 as a 1-hour infusion every 3 weeks. Given in combination with oral prednisone 10 mg administered daily throughout cabazitaxel treatment.

DOSE ADJUSTMENTS
Recommendations for dose adjustment for adverse reactions are listed in the following chart.

Recommended Cabazitaxel Dose Modifications for Adverse Reactions	
Toxicity*	Dose Modification
Prolonged Grade ≥3 neutropenia (greater than 1 week) despite appropriate medication, including G-CSF	Delay treatment until neutrophil count is >1,500 cells/mm^3, then reduce dose of cabazitaxel to 20 mg/M^2. Use G-CSF for secondary prophylaxis.
Febrile neutropenia or neutropenic infection	Delay treatment until improvement or resolution and until neutrophil count is >1,500 cells/mm^3, then reduce dose of cabazitaxel to 20 mg/M^2. Use G-CSF for secondary prophylaxis.
Grade ≥3 diarrhea or persisting diarrhea despite appropriate medication and fluid and electrolytes replacement.	Delay treatment until improvement or resolution, then reduce dose of cabazitaxel to 20 mg/M^2.
Grade 2 peripheral neuropathy	Delay treatment until improvement or resolution, then reduce dose of cabazitaxel to 20 mg/M^2.
Grade ≥3 peripheral neuropathy	Discontinue cabazitaxel.

*Toxicities graded in accordance with National Cancer Institute (NCI) Common Terminology Criteria for Adverse Events (CTCAE), version 4.0.

Discontinue if any of these reactions continue at a cabazitaxel dose of 20 mg/M^2. ▪ Dosage modifications based on the degree of hepatic impairment are outlined in the following chart.

Dose Modification for Hepatic Impairment	
Degree of Impairment	Dosage Modification
Mild hepatic impairment (total bilirubin >1 to ≤1.5 ULN or AST >1.5 × ULN)	Reduce starting dose of cabazitaxel to 20 mg/M^2.
Moderate hepatic impairment (total bilirubin >1.5 to ≤3 ULN or AST = Any value)	Reduce starting dose of cabazitaxel to 15 mg/M^2 based on tolerability data in these patients; however, the efficacy of this dose is unknown.
Severe hepatic impairment (total bilirubin >3 × ULN	Cabazitaxel is contraindicated; do not administer.

■ Avoid coadministration with strong CYP3A inhibitors. If coadministration is required, consider a 25% cabazitaxel dose reduction; see Drug/Lab Interactions.

DILUTION

Specific techniques required; see Precautions. Improper preparation has resulted in overdose. Must be diluted by a specific 2-step process and given as an infusion. Do not use PVC infusion containers and polyurethane infusion sets for preparation or administration. A clear yellow to brownish-yellow viscous solution.

Step 1: Initially withdraw the **entire contents** of the provided diluent and inject into the vial of cabazitaxel (60 mg/1.5 mL). When transferring the diluent, direct the needle onto the inside wall of the cabazitaxel vial to limit foaming. Gently mix by repeated inversions for at least 45 seconds to ensure full mixing of drug and diluent. Do not shake. Allow to stand for a few seconds to allow most of the foam to dissipate. Should not contain visible particulate matter. Concentration of the resultant dilution is 10 mg/mL. This initially diluted solution should be used immediately but must be used within 30 minutes of entry into the vial.

Step 2: Withdraw the recommended dose from the 10-mg/mL vial of cabazitaxel. Further dilute into a sterile 250-mL PVC-free container of either NS or D5W for infusion. If a dose greater than 65 mg is required, use a larger volume of NS or D5W infusion so a concentration of 0.26 mg/mL is not exceeded. Concentration of the final solution should be between 0.10 and 0.26 mg/mL. Thoroughly mix by gently inverting the bag or bottle.

Filters: Use of a 0.22-micron in-line filter is required for administration (not supplied).

Storage: Before use, store at 25° C (77° F), with excursions permitted between 15° to 30° C (59° to 86° F). Do not refrigerate. Initial diluted solution should be used immediately but must be used within 30 minutes; discard any unused portion. Final infusion solution should be used within 8 hours (including infusion time) at RT or within 24 hours (including infusion time) if refrigerated. Both solutions are supersaturated and may crystallize over time. Discard if crystallization occurs. Discard if either the initial diluted solution or final solution is not clear or appears to have precipitation.

COMPATIBILITY

Manufacturer states, "Do not use PVC infusion containers and polyurethane infusion sets for preparation or administration. Should not be mixed with any other drugs."

RATE OF ADMINISTRATION

A single dose properly diluted as an infusion over 1 hour. Use of a 0.22-micron in-line filter required for administration. See Dilution and Compatibility.

ACTIONS

An antineoplastic belonging to the taxane class. Prepared by semi-synthesis with a precursor extracted from yew needles. A microtubule inhibitor, it binds to tubulin and promotes its assembly into microtubules while simultaneously inhibiting disassembly. This leads to the stabilization of microtubules, which results in the inhibition of mitotic and interphase cellular functions. Highly protein bound (89% to 92%). Equally distributed between blood and plasma. Extensively metabolized in the liver, mainly by the CYP3A4/5 isoenzyme and to a lesser extent by CYP2C8. Terminal half-life is approximately 95 hours. Mainly excreted in feces as numerous metabolites with minimal excretion of unchanged drug in urine.

INDICATIONS AND USES

Treatment of patients with hormone-refractory metastatic prostate cancer previously treated with a docetaxel-containing treatment regimen. Used in combination with oral prednisone.

CONTRAINDICATIONS

Patients with neutrophil counts of equal to or less than 1,500/mm^3. ■ Patients with a history of severe hypersensitivity reactions to cabazitaxel or other drugs formulated with polysorbate 80. ■ Patients with severe hepatic impairment (total bilirubin greater than 3 times the ULN); see Dose Adjustments and Precautions.

PRECAUTIONS

Follow guidelines for handling cytotoxic agents. See Appendix A, p. 1331. ▪ Usually administered by or under the direction of the physician specialist in a facility with adequate diagnostic and treatment facilities to monitor the patient and respond to any medical emergency. ▪ If initial or fully diluted solution should come into contact with the skin or mucus, immediately and thoroughly wash with soap and water. ▪ Bone marrow suppression manifested as neutropenia, anemia, thrombocytopenia, and/or pancytopenia may occur. Neutropenic deaths have been reported. Primary prophylaxis with G-CSF should be considered in high-risk patients (e.g., extensive prior radiation ports, over 65 years of age, poor nutritional status, poor performance status, previous episodes of febrile neutropenia, or other serious comorbidities that may result in increased complications from prolonged neutropenia). Therapeutic use of G-CSF and secondary prophylaxis should be considered in all patients considered to be at increased risk for neutropenia complications. ▪ Use caution in patients with a hemoglobin less than 10 Gm/dL. ▪ Severe hypersensitivity reactions have occurred; all patients are premedicated to reduce the risk and/or severity of a hypersensitivity reaction. Patients with a history of severe hypersensitivity reactions should not be rechallenged with cabazitaxel. ▪ Nausea, vomiting, and severe diarrhea may occur. Deaths related to diarrhea and electrolyte imbalance have occurred. GI hemorrhage and perforation, ileus, enterocolitis, and neutropenic enterocolitis, including fatal outcome, have also been reported. Risk may be increased with neutropenia; age; steroid use; concomitant use of NSAIDs, antiplatelet therapy, or anticoagulants; and patients with a prior history of pelvic radiotherapy, adhesions, ulceration, and GI bleeding; see Drug/Lab Interactions. ▪ Deaths due to renal failure have occurred, and most occurred in association with sepsis, dehydration, or obstructive uropathy. ▪ Use with caution in patients with ESRD. ▪ Use with caution in patients with mild to moderate hepatic impairment; see Dose Adjustments and Contraindications.

Monitor: Obtain baseline CBC with differential and platelets. Monitor weekly during Cycle 1 and before each treatment cycle thereafter. ▪ If febrile neutropenia or prolonged neutropenia (greater than 1 week) occurs despite appropriate medications (e.g., G-CSF), dose reduction is indicated. May not be restarted until the neutrophil count recovers to a level greater than 1,500 cells/mm^3; see Contraindications and Dose Adjustments. ▪ G-CSF may be administered to reduce the risks of neutropenia complications; see Precautions. ▪ Monitor closely for hypersensitivity reactions, especially during the first and second infusions. May occur within the first few minutes, and beginning symptoms may include bronchospasm, generalized rash/erythema, and hypotension. ▪ Obtain baseline and periodic bilirubin and liver function tests. Patients with mild to moderate hepatic impairment should be monitored closely. ▪ Monitor for nausea, vomiting, and diarrhea. Use prophylactic antiemetics to reduce nausea and vomiting and increase patient comfort. Rehydrate and use antidiarrheal medications as indicated. ▪ Monitor for S/S that may indicate serious GI toxicity (e.g., abdominal pain and tenderness, fever, persistent constipation, diarrhea, with or without neutropenia). Evaluate and treat promptly; see Antidote. ▪ Monitor for S/S of impending renal failure (dehydration, reduced urine output). Monitoring of CrCl or SCr may be indicated. ▪ Observe closely for signs of infection. Prophylactic antibiotics may be indicated pending results of C/S in a febrile neutropenic patient. ▪ Monitor for thrombocytopenia (platelet count less than 50,000/mm^3). Initiate precautions to prevent excessive bleeding (e.g., inspect IV sites, skin, and mucous membranes; use extreme care during invasive procedures; test urine, emesis, stool, and secretions for occult blood).

Patient Education: Avoid pregnancy; nonhormonal birth control recommended. ▪ Routine monitoring of blood counts imperative. ▪ Oral prednisone must be taken as prescribed. ▪ Promptly report S/S of a hypersensitivity reaction (e.g., hives, rash, shortness of breath or troubled breathing, swelling of eyelids, lips, or face). ▪ May cause severe and/or fatal infections, dehydration, and renal failure. Take your temperature often and promptly report a fever. ▪ Promptly report burning on urination, cough, decreased urine output, hematuria, muscle aches, and/or significant diarrhea or vomiting. ▪ Drug interactions may occur; review prescription and nonprescription drugs with your physician. ▪ Certain side effects may be more frequent or severe in the elderly. ▪ See Appendix D, p. 1333.

Maternal/Child *(cabazitaxel is not indicated for female patients):* Category D: avoid pregnancy. Can cause fetal harm. ▪ Discontinue breast-feeding. ▪ Safety and effectiveness for use in pediatric patients not established.

Elderly: No overall differences in efficacy were observed. Patients over 65 years of age are more likely to experience fatal outcomes not related to disease progression and certain serious adverse reactions, including neutropenia and febrile neutropenia. The incidence of asthenia, dehydration, dizziness, fatigue, fever, and urinary tract infections was also increased in the elderly.

DRUG/LAB INTERACTIONS
Formal drug interaction studies have not been conducted. ▪ Prednisone administered at 10 mg daily did not affect the pharmacokinetics of cabazitaxel. ▪ Primarily metabolized through CYP3A. Concomitant administration with **strong CYP3A4 inhibitors** (e.g., atazanavir [Reyataz], clarithromycin [Biaxin], indinavir [Crixivan], itraconazole [Sporanox], ketoconazole [Nizoral], nefazodone, nelfinavir [Viracept], ritonavir [Norvir], saquinavir [Invirase], telithromycin [Ketek], and voriconazole [VFEND]) should be avoided if possible. Plasma concentration of cabazitaxel is expected to increase. If concomitant administration is required, consider dose reduction; see Dose Adjustments. ▪ Concomitant administration with **rifampin (Rifadin)**, a strong CYP3A4 inducer, decreased the plasma concentration of cabazitaxel. Although no formal drug interactions have been conducted, it has been recommended that coadministration with **strong CYP3A4 inducers** (e.g., carbamazepine [Tegretol], phenytoin [Dilantin], phenobarbital [Luminal], rifabutin [Mycobutin], rifampin [Rifadin], and rifapentine [Priftin]) be avoided. ▪ Avoid use of **St. John's wort;** may also decrease concentration of cabazitaxel. ▪ Cabazitaxel is not an inhibitor of CYP3A.

SIDE EFFECTS
Abdominal pain, alopecia, anorexia, arthralgia, asthenia, back pain, bone marrow suppression (e.g., anemia, leukopenia, neutropenia, thrombocytopenia), constipation, cough, diarrhea, dysgeusia, dyspnea, fatigue, fever, hematuria, nausea, peripheral neuropathy, and vomiting are most common. Serious side effects include gastrointestinal symptoms, hypersensitivity reactions, infection, neutropenia, febrile neutropenia, and renal failure. Cardiac arrhythmia, dehydration, dizziness, dyspepsia, dysuria, headache, hypotension, mucosal inflammation, muscle spasms, pain, peripheral edema, UTI, and weight loss have also occurred.

Post-Marketing: Gastritis and intestinal obstruction.

Overdose: Exacerbation of adverse reactions such as bone marrow suppression and GI disorders.

ANTIDOTE
Keep physician informed of all side effects. Most will be treated symptomatically as indicated. Minor hypersensitivity reactions may subside with temporary discontinuation of cabazitaxel and additional antihistamines, corticosteroids, or H₂ antagonists. Reduction in rate of administration may allow continued treatment. Discontinue immediately if severe hypersensitivity reactions occur, and administer appropriate therapy. Neutropenia can be profound but may be treated with filgrastim (Neupogen, Zarxio). Severe thrombocytopenia may require platelet transfusions. Severe anemia (less than 8 Gm/dL) may require packed cell transfusions; moderate anemia (less than 11 Gm/dL) may be treated with darbepoetin alfa (Aranesp) or epoetin alfa (Epogen). Severe GI toxicity may require cabazitaxel treatment delay or discontinuation. Discontinue cabazitaxel for Grade 3 or higher peripheral neuropathy or if adverse reactions continue after the dose adjustment to 20 mg/M². There is no specific antidote for overdose. Administer G-CSF as soon as possible and closely monitor chemistry, vital signs, and other functions. Resuscitate if indicated.

CAFFEINE CITRATE
(**KAF**-feen **SIT**-rayt)

Cafcit

CNS stimulant
Respiratory stimulant adjunct

pH 4.7

PEDIATRIC DOSE
The dose expressed as caffeine base is one half the dose when expressed as caffeine citrate. The recommended loading dose and maintenance dose are listed in the following chart.

Guidelines for Loading and Maintenance Doses of Caffeine Citrate		
	Dose of Cafcit (volume)	Dose Expressed as Caffeine Citrate
Loading dose	1 mL/kg	20 mg/kg for 1 dose
Maintenance dose	0.25 mL/kg	5 mg/kg every 24 hours

Begin maintenance dose 24 hours after loading dose. Maintenance dose may be given IV or orally. Duration of treatment beyond 10 to 12 days has not been studied. See Precautions.

DOSE ADJUSTMENTS
May adjust maintenance dose using serum concentrations of caffeine. ▪ To avoid toxicity in neonates with impaired renal or hepatic function, use with caution and monitor serum concentrations.

DILUTION
Both the IV and the oral doses are supplied in vials containing 60 mg/3 mL of caffeine citrate (30 mg/3 mL of caffeine base). Confirm vial is for IV use. Withdraw calculated dose and dilute with sufficient D5W to administer at the recommended rate of administration.

Storage: Store at CRT. Single-use vial. Discard any unused solution. Stable for 24 hours at room temperature when mixed with any of the solutions listed by the manufacturer in Compatibility.

COMPATIBILITY
Consider any drug NOT listed as compatible to be INCOMPATIBLE until consulting a pharmacist; specific conditions may apply.

Solution: Manufacturer lists D5W; another source adds D5/¹/4NS, D5/¹/4NS with 20 mEq KCl/L.

Additive: Manufacturer lists amino acid solution 8.5% (Aminosyn 8.5%), calcium gluconate 10%, D5W, dextrose 50%, dopamine 40 mg/mL diluted to 0.6 mg/mL with D5W, fentanyl 50 mcg/mL diluted to 10 mcg/mL with D5W, heparin sodium 1,000 units/mL diluted to 1 unit/mL with D5W, IV fat emulsion 20% (Intralipid 20%).

One source suggests the following **compatibilities:**

Y-site: Dopamine, doxapram (Dopram), fentanyl, heparin, levofloxacin (Levaquin).

RATE OF ADMINISTRATION
Use of a syringe pump infuser is recommended.

Loading dose: Infuse over 30 minutes.

Maintenance dose: Infuse over 10 minutes.

ACTIONS
A bronchial smooth muscle relaxant, a CNS and cardiac stimulant, and a diuretic. Structurally related to other methylxanthines (e.g., theophylline and theobromine). Exact mechanism of action in apnea of prematurity is not known. Postulated mechanisms include stimulation of the respiratory center, increased minute ventilation, decreased threshold to hypercapnia, increased response to hypercapnia, increased skeletal muscle

tone, decreased diaphragmatic fatigue, increased metabolic rate, increased oxygen consumption, blood vessel dilatation, central vessel vasoconstriction, and smooth muscle relaxation. Readily distributes into the brain. Caffeine levels in the CSF of preterm neonates approximate plasma levels. Metabolized in the liver by the cytochrome P_{450} system. Metabolism and elimination in the preterm neonate are much slower than in adults due to immature hepatic and/or renal function. Mean half-life and fraction excreted unchanged in the urine is inversely related to gestational/postconceptual age. In neonates, the half-life is approximately 3 to 4 days and the fraction excreted unchanged in the urine is approximately 86% (within 6 days). By 9 months of age, the metabolism of caffeine approximates that seen in adults (half-life is 5 hours and amount excreted unchanged is 1%). Interconversion between caffeine and theophylline has been reported in preterm neonates. After theophylline administration, caffeine levels are approximately 25% of theophylline levels. After caffeine administration, 3% to 5% of caffeine administered converts to theophylline.

INDICATIONS AND USES
Short-term treatment of apnea of prematurity in infants more than 28 but less than 33 weeks' gestational age. In one study apnea of prematurity was defined as having at least 6 apnea episodes of more than 20 seconds' duration in a 24-hour period with no other identifiable cause of apnea.
Unlabeled uses: Prevention of postoperative apnea in former preterm infants.

CONTRAINDICATIONS
Hypersensitivity to any of its components.

PRECAUTIONS
Reports in the literature suggest a possible association between the use of methylxanthines and the development of necrotizing enterocolitis. Necrotizing enterocolitis, resulting in death in some cases, has been reported in neonates receiving caffeine citrate. ▪ Apnea of prematurity is a diagnosis of exclusion. Other causes of apnea (e.g., CNS disorders, primary lung disease, anemia, sepsis, metabolic disturbances, cardiovascular abnormalities, or obstructive apnea) should be ruled out or properly treated before initiating therapy with caffeine citrate. ▪ Is a CNS stimulant. Use with caution in infants with seizure disorders. ▪ May increase heart rate, left ventricular output, and stroke volume. Use with caution in infants with cardiovascular disease. ▪ Duration of treatment of apnea of prematurity in trials has been limited to 10 to 12 days. Safety and efficacy of therapy beyond this time have not been established. ▪ Safety and efficacy for use in prophylactic treatment of sudden infant death syndrome (SIDS) or before extubation in mechanically ventilated infants have not been established. ▪ Use with caution in infants with impaired renal or hepatic function; see Dose Adjustments and Monitor. ▪ Patients sensitive to other xanthines (e.g., aminophylline) may also be sensitive to caffeine.
Monitor: Obtain baseline serum caffeine levels in infants previously treated with theophylline because preterm infants metabolize theophylline to caffeine; see Actions. Levels should also be obtained in infants born to mothers who ingested caffeine before delivery, as caffeine readily crosses the placenta. Caffeine levels ranged from 8 to 40 mg/L in clinical trials. A therapeutic plasma concentration range has not been determined, but one source suggests 5 to 25 mcg/mL. Serious toxicity has been reported at levels exceeding 50 mg/L. Monitor levels periodically during treatment to avoid toxicity. Monitoring is especially important in infants with impaired renal or hepatic function; see Dose Adjustments. ▪ Monitor serum glucose periodically. Hypoglycemia and hyperglycemia have been reported. ▪ Monitor for S/S of necrotizing enterocolitis (e.g., gastric distension, vomiting, bloody stools). Screening stools for occult blood may be helpful in identifying early-onset necrotizing enterocolitis.
Patient Education: Caregivers should be instructed to consult physician if infant continues to have apnea events and to not increase the dose of caffeine citrate without consulting a physician. ▪ Contact physician at the first sign of lethargy or GI intolerance (e.g., ab-

dominal distension, vomiting, or bloody stools). ▪ Dose must be accurately measured, and any unused solution must be discarded.

Maternal/Child: Category C: no controlled studies; benefits should outweigh risks. ▪ Half-life is increased in pregnant women. ▪ Half-life may be in excess of 100 hours in infants under 6 months of age due to immature liver function.

DRUG/LAB INTERACTIONS

Metabolized by the cytochrome P_{450} system. Lower caffeine doses may be required with coadministration of medications that **inhibit the P_{450} system,** decreasing the elimination of caffeine (e.g., cimetidine [Tagamet] and ketoconazole [Nizoral]). Higher caffeine doses may be needed with coadministration of medications that **induce the P_{450} system,** increasing the elimination of caffeine (e.g., phenobarbital and phenytoin). ▪ Interconversion between caffeine and **theophylline** has been reported. Concurrent use of these drugs is not recommended; see Actions.

SIDE EFFECTS

Cardiovascular effects (e.g., tachycardia, increased left ventricular output, and increased stroke volume), CNS stimulation (e.g., irritability, jitteriness, restlessness), GI effects (e.g., feeding intolerance, gastritis, increased gastric aspirate, and necrotizing enterocolitis), hyperglycemia, hypoglycemia, renal effects (e.g., increased urine output, increased CrCl, and increased sodium and calcium excretion).

Overdose: Signs and symptoms of caffeine overdose in the preterm infant may include: elevated BUN, elevated total leukocyte concentration, fever, fine tremor of extremities, hyperglycemia, hypertonia, insomnia, jitteriness, nonpurposeful jaw and lip movements, opisthotonos, seizures, tachypnea, tonic-clonic movements, or vomiting.

ANTIDOTE

Notify the physician of any side effects. Treatment of overdose is primarily symptomatic and supportive. Seizures may be treated with intravenous administration of diazepam (Valium) or a barbiturate such as pentobarbital (Nembutal). Caffeine levels have been shown to decrease after exchange transfusions. Resuscitate as necessary.

CALCITRIOL   Vitamin D
(kal-si-**TRYE**-ole)

Calcijex   pH 5.9 to 7

USUAL DOSE

Effectiveness of calcitriol therapy is dependent on adequate daily intake of calcium. The RDA of calcium in adults is 800 mg. Calcium supplementation or proper dietary measures must be initiated and maintained.

Hypocalcemia and/or secondary hyperparathyroidism: Recommended initial dose, depending on the severity of hypocalcemia and/or secondary hyperparathyroidism, is 1 mcg (0.02 mcg/kg) to 2 mcg administered at each hemodialysis treatment (three times weekly, approximately every other day). Initial doses have ranged from 0.5 to 4 mcg three times weekly.

Information supplied by the manufacturer suggests that the relative dosing of paricalcitol to calcitriol is 4:1. When converting a patient from calcitriol to paricalcitol, the initial dose of paricalcitol should be four times greater than the patient's dose of calcitriol.

PEDIATRIC DOSE

Hypocalcemia in end-stage renal disease (ESRD) (unlabeled): 0.01 to 0.05 mcg/kg/dose given 3 times a week; see Maternal/Child. See all comments under Usual Dose.

DOSE ADJUSTMENTS

Adjust dosing based on patient response. Begin dosing at lower end of dose range in the elderly; see Elderly. If a satisfactory response is not observed, dose may be increased by 0.5 to 1 mcg at 2- to 4-week intervals. Monitor serum calcium, phosphorus, and calcium $\times$ phosphorus product (Ca $\times$ P) frequently during any dose adjustment period; see Monitor. ■ Discontinue therapy if elevated calcium level or a Ca $\times$ P product of greater than 70 is noted. Re-initiate therapy at a lower dose when parameters normalize. ■ Calcitriol dose may need to be reduced as the parathyroid hormone (PTH) levels decrease in response to therapy. The currently accepted target range for intact parathyroid hormone (iPTH) in chronic renal failure (CRF) patients is no more than 1.5 to 3 times the non-uremic upper limit of normal. Incremental dosing must be individualized and commensurate with PTH, serum calcium, and phosphorus levels. The following chart is a suggested approach to dose titration.

Calcitriol Suggested Dosing Guidelines	
PTH Levels	Calcitriol Dose
The same or increasing	Increase
Decreasing by <30%	Increase
Decreasing by >30% but <60%	Maintain
Decreasing by >60%	Decrease
One and one-half to three times the upper limit of normal	Maintain

DILUTION

May be given undiluted. Available in 1-mcg/mL ampules.

Storage: Store ampules at CRT. Protect from light. Calcitriol may be drawn up into a syringe up to 8 hours before administration but must be protected from direct sunlight.

COMPATIBILITY

Y-site: D5W, NS, SWFI.

RATE OF ADMINISTRATION

Administer as a bolus dose into the venous line at the end of hemodialysis.

ACTIONS

The active form of vitamin D_3 (cholecalciferol). Must be metabolically activated in liver and kidney before it is fully active on its target tissues. In bone, acts with PTH to stimulate resorption of calcium. In kidneys, increases tubular reabsorption of calcium. Stimulates intestinal calcium transport and directly suppresses synthesis and release of PTH from the parathyroid gland. A vitamin D–resistant state may exist in uremic patients because of the failure of the kidney to adequately convert precursors to the active compound, calcitriol. Duration of action is 3 to 5 days.

INDICATIONS AND USES

Management of hypocalcemia in patients undergoing chronic renal dialysis. Has been shown to significantly reduce elevated PTH levels, which results in improvement in renal osteodystrophy.

CONTRAINDICATIONS

Patients with hypercalcemia or evidence of vitamin D toxicity.

PRECAUTIONS

Because calcitriol is the most potent form of vitamin D available, oral vitamin D supplements should be discontinued during treatment. ■ Dietary phosphorus should be restricted and a non–aluminum phosphate–binding compound (e.g., calcium acetate [PhosLo], sevelamer [Renagel]) should be administered to control serum phosphorus levels in patients undergoing dialysis.

Monitor: Obtain baseline serum calcium, phosphorus, aluminum, albumin, and PTH assays. ■ Serum calcium levels should be corrected for serum albumin using the following equation: Corrected Ca = observed Ca + 0.8 × (normal albumin − observed albumin). For example: If serum calcium is 7 mg/dL and observed albumin is 2.5 Gm/dL, Corrected Ca = 7 + 0.8 × (4 − 2.5) = 8.2 mg/dL. All decisions regarding therapy should be based on corrected calcium values. ▪ Monitor magnesium, alkaline phosphatase, and 24-hour urinary calcium and phosphorus periodically. ▪ Criteria used to determine if calcitriol should be administered include: serum calcium less than 11.5 mg/dL, Ca × P less than 70, serum albumin less than 60 mcg/L (within normal limits), and PTH more than 3 times the upper limit of normal. ▪ Serum calcium, phosphorus, and the Ca × P product should be monitored twice weekly during dose titration. Once stable, decrease monitoring to once monthly. See Dose Adjustments. ▪ PTH levels, once stable, should be monitored every 3 months. Adynamic bone lesions may develop if PTH levels are suppressed to abnormal levels. If PTH levels fall below the target range (1.5 to 3 times the upper limit of normal), the calcitriol dose should be reduced. Discontinuation may result in rebound effect. Therefore gradual titration downward to a new maintenance dose is recommended; see Dose Adjustments. ▪ Overdosage of vitamin D is dangerous. May induce hypercalcemia and/or hypercalciuria. If clinically significant hypercalcemia develops, dose should be reduced or held. Chronic hypercalcemia can lead to generalized vascular calcification, nephrocalcinosis, and other soft-tissue calcification. The serum Ca × P product should not be allowed to exceed 70. Radiographic evaluation of suspect anatomic regions may be useful in early detection of this condition; see Side Effects and Antidote. ▪ Use with caution in patients receiving digoxin. Hypercalcemia may precipitate cardiac arrhythmias; see Drug/Lab Interactions.

Patient Education: Report symptoms of hypercalcemia promptly. Dose adjustment or treatment may be required. Strict adherence to dietary supplementation of calcium and restriction of phosphorus is required to ensure optimal effectiveness of therapy. Phosphate-binding compounds (e.g., calcium acetate [PhosLo]) may be needed to control serum phosphorus levels in patients with CRF, but excessive use of aluminum-containing products (e.g., aluminum hydroxide gel [Alternagel]) should be avoided. ▪ Avoid use of unapproved nonprescription medications, including magnesium-containing antacids.

Maternal/Child: Category C: safety for use in pregnancy not established. Benefits must outweigh risks. ▪ Safety for use in breast-feeding not established. A decision should be made whether to discontinue nursing or to discontinue the drug. ▪ Safety and effectiveness have been studied in a small number of pediatric patients, ages 13 to 18 years, with ESRD on hemodialysis. The mean weekly dose ranged from 1 to 1.4 mcg. Use in this study program appeared to be safe and effective. See package insert for study information.

Elderly: Begin dosing at lower end of dose range. Consider age-related organ impairment, concomitant disease, and/or drug therapy; see Dose Adjustments.

DRUG/LAB INTERACTIONS

Specific interaction studies have not been performed. ▪ **Digoxin** toxicity is potentiated by hypercalcemia. Use caution when calcitriol is prescribed concomitantly with digoxin compounds. ▪ **Phosphate or vitamin D–related compounds** should not be taken concomitantly with calcitriol. ▪ **Magnesium-containing antacids** and calcitriol should not be used concomitantly. Hypermagnesemia may result.

SIDE EFFECTS

Overdose or chronic administration may lead to hypercalcemia, hypercalciuria, and hyperphosphatemia. High intake of calcium and phosphate concomitant with calcitriol therapy may lead to similar abnormalities. Signs and symptoms of vitamin D intoxication associated with hypercalcemia include *Early:* bone pain, constipation, dry mouth, headache, metallic taste, muscle pain, nausea, somnolence, vomiting, and weakness. *Late:* albuminuria, anorexia, cardiac arrhythmias, conjunctivitis (calcific), decreased libido, ectopic calcification, elevated AST and ALT, elevated BUN, hypercholesterolemia, hypertension, hyperthermia, nocturia, overt psychosis (rare), pain at injection site, pancreatitis, photophobia, polydipsia, polyuria, pruritus, rhinorrhea, and weight loss. Rare cases of hypersensitivity reactions, including anaphylaxis, have been reported.

ANTIDOTE

Notify physician of any side effects. Treatment of patients with clinically significant hypercalcemia (more than 1 mg/dL above the upper limit of normal range) consists of supportive measures, immediate dose reduction or interruption of therapy, initiation of a low-calcium diet, withdrawal of calcium supplements, patient mobilization, attention to fluid and electrolyte imbalances, assessment of electrocardiographic abnormalities (critical in patients receiving digoxin), and hemodialysis or peritoneal dialysis against a calcium-free dialysate, as warranted. Hypercalcemia usually resolves in 2 to 7 days. Monitor serum calcium levels frequently until calcium levels return to within normal limits. May re-initiate calcitriol therapy at a dose 0.5 mcg less than prior dose. See Dose Adjustments.

CALCIUM CHLORIDE
(**KAL**-see-um **KLOR**-eyed)

Electrolyte replenisher
Antihypocalcemic
Cardiotonic
Antihyperkalemic
Antihypermagnesemic

pH 5.5 to 7.5

USUAL DOSE

*In a 10% solution, 10 mL (1 Gm) contains 13.6 mEq (272 mg) of calcium; 1 mL (100 mg), 1.36 mEq (27.2 mg). **All doses based on a 10% solution.***

Hypocalcemic disorders (prophylaxis, treatment, electrolyte replacement, maintenance): 5 to 10 mL (500 mg to 1 Gm) at intervals of 1 to 3 days. Repeat doses may be required and are based on patient response or serum calcium levels. May be given as part of a TPN program.

Magnesium intoxication: 5 mL (500 mg). Observe for signs of recovery before giving any additional calcium.

Hyperkalemia ECG disturbances of cardiac function: 1 to 10 mL (100 mg to 1 Gm); titrate dose by monitoring ECG changes. AHA guidelines recommend 5 to 10 mL of a 10% solution (500 mg to 1 Gm). Repeat as needed.

Cardiac resuscitation (see Indications for specific uses): 0.02 to 0.04 mL/kg (2 to 4 mg/kg); repeat at 10-minute intervals as indicated or as measured by serum deficits of calcium. Consider need for calcium (usually gluconate or gluceptate) for every 500 mL of whole blood if arrest occurs in a situation requiring copious blood replacement.

Overdose of calcium channel blockers or beta adrenergic blockers (unlabeled): AHA guidelines recommend 5 to 10 mL of a 10% solution (500 mg to 1 Gm). May repeat as needed.

PEDIATRIC DOSE

Do not administer into a scalp vein in pediatric patients; see Precautions, Monitor, and Maternal/Child.

Hypocalcemic disorders: 0.027 to 0.05 mL/kg of body weight (2.7 to 5 mg/kg) of a 10% solution. Up to 10 mL (1 Gm)/day may be required. No data from clinical trials are available regarding repeat doses. Sources suggest repeat doses every 4 to 6 hours based on patient response or serum calcium levels.

Cardiac resuscitation (see Indications for specific uses): 0.2 mL/kg of a 10% solution (20 mg/kg). Repeat as indicated at 10-minute intervals. AHA guidelines recommend consideration of this dose for documented or suspected hypocalcemia or hyperkalemia as well as for hypomagnesemia and calcium channel blocker overdose.

DILUTION

May be given undiluted, but preferably diluted with an equal amount of SWFI or NS for injection to make a 5% solution. Solution should be warmed to body temperature. May be further diluted with most common infusion solutions and given as an intermittent or continuous infusion.

COMPATIBILITY (Underline Indicates Conflicting Compatibility Information)
Consider any drug NOT listed as compatible to be INCOMPATIBLE until consulting a pharmacist; specific conditions may apply.

Calcium salts not generally mixed with carbonates, phosphates, sulfates, or tartrates. *Extreme caution and a specific multistep process are required when calcium and phosphates are combined in parenteral nutrition solutions. Consult pharmacist.*

One source suggests the following **compatibilities:**

Additive: Amikacin, ascorbic acid, chloramphenicol (Chloromycetin), dobutamine, dopamine, hydrocortisone sodium succinate (Solu-Cortef), isoproterenol (Isuprel), lidocaine, magnesium sulfate, norepinephrine (Levophed), penicillin G potassium and sodium, pentobarbital (Nembutal), phenobarbital (Luminal), sodium bicarbonate, verapamil.

Y-site: Amiodarone (Nexterone), ceftaroline (Teflaro), dobutamine, doxapram (Dopram), epinephrine (Adrenalin), esmolol (Brevibloc), 6% hydroxyethyl starch (Voluven), micafungin (Mycamine), milrinone (Primacor), morphine, nitroprusside sodium (Nitropress), paclitaxel (Taxol).

RATE OF ADMINISTRATION
0.5 to 1 mL of solution over 1 minute. Administration into a central or deep vein is preferred; see Monitor. Stop or slow infusion rate if patient complains of discomfort. Do not exceed the equivalent of 1 mL calcium chloride/minute by IV injection or infusion. Rapid administration may cause bradycardia; heat waves; local burning sensation; metallic, calcium, or chalky taste; moderate drop in BP; peripheral vasodilation; or a sense of oppression.

ACTIONS
Calcium is a basic element prevalent in the human body. It affects bones, nerves, muscles, glands, cardiac and vascular tone, and normal coagulation of the blood. It is excreted in the urine and feces.

INDICATIONS AND USES
Calcium preparations other than calcium chloride are often preferred except in cardiac resuscitation or calcium channel blocker toxicity. ■ Increase plasma calcium levels in hypocalcemic disorders (e.g., tetany [neonatal, parathyroid deficiency], vitamin D deficiency, alkalosis, conditions associated with intestinal malabsorption). ■ Treat ECG disturbances caused by hyperkalemia. ■ Adjunctive therapy in sensitivity reactions (especially with urticaria), insect bites or stings (relieve muscle cramping), acute symptoms of lead colic, rickets, or osteomalacia. ■ Cardiac resuscitation only to treat hypocalcemia, hyperkalemia, or calcium-channel blocker toxicity (verapamil, diltiazem), or after open heart surgery if epinephrine does not produce effective myocardial contractions. ■ Antidote for cardiac and respiratory depression of magnesium sulfate toxicity.

Unlabeled uses: Treatment of arrhythmias and/or hypotension caused by an overdose of calcium channel blockers (e.g., diltiazem [Cardizem], verapamil) or beta-adrenergic blockers (e.g., atenolol [Tenormin], metoprolol [Lopressor], propranolol). ■ Prevention of hypotension caused by calcium channel blockers.

CONTRAINDICATIONS
Digitalized patients, hypercalcemia, ventricular fibrillation. Not recommended in the treatment of asystole and electromechanical dissociation.

PRECAUTIONS
Three times more potent than calcium gluconate. ■ For IV use only. ■ See Drug/Lab Interactions.

Monitor: Confirm patency of vein; select a large vein and use a small needle to reduce vein irritation. Administration into a central or deep vein is preferred. Necrosis and sloughing will occur with IM or SC injection or extravasation. ■ Keep patient recumbent after injection to prevent postural hypotension. ■ Monitor vital signs carefully. ■ Monitor serum calcium levels as indicated. May cause hyperchloremic acidosis.

Maternal/Child: Category C: safety for use in pregnancy and breast-feeding not established. Use only when clearly needed. ▪ Rarely used IV in pediatric patients. Use of a less irritating salt preferred because of small vein size.

DRUG/LAB INTERACTIONS

Will increase **digoxin** toxicity and may cause arrhythmias. If necessary, give small amounts very slowly. ▪ Potentiated by **thiazide diuretics** (e.g., chlorothiazide [Diuril]); may cause hypercalcemia or calcium toxicity. ▪ May reduce plasma levels of **atenolol** (Tenormin). ▪ Can reduce neuromuscular paralysis and respiratory depression produced by **antibiotics such as kanamycin.** ▪ Antagonizes **verapamil;** can reverse clinical effects. ▪ May cause metabolic alkalosis and inhibit binding of potassium with **sodium polystyrene sulfonate.**

SIDE EFFECTS

Usual doses will produce a local burning sensation, moderate drop in BP, and peripheral vasodilation. May cause bradycardia; cardiac arrest; heat waves; metallic, calcium, or chalky taste; prolonged state of cardiac contraction; sense of oppression; or tingling sensation, especially with a too-rapid rate of administration.

Overdose: Coma, intractable nausea and vomiting, lethargy, markedly elevated plasma calcium level, weakness, and sudden death.

ANTIDOTE

If side effects occur, further dilution and decrease in the rate of administration may be necessary. If side effects persist, discontinue the drug and notify the physician. IV infusion of sodium chloride (to maintain normovolemia) and furosemide (Lasix) 80 to 100 mg IV every 2 to 4 hours (with caution) is recommended in overdose. Sodium chloride competes with calcium for reabsorption in the renal tubules; furosemide enhances the activity. Together they will reduce hypercalcemia by causing a marked increase in calcium excretion. Monitoring of fluid, electrolytes, and cardiac and respiratory status is imperative. Disodium edetate may be used with extreme caution as a calcium chelating agent if overdose is critical. For extravasation inject affected area with 1% procaine hydrochloride and hyaluronidase to reduce venospasm and dilute calcium. Use a 27- or 25-gauge needle. Warm, moist compresses may be helpful. Resuscitate as necessary.

CALCIUM GLUCONATE
(**KAL**-see-um **GLOO**-koh-nayt)

Electrolyte replenisher
Antihypocalcemic
Cardiotonic
Antihyperkalemic
Antihypermagnesemic

pH 6 to 8.2

USUAL DOSE
All doses based on a 10% solution, which yields 10 Gm/100 mL or 100 mg/mL.
Hypocalcemia disorders/maintenance: 2 to 15 Gm/24 hr in divided doses every 6 hours (0.5 to 3.75 Gm every 6 hours). Larger amounts may be given as an intermittent or continuous IV infusion. 10 mL (1 Gm in a 10% solution) contains 4.65 mEq (93 mg) of calcium.
Cardiac resuscitation (see Indications for specific uses): 500 to 800 mg/dose. Repeat at 10-minute intervals as indicated by clinical condition or serum calcium level.
Hypocalcemic tetany: 1 to 3 Gm IV over 10 to 30 minutes; repeat in 6 hours if indicated.
Magnesium intoxication: 500 to 800 mg/dose (maximum dose 3 Gm). Repeat as indicated by patient response; observe for signs of recovery before giving additional calcium.
Hypocalcemia secondary to citrated blood infusion: 500 mg to 1 Gm/500 mL of citrated blood (infuse into another vein).

PEDIATRIC DOSE
Do not administer into a scalp vein in pediatric patients; see Precautions/Monitor. *All doses based on a 10% solution.*
Hypocalcemia disorders/maintenance: 200 to 500 mg/kg/24 hr in divided doses every 6 hours (50 to 125 mg/kg [0.5 to 1.25 mL/kg] every 6 hours).
Hypocalcemic tetany: 100 to 200 mg/kg/dose (1 to 2 mL/kg) IV over 5 to 10 minutes. Repeat dose 6 hours later if indicated. Maximum dose 500 mg/kg/24 hr.
Cardiac resuscitation (see Indications for specific uses): 100 mg/kg/dose (1 mL/kg/dose) IV every 10 minutes. AHA guidelines recommend 0.6 to 1 mL/kg of a 10% solution (60 to 100 mg/kg). Repeat if indicated. AHA guidelines recommend consideration of this dose for documented or suspected hypocalcemia or hyperkalemia as well as for hypomagnesemia and calcium channel blocker overdose.

NEONATAL DOSE
Do not administer into a scalp vein in neonates; see Precautions/Monitor.
Hypocalcemia disorders/maintenance: 200 to 800 mg/kg/24 hr in divided doses every 6 hours (50 to 200 mg/kg/dose [0.5 to 2 mL/kg/dose] every 6 hours).
Hypocalcemic tetany: 100 to 200 mg/kg/dose (1 to 2 mL/kg) IV over 5 to 10 minutes. Repeat dose 6 hours later if indicated; maximum dose 500 mg/kg/24 hr.

DILUTION
May be given undiluted or may be further diluted in up to 1,000 mL of NS for infusion. Solution should be warmed to body temperature. Solution must be clear and free of crystals. Crystals can be dissolved by heating to 80° C (146° F) in a dry heat oven for at least 1 hour. Shake vigorously; cool to room temperature. Discard if crystals persist.
Pediatric and neonatal dilution: Must be further diluted with NS.

COMPATIBILITY
(Underline Indicates Conflicting Compatibility Information)
Consider any drug NOT listed as compatible to be INCOMPATIBLE until consulting a pharmacist; specific conditions may apply.
Calcium salts not generally mixed with carbonates, phosphates, sulfates, or tartrates.
Extreme caution and a specific multistep process are required when calcium and phosphates are combined in parenteral nutrition solutions. Consult pharmacist.
    One source suggests the following **compatibilities:**
Additive: Amikacin, aminophylline, ascorbic acid, chloramphenicol (Chloromycetin), furosemide (Lasix), heparin, hydrocortisone sodium succinate (Solu-Cortef), lidocaine,

magnesium sulfate, norepinephrine (Levophed), penicillin G potassium and sodium, phenobarbital (Luminal), potassium chloride (KCl), prochlorperazine (Compazine), to-bramycin, vancomycin, verapamil.

Y-site: Aldesleukin (Proleukin), allopurinol (Aloprim), amifostine (Ethyol), amiodarone (Nexterone), ampicillin, aztreonam (Azactam), bivalirudin (Angiomax), cefazolin (Ancef), ceftaroline (Teflaro), ciprofloxacin (Cipro IV), cisatracurium (Nimbex), cladribine (Leustatin), dexmedetomidine (Precedex), dobutamine, docetaxel (Taxotere), doripenem (Doribax), doxapram (Dopram), doxorubicin liposomal (Doxil), enalaprilat (Vasotec IV), epinephrine (Adrenalin), etoposide phosphate (Etopophos), famotidine (Pepcid IV), fenoldopam (Corlopam), filgrastim (Neupogen), gemcitabine (Gemzar), granisetron (Kytril), heparin, hetastarch in electrolytes (Hextend), hydrocortisone sodium succinate (Solu-Cortef), 6% hydroxyethyl starch (Voluven), labetalol, linezolid (Zyvox), melpha-lan (Alkeran), meropenem (Merrem IV), micafungin (Mycamine), midazolam (Versed), milrinone (Primacor), nicardipine (Cardene IV), oxaliplatin (Eloxatin), piperacillin/tazobactam (Zosyn), potassium chloride (KCl), prochlorperazine (Compazine), propofol (Diprivan), remifentanil (Ultiva), sargramostim (Leukine), tacrolimus (Prograf), tela-vancin (Vibativ), teniposide (Vumon), thiotepa, vinorelbine (Navelbine).

RATE OF ADMINISTRATION

In all situations stop or slow infusion rate if patient complains of discomfort. Rapid ad-ministration may cause vasodilation, decreased BP, cardiac arrhythmias, syncope, and cardiac arrest.

IV injection: Undiluted, each 0.5 mL or fraction thereof over 1 minute. Do not exceed 1 mL/min (100 mg). 100 mg over 10 to 20 seconds in cardiac arrest.

Intermittent IV: Do not exceed a rate of 100 mg/min (IV injection rate).

Infusion: Do not exceed 120 to 240 mg/kg/hr with a maximum concentration of 50 mg/mL.

Pediatric and neonatal rate of administration: Slow rate of administration considerably. Ob-serve continuously.

ACTIONS

Calcium is a basic element prevalent in the human body. It affects bones, nerves, glands, cardiac and vascular tone, and normal coagulation of the blood. It crosses the placental barrier and is secreted in breast milk. It is excreted in the urine and feces.

INDICATIONS AND USES

Increase plasma calcium levels in hypocalcemic disorders (e.g., tetany [neonatal, para-thyroid deficiency], vitamin D deficiency, alkalosis, conditions associated with intestinal malabsorption). ▪ Adjunctive therapy in sensitivity reactions (especially with urticaria), insect bites or stings (relieves muscle cramping), acute symptoms of lead colic, rickets, or osteomalacia. ▪ Cardiac resuscitation only to treat hypocalcemia, hyperkalemia, or calcium-channel blocker overdose (verapamil, diltiazem). ▪ Antidote for cardiac and respiratory depression of magnesium sulfate toxicity. ▪ Prevention of hypocalcemia during exchange transfusions. ▪ Decrease capillary permeability in allergic conditions, nonthrombocytopenic purpura, and exudative dermatoses (e.g., dermatitis herpetifor-mis). ▪ Treat pruritus of eruptions caused by drugs. ▪ Treat ECG disturbances caused by hyperkalemia or verapamil-induced hypotension.

Unlabeled uses: Treatment of verapamil overdose, acute hypotension from verapamil, and prevention of initial hypotension when it could be detrimental to a specific patient and verapamil is required.

CONTRAINDICATIONS

IM use in infants and small children. Digitalized patients, hypercalcemia, ventricular fibrillation.

PRECAUTIONS

Has only one third the potency of calcium chloride. ▪ For IV use only; IM use permitted in adults only if IV administration cannot be accomplished; see Monitor.

Monitor: Confirm patency of vein; select a large vein and use a small needle to reduce vein irritation. Local necrosis and abscess formation can occur with IM or SC injection or

extravasation. ▪ Keep patient recumbent after injection to prevent postural hypotension. ▪ Monitor vital signs carefully.
Maternal/Child: Category C: safety for use in pregnancy not established; benefits must outweigh risk. ▪ See Contraindications.

DRUG/LAB INTERACTIONS
Will increase **digoxin** toxicity and may cause arrhythmias. If necessary, give small amounts very slowly. ▪ Potentiated by **thiazide diuretics** (e.g., chlorothiazide [Diuril]); may cause hypercalcemia or calcium toxicity. ▪ May reduce plasma levels of **atenolol** (Tenormin). ▪ Antagonizes **verapamil;** can reverse clinical effects. ▪ May cause metabolic alkalosis and inhibit binding of potassium with **sodium polystyrene sulfonate.**

SIDE EFFECTS
Rare when given as recommended: bradycardia; cardiac arrest; cardiac arrhythmias; heat waves; hypotension; metallic, calcium, or chalky taste; sense of oppression; syncope; tingling; and vasodilation can occur with too-rapid rate of administration. Depression of neuromuscular function, flushing, prolonged state of cardiac contraction can occur.
Overdose: Coma, intractable nausea and vomiting, lethargy, markedly elevated plasma calcium level, weakness, and sudden death.

ANTIDOTE
If side effects occur, further dilution and decrease in the rate of administration may be necessary. If side effects persist, discontinue the drug and notify the physician. IV infusion of sodium chloride (to maintain normovolemia) and furosemide (Lasix) 80 to 100 mg IV every 2 to 4 hours (with caution) is recommended in overdose. Sodium chloride competes with calcium for reabsorption in the renal tubules; furosemide enhances the activity. Together they will reduce hypercalcemia by causing a marked increase in calcium excretion. Monitoring of fluid, electrolytes, and cardiac and respiratory status is imperative. Disodium edetate may be used with extreme caution as a calcium chelating agent if overdosage is critical. For extravasation inject affected area with 1% procaine hydrochloride and hyaluronidase to reduce venospasm and dilute calcium. Use a 27- or 25-gauge needle. Warm, moist compresses may be helpful. Resuscitate as necessary.

CANGRELOR

Antiplatelet agent

(**KAN**-grel-or)

Kengreal

USUAL DOSE

Cangrelor: 30 mcg/kg as an IV *bolus* followed immediately by a 4 mcg/kg/min IV infusion. Initiate the bolus infusion prior to percutaneous coronary intervention (PCI). The maintenance infusion should ordinarily be continued for at least 2 hours or for the duration of PCI, whichever is longer.

Transitioning to oral P2Y$_{12}$ therapy: To maintain platelet inhibition after discontinuation of cangrelor infusion, an oral P2Y$_{12}$ platelet inhibitor should be administered. Administer one as described below:

Ticagrelor (Brilinta): 180 mg at any time during cangrelor infusion or immediately after discontinuation.

Prasugrel (Effient): 60 mg immediately after discontinuation of cangrelor. Do not administer prasugrel before discontinuation of cangrelor.

Clopidogrel (Plavix): 600 mg immediately after discontinuation of cangrelor. Do not administer clopidogrel before discontinuation of cangrelor.

DOSE ADJUSTMENTS

No dose adjustments needed based on sex, age, renal status, or hepatic function. ▪ The impact of weight on drug exposure is accounted for by the use of weight-based dosing.

DILUTION

Available as a sterile lyophilized powder in single-use 10-mL vials containing 50 mg cangrelor. Reconstitute each 50-mg vial with 5 mL of SWFI. Swirl gently until all material is dissolved. Avoid vigorous mixing. Allow any foam to settle. Ensure that the contents of the vial are fully dissolved and the reconstituted material is a clear, colorless to pale yellow solution. Before administration, each reconstituted vial must be further diluted with NS or D5W. Withdraw the contents from the reconstituted vial and add to a 250-mL bag of NS or D5W. Mix the bag thoroughly. Final concentration is 200 mcg/mL and should be sufficient for at least 2 hours of dosing. Patients 100 kg and over will require a minimum of 2 bags.

Storage: Store vials of cangrelor at CRT (20° to 25° C [68° to 77° F]), with excursions between 15° and 30° C (59° and 86° F) permitted. Reconstituted cangrelor should be further diluted immediately. Cangrelor is stable at RT for 12 hours diluted in D5W and for 24 hours diluted in NS. Discard any unused portion of reconstituted solution remaining in the vial.

COMPATIBILITY

Manufacturer states, "Administer cangrelor via a dedicated IV line."

RATE OF ADMINISTRATION

Administer cangrelor via a dedicated IV line.

Bolus: Administer the bolus volume rapidly (less than 1 minute) from the diluted bag via manual IV push or pump. Ensure the bolus is completely administered before the start of PCI. Start the infusion immediately after administration of the bolus.

Infusion: Administer at 4 mcg/kg/min. Continue for at least 2 hours or for the duration of PCI, whichever is longer.

ACTIONS

A direct P2Y$_{12}$ platelet receptor inhibitor that blocks adenosine diphosphate (ADP)–induced platelet activation and aggregation. It binds selectively and reversibly to the P2Y$_{12}$ receptor to prevent further signaling and platelet activation. When given according to the recommended regimen, platelet inhibition occurs within 2 minutes. Metabolism of cangrelor is independent of hepatic function and does not interfere with other drugs metabolized by hepatic enzymes. It is deactivated rapidly in the circulation by dephosphorylation to its primary metabolite, a nucleoside that has negligible antiplatelet activity. After discontinuation of the infusion, the antiplatelet effect decreases rapidly and platelet function returns to normal within 1 hour. The average elimination half-life is about 3 to 6 minutes. Excreted in urine and feces.

INDICATIONS AND USES

An adjunct to percutaneous coronary intervention (PCI) to reduce the risk of periprocedural myocardial infarction (MI), repeat coronary revascularization, and stent thrombosis (ST) in patients who have not been treated with a $P2Y_{12}$ platelet inhibitor and are not being given a glycoprotein IIb/IIIa inhibitor.

CONTRAINDICATIONS

Patients with significant active bleeding. ▪ Known hypersensitivity (e.g., anaphylaxis) to cangrelor or any component of the product.

PRECAUTIONS

For IV use only. ▪ Bleeding is the most common complication encountered during therapy. ▪ Drugs that inhibit platelet $P2Y_{12}$ function, including cangrelor, increase the risk of bleeding. ▪ Once cangrelor is discontinued, there is no antiplatelet effect after 1 hour. ▪ Serious hypersensitivity reactions have been reported.

Monitor: Monitor for S/S of bleeding. ▪ Monitor for S/S of hypersensitivity reactions (e.g., anaphylaxis, hypotension, pruritus, rash, urticaria, or wheezing).

Patient Education: Promptly report S/S of a hypersensitivity reaction (e.g., hives, rash, shortness of breath or troubled breathing, swelling of eyelids, lips, or face).

Maternal/Child: Category C: use during pregnancy only if clearly needed. ▪ It is not known if cangrelor is excreted in human milk. ▪ Safety and effectiveness for use in pediatric patients not established.

Elderly: No overall difference in safety or effectiveness between older and younger patients has been observed.

DRUG/LAB INTERACTIONS

If **clopidogrel** or **prasugrel** is administered during cangrelor infusion, it will have no antiplatelet effect until the next dose is administered. Therefore **clopidogrel** and **prasugrel** should not be administered until cangrelor infusion is discontinued. ▪ Administration of **ticagrelor** during cangrelor infusion does not attenuate the antiplatelet effect of ticagrelor. ▪ Coadministration of cangrelor with unfractionated **heparin, aspirin,** and **nitroglycerin** was formally studied in healthy subjects, with no evidence of an effect on the pharmacokinetics and pharmacodynamics of cangrelor. ▪ Cangrelor has been coadministered with bivalirudin, low-molecular-weight heparin, clopidogrel, prasugrel, and ticagrelor without clinically detectable interactions.

SIDE EFFECTS

The most common adverse reaction is bleeding.

Coronary artery dissection, coronary artery perforation, and dyspnea were the most frequent events leading to discontinuation of cangrelor. Serious cases of hypersensitivity, including angioedema, anaphylactic reactions, anaphylactic shock, bronchospasm, and stridor, have occurred. Decreased renal function was reported in a small number of patients with severe renal impairment (creatinine clearance less than 30 mL/min).

ANTIDOTE

There is no specific treatment to reverse the antiplatelet effect of cangrelor, but the effect is gone within 1 hour after discontinuation of the drug. Treat anaphylaxis immediately with oxygen, epinephrine (Adrenalin), antihistamines (e.g., diphenhydramine [Benadryl]), vasopressors (e.g., dopamine), corticosteroids, albuterol, IV fluids, and ventilation equipment as indicated. Resuscitate as necessary.

CAPREOMYCIN `BBW`
(kap-ree-oh-**MYE**-sin)

Capastat

Antibacterial
(antituberculosis)

USUAL DOSE
1 Gm daily, not to exceed 20 mg/kg/day. Give for 60 to 120 days, followed by 1 Gm two or three times weekly. Therapy for tuberculosis should be maintained for 12 to 24 months. Administered in combination with at least one other antituberculosis agent to which the patient's strain of tubercle bacilli is susceptible.

DOSE ADJUSTMENTS
The elderly and patients with reduced renal function should have dosage reduction based on CrCl using the guidelines in the following chart. These dosages are designed to achieve a mean steady-state capreomycin level of 10 mcg/mL. Elevation of BUN above 30 mg/dL or any other evidence of decreasing renal function warrants evaluation of patient. Dose reduction or discontinuation of therapy may be required.

Estimated Dosages to Attain Mean Steady-State Serum Capreomycin Concentration of 10 mcg/mL Based on CrCl			
	Dose* (mg/kg) Based on Dosing Intervals		
CrCl (mL/min)	24 hr	48 hr	72 hr
0 mL/min	1.29 mg/kg	2.58 mg/kg	3.87 mg/kg
10 mL/min	2.43 mg/kg	4.87 mg/kg	7.30 mg/kg
20 mL/min	3.58 mg/kg	7.16 mg/kg	10.7 mg/kg
30 mL/min	4.72 mg/kg	9.45 mg/kg	14.2 mg/kg
40 mL/min	5.87 mg/kg	11.7 mg/kg	
50 mL/min	7.01 mg/kg	14.0 mg/kg	
60 mL/min	8.16 mg/kg		
80 mL/min	10.4 mg/kg†		
100 mL/min	12.7 mg/kg†		
110 mL/min	13.9 mg/kg†		

*Optional dosing intervals are given. Longer intervals are expected to provide greater peaks and lower trough serum levels than shorter intervals.
†See Usual Dose.

DILUTION
Reconstitute each 1-Gm vial with 2 mL of NS or SWFI. Allow 2 to 3 minutes for complete dissolution. Withdraw calculated dose and further dilute in 100 mL NS.
Filters: No data available from manufacturer.
Storage: Store at CRT before reconstitution. After reconstitution, stable for 24 hours if refrigerated.

COMPATIBILITY
Specific information not available; consult pharmacist.

RATE OF ADMINISTRATION
A single dose as an infusion over 60 minutes. Neuromuscular blockade or respiratory paralysis may occur following rapid intravenous infusion. See Precautions and Side Effects.

ACTIONS

A polypeptide antibiotic isolated from *Streptomyces capreolus*. Active against strains of *Mycobacterium tuberculosis*. Half-life is 4 to 6 hours in patients with normal renal function. Excreted primarily unchanged in urine. Small amounts excreted in bile. Crosses the placenta. Does not penetrate into CSF.

INDICATIONS AND USES

Used concomitantly with other appropriate antituberculosis agents to treat pulmonary infections caused by capreomycin-susceptible strains of *M. tuberculosis* when the primary agents (isoniazid, rifampin, ethambutol, aminosalicylic acid, and streptomycin) have been ineffective or cannot be used because of toxicity or the presence of resistant tubercle bacilli.

CONTRAINDICATIONS

Hypersensitivity to capreomycin.

PRECAUTIONS

Usually given IM; IV used in patients with limited muscle mass. ▪ Sensitivity studies necessary to determine susceptibility of causative organism to capreomycin. ▪ To reduce the development of drug-resistant bacteria and maintain its effectiveness, capreomycin should be used to treat or prevent only those infections proven or strongly suspected to be caused by bacteria. ▪ Use with caution in patients with pre-existing auditory impairment, dehydration, or renal insufficiency or when used concomitantly with other potentially ototoxic or nephrotoxic drugs (e.g., aminoglycosides [e.g., amikacin, gentamicin, tobramycin], colistin sulfate, polymyxin A, vancomycin). Must weigh risk of additional cranial nerve VIII (auditory and vestibular) damage or renal injury against benefit of therapy. ▪ Coadministration with other parenteral antituberculosis agents (e.g., streptomycin) is not recommended. Toxicity is additive. ▪ Renal injury, with tubular necrosis, elevation of BUN or SCr, and abnormal urinary sediment (casts, RBCs, WBCs), has been reported. Elderly patients, patients with abnormal renal function or dehydration, and patients receiving other nephrotoxic drugs are at increased risk for developing acute tubular necrosis. ▪ Elevation of BUN above 30 mg/dL or other evidence of decreasing renal function warrants evaluation of patient. Dose reduction or discontinuation of drug may be necessary; see Dose Adjustments. Clinical significance of abnormal urine sediment and slight increase in BUN or SCr during long-term therapy is not known. ▪ The peripheral neuromuscular blocking action seen with other polypeptide antibiotics (colistin sulfate, polymyxin A sulfate) and aminoglycosides (e.g., kanamycin, neomycin, streptomycin) has been reported with capreomycin. ▪ Cross-resistance between capreomycin and kanamycin, neomycin and viomycin reported. No cross-resistance observed between capreomycin and aminosalicylic acid, cycloserine, ethambutol, ethionamide, isoniazid, and streptomycin. ▪ Use with caution in patients with allergies (especially drug allergies).

Monitor: Audiometric measurements and assessment of vestibular function should be performed before initiation of therapy and at regular intervals during treatment. ▪ Obtain baseline SCr, BUN, liver function tests, and electrolytes before initiating therapy. Reduced dosage required for patients with impaired renal function; see Dose Adjustments. Weekly monitoring of renal function and periodic monitoring of electrolytes and liver function tests are recommended. ▪ Obtain serum calcium, potassium, and magnesium levels frequently; hypocalcemia, hypokalemia, and hypomagnesemia may occur during therapy. ▪ Monitor for S/S of hypersensitivity.

Patient Education: Compliance with full course of therapy is imperative. Report any side effects promptly.

Maternal/Child: Category C: safety for use during pregnancy and breast-feeding not established. Benefits must outweigh risks. Crosses the placenta. ▪ Safety and effectiveness for use in pediatric patients not established.

Elderly: Response similar to younger adults; however, dosing should be cautious; see Dose Adjustments. ▪ May be at increased risk of toxicity because of age-related decrease in renal function; monitor renal function. ▪ More likely to have impaired hearing at baseline. Initial and periodic audiometric measurement and assessment of vestibular function are recommended. See Precautions.

DRUG/LAB INTERACTIONS

Neuromuscular blockade of **nondepolarizing neuromuscular blocking agents** (e.g., vecuronium) may be enhanced with concurrent use of capreomycin because of synergistic effects and may be further enhanced by **ether or methoxyflurane anesthesia.** ▪ Risk of neuromuscular blockade increased when administered concurrently or sequentially with **polymyxins or aminoglycosides** (e.g., kanamycin, neomycin, streptomycin); see Precautions. ▪ Neuromuscular blockade antagonized by **neostigmine.** ▪ Risk of ototoxicity, nephrotoxicity, and respiratory paralysis increased when administered concurrently or sequentially with **other potentially ototoxic or nephrotoxic medications** (e.g., aminoglycosides [e.g., amikacin, gentamicin, streptomycin, tobramycin], colistin sulfate, polymyxin A, vancomycin); see Precautions.

SIDE EFFECTS

Abnormal liver function tests; abnormal urine sediment; dizziness; electrolyte disturbances resembling Bartter's syndrome, as well as hypocalcemia, hypokalemia, and hypomagnesemia; elevated BUN or SCr; eosinophilia; febrile reactions; hypersensitivity; leukocytosis; leukopenia; maculopapular skin rash; pain and induration at injection site; subclinical auditory loss (high-tone acuity); thrombocytopenia; tinnitus; toxic nephritis; urticaria; vertigo.

ANTIDOTE

Protect airway and support ventilation and perfusion. Hydrate patient to maintain urine output of 3 to 5 mL/kg/hr. Monitor fluid balance, electrolytes, renal function, vital signs, and blood gases; treat abnormalities as indicated. Hemodialysis may be useful. Resuscitate as necessary.

CARBOPLATIN BBW
(**KAR**-boh-plah-tin)

Paraplatin

Antineoplastic
(alkylating agent)

pH 5 to 7

USUAL DOSE

Before giving a dose in a cycle, it is recommended that platelets be above 100,000/mm³ and neutrophils above 2,000/mm³; see Dose Adjustments. The Calvert formula for carboplatin dosing based on pre-existing renal function and/or desired platelet nadir determines the patient's dose.

$$\text{Total dose (mg)} = (\text{Target AUC}) \times (\text{GFR} + 25)$$

Dose is calculated in milligrams, not mg/M². The ordering physician determines the target AUC (area under the curve) and supplies the required information on the GFR (glomerular filtration rate) or CrCl, as well as the desired response. The pharmacist calculates the correct dose. See package insert for additional information.

Initial treatment of advanced ovarian cancer in combination with cyclophosphamide: Carboplatin 300 mg/M² plus cyclophosphamide 600 mg/M² on Day 1 every 4 weeks for 6 cycles or carboplatin dose targeted by Calvert equation to an AUC of 6 to 7 plus cyclophosphamide 600 mg/M² on Day 1 every 4 weeks.

Palliative treatment of recurrent ovarian cancer after prior chemotherapy: *As a single agent:* With normal renal function (CrCl greater than 60 mL/min), give 360 mg/M² on Day 1 every 4 weeks or, alternately, a dose targeted by Calvert equation to an AUC of 4 to 6 appears to provide an appropriate dose range in these patients.

DOSE ADJUSTMENTS

Single agent or combination therapy. Dose adjustment is based on nadir after prior dose according to the following chart.

Carboplatin Dose Based on Bone Marrow Suppression		
Platelets/mm³	Neutrophils/mm³	Adjusted Dose (from Prior Course)*
>100,000	>2,000	Increase to 125%
50,000-100,000	500-2,000	No adjustment
<50,000	<500	Decrease to 75%

*Percentages apply to carboplatin as a single agent or to both carboplatin and cyclophosphamide in combination.

Once the dose has been increased to 125% of the starting dose, no further dose increases are indicated. ▪ With impaired renal function (CrCl 16 to 40 mL/min), give 200 mg/M²; CrCl 41 to 59 mL/min, give 250 mg/M². Dose recommendation not available for patients with a CrCl less than 16 mL/min. ▪ Bone marrow suppression is more severe in patients who have had prior therapy, especially with cisplatin and when carboplatin is used with other bone marrow–suppressing therapies or radiation, and may be more severe in the elderly. Reduced dose may be indicated. Monitor carefully and manage dose and timing to reduce additive effects.

DILUTION

Specific techniques required; see Precautions. Available as a premixed solution (10 mg/mL) and as a lyophilized powder. Immediately before use, reconstitute each 10 mg of carboplatin lyophilized powder with 1 mL of SWFI, D5W, or NS (50 mg with 5 mL, 150 mg with 15 mL, 450 mg with 45 mL). All yield 10 mg/mL. Both preparations may be further diluted with NS or D5W to concentrations as low as 0.5 mg/mL. Do not use needles or IV tubing with aluminum parts to mix or administer; a precipitate will form and decrease potency. Best to mix lyophilized preparation immediately before use.

Storage: *Premixed solutions:* Stable to the date indicated on the package stored at CRT and protected from light. Multidose vials maintain microbial, chemical, and physical stability for up to 14 days at RT (25° C [77° F]) following multiple-needle entries. *Lyophilized powder:* Store unopened vials at CRT. Protect from light. Reconstituted solutions are stable for 8 hours at RT (25° C [77° F]). Discard 8 hours after dilution.

COMPATIBILITY (Underline Indicates Conflicting Compatibility Information)

Consider any drug NOT listed as compatible to be INCOMPATIBLE until consulting a pharmacist; specific conditions may apply.

Forms a precipitate if in contact with aluminum (e.g., needles, syringes, catheters).

One source suggests the following **compatibilities:**

Additive: Cisplatin, etoposide (VePesid), ifosfamide (Ifex), paclitaxel (Taxol).

Y-site: Allopurinol (Aloprim), amifostine (Ethyol), anidulafungin (Eraxis), aztreonam (Azactam), caspofungin (Cancidas), cladribine (Leustatin), doripenem (Doribax), doxorubicin liposomal (Doxil), etoposide phosphate (Etopophos), filgrastim (Neupogen), fludarabine (Fludara), gemcitabine (Gemzar), granisetron (Kytril), linezolid (Zyvox), melphalan (Alkeran), micafungin (Mycamine), ondansetron (Zofran), oxaliplatin (Eloxatin), paclitaxel (Taxol), palonosetron (Aloxi), pemetrexed (Alimta), piperacillin/tazobactam (Zosyn), propofol (Diprivan), sargramostim (Leukine), teniposide (Vumon), thiotepa, topotecan (Hycamtin), vinorelbine (Navelbine).

RATE OF ADMINISTRATION

A single dose as an infusion over a minimum of 15 minutes. Extend administration time based on amount of diluent and patient condition.

ACTIONS

An alkylating agent. Better tolerated by patients, carboplatin causes less nausea and vomiting, less neurotoxicity, and less nephrotoxicity than cisplatin. Myelosuppression is generally reversible and manageable with antibiotics and transfusions. Produces interstrand DNA cross-links and is cell-cycle nonspecific. Not bound to plasma proteins. Half-life is 2.6 to 5.9 hours. Majority of carboplatin is excreted in the urine within 24 hours.

INDICATIONS AND USES

Initial treatment of advanced ovarian cancer in combination with other approved chemotherapeutic agents (e.g., cyclophosphamide). ▪ Palliative treatment of recurrent ovarian cancer after prior chemotherapy, including patients treated with cisplatin.

Unlabeled uses: Treatment of bladder cancer, non–small-cell lung cancer, and small-cell lung cancer.

CONTRAINDICATIONS

Hypersensitivity to cisplatin or other platinum-containing compounds or mannitol; severe bone marrow suppression; significant bleeding.

PRECAUTIONS

Follow guidelines for handling cytotoxic agents. See Appendix A, p. 1331. ▪ Usually administered by or under the direction of the physician specialist in a facility with adequate diagnostic and treatment facilities to monitor the patient and respond to any medical emergency. ▪ Bone marrow suppression is dose related and may be severe, resulting in infection and/or bleeding. Anemia may be cumulative and may require transfusion support. Bone marrow suppression increased in patients who have received prior therapy, especially regimens including cisplatin, and in patients with impaired kidney function. ▪ Anaphylaxis has been reported and may occur within minutes of administration. ▪ Risk of hypersensitivity increased in patients previously exposed to platinum therapy. Patients sensitive to other platinum compounds (e.g., cisplatin) may be sensitive to carboplatin; see Contraindications. ▪ Peripheral neurotoxicity is uncommon, but risk may be increased in patients over 65 years of age and in patients previously treated with cisplatin. ▪ Secondary malignancies, including acute nonlymphocytic leukemia, myeloproliferation syndrome, and carcinoma have been reported in patients treated with alkylating agents. ▪ See Drug/Lab Interactions.

Monitor: BUN and SCr should be done before each dose. CrCl, WBC, platelet count, and hemoglobin are recommended before each dose and weekly thereafter. Platelet count recommended to be 100,000/mm³ and neutrophils 2,000/mm³ before a dose can be re-peated; see Dose Adjustments. Anemia is frequent and cumulative. Transfusion is often indicated. ▪ Excessive hydration or forced diuresis not required, but maintain adequate hydration and urinary output. ▪ Nausea and vomiting are frequently severe but less than with cisplatin; generally last 24 hours. Prophylactic administration of antiemetics is indicated. Various protocols are used. ▪ Observe for symptoms of hypersensitivity reactions during administration; epinephrine, corticosteroids, and antihistamines should be available. ▪ Observe closely for symptoms of infection. Prophylactic antibiotics may be indicated pending results of C/S in a febrile neutropenic patient. ▪ Monitor for thrombocytopenia (platelet count less than 50,000/mm³). Initiate precautions to prevent excessive bleeding (e.g., inspect IV sites, skin, and mucous membranes; use extreme care during invasive procedures; test urine, emesis, stool, and secretions for occult blood).

Patient Education: Nonhormonal birth control recommended. Manufacturer provides a patient information booklet. ▪ See Appendix D, p. 1333.

Maternal/Child: Category D: avoid pregnancy. ▪ Discontinue breast-feeding. ▪ Safety and effectiveness for use in pediatric patients not established. ▪ Significant hearing loss has been reported in pediatric patients; occurred with higher-than-recommended doses of carboplatin in combination with other ototoxic agents.

Elderly: Neurotoxicity and myelotoxicity may be more severe. ▪ Consider possibility of decreased renal function. ▪ See Dose Adjustments and Precautions.

DRUG/LAB INTERACTIONS

Nephrotoxicity and ototoxicity are additive when used with other **ototoxic or nephrotoxic agents** (e.g., acyclovir [Zovirax], aminoglycosides [e.g., gentamicin], cisplatin, rifampin [Rifadin], quinidine). Use with caution. ▪ Bone marrow toxicity increased with other **antineoplastic agents, radiation therapy, and/or other agents that may cause blood dyscrasias** (e.g., anticonvulsants [e.g., phenytoin (Dilantin)], cephalosporins, mycophenolate [Cell-Cept], rituximab [Rituxan]). Dose adjustment of either or both drugs may be indicated. ▪ Do not administer **live virus vaccines** to patients receiving antineoplastic drugs. ▪ See Dose Adjustments.

SIDE EFFECTS

Allergic reactions, including anaphylaxis, can occur during administration. Alopecia (rare), anemia, anorexia, bleeding, bone marrow suppression (usually reversible), bronchospasm, bruising, changes in taste, constipation, death, decreased urine output, decreased serum electrolytes, dehydration, diarrhea, erythema, fatigue, fever, hemolytic uremic syndrome (rare, cancer-associated), hypotension, infection, laboratory test abnormalities (alkaline phosphatase, aspartate aminotransferase [AST], BUN, SCr, total bilirubin), nausea and vomiting (severe), neutropenia, ototoxicity, peripheral neuropathies, pruritus, rash, stomatitis, thrombocytopenia, urticaria, visual disturbances, weakness.

ANTIDOTE

Notify physician of all side effects. Symptomatic and supportive treatment is indicated. Withhold carboplatin until myelosuppression has resolved. Administration of whole blood products (e.g., packed RBCs, platelets, leukocytes) may be required. Blood modifiers (e.g., darbepoetin alfa [Aranesp], epoetin alfa [Epogen], filgrastim [Neupogen, Zarxio], pegfilgrastim [Neulasta], sargramostim [Leukine]) may be indicated to treat bone marrow toxicity. Treat anaphylaxis with epinephrine, corticosteroids, oxygen, and antihistamines. There is no specific antidote.

CARFILZOMIB
(kar-**FILZ**-oh-mib)

Kyprolis

Antineoplastic
Proteasome inhibitor

pH 3.5

USUAL DOSE

Hydration: Hydration is indicated, especially in patients at high risk for renal toxicity and tumor lysis syndrome (TLS). Recommended hydration includes both oral fluids (30 mL/kg at least 48 hours before Cycle 1, Day 1) and intravenous fluids (250 to 500 mL of appropriate intravenous fluids before each dose in Cycle 1). Administer an additional 250 to 500 mL of intravenous fluid as needed after carfilzomib administration. Monitor fluid status and continue oral and/or intravenous hydration as needed in subsequent cycles.

Premedication: To reduce the incidence and severity of infusion reactions, premedicate with *dexamethasone.* Dexamethasone dose depends on regimen used. Administer 4 mg IV or PO for 20/27 mg/M^2 monotherapy, 8 mg IV or PO for 20/56 mg/M^2 monotherapy, or the recommended dexamethasone dose if undergoing combination therapy. Administer at least 30 minutes before but no more than 4 hours before all doses of carfilzomib during Cycle 1. If infusion reactions occur during subsequent cycles, premedication with dexamethasone should be continued.

Thromboprophylaxis: Thromboprophylaxis is recommended for patients being treated with a combination of carfilzomib with dexamethasone or of carfilzomib with lenalidomide plus dexamethasone. The regimen should be based on an assessment of the patient's underlying risks; see Precautions.

Infection prophylaxis: Consider antiviral prophylaxis in patients being treated with carfilzomib to decrease the risk of herpes zoster reactivation.

Carfilzomib: Dose is calculated using actual body surface area (BSA) at baseline. Patients with a BSA greater than 2.2 M^2 should receive a dose based on a BSA of 2.2 M^2. Dose adjustments do not need to be made for weight changes less than or equal to 20%.

Combination therapy with lenalidomide and dexamethasone: Administer over 10 minutes on 2 consecutive days each week for 3 weeks (Days 1, 2, 8, 9, 15, and 16), followed by a 12-day rest period (Days 17 to 28). Each 28-day period is considered 1 treatment cycle. The recommended starting dose of carfilzomib is 20 mg/M^2 in Cycle 1 on Days 1 and 2. If tolerated, escalate to a target dose of 27 mg/M^2 on Day 8 of Cycle 1. Beginning with Cycle 13, omit Days 8 and 9 doses of carfilzomib. Discontinue carfilzomib after Cycle 18. Administer lenalidomide (Revlimid) 25 mg PO on Days 1 to 21 and dexamethasone (Decadron) 40 mg PO or IV on Days 1, 8, 15, and 22 of the 28-day cycles. A summary of the combination dosing regimen for carfilzomib is outlined in the following chart.

Continued

Carfilzomib (10-Minute Infusion) in Combination with Lenalidomide and Dexamethasone										
Cycle 1										
Week 1			Week 2			Week 3			Week 4	
Day 1	Day 2	Days 3-7	Day 8	Day 9	Days 10-14	Day 15	Day 16	Days 17-21	Day 22	Days 23-28
Carfilzomib (mg/M²)										
20 mg/M²	20 mg/M²	—	27 mg/M²	27 mg/M²	—	27 mg/M²	27 mg/M²	—	—	—
Dexamethasone (mg)										
40 mg	—	—	40 mg	—	—	40 mg	—	—	40 mg	—
Lenalidomide (mg)										
25 mg daily on Days 1-21									—	—
Cycles 2 to 12										
Week 1			Week 2			Week 3			Week 4	
Day 1	Day 2	Days 3-7	Day 8	Day 9	Days 10-14	Day 15	Day 16	Days 17-21	Day 22	Days 23-28
Carfilzomib (mg/M²)										
27 mg/M²	27 mg/M²	—	27 mg/M²	27 mg/M²	—	27 mg/M²	27 mg/M²	—	—	—
Dexamethasone (mg)										
40 mg	—	—	40 mg	—	—	40 mg	—	—	40 mg	—
Lenalidomide (mg)										
25 mg daily on Days 1-21									—	—
Cycle 13 on*										
Week 1			Week 2			Week 3			Week 4	
Day 1	Day 2	Days 3-7	Day 8	Day 9	Days 10-14	Day 15	Day 16	Days 17-21	Day 22	Days 23-28
Carfilzomib (mg/M²)										
27 mg/M²	27 mg/M²	—	—	—	—	27 mg/M²	27 mg/M²	—	—	—
Dexamethasone (mg)										
40 mg	—	—	40 mg	—	—	40 mg	—	—	40 mg	—
Lenalidomide (mg)										
25 mg daily on Days 1-21									—	—

*Carfilzomib is administered through Cycle 18; lenalidomide and dexamethasone continue thereafter.

Continue treatment until disease progression or unacceptable toxicity occurs. See prescribing information for lenalidomide and dexamethasone for other concomitant medications that may be required with those agents, such as anticoagulants or antacid prophylactic agents.

Combination therapy with dexamethasone: Administer over 30 minutes on 2 consecutive days each week for 3 weeks (Days 1, 2, 8, 9, 15, and 16), followed by a 12-day rest period (Days 17 to 28). Each 28-day period is considered 1 treatment cycle. The recommended starting dose of carfilzomib is 20 mg/M² on Days 1 and 2 of Cycle 1. If tolerated, escalate to a target dose of 56 mg/M² on Days 8, 9, 15, and 16 of Cycle 1. Administer dexamethasone (Decadron) 20 mg PO or IV on Days 1, 2, 8, 9, 15, 16, 22, and 23 of each

28-day cycle. A summary of the combination dosing regimen for carfilzomib is outlined in the following chart.

Carfilzomib (30-Minute Infusion) in Combination with Dexamethasone											
Cycle 1											
Week 1			Week 2			Week 3			Week 4		
Day 1	Day 2	Days 3-7	Day 8	Day 9	Days 10-14	Day 15	Day 16	Days 17-21	Day 22	Day 23	Days 24-28
Carfilzomib (mg/M^2)											
20 mg/M^2	20 mg/M^2	—	56 mg/M^2	56 mg/M^2	—	56 mg/M^2	56 mg/M^2	—	—	—	—
Dexamethasone (mg)											
20 mg	20 mg	—	20 mg	20 mg	—	20 mg	20 mg	—	20 mg	20 mg	—
Cycle 2 on											
Week 1			Week 2			Week 3			Week 4		
Day 1	Day 2	Days 3-7	Day 8	Day 9	Days 10-14	Day 15	Day 16	Days 17-21	Day 22	Day 23	Days 24-28
Carfilzomib (mg/M^2)											
56 mg/M^2	56 mg/M^2	—	56 mg/M^2	56 mg/M^2	—	56 mg/M^2	56 mg/M^2	—	—	—	—
Dexamethasone (mg)											
20 mg	20 mg	—	20 mg	20 mg	—	20 mg	20 mg	—	20 mg	20 mg	—

Continue treatment until disease progression or unacceptable toxicity occurs. See prescribing information for dexamethasone for other concomitant medications.

Monotherapy: Administer over 10 or 30 minutes, depending on the regimen as described in the following sections.

20/27 mg/M^2 regimen by 10-minute infusion: Administer over 10 minutes on 2 consecutive days each week for 3 weeks (Days 1, 2, 8, 9, 15, and 16), followed by a 12-day rest period (Days 17 to 28). Each 28-day period is considered 1 treatment cycle. The recommended starting dose of carfilzomib is 20 mg/M^2 on Days 1 and 2 of Cycle 1. If tolerated, escalate to a target dose of 27 mg/M^2 on Days 8, 9, 15, and 16 of Cycle 1. Beginning with Cycle 13, omit Days 8 and 9 doses of carfilzomib. Continue treatment until disease progression or unacceptable toxicity occurs. A summary of this dosing regimen for carfilzomib is outlined in the following chart.

Continued

Carfilzomib Monotherapy (20/27 mg/M² 10-Minute Infusion)									
Cycle 1									
Carfilzomib* (mg/M²)	Week 1			Week 2			Week 3		Week 4
	Day 1	Day 2	Days 3-7	Day 8	Day 9	Days 10-14	Day 15	Day 16	Days 17-21	Days 22-28
	20 mg/M²	20 mg/M²	—	27 mg/M²	27 mg/M²	—	27 mg/M²	27 mg/M²	—	—
Cycles 2 to 12									
Carfilzomib (mg/M²)	Week 1			Week 2			Week 3		Week 4
	Day 1	Day 2	Days 3-7	Day 8	Day 9	Days 10-14	Day 15	Day 16	Days 17-21	Days 22-28
	27 mg/M²	27 mg/M²	—	27 mg/M²	27 mg/M²	—	27 mg/M²	27 mg/M²	—	—
Cycle 13 on									
Carfilzomib (mg/M²)	Week 1			Week 2			Week 3		Week 4
	Day 1	Day 2	Days 3-7	Day 8	Day 9	Days 10-14	Day 15	Day 16	Days 17-21	Day 22-28
	27 mg/M²	27 mg/M²	—	—	—	—	27 mg/M²	27 mg/M²	—	—

*Dexamethasone premedication is required for each carfilzomib dose in Cycle 1.

20/56 mg/M² regimen by 30-minute infusion: Administer over 30 minutes on 2 consecutive days each week for 3 weeks (Days 1, 2, 8, 9, 15, 16), followed by a 12-day rest period (Days 17 to 28). Each 28-day period is considered 1 treatment cycle. The recommended starting dose of carfilzomib is 20 mg/M² on Days 1 and 2 of Cycle 1. If tolerated, escalate to a target dose of 56 mg/M² on Day 8 of Cycle 1. Beginning with Cycle 13, omit Days 8 and 9 doses of carfilzomib. Continue treatment until disease progression or unacceptable toxicity occurs. A summary of this dosing regimen for carfilzomib is outlined in the following chart.

Carfilzomib Monotherapy (20/56 mg/M² 30-Minute Infusion)									
Cycle 1									
Carfilzomib* (mg/M²)	Week 1			Week 2			Week 3		Week 4
	Day 1	Day 2	Days 3-7	Day 8	Day 9	Days 10-14	Day 15	Day 16	Days 17-21	Days 22-28
	20 mg/M²	20 mg/M²	—	56 mg/M²	56 mg/M²	—	56 mg/M²	56 mg/M²	—	—
Cycles 2 to 12									
Carfilzomib (mg/M²)	Week 1			Week 2			Week 3		Week 4
	Day 1	Day 2	Days 3-7	Day 8	Day 9	Days 10-14	Day 15	Day 16	Days 17-21	Days 22-28
	56 mg/M²	56 mg/M²	—	56 mg/M²	56 mg/M²	—	56 mg/M²	56 mg/M²	—	—
Cycle 13 on									
Carfilzomib (mg/M²)	Week 1			Week 2			Week 3		Week 4
	Day 1	Day 2	Days 3-7	Day 8	Day 9	Days 10-14	Day 15	Day 16	Days 17-21	Day 22-28
	56 mg/M²	56 mg/M²	—	—	—	—	56 mg/M²	56 mg/M²	—	—

*Dexamethasone premedication is required for each carfilzomib dose in Cycle 1.

DOSE ADJUSTMENTS

Dose is calculated using actual body surface area (BSA) at baseline. Patients with a BSA greater than 2.2 M^2 should receive a dose based on a BSA of 2.2 M^2. Dose adjustments do not need to be made for weight changes less than or equal to 20%. ▪ Pharmacokinetics and safety of carfilzomib are not influenced by renal impairment. Because dialysis clearance of carfilzomib has not been studied, patients undergoing dialysis should receive carfilzomib after the dialysis procedure. ▪ The pharmacokinetics of carfilzomib is not affected by age or gender.

Recommended actions/dose modifications based on toxicities are in the following chart.

Dose Modifications for Toxicity During Carfilzomib Treatment	
Hematologic Toxicity	**Recommended Action**
Absolute neutrophil count <0.5 × 10^9/L (500 cells/mm³)	• Withhold dose. • If recovered to ≥0.5 x 10^9/L, continue at same dose level. • For subsequent drops to <0.5 × 10^9/L, follow the same recommendations as above and consider 1 dose level reduction when restarting carfilzomib.*
Febrile neutropenia: ANC <0.5 × 10^9/L and an oral temperature more than 38.5° C or two consecutive readings of more than 38.0° C for 2 hours	• Withhold dose. • If ANC returns to baseline grade and fever resolves, resume at the same dose level.
Platelets <10 × 10^9/L (10,000 cells/mm³) or evidence of bleeding with thrombocytopenia	• Withhold dose. • If recovered to ≥10 × 10^9/L and/or bleeding is controlled, continue at the same dose level. • For subsequent drops to <10 × 10^9/L, follow the same recommendations as above and consider 1 dose level reduction when restarting carfilzomib.*
Renal Toxicity	

Serum creatinine ≥2 × baseline OR Creatinine clearance <15 mL/min OR Creatinine clearance decreases to ≤50% of baseline OR Need for dialysis	• Withhold dose and continue monitoring renal function (serum creatinine or creatinine clearance).
	  • If attributable to carfilzomib, resume when renal function has recovered to within 25% of baseline; start at 1 dose level reduction.*
	  • If not attributable to carfilzomib, dosing may be resumed at the discretion of the physician.
	• For patients on dialysis receiving carfilzomib, the dose is to be administered after the dialysis procedure.

Other Nonhematologic Toxicity	
All other severe or life-threatening† non-hematologic toxicities	• Withhold until resolved or returned to baseline. • Consider restarting the next scheduled treatment at 1 dose level reduction.*

*See the following chart for dose level reductions.
†CTCAE Grades 3 and 4.

Dose Level Reductions for Carfilzomib				
Regimen	Dose	First Dose Reduction	Second Dose Reduction	Third Dose Reduction
Carfilzomib, lenalidomide, and dexamethasone OR Monotherapy (20/27 mg/M²)	27 mg/M^2	20 mg/M^2	15 mg/M^2*	—
Carfilzomib and dexamethasone OR Monotherapy (20/56 mg/M²)	56 mg/M^2	45 mg/M^2	36 mg/M^2	27 mg/M^2*

NOTE: Infusion times remain unchanged during dose reduction(s).
*If toxicity persists, discontinue carfilzomib treatment.

DILUTION

Specific techniques required; see Precautions. Available in a 60-mg single-use vial. Remove from refrigerator just before use. Reconstitute each vial with 29 mL of SWFI. Direct the solution onto the inside wall of the vial to minimize foaming. Gently swirl and/or invert vial slowly for about 1 minute or until complete dissolution occurs. *Do not shake.* If foaming occurs, allow solution to rest in vial for about 5 minutes, until foaming subsides. Final concentration of reconstituted solution is 2 mg/mL. May withdraw reconstituted calculated dose from vial and administer without further dilution directly into the port of an IV set. Alternately, may withdraw calculated dose and dilute in 50 mL of D5W and administer as an infusion; see Rate of Administration.

Filters: No data available from manufacturer.

Storage: Unopened vials should be refrigerated at 2° to 8° C (36° to 46° F). Retain in original package to protect from light. Both the reconstituted solution stored in the vial or a syringe and the solution diluted in D5W are stable for 24 hours when refrigerated and for 4 hours when stored at RT. Total time from reconstitution to administration should not exceed 24 hours. Discard any unused portion.

COMPATIBILITY

Manufacturer states, "Do not mix with or administer as an infusion with other medicinal products."

RATE OF ADMINISTRATION

Administer intravenously over 10 or 30 minutes depending on the carfilzomib regimen. **Do not** administer as a bolus. Flush line with NS or D5W immediately before and after carfilzomib administration.

ACTIONS

Carfilzomib is a proteasome inhibitor that irreversibly binds to specific sites on the 20S proteasome. Has antiproliferative and pro-apoptotic activities in vitro in solid and in hematologic tumor cells. Actions result in cell-cycle arrest and apoptosis. Highly protein bound. Extensively metabolized via peptidase and epoxide hydrolase activities. Metabolites have no known biologic activity. Has a half-life of ≤1 hour on Day 1 of Cycle 1. The pathways of carfilzomib elimination have not been characterized in humans. Partially excreted in the urine as metabolites.

INDICATIONS AND USES

Treatment of patients with relapsed or refractory multiple myeloma who have received one to three prior lines of therapy. Given in combination with dexamethasone or with lenalidomide plus dexamethasone. ▪ As a single agent for treatment of patients with relapsed or refractory multiple myeloma who have received one or more lines of therapy.

CONTRAINDICATIONS

Manufacturer states, "None."

PRECAUTIONS

Follow guidelines for handling cytotoxic agents. See Appendix A, p. 1331. ▪ For IV use only; see Rate of Administration. ▪ Administered by or under the direction of the physician specialist in a facility with adequate diagnostic and treatment facilities to monitor the patient and respond to any medical emergency. ▪ New onset or worsening of pre-existing cardiac failure (e.g., congestive heart failure, pulmonary edema, decreased ejection fraction), restrictive cardiomyopathy, myocardial ischemia, and myocardial infarction, including fatalities, have been reported and have occurred throughout the course of therapy. Death from cardiac arrest has occurred within a day of administration. Patients with New York Heart Association Class III and IV heart failure, recent myocardial infarction, conduction abnormalities, or angina or arrhythmias uncontrolled by medications may be at greater risk for cardiac complications and were not eligible for the clinical trials. ▪ Renal adverse events, including renal impairment and acute renal failure, have been reported. Acute renal failure was reported more frequently in patients with advanced relapsed and refractory multiple myeloma who received carfilzomib monotherapy. This risk was greater in patients with existing renal impairment. ▪ Acute respiratory distress syndrome (ARDS), acute respiratory failure, and acute diffuse infiltrative pulmonary disease such as pneumonitis and interstitial lung disease have been reported. ▪ Pulmonary arterial hypertension has been reported. ▪ Dyspnea was reported in close to one third of patients in clinical trials. ▪ Hypertension, including hypertensive crisis and hypertensive emergency, has been observed. Some events have been fatal. ▪ Venous thromboembolic events (including deep venous thrombosis [DVT] and pulmonary embolism [PE]) have been observed. Incidence of events was higher with combination therapy. Thromboprophylaxis is recommended and should be based on an assessment of the patient's underlying risk factors, treatment regimen, and clinical status. ▪ Infusion reactions, including life-threatening reactions, can occur immediately after or up to 24 hours after administration of carfilzomib. Premedication with dexamethasone may reduce the incidence and severity of reaction. ▪ Cases of TLS, some with fatal outcome, have been reported. Patients with multiple myeloma and a high tumor burden may be at increased risk for developing TLS. ▪ Carfilzomib may cause elevations of serum transaminases and bilirubin. Cases of hepatic failure have been reported. Fatalities have occurred. Safety, efficacy, and pharmacokinetics have not been studied in patients with hepatic impairment. Use caution. ▪ Cases of thrombotic microangiopathy, including thrombotic thrombocytopenic purpura/hemolytic uremic syndrome (TTP/HUS), have been reported. Some cases have been fatal. ▪ Cases of posterior reversible encephalopathy syndrome (PRES) have been reported. ▪ See Dose Adjustments.

Monitor: Obtain baseline CBC with differential and platelets. Obtain baseline AST, ALT, bilirubin, and SCr. ▪ Monitor fluid status, blood chemistries, and serum potassium closely throughout treatment. Avoid fluid overload, especially in patients at risk for cardiac failure. ▪ Monitor for cardiac complications (e.g., cardiac failure, pulmonary edema, decrease in ejection fraction, ischemia) and treat promptly. Patients with pre-existing cardiovascular disease may be at greater risk for cardiac complications. A comprehensive medical assessment (including BP and fluid management) should be performed before starting treatment. Close follow-up is required during therapy. ▪ Monitor for S/S of pulmonary hypertension. Evaluate with cardiac imaging and/or other tests as indicated. ▪ Monitor pulmonary function with new or worsening pulmonary symptoms (e.g., dyspnea). Evaluate dyspnea to exclude cardiopulmonary conditions, including cardiac failure and pulmonary syndromes. ▪ Monitor BP regularly. ▪ Monitor for S/S of DVT and/or PE (e.g., swelling, pain, and/or warmth of extremity, shortness of breath). ▪ Monitor for S/S of an infusion reaction (e.g., angina, arthralgia, chest tightness, chills, facial edema, facial flushing, fever, hypotension, myalgia, shortness of breath, syncope, vomiting, and weakness). ▪ Monitor uric acid levels as indicated. Prevention and treatment of hyperuricemia due to TLS may be accomplished with adequate hydration and, if necessary, with allopurinol and alkalinization of urine. ▪ Carfilzomib causes thrombocytopenia. Monitor platelet counts frequently. Nadir occurs between Day 8 and Day 15 of each 28-day cycle. Recovery to baseline should occur by the start of the next 28-day cycle. Initiate precautions to prevent excessive bleeding (e.g., inspect IV sites, skin, and mucous membranes; use extreme care during invasive procedures; test urine, emesis, stool, and secretions for occult blood). ▪ Monitor serum transaminases and bilirubin frequently. ▪ Monitor for S/S of TTP/HUS. The safety of re-initiating carfilzomib therapy in patients previously experiencing TTP/HUS is not known. ▪ Monitor for S/S of PRES (e.g., altered consciousness, blindness, confusion, headache, lethargy, seizure, and other visual and neurologic disturbances along with hypertension. Diagnosis is confirmed by neuroradiologic imaging (MRI). The safety of re-initiating carfilzomib therapy in patients previously experiencing PRES is not known. ▪ See Dose Adjustments.

Patient Education: Avoid pregnancy. Female patients with reproductive potential must use effective contraceptive measures during treatment with carfilzomib and for at least 30 days after completion of therapy. Patients using oral contraceptives or a hormonal method of contraception associated with a risk of thrombosis should consider an alternative method of effective contraception during treatment with carfilzomib in combination with dexamethasone or with lenalidomide plus dexamethasone. ▪ Male patients with reproductive potential should avoid fathering a child while being treated with carfilzomib and for at least 90 days after completion of therapy. ▪ Promptly report symptoms such as bleeding, bruising, chest pain, chills, confusion, cough, dyspnea, fever, headaches, rigors, seizures, swelling of the feet or legs, visual loss, or weakness. ▪ May cause fatigue, dizziness, fainting, and/or a drop in blood pressure. Use caution in tasks that require alertness. ▪ Avoid dehydration. Seek medical advice if dizziness, lightheadedness, or fainting spells are experienced. ▪ Review all medications with a physician or pharmacist. ▪ See Appendix D, p. 1333.

Maternal/Child: Can cause fetal harm when administered to a pregnant woman. ▪ Use caution with breast-feeding; no information available. ▪ Safety and effectiveness of carfilzomib in pediatric patients have not been established.

Elderly: Differences in efficacy between patients less than 65 years of age and patients 65 years of age and older have not been identified. The incidence of serious adverse events is higher in patients 65 years of age or older. The risk of cardiac failure is increased in patients 75 years of age or older.

DRUG/LAB INTERACTIONS

Carfilzomib is primarily metabolized via peptidase and epoxide hydrolase activities and, as a result, is unlikely to be affected by concomitant administration of cytochrome P_{450} inhibitors and inducers. ▪ Because of IV administration and extensive metabolism, carfilzomib should not be affected by P-gp inhibitors or inducers. ▪ Carfilzomib is not expected to influence exposure of other drugs.

SIDE EFFECTS

The most commonly reported adverse reactions occurring in at least 20% of patients treated with *carfilzomib in monotherapy* are anemia, cough, diarrhea, dyspnea, fatigue, fever, headache, nausea, peripheral edema, and thrombocytopenia. The most common serious adverse reactions are acute renal failure, anemia, congestive heart failure, dyspnea, fever, hypercalcemia, and pneumonia. The most commonly reported adverse reactions occurring in at least 20% of patients treated with *carfilzomib combination therapy* are anemia, cough, diarrhea, dyspnea, fatigue, fever, hypokalemia, insomnia, muscle spasm, neutropenia, thrombocytopenia, and upper respiratory tract infection. The most common serious adverse reactions are fever, pneumonia, pulmonary embolism, and respiratory tract infection. Additional adverse reactions reported in at least 10% of patients receiving carfilzomib as either monotherapy or combination therapy include anorexia; arthralgia; asthenia; back pain; bronchitis; chills; constipation; decreased absolute neutrophil count, lymphocytes, and total white blood cell count; dizziness; elevated aspartate aminotransferase (AST); elevated serum creatinine; epistaxis; hyperglycemia; hyperkalemia; hypertension; hyperuricemia; hypocalcemia; hypoesthesia; hypomagnesemia; hyponatremia; hypophosphatemia; insomnia; nasopharyngitis; pain; peripheral neuropathy; pneumonia; rash; venous embolic and thrombotic events; and vomiting. Serious but less commonly reported adverse reactions include acute kidney injury, cardiac toxicities (cardiac arrest, congestive heart failure, myocardial ischemia), hepatic toxicity and hepatic failure, infusion reactions, PRES, pulmonary toxicity, pulmonary hypertension, TTP/HUS, and TLS. Several other adverse reactions have been reported; see manufacturer's prescribing information.

Post-Marketing: GI perforation, pericarditis.

ANTIDOTE

Notify physician of all side effects. Most will be treated symptomatically. If signs of an infusion reaction occur, slow or interrupt the infusion and treat appropriately. Monitor patients carefully until symptoms resolve. Discontinue immediately for a serious hypersensitivity reaction. Discontinue for any drug-induced pulmonary toxicity. Discontinue therapy if TTP/HUS or PRES is suspected. There is no specific antidote for carfilzomib.

In the event of an overdose or with the occurrence of a serious adverse reaction, discontinue carfilzomib; see Dose Adjustments. Notify the physician and provide supportive care as indicated. Administration of whole blood products (e.g., packed RBCs, platelets, leukocytes) and/or blood modifiers (e.g., darbepoetin alfa [Aranesp], epoetin alfa [Epogen], filgrastim [Neupogen, Zarxio], pegfilgrastim [Neulasta], sargramostim [Leukine]) may be indicated to treat bone marrow toxicity. Treat hypersensitivity reactions with epinephrine, antihistamines, corticosteroids, bronchodilators, and oxygen. Resuscitate as indicated.

CARMUSTINE (BCNU) BBW

(kar-**MUS**-teen)

BiCNU

Antineoplastic
(alkylating agent/nitrosourea)

pH 5.6 to 6

USUAL DOSE

Initial dose as a single agent in previously untreated patients is 150 to 200 mg/M². May be given as a single dose, or one half of the calculated dose may be given initially and repeated the next day. Repeat every 6 weeks if bone marrow is sufficiently recovered. Repeat course should not be administered until leukocytes are above 4,000/mm³ and platelets are above 100,000/mm³. Repeat doses adjusted according to hematologic response of previous dose (see Dose Adjustments).

DOSE ADJUSTMENTS

Bone marrow toxicity is cumulative. Dose adjustments must be considered *based on the nadir blood counts from the prior dose* according to the following chart.

Carmustine Dose Adjustment Based on Bone Marrow Suppression		
Nadir After Prior Dose		Percentage of Prior Dose to Be Given
Leukocytes/mm³	Platelets/mm³	%
≥4,000	≥100,000	100%
3,000-3,999	75,000-99,999	100%
2,000-2,999	25,000-74,999	70%
<2,000	<25,000	50%

Adjust doses accordingly when carmustine is used in combination with other myelosuppressive drugs or in patients with depleted bone marrow reserve. ▪ Dosing should be cautious in the elderly. Lower-end initial doses may be indicated. Consider decrease in cardiac, hepatic, and renal function; concomitant disease; or other drug therapy; see Elderly.

DILUTION

Specific techniques required; see Precautions. Initially dilute 100-mg vial with supplied sterile diluent (3 mL of dehydrated alcohol injection). Further dilute with 27 mL of SWFI. Each mL will contain 3.3 mg carmustine. Withdraw desired dose and further dilute in 100 mL or more of D5W and give as an infusion. Use glass containers; loss of potency occurs in PVC containers and IV tubing.

Filters: No significant loss of potency with any size cellular ester membrane filter when reconstituted or diluted as recommended.

Storage: Must be protected from light in all forms. Store unopened vials of the dry drug (carmustine) and supplied diluent in refrigerator (2° to 8° C [35° to 46° F]). After reconstitution as directed, carmustine is stable for 24 hours under refrigeration. Reconstituted vials should be examined for crystal formation before use. If crystals have formed, they may be redissolved by warming the vial to RT with agitation. After reconstitution and after further dilution to a concentration of 0.2 mg/mL in D5W, may be stored at RT but must be used within 8 hours. Temperatures above 27° C (80° F) will cause liquefaction of the drug powder; discard immediately.

COMPATIBILITY
Consider any drug NOT listed as compatible to be INCOMPATIBLE until consulting a pharmacist; specific conditions may apply.
Manufacturer lists as **incompatible** with polyvinyl chloride infusion bags; use only glass containers.

One source suggests the following **compatibilities:**
Y-site: Amifostine (Ethyol), aztreonam (Azactam), etoposide phosphate (Etopophos), filgrastim (Neupogen), fludarabine (Fludara), gemcitabine (Gemzar), granisetron (Kytril), melphalan (Alkeran), ondansetron (Zofran), piperacillin/tazobactam (Zosyn), sargramostim (Leukine), teniposide (Vumon), thiotepa, vinorelbine (Navelbine).

RATE OF ADMINISTRATION
Each single dose must be given as a slow IV infusion. Administration over fewer than 2 hours can lead to pain and burning at the injection site. Reduce rate for pain or burning at injection site, flushing of the skin, or suffusion of the conjunctiva.

ACTIONS
An alkylating agent of the nitrosourea group with antitumor activity, cell-cycle phase nonspecific. Degraded to metabolites within 15 minutes of administration. It is thought that the antineoplastic and toxic activities may be due to metabolites. Effectively crosses the blood-brain barrier. Excreted in changed form in urine. Small amounts excreted as respiratory CO_2.

INDICATIONS AND USES
Palliative therapy as a single agent or in established combination therapies in the treatment of brain tumors; multiple myeloma; Hodgkin's disease; and some non-Hodgkin's lymphomas.

CONTRAINDICATIONS
Hypersensitivity to carmustine.

PRECAUTIONS
Follow guidelines for handling cytotoxic agents. See Appendix A, p. 1331. ▪ Administered by or under the direction of the physician specialist. ▪ Delayed bone marrow suppression may be severe, especially in an already compromised patient, and result in infection and/or bleeding. Anemia may be cumulative and may require transfusion support. ▪ Pulmonary toxicity is dose related. Risk is increased with a cumulative dose greater than 1,400 mg/M². Delayed-onset pulmonary fibrosis has occurred up to 17 years after treatment with injectable carmustine in patients who received it in childhood or early adolescence. ▪ Often used with other antineoplastic drugs in reduced doses to achieve tumor remission. ▪ Secondary malignancies, including acute nonlymphocytic leukemia, myeloproliferation syndrome, and carcinoma have been reported in patients treated with alkylating agents.
Monitor: Determine absolute patency and quality of vein and adequate circulation of extremity. Severe cellulitis may result from extravasation. ▪ Delayed toxicity probable in 4 to 6 weeks; wait at least 6 weeks between doses; obtain baseline CBC, including leukocyte and platelet counts, and monitor weekly. ▪ Obtain baseline pulmonary function studies and monitor pulmonary function frequently during treatment. Risk of pulmonary toxicity is increased in patients with a baseline below 70% of the predicted forced vital capacity (FVC) or carbon monoxide diffusing capacity (DLco). ▪ Periodic monitoring of liver and renal function tests is recommended. ▪ Nausea and vomiting can be severe. Prophylactic administration of antiemetics recommended. ▪ Avoid contact of carmustine solution with the skin. ▪ Observe for any signs of infection. Prophylactic antibiotics may be

indicated pending results of C/S in a febrile neutropenic patient. ■ Maintain hydration. ■ Monitor for thrombocytopenia (platelet count less than 50,000/mm³). Initiate precautions to prevent excessive bleeding (e.g., inspect IV sites, skin, and mucous membranes; use extreme care during invasive procedures; test urine, emesis, stool, and secretions for occult blood).

Patient Education: Nonhormonal birth control recommended. ■ Report stinging or burning at IV site promptly. ■ See Appendix D, p. 1333.

Maternal/Child: Category D: avoid pregnancy; embryotoxic and teratogenic in rats; has mutagenic potential. ■ Discontinue breast-feeding. ■ Safety and effectiveness for use in pediatric patients not established. Risk versus benefit must be carefully considered due to a high risk of pulmonary toxicity occurring years after treatment and resulting in death.

Elderly: Dose selection should be cautious; see Dose Adjustments. ■ Toxicity may be increased. ■ Monitoring of renal function is suggested.

DRUG/LAB INTERACTIONS

Potentiated by **cimetidine** (Tagamet); increased myelosuppression (e.g., leukopenia and neutropenia) have been reported with concurrent use. ■ Inhibits **digoxin and phenytoin** (Dilantin); may reduce serum levels. ■ Do not administer **vaccines or chloroquine** to patients receiving antineoplastic drugs. ■ See Dose Adjustments.

SIDE EFFECTS

Most are dose related and can be reversed. Bone marrow toxicity (especially leukopenia and thrombocytopenia) is most pronounced at 4 to 6 weeks; can be severe and cumulative with repeated dosage. Anemia, chest pain, elevated liver function test results, flushing of skin and suffusion of conjunctiva from too-rapid infusion rate, headache, hyperpigmentation and burning of skin (from actual contact with solution), hypersensitivity reactions, hypotension, nausea and vomiting, neuroretinitis, pulmonary infiltrates or fibrosis with long-term therapy, renal abnormalities, retinal hemorrhage, and tachycardia.

ANTIDOTE

Notify physician of all side effects. Most will decrease in severity with reduced dosage, increased time span between doses, or symptomatic treatment. May reduce therapeutic effectiveness. Bone marrow suppression may require withholding carmustine until recovery occurs. Administration of whole blood products (e.g., packed RBCs, platelets, leukocytes) may be required. Blood modifiers (e.g., darbepoetin alfa [Aranesp], epoetin alfa [Epogen], filgrastim [Neupogen, Zarxio], pegfilgrastim [Neulasta], sargramostim [Leukine]) may be indicated to treat bone marrow toxicity. There is no specific antidote. Supportive therapy as indicated will help sustain the patient in toxicity.

CASPOFUNGIN ACETATE

(**kas**-po-**FUN**-jin **AS**-ah-tayt)

Cancidas

Antifungal
(echinocandin)

pH 6.6

USUAL DOSE

Empirical therapy: 70 mg as an infusion on Day 1. Beginning on Day 2, reduce subsequent doses to 50 mg/day. Duration of empiric therapy is based on clinical response and should continue at least until resolution of neutropenia. Patients found to have a fungal infection should be treated for a minimum of 14 days; treatment should continue for at least 7 days after both neutropenia and clinical symptoms have resolved.

Candidemia and other *Candida* infections: 70 mg as an infusion on Day 1. Beginning on Day 2, reduce subsequent doses to 50 mg/day. Duration of treatment is based on clinical and microbiologic response. Usually continued for at least 14 days after the last positive culture. Persistently neutropenic patients may require a longer course of therapy pending resolution of the neutropenia. A 150-mg dose has been studied in a small number of adult patients. Efficacy of this higher dose was not significantly better than the 50-mg dose.

Esophageal candidiasis: 50 mg daily as an infusion. Continue for 7 to 14 days after symptom resolution. A 70-mg loading dose has not been studied for this indication. Suppressive oral therapy following treatment with caspofungin may be considered to decrease the risk of relapse of oropharyngeal candidiasis in patients with HIV infections.

Invasive aspergillosis: 70 mg as an infusion on Day 1. Beginning on Day 2, reduce subsequent doses to 50 mg/day. Duration of treatment is based on severity of the underlying disease, recovery from immunosuppression, and clinical response.

PEDIATRIC DOSE

Pediatric patients 3 months to 17 years of age (for all indications): 70 mg/M^2 as an infusion on Day 1. Beginning on Day 2, reduce subsequent doses to 50 mg/M^2/day. Regardless of the patient's calculated dose, the loading dose and/or the daily maintenance dose should not exceed a maximum of 70 mg. Duration of therapy for each indication should be individualized as outlined in Usual Dose.

DOSE ADJUSTMENTS

All diagnoses: *Adult and pediatric patients:* Dose adjustment is not indicated based on age, gender, or race. ▪ See Drug/Lab Interactions.

Adults: Dose adjustment is not indicated in patients with impaired renal function or in patients with mild impaired hepatic function (Child-Pugh score 5 to 6). ▪ In patients with moderate hepatic insufficiency (Child-Pugh score 7 to 9), reduce daily doses to 35 mg after the initial dose of 50 or 70 mg. ▪ Dose may be increased from 50 to 70 mg daily in patients not clinically responding to the 50-mg dose; experience limited. ▪ In patients receiving concurrent administration of rifampin (Rifadin), increase the daily dose to 70 mg. An increase in the daily dose to 70 mg/day should be considered in patients who are not clinically responding and are taking other inducers and/or mixed inducers/inhibitors of caspofungin clearance, specifically carbamazepine (Tegretol), dexamethasone (Decadron), efavirenz (Sustiva), nevirapine (Viramune), and phenytoin (Dilantin).

Pediatric patients: If the 50-mg/M^2 daily dose is well tolerated but does not provide adequate clinical response, it may be increased to 70 mg/M^2 (not to exceed a total dose of 70 mg). ▪ There is no experience in pediatric patients with any degree of hepatic insufficiency. ▪ Consider a dose of 70 mg/M^2 (not to exceed a total dose of 70 mg) in pediatric patients receiving inducers of caspofungin clearance, specifically carbamazepine (Tegretol), dexamethasone (Decadron), efavirenz (Sustiva), nevirapine (Viramune), phenytoin (Dilantin), and rifampin (Rifadin).

DILUTION

Available in 70-mg and 50-mg vials. Select appropriate dose and allow vial of caspofungin to come to room temperature. Reconstitute selected dose with 10.8 mL of NS, SWFI, or BWFI. Mix gently to achieve a clear solution; should dissolve completely. The 70-mg vial will yield 7 mg/mL, and the 50-mg vial will yield 5 mg/mL.

Adults: Withdraw 10 mL of reconstituted solution and add to 250 mL of NS, $^1/_2$NS, $^1/_4$NS, or LR for infusion. If a 70-mg vial is not available, reconstitute two 50-mg vials and withdraw a total of 14 mL to be further diluted in 250 mL of the above solutions. When preparing a 35-mg dose, withdraw 7 mL from the reconstituted 50-mg vial and further dilute in 250 mL of the previously listed solutions. In fluid-restricted or pediatric patients, the appropriate volume of caspofungin may be added to reduced volumes of the above solutions, not to exceed a final concentration of 0.5 mg/mL.

Pediatric patients: The choice of vial used should be based on the total dose to be administered. Pediatric doses less than 50 mg should be withdrawn from a 50-mg vial to ensure accuracy. After reconstitution, withdraw the volume required to provide the correct dose, and add to a volume of NS, $^1/_2$NS, $^1/_4$NS, or LR for infusion to achieve a final concentration not to exceed 0.5 mg/mL.

Storage: Refrigerate unopened vials. Reconstituted vials may be kept at less than or equal to 25° C (77° F) for 1 hour before preparing as an infusion solution. Discard any unused reconstituted solution. Fully diluted solutions may be stored at less than or equal to 25° C (77° F) for 24 hours or refrigerated for 48 hours.

COMPATIBILITY
(Underline Indicates Conflicting Compatibility Information)

Manufacturer states, "Do not mix or co-infuse caspofungin with other medications. Do not use diluents containing dextrose."

One source suggests the following **compatibilities:**

Y-site: Acyclovir (Zovirax), amikacin, amiodarone (Nexterone), azithromycin (Zithromax), aztreonam (Azactam), bumetanide, carboplatin (Paraplatin), ciprofloxacin (Cipro IV), cisplatin, cyclosporine (Sandimmune), daptomycin (Cubicin), daunorubicin (Cerubidine), diltiazem (Cardizem), diphenhydramine (Benadryl), dobutamine, dolasetron (Anzemet), dopamine, doripenem (Doribax), doxorubicin (Adriamycin), epinephrine (Adrenalin), etoposide phosphate (Etopophos), famotidine (Pepcid IV), fentanyl, fluconazole (Diflucan), ganciclovir (Cytovene IV), gentamicin, hydralazine, hydrocortisone sodium succinate (Solu-Cortef), hydromorphone (Dilaudid), ifosfamide (Ifex), imipenem-cilastatin (Primaxin), insulin (regular), levofloxacin (Levaquin), linezolid (Zyvox), lorazepam (Ativan), magnesium sulfate, melphalan (Alkeran), meperidine (Demerol), meropenem (Merrem IV), metronidazole (Flagyl IV), midazolam (Versed), milrinone (Primacor), mitomycin (Mutamycin), morphine, mycophenolate (CellCept IV), norepinephrine (Levophed), ondansetron (Zofran), pantoprazole (Protonix IV), phenylephrine (Neo-Synephrine), potassium chloride, quinupristin/dalfopristin (Synercid), tacrolimus (Prograf), telavancin (Vibativ), tobramycin, vancomycin, vasopressin, vincristine, voriconazole (VFEND IV).

RATE OF ADMINISTRATION

A single dose as an infusion evenly distributed over 1 hour.

ACTIONS

An antifungal. An echinocandin or glucan synthesis inhibitor. It attacks the fungal cell wall and inhibits the synthesis of beta (1,3)-D-glucan, an essential component of the cell wall of susceptible *Aspergillus* and *Candida* species. Beta (1,3)-D-glucan is not found in human cells. Extensively bound to albumin (97%). After completion of an IV infusion, plasma concentrations decline in several phases, each with its own half-life (e.g., 9 to 11 hours, 40 to 50 hours). Distribution, rather than excretion or biotransformation, is the primary mechanism influencing plasma clearance. Slowly metabolized by hydrolysis and *N*-acetylation, eventually breaking down to amino acids and their degradates. Excreted in urine and feces.

INDICATIONS AND USES

Empirical therapy for presumed fungal infections in febrile, neutropenic patients. ▪ Treatment of invasive aspergillosis in patients who are refractory to or intolerant of other therapies (i.e., amphotericin B [conventional], lipid formulations of amphotericin B [e.g., Abelcet, AmBisome, Amphotec], and/or itraconazole [Sporanox]). Has not been studied for initial therapy for invasive aspergillosis. ▪ Treatment of esophageal candidiasis. ▪ Treatment of candidemia and the following *Candida* infections: intra-abdominal abscesses, peritonitis, and pleural space infections. Has not been studied in endocarditis, osteomyelitis, and meningitis due to *Candida*.

CONTRAINDICATIONS

Known hypersensitivity to caspofungin or any of its components.

PRECAUTIONS

Concomitant use with cyclosporine is not recommended unless the potential benefit outweighs the risk; see Monitor and Drug/Lab Interactions. ▪ Abnormal LFTs have been seen in healthy volunteers and in adult and pediatric patients treated with caspofungin. In some patients with serious underlying conditions who were receiving multiple concomitant medications with caspofungin, isolated cases of clinically significant hepatic dysfunction, hepatitis, and hepatic failure have been reported. A causal relationship to caspofungin has not been established. ▪ There is no clinical experience in adult patients with severe hepatic insufficiency (Child-Pugh score greater than 9) or in pediatric patients with any degree of hepatic impairment. ▪ Possible histamine-mediated reactions and hypersensitivity reactions, including anaphylaxis, have been reported. ▪ Clinical failures due to drug resistance in patients receiving caspofungin therapy have been reported.

Monitor: Most patients have serious underlying medical conditions (e.g., bone marrow transplant, HIV, malignancies) requiring multiple concomitant medications. Obtain baseline studies as required and repeat as indicated. ▪ Monitor vital signs. ▪ Observe for S/S of a histamine-mediated reaction (e.g., angioedema, bronchospasm, facial swelling, pruritus, rash, sensation of warmth) or a hypersensitivity reaction (e.g., chills, difficulty breathing, hypotension, rash). ▪ Encourage fluids to maintain hydration. ▪ Effects of severe hepatic impairment unknown; monitor liver function tests (e.g., AST, ALT) in patients with pre-existing impaired hepatic function and any time S/S suggestive of liver dysfunction develop (e.g., jaundice, lethargy). ▪ Monitor liver function in patients receiving therapy with both caspofungin and cyclosporine. Monitor closely in patients who develop abnormal liver function tests. The risk/benefit of continued therapy should be evaluated. ▪ See Drug/Lab Interactions.

Patient Education: Review all medical conditions and medications before beginning treatment. ▪ Promptly report pain at infusion site, symptoms of histamine reactions (e.g., facial swelling, pruritus, rash, sensation of warmth), hypersensitivity reactions (e.g., chills, difficulty breathing, hypotension, rash), or hepatic toxicity (e.g., jaundice).

Maternal/Child: Category C: use during pregnancy only if benefits outweigh potential risks to fetus. Based on animal studies, may cause fetal harm. ▪ Has been found in the milk of lactating, drug-treated rats; use caution if required during breast-feeding, or discontinue breast-feeding. ▪ Safety and effectiveness for use in neonates and infants under 3 months of age not studied.

Elderly: Response similar to that in younger patients. Dose adjustment is not recommended; however, use caution; may have greater sensitivity to its effects.

DRUG/LAB INTERACTIONS

Concomitant use with **cyclosporine** (Sandimmune) is not recommended unless benefit outweighs risk. By Day 10 of concomitant administration some patients had a transient ALT 2 to 3 times the upper limit of normal, and the AUC of caspofungin had increased by about 35%. ▪ Pharmacokinetics of caspofungin are not altered by **amphotericin B**, **itraconazole** (Sporanox), **mycophenolate** (CellCept), **nelfinavir** (Viracept), **or tacrolimus** (Prograf). ▪ Serum concentrations of tacrolimus may be somewhat decreased with concomitant administration; monitor tacrolimus concentrations and adjust dose as indicated. ▪ **Inducers and/or mixed inducers/inhibitors of caspofungin clearance** (e.g., carbamazepine [Tegretol], dexamethasone [Decadron], efavirenz [Sustiva], nevirapine [Viramune], phenytoin [Dilantin], rifampin [Rifadin]) may significantly increase caspofungin clearance and require an increase in dose; see Dose Adjustments. ▪ Although its clearance may be affected by the enzyme inducers previously mentioned, caspofungin is not an inhibitor or inducer of any enzyme in the cytochrome P_{450} (CPY) system. It is not a substrate (a substance on which an enzyme acts) for P-glycoprotein and is a poor substrate for cytochrome P_{450} enzymes. It is not expected to interact with drugs metabolized by this system (e.g., amiodarone [Nexterone], calcium channel blockers [e.g., diltiazem (Cardizem), verapamil], cimetidine [Tagamet], MAO inhibitors [e.g., selegiline (Eldepryl)]).

SIDE EFFECTS

Side effect profile is similar in both adult and pediatric patients. Incidence difficult to assess because of multiple medical conditions and multiple medications. Most commonly reported side effects include chills, diarrhea, elevated liver function tests (e.g., alkaline phosphatase, ALT, AST), fever, hypokalemia, hypotension, and rash. Other side effects reported include abdominal pain, ARDS, cough, diaphoresis, flushing, headache, hyperbilirubinemia, hypercalcemia, hyperglycemia, hypertension, hypomagnesemia, increased RBCs and protein in urine, infusion-related reactions, injection site reactions, nausea, peripheral edema, phlebitis, pneumonia, pulmonary edema, radiographic infiltrates, tachycardia, and vomiting. Possible histamine-mediated symptoms (e.g., angioedema, bronchospasm, facial swelling, pruritus, rash, sensation of warmth) and hypersensitivity reactions with dyspnea, stridor, worsening of rash, and anaphylaxis have been reported.

Post-Marketing: Erythema multiforme, hepatic necrosis, hepatobiliary adverse reactions (e.g., clinically significant hepatic dysfunction, hepatitis, hepatic failure) in adult and pediatric patients with serious underlying medical conditions, increased gamma-glutamyl transferase, pancreatitis, renal dysfunction (clinically significant), skin exfoliation, and Stevens-Johnson syndrome.

ANTIDOTE

Notify physician of all side effects; most will be treated symptomatically. Discontinue caspofungin and notify physician of abnormal liver function tests progressing to clinical S/S of liver disease. Rash may be the first sign of an exfoliative skin disorder in immunocompromised patients; discontinue caspofungin and notify physician. Histamine-mediated reactions may require discontinuation of caspofungin and appropriate treatment. Not removed by hemodialysis. Discontinue caspofungin and treat anaphylaxis as indicated and/or resuscitate as necessary.

CEFAZOLIN SODIUM
(sef-**AYZ**-oh-lin **SO**-dee-um)

Ancef, Kefzol

Antibacterial
(cephalosporin)

pH 4.5 to 7

USUAL DOSE
250 mg to 1.5 Gm every 6 to 8 hours. Up to 6 Gm is usual, but 12 Gm in 24 hours has been used, depending on severity of infection.

Mild infections: 250 to 500 mg every 8 hours.

Moderate to severe infections: 500 mg to 1 Gm every 6 to 8 hours.

Life-threatening infections (e.g., endocarditis, septicemia): 1 to 1.5 Gm every 6 hours.

Pneumococcal pneumonia: 500 mg every 12 hours.

Acute, uncomplicated urinary tract infections: 1 Gm every 12 hours.

Perioperative prophylaxis: 1 to 2 Gm 30 minutes to 1 hour before incision. For lengthy procedures (e.g., 2 hours or more), 0.5 to 1 Gm may be repeated in the OR. Administer every 6 to 8 hours for 24 hours postoperatively.

Endocarditis prophylaxis (unlabeled): 1 Gm 30 minutes before surgery.

PEDIATRIC DOSE
Mild to moderately severe infections: 25 to 50 mg/kg/day, divided into 3 or 4 doses (6.25 to 12.5 mg/kg every 6 hours, or 8.3 to 16.6 mg/kg every 8 hours).

Severe infections: 100 mg/kg/day, divided into 3 or 4 doses (25 mg/kg every 6 hours or 33.3 mg/kg every 8 hours. Do not exceed adult dose.

Perioperative prophylaxis: The manufacturer does not provide dosage recommendations in pediatric patients. However, one source recommends 30 mg/kg (not to exceed 2 Gm) administered within 60 minutes of the surgical incision.

Endocarditis prophylaxis (unlabeled): 50 mg/kg 30 minutes before the start of surgery. Do not exceed 1 Gm.

NEONATAL DOSE
See Maternal/Child. American Academy of Pediatrics (AAP) recommends:

7 days of age or younger regardless of weight: 25 mg/kg every 12 hours.

8 to 28 days of age; weight 2 kg or less: 25 mg/kg every 12 hours.

8 to 28 days of age; weight more than 2 kg: 25 mg/kg every 8 hours.

DOSE ADJUSTMENTS
Reduced doses or extended intervals may be indicated in the elderly; consider age-related impaired organ function, nutritional status, and concomitant disease or drug therapy. In impaired renal function, the initial dose in adults and pediatric patients should be as above. Reduce all subsequent doses according to the following charts.

Cefazolin Dose Guidelines in Impaired Renal Function for Adults		
CrCl	Dose	Frequency
CrCl >55 mL/min	Full	Normal
CrCl 35-54 mL/min	Full	q 8 hr or less frequently
CrCl 11-34 mL/min	$^1/_2$ Usual dose	q 12 hr
CrCl 10 mL/min	$^1/_2$ Usual dose	q 18-24 hr

Cefazolin Dose Guidelines in Impaired Renal Function for Pediatric Patients		
Creatinine Clearance (mL/min)	Dose	Frequency
>70 mL/min	Full	Normal
40-70 mL/min	60% of normal daily dose*	q 12 hr
20-40 mL/min	25% of normal daily dose*	q 12 hr
5-20 mL/min	10% of normal daily dose*	q 24 hr

*In equally divided doses.

DILUTION

Each 1 Gm or fraction thereof of the lyophilized powder must be reconstituted with at least 2.5 mL of SWFI. Shake well. To reduce the incidence of thrombophlebitis, may be further diluted in 50 to 100 mL of D5W, NS, or other **compatible** infusion solutions (see chart on inside back cover or literature) and given as an intermittent infusion. Available in several forms (other than vials of lyophilized powder), including dual-chamber DUPLEX containers with dextrose, premixed with dextrose in a frozen Galaxy container, Add-Vantage vials, and pharmacy bulk vials. Refer to manufacturer's prescribing information for specific preparation and storage requirements.

Storage: Before reconstitution of the lyophilized powder, protect from light and store at CRT. Give within 24 hours of preparation if stored at CRT or within 10 days if under refrigeration. Discard pharmacy bulk vials within 4 hours after initial entry.

COMPATIBILITY   (Underline Indicates Conflicting Compatibility Information)

Consider any drug NOT listed as compatible to be INCOMPATIBLE until consulting a pharmacist; specific conditions may apply.

May be used concomitantly with aminoglycosides (e.g., amikacin, gentamicin), but these drugs must never be mixed in the same infusion (mutual inactivation). If given concurrently, administer separately and flush IV line before and after administration.

One source suggests the following **compatibilities:**

Additive: Aztreonam (Azactam), clindamycin (Cleocin), famotidine (Pepcid IV), fluconazole (Diflucan), linezolid (Zyvox), meperidine (Demerol), metronidazole (Flagyl IV), verapamil.

Y-site: Acyclovir (Zovirax), allopurinol (Aloprim), alprostadil, amifostine (Ethyol), amiodarone (Nexterone), anidulafungin (Eraxis), atracurium (Tracrium), aztreonam (Azactam), bivalirudin (Angiomax), calcium gluconate, cisatracurium (Nimbex), cyclophosphamide (Cytoxan), dexmedetomidine (Precedex), diltiazem (Cardizem), docetaxel (Taxotere), doxapram (Dopram), doxorubicin liposomal (Doxil), enalaprilat (Vasotec IV), esmolol (Brevibloc), etoposide phosphate (Etopophos), famotidine (Pepcid IV), fenoldopam (Corlopam), filgrastim (Neupogen), fluconazole (Diflucan), fludarabine (Fludara), foscarnet (Foscavir), gallium nitrate (Ganite), gemcitabine (Gemzar), granisetron (Kytril), heparin, hetastarch in electrolytes (Hextend), hetastarch in NS (Hespan), hydromorphone (Dilaudid), 6% hydroxyethyl starch (Voluven), insulin (regular), labetalol, lidocaine, linezolid (Zyvox), magnesium sulfate, melphalan (Alkeran), meperidine (Demerol), midazolam (Versed), milrinone (Primacor), morphine, multivitamins (M.V.I.), nicardipine (Cardene IV), ondansetron (Zofran), palonosetron (Aloxi), pancuronium, pantoprazole (Protonix IV), propofol (Diprivan), ranitidine (Zantac), remifentanil (Ultiva), sargramostim (Leukine), tacrolimus (Prograf), teniposide (Vumon), theophylline, thiotepa, vancomycin, vecuronium, warfarin (Coumadin).

RATE OF ADMINISTRATION

IV injection: Each 1 Gm or fraction thereof over 3 to 5 minutes.

Intermittent infusion: Extend administration time as indicated by amount of solution and condition of patient. Usually administered over 30 to 60 minutes.

ACTIONS

A semi-synthetic, first-generation cephalosporin antibiotic that is bactericidal through inhibition of cell wall synthesis to some gram-positive and gram-negative organisms, including staphylococci and streptococci. Peak serum levels achieved by end of infusion. Widely distributed in most tissues and body fluids (CSF minimal), including bone, gallbladder, myocardium, and skin and soft tissue. Serum half-life is 1.8 hours. Excreted rapidly in the urine. Crosses the placental barrier. Secreted in breast milk.

INDICATIONS AND USES
Treatment of serious infections of the bone, joints, skin, soft tissue, respiratory tract, biliary tract, and GU tract; septicemia; and endocarditis. Effective only if the causative organism is susceptible. ▪ Perioperative prophylaxis.

Unlabeled uses: Prophylaxis of bacterial endocarditis.

CONTRAINDICATIONS
Previous immediate hypersensitivity reaction (e.g., anaphylaxis, serious skin reactions) to cefazolin or the cephalosporin class of antibiotics, penicillins, or other beta-lactams; see Precautions. ▪ Premixed solutions containing dextrose may be contraindicated in patients with known allergies to corn or corn products.

PRECAUTIONS
Hypersensitivity reactions, including fatalities, have been reported and include reports of individuals with a history of penicillin hypersensitivity or sensitivity to multiple allergens experiencing severe reactions when treated with cephalosporins. Check history of previous hypersensitivity reactions to penicillins, cephalosporins, or other allergens. Actual incidence of cross-allergenicity not established but may be more common with first-generation cephalosporins. ▪ Hypersensitivity reactions have been reported with administration of corn-derived, dextrose-containing products to patients with or without a history of hypersensitivity to corn products. Cefazolin in the DUPLEX and Galaxy containers contains dextrose. ▪ Sensitivity studies indicated to determine susceptibility of the causative organisms to cefazolin. ▪ To reduce the development of drug-resistant bacteria and maintain its effectiveness, cefazolin should be used to treat or prevent only those infections proven or strongly suspected to be caused by bacteria. ▪ Continue antibiotic therapy for at least 2 to 3 days after all symptoms of infection subside. ▪ Avoid prolonged use of drug; superinfection caused by overgrowth of nonsusceptible organisms may result. ▪ Use caution in patients with impaired renal function, allergies, or a history of GI disease (especially colitis). ▪ With inappropriately high doses, seizures may occur in patients with impaired renal function. ▪ May be associated with an elevated INR, especially in patients with impaired renal or hepatic function, those with a poor nutritional state, and those receiving extended courses of antimicrobial therapy. ▪ *Clostridium difficile*–associated diarrhea (CDAD) has been reported. May range from mild diarrhea to fatal colitis. Consider in patients who present with diarrhea during or after treatment with cefazolin.

Monitor: Watch for early symptoms of hypersensitivity reactions. ▪ Obtain baseline PT/INR and monitor, especially in at-risk patients (see Precautions); vitamin K may be indicated. ▪ See Drug/Lab Interactions; additional monitoring may be indicated (e.g., renal function, drug serum levels, PT/INR).

Patient Education: Report promptly any bleeding or bruising, diarrhea, or symptoms of allergy (e.g., difficulty breathing, hives, itching, rash). ▪ Promptly report diarrhea or bloody stools that occur during treatment or up to several months after an antibiotic has been discontinued; may indicate CDAD and require treatment.

Maternal/Child: Category B: safety for use during pregnancy and breast-feeding not established. No problems documented. ▪ Safety for use in premature infants and neonates under 1 month of age not established; immature renal function will increase blood levels. See Pediatric Dose.

Elderly: No specific problems documented. ▪ See Usual Dose and Dose Adjustments.

DRUG/LAB INTERACTIONS
Risk of nephrotoxicity may be increased with **aminoglycosides and other nephrotoxic agents** (e.g., loop diuretics [e.g., furosemide (Lasix)]). ▪ **Probenecid** inhibits excretion, resulting in elevated cefazolin levels. Dose reduction of cefazolin may be necessary. ▪ May be antagonized by **bacteriostatic antibiotics** (e.g., chloramphenicol, erythromycin,

tetracyclines); may interfere with bactericidal action. ▪ May result in false-positive reaction for **urine glucose** except with enzyme-based tests (e.g., Clinistix). ▪ Positive direct Coombs' tests have been reported. ▪ See Compatibility and Side Effects.

SIDE EFFECTS

Anorexia; CDAD; diarrhea; elevated BUN and creatinine levels; elevated PT/INR; hypersensitivity reactions, including anaphylaxis; leukopenia; local site pain; nausea and vomiting; neutropenia; oral thrush; phlebitis; positive direct and indirect Coombs' test; pruritis; transient elevation of AST, ALT, and alkaline phosphatase; seizures (large doses); thrombophlebitis; vaginal itching or discharge. Hypoprothrombinemia (rare) and hemolytic anemia may occur. Hepatitis and renal failure have been reported. Aplastic anemia, erythema multiforme, hemolytic anemia, hemorrhage, hepatic impairment (including cholestasis), pancytopenia, renal impairment, Stevens-Johnson syndrome, toxic epidermal necrolysis, and toxic nephropathy have been reported with cephalosporin-class antibiotics.

ANTIDOTE

Notify the physician of any side effects. Discontinue the drug if indicated. Mild cases of CDAD may respond to discontinuation of cefazolin. Treat CDAD with fluids, electrolytes, protein supplements, and oral vancomycin (Vancocin) or metronidazole (Flagyl) as indicated. In severe cases, surgical evaluation may be indicated. Discontinue cefazolin and treat hypersensitivity reaction as indicated (airway, oxygen, IV fluids, antihistamines [e.g., diphenhydramine], corticosteroids [e.g., hydrocortisone sodium succinate (Solu-Cortef)], epinephrine, pressor-amines [e.g., dopamine]) and resuscitate as necessary. Hemodialysis may be useful in overdose.

CEFEPIME HYDROCHLORIDE

(SEF-eh-pim hy-droh-**KLOR**-eyed)

Antibacterial
(cephalosporin)

Maxipime

pH 4 to 6

USUAL DOSE

Adults: Range is from 0.5 Gm to 2 Gm. Usually given every 12 hours. Dose based on severity of disease and/or specific susceptibility of the causative organism according to the following chart.

Cefepime Dose Guidelines			
Site and Type of Infection	Dose	Frequency	Duration (days)
Mild to Moderate Uncomplicated or complicated urinary tract infections, including pyelonephritis	0.5-1 Gm IV/IM	q 12 hr	7-10
Severe Uncomplicated or complicated urinary tract infections, including pyelonephritis	2 Gm IV	q 12 hr	10
Moderate to Severe Pneumonia*	1-2 Gm IV	q 8-12 hr	10
Moderate to Severe Uncomplicated skin and skin structure infections	2 Gm IV	q 12 hr	10
Empiric Therapy For febrile neutropenic patients	2 Gm IV	q 8 hr	7 or until neutropenia resolves
Complicated Intra-abdominal infections	Cefepime 2 Gm IV q 8-12 hr in combination with metronidazole 500 mg or 7.5 mg/kg q 6 hr, not to exceed 4 Gm/24 hr of metronidazole		7-10

*For *Pseudomonas aeruginosa,* use 2 Gm q 8 h.

PEDIATRIC DOSE

Pediatric patients 2 months to 16 years; weight up to 40 kg: 50 mg/kg every 12 hours with the duration of therapy as outlined under Usual Dose. Increase frequency to every 8 hours for empiric monotherapy in febrile neutropenia and for treatment of pneumonia due to *Pseudomonas aeruginosa.* Do not exceed adult dose.

DOSE ADJUSTMENTS

In impaired renal function, the initial dose should be as stated earlier (except in patients undergoing hemodialysis). All remaining doses should be reduced based on CrCl according to the following chart (e.g., if the normal dose is 1 Gm every 12 hours with a CrCl greater than 60, the maintenance dose would be reduced to 1 Gm every 24 hours with a CrCl between 30 and 60 mL/min). Dose reductions should be comparable in *pediatric patients.*

Cefepime Dose Guidelines in Impaired Renal Function				
Creatinine Clearance (mL/min)	Recommended Maintenance Schedule (relative to normal dosing schedule)			
Normal Recommended Dosing Schedule (>60 mL/min)	500 mg q 12 hr	1 Gm q 12 hr	2 Gm q 12 hr	2 Gm q 8 hr
30-60 mL/min	500 mg q 24 hr	1 Gm q 24 hr	2 Gm q 24 hr	2 Gm q 12 hr
11-29 mL/min	500 mg q 24 hr	500 mg q 24 hr	1 Gm q 24 hr	2 Gm q 24 hr
<11 mL/min	250 mg q 24 hr	250 mg q 24 hr	500 mg q 24 hr	1 Gm q 24 hr
CAPD	500 mg q 48 hr	1 Gm q 48 hr	2 Gm q 48 hr	2 Gm q 48 hr
*Hemodialysis	1 Gm on Day 1, then 500 mg q 24 hr. Increase to 1 Gm q 24 hr in febrile neutropenia.			1 Gm q 24 hr

*On hemodialysis days, cefepime should be administered following hemodialysis. Whenever possible, administer at the same time each day.

Consult literature or Important IV Therapy Facts, p. xx, for conversion formula if dose is to be based on SCr. ▪ Reduced dose may be required in the elderly based on renal function. ▪ Dose adjustment not required in impaired hepatic function.

DILUTION
Vials of the lyophilized powder for IM/IV use may be reconstituted (see the following chart) and then further diluted with NS, D5W, D10W, D5NS, D5LR, $^1/_6$ M sodium lactate, Normosol-R, or D5/Normosol M. Concentrations between 1 mg/mL and 40 mg/mL are acceptable. (500 mg reconstituted with 5 mL = 100 mg/mL, further diluted with 95 mL = 5 mg/mL, with 45 mL = 10 mg/mL.) Available in several forms (other than vials of lyophilized powder), including Add-Vantage vials, dual-chamber DUPLEX containers with dextrose, and premixed with dextrose in a frozen Galaxy container. Refer to manufacturer's prescribing information for specific preparation and storage requirements.

Cefepime Dilution Guidelines			
Single-Dose Vials for Intravenous Administration	Amount of Diluent to Be Added (mL)	Approximate Available Volume (mL)	Approximate Cefepime Concentration (mg/mL)
CEFEPIME VIAL CONTENT			
500 mg (IV)	5 mL	5.6 mL	100 mg/mL
1 Gm (IV)	10 mL	11.3 mL	100 mg/mL
2 Gm (IV)	10 mL	12.5 mL	160 mg/mL
ADD-VANTAGE			
1-Gm vial	50 mL	50 mL	20 mg/mL
1-Gm vial	100 mL	100 mL	10 mg/mL
2-Gm vial	50 mL	50 mL	40 mg/mL
2-Gm vial	100 mL	100 mL	20 mg/mL

Filters: Specific information from studies not available; contact manufacturer for further information.

Storage: See manufacturer's directions. Recommendations for storing vary from CRT (20° to 25° C [68° to 77° F]) to 2° to 25° C (36° to 77° F) in the dry state; protect from light. Most reconstituted or diluted solutions are stable for 24 hours at CRT and 7 days if refrigerated (recommendations may vary with diluent).

COMPATIBILITY   (Underline Indicates Conflicting Compatibility Information)
Consider any drug NOT listed as compatible to be INCOMPATIBLE until consulting a pharmacist; specific conditions may apply.

Manufacturer recommends temporarily discontinuing other solutions infusing at the same site during intermittent infusion. May be used concomitantly with aminoglycosides (e.g., gentamicin, tobramycin), aminophylline, metronidazole (Flagyl IV), and vancomycin, but these drugs must never be mixed in the same infusion (mutual inactivation or other potential interactions). If concurrent therapy with cefepime is indicated, each of these antibiotics can be administered separately. Flush IV line before and after administration.

Sources suggest the following **compatibilities:**
Additive: Manufacturer lists specific concentrations of amikacin, ampicillin, clindamycin (Cleocin), heparin, potassium chloride (KCl), theophylline, Aminosyn II 4.25% with electrolytes and calcium, and Inpersol with 4.25% dextrose. Other sources add metronidazole (Flagyl IV) and vancomycin. Do not introduce additives into Add-Vantage vials, DUPLEX containers, or Galaxy containers.
Y-site: Amikacin, anidulafungin (Eraxis), bivalirudin (Angiomax), dexmedetomidine (Precedex), dobutamine, docetaxel (Taxotere), dopamine, doxorubicin liposomal (Doxil), fenoldopam (Corlopam), fluconazole (Diflucan), furosemide (Lasix), gentamicin, granisetron (Kytril), hetastarch in electrolytes (Hextend), insulin (regular), ketamine (Ketalar), methylprednisolone (Solu-Medrol), milrinone (Primacor), morphine, mycophenolate (CellCept IV), remefentanil (Ultiva), sufentanil (Sufenta), telavancin (Vibativ), tigecycline (Tygacil), tobramycin, valproate (Depacon), vancomycin.

RATE OF ADMINISTRATION
Do not use plastic containers in a series connection; could result in air embolism. May be given through Y-tube or three-way stopcock of infusion set; see Compatibility.
Intermittent infusion: A single dose equally distributed over 30 minutes.

ACTIONS
A semi-synthetic, broad-spectrum, fourth-generation cephalosporin antibiotic. Bactericidal to both gram-positive and gram-negative organisms, including many strains resistant to third-generation cephalosporins and aminoglycosides. Acts by inhibition of bacterial wall synthesis. Has a well-balanced spectrum with good antistaphylococcal activity, enhanced activity against gram-negative organisms, and good antipseudomonal activity. Peak serum levels achieved by end of infusion; half-life is 1.7 to 2.3 hours. Therapeutic levels last for 12 hours, allowing for twice-daily dosing. Well distributed into many body fluids and tissues. Partially metabolized; 85% excreted unchanged in urine. Secreted in breast milk.

INDICATIONS AND USES
Treatment of moderate to severe pneumonia caused by susceptible organisms, including cases associated with concurrent bacteremia. ▪ Treatment of uncomplicated and complicated urinary tract infections caused by susceptible organisms, including pyelonephritis and cases associated with concurrent bacteremia. ▪ Treatment of uncomplicated skin and skin structure infections caused by susceptible organisms. ▪ Empiric monotherapy in the treatment of febrile neutropenic patients. ▪ Treatment of complicated intraabdominal infections in adults; used in combination with metronidazole (Flagyl). ▪ See literature for list of susceptible organisms.

CONTRAINDICATIONS
Patients who have shown immediate hypersensitivity reactions to cefepime, any cephalosporin, penicillins, or other beta-lactam antibiotics; see Precautions. ▪ Premixed solutions containing dextrose may be contraindicated in patients with known allergies to corn or corn products.

PRECAUTIONS
Hypersensitivity reactions, including fatalities, have been reported and include reports of individuals with a history of penicillin hypersensitivity or sensitivity to multiple allergens experiencing severe reactions when treated with cephalosporins. Check history of previ-

ous hypersensitivity reactions to penicillins, cephalosporins, or other allergens. Actual incidence of cross-allergenicity not established but may be more common with first-generation cephalosporins. ▪ Specific sensitivity studies are indicated to determine susceptibility of the causative organism to cefepime. ▪ To reduce the development of drug-resistant bacteria and maintain its effectiveness, cefepime should be used to treat or prevent only those infections proven or strongly suspected to be caused by bacteria. ▪ Generally more resistant to hydrolysis by beta-lactamases than third-generation cephalosporins are. ▪ IM injection is used only for mild to moderate urinary tract infections. ▪ Avoid prolonged use of drug; superinfection caused by overgrowth of nonsusceptible organisms may result. ▪ Continue for at least 2 days after all symptoms of infection subside. ▪ May decrease prothrombin activity, especially in patients with impaired renal or hepatic function, those in a poor nutritional state, and those receiving extended courses of antimicrobial therapy. ▪ Use caution in patients with a history of GI disease (especially colitis). ▪ Serious adverse events, including aphasia, encephalopathy (changes in consciousness, including coma, confusion, hallucinations, and stupor), myoclonus, nonconvulsive status epilepticus, seizures, and other life-threatening or fatal events, have occurred. Patients with impaired renal function may be at greater risk, especially if doses are not properly adjusted; see Dose Adjustments and monitor closely. In most cases, neurotoxicity was reversible and resolved after cefepime was discontinued and/or after hemodialysis. ▪ *Clostridium difficile*–associated diarrhea (CDAD) has been reported. May range from mild diarrhea to fatal colitis. Consider in patients who present with diarrhea during or after treatment with cefepime. ▪ Contains arginine, which may alter glucose metabolism and elevate serum potassium. ▪ Higher-end doses may increase incidence and severity of rash and require cefepime to be discontinued. ▪ Insufficient data exist for monotherapy of febrile neutropenia in patients at high risk for severe infection (e.g., history of recent bone marrow transplant, hypotension on presentation, underlying hematologic malignancy, severe or prolonged neutropenia). No data are available for patients with septic shock. ▪ If meningitis is suspected or documented, an alternate agent with demonstrated clinical effectiveness should be used.

Monitor: Watch for early symptoms of a hypersensitivity reaction. ▪ Obtain baseline CBC with differential and platelets and SCr. ▪ Obtain baseline PT and monitor, especially in at-risk patients (see Precautions); vitamin K may be indicated. ▪ Monitoring of serum glucose and electrolytes (e.g., potassium, calcium) may be indicated. ▪ May cause thrombophlebitis. ▪ Monitor and re-evaluate frequently the need for continued antimicrobial treatment in patients whose fever resolves but who remain neutropenic for more than 7 days. ▪ See Drug/Lab Interactions.

Patient Education: Promptly report any bleeding or bruising or symptoms of hypersensitivity (e.g., difficulty breathing, hives, itching, rash). ▪ Promptly report diarrhea or bloody stools that occur during treatment or up to several months after an antibiotic has been discontinued; may indicate CDAD and require treatment. ▪ Promptly report neurologic S/S (e.g., change in consciousness, confusion, hallucinations, seizures, stupor).

Maternal/Child: Category B: safety for use during pregnancy, labor and delivery, and breast-feeding not established; use only if clearly needed. ▪ Safety and effectiveness have not been established for use in infants under 2 months of age, in pediatric patients for treatment of complicated intra-abdominal infections, or for treatment of serious infections in pediatric patients in whom the suspected or proven pathogen is *Haemophilus influenzae* type b. ▪ Pharmacokinetics in pediatric patients and adults are similar. Dose modification similar to adults is indicated in impaired renal function; see Dose Adjustments. ▪ Immature renal function of infants and small children will increase blood levels of all cephalosporins.

Elderly: Consider age-related impaired organ function, nutritional status, and concomitant disease or drug therapy; reduced dose or extended intervals may be indicated. Serious adverse reactions (e.g., aphasia, encephalopathy, myoclonus, nonconvulsive status epilepticus, seizures) have occurred in elderly patients with renal impairment given unadjusted doses of cefepime; see Dose Adjustments. Monitor for hypocalcemia.

DRUG/LAB INTERACTIONS

Risk of nephrotoxicity may be increased with **aminoglycosides and other nephrotoxic agents** (e.g., loop diuretics [e.g., furosemide (Lasix)]); monitor renal function closely. ▪ Risk of ototoxicity may be increased when administered with aminoglycosides (e.g., gentamicin). ▪ May cause a false-positive **direct Coombs' test.** ▪ May have a false-positive reaction for **urine glucose** except with enzyme-based tests (e.g., Clinistix). ▪ See Side Effects. ▪ Although it has not been specifically studied with cefepime, other cephalosporins have the following drug interactions. May be antagonized by **bacteriostatic antibiotics** (e.g., chloramphenicol, erythromycin, tetracyclines); may interfere with bactericidal action. ▪ Large amounts of **cephalosporins and/or salicylates** may induce hypoprothrombinemia (deficiency of prothrombin [factor II]). The addition of **agents that affect platelet aggregation and/or may have GI ulcerative potential** (e.g., NSAIDs [ibuprofen (Advil, Motrin), naproxen (Aleve, Naprosyn)] or sulfinpyrazone [Anturane]) may increase risk of hemorrhage. ▪ See Compatibility.

SIDE EFFECTS

Local reactions (including phlebitis), pain and/or inflammation, and rash are most common. Full scope of hypersensitivity reactions (e.g., anaphylaxis, itching, rash, shock, urticaria). Abnormal PT and PTT; bone marrow suppression (e.g., agranulocytosis, anemia, leukopenia, neutropenia, thrombocytopenia); CDAD; decreased calcium (more common in elderly) and phosphorus; diarrhea; elevated alkaline phosphatase, AST, ALT, BUN, calcium, creatinine, eosinophils, phosphorus, potassium, and total bilirubin; erythema; fever; headache; nausea and vomiting; neurotoxicity (e.g., seizures [large doses, or standard doses in renally impaired patients]); oral moniliasis; prolonged PT; positive Coombs' test (without hemolysis); vaginitis. Aplastic anemia, erythema multiforme, hemolytic anemia, hemorrhage, hepatic dysfunction (including cholestasis), pancytopenia, renal dysfunction, Stevens-Johnson syndrome, toxic epidermal necrolysis, and toxic nephropathy have been reported with cephalosporin-class antibiotics.

Overdose: Aphasia, encephalopathy (disturbances of consciousness, including confusion, hallucinations, stupor, and coma), myoclonus, neuromuscular excitability, seizures.

Post-Marketing: Agranulocytosis, anaphylaxis, aphasia, encephalopathy, myoclonus, seizures, nonconvulsive status epilepticus.

ANTIDOTE

Notify physician of any side effects. Discontinue cefepime and treat hypersensitivity reactions as indicated (airway, oxygen, IV fluids, epinephrine, corticosteroids, pressor amines [e.g., dopamine], antihistamines [e.g., diphenhydramine]). Resuscitate as necessary. Discontinue cefepime if seizures occur and treat with anticonvulsants (e.g., diazepam [Valium]). Mild cases of CDAD may respond to discontinuation of cefepime. Treat CDAD with fluids, electrolytes, protein supplements, and oral vancomycin (Vancocin) or metronidazole (Flagyl) as indicated. In severe cases, surgical evaluation may be indicated. Hemodialysis may be useful in overdose.

CEFOTAXIME SODIUM
(sef-oh-**TAX**-eem **SO**-dee-um)

Claforan

Antibacterial
(cephalosporin)

pH 5 to 7.5

USUAL DOSE
Range is 2 to 12 Gm/24 hr. Depends on seriousness of infection. Maximum daily dose is 12 Gm. Duration of treatment depends on the organism and infection being treated. A minimum of 10 days is recommended for infections caused by *group A beta-hemolytic streptococci* to guard against the risk of rheumatic fever or glomerulonephritis.

Uncomplicated infections: 1 Gm every 12 hours.

Moderate to severe infections: 1 to 2 Gm every 8 hours.

Serious infections and septicemia: 2 Gm every 6 to 8 hours.

Life-threatening infections: 2 Gm every 4 hours.

For moderate to life-threatening infections, higher doses are often reduced after a positive clinical response.

Disseminated gonococcal infections: 1 Gm every 8 hours; continue for 24 to 48 hours after symptoms improve. Transfer to oral cefixime to complete a minimum of 1 week of treatment.

Perioperative prophylaxis: 1 Gm 30 to 90 minutes before incision. Equal to or less than 60 minutes is recommended. May be repeated in a lengthy procedure. In *cesarean section* give initial dose after cord is clamped, then 1 Gm at 6 and 12 hours postoperatively.

PEDIATRIC DOSE
Maximum daily dose 12 Gm/24 hr. Differentiation between premature and normal gestational age is not necessary.

0 to 1 week of age: 50 mg/kg/dose every 12 hours.

1 to 4 weeks of age: 50 mg/kg/dose every 8 hours. One source increases the interval to every 12 hours in infants weighing less than 1,200 Gm.

1 month to 12 years, weight less than 50 kg: 50 to 180 mg/kg/24 hr equally divided into 4 to 6 doses (8.3 to 30 mg/kg/dose every 4 hours or 12.5 to 45 mg/kg/dose every 6 hours). Use higher-end doses for serious infections, including meningitis.

Weight 50 kg or more: See Usual Dose.

DOSE ADJUSTMENTS
In impaired renal function with a CrCl less than 20 mL/min/1.73 M^2, reduce dose by one half and maintain same dosing interval. ▪ Reduced doses or extended intervals may be indicated in the elderly. Consider age-related impaired organ function, nutritional status, and concomitant disease or drug therapy. ▪ See Usual Dose and Drug/Lab Interactions.

DILUTION
Each dose of the lyophilized powder (500 mg, 1 Gm, 2 Gm) must be reconstituted with 10 mL SWFI, D5W, NS, or other **compatible** infusion solution (see chart on inside back cover or literature). Do not prepare with diluents having a pH above 7.5; see Compatibility. Solution color ranges from pale yellow to light amber. May be further diluted with 50 to 100 mL of **compatible** solutions and given as an intermittent infusion or added to larger volumes and given as a continuous infusion. (1 Gm in 14 mL of SWFI is isotonic.)

Available in several forms (other than vials of lyophilized powder), including premixed with dextrose in a frozen Galaxy container, in ADD-Vantage vials for use with ADD-Vantage infusion containers, and in pharmacy bulk vials. Refer to manufacturer's prescribing information for specific preparation and storage requirements.

Storage: Store unopened cartons at CRT. Protect from excessive light. Stability of reconstituted solutions ranges from 12 hours at RT to 10 days refrigerated depending on concentration, diluent, and infusion container; see prescribing information.

COMPATIBILITY   (Underline Indicates Conflicting Compatibility Information)

Consider any drug NOT listed as compatible to be INCOMPATIBLE until consulting a pharmacist; specific conditions may apply.

May be used concomitantly with aminoglycosides (e.g., amikacin, gentamicin), but these drugs must never be mixed in the same infusion (mutual inactivation). If given concurrently, administer separately and flush the IV line before and after administration. Manufacturer recommends temporarily discontinuing other solutions infusing at the same site during intermittent infusion and states, "Do not add supplementary medications to premixed plastic IV containers." Manufacturer also states, "Should not be prepared with solutions having a pH above 7.5, such as sodium bicarbonate."

One source suggests the following **compatibilities:**

Additive: Clindamycin (Cleocin), metronidazole (Flagyl IV), verapamil.

Y-site: Acyclovir (Zovirax), alprostadil, amifostine (Ethyol), aztreonam (Azactam), bivalirudin (Angiomax), cisatracurium (Nimbex), cyclophosphamide (Cytoxan), dexmedetomidine (Precedex), diltiazem (Cardizem), docetaxel (Taxotere), etoposide phosphate (Etopophos), famotidine (Pepcid IV), fenoldopam (Corlopam), fludarabine (Fludara), granisetron (Kytril), hetastarch in electrolytes (Hextend), hydromorphone (Dilaudid), levofloxacin (Levaquin), lorazepam (Ativan), magnesium sulfate, melphalan (Alkeran), meperidine (Demerol), midazolam (Versed), milrinone (Primacor), morphine, ondansetron (Zofran), propofol (Diprivan), remifentanil (Ultiva), sargramostim (Leukine), teniposide (Vumon), thiotepa, tigecycline (Tygacil), vancomycin, vinorelbine (Navelbine).

RATE OF ADMINISTRATION

See Compatibility. Injection and intermittent infusion may be given through Y-tube or three-way stopcock of infusion set.

IV injection: A single dose equally distributed over a minimum of 3 to 5 minutes. Rapid bolus injections (less than 60 seconds) have caused life-threatening arrhythmias.

Intermittent IV: A single dose over 30 minutes.

Continuous infusion: 500 to 1,000 mL over 6 to 24 hours, depending on total dose and concentration.

ACTIONS

A broad-spectrum, third-generation cephalosporin antibiotic. Bactericidal to many gram-negative, gram-positive, and anaerobic organisms. Effective against many otherwise resistant organisms. Inhibits bacterial cell wall synthesis. Distributed into most body tissues and fluids, including inflamed meninges. Some metabolites formed. Half-life is approximately 1 hour. Excreted in the urine. Crosses placental barrier. Secreted in breast milk.

INDICATIONS AND USES

Treatment of serious lower respiratory tract, urinary tract, skin and skin structure, intra-abdominal, bone and joint, CNS, gynecologic infections, and bacteremia/septicemia. Most effective against specific organisms (see literature). ▪ Perioperative prophylaxis.

Unlabeled uses: Treatment of disseminated gonococcal infections and Lyme disease.

CONTRAINDICATIONS

Previous hypersensitivity reaction to cephalosporins; see Precautions. ▪ Premixed solutions containing dextrose may be contraindicated in patients with known allergies to corn or corn products.

PRECAUTIONS

Hypersensitivity reactions, including fatalities, have been reported and include reports of individuals with a history of penicillin hypersensitivity or sensitivity to multiple allergens experiencing severe reactions when treated with cephalosporins. Check history of previous hypersensitivity reactions to penicillins, cephalosporins, or other allergens. Actual incidence of cross-allergenicity not established but may be more common with first-generation cephalosporins. ▪ Sensitivity studies indicated to determine susceptibility of the causative organism to cefotaxime. ▪ To reduce the development of drug-resistant bacteria and maintain its effectiveness, cefotaxime should be used to treat or prevent only those infections proven or strongly suspected to be caused by bacteria. ▪ Continue for 2 to 3 days after all symptoms of infection subside. ▪ Avoid prolonged use of drug; super-infection caused by overgrowth of nonsusceptible organisms may result. ▪ Use caution in patients with impaired renal function, allergies, or a history of GI disease (especially colitis). ▪ *Clostridium difficile*–associated diarrhea (CDAD) has been reported. May range from mild diarrhea to fatal colitis. Consider in patients who present with diarrhea during or after treatment with cefotaxime. ▪ Granulocytopenia and, rarely, agranulocy-tosis can occur, especially during prolonged therapy; see Monitor.

Monitor: Watch for early symptoms of a hypersensitivity reaction. ▪ Monitor CBC if duration of treatment is more than 10 days. ▪ May cause thrombophlebitis. Use small needles and large veins, and rotate infusion sites. ▪ See Drug/Lab Interactions; addi-tional monitoring may be indicated (e.g., renal function, drug serum levels, PT).

Patient Education: Report promptly any bleeding or bruising or symptoms of hypersensi-tivity (e.g., difficulty breathing, hives, itching, rash). ▪ Promptly report diarrhea or bloody stools that occur during treatment or up to several months after an antibiotic has been discontinued; may indicate CDAD and require treatment.

Maternal/Child: Category B: safety for use during pregnancy and breast-feeding not estab-lished. No problems documented. ▪ Immature renal function of infants and small chil-dren will increase blood levels of all cephalosporins.

Elderly: No specific problems documented; see Dose Adjustments.

DRUG/LAB INTERACTIONS

Risk of nephrotoxicity may be increased with **aminoglycosides and other nephrotoxic agents** (e.g., loop diuretics [e.g., furosemide (Lasix)], NSAIDs [e.g., ibuprofen (Advil, Motrin), ketoprofen, naproxen (Aleve, Naprosyn)]). ▪ **Probenecid** inhibits excretion of cefotaxime, decreasing clearance by approximately 50%. Limit administration of cef-otaxime to no more than 6 Gm/day when given concurrently with probenecid. ▪ May be antagonized by **bacteriostatic antibiotics** (e.g., chloramphenicol, erythromycin, tetracy-clines); may interfere with bactericidal action. ▪ See Compatibility and Side Effects. ▪ May cause a positive direct **Coombs' test.** ▪ May produce a false-positive reaction for **urine glucose** except with enzyme-based tests (e.g., Clinistix).

SIDE EFFECTS

Generally well tolerated. Most common side effect is a local reaction at the injection site. Less frequent reactions include full scope of hypersensitivity reactions, including ana-phylaxis; CDAD; colitis; decreased hemoglobin or decreased hematocrit; decreased platelet functions; diarrhea; dyspnea; elevation of AST, ALT, total bilirubin, alkaline phosphatase, LDH, and BUN (transient); eosinophilia; fever; leukopenia; local site pain; nausea; oral thrush; positive direct Coombs' test; prolonged PT; seizures (large doses); thrombophlebitis; transient neutropenia; vaginitis; vomiting. Generally resolve after cephalosporins are discontinued. Aplastic anemia, erythema multiforme, hemolytic ane-mia, hemorrhage, hepatic dysfunction (including cholestasis), pancytopenia, renal dys-function, Stevens-Johnson syndrome, toxic epidermal necrolysis, and toxic nephropathy have been reported with cephalosporin-class antibiotics.

Post-Marketing: Arrhythmia (with rapid injection), cutaneous reactions (e.g., isolated cases of erythema multiforme, Stevens-Johnson syndrome, toxic epidermal necrolysis), encephalopathy (e.g., impairment of consciousness, abnormal movements and seizures), hematologic reactions (e.g., agranulocytosis, hemolytic anemia, thrombocytopenia), he-patic reactions (e.g., cholestasis, elevated gamma-glutamyl transferase (GGT) and biliru-bin, hepatitis, jaundice), renal reactions (e.g., interstitial nephritis and transient elevations in SCr).

ANTIDOTE

Notify the physician of any side effects. Discontinue the drug if indicated. Mild cases of CDAD may respond to discontinuation of cefotaxime. Treat CDAD with fluids, elec-trolytes, protein supplements, and oral vancomycin (Vancocin) or metronidazole (Flagyl) as indicated. In severe cases, surgical evaluation may be indicated. Treat hypersensitivity reactions as indicated and resuscitate as necessary. Hemodialysis may be useful in overdose.

CEFOTETAN DISODIUM
(sef-oh-**TEE**-tan dye-**SO**-dee-um)

Antibacterial
(cephalosporin)

pH 4.5 to 6.5

USUAL DOSE
Range is 1 to 6 Gm/24 hr for 5 to 10 days. Do not exceed 6 Gm/24 hr.

Urinary tract infections: 500 mg to 2 Gm every 12 hours or 1 to 2 Gm every 12 to 24 hours.

Moderate infections: 1 or 2 Gm every 12 hours.

Moderate infections of skin and skin structure: 2 Gm every 24 hours or 1 Gm every 12 hours. Give 1 or 2 Gm every 12 hours if *Klebsiella pneumoniae* is the causative organism.

Serious infections: 2 Gm every 12 hours.

Life-threatening infections: 3 Gm every 12 hours.

Pelvic inflammatory disease: 2 Gm every 12 hours for 14 days. Transfer to oral therapy at any time it is clinically appropriate, usually 48 hours after clinical improvement.

Perioperative prophylaxis: 1 to 2 Gm IV 30 to 60 minutes before incision except during cesarean section. Given only after clamping the umbilical cord in *cesarean section.*

PEDIATRIC DOSE
Unlabeled: 20 to 40 mg/kg of body weight every 12 hours; see Maternal/Child.

DOSE ADJUSTMENTS
Reduced doses or extended intervals may be indicated in the elderly; consider age-related impaired organ function, nutritional status, and concomitant disease or drug therapy.

- Reduce total daily dose if renal function impaired according to the following chart.

Cefotetan Dose Guidelines in Impaired Renal Function	
Creatinine Clearance (mL/min)	Dose/Frequency
>30 mL/min	Usual recommended dose q 12 hr
10-30 mL/min	Usual recommended dose q 24 hr or $^1/_2$ usual recommended dose q 12 hr
<10 mL/min	Usual recommended dose q 48 hr or $^1/_4$ usual recommended dose q 12 hr
Hemodialysis patients	$^1/_4$ usual adult dose q 24 hr on days between dialysis sessions $^1/_2$ usual adult dose on the day of dialysis

DILUTION
IV injection: Reconstitute each 1 Gm of the lyophilized powder with 10 mL of SW for injection (2 Gm with 20 mL). Shake well and let stand until clear.

Intermittent IV: *Vials:* A single dose may be further diluted or initially diluted with 50 to 100 mL of D5W or NS. Also available in dual-chamber DUPLEX containers and pharmacy bulk packaging. Refer to manufacturer's prescribing information for specific preparation and storage requirements.

Filters: No data available from manufacturer.

Storage: Store vials below 22° C (72° F); protect from light. Administer within 24 hours of preparation or within 96 hours if refrigerated. Stable after dilution for 1 week if frozen; thaw at room temperature before use; discard remaining solution; do not refreeze. Slight yellowing does not affect potency.

COMPATIBILITY

Consider any drug NOT listed as compatible to be INCOMPATIBLE until consulting a pharmacist; specific conditions may apply.

May be used concomitantly with aminoglycosides (e.g., amikacin, gentamicin), but these drugs must never be mixed in the same infusion (mutual inactivation). If given concurrently, administer separately and flush the IV line before and after administration. Manufacturer recommends temporarily discontinuing other solutions infusing at the same site during intermittent infusion and states, "Do not add supplementary medications to premixed plastic IV containers" (e.g., Galaxy).

One source suggests the following **compatibilities:**

Y-site: Allopurinol (Aloprim), amifostine (Ethyol), aztreonam (Azactam), bivalirudin (Angiomax), dexmedetomidine (Precedex), diltiazem (Cardizem), docetaxel (Taxotere), etoposide phosphate (Etopophos), famotidine (Pepcid IV), fenoldopam (Corlopam), filgrastim (Neupogen), fluconazole (Diflucan), fludarabine (Fludara), gemcitabine (Gemzar), granisetron (Kytril), heparin, hetastarch in electrolytes (Hextend), insulin (regular), linezolid (Zyvox), melphalan (Alkeran), meperidine (Demerol), morphine, paclitaxel (Taxol), palonosetron (Aloxi), propofol (Diprivan), remifentanil (Ultiva), sargramostim (Leukine), tacrolimus (Prograf), teniposide (Vumon), theophylline, thiotepa, vancomycin.

RATE OF ADMINISTRATION

See Compatibility. May be given through Y-tube or three-way stopcock of infusion set.

IV injection: A single dose equally distributed over 3 to 5 minutes.

Intermittent IV: A single dose equally distributed over 30 minutes.

ACTIONS

A broad-spectrum, second-generation cephalosporin antibiotic. Bactericidal to selected gram-negative, gram-positive, and anaerobic organisms. Inhibits bacterial cell wall synthesis. Effective against many otherwise resistant organisms. Peak serum levels achieved at end of infusion. Widely distributed in most tissues, body fluids (CSF minimal), bone, gallbladder, myocardium, and skin and soft tissue. Half-life is from 3 to 4.6 hours. Primarily excreted in the urine. Crosses placental barrier. Secreted in breast milk.

INDICATIONS AND USES

Treatment of serious lower respiratory tract, urinary tract, skin and skin structure, gynecologic, intra-abdominal, and bone and joint infections. Most effective against specific organisms (see literature). ▪ Perioperative prophylaxis.

CONTRAINDICATIONS

Previous hypersensitivity reaction to cephalosporins or related antibiotics (penicillins). Absolute only if reaction was serious and in patients who have experienced a cephalosporin-associated hemolytic anemia. ▪ Premixed solutions containing dextrose may be contraindicated in patients with known allergies to corn or corn products.

PRECAUTIONS

Specific sensitivity studies are indicated to determine susceptibility of the causative organism to cefotetan. ▪ To reduce the development of drug-resistant bacteria and maintain its effectiveness, cefotetan should be used to treat or prevent only those infections proven or strongly suspected to be caused by bacteria. ▪ Continue for at least 2 or 3 days after all symptoms of infection subside. ▪ Avoid prolonged use of drug; superinfection caused by overgrowth of nonsusceptible organisms may result. ▪ Use caution in patients with impaired renal function, a history of GI disease (especially colitis), bleeding disorders or allergies, and those receiving an extended course of cephalosporins. ▪ *Clostridium difficile*–associated diarrhea (CDAD) has been reported. May range from mild diarrhea to fatal colitis. Consider in patients who present with diarrhea during or after treatment with cefotetan. ▪ Hemolytic anemia, including fatalities, has been reported. Discontinue cefotetan immediately if anemia develops during the course of therapy. May present during treatment or up to 2 to 3 weeks following therapy completion.

Monitor: Watch for early symptoms of a hypersensitivity reaction. ▪ Use extreme caution in the penicillin-sensitive patient; incidence of cross-sensitivity may be up to 10%. ▪ May cause hypoprothrombinemia (deficiency of prothrombin [factor II]); 10 mg/week of prophylactic vitamin K may be indicated in elderly, debilitated, or other patients with vitamin K deficiency. Monitor PT. ▪ May cause thrombophlebitis. Use small needles and large veins, and rotate infusion sites. ▪ Observe for electrolyte imbalance and cardiac irregularities. Contains 3.5 mEq sodium per Gm. ▪ Monitor for S/S of hemolytic anemia, including CBC if indicated. ▪ See Drug/Lab Interactions; additional monitoring may be indicated (e.g., renal function, drug serum levels, PT).

Patient Education: Avoid alcohol or alcohol-containing preparations; may cause abdominal cramps, flushing, headache, nausea and vomiting, shortness of breath, sweating, and tachycardia. ▪ Report promptly any bleeding or bruising or symptoms of allergy (e.g., difficulty breathing, hives, itching, rash). ▪ Promptly report diarrhea or bloody stools that occur during treatment or up to several months after an antibiotic has been discontinued; may indicate CDAD and require treatment.

Maternal/Child: Category B: safety for use during pregnancy not established. Use only if clearly needed. ▪ Use caution if breast-feeding. ▪ Safety for use in pediatric patients not established. Immature renal function of infants and small children will increase blood levels of all cephalosporins.

Elderly: See Dose Adjustments. ▪ Safety and effectiveness similar to younger adults; however, greater sensitivity of some older individuals cannot be ruled out. ▪ Monitoring of renal function suggested.

DRUG/LAB INTERACTIONS

May produce symptoms of acute intolerance with **alcohol** (a disulfiram-like reaction with abdominal cramps, headache, flushing, nausea and vomiting, shortness of breath, sweating, tachycardia). Patient must abstain from alcohol during treatment and until at least 72 hours after discontinuation. ▪ Risk of nephrotoxicity may be increased with **aminoglycosides and other nephrotoxic agents** (e.g., loop diuretics [furosemide (Lasix)]). ▪ Sources differ on inhibition of excretion by **probenecid.** ▪ May be antagonized by **bacteriostatic antibiotics** (e.g., chloramphenicol, erythromycin, tetracyclines); may interfere with bactericidal action. ▪ Bleeding tendency increased with **any medicine that affects blood clotting** (e.g., heparin and oral anticoagulants [warfarin (Coumadin)], thrombolytic agents [e.g., alteplase (tPA)], salicylates, NSAIDs [e.g., ibuprofen (Advil, Motrin), naproxen (Aleve, Naprosyn)], sulfinpyrazone [Anturane]). ▪ Large amounts of cephalosporins and/or salicylates may induce **hypoprothrombinemia.** ▪ **False increases in creatinine levels** with Jaffe method. ▪ **False-positive for urine glucose** except with enzyme-based tests (e.g., Clinistix). ▪ **Positive direct Coombs' test.** ▪ See Compatibility and Side Effects.

SIDE EFFECTS

Full scope of hypersensitivity reactions, including anaphylaxis. Bleeding episodes; burning, discomfort, and pain at injection site; CDAD; diarrhea; elevated alkaline phosphatase, AST, ALT, and LDH; eosinophilia; nausea; prolonged PT; seizures (large doses); thrombocytosis. Hypoprothrombinemia (rare) and hemolytic anemia may occur.

ANTIDOTE

Notify physician of any side effects. Discontinue the drug if indicated. Treat hypersensitivity reactions as indicated and resuscitate as necessary. Mild cases of CDAD may respond to discontinuation of cefotetan. Treat CDAD with fluids, electrolytes, protein supplements, and oral vancomycin (Vancocin) or metronidazole (Flagyl) as indicated. In severe cases, surgical evaluation may be indicated. Bleeding episodes may respond to vitamin K or require discontinuation of drug. Fresh-frozen plasma, packed red cells, or platelet concentrates may be indicated in abnormal bleeding tendencies confirmed by lab evaluations. If bleeding is due to platelet dysfunction, discontinue and use an alternate antibiotic. Blood transfusions (e.g., packed red cells) may be indicated if hemolytic anemia develops. Hemodialysis is only slightly useful in overdose.

CEFOXITIN SODIUM
(seh-**FOX**-ih-tin **SO**-dee-um)

Mefoxin

Antibacterial
(cephalosporin)

pH 4.2 to 7

USUAL DOSE

Range is 1 to 2 Gm every 6 to 8 hours. Dose based on severity of disease, susceptibility of pathogens, and condition of patient.

Cefoxitin Dosing Guidelines		
Type of Infection	Dose and Frequency	Total Daily Dose
Uncomplicated forms* of infections such as pneumonia, urinary tract infection, cutaneous infection	1 Gm every 6 to 8 hr	3 to 4 Gm
Moderately severe or severe infections	1 Gm every 4 hr or 2 Gm every 6 to 8 hr	6 to 8 Gm
Infections commonly needing antibiotics in higher doses (e.g., gas gangrene)	2 Gm every 4 hr or 3 Gm every 6 hr	12 Gm

*Including patients in whom bacteremia is absent or unlikely.

Perioperative prophylaxis: 2 Gm 30 minutes to 1 hour before incision. Follow with 2 Gm every 6 hours for 24 hours.

Prophylaxis during cesarean section: Either a single 2-Gm dose after clamping the umbilical cord or a 3-dose regimen consisting of 2 Gm given as soon as the umbilical cord is clamped followed by 2 Gm in 4 hours and again in 8 hours.

PEDIATRIC DOSE

Pediatric patients over 3 months of age: *Mild to moderate infections:* 80 to 100 mg/kg/24 hr in equally divided doses every 6 to 8 hours (20 to 25 mg/kg every 6 hours or 26.66 to 33.33 mg/kg every 8 hours). *Severe infections:* 100 to 160 mg/kg/24 hr in equally divided doses every 4 to 6 hours (16.66 to 26.66 mg/kg every 4 hours or 25 to 40 mg/kg every 6 hours). Do not exceed adult dose and/or 12 Gm.

Perioperative prophylaxis in pediatric patients over 3 months of age: 30 to 40 mg/kg 30 minutes to 1 hour before incision and every 6 hours for 24 hours.

NEONATAL DOSE (unlabeled)

Use sterile cefoxitin sodium USP only. Other formulations may contain benzyl alcohol.

90 to 100 mg/kg/24 hr in equally divided doses every 8 hours (30 to 33.3 mg/kg every 8 hours).

DOSE ADJUSTMENTS

Reduced dose or extended intervals may be indicated in the elderly; consider age-related impaired organ function, nutritional status, and concomitant disease or drug therapy. ■ In impaired renal function, the initial dose should be as previously listed, but all remaining doses should be based on CrCl according to the following chart. See Drug/Lab Interactions.

Cefoxitin Maintenance Dose in Adults with Impaired Renal Function		
Creatinine Clearance (mL/min)	Dose (Gm)	Frequency
30-50 mL/min	1-2 Gm	q 8-12 hr
10-29 mL/min	1-2 Gm	q 12-24 hr
5-9 mL/min	0.5-1 Gm	q 12-24 hr
<5 mL/min	0.5-1 Gm	q 24-48 hr

Hemodialysis patients should receive a loading dose of 1 to 2 Gm after each dialysis in addition to the maintenance dose listed in the previous chart.

In pediatric patients, **the manufacturer recommends reducing the dose and frequency consistent with the recommendations for adults.**

DILUTION

1 Gm of the lyophilized solution must be reconstituted with at least 10 mL, and 2 Gm with 10 or 20 mL, of SWFI, BWFI, D5W, or NS. A single dose may be further diluted in 50 to 100 mL of most common infusion solutions (see chart on inside back cover and literature). The use of butterfly needles and dilution in up to 1,000 mL of D5W, D5NS, or NS are preferred when administering larger doses as a continuous infusion. Also available in dual-chamber DUPLEX containers and as a frozen, premixed solution. Refer to manufacturer's prescribing information for specific preparation and storage requirements. May be given through a Y-tube, three-way stopcock, additive infusion set, or as a continuous infusion.

Storage: Storage before use is dependent on product. Reconstituted solutions are stable at RT for 6 hours and 7 days if refrigerated. Solutions diluted in 50 to 1,000 mL diluent are stable for an additional 18 hours at RT and an additional 48 hours if refrigerated.

COMPATIBILITY   (Underline Indicates Conflicting Compatibility Information)

Consider any drug NOT listed as compatible to be INCOMPATIBLE until consulting a pharmacist; specific conditions may apply.

May be used concomitantly with aminoglycosides (e.g., amikacin, gentamicin), but these drugs must never be mixed in the same infusion (mutual inactivation). If given concurrently, administer separately and flush the IV line before and after administration. Manufacturer recommends temporarily discontinuing other solutions infusing at the same site during intermittent infusion.

One source suggests the following **compatibilities:**

Additive: Aztreonam (Azactam), clindamycin (Cleocin), mannitol, metronidazole (Flagyl IV), multivitamins (M.V.I.), sodium bicarbonate (Neut), verapamil.

Y-site: Acetaminophen (Ofirmev), acyclovir (Zovirax), amifostine (Ethyol), amphotericin B cholesteryl (Amphotec), anidulafungin (Eraxis), aztreonam (Azactam), bivalirudin (Angiomax), cisatracurium (Nimbex), cyclophosphamide (Cytoxan), dexmedetomidine (Precedex), diltiazem (Cardizem), docetaxel (Taxotere), doxorubicin liposomal (Doxil), etoposide phosphate (Etopophos), famotidine (Pepcid IV), fluconazole (Diflucan), foscarnet (Foscavir), gemcitabine (Gemzar), granisetron (Kytril), hetastarch in electrolytes (Hextend), hydromorphone (Dilaudid), linezolid (Zyvox), magnesium sulfate, meperidine (Demerol), morphine, ondansetron (Zofran), propofol (Diprivan), ranitidine (Zantac), remifentanil (Ultiva), teniposide (Vumon), thiotepa, vancomycin.

RATE OF ADMINISTRATION

See Compatibility. Each 1 Gm or fraction thereof over 3 to 5 minutes or longer as indicated by amount of solution and condition of the patient. Rate of continuous infusion should be by physician order.

ACTIONS

A semi-synthetic, second-generation cephalosporin antibiotic that is bactericidal to many gram-positive, gram-negative, and anaerobic organisms. Inhibits bacterial cell wall synthesis. Has activity in the presence of some beta-lactamases, both penicillinases and cephalosporinases, of gram-negative and gram-positive bacteria. Peak serum levels achieved by end of infusion. Widely distributed into many body tissues and fluids (CSF minimal). Passes into pleural and joint fluids and is detectable in antibacterial concentrations in bile. Half-life is 41 to 59 minutes. Excreted rapidly in the urine. Crosses the placental barrier. Secreted in breast milk.

INDICATIONS AND USES

Treatment of serious lower respiratory, urinary, intra-abdominal, gynecologic, bone and joint, skin and skin structure infections and septicemia. Effective only if the causative organism is susceptible. If *C. trachomatis* is a suspected pathogen, antichlamydial coverage is indicated. ▪ Perioperative prophylaxis in patients undergoing uncontaminated gastrointestinal surgery, vaginal or abdominal hysterectomy, or cesarean section.

Unlabeled uses: Treatment of acute pelvic inflammatory disease (CDC recommendation). ▪ Treatment of oral bacterial *Eikenella corrodens.*

CONTRAINDICATIONS

Previous hypersensitivity reaction to cephalosporins; see Precautions. ▪ Premixed solutions containing dextrose may be contraindicated in patients with known allergies to corn or corn products.

PRECAUTIONS

Hypersensitivity reactions, including fatalities, have been reported and include reports of individuals with a history of penicillin hypersensitivity or sensitivity to multiple allergens experiencing severe reactions when treated with cephalosporins. Check history of previous hypersensitivity reactions to penicillins, cephalosporins, or other allergens. Actual incidence of cross-allergenicity not established but may be more common with first-generation cephalosporins. ▪ Sensitivity studies indicated to determine susceptibility of the causative organism to cefoxitin. ▪ To reduce the development of drug-resistant bacteria and maintain its effectiveness, cefoxitin should be used to treat or prevent only those infections proven or strongly suspected to be caused by bacteria. ▪ Continue for at least 2 to 3 days after all symptoms of infection subside. ▪ Avoid prolonged use of drug; superinfection caused by overgrowth of nonsusceptible organisms may result. ▪ Use caution in patients with impaired renal function, allergies, or a history of GI disease (especially colitis). ▪ *Clostridium difficile*–associated diarrhea (CDAD) has been reported. May range from mild diarrhea to fatal colitis. Consider in patients who present with diarrhea during or after treatment with cefoxitin. ▪ Continue treatment for group A beta-hemolytic streptococcal infections for 10 days or more to decrease the risk of rheumatic fever or glomerulonephritis.

Monitor: Watch for early symptoms of a hypersensitivity reaction. ▪ Use extreme caution in the penicillin-sensitive patient; cross-sensitivity has been reported. ▪ Thrombophlebitis may result from prolonged or high dosage; use small needles and larger veins, and rotate infusion sites. ▪ Periodic monitoring of CBC, SCr, and liver function tests is recommended during prolonged therapy. ▪ See Drug/Lab Interactions; additional monitoring may be indicated (e.g., renal function, drug serum levels, PT).

Patient Education: Report promptly any bleeding or bruising or symptoms of allergy (e.g., difficulty breathing, hives, itching, rash). ▪ Promptly report diarrhea or bloody stools that occur during treatment or up to several months after an antibiotic has been discontinued; may indicate CDAD and require treatment.

Maternal/Child: Category B: safety for use during pregnancy and breast-feeding not established. No problems documented. ▪ Safety and effectiveness for use in pediatric patients from birth to 3 months of age not established. ▪ Do not use formulations containing benzyl alcohol in infants and children under 3 months. ▪ Immature renal function will increase blood levels. ▪ Eosinophilia and elevated AST associated with higher doses in infants and children.

Elderly: Response similar to that seen in younger adults. Dose selection should be cautious; see Dose Adjustments. Monitoring of renal function suggested.

DRUG/LAB INTERACTIONS

Risk of nephrotoxicity may be increased with **aminoglycosides and other nephrotoxic agents** (e.g., loop diuretics such as furosemide [Lasix]). ▪ **Probenecid** inhibits excretion. Reduced dose of cefoxitin may be required with concomitant use. ▪ May be antagonized by **bacteriostatic antibiotics** (e.g., chloramphenicol, erythromycin, tetracyclines); may interfere with bactericidal action. ▪ False-positive reaction for **urine glucose** except with enzyme-based tests (e.g., Clinistix). ▪ Positive **Coombs' test.** ▪ False increases in **creatinine levels** with Jaffe method. ▪ See Compatibility and Side Effects.

SIDE EFFECTS

Local site reactions are most common. Anorexia; CDAD; colitis; flushing; hypersensitivity reactions, including anaphylaxis; eosinophilia; leukopenia; nausea and vomiting;

neutropenia; oral thrush; phlebitis; prolonged PT; proteinuria; seizures (large doses); thrombophlebitis; transient elevation of AST, ALT, BUN, and alkaline phosphatase; and urticaria have occurred. Hypoprothrombinemia (rare) and hemolytic anemia may occur. Aplastic anemia, erythema multiforme, hemolytic anemia, hemorrhage, hepatic dysfunction (including cholestasis), pancytopenia, renal dysfunction, Stevens-Johnson syndrome, toxic epidermal necrolysis, and toxic nephropathy have been reported with cephalosporin-class antibiotics.

ANTIDOTE
Notify physician of any side effects. Discontinue the drug if indicated. Treat CDAD with fluids, electrolytes, protein supplements, and oral vancomycin (Vancocin) or metronidazole (Flagyl) as indicated. In severe cases, surgical evaluation may be indicated. Treat hypersensitivity reactions as indicated and resuscitate as necessary. Hemodialysis may be useful in overdose.

CEFTAROLINE FOSAMIL
(cef-**TAR**-oh-leen **FOS**-a-mil)

Teflaro

Antibacterial
(cephalosporin)

pH 4.8 to 6.5

USUAL DOSE
600 mg every 12 hours as an IV infusion. Duration of therapy should be guided by the severity and the site of infection and the patient's clinical and bacteriologic progress as shown in the following chart.

Dosage of Ceftaroline				
Infection	Dosage	Frequency	Infusion Time (minutes)	Recommended Duration of Total Antimicrobial Therapy
Acute bacterial skin and skin structure infection (ABSSSI)	600 mg	q 12 hr	5-60 minutes	5-14 days
Community-acquired bacterial pneumonia (CABP)	600 mg	q 12 hr	5-60 minutes	5-7 days

DOSE ADJUSTMENTS
Dose adjustment required with renal impairment as outlined in the following chart.

Dosage of Ceftaroline in Patients with Renal Impairment	
Estimated CrCl* (mL/min)	Recommended Dosage Regimen
>50 mL/min	600 mg q 12 hr
>30 to ≤50 mL/min	400 mg q 12 hr
≥15 to ≤30 mL/min	300 mg q 12 hr
End-stage renal disease, including hemodialysis†	200 mg q 12 hr‡

*CrCl as calculated by Cockcroft-Gault formula.
†End-stage renal disease is defined as CrCl <15 mL/min.
‡Ceftaroline is hemodialyzable; administer after hemodialysis on hemodialysis days.

- Dose adjustment is not indicated based on gender, race, or hepatic function. ■ Reduced dose may be indicated in the elderly based on age-related renal impairment.

DILUTION

Reconstitute with 20 mL of SWFI, NS, D5W, or LR as shown in the following chart. Mix gently. Time to dissolution is less than 2 minutes.

Preparation of Ceftaroline for Intravenous Use			
Dosage Strength (mg)	Volume of Diluent to Be Added (mL)	Approximate Ceftaroline Concentration (mg/mL)	Amount to Be Withdrawn
400	20 mL	20 mg/mL	Total volume
600	20 mL	30 mg/mL	Total volume

Further dilute the reconstituted solution in 50 to 250 mL of NS, D5W, D2.5/0.45NS, or LR. Use the same diluent for further dilution unless SWFI was used. If SWFI was used as the initial diluent, further dilute the reconstituted solution in NS, D5W, D2.5/0.45NS, or LR. When preparing a ceftaroline dose in a 50-mL infusion bag, withdraw 20 mL of the infusion solution before injecting the reconstituted drug into the bag. Infusion solution ranges from clear light yellow to dark yellow depending on the concentration and the storage conditions.

Filter: Data not available.

Storage: Store unopened vials at CRT. Diluted solution should be used within 6 hours when stored at RT or within 24 hours when refrigerated.

COMPATIBILITY   (Underline Indicates Conflicting Compatibility Information)

Consider any drug NOT listed as compatible to be INCOMPATIBLE until consulting a pharmacist; specific conditions may apply.

Manufacturer states, "Should not be mixed with or physically added to solutions containing other drugs." **Compatibility** with other drugs has not been established.

One source suggests the following **compatibilities** for specific time frames; consult pharmacist:

Y-site: Acyclovir (Zovirax), amikacin, aminophylline, amiodarone (Nexterone), azithromycin (Zithromax), bumetanide, calcium chloride, calcium gluconate, ciprofloxacin (Cipro IV), cisatracurium (Nimbex), clindamycin (Cleocin), cyclosporine (Sandimmune), dexamethasone (Decadron), digoxin (Lanoxin), diltiazem (Cardizem), diphenhydramine (Benadryl), dobutamine, dopamine, doripenem (Doribax), enalaprilat (Vasotec IV), esomeprazole (Nexium IV), famotidine (Pepcid IV), fentanyl, fluconazole (Diflucan), furosemide (Lasix), gentamicin, granisetron (Kytril), heparin, hydrocortisone sodium succinate (Solu-Cortef), hydromorphone (Dilaudid), insulin (regular), levofloxacin (Levaquin), lidocaine, lorazepam (Ativan), magnesium sulfate, mannitol (Osmitrol), meperidine (Demerol), methylprednisolone sodium succinate (Solu-Medrol), metoclopramide (Reglan), metoprolol (Lopressor), metronidazole (Flagyl IV), midazolam (Versed), milrinone (Primacor), morphine, moxifloxacin (Avelox), multivitamin infusion (M.V.I.), norepinephrine (Levophed), ondansetron (Zofran), pantoprazole (Protonix IV), potassium chloride, promethazine (Phenergan), propofol (Diprivan), ranitidine (Zantac), remifentanil (Ultiva), sodium bicarbonate, sulfamethoxazole/trimethoprim (SMZ-TMP), tobramycin, vasopressin, voriconazole (VFEND IV).

RATE OF ADMINISTRATION

A single dose equally distributed over 5 to 60 minutes.

ACTIONS

A semi-synthetic, broad-spectrum cephalosporin. Ceftaroline fosamil, a prodrug, is converted into the bioactive ceftaroline in plasma by a phosphatase enzyme. Bactericidal to many gram-negative and gram-positive organisms. Inhibits bacterial cell wall synthesis. Protein binding is minimal (20%). Ceftaroline undergoes hydrolysis, forming an inactive metabolite. Half-life is approximately 2.2 to 3 hours. Both ceftaroline and its metabolites are primarily eliminated by the kidneys.

INDICATIONS AND USES

Treatment of adults with infections caused by susceptible strains of microorganisms in conditions that include acute bacterial skin and skin structure infections (ABSSSI) and community-acquired bacterial pneumonia (CABP).

CONTRAINDICATIONS

Known serious hypersensitivity to ceftaroline or other members of the cephalosporin class.

PRECAUTIONS

Hypersensitivity reactions, some fatal, and serious skin reactions have been reported in patients receiving beta-lactam antibiotics and include reports of individuals with a history of penicillin hypersensitivity or sensitivity to multiple allergens experiencing severe reactions when treated with cephalosporins. Check history of previous hypersensitivity reactions to penicillins, cephalosporins, carbapenems, or other allergens. Actual incidence of cross-allergenicity not established but may be more common with first-generation cephalosporins. ▪ Specific sensitivity studies are indicated to determine susceptibility of the causative organism to ceftaroline. ▪ To reduce the development of drug-resistant bacteria and maintain its effectiveness, ceftaroline should be used to treat only those infections proven or strongly suspected to be caused by bacteria. ▪ Although cross-resistance may occur, some isolates resistant to other cephalosporins may be susceptible to ceftaroline. ▪ *Clostridium difficile*–associated diarrhea (CDAD) has been reported. May range from mild diarrhea to fatal colitis. Consider in patients who present with diarrhea during or after treatment with ceftaroline. ▪ Seroconversion from a negative to a positive direct Coombs' test occurred in approximately 10% of patients in Phase 3 trials. No adverse reactions representing hemolytic anemia were reported. If anemia develops during or after treatment with ceftaroline, drug-induced hemolytic anemia should be considered and diagnostic studies, including a direct Coombs' test, should be performed.

Monitor: Watch for early symptoms of a hypersensitivity reaction. ▪ Obtain baseline CBC with differential and platelet count and SCr.

Patient Education: Promptly report S/S of a hypersensitivity reaction (e.g., rash, hives, wheezing, shortness of breath). ▪ Promptly report diarrhea or bloody stools that occur during treatment or up to several months after an antibiotic has been discontinued; may indicate CDAD and require treatment.

Maternal/Child: Category B: safety for use during pregnancy and breast-feeding not established; use only if clearly needed. ▪ Safety and effectiveness for use in pediatric patients not established.

Elderly: No specific problems documented. Efficacy and safety appear similar to that seen in younger patients. Consider age-related renal impairment; see Dose Adjustments.

DRUG/LAB INTERACTIONS

No clinical drug-drug interaction studies have been conducted. There is minimal potential for drug-drug interactions between ceftaroline and CYP450 substrates, inhibitors, or inducers; drugs known to undergo active renal secretion; and drugs that may alter renal blood flow. ▪ In vitro studies have not demonstrated any antagonism between ceftaroline and other commonly used antibiotics (e.g., amikacin, azithromycin, aztreonam, daptomycin, levofloxacin, linezolid, meropenem, tigecycline, vancomycin).

SIDE EFFECTS

The most common side effects were diarrhea, nausea, and rash. Hypersensitivity reactions were the most frequently reported serious side effects leading to discontinuation of therapy. Other less frequently reported side effects included CDAD, constipation, hypokalemia, increased transaminases (ALT, AST), phlebitis, seroconversion from a negative to a positive direct Coombs' test, and vomiting. Several other side effects were reported in less than 2% of the population studied.

Post-Marketing: Agranulocytosis.

ANTIDOTE

Notify physician of any side effects. Discontinue the drug if indicated. Treat hypersensitivity reactions as indicated (e.g., diphenhydramine [Benadryl], epinephrine [Adrenalin], albuterol) and resuscitate as necessary. Discontinue ceftaroline for suspected drug-induced hemolytic anemia and initiate supportive therapy as indicated (e.g., transfusion). Mild cases of CDAD may respond to discontinuation of ceftaroline. Treat CDAD with fluids, electrolytes, protein supplements, and oral vancomycin (Vancocin) or metronidazole (Flagyl) as indicated. In severe cases, surgical evaluation may be indicated. Ceftaroline is removed by hemodialysis.

CEFTAZIDIME

(sef-**TAY**-zih-deem)

Fortaz, Tazicef

Antibacterial

(cephalosporin)

pH 5 to 8

USUAL DOSE

Range is from 250 mg to 2 Gm every 8 to 12 hours. Dosage based on severity of infection, condition and renal function of the patient, and susceptibility of the causative organism.

Uncomplicated GU infections: 250 mg every 12 hours.

Complicated GU infections: 500 mg every 8 to 12 hours.

Uncomplicated pneumonia; skin and skin structure infections: 500 mg to 1 Gm every 8 hours.

Bone and joint infections: 2 Gm every 12 hours.

Severe or life-threatening infections (especially in immunocompromised patients), meningitis, serious gynecologic and intra-abdominal infections: 2 Gm every 8 hours.

Pseudomonal lung infections in cystic fibrosis patients (must have normal renal function): 30 to 50 mg/kg of body weight every 8 hours. Do not exceed 6 Gm/24 hr.

Melioidosis (unlabeled): 50 mg/kg (maximum dose: 2 Gm) every 8 hours.

PEDIATRIC DOSE

Pediatric patients 1 month to 12 years of age: 30 to 50 mg/kg of body weight every 8 hours. Reserve higher doses for immunocompromised pediatric patients or for those with cystic fibrosis or meningitis. Do not exceed 6 Gm/24 hr.

NEONATAL DOSE

Neonates up to 4 weeks of age: 30 mg/kg every 12 hours.

The American Academy of Pediatrics suggests the following doses:

Neonates 7 days of age or younger regardless of weight: 50 mg/kg every 12 hours.

Neonates from 8 to 28 days of age weighing 2 kg or less: 50 mg/kg every 8 to 12 hours.

Neonates from 8 to 28 days of age weighing more than 2 kg: 50 mg/kg every 8 hours.

DOSE ADJUSTMENTS

Reduced dose or extended intervals may be indicated in the elderly; consider age-related impaired organ function, nutritional status, and concomitant disease or drug therapy. ▪ In impaired renal function, an initial loading dose of 1 Gm may be given, but all remaining doses should be based on CrCl according to the following chart. If the normal dose would be lower than the doses in the chart, use the lower dose. Adjustment for pediatric patients is similar to adults; consider body surface area or lean body mass and reduce dosing frequency.

Ceftazidime Maintenance Dose in Impaired Renal Function		
Creatinine Clearance (mL/min)	Dose	Frequency
31-50 mL/min	1 Gm	q 12 hr
16-30 mL/min	1 Gm	q 24 hr
6-15 mL/min	500 mg	q 24 hr
<5 mL/min	500 mg	q 48 hr
Hemodialysis patients	1 Gm	After each dialysis session
Peritoneal dialysis patients	500 mg	q 24 hr

In patients with impaired renal function who have severe infection (normally requiring a 6 Gm/24 hr dose), the dose in the previous chart may be increased by 50% or the dosing frequency may be increased. In patients undergoing hemodialysis, give a loading dose of 1 Gm followed by 1 Gm after each dialysis. ▪ In peritoneal dialysis patients (CAPD), give a loading dose of 1 Gm followed by 500 mg every 24 hours. In addition to IV use, ceftazidime can be incorporated in the dialysis fluid at a concentration of 250 mg for 2 L of dialysis fluid. ▪ Dose reduction not required in impaired hepatic function.

DILUTION
IV injection: Directions for the initial preparation of ceftazidime solutions are outlined in the following chart.

Preparation of Ceftazidime Solutions			
Size	Amount of Diluent to Be Added (mL)	Approximate Available Volume (mL)	Approximate Ceftazidime Concentration (mg/mL)
500-mg vial	5.3	5.7*	100
1-Gm vial	10	10.8†	100
2-Gm vial	10	11.5‡	170

*To obtain a dose of 500 mg, withdraw 5 mL from vial after reconstitution.
†To obtain a dose of 1 Gm, withdraw 10 mL from vial after reconstitution.
‡To obtain a dose of 2 Gm, withdraw 11.5 mL from vial after reconstitution.

Reconstitute with SWFI as outlined in the chart. Shake well. Dilution generates CO_2. Invert vial and completely depress plunger of syringe. Insert needle through stopper and keep it within the solution. Expel bubbles from solution in syringe before injection.

Intermittent IV infusion: A single dose may be further diluted in 50 to 100 mL of D5W, NS, or other **compatible** infusion solutions for injection (see literature or chart on inside back cover). Also available in dual-chamber DUPLEX containers, in ADD-Vantage vials, in Twist vials, premixed in frozen Galaxy bags, and in pharmacy bulk packaging. Refer to manufacturer's prescribing information for specific preparation and storage requirements.

Storage: Store unopened vials in carton at CRT. Protect from light. Administer within 12 hours of preparation if stored at CRT, or refrigerate for up to 3 days. May be frozen for up to 3 months after initial dilution; thaw at room temperature (see instructions); do not refreeze. Will be light yellow to amber in color depending on concentration and diluent.

COMPATIBILITY   (Underline Indicates Conflicting Compatibility Information)
Consider any drug NOT listed as compatible to be INCOMPATIBLE until consulting a pharmacist; specific conditions may apply.

May be used concomitantly with aminoglycosides (e.g., amikacin, gentamicin, and tobramycin), but these drugs must never be mixed in the same infusion (mutual inactivation). If given concurrently, administer separately and flush IV line before and after administration. Manufacturer recommends temporarily discontinuing other solutions infusing at the same site during intermittent infusion and states, "Do not add supplementary medications to premixed plastic IV containers."

One source suggests the following **compatibilities:**

Additive: Clindamycin (Cleocin), fluconazole (Diflucan), heparin, linezolid (Zyvox), metronidazole (Flagyl IV), potassium chloride, sodium bicarbonate.

Y-site: Acyclovir (Zovirax), allopurinol (Aloprim), amifostine (Ethyol), aminophylline, anidulafungin (Eraxis), aztreonam (Azactam), bivalirudin (Angiomax), ciprofloxacin (Cipro IV), cisatracurium (Nimbex), daptomycin (Cubicin), dexmedetomidine (Precedex), diltiazem (Cardizem), dobutamine, docetaxel (Taxotere), dopamine, doxapram (Dopram), enalaprilat (Vasotec IV), epinephrine (Adrenalin), esmolol (Brevibloc), etoposide phosphate (Etopophos), famotidine (Pepcid IV), fenoldopam (Corlopam), filgrastim (Neupogen), fluconazole (Diflucan), fludarabine (Fludara), foscarnet (Foscavir), furosemide (Lasix), gallium nitrate (Ganite), gemcitabine (Gemzar), granisetron (Kytril), heparin, hetastarch in electrolytes (Hextend), hydromorphone (Dilaudid), insulin (regular), ketamine (Ketalar), labetalol, linezolid (Zyvox), melphalan (Alkeran), meperidine (Demerol), methylprednisolone (Solu-Medrol), milrinone (Primacor), morphine, nicardipine (Cardene IV), ondansetron (Zofran), paclitaxel (Taxol), propofol (Diprivan), ranitidine (Zantac), remifentanil (Ultiva), sargramostim (Leukine), sufentanil (Sufenta), tacrolimus (Prograf), telavancin (Vibativ), teniposide (Vumon), theophylline, thiotepa, tigecycline (Tygacil), valproate (Depacon), vancomycin, vinorelbine (Navelbine), zidovudine (AZT, Retrovir).

RATE OF ADMINISTRATION

See Compatibility. May be given through Y-tube or three-way stopcock of infusion set.

IV injection: A single dose equally distributed over 3 to 5 minutes.

Intermittent IV: A single dose over 15 to 30 minutes.

ACTIONS

A broad-spectrum, third-generation cephalosporin antibiotic. Bactericidal to selected gram-negative, gram-positive, and anaerobic organisms. Effective against many otherwise resistant organisms, including *Pseudomonas aeruginosa*. Inhibits bacterial cell wall synthesis. Peak serum levels achieved by end of infusion. Therapeutic levels distributed into many body fluids and tissues, including CSF and aqueous humor. Half-life is 1.9 hours. Excreted unchanged in the urine. Crosses placental barrier. Secreted in breast milk.

INDICATIONS AND USES

Treatment of the following infections caused by susceptible isolates of the designated microorganisms (see prescribing information): lower respiratory tract, urinary tract, skin and skin structure, bone and joint, gynecologic, intra-abdominal, and CNS infections (including meningitis), and bacterial septicemia.

Unlabeled uses: Treatment of melioidosis; empiric treatment of febrile neutropenia.

CONTRAINDICATIONS

History of immediate hypersensitivity reaction (e.g., anaphylaxis, serious skin reactions) to ceftazidime or the cephalosporin class of antibiotics, penicillins, or other beta-lactam antibiotics; see Precautions. ▪ Premixed solutions containing dextrose may be contraindicated in patients with known allergies to corn or corn products.

PRECAUTIONS

Hypersensitivity reactions, including fatalities, have been reported and include reports of individuals with a history of penicillin hypersensitivity or sensitivity to multiple allergens experiencing severe reactions when treated with cephalosporins. Check history of previous hypersensitivity reactions to penicillins, cephalosporins, or other allergens. Actual incidence of cross-allergenicity not established but may be more common with first-generation cephalosporins. ▪ Hypersensitivity reactions have been reported with administration of corn-derived, dextrose-containing products in patients with or without a history of hypersensitivity to corn products. Ceftazidime in the DUPLEX container contains dextrose. ▪ Specific sensitivity studies indicated to determine susceptibility of causative organism to ceftazidime. Inducible type I beta-lactamase resistance has been noted with some organisms and can develop during therapy, leading to clinical failure. Periodic susceptibility testing may be indicated. ▪ To reduce the development of drug-resistant bacteria and maintain its effectiveness, ceftazidime should be used to treat or prevent only those infections proven or strongly suspected to be caused by bacteria. ▪ An immune-mediated hemolytic anemia has been observed in patients receiving cephalosporin antibiotics, including ceftazidime. Fatalities have been reported. ▪ Use with caution in patients with renal impairment. Elevated levels of ceftazidime in these patients can lead to asterixis, coma, encephalopathy, myoclonus, neuromuscular excitability, and seizures; see Dose Adjustments. ▪ May be associated with a fall in prothrombin activity. Patients at risk include those with renal or hepatic impairment, those with poor nutritional status, those receiving a protracted course of antimicrobial therapy, and/or those previously stabilized on anticoagulant therapy; see Monitor. ▪ Avoid prolonged use of drug; superinfection caused by overgrowth of nonsusceptible organisms may result. ▪ Use caution in patients with allergies or a history of GI disease (especially colitis). ▪ *Clostridium difficile*–associated diarrhea (CDAD) has been reported. May range from mild diarrhea to fatal colitis. Consider in patients who present with diarrhea during or after treatment with ceftazidime. ▪ Continue for at least 2 days after all symptoms of infection subside.

Monitor: Obtain baseline CBC and SCr. ▪ Watch for early symptoms of a hypersensitivity reaction. ▪ Monitor CBC. If a patient develops anemia while taking ceftazidime, consider the diagnosis of a cephalosporin-associated anemia. Ceftazidime should be held until the etiology is determined. ▪ May cause thrombophlebitis. Use small needles and large veins, and rotate infusion sites. ▪ Monitor PT and administer vitamin K as indicated; see Precautions. ▪ See Drug/Lab Interactions; additional monitoring may be indicated (e.g., renal function, drug serum levels, PT).

Patient Education: Report promptly any bleeding or bruising, symptoms of allergy (e.g., difficulty breathing, hives, itching, rash), or neurologic symptoms (e.g., confusion, myoclonus, seizures). ▪ Promptly report diarrhea or bloody stools that occur during treatment or up to several months after an antibiotic has been discontinued; may indicate CDAD and require treatment.

Maternal/Child: Category B: safety for use during pregnancy and breast-feeding not established. No problems documented. Use caution. ▪ Immature renal function of infants and small children will increase blood levels of all cephalosporins. ▪ Only specific solutions can be used in pediatric patients.

Elderly: No specific problems documented. ▪ See Usual Dose and Dose Adjustments.

DRUG/LAB INTERACTIONS

Risk of nephrotoxicity and ototoxicity may be increased with **aminoglycosides and other nephrotoxic and/or ototoxic agents** (e.g., loop diuretics such as furosemide [Lasix]). ▪ May be antagonized by **bacteriostatic antibiotics** (e.g., chloramphenicol, erythromycin, tetracyclines); may interfere with bactericidal action. ▪ May reduce the effectiveness of **oral estrogen/progesterone contraceptives.** ▪ False-positive **Coombs' test.** ▪ May have a false-positive reaction for **urine glucose** except with enzyme-based tests (e.g., Clinistix). ▪ See Compatibility and Side Effects.

SIDE EFFECTS

The most common adverse reactions occurring in fewer than 2% of patients include hypersensitivity reactions, GI symptoms, and CNS reactions. Full scope of hypersensitivity reactions (including anaphylaxis and cardiopulmonary arrest); abdominal pain; angioedema; burning, discomfort, and pain at injection site; candidiasis; CDAD; colitis; diarrhea; dizziness; elevated alkaline phosphatase, AST, ALT, GGT, and BUN/SCr; erythema multiforme; fever; headache; jaundice; nausea and vomiting; paresthesia; prolonged PT; pruritus; rash; renal impairment; seizures (large doses or in patients with renal impairment); Stevens-Johnson syndrome; toxic epidermal necrolysis; toxic nephropathy; urticaria; vaginitis. Hypoprothrombinemia (rare) and hemolytic anemia may occur. Aplastic anemia, erythema multiforme, hemolytic anemia, hemorrhage, hepatic dysfunction (including cholestasis), pancytopenia, renal dysfunction, Stevens-Johnson syndrome, toxic epidermal necrolysis, and toxic nephropathy have been reported with cephalosporin-class antibiotics.

Overdose: Asterixis, coma, encephalopathy, neuromuscular excitability, and seizures may occur in patients with renal impairment; see Precautions.

Post-Marketing: Hemorrhage, hyperbilirubinemia, jaundice, toxic nephropathy.

ANTIDOTE

Notify physician of any side effects. Discontinue the drug if indicated. Treat hypersensitivity reaction as indicated and resuscitate as necessary. Mild cases of CDAD may respond to discontinuation of ceftazidime. Treat CDAD with fluids, electrolytes, protein supplements, and oral vancomycin (Vancocin) or metronidazole (Flagyl) as indicated. In severe cases, surgical evaluation may be indicated. Hemodialysis may be useful in overdose.

CEFTAZIDIME/AVIBACTAM

(sef-**TAY**-zih-deem a-vih-**BAK**-tam)

Avycaz

Antibacterial
(cephalosporin/beta-lactamase inhibitor)

USUAL DOSE

2.5 Gm (2 Gm ceftazidime/0.5 Gm avibactam) every 8 hours as an infusion over 2 hours.

Ceftazidime-Avibactam Dosing in Patients with Normal Renal Function				
Infection	Dose	Frequency	Infusion Time (hours)	Recommended Duration of Total Antimicrobial Treatment
Complicated intra-abdominal infections (cIAI)*	2.5 Gm (2 Gm/0.5 Gm)	Every 8 hours	2 hours	5 to 14 days
Complicated urinary tract infections (cUTI), including pyelonephritis	2.5 Gm (2 Gm/0.5 Gm)	Every 8 hours	2 hours	7 to 14 days

*Use in conjunction with metronidazole (Flagyl) 500 mg intravenously every 8 hours.

DOSE ADJUSTMENTS

No dose adjustment is recommended based on age, gender, or hepatic impairment. ■ Dose adjustment required for patients with moderate and severe renal impairment and end-stage renal disease according to the following chart.

Ceftazidime-Avibactam Dosing in Patients with Renal Impairment and cIAI or cUTI	
Estimated CrCl (mL/min)	Recommended Dose Regimen
>50 mL/min	2.5 Gm (2 Gm/0.5 Gm) IV (over 2 hours) every 8 hours.
31 to 50 mL/min	1.25 Gm (1 Gm/0.25 Gm) IV (over 2 hours) every 8 hours.
16 to 30 mL/min	0.94 Gm (0.75 Gm/0.19 Gm) IV (over 2 hours) every 12 hours.
6 to 15 mL/min*	0.94 Gm (0.75 Gm/0.19 Gm) IV (over 2 hours) every 24 hours.
≤5 mL/min*	0.94 Gm (0.75 Gm/0.19 Gm) IV (over 2 hours) every 48 hours.

*Both ceftazidime and avibactam are hemodialyzable; administer after hemodialysis on hemodialysis days.

DILUTION
Available as single-use vials containing 2 Gm ceftazidime and 0.5 Gm avibactam. Reconstitute each vial with 10 mL of SWFI, NS, D5W, all combinations of dextrose and sodium chloride injection containing up to 2.5% dextrose and 0.45% NS, or LR injection. Mix gently. Reconstituted solution will have an approximate final volume of 12 mL, an approximate ceftazidime concentration of 0.167 Gm/mL, and an approximate avibactam concentration of 0.042 Gm/mL. Must be further diluted before infusion. Withdraw the required dose from the vial according to the following chart and transfer into an infusion bag containing the same diluent used for reconstitution of the powder (except SWFI) to achieve a total volume between 50 and 250 mL. If SWFI was used for reconstitution, use any of the other appropriate diluents listed previously for dilution.

Preparation of Ceftazidime-Avibactam to Achieve Required Doses	
Ceftazidime-Avibactam Dose	Volume to Withdraw from Reconstituted Vial
2.5 Gm (2 Gm/0.5 Gm)	Entire contents (12 mL)
1.25 Gm (1 Gm/0.25 Gm)	$^1/_2$ of vial contents (6 mL)
0.94 Gm (0.75 Gm/0.19 Gm)	4.5 mL

Ensure contents are completely dissolved. Infusion solution ranges from clear to light yellow.

Filters: Specific information not available.

Storage: Before use, store at CRT in original carton to protect from light. The reconstituted solution may be held for no longer than 30 minutes before dilution in a suitable infusion solution. Fully diluted solutions may be stored for 12 hours at room temperature or for 24 hours refrigerated at 2° to 8° C (36° to 46° F). Use refrigerated solution within 12 hours of subsequent storage at RT.

COMPATIBILITY
Compatibility with other drugs not established. Manufacturer states **compatible** with the more commonly used IV infusion fluids in infusion bags (including Baxter Mini-Bag Plus); see Dilution.

RATE OF ADMINISTRATION
A single dose as an infusion equally distributed over 2 hours.

ACTIONS
Ceftazidime-avibactam is an antibacterial combination product consisting of the cephalosporin ceftazidime pentahydrate and the beta-lactamase inhibitor avibactam sodium. Ceftazidme is a cephalosporin antibacterial drug with in vitro activity against certain gram-negative and gram-positive bacteria. Active against several gram-negative bacteria in clinical infections. Its bactericidal action results from inhibition of cell wall biosynthesis and is mediated through binding to penicillin-binding proteins (PBPs). Avibactam is a non–beta-lactam beta-lactamase inhibitor that inactivates some beta-lactamases and protects ceftazidime from degradation by certain beta-lactamases. Less than 10% of ceftazidime is protein bound. Both ceftazidime and avibactam are excreted mainly by the kidneys, primarily as unchanged drug. Terminal half-life is approximately 2.8 hours. Ceftazidime is excreted in human milk in low concentrations.

INDICATIONS AND USES
Used in combination with metronidazole (Flagyl) for the treatment of patients 18 years or older with complicated intra-abdominal infections (cIAI) caused by designated susceptible microorganisms. ▪ Treatment of patients 18 years or older with complicated urinary tract infections (cUTI), including pyelonephritis caused by designated susceptible microorganisms. ▪ Reserve ceftazidime-avibactam for use in patients who have limited or no alternative treatment options. Limited clinical safety and efficacy data currently available.

CONTRAINDICATIONS

Known serious hypersensitivity to ceftazidime-avibactam, ceftazidime, avibactam-containing products, or other members of the cephalosporin class.

PRECAUTIONS

For IV infusion only; do not administer as an IV bolus. ▪ In a cIAI trial, clinical cure rates were lower in a subgroup of patients with a baseline CrCl of 30 mL/min to less than or equal to 50 mL/min compared with patients with a CrCl of greater than 50 mL/min. Reduction in clinical cure rates was more marked in patients treated with ceftazidime-avibactam plus metronidazole compared with meropenem-treated patients. Within this subgroup, patients treated with ceftazidime/avibactam received a 33% lower daily dose than is currently recommended for patients with a CrCl of 30 mL/min to less than or equal to 50 mL/min; see Monitor. ▪ Serious and occasionally fatal hypersensitivity (anaphylactic) reactions and serious skin reactions have been reported in patients receiving beta-lactam antibacterial drugs. Check history of previous hypersensitivity reactions to other cephalosporins, penicillins, or carbapenems. Cross-sensitivity among beta-lactam antibacterial drugs has been established. ▪ Specific sensitivity studies are indicated to determine susceptibility of the causative organism to ceftazidime-avibactam. ▪ To reduce the development of drug-resistant bacteria and maintain its effectiveness, ceftazidime-avibactam should be used to treat only those infections proven or strongly suspected to be caused by susceptible bacteria. ▪ No cross-resistance with other classes of antimicrobials has been identified. Some isolates resistant to other cephalosporins (including ceftazidime) and to carbapenems may be susceptible to ceftazidime-avibactam. ▪ *Clostridium difficile*–associated diarrhea (CDAD) has been reported for nearly all systemic antibacterial agents and may range in severity from mild diarrhea to fatal colitis. Consider in patients who present with diarrhea during or after treatment with ceftazidime-avibactam. ▪ Central nervous system reactions (e.g., asterixis, coma, encephalopathy, myoclonia, neuromuscular excitability, nonconvulsive status epilepticus, and seizures) have been reported in patients treated with ceftazidime, particularly in patients with renal impairment. Adjust dose based on CrCl. ▪ Seroconversion from a negative to a positive direct Coombs' test result has occurred. No adverse reactions representing hemolytic anemia were reported.

Monitor: Monitor CrCl at least daily in patients with changing renal function. Adjust dose of ceftazidime-avibactam accordingly; see Dose Adjustments. ▪ Monitor for S/S of a hypersensitivity reaction (e.g., hypotension, rash, urticaria, tightness of the chest, wheezing).

Patient Education: Promptly report S/S of a hypersensitivity reaction (e.g., hives, rash, shortness of breath, wheezing). ▪ Promptly report diarrhea or bloody stools that occur during treatment or up to several months after an antibiotic has been discontinued; may indicate CDAD and require treatment. ▪ Promptly report neurologic S/S (e.g., encephalopathy [disturbance of consciousness including confusion, hallucinations, stupor, and coma], myoclonus, and seizures). ▪ Full course of therapy must be completed.

Maternal/Child: Category B: use during pregnancy only if clearly needed. ▪ Use caution during breast-feeding. ▪ Safety and effectiveness for use in patients less than 18 years of age not established.

Elderly: Because of limited data, differences in outcomes or specific risks with ceftazidime-avibactam cannot be ruled out for patients 65 years of age and older. ▪ Consider age-related renal impairment, monitoring of renal function, and dose with caution; see Dose Adjustments.

DRUG/LAB INTERACTIONS

Formal drug interaction studies have not been conducted. ▪ In vitro, avibactam is a substrate of OAT1 and OAT3. Coadministration with the OAT1/OAT3 inhibitor **probenecid** prolongs the half-life of avibactam and is not recommended. ▪ In vitro studies have not demonstrated antagonism between ceftazidime-avibactam and colistin, levofloxacin (Levaquin), linezolid (Zyvox), metronidazole (Flagyl), tigecycline (Tygacil), tobramycin, or vancomycin. ▪ May have a false-positive reaction for **urine glucose** except with enzyme-based tests (e.g., Clinistix).

SIDE EFFECTS
Most common side effects reported are anxiety, constipation, nausea, and vomiting. Hypersensitivity reactions, skin reactions, central nervous system reactions, and CDAD may be severe. Other reported side effects include abdominal pain, dizziness, increased ALT, increased alkaline phosphatase, and upper abdominal pain. Other side effects have been reported in fewer than 5% of patients.

ANTIDOTE
Notify physician of any side effects. Discontinue the drug if indicated. Treat hypersensitivity reactions as indicated (e.g., diphenhydramine [Benadryl], epinephrine [Adrenalin], albuterol) and resuscitate as necessary. Mild cases of CDAD may respond to discontinuation of ceftazidime-avibactam. Treat CDAD with fluids, electrolytes, protein supplements, and oral vancomycin (Vancocin) or metronidazole (Flagyl) as indicated. In severe cases, surgical evaluation may be indicated. Both ceftazidime and avibactam can be removed from the circulation by hemodialysis.

CEFTOLOZANE/TAZOBACTAM
(sef-**TOL**-oh-zane/**TAZ**-oh-**BAK**-tam)

Zerbaxa

Antibacterial
(cephalosporin/
beta-lactamase inhibitor)

USUAL DOSE
1.5 Gm (ceftolozane 1 Gm and tazobactam 0.5 Gm) every 8 hours as an infusion over 1 hour. Guide duration of treatment by the severity and site of the infection and the patient's clinical and bacteriologic progress.

Ceftolozane/Tazobactam Dosing in Patients with a CrCl Greater Than 50 mL/min				
Infection	Dose	Frequency	Infusion Time (hours)	Duration of Treatment
Complicated intra-abdominal infections*	1.5 Gm	Every 8 hours	1 hour	4 to 14 days
Complicated urinary tract infections, including pyelonephritis	1.5 Gm	Every 8 hours	1 hour	7 days

*Use in conjunction with metronidazole (Flagyl) 500 mg intravenously every 8 hours.

DOSE ADJUSTMENTS
No dose adjustment is recommended based on age, gender, hepatic impairment, or race.
- Dose adjustment is required for patients with a CrCl of 50 mL/min or less according to the following chart.

Ceftolozane/Tazobactam Dosing in Patients with Renal Impairment	
Estimated CrCl (mL/min)	Recommended Dose Regimen for Ceftolozane 1 Gm and Tazobactam 0.5 Gm
30 to 50 mL/min	750 mg (500 mg and 250 mg) IV every 8 hours
15 to 29 mL/min	375 mg (250 mg and 125 mg) IV every 8 hours
End-stage renal disease (ESRD) on hemodialysis (HD)	A single loading dose of 750 mg (500 mg and 250 mg) followed by a 150 mg (100 mg and 50 mg) maintenance dose administered every 8 hours for the remainder of the treatment period (on hemodialysis days, administer the dose at the earliest possible time following completion of dialysis)

DILUTION

Available as single-dose vials containing 1 Gm ceftolozane and 0.5 Gm tazobactam. Reconstitute each vial with 10 mL of SWFI or NS and gently shake to dissolve. Final volume is approximately 11.4 mL. Reconstituted solution is **NOT** for direct injection.

Withdraw the required dose from the vial according to the following chart and transfer to an infusion bag containing 100 mL of NS or D5W.

Preparation of Ceftolozane/Tazobactam to Achieve Required Doses	
Ceftolozane/Tazobactam Dose	Volume to Withdraw from Reconstituted Vial
1.5 Gm (1 Gm and 0.5 Gm)	11.4 mL (entire contents)
750 mg (500 mg and 250 mg)	5.7 mL
375 mg (250 mg and 125 mg)	2.9 mL
150 mg (100 mg and 50 mg)	1.2 mL

Infusion solutions range from clear, colorless solutions to clear and slightly yellow.

Filters: Specific information not available.

Storage: Refrigerate vials at 2° to 8° C (36° to 46° F) in original carton to protect from light. Solutions reconstituted with SWFI or NS may be held for 1 hour before transfer and dilution. Fully diluted solutions may be stored for 24 hours at room temperature or for 7 days if refrigerated. Do not freeze.

COMPATIBILITY

Compatibility with other drugs not established. Manufacturer states, "Ceftolozane/tazobactam should not be mixed with other drugs or physically added to solutions containing other drugs."

RATE OF ADMINISTRATION

A single dose as an infusion equally distributed over 1 hour.

ACTIONS

Ceftolozane/tazobactam is an antibacterial combination product consisting of the cephalosporin antibacterial drug ceftolozane sulfate and the beta-lactamase inhibitor tazobactam sodium. Its bactericidal action results from inhibition of cell wall biosynthesis and is mediated through binding to penicillin-binding proteins (PBPs). Tazobactam sodium is an irreversible inhibitor of some beta-lactamases (enzymes [e.g., certain penicillinases and cephalosporinases] produced by bacteria and capable of hydrolyzing/inactivating penicillins and cephalosporins). Active against a variety of gram-negative, gram-positive, and anaerobic bacteria. Protein binding of ceftolozane and tazobactam is approximately 16% to 21% and 30%, respectively. Ceftolozane does not appear to be metabolized to an appreciable extent. Tazobactam is hydrolyzed to an inactive metabolite. Half-life of ceftolozane is approximately 3 hours. Half-life of tazobactam is approximately 1 hour. Both ceftolozane and tazobactam are eliminated by the kidneys—ceftolozane as the unchanged parent drug and tazobactam as the unchanged parent drug and its inactive metabolite.

INDICATIONS AND USES

Treatment of patients 18 years or older with complicated intra-abdominal infections or complicated urinary tract infections, including pyelonephritis caused by designated susceptible microorganisms.

CONTRAINDICATIONS

Known serious hypersensitivity to ceftolozane/tazobactam, piperacillin/tazobactam, or other members of the beta-lactam class.

PRECAUTIONS

For IV infusion only; do not administer as an IV bolus. ▪ Effectiveness is decreased in patients with a baseline CrCl of 30 to 50 mL/min; see Monitor. ▪ Serious and occasionally fatal hypersensitivity (anaphylactic) reactions have been reported in patients receiving beta-lactam antibacterial drugs. Check the history of previous hypersensitivity reactions to penicillins, cephalosporins, or other beta-lactam antibacterial drugs. Cross-sensitivity has been established. ▪ Specific sensitivity studies are indicated to determine susceptibility of the causative organism to ceftolozane/tazobactam. ▪ Bacteria resistant to other cephalosporins may be susceptible to ceftolozane/tazobactam, although cross-resistance may occur. ▪ To reduce the development of drug-resistant bacteria and maintain its effectiveness, ceftolozane/tazobactam should be used to treat only those infections proven or strongly suspected to be caused by bacteria. ▪ *Clostridium difficile*–associated diarrhea (CDAD) has been reported for nearly all systemic antibacterial agents and may range in severity from mild diarrhea to fatal colitis. Consider in patients who present with diarrhea during or after treatment with ceftolozane/tazobactam.

Monitor: Monitor the CrCl at least daily in patients with changing renal function. Adjust dose of ceftolozane/tazobactam accordingly. ▪ Monitor for S/S of a hypersensitivity reaction (e.g., hypotension, rash, urticaria, tightness of the chest, wheezing).

Patient Education: Promptly report S/S of a hypersensitivity reaction (e.g., hives, rash, shortness of breath, wheezing). ▪ Promptly report diarrhea or bloody stools that occur during treatment or up to several months after an antibiotic has been discontinued; may indicate CDAD and require treatment.

Maternal/Child: Category B: use during pregnancy only if the potential benefit outweighs the possible risk. ▪ Use caution during breast-feeding. ▪ Safety and effectiveness for use in pediatric patients not established.

Elderly: A higher incidence of adverse reactions occurs in patients 65 years of age and older. ▪ In the complicated intra-abdominal infection clinical trial, cure rates were lower in patients 65 years of age or older in the ceftolozane/tazobactam group compared with the comparator group. This finding in the elderly population was not seen in the complicated UTI trial. ▪ Consider age-related renal impairment, monitoring of renal function, and dose with caution; see Dose Adjustments.

DRUG/LAB INTERACTIONS

Ceftolozane/tazobactam is not metabolized in the liver. No significant drug-drug interactions are anticipated between ceftolozane/tazobactam and substrates, inhibitors, and inducers of cytochrome P_{450} enzymes. ▪ It is not a substrate for P-glycoprotein (P-gp). ▪ Tazobactam is a known substrate for OAT1 and OAT3. Coadministration with the OAT1/OAT3 inhibitor **probenecid** prolongs the half-life of tazobactam by 71%.

SIDE EFFECTS

Most common side effects reported are diarrhea, fever, headache, and nausea. Hypersensitivity reactions and CDAD may be severe. Other reported side effects include abdominal pain, anemia, anxiety, atrial fibrillation, constipation, dizziness, hypokalemia, hypotension, increased ALT and AST, insomnia, rash, thrombocytosis, and vomiting. Other side effects have been reported in fewer than 1% of patients.

ANTIDOTE

Notify physician of any side effects. Discontinue the drug if indicated. Treat hypersensitivity reactions as indicated (e.g., diphenhydramine [Benadryl], epinephrine [Adrenalin], albuterol) and resuscitate as necessary. Mild cases of CDAD may respond to discontinuation of ceftolozane/tazobactam. Treat CDAD with fluids, electrolytes, protein supplements, and oral vancomycin (Vancocin) or metronidazole (Flagyl) as indicated. In severe cases, surgical evaluation may be indicated. Both ceftolozane and tazobactam are partially removed by hemodialysis.

CEFTRIAXONE SODIUM
(sef-try-**AX**-ohn **SO**-dee-um)

Antibacterial
(cephalosporin)

Rocephin

pH 6.6 to 6.7

USUAL DOSE

Adults and pediatric patients over 12 years: 1 to 2 Gm/24 hr. May be given as a single dose every 24 hours or equally divided into 2 doses and given every 12 hours depending on the type and severity of the infection. Do not exceed a total dose of 4 Gm/24 hr.

Meningitis: 2 Gm every 12 hours.

Disseminated gonococcal infections (unlabeled): 1 Gm daily for 24 to 48 hours. Transfer to oral dosing after improvement is noted, and continue for a total of 7 days of therapy.

Perioperative prophylaxis: 1 Gm IV 30 minutes to 2 hours before incision. Used primarily in patients undergoing coronary artery bypass surgery and in contaminated or potentially contaminated surgeries.

Lyme disease (unlabeled): 2 Gm daily for 14 days (range 14 to 28 days).

PEDIATRIC DOSE

Pediatric patients 1 month to 12 years of age: See Maternal/Child.

Skin and soft tissue: 50 to 75 mg/kg of body weight/24 hr as a single dose or in equally divided doses every 12 hours (25 to 37.5 mg/kg every 12 hours). Do not exceed a total dose of 2 Gm/24 hr.

Other serious infections (other than meningitis): 50 to 75 mg/kg of body weight/24 hr in equally divided doses every 12 hours (25 to 37.5 mg/kg every 12 hours). Do not exceed a total dose of 2 Gm/24 hr.

Bacterial meningitis: Begin with a loading dose of 100 mg/kg on day 1 (do not exceed a total dose of 4 Gm), follow with 100 mg/kg/day (not to exceed 4 Gm) as a single dose or in equally divided doses every 12 hours (50 mg/kg every 12 hours). Continue for 7 to 14 days depending on the causative organism.

Lyme disease (unlabeled): 50 to 75 mg/kg/day for 14 days (range 10 to 28 days). Maximum dose is 2 Gm.

NEONATAL DOSE

See Contraindications, Rate of Administration, and Maternal/Child before administration to neonates.

Neonatal doses may also be given IM.

The American Academy of Pediatrics (AAP) recommends the following:

28 days of age or younger regardless of weight: 50 mg/kg/day as a single daily dose.

Bacterial meningitis: Same as Pediatric Dose.

Infants born to mothers with gonococcal infections: 25 to 50 mg/kg one time only (do not exceed 125 mg).

DOSE ADJUSTMENTS

In adults with both hepatic and renal impairment, dose should not exceed 2 Gm daily.

■ Dose adjustment not required for elderly patients with doses up to 2 Gm/day provided there is no severe renal and hepatic impairment. ■ See Drug/Lab Interactions.

DILUTION

Initially reconstitute each 250 mg of sterile powder with 2.4 mL (500 mg with 4.8 mL, 1 Gm with 9.6 mL, 2 Gm with 19.2 mL) of SWFI, NS, D5W, D10W, D5NS, or D5/½NS for injection (see chart on inside back cover or literature for additional diluents). Each mL will contain 100 mg. A single dose must be further diluted to the desired concentration with the same solution and given as an intermittent infusion. Shake well. Concentrations of 10 mg/mL to 40 mg/mL are recommended for intermittent infusion. Color of solution ranges from light yellow to amber depending on length of storage, concentration, and diluent used. Should not be reconstituted, further diluted, or simultaneously administered with calcium-containing IV solutions. A precipitate can form; see Compatibility. Also available in a premixed frozen Galaxy container, in dual-chamber DUPLEX containers, in ADD-Vantage vials for use with ADD-Vantage infusion containers, and in pharmacy bulk packages. Refer to manufacturer's prescribing information for specific preparation and storage requirements.

Storage: See manufacturer's directions. Recommendations for storing vary from CRT (20° to 25° C [68° to 77° F]) to RT (25° C [77° F]) or below and protect from light. Stable at RT for at least 24 hours in stated solutions or selected solutions up to 10 days if refrigerated (see prescribing information). D5NS and D5/¹/₂NS should not be refrigerated. Stability and color (light yellow to amber) depend on concentration and diluent. Solutions reconstituted in D5W or NS in concentrations between 10 and 40 mg/mL and then frozen at −20° C in PVC or polyolefin containers remain stable for 26 weeks.

COMPATIBILITY (Underline Indicates Conflicting Compatibility Information)
Consider any drug NOT listed as compatible to be INCOMPATIBLE until consulting a pharmacist; specific conditions may apply.
Manufacturer states, "Do not use diluents containing calcium, such as Ringer's solution or Hartmann's solution, to reconstitute or further dilute ceftriaxone. Particulate formation can result. Ceftriaxone and calcium-containing solutions, including continuous calcium-containing infusions such as parenteral nutrition, should not be mixed or coadministered simultaneously via a **Y-site**." However, in patients other than neonates, ceftriaxone and calcium-containing solutions may be administered sequentially if the infusion lines are thoroughly flushed between infusions with a **compatible** fluid; see Contraindications and Precautions. Manufacturer lists as **compatible** with metronidazole (Flagyl IV) as an **additive** in NS or D5W if the concentration of metronidazole does not exceed 5 to 7.5 mg/mL with ceftriaxone 10 mg/mL as an admixture. Mixture is stable at RT for 24 hours. Precipitation will occur if refrigerated or if concentration of metronidazole exceeds 8 mg/mL. No studies have been done with Flagyl IV RTU. Manufacturer lists aminoglycosides (e.g., gentamicin), amsacrine (Amsidyl), fluconazole (Diflucan), and vancomycin as **incompatible** and states, "May be given sequentially with thorough flushing of the IV line with **compatible** solution between the administrations."

One source suggests the following **compatibilities:**
Additive: Mannitol (Osmitrol).
Y-site: Acetaminophen (Ofirmev), acyclovir (Zovirax), allopurinol (Aloprim), amifostine (Ethyol), amiodarone (Nexterone), anidulafungin (Eraxis), aztreonam (Azactam), bivalirudin (Angiomax), cisatracurium (Nimbex), daptomycin (Cubicin), dexmedetomidine (Precedex), diltiazem (Cardizem), docetaxel (Taxotere), doxorubicin liposomal (Doxil), etoposide phosphate (Etopophos), famotidine (Pepcid IV), fenoldopam (Corlopam), fludarabine (Fludara), foscarnet (Foscavir), gallium nitrate (Ganite), gemcitabine (Gemzar), granisetron (Kytril), heparin, 6% hydroxyethyl starch (Voluven), linezolid (Zyvox), melphalan (Alkeran), meperidine (Demerol), methotrexate, morphine, paclitaxel (Taxol), pantoprazole (Protonix IV), pemetrexed (Alimta), propofol (Diprivan), remifentanil (Ultiva), sargramostim (Leukine), sodium bicarbonate, tacrolimus (Prograf), telavancin (Vibativ), teniposide (Vumon), theophylline, thiotepa, tigecycline (Tygacil), vancomycin, warfarin (Coumadin), zidovudine (AZT, Retrovir).

RATE OF ADMINISTRATION
Intermittent IV: A single dose over 30 minutes.
Neonates: Intravenous doses should be given over 60 minutes to reduce the risk of bilirubin encephalopathy.

ACTIONS
A broad-spectrum, third-generation cephalosporin antibiotic. Bactericidal to selected gram-negative, gram-positive, and anaerobic organisms. Effective against many otherwise resistant organisms. Inhibits bacterial cell wall synthesis. Therapeutic concentrations achieved in many body fluids and tissues, including CSF. Highly protein bound. Has a long half-life (range is 5.8 to 8.7 hours), allowing once-a-day dosing for many indications. Peak serum levels achieved by end of infusion. Excreted through urine, bile, and feces. Crosses placental barrier. Secreted in breast milk.

INDICATIONS AND USES
Treatment of serious lower respiratory tract, urinary tract, skin and skin structure, bone and joint, and intra-abdominal infections. ▪ Bacterial septicemia. ▪ Meningitis. ▪ Most effective against specific organisms (see literature). ▪ Perioperative prophylaxis. ▪ Given IM for additional indications (e.g., acute bacterial otitis, uncomplicated gonorrhea, and pelvic inflammatory disease).
Unlabeled uses: Treatment of Lyme disease and numerous other infections. ▪ Disseminated gonococcal infections. ▪ IM for CDC recommendation for chancroid.

CONTRAINDICATIONS
Known hypersensitivity to ceftriaxone, any of its excipients, or other cephalosporins; see Precautions. ▪ Premature neonates up to a postmenstrual age of 41 weeks (gestational age + chronological age). ▪ Hyperbilirubinemic neonates; see Maternal/Child. ▪ Co-administration with calcium-containing IV solutions, including parenteral nutrition, in infants up to 28 days of age is contraindicated because of the risk of precipitation of ceftriaxone-calcium salt. Cases of fatal outcomes in which a crystalline material was observed in the lungs and kidneys on autopsy have been reported in neonates receiving ceftriaxone and calcium-containing fluids; see Precautions and Compatibility. ▪ Intravenous administration of ceftriaxone solutions containing lidocaine is contraindicated. When lidocaine solution is used as a solvent with ceftriaxone for intramuscular injection, these contraindications do not apply; see IM prescribing information. ▪ Solutions containing dextrose may be contraindicated in patients with hypersensitivity to corn products.

PRECAUTIONS
Hypersensitivity reactions, including fatalities, have been reported. Obtain history of previous hypersensitivity reactions to penicillins, cephalosporins, other beta-lactam agents, or other allergens. Ceftriaxone should be administered with caution to any patient with such a history. Actual incidence of cross-allergenicity not established but may be more common with first-generation cephalosporins. ▪ Sensitivity studies are indicated to determine susceptibility of the causative organism to ceftriaxone. ▪ To reduce the development of drug-resistant bacteria and maintain its effectiveness, ceftriaxone should be used to treat or prevent only those infections proven or strongly suspected to be caused by bacteria. ▪ Continue for at least 2 days after all symptoms of infection subside. Usual course of therapy is 4 to 14 days; *S. pyogenes* requires treatment for 10 days. ▪ Should not be reconstituted, further diluted, or simultaneously administered with calcium-containing IV solutions. A precipitate can form; see Compatibility. There have been no reports of an interaction between ceftriaxone and oral calcium-containing products or between IM ceftriaxone and oral or IV calcium-containing products. ▪ May be associated with an alteration in prothrombin time. Patients at risk include those with impaired vitamin K synthesis or low vitamin K stores (e.g., chronic hepatic disease and malnutrition). Vitamin K administration (10 mg weekly) may be necessary if the prothrombin time is prolonged before or during therapy. ▪ Avoid prolonged use of drug; superinfection caused by overgrowth of nonsusceptible organisms may result. ▪ Use caution in patients with both impaired renal and hepatic function, allergies, or a history of GI disease (especially colitis). ▪ *Clostridium difficile*–associated diarrhea (CDAD) has been reported. May range from mild diarrhea to fatal colitis. Consider in patients who present with diarrhea during or after treatment with ceftriaxone. ▪ Immune-mediated hemolytic anemia has been reported in both adults and pediatric patients. Fatalities have occurred. ▪ Ceftriaxone-calcium precipitates in the gallbladder have been observed in patients receiving ceftriaxone. These precipitates appear on sonogram and may be misinterpreted as gallstones. Patients may be asymptomatic or may develop symptoms of gallbladder disease. The abnormalities appear to be transient and reversible with the discontinuation of ceftriaxone; see Antidote. ▪ Ceftriaxone-calcium precipitates in the urinary tract have been observed in patients receiving ceftriaxone and may be detected as sonographic abnormalities. Patients may be asymptomatic or may develop symptoms of urolithiasis, ureteral obstruction, and postrenal acute renal failure. The condition

appears to be reversible with discontinuation of ceftriaxone and institution of appropriate management; see Antidote. ▪ Pancreatitis, possibly secondary to biliary obstruction, has been reported.

Monitor: Watch for early symptoms of a hypersensitivity reaction. ▪ Monitor PT/INR and administer vitamin K as indicated; see Precautions. ▪ Monitor CBC for development of cephalosporin-induced anemia. ▪ Ensure adequate hydration and monitor renal function. ▪ See Dose Adjustments and Drug/Lab Interactions; additional monitoring may be indicated (e.g., renal function, drug serum levels, PT).

Patient Education: Report promptly any bleeding or bruising or symptoms of allergy (e.g., difficulty breathing, hives, itching, rash). ▪ Promptly report diarrhea or bloody stools that occur during treatment or up to several months after an antibiotic has been discontinued; may indicate CDAD and require treatment.

Maternal/Child: Category B: safety for use during pregnancy not established. No problems documented. ▪ Use caution during breast-feeding. Low concentrations of ceftriaxone are excreted in human milk. ▪ Safety and effectiveness of ceftriaxone in neonates, infants, and pediatric patients have been established. Immature renal function of infants and small children will increase blood levels of all cephalosporins. ▪ Use is contraindicated in hyperbilirubinemic neonates. Ceftriaxone can displace bilirubin from its binding sites on albumin. Risk of bilirubin encephalopathy exists; see Contraindications and Precautions. ▪ Ceftriaxone is also contraindicated in premature neonates up to a postmenstrual age of 41 weeks and in neonates less than or equal to 28 days of age if they require calcium-containing IV solutions; see Contraindications. ▪ The probability of ceftriaxone-calcium precipitates in the gallbladder or urinary tract appears to be greatest in pediatric patients.

Elderly: Response similar to other age-groups; however, greater sensitivity of the elderly cannot be ruled out; see Dose Adjustments.

DRUG/LAB INTERACTIONS
Risk of nephrotoxicity may be increased with **aminoglycosides and other nephrotoxic agents** (e.g., loop diuretics such as furosemide [Lasix]). ▪ **Probenecid** does not alter the elimination of ceftriaxone. ▪ May be antagonized by **bacteriostatic antibiotics** (e.g., chloramphenicol, erythromycin, tetracyclines); may interfere with bactericidal action. ▪ Concomitant use with **vitamin K antagonists** (e.g., warfarin) may increase the risk of bleeding. Monitor coagulation parameters frequently, and adjust anticoagulant dose accordingly. ▪ May cause false-positive **Coombs' test.** ▪ The presence of ceftriaxone may falsely lower estimated blood glucose values obtained with some **blood glucose monitoring systems.** Consult manufacturer's instructions and use alternative testing methods if necessary. ▪ May produce false-positive reaction for **urine glucose** except with enzyme-based tests (e.g., Clinistix). ▪ See Compatibility and Side Effects.

SIDE EFFECTS
Full scope of hypersensitivity reactions (e.g., anaphylaxis with fatal outcome, chills, fever, and pruritus) has been reported. Agranulocytosis; allergic pneumonitis; "biliary sludge" or pseudolithiasis; bleeding episodes; burning, discomfort, and pain at injection site; casts in urine; CDAD; colitis; diarrhea; dizziness; dysgeusia; elevated alkaline phosphatase, bilirubin, BUN, creatinine, AST, and ALT; headache; leukopenia; nausea and vomiting; nephrolithiasis; pancreatitis; prolonged PT; renal precipitations; seizures; thrombophlebitis. Other hematologic reactions (e.g., anemia, eosinophilia, hemolytic anemia, leukopenia, lymphopenia, neutropenia, thrombocytopenia, thrombocytosis) may occur. Aplastic anemia, erythema multiforme, hemolytic anemia, hemorrhage, hepatic dysfunction (including cholestasis), pancytopenia, renal dysfunction, Stevens-Johnson syndrome, toxic epidermal necrolysis, and toxic nephropathy have been reported with cephalosporin-class antibiotics.

Post-Marketing: Dermatologic reactions (e.g., acute generalized exanthematous pustulosis, allergic dermatitis, exanthema, and isolated cases of Stevens-Johnson syndrome and toxic epidermal necrolysis), genitourinary reactions (e.g., oliguria, postrenal acute renal failure, ureteric obstruction), kernicterus, stomatitis, symptomatic precipitation of ceftriaxone-calcium salt in the gallbladder. Fatal cases of ceftriaxone-calcium precipitates in lungs and kidneys of neonates have been reported; see Contraindications, Precautions, and Maternal/Child.

ANTIDOTE

Notify physician of any side effects. Discontinue the drug if indicated (e.g., CDAD, hypersensitivity reactions, seizures, S/S of gallbladder disease, or S/S suggestive of urolithiasis, oliguria, or renal failure). Treat hypersensitivity reactions as indicated and resuscitate as necessary. Mild cases of CDAD may respond to discontinuation of ceftriaxone. Treat CDAD with fluids, electrolytes, protein supplements, and oral vancomycin (Vancocin) or metronidazole (Flagyl) as indicated. In severe cases, surgical evaluation may be indicated. Vitamin K may be useful in bleeding episodes, or drug may need to be discontinued. Not removed by hemodialysis.

CEFUROXIME SODIUM

(sef-your-**OX**-eem **SO**-dee-um)

Zinacef

Antibacterial
(cephalosporin)

pH 5 to 8.5

USUAL DOSE

Dependent on seriousness of infection. Usual dose is 750 mg to 1.5 Gm every 8 hours for 5 to 10 days. Maximum dose is 3 Gm every 8 hours.

Uncomplicated infections (gonococcal, pneumonia, skin and soft tissue, urinary tract): 750 mg every 8 hours.

Severe or complicated infections and bone and joint infections: 1.5 Gm every 8 hours.

Life-threatening or infections due to less susceptible organisms: 1.5 Gm every 6 hours.

Bacterial meningitis: 3 Gm every 8 hours; see Precautions.

Perioperative prophylaxis: 1.5 Gm IV 30 minutes to 1 hour before incision; then 750 mg every 8 hours during prolonged procedures. 1.5 Gm at induction of anesthesia and every 12 hours to total dose of 6 Gm in open heart surgery.

PEDIATRIC DOSE

Do not exceed adult dose.

Pediatric patients 3 months of age or older: 50 to 100 mg/kg/day in equally divided doses every 6 to 8 hours (12.5 to 25 mg/kg every 6 hours or 16.7 to 33.3 mg/kg every 8 hours). Higher-end dosing used for more serious infections.

Bone and joint infections: 50 mg/kg every 8 hours. Up to 1.5 Gm/dose has been given.

Bacterial meningitis: 200 to 240 mg/kg/day in equally divided doses every 6 to 8 hours (50 to 60 mg/kg every 6 hours or 66.7 to 80 mg/kg every 8 hours); see Precautions.

NEONATAL DOSE

Neonatal doses are unlabeled; see Precautions and Maternal/Child.

The American Academy of Pediatrics suggests the following doses:

Neonates: 7 days of age or younger regardless of weight: 50 mg/kg every 12 hours.

Neonates from 8 to 28 days of age weighing 2 kg or less: 50 mg/kg every 8 to 12 hours.

Neonates from 8 to 28 days of age weighing more than 2 kg: 50 mg/kg every 8 hours.

DOSE ADJUSTMENTS

Reduced doses or extended intervals may be indicated in the elderly; consider age-related impaired organ function, nutritional status, and concomitant disease or drug therapy.

Adults: Reduce total daily dose if renal function impaired according to the following chart. ■ See Drug/Lab Interactions.

Cefuroxime Dose Guidelines in Impaired Renal Function in Adults		
Creatinine Clearance (mL/min)	Dose	Frequency
>20 mL/min	750 mg-1.5 Gm	q 8 hr
10-20 mL/min	750 mg	q 12 hr
<10 mL/min	750 mg	q 24 hr
Hemodialysis patients	An additional dose of 750 mg at end of each dialysis session	

Pediatric patients: In pediatric patients with impaired renal function, reduce frequency as indicated in the chart for adults.

DILUTION

Reconstitute 750 mg with 8.3 mL SWFI. Reconstitute 1.5 Gm with 16 mL SWFI. Shake well. May be further diluted to 50 or 100 mL with D5W, NS, or other **compatible** infusion solution (see chart on inside back cover or literature) and given as an intermittent infusion, or added to 500 to 1,000 mL and given as a continuous infusion. Also available in dual-chamber DUPLEX containers, ADD-Vantage vials, Twist vials, premixed frozen Galaxy bags, and pharmacy bulk packaging. Refer to manufacturer's prescribing information for specific preparation and storage requirements.

Storage: In dry state, store between 15° and 30° C (59° to 86° F); protect from light. Reconstituted vials are stable for 24 hours at CRT or 48 hours if refrigerated. Diluted solutions may be stable for up to 7 days if refrigerated.

COMPATIBILITY   (Underline Indicates Conflicting Compatibility Information)

Consider any drug NOT listed as compatible to be INCOMPATIBLE until consulting a pharmacist; specific conditions may apply.

May be used concomitantly with aminoglycosides (e.g., amikacin, gentamicin), but these drugs must never be mixed in the same infusion (mutual inactivation). If given concurrently, administer separately and flush the IV line before and after administration. Manufacturer recommends temporarily discontinuing other solutions infusing at the same site during intermittent infusion and lists sodium bicarbonate **incompatible** as a diluent.

Sources suggest the following **compatibilities:**

Additive: Manufacturer lists heparin (10 and 50 units/mL in NS) and potassium chloride (10 and 40 mEq/L in NS). Other sources list clindamycin (Cleocin), furosemide (Lasix), metronidazole (Flagyl IV), midazolam (Versed).

Y-site: Acyclovir (Zovirax), allopurinol (Aloprim), amifostine (Ethyol), amiodarone (Nexterone), anidulafungin (Eraxis), atracurium (Tracrium), aztreonam (Azactam), bivalirudin (Angiomax), cisatracurium (Nimbex), cyclophosphamide (Cytoxan), dexmedetomidine (Precedex), diltiazem (Cardizem), docetaxel (Taxotere), etoposide phosphate (Etopophos), famotidine (Pepcid IV), fenoldopam (Corlopam), fludarabine (Fludara), foscarnet (Foscavir), gemcitabine (Gemzar), granisetron (Kytril), hetastarch in electrolytes (Hextend), hydromorphone (Dilaudid), linezolid (Zyvox), melphalan (Alkeran), meperidine (Demerol), milrinone (Primacor), morphine, ondansetron (Zofran), pancuronium, pemetrexed (Alimta), propofol (Diprivan), remifentanil (Ultiva), sargramostim (Leukine), tacrolimus (Prograf), teniposide (Vumon), thiotepa, vancomycin, vecuronium.

RATE OF ADMINISTRATION

See Compatibility. Injection or intermittent infusion may be given through Y-tube or three-way stopcock of infusion set.

IV injection: A single dose equally distributed over 3 to 5 minutes.

Intermittent IV: A single dose over 15 to 30 minutes.

Continuous infusion: 500 to 1,000 mL over 6 to 24 hours, depending on total dose and concentration.

ACTIONS

A broad-spectrum, second-generation cephalosporin antibiotic. Bactericidal to selected gram-negative and gram-positive organisms. Effective against many otherwise resistant organisms. Inhibits bacterial cell wall synthesis. Peak serum levels achieved by end of infusion. Widely distributed. 50% bound to serum proteins. Therapeutic concentrations found in pleural fluid, joint fluid, bile, sputum, bone, aqueous humor, and CSF. Half-life is 80 minutes. Excreted in the urine. Crosses placental barrier. Secreted in breast milk.

INDICATIONS AND USES

Treatment of patients with infections caused by susceptible strains of designated organisms in the following diseases: serious lower respiratory tract, urinary tract, bone and joint, skin and skin structure infections, septicemia, and meningitis. ▪ Perioperative prophylaxis. ▪ Used IM to treat gonorrhea.

CONTRAINDICATIONS

Previous hypersensitivity reaction to cephalosporins; see Precautions. ▪ Premixed solutions containing dextrose may be contraindicated in patients with known allergies to corn or corn products.

PRECAUTIONS

Hypersensitivity reactions, including fatalities, have been reported and include reports of individuals with a history of penicillin hypersensitivity or sensitivity to multiple allergens experiencing severe reactions when treated with cephalosporins. Check history of previous hypersensitivity reactions to penicillins, cephalosporins, or other allergens. Actual incidence of cross-allergenicity not established but may be more common with first-generation cephalosporins. ▪ Sensitivity studies indicated to determine susceptibility of the causative organism to cefuroxime. ▪ To reduce the development of drug-resistant bacteria and maintain its effectiveness, cefuroxime should be used to treat or prevent only those infections proven or strongly suspected to be caused by bacteria. ▪ Continue for at least 2 to 3 days after all symptoms of infection subside. ▪ Continue treatment of *Streptococcus pyogenes* infections for a minimum of 10 days to decrease the risk of rheumatic fever or glomerulonephritis. ▪ Avoid prolonged use of drug; superinfection caused by overgrowth of nonsusceptible organisms may result. ▪ Use caution in patients with impaired renal function, allergies, or a history of GI disease (especially colitis). ▪ *Clostridium difficile*–associated diarrhea (CDAD) has been reported. May range from mild diarrhea to fatal colitis. Consider in patients who present with diarrhea during or after treatment with cefuroxime. ▪ May be associated with a fall in prothrombin activity. Patients at risk include those with renal or hepatic impairment, patients with poor nutritional status, patients receiving a protracted course of antimicrobial therapy, and patients previously stabilized on anticoagulant therapy; see Monitor. ▪ Mild to moderate hearing loss has been reported in a few pediatric patients treated for meningitis.

Monitor: Watch for early symptoms of a hypersensitivity reaction. ▪ May cause thrombophlebitis. Use small needles and large veins, and rotate infusion sites. ▪ Obtain baseline SCr and monitor renal function periodically during therapy. ▪ Monitor PT and administer vitamin K as indicated. ▪ See Drug/Lab Interactions; additional monitoring may be indicated (e.g., renal function, drug serum levels).

Patient Education: Report promptly any bleeding or bruising or symptoms of allergy (e.g., difficulty breathing, hives, itching, rash). ▪ Promptly report diarrhea or bloody stools that occur during treatment or up to several months after an antibiotic has been discontinued; may indicate CDAD and require treatment.

Maternal/Child: Category B: safety for use during pregnancy and breast-feeding not established. No problems documented. ▪ Is used in infants under 3 months of age, but safety not established; immature renal function will increase blood levels.

Elderly: See Dose Adjustments. ▪ Response similar to other age-groups; however, greater sensitivity of the elderly cannot be ruled out.

DRUG/LAB INTERACTIONS

Risk of nephrotoxicity may be increased with **aminoglycosides and other nephrotoxic agents** (e.g., loop diuretics such as furosemide [Lasix]). ▪ **Probenecid** inhibits excretion.

Reduced dose of cefuroxime may be required with concomitant use. ▪ May be antagonized by **bacteriostatic antibiotics** (e.g., chloramphenicol, erythromycin, tetracyclines); bactericidal action may be negated. ▪ May reduce effectiveness of **estrogen/progesterone oral contraceptives.** ▪ May cause a false-negative reaction in specific **blood glucose** tests (ferricyanide). ▪ False-positive reaction for **urine glucose** except with enzyme-based tests (e.g., Clinistix). ▪ False-positive **Coombs' test.** ▪ See Compatibility and Side Effects.

SIDE EFFECTS

Full scope of hypersensitivity reactions, including anaphylaxis, drug fever, erythema multiforme, interstitial nephritis, positive Coombs' test, pruritus, rash, Stevens-Johnson syndrome, toxic epidermal necrolysis, and urticaria. CDAD; decreased hemoglobin, hematocrit, or platelet functions; diarrhea; elevation of AST, ALT, total bilirubin, alkaline phosphatase, LDH, and BUN/SCr (transient); eosinophilia; fever; leukopenia; local site pain; nausea; oral thrush; seizures (large doses and decreased renal function); transient neutropenia; thrombocytopenia; thrombophlebitis. Abdominal pain, agranulocytosis, aplastic anemia, colitis, hemolytic anemia, hemorrhage, hepatic dysfunction (including cholestasis), pancytopenia, prolonged prothrombin time, renal dysfunction, toxic nephropathy, and vaginitis, including vaginal candidiasis, have been reported with cephalosporin-class antibiotics.

Post-Marketing: Angioedema, cutaneous vasculitis, seizures.

ANTIDOTE

Notify physician of any side effects. Discontinue the drug if indicated. Mild cases of CDAD may respond to discontinuation of drug. Treat CDAD with fluids, electrolytes, protein supplements, and oral vancomycin (Vancocin) or metronidazole (Flagyl) as indicated. In severe cases, surgical evaluation may be indicated. Treat hypersensitivity reactions and resuscitate as necessary. Hemodialysis or peritoneal dialysis may be somewhat useful in overdose.

CENTRUROIDES (SCORPION) IMMUNE F(ab')₂ (EQUINE) INJECTION

Antivenin

(**SEN**-troo-roy-deez [**SKOR**-pee-on] i-**MUNE**-fab-too)

Anascorp

USUAL DOSE

Initiate as soon as possible after scorpion sting in patients who develop clinically important signs of scorpion envenomation (e.g., loss of muscle control, roving or abnormal eye movements, slurred speech, respiratory distress, excessive salivation, frothing at the mouth, and vomiting).

Initial dose: Entire contents of 3 vials is the recommended initial dose based on clinical experience. Observe during and for up to 1 hour after the initial dose is administered. Desired outcome is resolution of signs of envenomation.

Repeat doses: If control of symptoms is not accomplished by the initial dose, infuse one vial at a time at intervals of 30 to 60 minutes. Observe as above for resolution of S/S of envenomation. This dose may be repeated until initial control has been established. Maximum number of doses that can be administered safely is unknown.

Summary of Dosing for Centruroides (Scorpion) Immune F(ab')₂ Equine Injection		
Initial dose	3 vials	Reconstitute each vial with 5 mL of NS. Combine and further dilute to a total of 50 mL with NS. Infuse IV over 10 minutes.
Additional dose(s)	As needed	Administer one vial at a time at 30- to 60-minute intervals. Dilute to a total of 50 mL with NS. Infuse IV over 10 minutes.

PEDIATRIC DOSE

See Usual Dose. Absolute venom dose following scorpion sting is expected to be the same in pediatric patients and adults; no dose adjustment for age is required. See Maternal/Child.

DILUTION

Initial dose: Reconstitute each of the 3 vials with 5 mL NS. Mix by continuous gentle swirling. Combine the contents of the reconstituted vials and further dilute to a total volume of 50 mL with NS. For initial and repeat doses, the solution should be clear; do not use if turbidity is present.

Repeat doses: Reconstitute each single vial with 5 mL NS. Mix by continuous gentle swirling. Further dilute the contents of the reconstituted vial to a total volume of 50 mL with NS.

Filters: Specific information not available.

Storage: Store at RT (up to 25° C [77° F]). Temperature excursions are permitted up to 40° C (104° F). Do not freeze. Discard partially used vials.

COMPATIBILITY

Specific information not available. Consider administration through a separate line without mixing with other IV fluids or medications due to specific use and potential for anaphylaxis.

RATE OF ADMINISTRATION

A single dose equally distributed over 10 minutes.

ACTIONS

A venom-specific F(ab')₂ fragment of equine immune globulin G (IgG) obtained from horse plasma immunized with scorpion venom. Obtained by pepsin digestion of horse plasma to remove the F_c portion of immune globulin, followed by fractionation and purification steps. Binds and neutralizes venom toxins, facilitating redistribution away from target tissues and elimination from the body. Half-life ranges from 102 to 216 hours. Time from the start of injection to resolution of clinical S/S averages 1.42 hours (range 0.2 to 20.5 hours).

INDICATIONS AND USES
Treatment of adult and pediatric patients with clinical signs of scorpion envenomation.

CONTRAINDICATIONS
Manufacturer states, "None."

PRECAUTIONS
Administer under the direction of a physician knowledgeable in its use in a facility with adequate diagnostic and treatment facilities and appropriate emergency drugs to monitor the patient and respond to any medical emergency. ▪ Severe hypersensitivity reactions, including anaphylaxis, may occur. Patients with a known allergy to horse protein are particularly at risk for anaphylaxis. Patients who have had a previous equine antivenom/antitoxin may be sensitized to equine proteins and be at risk for severe hypersensitivity reactions. ▪ Delayed hypersensitivity reactions (e.g., serum sickness) have been reported. ▪ Made from equine (horse) plasma; may carry and transmit infectious agents (e.g., viruses). ▪ Contains trace amounts of cresol; may cause localized reactions and generalized myalgias.

Monitor: Observe closely for S/S of a hypersensitivity reaction (e.g., chest pain, dizziness, dyspnea, fever, flushing, hypotension, nausea, pruritus, rash, rigors, urticaria); see Antidote. ▪ Monitor closely during infusion and for a minimum of 1 hour to assess if clinically important signs of envenomation have resolved. ▪ Follow-up visits are recommended to monitor for S/S of serum sickness (e.g., arthralgia, fever, myalgia, rash).

Patient Education: Promptly report any S/S of delayed hypersensitivity reactions or serum sickness (e.g., arthralgia, fever, joint pain, lymphadenopathy, malaise, pruritus, rash). May occur up to 14 days following discharge.

Maternal/Child: Category C: use during pregnancy only if clearly needed. ▪ Use caution; safety for use during breast-feeding not established. ▪ Safety and effectiveness comparable in pediatric and adult patients. Pediatric patients generally experienced a slightly faster time to resolution (1.28 ± 0.8 hours) compared with adults (1.91 ± 1.4 hours).

Elderly: Safety and effectiveness comparable to overall patient population.

DRUG/LAB INTERACTIONS
Drug interaction studies have not been conducted. ▪ Time to resolution of symptoms was not affected by the use of sedatives.

SIDE EFFECTS
The most common side effects were fever, nausea, pruritus, rash, and vomiting. Hypersensitivity reactions, including anaphylaxis, have occurred. Less common side effects included cough, diarrhea, fatigue, headache, lethargy, myalgia, and rhinorrhea. Other rarely reported side effects included aspiration, ataxia, hypoxia, pneumonia, respiratory distress, serum sickness, and swelling of the eyes.

Post-Marketing: Chest tightness, palpitations.

ANTIDOTE
Keep the physician informed of all side effects and the extent or progression of envenomation. Discontinue the drug and treat hypersensitivity reactions and/or anaphylaxis immediately with oxygen, epinephrine (Adrenalin), antihistamines (e.g., diphenhydramine [Benadryl]), vasopressors (e.g., dopamine), corticosteroids, albuterol, IV fluids, and ventilation equipment as indicated. Resuscitate as necessary.

CETUXIMAB BBW
(seh-**TUX**-ih-mab)

Recombinant monoclonal antibody
Antineoplastic

Erbitux

pH 7 to 7.4

USUAL DOSE
Premedication: To prevent or attenuate severe infusion reactions, premedicate with diphenhydramine 50 mg IV 30 to 60 minutes before the first dose. Premedication for subsequent infusions should be based on clinical judgment and the presence/severity of previous infusion reactions.

Squamous cell carcinoma of the head and neck (SCCHN) in combination with radiation therapy or in combination with platinum-based therapy with 5-FU: *First infusion:* 400 mg/M^2 as an initial loading dose 1 week **before the initiation** of a course of radiation therapy or on the day of initiation of platinum-based therapy with 5-FU. Complete cetuximab administration 1 hour before beginning platinum-based therapy with 5-FU.

Subsequent infusions: 250 mg/M^2 once each week for the duration of radiation therapy (6 to 7 weeks) or until disease progression or unacceptable toxicity when administered with platinum-based therapy with 5-FU. Complete infusion 1 hour before radiation therapy or platinum-based therapy with 5-FU.

Squamous cell carcinoma of the head and neck as monotherapy:
First infusion: 400 mg/M^2 as an initial loading dose. Complete infusion 1 hour before FOLFIRI (irinotecan, 5-FU, leucovorin) for both first and subsequent infusions.

Subsequent infusions: 250 mg/M^2 once each week as a maintenance dose. Continue until disease progression or unacceptable toxicity.

Colorectal cancer in combination with irinotecan, FOLFIRI, or as monotherapy: Determine K-Ras mutation and epidermal growth factor receptor (EGFR)-expression status before initiating treatment; see Indications.

First infusion: 400 mg/M^2 as an initial loading dose.

Subsequent infusions: 250 mg/M^2 once each week as a maintenance dose. Continue until disease progression or unacceptable toxicity.

DOSE ADJUSTMENTS
No dose adjustment required based on age, gender, race, or hepatic or renal function. ▪ No dose adjustment indicated for mild to moderate skin toxicity. ▪ If a mild or moderate (Grade 1 or 2) or nonserious (Grade 3) infusion reaction occurs (e.g., chills, dyspnea, fever), reduce the infusion rate by 50% for the balance of that infusion and for all further infusions. ▪ Permanently discontinue cetuximab therapy if a serious infusion reaction requiring medical intervention and/or hospitalization occurs. ▪ If a severe acneiform rash is experienced, adjust infusion schedule according to the following chart. **Dose modification is not recommended for severe radiation dermatitis.**

Cetuximab Dose Modification Guidelines for Occurrences of Severe Acneiform Rash			
Severe Acneiform Rash	Cetuximab	Outcome	Cetuximab Dose Modification
1st occurrence	Delay infusion 1 to 2 weeks	Improvement	Continue at 250 mg/M^2
		No improvement	Discontinue cetuximab
2nd occurrence	Delay infusion 1 to 2 weeks	Improvement	Reduce dose to 200 mg/M^2
		No improvement	Discontinue cetuximab
3rd occurrence	Delay infusion 1 to 2 weeks	Improvement	Reduce dose to 150 mg/M^2
		No improvement	Discontinue cetuximab
4th occurrence	Discontinue cetuximab		

DILUTION
Available in 100 mg/50 mL and 200 mg/100 mL vials (2 mg/mL). Multiple vials may be needed for each dose. May pool volume required to provide calculated dose into an empty evacuated container. Solution is clear and may contain small amounts of easily visible white particulates. *Do not shake or dilute.*

Filters: Use of a low–protein binding, 0.22-micron in-line filter is required; see Rate of Administration.

Storage: Refrigerate vials at 2° to 8° C (36° to 46° F). Do not freeze. Preparations in infusion containers are chemically and physically stable for 12 hours if refrigerated or 8 hours at CRT. Discard remaining solution in the infusion container after 8 hours at CRT. Discard any unused portion of the vial.

COMPATIBILITY
Specific information not available; however, manufacturer states, "Cetuximab should be piggybacked to the patient's infusion line." Manufacturer recommends flushing the infusion line with NS before the infusion and at the end of the infusion to ensure delivery of the entire dose.

RATE OF ADMINISTRATION
Do not administer as an IV push or bolus. Must be given as an infusion via an infusion pump or a syringe pump. Must be administered through a low–protein binding, 0.22-micron in-line filter placed as proximal to the patient as is practical and piggybacked to the patient's infusion line. Prime infusion line with cetuximab. Flush the infusion line with NS after the infusion.

First infusion: The initial loading dose should be infused evenly distributed over 2 hours (120 minutes). Do not exceed a rate of 10 mg/min (5 mL/min). In patients who have mild to moderate infusion reactions, decrease the rate of administration by 50% and continue this reduced rate for all subsequent infusions. See Dose Adjustments.

Subsequent infusions: Weekly maintenance doses should be infused evenly distributed over 1 hour (60 minutes). Do not exceed a rate of 10 mg/min (5 mL/min). In patients who have mild to moderate infusion reactions, decrease the rate of administration by 50% and continue this reduced rate for all subsequent infusions. See Dose Adjustments.

ACTIONS
An antineoplastic agent. A humanized IgG_1 monoclonal antibody produced by recombinant DNA technology. Designed to bind to the epidermal growth factor receptor (EGFR) found on the surface of both normal cells and malignant tumor cells. It interferes with the growth and survival of cancer cells by binding to tumor cells that overexpress the EGFR so that the normal (natural) EGFR cannot bind to the tumor cells and stimulate them to grow. Antitumor effects were not observed in tumor cells that did not express the EGFR. With the recommended dose regimen, cetuximab concentrations reached steady-state levels by the third weekly infusion with a mean half-life of 112 hours (range 63 to 230 hours). IgG antibodies may cross the placental barrier and may be secreted in breast milk.

INDICATIONS AND USES
Treatment of locally or regionally advanced SCCHN in combination with radiation therapy. ■ First-line treatment of patients with recurrent locoregional disease or metastatic SCCHN in combination with platinum-based therapy with 5-FU. ■ Used as a single agent for the treatment of patients with recurrent or metastatic SCCHN in whom platinum-based chemotherapy has failed. ■ Treatment of K-*Ras* wild type, epidermal growth factor receptor (EGFR)–expressing metastatic colorectal cancer (mCRC) as determined by FDA-approved tests for this use. Used in combination with FOLFIRI (irinotecan, 5-fluorouracil, leucovorin) for first-line treatment. Used in combination with irinotecan (Camptosar) in patients who are refractory to irinotecan-based chemotherapy. Used as a single agent in patients who cannot tolerate irinotecan or in those who have failed treatment with both irinotecan (Camptosar) and oxaliplatin (Eloxatin) based regimens.

Limitation of use: Not recommended for treatment of *Ras* mutant colorectal cancer or when the results of the *Ras* mutation tests are unknown.

CONTRAINDICATIONS

Manufacturer states, "None." However, a repeat dose is contraindicated in any patient who has a severe infusion reaction (Grade 3 or 4). ▪ Use with caution in patients with known hypersensitivity to murine proteins, cetuximab, or any of its components.

PRECAUTIONS

Do not administer as an IV push or bolus. Must be given as an infusion via an infusion pump or a syringe pump. ▪ Should be administered by or under the direction of the physician specialist in a facility equipped to monitor the patient and respond to any medical emergency. ▪ Severe infusion reactions and hypersensitivity reactions have occurred, and some have been fatal (less than 1 in 1,000). Most severe reactions occur with the first infusion and have occurred even with the use of prophylactic antihistamines. S/S of severe reactions may include hypotension, rapid onset of airway obstruction (e.g., bronchospasm, hoarseness, stridor), urticaria, and/or cardiac arrest. Some patients experienced their first infusion reaction during later infusions. ▪ Cardiopulmonary arrest and/or sudden death has been reported in patients with SCCHN treated with cetuximab and radiation and in patients with SCCHN treated with cetuximab and a combination of platinum-based therapy with 5-FU. Carefully consider the use of cetuximab in combination with radiation therapy or platinum-based therapy with 5-FU in patients with head and neck cancer who have a history of arrhythmias, coronary artery disease, or congestive heart failure. ▪ Pulmonary toxicity, including interstitial lung disease (ILD), has been reported. Interstitial pneumonitis with noncardiogenic pulmonary edema resulted in the death of a patient. Use caution in patients with pre-existing fibrotic lung disease. ▪ Severe dermatologic toxicities, including acneiform rash, skin drying and fissuring, and inflammatory and infectious sequelae (e.g., blepharitis [inflammation of the eyelids], cellulitis [diffuse subcutaneous inflammation of connective tissues], cheilitis [inflammation of the lip], conjunctivitis, cyst, hypertrichosis, and keratitis/ulcerative keratitis with decreased visual acuity), have occurred and may be dose limiting. Complications involving *S. aureus* sepsis and abscesses requiring incision and drainage have been reported. ▪ Safety for use in combination with radiation therapy and cisplatin has not been established. Death and serious cardiotoxicity have been seen in trials. ▪ A protein substance, it has the potential for producing immunogenicity. However, there does not appear to be a relationship between the appearance of antibodies to cetuximab and the safety or antitumor activity of the molecule. ▪ See Monitor and Antidote.

Monitor: Expression of EGFR has been detected in nearly all patients with SCCHN. Determine EGFR-expression status and the absence of a *Ras* mutation in patients with metastatic colorectal cancer (mCRC) using FDA-approved tests before initiating treatment. See prescribing information for access to FDA-approved tests. Use of cetuximab in patients with *Ras* mutant mCRC resulted in increased tumor progression, increased mortality, or lack of clinical benefit. ▪ Monitor VS frequently. ▪ Observe patient closely during every infusion and for at least 1 hour after each infusion. Infusion reactions can occur at any time, even in patients who are premedicated with diphenhydramine and/or who have not had infusion reactions with previous doses; see Precautions. S/S of Grade 1 and 2 infusion reactions include chills, fever, and dyspnea. S/S of severe reactions may include hypotension, rapid onset of airway obstruction (e.g., bronchospasm, hoarseness, stridor), loss of consciousness, MI, shock, urticaria, and/or cardiac arrest. Increase observation period for patients who experience infusion reactions. ▪ Monitor magnesium, calcium, and potassium periodically during therapy and for 8 weeks following completion. Electrolyte loss may occur from days to months after initiating cetuximab. Oral or parenteral electrolyte replacement may be indicated. ▪ Monitor for S/S of dermatologic toxicity such as acneiform rash (e.g., multiple follicular-pustular–appearing lesions on the face, upper chest, back, and extremities), skin drying, and fissuring. Dose adjustments or termination of therapy may be indicated; see Dose Adjustments and Precautions. The first onset of acneiform rash may occur within the first 2 weeks, may subside when treatment is discontinued, or may persist for longer periods. Inflammatory or infectious sequelae (e.g., blepharitis, cellulitis, cheilitis, cyst) may develop and should be treated promptly. ▪ Monitor for S/S of interstitial lung disease (e.g., dyspnea on exertion, nonproductive cough, inspiratory crackles on chest examination). Worsening symptoms may require interruption or discontinuation of cetuximab therapy. ▪ See Dose Adjustments, Rate of Administration, Precautions, and Antidote.

Patient Education: Avoid pregnancy; nonhormonal birth control recommended for both females and males during therapy and for 6 months following the last dose. See Maternal/Child. Women should report a suspected pregnancy immediately. ▪ Review potential side effects before therapy. ▪ Report any unusual or unexpected symptoms or side effects promptly, especially infusion-related reactions (e.g., dyspnea, feeling of faintness, hives, wheezing). ▪ Sunlight can worsen the skin reactions that may occur. Limit exposure to the sun, and wear sunscreen, protective clothing, and hats when outdoors. ▪ See Appendix D, p. 1333.

Maternal/Child: Category C: has the potential to be transferred from the mother to the developing fetus; avoid pregnancy. Use during pregnancy or in any woman not using adequate contraception methods only if benefit justifies the potential risk to the fetus. ▪ Discontinue breast-feeding during treatment with cetuximab and for 60 days following the last dose. ▪ Safety and effectiveness for use in pediatric patients not established.

Elderly: Safety and effectiveness similar to younger adults.

DRUG/LAB INTERACTIONS

No evidence of pharmacokinetic interactions between cetuximab and irinotecan. ▪ No other drug interaction studies have been completed. ▪ The safety of combination use with **cisplatin** has not been established. Death and serious cardiotoxicity have been observed when **cetuximab, cisplatin, and radiation therapy** have been used concomitantly.

SIDE EFFECTS

The most common side effects are cutaneous adverse reactions (e.g., nail changes, pruritus, rash), diarrhea, headache, and infection. The most serious side effects are cardiopulmonary arrest, dermatologic toxicity, infusion reactions, interstitial lung disease, pulmonary embolus, radiation dermatitis, renal failure, and sepsis.

SCCHN: Confusion; dehydration; diarrhea; dry mouth; elevated ALT, AST, and alkaline phosphatase; mucositis/stomatitis/pharyngitis; and radiation dermatitis/toxicities occurred with more frequency in this group and were considered serious.

Colorectal cancer: Dehydration, diarrhea, fatigue, fever, kidney failure, neutropenia, pulmonary embolus, rash, and sepsis occurred with more frequency in this group and were considered serious.

All diagnoses: Acneiform rash, asthenia, chills, constipation, dysphagia, electrolyte abnormalities (e.g., hypocalcemia, hypokalemia, hypomagnesemia), fever, malaise, nausea and vomiting, and weight loss occur frequently. Other side effects reported include alopecia, anemia, anorexia, back pain, conjunctivitis, cough (increased), depression, dyspepsia, dyspnea, headache, insomnia, leukopenia, nail disorders (paronychial inflammation of the toes and fingers), pain, peripheral edema, pruritus, skin disorders, stomatitis.

Post-Marketing: Aseptic meningitis, Stevens-Johnson syndrome, toxic epidermal necrolysis, life-threatening and fatal bullous mucocutaneous disease.

ANTIDOTE

Keep physician informed of all side effects. May constitute a medical emergency or will be treated symptomatically as indicated. Hypersensitivity or infusion-related side effects may resolve with reduction in the rate of infusion by 50% and by continued use of premedication with diphenhydramine (Benadryl). Discontinue cetuximab immediately for severe infusion reactions; *do not rechallenge.* Treat hypersensitivity or infusion reactions as indicated; may require use of epinephrine, corticosteroids, diphenhydramine, bronchodilators (e.g., albuterol, aminophylline), IV saline, oxygen, and/or acetaminophen. Dermatologic toxicities may be dose limiting (see Dose Adjustments) or may be treated with topical and/or oral antibiotics as appropriate. Use of topical corticosteroids is not recommended. Interrupt cetuximab with the onset of acute or worsening pulmonary symptoms. Treat as indicated; permanently discontinue cetuximab for confirmed interstitial lung disease. Replace electrolytes as indicated. Resuscitate if indicated.

CHLORAMPHENICOL SODIUM SUCCINATE BBW
Antibacterial

(klor-am-**FEN**-ih-kohl **SO**-dee-um **SUK**-suh-nayt)

Chloromycetin
pH 6.4 to 7

USUAL DOSE
For all age levels, determine baseline blood studies before administration. Avoid repeated courses of this drug if at all possible. Treatment should not be continued longer than the time required to produce a cure with little or no risk of relapse of disease.

Adults and pediatric patients with mature metabolic processes (e.g., normal kidney and liver function): 12.5 mg/kg every 6 hours. In exceptional cases, infections due to moderately resistant organisms may require up to 25 mg/kg every 6 hours. Severe infections (e.g., bacteremia or meningitis), especially when adequate cerebrospinal fluid concentrations are desired, may require up to 25 mg/kg every 6 hours. These increased doses must be reduced to 12.5 mg/kg every 6 hours as soon as possible. Maximum dose is 4 Gm/24 hr for all ages. Change to oral form as soon as practical.

NEONATAL DOSE
When kidney or liver function is immature in infants (or seriously impaired in adults), high concentrations of chloromycetin are found and tend to increase with succeeding doses. See Maternal/Child.

Infants under 2 weeks of age or older infants with immature metabolic processes (e.g., premature infants): 6.25 mg/kg every 6 hours. Increased doses demanded by severe infections should be given only to maintain the blood concentration within a therapeutically effective range. Close monitoring of blood concentrations by microtechniques is recommended (information available from manufacturer).

Infants 2 weeks of age or older with mature metabolic processes: 12.5 mg/kg every 6 hours may ordinarily be administered. See comments under Usual Dose.

Another source suggests a *loading dose* followed by *maintenance doses* based on age and weight.

Loading dose: 20 mg/kg.

Maintenance dose: Administer the first maintenance dose 12 hours after the loading dose.

7 days of age or younger and over 7 days of age if weight is 2 kg or less: 25 mg/kg of body weight once daily.

Over 7 days of age and over 2 kg: 25 mg/kg every 12 hours.

DOSE ADJUSTMENTS
Reduce dose and/or initiate oral therapy as soon as feasible. ▪ Reduce dose and/or extend intervals in infants and children with immature metabolic processes. See specific dose recommendations. Close monitoring of blood concentrations by microtechniques is recommended. ▪ In patients with immature or impaired hepatic or renal function, dose reduction may be required. ▪ Dosing should be cautious in the elderly. Consider decreased organ function and concomitant disease or drug therapy.

DILUTION
Each 1 Gm should be reconstituted with 10 mL of SWFI or D5W to prepare a 10% solution (100 mg/mL). May be further diluted in 50 to 100 mL of D5W for intermittent infusion. Give through Y-tube, three-way stopcock, or additive infusion set.

Storage: Store at CRT. Administer within 24 hours of preparation.

COMPATIBILITY
(Underline Indicates Conflicting Compatibility Information)

Consider any drug NOT listed as compatible to be INCOMPATIBLE until consulting a pharmacist; specific conditions may apply.

One source suggests the following **compatibilities:**

Solution: Most common infusion solutions.

Additive: Amikacin, aminophylline, ascorbic acid, calcium chloride, calcium gluconate, colistimethate (Coly-Mycin M), dimenhydrinate, dopamine, ephedrine, fat emulsion IV, heparin, hydrocortisone sodium succinate (Solu-Cortef), lidocaine, lincomycin (Linco-cin), magnesium sulfate, methyldopate, methylprednisolone (Solu-Medrol), nafcillin (Nallpen), oxacillin (Bactocill), oxytocin (Pitocin), penicillin G potassium and sodium, pentobarbital (Nembutal), phenylephrine (Neo-Synephrine), phytonadione (vitamin K_1), potassium chloride (KCl), ranitidine (Zantac), sodium bicarbonate, verapamil.

Y-site: Acyclovir (Zovirax), cyclophosphamide (Cytoxan), enalaprilat (Vasotec IV), es-molol (Brevibloc), foscarnet (Foscavir), hydromorphone (Dilaudid), labetalol, magne-sium sulfate, meperidine (Demerol), morphine, nicardipine (Cardene IV), tacrolimus (Prograf).

RATE OF ADMINISTRATION

IV injection: 1 Gm or fraction thereof over a minimum of 1 minute.

Intermittent infusion: A single dose over 10 to 30 minutes.

ACTIONS

Effective against a wide range of gram-positive and gram-negative bacteria. Primarily bacteriostatic. May be bactericidal at high concentrations or against highly susceptible organisms. Acts by inhibiting protein synthesis. Well distributed in therapeutic doses throughout the body, especially in the liver and kidneys. Lowest concentrations are found in the brain and spinal fluid; however, chloramphenicol enters cerebrospinal fluid even in the absence of meningeal inflammation, appearing in concentrations about half of those found in the blood. Partially metabolized. Excreted in urine, bile, and feces. Crosses the placental barrier. Secreted in breast milk.

INDICATIONS AND USES

Only in serious infections in which potentially less dangerous drugs are ineffective or contraindicated; acute *Salmonella typhi* infections, meningeal infections (e.g., *Haemophilus influenzae*), bacteremia, rickettsia, lymphogranuloma psittacosis, and other serious gram-negative infections. ▪ Cystic fibrosis regimens.

CONTRAINDICATIONS

Known chloramphenicol sensitivity. Must not be used in the treatment of trivial infec-tions.

PRECAUTIONS

Serious blood dyscrasias (e.g., aplastic anemia, hypoplastic anemia, thrombocytopenia, and granulocy-topenia) resulting in irreversible bone marrow suppression and death are known to occur. Aplastic anemia resulting in leukemia has been reported. Blood dyscrasias have occurred after both short-term and longer-term therapy. Do not use if potentially less dangerous agents would be effective. ▪ Admin-istration in a hospital with facilities for monitoring the patient and responding to any medical emergency is preferred. ▪ Sensitivity studies mandatory to determine susceptibility of the causative organism not only to chloramphenicol but also to other less dangerous drugs. ▪ Super-infection caused by overgrowth of nonsusceptible organisms, including fungi, is possi-ble. Treatment should not be continued longer than required to produce a cure with little or no risk of relapse of the disease. ▪ For IV use only. ▪ A reversible type of bone marrow suppression characterized by vacuolization of the erythroid cells, reduction of reticulocytes, and leukopenia is dose related and usually responds to withdrawal of chlor-amphenicol. ▪ *Clostridium difficile*–associated diarrhea (CDAD) has been reported. May range from mild diarrhea to fatal colitis. Consider in patients who present with diar-rhea during or after treatment with chloramphenicol. ▪ Use caution in patients with impaired hepatic and/or renal function.

Monitor: Obtain blood studies (CBC) before initiating therapy and approximately every 2 days during therapy; discontinue drug if blood studies show any indication of anemia, leukopenia, reticulocytopenia, thrombocytopenia, or any blood study findings attributable to chlor-amphenicol. ▪ Monitor chloramphenicol serum levels at least weekly, and more often if indicated (e.g., impaired liver or kidney function, immature metabolic processes, suspi-cion of beginning blood dyscrasias). ▪ Therapeutic levels range between 15 and 25 mcg/mL for meningitis; 10 and 20 mcg/mL for other infections. Trough levels should range between 5 and 15 mcg/mL for meningitis; 5 and 10 mcg/mL for other infections. ▪ Monitor hepatic and renal function as indicated; see Dose Adjustments. ▪ See Drug/Lab Interactions.

Patient Education: Promptly report fever, sore throat, tiredness, unusual bleeding, or bruising. ▪ Promptly report diarrhea or bloody stools that occur during treatment or up to several months after an antibiotic has been discontinued; may indicate CDAD and require treatment.

Maternal/Child: Category C: no studies documented. Use during pregnancy with extreme caution; may have toxic effects on fetus. ▪ Discontinue breast-feeding. ▪ Blood concentration in all premature and full-term neonates under 2 weeks of age differs from that of other neonates. Use caution, lower doses, and/or extended intervals in premature infants and newborns. May cause gray syndrome (e.g., abdominal distension with or without emesis, progressive pallid cyanosis, vasomotor collapse, irregular respiration, death within a few hours of onset of symptoms); monitor serum levels; see Precautions/Monitor.

Elderly: See Dose Adjustments. ▪ Response similar to that seen in younger patients. ▪ Monitor renal function.

DRUG/LAB INTERACTIONS

May cause irreversible bone marrow suppression. Avoid concurrent therapy with **drugs that cause blood dyscrasias** (e.g., penicillins, hydantoins [phenytoin (Dilantin)]), **other bone marrow suppressants** (e.g., cytotoxic drugs, radiation therapy). ▪ Increases serum levels of **oral antidiabetics** (e.g., chlorpropamide [Diabinase]) and increases hypoglycemic effects; dose reduction may be required. ▪ May be synergistic with or antagonize effects of **aminoglycosides, cephalosporins, and penicillins.** (Is used with ampicillin in pediatric patients.) ▪ Chloramphenicol can inhibit specific P_{450} enzymes; reduced metabolism and increased serum levels may occur in agents also metabolized by that route (e.g., **chlorpropamide** [Diabinese], **phenobarbital, phenytoin** [Dilantin], **tolbutamide, warfarin** [Coumadin]). ▪ Concurrent use with **hydantoins** (e.g., phenytoin [Dilantin]) may decrease or increase the effectiveness of chloramphenicol. Hydantoin levels may be increased, resulting in toxicity. ▪ Concurrent use with **phenobarbital** may decrease chloramphenicol serum levels and increase phenobarbital serum levels, resulting in phenobarbital toxicity. Monitor serum levels of both drugs if concurrent use is indicated. ▪ Concurrent administration with **anticoagulants** (e.g., heparin, warfarin [Coumadin]) may prolong PT. ▪ May increase **serum iron** levels. ▪ May delay response to **antianemia drugs** (e.g., iron preparations, vitamin B_{12}, folic acid). Avoid concurrent use in patients with anemia if possible. ▪ **Rifampin** increases chloramphenicol metabolism and decreases its effects.

SIDE EFFECTS

Blood dyscrasias (e.g., aplastic anemia, hypoplastic anemia, granulocytopenia, thrombocytopenia) may result in irreversible bone marrow suppression and death. CDAD, confusion, depression, diarrhea, fever, gray syndrome of newborns and infants, headache, hypersensitivity reactions (e.g., angioedema, anaphylaxis, fever, rashes, urticaria), leukemia, nausea, optic and peripheral neuritis, paroxysmal nocturnal hemoglobinuria, pseudomembranous colitis, rashes, stomatitis, vomiting, and many others. *May be fatal.*

ANTIDOTE

Notify the physician immediately of any adverse symptoms. Discontinue the drug upon appearance of anemia, leukopenia, reticulocytopenia, thrombocytopenia, or any other blood study findings attributable to chloramphenicol. Discontinue the drug for symptoms of optic and peripheral neuritis. Monitoring of plasma levels is imperative in all patients and especially in neonates. Treat hypersensitivity reactions as indicated. Treat CDAD with fluids, electrolytes, protein supplements, and oral vancomycin (Vancocin) or metronidazole (Flagyl) as indicated. In severe cases, surgical evaluation may be indicated. Resuscitate as necessary.

CHLORPROMAZINE HYDROCHLORIDE BBW

(klor-**PROH**-mah-zeen hy-droh-**KLOR**-eyed)

Phenothiazine
Antipsychotic
Antiemetic

Thorazine

pH 3 to 5

USUAL DOSE

Use of the IV route is reserved for the treatment of acute nausea and vomiting in surgery, intractable hiccups, and tetanus.

Acute nausea and vomiting in surgery: 2 mg. May repeat at 2-minute intervals as indicated. Do not exceed 25 mg. Usually given as an infusion.

Intractable hiccups: 25 to 50 mg diluted in 500 to 1,000 mL of NS. Given as a slow IV infusion with patient flat in bed. Monitor BP closely.

Tetanus: 25 to 50 mg as an infusion of at least 1 mg/mL. Individualize dose to patient response and tolerance. Repeat every 6 to 8 hours. Usually given in conjunction with barbiturates.

PEDIATRIC DOSE

See Maternal/Child. IV route rarely used for pediatric patients. Not recommended for use in infants less than 6 months of age.

Acute nausea and vomiting in surgery, pediatric patients 6 months of age or older: 1 mg. May repeat at 2-minute intervals as indicated. Monitor for hypotension. Another source suggests 2.5 to 4 mg/kg/24 hr in equally divided doses every 6 to 8 hours (0.625 to 1 mg/kg every 6 hours or 0.83 to 1.33 mg/kg every 8 hours). Usual IV/IM dose does not exceed 2.5 to 4 mg/kg/24 hr or 40 mg/24 hr (whichever is less) in pediatric patients 6 months to 5 years of age or up to 50 lb, and 75 mg/24 hr in pediatric patients 5 to 12 years of age.

Tetanus: 0.55 mg/kg of body weight (0.25 mg/lb) every 6 to 8 hours. Do not exceed 40 mg/24 hr for up to 23 kg (50 lb) and 75 mg/24 hr for up to 50 kg (50 to 100 lb), except in severe cases.

DOSE ADJUSTMENTS

Adjust dose to the individual and severity of condition. Reduce dose of any medication potentiated by phenothiazines by one fourth to one half. See Drug/Lab Interactions. ▪ Reduce dose by one fourth to one half in the elderly, debilitated patients, or emaciated patients, and increase very gradually by response.

DILUTION

Each 25 mg (1 mL) must be diluted with 24 mL of NS for injection. 1 mL will equal 1 mg. May be further diluted in 500 to 1,000 mL of NS and given as an infusion. Handle carefully; may cause contact dermatitis. Sensitive to light. Slightly yellow color does not alter potency. Discard if markedly discolored.

Storage: Store at CRT. Protect from light and freezing.

COMPATIBILITY

(Underline Indicates Conflicting Compatibility Information)

Consider any drug NOT listed as compatible to be INCOMPATIBLE until consulting a pharmacist; specific conditions may apply.

One source suggests the following **compatibilities**:

Additive: Ascorbic acid, ethacrynic acid (Edecrin), theophylline.

Y-site: Cisatracurium (Nimbex), cladribine (Leustatin), dexmedetomidine (Precedex), docetaxel (Taxotere), doxorubicin liposomal (Doxil), famotidine (Pepcid IV), fenoldopam (Corlopam), filgrastim (Neupogen), fluconazole (Diflucan), gemcitabine (Gemzar), granisetron (Kytril), heparin, hetastarch in electrolytes (Hextend), hydrocortisone sodium succinate (Solu-Cortef), ondansetron (Zofran), oxaliplatin (Eloxatin), potassium chloride (KCl), propofol (Diprivan), remifentanil (Ultiva), teniposide (Vumon), thiotepa, vinorelbine (Navelbine).

RATE OF ADMINISTRATION

Titrate to symptoms and vital signs. See Precautions.

IV injection: Each 1 mg or fraction thereof over 1 minute.

Infusion: Given very slowly. Do not exceed 1 mg/min.

Pediatric rate: Do not exceed 1 mg or fraction thereof over 2 minutes.

ACTIONS

A phenothiazine derivative with effects on the central, autonomic, and peripheral nervous systems. A psychotropic agent. Decreases anxiety and tension, relaxes muscles, produces sedation, and tranquilizes. Has an antiemetic effect and potentiates CNS depressants. Has strong antiadrenergic and anticholinergic activity. Also possesses slight antihistaminic and antiserotonin activity. Onset of action is prompt and of short duration in small IV doses. Extensively metabolized in liver and kidney and excreted primarily in urine. Crosses the placental barrier. Secreted in breast milk.

INDICATIONS AND USES

The IV route is used only for the treatment of acute nausea and vomiting in surgery, the treatment of intractable hiccups, and as an adjunct in the treatment of tetanus. ▪ Used IM or PO for the treatment of schizophrenia and the management of psychotic disorders. ▪ Also indicated IM, PO, or rectally to relieve restlessness and apprehension before surgery, to manage acute intermittent porphyria, to control manic episodes in manic-depressive illness, and to treat severe behavioral problems in pediatric patients.

Unlabeled uses: Treatment of phencyclidine (PCP) psychosis. ▪ Treatment of migraine headaches (IV or IM). ▪ To reduce choreiform movements of Huntington's disease.

CONTRAINDICATIONS

Hypersensitivity to phenothiazines, comatose or severely depressed states, or the presence of large amounts of CNS depressants (e.g., alcohol, barbiturates, narcotics).

PRECAUTIONS

Not approved for dementia-related psychosis; mortality risk in elderly dementia patients taking conventional or atypical antipsychotics is increased; most deaths are due to cardiovascular or infectious events. ▪ Use of the IV route is reserved for the treatment of acute nausea and vomiting in surgery, intractable hiccups, and tetanus. IM injection preferred. ▪ Use caution in patients with bone marrow suppression; glaucoma; cardiovascular, liver, renal, and chronic respiratory diseases; and acute respiratory diseases of pediatric patients. ▪ Reexposure of patients who have experienced jaundice, skin reactions, or blood dyscrasias with a phenothiazine is not recommended. Cross-sensitivity may occur. ▪ May produce ECG changes (e.g., prolonged QT interval, changes in T waves). ▪ Use with caution in patients with a history of seizure disorders; may lower seizure threshold. ▪ Extrapyramidal symptoms caused by chlorpromazine may be confused with CNS signs of an undiagnosed disease (e.g., Reye's syndrome or encephalopathy). ▪ May mask diagnosis of brain tumor, drug intoxication, and intestinal obstruction. ▪ Tardive dyskinesia (potentially irreversible involuntary dyskinetic movements) may develop. Use smallest doses and shortest duration of therapy to minimize risk. ▪ Neuroleptic malignant syndrome (NMS) characterized by hyperpyrexia, muscle rigidity, altered mental status, and autonomic instability has been reported; see Antidote. ▪ May cause paradoxical excitation in pediatric patients and the elderly. ▪ Use phenothiazines with extreme caution in pediatric patients with a history of sleep apnea, a family history of SIDS, or in the presence of Reye's syndrome. ▪ May contain sulfites; use caution in patients with asthma. ▪ Taper dose gradually following high dose or extended therapy to prevent possible occurrence of withdrawal symptoms (e.g., dizziness, gastritis, nausea, tremors, and vomiting).

Monitor: Keep patient in supine position throughout treatment and for at least $^1/_2$ hour after treatment. Ambulate slowly and carefully; may cause postural hypotension. ▪ Monitor BP and pulse before and during administration and between doses. ▪ Cough reflex is often depressed; monitor closely if nauseated or vomiting to prevent aspiration. ▪ Anticholinergic and cardiac effects may be troublesome during anesthesia. For patients receiving phenothiazines, taper and discontinue preoperatively if they will not be continued after surgery. ▪ May discolor urine pink to reddish brown. ▪ Photosensitivity of skin is possible. ▪ See Drug/Lab Interactions.

Patient Education: Request assistance for ambulation; may cause dizziness or fainting. ▪ Observe caution when performing tasks that require alertness. ▪ Avoid use of alcohol and other CNS depressants (e.g., diazepam [Valium], narcotics). ▪ Possible eye and skin photosensitivity. Avoid unprotected exposure to sun. ▪ Urine may discolor to pink or reddish brown.

Maternal/Child: See Precautions and Contraindications. ▪ Category C: use during pregnancy only when clearly needed. Use near term may cause maternal hypotension and adverse neonatal effects (e.g., extrapyramidal syndrome, hyperreflexia, hyporeflexia, jaundice). ▪ Fetuses and infants have a reduced capacity to metabolize and eliminate; may cause embryo toxicity, increase neonatal mortality, or cause permanent neurologic damage. May contain benzyl alcohol; use not recommended in neonates. ▪ Not recommended during breast-feeding. Increases risk of dystonia and tardive dyskinesia. ▪ Children metabolize antipsychotic agents more rapidly than adults and are at increased risk to develop extrapyramidal actions, especially during acute illness (e.g., chickenpox, CNS infections, dehydration, gastroenteritis, measles); monitor closely.

Elderly: See Dose Adjustments and Precautions. ▪ Have a reduced capacity to metabolize and eliminate. May have increased sensitivity to postural hypotension, anticholinergic and sedative effects. ▪ Increased risk of extrapyramidal side effects (e.g., tardive dyskinesia, parkinsonism).

DRUG/LAB INTERACTIONS

Use with **epinephrine** not recommended; may cause precipitous hypotension. ▪ Use with **agents that produce hypotension** (e.g., antihypertensives, benzodiazepines, diuretics, lidocaine, paclitaxel) may produce severe hypotension. ▪ Increased CNS, respiratory depression, and hypotensive effects with **CNS depressants** (e.g., narcotics, alcohol, anesthetics, and barbiturates); reduced doses of these agents usually indicated. ▪ Chlorpromazine does not potentiate the anticonvulsant actions of **barbiturates.** Doses of **anticonvulsant barbiturates** should not be decreased if chlorpromazine is introduced. Instead begin chlorpromazine at a lower dose and titrate to effect. ▪ Chlorpromazine may lower the seizure threshold. It may also interfere with **phenytoin and valproic acid** clearance, increasing potential for toxicity. Dose adjustment of anticonvulsants may be necessary. ▪ Additive effects with **MAO inhibitors** (e.g., selegiline [Eldepryl]), **anticholinergics, antihistamines, antihypertensives, hypnotics, muscle relaxants, rauwolfia alkaloids, and thiazide diuretics;** dose adjustment may be necessary. ▪ **Barbiturates** may also increase metabolism of chlorpromazine and reduce its effects. ▪ Risk of cardiotoxicity increased with **pimozide** (Orap) **and sparfloxacin** (Zagam); concurrent use not recommended. ▪ Risk of additive QT interval prolongation, cardiac depressant effects, and cardiac arrhythmias increased with **cisapride** (Propulsid), **disopyramide** (Norpace), **erythromycin, probucol** (Lorelco), **procainamide** (Pronestyl), **and quinidine.** ▪ Concurrent use with **antidepressants** (e.g., fluoxetine [Prozac], paroxetine [Paxil]), **tricyclic antidepressants** (e.g., amitriptyline [Elavil], imipramine [Tofranil]), **or MAO inhibitors** (e.g., selegiline [Eldepryl]) may increase effects of both drugs; risk of NMS may be increased. ▪ Use with **antithyroid drugs** may increase risk of agranulocytosis. ▪ May inhibit antiparkinson effects of **levodopa.** ▪ May decrease pressor response to **ephedrine.** ▪ May increase anticholinergic effect of **orphenadrine** (Norflex). ▪ May decrease effects of **oral anticoagulants.** ▪ Concurrent use with **haloperidol, droperidol, or metoclopramide** may cause increased extrapyramidal effects. ▪ Use with **metrizamide** (Amipaque) may lower seizure threshold; discontinue chlorpromazine 48 hours before myelography and do not resume for 24 hours after test is completed. ▪ Metabolism and clearance of chlorpromazine is increased in cigarette **smokers;** decreased plasma levels and effectiveness may occur; dose adjustment of chlorpromazine may be indicated. ▪ Decreased drowsiness may occur in cigarette **smokers.** May be offset by increased doses of chlorpromazine. ▪ Use caution during anesthesia with **barbiturates** (e.g., methohexital, thiopental); may increase frequency and severity of hypotension and neuromuscular excitation. ▪ Encephalopathic syndrome has been reported with concurrent use of **lithium;** monitor for S/S of neurologic toxicity. ▪ Capable of innumerable other interactions. ▪ May cause false-positive **pregnancy test** and false-positive **amylase, PKU, and other urine tests.**

SIDE EFFECTS
Usually transient if drug is discontinued, but may require treatment if severe. Anaphylaxis, cardiac arrest, distorted Q and T waves, drowsiness, excitement, extrapyramidal symptoms (e.g., abnormal positioning, extreme restlessness, pseudoparkinsonism, weakness of extremities), fever, hematologic toxicities (e.g., agranulocytosis, aplastic anemia, leukopenia, thrombocytopenia), hypersensitivity reactions, hypertension, hypotension (occurs less frequently in smokers), melanosis, photosensitivity, tachycardia, tardive dyskinesia, and many others.

Overdose: Can cause convulsions, hallucinations, and death.

ANTIDOTE
Discontinue the drug at onset of any side effect and notify the physician. Discontinue chlorpromazine and all drugs not essential to concurrent therapy immediately if NMS occurs. Will require intensive symptomatic treatment, medical monitoring, and management of concomitant medical problems. Counteract hypotension with norepinephrine (Levophed) or phenylephrine (Neo-Synephrine) and IV fluids. Counteract extrapyramidal symptoms with benztropine (Cogentin) or diphenhydramine (Benadryl). Use diazepam (Valium) followed by phenytoin (Dilantin) for convulsions or hyperactivity. Maintain a clear airway and adequate hydration. Epinephrine is contraindicated for hypotension; further hypotension will occur. Phenytoin may be helpful in ventricular arrhythmias. Avoid analeptics such as caffeine and sodium benzoate in treating respiratory depression and unconsciousness; they may cause convulsions. Resuscitate as necessary. Not removed by dialysis.

CIDOFOVIR INJECTION BBW

(sih-**DOF**-oh-veer in-**JEK**-shun)

Vistide

Antiviral
(nucleotide analog)

pH 6.7 to 7.6

USUAL DOSE
Preliminary lab work required before each dose; see Monitor.

A specific protocol is required; see the following chart. A 4-Gm course of oral probenecid is required on the day of each infusion of cidofovir to reduce the risk of renal impairment. Hydration with 1 to 2 liters of NS is required to help reduce proteinuria and prevent increases in SCr. Infrequent dosing schedule may eliminate need for an indwelling IV catheter, reducing discomfort and potential for infection.

Induction: 5 mg/kg in 100 mL NS once weekly for 2 consecutive weeks.

Maintenance: 5 mg/kg in 100 mL NS once every other week.

Overview of the Treatment Regimen for Cidofovir		
Before Cidofovir Infusion	**During Cidofovir Infusion**	**After Cidofovir Infusion**
1. Patient takes 2 Gm of proben-ecid* (4 × 500 mg tablets) 3 hours before cidofovir infusion	1. Begin IV infusion of cidofo-vir (5 mg/kg body weight in 100 mL NS) at a con-stant rate over 1 hour)†	1. Patient takes 1 Gm of proben-ecid (2 × 500 mg tablets) 2 hours after the *end* of ci-dofovir infusion
2. Infuse first liter of NS over 1 to 2 hours immediately before starting cidofovir infusion	2. For patients who can tolerate the extra fluid load, infuse a second liter of NS. If ad-ministered, initiate either at the start of the cidofovir infusion or immediately afterward, and infuse over a 1- to 3-hour period	2. Patient takes 1 Gm of proben-ecid (2 × 500 mg tablets) 8 hours after the *end* of ci-dofovir infusion

*Patients receiving concomitant probenecid and zidovudine should temporarily discontinue zidovudine or decrease the zid-ovudine dose by 50% on days of combined zidovudine and probenecid administration.
†The recommended dosage, frequency, or infusion rate must not be exceeded.

DOSE ADJUSTMENTS
Reduce dose to 3 mg/kg for the remainder of therapy, if SCr increases by 0.3 to 0.4 mg/dL above baseline. ■ 5 mg/kg may be given to patients who develop a 2^+ pro-teinuria but have a stable SCr. Encourage oral hydration; additional IV hydration may be appropriate. ■ Discontinue cidofovir if the SCr increases by 0.5 mg/dL or more above baseline or if proteinuria 3^+ or more develops. ■ Restarting cidofovir in patients whose renal function has returned to baseline after a SCr elevation of more than 0.5 mg/dL is not recommended. ■ Discontinue cidofovir in any patient who requires therapy with a nephrotoxic agent; see Contraindications. Cidofovir may be restarted after other nephro-toxic therapy is complete, an adequate washout period of at least 7 days has passed, and adequate renal function (SCr less than 1.5 mg/dL) is confirmed.

DILUTION
Specific techniques required; see Precautions. A calculated dose must be diluted in 100 mL of NS.

Storage: Store unopened vials at CRT. May be refrigerated but must be used within 24 hours of dilution with NS. Allow to return to room temperature before administration. Discard partially used vials.

COMPATIBILITY
Manufacturer states, "**Compatibility** with Ringer's solution, LR, or bacteriostatic IV fluids not evaluated; no data available to support the addition of other drugs or supplements for concurrent administration."

RATE OF ADMINISTRATION
A single dose as an infusion at a constant rate over 1 hour. Use of an infusion pump is recommended.

ACTIONS
A nucleotide analog antiviral. Its active intracellular metabolite selectively inhibits CMV DNA synthesis. It is incorporated into the growing viral DNA chain, resulting in reduc-tions in the rate of viral DNA synthesis. This action is independent of virus infection (acyclovir or ganciclovir require activation by a virally encoded enzyme). Elimination half-life is short (2.6 hours), but it has a long intracellular half-life, which permits infre-quent dosing. Primarily excreted in urine (70% to 85% in 24 hours with concomitant doses of probenecid).

INDICATIONS AND USES
Treatment of newly diagnosed or relapsing CMV retinitis in patients with AIDS is the only approved indication.

CONTRAINDICATIONS

Pre-existing renal dysfunction (e.g., baseline SCr more than 1.5 mg/dL, calculated CrCl equal to or less than 55 mL/min, or a urine protein equal to or greater than 100 mg/dL [equivalent to a 2^+ or more proteinuria]). ▪ Patients receiving agents with nephrotoxic potential (e.g., aminoglycosides, amphotericin B, foscarnet [Foscavir], NSAIDs [ibuprofen (Advil, Motrin), naproxen (Aleve, Naprosyn)], IV pentamidine, vancomycin). No other nephrotoxic agent should be administered within 7 days of starting cidofovir or concomitantly during cidofovir therapy. ▪ Hypersensitivity to cidofovir and/or a history of clinically severe hypersensitivity (e.g., hypotension, respiratory distress) to probenecid or other sulfa-containing medications (e.g., sulfamethoxazole/trimethoprim).

PRECAUTIONS

Follow guidelines for handling cytotoxic agents. See Appendix A, p. 1331. ▪ Administered by or under the direction of the physician specialist, preferably in an environment where emergency treatment is available. ▪ This formulation is for IV use only; **DO NOT** use for intraocular injection. ▪ Safety and effectiveness have not been established for treatment of other CMV infections (e.g., pneumonitis, gastroenteritis, congenital or neonatal CMV disease) or for CMV disease in non–HIV-infected individuals. ▪ Calculated CrCl may not accurately estimate renal function in emaciated (e.g., patients with AIDS) or extremely muscular patients; a 24-hour urine collection may be required. ▪ CMV resistant to ganciclovir may also be resistant to cidofovir, but may be sensitive to foscarnet (Foscavir). ▪ CMV resistant to foscarnet (Foscavir) may be sensitive to cidofovir. ▪ Nephrotoxicity is dose limiting and is the major toxicity of cidofovir. Do not exceed recommended dose, frequency, or rate of administration; may cause increased risk of renal toxicity. Acute renal failure requiring dialysis or contributing to death has occurred with as few as 1 or 2 doses of cidofovir. ▪ Renal function may not return to baseline after treatment with cidofovir. ▪ Proteinuria is an early indicator of nephrotoxicity; continued administration of cidofovir may lead to additional proximal tubular cell injury resulting in glycosuria, decreased serum phosphate, uric acid, and bicarbonate; increased SCr; and/or acute renal failure, which may necessitate dialysis. ▪ May cause granulocytopenia (e.g., neutropenia). ▪ Although some reference sources have published doses for patients with impaired renal function, this drug is contraindicated in such patients and should be given only to those who meet specific dosing criteria; see Contraindications.

Monitor: 24 to 48 hours before each cidofovir infusion, obtain SCr, urine protein (via dipstick or quantitative urinalysis), and CBC with differential (absolute neutrophil count [ANC]). Repeat between doses if indicated. ▪ Administration of probenecid as ordered and adequate hydration (oral and IV) are imperative. ▪ Antiretroviral therapy may be continued with the exception of zidovudine; see Drug/Lab Interactions. ▪ Probenecid frequently causes fever, flushing, headache, nausea with or without emesis, and rash. Use acetaminophen for prophylaxis or treatment of fever or headache. Encourage ingestion of food before each dose of probenecid to reduce nausea; prophylactic antiemetics (e.g., ondansetron [Zofran]) are appropriate. Consider use of antihistamines (e.g., diphenhydramine [Benadryl]) for prophylaxis or treatment in patients who develop mild hypersensitivity reactions (e.g., rash). Severe hypersensitivity reactions (e.g., laryngospasm, hypotension) have occasionally been reported with probenecid. Usually occur within several hours after patients have received probenecid even though they have received it before with no adverse reactions. Observe patient carefully for hypersensitivity reactions. Treatment for anaphylaxis (e.g., epinephrine, corticosteroids, and antihistamines) must be readily available. ▪ Monitor intraocular pressure, visual acuity, and ocular symptoms with a baseline ophthalmologic exam and periodically during therapy. Uveitis or iritis has been reported; may be treated with topical steroids. Risk of increased intraocular pressure and other visual problems may be increased in patients with pre-existing diabetes mellitus. ▪ Use of the Cockcroft-Gault formula is recommended if a precise estimate of CrCl measurement is indicated.

Patient Education: Not a cure for CMV retinitis. Retinitis may recur during maintenance or after treatment; regular ophthalmologic exams imperative. ▪ Full compliance with regimen imperative (e.g., probenecid with food, increased IV and oral hydration, regular lab testing). ▪ Report diarrhea, eye pain or change in vision, fever, headache, loss of appetite, rash, nausea, and vomiting promptly. ▪ Report concomitant medication changes or additions. ▪ Notify all health care personnel of treatment with probenecid to avoid interactions. ▪ Consider birth control options; see Precautions/Maternal/Child.

Maternal/Child: Category C: should not be used during pregnancy; embryotoxic in animals. A potential carcinogen; knowledge of effects on women unknown. ▪ Women of childbearing age should use effective contraception during cidofovir therapy and for 1 month after completion. ▪ Men should use barrier contraception during cidofovir therapy and for 3 months after completion. ▪ Has caused reduced testicular weight and hypospermia in animals. ▪ Do not administer to nursing mothers. HIV-infected mothers are advised not to breast-feed to avoid transmission to an uninfected child. ▪ Safety and effectiveness for use in pediatric patients not established. Use in pediatric patients with extreme caution and only if the benefits of treatment outweigh the risks of long-term carcinogenicity and reproductive toxicity. Consult physician specialist for adjustments in probenecid and hydration.

Elderly: Effects have not been studied; monitor renal function carefully.

DRUG/LAB INTERACTIONS

Limited information available. Drug profile review by pharmacist imperative. ▪ Nephrotoxicity increased by other **nephrotoxic agents** (e.g., aminoglycosides [e.g., amikacin, gentamicin], amphotericin B [conventional, Abelcet], foscarnet [Foscavir], IV pentamidine, NSAIDs [e.g., ibuprofen (Motrin)], vancomycin); see Contraindications. ▪ Prior treatment with **foscarnet** (Foscavir) may also increase the risk of nephrotoxicity; monitor renal function carefully. ▪ **Probenecid** decreases clearance of zidovudine; temporarily discontinue or reduce dose of zidovudine by 50% on days of combined zidovudine and probenecid administration. ▪ **Probenecid** may have interactions with numerous other drugs (e.g., **acetaminophen, acyclovir** [Zovirax], **ACE inhibitors** [e.g., enalapril (Vasotec)], **aminosalicylic acid, barbiturates, benzodiazepines** [e.g., diazepam, lorazepam (Ativan), midazolam], **bumetamide, chlorpropamide** [Diabinese], **clofibrate, ddC, famotidine, furosemide, methotrexate, NSAIDs** [e.g., ketoprofen (Orudis), ibuprofen (Advil, Motrin), naproxen (Aleve, Naprosyn)], **theophyllines**), usually decreasing their rate of excretion and increasing toxicity. Consider withholding any drug that may interact with probenecid on the day of cidofovir administration.

SIDE EFFECTS

Nephrotoxicity is dose limiting. Metabolic acidosis (Fanconi's syndrome), neutropenia, and ocular hypotony may be dose limiting and require prompt treatment. Anorexia, asthenia, chills, decreased intraocular pressure, decreased serum bicarbonate, diarrhea, dyspnea, fever, headache, increased creatinine, infection, nausea and vomiting, ophthalmic effects (e.g., change in vision, eye pain, increased sensitivity to light, reddened eyes), pneumonia, proteinuria, rash, and unusual tiredness or weakness may occur.

ANTIDOTE

There is no specific antidote. Keep physician informed. Adequate hydration, use of probenecid, and careful monitoring will help to reduce potential for renal impairment and may minimize other side effects. Filgrastim (Neupogen, Zarxio) may be used to treat neutropenia. See Monitor for management of probenecid side effects. Discontinue cidofovir based on criteria in Dose Adjustments. Treat overdose for 3 to 5 days with probenecid 1 Gm three times daily and vigorous IV hydration to tolerance. Treat anaphylaxis and resuscitate as indicated. Hemodialysis may be helpful in overdose. High-flux hemodialysis has reduced serum level of cidofovir by up to 75%.

CIPROFLOXACIN BBW

(sip-row-**FLOX**-ah-sin)

Cipro IV

Antibacterial
(fluoroquinolone)

pH 3.5 to 4.6

USUAL DOSE

Dose based on severity and nature of the infection, susceptibility of the causative organism, integrity of host-defense mechanisms, and renal and hepatic status. Range is from 200 to 400 mg according to the following chart. Continue for 7 to 14 days (at least 2 days after all symptoms of infection subside). Bone and joint infections may require treatment for 4 to 6 weeks or more. May be transferred to oral dosing when appropriate; see Monitor.

Ciprofloxacin Dose Guidelines				
Infection	Type of Severity	Unit Dose	Frequency	Duration
Urinary tract	Mild/moderate	200 mg	q 12 hr	
	Severe/complicated	400 mg	q 12 hr or q 8 hr	7-14 days
Lower respiratory tract	Mild/moderate	400 mg	q 12 hr	7-14 days
	Severe/complicated	400 mg	q 8 hr	
Nosocomial pneumonia	Mild/moderate/ severe	400 mg	q 8 hr	10-14 days
Skin and skin structure	Mild/moderate	400 mg	q 12 hr	7-14 days
	Severe/complicated	400 mg	q 8 hr	
Bone and joint	Mild/moderate	400 mg	q 12 hr	≥4-6 weeks
	Severe/complicated	400 mg	q 8 hr	
Septicemia (Canada)		400 mg	q 12 hr	
Acute sinusitis	Mild/moderate	400 mg	q 12 hr	10 days
Chronic bacterial prostatitis	Mild/moderate	400 mg	q 12 hr	28 days
Inhalation anthrax*	Postexposure	400 mg	q 12 hr	60 days
Intra-abdominal, complicated	Ciprofloxacin + metronidazole	400 mg 500 mg	q 12 hr q 6 hr	7-14 days
Empirical therapy in febrile neutropenic patients	Ciprofloxacin + piperacillin	400 mg 50 mg/kg	q 8 hr q 4 hr	7-14 days

*Begin drug administration as soon as possible after suspected or confirmed exposure.

PEDIATRIC DOSE

Used only when alternate therapy cannot be used; see Precautions and Maternal/Child.
In all situations, do not exceed an IV dose of 400 mg.
Inhalation anthrax (postexposure): 10 mg/kg every 12 hours IV. Do not exceed 400 mg/dose IV. May transfer to oral therapy when appropriate. Dose is 15 mg/kg PO every 12 hours. Do not exceed a 500-mg dose PO. Administer for 60 days.
Complicated UTIs or pyelonephritis in patients from 1 to 17 years of age: Dosing and initial route (IV or PO) should be determined by severity of infection. 6 to 10 mg/kg IV every 8 hours. Do not exceed 400 mg/dose IV. May transfer to oral therapy with a dose of 10 to 20 mg/kg PO every 12 hours at discretion of physician. Do not exceed a 750-mg dose PO. Total duration of treatment is 10 to 21 days.

Pulmonary exacerbations of cystic fibrosis in patients from 5 to 17 years of age (unlabeled): 10 mg/kg/dose IV every 8 hours for 1 week. Do not exceed 1.2 Gm/24 hr. Follow with 20 mg/kg/dose PO every 12 hours for 3 to 14 additional days to complete a 10- to 21-day regimen; see Monitor.

DOSE ADJUSTMENTS

Increase interval between doses (200 to 400 mg every 18 to 24 hours) if CrCl is less than 30 mL/min (see literature for additional information). ▪ Information on dosing adjustments for pediatric patients with renal insufficiency is not available. ▪ Dose reduction not required based on age; see Elderly. ▪ See Drug/Lab Interactions.

DILUTION

Available prediluted in D5W in latex-free plastic infusion containers ready for use. A clear, colorless to slightly yellow solution. Do not hang plastic containers in a series; may cause air embolism. Also available in 20- and 40-mL vials containing 10 mg/mL (1% solution), which must be diluted with NS, D5W, SWFI, D10W, D5/^{1}/$_4$NS, D5/^{1}/$_2$NS, or LR to a final concentration of 1 to 2 mg/mL.

Filters: No recommendations available from manufacturer.

Storage: Store flexible containers and vials between 5° and 25° C (41° and 77° F); protect from light, excessive heat, and freezing. Vials diluted in recommended solutions are stable for up to 14 days refrigerated or at room temperature if the final diluted concentration is between 0.5 and 2 mg/mL.

COMPATIBILITY   (Underline Indicates Conflicting Compatibility Information)

Consider any drug NOT listed as compatible to be INCOMPATIBLE until consulting a pharmacist; specific conditions may apply.

Manufacturer recommends temporarily discontinuing other solutions infusing at the same site during intermittent infusion through a **Y-site** or volume control and that ciprofloxacin be administered separately and the IV line be flushed before and after administration of any other drug.

One source suggests the following **compatibilities:**

Additive: Amikacin, atracurium (Tracrium), aztreonam (Azactam), cyclosporine (Sandimmune), dobutamine, dopamine, fluconazole (Diflucan), gentamicin, lidocaine, linezolid (Zyvox), metronidazole (Flagyl IV), midazolam (Versed), norepinephrine (Levophed), pancuronium, potassium chloride (KCl), ranitidine (Zantac), tobramycin, vecuronium.

Y-site: Amifostine (Ethyol), amino acids with dextrose, amiodarone (Nexterone), anidulafungin (Eraxis), aztreonam (Azactam), bivalirudin (Angiomax), calcium gluconate, caspofungin (Cancidas), ceftaroline (Teflaro), ceftazidime (Fortaz), cisatracurium (Nimbex), dexmedetomidine (Precedex), digoxin (Lanoxin), diltiazem (Cardizem), dimenhydrinate, diphenhydramine (Benadryl), dobutamine, docetaxel (Taxotere), dopamine, doripenem (Doribax), doxorubicin liposomal (Doxil), etoposide phosphate (Etopophos), fenoldopam (Corlopam), gallium nitrate (Ganite), gemcitabine (Gemzar), gentamicin, granisetron (Kytril), hetastarch in electrolytes (Hextend), 6% hydroxyethyl starch (Voluven), lidocaine, linezolid (Zyvox), lorazepam (Ativan), magnesium sulfate, metoclopramide (Reglan), midazolam (Versed), milrinone (Primacor), potassium acetate, potassium chloride (KCl), promethazine (Phenergan), quinupristin/dalfopristin (Synercid [1 mg/mL]), ranitidine (Zantac), remifentanil (Ultiva), sodium bicarbonate, sodium chloride, tacrolimus (Prograf), telavancin (Vibativ), teniposide (Vumon), thiotepa, tigecycline (Tygacil), tobramycin, vasopressin, verapamil.

RATE OF ADMINISTRATION

A single dose must be equally distributed over 60 minutes as an infusion. Too-rapid administration and/or the use of a small vein may increase incidence of local site inflammation and other side effects. May be given through a Y-tube or three-way stopcock of infusion set. Temporarily discontinue other solutions infusing at the same site.

ACTIONS

A synthetic, broad-spectrum antimicrobial agent, a fluoroquinolone. Bactericidal to a wide range of aerobic gram-negative and gram-positive organisms through interference with the enzymes needed for synthesis of bacterial DNA. Onset of action is prompt, and serum levels are dose related. Half-life averages 5 to 6 hours. Readily distributed to body fluids (saliva, nasal and bronchial secretions, sputum, skin blister fluid, lymph, peritoneal fluid, bile and prostatic secretions). Found in lung, skin, fat, muscle, cartilage, and bone. Levels in cerebrospinal fluid and eye fluids are lower than plasma levels. Limited metabolism. Excreted primarily as unchanged drug in the urine, usually within 24 hours. A small amount is excreted in the bile and feces. Crosses placental barrier. Secreted in breast milk.

INDICATIONS AND USES
Treatment of infections caused by susceptible isolates of designated organisms in the conditions and patient populations listed below. ▪ Treatment in adults of mild, moderate, severe, and complicated infections of the urinary tract and skin and skin structure. ▪ Treatment in adults of lower respiratory infections (*not* the drug of first choice in treatment of pneumonia secondary to *Streptococcus pneumoniae*). ▪ Treatment in adults of mild, moderate, and severe nosocomial pneumonia. ▪ Treatment in adults of acute sinusitis, bone and joint infections, chronic bacterial prostatitis, and septicemia (Canada). ▪ Treatment in adults of complicated intra-abdominal infections in combination with metronidazole (Flagyl). ▪ Empirical therapy in adult febrile neutropenic patients in combination with piperacillin. ▪ Reduce the incidence or progression of disease in adults or pediatric patients following exposure to aerosolized *Bacillus anthracis* (Anthrax). ▪ Treatment of complicated UTI and pyelonephritis due to *Escherichia coli* in pediatric patients 1 to 17 years of age; see Maternal/Child. ▪ Treatment of plague, including pneumonic and septicemic plague due to *Yersinia pestis*, and prophylaxis for plague in adults and pediatric patients from birth to 17 years of age. ▪ Additional appropriate therapy required if anaerobic organisms are suspected of contributing to the infection. ▪ Oral route of administration indicated for treatment of other infections (e.g., infectious diarrhea, typhoid fever, urethral and cervical gonococcal infections).
Unlabeled uses: Cystic fibrosis. ▪ Infective endocarditis. ▪ Surgical prophylaxis. ▪ Tularemia.

CONTRAINDICATIONS
Known hypersensitivity to ciprofloxacin or any other quinolone antimicrobial agent (e.g., levofloxacin [Levaquin], norfloxacin [Noroxin]) or any of the product components. ▪ Concomitant administration with tizanidine (Zanaflex) is contraindicated.

PRECAUTIONS
Specific culture and sensitivity studies indicated to determine susceptibility of the causative organism to ciprofloxacin. ▪ The emergence of bacterial resistance to fluoroquinolones and the occurrence of cross-resistance with other fluoroquinolones have been observed and are of concern. Proper use of fluoroquinolones and other classes of antibiotics is encouraged to avoid the emergence of resistant bacteria from overuse. ▪ *Pseudomonas aeruginosa* may develop resistance during treatment. Ongoing culture and sensitivity studies indicated. ▪ Prolonged use may cause superinfection because of overgrowth of nonsusceptible organisms. Monitor carefully. ▪ *Clostridium difficile*–associated diarrhea (CDAD) has been reported. May range from mild diarrhea to fatal colitis. Consider in patients who present with diarrhea during or after treatment with ciprofloxacin. ▪ Convulsions, increased intracranial pressure (including pseudotumor cerebri), and toxic psychosis have been reported in patients receiving quinolones, including ciprofloxacin. Ciprofloxacin may also cause CNS events, including confusion, depression, dizziness, hallucinations, tremors and, rarely, suicidal thoughts or acts. ▪ Use caution in patients with epilepsy or known or suspected CNS disorders (e.g., severe cerebral arteriosclerosis, previous history of convulsion), reduced cerebral blood flow, altered brain structure, stroke, drugs that may lower the seizure threshold, and renal dysfunction. ▪ Tendinitis and tendon rupture that required surgical repair or resulted in prolonged disability have been reported in patients receiving quinolones. Most frequently involves the Achilles tendon but has also been reported with the shoulder, hand, biceps,

thumb, and other tendon sites. ■ Inflammation and tendon rupture may occur during or up to months after fluoroquinolone therapy. Has been reported within the first 48 hours of therapy and may occur bilaterally. Use caution in patients with a history of tendon disorders. Risk may be increased in patients over 60 years of age; in patients taking corticosteroids; in patients with heart, kidney, or lung transplants; with strenuous physical activity; and in patients with renal failure or previous tendon disorders such as rheumatoid arthritis. ■ Fluoroquinolones have neuromuscular blocking activity. Serious adverse events, including requirement for ventilatory support and deaths, have been reported in patients with myasthenia gravis. Avoid use in patients with a known history of myasthenia gravis; may exacerbate muscle weakness. ■ Rare cases of peripheral neuropathy (e.g., paresthesias, hypoesthesias, dysesthesias [impairment of sensitivity or touch], or weakness) have been reported. Symptoms may occur soon after initiation of therapy and may be irreversible. ■ Prolongation of the QT interval on ECG and infrequent cases of arrhythmia (including torsades de pointes) have been reported with the use of some fluoroquinolones. The risk of arrhythmia may be reduced by avoiding their use in patients with known prolongation of the QT interval or in the presence of uncorrected electrolyte imbalances (e.g., hypokalemia, hypomagnesemia), significant bradycardia, cardiomyopathy, or concurrent treatment with Class 1A antiarrhythmic agents (e.g., quinidine, procainamide [Pronestyl]) or with Class III antiarrhythmic agents (e.g., amiodarone [Nexterone], sotalol [Betapace]). ■ Other serious events (sometimes fatal) due to hypersensitivity or uncertain etiology have been reported with fluoroquinolones, including ciprofloxacin; see Side Effects, Post-Marketing. Discontinue ciprofloxacin at the first appearance of a skin rash, jaundice, or other signs of hypersensitivity. ■ Cases of severe hepatic toxicity, including necrosis, life-threatening hepatic failure, and fatal events have been reported. Acute liver injury is rapid in onset (range 1 to 39 days) and is often associated with hypersensitivity. ■ Moderate to severe photosensitivity/phototoxicity reactions have been reported in patients receiving quinolones; see Patient Education.

Monitor: May cause anaphylaxis with the first or succeeding doses, even in patients without known hypersensitivity. Emergency equipment must always be available. ■ Monitor for S/S of peripheral neuropathy. Discontinue ciprofloxacin at the first symptoms of neuropathy (e.g., pain, burning, tingling, numbness and/or weakness) or if patient is found to have deficits in light touch, pain, temperature, position sense, vibratory sensation, and/or motor strength. ■ Maintain adequate hydration and acidity of urine throughout treatment. Will form crystals in alkaline urine. ■ Monitor hematopoietic, hepatic, and renal systems during prolonged treatment. ■ Use of large veins recommended to reduce incidence of local irritation. Symptoms of local irritation do not preclude further administration of ciprofloxacin unless they recur or worsen. Generally resolve when infusion complete. ■ Concomitant use with theophylline may cause cardiac arrest, respiratory failure, seizures, and/or status epilepticus. If concomitant use cannot be avoided, monitor serum levels of theophylline and adjust dose as indicated. ■ Doses will increase slightly with transfer to oral ciprofloxacin (e.g., 200 mg IV every 12 hours equals 250 mg PO every 12 hours; 400 mg IV every 12 hours equals 500 mg PO every 12 hours; 400 mg IV every 8 hours equals 750 mg PO every 12 hours). ■ See Drug/Lab Interactions.

Patient Education: A patient medication guide is available from the manufacturer. ■ Review all prescription and nonprescription medications with your health care provider. ■ Inform physician of any history of myasthenia gravis. Patients with a history of myasthenia gravis should avoid using ciprofloxacin. ■ Consider birth control options. ■ Photosensitivity has occurred in a minimum number of patients, but it is best to avoid excessive sunlight or artificial ultraviolet light. May cause severe sunburn; wear protective clothing, use sunscreen, and wear dark glasses outdoors. Report a sunburn-like reaction or skin eruption promptly. ■ Request assistance for ambulation; may cause dizziness and light-headedness. Use caution in tasks that require alertness. ■ Effects of caffeine- or theophylline-containing preparations may be increased; promptly report difficulty breathing and/or seizures. Limit or eliminate concurrent use. Monitor if concurrent use is necessary. ■ Report tendon pain or inflammation promptly; rest and refrain from exercise. ■ Promptly report skin rash or any other hypersensitivity reaction. ■ Promptly report pain, burning, tingling, numbness, and/or weakness. Nerve damage can be permanent. ▪ Inform physician of any history of seizures. ▪ Parents should inform physician of any history of joint-related problems and should promptly report any joint-related problems that develop during or after therapy. ▪ Promptly report diarrhea or bloody stools that occur during treatment or up to several months after an antibiotic has been discontinued; may indicate CDAD and require treatment.

Maternal/Child: Category C: use during pregnancy only if benefits justify potential risk to fetus and mother. ▪ Discontinue breast-feeding. ▪ Safety for use in pediatric patients under 18 years of age not established except for use postexposure of inhalation anthrax and UTIs or pyelonephritis. Appropriateness based on risk/benefit assessment. ▪ May erode cartilage of weight-bearing joints or cause other signs of arthropathy in infants and children. ▪ Has been used in infants and children to treat serious infections unresponsive to other antibiotic regimens.

Elderly: Safety and effectiveness similar to younger adults. ▪ May be at increased risk of experiencing side effects (e.g., CNS effects, drug-associated effects on the QT interval, tendinitis, tendon rupture); see Precautions. Half-life may be slightly extended because of age-related renal impairment; see Dose Adjustments. Monitoring of renal function may be useful.

DRUG/LAB INTERACTIONS

Ciprofloxacin is an inhibitor of the hepatic CYP1A2 enzyme pathway. Coadministration with other drugs metabolized by this route, such as **clozapine** (Clozaril), **methylxanthines** (e.g., theophylline), **olanzapine** (Zyprexa), **ropinirole** (Requip), **or tizanidine** (Zanaflex), results in increased plasma concentrations of these drugs, which may cause significant toxicity. **Concomitant administration with tizanidine (Zanaflex) is contraindicated** (hypotensive and sedative effects potentiated). ▪ May cause serious or fatal reactions with **theophylline** (e.g., cardiac arrhythmias or arrest, respiratory failure, or seizures). If must be used concomitantly, monitor serum levels of theophylline and decrease dose as appropriate. Observe closely with **caffeine** intake; has caused similar problems. Elevated serum levels of other xanthine derivatives (e.g., pentoxifylline-containing products [e.g., Trental]) have also been seen with concurrent use. ▪ Use with **cyclosporine** may cause an increase in SCr and nephrotoxic effects. ▪ May potentiate **oral anticoagulants** (e.g., warfarin [Coumadin]); monitor PT/INR. ▪ Potentiated by **probenecid;** may require dose adjustment based on ciprofloxacin serum levels. ▪ Severe hypoglycemia has been reported with concomitant use of **oral antidiabetic agents** (e.g., glyburide [DiaBeta], glimepiride [Amaryl]); monitor serum glucose levels. ▪ May increase or decrease serum **phenytoin** levels; monitor phenytoin levels with concurrent use and repeat phenytoin levels shortly after completion of ciprofloxacin therapy. ▪ Two case reports suggest concurrent administration with **foscarnet** (Foscavir) may cause seizures; monitor patient carefully. ▪ Risk of CNS stimulation and seizures may be increased with concurrent use of **NSAIDs** (e.g., ibuprofen [Advil, Motrin], naproxen [Aleve, Naprosyn]) with high doses of quinolones. ▪ Concurrent use with **methotrexate** requires close monitoring. May inhibit renal tubular transport of methotrexate, thereby increasing methotrexate serum levels and the risk of toxicity. ▪ Coadministration with **drugs that prolong the QT interval** such as **Class IA or III antiarrhythmic agents** (e.g., amiodarone [Nexterone], disopyramide [Norpace], procainamide [Pronestyl], quinidine), **tricyclic antidepressants** (e.g., amitriptyline [Elavil], imipramine [Tofranil]), **macrolide antibiotics** (e.g., azithromycin [Zithromax]), and **antipsychotics** (e.g., iloperidone [Fanapt], paliperidone [Invega], phenothiazines [e.g., chlorpromazine, thioridazine], ziprasidone [Geodon]) may increase the risk of QT prolongation and life-threatening arrhythmias. ▪ Pharmacologic effects of **metoprolol** (Lopressor) may be increased. Monitor cardiac function when initiating or discontinuing ciprofloxacin. ▪ May increase serum concentrations of many drugs (e.g., **duloxetine** [Cymbalta], **lidocaine, methadone** [Dolophine], **mexiletine, MAO inhibitors** [e.g., rasagiline (Azilect)], **ropivacaine** [Naropin], **sildenafil** [Revatio, Viagra]). Therapeutic effects and/or side effects may be increased; dose reductions of these drugs may be indicated. ▪ May cause a false-positive when **testing urine for opiates;** more specific testing methods may be indicated. ▪ See Side Effects.

SIDE EFFECTS

Diarrhea, hepatic enzyme abnormalities (elevation of alkaline phosphatase, AST, ALT, LDH, serum bilirubin), nausea and vomiting, and rash are reported most frequently. Other less frequent reactions include allergic reactions (anaphylaxis, cardiovascular collapse, death, dyspnea, edema [facial, pharyngeal, or pulmonary], eosinophilia, fever, itching, loss of consciousness, rash, urticaria); cardiovascular effects (e.g., cardiac arrest, palpitations, QT interval prolongation, tachycardia, torsades de pointes, vasodilation, ventricular tachyarrhythmias); CDAD; CNS stimulation (confusion, hallucinations, light-headedness, restlessness, seizures, tingling, toxic psychosis, tremors); decreased hemoglobin, hematocrit, and platelet count; elevation of eosinophil and platelet counts, BUN, serum amylase, serum creatinine, serum creatine phosphokinase, serum potassium, uric acid, and triglycerides; headache; hyperglycemia; hypoglycemia; increased intracranial pressure; local site reactions; myalgias; nausea; peripheral neuropathy (e.g., pain, burning, tingling, numbness and/or weakness [see Precautions, Monitor]); photosensitivity/phototoxicity and vision changes; postural hypotension; respiratory failure; status epilepticus; tendinitis; and tendon rupture. Capable of numerous other reactions in fewer than 1% of patients.

Post-Marketing: Acute generalized exanthematous pustulosis (AGEP), allergic pneumonitis, arthralgia, hematologic abnormalities (agranulocytosis, anemia [hemolytic and aplastic], leukopenia, pancytopenia, thrombocytopenia, thrombotic thrombocytopenic purpura), increased INR in patients treated with vitamin K antagonists, interstitial nephritis, jaundice, liver abnormalities (e.g., acute hepatic necrosis or failure, hepatitis, jaundice), myalgia, polyneuropathy, rash, serum sickness, severe dermatologic reactions (e.g., toxic epidermal necrolysis [Lyell's syndrome], Stevens-Johnson syndrome), vasculitis.

ANTIDOTE

Death may result from some of these side effects. Discontinue ciprofloxacin at the first appearance of a skin rash or major side effect (hypersensitivity, CDAD, CNS symptoms, dermatologic reactions, phototoxicity, or tendon rupture). Treat hypersensitivity reactions with epinephrine (Adrenalin), airway management, oxygen, IV fluids, antihistamines (diphenhydramine [Benadryl]), corticosteroids (hydrocortisone sodium succinate [Solu-Cortef]), and pressor amines (dopamine) as indicated. Treat CNS symptoms as indicated. May require diazepam (Valium) for seizures. Mild cases of CDAD may respond to discontinuation of ciprofloxacin. Treat CDAD with fluids, electrolytes, protein supplements, and oral vancomycin (Vancocin) or metronidazole (Flagyl) as indicated. In severe cases, surgical evaluation may be indicated. Drugs that inhibit peristalsis should be avoided. Keep physician informed of all side effects. Many will require symptomatic treatment; monitor closely. In overdose, observe carefully, provide supportive treatment, maintain hydration, and monitor renal function and urinary pH and acidify, if required, to prevent crystalluria. No specific antidote; up to 10% may be removed by hemodialysis or peritoneal dialysis. Maintain patient until drug excreted.

CISATRACURIUM BESYLATE BBW

(sis-ah-trah-**KYOU**-ree-um **BES**-ih-layt)

Neuromuscular blocking agent
(nondepolarizing)
Anesthesia adjunct

Nimbex, Nimbex PF

pH 3.25 to 3.65

USUAL DOSE
Must be individualized based on previous drugs administered (e.g., fentanyl, midazolam [Versed]), desired time to intubation, and anticipated length of surgery. Must be used with adequate anesthesia and/or sedation and after unconsciousness induced. Use of a peripheral nerve stimulator is indicated in all situations.

ADJUNCT TO PROPOFOL/N_2O/O_2 ANESTHESIA FOR ADULTS (IV BOLUS)
Initial dose: 0.15 to 0.2 mg/kg. 0.15 mg/kg should provide good to excellent conditions for intubation within 2 minutes and adequate muscle relaxation for 55 minutes (range 44 to 74 min). 0.2 mg/kg (7 mL [of a 2 mg/mL conc] for a 70-kg patient) should be effective within 1.5 minutes and last for 61 minutes (range 41 to 81 min). Up to 0.4 mg/kg has been used; has a dose-related length of effectiveness.

Maintenance dose: May be given by IV bolus or as a continuous infusion. Determine need for maintenance dose based on beginning symptoms of neuromuscular blockade reversal determined by a peripheral nerve stimulator. Usually required 40 to 60 minutes after a bolus dose. Do not administer before recovery begins. Repeated doses have no cumulative effect if recovery is allowed to begin before administration. See Dose Adjustments.

IV bolus: 0.03 mg/kg (1 mL [of a 2 mg/mL conc] for a 70-kg patient) should provide an additional 20 minutes of muscle relaxation. Smaller or larger doses may be given based on expected duration of procedure.

Continuous infusion: Begin infusion with 3 mcg/kg/min to rapidly counteract the spontaneous recovery, then decrease to 1 to 2 mcg/kg/min. Monitor maintenance infusion with a peripheral nerve stimulator.

SUPPORT OF INTUBATED, MECHANICALLY VENTILATED, OR RESPIRATORY CONTROLLED ADULT ICU PATIENTS
After intubation is accomplished (usually with succinylcholine), an initial bolus dose of 0.1 mg/kg provides adequate neuromuscular blockade. Maintain with 3 mcg/kg/min (range 0.5 to 10.2 mcg/kg/min). Published reports describe a wide interpatient variability in dosing requirements that may change from day to day. Adjust infusion rate according to clinical assessment of the patient's response. Use of a peripheral nerve stimulator is recommended. Do not increase dose until there is a definite response to nerve stimulation. If recovery from neuromuscular block has progressed, readministration of a bolus dose may be necessary. Long-term use (beyond 6 days) has not been studied.

PEDIATRIC DOSE
See all comments under Usual Dose and Maternal/Child.

ADJUNCT TO HALOTHANE OR OPIOID ANESTHESIA FOR PEDIATRIC PATIENTS 1 MONTH TO 23 MONTHS OF AGE
0.15 mg/kg. Should produce maximum block in 2 minutes and adequate muscle relaxation for 43 minutes (range is 34 to 58 minutes).

ADJUNCT TO HALOTHANE OR OPIOID ANESTHESIA FOR PEDIATRIC PATIENTS 2 TO 12 YEARS OF AGE
Initial dose: 0.1 to 0.15 mg/kg as an IV bolus. 0.1 mg/kg should provide good to excellent conditions for intubation within 2.8 minutes and adequate muscle relaxation for 28 minutes (range 21 to 38 minutes). 0.15 mg/kg should produce maximum block in 3 minutes and adequate muscle relaxation for 36 minutes (range 29 to 46 minutes).

Maintenance dose: Same as adult dosing; see all comments.

DOSE ADJUSTMENTS
Reduce initial dose to 0.02 mg/kg in any condition that may result in a prolonged neuromuscular blockade (e.g., myasthenia gravis, myasthenic syndrome, carcinomatosis, debilitation, other drugs). Use a peripheral nerve stimulator to assess the level of neuromus-

cular block and to monitor dose requirements. See Drug/Lab Interactions. ▪ Increased initial and maintenance doses may be required in burn patients. Duration of action may be shortened. ▪ Half-life is extended but no dose adjustment is required in patients with renal or hepatic disease or in the elderly. Time of onset may be slightly faster in patients with liver disease and slower in the elderly and patients with renal disease. Slower onset may require a delay of an additional minute before intubation. ▪ Reduce maintenance dose by 30% to 40% in the presence of isoflurane or enflurane anesthesia. Larger reductions may be indicated in prolonged anesthesia. ▪ May need to reduce maintenance dose by 50% in patients undergoing coronary artery bypass surgery with induced hypothermia.

DILUTION
IV bolus: May be given undiluted.

Infusion: Further dilute in NS, D5W, or D5NS to a 0.1 mg/mL or 0.4 mg/mL solution. Using the 2 mg/mL solution, 10 mg diluted in 95 mL yields 0.1 mg/mL; 40 mg diluted in 80 mL yields 0.4 mg/mL.

ICU infusion: A 20-mL vial (10 mg/mL concentration) is available for use in ICU (200 mg/vial). 200 mg in 1,000 mL yields 0.2 mg/mL, in 500 mL yields 0.4 mg/mL.

Storage: Refrigerate in carton before use; protect from light; do not freeze. Use within 21 days if at room temperature even if it was re-refrigerated. Most diluted solutions are stable refrigerated or at room temperature for 24 hours.

COMPATIBILITY   (Underline Indicates Conflicting Compatibility Information)
Consider any drug NOT listed as compatible to be INCOMPATIBLE until consulting a pharmacist; specific conditions may apply.

Manufacturer lists propofol (Diprivan) and ketorolac (Toradol) as **incompatible**. Has an acid pH and may be **incompatible** with alkaline solutions having a pH greater than 8.5 (e.g., aminophylline, barbiturates, sodium bicarbonate).

Manufacturer lists alfentanil, droperidol (Inapsine), fentanyl, midazolam (Versed), and sufentanil (Sufenta) as **compatible** but does not specify **additive** or **Y-site.**

Another source suggests the following **compatibilities:**

Y-site: <u>Acyclovir (Zovirax)</u>, alfentanil, amikacin, <u>aminophylline</u>, <u>amphotericin B (conventional)</u>, ampicillin, <u>ampicillin/sulbactam (Unasyn)</u>, aztreonam (Azactam), bumetanide, buprenorphine (Buprenex), butorphanol (Stadol), calcium gluconate, <u>cefazolin (Ancef)</u>, <u>cefotaxime (Claforan)</u>, <u>cefoxitin (Mefoxin)</u>, ceftaroline (Teflaro), <u>ceftazidime (Fortaz)</u>, ceftriaxone (Rocephin), <u>cefuroxime (Zinacef)</u>, chlorpromazine (Thorazine), ciprofloxacin (Cipro IV), clindamycin (Cleocin), dexamethasone (Decadron), dexmedetomidine (Precedex), <u>diazepam (Valium)</u>, digoxin (Lanoxin), diphenhydramine (Benadryl), dobutamine, dopamine, doxycycline, droperidol (Inapsine), enalaprilat (Vasotec IV), epinephrine (Adrenalin), esmolol (Brevibloc), famotidine (Pepcid IV), fenoldopam (Corlopam), fentanyl, fluconazole (Diflucan), <u>furosemide (Lasix)</u>, <u>ganciclovir (Cytovene IV)</u>, gentamicin, <u>heparin</u>, hetastarch in electrolytes (Hextend), hydrocortisone sodium succinate (Solu-Cortef), hydromorphone (Dilaudid), imipenem-cilastatin (Primaxin), isoproterenol (Isuprel), lidocaine, linezolid (Zyvox), lorazepam (Ativan), magnesium sulfate, mannitol, meperidine (Demerol), <u>methylprednisolone (Solu-Medrol)</u>, metoclopramide (Reglan), metronidazole (Flagyl IV), midazolam (Versed), morphine, nalbuphine, nitroglycerin IV, <u>nitroprusside sodium</u>, norepinephrine (Levophed), ondansetron (Zofran), <u>palonosetron (Aloxi)</u>, phenylephrine (Neo-Synephrine), <u>piperacillin/tazobactam (Zosyn)</u>, potassium chloride (KCl), procainamide (Pronestyl), prochlorperazine (Compazine), promethazine (Phenergan), <u>propofol (Diprivan)</u>, ranitidine (Zantac), remifentanil (Ultiva), <u>sodium bicarbonate</u>, sufentanil (Sufenta), <u>sulfamethoxazole/trimethoprim</u>, theophylline, <u>ticarcillin/clavulanate (Timentin)</u>, tobramycin, vancomycin, zidovudine (AZT, Retrovir).

RATE OF ADMINISTRATION
IV bolus: A single dose over 5 to 10 seconds.

Infusion for anesthesia adjunct or ICU: Use of a microdrip (60 gtt/mL) or volume infusion pump required. Adjust rate to desired dose based on the following charts for 0.1 mg/mL and 0.4 mg/mL. For 0.2 mg/mL solution in ICU, multiply rates (mL/hr) of 0.1 mg/mL solution by 2 or divide rates (mL/hr) of 0.4 mg/mL solution in half.

Cisatracurium Infusion Rates for a Concentration of 0.1 mg/mL					
Patient Weight (kg)	Drug Delivery Rate (mcg/kg/min)				
	1	1.5	2	3	5
	Infusion Delivery Rate (mL/hr)				
10 kg	6 mL/hr	9 mL/hr	12 mL/hr	18 mL/hr	30 mL/hr
45 kg	27 mL/hr	41 mL/hr	54 mL/hr	81 mL/hr	135 mL/hr
70 kg	42 mL/hr	63 mL/hr	84 mL/hr	126 mL/hr	210 mL/hr
100 kg	60 mL/hr	90 mL/hr	120 mL/hr	180 mL/hr	300 mL/hr

Cisatracurium Infusion Rates for a Concentration of 0.4 mg/mL					
Patient Weight (kg)	Drug Delivery Rate (mcg/kg/min)				
	1	1.5	2	3	5
	Infusion Delivery Rate (mL/hr)				
10 kg	1.5 mL/hr	2.3 mL/hr	3 mL/hr	4.5 mL/hr	7.5 mL/hr
45 kg	6.8 mL/hr	10.1 mL/hr	13.5 mL/hr	20.3 mL/hr	33.8 mL/hr
70 kg	10.5 mL/hr	15.8 mL/hr	21 mL/hr	31.5 mL/hr	52.5 mL/hr
100 kg	15 mL/hr	22.5 mL/hr	30 mL/hr	45 mL/hr	75 mL/hr

ACTIONS

A nondepolarizing skeletal muscle relaxant with intermediate onset and duration of action. An isomer of atracurium (Tracrium) with three times its potency at a mg-for-mg dose. In contrast to most of the other neuromuscular blocking agents, cisatracurium has no clinically significant effect on HR or BP with usual doses even in patients with serious cardiovascular disease, and it also does not produce a dose-related histamine release. Causes paralysis by interfering with neural transmission at the myoneural junction. Produces maximum neuromuscular blockade within 1.5 to 3 minutes and lasts about 50 minutes in adults. Recovery to 75% usually occurs within 30 minutes. Metabolized by a process that mostly bypasses both the kidney and the liver. Forms specific metabolites (e.g., alcohol, laudanosine) that do not have neuromuscular blocking activity. Because of reduced dose requirements, laudanosine accumulation is lower than with atracurium, lowering the potential of seizures. Eliminated renally, primarily as metabolites.

INDICATIONS AND USES

Adjunctive to general anesthesia for inpatients and outpatients to facilitate endotracheal intubation and to relax skeletal muscles during surgery. ▪ Relax skeletal muscles during mechanical ventilation in ICU.

CONTRAINDICATIONS

Known hypersensitivity to cisatracurium, other bis-benzylisoquinolinium compounds (e.g., atracurium), and benzyl alcohol (some preparations contain benzyl alcohol).

PRECAUTIONS

For IV use only. ▪ Administered by or under the observation of the anesthesiologist. Adequate facilities, emergency resuscitation drugs and equipment, neuromuscular blocking antagonists (e.g., anticholinesterase agents [e.g., neostigmine, edrophonium]), and atropine must always be available. ▪ Not recommended for rapid sequence intubation; succinylcholine is usually the drug of choice. ▪ Severe anaphylactic reactions have been reported with neuromuscular blocking agents; some have been fatal. Use caution in patients who have had an anaphylactic reaction to another neuromuscular blocking agent (depolarizing or nondepolarizing); cross-reactivity has occurred. ▪ Myasthenia gravis and other neuromuscular diseases increase sensitivity to cisatracurium. Can cause critical reactions. ▪ Sensitivity may be decreased in patients with burns or paralysis. See Dose Adjustments and Monitor. ▪ In patients with renal or hepatic disease, half-life of metabolites is longer, and concentrations may be higher with long-term administration. ▪ Did not trigger malignant hypertension (MH) in susceptible pigs at doses above those required for humans, but has not been studied in MH-susceptible humans. ▪ Respiratory depression with propofol (Diprivan) or morphine may be preferred in some patients requiring mechanical ventilation. ▪ Will not counteract the bradycardia produced by many anesthetic agents or vagal stimulation. ▪ Transient hypotension and CNS excitation (generalized muscle twitching to seizures) have been reported rarely in ICU patients undergoing prolonged therapy.

Monitor: This drug produces apnea. Controlled artificial ventilation with oxygen must be continuous and under direct observation at all times. Maintain a patent airway. ▪ Use a peripheral nerve stimulator to monitor drug effect, determine the need for additional doses, confirm recovery from neuromuscular block, and avoid overdose. Place on a non-paralyzed limb in patients with paralysis. ▪ Monitor vital signs and ECG continuously. ▪ Has no analgesic properties or effect on consciousness. Use in conjunction with anesthesia, sedation, or analgesia as indicated. ▪ Action potentiated by hypokalemia and some carcinomas. ▪ Action may be potentiated or antagonized by dehydration, electrolyte imbalance, body temperature, or acid-base imbalance.

Maternal/Child: Category B: use in pregnancy only if clearly needed. Safety for use during labor and delivery not established. ▪ Use caution during breast-feeding; probably best to defer breast-feeding until after full recovery. ▪ Safety for use in infants under 1 month of age not established. ▪ 10 mL (2 mg/mL) multiple-dose vials contain benzyl alcohol; do not use in newborns. ▪ In pediatric patients 2 to 12 years of age, onset is faster, duration shorter, and recovery faster than in adults. In infants 1 month to 23 months of age, onset is faster; however, duration and recovery are similar to adults. ▪ For induction of anesthesia in pediatric patients 1 month to 12 years of age, intubation was facilitated more reliably when cisatracurium was used in combination with halothane anesthesia than when used in combination with opioids and nitrous oxide. ▪ Rare incidences of wheezing, laryngospasm, bronchospasm, rash, and itching have been reported in pediatric patients.

Elderly: Safely administered even in patients with significant cardiac disease. ▪ Response similar to that seen in younger adults; however, greater sensitivity of some older individuals cannot be ruled out. ▪ Onset to complete neuromuscular block slightly slower; delay intubation until fully effective. Recovery may be slower.

DRUG/LAB INTERACTIONS

Potentiated by **general anesthetics** (e.g., enflurane, isoflurane), many **antibiotics** (e.g., aminoglycosides [kanamycin, gentamicin], lincosamides [clindamycin (Cleocin)], polypeptides [bacitracin, colistimethate], tetracyclines), **muscle relaxants, diuretics, lithium, local anesthetics, magnesium sulfate, procainamide** (Pronestyl), **quinidine, succinylcholine, and others.** May need to reduce initial or maintenance dose of cisatracurium; use with caution. ▪ Antagonized by **acetylcholine and anticholinesterases.** ▪ Duration of neuromuscular block may be shorter and dose requirements may be higher during maintenance infusion in patients stabilized on **carbamazepine** (Tegretol) **or phenytoin** (Dilantin). ▪ Time to onset of maximum block is faster when **succinylcholine** is given before cisatracurium. Succinylcholine must show signs of wearing off before cisatracurium is given. Use caution.

SIDE EFFECTS

Bradycardia, bronchospasm, flushing, hypotension, and rash occurred in fewer than 1% of patients. Both inadequate and/or prolonged neuromuscular blocks have been reported. Rare reports of seizures with similar agents in ICU could be caused by accumulated laudanosine, other conditions, or medications. Excessive dosing or prolonged action may result in respiratory insufficiency or apnea. Airway closure may be caused by relaxation of epiglottis, pharynx, and tongue muscles. Hypersensitivity reactions have been reported.

ANTIDOTE

Side effects can be medical emergencies. Treat symptomatically. Maintain a patent airway and continuous controlled artificial ventilation and oxygenation until full recovery is ensured. The more profound the neuromuscular block, the longer it will take until recovery begins. Recovery from neuromuscular block must be confirmed by a peripheral nerve stimulator before anticholinesterase agents (e.g., neostigmine or edrophonium [Enlon]) can be given with an anticholinergic agent (e.g., atropine) to reverse the muscle relaxation. Neostigmine 0.04 to 0.07 mg/kg at 10% recovery in conjunction with atropine should be effective in 9 to 10 minutes. Edrophonium 1 mg/kg at 25% recovery in conjunction with atropine (Enlon-Plus is edrophonium and atropine combined) should be effective in 3 to 5 minutes. Confirm recovery by 5-second head lift and grip strength. Recovery may be inhibited by cachexia, carcinomatosis, debilitation, or the concomitant use of certain drugs; see Drug/Lab Interactions. Resuscitate as necessary.

CISPLATIN BBW
(sis-**PLAH**-tin)

CDDP

Antineoplastic
(alkylating agent)

pH 3.5 to 6

USUAL DOSE

Prehydration required; see Precautions and Monitor. See Dose Adjustments. May be given in combination with amifostine (Ethyol) to reduce nephrotoxicity and neurotoxicity of cisplatin. See amifostine monograph. Administration as a 6- to 8-hour infusion with intravenous hydration and mannitol has been used to reduce nephrotoxicity. Doses greater than 100 mg/M^2 once every 3 to 4 weeks are rarely used.

Metastatic testicular tumors: Used in combination with other approved chemotherapeutic agents. 20 mg/M^2 daily for 5 days per cycle.

Metastatic ovarian tumors: 75 to 100 mg/M^2 on Day 1 every 4 weeks. Used in combination with cyclophosphamide (Cytoxan) 600 mg/M^2 IV on Day 1 every 4 weeks. Another regimen (unlabeled in cisplatin prescribing information) uses paclitaxel 135 mg/M^2 (as a 24-hour infusion) followed by cisplatin 75 mg/M^2. Both agents are given once every 3 weeks for 6 courses. See paclitaxel monograph; premedication required. Used as a *single agent,* the dose of cisplatin is 100 mg/M^2 every 4 weeks.

First-line treatment of ovarian cancer (unlabeled in cisplatin prescribing information): Given in combination with paclitaxel as follows: give paclitaxel (Taxol) 135 mg/M^2 as an infusion over 24 hours. Follow with cisplatin 75 mg/M^2 as an infusion over 6 to 8 hours. Repeat every 3 weeks. See paclitaxel monograph; premedication required. Other dose combinations and infusion times are being used.

Advanced bladder cancer: 50 to 70 mg/M^2 once every 3 to 4 weeks. 50 mg/M^2 is recommended once every 4 weeks for patients heavily pretreated with radiation or chemotherapy. Numerous other doses and combinations are used.

Non–small-cell lung cancer (unlabeled in cisplatin prescribing information): Given in combination with gemcitabine as follows: gemcitabine (Gemzar) 1,000 mg/M^2 as an infusion on Days 1, 8, and 15 of each 28-day cycle. Follow the gemcitabine infusion on Day 1 with cisplatin 100 mg/M^2. See gemcitabine monograph; other dosing schedules are in use. Another regimen uses a combination of paclitaxel and cisplatin as follows: paclitaxel 135 mg/M^2 as an infusion over 24 hours followed by cisplatin 75 mg/M^2 over 6 to 8 hours. Repeat every 3 weeks. See paclitaxel monograph; premedication required. Also used with docetaxel 75 mg/M^2 infused over 1 hour followed immediately by an infusion of cisplatin 75 mg/M^2 over 30 to 60 minutes. Repeat every 3 weeks. See docetaxel monograph; premedication required.

DOSE ADJUSTMENTS

All doses adjusted based on prior radiation therapy or chemotherapy. ▪ Repeat doses may not be given unless SCr is below 1.5 mg/100 mL and/or BUN is below 25 mg/100 mL. Renal toxicity becomes more prolonged and severe with repeated courses. Renal function must return to normal before next dose is given. ▪ Platelets should be 100,000/mm^3 and leukocytes 4,000/mm^3; verify auditory acuity as within normal limits. ▪ Dosing should be cautious in the elderly. Lower-end initial doses may be indicated. Consider decrease in cardiac, hepatic, and renal function; concomitant disease; or other drug therapy; see Elderly.

DILUTION

Specific techniques required; see Precautions. Available in liquid form, 1 mg/mL. Withdraw desired dose. Immediately before use, manufacturer recommends diluting a single dose in 2 liters of D5½NS or D5⅓NS containing 37.5 Gm of mannitol. Do not use D5W. Will decompose if adequate chloride ion not available. Is also diluted in smaller amounts of NS (100 to 500 mL). Do not use needles or IV tubing with aluminum parts to administer; a precipitate will form, and potency will decrease. See Monitor for additional optional additives.

Storage: Cisplatin remaining in multidose vial is stable at CRT for 28 days protected from light or 7 days under fluorescent light. Do not refrigerate. Protect from light if it will not be used within 6 hours.

COMPATIBILITY   (Underline Indicates Conflicting Compatibility Information)

Consider any drug NOT listed as compatible to be INCOMPATIBLE until consulting a pharmacist; specific conditions may apply.

Manufacturer states, "Do not use needles, IV sets, or equipment containing aluminum." Aluminum reacts with cisplatin, causing precipitate formation and loss of potency. A precipitate will form if reconstituted solutions are refrigerated.

One source suggests the following **compatibilities:**

Additive: Carboplatin (Paraplatin), cyclophosphamide (Cytoxan), etoposide (VePesid), ifosfamide (Ifex), leucovorin calcium, magnesium sulfate, mannitol, ondansetron (Zofran), paclitaxel (Taxol). Another source adds carmustine (BiCNU).

Y-site: Allopurinol (Aloprim), anidulafungin (Eraxis), aztreonam (Azactam), bleomycin (Blenoxane), caspofungin (Cancidas), cladribine (Leustatin), cyclophosphamide (Cytoxan), doripenem (Doribax), doxorubicin (Adriamycin), doxorubicin liposomal (Doxil), droperidol (Inapsine), etoposide phosphate (Etopophos), filgrastim (Neupogen), fludarabine (Fludara), fluorouracil (5-FU), furosemide (Lasix), gemcitabine (Gemzar), granisetron (Kytril), heparin, leucovorin calcium, linezolid (Zyvox), melphalan (Alkeran), methotrexate, metoclopramide (Reglan), mitomycin (Mutamycin), ondansetron (Zofran), paclitaxel (Taxol), palonosetron (Aloxi), pemetrexed (Alimta), propofol (Diprivan), sargramostim (Leukine), teniposide (Vumon), topotecan (Hycamtin), vinblastine, vincristine, vinorelbine (Navelbine).

RATE OF ADMINISTRATION

Administer as a slow IV infusion; *should not be given as a rapid IV injection.* Rates vary based on protocol. Manufacturer suggests administering each 1 liter of infusion solution over 3 to 4 hours. Give total dose (2 liters) over 6 to 8 hours. Rate must be sufficient to maintain hydration and diuresis. Infusion times of 30 to 120 minutes are common, but infusion time has also been extended to 24 hours/dose. One source recommends a maximum rate not to exceed 1 mg/min. Too-rapid administration increases nephrotoxicity and ototoxicity.

ACTIONS

A heavy metal complex (platinum and chloride atoms). Has properties similar to alkylating agents and is cell-cycle nonspecific. Inhibits DNA synthesis by formation of DNA cross-links. Concentration is highest in liver, prostate, and kidney; somewhat lower in bladder, muscle, testicle, pancreas, and spleen. Heavily protein bound. Only one fourth to one half of the drug is excreted in the urine by the end of 5 days. Platinum may be present in tissues for as long as 180 days after the last administration. Secreted in breast milk.

INDICATIONS AND USES

Treatment of metastatic testicular tumors; used in combination therapy with other approved chemotherapy agents in patients who have already received appropriate surgical and/or radiotherapeutic procedures. ▪ Treatment of metastatic ovarian tumors; used in combination therapy with other approved chemotherapy agents in patients who have already received appropriate surgical and/or radiotherapeutic procedures. ▪ Used as a single agent as secondary treatment in patients with metastatic ovarian tumors refractory to standard chemotherapy who have not previously received cisplatin therapy. ▪ Used as a single agent for treatment of patients with transitional cell bladder cancer that is no longer amenable to local treatment such as surgery and/or radiotherapy. ▪ Is used in specific combinations with other chemotherapeutic drugs.

Unlabeled uses: First-line therapy for treatment of advanced cancer of the ovary in combination with paclitaxel. ▪ First-line treatment of patients with inoperable, locally advanced, or metastatic non–small-cell lung cancer (NSCLC) in combination with gemcitabine, paclitaxel, or docetaxel. ▪ Treatment of cancers of the brain, adrenal cortex, breast, cervix, uterus, endometrium, head and neck, esophagus, lung, and liver; osteogenic sarcomas; and numerous other malignancies.

CONTRAINDICATIONS

Hypersensitivity to cisplatin or other platinum-containing compounds, myelosuppressed patients, pre-existing impaired renal function, or hearing deficit.

PRECAUTIONS

Follow guidelines for handling cytotoxic agents. See Appendix A, p. 1331. ▪ Administered by or under the direction of the physician specialist. ▪ Adequate facilities and emergency resuscitation equipment and supplies must always be available. ▪ Renal toxicity can be cumulative and may be severe. ▪ Other major dose-related toxicities include myelosuppression, nausea, and vomiting. ▪ Ototoxicity (tinnitus, loss of high-frequency hearing, and/or deafness) can be significant and may be more pronounced in pediatric patients. ▪ Anaphylaxis has been reported and may occur within minutes of cisplatin administration. ▪ Labeling changed to read, "Doses greater than 100 mg/M^2/cycle once every 3 to 4 weeks are rarely used." This is an effort to eliminate serious errors resulting from confusion with carboplatin (Paraplatin). Flip-off seal on vial now says, "Call Dr. if dose greater than 100 mg/M^2/cycle." ▪ Neuropathies may occur with higher doses, greater frequency of average doses, or prolonged therapy. Usually occur after prolonged therapy but have been reported after a single dose. If symptoms of neuropathy are observed, discontinue cisplatin. ▪ See Elderly.

Monitor: Obtain baseline CBC, SCr, BUN, CrCl and calcium, magnesium, potassium, and sodium levels. Repeat CBC weekly and other listed labs before each subsequent cycle. ▪ Hydrate patient with 1 to 2 L of infusion fluid for 8 to 12 hours before cisplatin administration. Urine output should exceed 100 to 150 mL/hr. ▪ Maintain adequate hydration and urine output of at least 100 to 200 mL/hr for 24 hours after each dose. ▪ Nausea and vomiting are frequently severe and prolonged (up to a week). May begin within 1 to 4 hours of administration or may be delayed. Prophylactic administration of antiemetics recommended. Fosaprepitant (Emend), ondansetron (Zofran), metoclopramide (Reglan), or dexamethasone are effective in most patients. ▪ Ototoxicity is cumulative; test hearing before administration and regularly during treatment. Ototoxicity increased in pediatric patients. ▪ Monitor uric acid levels before and during treatment and maintain hydration. Allopurinol and alkalinization of urine may be indicated. ▪ Monitor for anaphylactic-like reactions (e.g., bronchoconstriction, facial edema, hypotension, tachycardia). ▪ Monitor liver function periodically. ▪ Perform neurologic exams on a regular basis. Neuropathy may present as paresthesias, areflexia, and loss of proprioception and vibratory sensation. ▪ Replace depleted electrolytes as necessary. ▪ Observe closely for signs of infection. Prophylactic antibiotics may be indicated pending results of C/S in a febrile neutropenic patient. ▪ Monitor infusion site carefully during infusion; local soft tissue toxicity has been reported with extravasation. ▪ Monitor for thrombocytopenia (platelet count less than 50,000/mm^3). Initiate precautions to prevent excessive bleeding (e.g., inspect IV sites, skin, and mucous membranes; use extreme care during invasive procedures; test urine, emesis, stool, and secretions for occult blood).

Patient Education: Nonhormonal birth control recommended. ▪ See Appendix D, p. 1333.

Maternal/Child: Category D: avoid pregnancy; can cause fetal harm. Has a mutagenic potential. ▪ Discontinue breast-feeding. ▪ Safety and effectiveness for use in pediatric patients not established. ▪ Ototoxicity increased in pediatric patients. All pediatric patients should have audiometric monitoring performed before initiation of therapy, before each dose, and for several years after therapy.

Elderly: Dose selection should be cautious; see Dose Adjustments. ▪ Response (e.g., effectiveness) is similar to younger adults, but length of survival may be shorter. ▪ Incidence of myelosuppression (e.g., severe leukopenia, neutropenia, thrombocytopenia), infectious complications, nephrotoxicity, and peripheral neuropathy may be increased.

DRUG/LAB INTERACTIONS

Ototoxicity and nephrotoxicity are potentiated with other **ototoxic or nephrotoxic agents** (e.g., aminoglycosides [e.g., gentamicin] and loop diuretics [e.g., furosemide (Lasix), ethacrynic acid (Edecrin)]). Concurrent use not recommended (Lasix is used to control fluid overload; use caution). ▪ Serum levels of **anticonvulsant agents** (e.g., phenytoin [Dilantin]) may become subtherapeutic when used concurrently with cisplatin. Monitor anticonvulsant levels; increased doses may be indicated. ▪ Bone marrow toxicity increased with **other antineoplastic agents and/or radiation therapy.** ▪ Synergistic with **etoposide** (VePesid); may be beneficial. ▪ May affect renal excretion and increase toxicity of many drugs **(e.g., bleomycin, methotrexate).** ▪ Response duration may be shortened with concurrent use of **pyridoxine (vitamin B$_6$) and altretamine (Hexalen).** ▪ Do not administer **live virus vaccines** to patients receiving antineoplastic agents.

SIDE EFFECTS

Are frequent; can occur with the initial dose and will become more severe with succeeding doses. Dose-related and cumulative renal insufficiency, including renal failure, is the major dose-limiting toxicity (often noted during the second week following a dose). Acute leukemia, alopecia, anaphylaxis (facial edema, hypotension, tachycardia, and wheezing within minutes of administration), asthenia, cardiac abnormalities, dehydration, diarrhea, electrolyte disturbances (hypocalcemia, hypokalemia, hypomagnesemia, hyponatremia, hypophosphatemia), elevated serum amylase, hemolytic anemia, hepatotoxicity, hyperuricemia, malaise, myelosuppression, nausea and vomiting (acute or delayed), syndrome of inappropriate antidiuretic hormone (SIADH), neurotoxicity (including peripheral neuropathy that may be reversible, leukoencephalopathy, and reversible posterior leukoencephalopathy syndrome [RPLS]), ocular toxicity (e.g., blurred vision, cerebral blindness, optic neuritis, papilledema), ototoxicity including tinnitus and hearing loss in the high-frequency range, peripheral neuropathy (may be irreversible), vascular toxicities (e.g., cerebral arteritis, CVA, MI, or thrombotic microangiopathy [hemo-lytic-uremic syndrome (HUS)]), and vestibular toxicity.

Overdose: Deafness, intractable nausea and vomiting, kidney failure, liver failure, neuritis, ocular toxicity, significant myelosuppression, and death.

ANTIDOTE
Notify physician of all side effects. Cisplatin may have to be discontinued permanently or until recovery. Symptomatic and supportive treatment is indicated. Administration of whole blood products (e.g., packed RBCs, platelets, leukocytes) and/or blood modifiers (e.g., darbepoetin alfa [Aranesp], epoetin alfa [Epogen], filgrastim [Neupogen, Zarxio], pegfilgrastim [Neulasta], sargramostim [Leukine]) may be indicated to treat bone marrow toxicity. Pretreatment with amifostine may reduce nephrotoxic, neurotoxic, and hematologic effects. Treat anaphylaxis with epinephrine, corticosteroids, oxygen, and antihistamines. There is no specific antidote. Hemodialysis appears to have little effect on removing platinum from the body because of the rapid and high degree of protein binding.

CLADRIBINE BBW
(**KLAD**-rih-bean)

Leustatin

Antineoplastic
(antimetabolite)

pH 6 to 6.6

USUAL DOSE
In all situations, may be administered on an outpatient basis with an appropriate pump and a central venous line in place. Administer any subsequent course with extreme caution. Hematologic recovery must be considered.

Hairy cell leukemia: 0.09 mg/kg/day equally distributed as a continuous infusion over 24 hours. Repeat daily for 7 consecutive days.

Chronic lymphocytic leukemia and Waldenström's macroglobulinemia (unlabeled): 0.1 mg/kg/day equally distributed as a continuous infusion over 24 hours for 7 consecutive days.

Acute myeloid leukemia and mantle cell lymphoma (unlabeled): 5 mg/M²/day over 2 hours for 5 days.

DOSE ADJUSTMENTS
May be required with severe bone marrow impairment, with prior radiation or myelosuppressive agents. ▪ May be required in severe renal insufficiency; effects of renal or hepatic impairment on excretion of cladribine not yet clarified for humans. ▪ See Drug/Lab Interactions.

DILUTION
Specific techniques required; see Precautions. Available in single-use 10-mL vials containing 10 mg (1 mg/mL). Contains no preservatives; aseptic technique imperative. May develop a precipitate at low temperatures. Warm naturally to room temperature and shake vigorously. Do not heat or microwave.

Inpatient continuous infusion: Add the calculated daily dose of cladribine through a sterile 0.22-micron disposable hydrophilic syringe filter to an infusion bag containing 500 mL of NS.

Outpatient continuous infusion: A total 7-day dose is added to a calculated amount of bacteriostatic NS to make a total volume of 100 mL. Add the calculated dose of cladribine (7 days × 0.09 mg/kg or 0.09 mL/kg) to the infusion reservoir through the sterile 0.22-micron disposable hydrophilic syringe filter, then add the calculated amount of bacteriostatic NS to the reservoir through the filter. Total volume in the reservoir should equal 100 mL. Specific equipment (i.e., a sterile medication reservoir and pump capable of delivering accurate minute amounts into a central venous line [presently using SIMS

Deltec medication cassette with SIMS Deltec pump]) and a specific process including the use of a 0.22-micron syringe filter are required. Preparation of cassette usually done by pharmacist. Line of cassette remains clamped until attached to central venous line and pump is functional. See literature for details, and follow all specific instructions for medication pump.

Filters: To minimize the risk of microbial contamination, a 0.22-micron hydrophilic syringe filter is required in the preparation of the outpatient continuous infusion.

Storage: Protect from light. Refrigerate before reconstitution. Never refreeze. Discard any unused concentrate. *500 mL dilution* is stable for at least 24 hours at RT under normal fluorescent light; may be refrigerated for up to 8 hours after dilution. Immediate use preferred. *100 mL dilution* is stable in reservoir of medication cassette for 7 days if correctly diluted.

COMPATIBILITY
Consider any drug NOT listed as compatible to be INCOMPATIBLE until consulting a pharmacist; specific conditions may apply.

D5W will cause degradation of cladribine. Manufacturer states, "Adherence to the recommended diluents and infusion systems is advised."

One source suggests the following **compatibilities:**

Y-site: Aminophylline, bumetanide, buprenorphine (Buprenex), butorphanol (Stadol), calcium gluconate, carboplatin (Paraplatin), chlorpromazine (Thorazine), cisplatin, cyclophosphamide (Cytoxan), cytarabine (ARA-C), dexamethasone (Decadron), diphenhydramine (Benadryl), dobutamine, dopamine, doxorubicin (Adriamycin), droperidol (Inapsine), enalaprilat (Vasotec IV), etoposide (VePesid), famotidine (Pepcid IV), furosemide (Lasix), gallium nitrate (Ganite), granisetron (Kytril), heparin, hydrocortisone sodium succinate (Solu-Cortef), hydromorphone (Dilaudid), idarubicin (Idamycin), leucovorin calcium, lorazepam (Ativan), mannitol, meperidine (Demerol), mesna (Mesnex), methylprednisolone (Solu-Medrol), metoclopramide (Reglan), mitoxantrone (Novantrone), morphine, nalbuphine, ondansetron (Zofran), paclitaxel (Taxol), potassium chloride (KCl), prochlorperazine (Compazine), promethazine (Phenergan), ranitidine (Zantac), sodium bicarbonate, teniposide (Vumon), vincristine.

RATE OF ADMINISTRATION
Inpatient continuous infusion: A single dose properly diluted evenly distributed as an infusion over 24 hours.

Outpatient continuous infusion: Administered through a central venous line (very concentrated solution). Medication reservoir and pump required (presently using Pharmacia Deltec medication cassette and pump worn as a portable pack). Set rate for equal distribution of 100 mL over 7 days. Follow all specific instructions for pump.

ACTIONS
A chlorinated purine nucleoside analog and synthetic antineoplastic agent. Mechanism of action is not known, but it is believed to be cytotoxic by inhibiting both DNA synthesis and repair. Affects both dividing and resting cells. The 7-day course for hairy cell leukemia has resulted in complete response in a majority of patients with no evidence of persistent bone marrow disease. Crosses the blood-brain barrier. Average half-life is 4.2 to 9.2 hours. Specific methods of metabolism and routes of excretion are not known. Some drug does appear in urine.

INDICATIONS AND USES
Treatment of active hairy cell leukemia (HCL) as defined by clinically significant anemia, neutropenia, thrombocytopenia, or disease-related symptoms.

Unlabeled uses: Treatment of acute myeloid leukemia, chronic lymphocytic leukemia, mantle cell lymphoma, and Waldenström's macroglobulinemia.

CONTRAINDICATIONS
Hypersensitivity to cladribine or any of its components; neonates (7-day dilution contains benzyl alcohol).

PRECAUTIONS

Follow guidelines for handling cytotoxic agents. See Appendix A, p. 1331. ▪ Administered by or under the direction of the physician specialist. ▪ Anticipate severe suppression of bone marrow function, including neutropenia, anemia, and thrombocytopenia; usually reversible and appears to be dose dependent. ▪ Myelosuppressive effects are most notable during the first month after therapy. ▪ Serious, sometimes fatal, infections have been reported (e.g., respiratory tract infections, pneumonia, viral skin infections, sepsis). ▪ Neurologic toxicity, including paraparesis and quadriparesis, has been reported. Usually occurs with higher doses but has been seen with standard dosing regimens. ▪ Because of the possibility of increased toxicity, use caution in known or suspected renal or hepatic insufficiency, or any severe bone marrow impairment, or prior cytoxic or radiation therapy. ▪ Acute nephrotoxicity has been observed with high doses (4 to 9 times the recommended dose for HCL). Risk of toxicity increased when given concurrently with other nephrotoxic agents and/or therapies. ▪ Rare cases of tumor lysis syndrome have been reported. ▪ Appears to be no relationship between serum concentrations and ultimate clinical outcome. ▪ Additional courses did not improve overall response. ▪ Current studies suggest that overall response rate may be decreased in patients previously treated with splenectomy, deoxycoformycin (pentostatin), and in patients refractory to alpha-interferon. ▪ May cause prolonged bone marrow hypocellularity; clinical significance not known.

Monitor: Obtain baseline CBC with differential and platelets before therapy. May be repeated as indicated, but usually not required again until 7 or 8 days after treatment begins; then monitor as indicated for at least 4 to 8 weeks (anemia, neutropenia, thrombocytopenia, infection [bacterial, fungal, or viral], and bleeding are common and must be treated promptly). Monitoring schedule facilitates outpatient treatment; keep in close contact with patient. ▪ Consider possibility of infection if fever occurs; appropriate lab tests, x-rays, and broad-spectrum antibiotics may be indicated, especially in a febrile neutropenic patient. ▪ Monitor uric acid levels before and during treatment; maintain hydration; allopurinol may be indicated (preferred agent). Alkalinization of urine may also be indicated. ▪ Monitor renal and hepatic function periodically. ▪ Platelet count usually returns to normal in 12 days (may be delayed if severe baseline thrombocytopenia was present), absolute neutrophil count (ANC) usually returns to normal in 5 weeks, and hemoglobin in 8 weeks. All should be normal by 9 weeks. ▪ Complete response is indicated by an absence of hairy cells in bone marrow and peripheral blood and normalization of peripheral blood parameters. Confirm response with bone marrow aspiration and biopsy between 9 weeks and 4 months. ▪ Prophylactic antiemetics may improve patient comfort. ▪ Monitor for thrombocytopenia (platelet count less than $50,000/mm^3$). Initiate precautions to prevent excessive bleeding (e.g., inspect IV sites, skin, and mucous membranes; use extreme care during invasive procedures; test urine, emesis, stool, and secretions for occult blood). Avoid constipation and avoid alcohol and aspirin (risk of GI bleeding).

Patient Education: Avoid pregnancy; consider birth control options and future fertility. ▪ Report fever, bleeding, cough, edema, injection site reactions, malaise, mouth sores, rashes, shortness of breath, stomach pain, and tachycardia promptly. Maintain hydration. ▪ Manufacturer supplies a patient education booklet; review thoroughly and discuss with physician and nurse. ▪ Review all literature provided with pump to deliver outpatient dosing. ▪ See Appendix D, p. 1333.

Maternal/Child: Category D: avoid pregnancy; has potential to cause fetal harm. Has caused suppression of testicular cells in monkeys; effect on human fertility unknown. ▪ Discontinue breast-feeding. ▪ Safety for use in pediatric patients not established. Investigationally used in higher doses to treat relapsed acute leukemia. Dose-limiting toxicity occurred.

Elderly: Geriatric-specific problems not encountered in studies to date. Consider age-related organ impairment.

DRUG/LAB INTERACTIONS
Increased toxicity with other **myelosuppressive agents** (e.g., methotrexate). ▪ May raise concentration of blood uric acid; increased doses of **antigout agents** (e.g., allopurinol [Aloprim]) may be indicated; **avoid uricosurics** (e.g., probenecid, sulfinpyrazone [Anturane]). ▪ Do not administer **live attenuated vaccines** to patients receiving antineoplastic agents.

SIDE EFFECTS
Fever occurs first. Onset of thrombocytopenia begins in 7 to 10 days followed by anemia (severe) and neutropenia (severe). Fatigue, headache, injection site reactions, infection, nausea, and rash are common. Many other side effects may or may not be related to cladribine: abdominal pain, abnormal breath sounds, abnormal chest sounds, anorexia, arthralgia, asthenia, chills, constipation, cough, diaphoresis, diarrhea, dizziness, edema, epistaxis, erythema, insomnia, malaise, myalgia, pain, petechiae, pruritus, purpura, shortness of breath, tachycardia, trunk pain, weakness, vomiting.

Post-Marketing: Most of these additional side effects occurred in patients who received multiple courses of cladribine and include altered level of consciousness, aplastic anemia, conjunctivitis, elevated bilirubin and transaminases, hemolytic anemia, hypereosinophilia, hypersensitivity, myelodysplastic syndrome, neurologic toxicity, opportunistic infections, pulmonary interstitial infiltrates (usually with an infectious etiology), renal impairment, Stevens-Johnson syndrome, toxic epidermal necrolysis, and tumor lysis syndrome.

Overdose: Acute nephrotoxicity, irreversible neurologic toxicity (paraparesis/quadriparesis), severe bone marrow suppression (anemia, neutropenia, and thrombocytopenia).

ANTIDOTE
Keep physician informed of all side effects; many will be treated symptomatically as indicated. Platelet or RBC transfusions are frequently required to treat anemia or thrombocytopenia, especially during the first month. Filgrastim (Neupogen, Zarxio) or pegfilgrastim (Neulasta) may be used to increase neutrophil count, although recovery is usually spontaneous. Use specific antibiotics to combat infection. Discontinue cladribine if renal toxicity, neurotoxicity, or overdose occurs. No specific antidote for overdose. Supportive therapy as indicated will help sustain the patient in toxicity. Resuscitate if indicated.

CLEVIDIPINE BUTYRATE
(klev-**ID**-i-peen **BUE**-tih-rate)

Calcium channel blocker
Antihypertensive

Cleviprex

pH 6 to 8

USUAL DOSE
Must be individualized to achieve the desired BP reduction. Titrate to patient response and BP goal.

Initial dose: 1 to 2 mg/hr (2 to 4 mL/hr) as a continuous infusion.

Dose titration: Initially, double the dose at 90-second intervals. As the BP approaches goal, increase the dose by less than doubling and lengthen the time between dose adjustments to every 5 to 10 minutes. In general, a 1- to 2-mg/hr increase in dose will produce an additional 2- to 4-mm Hg decrease in systolic pressure. The maximum dose used for most patients in studies was 16 mg/hr.

Maintenance dose: The desired therapeutic response for most patients occurs at 4 to 6 mg/hr (8 to 12 mL/hr). Doses as high as 32 mg/hr (64 mL/hr) have been administered. Data are limited. Because of lipid-load restrictions, no more than 1,000 mL or an average of 21 mg/hr (42 mL/hr) is recommended per 24-hour period. In studies, most infusions were administered for less than 24 hours. There is little experience with infusions lasting more than 72 hours at any dose.

Transition to oral therapy: Discontinue or titrate the infusion downward while establishing appropriate oral therapy. Consider the lag time of onset of oral agent's effect. See Monitor.

DOSE ADJUSTMENTS
Lower-end initial doses may be indicated in the elderly. Consider the potential for decreased organ function and concomitant disease or drug therapy. ■ Patients with abnormal hepatic or renal function may receive the initial dose listed under Usual Dose.

DILUTION
Strict aseptic technique is imperative. Available as a single-dose, ready-to-use vial containing a 0.5-mg/mL phospholipid emulsion that can support microbial growth. Invert vial gently several times before use to ensure uniformity of emulsion.

Filter: No data available from manufacturer.

Storage: Refrigerate unopened vials at 2° to 8° C (36° to 46° F) or store at 25° C (77° F) for up to 2 months. Vials stored at RT should not be returned to the refrigerator. Do not freeze. Protect from light until administration. Once vial is punctured, use within 4 hours and discard any unused portion, including that which is currently being infused.

COMPATIBILITY
Manufacturer states, "Should not be administered in the same line as other medications. Should not be diluted, but can be administered via a Y-tube or medication port with SWFI, NS, D5W, D5NS, D5LR, LR, and 10% amino acid."

RATE OF ADMINISTRATION
Administer as a continuous infusion as outlined in Usual Dose. Use of an infusion device required. May be given through a central or peripheral line.

ACTIONS
A dihydropyridine calcium channel blocker. Mediates the influx of calcium during depolarization in arterial smooth muscle. Reduces mean arterial BP by decreasing systemic vascular resistance in a dose-dependent manner. Does not reduce cardiac filling pressure (preload), confirming the lack of effect on venous capacitance vessels. Vasodilation and the resulting decrease in BP may produce a reflex increase in heart rate. Onset of effects begins within 2 to 4 minutes. Evidence of tolerance or hysteresis has not been observed in patients receiving infusions of up to 72 hours' duration. Full recovery of BP is achieved 5 to 15 minutes after the infusion is stopped. Rapidly distributed. Highly protein bound. Metabolized by hydrolysis in the blood and extravascular tissues, making its

elimination unlikely to be affected by hepatic or renal dysfunction. Half-life is approximately 15 minutes. Excreted primarily in urine and, to a lesser extent, in feces.

INDICATIONS AND USES
Reduction of BP when oral therapy is not feasible or not desirable.

CONTRAINDICATIONS
Allergies to soybeans, soy products, eggs, or egg products. ■ Defective lipid metabolism such as pathologic hyperlipidemia, lipoid nephrosis, or acute pancreatitis if accompanied by hyperlipidemia. ■ Severe aortic stenosis (afterload reduction can be expected to reduce myocardial oxygen delivery).

PRECAUTIONS
For IV use only. ■ Strict aseptic technique required; see Dilution. ■ May produce systemic hypotension and reflex tachycardia. Dose reduction may be indicated. ■ Use caution in patients with lipid metabolism disorders. Contains approximately 0.2 Gm of lipid per mL. Lipid intake restrictions may be necessary in these patients. A reduction in the quantity of concurrently administered lipids (e.g., propofol, IV fat) may be necessary to compensate for the amount of lipid infused as part of the clevidipine formulation. See Usual Dose. ■ May produce a negative inotropic effect and exacerbate heart failure. ■ Rebound hypertension may occur in patients undergoing prolonged therapy; see Monitor. ■ Has not been studied for the treatment of hypertension associated with pheochromocytoma.

Monitor: Monitor BP and HR during infusion and until vital signs are stable. ■ Rebound hypertension may occur in patients who receive a prolonged infusion and are not transitioned to other antihypertensive therapies. Monitor BP for at least 8 hours after the infusion is discontinued. ■ During transition to oral therapy, continue BP monitoring until patient is stabilized. ■ Monitor heart failure patients closely.

Patient Education: Promptly report signs of a hypertensive emergency (e.g., neurologic symptoms, vision changes, evidence of CHF). ■ Continued follow-up and treatment of pre-existing hypertension required.

Maternal/Child: Category C: use during pregnancy only if potential benefit justifies potential risk to the fetus. ■ Safety in labor and delivery not established. Other calcium channel blockers suppress uterine contractions in humans. ■ Safety for use in breast-feeding not established; effects unknown. ■ Safety and effectiveness for use in pediatric patients not established.

Elderly: Response similar to that seen in younger adults; however, greater sensitivity in the elderly cannot be ruled out. ■ See Dose Adjustments.

DRUG/LAB INTERACTIONS
Formal studies have not been conducted. ■ Does not have the potential for inducing or inhibiting the cytochrome P_{450} system. ■ Use of **beta-blockers** as treatment for clevidipine-induced reflex tachycardia is not recommended. Experience is limited. ■ If used concomitantly with **beta-blockers** and beta-blockers are to be discontinued, withdraw beta-blocker therapy gradually. Clevidipine will not protect against the effects of abrupt beta-blocker withdrawal.

SIDE EFFECTS
Acute renal failure, atrial fibrillation, cardiac arrest, dyspnea, flushing, headache, hypotension, myocardial infarction, nausea, peripheral edema, rebound hypertension, reflex tachycardia, syncope, and vomiting.

Post-Marketing: Decreased oxygen saturation (possible pulmonary shunting), hypersensitivity reactions, increased blood triglycerides, ileus.

ANTIDOTE
Notify physician of any side effects; most will be treated symptomatically. Reduce dose for systemic hypotension or reflex tachycardia. Discontinue for suspected overdose. Reduction in antihypertensive effects should be seen within 5 to 15 minutes. Monitor BP and support if needed. Resuscitate as necessary.

CLINDAMYCIN PHOSPHATE BBW
(klin-dah-**MY**-cin **FOS**-fayt)

Antibacterial
Antiprotozoal
(lincosamide)

Cleocin Phosphate

pH 5.5 to 7

USUAL DOSE
Doses based on susceptibility of specific organisms; see literature.

Serious infections: 600 to 1,200 mg/24 hr in 2, 3, or 4 equally divided doses (300 to 600 mg every 12 hours, 200 to 400 mg every 8 hours, or 150 to 300 mg every 6 hours).

More severe infections: 1,200 to 2,700 mg/24 hr in 2, 3, or 4 equally divided doses (600 to 1,350 mg every 12 hours, 400 to 900 mg every 8 hours, or 300 to 675 mg every 6 hours).

Life-threatening infections: Up to 4,800 mg/24 hr has been given.

Acute pelvic inflammatory disease (unlabeled): 900 mg every 8 hours. Used in combination with gentamicin. Continue both drugs for at least 24 hours after patient improves. Complete 14-day treatment program with oral doxycycline or clindamycin.

CNS toxoplasmosis in AIDS (unlabeled): 600 mg every 6 hours. Used in combination with pyrimethamine (Daraprim) and leucovorin.

***Pneumocystis jiroveci* pneumonia (unlabeled):** 600 mg every 6 hours or 900 mg every 8 hours. Used in combination with primaquine.

Babesiosis (unlabeled): 1,200 to 2,400 mg/24 hr in 4 equally divided doses (300 to 600 mg every 6 hours). Continue for 7 to 10 days. Used in combination with quinine.

Prophylaxis of bacterial endocarditis: 600 mg IV or PO 30 minutes before procedure.

PEDIATRIC DOSE
Pediatric patients over 1 month of age: 20 to 40 mg/kg of body weight/24 hr in 3 or 4 equally divided doses based on the seriousness of the infection (5 to 10 mg/kg every 6 hours or 6.66 to 13.3 mg/kg every 8 hours). Alternately 350 mg/M^2/24 hr may be used (87.5 mg/M^2 every 6 hours or 116.6 mg/M^2 every 8 hours). 450 mg/M^2/24 hr may be used for more serious infections if necessary (112.5 mg/M^2 every 6 hours or 150 mg/M^2 every 8 hours).

Prophylaxis of bacterial endocarditis: 20 mg/kg IV or PO 30 minutes before procedure. Do not exceed adult dose.

NEONATAL DOSE
See Maternal/Child.

Under 1 month of age, full term: 3.75 to 5 mg/kg every 6 hours or 5 to 6.7 mg/kg every 8 hours. Another source suggests:

Neonates 7 days of age or less weighing less than or equal to 2 kg: 5 mg/kg every 12 hours.

Neonates 7 days of age or less weighing over 2 kg: 5 mg/kg every 8 hours.

Neonates over 7 days of age weighing less than 1.2 kg: 5 mg/kg every 12 hours.

Neonates over 7 days of age weighing 1.2 to 2 kg: 5 mg/kg every 8 hours.

Neonates over 7 days of age weighing over 2 kg: 5 mg/kg every 6 hours.

DOSE ADJUSTMENTS
Dose adjustments are not required in the presence of mild to moderate renal or hepatic disease and should not be required in severe disease; see Monitor.

DILUTION
Available prediluted in 300-, 600-, and 900-mg doses, in ADD-Vantage vials for use with ADD-Vantage infusion containers, as a 150 mg/mL solution in flip-top vials, in ready-to-use Galaxy bags, and in pharmacy bulk packages (for use only by the pharmacy). Dilute ADD-Vantage vials with 50 to 100 mL of D5W or NS. Doses prepared using the 150 mg/mL solutions are most commonly diluted in 50 to 100 mL of D5W, NS, or other **compatible** infusion solution. Concentration of clindamycin in diluent should not exceed 18 mg/mL. See chart on inside back cover or product insert for additional diluents. May

be further diluted in larger amounts of **compatible** infusion solutions and given as a continuous infusion after the initial dose.

Storage: Store vials at CRT before use. Administration as soon as possible after dilution is recommended. Stable at CRT for at least 24 hours in **compatible** infusion solutions. See manufacturer's literature for additional stability data if diluted solutions are kept at RT, refrigerated, or frozen. Frozen solutions should be thawed at room temperature and not refrozen.

COMPATIBILITY   (Underline Indicates Conflicting Compatibility Information)

Consider any drug NOT listed as compatible to be INCOMPATIBLE until consulting a pharmacist; specific conditions may apply.

Manufacturer lists as **compatible** for 24 hours at RT with IV solutions containing sodium chloride, glucose, calcium, or potassium and with solutions containing vitamin B complex in concentrations usually used clinically. Manufacturer states, "No **incompatibility** has been demonstrated with the antibiotics gentamicin, kanamycin, or penicillin."

Manufacturer lists as **incompatible** with aminophylline, ampicillin, barbiturates, calcium gluconate, magnesium sulfate, phenytoin (Dilantin).

Sources suggest the following **compatibilities:**

Solution: Isolyte H, D5/Isolyte M, D5/Isolyte P, Normosol R; see chart on inside back cover.

Additive: Manufacturer states no **incompatibility** has been demonstrated with gentamicin or penicillin. Other sources list amikacin, ampicillin, aztreonam (Azactam), cefazolin (Ancef), cefepime (Maxipime), cefotaxime (Claforan), cefoxitin (Mefoxin), ceftazidime (Fortaz), cefuroxime (Zinacef), fluconazole (Diflucan), heparin, hydrocortisone sodium succinate (Solu-Cortef), methylprednisolone (Solu-Medrol), metoclopramide (Reglan), potassium chloride (KCl), ranitidine (Zantac), sodium bicarbonate, tobramycin, verapamil.

Y-site: Acyclovir (Zovirax), amifostine (Ethyol), amiodarone (Nexterone), amphotericin B cholesteryl (Amphotec), anidulafungin (Eraxis), aztreonam (Azactam), bivalirudin (Angiomax), ceftaroline (Teflaro), cisatracurium (Nimbex), cyclophosphamide (Cytoxan), dexmedetomidine (Precedex), diltiazem (Cardizem), docetaxel (Taxotere), doxorubicin liposomal (Doxil), enalaprilat (Vasotec IV), esmolol (Brevibloc), etoposide phosphate (Etopophos), fenoldopam (Corlopam), fludarabine (Fludara), foscarnet (Foscavir), gemcitabine (Gemzar), granisetron (Kytril), heparin, hetastarch in electrolytes (Hextend), hydromorphone (Dilaudid), 6% hydroxyethyl starch (Voluven), labetalol, levofloxacin (Levaquin), linezolid (Zyvox), magnesium sulfate, melphalan (Alkeran), meperidine (Demerol), midazolam (Versed), milrinone (Primacor), morphine, multivitamins (M.V.I.), nicardipine (Cardene IV), ondansetron (Zofran), pemetrexed (Alimta), piperacillin/tazobactam (Zosyn), propofol (Diprivan), remifentanil (Ultiva), sargramostim (Leukine), tacrolimus (Prograf), teniposide (Vumon), theophylline, thiotepa, vinorelbine (Navelbine), zidovudine (AZT, Retrovir).

RATE OF ADMINISTRATION

Should not be administered intravenously undiluted as a bolus. Severe hypotension and cardiac arrest can occur with too-rapid injection.

Intermittent infusion: 30 mg or fraction thereof over at least 1 minute (each 300 mg over a minimum of 10 minutes/1,200 mg over a minimum of 40 to 60 minutes). Do not give more than 1,200 mg in single 1-hour infusion.

Continuous infusion: Administer initial dose at 10 (15 or 20) mg/min over 30 minutes (rapid infusion rate). Will result in serum levels above 4 (5 or 6) mg/mL. To maintain these serum levels, continue infusion at 0.75 (1 or 1.25) mg/min.

ACTIONS

A semi-synthetic antibiotic that quickly converts to active clindamycin. Bacteriostatic with activity against gram-positive aerobes and anaerobes, as well as some gram-negative anaerobes. It inhibits bacterial protein synthesis by binding to the 50S subunit of the ribosome. Widely distributed in most body fluids and tissues. There is no clinically effective distribution to cerebrospinal fluid. Half-life is approximately 3 hours. Excreted in urine and feces in small amounts. Crosses placental barrier. Secreted in breast milk.

INDICATIONS AND USES

Treatment of serious infections caused by susceptible anaerobic bacteria; treatment of infections due to susceptible strains of streptococcal, pneumococcal, and staphylococcal bacteria in penicillin-allergic patients; or treatment of infections that do not respond or are resistant to other less toxic antibiotics, such as erythromycin. Conditions indicated include septicemia, lower respiratory tract infections (including pneumonia), and skin and skin structure, gynecologic, intra-abdominal, and bone and joint infections.

Unlabeled uses: Alternative to sulfonamides with pyrimethamine to treat CNS toxoplasmosis in AIDS patients. ▪ Treat *Pneumocystis jiroveci* pneumonia in combination with primaquine. ▪ Treatment of babesiosis. ▪ Prophylaxis of bacterial endocarditis. ▪ Treatment of acute pelvic inflammatory disease.

CONTRAINDICATIONS

Known hypersensitivity to clindamycin or lincomycin.

PRECAUTIONS

To reduce the development of drug-resistant bacteria and maintain its effectiveness, clindamycin should be used to treat or prevent only those infections proven or strongly suspected to be caused by bacteria. ▪ Sensitivity studies are indicated to determine susceptibility of the causative organism to clindamycin. ▪ Avoid prolonged use; superinfection caused by overgrowth of nonsusceptible organisms may result. ▪ Because its use has been associated with severe colitis, it should be reserved for serious infections in which less toxic antimicrobial agents are inappropriate. ▪ *Clostridium difficile*–associated diarrhea (CDAD) has been reported. May range from mild diarrhea to fatal colitis. Consider in patients who present with diarrhea during or after treatment with clindamycin. ▪ Use caution with a history of GI, severe renal, or liver disease, and in patients with a history of asthma or significant allergies. ▪ Severe skin reactions such as toxic epidermal necrolysis, some with fatal outcome, have been reported. ▪ Serious anaphylactoid reactions have been reported. ▪ Certain infections may require incision and drainage or other indicated surgical procedures in addition to antibiotic therapy. ▪ Not appropriate to treat meningitis.

Monitor: Capable of causing severe, even fatal, colitis; observe for symptoms of diarrhea. ▪ Periodic blood cell counts and liver and kidney studies are indicated in prolonged therapy. ▪ Monitor liver enzymes periodically in patients with severe liver disease. ▪ Monitor for S/S of hypersensitivity reactions, including severe skin and anaphylactoid reactions.

Patient Education: Promptly report diarrhea or bloody stools that occur during treatment or up to several months after an antibiotic has been discontinued; may indicate CDAD and require treatment. ▪ Do not treat diarrhea without notifying physician.

Maternal/Child: Category B: in clinical trials with pregnant women, the systemic administration of clindamycin during the second or third trimesters has not been associated with an increased frequency of congenital abnormalities. Should be used during the first trimester only if clearly needed. ▪ Discontinue breast-feeding. ▪ Contains benzyl alcohol, which has been associated with a fatal "gasping syndrome" in neonates. ▪ Benzyl alcohol can cross the placenta. ▪ Monitor organ system functions if used in pediatric patients.

Elderly: CDAD may occur more frequently in elderly patients (greater than 60 years of age) and may be more severe. Monitor carefully for changes in bowel frequency; may not tolerate diarrhea well.

DRUG/LAB INTERACTIONS

May potentiate **neuromuscular blocking agents** (e.g., atracurium [Tracrium]) and cause profound respiratory depression. ▪ Antagonized by **erythromycin.** ▪ May decrease **cyclosporine** (Sandimmune) levels. Monitor and adjust dose if necessary.

SIDE EFFECTS

Abdominal pain, abnormal liver function tests, agranulocytosis, anaphylaxis, azotemia, cardiac arrest, CDAD, diarrhea, drug reaction with eosinophilia and systemic symptoms

(DRESS), eosinophilia (transient), esophagitis, hypersensitivity reactions, hypotension, injection site reactions, jaundice, leukopenia, metallic taste, nausea, neutropenia (transient), oliguria, polyarthritis (rare), proteinuria, pruritus, pseudomembranous colitis, severe skin reactions (e.g., toxic epidermal necrolysis, acute generalized exanthematous pustulosis [AGEP], erythema multiforme), skin rashes, thrombophlebitis, urticaria, vaginitis, vomiting.

ANTIDOTE

Notify the physician of any side effects. Discontinue the drug if indicated (e.g., CDAD, diarrhea, hypersensitivity reactions, severe skin reaction), treat hypersensitivity reactions as indicated, and resuscitate as necessary. Mild cases of CDAD may respond to discontinuation of drug. Treat CDAD with fluids, electrolytes, protein supplements, and oral vancomycin (Vancocin) or metronidazole (Flagyl) as indicated. In severe cases, surgical evaluation may be indicated. Hemodialysis or CAPD will not decrease blood levels in toxicity.

CLOFARABINE

(kloh-**FARE**-ah-bean)

Clolar

Antineoplastic
(metabolic inhibitor)

pH 4.5 to 7.5

PEDIATRIC DOSE

Premedication: Consider prophylactic antiemetic medications. Consider use of prophylactic steroids (e.g., hydrocortisone 100 mg/M^2 on Days 1 through 3) to mitigate or prevent the development of systemic inflammatory response syndrome (SIRS) or capillary leak syndrome (e.g., hypotension, pulmonary edema, tachycardia, tachypnea). See Drug/Lab Interactions.

Clofarabine: 52 mg/M^2 as an infusion each day for 5 consecutive days. Dose is based on body surface area (BSA), which is calculated using the actual height and weight before the start of each cycle. Repeat every 2 to 6 weeks; see Dose Adjustments. Frequency is based on recovery or return to baseline organ function. Median time between cycles during clinical studies was 28 days (range 12 to 55 days).

DOSE ADJUSTMENTS

Administer subsequent cycles no sooner than 14 days from the starting day of the previous cycle provided the patient's ANC is greater than or equal to 0.75 × 10^9/L. ▪ Reduce dose by 50% in patients with a CrCl between 30 and 60 mL/min. Information is insufficient to make a dose recommendation in patients with a CrCl less than 30 mL/min or in patients on dialysis. ▪ Reduce the dose of the next cycle by 25% in patients experiencing a Grade 4 neutropenia (ANC less than 0.5 × 10^9/L) that lasts 4 or more weeks. ▪ Withhold clofarabine if a clinically significant infection develops. When the infection is clinically controlled, restart therapy at full dose. ▪ Discontinue if hypotension develops at any time during the 5 days of administration. ▪ Discontinue drug immediately if Grade 3 or higher increases in SCr, liver enzymes, or bilirubin occur; see Monitor and Antidote. May be restarted (generally with a 25% dose reduction) when the patient is stable and organ function has returned to baseline. ▪ Discontinue drug immediately if S/S of SIRS or capillary leak syndrome occur; see Monitor and Antidote. May be restarted (generally with a 25% dose reduction) when the patient is stable. ▪ Withhold clofarabine if a Grade 3 noninfectious nonhematologic toxicity occurs (excluding transient elevations in serum transaminases and/or serum bilirubin and/or nausea and vomiting that is controlled by antiemetics). With resolution or a return to baseline, restart clofarabine at a 25% dose reduction. ▪ Discontinue therapy if a Grade 4 noninfectious nonhematologic toxicity occurs.

DILUTION

Specific techniques required; see Precautions. Available in single-use 20-mL vials containing 20 mg (1 mg/mL). Contains no preservatives; aseptic technique is imperative.
Calculate the exact number of vials needed to achieve the total dosing volume required.

$$\text{Total number of vials required} = \text{Total dose (mg)} \div 20 \text{ mg}$$

$$\text{Dosing volume (mL)} = \text{Total dose (mg)}$$

For example, a child with a body surface area (BSA) of 0.75 M^2 would need a dose of 39 mg of clofarabine (39 ÷ 20 mg = 1.95 vials, so 2 vials of clofarabine would be needed; 39 mg equals a dosing volume of 39 mL).

Withdraw the calculated dose from the vial(s). Using a 0.2-micron syringe filter, add the calculated dose to a sufficient volume of D5W or NS to provide a final concentration between 0.15 mg/mL and 0.4 mg/mL (e.g., 39 mg [39 mL in the example above] added to 100 mL of D5W or NS will provide a final concentration of approximately 0.28 mg/mL).

Filters: Use of a 0.2-micron syringe filter is recommended for use during dilution in D5W or NS.

Storage: Store unopened vials at CRT. Diluted solutions may be stored at CRT but must be used within 24 hours.

COMPATIBILITY

Manufacturer states, "To prevent drug **incompatibilities,** no other medications should be administered through the same IV line."

RATE OF ADMINISTRATION

A single dose properly diluted and evenly distributed as an infusion over 2 hours.

ACTIONS

A purine nucleoside metabolic inhibitor. Acts by inhibiting DNA synthesis. Also disrupts the mitochondrial membrane, causing the release of mitochondrial proteins, cytochrome C, and apoptosis-inducing factor, which leads to cell death. Is cytotoxic to rapidly proliferating and quiescent cancer cell types in vitro. Results in a rapid reduction of peripheral leukemia cells. Metabolism in the liver is very limited. Pathways of nonhepatic elimination not known. Estimated half-life is 5.2 hours. Excreted primarily in the urine.

INDICATIONS AND USES

Treatment of pediatric patients 1 to 21 years of age with relapsed or refractory acute lymphoblastic leukemia (ALL) after treatment with at least two prior regimens. This indication is based on response rate. There are no trials verifying an improvement in disease-related symptoms or increased survival with clofarabine.

Unlabeled uses: Treatment of other relapsed or refractory leukemias, including acute myelocytic leukemia (AML), myelodysplastic syndrome (MDS), and chronic myeloid leukemia in blast phase.

CONTRAINDICATIONS

Manufacturer states, "None."

PRECAUTIONS

Follow guidelines for handling cytotoxic agents. See Appendix A, p. 1331. ▪ Administered by or under the direction of the physician specialist in a facility with adequate diagnostic and treatment facilities to monitor the patient and respond to any medical emergency. ▪ At the initiation of treatment, most patients have hematologic impairment as a manifestation of the leukemia. Clofarabine causes myelosuppression, which may be severe and prolonged. Treatment may result in prolonged and severe neutropenia, including febrile neutropenia. Patients may be at an increased risk for infection, including severe and fatal sepsis and opportunistic infections. ▪ Use with great caution in patients with impaired hepatic or renal function. ▪ May develop tumor lysis syndrome, cytokine release syndrome, systemic inflammatory response syndrome, capillary leak syndrome, and organ dysfunction; deaths have been reported; see Monitor. ▪ Serious and fatal hemorrhage, including cerebral, GI, and pulmonary hemorrhage, has occurred. Most cases were associated with thrombocytopenia; see Monitor. ▪ Patients who have previously received a hematopoietic stem cell transplant (HSCT) are at higher risk for hepatotoxicity suggestive of veno-occlusive disease (VOD) following treatment with clofarabine (40 mg/M^2) used in combination with etoposide (VePesid 100 mg/M^2) and cyclophosphamide (Cytoxan 440 mg/M^2); has also been reported with monotherapy. ▪ Severe and fatal hepatotoxic events, including hepatitis and hepatic failure, have been reported; see Monitor. ▪ Renal toxicity, including Grade 3 or 4 elevated creatinine, acute renal failure, and hematuria, have been reported; see Monitor and Dose Adjustments. ▪ Fatal and serious cases of enterocolitis (neutropenic colitis, cecitis, and *C. difficile* colitis) have been reported. Occurs more frequently within 30 days of treatment and in the setting of combination chemotherapy. May lead to necrosis, perforation, hemorrhage, or sepsis complications. ▪ Serious and fatal skin reactions (Stevens-Johnson syndrome [SJS] and toxic epidermal necrolysis [TEN]) have been reported. ▪ Safety and effectiveness in adults not established. In a Phase 1 study of adults with refractory and/or relapsed hematologic malignancies, the pediatric dose of 52 mg/M^2 was not tolerated.

Monitor: Obtain baseline CBC with differential and platelets and serum electrolytes. Bone marrow suppression is expected. Appears to be dose-dependent and is usually reversible (with interruption of clofarabine treatment) but can be severe; monitor regularly and more frequently in patients who develop cytopenias. Monitoring of CBC and platelets is recommended daily during the 5 days of clofarabine administration, then 1 to 2 times weekly or as clinically indicated. ▪ Obtain baseline renal and hepatic function studies (e.g., SCr, bilirubin, ALT, AST), and uric acid levels. Monitor renal and hepatic function closely during the 5 days of clofarabine administration. Monitor for S/S of hepatitis and hepatic failure. Discontinue drug immediately if Grade 3 or higher increases in SCr, liver enzymes, or bilirubin occur; see Antidote. ▪ Monitor HR, BP, and respiratory status closely during infusion. Hypotension should be reported immediately; see Antidote. ▪ Monitor for S/S of tumor lysis syndrome (e.g., hyperkalemia, hyperphosphatemia, hyperuricemia, hypocalcemia, metabolic acidosis, urate crystalluria, and renal failure). Adequate hydration, antihyperuricemics (e.g., allopurinol), and alkalinization of urine are indicated to prevent and/or treat hyperuricemia due to tumor lysis syndrome. ▪ Monitor for S/S of cytokine release syndrome (e.g., hypotension, pulmonary edema, tachycardia, tachypnea); may develop into systemic inflammatory response syndrome (SIRS)/ capillary leak syndrome (rapid onset of respiratory distress, hypotension, pleural and pericardial effusion, and multiorgan failure). Close monitoring and early intervention may reduce risk; see Pediatric Dose and Antidote. To reduce the effects of tumor lysis and other adverse events (e.g., SIRS), the continuous administration of IV fluids throughout the 5 days of clofarabine treatment is recommended. ▪ Observe closely for signs of infection. Prophylactic antibiotics may be indicated pending the result of C/S in a febrile neutropenic patient. ▪ Use prophylactic antiemetics to reduce nausea and vomiting and increase patient comfort. ▪ Monitor for thrombocytopenia (platelet count less than 50,000/mm^3). Initiate precautions to prevent excessive bleeding (e.g., inspect IV sites, skin, and mucous membranes; use extreme care during invasive procedures; test urine, emesis, stool, and secretions for occult blood). ▪ Monitor patients for S/S of enterocolitis and treat promptly. ▪ Monitor for development of skin reactions.

Patient Education: Avoid pregnancy; nonhormonal birth control recommended for men and women. Report a suspected pregnancy immediately. ▪ Drink plenty of fluids and avoid dehydration that may be caused by diarrhea and vomiting; report promptly if significant. ▪ Laboratory monitoring required. ▪ Promptly report bleeding, decreased urine output, dizziness, fainting spells, infection, jaundice, light-headedness, rapid respiratory rate, or a rapid heart rate. ▪ Review medications with pharmacist or physician. Avoid medications that may be hepatotoxic or nephrotoxic, including OTC or herbal medications. ▪ Skin rash may occur; report promptly if significant. ▪ See Appendix D, p. 1333.

Maternal/Child: Category D: avoid pregnancy; may cause fetal harm. Also has dose-related effects on male reproductive organs in animals. ▪ Discontinue breast-feeding.
Elderly: Not indicated in this patient population.

DRUG/LAB INTERACTIONS

Clinical drug-drug interactions have not been studied; however, the following cautions should be considered. ▪ Primarily excreted by the kidneys; minimize exposure to drugs with known renal toxicity during the 5 days of clofarabine administration (e.g., **aminoglycosides** [e.g., gentamicin], **amphotericin B, NSAIDs** [e.g., ibuprofen (Advil, Motrin), naproxen (Aleve, Naprosyn)], **rifampin** [Rifadin]). Risk of renal toxicity may be increased. ▪ The liver is a known target organ for toxicity; consider avoiding drugs known to induce hepatic toxicity (e.g., **amiodarone** [Nexterone], **NSAIDs** [e.g., ibuprofen (Advil, Motrin), naproxen (Aleve, Naprosyn)], **phenothiazines** [e.g., prochlorperazine (Compazine)], **zidovudine** [AZT, Retrovir]). ▪ Close monitoring is required with concomitant administration of medications affecting blood pressure or cardiac function (e.g., **diuretics** [furosemide (Lasix)], **calcium channel blockers** [diltiazem (Cardizem)], **and other antihypertensives**). ▪ Cytochrome P_{450} inhibitors (e.g., cimetidine [Tagamet], erythromycins, antifungal agents [e.g., itraconazole (Sporanox)], ritonavir [Norvir], verapamil) and cytochrome P_{450} inducers (e.g., carbamazepine [Tegretol], phenobarbital, phenytoin [Dilantin], rifampin [Rifadin]) are unlikely to affect the metabolism of clofarabine. The effect on cytochrome P_{450} substrates has not been studied.

SIDE EFFECTS

Bone marrow suppression (e.g., anemia, leukopenia, neutropenia, thrombocytopenia) is anticipated, appears to be dose dependent, and is usually reversible. Anxiety, diarrhea, fatigue, febrile neutropenia, fever, flushing, headache, mucosal inflammation, nausea and vomiting, palmar-plantar erythrodysesthesia syndrome, pruritus, and rash occur most frequently. SIRS/capillary leak syndrome (e.g., rapid onset of respiratory distress, hypotension, pleural and pericardial effusion, and multiorgan failure) has occurred and can be fatal. Hepatotoxicity (elevated AST, ALT, bilirubin), renal toxicity (elevated SCr, acute renal failure), and veno-occlusive disease of the liver have occurred. Serious and fatal hemorrhage (cerebral, GI, and pulmonary), enterocolitis (neutropenic colitis, cecitis, and *C. difficile* colitis), and skin reactions (SJS and TEN) have been reported. Numerous additional side effects may occur and include abdominal pain, anorexia, arthralgia, back pain, cardiac toxicity (e.g., pericardial effusion, tachycardia), confusion, constipation, cough, depression, dermatitis, dizziness, dyspnea, edema, elevated creatinine, epistaxis, erythema, gingival bleeding, hematuria, hepatobiliary toxicity (e.g., elevated AST, ALT, bilirubin), hepatomegaly, hypertension, hypotension, infections (e.g., bacteremia, cellulitis, herpes simplex, oral candidiasis, pneumonia, sepsis, staphylococcal), injection site pain, irritability, jaundice, lethargy, myalgia, pain, petechiae, pleural effusion, renal toxicity, respiratory distress, rigors, somnolence, sore throat, transfusion reaction, tremor, weight loss.
Post-Marketing: Bone marrow failure, GI hemorrhage (including fatalities), hepatic failure, hepatitis, hyponatremia, Stevens-Johnson syndrome, toxic epidermal necrolysis, and veno-occlusive disease.

ANTIDOTE

Keep physician informed of all side effects; most will be treated symptomatically as indicated. Discontinue if hypotension develops at any time during the 5 days of administration. Discontinue clofarabine immediately if early S/S of SIRS or capillary leak (e.g., hypotension) appear. Use of albumin, diuretics, and steroids may be indicated. May consider restarting (usually at a lower dose) after the patient is stabilized and organ function has returned to baseline. Discontinue clofarabine immediately if substantial increases in SCr, liver enzymes, or bilirubin occur. May be restarted (possibly at a lower dose) when the patient is stable and organ function has returned to baseline. Discontinue clofarabine for exfoliative or bullous rash or if SJS or TEN is suspected. Bone marrow suppression must be resolved before additional doses can be given. Administration of whole blood products (e.g., packed RBCs, platelets, or leukocytes) and/or blood modifiers (e.g., darbepoetin alfa [Aranesp], epoetin alfa [Epogen], filgrastim [Neupogen, Zarxio], pegfilgrastim [Neulasta], sargramostim [Leukine]) may be indicated to treat bone marrow toxicity. Use specific antibiotics to combat infection. No specific antidote for overdose. Supportive therapy as indicated will help sustain the patient in toxicity. Should a hypersensitivity reaction occur, treat with antihistamines, corticosteroids, epinephrine, and oxygen as indicated. Resuscitate if indicated.

COAGULATION FACTOR VIIa (RECOMBINANT) RTS BBW

Antihemorrhagic

(ko-ag-yew-**LA**-shun **FAK**-ter 7a [re-**KOM**-be-nant])

NovoSeven RT   pH 5.5

USUAL DOSE

HEMOPHILIA A OR B PATIENTS WITH INHIBITORS

Bleeding episodes: 90 mcg/kg every 2 hours until hemostasis is achieved or until the treatment has been judged to be ineffective. Doses between 35 and 120 mcg/kg have been used successfully. Minimum effective dose has not been established. The dose and dosing interval may be adjusted based on the severity of the bleeding and the degree of homeostasis achieved. In clinical studies, a decision on outcome was reached for a majority of patients with joint or muscle bleeds within 8 doses, although more doses were required for severe bleeds. For severe bleeds, dosing should continue at 3- to 6-hour intervals after hemostasis is achieved to maintain the hemostatic plug. The appropriate duration of post-hemostatic dosing has not been studied and should be minimized; see Precautions. If a new bleeding episode or rebleeding occurs, return to 2-hour dosing intervals.

Surgical intervention: 90 mcg/kg immediately before the intervention. Repeat every 2 hours during intervention. *For minor surgery,* postsurgical dosing should be administered every 2 hours for 48 hours and then every 2 to 6 hours until healing has occurred. *For major surgery,* postsurgical dosing should be administered every 2 hours for 5 days and then every 4 hours until healing has occurred. Additional doses may be given if required.

CONGENITAL FACTOR VII DEFICIENCY PATIENTS

Bleeding episodes and surgical intervention: 15 to 30 mcg/kg every 4 to 6 hours until hemostasis is achieved. Doses as low as 10 mcg/kg have been effective. Dose and dosing interval should be adjusted to each individual based on the severity of bleeding and the degree of hemostasis achieved. Minimal effective dose has not been determined.

ACQUIRED HEMOPHILIA

70 to 90 mcg/kg every 2 to 3 hours until hemostasis is achieved. Minimum effective dose has not been determined.

PEDIATRIC DOSE

See Usual Dose. Clinical studies were conducted with dosing determined according to body weight and not according to age. See Maternal/Child.

DOSE ADJUSTMENTS

Dose and administration interval may be adjusted based on the severity of the bleeding and the degree of hemostasis achieved. If patient develops intravascular coagulation or thrombosis, dosage should be reduced or treatment stopped; see Monitor.

DILUTION

NovoSeven RT is room temperature stable (RTS); aseptic technique is imperative. Available in packages that contain 1-, 2-, or 5-mg vials with a specified volume of histidine diluent. Select the appropriate vial package based on the calculated dose. Bring vial and diluent to RT. Do not exceed 37° C (98.6° F). Reconstitute powder with provided diluent, aiming the needle (20- to 26-gauge needle recommended) and the stream of diluent against the side of the vial. Do not inject the diluent directly on the powder. Do not use SWFI or other diluents. Gently swirl vial until powder is completely dissolved. Final concentration of reconstituted solution is 1 mg/mL (1,000 mcg/mL).

Storage: Before reconstitution, refrigerate or store between 2° and 25° C (36° and 77° F). Avoid exposure to direct sunlight. Do not freeze. After reconstitution, store at RT or refrigerate. Should be used within 3 hours. Do not freeze reconstituted product or store in syringe. Discard unused product.

COMPATIBILITY
Manufacturer states, "Intended for IV injection only and should not be mixed with infusion solutions. Do not store reconstituted solution in syringes." If line needs to be flushed before or after NovoSeven RT administration, use NS.

RATE OF ADMINISTRATION
A single dose as a slow IV injection over 2 to 5 minutes, depending on dose administered.

ACTIONS
A vitamin K–dependent glycoprotein structurally similar to human plasma–derived factor VIIa. Produced by recombinant DNA technology. Promotes hemostasis by activating the extrinsic pathway of the coagulation cascade. When complexed with tissue factor, can activate coagulation factor X to factor Xa, and coagulation factor IX to factor IXa. Factor Xa, in complex with other factors, then converts prothrombin to thrombin. This leads to the formation of a hemostatic plug by converting fibrinogen to fibrin. Half-life is 2.3 hours. Duration of action is 3 hours.

INDICATIONS AND USES
Treatment of bleeding episodes or prevention of bleeding in surgical interventions or invasive procedures in hemophilia A or B patients with inhibitors to factor VIII or factor IX and in patients with acquired hemophilia. ■ Treatment of bleeding episodes or prevention of bleeding in surgical interventions or invasive procedures in patients with congenital FVII deficiency.

CONTRAINDICATIONS
Manufacturer states, "None." Use with caution in patients with known hypersensitivity to coagulation factor VIIa (recombinant), any of its components, and in patients with known hypersensitivity to mouse, hamster, or bovine proteins.

PRECAUTIONS
For intravenous bolus administration only. ■ Should be administered to patients only under the direct supervision of a physician experienced in the treatment of bleeding disorders. ■ Thrombotic events have been reported in clinical trials as well as through post-marketing surveillance following coagulation factor VIIa (recombinant) RTS use for each of the approved indications. Patients with disseminated intravascular coagulation (DIC), advanced atherosclerotic disease, crush injury, septicemia, or concomitant treatment with aPCCs/PCCs (activated or nonactivated prothrombin complex concentrates) may have an increased risk of developing thrombotic events due to circulating tissue factor or predisposing coagulopathy. Use caution in patients with an increased risk of thromboembolic complications. These include, but are not limited to, patients with a history of coronary artery disease (CAD), liver disease, DIC, or postoperative immobilization; elderly patients; and neonates. ■ Coagulation factor VIIa has been studied in placebo-controlled trials outside the approved indications to control bleeding in intracranial hemorrhage, advanced liver disease, trauma, cardiac surgery, spinal surgery, and other therapeutic areas. Safety and effectiveness have not been established in these settings, and the use is not approved by the FDA. Arterial and venous thrombotic and thromboembolic events have been reported during post-marketing surveillance. Studies have shown an increased risk of arterial thromboembolic adverse events (e.g., MI, myocardial ischemia, cerebral infarction, and cerebral ischemia) with coagulation factor VIIa when administered outside the current approved guidelines. ■ Biologic and clinical effects of prolonged elevated levels of factor VIIa have not been studied; there-

fore, the duration of posthemostatic dosing should be minimized, and patients should be appropriately monitored by a physician experienced in the treatment of hemophilia during this time period.

Monitor: Evaluation of hemostasis should be used to determine the effectiveness of therapy and to provide a basis for modification of the treatment schedule; coagulation parameters do not necessarily correlate with or predict the effectiveness of therapy. Coagulation parameters (e.g., PT, aPTT, plasma FVII clotting activity [FVII:C]) may be used as an adjunct to the clinical evaluation of hemostasis in monitoring the effectiveness and treatment schedule, although these parameters have shown no direct correlation to achieving hemostasis. ▪ Patients with factor VII deficiency should be monitored for PT and factor VII coagulant activity before and after treatment. If the factor VIIa activity fails to reach the expected level, if PT is not corrected, or if bleeding is not controlled after treatment with the recommended doses, antibody formation should be suspected and analysis for antibodies should be performed. ▪ The normal factor VII plasma concentration is 0.5 mcg/mL. Factor VIIa levels of 15% to 25% (0.075 to 0.125 mcg/mL) are generally sufficient to achieve normal hemostasis. ▪ Monitor patients for the development of signs or symptoms of activation of the coagulation system or thrombosis. When there is laboratory confirmation of intravascular coagulation or presence of clinical thrombosis, dosage should be reduced or the treatment stopped, depending on the patient's symptoms; see Dose Adjustments.

Patient Education: Discuss benefits versus risk of therapy and signs of hypersensitivity reactions including hives, urticaria, chest tightness, wheezing, hypotension, and anaphylaxis. ▪ Signs of bleeding may be similar to signs of thrombosis and can include new-onset swelling and pain in the limbs or abdomen, new-onset chest pain, shortness of breath, loss of sensation or motor power, or altered consciousness or speech.

Maternal/Child: Category C: safety for use during pregnancy not established. Use only if clearly indicated and benefit justifies potential risk to the fetus. ▪ Discontinue breastfeeding. ▪ Thrombotic events have been reported in women without a prior diagnosis of bleeding disorders who have received coagulation factor VIIa for uncontrolled postpartum hemorrhage. ▪ A decision should be made whether to discontinue nursing or to discontinue the drug. ▪ The safety and effectiveness have not been studied to determine if there are differences among various age-groups from infants to adolescents (0 to 16 years of age); see Pediatric Dose.

Elderly: Numbers in clinical studies insufficient to determine if the elderly respond differently than younger subjects.

DRUG/LAB INTERACTIONS

The risk of potential interaction between factor VIIa and coagulation factor concentrates has not been adequately evaluated. Simultaneous use of **activated prothrombin complex concentrates** (e.g., anti-inhibitor coagulant complex [Feiba]) or **prothrombin complex concentrates** (e.g., factor IX [AlphaNine SD, Benefix]) should be avoided.

SIDE EFFECTS

Generally well tolerated. The majority of patients reporting side effects received more than 12 doses. The most common side effects are arthralgia, edema, fever, headache, hemorrhage, hypertension, hypotension, injection site reaction, nausea, pain, rash, and vomiting. Most serious adverse reactions are thrombotic events; however, the risk in patients with hemophilia and inhibitors is considered to be low. Fatal and nonfatal thrombotic events have been reported when used for both labeled and off-label indications. Other side effects include arthrosis, bradycardia, coagulation disorder, DIC, decreased fibrinogen plasma, decreased prothrombin, decreased therapeutic response, hemarthrosis, hypersensitivity reactions, increased fibrinolysis, pneumonia, pruritus, purpura, renal function abnormalities, shock, subdural hematoma, thrombosis, urticaria.

Post-Marketing: High D-dimer levels and consumptive coagulopathy; thromboembolic events, including myocardial ischemia and/or infarction, cerebral ischemia and/or infarction, thrombophlebitis, arterial thrombosis, deep vein thrombosis, and related pulmonary embolism; and isolated cases of hypersensitivity reactions (including anaphylaxis) have occurred following use in both labeled and unlabeled indications.

ANTIDOTE

Discontinue drug and notify physician of any major side effects. Treat hypersensitivity reactions as indicated. For thrombosis or DIC, anticoagulation with heparin may be indicated.

COAGULATION FACTOR X (HUMAN)   Antihemorrhagic
(ko-ag-yew-**LA**-shun **FAK**-ter X)

Coagadex

USUAL DOSE   (INTERNATIONAL UNITS [IU])

Dose, frequency, and duration must be individualized based on the severity of the factor X deficiency, location and extent of bleeding, patient's clinical condition, and individual clinical response. Each vial is labeled with the actual factor X potency/content in international units (IU). The dose to achieve a desired in vivo peak increase in factor X level can be calculated with the following formula.

$$\text{Dose (IU)} = \text{Body weight (kg)} \times \text{Desired factor X rise (IU/dL)} \times 0.5$$

The desired factor X rise is the difference between the patient's plasma factor X level and the desired level. The dosing formula is based on the observed recovery of 2 IU/dL per IU/kg (i.e., for each 1 IU/kg of factor X administered, the circulating factor X level increases by approximately 2 IU/dL).

On-demand treatment and control of bleeding episodes: 25 IU/kg at the first sign of bleeding. Repeat every 24 hours until the bleed stops. Do not administer more than 60 IU/kg daily.

Perioperative management of bleeding: Do not administer more than 60 IU/kg daily.

Presurgery: Calculate the dose of coagulation factor X required to raise plasma factor X levels to 70 to 90 IU/dL using the following formula.

$$\text{Required dose (IU)} = \text{Body weight (kg)} \times \text{Desired factor X rise (IU/dL)} \times 0.5$$

Postsurgery: Repeat dose as necessary to maintain plasma factor X levels at a minimum of 50 IU/dL until there is no longer a risk of bleeding due to surgery.

DOSE ADJUSTMENTS

Adjust dose and duration based on factor X levels, location and extent of bleeding, patient's clinical condition, and clinical response to therapy.

DILUTION

Supplied in single-use glass vials containing approximately 250 or 500 IU (approximately 100 IU/mL after reconstitution) of factor X activity, packaged with 2.5 or 5 mL of SWFI, respectively, and a Mix2Vial transfer device. The total number of IUs available is clearly marked on each vial. Record the batch number of each vial. Consult instructions for reconstitution and administration in the package insert. If stored in the refrigerator, warm to room temperature (25° C) before reconstitution. If more than 1 vial is required, use a new Mix2Vial transfer set for each vial of drug. Solution from multiple vials can be pooled into a single syringe. Do not shake. Do not use if the reconstituted solution is cloudy or contains any particles. The reconstituted solution should be clear or a slightly pearl-like solution.

Filters: Incorporated into the Mix2Vial.

Storage: Store in refrigerator or at RT (2° to 30° C [36° to 86° F]) in original carton to protect from light until ready to use. Do not freeze. Do not use beyond the expiration date on the product vial. Should be used immediately but must be used within 1 hour of reconstitution.

COMPATIBILITY

Specific information not available; consider specific use and contact pharmacist.

RATE OF ADMINISTRATION

A single dose may be administered as an infusion at a rate of 10 mL/min up to a maximum rate of 20 mL/min; consider patient comfort. Reduce rate of administration or interrupt the infusion if a marked increase in pulse occurs.

ACTIONS

Coagulation factor X is a plasma-derived, purified concentrate of human coagulation factor X. It temporarily replaces the missing factor X needed for effective hemostasis. After conversion to its active form (factor Xa), it associates with factor Va to form the prothrombinase complex, which activates prothrombin to thrombin. Thrombin then acts on soluble fibrinogen and factor XIII to generate a cross-linked fibrin clot. Mean half-life is approximately 30.3 hours.

INDICATIONS AND USES

Treatment of adults and pediatric patients (12 years of age and above) with hereditary factor X deficiency for on-demand treatment and control of bleeding episodes and perioperative management of bleeding in patients with mild hereditary factor X deficiency. **Limitation of use:** Perioperative management of bleeding in major surgery in patients with moderate and severe hereditary factor X deficiency has not been studied.

CONTRAINDICATIONS

Life-threatening hypersensitivity reactions to coagulation factor X or any of the product components.

PRECAUTIONS

For IV use only. ▪ Administered under the direction of a physician knowledgeable in the treatment of coagulation disorders in a facility with adequate diagnostic and treatment facilities to monitor the patient and respond to any medical emergency. ▪ Hypersensitivity reactions, including anaphylaxis, have occurred; see Monitor ▪ Manufactured from human plasma. Risk of transmitting infectious agents (e.g., HIV, hepatitis and, theoretically, Creutzfeldt-Jakob disease) has been greatly reduced by screening, testing, and manufacturing techniques. However, risk of transmission cannot be totally eliminated. Health care professionals should use caution during administration; may have risk of exposure to viral infection. ▪ Contains trace human proteins other than factor X. ▪ Neutralizing antibodies (inhibitors) to factor X may occur; see Monitor.

Monitor: Monitor BP and pulse during infusion. If a marked increase in pulse occurs, either reduce rate of infusion or interrupt the infusion. ▪ Throughout the infusion, monitor for S/S of a hypersensitivity reaction (e.g., angioedema, chest tightness, chills, fever, headache, hypotension, lethargy, nausea, pruritus, rash, restlessness, tachycardia, urticaria, wheezing). ▪ Monitor plasma factor X activity by performing a validated test (e.g., one-stage clotting assay) to confirm that adequate factor X levels have been achieved and maintained. ▪ In surgery patients, monitor postinfusion plasma factor X levels before and after surgery to ensure that hemostatic levels are obtained and maintained. ▪ Monitor for the development of factor X inhibitors. Perform a Nijmegen-Bethesda inhibitor assay if expected factor X plasma levels are not attained or if bleeding is not controlled with the expected dose of coagulation factor X.

Patient Education: Review manufacturer's medication guide. ▪ Promptly report S/S of a hypersensitivity reaction (e.g., dizziness, hives, itching, rash, tightness of the chest, wheezing). ▪ Report a lack of clinical response to therapy; may be a manifestation of an inhibitor. ▪ Report symptoms of possibly transmitted viral infections immediately. Symptoms may include anorexia, arthralgias, fatigue, jaundice, low-grade fever, nausea, or vomiting. ▪ If traveling, bring an adequate supply of medication based on current treatment regimen.

Maternal/Child: Use during pregnancy or labor and delivery only if clearly needed. ▪ Safety for use during breast-feeding not known; consider benefit versus risk. ▪ Safety and effectiveness for use in pediatric patients under 12 years of age not established.

Elderly: Numbers insufficient to determine differences in response between older and younger patients.

DRUG/LAB INTERACTIONS

Drug interaction studies have not been performed. ▪ Use with caution in patients who are receiving other plasma products that may contain factor X (e.g., fresh frozen plasma, prothrombin complex concentrates [e.g., Kcentra]). ▪ Based on its mechanism of action, coagulation factor X is likely to be counteracted by direct and indirect factor Xa inhibitors (e.g., apixaban [Eliquis], edoxaban [Savaysa], rivaroxaban [Xarelto]).

SIDE EFFECTS

The most common side effects observed are back pain, fatigue, infusion site erythema, and infusion site pain. Hypersensitivity reactions have occurred.

ANTIDOTE

Keep the physician informed of side effects. Slow or interrupt infusion for a marked increase in pulse rate or a mild hypersensitivity reaction. Discontinue the infusion immediately if a severe hypersensitivity reaction occurs. Treat hypersensitivity as necessary (e.g., antihistamines, epinephrine, corticosteroids). Resuscitate as necessary.

COAGULATION FACTOR XIII A-SUBUNIT (RECOMBINANT)   Antihemorrhagic

(ko-ag-yew-**LA**-shun **FAK**-ter XIII [re-**KOM**-be-nant])

Tretten   pH 8

USUAL DOSE   (International units [IU])

Adult and pediatric patients: 35 IU/kg once monthly to achieve a target trough level of factor XIII activity at or above 10% using a validated assay.

DOSE ADJUSTMENTS

Consider increasing dose if adequate trough levels are not achieved.

DILUTION

Available as a white lyophilized powder in single-use vials. May contain from 2,000 to 3,125 IU. Actual amount is stated on each vial and each carton. Can be reconstituted using the vial adapter and diluent included with the packaging (see prescribing information) **or** using a needle and syringe with SWFI as a diluent. Bring vial and diluent to RT (not to exceed 25° C (77° F). Withdraw 3.2 mL of SWFI and inject into the powder by aiming the needle and stream of diluent against the side of the vial. To avoid foaming, do not inject the diluent directly on the powder. Gently swirl to dissolve. **Do not shake.** A clear and colorless solution. After reconstitution, each mL contains 667 to 1,042 IU.

If a large dose requires the use of multiple vials, reconstitute each additional vial with a separate syringe. For a smaller dose that requires less than the full volume in the vial, the reconstituted solution may be further diluted with NS to facilitate measurement and administration; discard remaining product. Must be used within 3 hours.

Filters: Specific information not available.

Storage: Refrigerate at 2° to 8° C (36° to 46° F) in original carton to protect from light. Do not freeze. Stable until expiration date on carton. Immediate use of reconstituted solution is preferred but may be refrigerated or kept at RT (not to exceed 25° C [77° F]) for up to 3 hours. Discard after 3 hours.

COMPATIBILITY
Manufacturer states, "Do not administer with other infusion solutions."

RATE OF ADMINISTRATION
A single dose as an IV injection at a rate not to exceed 1 to 2 mL/min. Do not administer as a drip infusion.

ACTIONS
A human factor XIII-A_2 homodimer produced by recombinant DNA technology. Factor XIII is the terminal enzyme in the blood coagulation cascade. When activated by thrombin at the site of vessel wall injury, factor XIII plays an important role in the maintenance of hemostasis through cross-linking of fibrin and other proteins in the fibrin clot. After combining with available factor XIII B-subunits, it has been shown to have the same pharmacodynamics properties in plasma as endogenous factor XIII. Increases the mechanical strength of fibrin clots, retards fibrinolysis, and enhances platelet adhesion to the site of injury. Mean half-life based on baseline (trough) adjusted factor XIII activity was 5.1 days in patients 7 to 58 years of age and 7.1 days in pediatric patients 1 to less than 6 years of age.

INDICATIONS AND USES
Routine prophylaxis for bleeding in patients with congenital factor XIII A-subunit deficiency.

Limitation of use: Not for use in patients with congenital factor XIII B-subunit deficiency.

CONTRAINDICATIONS
Known hypersensitivity to the active substance or any of its excipients.

PRECAUTIONS
For IV injection only. Do not administer as a drip infusion. ▪ Should be administered under the supervision of a physician experienced in the treatment of rare bleeding disorders. ▪ Hypersensitivity reactions (including anaphylaxis) may occur. ▪ Thrombotic events may occur. Use caution in patients with an increased risk of thromboembolic complications. These include, but are not limited to, patients with a history of coronary artery disease (CAD), liver disease, DIC, or postoperative immobilization; elderly patients; and neonates. ▪ Inhibitory antibodies may occur and should be considered if there is an inadequate response or a reduced therapeutic effect to treatment.

Monitor: Confirm factor XIII A-subunit deficiency. ▪ Evaluate effectiveness of treatment to achieve a target trough level of factor XIII activity at or above 10% using a validated assay at least monthly or more frequently if indicated. Adjust dose as indicated. ▪ Monitor for S/S of hypersensitivity (e.g., hypotension, rash, urticaria, tightness of the chest, wheezing). ▪ Monitor for S/S of thromboembolic complications (e.g., chest pain, limb or abdominal swelling and/or pain, shortness of breath, loss of sensation or motor power, altered consciousness, vision, or speech). ▪ Monitor for S/S of inhibitory antibodies (e.g., expected plasma factor XIII activity levels are not attained, or breakthrough bleeding occurs during prophylactic treatment). Confirm with an assay that measures factor XIII inhibitory antibody concentrations.

Patient Education: Review manufacturer's medication guide. ▪ Promptly report S/S of a hypersensitivity reaction (e.g., light-headedness, rash, urticaria, tightness of the chest, wheezing). ▪ Signs of bleeding may be similar to signs of thrombosis and can include new-onset swelling and pain in the limbs or abdomen, new-onset chest pain, shortness of breath, loss of sensation or motor power, or altered consciousness, vision, or speech. Promptly report any of these signs. ▪ Report breakthrough bleeding; it may be a symptom of inhibitor formation and require further testing.

Maternal/Child: Category C: safety for use during pregnancy not established. Use only if clearly needed. ▪ Use caution during breast-feeding. ▪ Clinical studies included small numbers of pediatric patients from neonates to adolescents who were treated with multiple exposures. Side effects were reported more frequently in pediatric patients 6 to less than 18 years of age.

Elderly: Numbers in clinical studies insufficient to determine if the elderly respond differently from younger subjects.

DRUG/LAB INTERACTIONS

Concomitant administration with coagulation factor VIIa may cause thrombosis.

SIDE EFFECTS

Headache, increase in fibrin D-dimer levels, injection site pain, and pain in the extremities were most commonly reported and were reported more frequently in pediatric patients 6 to less than 18 years of age. Hypersensitivity reactions (including anaphylaxis) and thromboembolic events are the most serious side effects. Formation of inhibitory antibodies has occurred.

ANTIDOTE

Discontinue drug and notify physician of any major side effect. Treat hypersensitivity reactions with oxygen, epinephrine (Adrenalin), antihistamines (e.g., diphenhydramine [Benadryl]), vasopressors (e.g., dopamine), corticosteroids, albuterol, IV fluids, and ventilation equipment as indicated. Resuscitate as necessary.

CONIVAPTAN HYDROCHLORIDE

Arginine vasopressin antagonist

(kon-ih-**VAP**-tan hy-droh-**KLOR**-eyed)

Vaprisol

pH 3 to 3.8

USUAL DOSE

Loading dose: 20 mg as an IV infusion over 30 minutes. Follow with 20 mg administered as a **continuous infusion** evenly distributed over 24 hours. May be administered for an additional 1 to 3 days as a continuous infusion of 20 mg/day. The total duration of infusion (after the loading dose) should not exceed 4 days.

DOSE ADJUSTMENTS

If the serum sodium does not rise at the desired rate, the dose may be titrated up to 40 mg as a continuous infusion over 24 hours. 40 mg is the maximum daily dose. ▪ A reduced dose may be required if the patient experiences an undesirably rapid rate of rise of serum sodium; see Precautions. ▪ If hyponatremia persists or recurs (after initial interruption of therapy) and the patient has no evidence of neurologic sequelae, conivaptan may be resumed at a reduced dose; see Monitor. ▪ A reduced dose may also be required in patients who develop hypotension or hypovolemia; see Monitor. ▪ No dose adjustment indicated in patients with mild hepatic impairment. ▪ Reduced dose required in patients with moderate hepatic impairment. Initiate with a loading dose of 10 mg. Follow with a continuous infusion of 10 mg over 24 hours for 2 days to a maximum of 4 days. If sodium is not rising at the desired rate, the conivaptan dose may be titrated up to 20 mg/day. ▪ Use in patients with severe renal impairment (CrCl less than 30 mL/min) is not recommended; see Contraindications.

DILUTION

Available in a single-use, ready-to-use (RTU) plastic container containing 20 mg conivaptan in 100 mL D5W. If the RTU container is being administered as a 40-mg dose, administer two consecutive 20 mg/100 mL containers over 24 hours.

Storage: Store in carton at CRT. Protect from light and freezing. Do not remove container from overwrap until ready to use. Overwrap is a moisture and light barrier.

COMPATIBILITY

Manufacturer states, "Should not be mixed or administered with lactated Ringer's or furosemide (Lasix). Should not be combined with any other product in the same intravenous line or bag."

RATE OF ADMINISTRATION

Loading dose: A single dose equally distributed over 30 minutes as an infusion.

Continuous infusion: A single dose equally distributed over 24 hours.

ACTIONS

A nonpeptide, dual antagonist of arginine vasopressin (AVP) V_{1A} and V_2 receptors. The level of AVP in the blood is critical for the regulation of water and electrolyte balance and is usually elevated in both euvolemic and hypervolemic hyponatremia (in euvolemic hyponatremia there is an increase in total body water, but the sodium content remains the same; in hypervolemic hyponatremia both sodium and water content in the body increase, but the water gain is greater). AVP excess is associated with hyponatremia without edema. The AVP effect is mediated through V_2 receptors that help maintain plasma osmolality. Conivaptan blocks V_2 receptors in the renal collecting ducts, resulting in aquaresis (excretion of free water). This is generally accompanied by increased net fluid loss, increased urine output, and decreased urine osmolality. Conivaptan is highly protein bound. It is metabolized in the liver by the cytochrome P_{450} isoenzyme, CYP3A. Its half-life is 5.3 to 8.1 hours, depending on dose. Primarily excreted in the feces and, to a lesser extent, in urine. Crosses the placenta in animals.

INDICATIONS AND USES

For use in the hospitalized patient to treat euvolemic and hypervolemic hyponatremia. Euvolemic hyponatremia may occur in the syndrome of inappropriate secretion of antidiuretic hormone (SIADH, an inability of the body to excrete dilute urine) or in the setting of certain conditions, including hypothyroidism, adrenal insufficiency, and pulmonary disorders. ▪ Not indicated for the treatment of the S/S of heart failure. Raising serum sodium with conivaptan has not been shown to provide a symptomatic benefit.

CONTRAINDICATIONS

Patients with hypovolemic hyponatremia. ▪ Hypersensitivity to conivaptan or any of its components (propylene glycol, ethanol, lactic acid). ▪ Coadministration with potent CYP3A inhibitors, such as clarithromycin, indinavir, itraconazole, ketoconazole, and ritonavir; see Drug Interactions. ▪ Premixed solution contains dextrose, which may be contraindicated in patients with a known allergy to corn or corn products. ▪ Anuria (no benefit expected).

PRECAUTIONS

For IV use only. ▪ Use only in hospitalized patients. ▪ Safety for use in hypovolemic hyponatremic patients with underlying CHF has not been established. Should be used to raise sodium in these patients only after other treatment options have been considered. Incidence of adverse cardiac events may be increased. ▪ An overly rapid increase in serum sodium concentration (more than 12 mEq/L/24 hr) may result in serious sequelae. Although not observed in clinical trials, osmotic demyelination syndrome (brain cell dehydration) has been reported following rapid correction of low serum sodium concentration. Osmotic demyelination results in dysarthria, lethargy, affective changes, spastic quadriparesis, seizures, coma, or death. Patients with severe malnutrition, alcoholism, or advanced liver disease may be at increased risk; use slower rates of correction; see Monitor. ▪ Reduced doses required in patients with moderate hepatic impairment; see Dose Adjustments. Impact of severe hepatic impairment has not been studied. ▪ May cause significant infusion site reaction; see Monitor.

Monitor: Administer via a large vein. Monitor infusion site and rotate every 24 hours. ▪ Monitor serum sodium concentration and neurologic status closely during therapy. If an overly rapid increase in serum sodium concentration occurs (greater than 12 mEq/L/24 hr), administration should be discontinued. If the sodium continues to rise, administration should not be resumed. If hyponatremia persists or recurs (after initial interruption of therapy) and the patient has no evidence of neurologic sequelae, conivaptan may be resumed at a reduced dose. ▪ Monitor vital signs, urine output and osmolality, and volume status of patient. Discontinue therapy in patients who develop hypotension or hypovolemia. Once the patient is again euvolemic and is no longer hypotensive, therapy may be resumed at a reduced dose; see Dose Adjustments.

Patient Education: Promptly report any burning at the infusion site or other side effects. ▪ Request assistance for ambulation. ▪ Review list of allergies and medications with physician or pharmacist.

Maternal/Child: Category C: use during pregnancy only if benefits justify risk to the fetus. Has been shown to cause fetal harm in animals. ▪ Discontinue breast-feeding. ▪ Safety and effectiveness for use in pediatric patients have not been studied.

Elderly: Response similar to that seen in the general study population.

DRUG/LAB INTERACTIONS

A substrate of CYP3A. Coadministration with inhibitors of this enzyme could lead to an increase in conivaptan concentrations, the effect of which is unknown. Concomitant use with **potent CYP3A4** inhibitors such as clarithromycin (Biaxin), indinavir (Crixivan), itraconazole (Sporanox), ketoconazole (Nizoral), and ritonavir (Norvir) is contraindicated. ▪ A potent inhibitor of CYP3A. May increase plasma concentrations of drugs that are primarily metabolized by this enzyme. Coadministration with **amlodipine** (Norvasc), **midazolam** (Versed), **and simvastatin** (Zocor) resulted in increased concentrations of each of the drugs. Two cases of rhabdomyolysis occurred in patients who were receiving a **CYP3A4-metabolized HMG-CoA reductase inhibitor** (e.g., simvastatin [Zocor]). Avoid concomitant use with drugs eliminated primarily by **CYP3A4-mediated metabolism.** Do not initiate subsequent therapy with **CYP3A4 substrate drugs** until at least 1 week after an infusion of conivaptan. ▪ May decrease clearance and increase serum concentration of **digoxin.** Monitor digoxin levels. ▪ Captopril and furosemide (Lasix) do not appear to affect the pharmacokinetics of conivaptan. ▪ Does not appear to affect PT/INR when coadministered with warfarin (Coumadin). ▪ Does not appear to affect the QT interval.

SIDE EFFECTS

The most common adverse reactions are infusion site reactions (e.g., erythema, pain, phlebitis), fever, headache, hypokalemia, orthostatic hypotension, peripheral edema. Other reactions that occurred in more than 2% of patients include anemia, atrial fibrillation, confusion, constipation, diarrhea, hypertension, hypomagnesemia, hyponatremia, hypotension, insomnia, nausea, pharyngolaryngeal pain, pneumonia, pruritus, pyrexia, ST segment depression on ECG, thirst, urinary tract infection, and vomiting.

ANTIDOTE

Notify physician of any side effects. Most will be treated symptomatically. Discontinue therapy if there is an overly rapid increase in serum sodium concentration or if the patient experiences hypotension or hypovolemia. Discontinue therapy permanently if neurologic sequelae are present; see Precautions, Monitor, and Dose Adjustments. Resuscitate as necessary.

CONJUGATED ESTROGENS BBW
(**KON**-jyou-**gay**-ted **ES**-troh-jens)

Hormone (estrogen)
Antihemorrhagic

Premarin Intravenous

pH 7.2 to 7.4

USUAL DOSE
25 mg in 1 injection. May be repeated in 6 to 12 hours if indicated.

DILUTION
Reconstitute with 5 mL SWFI, directing the flow of diluent gently against the side of the vial. Agitate gently. Do not shake violently. Do not use if discolored or if precipitate is present. Dilution in an IV infusion is not recommended.
Storage: Refrigerate prior to use. Use immediately after reconstitution.

COMPATIBILITY
Consider any drug NOT listed as compatible to be INCOMPATIBLE until consulting a pharmacist; specific conditions may apply.
Manufacturer lists as **incompatible** with ascorbic acid, protein hydrolysate, or any solution with an acid pH.

According to the manufacturer, infusion with other agents is not generally recommended. May be given at Y-tube if **compatible** solutions are infusing (NS, dextrose, and invert sugar solutions). According to one source, it is **compatible** at the **Y-site** with heparin, hydrocortisone sodium succinate (Solu-Cortef), and potassium chloride (KCl).

RATE OF ADMINISTRATION
5 mg or fraction thereof over 1 minute. Must be given direct IV or through IV tubing close to needle site. Infusion solution must be **compatible.** Too-rapid injection may cause flushing.

ACTIONS
A mixture of conjugated estrogens obtained from natural sources. Administration provides a rapid and temporary increase in estrogen levels. Acts at several points on the clotting cascade, enhancing coagulability of the blood, especially in the capillary beds. Promptly corrects bleeding due to estrogen deficiency. Widely distributed in the body. Metabolized primarily in the liver and excreted in the urine. Secreted in breast milk.

INDICATIONS AND USES
Treatment of abnormal uterine bleeding caused by hormonal imbalance in the absence of organic pathology. Indicated for short-term use only to provide a rapid and temporary increase in estrogen levels.
Unlabeled uses: Postcoital contraception.

CONTRAINDICATIONS
Known, suspected, or history of breast cancer, active deep venous thrombosis, or pulmonary embolism. ▪ A history of or active arterial thromboembolic disease (e.g., stroke, MI). ▪ Known or suspected estrogen-dependent neoplasia, pregnancy, undiagnosed abnormal genital bleeding, liver dysfunction or disease. ▪ Hypersensitivity to this product or its ingredients (e.g., known anaphylactic reaction and angioedema). ▪ Known protein C, protein S, or antithrombin deficiency, or other known thrombophilic disorders. ▪ Other specific contraindications for estrogens must be considered.

PRECAUTIONS
IV therapy with conjugated estrogens is indicated for short-term use. However, warnings and precautions associated with oral therapy should be considered (e.g., changes in vaginal bleeding, headache, hypersensitivity reactions, skin reactions, and many more); see Precautions and prescribing information. ▪ Estrogens with or without progestins should not be used for the prevention of cardiovascular disease or dementia. ▪ Even though bleeding is controlled, the etiology of the bleeding must be determined and definitive therapy instituted. ▪ May cause fluid retention. Use with caution in patients with cardiac or renal dysfunction. ▪ Use with caution in asthma, diabetes, endometriosis, epilepsy, hepatic

hemangiomas, hepatic or gallbladder disease, hypercalcemia or hypocalcemia, hypercholesterolemia, hypertension, hypertriglyceridemia, hypoparathyroidism, migraines, obesity, porphyria, systemic lupus erythematosus, or tobacco use; may exacerbate condition. ■ May induce or exacerbate symptoms of angioedema, particularly in women with hereditary angioedema. ■ Retinal vascular thrombosis has been reported in patients receiving estrogen therapy. Discontinue therapy and obtain ophthalmologic exam if visual disturbances occur. ■ Patients dependent on thyroid hormone replacement therapy (e.g., levothyroxine [Synthroid]) who are also receiving estrogen may require dose adjustment of thyroid replacement medication. ■ Estrogens may increase the risk of deep venous thrombosis, MI, pulmonary embolism, stroke, breast cancer, endometrial cancer, and dementia. ■ Follow immediately with oral estrogens as recommended for dysfunctional uterine bleeding.

Monitor: Monitor VS; may cause a temporary BP elevation.

Patient Education: Review health history and disease states with physician before beginning treatment with conjugated estrogens. ■ Review possible side effects with physician and report any side effects promptly.

Maternal/Child: Category X: avoid pregnancy. ■ Use caution during breast-feeding. Detectable amounts have been found in breast milk and may decrease quantity and quality of milk. ■ Safety for use in pediatric patients not established. Extended use may accelerate epiphyseal closure, which could result in short adult stature.

Elderly: Differences in response compared to younger adults not identified.

DRUG/LAB INTERACTIONS

May decrease effects of **oral antidiabetics.** ■ **Barbiturates** (e.g., phenobarbital), **carbamazepine** (Tegretol), **phenytoin** (Dilantin), **rifampin** (Rifadin), **and St. John's wort** increase metabolism and decrease serum levels and effects. ■ Plasma concentrations may be increased with coadministration of **clarithromycin** (Biaxin), **erythromycin, itraconazole** (Sporanox), **ketoconazole** (Nizoral), **ritonavir** (Norvir), **and grapefruit juice.** ■ May decrease metabolism and increase serum levels of **cyclosporine.** May increase risk of cyclosporine toxicity. ■ Increased risk of hepatotoxicity with **other hepatotoxic agents** (e.g., dantrolene [Dantrium]). ■ May increase **blood glucose** levels and **serum lipids.** ■ May reduce response to **metyrapone test.** ■ May alter numerous **coagulation tests, glucose tolerance, and thyroid and other protein-binding tests.**

SIDE EFFECTS

Rare when used as directed; flushing, nausea, vomiting. IV therapy with conjugated estrogens is indicated for short-term use. However, the numerous adverse reactions associated with oral therapy should be considered (e.g., changes in vaginal bleeding, headache, hypersensitivity reactions, skin reactions, and many more); see Precautions and prescribing information.

Post-Marketing: Anaphylaxis within minutes to hours of infusion; angioedema involving the face, tongue, larynx, hands, and feet.

ANTIDOTE

No toxicity has been reported throughout years of clinical use. Discontinue if jaundice occurs. Discontinue immediately if DVT, MI, PE, stroke, or venous thromboembolism occurs.

COSYNTROPIN
(koh-**SIN**-troh-pin)

Cortrosyn

USUAL DOSE
250 mcg (0.25 mg). Up to 750 mcg (0.75 mg) has been used.

PEDIATRIC DOSE
Pediatric patients over 2 years of age: May use adult dose, but 125 mcg (0.125 mg) is usually adequate.

Pediatric patients 2 years of age or less: 125 mcg (0.125 mg). Usually given IM.

DILUTION
Available as a lyophilized powder or as a solution. Reconstitute powder with 1 mL NS. For IV use, both formulations should be diluted with 2 to 5 mL of NS. May be given directly IV after this initial dilution or further diluted in D5W or NS and given as an infusion (250 mcg in 250 mL equals 1 mcg/mL).

Storage: *Lyophilized powder:* Store at CRT. *Liquid formulation:* Store at 2° to 8° C (36° to 46° F); protect from light and freezing. Discard any unused drug.

COMPATIBILITY
Manufacturer states, "Should not be added to blood or plasma; may be inactivated by enzymes." Consider specific use.

RATE OF ADMINISTRATION
IV injection: A single dose over 2 minutes.

Infusion: A single dose at a rate of approximately 40 mcg/hr over 6 hours.

ACTIONS
A synthetic form of adrenocorticotropic hormone (ACTH). Stimulates the adrenal cortex to secrete adrenocortical hormone. Does not increase cortisol secretion in patients with primary adrenocortical insufficiency. Peak plasma cortisol levels occur in 1 to 2 hours depending on formulation used.

INDICATIONS AND USES
Diagnostic aid for adrenocortical insufficiency.

CONTRAINDICATIONS
Hypersensitivity to cosyntropin.

PRECAUTIONS
The liquid formulation of cosyntropin is for IV use only. Cortrosyn may be used IV or IM. ▪ Preferable to ACTH because it is less likely to cause hypersensitivity reactions; however, hypersensitivity reactions have occurred. Administer in a facility equipped to monitor the patient and respond to any medical emergency. ▪ May be used in patients who have had a hypersensitivity reaction to ACTH.

Monitor: Continuous observation for at least the first 30 minutes is mandatory. Observe frequently thereafter. ▪ Check BP frequently; may cause elevated BP and salt and water retention. ▪ Monitor correct collection of specimens; see prescribing information for specific details. ▪ See Drug/Lab Interactions.

Patient Education: Promptly report S/S of a hypersensitivity reaction (e.g., hives, rash, shortness of breath or troubled breathing, swelling of eyelids, lips, or face).

Maternal/Child: Category C: use during pregnancy only if benefits outweigh risks. ▪ Use with caution during breast-feeding.

DRUG/LAB INTERACTIONS
Plasma cortisol may be falsely elevated with **cortisone, hydrocortisone, or spironolactone.** Patients receiving cortisone, hydrocortisone, or spironolactone should omit their pretest doses on the day of testing. ▪ Abnormally high basal plasma cortisol levels may also occur in patients taking inadvertent doses of **cortisone or hydrocortisone** on the test day

and in women taking drugs that contain **estrogen.** ▪ Many drug reactions are possible with corticosteroids, but usually not a concern with specific diagnostic use. ▪ May accentuate electrolyte loss associated with **diuretic therapy.**

SIDE EFFECTS
Bradycardia, hypertension, peripheral edema, rash, and tachycardia have been reported. Hypersensitivity reactions, including anaphylaxis (rare), have occurred.

ANTIDOTE
Notify the physician of any side effect. Keep epinephrine and diphenhydramine available to treat anaphylaxis. Resuscitate as necessary.

CYCLOPHOSPHAMIDE
(sye-kloh-**FOS**-fah-myd)

Antineoplastic
(alkylating agent/
nitrogen mustard)

Lyophilized Cytoxan, ✦Procytox

pH 3 to 7.5

USUAL DOSE
Although effective alone in susceptible malignancies, cyclophosphamide is more frequently used concurrently or sequentially with other antineoplastic agents. **Doses may be expressed in mg/kg or mg/M².** During or immediately after administration, adequate amounts of fluid should be ingested or infused to force diuresis and thus reduce the risk of urinary toxicity. Cyclophosphamide should be administered in the morning; see Monitor.

Malignant diseases (adult and pediatric patients): *As a single agent:* The initial dose may be 40 to 50 mg/kg of body weight, usually given in divided doses over 2 to 5 days. Alternate dosing schedules are 3 to 5 mg/kg twice weekly or 10 to 15 mg/kg every 7 to 10 days. Higher doses have been used with some protocols based on the condition being treated. Adequate hydration is indicated, and the use of mesna can be considered to attenuate or reduce the incidence of hemorrhagic cystitis. **Combination protocols:** Numerous combination therapies are in use. Has been used with bleomycin, bortezomib, carboplatin, cisplatin, dacarbazine, dexamethasone, docetaxel, doxorubicin, epirubicin, etoposide, fludarabine, fluorouracil, methotrexate, prednisone, procarbazine, rituximab, topotecan, vinblastine, and vincristine. See literature for various regimens.

Adjuvant treatment of operable node-positive breast cancer: Treatment protocol includes cyclophosphamide, doxorubicin, and docetaxel. Administer cyclophosphamide 500 mg/M² and doxorubicin 50 mg/M². One hour later, give docetaxel 75 mg/M². Repeat every 3 weeks for 6 cycles. See docetaxel (Taxotere) and doxorubicin (Adriamycin) monographs.

PEDIATRIC DOSE
Malignant diseases: See Usual Dose.

DOSE ADJUSTMENTS
Dosages must be adjusted based on antitumor activity and/or leukopenia. Total leukocyte count is a good, objective guide for regulating dosage. Withhold therapy in patients with neutrophils less than or equal to 1,500/mm³ and platelets less than 50,000/mm³. ▪ When used as a component of a multidrug regimen, it may be necessary to reduce the dose of cyclophosphamide as well as the doses of the other drugs. ▪ Dosing should be cautious in the elderly. Lower-end initial doses may be indicated. Consider decrease in cardiac, hepatic, and renal function; concomitant disease; or other drug therapy; see Elderly.

DILUTION
Specific techniques required; see Precautions. Contains no preservatives; aseptic technique imperative. Each 100 mg must be diluted with 5 mL of NS or SWFI; yields 20 mg/mL

(a 2% solution). Shake solution gently and allow to stand until clear. A 2% solution reconstituted with NS may be injected directly or further diluted to a minimum concentration of 0.2% (2 mg/mL) for infusion. A 2% solution reconstituted with SWFI is hypotonic and should not be injected directly. It *must* be further diluted to a minimum concentration of 0.2% (2 mg/mL). D5W, ¹/₂NS, and D5NS are **compatible** diluents. Do not use heat to facilitate dilution. See Monitor.

Filters: May be filtered through available micron sizes of cellulose ester membrane filters.
Storage: Store unopened vials at or below 25° C (77° F). Cyclophosphamide that is reconstituted in SWFI must be used immediately. Do not store. If reconstituted in NS or further diluted, it must be used within 24 hours when stored at RT. Solutions reconstituted in NS or further diluted in ¹/₂NS are stable up to 6 days if refrigerated. Solutions further diluted in D5W or D5NS are stable for 36 hours if refrigerated. Do not use cyclophosphamide vials if there are signs of melting (clear or yellowish viscous liquid or droplets).

COMPATIBILITY   (Underline Indicates Conflicting Compatibility Information)
Consider any drug NOT listed as compatible to be INCOMPATIBLE until consulting a pharmacist; specific conditions may apply.
One source suggests the following **compatibilities:**
Additive: Bleomycin (Blenoxane), cisplatin, fluorouracil (5-FU), mesna (Mesnex), methotrexate, mitoxantrone (Novantrone), ondansetron (Zofran).
Y-site: Allopurinol (Aloprim), amifostine (Ethyol), amikacin, ampicillin, anidulafungin (Eraxis), aztreonam (Azactam), bleomycin (Blenoxane), cefazolin (Ancef), cefotaxime (Claforan), cefoxitin (Mefoxin), cefuroxime (Zinacef), chloramphenicol (Chloromycetin), cisplatin, cladribine (Leustatin), clindamycin (Cleocin), doripenem (Doribax), doxorubicin (Adriamycin), doxorubicin liposomal (Doxil), doxycycline, droperidol (Inapsine), erythromycin (Erythrocin), etoposide phosphate (Etopophos), filgrastim (Neupogen), fludarabine (Fludara), fluorouracil (5-FU), furosemide (Lasix), gallium nitrate (Ganite), gemcitabine (Gemzar), gentamicin, granisetron (Kytril), heparin, idarubicin (Idamycin), leucovorin calcium, linezolid (Zyvox), melphalan (Alkeran), methotrexate, metoclopramide (Reglan), metronidazole (Flagyl IV), mitomycin (Mutamycin), nafcillin (Nallpen), ondansetron (Zofran), oxacillin (Bactocill), oxaliplatin (Eloxatin), paclitaxel (Taxol), palonosetron (Aloxi), pemetrexed (Alimta), penicillin G potassium, piperacillin/tazobactam (Zosyn), propofol (Diprivan), sargramostim (Leukine), sodium bicarbonate, sulfamethoxazole/trimethoprim, teniposide (Vumon), thiotepa, ticarcillin/clavulanate (Timentin), tobramycin, topotecan (Hycamtin), vancomycin, vinblastine, vincristine, vinorelbine (Navelbine).

RATE OF ADMINISTRATION
Rate may vary depending on protocol. May be given by IV push or as an intermittent or continuous infusion. Inject or infuse very slowly to reduce the likelihood of adverse reactions that may be administration rate–dependent (e.g., facial swelling, headache, nasal congestion, scalp burning). Duration of infusion should be appropriate for the volume to be infused.

ACTIONS
An alkylating agent of the nitrogen mustard group with antitumor activity; cell cycle phase nonspecific, but most effective in S phase. Cyclophosphamide is a prodrug that is activated by hepatic microsomal enzymes. It is thought to prevent cell division by cross-linking DNA strands and preventing DNA synthesis. Elimination half-life is 3 to 12 hours. Metabolized in the liver, it or its metabolites are excreted in the urine. Secreted in breast milk.

INDICATIONS AND USES
Although effective alone in susceptible malignancies, cyclophosphamide is more frequently used concurrently or sequentially with other antineoplastic agents. Cyclophosphamide has been used in the treatment of the following malignancies: malignant lymphomas (e.g., Hodgkin's disease, lymphocytic lymphoma, mixed-cell–type lymphomas, histiocytic lymphoma, Burkitt's lymphoma), multiple myeloma, leukemias (e.g., chronic

lymphocytic leukemia, chronic granulocytic leukemia, acute myelogenous and mono-cytic leukemia, acute lymphoblastic [stem cell] leukemia in children), mycosis fungoi-des, neuroblastoma, adenocarcinoma of the ovary, retinoblastoma, and carcinoma of the breast. ▪ Adjuvant treatment of operable node-positive breast cancer in combination with doxorubicin and docetaxel. ▪ Used orally to treat many other indications, including biopsy-proven nephrotic syndrome, in pediatric patients when disease fails to respond to primary therapy or when primary therapy causes intolerable side effects.

Limitations of use: Safety and effectiveness for the treatment of nephrotic syndrome in adults or of other renal disease have not been established.

Unlabeled uses: Ewing's sarcoma, granulomatosis with polyangiitis (GPA, Wegener's granulomatosis), lupus nephritis, non-Hodgkin's lymphoma, severe rheumatologic con-ditions. ▪ Transplant conditioning and many others; see literature.

CONTRAINDICATIONS

Hypersensitivity to cyclophosphamide, any of its metabolites, or to other components of the product. ▪ Urinary outflow obstruction.

PRECAUTIONS

Follow guidelines for handling cytotoxic agents. See Appendix A, p. 1331. ▪ Adminis-tered by or under the direction of the physician specialist. ▪ Myelosuppression (leuko-penia, neutropenia, thrombocytopenia, and anemia), bone marrow failure, and severe immunosuppression may lead to serious and sometimes fatal infections. Sepsis and sep-tic shock can occur. Latent infections (e.g., tuberculosis, viral hepatitis) can be reacti-vated. ▪ Hemorrhagic cystitis, pyelitis, ureteritis, and hematuria have been reported. Urotoxicity can be fatal. ▪ Exclude or correct any urinary tract obstructions before starting treatment; see Contraindications. ▪ Use with caution, if at all, in patients with active urinary tract infections. ▪ Myocarditis, myopericarditis, pericardial effusions in-cluding cardiac tamponade, and congestive heart failure have been reported and may be fatal. Supraventricular and ventricular arrhythmias (including severe QT prolongation) have been reported. Risk of cardiotoxicity may be increased with high doses, in the el-derly, in patients with pre-existing cardiac disease, and in patients with previous radiation treatment to the cardiac region and/or previous or concomitant treatment with other cardiotoxic drugs (e.g., bleomycin, doxorubicin). ▪ Pneumonitis, pulmonary fibrosis, pulmonary veno-occlusive disease, and other forms of pulmonary toxicity leading to respiratory failure have been reported during and after treatment with cyclophosphamide. Late-onset pneumonitis (greater than 6 months after the start of therapy) appears to be associated with increased mortality. Pneumonitis may develop years after treat-ment. ▪ Development of secondary malignancies has been reported in patients treated with cyclophosphamide used alone or in association with other antineoplastic agents. May develop several years after treatment has been discontinued. ▪ Risk of bladder cancer may be reduced by prevention of hemorrhagic cystitis. ▪ Veno-occlusive liver disease (VOD) has been reported. Fatalities have occurred. A cytoreductive regimen in preparation for bone marrow transplantation that consists of cyclophosphamide in com-bination with whole-body irradiation, busulfan, or other agents has been identified as a major risk factor. VOD has also been reported to develop gradually in patients receiving long-term, low-dose, immunosuppressive doses of cyclophosphamide; in patients with pre-existing hepatic impairment; in patients who have received abdominal radiation; and in patients with low performance status. ▪ Hyponatremia associated with increased total body water, acute water intoxication, and a syndrome that resembles syndrome of inap-propriate secretion of antidiuretic hormone (SIADH) has been reported. ▪ Use caution in patients with impaired renal function. ▪ Use with caution in patients with impaired hepatic function. Reduced conversion to active metabolite may cause decreased effi-cacy. ▪ May interfere with normal wound healing. ▪ Do not administer any live virus vaccine to patients receiving antineoplastic drugs. ▪ Anaphylaxis resulting in death has been reported.

Monitor: Monitor CBC and platelets and SCr frequently; see Dose Adjustments. ▪ Check urinary sediment regularly for presence of erythrocytes and other signs of urotoxicity and/or nephrotoxicity. ▪ Aggressive hydration with forced diuresis and frequent bladder emptying can reduce the frequency and severity of bladder toxicity. Mesna has been used to prevent severe bladder toxicity. ▪ Monitor patients with severe renal impairment (CrCl 10 to 24 mL/min) for signs and symptoms of toxicity. ▪ Observe continuously for infection. Prophylactic antibiotics may be indicated pending results of C/S in a febrile neutropenic patient. Antimycotics and/or antivirals may also be indicated. ▪ Monitor patients with risk factors for cardiotoxicity. ▪ Monitor patients for signs and symptoms of pulmonary toxicity. ▪ Use antiemetics for patient comfort. ▪ Monitor for thrombocytopenia (platelet count less than 50,000/mm^3). Initiate precautions to prevent excessive bleeding (e.g., inspect IV sites, skin, and mucous membranes; use extreme care during invasive procedures; test urine, emesis, stool, and secretions for occult blood).

Patient Education: Nonhormonal birth control recommended. Female patients should use highly effective contraception during and for up to 1 year after completion of treatment. Male patients with a female partner who is or may become pregnant should use a condom during and for at least 4 months after treatment. ▪ Male and female reproductive function and fertility may be impaired. ▪ Interferes with oogenesis and spermatogenesis. May cause sterility in both sexes. ▪ Increase fluid intake and void frequently. ▪ Promptly report any signs or symptoms of infection, any urinary symptoms, new or worsening shortness of breath, cough, swelling of the ankles/legs, palpitations, weight gain, dizziness, loss of consciousness, or other side effects. ▪ See Appendix D, p. 1333.

Maternal/Child: Category D: may produce fetal harm. ▪ Discontinue breast-feeding. ▪ Safety profile in pediatric patients similar to that of adults. ▪ See Patient Education.

Elderly: Consider age-related organ impairment. Dose selection should be cautious; see Dose Adjustments. Toxicity may be increased. Monitoring of renal function is suggested.

DRUG/LAB INTERACTIONS

Severe myelosuppression may be expected in patients pretreated with and/or receiving concomitant chemotherapy and/or radiation therapy. ▪ Concomitant use of **protease inhibitors** (e.g., atazanavir [Reyataz], indinavir [Crixivan], nelfinavir [Viracept], ritonavir [Norvir], saquinavir [Invirase]) may increase the concentration of cytotoxic metabolites. Use of protease inhibitor–based regimens was found to be associated with a higher incidence of infections and neutropenia in patients receiving cyclophosphamide, doxorubicin, and etoposide (CDE) than in patients receiving a nonnucleoside reverse transcriptase inhibitor–based regimen (e.g., delavirdine [Rescriptor], nevirapine [Viramune]). ▪ Increased hematotoxicity and/or immunosuppression may result from the combined effect of cyclophosphamide and **ACE inhibitors** (e.g., enalapril [Vasotec], lisinopril [Prinivil, Zestril]), **allopurinol** (Aloprim), **natalizumab** (Tysabri), **paclitaxel** (Taxol), **thiazide diuretics** (e.g., hydrochlorothiazide), and **zidovudine** (AZT, Retrovir). ▪ Cardiotoxicity may result from a combined effect of cyclophosphamide and **anthracyclines** (e.g., doxorubicin [Adriamycin], liposomal doxorubicin [Doxil], epirubicin [Ellence]), **cytarabine** (ARA-C), **pentostatin** (Nipent), **radiation therapy** of the cardiac region, and **trastuzumab** (Herceptin). ▪ Increased pulmonary toxicity may result from a combined effect of cyclophosphamide and **amiodarone** (Nexterone), **filgrastim** (Neupogen), and **sargramostim** (Leukine). ▪ Increased nephrotoxicity may result from the combined effect of cyclophosphamide and **amphotericin B and indomethacin**. ▪ Risk of hepatotoxicity is increased when administered with **azathioprine**. ▪ Increased incidence of hepatic VOD and mucositis when administered with **busulfan** (Busulfex, Myleran). ▪ Increased incidence of mucositis when administered with **protease inhibitors** (e.g., atazanavir [Reyataz], indinavir [Crixivan], nelfinavir [Viracept], ritonavir [Norvir], saquinavir [Invirase]). ▪ Increased risk of hemorrhagic cystitis may result from a combined effect of cyclophosphamide and past or concomitant **radiation treatment**. ▪ Higher incidence of noncutaneous malignant solid tumors in patients with Wegener's granulomatosis when administered with **etanercept** (Enbrel). ▪ Acute encephalopathy has been reported in patients receiving **metronidazole** (Flagyl) and cyclophosphamide. ▪ Concomitant use with **tamoxifen** (Soltamox) may increase the risk of thromboembolic complications. ▪ May increase or decrease activity of

anticoagulants (e.g., warfarin [Coumadin]); monitor INR and adjust dose as indicated. ▪ May reduce serum **digoxin** (Lanoxin) and **cyclosporine** (Sandimmune, Neoral) levels. ▪ May prolong neuromuscular blockade and prolonged respiratory depression caused by **succinylcholine.** These effects are dose dependent and may occur up to several days after cyclophosphamide is discontinued. Alert the anesthesiologist. ▪ May decrease effectiveness of oral **quinolone antibiotics** (e.g., ciprofloxacin [Cipro], levofloxacin [Levaquin]). ▪ Capable of many other interactions.

SIDE EFFECTS

The most commonly reported side effects are alopecia (regrowth may be slightly darker), diarrhea, febrile neutropenia, fever, nausea, neutropenia, and vomiting. Other side effects include abdominal pain, amenorrhea, anorexia, gonadal suppression, impaired wound healing, leukopenia (see Precautions), malaise, mucosal ulcerations, darkening of skin and fingernails, susceptibility to infection, including opportunistic infections.

Major: Anaphylaxis, bone marrow suppression (anemia, leukopenia, thrombocytopenia) or failure, hemorrhagic cystitis or ureteritis (reversible), infection, pneumonitis, pulmonary fibrosis, rash, renal tubular necrosis (reversible), secondary neoplasia, SIADH, urinary tract and renal toxicity (e.g., bladder fibrosis, hemorrhagic cystitis, ureteritis), veno-occlusive disease.

Post-Marketing: Numerous side effects have been identified from post-marketing surveillance. These include acute respiratory distress syndrome, arthralgia, ascites, asthenia, bronchospasm, cardiotoxicity (e.g., arrhythmias, cardiac arrest, cardiac failure, cardiogenic shock, cardiomyopathy, myocardial infarction, myocarditis, pericarditis), chest pain, chills, cholestasis, colitis, convulsions, disseminated intravascular coagulation, dizziness, dyspnea, edema, encephalopathy, fatigue, fever, fluid retention, headache, hemolytic-uremic syndrome, hepatic encephalopathy, hepatitis, hepatotoxicity with hepatic failure, hyperglycemia, hypertension, hypoglycemia, hyponatremia, hypotension, increased liver function tests, infusion site reactions, interstitial pneumonitis, malaise, muscle spasms, myalgia, pancreatitis, paresthesia, peripheral neuropathy, pruritus, pulmonary edema, radiation recall dermatitis, reversible posterior leukoencephalopathy syndrome, rhabdomyolysis, Stevens-Johnson syndrome, stomatitis, toxic epidermal necrolysis, visual impairment, and many others.

ANTIDOTE

No specific antidote available. Minor side effects will be treated symptomatically if necessary. Discontinue the drug in cases of severe hemorrhagic cystitis. Urotoxicity may require interruption of treatment or cystectomy. Mesna has been used to decrease the incidence of cystitis. Interrupt therapy, reduce dose, or discontinue in patients who have or who develop potentially serious infections. Administration of whole blood products (e.g., packed RBCs, platelets, leukocytes) and/or blood modifiers (e.g., darbepoetin alfa [Aranesp], epoetin alfa [Epogen], filgrastim [Neupogen, Zarxio], pegfilgrastim [Neulasta], sargramostim [Leukine]) may be indicated to treat bone marrow toxicity. Leukocyte and thrombocyte nadirs are usually reached in the first or second week of treatment. Peripheral blood cell counts are expected to normalize after approximately 20 days. Supportive therapy as indicated will help sustain the patient in toxicity. Cyclophosphamide and its metabolites are dialyzable.

CYCLOSPORINE BBW

(sye-kloh-**SPOR**-een)

Immunosuppressant

Sandimmune

C

USUAL DOSE
5 to 6 mg/kg of body weight as a single dose 4 to 12 hours before transplantation. Repeat once each day until oral dosage form can be tolerated. Individualized adjustment is imperative and may be required on a daily basis. Administered at $^1/_3$ of the oral dose in patients temporarily unable to take oral cyclosporine. Administered in conjunction with adrenal corticosteroids; different regimens used; see prescribing information.

PEDIATRIC DOSE
Same as adult dose; however, higher doses may be required. See Maternal/Child.

DOSE ADJUSTMENTS
Reduced dose may be required in impaired renal function and in patients with severe hepatic impairment. ▪ Higher doses may be required in pediatric patients. ▪ Lower-end doses may be indicated in the elderly. Consider impaired organ function and concomitant disease or other drug therapy. ▪ Cyclosporine (Sandimmune) is not bioequivalent to Neoral (a brand of cyclosporine oral solution). Conversion from Neoral dosing to Sandimmune may result in lower cyclosporine blood concentrations. Blood concentration monitoring is indicated to avoid potential underdosing. ▪ See Monitor and Drug/Lab Interactions.

DILUTION
Each 50 mg should be diluted immediately before use with 20 to 100 mL of NS or D5W and given as an infusion. May leach phthalate from polyvinylchloride containers; use diluents in glass infusion bottles. Dilute immediately before use and discard unused portion.

Filters: Filtered through a 0.45-micron polyprolene filter during manufacturing. Has a high ethanol content, which the filter must accommodate. A large-bore needle filter may be used when withdrawing cyclosporine from an ampule. Adsorption should be negligible, but if there is concern, draw diluent through the same filter. In-line filtering is acceptable. Manufacturer indicates that cyclosporine molecules are small enough to pass through an in-line filter as small as 0.22 microns. Loss of potency is not expected. Another source used 0.22- and 0.45-micron filters and indicates an initial loss of potency that recovered to full concentration.

Storage: Before use, store ampules at CRT. Protect from light. Discard diluted solution after 24 hours.

COMPATIBILITY
(Underline Indicates Conflicting Compatibility Information)

Consider any drug NOT listed as compatible to be INCOMPATIBLE until consulting a pharmacist; specific conditions may apply.

Leaches out plasticizers, including DEHP from PVC infusion bags and IV tubing; use of non-PVC containers and IV tubing recommended.

One source suggests the following **compatibilities:**

Additive: Ciprofloxacin (Cipro IV), fat emulsion IV.

Y-site: Anidulafungin (Eraxis), caspofungin (Cancidas), ceftaroline (Teflaro), doripenem (Doribax), linezolid (Zyvox), meropenem (Merrem IV), micafungin (Mycamine), propofol (Diprivan), sargramostim (Leukine), telavancin (Vibativ).

RATE OF ADMINISTRATION
A single dose properly diluted as a slow IV infusion equally distributed over 2 to 6 hours.

ACTIONS
A potent immunosuppressive agent. Interferes with IL-2 production and blocks T-cell proliferative signals during early T-cell activation. Prolongs survival of kidney, liver, and heart allogeneic transplants in the human. Measured by specific or nonspecific assays.

Extensively metabolized by the cytochrome P_{450} hepatic enzyme system. Half-life is 19 hours (range 10 to 27 hours). Primarily excreted in bile and to a small extent in urine. Crosses the placental barrier. Secreted in breast milk.

INDICATIONS AND USES

Prophylaxis of organ rejection in kidney, liver, and heart allogeneic transplants in conjunction with adrenocortical steroids. ▪ Treatment of chronic rejection in patients previously treated with other immunosuppressive agents. Reserve parenteral formulation for when oral administration not feasible.

Unlabeled uses: Decrease frequency of pancreatic or corneal allograft rejection. ▪ Prevention of acute graft-versus-host disease. ▪ Crohn's disease.

CONTRAINDICATIONS

Hypersensitivity to cyclosporine or to Cremophor EL (polyoxyethylated castor oil).

PRECAUTIONS

Anaphylactic reactions have been reported with the IV formulation. These reactions may be related to the IV vehicle Cremophor EL; patients who experienced these reactions have subsequently been treated with the oral formulation of cyclosporine without incident. Because of the risk of anaphylaxis, IV cyclosporine should be reserved for patients who are unable to take oral therapy. ▪ Usually administered in the hospital by or under the direction of a physician experienced in immunosuppressive therapy and management of organ transplant patients. ▪ Adequate laboratory and supportive medical resources must be available. ▪ All formulations may be given concomitantly with adrenocortical steroids. Manufacturer has a Black Box Warning. *Do not administer cyclosporine with any other immunosuppressive agent except adrenocortical steroids.* ▪ Can cause hepatotoxicity and nephrotoxicity; see Monitor. In impaired renal function, if rejection is severe, try other immunosuppressive therapy or allow rejection and removal of the kidney rather than increase dose of cyclosporine. ▪ May cause lymphomas and other malignancies, particularly those of the skin. Increased risk of developing a malignancy appears to be related to the intensity and duration of immunosuppression. Some malignancies may be fatal. ▪ Patients receiving immunosuppressive therapies, including cyclosporine and cyclosporine-containing regimens, are at increased risk for infections (viral, bacterial, fungal, protozoal). Both generalized and localized infections can occur. Opportunistic infections include polyomavirus infections (e.g., JC virus–associated progressive multifocal leukoencephalopathy [PML]; polyoma virus–associated nephropathy [PVAN], especially due to BK virus infection). Pre-existing infections may be aggravated. Latent infections may be reactivated. Fatal outcomes have been reported. ▪ Encephalopathy has been reported, including posterior reversible encephalopathy syndrome (PRES). May be manifest as impaired consciousness, convulsions, visual disturbances (including blindness), loss of motor function, movement disorders, and psychiatric disturbances. Predisposing factors may include hypertension, hypomagnesemia, hypocholesterolemia, high-dose corticosteroids, high cyclosporine blood levels, and graft-versus-host disease. Patients receiving liver transplants may be more susceptible to encephalopathy than patients receiving kidney transplants. Reversal of encephalopathy has occurred after discontinuation or dose reduction of cyclosporine. ▪ Convulsions have been reported, particularly in patients receiving concomitant therapy with high-dose methylprednisolone. ▪ Significant hyperkalemia (sometimes associated with hyperchloremic acidosis) and hyperuricemia have been reported. ▪ A syndrome of thrombocytopenia and microangiopathic hemolytic anemia that may result in graft failure has been reported. ▪ Optic disc edema, including papilledema, with possible visual impairment secondary to benign intracranial hypertension has been reported. ▪ See Drug/Lab Interactions.

Monitor: Observe for S/S of an anaphylactic reaction (e.g., blood pressure changes; bronchospasm; dyspnea; edema of face, tongue, or throat; itching; rash; tachycardia; wheezing). Monitor continuously for the first 30 minutes of the infusion and frequently thereafter. ▪ Can cause hepatotoxicity and nephrotoxicity. Monitor BUN, SCr, serum bilirubin, and liver enzymes frequently. Timing and amount of rise in BUN and creatinine and degree of nephrotoxicity or hepatotoxicity distinguish between need for dose reduction or symptoms of organ rejection. ▪ May be difficult to distinguish between nephrotoxicity and rejection. Up to 20% of patients may have simultaneous nephrotoxicity and rejection. See package insert for a chart discussing differential diagnoses for each. ▪ Monitor cyclosporine blood levels. Measured by specific or nonspecific assay. 24-hour specific trough values of 100 to 200 ng/mL of whole blood or 24-hour nonspecific trough values of 250 to 800 ng/mL of whole blood minimize side effects and rejection events. Nonspecific assays trough values are higher because they include metabolites. Plasma levels may range from $^1/_2$ to $^1/_5$ of whole blood levels. Consistent use of one assay is recommended. Confirm assay method to evaluate appropriately. ▪ Observe constantly for signs of infection (fever, sore throat, tiredness) or unusual bleeding or bruising. ▪ Prophylactic antibiotics may be indicated pending results of C/S. ▪ Monitor for development of PVAN and BK virus–associated nephropathy (e.g., deteriorating renal function and renal graft loss). Dose reduction may be indicated. ▪ Monitor for development of PML (e.g., apathy, ataxia, cognitive deficiencies, confusion, hemiparesis). If symptoms appear, consultation with a neurologist may be indicated. ▪ Monitor BP. Hypertension is a common side effect. Initiation or modification of antihypertensive therapy may be indicated; do not use potassium-sparing diuretics (e.g., spironolactone [Aldactone]); may increase risk of hyperkalemia. ▪ Monitor for S/S of encephalopathy and/or PRES. ▪ See Precautions and Drug/Lab Interactions.

Patient Education: Use nonhormonal birth control. Do not use oral contraceptives. See Appendix D, p. 1333. ▪ Do not make any changes in formulation (e.g., IV, capsules, oral solution) without physician direction; products are not equivalent. May require dose adjustment. ▪ Review side effects with a health care professional and report all side effects promptly. ▪ Capable of multiple drug-drug interactions; obtain physician approval before adding or stopping medications. ▪ Compliance with frequent laboratory tests is imperative.

Maternal/Child: Category C: safety for use in pregnancy not established. Should not be used unless benefit to the mother justifies potential risk to the fetus. Use in men and women capable of conception not established. Reported outcomes of pregnancies in women who received cyclosporine are difficult to evaluate. It is not possible to separate the effects of cyclosporine from the effects of other medications, underlying maternal disorders, or other aspects of the transplantation process. Negative outcomes included prematurity, low birth weight, fetal loss, and various malformations. ▪ Discontinue breast-feeding. ▪ Safety for use in pediatric patients not established but has been used in patients as young as 6 months. Accidental parenteral overdose in premature neonates has caused serious symptoms of intoxication.

Elderly: Dose selection should be cautious; see Dose Adjustments. ▪ Differences in response compared to younger adults not identified.

DRUG/LAB INTERACTIONS
Interactions are numerous and potentially life threatening. Review of drug profile by pharmacist imperative. ▪ Risk of nephrotoxicity increased when given with other drugs that may potentiate renal dysfunction. Use extreme caution and monitor renal function closely. If impairment of renal function is significant, either reduce the dose of cyclosporine and/or the coadministered drug, or consider an alternative treatment. Manufacturer lists **antibiotics** (e.g., ciprofloxacin [Cipro], gentamicin, tobramycin, sulfamethoxazole/trimethoprim, vancomycin), **antifungals** (e.g., amphotericin B, ketoconazole [Nizoral]), **anti-inflammatory drugs** (e.g., azapropazon [Rheumox], colchicine, diclofenac [Voltaren, Cataflam], naproxen [Aleve, Naprosyn], sulindac [Clinoril]), **H$_2$ antagonists** (e.g., cimetidine [Tagamet], ranitidine [Zantac]), **immunosuppressives** (e.g., tacrolimus [Prograf]), **antineoplastics** (e.g., melphalan [Alkeran], methotrexate), **and fibric acid derivatives** (e.g., fenofibrate [Tricor]). Other sources list **acyclovir** (Zovirax), **foscarnet** (Foscavir), **selected quinolones** (e.g., norfloxacin [Noroxin]), **and numerous other nephrotoxic drugs.** ▪ Concurrent administration with **colchicine** may cause cyclosporine toxicity (e.g., GI, hepatic, renal, and neuromuscular toxicity). Cyclosporine may decrease the clearance and in-

crease the toxic effects of colchicine (e.g., myopathy, neuropathy), especially in patients with renal impairment. With concurrent use, close clinical observation is required. Reduce colchicine dose or discontinue as indicated. ▪ May increase **diclofenac** (Voltaren) serum levels with concomitant administration; initiate diclofenac dose at the lower end of the therapeutic range. ▪ Cyclosporine is extensively metabolized by CYP3A4 and is a substrate of the multidrug efflux transporter P-glycoprotein. **Drugs that inhibit or induce CYP3A4, P-glycoprotein transporter, or organic anion transporter proteins** will result in an alteration of cyclosporine concentrations. Toxicity or allograft rejection may occur. Compounds that decrease cyclosporine absorption, such as **orlistat** (Alli), should be avoided. ▪ Cyclosporine plasma levels may be increased with concurrent use of **protease inhibitors** (e.g., boceprevir [Victrelis], indinavir [Crixivan], nelfinavir [Viracept], ritonavir [Norvir], saquinavir [Invirase], telaprevir [Incivek]), which are metabolized by cytochrome P_{450} 3A; use caution. ▪ Drugs that inhibit the cytochrome P_{450} system may decrease the metabolism of cyclosporine and increase its serum concentrations. Manufacturer lists **allopurinol** (Aloprim), **amiodarone** (Nexterone), **antibiotics** (e.g., azithromycin [Zithromax], clarithromycin, erythromycin, quinupristin/dalfopristin [Synercid]), **antifungals** (e.g., fluconazole [Diflucan], itraconazole [Sporanox], ketoconazole [Nizoral], voriconazole [VFEND]), **bromocriptine** (Parlodel), **calcium channel blockers** (e.g., diltiazem [Cardizem], nicardipine [Cardene], verapamil), **danazol** (Danocrine), **glucocorticoids** (e.g., methylprednisolone [Solu-Medrol]), **imatinib** (Gleevec), **metoclopramide** (Reglan), **nefazodone, and oral contraceptives.** Monitor blood levels with concurrent use to avoid cyclosporine toxicity. ▪ Drugs that decrease cyclosporine concentrations should be avoided. Manufacturer lists **antibiotics** (e.g., nafcillin [Nallpen], rifampin [Rifadin]), **anticonvulsants** (e.g., carbamazepine [Tegretol], oxcarbazepine [Trileptal], phenobarbital [Luminal], phenytoin [Dilantin]), **bosentan** (Tracleer), **octreotide** (Sandostatin), **orlistat** (Alli, Xenical), **terbinafine** (Lamisil), **ticlopidine** (Ticlid), **St. John's wort, and sulfinpyrazone** (Anturane). Other sources list **sulfamethoxazole/trimethoprim;** monitor levels and adjust cyclosporine dose as indicated to avoid transplant rejection. ▪ **Rifabutin** (Mycobutin) may increase metabolism of cyclosporine; use care with concomitant use. ▪ Cyclosporine inhibits CYP3A4 and the multidrug efflux transporter P-glycoprotein and may increase plasma concentrations of co-medications that are substrates of CYP3A4, P-glycoprotein, or organic anion transporter proteins. Cyclosporine reduces clearance and may increase blood levels of **ambrisentan** (Letairis), **bosentan** (Tracleer), **dabigatran** (Pradaxa), **digoxin** (Lanoxin), **etoposide** (VePesid), **methotrexate, NSAIDs, prednisolone, repaglinide** (Prandin), **sirolimus** (Rapamune), **and other drugs.** May decrease the volume distribution of **digoxin** and cause toxicity rather quickly. With concurrent use, monitor digoxin levels, reduce digoxin dose, or discontinue as indicated. ▪ Concomitant use with **NSAIDs,** particularly in dehydrated patients, may potentiate renal dysfunction. ▪ Avoid concurrent use with **bosentan.** ▪ When coadministering **ambrisentan** with cyclosporine, the ambrisentan dose should *not* be titrated to the recommended maximum daily dose. ▪ Cyclosporine may decrease the clearance of **HMG-CoA reductase inhibitors (statins)** such as atorvastatin (Lipitor), lovastatin (Mevacor), pravastatin (Pravachol), simvastatin (Zocor) and, rarely, fluvastatin (Lescol). Cases of myotoxicity (including muscle pain and weakness, myositis, and rhabdomyolysis) have been reported with concomitant use. Dose reduction of statins is indicated. Statins may be temporarily withheld or discontinued in patients with S/S of myopathy or potential for renal injury, including renal failure, secondary to rhabdomyolysis. ▪ Coadministration with **aliskiren** (Tekturna) is not recommended. ▪ May decrease **mycophenolate** (CellCept) levels. Monitor levels closely when cyclosporine is added or removed from a drug regimen containing mycophenolate. ▪ Concurrent use of cyclosporine with **imipenem-cilastatin** (Primaxin) may increase CNS toxicity of both agents. ▪ Potentiates **nondepolarizing muscle relaxants** (e.g., atracurium [Tracrium]); will prolong neuromuscular blockade. ▪ Do not use **potassium-sparing diuretics** (e.g., spironolactone [Aldactone]); may increase risk of hyperkalemia. Use caution when coadministered with **other potassium-sparing drugs** (e.g., angiotensin-converting inhibitors [e.g., enalapril (Vasotec), lisinopril (Zestril)], angiotensin II receptor antagonists [e.g., losartan (Cozaar), valsartan (Diovan)]), **potassium-containing drugs,** and/or in patients on a **potassium-rich diet.** Hyperkalemia can occur. ▪ May cause convulsions with high doses of **methylprednisolone.** ▪ May be given in combination with **steroids** but has additive effects with other **immunosuppressive agents;** may increase risk of lymphoma. ▪ Concurrent administration with **sirolimus** (Rapamune) increases blood levels of sirolimus. To minimize the effect on blood levels, administer sirolimus 4 hours after cyclosporine dose. ▪ Elevations in SCr have been reported with coadministration of **sirolimus** and cyclosporine. Effect is usually reversible with cyclosporine dose reduction. ▪ Serum levels may increase with **chloroquine** (Aralen). ▪ Avoid use in psoriasis patients receiving **other immunosuppressive agents or radiation therapy, including PUVA and UVB.** Immunosuppression may be excessive. ▪ May increase the plasma concentrations of **repaglinide** (Prandin), which increases the risk for hypoglycemia. Monitor blood glucose levels closely. ▪ Concurrent use with **nifedipine** (Procardia) has caused gingival hyperplasia; avoid use in patients who develop gingival hyperplasia. ▪ High doses of cyclosporine (e.g., IV doses of 16 mg/kg/day) may increase the exposure to **anthracycline antibiotics** (e.g., daunorubicin, doxorubicin, mitoxantrone) in cancer patients. ▪ Monitor serum creatinine when used with **NSAIDs** in rheumatoid arthritis patients. ▪ Vaccinations may be less effective. Avoid use of **live virus vaccines** in patients receiving cyclosporine. ▪ **Grapefruit juice** may affect certain enzymes of the P_{450} enzyme system and should be avoided.

SIDE EFFECTS
The most common side effects include gum hyperplasia, hirsutism, hypertension, renal dysfunction, and tremor. Other side effects include acne, convulsions, cramps, diarrhea, encephalopathy, glomerular capillary thrombosis, headache, hepatotoxicity, hyperkalemia, hyperuricemia, hypomagnesemia, infection, leukopenia, lymphoma, microangiopathic hemolytic anemia, nausea and vomiting, paresthesia, skin rash, and thrombocytopenia. Hypersensitivity reactions including anaphylaxis have occurred. Stevens-Johnson syndrome and toxic epidermal necrolysis have occurred rarely.

Post-Marketing: Headache, including migraine; hepatotoxicity and liver injury, including cholestasis, hepatitis, jaundice, and liver failure with serious and/or fatal outcomes; isolated cases of pain in the lower extremities; JC virus–associated PML, sometimes fatal; and PVAN, especially due to BK virus infection, resulting in graft loss.

ANTIDOTE
Notify physician of all side effects. Most can be treated symptomatically. Drug may be decreased or discontinued or other immunosuppressive agents utilized. Consider reducing total immunosuppression in transplant patients who develop PML or PVAN; may place graft at risk. Discontinue infusion at the first sign of a severe hypersensitivity reaction. Treat hypersensitivity as indicated; may require oxygen, epinephrine (Adrenalin), antihistamines (e.g., diphenhydramine [Benadryl]), vasopressors (e.g., dopamine), corticosteroids, albuterol, IV fluids, and/or ventilation equipment. Nephrotoxicity, hepatotoxicity, encephalopathy (including PRES), or hematopoietic depression may require temporary reduction of dosage or permanent withholding of treatment. Dialysis is not effective in overdose.

CYTARABINE BBW

(sye-**TAIR**-ah-bean)

ARA-C, Cytosar♦, Cytosar-U♦

Antineoplastic
(antimetabolite)

pH 5

USUAL DOSE

Acute nonlymphocytic leukemia in adult and pediatric patients: *Single agent:* 200 mg/M^2/24 hr as a continuous infusion for 5 days. Repeat every 2 weeks. **Combination chemotherapy:** Dose is variable depending on specific regimen or protocol. Examples are 100 mg/M^2/24 hr as a continuous infusion or 100 mg/M^2 as an IV injection every 12 hours. Repeat daily on days 1 through 7. Another regimen uses 100 to 200 mg/M^2 or 2 to 6 mg/kg/24 hr as a continuous infusion or equally divided into 2 or 3 doses and given by IV injection or intermittent infusion. Given for 5 to 10 days. Maintain treatment until therapeutic effect or toxicity occurs. Modify on a day-to-day basis for maximum individualized effectiveness.

Acute myelocytic leukemia or erythroleukemia in adult and pediatric patients: As a single agent, 100 to 200 mg/M^2/24 hr or 3 mg/kg/24 hr for 5 to 10 days as a continuous infusion or in divided doses by IV injection. Total dose is 1,000 mg/M^2. Repeat every 2 weeks.

DOSE ADJUSTMENTS

Dose (mg/kg) based on average weight in presence of edema or ascites. ▪ Dose reduction may be indicated in impaired hepatic or renal function. ▪ See Precautions/Monitor. ▪ Usually used with other antineoplastic drugs in specific doses to achieve tumor remission. ▪ Withhold or modify dose based on degree of bone marrow suppression; see Monitor.

DILUTION

Specific techniques required; see Precautions. Some preparations are liquid and do not require reconstitution or each 100 mg must be reconstituted with 5 mL (500 mg with 10 mL) of SWFI with benzyl alcohol 0.9%. Solution pH about 5. May be given by IV injection as is or further diluted in NS or D5W and given as an infusion. IV injection should be through a free-flowing IV tubing. Use only clear solutions.

Storage: Stable at room temperature for 48 hours.

COMPATIBILITY
(Underline Indicates Conflicting Compatibility Information)

Consider any drug NOT listed as compatible to be INCOMPATIBLE until consulting a pharmacist; specific conditions may apply.

One source suggests the following **compatibilities:**

Additive: Daunorubicin (Cerubidine), gentamicin, hydrocortisone sodium succinate (Solu-Cortef), lincomycin (Lincocin), methotrexate, methylprednisolone (Solu-Medrol), mitoxantrone (Novantrone), ondansetron (Zofran), potassium chloride (KCl), sodium bicarbonate, vincristine.

Y-site: Amifostine (Ethyol), amphotericin B cholesteryl (Amphotec), anidulafungin (Eraxis), aztreonam (Azactam), cladribine (Leustatin), doxorubicin liposomal (Doxil), etoposide phosphate (Etopophos), filgrastim (Neupogen), fludarabine (Fludara), gemcitabine (Gemzar), gentamicin, granisetron (Kytril), hydrocortisone sodium succinate (Solu-Cortef), idarubicin (Idamycin), linezolid (Zyvox), melphalan (Alkeran), methotrexate, methylprednisolone (Solu-Medrol), ondansetron (Zofran), paclitaxel (Taxol), pemetrexed (Alimta), piperacillin/tazobactam (Zosyn), propofol (Diprivan), sargramostim (Leukine), sodium bicarbonate, teniposide (Vumon), thiotepa, vinorelbine (Navelbine).

RATE OF ADMINISTRATION

IV injection: Each 100 mg or fraction thereof over 1 to 3 minutes.

IV infusion: Single daily dose properly diluted over 30 minutes to 24 hours, depending on amount of infusion solution and dosage regimen.

ACTIONS

An antimetabolite and pyrimidine antagonist that interferes with the synthesis of DNA. Cell cycle specific for S phase. Through various chemical processes this deprivation acts more quickly on rapidly growing cells and causes their death. Cytotoxic and cytostatic. A potent bone marrow suppressant. Crosses the blood-brain barrier. Serum half-life averages 1 to 3 hours. Metabolized in the liver and excreted in the urine.

INDICATIONS AND USES

Induction and maintenance of remission in acute nonlymphocytic leukemia in adults and pediatric patients. Also used for treatment of acute lymphocytic leukemia (ALL), the blast phase of chronic myelocytic leukemia, and acute myelocytic leukemia (AML). ▪ Is used intrathecally in the treatment of meningeal leukemia. A liposomal formulation (DepoCyt) is available for intrathecal use only; lipofoam molecules contained in this product are much too large for IV use.

CONTRAINDICATIONS

Hypersensitivity to cytarabine, pre-existing drug-induced bone marrow suppression.

PRECAUTIONS

Follow guidelines for handling cytotoxic agents. See Appendix A, p. 1331. ▪ Administered by or under the direction of a physician specialist in a facility with adequate diagnostic and treatment facilities to monitor the patient and respond to any medical emergency. ▪ Remissions induced by cytarabine are brief unless followed by maintenance therapy. ▪ Use caution with impaired liver or renal function. ▪ Severe GI, pulmonary, or CNS toxicity has occurred with experimental cytarabine regimens. Toxicities are different (e.g., reversible corneal toxicity, hemorrhagic conjunctivitis, cerebral and cerebellar dysfunction, severe GI ulceration) from those seen with conventional therapy. Deaths have been reported. ▪ Benzyl alcohol may cause a fatal "gasping syndrome" in premature infants.

Monitor: Leukocyte and platelet counts should be monitored daily. ▪ During induction therapy, WBC depression is biphasic with the first nadir occurring at days 7 to 9 and a deeper fall at days 15 to 24. Platelet depression begins around day 5 and reaches a nadir at days 12 to 15. ▪ Hold or modify therapy for platelet count less than 50,000 or polymorphonuclear granulocytes less than 1,000 cells/mm³. Restart therapy when bone marrow recovery is confirmed. ▪ Monitor bone marrow, liver, and renal function at regular intervals during therapy. ▪ Higher doses tolerated by IV injection compared with IV infusion, but the incidence and intensity of nausea and vomiting are increased. ▪ Prophylactic administration of antiemetics recommended. ▪ Be alert for signs of bone marrow suppression, bleeding, infection, or neurotoxicity. These side effects are dose- and schedule-dependent. ▪ Monitor for thrombocytopenia (platelet count less than 50,000/mm³). Initiate precautions to prevent excessive bleeding (e.g., inspect IV sites, skin, and mucous membranes; use extreme care during invasive procedures; test urine, emesis, stool, and secretions for occult blood). ▪ Prophylactic antibiotics may be indicated pending results of C/S in a febrile neutropenic patient. ▪ Monitor uric acid levels; maintain hydration; allopurinol may be indicated.

Patient Education: Nonhormonal birth control recommended. ▪ See Appendix D, p. 1333. ▪ Promptly report early signs of neurotoxicity (e.g., ataxia, confusion, lethargy).

Maternal/Child: Category D: avoid pregnancy. May produce teratogenic effects on the fetus, especially during the first trimester. ▪ Discontinue breast-feeding. ▪ See Drug/Lab Interactions.

Elderly: Consider age-related organ impairment; toxicity may be increased.

DRUG/LAB INTERACTIONS

May inhibit **digoxin** absorption. ▪ Do not administer any **live virus vaccines** to patients receiving antineoplastic drugs. ▪ May cause acute pancreatitis in patients who previously received **L-asparaginase.** ▪ May antagonize action of **gentamicin** against *Klebsiella*. ▪ May antagonize antifungal actions of **flucytosine** (Ancobon). ▪ Clearance decreased and toxicity increased with **nephrotoxic agents** (e.g., aminoglycosides [gentamicin]); may cause neurotoxic symptoms (e.g., ataxia, confusion, lethargy). ▪ Concurrent use of high doses of **cytarabine** with cisplatin may increase ototoxicity.

SIDE EFFECTS

Abdominal pain, bone marrow suppression (e.g., anemia, leukopenia, thrombocytopenia), bone pain, cardiomyopathy, chest pain, conjunctivitis, diarrhea, esophagitis, fever, hepatic dysfunction, hypersensitivity reactions, hyperuricemia, malaise, megaloblastosis, mucosal bleeding, myalgia, nausea, oral ulceration, pancreatitis, peripheral motor and sensory neuropathies, rash, stomatitis, thrombophlebitis, vomiting. Higher than usual dose regimens may cause severe coma, GI ulcerations and peritonitis, personality changes, pulmonary toxicity, somnolence, or death.

ANTIDOTE

Notify the physician of all side effects. Most will be treated symptomatically. Some toxicity is necessary to produce remission. Discontinue the drug for serious bone marrow suppression. Administration of whole blood products (e.g., packed RBCs, platelets, leukocytes) and/or blood modifiers (e.g., darbepoetin alfa [Aranesp], epoetin alfa [Epogen], filgrastim [Neupogen, Zarxio], pegfilgrastim [Neulasta], sargramostim [Leukine]) may be indicated to treat bone marrow toxicity. Drug must be restarted as soon as signs of bone marrow recovery occur, or its effectiveness will be lost. Use corticosteroids for cytarabine syndrome (fever, myalgia, bone pain, occasional chest pain, maculopapular rash, conjunctivitis, malaise). Usually occurs in 6 to 12 hours after administration. Continue cytarabine if patient responds to corticosteriods. There is no specific antidote; supportive therapy as indicated will help to sustain the patient in toxicity.

CYTOMEGALOVIRUS IMMUNE GLOBULIN INTRAVENOUS (HUMAN) BBW*

Passive immunizing agent
Antibacterial
Antiviral

(**sigh**-toh-**meg**-ah-lo-**VIGH**-rus ih-**MUNE** GLAW-byoo-lin)

CMV-IGIV, CytoGam

*This drug is on the Black Box Warning list; however, a BBW is not provided in the parenteral prescribing information.

USUAL DOSE

150 mg/kg is the maximum recommended dose per infusion.

Kidney transplant: 150 mg/kg of body weight as an IV infusion. This initial dose must be given within 72 hours of transplant. Additional infusions of 100 mg/kg are given at 2, 4, 6, and 8 weeks posttransplant, then reduced to 50 mg/kg at 12 and 16 weeks posttransplant.

Heart, liver, lung, and pancreas transplants: 150 mg/kg of body weight as an IV infusion. This initial dose must be given within 72 hours of transplant. Consider use in combination with ganciclovir (Cytovene) 10 mg/kg/day for 14 days. Additional infusions of cytomegalovirus IGIV containing 150 mg/kg are given at 2, 4, 6, and 8 weeks posttransplant, then reduced to 100 mg/kg at 12 and 16 weeks posttransplant.

DILUTION

Absolute sterile technique required; contains no preservatives. Available in 20- and 50-mL vials (50 mg/mL); multiple vials may be required. Use only if clear and colorless. Enter vial only once and initiate infusion within 6 hours. Must be completely infused within 12 hours of dilution. See Rate of Administration.

Filters: Use of an in-line filter (pore size 15 microns [0.2 microns acceptable]) is required; see Rate of Administration.

Storage: Store dry powder in refrigerator between 2° and 8° C (35° to 46° F).

COMPATIBILITY

Administration through a separate infusion line recommended. If absolutely necessary, may be piggybacked in a pre-existing line containing NS, 1/2NS, dextrose 2.5%, 5%, 10%, or 20% in water or saline. Do not dilute CMV-IGIV more than one part to two parts of any of these solutions.

RATE OF ADMINISTRATION

Use of an in-line filter (pore size 15 microns [0.2 microns acceptable]) and a constant infusion pump (e.g., IVAC) is required. Begin with a rate of 15 mg/kg/hr. May be increased to 30 mg/kg/hr in 30 minutes if no discomfort or adverse effects. May be increased in another 30 minutes to 60 mg/kg/hr if no discomfort or adverse effects. Do not exceed the 60 mg/kg/hr rate or allow the volume infused to exceed 75 mL/hr regardless of mg/kg/hr dose. Slow rate of infusion at onset of patient discomfort or any adverse reactions. Infusion must be complete within 12 hours of dilution. Subsequent doses may be increased at 15-minute intervals using the same mg/kg/hr rates and adhering to the volume maximum of 75 mL/hr.

ACTIONS

A sterile solution of immunoglobulin G (IgG). Derived from pooled adult human plasma selected for high titers of antibody for cytomegalovirus (CMV). Purified by a specific process. Can raise the relevant antibody levels sufficiently to attenuate or reduce the incidence of serious CMV disease. Antibody levels will last 2 to 3 weeks. Recent studies of combined prophylaxis with CMV-IGIV and ganciclovir have shown reductions in the incidence of serious CMV-associated disease in CMV-seronegative recipients of CMV-seropositive organs below that expected from one drug alone.

INDICATIONS AND USES

Prophylaxis of CMV disease associated with transplantation of kidney, heart, liver, lung, and pancreas. In transplants of these organs other than kidney from CMV-seropositive donors to seronegative recipients, prophylactic CMV-IGIV should be considered in combination with ganciclovir.

CONTRAINDICATIONS

History of a prior severe reaction associated with any human immunoglobulin preparations. Individuals with selective immunoglobulin A deficiency may develop antibodies to IgA and are at risk for anaphylaxis.

PRECAUTIONS

75% of untreated recipients would be expected to develop CMV disease. Use of CMV-IGIV has effected a 50% reduction in this disease rate. Effective results have been obtained with a variety of immunosuppressive regimens (e.g., combinations of azathioprine, cyclosporine, prednisone). ▪ A fatal CMV infection occurred even with ganciclovir treatment in one patient, who inadvertently missed a single injection.

Monitor: Continuous monitoring of vital signs is preferred. Must be monitored before infusion, at every rate change, at the midpoint, at the conclusion, and several times after completion. ▪ All supplies for emergency treatment of acute anaphylatic reaction must be available; see Antidote.

Patient Education: Adherence to the prescribed regimen is imperative.

Maternal/Child: Category C: safety for use during pregnancy or breast-feeding not established. Use only if clearly needed.

DRUG/LAB INTERACTIONS

Defer vaccination with any **live virus vaccine** (e.g., measles, mumps, rubella) until 3 months after CMV-IGIV administration.

SIDE EFFECTS

Incidence related to rate of administration; back pain, chills, fever, flushing, hypotension, muscle cramps, nausea, vomiting, wheezing. Hypersensitivity reactions, including anaphylaxis, are possible.

ANTIDOTE

With onset of any minor side effect, reduce rate of infusion immediately or discontinue temporarily. Discontinue CMV-IGIV if symptoms persist, and notify the physician. May be treated symptomatically and infusion resumed at a slower rate if symptoms subside. Discontinue CMV-IGIV if hypotension or anaphylaxis occur and treat immediately. Epinephrine (Adrenalin), diphenhydramine (Benadryl), oxygen, vasopressors (e.g., dopamine), corticosteroids, and ventilation equipment must always be available. Resuscitate as necessary.

DACARBAZINE BBW
(dah-**KAR**-bah-zeen)

Antineoplastic
(alkylating agent)

DTIC, DTIC-Dome

pH 3 to 4

USUAL DOSE
Malignant melanoma: 2 to 4.5 mg/kg of body weight/24 hr for 10 days. May be repeated at 4-week intervals. May administer 250 mg/M² daily for 5 days. Repeat in 3 weeks. Has proved as effective in lesser doses as in larger doses. Individualized response determines dosage of subsequent treatments.

Hodgkin's disease: 150 mg/M²/24 hr for 5 days. Repeat every 4 weeks. Used in combination with other drugs in a specific regimen. An alternate regimen is 375 mg/M² on Days 1 and 15 every 4 weeks or 100 mg/M²/day for 5 days. Given as part of a specific protocol.

DOSE ADJUSTMENTS
Dose (mg/kg) based on average weight in presence of edema or ascites. ▪ Used with other antineoplastic drugs and radiation therapy in reduced doses to achieve tumor remission. ▪ Dose reduction may be required in impaired liver and renal function.

DILUTION
Specific techniques required; see Precautions. Each 100-mg vial is diluted with 9.9 mL (200 mg with 19.7 mL) of SWFI (10 mg/mL). Further dilution in 50 to 250 mL of D5W or NS for infusion is preferred. May be given through Y-tube or three-way stopcock of infusion set through a free-flowing IV.

Storage: Discard in 6 to 8 hours if kept at room temperature. Reconstituted solution stable for 72 hours, diluted solution for 24 hours if refrigerated at 4° C (39° F).

COMPATIBILITY
(Underline Indicates Conflicting Compatibility Information)
Consider any drug NOT listed as compatible to be INCOMPATIBLE until consulting a pharmacist; specific conditions may apply.
One source suggests the following **compatibilities:**
Additive: Ondansetron (Zofran).
Y-site: Amifostine (Ethyol), aztreonam (Azactam), doxorubicin liposomal (Doxil), etoposide phosphate (Etopophos), filgrastim (Neupogen), fludarabine (Fludara), granisetron (Kytril), heparin, melphalan (Alkeran), ondansetron (Zofran), paclitaxel (Taxol), palonosetron (Aloxi), sargramostim (Leukine), teniposide (Vumon), thiotepa, vinorelbine (Navelbine).

RATE OF ADMINISTRATION
Total dose over 30 to 60 minutes. More rapid rate may cause severe venous irritation.

ACTIONS
An antineoplastic agent. Exact mechanism of action is not known; may inhibit DNA and RNA synthesis. It is an alkylating agent, cell cycle phase nonspecific. Probably localizes in the liver and is excreted in the urine.

INDICATIONS AND USES
Metastatic malignant melanoma. ▪ Hodgkin's disease. ▪ Soft-tissue sarcomas.
Unlabeled uses: Treatment of malignant pheochromocytoma with cyclophosphamide and vincristine. ▪ Treatment of metastatic malignant melanoma with tamoxifen.

CONTRAINDICATIONS
Known hypersensitivity to dacarbazine.

PRECAUTIONS
Follow guidelines for handling cytotoxic agents. See Appendix A, p. 1331. ▪ Administered by or under the direction of the physician specialist. ▪ Bone marrow suppression is the most common toxicity. ▪ Hepatic necrosis has been reported. ▪ Consider potential for therapeutic benefit versus risk for toxicity. ▪ Use caution in impaired liver and renal function.

Monitor: Determine absolute patency of vein; a stinging or burning sensation indicates extravasation; severe cellulitis and tissue necrosis will result. Discontinue injection; use another vein. ▪ Monitor bone marrow function, white and RBC count, and platelet count frequently. ▪ Nausea and vomiting may be reduced by restricting oral intake of fluid and foods for 4 to 6 hours before administration. Use prophylactic antiemetics. ▪ Be alert for signs of bone marrow suppression, bleeding, or infection. ▪ Monitor for thrombocytopenia (platelet count less than 50,000/mm^3). Initiate precautions to prevent excessive bleeding (e.g., inspect IV sites, skin, and mucous membranes; use extreme care during invasive procedures; test urine, emesis, stool, and secretions for occult blood). ▪ Prophylactic antibiotics may be indicated pending results of C/S in a febrile neutropenic patient.

Patient Education: Protect skin surfaces; may cause photosensitive skin reactions. ▪ Nonhormonal birth control recommended. ▪ Report burning or stinging at IV site promptly. ▪ See Appendix D, p. 1333.

Maternal/Child: Category C: safety for use in pregnancy or breast-feeding and in men and women capable of conception not established. ▪ Carcinogenic and teratogenic in animals. ▪ Discontinue breast-feeding.

Elderly: Consider age-related organ impairment; toxicity may be increased.

DRUG/LAB INTERACTIONS

Do not administer any **live virus vaccines** to patients receiving antineoplastic drugs. ▪ Inhibited by **phenobarbital and phenytoin** (Dilantin). ▪ Potentiates **allopurinol**. ▪ Effects of dacarbazine may be increased with **ciprofloxacin** (Cipro), **isoniazid** (INH), **fluvoxamine** (Luvox), **ketoconazole** (Nizoral), **miconazole** (Monistat), **and norfloxacin** (Noroxin). Effects may be decreased with **carbamazepine** (Tegretol), **phenobarbital, and rifampin** (Rifadin).

SIDE EFFECTS

Leukopenia and thrombocytopenia may be serious enough to cause death. Alopecia, anaphylaxis, anorexia, facial flushing, facial paresthesias, fever, hepatotoxicity, malaise, myalgia, nausea, skin necrosis, vomiting.

ANTIDOTE

Notify physician of all side effects. Most will be treated symptomatically. Bone marrow suppression may require temporary or permanent withholding of treatment. Administration of whole blood products (e.g., packed RBCs, platelets, leukocytes) and/or blood modifiers (e.g., darbepoetin alfa [Aranesp], epoetin alfa [Epogen], filgrastim [Neupogen, Zarxio], pegfilgrastim [Neulasta], sargramostim [Leukine]) may be indicated to treat bone marrow toxicity. There is no specific antidote. Supportive therapy as indicated will help sustain the patient in toxicity. For extravasation, elevate extremity; consider injection of long-acting dexamethasone (Decadron LA) throughout extravasated tissue. Use a 27- or 25-gauge needle. Apply moist, warm compresses.

DACTINOMYCIN BBW

(dack-tin-oh-**MY**-sin)

Cosmegen

Antineoplastic
(antibiotic)

pH 5.5 to 7

USUAL DOSE

Dose will depend on tolerance of the patient, the size and location of the tumor, and the use of other forms of therapy. Calculate each dose carefully before administration. Calculation of the dose for obese or edematous patients should be based on body surface area. The dose intensity per 2-week cycle for adult and pediatric patients should not exceed 15 mcg/kg/day (0.015 mg/kg/day) or 400 to 600 mcg/M^2/day (0.4 to 0.6 mg/M^2/day) for 5 days.

Wilms' tumor, childhood rhabdomyosarcoma, and Ewing's sarcoma: 15 mcg/kg/day for 5 days, not to exceed 0.5 mg/day (500 mcg/day). May be administered in various combinations and schedules with other chemotherapeutic agents.

Metastatic nonseminomatous testicular cancer: 1,000 mcg/M^2 (1 mg/M^2) on Day 1 as part of a combination regimen with cyclophosphamide, bleomycin, vinblastine, and cisplatin.

Gestational trophoblastic neoplasia: 12 mcg/kg/day for 5 days as a single agent or 500 mcg on Days 1 and 2 as part of a combination regimen with etoposide, methotrexate, folinic acid, vincristine, cyclophosphamide, and cisplatin.

PEDIATRIC DOSE

Same as Usual Dose for adults; see Contraindications.

DOSE ADJUSTMENTS

Calculate dose based on body surface area in presence of edema or ascites. ▪ Used with other antineoplastic drugs in reduced doses to achieve tumor remission. ▪ Reduce dose of dactinomycin and radiation therapy when used concurrently, if either has been used previously, or if previous chemotherapy has been employed. ▪ Dose selection should be cautious in the elderly. Consider potential for decreased cardiac, hepatic, and renal function, and concomitant disease or drug therapy; see Elderly.

DILUTION

Specific techniques required; see Precautions. Highly toxic. Both powder and solution must be handled with care. Dilute each 0.5-mg vial with 1.1 mL of preservative-free SWFI (0.5 mg/mL). Reconstituted product is a clear, gold-colored solution. SWFI with preservative (benzyl alcohol or paraben) will cause precipitation. Very corrosive to soft tissue. Use sterile two-needle technique if given by IV injection; one needle to dilute and withdraw and one needle to inject into the vein (rinse with blood or IV solution before removing). May be given by IV injection, through the Y-tube or three-way stopcock of a free-flowing infusion of D5W or NS, or further diluted in one of the above solutions for infusion to a final concentration of 10 mcg/mL or higher.

Filters: Manufacturer states, "Use of some in-line cellulose ester membrane filters have resulted in loss of potency." Another source suggests no loss of drug potency with a 5-micron stainless steel depth filter.

Storage: Store at 25° C (77° F). Protect from light and humidity. Prepared product must be used within 4 hours of initial reconstitution when stored at ambient RT. Discard any unused portion.

COMPATIBILITY

Consider any drug NOT listed as compatible to be INCOMPATIBLE until consulting a pharmacist; specific conditions may apply.

Forms a precipitate with SWFI that contains preservatives. Cellulose ester membrane filters may reduce dose by partial removal of dactinomycin.

One source suggests the following **compatibilities:**

Y-site: Allopurinol (Aloprim), amifostine (Ethyol), aztreonam (Azactam), etoposide phosphate (Etopophos), fludarabine (Fludara), gemcitabine (Gemzar), granisetron (Kytril), melphalan (Alkeran), ondansetron (Zofran), sargramostim (Leukine), teniposide (Vumon), thiotepa, vinorelbine (Navelbine).

RATE OF ADMINISTRATION

IV injection: A single dose over 2 to 3 minutes.

IV infusion: A single dose over 10 to 15 minutes.

ACTIONS

A highly toxic antibiotic antineoplastic agent, cell cycle phase nonspecific. Cytotoxic, it interferes with cell division by binding DNA to slow production of RNA. Found in high concentrations in the kidney, liver, and spleen. Does not penetrate the blood-brain barrier. Minimally metabolized. Elimination half-life is approximately 36 hours. Excreted as unchanged drug in bile and urine.

INDICATIONS AND USES

As part of a combination chemotherapy and/or multimodality regimen for treatment of Wilms' tumor, childhood rhabdomyosarcoma, Ewing's sarcoma, and metastatic non-seminomatous testicular cancer. ■ Alone or in combination with other chemotherapeutic agents for the treatment of gestational trophoblastic neoplasia.

Unlabeled uses: Treatment of osteosarcoma, malignant melanoma, Paget's disease of the bone.

CONTRAINDICATIONS

Exposure to chickenpox, herpes zoster, known sensitivity to dactinomycin, infants under 6 to 12 months of age.

PRECAUTIONS

Follow guidelines for handling cytotoxic agents. Review guidelines before handling, and follow diligently. See Appendix A, p. 1331. ■ For IV use only. Do not administer IM or SC. ■ Highly toxic; both the powder and solution must be handled and administered with care. Inhalation of dust or vapors and contact with skin or mucous membranes, especially those of the eyes, must be avoided. If eye contact occurs, rinse for at least 15 minutes with water, saline or a balanced salt ophthalmic solution and then seek immediate ophthalmologic consultation. If skin contact occurs, remove contaminated clothing and rinse area for 15 minutes. Medical attention should be sought immediately and clothes should be destroyed. ■ Administered by or under the direction of a physician specialist. ■ In general, dactinomycin should not be administered concomitantly with radiation therapy in the treatment of Wilms' tumor unless the benefit outweighs the risk. Hepatomegaly and elevated AST levels have been reported. ■ Hepatic veno-occlusive disease that may be associated with intravascular clotting disorder and multiorgan failure has been reported. Pediatric patients younger than 48 months of age may be at increased risk. ■ May have increased incidence of second primary tumors following treatment with dactinomycin and radiation. Long-term follow-up of cancer survivors is indicated.

Monitor: Very corrosive to soft tissue; determine absolute patency of vein. If extravasation occurs, severe damage to soft tissue will result. A stinging or burning sensation indicates extravasation; severe cellulitis and tissue necrosis will result. Discontinue injection; use another vein. Close observation and reconstructive surgery consultation are recommended. ■ Monitor renal, hepatic, and bone marrow function frequently. ■ Except for immediate nausea and vomiting, side effects may not appear for 2 to 4 days and may not peak for 1 to 2 weeks. Always observe closely. Use prophylactic antiemetics. ■ If stomatitis, diarrhea, or severe hematopoietic depression appears, discontinue therapy until the patient has recovered. ■ An increased incidence of GI toxicity, bone marrow suppression, and skin and mucosal reactions has been reported when dactinomycin is administered in combination with radiation therapy. ■ Monitor for thrombocytopenia (platelet count less than 50,000/mm^3). Initiate precautions to prevent excessive bleeding (e.g., inspect IV sites, skin, and mucous membranes; use extreme care during invasive procedures; test urine, emesis, stool, and secretions for occult blood). ■ Allopurinol, increased fluid intake, and alkalinization of urine may be required to reduce uric acid levels. ■ Observe closely for signs of infection. Prophylactic antibiotics may be indicated pending results of C/S in a febrile neutropenic patient.

Patient Education: Nonhormonal birth control recommended. ▪ Report burning or stinging at IV site promptly. ▪ See Appendix D, p. 1333.
Maternal/Child: Category D: avoid pregnancy. May produce teratogenic effects on the fetus; use caution in men and women capable of conception. ▪ Discontinue breast-feeding. ▪ Greater frequency of toxic effects seen in infants. See Contraindications and Precautions.
Elderly: Response similar to that in younger adults; however, recent studies suggest elderly may be at increased risk for myelosuppression; see Dose Adjustments.

DRUG/LAB INTERACTIONS

Dactinomycin potentiates the effects of **radiation therapy;** use with caution in patients receiving radiation therapy. Reduced doses are indicated with simultaneous use; risk of GI toxicity and myelosuppression increased. ▪ Dactinomycin alone may reactivate erythema from **previous radiation therapy.** ▪ Do not administer **live virus vaccines** to patients receiving antineoplastic drugs. ▪ Inhibits action of **penicillin.** ▪ See Dose Adjustments. ▪ May interfere with **bioassay procedures** used in determining antibacterial drug levels.

SIDE EFFECTS

Toxic reactions are frequent, may be severe, and may be dose limiting; however, the severity of toxicity varies markedly and is only partly dependent on the dose administered. Abdominal pain, acne, alopecia, anaphylaxis, anorexia, bone marrow suppression (e.g., anemia, aplastic anemia, agranulocytosis, febrile neutropenia, leukopenia, neutropenia, thrombocytopenia), cheilitis, diarrhea, dysphagia, erythema flare-up, erythema multiforme, esophagitis, fatigue, fever, GI ulceration, hypocalcemia, lethargy, liver toxicity (ascites, hepatitis, hepatic failure with reports of death, hepatic veno-occlusive disease, hepatomegaly, and liver function test abnormalities), malaise, myalgia, nausea, pharyngitis, pneumonitis, proctitis, sepsis (including neutropenic sepsis), skin eruptions, ulcerative stomatitis, vomiting.
Post-Marketing: Stevens-Johnson syndrome, toxic epidermal necrolysis.

ANTIDOTE

Any side effect can result in death. Notify the physician of all side effects. Most will be treated symptomatically. Bone marrow suppression may require withholding dactinomycin until recovery occurs. No specific antidote. Supportive therapy as indicated will help sustain the patient in toxicity. Administration of whole blood products (e.g., packed RBCs, platelets, leukocytes) and/or blood modifiers (e.g., darbepoetin alfa [Aranesp], epoetin alfa [Epogen], filgrastim [Neupogen, Zarxio], pegfilgrastim [Neulasta], sargramostim [Leukine]) may be indicated to treat bone marrow toxicity. For extravasation, discontinue immediately and elevate extremity. Apply ice to site four times daily for 3 days. Close observation and reconstructive surgery consultation recommended.

DALBAVANCIN
(**DAL**-ba-**VAN**-sin)

Dalvance

USUAL DOSE

1,500 mg. May be administered as a single dose or as a two-dose regimen with an initial dose of 1,000 mg followed 1 week later by 500 mg. Administer as an infusion over 30 minutes.

DOSE ADJUSTMENTS

Dosage should be adjusted in patients with renal impairment as outlined in the following chart.

Dosage of Dalbavancin in Patients with Renal Impairment		
Estimated CrCl*	Dalbavancin Single-Dose Regimen†	Dalbavancin Two-Dose Regimen†
≥30 mL/min or on regular hemodialysis	1,500 mg	1,000 mg followed 1 week later by 500 mg
<30 mL/min and not on regular hemodialysis	1,125 mg	750 mg followed 1 week later by 375 mg

*As calculated using the Cockcroft-Gault formula.
†Administered IV over 30 minutes.

- No dose adjustment is recommended for patients receiving regularly scheduled hemodialysis, and dalbavancin can be administered without regard to the timing of hemodialysis. ■ No dose adjustment is recommended for patients with mild hepatic impairment (Child-Pugh Class A). ■ Use caution when prescribed for patients with moderate or severe hepatic impairment (Child-Pugh Class B or C). No data are available to determine appropriate dosing in these patients. ■ No dose adjustment based on age or gender; see Elderly.

DILUTION

Available in single-use vials containing 500 mg of dalbavancin as a lyophilized powder. Reconstitute each 500-mg vial with 25 mL of SWFI or D5W. To avoid foaming, alternate between gentle swirling and inversion of the vial until contents are completely dissolved. **Do not shake.** Concentration is 20 mg/mL. Solution should be clear and colorless to yellow. Do not use if particulate matter remains. Transfer the required dose to an IV bag or bottle containing D5W. Diluted solution must have a final concentration of 1 mg/mL to 5 mg/mL.

Filters: Specific information not available.

Storage: Vials may be stored at CRT. Reconstituted vials and/or fully diluted solutions may be stored at RT or refrigerated at 2° to 8° C (36° to 46° F). Do not freeze. Total time from reconstitution to dilution to administration should not exceed 48 hours.

COMPATIBILITY

Manufacturer states, "Do not co-infuse dalbavancin with other medications or electrolytes. Saline-based infusion solutions may cause precipitation and should not be used. The **compatibility** of reconstituted dalbavancin with IV medications, additives, or substances other than D5W has not been established."

RATE OF ADMINISTRATION

A single dose as an infusion equally distributed over 30 minutes. If a common IV line is used to administer other drugs in addition to dalbavancin, flush the IV line before and after each dalbavancin infusion with D5W. Too-rapid infusion may cause "red-man syndrome," including flushing of the upper body, pruritus, rash, and/or urticaria. Temporarily stop or slow the infusion as indicated.

ACTIONS

Dalbavancin is a semi-synthetic lipoglycopeptide antibacterial drug. It interferes with cell wall synthesis by binding to the D-alanyl-D-alanine terminus of the stem pentapeptide in nascent cell wall peptidoglycan, thus preventing cross-linking. In vitro, dalbavancin is bactericidal against *Staphylococcus aureus* and *Streptococcus pyogenes* at concentrations similar to those sustained throughout treatment; see Indications. 93% bound to plasma proteins, primarily to albumin. Mean concentrations achieved in skin blister fluid remain above 30 mg/L up to 7 days after dosing. Effective half-life is approximately 346 hours. Excreted in feces and urine as unchanged drug and as a metabolite.

INDICATIONS AND USES

Treatment of adult patients with acute bacterial skin and skin structure infections (ABSSSI) caused by susceptible isolates of designated gram-positive microorganisms, including *Staphylococcus aureus* (both methicillin-susceptible [MSSA] and methicillin-resistant [MRSA] strains).

CONTRAINDICATIONS

Known hypersensitivity to dalbavancin. No data available on cross-reactivity between dalbavancin and other glycopeptides, including vancomycin.

PRECAUTIONS

Serious hypersensitivity (anaphylactic) and skin reactions have been reported. Check history of previous hypersensitivity reactions to glycopeptides (e.g., oritavancin [Orbactiv], telavancin [Vibativ], vancomycin). Exercise caution in patients with a history of glycopeptide allergy; cross-sensitivity is possible. ▪ Infusion-related reactions have been reported; see Rate of Administration. ▪ Specific sensitivity studies are indicated to determine susceptibility of the causative organism to dalbavancin. ▪ To reduce the development of drug-resistant bacteria and maintain its effectiveness, dalbavancin should be used to treat only those infections proven or strongly suspected to be caused by bacteria. ▪ *Clostridium difficile*–associated diarrhea (CDAD) has been reported for nearly all systemic antibacterial agents and may range in severity from mild diarrhea to fatal colitis. Consider in patients who present with diarrhea during or after treatment with dalbavancin. ▪ ALT elevations greater than three times the ULN occurred in some patients with normal baseline transaminase levels before treatment.

Monitor: Obtain baseline SCr. ▪ Monitor for S/S of hypersensitivity (e.g., hypotension, rash, urticaria, tightness of the chest, wheezing). ▪ Monitor for S/S of an infusion reaction; see Rate of Administration. ▪ See Precautions; baseline liver function studies may be indicated.

Patient Education: Promptly report S/S of a hypersensitivity reaction (e.g., hives, rash, shortness of breath, wheezing) or an infusion reaction (e.g., flushing of the upper body, pruritus, rash, and/or urticaria). ▪ Promptly report diarrhea or bloody stools that occur during treatment or up to several months after an antibiotic has been discontinued; may indicate CDAD and require treatment.

Maternal/Child: Use during pregnancy only if the potential benefit outweighs the possible risk to the fetus. ▪ Use caution during breast-feeding. ▪ Safety and effectiveness for use in pediatric patients not established.

Elderly: Consider age-related renal impairment, monitoring of renal function, and dose with caution; see Dose Adjustments.

DRUG/LAB INTERACTIONS

Clinical drug-drug interaction studies have not been conducted. ▪ There is minimal potential for drug-drug interactions between dalbavancin and substrates, inhibitors, and inducers of cytochrome P_{450} enzymes. ▪ Dalbavancin pharmacokinetics were not affected by coadministration of acetaminophen (Ofirmev), aztreonam (Azactam), fentanyl, furosemide (Lasix), metronidazole (Flagyl), midazolam (Versed), proton pump inhibitors (e.g., esomeprazole [Nexium], lansoprazole [Prevacid], omeprazole [Prilosec], pantoprazole [Protonix]), and simvastatin (Zocor). ▪ In vitro, dalbavancin demonstrated synergistic interactions with **oxacillin** and did not demonstrate antagonistic or synergistic interactions with aztreonam (Azactam), clindamycin (Cleocin), daptomycin (Cubicin), gentamicin, levofloxacin (Levaquin), linezolid (Zyvox), quinupristin/dalfopristin (Synercid), rifampin (Rifadin), or vancomycin. Clinical significance unknown.

SIDE EFFECTS

Most common side effects reported are diarrhea, headache, and nausea. Hypersensitivity and/or infusion reactions may be severe. Increased ALT levels (reversible), pruritus, rash, and vomiting were also reported. Many other side effects occurred in fewer than 2% of patients.

ANTIDOTE

Notify physician of any side effects. Discontinue the drug if indicated. Treat hypersensitivity reactions as indicated (e.g., diphenhydramine [Benadryl], epinephrine [Adrenalin], albuterol) and resuscitate as necessary. Temporarily discontinue or slow infusion for infusion-related reactions. Mild cases of CDAD may respond to discontinuation of dalbavancin. Treat CDAD with fluids, electrolytes, protein supplements, and oral vancomycin (Vancocin) or metronidazole (Flagyl) as indicated. In severe cases, surgical evaluation may be indicated. Less than 6% of the recommended dose of dalbavancin is removed by hemodialysis.

DANTROLENE SODIUM
(DAN-troh-leen SO-dee-um)

Dantrium, Revonto ▪ Ryanodex

Skeletal muscle relaxant
(direct acting)

pH 9.5 ▪ 10.3

USUAL DOSE

In patients known to be susceptible to malignant hyperthermia (MH), oral dantrolene may be used prophylactically preoperatively. Oral or IV therapy should be used postoperatively for 1 to 3 days following IV treatment for MH crisis. Postoperative dosing is indicated after emergency treatment to prevent recurrence of the manifestations of MH.

Prophylactic dose: DANTRIUM, REVONTO: 2.5 mg/kg as an infusion. Begin administration 1¼ hours before anesthesia, and administer over 1 hour. Oral dantrolene may be used.

RYANODEX: 2.5 mg/kg as an IV injection over at least 1 minute. Begin administration 1¼ hours before surgery. If surgery is prolonged, administer additional individualized doses during anesthesia and surgery as needed.

ALL FORMULATIONS: Avoid agents that trigger MH (e.g., general anesthetics and depolarizing neuromuscular blocking agents [succinylcholine]).

Therapeutic or emergency dose: ALL FORMULATIONS: Discontinue all anesthetic agents at the first sign of a malignant hyperthermia reaction. Administration of 100% oxygen is recommended.

1 mg/kg of body weight as an initial dose as a rapid IV push. Repeat as necessary until symptoms subside or a cumulative dose of 10 mg/kg is reached. Entire regimen may be repeated if symptoms reappear. Dose required depends on degree of susceptibility to malignant hyperthermia, length of time of exposure to triggering agent, and time lapse between onset of crisis and beginning of treatment.

Post-crisis follow-up: An oral dose of 4 to 8 mg/kg/day for 1 to 3 days to prevent recurrences. If oral dosing not feasible, begin IV dose at 1 mg/kg and individualize by increasing based on patient response.

PEDIATRIC DOSE

Prophylactic, therapeutic, and post-crisis follow-up doses are the same as for adults; see Maternal/Child.

DOSE ADJUSTMENTS

Dose selection should be cautious in the elderly. Reduced doses may be indicated based on the potential for decreased organ function and concomitant disease or drug therapy.

DILUTION

DANTRIUM, REVONTO: Each 20 mg must be diluted with 60 mL SWFI without a bacteriostatic agent. Shake until solution is clear. May be administered through a Y-tube or three-way stopcock of infusion tubing. If large volumes will be used, transfer to plastic infusion bags; do not use glass bottles; see Compatibility.

RYANODEX: Reconstitute each 250-mg vial with 5 mL of SWFI without a bacteriostatic agent. Shake the vial to ensure an orange-colored uniform suspension. Do not reconstitute with D5W or NS; see Compatibility. May be administered directly into an indwelling catheter or through a Y-tube or three-way stopcock of a free-flowing infusion of D5W or NS.

Storage: ALL FORMULATIONS: Store undiluted vials at CRT and protect from light. Store diluted solution at CRT and protect from direct light. Discard after 6 hours.

COMPATIBILITY

DANTRIUM, REVONTO: Manufacturer states, "D5W, NS, and acidic solutions are **not compatible** and should not be used." May form a precipitate with glass bottles; use of plastic IV bags recommended.

RYANODEX: Do not dilute or transfer the reconstituted suspension to another container to infuse the product.

RATE OF ADMINISTRATION
Prophylactic dose: DANTRIUM, REVONTO: A single dose as an infusion distributed over 1 hour. **RYANODEX:** A single dose as an IV injection over at least 1 minute. If administering into an indwelling catheter without a free-flowing IV, flush line after administration of Ryanodex to ensure there is no residual drug left in the catheter.

Therapeutic or emergency dose: ALL FORMULATIONS: Each single dose should be given by rapid continuous IV push. Follow immediately with subsequent doses as indicated.

ACTIONS
A direct-acting skeletal muscle relaxant. Inhibits excitation-contraction coupling by interfering with the release of the calcium ion from the sarcoplasmic reticulum to reverse the physiologic cause of malignant hyperthermia and produce relaxation. The addition of dantrolene to the "triggered" malignant hyperthermic muscle cell may re-establish a normal level of ionized calcium in the myoplasm. Physiologic, metabolic, and biochemical changes associated with the malignant hyperthermia crisis may be reversed or attenuated. Has no appreciable effect on cardiovascular or respiratory function. Onset of action is prompt. Half-life of **Dantrium** and **Revonto** is 4 to 8 hours. Half-life of **Ryanodex** is 8.5 to 11.4 hours. Metabolized in the liver and excreted in urine. Readily crosses the placental barrier. Secreted in breast milk.

INDICATIONS AND USES
Treatment of malignant hyperthermia in conjunction with appropriate supportive measures. ▪ Prevention of malignant hyperthermia in patients at high risk.

CONTRAINDICATIONS
None.

PRECAUTIONS
Use caution in patients with impaired pulmonary or cardiac function or history of liver disease. ▪ Discontinue all anesthetic agents immediately when onset of malignant hyperthermia is recognized. Administration of 100% oxygen is recommended. ▪ Hepatotoxicity has been reported with oral dantrolene. ▪ Not indicated for use in patients with neuroleptic malignant syndrome (NMS).

Monitor: S/S of malignant hyperthermia crises include central venous desaturation, cyanosis and mottling of the skin, hypercarbia, increased utilization of anesthesia circuit carbon dioxide absorber, metabolic acidosis, skeletal muscle rigidity, tachycardia, tachypnea and, in many cases, fever. ▪ Monitor ECG, vital signs, electrolytes, and urine output continuously. ▪ Oxygen needs are increased. ▪ Manage metabolic acidosis. ▪ Institute cooling measures. ▪ Diuretics may be required to prevent or treat late kidney injury due to myoglobinuria. Consider amount of mannitol present in **Dantrium** or **Revonto** formulations. (**Ryanodex** does not contain a sufficient amount of mannitol to maintain diuresis.) ▪ Confirm absolute patency of vein; avoid extravasation. High pH may cause tissue necrosis. ▪ Associated with skeletal muscle weakness; see Patient Education. ▪ Ensure adequate ventilation; has been associated with dyspnea, respiratory muscle weakness, and decreased inspiratory capacity. ▪ Assess patients for difficulty swallowing and choking. ▪ Monitor hepatic function, including ALT, AST. ▪ Somnolence and dizziness may persist for up to 48 hours postdose. Ambulate with assistance.

Patient Education: May experience decreased grip strength, weakness in leg muscles, and light-headedness postoperatively. May persist for 48 hours. ▪ Request assistance for ambulation. ▪ Use caution when eating; choking and difficulty swallowing have been reported on day of administration. ▪ Avoid alcohol and other CNS depressants (e.g., diazepam [Valium]). ▪ Avoid tasks that require alertness. ▪ Promptly report bloody or tarry stools, itching, jaundice (yellow color) of eyes and skin, or skin rash.

Maternal/Child: Category C: embryocidal in animal studies. Use during pregnancy only if potential benefit justifies potential risk to the fetus. ▪ Discontinue breast-feeding. ▪ Safety and effectiveness for use in pediatric patients have been established. Dose is the same as for adults.

Elderly: Differences in responses between the elderly and younger patients have not been identified. Dose selection should be cautious; see Dose Adjustments.

DRUG/LAB INTERACTIONS

ALL FORMULATIONS: Avoid concurrent use of **calcium channel blockers** (e.g., diltiazem [Cardizem]) **and dantrolene**. Cardiovascular collapse, arrhythmias, and hyperkalemia have been reported. ■ Ability to bind to plasma proteins inhibited by **warfarin** (Coumadin) **and clofibrate** (Atromid-S); increased by **tolbutamide** (Orinase). ■ Phenobarbital (Luminal) and diazepam (Valium) do not affect dantrolene sodium metabolism.

DANTRIUM AND REVONTO: May potentiate **vecuronium**-induced neuromuscular blockade. ■ Binding to plasma protein is not significantly altered by diazepam [Valium], diphenylhydantoin, or phenylbutazone (Butazolidin).

RYANODEX: May potentiate the neuromuscular block when given with **muscle relaxants**. ■ May potentiate the effects of **antipsychotic agents** (e.g., pimozide [Orap], clozapine [Clozaril]) and **antianxiety agents** (e.g., diazepam [Valium]) on the central nervous system. ■ Concomitant use of **sedative agents** may increase the risk of somnolence and dizziness.

SIDE EFFECTS

Dizziness, drowsiness, loss of grip strength, and weakness in the legs are most common. Other reported side effects include erythema, hypersensitivity reactions (including anaphylaxis), injection site reactions, nausea, pulmonary edema, thrombophlebitis, tissue necrosis secondary to extravasation, urticaria.

ANTIDOTE

No specific antidote is available or needed when used correctly. Notify physician and initiate supportive measures (ensure adequate airway and ventilation, monitor ECG) in overdosage. Large amounts of IV fluids may be needed to prevent crystalluria. Treat anaphylaxis and resuscitate as necessary. Value of dialysis in overdose is not known.

DAPTOMYCIN
(**dap**-toe-**MY**-sin)

Antibacterial
(cyclic lipopeptide)

Cubicin

USUAL DOSE

Complicated skin and skin structure infections: 4 mg/kg once every 24 hours for 7 to 14 days. Do not administer more frequently than once daily.

***Staphylococcus aureus* bloodstream infections (bacteremia), including those with right-sided endocarditis:** 6 mg/kg once every 24 hours for 2 to 6 weeks. Duration of treatment is dependent on diagnosis. Safety data for use more than 28 days is limited. Do not administer more frequently than once daily.

DOSE ADJUSTMENTS

Dose adjustment required in patients with severe renal impairment. In patients with CrCl less than 30 mL/min, including patients undergoing hemodialysis or CAPD, administer a single dose (4 or 6 mg/kg) every 48 hours. If possible, administer dose following completion of hemodialysis on hemodialysis days. ■ No specific dose adjustments required based on age, gender, obesity, or mild to moderate hepatic impairment. Has not been studied in patients with severe hepatic impairment.

DILUTION

Available in 500-mg vials. Reconstitute each 500-mg vial by slowly directing 10 mL of NS to vial sides (50 mg/mL). Ensure wetting of entire daptomycin product. Allow vial to stand for 10 minutes, then gently rotate to ensure complete dilution. *To minimize foaming, avoid vigorous agitation or shaking during or after reconstitution.* Freshly reconstituted solutions range in color from pale yellow to light brown. May be administered as a

50 mg/mL reconstituted solution or may be further diluted with 50 mL of NS before administration and given as an infusion.

Filters: No data available from manufacturer.

Storage: Refrigerate unopened vials at 2° to 8° C (36° to 46° F). Both reconstituted and diluted solutions are stable for 12 hours at RT or up to 48 hours refrigerated. The combined time (vial and infusion bag) at RT should not exceed 12 hours. Combined refrigeration time (vial and infusion bag) should not exceed 48 hours.

COMPATIBILITY   (Underline Indicates Conflicting Compatibility Information)

Consider any drug NOT listed as compatible to be INCOMPATIBLE until consulting a pharmacist; specific conditions may apply.

Manufacturer states, "Additives or other medications should not be added to daptomycin single-use vials or infused simultaneously through the same intravenous line. If the same intravenous line is used for sequential infusion of several different drugs, the line should be flushed with a **compatible** infusion solution before and after infusion with daptomycin." ▪ Manufacturer states, "Daptomycin is **compatible** with NS and LR but is **incompatible** with dextrose-containing diluents." ▪ Do not use in conjunction with ReadyMED® elastomeric infusion pumps; an **incompatibility** occurs because of an impurity leaching from this pump system into the daptomycin solution.

One source suggests the following **compatibilities:**

Y-site: Aztreonam (Azactam), <u>caspofungin (Cancidas)</u>, ceftazidime (Fortaz), ceftriaxone (Rocephin), dopamine, doripenem (Doribax), fluconazole (Diflucan), gentamicin, heparin, levofloxacin (Levaquin), lidocaine.

RATE OF ADMINISTRATION

See Compatibility. Flushing of the IV line before and after infusion may be indicated.

Injection: A single dose properly reconstituted and administered over 2 minutes.

Infusion: A single dose properly diluted and administered over 30 minutes.

ACTIONS

A cyclic lipopeptide antibacterial agent. Binds to bacterial membranes and causes a rapid depolarization of the membrane potential. Loss of the membrane potential leads to inhibition of protein, DNA, and RNA synthesis, which results in bacterial cell death. Exhibits bactericidal activity against aerobic gram-positive bacteria and has been shown to retain potency against antibiotic-resistant, gram-positive bacteria, including isolates resistant to methicillin. Cross-resistance between daptomycin and other antibacterial agents has not been reported. Highly protein bound, primarily to albumin. Site of metabolism has not been identified. Half-life is approximately 7 to 9 hours. Is excreted primarily by the kidney. A small fraction is excreted through the feces. Secreted in breast milk.

INDICATIONS AND USES

Treatment of complicated skin and skin structure infections caused by susceptible strains of several aerobic gram-positive microorganisms and *Staphylococcus aureus* bloodstream infections (bacteremia), including those with right-sided infective endocarditis caused by methicillin-susceptible and methicillin-resistant isolates.

Limitation of use: Daptomycin is not indicated for treatment of left-sided infective endocarditis due to *S. aureus* and has not been studied in patients with prosthetic valve endocarditis. ▪ **Not** indicated for treatment of pneumonia. In Phase 3 studies of community-acquired pneumonia, the death rate and rates of serious cardiorespiratory adverse events were higher in daptomycin-treated patients than in patients treated with a comparator agent. These differences resulted from the lack of therapeutic effectiveness of daptomycin in the treatment of community-acquired pneumonia.

CONTRAINDICATIONS

Known hypersensitivity to daptomycin.

PRECAUTIONS

C/S indicated to determine susceptibility of causative organism to daptomycin. ▪ To reduce the development of drug-resistant bacteria and maintain its effectiveness, daptomycin should be used to treat only those infections that are proven or strongly suspected to be caused by susceptible bacteria. ▪ Combination therapy may be clinically indicated if the documented or presumed pathogens include gram-negative or anaerobic organisms. ▪ Eosinophilic pneumonia has been reported. Onset is usually 2 to 4 weeks after initiation of daptomycin and improves when therapy is discontinued. Patient may present with fever, dyspnea with hypoxic respiratory insufficiency, and diffuse pulmonary infiltrates. ▪ Superinfection caused by the overgrowth of nonsusceptible organisms may occur with antibiotic use. Treat as indicated. ▪ *Clostridium difficile*–associated diarrhea (CDAD) has been reported. May range from mild diarrhea to fatal colitis. Consider in patients who present with diarrhea during or after treatment with daptomycin. ▪ Skeletal muscle effects associated with daptomycin have been observed. Elevations in serum creatine phosphokinase (CPK); myopathy; and rhabdomyolysis, with or without acute renal failure, have been reported. Some cases involved patients treated concurrently with daptomycin and HMG-CoA reductase inhibitors; see Drug/Lab Interactions. ▪ Cases of peripheral neuropathy have been reported. ▪ Hypersensitivity reactions, including anaphylaxis, have been reported. ▪ In clinical trials, decreased efficacy was observed in patients with moderate baseline renal impairment (CrCl less than 50 mL/min).

Monitor: Obtain baseline and weekly SCr, BUN, and CPK levels. Patients who received recent, prior, or concomitant therapy with an HMG-CoA reductase inhibitor (e.g., simvastatin [Zocor], lovastatin [Mevacor]), patients with renal insufficiency, and patients who develop unexplained elevations in CPK while receiving daptomycin should be monitored more frequently. See Precautions and Antidote. ▪ Monitor for S/S of hypersensitivity reactions (e.g., dyspnea, fever, flushing, hypotension, nausea, pruritus, rash, urticaria). ▪ Monitor for the development of muscle pain or weakness, particularly in the distal extremities. ▪ Monitor for S/S of neuropathy. ▪ Repeat blood cultures indicated in patients with persisting or relapsing *S. aureus* infection or poor clinical response. MIC (minimum inhibitory concentration) susceptibility testing and diagnostic evaluation to rule out sequestered foci of infection may be indicated. Surgical intervention (e.g., débridement, removal of prosthetic device) and/or consideration of a change in antibacterial regimen may be required. ▪ Monitor for S/S of eosinophilic pneumonia (e.g., cough, fever, difficulty breathing, shortness of breath, diffuse pulmonary infiltrates). Treatment with systemic steroids is recommended.

Patient Education: Review side effects with physician. Promptly report muscle pain or weakness, S/S of a hypersensitivity reaction (e.g., hives, rash, shortness of breath or troubled breathing, swelling of eyelids, lips, or face), S/S of neuropathy (e.g., tingling or numbness, especially in the forearm or lower leg), or new or worsening cough or fever. ▪ Review medications (prescription and nonprescription) with health care provider. ▪ Promptly report diarrhea or bloody stools that occur during treatment or up to several months after an antibiotic has been discontinued; may indicate CDAD and require treatment.

Maternal/Child: Category B: use during pregnancy only if clearly needed. ▪ Use caution during breastfeeding. Is present in breast milk, but oral bioavailability is poor. ▪ Safety and effectiveness for use in pediatric patients under 18 years of age not established. Avoid use in pediatric patients younger than 12 months of age. Animal studies suggest risk of potential effects on muscular, neuromuscular, and/or nervous systems (either peripheral and/or central).

Elderly: Lower clinical success rates were seen in patients 65 years of age or older. In addition, adverse events were more common in this age-group. Consider age-related renal impairment. See Dose Adjustment.

DRUG/LAB INTERACTIONS

Daptomycin does not appear to inhibit or induce the activities of the cytochrome P_{450} isoforms: 1A2, 2A6, 2C9, 2C19, 2D6, 2E1, and 3A4. It is unlikely that it will inhibit or induce the metabolism of drugs metabolized by this system. ▪ In vitro synergistic interactions occurred with **aminoglycosides, beta-lactam antibiotics, and rifampin** (Rifadin) against some isolates of staphylococci and enterococci, including some methicillin-resistant *Staphylococcus aureus* (MRSA) isolates and some vancomycin-resistant enterococci isolates. ▪ Has been administered with **warfarin.** Does not appear to affect the pharmacokinetics of either drug. However, daptomycin can cause a significant concentration-dependent false prolongation of PT and elevation of INR when certain recombinant thromboplastin reagents are used for the assay. This drug-lab interaction can be minimized by drawing specimens for PT/INR near the time of trough plasma concentrations of daptomycin. Evaluation of PT/INR using an alternative method may be required. ▪ Inhibitors of **HMG-CoA reductase** (e.g., simvastatin [Zocor], atorvastatin [Lipitor]) may cause myopathy, which is manifested as muscle pain or weakness associated with elevated levels of CPK and possible rhabdomyolysis. Consider temporarily suspending the use of HMG-CoA reductase inhibitors in patients receiving daptomycin. ▪ Has been used concomitantly with aztreonam (Azactam). No dose adjustment for either antibiotic was required. ▪ No dose adjustment is required when given concomitantly with probenecid.

SIDE EFFECTS

Most side effects are mild to moderate in intensity. The most frequently reported side effects were abnormal liver function tests, dyspnea, and elevated CPK. Side effects occurring in 2% or more of patients include abdominal pain, bacteremia, chest pain, diarrhea, dizziness, edema, headache, hypertension, hypotension, insomnia, pharyngolaryngeal pain, pruritus, rash, sepsis, sweating, and urinary tract infections. Less frequently reported side effects include anxiety, back pain, *Candida* infections, cardiac failure, CDAD, cellulitis, confusion, cough, decreased appetite, elevated alkaline phosphatase, hyperglycemia, hypoglycemia, hypokalemia, and sore throat. Muscle pain or weakness, rhabdomyolysis (with or without renal failure), and peripheral neuropathy have been reported rarely. See Precautions. Hypersensitivity reactions including anaphylaxis, difficulty swallowing, hives, pruritus, shortness of breath, and truncal erythema have been reported. Other reactions have been reported in fewer than 1% of study patients. See manufacturer's literature.

Post-Marketing: Angioedema, drug rash with eosinophilia and systemic symptoms (DRESS), eosinophilic pneumonia, nausea and vomiting, serious skin reactions including Stevens-Johnson syndrome, vesiculobullous rash, and visual disturbances.

ANTIDOTE

Notify physician of any side effects. Discontinue drug in patients with unexplained S/S of myopathy in conjunction with CPK elevation greater than 1,000 units/L (approximately 5 times the upper limit of normal) or in patients without reported symptoms who have marked elevation in CPK, with levels of greater than 2,000 units/L (equal to or greater than 10 times the upper limit of normal). In animal studies, skeletal muscle effects and neuropathies were reversible with discontinuation of the drug. Discontinue daptomycin at the first sign of eosinophilic pneumonia. Treatment with systemic steroids is recommended. Treat CDAD with fluids, electrolytes, protein supplements, and oral vancomycin (Vancocin) or metronidazole (Flagyl) as indicated. In severe cases, surgical evaluation may be indicated. Treat hypersensitivity reactions as indicated (e.g., oxygen, diphenhydramine, epinephrine, corticosteroids, vasopressors, and/or fluids). Approximately 15% of daptomycin is removed during a 4-hour hemodialysis run. Approximately 11% is recovered over 48 hours with peritoneal dialysis. Use of a high-flux dialysis membrane may increase the amount of drug removal. Resuscitate as necessary.

DARATUMUMAB
(**DAR**-a-**TOOM**-ue-mab)

Darzalex

Monoclonal antibody
Antineoplastic

pH 5.5

USUAL DOSE
Premedication: To reduce the risk of infusion reactions, administer an IV corticosteroid (methylprednisolone 100 mg or equivalent intermediate- or long-acting corticosteroid), an oral antipyretic (acetaminophen 650 to 1,000 mg), and an oral or IV antihistamine (diphenhydramine 25 to 50 mg or equivalent) 1 hour before every infusion of daratumumab. Following the second infusion, the dose of corticosteroid may be reduced (methylprednisolone 60 mg IV).

Daratumumab: 16 mg/kg as an infusion at a specified rate; see Rate of Administration. Repeat dose weekly for Weeks 1 through 8, every 2 weeks for Weeks 9 through 24, and every 4 weeks from Week 25 onward until disease progression. If a planned dose is missed, administer as soon as possible and adjust the dosing schedule accordingly, maintaining the treatment interval.

Postinfusion medication: To reduce the risk of delayed infusion reactions, administer an oral corticosteroid (20 mg methylprednisolone or equivalent) after all infusions on the first and second day. For patients with a history of obstructive pulmonary disorder, consider postinfusion short- and long-acting bronchodilators and inhaled corticosteroids after the first four infusions. These additional inhaled postinfusion medications may be discontinued if no major infusion reactions occur.

Herpes zoster reactivation prophylaxis: Initiate within 1 week of starting daratumumab and continue for 3 months following treatment.

DOSE ADJUSTMENTS
Upon resolution of Grade 1 or 2 (mild to moderate) infusion reactions, resume the infusion at no more than half the rate at which the reaction occurred. If no further reactions occur, infusion rate escalation may resume at increments and intervals as appropriate; see Rate of Administration. ▪ Upon resolution to Grade 2 or lower from a Grade 3 (severe) reaction, consider restarting the infusion at no more than half the rate at which the reaction occurred. If no further reactions occur, resume rate escalation at increments and intervals as appropriate; see Rate of Administration. ▪ If Grade 3 reactions occur for a second time, repeat the protocol as outlined. ▪ Permanently discontinue daratumumab if a third Grade 3 or a Grade 4 (life-threatening) reaction occurs. ▪ No dose adjustment required for renal impairment or mild hepatic impairment.

DILUTION
Available as a 100 mg/5 mL or a 400 mg/20 mL single-dose vial (20 mg/mL). Calculate the dose (mg) based on actual body weight, total volume (mL) of daratumumab solution required, and the number of vials required using the following calculations:

$$\text{Dose (mg)} = \text{Weight (kg)} \times \text{Dose (mg/kg)}$$

$$\text{\# of vials required} = \text{Dose (mg)} \div 100\ (400)\ \text{mg/vial}$$

$$\text{\# of mL required} = \text{Dose (mg)} \div 20\ \text{mg/mL}$$

For a 60-kg patient: [(60 kg) × (16 mg/kg)] ÷ 100 (400) mg/vial = 9.6 vials of the 100-mg/vial solution and 2.4 vials of the 400-mg/vial solution. After patient is weighed and appropriate dose is calculated, remove sufficient vials from the refrigerator. Aseptic technique imperative. Solution should be colorless to pale yellow. Do not use if opaque particles, discoloration, or other foreign particles are present. Withdraw the calculated dose (48 mL in both of the previous examples) from the required number of vials. This calculated dose must be further diluted in NS. Withdraw and discard a volume of NS equal to the calculated volume of daratumumab from a bag/container of NS based on the chart in Rate of Administration (1,000 or 500 mL) and slowly add daratumumab solution. Gently invert the bag/bottle to mix the solution. Infusion bags/containers must be made of polyvinylchloride (PVC), polypropylene (PP), polyethylene (PE), or polyolefin blend (PP+PE).

Filters: Must be administered through an infusion set with a flow regulator and an in-line, sterile, nonpyrogenic, low–protein binding polyethersulfone (PES) filter (pore size 0.22 or 0.2 micrometer). Polyurethane (PU), polybutadiene (PBD), PVC, PP, or PE administration sets must be used.

Storage: Refrigerate at 2° to 8° C (36° to 46° F) in original carton to protect from light. Do not freeze or shake. The diluted product may be stored for up to 24 hours if refrigerated and protected from light. Do not freeze. Bring to room temperature before infusion and use immediately. Diluted solution may develop very small, translucent to white proteinaceous particles because daratumumab is a protein. Do not use if opaque particles, discoloration, or other foreign particles are present. Infusion should be completed within 15 hours. Discard any unused product remaining in vials.

COMPATIBILITY

Manufacturer states, "Do not infuse concomitantly in the same IV line with other agents." **Compatible** only with IV bags/containers of polyvinylchloride (PVC), polypropylene (PP), polyethylene (PE), or polyolefin blend (PP+PE); filters of polyethersulfone (PES); and administration sets of polyurethane (PU), polybutadiene (PBD), PVC, PP, or PE.

RATE OF ADMINISTRATION

For IV infusion only. Interrupt daratumumab infusion for infusion reactions of any severity and manage symptoms. See the following chart for daratumumab infusion rates.

Infusion Rates for Daratumumab Administration				
	Dilution Volume	Initial Rate (First Hour)	Rate Increment	Maximum Rate
First infusion	1,000 mL	50 mL/hr	50 mL/hr every hour	200 mL/hr
Second infusion*	500 mL	50 mL/hr	50 mL/hr every hour	200 mL/hr
Subsequent infusions†	500 mL	100 mL/hr	50 mL/hr every hour	200 mL/hr

*Escalate only if there were no Grade 1 (mild) or greater infusion reactions during the first 3 hours of the first infusion.
†Escalate only if there were no Grade 1 (mild) or greater infusion reactions during a final infusion rate of equal to or greater than 100 mL/hr in the first two infusions. See Dose Adjustments.

ACTIONS

CD38 is a transmembrane glycoprotein expressed on the surface of hematopoietic cells, including multiple myeloma and other cell types and tissues, and has multiple functions. Daratumumab is an $IgG1_k$ human monoclonal antibody that binds to CD38 and inhibits the growth of CD38-expressing tumor cells by inducing apoptosis. Steady state is achieved approximately 5 months into the every-4-week dosing period (by the 21st infusion). Half-life is approximately 18 days.

INDICATIONS AND USES

Treatment of patients with multiple myeloma who have received at least 3 prior lines of therapy, including a proteasome inhibitor (PI) and an immunomodulatory agent, or who are double-refractory to a PI and an immunomodulatory agent. Accelerated approval is based on response rate; continued approval may be contingent on verification of clinical benefit.

CONTRAINDICATIONS

Manufacturer states, "None."

PRECAUTIONS

For IV infusion only. ▪ Administered under the direction of a physician knowledgeable in its use in a facility with adequate diagnostic and treatment facilities to monitor the patient and respond to any medical emergency. ▪ Can cause severe infusion reactions.

Approximately half of all patients experienced a reaction, most during the first infusion. Reactions can also occur with subsequent infusions. Most reactions occur during the infusion or within 4 hours of administration. ▪ Interferes with serologic testing (compatibility testing, including cross-matching and antibody screening) for up to 6 months after the last infusion; see Drug/Lab Interactions. ▪ Can be detected on assays used for monitoring endogenous M protein. Interference with these assays can affect the determination of complete response and of disease progression in some patients with IgG kappa myeloma protein; see Drug/Lab Interactions. ▪ Has not been studied in patients with moderate to severe hepatic impairment. ▪ A therapeutic protein; has the potential for immunogenicity.

Monitor: Premedication required; see Usual Dose. ▪ Type and screen patients' blood before starting daratumumab. ▪ Obtain baseline CBC and differential and monitor as indicated during therapy. ▪ Monitor vital signs. ▪ Monitor for S/S of infusion reactions (e.g., bronchospasm, cough, chills, dyspnea, headache, hypertension, hypotension, hypoxia, laryngeal edema, larynx and throat tightness and irritation, nasal congestion, nausea, pruritus, pulmonary edema, rash, rhinitis, urticaria, vomiting, wheezing). Immediately interrupt the infusion for infusion reactions of any grade/severity; see Dose Adjustments and Antidote.

Patient Education: Review manufacturer's medication guide. ▪ Effective contraception required for women of reproductive potential during treatment with and for 3 months after the last dose of daratumumab. ▪ Immediately report any S/S of infusion-related reactions (e.g., chills, cough, difficulty breathing, headache; itchy, runny, or blocked nose). ▪ Some side effects may require corticosteroid treatment and interruption or discontinuation of daratumumab. ▪ Daratumumab can affect the results of some tests, including testing for complete response, and additional testing may be indicated to evaluate response to therapy. ▪ Inform all health care providers, including blood transfusion centers, of daratumumab use in the event of a planned blood transfusion.

Maternal/Child: Has the potential to be transmitted from the mother to the developing fetus. Based on its mechanism of action, daratumumab may cause fetal myeloid or lymphoid-cell depletion and decreased bone density. Effective contraception required; see Patient Education. ▪ Administration of live vaccines to neonates and infants exposed to daratumumab in utero should be deferred until a hematology evaluation is completed. ▪ Safety for use during breast-feeding is unknown. ▪ Safety and effectiveness for use in pediatric patients not established.

Elderly: No overall differences in safety or efficacy were reported between elderly patients and younger adults.

DRUG/LAB INTERACTIONS

No drug interaction studies have been performed. ▪ Interferes with serologic testing. Daratumumab binds to CD38 on the RBCs and results in a positive indirect antiglobulin test (Coombs test). This effect may last for up to 6 months after the final daratumumab infusion. Daratumumab bound to RBCs masks detection of antibodies to minor antigens in the patient's serum. A patient's ABO and Rh blood type are not affected. Notify blood transfusion centers of this interference. ▪ Administration of live vaccines to neonates and infants exposed to daratumumab in utero should be deferred until a hematology evaluation is completed.

SIDE EFFECTS

The most frequently reported side effects included back pain, cough, fatigue, fever, infusion reactions, nausea, and upper respiratory tract infections. The most frequent serious side effects were fever, general physical health deterioration, infusion reactions, and pneumonia. Treatment-emergent Grade 3 to 4 laboratory abnormalities included anemia, lymphopenia, neutropenia, and thrombocytopenia. Arthralgia, chills, constipation, decreased appetite, diarrhea, dyspnea, extremity pain, headache, herpes zoster reactivation, hypertension, musculoskeletal chest pain, nasal congestion, nasopharyngitis, and vomiting have occurred.

ANTIDOTE
Notify physician of any side effects; most will be treated symptomatically. Interrupt daratumumab infusion for infusion reactions of any severity. Permanently discontinue daratumumab if a third Grade 3 or a Grade 4 (life-threatening) hypersensitivity/infusion reaction occurs. Treat a hypersensitivity/infusion reaction with oxygen, epinephrine (Adrenalin), antihistamines (e.g., diphenhydramine [Benadryl]), vasopressors (e.g., dopamine), corticosteroids, albuterol, IV fluids, and ventilation equipment as indicated.

DARBEPOETIN ALFA BBW
(DAR-beh-poh-eh-tin AL-fah)

Erythropoiesis-stimulating agent (ESA)

Aranesp

pH 6 to 6.4

USUAL DOSE
Adult and pediatric patients: Rate of hemoglobin increase is dose dependent and varies among patients. Availability of iron stores, baseline hemoglobin, and concurrent medical problems affect the rate and extent of response. In controlled clinical trials, patients experienced greater risks for death, serious adverse cardiovascular reactions, and stroke when administered erythropoiesis-stimulating agents (ESAs) to target a hemoglobin level of greater than 11 Gm/dL. Use the lowest dose for each patient that will gradually increase the hemoglobin concentration to avoid the need for RBC transfusion. If a patient fails to respond or maintain a response, other etiologies should be considered and evaluated. See Monitor, Precautions, and Maternal/Child.
Anemia associated with chronic kidney disease (CKD) for patients on dialysis: Initiate darbepoetin when the hemoglobin level is less than 10 Gm/dL: *Starting dose:* 0.45 mcg/kg of body weight once per week or 0.75 mcg/kg once every 2 weeks as appropriate. May be given by IV or SC injection. The IV route is recommended for patients on hemodialysis; see Precautions. See Dose Adjustments and Maternal/Child.
Anemia associated with chronic kidney disease (CKD) for patients NOT on dialysis: Consider initiating darbepoetin only when the hemoglobin level is less than 10 Gm/dL and the following two considerations apply: (1) the rate of hemoglobin decline indicates the likelihood of requiring a RBC transfusion, and (2) reducing the risk of alloimmunization and/or other RBC transfusion-related risks is a goal. *Starting dose:* 0.45 mcg/kg of body weight IV or SC given once every 4 weeks as appropriate.
Conversion from epoetin alfa to darbepoetin alfa in patients with CKD on dialysis: Estimate starting weekly dose of darbepoetin for adult and pediatric patients based on the weekly dose of epoetin alfa at the time of substitution as shown in the following chart. Administer darbepoetin once per week in patients who were receiving epoetin alfa 2 to 3 times

Continued

a week and once every 2 weeks in patients who were receiving epoetin alfa once per week. The route of administration (IV or SC) should remain the same.

Estimated Darbepoetin Alfa Starting Dose Based on Previous Epoetin Alfa Dose for Patients with CKD on Dialysis		
Previous Weekly Epoetin Alfa Dose (units/week)	Weekly Darbepoetin Alfa Dose (mcg/week)	
	Adult	Pediatric
<1,500 units/week	6.25 mcg/week	See *
1,500 to 2,499 units/week	6.25 mcg/week	6.25 mcg/week
2,500 to 4,999 units/week	12.5 mcg/week	10 mcg/week
5,000 to 10,999 units/week	25 mcg/week	20 mcg/week
11,000 to 17,999 units/week	40 mcg/week	40 mcg/week
18,000 to 33,999 units/week	60 mcg/week	60 mcg/week
34,000 to 89,999 units/week	100 mcg/week	100 mcg/week
≥90,000 units/week	200 mcg/week	200 mcg/week

*Data insufficient to determine a darbepoetin alfa conversion dose in pediatric patients receiving a weekly epoetin alfa dose of less than 1,500 units/week.

Conversion from epoetin alfa to darbepoetin alfa in patients with CKD NOT on dialysis: The dose conversion shown in the previous chart (for patients with CKD on dialysis) does not accurately estimate the once-monthly dose of darbepoetin.

Anemia associated with chemotherapy in cancer patients: ESAs shortened overall survival and/or increased the risk of tumor progression or recurrence in clinical studies of patients with certain types of cancer; see Precautions. Initiate darbepoetin in patients undergoing cancer chemotherapy only if the hemoglobin is less than 10 Gm/dL and there is a minimum of 2 additional months of planned chemotherapy. Use the lowest dose necessary to avoid RBC transfusions. *Starting dose:* 2.25 mcg/kg of body weight SC every week until completion of chemotherapy course. An alternative schedule is 500 mcg SC every 3 weeks until completion of chemotherapy course.

PEDIATRIC DOSE

Pediatric patients with CKD (less than 18 years of age): Initiate darbepoetin when the hemoglobin level is less than 10 Gm/dL. *Starting dose:* 0.45 mcg/kg of body weight once per week as an IV or SC injection. Patients not receiving dialysis may also be initiated at a dose of 0.75 mcg/kg once every 2 weeks. If the hemoglobin level approaches or exceeds 12 Gm/dL, reduce or interrupt the dose of darbepoetin.

DOSE ADJUSTMENTS

All patients with CKD: When adjusting therapy, consider hemoglobin rate of rise, hemoglobin rate of decline, ESA responsiveness, and hemoglobin variability. A single hemoglobin excursion may not require a dose adjustment. Dose should be started slowly and adjusted for each patient to achieve and maintain the lowest hemoglobin level sufficient to avoid the need for RBC transfusion. Allow sufficient time before adjusting a dose; increased hemoglobin levels may not be observed for 2 to 6 weeks. ▪ Do not increase the dose more frequently than once every 4 weeks. Decreases in dose can occur more frequently. ▪ If the hemoglobin rises rapidly (e.g., more than 1 Gm/dL in any 2-week period), reduce the dose by 25% or more as needed to reduce rapid responses. ▪ For patients who do not respond adequately (e.g., the hemoglobin has not increased by more than 1 Gm/dL) after 4 weeks of therapy, increase the dose by 25%. ▪ For patients who do not respond adequately over a 12-week escalation period, increasing the dose further is unlikely to improve response and may increase risks. Discontinue darbepoetin if responsiveness does not improve.

Patients with CKD on dialysis: If the hemoglobin level approaches or exceeds 11 Gm/dL, reduce or interrupt the dose of darbepoetin.

Patients with CKD NOT on dialysis: If the hemoglobin level exceeds 10 Gm/dL, reduce or interrupt the dose of darbepoetin.

Anemia associated with chemotherapy in cancer patients:

Dose Adjustment in Patients Undergoing Cancer Chemotherapy		
Dose Adjustment	Weekly Schedule	Every-3-Week Schedule
If hemoglobin increases greater than 1 Gm/dL in any 2-week period or If hemoglobin reaches a level needed to avoid RBC transfusion	Reduce dose by 40%	Reduce dose by 40%
If hemoglobin exceeds a level needed to avoid RBC transfusion	Withhold dose until hemoglobin approaches a level at which RBC transfusions may be required Reinitiate at a dose 40% below the previous dose	Withhold dose until hemoglobin approaches a level at which RBC transfusions may be required Reinitiate at a dose 40% below the previous dose
If hemoglobin increases by less than 1 Gm/dL **and** remains below 10 Gm/dL after 6 weeks of therapy	Increase dose to 4.5 mcg/kg/week	No dose adjustment
If there is no response as measured by hemoglobin levels or if RBC transfusions are still required after 8 weeks of therapy Following completion of a chemotherapy course	Discontinue darbepoetin	Discontinue darbepoetin

DILUTION
Available in numerous concentrations. Supplied in vials or prefilled syringes with needle guards (needle cover contains a derivative of latex). Must be given undiluted as an IV injection. Do not administer in conjunction with other drug solutions. ***Do not shake*** and keep covered to protect from room light until administration. Vigorous shaking or exposure to light will render solution biologically inactive. Single-dose vial contains no preservatives. Use only 1 dose per vial, then discard.

Filters: Not required; however, it was filtered during manufacturing with 0.2-micron filters. No significant loss of potency expected with use of non–protein binding filters of a similar size or larger.

Storage: Store in carton at 2° to 8° C (36° to 46° F). Do not freeze or shake. Protect from light.

COMPATIBILITY
Manufacturer states, "Do not administer in conjunction with other drug solutions."

RATE OF ADMINISTRATION
A single dose over at least 1 minute.

ACTIONS
An erythropoiesis-stimulating protein produced by recombinant DNA technology. Closely related to human erythropoietin. Production of endogenous erythropoietin is impaired in patients with chronic renal failure, and erythropoietin deficiency is the primary cause of their anemia. Darbepoetin has the same biologic effects as erythropoietin produced naturally by the kidneys. Stimulates bone marrow to produce RBCs, increasing the reticulocyte count within 10 days and the red cell count, hemoglobin, and hematocrit within 2 to 6 weeks. Normal iron stores are necessary because it steps up RBC production to a rate above what the body usually makes. New cells need iron, which is quickly

depleted. Distribution is confined to the vascular space. Half-life is approximately 21 hours. Continued therapy will maintain improved RBC levels and decrease the need for transfusions.

INDICATIONS AND USES

Treatment of anemia associated with chronic kidney disease, including patients receiving dialysis and patients not receiving dialysis. ▪ As a SC injection to treat chemotherapy-induced anemia in adult cancer patients who have nonmyeloid malignancies in which anemia is a result of the effect of concomitant myelosuppressive chemotherapy and who, upon initiation of therapy, have a minimum of 2 additional months of planned chemotherapy.

Limitation of use: Not indicated for use in patients with cancer receiving hormonal agents, therapeutic biologic products, or radiotherapy unless receiving concomitant myelosuppressive chemotherapy. ▪ Not indicated for patients receiving myelosuppressive therapy when the anticipated outcome is cure; see Precautions. ▪ Has not been shown to improve symptoms of anemia, quality of life, fatigue, or patient well-being; see Precautions. ▪ Not indicated for reduction in allogeneic RBC transfusions in patients scheduled for surgical procedures. ▪ Not indicated as a substitute for a RBC transfusion in patients who require immediate correction of anemia.

CONTRAINDICATIONS

Known hypersensitivity to darbepoetin. ▪ Uncontrolled hypertension. ▪ Pure red cell aplasia (PRCA) that begins after treatment with darbepoetin or other erythropoietin agents.

PRECAUTIONS

May be given IV or SC to patients not receiving dialysis. ▪ Erythropoiesis-stimulating agents (ESAs) increase the risk of death, MI, stroke, venous thromboembolism, and thrombosis of vascular access. Patients experienced greater risks of these adverse events when ESAs were administered to target a hemoglobin of greater than 11 Gm/dL. No trial has identified a hemoglobin target level, a darbepoetin dose, or a dosing strategy that does not increase these risks. Use the lowest darbepoetin dose sufficient to reduce the need for RBC transfusions. ▪ Use with caution in patients with coexistent cardiovascular disease and stroke. Patients with CKD and an insufficient hemoglobin response to ESA therapy may be at even greater risk for cardiovascular reactions and mortality than other patients. ▪ In clinical trials, ESAs increased the risk of death in patients undergoing CABG surgery and the risk of deep venous thrombosis in patients undergoing orthopedic procedures. ▪ Increases in hemoglobin of greater than 1 Gm/dL during any 2-week period have been associated with an increased incidence of cardiac arrest, neurologic events (e.g., seizures, stroke), exacerbations of hypertension, congestive heart failure (CHF), vascular thrombosis/ischemia/infarction, acute MI, deep vein thrombosis (DVT), pulmonary embolus, hemodialysis graft occlusion, and fluid overload/edema. See Dose Adjustments. ▪ Administration of erythropoiesis-stimulating agents (ESAs) to cancer patients shortened the overall survival time and/or increased the risk of tumor progression or recurrence in clinical studies of some patients with breast, cervical, head and neck, lymphoid, and non–small-cell lung malignancies. To minimize these risks, as well as the risks of serious cardiovascular and thrombovascular events, use the lowest dose needed to avoid a red blood cell transfusion. Use only to treat anemia due to concomitant myelosuppressive chemotherapy, and discontinue after completion of a chemotherapy course. Prescribers and hospitals are now required to enroll in and comply with the ESA APPRISE Oncology Program to prescribe and/or dispense ESAs to patients with cancer. See prescribing information Black Box Warning. ▪ BP may increase during therapy with darbepoetin. Hypertensive encephalopathy and seizures have been observed. ▪ Patients with uncontrolled hypertension should not be treated with darbepoetin until BP has been adequately controlled. ▪ In addition to low baseline hemoglobin and inadequate iron stores, delayed or diminished response may result from concurrent medical problems (e.g., infections, inflammatory or malignant processes, occult blood loss, underlying hematologic disease, folic acid or vitamin B_{12} deficiency, hemolysis, aluminum intoxication, osteofibrosis cystica, bone marrow fibrosis, pure red cell aplasia [PRCA], or anti-erythropoietin antibody–associated anemia). Correct or exclude other causes of anemia before initiating therapy. Not intended for use in anemia caused by iron or folate deficiencies, hemolysis, or GI bleeding or for use in treating symptoms of anemia, including dizziness, fatigue, low energy, poor quality of life, or shortness of breath. ▪ Safety and efficacy have not been established in patients with underlying hematologic diseases (e.g., hemolytic anemia, sickle cell anemia, thalassemia, porphyria). ▪ Therapy results in an increase in RBCs and a decrease in plasma volume, which could reduce dialysis efficiency; adjustment of dialysis prescription may be necessary. ▪ Darbepoetin increases the risk of seizures in patients with CKD. Use with caution in patients with epilepsy. ▪ As with all proteins, there is a potential for immunogenicity. The incidence of antibody development in patients receiving darbepoetin has not been determined. Use caution; hypersensitivity reactions and/or anaphylaxis can occur. ▪ Pure red cell aplasia (PRCA) and severe anemia, with or without other cytopenias, in association with neutralizing antibodies to erythropoietin have been observed. Most often reported in CKD patients receiving epoetin alfa by SC injection. Evaluate any patient who develops a sudden loss of response to darbepoetin alfa accompanied by severe anemia and low reticulocyte count. Physicians may contact the manufacturer (Amgen) for help with evaluation of these patients. ▪ Darbepoetin is a growth factor that stimulates RBC production. Erythropoetin receptors are also found on the surfaces of normal, nonhematopoietic tissue and some malignant cell lines. The possibility that darbepoetin can act as a growth factor for any tumor type cannot be ruled out.

Monitor: Monitor hemoglobin weekly in patients who are initiating therapy. Continue until stable and the maintenance dose has been established, then monitor at regular intervals (at least monthly). ▪ Monitor hemoglobin weekly for at least 4 weeks following adjustment of therapy. Once stabilized, continue to monitor at regular intervals (at least monthly). ▪ Monitor BP routinely. Initiation or intensification of antihypertensive therapy and dietary restrictions may be necessary. If BP is difficult to control by pharmacologic or dietary measures, the dose of darbepoetin should be reduced or withheld. ▪ Monitor for the presence of premonitory neurologic symptoms during initiation of therapy or when dose is adjusted. Seizures have been reported; see Precautions. ▪ Monitor for S/S of hypersensitivity reactions (e.g., anaphylaxis, angioedema, bronchospasm, rash, urticaria). ▪ Normal iron stores required to support epoetin-stimulated erythropoiesis. Transferrin saturation should be at least 20% and ferritin at least 100 ng/mL (100 mcg/L). Monitor before and during therapy. Supplemental iron is usually required to increase and maintain transferrin saturation. Administration of parenteral iron may be necessary in some patients.

Patient Education: Risk of seizures, especially for first several months of therapy. Do not drive or operate heavy equipment. ▪ Stress the importance of compliance with diet, iron and vitamin (e.g., folic acid, B_{12}) supplementation, BP control, and dialysis regimen. ▪ Close monitoring of BP and hemoglobin is imperative. ▪ Promptly report S/S of a hypersensitivity reaction, pain or swelling in the legs, shortness of breath (SOB), increase in BP, dizziness, or loss of consciousness. ▪ Menses may resume; possibility of pregnancy. Contraception may be indicated. ▪ Additional instruction (e.g., equipment, techniques) will be required in patients who will self-administer (manufacturer supplies brochure). ▪ Increased risk of mortality, serious cardiovascular events, thromboembolic events, and tumor progression or recurrence. ▪ Read medication guide carefully. All patients should discuss the risks of using an ESA with a health care professional. ▪ Cancer patients must sign a patient–health care provider acknowledgment form through the APPRISE Oncology Program before initiating therapy; see Precautions.

Maternal/Child: Category C: may present risk to fetus; benefits must justify risk. ▪ Use caution in nursing mothers. ▪ Safety and effectiveness were similar between adult and pediatric patients with CKD when darbepoetin was used for the initial treatment of anemia or when patients were transitioned from another erythropoietin to darbepoetin. ▪ Safety and effectiveness for use in pediatric cancer patients not established. ▪ Half-life and plasma concentrations in pediatric patients 3 years of age and older are similar to those seen in adults. See package insert.

Elderly: No differences in safety or efficacy were observed between older and younger patients.

DRUG/LAB INTERACTIONS

Specific information not available.

SIDE EFFECTS

Adult chronic kidney disease patients: Commonly reported adverse reactions include cough, dyspnea, hypertension, peripheral edema, and procedural hypotension. *Serious* adverse reactions include hypertension, increased mortality, MI, PRCA, seizures, serious hypersensitivity reactions, stroke, and thromboembolism. Other reported adverse reactions include angina, arteriovenous graft thrombosis, fluid overload, rash, and vascular access complications.

Pediatric chronic kidney disease patients: Commonly reported adverse reactions include convulsions, hypertension, injection site pain, and rash. *Serious* adverse reactions include convulsions and hypertension.

Cancer patients receiving chemotherapy: Commonly reported adverse reactions include abdominal pain, edema, and thrombovascular events. *Serious* adverse reactions include hypertension, increased mortality, increased risk of tumor progression or recurrence, MI, PRCA, seizures, serious hypersensitivity reactions, stroke, and thromboembolism.

Post-Marketing: PRCA and severe anemia, with or without other cytopenias, in association with neutralizing antibodies have been reported; see Precautions. Seizures and serious hypersensitivity reactions have also been reported.

ANTIDOTE

Notify physician of all side effects; most will be treated symptomatically. Excessive hypertension may require discontinuation of darbepoetin until BP is controlled or may respond to a reduction in dose of darbepoetin or to an increase in antihypertensive therapy. Reduce dose of darbepoetin in patients with an increase in hemoglobin of more than 1 Gm/dL in 2 weeks. May need to withhold darbepoetin until hemoglobin falls to desired goal. Consider phlebotomy in the event of overdose or polycythemia. If overdose or polycythemia does occur, monitor closely for cardiovascular events and hematologic abnormalities. When resuming therapy, monitor closely for evidence of rapid increases in hemoglobin concentration (greater than 1 Gm/dL within 14 days) and reduce dose as indicated. Adjustments in dialysis prescription may be required during dialysis to prevent clotting. Permanently discontinue therapy in patients with antibody-mediated anemia. Patients should not be switched to other erythropoietic proteins, because antibodies may cross-react. Treat minor hypersensitivity reactions symptomatically. Discontinue drug and treat anaphylaxis as indicated; resuscitate as necessary.

387

DAUNORUBICIN HYDROCHLORIDE BBW ▪
DAUNORUBICIN CITRATE
LIPOSOMAL INJECTION BBW
(daw-noh-**ROO**-bih-sin hy-droh-**KLOR**-eyed)
(daw-noh-**ROO**-bih-sin **SIH**-trate **LIP**-oh-sohm-ul)

Antineoplastic
(anthracycline)

Cerubidine ▪ DaunoXome

pH 4.5 to 6.5 ▪ 4.9 to 6

USUAL DOSE
CONVENTIONAL DAUNORUBICIN
Adult acute nonlymphocytic leukemia: 45 mg/M^2/day on Days 1, 2, and 3 in adults under age 60 (adults over age 60 may require reduction to 30 mg/M^2/day). Used in specific protocol combination therapy (e.g., cytarabine 100 mg/M^2/day for 7 days). Regimen repeated every 3 to 4 weeks. In these subsequent courses, repeat daunorubicin, 30 to 45 mg/M^2/day (depending on age) for only 2 days and cytarabine for only 5 days. To obtain a normal-appearing bone marrow may require up to 3 courses.
Adult acute lymphocytic leukemia: 45 mg/M^2/day on Days 1, 2, and 3. Used in combination therapy (e.g., vincristine, prednisone, and L-asparaginase). In all situations, when remission is complete, an individual maintenance program should be established.
DAUNOXOME (LIPOSOMAL INJECTION)
Advanced, HIV-associated Kaposi's sarcoma: 40 mg/M^2 as an IV infusion. Repeat every 2 weeks. Continue treatment until there is evidence of disease progression (specifics outlined in package insert).
PEDIATRIC DOSE
CONVENTIONAL DAUNORUBICIN
See Maternal/Child.
Acute lymphocytic leukemia in pediatric patients 2 years of age and older: 25 mg/M^2/day on Day 1 each week, vincristine 1.5 mg/M^2 on Day 1 each week, and prednisone 40 mg/M^2 PO daily. Remission should be obtained in 4 weeks. If a partial remission is obtained after 4 weeks, 1 or 2 more weeks of treatment may produce a complete remission.
Acute lymphocytic leukemia in infants and children less than 2 years of age or less than 0.5 M^2 body surface: Calculate dose based on weight instead of body surface area: 1 mg/kg.
DAUNOXOME: Safety for use in pediatric patients not established.
DOSE ADJUSTMENTS
ALL DAUNORUBICINS: See Precautions/Monitor.
CONVENTIONAL DAUNORUBICIN: Profound bone marrow suppression is usually required to eradicate the leukemic cells and induce a complete remission. Evaluate bone marrow and peripheral blood to determine need for additional courses. ▪ See Usual Dose for adults over 60 years of age. ▪ Reduce dose in impaired hepatic or renal function according to the following chart.

Daunorubicin Dosing in Impaired Hepatic or Renal Function		
Serum Bilirubin	Serum Creatinine	Dose Reduction
1.2 to 3.0 mg	—	25%
>3 mg	—	50%
—	>3 mg	50%

DAUNOXOME: Reduce dose to 75% of normal (30 mg/M^2) if serum bilirubin is 1.2 to 3 mg/dL. Reduce dose to 50% of normal (20 mg/M^2) if serum bilirubin or creatinine is greater than 3 mg/dL. ▪ Withhold dose if absolute granulocyte count is less than 750 cells/mm^3.

DILUTION
Specific techniques required; see Precautions.
Conventional daunorubicin: Each 20 mg must be diluted with 4 mL of SWFI (5 mg/mL). Agitate gently to dissolve completely. Further dilute each dose with 10 to 15 mL of NS. Must be given through Y-tube or three-way stopcock of a free-flowing infusion of D5W or NS. May be added to 100 mL NS and given as an infusion. Use extreme caution.
DaunoXome: Dilute each single dose with an equal amount of D5W. Available as a 2 mg/mL preservative-free solution. Withdraw calculated volume (dose of DaunoXome) from vial; transfer to a sterile infusion bag that contains an equal volume of D5W. Desired concentration is 1 mg/mL. Do not use any other diluent. A translucent red liposomal dispersion; do not use if opaque. Do not use in-line filters for infusion. See Compatibility.
Filters: *DaunoXome:* Manufacturer states, "Do not use in-line filters for infusion."
Storage: *Conventional daunorubicin:* Protect from sunlight. Diluted solution stable 24 hours at room temperature, 48 hours if refrigerated; then discard.
DaunoXome: Refrigerate unopened vials; avoid freezing. Protect from light. Discard unused drug. Reconstituted solutions may be refrigerated for a maximum of 6 hours.

COMPATIBILITY   (Underline Indicates Conflicting Compatibility Information)
Consider any drug NOT listed as compatible to be INCOMPATIBLE until consulting a pharmacist; specific conditions may apply.
CONVENTIONAL DAUNORUBICIN
Manufacturer states, "Should not be administered mixed with other drugs or heparin."
One source suggests the following **compatibilities:**
Additive: *Not recommended by manufacturer.* Cytarabine (ARA-C), etoposide (VePesid), hydrocortisone sodium succinate (Solu-Cortef).
Y-site: Amifostine (Ethyol), anidulafungin (Eraxis), caspofungin (Cancidas), etoposide phosphate (Etopophos), filgrastim (Neupogen), gemcitabine (Gemzar), granisetron (Kytril), melphalan (Alkeran), methotrexate, ondansetron (Zofran), sodium bicarbonate, teniposide (Vumon), thiotepa, vinorelbine (Navelbine).
DAUNOXOME
Manufacturer states, "The only fluid that may be mixed with DaunoXome is D5W. Must not be mixed with saline, bacteriostatic agents such as benzyl alcohol, or any other solution."

RATE OF ADMINISTRATION
CONVENTIONAL DAUNORUBICIN
IV injection: A single dose of properly diluted medication over 3 to 5 minutes.
IV infusion: A single dose evenly distributed over 30 to 45 minutes.
DAUNOXOME
A single dose as an infusion evenly distributed over 60 minutes. Do not use an in-line filter. Back pain, flushing, and chest tightness may occur. Usually subsides if infusion is stopped, and usually does not recur if infusion is restarted at a slower rate after symptoms subside.

ACTIONS
CONVENTIONAL DAUNORUBICIN: A highly toxic antibiotic antineoplastic agent. Rapidly cleared from plasma, it inhibits synthesis of DNA. Cell-cycle specific for S phase; exact method of action is unknown; antimitotic, cytotoxic, and immunosuppressive. Widely distributed in tissues, with the highest concentrations occurring in the spleen, kidneys, liver, lungs, and heart. Does not cross blood-brain barrier. Metabolized in the liver and other tissues. Elimination half-life is 18 to 30 hours. Slowly excreted in bile and urine.
DAUNOXOME: A liposomal preparation of daunorubicin formulated to maximize selectivity for solid tumors. In the circulation, the liposomal preparation protects the entrapped daunorubicin from chemical and enzymatic degradation, minimizes protein binding, and generally decreases uptake by normal (non–reticuloendothelial system) tissues. The mechanism of delivery is not known, but may be through the often altered and/or compromised vasculature of tumors. In animals, it has been shown to accumulate in tumors to a greater extent than conventional daunorubicin. Released over time within the cells of the solid tumor. Persists at high levels within tumor tissue for several days. It differs

from conventional daunorubicin because it mostly confines itself to vascular fluid volume. Plasma clearance is slower and the AUC (area under the curve) is larger.

INDICATIONS AND USES

CONVENTIONAL DAUNORUBICIN: Treatment of acute nonlymphocytic leukemia in adults (myelogenous, monocytic, erythroid). ▪ Combination therapy for induction of remission in acute lymphocytic leukemia in adults and pediatric patients.

DAUNOXOME: Currently approved only for first-line cytotoxic therapy for advanced HIV-associated Kaposi's sarcoma.

CONTRAINDICATIONS

CONVENTIONAL DAUNORUBICIN: Hypersensitivity to daunorubicin or any of its components. *Not absolute:* pre-existing bone marrow suppression, impaired cardiac function, pre-existing infection; see Precautions.

DAUNOXOME: History of hypersensitivity reaction to previous treatment with DaunoXome or any of its components (includes conventional daunorubicin). Not recommended in patients with less than advanced HIV-related Kaposi's sarcoma.

PRECAUTIONS

ALL DAUNORUBICINS: Follow guidelines for handling cytotoxic agents. See Appendix A, p. 1331. ▪ Administered by or under the direction of the physician specialist with facilities for monitoring the patient and responding to any medical emergency. ▪ For IV use only; do not give IM or SC. ▪ Severe myelosuppression may occur and may lead to infection or hemorrhage. ▪ Use extreme caution in pre-existing drug-induced bone marrow suppression, existing heart disease, previous treatment with other anthracyclines (e.g., doxorubicin [Adriamycin]), or radiation therapy encompassing the heart. ▪ Incidence of myocardial toxicity increases after a total cumulative dose that exceeds 400 to 550 mg/M^2 in adults, 300 mg/M^2 in pediatric patients more than 2 years of age, or 10 mg/kg in pediatric patients less than 2 years of age. Potentially fatal congestive heart failure may occur either during therapy or months to years after therapy is complete. ▪ Urine may be reddish color (from dye, not hematuria).

Monitor: ALL DAUNORUBICINS: Monitor CBC including differential and platelet count before each dose. ▪ Monitoring of liver function, kidney function, ECG, chest x-ray, echocardiography, and systolic ejection fraction indicated before and during therapy; recommended before each course. ▪ Evaluation of cardiac function by medical history and physical exam is recommended before each dose; see Precautions. ▪ Monitor closely for S/S of hemorrhage or infection; may be life threatening. ▪ Prophylactic antibiotics may be indicated pending results of C/S in a febrile neutropenic patient. ▪ Determine absolute patency of vein. A stinging or burning sensation indicates extravasation; discontinue injection and use another vein. Severe cellulitis and tissue necrosis will result from extravasation with conventional daunorubicins; has not been observed with DaunoXome. ▪ Prophylactic antiemetics may reduce nausea and vomiting and increase patient comfort. ▪ Monitor uric acid levels; maintain hydration; alkalinization of urine or allopurinol may be indicated. ▪ Monitor for thrombocytopenia (platelet count less than 50,000/mm^3). Initiate precautions to prevent excessive bleeding (e.g., inspect IV sites, skin, and mucous membranes; use extreme care during invasive procedures; test urine, emesis, stool, and secretions for occult blood).

CONVENTIONAL DAUNORUBICIN: May cause acute congestive heart failure with total cumulative doses over 550 mg/M^2 in adults (400 mg/M^2 if previous treatment with doxorubicin or radiation therapy in area of heart), 300 mg/M^2 in pediatric patients over 2 years, and 10 mg/kg in pediatric patients under 2 years.

DAUNOXOME: May also cause cardiomyopathy. Monitoring of LVEF recommended at total cumulative doses of 320 mg/M^2, 480 mg/M^2, and every 240 mg/M^2 thereafter.

Patient Education: Nonhormonal birth control recommended. ▪ Report IV site burning or stinging promptly. ▪ Secondary leukemias have been reported. ▪ See Appendix D, p. 1333.

Maternal/Child: ALL DAUNORUBICINS: Category D: can cause fetal harm. Avoid pregnancy. ▪ Safety for use in breast-feeding not established; discontinue breast-feeding. ▪ Cardiotoxicity may be more frequent and occur at lower cumulative doses in pediatric patients. ▪ See Monitor.

DAUNOXOME: Safety for use in pediatric patients not established.

Elderly: Cardiotoxicity and myelotoxicity may be more severe. Consider age-related renal impairment. Safety of DaunoXome for use in the elderly has not been established.

DRUG/LAB INTERACTIONS

Concurrent use with **cyclophosphamide** (Cytoxan) may increase cardiotoxicity. ▪ Dose reduction may be required with concurrent use of **other myelosuppressive agents.** ▪ Concurrent use with **hepatotoxic agents** (e.g., high-dose methotrexate) may increase risk of toxicity. ▪ Risk of cardiotoxicity increased in patients previously treated with maximum cumulative doses of **other anthracyclines** (e.g., doxorubicin [Adriamycin], idarubicin [Idamycin]) **and/or radiation encompassing the heart.** ▪ Do not administer **vaccines or chloroquine** to patients receiving antineoplastic drugs. ▪ See Precautions.

SIDE EFFECTS

ALL DAUNORUBICINS: Bone marrow suppression and cardiotoxicity are dose related and dose limiting.

CONVENTIONAL DAUNORUBICIN: Acute congestive heart failure, alopecia (reversible), bone marrow suppression (marked with average doses), chills, decrease in systolic ejection fraction, depressed QRS voltage, diarrhea, fever, gonadal suppression, mucositis, myocarditis, nausea, pericarditis, skin rash, vomiting.

DAUNOXOME: Granulocytopenia is most common. Symptoms common to conventional daunorubicin may also occur. Infusion-related back pain, chest tightness, and flushing may be related to liposomal formulation.

Overdose: Will cause increased severity of myelosuppression, fatigue, nausea, and vomiting.

ANTIDOTE

Most side effects will be tolerated or treated symptomatically. Keep physician informed. Close monitoring of cumulative dosage, bone marrow, ECG, chest x-ray, echocardiography, and systolic ejection fraction may prevent most serious and potentially fatal side effects. There is no specific antidote. Supportive therapy as indicated will help sustain the patient in toxicity. Administration of whole blood products (e.g., packed RBCs, platelets, leukocytes) and/or blood modifiers (e.g., darbepoetin alfa [Aranesp], epoetin alfa [Epogen], filgrastim [Neupogen, Zarxio], pegfilgrastim [Neulasta], sargramostim [Leukine]) may be indicated to treat bone marrow toxicity. For extravasation, aspirate as much infiltrated drug as possible, flood site with normal saline, and inject hydrocortisone sodium succinate (Solu-Cortef) or hyaluronidase (Wydase) throughout extravasated tissue. Use a 27- or 25-gauge needle. Cold, moist compresses may be helpful; elevate extremity. Site should be observed promptly by a reconstructive surgeon.

DECITABINE FOR INJECTION
(deh-**SIGHT**-ah-been for in-**JEK**-shun)

Dacogen

Antineoplastic
(miscellaneous)

pH 6.7 to 7.3

USUAL DOSE
There are two treatment options. With either regimen, treatment for a minimum of 4 cycles is recommended. A complete or partial response may take longer than 4 cycles.
Premedication: Standard antiemetic therapy is indicated.
Decitabine: *Option 1:* 15 mg/M^2 as an infusion over 3 hours. Repeat every 8 hours for 3 days. Repeat this complete cycle every 6 weeks. See Dose Adjustments and Monitor.
Option 2: 20 mg/M^2 as an infusion over 1 hour. Repeat once each day for 5 days. Repeat this complete cycle every 4 weeks. See Dose Adjustments and Monitor.

DOSE ADJUSTMENTS
Option 1 and Option 2: Hematologic recovery to at least an ANC equal to or greater than 1,000 cells/mm^3 and platelets equal to or greater than 50,000 cells/mm^3 is required before subsequent cycles are administered. ▪ If a SCr equal to or greater than 2 mg/dL, an ALT or a total bilirubin equal to or greater than 2 times the ULN, and/or an active or uncontrolled infection occur, do not restart decitabine therapy until the toxicity is resolved. ▪ No additional dose reductions are indicated based on age, gender, or race; see Precautions and Elderly.
Option 1: If hematologic recovery requires more than 6 weeks but less than 8 weeks, delay repeat cycle of decitabine for up to 2 weeks. When therapy is restarted, reduce dose for that cycle to 11 mg/M^2 every 8 hours (33 mg/M^2/day, 99 mg/M^2/cycle). ▪ If hematologic recovery requires more than 8 weeks but less than 10 weeks, assess the patient for disease progression (by bone marrow aspirates). If disease progression has not occurred, delay repeat cycle of decitabine for up to 2 more weeks to allow for hematologic recovery. When therapy is restarted, reduce dose for that cycle to 11 mg/M^2 every 8 hours (33 mg/M^2/day, 99 mg/M^2/cycle). In subsequent cycles, maintain or increase dose based on hematologic recovery.

DILUTION
Specific techniques required; see Precautions. Reconstitute a single vial (50 mg) with 10 mL SWFI (each mL contains 5 mg of decitabine at a pH of 6.7 to 7.3). Further dilute immediately with NS, D5W, or LR to a final concentration of 0.1 to 1 mg/mL (further dilute each mL with 4 mL additional diluent for a 1 mg/mL concentration or 49 mL for a 0.1 mg/mL concentration). Must be used within 15 minutes of reconstitution. If decitabine will not be used within 15 minutes of reconstitution, it must be diluted using cold (2° C to 8° C) infusion fluids and stored at 2° C to 8° C (36° F to 46° F) for up to a maximum of 7 hours.
Filters: Specific information not available.
Storage: Store unopened vials at 25° C (77° F); excursions permitted to 15° to 30° C (59° to 86° F). Use of reconstituted and/or diluted solution within 15 minutes of reconstitution is preferred or a specific process is required; see Dilution.

COMPATIBILITY
Specific information not available. Consider specific use; consult pharmacist.

RATE OF ADMINISTRATION
Option 1: A single dose as an infusion equally distributed over 3 hours.
Option 2: A single dose as an infusion equally distributed over 1 hour.

ACTIONS
A hypomethylating antineoplastic agent. Cytotoxic to proliferating cells through a process that incorporates it into DNA, inhibits the enzyme DNA methyltransferase, and causes hypomethylation of DNA, leading to cell disintegration and/or death. This hypomethylation in neoplastic cells may restore normal function to genes that are critical for

the control of cellular differentiation and proliferation and allow the formation of normal RBCs and platelets. Patients with myelodysplastic syndromes who have responded to decitabine have become transfusion independent. Terminal half-life range is 0.21 to 0.82 hours. Extensively metabolized by an unknown route(s). Protein binding is negligible.

INDICATIONS AND USES
Treatment of patients with myelodysplastic syndromes (MDS), including previously treated and untreated *de novo* and secondary MDS of all French-American-British subtypes (refractory anemia, refractory anemia with ringed sideroblasts, refractory anemia with excess blasts, refractory anemia with excess blasts in transformation, and chronic myelomonocytic leukemia) and intermediate-1, intermediate-2, and high-risk International Prognostic Scoring System groups.

CONTRAINDICATIONS
Manufacturer states, "None."

PRECAUTIONS
Follow guidelines for handling cytotoxic agents. See Appendix A, p. 1331. ▪ Administered by or under the direction of a physician specialist in a facility with adequate diagnostic and treatment facilities to monitor the patient and respond to any medical emergency. ▪ The effects of age, gender, race, or renal or hepatic impairment on the pharmacokinetics of decitabine have not been studied. ▪ Myelosuppression and worsening neutropenia may occur more frequently in the first or second treatment cycles and may not indicate progression of underlying MDS. Neutropenia and thrombocytopenia may be dose-limiting toxicities. ▪ Patients with MDS produce poorly functioning and immature blood cells and experience anemia, bleeding, fatigue, infection, and weakness. High-risk MDS patients may experience bone marrow failure, which may lead to death from bleeding and infection. ▪ MDS can progress to acute leukemia (AML). ▪ Use caution in patients with renal or hepatic impairment. Use has not been studied.

Monitor: Obtain a baseline CBC with platelets and monitor before each dosing cycle and as indicated between cycles. ▪ Consider early institution of growth factors as indicated. ▪ Obtain a baseline and monitor renal and hepatic function (BUN, SCr, bilirubin) as indicated. ▪ Use prophylactic antiemetics to reduce nausea and vomiting and increase patient comfort. ▪ Monitor for S/S of infection. Prophylactic antibiotics may be indicated pending results of C/S in a febrile neutropenic patient. ▪ Monitor for thrombocytopenia (platelet count less than 50,000/mm^3). Initiate precautions to prevent excessive bleeding (e.g., inspect IV sites, skin, and mucous membranes; use extreme care during invasive procedures; test urine, emesis, stool, and secretions for occult blood). ▪ Avoid administration of live virus vaccine to immunocompromised patients. ▪ Observe for S/S of a hypersensitivity reaction; specific information not available. ▪ See Precautions and Antidote.

Patient Education: Avoid pregnancy; nonhormonal birth control recommended for both males and females; see Maternal/Child. Women should report a suspected pregnancy immediately. ▪ Discuss possible liver or kidney disease with a health care professional. ▪ Report S/S of infection (e.g., fever, sore throat), bruising, bleeding, or other suspected side effects.

Maternal/Child: Category D: avoid pregnancy; may cause fetal harm. Females should use birth control until at least 1 month after treatment with decitabine is discontinued. Males should not father a child until at least 2 months after treatment with decitabine is discontinued. ▪ Discontinue breast-feeding; has potential for serious harm to nursing infants. ▪ Safety and effectiveness for use in pediatric patients not established.

Elderly: The majority of patients in clinical trials were over 65 years of age. Safety and effectiveness similar to younger adults; however, greater sensitivity of some older individuals should be considered.

DRUG/LAB INTERACTIONS
Formal drug interactions studies have not been completed. In vitro studies suggest that decitabine is unlikely to inhibit or induce the activities of cytochrome P$_{450}$ isoenzymes.

- Plasma protein binding is negligible; interactions due to displacement of more highly protein bound drugs from plasma proteins are not expected. ■ Do not administer **live virus vaccines** to immunocompromised patients who are receiving antineoplastic agents.

SIDE EFFECTS

Cough, constipation, diarrhea, fatigue, fever, hyperglycemia, nausea, and petechiae have been reported most commonly. Bone marrow suppression (anemia, neutropenia, thrombocytopenia) was the most frequent cause of dose reduction, delay, and discontinuation. Grade 3 or 4 adverse events included febrile neutropenia, leukopenia, neutropenia, and thrombocytopenia. During clinical trials, therapy was also discontinued because of abnormal liver function tests, cardiopulmonary arrest, intracranial hemorrhage, *Mycobacterium avium* complex infection, and pneumonia. Atrial fibrillation, central line infection, febrile neutropenia, neutropenia, and pulmonary edema also resulted in delayed doses; bone marrow suppression (anemia, neutropenia, thrombocytopenia), depression, edema, lethargy, pharyngitis, and tachycardia resulted in reduced doses. Numerous other side effects may occur.

Post-Marketing: Acute febrile neutrophilic dermatosis (Sweet's syndrome) has been reported.

Overdose: Increased myelosuppression, including prolonged neutropenia and thrombocytopenia.

ANTIDOTE

Notify physician of any side effects. Most will be treated symptomatically. Dosage may be delayed for hematologic toxicity. Hematologic recovery to at least an ANC equal to or greater than 1,000 cells/mm^3 and platelets equal to or greater than 50,000 cells/mm^3 between cycles is required; see Dose Adjustments. If a SCr equal to or greater than 2 mg/dL, an ALT or a total bilirubin equal to or greater than 2 times the ULN, and/or an uncontrolled infection occur, discontinue decitabine therapy until the toxicity is resolved. Blood and blood products, antibiotics, and other adjunctive therapies must be available. Blood modifiers (e.g., darbepoetin alfa [Aranesp], epoetin alfa [Epogen], filgrastim [Neupogen, Zarxio], pegfilgrastim [Neulasta], sargramostim [Leukine]) may be indicated to treat bone marrow toxicity. No known antidote; provide supportive care in overdose. ■ Resuscitate as necessary.

DENILEUKIN DIFTITOX BBW

(den-ih-**LOO**-kin **DIF**-tih-tox)

Antineoplastic
Biological response modifier

Ontak

pH 6.9 to 7.2

USUAL DOSE

Pretesting indicated; see Monitor.

Premedication: Premedicate with an antihistamine (e.g., diphenhydramine [Benadryl]) and acetaminophen (Tylenol) before each infusion.

Denileukin diftitox: 9 or 18 mcg/kg/day administered as an IV infusion for 5 consecutive days. Repeat course every 21 days for 8 cycles.

DOSE ADJUSTMENTS

In patients with hypoalbuminemia, administration of denileukin diftitox should be delayed until serum albumin levels are at least 3 Gm/dL; see Monitor.

DILUTION

Each 2-mL vial contains 300 mcg (150 mcg/mL) of frozen recombinant denileukin diftitox. Thaw in refrigerator (2° to 8° C [36° to 46° F]) for not more than 24 hours or at CRT for 1 to 2 hours. Bring to CRT before preparing dose. Do not heat. Gently swirl contents of vial. Do not shake. Solution may be hazy initially. Haze should clear as solution reaches CRT. The concentration of denileukin diftitox must be at least 15 mcg/mL during all steps in the preparation of the infusion solution. This is best accomplished by aseptically withdrawing the calculated dose of denileukin diftitox and injecting it into an empty infusion bag. For each 1 mL of denileukin diftitox from the vial(s), no more than 9 mL of sterile NS without preservative should then be added to the bag. For example: A 70-kg patient receiving a 9-mcg/kg dose would require 630 mcg of denileukin diftitox (or 4.2 mL). Withdraw 4.2 mL of denileukin diftitox from vials and inject into an empty infusion bag. Add no more than 37.8 mL (9 × 4.2 mL) of preservative-free NS to infusion bag. The final solution will be 630 mcg in 42 mL of solution, which equals the desired concentration of 15 mcg/mL. Diluted denileukin diftitox must be prepared and stored in a plastic syringe or soft plastic IV infusion bag. Do not use a glass container; see Compatibility.

Filters: Manufacturer states, "Do not administer through an in-line filter."

Storage: Store unopened vials in freezer at or below −10° C (14° F). Prepared solutions should be administered within 6 hours. Discard unused solution. Do not refreeze.

COMPATIBILITY

Manufacturer states, "Do not physically mix denileukin diftitox with other drugs." Do not mix in glass. Adsorption to glass may occur in the dilute state.

RATE OF ADMINISTRATION

A single dose evenly distributed over 30 to 60 minutes. Administer via peripheral or central vein by a pump device or IV infusion bag. Do not administer as a bolus injection. Do not administer through an in-line filter. If adverse reactions occur during the infusion, the infusion should be discontinued or the rate should be reduced depending on the severity of the reaction. There is no clinical experience with infusion times lasting more than 80 minutes.

ACTIONS

A recombinant DNA–derived cytotoxic protein. A fusion protein that utilizes both the cytotoxic action of diphtheria toxin and the cell-targeting ability of human interleukin-2 (IL-2) to kill certain leukemia and lymphoma cells. Targets specific receptors (IL-2 receptors) on malignant cells while minimizing damage to normal cells that do not express the receptor. Ex vivo studies suggest that denileukin diftitox interacts with the high-affinity IL-2 receptor on the cell surface and inhibits cellular protein synthesis, resulting in cell death within hours. No differences in pharmacologic action noted based on age, gender, and/or race. Half-life in lymphoma patients is 70 to 80 minutes. Development of antibodies to denileukin diftitox has been shown to increase clearance; see Precautions.

INDICATIONS AND USES

Treatment of patients with persistent or recurrent cutaneous T-cell lymphoma (CTCL) whose malignant cells express the CD25 component of the IL-2 receptor. The safety and efficacy of denileukin diftitox in patients with CTCL whose malignant cells do not express the CD25 component of the IL-2 receptor have not been examined.

CONTRAINDICATIONS

Hypersensitivity to denileukin diftitox, any of its components, diphtheria toxin, or interleukin-2.

PRECAUTIONS

Administered under the supervision of a physician experienced in the use of antineoplastic therapy and the management of patients with cancer. ▪ Administer in a facility equipped and staffed for cardiopulmonary resuscitation and in which the patient can be properly monitored. ▪ Infusion and/or hypersensitivity reactions, defined as symptoms occurring within 24 hours of infusion and resolving within 48 hours of the last infusion in that course, have been reported and may be serious or life threatening. Deaths have occurred. Incidence of infusion reactions appears to decrease after the first 2 courses of therapy. ▪ Capillary leak syndrome (CLS) has resulted in death. CLS characterized by at least two of the following three symptoms (edema, hypoalbuminemia [3 Gm/dL or less], hypotension) has been reported. Symptoms are not required to occur simultaneously to be described as capillary leak syndrome. Onset can occur at any time. Usually occurs within 2 weeks of the infusion but may be delayed. Patients with edema or pre-existing low serum albumin levels may be predisposed to this syndrome. Symptoms may persist or worsen after denileukin diftitox is discontinued; treatment and/or hospitalization may be required; deaths have been reported. Use special caution in patients with pre-existing cardiovascular disease. ▪ A significant percentage of patients treated with denileukin diftitox tested positive for antibodies at baseline, probably due to a prior exposure to diphtheria toxin or its vaccine. With each subsequent course, the percent of patients who tested positive increased, C_{max} and AUC decreased, and clearance increased with increasing antibody formation. The formation of neutralizing antibodies was assessed in a number of patients. Evidence of inhibited functional activity in the cellular assay was seen. ▪ Loss of visual acuity (usually with loss of color vision, with or without retinal pigment mottling) has been reported. Some patients recover; however, most report persistent visual impairment.

Monitor: Before administration of denileukin diftitox, the patient's malignant cells should be tested for CD25 expression. A testing service for the assay of CD25 on skin biopsy samples is available; see manufacturer's prescribing information. ▪ Consider baseline and periodic monitoring of CBC and a blood chemistry panel, including liver and renal function, before therapy and weekly during therapy. ▪ Monitor serum albumin levels before each course of therapy. Nadir occurs 1 to 2 weeks after administration. Delay administration if necessary until serum albumin levels are at least 3 Gm/dL. Note Dose Adjustments. ▪ Observe for capillary leak syndrome. Monitor weight, edema, BP, and serum albumin levels on an outpatient basis. ▪ Monitor for signs and symptoms of infection. Patients with CTCL have a predisposition to cutaneous infections, and binding of denileukin diftitox to activated lymphocytes and macrophages may lead to cell death and may impair patient's immune system. ▪ Monitor for thrombocytopenia (platelet count less than 50,000/mm³). Initiate precautions to prevent excessive bleeding (e.g., inspect IV sites, skin, and mucous membranes; use extreme care during invasive procedures; test urine, emesis, stool, and secretions for occult blood). ▪ Monitor injection site. To minimize occurrence or phlebitis, change the injection site frequently. ▪ See Precautions, Side Effects, and Antidote.

Patient Education: Promptly report orthostatic hypotension (dizziness), weight gain, or edema following infusion. ▪ Weigh self daily. ▪ Report breathing problems, chest pain, chills, fever, tachycardia, and/or urticaria following infusion. ▪ Report vision changes. ▪ Keep physician informed of all side effects.

Maternal/Child: Safety for use in pregnancy not established. Use only if clearly needed. ▪ Discontinue breast-feeding. ▪ Safety and effectiveness in pediatric patients not established.

Elderly: Numbers in clinical studies insufficient to determine if the elderly respond differently than do younger adults.

DRUG/LAB INTERACTIONS
Drug interaction studies have not been conducted.

SIDE EFFECTS
All patients experienced at least one adverse event. The occurrence of side effects tended to diminish in frequency and severity after the first two courses of therapy. ▪ The most common side effects were cough, diarrhea, dyspnea, edema, fatigue, fever, headache, nausea, peripheral edema, pruritus, and rigors. The most common serious side effects were capillary leak syndrome, infusion reactions, and vision changes, including loss of visual acuity. During initial studies the most common reasons for discontinuation of therapy were systemic flu-like symptoms (e.g., anorexia, asthenia, chills, fever, malaise, nausea, and vomiting), hypoalbuminemia, infection, rash, respiratory events (e.g., dyspnea, apnea, pulmonary edema, or pneumonia), and capillary leak syndrome. The most common reasons for therapy-related hospitalization were evaluation of fever, management of capillary leak syndrome, or dehydration secondary to gastrointestinal toxicity. ▪ Other reported side effects include anorexia, arthralgia, asthenia, back pain, chest pain, dizziness, dysgeusia, hypotension, myalgia, pain, rash, upper respiratory tract infection, and vomiting.

Post-Marketing: Hyperthyroidism, hypothyroidism, thyroiditis, thyrotoxicosis, visual acuity loss.

ANTIDOTE

Notify physician of any side effects. If adverse reactions occur during administration, the infusion should be discontinued or the rate should be reduced depending on the severity of the reaction. If a serious infusion reaction occurs, immediately stop and permanently discontinue denileukin diftitox. IV antihistamines, corticosteroids, and/or epinephrine may be required. Most symptoms of the flu-like syndrome will respond to treatment with antipyretics and/or antiemetics (e.g., promethazine [Phenergan] or prochlorperazine [Compazine]). Premedication with acetaminophen and an antihistamine 30 to 60 minutes before each infusion may help reduce the frequency and/or severity of symptoms. While on therapy, patients may continue to receive acetaminophen every 4 to 6 hours while awake. Fever, chills, and/or pain not controlled with acetaminophen alone may be treated with an NSAID. Rigors may be treated with meperidine. Skin rashes may require treatment with topical and/or oral corticosteroids. Treatment of capillary leak syndrome depends on whether edema or hypotension is the primary clinical problem. Patients who present with dehydration should be considered for IV fluid replacement therapy. If BP is still not adequate after replacement therapy, pressor agents (e.g., dopamine) should be considered. Use of diuretics should be avoided in patients whose intravascular depletion has not been corrected. However, patients who present primarily with edema may benefit from diuretic therapy. Continuous monitoring of fluid status, weight, and BP is essential. If overdose occurs, hepatic and renal function and overall fluid status should be closely monitored. Resuscitate as necessary.

DESMOPRESSIN ACETATE
(des-moh-**PRESS**-in **AS**-ah-tayt)

DDAVP, 1-Deamino-8-D-Arginine Vasopressin

Hormone
Antidiuretic
Antihemorrhagic

pH 3.5 to 4

USUAL DOSE

Diabetes insipidus: 2 to 4 mcg daily in 2 divided doses. Adjust each dose individually for an adequate diurnal rhythm of water turnover. IV dose has 10 times the antidiuretic effect of intranasal desmopressin.

Hemophilia A and von Willebrand's disease (Type 1): 0.3 mcg/kg of body weight. If used preoperatively, administer 30 minutes before the scheduled procedure. The necessity for repeat administration of desmopressin or the use of any blood products for hemostasis should be determined by laboratory response and the clinical condition of the patient; see Monitor.

DOSE ADJUSTMENTS

Many specific requirements depending on diagnosis; see Limitations of Use, Precautions, and Monitor. ▪ Dosing should be cautious in the elderly. Consider potential for decreased organ function and concomitant disease or drug therapy. See Elderly and Contraindications. ▪ Reduce dose accordingly (to ¹/₁₀ of the intranasal dose) when transferring from intranasal to IV administration.

DILUTION

Diabetes insipidus: May be given undiluted.

Hemophilia A and von Willebrand's disease (Type 1): Dilute a single dose in 10 mL of NS for pediatric patients under 10 kg; 50 mL for adults and pediatric patients over 10 kg. Must be given as an infusion.

Storage: Refrigerate at 2° to 8° C (36° to 46° F). Use diluted product promptly.

COMPATIBILITY
Specific information not available. Consider specific use; consult pharmacist.

RATE OF ADMINISTRATION
Diabetes insipidus: A single dose by IV injection over 1 minute.
Hemophilia A and von Willebrand's disease (Type 1): A single dose as an infusion over 15 to 30 minutes.

ACTIONS
A synthetic analog of the natural hormone arginine vasopressin, an antidiuretic hormone affecting renal water conservation (human antidiuretic hormone—ADH). Has been shown to be more potent than arginine vasopressin in increasing plasma levels of factor VIII activity in patients with hemophilia A and von Willebrand's disease (Type 1). Produces dose-related increase in factor VIII levels within 30 minutes and peaks in 90 to 120 minutes. Onset of action as an antidiuretic is prompt. When administered by IV injection, desmopressin has an antidiuretic effect about 10 times that of an equivalent dose administered intranasally. Half-life is biphasic (7.8 minutes for fast phase and 75.5 minutes for slow phase). Increases water resorption in the kidney, increases urine osmolality, and decreases urine output. Increases plasma levels of von Willebrand factor, factor VIII, and t-PA, thereby contributing to a shortened activated partial thromboplastin time (aPTT) and bleeding time. Clinically effective antidiuretic doses are usually below the threshold levels for effects on vascular or visceral smooth muscle. Excreted in urine.

INDICATIONS AND USES
Diabetes insipidus: Antidiuretic replacement therapy in the management of central (cranial) diabetes insipidus and for the management of temporary polyuria and polydipsia following head trauma or surgery in the pituitary region.
Hemophilia A and von Willebrand's disease (Type 1): Maintenance of hemostasis in patients with hemophilia A and in patients with mild to moderate classic von Willebrand's disease (Type I) with factor VIII coagulant activity levels greater than 5%. Will often maintain hemostasis during surgical procedures and postoperatively when administered 30 minutes before a scheduled procedure and will also stop bleeding in episodes of spontaneous or trauma-induced injuries such as hemarthroses, intramuscular hematomas, or mucosal bleeding.
Limitations of use: Ineffective for the treatment of nephrogenic diabetes insipidus. ▪ Not indicated for the treatment of hemophilia A or von Willebrand's disease (Type I) with factor VIII coagulant activity levels equal to or less than 5%; see Monitor. ▪ Not indicated for the treatment of hemophilia B. ▪ Not indicated in patients who have factor VIII antibodies. ▪ Not indicated for the treatment of severe classic von Willebrand's disease (Type I) and when there is evidence of an abnormal molecular form of factor VIII antigen. ▪ Should not be used to treat Type IIB von Willebrand's disease; platelet aggregation may be induced.

CONTRAINDICATIONS
Infants under 3 months of age with hemophilia A or von Willebrand's disease, known hypersensitivity to desmopressin, patients with moderate to severe renal impairment (CrCl less than 50 mL/min), and patients with hyponatremia or a history of hyponatremia.

PRECAUTIONS
A potent antidiuretic. Administration may lead to water intoxication and/or hyponatremia, which can be fatal. Fluid restriction is recommended. ▪ When administered to patients who do not have a need for the antidiuretic effect, fluid intake should be adjusted downward to decrease the potential occurrence of water intoxication and hyponatremia. S/S may include headache, nausea and vomiting, decreased serum sodium, weight gain, restlessness, fatigue, lethargy, disorientation, depressed reflexes, loss of appetite, irritability, muscle weakness, muscle spasms, and abnormal mental status (e.g., confusion, decreased consciousness, hallucinations). Severe symptoms may include seizure, coma, and respiratory arrest caused by an extreme decrease in plasma osmolality. Pediatric and elderly patients may be at increased risk. ▪ Use with caution in patients with habitual or psychogenic polydipsia. May be more likely to drink excessive amounts of water, in-

creasing their risk of hyponatremia. ▪ Use caution in patients with coronary artery insufficiency or hypertension; has infrequently produced hypertension or hypotension, with a reflex increase in heart rate. ▪ Use with caution in patients predisposed to thrombus formation. There have been rare reports of thrombotic events following administration of desmopressin. ▪ Patients with conditions associated with fluid and electrolyte imbalance (e.g., cystic fibrosis, CHF, renal disorders) are prone to hyponatremia; use with caution. ▪ Severe hypersensitivity reactions, including anaphylaxis, have been reported. ▪ See Drug Interactions.

Monitor: *All diagnoses:* Monitor fluid intake and urine volume. Monitor for S/S of hyponatremia, especially in high-risk patient populations (pediatric patients, the elderly, and patients with CHF).

Diabetes insipidus: Confirm diagnosis of diabetes insipidus with urinalysis, the water deprivation test, or the hypertonic saline infusion test. ▪ Fluid restriction indicated; see Precautions. ▪ Monitor continued response by measuring urine output and osmolality. ▪ Monitoring of plasma osmolality may be indicated. ▪ Accuracy and effectiveness of dose measured by duration of sleep and adequate, not excessive, water turnover.

Hemophilia A: Determine factor VIII coagulant activity before administration for hemostasis. ▪ Monitor factor VIII coagulant, factor VIII antigen, factor VIII ristocetin cofactor (von Willebrand factor), and aPTT to assess patient status during treatment. ▪ Do not rely on desmopressin, but it may be considered for use in patients with factor VIII activity levels from 2% to 5% with careful monitoring. Generally used only when the factor VIII activity level is above 5%.

von Willebrand's disease (Type 1): Most effective when factor VIII activity level above 5%. ▪ Monitor bleeding time, factor VIII coagulant activity levels, ristocetin cofactor activity, and von Willebrand factor antigen during therapy to assess patient status. Patients with severe homozygous von Willebrand's disease with factor VIII coagulant activity and factor VIII von Willebrand factor antigen levels less than 1% are least likely to respond to treatment with desmopressin.

Hemophilia and von Willebrand's disease: Monitor BP and pulse during infusion. ▪ Fluid restriction indicated; see Precautions. ▪ Determine need for repeat administration of desmopressin or use of blood products by laboratory response as well as the clinical condition of the patient. Tachyphylaxis (lessening of response; i.e., a gradual diminution of the factor VIII activity increase) has been seen when given more frequently than every 48 hours.

Patient Education: Careful monitoring of fluid intake indicated in patients with diabetes insipidus. ▪ When antidiuretic effect is not needed, caution patients (especially the young and the elderly) to limit fluid intake to satisfy thirst needs only; this decreases potential occurrence of water intoxication and hyponatremia.

Maternal/Child: Category B: use only when clearly indicated in pregnancy and breastfeeding. ▪ Risk of hyponatremia and water intoxication increased in pediatric patients. Restrict fluid intake. ▪ Safety for use in pediatric patients under 12 years of age with diabetes insipidus not established. ▪ See Contraindications.

Elderly: Risk of hyponatremia and water intoxication increased. Use caution and restrict fluid intake. ▪ Response similar to that seen in younger adults. Dosing should be cautious in the elderly. Monitor renal function; see Dose Adjustments.

DRUG/LAB INTERACTIONS

Has been used with aminocaproic acid without adverse effects. ▪ May produce hypertension with other **vasopressors** (e.g., dopamine). ▪ Use caution when administered concurrently with other medications that can increase the risk of water intoxication with hyponatremia (e.g., **carbamazepine** [Tegretol], **chlorpromazine** [Thorazine], **lamotrigine** [Lamictal], **NSAIDs** [e.g., ibuprofen (Advil, Motrin), naproxen (Aleve, Naprosyn)], **opiate analgesics, selective serotonin reuptake inhibitors** [e.g., sertraline (Zoloft)], **tricyclic antidepressants** [e.g., imipramine (Tofranil)]). ▪ Hyponatremic convulsions have been reported with concomitant use with **oxybutynin** (Ditropan) **and imipramine** (Tofranil-PM).

SIDE EFFECTS

Mild abdominal cramps, nausea, transient headache, and vulval pain are most common and may disappear with reduced doses. Facial flushing, hypertension (slight), and/or hypotension with a compensatory tachycardia have occurred. May cause burning, local erythema, and swelling at site of injection. Most serious side effects include hyponatremia with resultant sequelae (see Precautions), water intoxication, and thrombotic events (cerebrovascular thrombosis, MI). Anaphylaxis has been reported.

Overdose: Confusion, continuing headache, drowsiness, problems passing urine, rapid weight gain due to fluid retention.

Post-Marketing: Hyponatremia (can be fatal), hyponatremic convulsions associated with concomitant use of oxybutinin (Ditropan) and imipramine (Tofranil-PM), thrombotic events (e.g., acute MI, cerebrovascular thrombosis).

ANTIDOTE

Notify physician of all side effects. Most will respond to reduction of dose or rate of administration, or symptomatic treatment. May need to discontinue drug. If overdose occurs, treat by reducing dose or frequency of administration, or discontinue drug if indicated. Treat hypersensitivity with oxygen, epinephrine (Adrenalin), antihistamines (e.g., diphenhydramine [Benadryl]), vasopressors (e.g., dopamine), corticosteroids, albuterol, IV fluids, and ventilation equipment as indicated. Resuscitate as necessary.

DEXAMETHASONE SODIUM PHOSPHATE
(dex-ah-**METH**-ah-zohn **SO**-dee-um **FOS**-fayt)

Hormone (corticosteroid)
Anti-inflammatory
Antiemetic
Immunosuppressant
Diagnostic agent

Decadron, Decadron Phosphate

pH 7 to 8.5

USUAL DOSE

Average dose range is 0.5 to 24 mg daily. May be divided into 2 to 4 doses. IV dexamethasone is usually given in an emergency situation or when oral dosing is not feasible. Larger doses may be justified by patient condition. Repeat until adequate response, then decrease dose as indicated. Total dose usually does not exceed 80 mg/24 hr. Dosage must be individualized. High-dose treatment is utilized until patient condition stabilizes, usually no longer than 48 to 72 hours. Doses similar by IV or oral route.

Anti-inflammatory: See average dose range above.

Shock: Several regimens have been suggested:

1 to 6 mg/kg as a single injection; *or*

40 mg. Repeat every 2 to 6 hours as needed; *or*

20 mg as a *loading dose,* followed by a continuous infusion of 3 mg/kg equally distributed over 24 hours.

Cerebral edema: *Loading dose:* 10 mg. *Maintenance dose:* 4 mg every 6 hours (usually given IM). Reduce dose after 2 to 4 days. Discontinue gradually over 5 to 7 days. A brain tumor requiring treatment before dexamethasone can be discontinued is the exception.

Cerebral edema (ICP) in recurrent or inoperable brain tumors: 2 mg every 8 to 12 hours (usually given IM). Adjust based on patient response.

Antiemetic in management of emesis-inducing chemotherapy: Several regimens have been used:

10 to 20 mg before chemotherapy. Lower doses may be given over the next 24 to 72 hours if necessary; *or*

Give a loading dose of 4 to 8 mg/M^2. May repeat 2 to 4 mg/M^2 every 6 hours; *or*

20 mg combined with 8 mg of ondansetron (Zofran) in 50 mL D5W before chemotherapy; *or*

20 mg 40 minutes before administration of chemotherapeutic agent. Given concurrently with metoclopramide and lorazepam or diphenhydramine; *or*

10 mg 30 minutes before administration of chemotherapeutic agent. Given concurrently with oral dexamethasone 8 mg beginning prior evening, 4 mg every 4 to 6 hours continuing through treatment day, with droperidol or haloperidol.

Airway edema: *Adult and pediatric patients:* 0.5 to 2 mg/kg/24 hr in equally divided doses every 6 hours (0.125 to 0.5 mg/kg every 6 hours) for croup or beginning 24 hours before elective extubation. Repeat for 4 to 6 doses. Up to 1 mg/kg/24 hr may be given in divided doses before and after extubation.

Allergic conditions: (Usually given IM or PO) 4 to 8 mg on the first day, then PO in decreasing doses (1.5 mg every 12 hours on Days 2 and 3; 0.75 mg every 12 hours on Day 4; and 0.75 mg on Days 5 and 6).

Meningitis: *Adult and pediatric patients:* 0.15 mg/kg/dose every 6 hours for 4 days.

Primary or secondary adrenocortical insufficiency (physiologic replacement): 0.03 to 0.15 mg/kg/24 hr or 0.6 to 0.75 mg/M^2/24 hr given in divided doses every 6 to 12 hours (0.015 to 0.075 mg/kg every 12 hours, or 0.0075 to 0.0375 mg/kg every 6 hours, or 0.3 to 0.375 mg/M^2 every 12 hours, or 0.15 to 0.1875 mg/M^2 every 6 hours). Usually given IM. Dexamethasone has minimal mineralocorticoid properties; may require a concomitant mineralocorticoid (e.g., hydrocortisone IV or PO). Hydrocortisone is the drug of choice for this indication.

PEDIATRIC DOSE
See Maternal/Child.
Cerebral edema: *Loading dose:* 1 to 2 mg/kg of body weight for 1 dose.
Maintenance dose: 1 to 1.5 mg/kg/24 hr in equally divided doses every 4 to 6 hours (0.17 to 0.25 mg/kg every 4 hours or 0.25 to 0.375 mg/kg every 6 hours) for 5 days, then gradually decrease. Maximum dose is 16 mg/24 hr.
Airway edema: See Usual Dose.
Antiemetic: *Loading dose:* 4 to 8 mg/M^2. May repeat 2 to 4 mg/M^2 every 6 hours.
Anti-inflammatory: 0.03 to 0.15 mg/kg/24 hr in equally divided doses every 6 to 12 hours (0.015 to 0.075 mg/kg every 12 hours or 0.0075 to 0.0375 mg/kg every 6 hours).
Meningitis: See Usual Dose.

DOSE ADJUSTMENTS
Reduced dose may be required in the elderly and with cyclophosphamide. ■ See Drug/Lab Interactions.

DILUTION
May be given undiluted or added to IV glucose or saline solutions and given as an infusion. 24 mg/mL product for IV use only; 4 mg/mL may be used IM/IV.
Storage: Use diluted solutions within 24 hours. Sensitive to heat. Protect from freezing.

COMPATIBILITY (Underline Indicates Conflicting Compatibility Information)
Consider any drug NOT listed as compatible to be INCOMPATIBLE until consulting a pharmacist; specific conditions may apply.
One source suggests the following **compatibilities:**
Additive: <u>Amikacin</u>, aminophylline, bleomycin (Blenoxane), furosemide (Lasix), granisetron (Kytril), lidocaine, meropenem (Merrem IV), mitomycin (Mutamycin), nafcillin (Nallpen), <u>ondansetron (Zofran)</u>, <u>palonosetron (Aloxi)</u>, prochlorperazine (Compazine), ranitidine (Zantac), verapamil.
Y-site: Acetaminophen (Ofirmev), acyclovir (Zovirax), allopurinol (Aloprim), amifostine (Ethyol), amikacin, amphotericin B cholesteryl (Amphotec), <u>anidulafungin (Eraxis)</u>, aztreonam (Azactam), bivalirudin (Angiomax), ceftaroline (Teflaro), cisatracurium (Nimbex), cladribine (Leustatin), dexmedetomidine (Precedex), docetaxel (Taxotere), doripenem (Doribax), doxorubicin liposomal (Doxil), etoposide phosphate (Etopophos), famotidine (Pepcid IV), fentanyl, filgrastim (Neupogen), fluconazole (Diflucan), fludarabine (Fludara), foscarnet (Foscavir), gallium nitrate (Ganite), gemcitabine (Gemzar), granisetron (Kytril), heparin, hetastarch in electrolytes (Hextend), hydrocortisone sodium succinate (Solu-Cortef), hydromorphone (Dilaudid), levofloxacin (Levaquin), linezolid (Zyvox), lorazepam (Ativan), melphalan (Alkeran), meperidine (Demerol), meropenem (Merrem IV), methadone (Dolophine), milrinone (Primacor), morphine, ondansetron (Zofran), oxaliplatin (Eloxatin), paclitaxel (Taxol), pemetrexed (Alimta), piperacillin/tazobactam (Zosyn), potassium chloride (KCl), propofol (Diprivan), remifentanil (Ultiva), sargramostim (Leukine), sodium bicarbonate, tacrolimus (Prograf), <u>telavancin (Vibativ)</u>, teniposide (Vumon), theophylline, thiotepa, vinorelbine (Navelbine), zidovudine (AZT, Retrovir).

RATE OF ADMINISTRATION
A single dose over 1 minute or less if necessary. As an IV infusion, give at prescribed rate.

ACTIONS
An anti-inflammatory glucocorticoid. A synthetic adrenocortical steroid with little sodium retention. Very soluble in water. Seven times as potent as prednisolone and 20 to 30 times as potent as hydrocortisone. Has minimal mineralocorticoid activity. Primarily used for anti-inflammatory and immunosuppressive effects. May be used in conjunction with other forms of therapy, such as epinephrine for acute hypersensitivity reactions or antibiotics for acute infections. Metabolized primarily in the liver and excreted as inactive metabolites in urine. Crosses the placental barrier. Excreted in urine and breast milk.

INDICATIONS AND USES

Supplementary therapy for severe allergic/hypersensitivity reactions. ▪ Reduction of acute edematous states (cerebral edema, airway edema). ▪ Shock unresponsive to conventional therapy. ▪ Acute exacerbations of disease for patients receiving steroid therapy. ▪ Adrenocortical insufficiency; total, relative, and operative. ▪ Antiemetic for chemotherapy-induced vomiting (e.g., cisplatin). Has numerous other uses by other routes of administration (e.g., IM, intra-articular, intralesional, intrasynovial, soft-tissue injection, oral inhalant).

Unlabeled uses: Adjunct to treatment of meningitis with antibiotics (to reduce incidence of ototoxicity). ▪ Dexamethasone or betamethasone is given IM to the mother to accelerate the production of lung surfactant in utero in the prevention of respiratory distress syndrome of premature infants.

CONTRAINDICATIONS

Hypersensitivity to any product component including sulfites, cerebral malaria, systemic fungal infections.

Relative contraindications: Active or latent peptic ulcer, acute or healed tuberculosis, acute or chronic infections (especially chickenpox), acute psychoses, diabetes mellitus, diverticulitis, fresh intestinal anastomoses, myasthenia gravis, ocular herpes simplex, osteoporosis, pregnancy, psychotic tendencies, renal insufficiency, thromboembolic tendencies.

PRECAUTIONS

Withdrawal from therapy should be gradual to avoid precipitation of symptoms of adrenal insufficiency. The patient is observed, especially under stress, for up to 2 years. ▪ Prophylactic antacids may prevent peptic ulcer complications. ▪ Use with caution in hypothyroidism and cirrhosis.

Monitor: May increase insulin needs in diabetes. ▪ Monitor electrolytes periodically. May cause sodium retention and potassium and calcium excretion. May cause hypertension secondary to fluid and electrolyte disturbances. ▪ May mask signs of infection. ▪ Administer a single dose before 9 AM to reduce suppression of individual's adrenocortical activity. ▪ Periodic ophthalmic exams may be necessary with prolonged treatment. ▪ See Drug/Lab Interactions.

Patient Education: Promptly report edema, tarry stools, or weight gain. Promptly report anorexia, diarrhea, dizziness, fatigue, low blood sugar, nausea, weakness, weight loss, and vomiting. May indicate adrenal insufficiency after dose reduction or discontinuing therapy. ▪ May mask signs of infection and/or decrease resistance. ▪ Patients with diabetes may have an increased requirement for insulin or oral hypoglycemics. ▪ Avoid immunization with live virus vaccines. ▪ Carry ID stating steroid dependent if receiving prolonged therapy.

Maternal/Child: Category C: has caused birth defects; benefits must outweigh risks. ▪ Observe newborn for hypoadrenalism if mother has received large doses. ▪ Monitor growth and development of pediatric patients receiving prolonged treatment. ▪ Use of a preservative-free solution recommended for neonates.

Elderly: Reduced muscle mass and plasma volume may necessitate a reduced dose. Monitor BP, blood glucose, and electrolytes carefully. ▪ Increased risk of hypertension. ▪ Higher risk of glucocorticoid-induced osteoporosis. ▪ Avoid aluminum-based antacids (risk of Alzheimer's disease).

DRUG/LAB INTERACTIONS

Some sources list additional interactions; review drug profile with pharmacist.

Aminoglutethimide (Cytadren) **and mitotane** (Lysodren) suppress adrenal function and increase metabolism of dexamethasone twofold. Not recommended for concurrent use, or dexamethasone dose may require doubling to be effective. Use of hydrocortisone suggested. ▪ Metabolism increased and effects reduced by **hepatic enzyme–inducing agents** (e.g., alcohol, barbiturates [e.g., phenobarbital], hydantoins [e.g., phenytoin (Dilantin)], rifampin [Rifadin]); dose adjustments may be required when adding or deleting from drug profile. ▪ Risk of hypokalemia increased with **amphotericin B or potassium-depleting diuretics** (e.g., thiazides, furosemide, ethacrynic acid). Monitor potassium levels and cardiac function. ▪ Increased risk of **digoxin** toxicity secondary to hypokalemia. ▪ May also decrease effectiveness of **potassium supplements;** monitor serum potassium. ▪ **Diuretics** decrease sodium and fluid retention effects of corticosteroids; corticosteroids decrease sodium excretion and diuretic effects of diuretics. ▪ Clearance increased and effects decreased with **ephedrine.** ▪ May antagonize effects of **anticholinesterases** (e.g., neostigmine), **isoniazid** (INH), **salicylates, and somatrem;** dose adjustments may be required. ▪ Clearance decreased and effects increased with **estrogens, oral contraceptives, and ketoconazole** (Nizoral). ▪ May interact with **anticoagulants, nondepolarizing muscle relaxants** (e.g., atracurium [Tracrium]), **or theophyllines;** may inhibit or potentiate action; monitor carefully. ▪ Monitor patients receiving **insulin or thyroid hormones** carefully; dose adjustments of either or both agents may be required. ▪ Do not vaccinate with **attenuated virus vaccines** (e.g., smallpox) during therapy. ▪ **Altered protein-binding capacity** will impact effectiveness of this drug. ▪ **Smoking** may antagonize therapeutic effects. ▪ See Precautions. ▪ Decreases uptake of **radioactive material** in cerebral edema; will alter brain scan.

SIDE EFFECTS
Do occur but are usually reversible: burning, Cushing's syndrome, electrolyte imbalance, euphoria, glycosuria, headache, hyperglycemia, hypersensitivity reactions including anaphylaxis, hypertension, insomnia, menstrual irregularities, mood swings, peptic ulcer, perforation and hemorrhage, protein catabolism, sweating, thromboembolism, tingling, weakness, and many others.

ANTIDOTE
Notify the physician of any side effect. Treat side effects as indicated. Resuscitate as necessary for anaphylaxis and notify physician. Keep epinephrine immediately available.

DEXMEDETOMIDINE HYDROCHLORIDE

(dex-**med**-ih-**TOM**-ih-deen hy-droh-**KLOR**-eyed)

Alpha$_2$-adrenoceptor agonist
Sedative-hypnotic

Precedex

pH 4.5 to 7.0

USUAL DOSE

Dosing should be individualized and titrated to desired clinical response.

ICU sedation: *Loading dose:* 1 mcg/kg as an infusion over 10 minutes. A loading dose may not be necessary in patients who are being converted from alternate sedative therapy. See Dose Adjustments.

Maintenance infusion: 0.2 to 0.7 mcg/kg/hr. Adjust rate to achieve the desired level of sedation; see Monitor. Dexmedetomidine is *not* indicated for infusions lasting longer than 24 hours. Has been infused in mechanically ventilated patients before, during, and after extubation provided the infusion does not exceed 24 hours. See Dose Adjustments.

Procedural sedation: *Loading dose for both adult and/or awake fiber optic intubation patients:* 1 mcg/kg as an infusion over 10 minutes. For less invasive procedures (e.g., ophthalmic surgery), a loading dose of 0.5 mcg/kg as an infusion over 10 minutes may be sufficient. See Dose Adjustments.

Maintenance infusion for adult patients: Begin with 0.6 mcg/kg/hr. Titrate to achieve desired level of sedation. Usual range is 0.2 to 1 mcg/kg/hr. See Dose Adjustments.

Maintenance infusion for awake fiber optic intubation patients: A dose of 0.7 mcg/kg/hr is recommended until the endotracheal tube is secured. See Dose Adjustments.

DOSE ADJUSTMENTS

Reduced doses may be required in patients with hepatic impairment and in the elderly. ▪ For patients over 65 years of age, reduce the loading dose for procedural sedation to 0.5 mcg/kg over 10 minutes. ▪ Dose reduction of either or both agents may be required when coadministered with anesthetics, sedatives, hypnotics, or opioids; see Drug Interactions.

DILUTION

Supplied in single-use vials containing 200 mcg/2 mL. Must be diluted before administration. Preparation of the solution is the same, whether for loading dose or maintenance infusion. Withdraw 2 mL of dexmedetomidine and add to 48 mL of NS for a final concentration of 4 mcg/mL. Shake gently. Also available in premixed, ready-to-use, single-use containers containing 80 mcg/20 mL, 200 mcg/50 mL, or 400 mcg/100 mL of dexmedetomidine in NS. No further dilution is required.

Storage: Store unopened vials and premixed solutions at CRT.

COMPATIBILITY

Consider any drug NOT listed as compatible to be INCOMPATIBLE until consulting a pharmacist; specific conditions may apply.

According to the manufacturer, the **compatibility** of dexmedetomidine with blood or plasma has not been established; avoid coadministration. Manufacturer lists as **incompatible** with amphotericin B and diazepam (Valium). Absorption of dexmedetomidine to some types of natural rubbers may occur. Although dexmedetomidine is dosed to effect, it is advisable to use administration components that are made with synthetic or coated natural rubber gaskets.

Manufacturer lists the following **compatibilities:** NS, D5W, 20% mannitol, LR, magnesium sulfate (100 mg/mL), and 0.3% potassium chloride solution.

One source suggests the following **compatibilities:**

Y-site: Alfentanil, amikacin, aminophylline, amiodarone (Nexterone), ampicillin, ampicillin/sulbactam (Unasyn), atracurium (Tracrium), atropine, azithromycin (Zithromax), aztreonam (Azactam), bumetanide, butorphanol (Stadol), calcium gluconate, cefazolin (Ancef), cefepime (Maxipime), cefotaxime (Claforan), cefotetan, cefoxitin (Mefoxin), ceftazidime (Fortaz), ceftriaxone (Rocephin), cefuroxime (Zinacef), chlorpromazine (Thorazine), ciprofloxacin (Cipro IV), cisatracurium (Nimbex), clindamycin (Cleocin), dexamethasone (Decadron), digoxin (Lanoxin), diltiazem (Cardizem), diphenhydramine (Benadryl), dobutamine, dolasetron (Anzemet), dopamine, doxycycline, droperidol (Inapsine), enalaprilat (Vasotec IV), ephedrine, epinephrine (Adrenalin), erythromycin (Erythrocin), esmolol (Brevibloc), etomidate (Amidate), famotidine (Pepcid IV), fenoldopam (Corlopam), fentanyl, fluconazole (Diflucan), furosemide (Lasix), gentamicin, glycopyrrolate (Robinul), granisetron (Kytril), heparin, hydromorphone (Dilaudid), isoproterenol (Isuprel), ketorolac (Toradol), labetalol, levofloxacin (Levaquin), lidocaine, linezolid (Zyvox), lorazepam (Ativan), magnesium, meperidine (Demerol), methylprednisolone (Solu-Medrol), metoclopramide (Reglan), metronidazole (Flagyl IV), midazolam (Versed), milrinone (Primacor), morphine, nalbuphine, nitroglycerin IV, nitroprusside sodium, norepinephrine (Levophed), ondansetron (Zofran), pancuronium, phenylephrine (Neo-Synephrine), piperacillin/tazobactam (Zosyn), potassium chloride, procainamide (Pronestyl), prochlorperazine (Compazine), promethazine (Phenergan), propofol (Diprivan), ranitidine (Zantac), remifentanil (Ultiva), rocuronium (Zemuron), sodium bicarbonate, succinylcholine (Anectine), sufentanil (Sufenta), sulfamethoxazole/trimethoprim, theophylline, ticarcillin/clavulanate (Timentin), tobramycin, vancomycin, vecuronium, verapamil.

RATE OF ADMINISTRATION

Administer using a controlled infusion device. Rapid IV or bolus administration may result in bradycardia and sinus arrest.

Loading dose: Infuse over 10 minutes. Increase infusion time (decrease infusion rate) if transient hypertension develops; see Monitor and Antidote.

Maintenance infusion: See Usual Dose. Titrate to desired clinical effect.

ACTIONS

A relatively selective alpha$_2$-adrenoceptor agonist with sedative properties. In animal studies, the desired alpha$_2$ selectivity is seen following slow IV infusions of low and medium doses (10 to 300 mcg/kg), but both alpha$_1$ and alpha$_2$ activity are seen following slow IV infusion of high doses (equal to or greater than 1,000 mcg/kg) or with rapid IV administration. Appears to have both sedative and moderate analgesic activity and may decrease the requirement for concomitant sedation and analgesia when used as a short-term infusion in the ICU setting. Other actions include reduced BP, HR, and reduced salivation. Highly protein bound. Almost completely metabolized in the liver via direct glucuronidation and cytochrome P$_{450}$-mediated metabolism. Metabolites excreted primarily in urine and to a small extent in feces. Half-life is approximately 2 hours. Pharmacokinetics not altered by age or gender.

INDICATIONS AND USES

Sedation of initially intubated and mechanically ventilated patients during treatment in an intensive care setting. Should be administered by continuous infusion not to exceed 24 hours. ▪ Sedation of nonintubated patients before and/or during surgical and other procedures.

CONTRAINDICATIONS

None noted.

PRECAUTIONS

Administered by persons skilled in the management of patients in the intensive care or operating room setting. ▪ Clinically significant episodes of bradycardia and sinus arrest have been reported in young, healthy volunteers with high vagal tone or with different routes of administration, including rapid intravenous or bolus administration; see Rate of Administration. ▪ Hypotension and bradycardia have been reported. Decreases sympathetic nervous system activity. Use caution in patients with advanced heart block, severe ventricular dysfunction, diabetes mellitus, chronic hypertension, hypovolemia, and in the elderly; hypotension and/or bradycardia may be more pronounced. Clinical intervention may be required; see Antidote. ▪ Patients may be arousable and alert when stimulated. This alone should not be considered as evidence of lack of effectiveness in the absence of other clinical signs and symptoms. ▪ The dependence potential of dexmedetomidine has not been studed in humans. May produce a clonidine-like withdrawal syndrome if discontinued abruptly. ▪ Dexmedetomidine should not be administered for longer than 24 hours. Adverse events related to withdrawal (e.g., agitation, hypertension, nausea and vomiting, tachycardia) have been reported with prolonged infusions. Most withdrawal-related events were seen 24 to 48 hours following discontinuation of the infusion. Withdrawal symptoms have not been seen with discontinuation of short-term infusions (less than 6 hours). ▪ Use beyond 24 hours has been associated with tolerance and tachyphylaxis and a dose-related increase in adverse reactions. ▪ Use with caution in patients with hepatic impairment. Clearance of dexmedetomidine is decreased; see Dose Adjustments.

Monitor: Continuous monitoring of VS, oxygenation, and cardiac and fluid status imperative. ▪ Hypovolemia may increase risk of hypotension. ▪ Use of a sedation scale (e.g., Ramsay) recommended for monitoring of sedative effect. ▪ Transient hypertension has been observed primarily during the loading dose in association with initial peripheral vasoconstrictive effects. Treatment is generally not required; see Rate of Administration and Antidote. ▪ See Precautions.

Patient Education: Report abdominal pain, agitation, confusion, constipation, diarrhea, dizziness, excessive sweating, headache, nervousness, salt cravings, weakness, or weight loss that occur within 48 hours.

Maternal/Child: Category C: safety for use in pregnancy not established. Studies suggest fetal exposure should be expected. ▪ Safety for use during labor and delivery and with breast-feeding not established. Use only when clearly indicated. ▪ Safety and effectiveness in pediatric patients under 18 years of age not established.

Elderly: In patients older than 65 years, a higher incidence of bradycardia and hypotension was observed following administration of dexmedetomidine. ▪ Consider age-related organ impairment and history of previous or concomitant disease or drug therapy. ▪ See Dose Adjustments.

DRUG/LAB INTERACTIONS

In vitro studies showed no evidence of cytochrome P_{450}-mediated drug interactions that are likely to be of clinical significance. ▪ Potentiated by **anesthetics** (e.g., enflurane, isoflurane, sevoflurane), **sedatives or hypnotics** (e.g., barbiturates, benzodiazepines [e.g., diazepam (Valium), midazolam (Versed)], propofol [Diprivan]), **and opioids** (e.g., alfentanil, meperidine, morphine). Reduced doses of both drugs may be indicated. See Dose Adjustments. ▪ Concurrent use with other **vasodilators** (e.g., nitroglycerin, nitroprusside sodium) **or negative chronotropic agents** (e.g., beta blockers [e.g., metoprolol (Lopressor)], calcium channel blockers [e.g., diltiazem (Cardizem)]) may have an additive effect; use with caution.

SIDE EFFECTS

The most common treatment-emergent side effects, occurring in more than 2% of patients in both ICU and procedural sedation studies, included bradycardia, dry mouth, and hypotension. Side effects associated with infusions greater than 24 hours in duration include agitation, ARDS, and respiratory failure. Other frequently reported side effects were anemia, fever, hypertension, hypoxia, nausea, tachycardia, and vomiting. Less frequently reported side effects include abnormal vision, acidosis, agitation, apnea, arrhythmia (e.g., atrial fibrillation), bronchospasm, confusion, delirium, dizziness, dyspnea, hallucination, headache, heart block, hypercapnia, hyperkalemia, hypoventilation, increased alkaline phosphatase, increased GGT (gamma glutamyltransferase), increased ALT, increased AST, increased sweating, infection, light anesthesia, neuralgia, neuritis, pain, pleural effusion, pulmonary edema, rigors, sinus arrest, somnolence, and speech disorder.

Overdose: Bradycardia, cardiac arrest, first-degree AV block, hypotension, second-degree heart block.

ANTIDOTE

Keep physician informed of all side effects. Hypotension and bradycardia may be treated by slowing or stopping the dexmedetomidine infusion, increasing the rate of IV fluid administration, elevation of the lower extremities, or use of pressor amines (e.g., dopamine). Administration of anticholinergic agents (e.g., atropine or glycopyrrolate) may be considered to modify vagal tone. Transient hypertension during loading dose may be treated by decreasing the rate of the infusion. Resuscitate as necessary.

DEXRAZOXANE
(dex-rah-**ZOX**-ayn)

Totect, Zinecard

Antidote
Antineoplastic adjunct
Chelating agent

pH 3.5 to 5.5

USUAL DOSE

TOTECT

Administer once daily for 3 consecutive days. Initiate treatment as soon as possible and within 6 hours of extravasation. Doses should be given 24 hours apart ($+$ or $-$ 3 hours); see Precautions. Recommended regimen is:

Day 1 and Day 2: 1,000 mg/M^2 not to exceed 2,000 mg.

Day 3: 500 mg/M^2 not to exceed 1,000 mg.

ZINECARD

Administered in conjunction with doxorubicin. Dose ratio of dexrazoxane to doxorubicin (Adriamycin) is 10:1 (e.g., 500 mg/M^2 dexrazoxane to 50 mg/M^2 doxorubicin). Doxorubicin dose must be given within 30 minutes of starting the dexrazoxane injection, but only after the full dose of dexrazoxane is administered.

DOSE ADJUSTMENTS

TOTECT AND ZINECARD

Decrease the recommended dose of dexrazoxane by 50% in patients with moderate to severe renal impairment (CrCl less than 40 mL/min). Ratio of Zinecard to doxorubicin will be 5:1 (e.g., 250 mg/M^2 dexrazoxane to 50 mg/M^2 doxorubicin). ■ Consider age-related impaired organ function and concomitant disease or drug therapy in the elderly; see Elderly. ■ See Antidote. ■ Has not been evaluated in hepatic insufficiency.

ZINECARD

When administering Zinecard, the dose of dexrazoxane is dependent on the dose of doxorubicin. When the dose of doxorubicin is reduced (e.g., patients with hyperbilirubinemia), adjust the dexrazoxane dose accordingly. Maintain a 10:1 ratio (dexrazoxane to doxorubicin) except in patients with CrCl less than 40 mL/min.

DILUTION

Specific techniques required; see Precautions.

TOTECT

Reconstitute each 500-mg vial with 50 mL of provided diluent (10 mg/mL). Further dilute the calculated dose in 1,000 mL of NS. Up to 10 vials of Totect and 10 vials of diluent may be needed to complete 3 days of treatment.

ZINECARD

Initially reconstitute each 250 mg (500 mg) with 25 mL (50 mL) of SWFI (10 mg/mL). This initial dilution has a pH of 1 to 3. Must be further diluted with LR. Concentration should range from 1.3 to 3 mg/mL. Further dilution of each 250-mg (500-mg) vial with 75 mL (150 mL) of LR would yield 2.5 mg/mL. Fully diluted solution has a pH of 3.5 to 5.5.

Storage: *Totect and Zinecard:* Store unopened vials at CRT. *Totect:* Protect unopened kit from light. Reconstituted solution should be used immediately (within 2 hours). Diluted product stable for 4 hours from time of reconstitution and dilution when stored below 25° C (77° F). *Zinecard:* Reconstituted solution stable for 30 minutes at RT or, if necessary, up to 3 hours from the time of reconstitution under refrigeration at 2° to 8° C (36° to 46° F). Fully diluted solutions in LR are stable for 1 hour at RT or up to 4 hours if refrigerated at 2° to 8° C (36° to 46° F). Discard unused solutions.

COMPATIBILITY

Consider any drug NOT listed as compatible to be INCOMPATIBLE until consulting a pharmacist; specific conditions may apply.

Manufacturer states, "Should not be mixed or administered with other drugs"; degrades rapidly at a pH above 7.

One source suggests the following **compatibilities:**

Y-site: Gemcitabine (Gemzar) and pemetrexed (Alimta).

RATE OF ADMINISTRATION

TOTECT

Administer a single dose as an IV infusion equally distributed over 1 to 2 hours. Infuse at RT with normal lighting.

ZINECARD

A single dose as a rapid infusion (given over 10 to 15 minutes in one study). Do not administer by IV push. Complete dexrazoxane dose but begin doxorubicin within 30 minutes of beginning dexrazoxane.

ACTIONS

DEXRAZOXANE

Rapidly distributed, at least partly metabolized. Elimination half-life is 2.5 hours. Primarily excreted in urine. See Drug/Lab Interactions.

TOTECT

Diminishes tissue damage resulting from extravasation of anthracycline drugs. Exact mode of action unknown. May inhibit topoisomerase II reversibly.

ZINECARD

A cardioprotective agent. A potent intracellular chelating agent that readily penetrates cell membranes and interferes with iron-mediated free radical generation thought to be, in part, responsible for anthracycline-induced cardiomyopathy. Reduces the incidence of doxorubicin cardiomyopathy.

INDICATIONS AND USES

TOTECT

Treatment of extravasation resulting from IV anthracycline chemotherapy.

ZINECARD

Reduce the incidence and severity of cardiomyopathy associated with cumulative doses of doxorubicin exceeding 300 mg/M². Currently approved only for use in women with metastatic breast cancer who would benefit from continuing doxorubicin therapy above this cumulative dose. Cardioprotective effect permits a greater number of patients to be treated with extended doxorubicin therapy. ▪ *Not recommended for use with the initiation of doxorubicin therapy.*

CONTRAINDICATIONS

TOTECT

None known.

ZINECARD

Do not use with chemotherapy regimens that do not contain an anthracycline or in the initiation of doxorubicin therapy.

PRECAUTIONS

TOTECT AND ZINECARD

Follow guidelines for handling cytotoxic agents. See Appendix A, p. 1331. ▪ Usually administered by or under the direction of the physician specialist. ▪ For IV infusion only; do not administer IV push. ▪ Use with caution in patients with renal or hepatic impairment; see Dose Adjustments.

TOTECT

Cytotoxic when administered to patients receiving anthracycline-containing chemotherapy; additive myelosuppression (leukopenia, neutropenia, thrombocytopenia) may occur. ▪ Administer in a large vein in an extremity/area other than the one affected by extravasation. Cooling procedures such as ice packs, if used, should be removed from the area at least 15 minutes before administration to allow sufficient blood flow to the extravasated area.

ZINECARD

May add to myelosuppression caused by chemotherapeutic agents. ▪ Evidence indicates that the use of dexrazoxane with the initiation of fluorouracil, doxorubicin, and cyclophosphamide (FAC) therapy interferes with the antitumor efficacy of the regimen. In one breast cancer trial, a lower response rate and a shorter time to progression were seen in patients who received dexrazoxane with their first cycle of FAC therapy. This use is not recommended; see Indications and Contraindications. ▪ Secondary malignancies (e.g., acute myeloid leukemia [AML] and myelodysplastic syndrome [MDS]) have been reported in pediatric patients and adults (not indicated for use in pediatric patients).

Monitor: TOTECT AND ZINECARD: Use of prophylactic antiemetics may be indicated.

TOTECT: Monitor CBC and differential and platelet count for increased bone marrow suppression. ▪ Obtain baseline and periodic renal and liver function tests as indicated.

ZINECARD: Obtain baseline ECG, serum levels of iron and zinc, and liver and renal function tests. Monitor at intervals. Baseline left ventricular ejection fraction (LVEF) helpful. ▪ Obtain baseline CBC and differential and platelet count. Monitor for increased bone marrow suppression. ▪ Reduces but does not eliminate the risk of doxorubicin-induced cardiotoxicity. Monitor for signs of congestive heart failure (e.g., basilar rales, S_3 gallop, paroxysmal nocturnal dyspnea, significant dyspnea on exertion, cardiomegaly by x-ray, or progressive decline from baseline of LVEF). A decline in QRS voltage on a 6-lead ECG of more than 30% may indicate cardiomyopathy.

Patient Education: Nonhormonal birth control recommended. Report a suspected pregnancy; see Maternal/Child. ▪ Report pain at injection site promptly.

Maternal/Child: TOTECT AND ZINECARD: Category D: avoid pregnancy. Can cause fetal harm. ▪ Embryotoxic and teratogenic in rats at doses lower than required for humans. May cause testicular atrophy. ▪ Discontinue breast-feeding. ▪ Safety for use in pediatric patients not established.

ELDERLY: Response similar to that seen in younger patients. ▪ Monitor renal function; see Dose Adjustments.

DRUG/LAB INTERACTIONS

TOTECT AND ZINECARD

May have additive bone marrow suppressant effects with **other bone marrow suppressants** (e.g., fluorouracil [5-FU], cyclophosphamide [Cytoxan]). ▪ Does not affect pharmacokinetics of **doxorubicin.**

TOTECT

Dimethylsulfoxide (DMSO) should not be used in patients who are receiving dexrazoxane for treatment of anthracycline-induced extravasation.

ZINECARD

Not indicated for use in initiation of doxorubicin therapy; may interfere with antitumor effects of combination regimens.

SIDE EFFECTS

Administered to patients receiving chemotherapeutic agents; side effect profile reflects a combination of dexrazoxane, underlying disease, and chemotherapy. Most common side effects are fever, injection site pain, nausea, and vomiting. Increased myelosuppression (e.g., granulocytopenia, leukopenia, and thrombocytopenia); may be dose limiting. Coagulation abnormalities, decreased serum zinc, increased serum iron, increased AST and

ALT, and increased serum triglycerides do occur. Alopecia, anorexia, diarrhea, and stomatitis, as well as other side effects, may occur.

ANTIDOTE

Keep physician informed of side effects; most will be treated symptomatically. Recovery from myelosuppression similar with or without dexrazoxane. A reduced dose may be indicated if coagulation abnormalities develop. Hemodialysis or peritoneal dialysis may be useful in overdose.

DEXTRAN HIGH MOLECULAR WEIGHT

Plasma volume expander

(**DEX**-tran hi mo-**LEK**-u-ler)

Dextran 70, Dextran 75, Gentran 75

pH 3 to 7

USUAL DOSE

Variable, depending on amount of fluid loss and resultant hemoconcentration. Initially 30 Gm (500 mL). Total dose should not exceed 1.2 Gm/kg (20 mL/kg) of body weight in the first 24 hours for adult and pediatric patients. May give 0.6 Gm/kg (10 mL/kg) every 24 hours thereafter if indicated. *Use of Dextran 1 is indicated for prophylaxis of serious anaphylactic reactions.*

DILUTION

Available as a 6% solution in 500-mL bottles properly diluted in NS or D5W and ready for use. Dextran 70 (Cutter) is available in a 250-mL bottle. Use only clear solution. Crystallization of dextran can occur at low temperatures. Submerge in warm water and dissolve all crystals before administration.

Storage: Store at constant temperature not above 25° C (76° F). Discard partially used solution; no preservative added.

COMPATIBILITY

One source suggests that drugs should not be added to a dextran solution.

RATE OF ADMINISTRATION

Variable, depending on indication, present blood volume, and patient response. Initial 500 mL may be given at 20 to 40 mL/min if hypovolemic. If additional high molecular weight dextran is required, reduce flow to lowest rate possible to maintain hemodynamic status desired. In normovolemic patients, rate should not exceed 4 mL/min.

ACTIONS

A glucose polymer that approximates colloidal properties of human albumin. Provides hemodynamically significant plasma volume expansion in excess of the amount infused for about 24 hours. Dilutes total serum proteins and hematocrit values. Smaller dextran molecules are eliminated in urine; larger molecules are degraded to glucose.

INDICATIONS AND USES

Adjunct in treatment of shock or impending shock caused by burns, hemorrhage, surgery, or trauma.

Unlabeled uses: Treatment of nephrosis, toxemia of late pregnancy, and prevention of postoperative deep vein thrombosis.

CONTRAINDICATIONS

Severe bleeding disorders; marked hemostatic defects (e.g., thrombocytopenia, hypofibrinogenemia), even if drug-induced (e.g., heparin, warfarin); known hypersensitivity to dextran; breast-feeding and pregnancy unless a lifesaving measure; severe congestive cardiac failure; renal failure.

PRECAUTIONS

For IV use only. ▪ Used when whole blood or blood products are not available. Not a substitute for whole blood or plasma proteins. ▪ Use extreme caution in heart disease, impaired hepatic or renal function, congestive heart failure, pulmonary edema, in patients with edema and sodium retention of pathologic abdominal conditions, and in patients receiving anticoagulants or corticosteroids.

Monitor: Monitor pulse, BP, central venous pressure, and urine output every 5 to 15 minutes for the first hour and hourly thereafter while indicated. ▪ Maintain hydration of patient with additional IV fluids; dextran promotes tissue dehydration. Avoid overhydration with dilution of electrolyte balance. ▪ Change IV tubing or flush well with normal saline before infusing blood. Dextran will promote coagulation of blood in the tubing (glucose content). ▪ May reduce coagulability of the circulating blood. Observe patient for increased bleeding; maintain hematocrit above 30%. ▪ Hemoglobin, hematocrit, electrolyte, and serum protein evaluations are necessary during therapy. ▪ 500 mL contains 77 mEq of sodium and chloride. ▪ See Drug/Lab Interactions.

Maternal/Child: Category C: safety for use in pregnancy and breast-feeding not established.

DRUG/LAB INTERACTIONS

Draw blood for **laboratory tests and type and cross-match** before giving dextran, or notify laboratory of its use. May alter type and cross-match, blood sugar, total protein, and total bilirubin evaluation. ▪ May produce elevated **urine specific gravity** (also symptom of dehydration) and increase **AST and ALT.** ▪ See Monitor for interaction with blood.

SIDE EFFECTS

Bleeding, dehydration, fever, hypotension, joint pain, nausea, overhydration, tightness of the chest, urticaria, vomiting, wheezing. Severe anaphylaxis and death have occurred. Excessive doses have caused wound hematoma, seroma, and bleeding; distant bleeding (hematuria, melena); and pulmonary edema.

ANTIDOTE

Notify physician of any side effect. Discontinue the drug immediately at the first sign of a hypersensitivity reaction, provided other means of sustaining the circulation are available. Use epinephrine (Adrenalin) and/or antihistamines (diphenhydramine [Benadryl]) as indicated. Factor VIII infusion may reverse excessive bleeding. Resuscitate as necessary.

DEXTRAN LOW MOLECULAR WEIGHT

Plasma volume expander

(**DEX**-tran lo mo-**LEK**-u-ler)

Dextran 40, Gentran 40, L.M.D. 10%, Rheomacrodex   pH 3 to 7

USUAL DOSE

Adjunct in shock: Variable, depending on amount of fluid loss and resultant hemoconcentration. Do not exceed 2 Gm/kg (20 mL) of body weight total over first 24 hours and 1 Gm/kg (10 mL) total over each succeeding 24 hours. Discontinue infusion after 5 days of therapy. *Dextran 1 is indicated for prophylaxis of serious anaphylactic reactions.*

Prophylaxis of venous thrombosis and/or pulmonary embolism: 10 mL/kg of body weight on day of surgery. 500 mL daily for 2 to 3 days, then 500 mL every 2 to 3 days up to 2 weeks. Length of treatment based on risk of thromboembolic complication. *Note previous comment on use of dextran 1.*

As priming fluid: 10 to 20 mL/kg of body weight. Do not exceed this dose. May be used in conjunction with other priming fluids.

DILUTION

Available as a 10% solution in 500-mL bottles properly diluted in NS or D5W and ready for use. Use only clear solution. Crystallization of dextran can occur at low temperatures. Submerge in warm water and dissolve all crystals before administration.

Storage: Store at constant temperature not above 25° C (76° F). Discard partially used solution; no preservative added.

COMPATIBILITY

Consider any drug NOT listed as compatible to be INCOMPATIBLE until consulting a pharmacist; specific conditions may apply.

One source suggests that drugs should not be added to a dextran solution. Another source suggests the following **compatibilities:**

Y-site: Enalaprilat (Vasotec IV), famotidine (Pepcid IV), and nicardipine (Cardene IV).

RATE OF ADMINISTRATION

Initial 500 mL may be given rapidly. Remainder of any desired daily dose should be evenly distributed over 8 to 24 hours depending on use. Slow rate or discontinue dextran for rapid increase of central venous pressure.

ACTIONS

A low-molecular-weight, rapid, but short-acting plasma volume expander. A colloid hypertonic solution, it increases plasma volume by once or twice its own volume. Helps to restore normal circulatory dynamics, increasing arterial and pulse pressure, central venous pressure, and cardiac output. Improves microcirculatory flow and prevents sludging in venous channels. Mobilizes water from body tissues and increases urine output.

INDICATIONS AND USES

Adjunctive therapy in the treatment of shock caused by hemorrhage, burns, trauma, or surgery. ■ Prophylaxis during surgical procedures with a high incidence of venous thrombosis and pulmonary embolism. ■ Pump priming during extracorporeal circulation.

CONTRAINDICATIONS

Severe bleeding disorders; marked hemostatic defects (e.g., thrombocytopenia, hypofibrinogenemia), even if drug-induced (e.g., heparin, warfarin); known hypersensitivity to dextran; breast-feeding and pregnancy unless a lifesaving measure; severe congestive cardiac failure; renal failure.

PRECAUTIONS

For IV use only. ■ Use caution in heart disease, renal shutdown, congestive heart failure, pulmonary edema, patients with edema and sodium retention, and patients taking corticosteroids.

Monitor: Monitor pulse, BP, central venous pressure (if possible), and urine output every 5 to 15 minutes for the first hour and hourly thereafter while indicated. ■ Slow rate or discontinue dextran for rapid increase of central venous pressure (normal 7 to 14 mm H_2O pressure). ■ If anuric or oliguric after 500 mL of dextran, discontinue the dextran. Mannitol may help increase urine flow. ■ Maintain hydration of patient with additional IV fluids; dextran promotes tissue dehydration. Avoid overhydration and dilution of serum electrolytes. ■ Change IV tubing or flush well with normal saline before superimposing blood. Dextran will promote coagulation of blood in the tubing (glucose content). ■ May reduce coagulability of the circulating blood slightly. Observe for bleeding complications, particularly following surgery or if patient is being anticoagulated. Maintain hematocrit above 30%. ■ 500 mL contains 77 mEq of sodium and chloride. ■ See Drug/Lab Interactions.

Maternal/Child: Category C: safety for use in pregnancy and breast-feeding not established.

DRUG/LAB INTERACTIONS

Draw blood for **laboratory tests and type and cross-match** before giving dextran, or notify laboratory of its use. May alter type and cross-match, blood sugar, total protein, and total bilirubin evaluation. ■ May produce elevated **urine specific gravity** (also a symptom of dehydration) and increase **AST and ALT.** ■ See Monitor for interaction with blood.

SIDE EFFECTS
Bleeding, dehydration, fever, hypotension, joint pain, nausea, overhydration, tightness of chest, urticaria, vomiting, wheezing. Severe anaphylaxis and death can occur. Excessive doses have caused wound hematoma, wound seroma, wound bleeding, distant bleeding (hematuria, melena), and pulmonary edema.

ANTIDOTE
Notify the physician of any side effect. Discontinue the drug immediately at the first sign of a hypersensitivity reaction, provided other means of sustaining the circulation are available. Use epinephrine (Adrenalin) and/or antihistamines (diphenhydramine [Benadryl]) as indicated. Factor VIII infusion may reverse excessive bleeding. Resuscitate as necessary.

DEXTROSE
(**DEX**-trohs)

Glucose

Nutritional (carbohydrate)
Antidote

pH 3.5 to 6.5

USUAL DOSE
Depends on indication for use, age, weight, and clinical condition of the patient. The average normal adult requires 2 to 3 L of fluid daily to replace water loss through perspiration and urine.

Treatment of hypoglycemia: 10 to 25 Gm (20 to 50 mL of 50% dextrose or 40 to 100 mL of 25% dextrose). Repeat as needed.

Nutritional support: Mixed with amino acid solution and/or SWFI with dose adjusted to meet individual patient requirements.

Treatment of hyperkalemia (unlabeled): 25 Gm (50 mL of 50% dextrose) administered with 5 to 10 units of regular insulin over 5 minutes. Repeat as needed.

PEDIATRIC DOSE
Dose is dependent on indication for use, weight, clinical condition, and laboratory results.

Treatment of hypoglycemia: *Infants 6 months of age or younger:* 0.25 to 0.5 Gm/kg/dose (1 to 2 mL/kg/dose of 25% dextrose); do not exceed 25 Gm/dose. *Infants over 6 months of age:* 0.5 to 1 Gm/kg/dose (2 to 4 mL/kg/dose of 25% dextrose). Do not exceed 25 Gm/dose. Repeat as needed.

Nutritional support: Mixed with amino acid solution and/or SWFI with dose adjusted to meet individual patient requirements.

Treatment of hyperkalemia (unlabeled): 0.5 Gm/kg (2 mL/kg of 25% dextrose) administered with 0.1 unit/kg of regular insulin. Repeat as needed.

See Rate of Administration, Precautions, Monitor, and Maternal/Child.

NEONATAL DOSE
Dose is dependent on indication for use, weight, clinical condition, and laboratory results. See Rate of Administration, Precautions, Monitor, and Maternal/Child.

DOSE ADJUSTMENTS
Dosing should be cautious in newborns, especially premature infants with low birth weight, and in the elderly. Lower-end initial doses may be indicated. Consider decrease in organ function, concomitant disease, or other drug therapy. See Rate of Administration, Precautions, and Maternal/Child.

DILUTION
Available in several concentrations. Final concentration for administration will depend on indication for use. May be given undiluted or further diluted to achieve desired concentration. Check label for aluminum content; see Precautions. Dextrose solutions are

excellent media for bacterial growth. Do not use unless the solution is entirely clear and the vial is sterile.

Filters: One manufacturer states, "Use of a final filter is recommended during administration of all parenteral solutions, where possible."

Storage: Store at 20° to 25° C (68° to 77° F). Protect from freezing.

COMPATIBILITY

Will cause pseudoagglutination of red blood cells if administered simultaneously with whole blood. Consult pharmacist or refer to individual drug monograph before admixing with other drugs or solutions. Mix thoroughly.

RATE OF ADMINISTRATION

Rate dependent on concentration and indication for use. A rate of 0.5 Gm/kg/hr will not cause glycosuria. At 0.8 Gm/kg/hr 95% is retained and will cause glycosuria. Excessively rapid administration may cause hyperosmolar syndrome.

Excessive or rapid administration in very-low-birth-weight infants may cause hyperglycemia, increased serum osmolality, and possible intracerebral hemorrhage. Infusion rate and volume depend on the age, weight, and clinical and metabolic conditions of the patient and on concomitant therapy and should be determined by a consulting physician experienced in pediatric IV fluid therapy.

When higher concentrations are given peripherally, administer slowly (preferably through a small-bore needle into a large vein) to minimize venous irritation; see Precautions.

Do not hang flexible plastic containers in series connection, do not pressurize to increase flow rates without first fully evacuating residual air from the container, and do not use vented IV administration sets. All may result in air embolism.

ACTIONS

A parenteral fluid and nutrient replenisher. A monosaccharide, it provides glucose calories for metabolic needs. Metabolized to CO_2 and water. Its oxidation provides water to sustain volume and may help lower excess ketone production. Restores blood glucose levels. May help minimize liver glycogen depletion and may exert a protein-sparing action. Hypertonic solutions (20% to 50%) act as diuretics. When given in conjunction with insulin for the treatment of hyperkalemia, dextrose stimulates the uptake of potassium into cells, lowering serum potassium levels. Readily excreted by the kidneys, producing diuresis.

INDICATIONS AND USES

Provide calories and fluid replacement by peripheral infusion when calories and fluid are required (2½%, 5%, 10%). ■ Provide calories by central IV infusion in combination with other amino acid solutions as total parenteral nutrition (10% to 70%). ■ Treatment of insulin-induced hypoglycemia (25% or 50%). ■ Treatment of acute symptomatic episodes of hypoglycemia in the neonate and infant (25%). ■ Adjunctive treatment of hyperkalemia (25% or 50% solution). ■ As a diluent for IV administration of medications (2½% to 10% solutions usually).

CONTRAINDICATIONS

Delirium tremens with dehydration; diabetic coma while blood sugar is excessive; intracranial or intraspinal hemorrhage. Solutions containing dextrose may be contraindicated in patients with known allergies to corn or corn products.

PRECAUTIONS

Administration of these solutions can cause fluid and/or solute overload, resulting in dilution of serum electrolyte concentrations, overhydration, congested states, or pulmonary edema. ■ Excessive administration of dextrose may result in significant hypokalemia and hypophosphatemia. ■ Use with caution in patients with subclinical or overt diabetes and in patients receiving corticosteroids. ■ Use dextrose with extreme caution in newborns, especially premature or low-birth-weight infants. Risk of developing hypoglycemia or hyperglycemia is increased; see Monitor. Hypoglycemia in the newborn can cause prolonged seizures, coma, and brain damage. Excessive or rapid administration may result in increased serum osmolality and possible intracerebral hemorrhage. Hyperglycemia has also been associated with late-onset bacterial and fungal infections, retinopathy of prematurity, necrotizing enterocolitis, bronchopulmonary dysplasia, prolonged length of hospital stay, and death. ▪ Some solutions may contain aluminum. In impaired kidney function, aluminum may reach toxic levels. Premature neonates are particularly at risk because of their immature kidneys and requirement for calcium and phosphate, which also contain aluminum. Research indicates that patients with impaired renal function who receive greater than 4 to 5 mcg/kg/day of parenteral aluminum are at risk for developing CNS or bone toxicity associated with aluminum accumulation. ▪ Concentrated dextrose solutions, if administered too rapidly, may result in significant hyperglycemia and possible hyperosmolar syndrome characterized by mental confusion and loss of consciousness. Fatty infiltration of the liver, acute respiratory failure, and difficulty in weaning hypermetabolic patients from the respirator may be caused by excessive carbohydrate calories. ▪ Concentrated dextrose solutions should not be withdrawn abruptly. May cause rebound hypoglycemia. Reduce rate of administration gradually and then follow with administration of 5% or 10% dextrose solution.

Monitor: Monitor changes in fluid balance, electrolyte concentrations, and acid-base balance during prolonged therapy or as indicated by patient condition. ▪ Electrolytes, vitamins, and minerals are readily depleted. Watch for any signs of beginning deficiency and replace as needed. ▪ A vesicant at concentrations greater than 10%. Ensure proper catheter or needle position, confirm patency of vein, and avoid extravasation. Administration through a central line is required for prolonged infusions of concentrations over 10%. ▪ Monitor blood glucose. Supplemental insulin may be required. ▪ See Rate of Administration and Precautions.

Pediatric patients: Monitor fluid intake, urine output, and serum electrolytes closely. Small volumes of fluid may affect fluid and electrolyte belance in very small infants and neonates. Renal function may be immature and the ability to excrete fluid and solute loads limited. ▪ Monitor serum glucose frequently in all pediatric patients but especially in infants, neonates, and low-birth-weight infants. Adequate glycemic control is imperative to avoid potential long-term adverse effects; see Precautions.

Maternal/Child: Category C: safety for use in pregnancy and breast-feeding not established. Benefits must outweigh risks. Use caution and monitor fluid balance, glucose and electrolyte concentrations, and acid-base balance of both mother and child. ▪ See Precautions.

Elderly: Lower-end initial doses may be indicated; see Dose Adjustments. Monitoring of renal function may be useful. Specific age-related differences in response have not been identified.

DRUG/LAB INTERACTIONS
See Monitor.

SIDE EFFECTS
Rare in small doses administered slowly: acidosis, alkalosis, febrile reactions, fluid overload (congested states, pulmonary edema, overhydration, dilution of serum electrolyte concentrations), hyperglycemia (during infusion), hyperosmolar syndrome (mental confusion, loss of consciousness), hypersensitivity reactions (e.g., anaphylaxis; coughing; difficulty breathing; periorbital, facial, and/or laryngeal edema; pruritus; sneezing; and uticaria), hypokalemia, hypovitaminosis, infection at injection site, rebound hypoglycemia (after infusion), venous thrombosis or phlebitis.

ANTIDOTE
Discontinue the drug and notify the physician of the side effect. Provide symptomatic treatment as required.

DIAZEPAM
(dye-**AYZ**-eh-pam)

Benzodiazepine
Sedative-hypnotic
Antianxiety agent
Anticonvulsant
Amnestic
Skeletal muscle relaxant (adjunct)

Valium ▪ Diazemuls ✦

pH 6.2 to 6.9 ▪ pH 8

USUAL DOSE
Maximum dose except in status epilepticus is 30 mg in 8 hours. Note some changes in times of administration between conventional diazepam (Valium) and emulsified forms (e.g., Diazemuls). The emulsified form is no longer available in the United States.

PREOPERATIVE MEDICATION
Conventional diazepam (Valium): 5 to 10 mg before surgery.
Emulsified diazepam (Diazemuls): 10 mg 1 to 2 hours before surgery.

MODERATE ANXIETY DISORDERS AND SYMPTOMS OF ANXIETY
All formulations: 2 to 5 mg. Repeat in 3 to 4 hours if necessary.

SEVERE ANXIETY DISORDERS AND SYMPTOMS OF ANXIETY
All formulations: 5 to 10 mg. Repeat in 3 to 4 hours if necessary.

ACUTE ALCOHOL WITHDRAWAL
All formulations: 10 mg initially, then 5 to 10 mg in 3 to 4 hours if necessary.

STATUS EPILEPTICUS
All formulations: 5 to 10 mg. May be repeated at intervals of 10 to 15 minutes up to a total dose of 30 mg. May repeat in 2 to 4 hours. Another source suggests 0.2 to 0.5 mg/kg every 15 to 30 minutes for 2 or 3 doses. Some specialists start with 20 mg and titrate the total dose over 10 minutes or until seizures stop. Maximum dose in 24 hours is 100 mg.

CARDIOVERSION
Conventional diazepam (Valium): 5 to 15 mg 5 to 10 minutes before procedure begins.
Emulsified diazepam (Diazemuls): 5 to 15 mg 10 to 20 minutes before procedure begins.

ENDOSCOPY
Conventional diazepam (Valium): 10 mg or less is usually effective given immediately before procedure begins; titrate to desired sedation (e.g., slurred speech). Up to 20 mg may be indicated if a narcotic is not used.
Emulsified diazepam (Diazemuls): 5 to 10 mg 30 minutes before the procedure begins; titrate to desired sedation (e.g., slurred speech). Up to 20 mg may be indicated if a narcotic is not used.

MUSCLE SPASM
All formulations: 5 to 10 mg. Repeat in 3 to 4 hours if necessary. Larger doses may be required in tetanus.

PEDIATRIC DOSE
Safety for use in neonates not established but is used. Neonates have reduced or immature organ function; may be susceptible to prolonged CNS depression. Avoid small veins (e.g., dorsum of hand or wrist); see Monitor. Use in infants and children is most frequent in tetany, status epilepticus, or hypersensitivity reactions. Use of longer-acting anticonvulsants (e.g., phenobarbital, phenytoin) following diazepam may be indicated. Not recommended but is used for other general indications.

SEDATIVE/MUSCLE RELAXANT
All formulations: 0.04 to 0.2 mg/kg every 2 to 4 hours. Maximum dose 0.6 mg/kg in 8 hours.

TETANUS IN PEDIATRIC PATIENTS FROM 30 DAYS OF AGE TO 5 YEARS OF AGE
Respiratory assistance must be available.
All formulations: 1 to 2 mg every 3 to 4 hours.

Conventional diazepam (Valium): One source suggests a maximum single dose not to exceed 0.25 mg/kg; repeat in 15 to 30 minutes if necessary. A third dose may be given, but if it does not relieve symptoms, consider alternative therapy.

TETANUS IN PEDIATRIC PATIENTS 5 YEARS OF AGE OR OLDER
Respiratory assistance must be available.

All formulations: 5 to 10 mg every 3 to 4 hours.

Conventional diazepam (Valium): One source suggests a maximum single dose not to exceed 0.25 mg/kg; repeat in 15 to 30 minutes if necessary. A third dose may be given, but if it does not relieve symptoms, consider alternative therapy.

STATUS EPILEPTICUS IN NEONATES (UNLABELED)
All formulations: 0.3 to 0.75 mg/kg every 15 to 30 minutes for 2 to 3 doses. Maximum total dose is 5 mg.

STATUS EPILEPTICUS IN PEDIATRIC PATIENTS FROM 30 DAYS OF AGE TO 5 YEARS OF AGE
All formulations: 0.2 to 0.5 mg every 2 to 5 minutes to a maximum 5-mg dose. May repeat in 2 to 4 hours. Another source suggests 0.2 to 0.5 mg/kg every 15 to 30 minutes to a maximum 5-mg dose.

STATUS EPILEPTICUS IN PEDIATRIC PATIENTS 5 YEARS OF AGE OR OLDER
All formulations: 1 mg every 2 to 5 minutes to a maximum 10-mg dose. May repeat in 2 to 4 hours. Another source suggests 0.2 to 0.5 mg/kg every 15 to 30 minutes to a maximum 10-mg dose.

DOSE ADJUSTMENTS
Reduce dose by one half for the elderly or debilitated, in impaired liver or renal function, in patients with limited pulmonary reserve, and in the presence of other CNS depressants. Begin with a small dose and increase in gradual increments. ■ See Drug/Lab Interactions.

DILUTION
All formulations: Do not dilute or mix with any other drug. Should be given directly into the vein. Inject into IV tubing close to vein site only when direct IV injection is not feasible. Consider heparin lock for frequent injection. Change site every 2 to 3 days. Some precipitation or adsorption into plastic tubing may occur.

Conventional diazepam: *Not soluble in any solution.* If dilution is imperative, add dilution solution to diazepam, not diazepam to solution; consult pharmacist. Direct IV administration is preferred but can be administered at a Y-tube injection site.

Emulsified diazepam: May be diluted with their emulsion base (Intralipid or Nutralipid). Mixture should be used within 6 hours. In any other solution, *emulsion may be destabilized and may not be visually apparent.* Incompatible with polyvinylchloride infusion sets. If a filter is used for emulsified forms, it must have a pore size of 5 microns or more so as not to break down the emulsion. Emulsified forms eliminate the use of nonphysiologic, potentially irritating solvents.

Filters: *Emulsified diazepam:* If a filter is used for emulsified forms, it must have a pore size of 5 microns or more to prevent breakdown of the emulsion.

Storage: *Conventional diazepam (Valium):* Store at CRT in cartons to protect from light. Do not freeze.

Emulsified diazepam (Diazemuls): Store below 25° C (77° F) unless manufacturer suggests refrigeration. Do not freeze. Protect from light. Note expiration date.

COMPATIBILITY   (Underline Indicates Conflicting Compatibility Information)
Consider any drug NOT listed as compatible to be INCOMPATIBLE until consulting a pharmacist; specific conditions may apply.

Manufacturers for all preparations recommend not mixing with any other drug or solution in syringe or solution. Precipitation can occur. Emulsified forms are **incompatible** with polyvinylchloride infusion sets. *Emulsion may be destabilized and may not be visually apparent.* See Dilution.

One source suggests the following **compatibilities:**

CONVENTIONAL DIAZEPAM
Additive: Levetiracetam (Keppra), verapamil.

Y-site: Cisatracurium (Nimbex), dobutamine, fentanyl, hydromorphone (Dilaudid), methadone (Dolophine), morphine, nafcillin (Nallpen), quinidine gluconate, remifentanil (Ultiva).

EMULSIFIED DIAZEPAM

Additive: Intralipid, Nutralipid; see Dilution.

RATE OF ADMINISTRATION

If a filter is used for emulsified forms, it must have a pore size of 5 microns or more so as not to break down the emulsion.

Adults: 5 mg (1 mL) or fraction thereof over 1 minute.

Infants and other pediatric patients: Give total dose over a minimum of 3 minutes, but do not exceed a rate of 0.25 mg/kg over 3 minutes.

ACTIONS

A benzodiazepine that depresses the central, autonomic, and peripheral nervous systems in an undetermined manner. Exerts antianxiety, sedative/hypnotic, amnesic, anticonvulsant, skeletal muscle relaxant, and antitremor effects. Diminishes patient recall. Metabolized in the liver; stays in the body in appreciable amounts for several days and is excreted very slowly in the urine. Crosses the placental barrier. Secreted in breast milk.

INDICATIONS AND USES

Management of moderate to severe anxiety disorders or short-term relief of symptoms of anxiety. ▪ Acute alcohol withdrawal. ▪ Acute stress reactions. ▪ Muscle spasm. ▪ Status epilepticus and severe recurrent convulsive seizures, including tetany. ▪ Preoperative medication, including endoscopic procedures. ▪ Cardioversion.

Unlabeled uses: Conscious sedation in dental procedures, treatment of panic disorders.

CONTRAINDICATIONS

Known hypersensitivity, open-angle glaucoma unless receiving appropriate therapy, shock, coma, acute alcoholic intoxication with depression of vital signs. Emulsion in Dizac contains soybean oil; do not use in patients with known hypersensitivity to soy protein.

PRECAUTIONS

Check label carefully. Some preparations are for IV use only (e.g., Diazemuls); others can be given IM/IV (e.g., Valium). ▪ Drug of choice for initial treatment of status epilepticus or seizures resulting from drug overdose or poisoning. Some specialists administer phenytoin simultaneously to facilitate long-term control (onset of action is not as immediate as diazepam). Oral phenytoin or phenobarbital may be used for maintenance. ▪ May not be effective if seizures are due to acute brain lesions. ▪ Not recommended for treatment of petit mal or petit mal variant seizures; may cause tonic state epilepticus. ▪ Use caution in the elderly, those who are very ill, and those with limited pulmonary reserve (e.g., chronic lung disease) or unstable cardiac status. ▪ Withdrawal symptoms will occur for several weeks after extended or large doses. ▪ Hypoalbuminemia may increase the incidence of side effects. ▪ Intended for short-term use only. ▪ Available PO and as a rectal gel.

Monitor: See Dilution. ▪ To reduce the incidence of thrombophlebitis, avoid smaller veins. Extravasation or arterial administration hazardous. ▪ Oxygen, respiratory assistance, and flumazenil (Romazicon) must always be available. ▪ Bed rest required for a minimum of 3 hours after IV injection.

Patient Education: May produce drowsiness or dizziness. Request assistance with ambulation and use caution performing tasks that require alertness. Do not drive or operate hazardous machinery until all effects have subsided. ▪ Avoid use of alcohol or other CNS depressants (e.g., antihistamines, barbiturates). ▪ May be habit-forming with long-term use or high-dose therapy. ▪ Has amnestic potential; may impair memory. ▪ Consider birth control options.

Maternal/Child: Category D: has caused birth deformities, especially in the first trimester. ▪ Not recommended during pregnancy, childbirth, or while breast-feeding.

Elderly: See Dose Adjustments. Start with a small dose and increase gradually based on response. ▪ More sensitive to therapeutic and adverse effects (e.g., ataxia, dizziness, oversedation). ▪ IV injection may be more likely to cause apnea, bradycardia, hypotension, and cardiac arrest. ▪ See Precautions and Drug/Lab Interactions.

DRUG/LAB INTERACTIONS

Concurrent use with other **CNS depressants** (e.g., alcohol, antihistamines, barbiturates, MAO inhibitors [e.g., selegiline (Eldepryl)], narcotics [e.g., morphine, meperidine (Demerol), fentanyl], phenothiazines [e.g., prochlorperazine (Compazine)], tricyclic antidepressants [e.g., imipramine (Tofranil-PM)]) may result in additive effects for up to 48 hours. Reduced doses of both drugs may be indicated. ▪ May increase serum concentrations of **digoxin and phenytoin** (Dilantin); monitor digoxin and phenytoin serum levels. ▪ **Ritonavir** (Norvir) may increase risk of prolonged sedation and respiratory depression. Concurrent use not recommended. Benzodiazepines metabolized by alternate routes may be safer (e.g., lorazepam [Ativan], oxazepam [Serax], temazepam [Restoril]). ▪ Concurrent use with **beta-blockers** (e.g., metoprolol [Lopressor], propranolol [Inderal]), **cimetidine** (Tagamet), **disulfiram** (Antabuse), **estrogen-containing oral contraceptives, fluoxetine** (Prozac), **isoniazid** (INH), **itraconazole** (Sporanox), **ketoconazole** (Nizoral), **omeprazole** (Prilosec), **probenecid, and valproic acid** (Depakene) may inhibit hepatic metabolism, resulting in increased plasma concentrations of benzodiazepines. ▪ Diazepam decreases clearance and increases toxicity of **zidovudine** (AZT, Retrovir). ▪ May increase clearance and decrease effectiveness of **levodopa.** ▪ Hypotensive effects of benzodiazepines may be increased by **any agent that induces hypotension** (e.g., antihypertensives, CNS depressants, diuretics, lidocaine, paclitaxel). ▪ Use with **rifampin** (Rifadin) increases clearance and reduces effects of diazepam. ▪ **Theophyllines** (e.g., Aminophylline) antagonize sedative effects of benzodiazepines. ▪ **Smoking** increases metabolism and clearance of diazepam, decreasing plasma levels and sedative effects. ▪ **Clozapine** (Leponex) has caused respiratory distress or cardiac arrest in a few patients; use concurrently with extreme caution. ▪ Decreased drowsiness may occur in cigarette **smokers,** especially if elderly. ▪ **Grapefruit juice** may affect certain enzymes of the P_{450} enzyme system and should be avoided.

SIDE EFFECTS

Apnea, ataxia, blurred vision, bradycardia, cardiac arrest, cardiovascular collapse, coma, confusion, coughing, depressed respiration, depression, diminished reflexes, drowsiness, dyspnea, headache, hiccups, hyperexcited states, hyperventilation, laryngospasm, neutropenia, nystagmus, somnolence, syncope, venous thrombosis and phlebitis at injection site, vertigo.

ANTIDOTE

Notify the physician of all side effects. Reduction of dosage may be required. Discontinue the drug for major side effects or paradoxical reactions, including hyperexcitability, hallucinations, and acute rage. Flumazenil (Romazicon) will reverse all sedative effects of benzodiazepines. A patent airway, artificial ventilation, oxygen therapy, and other symptomatic treatment must be instituted promptly. May cause emesis; observe closely. Treat hypersensitivity reaction, or resuscitate as necessary.

DICLOFENAC SODIUM BBW

NSAID

(dye-**KLOE**-fen-ak)

Dyloject

USUAL DOSE

To minimize the risk of serious adverse events, use the lowest effective dose for the shortest duration consistent with individual patient treatment goals. To reduce the risk of adverse renal reactions, patients must be well hydrated before administration.

Acute pain: 37.5 mg as an IV bolus injection over 15 seconds every 6 hours as needed. Total daily dose should not exceed 150 mg/day.

DOSE ADJUSTMENTS

No specific dose adjustments recommended.

DILUTION

Available as a solution containing 37.5 mg/mL in a single-dose vial. No further dilution required.

Filters: Specific information not available.

Storage: Store at CRT. Do not freeze. Protect from light.

COMPATIBILITY

Specific information not available; consult pharmacist.

RATE OF ADMINISTRATION

A single dose as an IV bolus over 15 seconds.

ACTIONS

A nonsteroidal anti-inflammatory drug (NSAID) that has anti-inflammatory, analgesic, and antipyretic activity. Mechanism of action is not completely understood but may involve inhibition of the cyclooxygenase (COX-1 and COX-2) pathways. May also be related to inhibition of prostaglandin synthetase. More than 99% bound to serum proteins, primarily albumin. Diffuses into and out of the synovial fluid. Metabolized into several metabolites. Terminal half-life is 1.4 hours. Excreted as metabolites in urine and bile.

INDICATIONS AND USES

A NSAID indicated in adults for management of mild to moderate pain and management of moderate to severe pain alone or in combination with opioid analgesics.

CONTRAINDICATIONS

Known hypersensitivity to diclofenac. ▪ History of asthma, urticaria, or allergic-type reactions after taking aspirin or other NSAIDs. ▪ Perioperative pain in the setting of coronary artery bypass graft (CABG) surgery. ▪ Patients with moderate to severe renal insufficiency in the perioperative period who are at risk for volume depletion.

PRECAUTIONS

For IV administration only. ▪ Nonsteroidal anti-inflammatory drugs (NSAIDs) may increase the risk of serious cardiovascular (CV) thrombotic events, myocardial infarction, and stroke, which can be fatal. This risk may increase with duration of use. Patients with cardiovascular disease or risk factors for cardiovascular disease may be at greater risk. In observational studies, patients treated with NSAIDs in the post-MI period were at increased risk for re-infarction, CV-related death, and all-cause mortality beginning in the first week of treatment. Avoid use in patients with recent MI unless benefits are expected to outweigh the risk of recurrent CV thrombotic events. ▪ No consistent evidence that concurrent use of aspirin mitigates the increased risk of serious CV thrombotic events associated with NSAID use. Concurrent use of aspirin and a NSAID does increase the risk of serious GI events. ▪ NSAIDs increase the risk of serious gastrointestinal (GI) adverse events, including inflammation, bleeding, ulceration, and perforation of the stomach or intestines, which can be fatal. These events can occur at any time during use and without warning symptoms. Elderly patients and patients with a prior history of peptic ulcer disease and/or GI bleeding are at greater risk for serious gastrointestinal events. ▪ Risk of GI events increases with longer duration of use; however, even short-term use is not without risk. Use with extreme caution in patients with a history of ulcer disease or GI bleeding. ▪ Other factors that increase the risk for GI bleeding include concomitant use of oral corticosteroids or anticoagulants, smoking, use of alcohol, and poor general health. Most reports of spontaneous fatal GI events are in elderly or debilitated patients. ▪ Use caution in patients with considerable dehydration; these patients are at increased risk for renal toxicity. Not recommended for patients with moderate to severe renal insufficiency; see Contraindications. ▪ Renal toxicity has also been seen in patients in whom renal prostaglandins have a compensatory role in the maintenance of renal perfusion. In these patients NSAIDs may cause a dose-dependent reduction in renal prostaglandin formation and, secondarily, in renal blood flow, which can precipitate renal failure. Patients with impaired renal function, heart failure, or liver dysfunction; elderly patients; and patients receiving ACE inhibitors (e.g., enalapril [Vasotec], lisinopril [Zestril]) or diuretics are at greatest risk. ▪ Elevations of one or more liver function tests may occur. Diclofenac injection is not indicated for long-term treatment. However, severe hepatotoxicity may develop at any time without a prodrome of distinguishing symptoms. ▪ Not recommended for patients with moderate or severe hepatic impairment. ▪ May precipitate new-onset hypertension or worsen pre-existing hypertension; see Drug/Lab Interactions. ▪ May cause fluid retention and edema; use caution in patients with CHF or edema. Avoid NSAID use in patients with severe heart failure unless the benefits are expected to outweigh the risk of worsening heart failure. NSAID use may increase the risk of MI, hospitalization for heart failure, and death. ▪ Hypersensitivity reactions, including anaphylaxis, have been reported. ▪ Use caution in patients with a history of asthma; see Contraindications. ▪ May cause serious skin reactions (e.g., exfoliative dermatitis, Stevens-Johnson syndrome, toxic epidermal necrolysis) without warning; some have been fatal. ▪ May cause anemia (due to fluid retention, occult or gross blood loss, or effects on erythropoiesis). ▪ NSAIDs inhibit platelet aggregation and may cause a prolonged bleeding time. ▪ May reduce inflammation and fever, making it difficult to detect infectious complications. ▪ Not a substitute for corticosteroids and cannot be used to treat corticosteroid insufficiency. If corticosteroids are discontinued in patients undergoing prolonged corticosteroid therapy, therapy should be tapered slowly. ▪ See Maternal/Child.

Monitor: Correct hypovolemia before administration and maintain adequate hydration. ▪ Obtain baseline blood pressure and monitor frequently during therapy. ▪ Baseline CBC, liver function tests, and SCr may be useful. Repeat as indicated if symptoms of toxicity develop. ▪ CV events (e.g., MI, stroke, other thrombotic events) may occur even in the absence of previous CV symptoms. Monitor patients with or without a previous history of CV disease for S/S of thromboembolic complications (e.g., altered consciousness, vision, or speech; chest pain; limb or abdominal swelling and/or pain; loss of sensation or motor power; shortness of breath). If used in patients with a recent MI, monitor for signs of cardiac ischemia. ▪ Monitor for edema or signs of worsening heart failure. ▪ Observe for S/S of GI ulceration or bleeding. ▪ Observe for S/S of liver dysfunction (e.g., abdominal pain, dark urine, diarrhea, elevated LFTs, eosinophilia, jaundice, rash). ▪ Monitor for S/S of hypersensitivity reactions (e.g., anaphylaxis, pruritus, rash, urticaria, or wheezing). ▪ Monitor for S/S of serious skin reactions (e.g., rash). ▪ Monitor patients who may be adversely affected by alterations in platelet function (e.g., patients with coagulation disorders or patients receiving anticoagulants).

Patient Education: Side effects have resulted in extended hospitalization and could be fatal. ▪ Promptly report any unusual S/S suggestive of thromboembolic events, GI toxicity, hepatotoxicity, hypersensitivity reactions, or fluid and electrolyte imbalance (e.g., abdominal pain, bloody emesis, changes in vision, chest pain, dark stools, diarrhea, dizziness, fatigue, flu-like symptoms, jaundice, lethargy, nausea, numbness of face or limbs, pruritus, rash, shortness of breath, unexplained weight gain or edema).

Maternal/Child: Category C before 30 weeks' gestation. Category D starting at 30 weeks' gestation. Avoid use of diclofenac and other NSAIDs starting at 30 weeks' gestation; premature closure of the ductus arteriosus in the fetus may occur. Use during pregnancy only if the potential benefit justifies the potential risk to the fetus. ▪ Do not use during labor and delivery. Inhibitory effects on prostaglandin synthesis may adversely affect fetal circulation, inhibit uterine contractions, and increase the risk of uterine bleeding. ▪ May be excreted in human milk; use caution during breast-feeding. ▪ Safety and effectiveness for use in pediatric patients not established.

Elderly: Use with caution in elderly patients. Consider the greater frequency of decreased hepatic, renal, or cardiac function and of concomitant disease or other drug therapy. Elderly patients are at increased risk for serious GI events and renal adverse events.

DRUG/LAB INTERACTIONS

Concurrent use with **aspirin** not recommended; may increase the risk of serious GI events. Aspirin also reduces the protein binding of diclofenac; clinical significance not known. ▪ The effects of **anticoagulants** (e.g., heparin, warfarin [Coumadin]) and NSAIDs on GI bleeding are synergistic; risk of GI bleeding increases with concomitant use. ▪ NSAIDs may decrease the antihypertensive effect of **ACE inhibitors** (e.g., enalapril [Vasotec], lisinopril [Zestril]). ▪ NSAIDs, including diclofenac, may affect renal prostaglandins and increase the toxicity of certain drugs. Use caution if administered concomitantly with **cyclosporine** (Sandimmune); cyclosporine nephrotoxicity may be increased. ▪ Diclofenac can reduce the natriuretic effects of **furosemide** (Lasix) and **thiazide diuretics** (e.g., hydrochlorothiazide). This response is thought to be due to inhibition of renal prostaglandin synthesis; observe for signs of renal failure and ensure diuretic effectiveness. ▪ Concurrent use of **lithium** with NSAIDs may decrease lithium clearance, increasing plasma levels of lithium; observe for signs of lithium toxicity. ▪ Concurrent use of NSAIDs with **methotrexate** may enhance methotrexate toxicity. ▪ Metabolized by cytochrome P_{450} enzymes, predominantly by CYP2C9. Coadministration with **CYP2C9 inhibitors** (e.g., voriconazole [Vfend]) may increase the toxicity of diclofenac, whereas coadministration with **CYP2C9 inducers** (e.g., rifampin [Rifadin]) may decrease the effectiveness of diclofenac. Use caution with concurrent use; dose adjustment may be indicated. ▪ Use with caution when administered concomitantly with **other potentially hepatotoxic drugs** (e.g., acetaminophen, certain antibiotics, antiepiletics).

SIDE EFFECTS

The most common side effects are constipation, dizziness, flatulence, headache, infusion site pain, insomnia, and nausea and vomiting. Serious side effects include CHF, CV thrombotic events, GI events, hypersensitivity reactions (including anaphylaxis), hypertension, renal and hepatic toxicity, and serious skin reactions; see Precautions. Other side effects occurring in 3% or more of patients receiving diclofenac injection include anemia, fever, hypotension, infusion site extravasation, and pruritus. Other frequently reported adverse reactions occurring in patients taking other formulations of diclofenac or other NSAIDs include edema, elevated liver enzymes, GI toxicity (e.g., abdominal pain, constipation, diarrhea, dyspepsia, gross bleeding/perforation, GI ulcers [gastric/duodenal], heartburn), increased bleeding time, pruritus, rashes, and tinnitus. In clinical trials, postoperative patients receiving diclofenac injection had more adverse reactions related to wound healing.

Overdose: Drowsiness, epigastric pain, GI bleeding, lethargy, nausea, vomiting.

ANTIDOTE

Keep the physician informed of side effects. With increasing severity or onset of symptoms of any major side effect (e.g., CHF; edema; GI bleeding, ulceration, or perforation; hepatic or renal toxicity; hypersensitivity reactions; hypertension; skin reactions; thrombotic events), discontinue the drug and notify the physician. A patent airway, artificial ventilation, oxygen therapy, and other symptomatic treatment must be instituted promptly if indicated. Treat anaphylaxis with epinephrine (Adrenalin), diphenhydramine (Benadryl), and corticosteroids as indicated. No specific antidote. Forced diuresis, alkalinization of urine, hemodialysis, or hemoperfusion may be used in an overdose situation but are unlikely to be useful due to high protein binding.

DIGOXIN
(dih-**JOX**-in)

Cardiac glycoside
Antiarrhythmic
Inotropic agent

Digoxin Pediatric, Lanoxin, Lanoxin Pediatric

pH 6.8 to 7.2

USUAL DOSE

Calculate dose based on lean body weight (LBW), CrCl, age, as well as concomitant disease states, concurrent medications, and other factors that may alter the effects of digoxin. In general, the dose of digoxin used should be determined on clinical grounds. Dosing can be either initiated with a loading dose followed by maintenance dosing (if rapid titration is desired) or initiated with maintenance dosing without a loading dose. Parenteral administration of digoxin should be reserved for when rapid digitalization is medically necessary or when the drug cannot be taken orally. When changing from IV to oral dosing, increase oral dose by 20% to 25% to allow for reduced bioavailability of the oral product.

Loading dosing regimen in adults and pediatric patients:

Recommended Digoxin Injection Loading Dose for Adult and Pediatric Patients	
Age	**Total IV Loading Dose (mcg/kg)** Administer half of the total loading dose initially, then $^1/_4$ of the loading dose every 6-8 hours twice
Premature	15 to 25 mcg/kg
Full-term	20 to 30 mcg/kg
1 to 24 months	30 to 50 mcg/kg
2 to 5 years	25 to 35 mcg/kg
5 to 10 years	15 to 30 mcg/kg
Adults and pediatric patients over 10 years	8 to 12 mcg/kg

Maintenance dosing in adults and pediatric patients over 10 years of age: 2.4 to 3.6 mcg/kg/day given once daily. Doses may be adjusted every 2 weeks according to clinical response, serum drug levels, and toxicity.

PEDIATRIC DOSE

Use 0.1 mg/mL pediatric injection (100 mcg/mL). If using a tuberculin syringe to measure a pediatric dose, do not flush syringe with parenteral solution after contents are injected; may result in an overdose. The recommended starting maintenance dose in pediatric patients less than 10 years of age is listed in the following chart. These recommendations assume the presence of normal renal function.

Recommended Starting Digoxin Maintenance Dosage in Pediatric Patients Less Than 10 Years of Age	
Age	**Dose Regimen (mcg/kg/dose)** Given twice daily
Premature	1.9 to 3.1 mcg/kg/dose
Full-term	3 to 4.5 mcg/kg/dose
1 to 24 months	4.5 to 7.5 mcg/kg/dose
2 to 5 years	3.8 to 5.3 mcg/kg/dose
5 to 10 years	2.3 to 4.5 mcg/kg/dose

Continued

DOSE ADJUSTMENTS

The following two charts provide recommended maintenance doses for specific patient populations based on lean body weight and renal function.

Digoxin Maintenance Dose (in mcg given once daily) in Adults and Pediatric Patients Over 10 Years of Age Based on Lean Body Weight and Renal Function

Corrected Creatinine Clearance*	Lean Body Weight (kg)‡							Number of Days Before Steady State Achieved†
	40	50	60	70	80	90	100	
10 mL/min	64	80	96	112	128	144	160	19
20 mL/min	72	90	108	126	144	162	180	16
30 mL/min	80	100	120	140	160	180	200	14
40 mL/min	88	110	132	154	176	198	220	13
50 mL/min	96	120	144	168	192	216	240	12
60 mL/min	104	130	156	182	208	234	260	11
70 mL/min	112	140	168	196	224	252	280	10
80 mL/min	120	150	180	210	240	270	300	9
90 mL/min	128	160	192	224	256	288	320	8
100 mL/min	136	170	204	238	272	306	340	7

*For adults, CrCl was corrected to a 70-kg body weight or 1.73 M² body surface area. For pediatric patients, the modified Schwartz equation may be used. The formula is based on height in cm and SCr in mg/dL where k is a constant and CCr is corrected to 1.73 M² body surface area. During the first year of life, the value of k is 0.33 for preterm infants and 0.45 for term infants. The k is 0.55 for pediatric patients and adolescent girls and 0.7 for adolescent boys:

$$GRF \ mL/min/1.73 \ M^2 = (k \times Height)/SCr$$

†If no loading dose administered.

‡The doses listed assume average body composition.

- Alternatively, the maintenance dose for adults and pediatric patients over 10 years of age may be estimated using the following formula:

$$Total \ maintenance \ dose \ (mcg) = Loading \ dose \ (mcg) \times \% \ Daily \ loss \div 100$$
$$Where \ \% \ daily \ loss = 14 + CrCl \div 5.$$

Digoxin Maintenance Dose* (in mcg given TWICE daily) in Pediatric Patients Under 10 Years of Age Based on Lean Body Weight and Renal Function

Corrected Creatinine Clearance‡	Lean Body Weight (kg)†							Number of Days Before Steady State Achieved§
	5	10	20	30	40	50	60	
10 mL/min	8	16	32	48	64	80	96	19
20 mL/min	9	18	36	54	72	90	108	16
30 mL/min	10	20	40	60	80	100	120	14
40 mL/min	11	22	44	66	88	110	132	13
50 mL/min	12	24	48	72	96	120	144	12
60 mL/min	13	26	52	78	104	130	156	11
70 mL/min	14	28	56	84	112	140	168	10
80 mL/min	15	30	60	90	120	150	180	9
90 mL/min	16	32	64	96	128	160	192	8
100 mL/min	17	34	68	102	136	170	204	7

*Recommended doses are to be given twice daily.

†The doses listed assume average body composition.

‡The modified Schwartz equation may be used to estimate creatinine clearance. See preceding chart.

§If no loading dose is administered.

▪ Reduce dose in patients whose lean weight is an abnormally small fraction of their total body mass because of obesity or edema. ▪ Monitor for S/S of digoxin toxicity and clinical response. Adjust dose based on toxicity, efficacy, and blood levels. ▪ Reduce dose in partially digitalized patients, in patients with impaired renal function, and in the elderly. ▪ Dose reduction may be required before cardioversion. ▪ See Drug/Lab Interactions; adjustments may be required with numerous drugs. ▪ Reduced doses may be indicated in advanced heart failure, myocardial infarction, severe carditis, or severe pulmonary disease. ▪ Renal clearance diminished in neonates, including premature infants; adjust dose as indicated. ▪ See Precautions.

DILUTION
Available as a 500 mcg (0.5 mg) in 2 mL injection (250 mcg [0.25 mg] per mL) and as a 100 mcg (0.1 mg) in 1 mL (pediatric) injection. May be given undiluted or each 1 mL may be diluted in 4 mL SWFI, NS, or D5W. Less diluent may cause precipitation. Use diluted solution immediately. Give through Y-tube or three-way stopcock of IV infusion set. See Pediatric Dose.

Storage: Store unopened vials at CRT protected from light.

COMPATIBILITY
(Underline Indicates Conflicting Compatibility Information)

Consider any drug NOT listed as compatible to be INCOMPATIBLE until consulting a pharmacist; specific conditions may apply.

Manufacturer recommends not mixing with other drugs in the same container and not administering simultaneously via the same IV line.

One source suggests the following **compatibilities** *(not recommended by manufacturer):*

Additive: Furosemide (Lasix), lidocaine, ranitidine (Zantac), verapamil.

Y-site: Anidulafungin (Eraxis), bivalirudin (Angiomax), ceftaroline (Teflaro), ciprofloxacin (Cipro IV), cisatracurium (Nimbex), dexmedetomidine (Precedex), diltiazem (Cardizem), doripenem (Doribax), famotidine (Pepcid IV), fenoldopam (Corlopam), heparin, hetastarch in electrolytes (Hextend), hydrocortisone sodium succinate (Solu-Cortef), insulin (regular), linezolid (Zyvox), meperidine (Demerol), meropenem (Merrem IV), midazolam (Versed), milrinone (Primacor), morphine, nesiritide (Natrecor), potassium chloride (KCl), remifentanil (Ultiva), tacrolimus (Prograf).

RATE OF ADMINISTRATION
Each single dose over a minimum of 5 minutes. Avoid bolus administration. Rapid administration may cause systemic and coronary arteriolar constriction.

ACTIONS
A cardiac glycoside obtained from *Digitalis lanata*. Inhibits Na-K ATPase, the "sodium pump" responsible for moving sodium ions out of cells and potassium ions into cells. The cardiologic consequences of this action are an increase in the force and velocity of myocardial systolic contraction (positive inotropic action), a slowing of the heart rate (negative chronotropic effect), decreased conduction velocity through the AV node, and a decrease in the degree of activation of the sympathetic nervous system and renin-angiotensin system (neurohormonal deactivating effect). Increases cardiac output and left ventricular ejection fraction and lowers pulmonary artery pressure, pulmonary capillary wedge pressure, and systemic vascular resistance. Widely distributed throughout the body. Onset of action is 5 to 30 minutes. Time to peak effect is 1 to 4 hours. Half-life is 1.5 to 2 days. Minimal metabolism. Rapidly excreted in urine, primarily as unchanged drug. Crosses the placenta and is secreted in breast milk.

INDICATIONS AND USES
Treatment of mild to moderate heart failure in adults. ▪ To increase myocardial contractility in pediatric patients with heart failure. ▪ Control of ventricular response rates in adult patients with chronic atrial fibrillation; see Precautions.

CONTRAINDICATIONS
Ventricular fibrillation and known hypersensitivity to digoxin or other digitalis preparations.

PRECAUTIONS

IV administration is the preferred parenteral route. Used only when oral therapy is not feasible or rapid therapeutic effect is necessary. ▪ Calcium channel blockers (e.g., diltiazem [Cardizem], verapamil) or beta blockers (e.g., atenolol [Tenormin], metoprolol [Lopressor]) are generally preferred for rate control in patients with atrial fibrillation; adenosine (Adenocard) is preferred to treat PSVT. ▪ Commonly prolongs the PR interval; may cause severe sinus bradycardia or sinoatrial block in patients with pre-existing sinus node disease and may cause advanced or complete heart block in patients with pre-existing incomplete AV block. Consider insertion of a pacemaker before treatment with digoxin in these patients. ▪ Use in patients with an accessory AV pathway (Wolff-Parkinson-White syndrome) increases risk of ventricular fibrillation and is not recommended. ▪ Avoid use in patients with heart failure associated with preserved left ventricular systolic function (e.g., acute cor pulmonale, amyloid heart disease, constrictive pericarditis, idiopathic hypertrophic subaortic stenosis, restrictive cardiomyopathy). Patients with these conditions may experience a decreased cardiac output. Has been used for ventricular rate control in a subgroup of these patients with atrial fibrillation. ▪ Avoid use in patients with myocarditis; may precipitate vasoconstriction. ▪ Use with caution in patients with impaired renal function; risk of toxicity increased; see Dose Adjustments. ▪ Use caution in patients with electrolyte disorders because potassium or magnesium depletion sensitizes the myocardium to digoxin; toxicity may occur with serum digoxin concentrations below 2 ng/mL. ▪ Patients with beriberi heart disease may fail to respond adequately to digoxin if the underlying thiamine deficiency is not treated concomitantly. ▪ Use with caution in patients with hypercalcemia. May increase risk of digoxin toxicity. Maintain normocalcemia. ▪ Hypocalcemia may nullify effect of digoxin. If calcium levels need to be restored to normal, give calcium slowly and in small amounts. Serious arrhythmias have occurred in digitalized patients receiving calcium. ▪ Hypothyroidism may reduce requirements for digoxin. Addressing the underlying condition is suggested in patients with heart failure and/or atrial arrhythmias resulting from hypermetabolic or hyperdynamic states (e.g., hyperthyroidism, hypoxia, or arteriovenous shunt). Atrial arrhythmias associated with hypermetabolic states are particularly resistant to digoxin treatment. ▪ Use is not recommended in patients with myocardial infarction. May cause an increase in myocardial oxygen demand and ischemia. ▪ Some clinicians suggest reducing or discontinuing the dose of digoxin for 1 to 2 days before an elective cardioversion to avoid the induction of ventricular arrhythmias, but physicians must consider the consequences of increasing the ventricular response if digoxin is decreased or withdrawn. If countershock is necessary (last-resort treatment of life-threatening arrhythmias), begin with low voltage levels and increase gradually to avoid ventricular arrhythmias. ▪ See Drug/Lab Interactions.

Monitor: Monitor for S/S of digoxin toxicity (anorexia, nausea, vomiting, vision changes, cardiac arrhythmias). ▪ Low body weight, advanced age, impaired renal function, hypomagnesemia, hypokalemia, and hypercalcemia may predispose patient to digoxin toxicity. Monitor electrolytes frequently during therapy. Avoid rapid changes. Supplements indicated to maintain normal serum electrolyte levels. ▪ Monitor renal function. ▪ Monitor digoxin levels. Draw at least 6 hours after the last dose, preferably just before the next dose. Serum digoxin levels less than 0.5 ng/mL have been associated with diminished efficacy, whereas levels above 2 ng/mL have been associated with increased toxicity without increased benefit. ▪ Monitor HR and BP. ▪ Baseline and periodic ECG monitoring suggested. May prolong the PR interval and cause depression of the ST segment on ECG. ▪ The earliest and most frequent manifestation of digoxin toxicity in infants and children is the appearance of cardiac arrhythmias, including sinus bradycardia. ECG monitoring recommended in pediatric patients to avoid intoxication. ▪ See Dose Adjustments, Precautions, and Drug/Lab Interactions.

Patient Education: Review all medications with pharmacist or physician. Capable of numerous drug interactions. ▪ Laboratory monitoring of digoxin levels and renal function required. ▪ Report any nausea, vomiting, persistent diarrhea, confusion, weakness, or vision disturbances.

Maternal/Child: Category C: use during pregnancy, labor, and delivery only if clearly needed. ▪ Use caution during breast-feeding. Digoxin does distribute into breast milk, but the estimated exposure of the nursing infant to digoxin via breast-feeding is far below the usual infant maintenance dose. ▪ Safety and effectiveness of digoxin in the control of ventricular rate in pediatric patients with atrial fibrillation have not been established. ▪ Safety and effectiveness in the treatment of heart failure in pediatric patients have not been established in well-controlled studies. However, in published literature of pediatric patients with heart failure of various etiologies, treatment with digoxin has been associated with improvements in hemodynamic parameters and in clinical S/S. ▪ Newborn infants display considerable variability in their tolerance to digoxin. Premature and immature infants are particularly sensitive. Dose must be reduced and individualized according to degree of maturity. ▪ Carefully titrate dose based on clinical response in pediatric patients with renal disease; see Dose Adjustments.

Elderly: Monitor carefully. Reduced dose may be indicated. Consider reduced body mass and reduced kidney function.

DRUG/LAB INTERACTIONS

Interactions are numerous. Careful monitoring required when initiating, adjusting, or discontinuing drugs that may interact with digoxin. Monitor serum levels carefully and adjust doses as indicated. ▪ Digoxin is a substrate for P-glycoprotein at the level of intestinal absorption, renal tubular secretion, and biliary-intestinal secretion. **Drugs that induce or inhibit P-glycoprotein** have the potential to alter digoxin pharmacokinetics. ▪ **Potassium-depleting diuretics** (e.g., furosemide [Lasix], chlorothiazide [Diuril]) are a major contributing factor to digitalis toxicity. ▪ **Calcium** may produce serious arrhythmias in digitalized patients, particularly with too-rapid IV administration. ▪ **Amiodarone** (Nexterone), **propafenone** (Rythmol), **quinine, spironolactone** (Aldactone), and **verapamil** may increase serum digoxin concentration. Reduce digoxin dose by 15% to 30% and monitor levels. ▪ **Quinidine** and **ritonavir** (Norvir) may increase serum levels. Decrease digoxin dose by 30% to 50% and monitor levels. ▪ Synergistic with **beta-blockers** (e.g., atenolol [Tenormin], metoprolol [Lopressor]) and **calcium channel blockers** (e.g., verapamil, diltiazem [Cardizem]). Additive effects on AV node conduction may result in bradycardia and/or advanced or complete heart block. ▪ **ACE inhibitors** (e.g., lisinopril [Prinivil, Zestril], enalapril [Vasotec]), **angiotensin receptor blockers** (e.g., valsartan [Diovan], irbesartan [Avapro]), **NSAIDs** (e.g., ibuprofen [Motrin, Advil], naproxen [Naprosyn, Aleve]), and **COX-2 inhibitors** (e.g., celecoxib [Celebrex]) may impair excretion of digoxin. ▪ Coadministration with **dofetilide** (Tikosyn) has been associated with a higher incidence of torsades de pointes. ▪ Coadministration with **sotalol** (Betapace) has been associated with more proarrhythmic events than when either drug was administered alone. ▪ Sudden death was more common in patients receiving digoxin with **dronedarone** (Multaq) than when either drug was given alone. ▪ **Teriparatide** (Forteo) transiently increases serum calcium, which may predispose patients to digoxin toxicity. ▪ **Succinylcholine** may cause a sudden extrusion of potassium from muscle cells; may cause arrhythmias in digitalized patients. ▪ Increased risk of arrhythmias with **sympathomimetic amines** (e.g., dopamine, epinephrine, norepinephrine). ▪ Initiation of **thyroid treatment** may require an increase in digoxin dose. ▪ No significant changes in digoxin exposure have been reported when IV digoxin is coadministered with **carvedilol** (Coreg), **clarithromycin** (Biaxin), **isradipine** (DynaCirc CR), **losartan** (Cozaar), and **rifampin** (Rifadin). ▪ Endogenous substances of unknown composition (**digoxin-like immunoreactive substances [DLIS]**) can interfere with standard radioimmunoassays for digoxin. This interference usually results in a falsely elevated level but sometimes causes results to be falsely reduced. DLIS are present in up to half of all neonates and in varying percentages of pregnant women, patients with hypertrophic cardiomyopathy, patients with renal or hepatic dysfunction, and other patients who are volume expanded for any reason. **Spironolactone and some traditional Chinese and Ayurvedic medicines** may also interfere with different assays; see manufacturer's prescribing information for further information. ▪ See Precautions and Monitor.

SIDE EFFECTS

The overall incidence of adverse reactions with digoxin has been reported as 5% to 20%, with 15% to 20% of adverse reactions considered serious. Cardiac toxicity accounts for about one half, GI disturbances for about one fourth, and CNS and other toxicity for about one fourth of these adverse reactions. *Cardiac:* Arrhythmias (e.g., first-degree, second-degree, or third-degree heart block [including asystole]; atrial tachycardia with block; AV dissociation; accelerated junctional [nodal] rhythm; unifocal or multiform ventricular premature contractions [especially bigeminy or trigeminy]; ventricular tachycardia; and ventricular fibrillation). *GI:* Abdominal pain, hemorrhagic necrosis of the intestines, intestinal ischemia, nausea and vomiting. *CNS:* Apathy, confusion, dizziness, headache, mental disturbances (e.g., anxiety, delirium, depression, hallucinations), and weakness. *Other:* Anorexia, gynecomastia, rash, thrombocytopenia, and visual changes.

Toxicity can cause death. The *most common manifestation of excessive dosing in pediatric patients* is the appearance of cardiac arrhythmias. Conduction disturbances or supraventricular tachyarrhythmias are the most common type of arrhythmia. Ventricular arrhythmias are less common.

Overdose: Anorexia, arrhythmias, CNS disturbances, fatigue, hyperkalemia, nausea and vomiting.

ANTIDOTE

Discontinue the drug at the first sign of toxicity, notify the physician, and place the patient on a cardiac monitor. Dosage may be decreased or discontinued. For severe toxicity, digoxin immune Fab is a specific antidote. Consider causes of toxicity (electrolyte disturbances, thyroid, concurrent medications) and correct/treat as indicated. Serum potassium must be obtained before administering potassium salts. See Precautions. Bradycardia and heart block caused by digoxin toxicity may respond to atropine. Ventricular arrhythmias may respond to lidocaine or phenytoin. A temporary pacemaker may also be used. With severe digoxin toxicity, potassium may be released from skeletal muscles, resulting in hyperkalemia. Hyperkalemia, if life-threatening, may be treated with D5W and insulin. Peritoneal dialysis or hemodialysis not effective in overdose.

DIGOXIN IMMUNE FAB (OVINE)
(dih-**JOX**-in im-**MYOUN** fab)

Antidote
(digoxin intoxication)

Digibind, DigiFab

pH 6 to 8

USUAL DOSE

Testing for sensitivity to sheep serum and/or premedication may be indicated; see Contraindications and Monitor.

Acute toxicity in adults and pediatric patients: Determine dose by symptoms and clinical findings. Serum concentration may not reflect actual toxicity for 6 to 12 hours. Symptoms of life-threatening toxicity due to digoxin overdose include severe arrhythmias (e.g., VT, VF), progressive bradycardia, second- or third-degree heart block not responsive to atropine, and/or serum potassium levels exceeding 5 to 5.5 mEq/L in adults and 6 mEq/L in pediatric patients.

Dose in numbers of vials based on ingested dose is calculated by dividing the body load of digoxin in milligrams by 0.5. Each vial of *Digibind* contains 38 mg/vial and will bind 0.5 mg digoxin. Each vial of *DigiFab* contains 40 mg/vial and will bind 0.5 mg of digoxin. Dose may also be based on serum digoxin levels (see package insert; has charts for adults and pediatric patients).

An initial dose of up to 20 vials has been used. 20 vials will bind approximately 50 (0.25 mg) tablets of Lanoxin and should provide adequate treatment of most life-threatening ingestions in adult and pediatric patients. If ingested substance is unknown, if serum digoxin level is not available, or if there is concern about sensitivity to the serum, consider giving 10 vials. Observe clinical response and repeat if indicated. In clinical trials of Digibind the average dose was 10 vials. A single dose may be repeated in several hours if toxicity has not reversed or appears to recur. Febrile reactions are dose related.

Toxicity in chronic therapy: *Adults:* 6 vials should be adequate to reverse most cases of toxicity in adults in acute distress or if a serum digoxin concentration is not available.

Pediatric patients: less than 20 kg: 1 vial should be adequate if signs of toxicity are present.

DILUTION
Each vial must be diluted with 4 mL of SWFI (results in 9.5 mg/mL for Digibind and 10 mg/mL for DigiFab). Mix gently. May be given in this initial dilution or may be further diluted with any desired amount of NS (with ***Digibind,*** 34 mL NS/vial yields 1 mg/mL; with ***DigiFab,*** 36 mL NS/vial yields 1 mg/mL). Consider volume overload in pediatric patients when further diluting in NS. Administer to infants after initial dilution using a tuberculin syringe to deliver an accurate dose with less volume; for extremely small doses, dilute to 1 mg/mL before administration.

Filters: *Digibind:* Must be given through a 0.22-micron membrane filter.

Storage: Refrigerate unreconstituted vials. Use reconstituted solution promptly or store in refrigerator for up to 4 hours.

COMPATIBILITY
Specific information not available. Consider specific use; consult pharmacist.

RATE OF ADMINISTRATION
Decrease the rate of infusion or discontinue temporarily if an infusion reaction occurs. Do not give as an IV bolus injection unless cardiac arrest is imminent. Be prepared to treat anaphylaxis.

Digibind: Must be given through a 0.22-micron membrane filter. A single dose as an IV infusion equally distributed over 15 to 30 minutes.

DigiFab: A single dose as an infusion over 30 minutes.

ACTIONS
Antigen-binding fragments (Fab) prepared from specific antidigoxin antibodies produced in sheep are isolated and purified. Fab fragments bind molecules of digoxin and make them unavailable for binding at their site of action. Freely distributed in extracellular space. Reduces the level of free digoxin in the serum. Onset of action is prompt, with improvement in symptoms of toxicity within 30 minutes. Fab-digoxin complexes are cleared by the kidney. DigiFab is also cleared in the reticuloendothelial system.

INDICATIONS AND USES
Digibind: Treatment of patients with life-threatening digoxin intoxication or overdose (digoxin).

DigiFab: Treatment of patients with life-threatening or potentially life-threatening digoxin toxicity or overdose. Not indicated for milder cases of digoxin toxicity.

All formulations: Indicated for known suicidal or accidental consumption of fatal doses of digoxin, including ingestion of 10 mg or more of digoxin in previously healthy adults, 4 mg (or more than 0.1 mg/kg) in previously healthy pediatric patients, or ingestion causing steady-state serum concentrations greater than 10 ng/mL. ▪ Indicated for chronic ingestions causing steady-state serum digoxin concentrations exceeding 6 ng/mL in adults or 4 ng/mL in pediatric patients. ▪ Indicated for manifestations of life-threatening toxicity due to digoxin overdose, including severe ventricular arrhythmias (such as VT or VF), progressive bradycardia, or third-degree heart block not responsive to atropine. ▪ Also indicated when potassium concentrations are above 5 to 5.5 mEq/L in adults or 6 mEq/L in pediatric patients with rapidly progressive S/S of digoxin toxicity. ▪ See Precautions and Maternal/Child.

CONTRAINDICATIONS

None known when used for specific indications. If hypersensitivity exists and treatment is necessary, premedicate with corticosteroids and diphenhydramine and prepare to treat anaphylaxis.

PRECAUTIONS

Administered under the direction of the physician specialist with facilities for monitoring the patient and responding to any medical emergency. Cardiac arrest can result from ingestion of more than 10 mg digoxin by healthy adults, 4 mg digoxin by healthy pediatric patients, or serum digoxin levels above 10 ng/mL. ▪ Larger doses of digoxin immune Fab act more quickly but increase the possibility of febrile or hypersensitivity reactions. ▪ Use caution in impaired cardiac function. Inability to use cardiac glycosides may endanger patient. Support with dopamine or vasodilators. ▪ The clinical problem may not be caused by digoxin toxicity if the patient fails to respond to digoxin immune Fab. ▪ Consider that multiple drugs may have been used and are producing toxicity in suicide attempts. ▪ See Monitor and Drug/Lab Interactions.

Monitor: Although allergy testing is not required before treating life-threatening digoxin toxicity, patients allergic to ovine proteins or those who have previously received antibodies or Fab fragments produced from sheep are at risk. Determine patient response to any previous injections of serum of any type and history of any allergic-type reactions. In addition, *DigiFab* considers that patients with allergies to papain, chymopapain, other papaya extracts, or the pineapple enzyme bromelain may be at risk. *Digibind* provides the information below on sensitivity testing; that information is not included in the package insert for *DigiFab*. ▪ Test for sensitivity if indicated. Make a 1:100 solution by diluting 0.1 mL of reconstituted solution (10 mg/mL) with 9.9 mL sterile NS (100 mcg/mL).

Scratch test: Make a ¼-inch skin scratch through a drop of 1:100 dilution in NS. Inspect the site in 20 minutes. An urticarial wheal surrounded by a zone of erythema is a positive reaction.

Skin test: Inject 0.1 mL (10 mcg) of 1:100 dilution intradermally. Inspect the site in 20 minutes. A urticarial wheal surrounded by a zone of erythema is a positive reaction. Concomitant use of antihistamines may interfere with sensitivity tests. If skin testing causes a systemic reaction, place a tourniquet above the testing site and treat anaphylaxis.

▪ Serum digoxin or digitoxin concentration should be obtained before administration if at all possible. These measurements may be difficult to interpret if drawn soon after the last digitalis dose because at least 6 to 8 hours are required for equilibration of digoxin between serum and tissue. ▪ Standard treatment of digoxin intoxication includes withdrawal of the intoxicating agent; correction of electrolyte disturbances (especially hyperkalemia), acid-base imbalances, and hypoxia; and treatment of cardiac arrhythmias. ▪ Monitor VS, ECG, and potassium concentration frequently during and after drug administration. ▪ Monitor for S/S of an acute hypersensitivity reaction (e.g., angioedema, bronchospasm with wheezing or cough, erythema, hypotension, laryngeal edema, pruritus, stridor, tachycardia, urticaria). ▪ Potassium may be shifted from inside to outside the cell, causing increased renal excretion. May appear to have hyperkalemia while there is a total body deficit of potassium. When the digoxin effect is reversed, hypokalemia may develop rapidly. ▪ Do not redigitalize until all Fab fragments have been eliminated from the body. May take several days. May take longer in severe renal impairment, and reintoxication may occur by release of newly unbound digoxin into the blood. ▪ See Precautions and Drug/Lab Interactions.

Maternal/Child: Category C: use only when clearly indicated and benefits outweigh risks in pregnancy, breast-feeding, and infants. ▪ *Digibind* indicates that it should be used in infants and children if more than 0.3 mg of digoxin is ingested, if serum digoxin levels are equal to or greater than 6.4 nmol/L, or if there is underlying heart disease.

Patient Education: Contact the physician immediately if S/S of a delayed hypersensitivity reaction or serum sickness occur (e.g., rash, pruritus, urticaria).

Elderly: Consider age-related impaired renal function; monitor closely for recurrent toxicity; see Monitor.

DRUG/LAB INTERACTIONS

Will cause a precipitous rise in **total serum digoxin,** but most will be bound to the Fab fragment. Will interfere with digoxin immunoassay measurements until Fab fragment is completely eliminated. ▪ **Catecholamines** (e.g., epinephrine) may aggravate digoxin arrhythmias. ▪ See skin test in Monitor.

SIDE EFFECTS

Acute anaphylaxis with urticaria, respiratory distress, and vascular collapse is possible. Exacerbation of congestive heart failure and low cardiac output states and increased ventricular response in atrial fibrillation may occur due to withdrawal of digoxin effects. Hypokalemia may be life threatening.

ANTIDOTE

Notify the physician of all side effects. Discontinue the drug and treat anaphylaxis immediately. Corticosteroids, epinephrine (Adrenalin [see Drug/Lab Interactions]), diphenhydramine (Benadryl), oxygen, IV fluids, vasopressors (dopamine), and ventilation equipment must always be available. Resuscitate as necessary. Treat hypokalemia cautiously when necessary. Support exacerbated cardiac conditions as necessary.

DIHYDROERGOTAMINE MESYLATE BBW

(dye-hy-droh-er-**GOT**-ah-meen **MES**-ih-layt)

D.H.E. 45

Ergot alkaloid
Migraine agent

pH 3.2 to 4

USUAL DOSE

Abort or prevent headaches: 1 mg (1 mL). May be repeated in 1 hour. No more than 2 doses (2 mg total) may be given IV in 24 hours. Do not exceed 6 mg in 1 week; see Precautions. Administration of an antiemetic (e.g., metoclopramide [Reglan] 10 mg) PO 1 hour before dihydroergotamine is recommended.

Chronic intractable headache: 0.5 mg (0.5 mL). Administer an antiemetic IV (e.g., metoclopramide) about 10 minutes before injection.

Prevention of orthostatic hypotension associated with spinal or epidural anesthesia (unlabeled): 0.5 mg (0.5 mL). Give a few minutes before anesthetic.

PEDIATRIC DOSE

See Maternal/Child. Administration of an antiemetic (e.g., metoclopramide, prochlorperazine), usually PO, 1 hour before dihydroergotamine is recommended.

Pediatric patients 6 to 9 years of age: 100 to 150 mcg (0.1 to 0.15 mg).

Pediatric patients 9 to 12 years of age: 200 mcg (0.2 mg).

Pediatric patients 12 to 16 years of age: 250 to 500 mcg (0.25 to 0.5 mg).

For all age ranges, repeat up to 2 doses at 20-minute intervals if necessary. Another source suggests 250 mcg (0.25 mg) at the start of the attack. Repeat in 1 hour if necessary.

DILUTION

May be given undiluted.

Storage: Protect ampules from light and heat.

COMPATIBILITY

Specific information not available. Consider specific use; consult pharmacist.

RATE OF ADMINISTRATION

1 mg or fraction thereof over 1 minute.

ACTIONS

An alpha-adrenergic blocking agent that causes constriction of both peripheral and cerebral blood vessels and produces depression of central vasomotor centers. Metabolized by the liver. Metabolites eliminated primarily in feces. Secreted in breast milk.

INDICATIONS AND USES

To abort or prevent vascular headaches (migraine, histamine cephalalgia). Used when rapid control is desired or other routes not feasible. ▪ Treatment of chronic intractable headache.

Unlabeled uses: To prevent orthostatic hypotension associated with spinal or epidural anesthesia. Use SC to enhance heparin effects in preventing postoperative deep vein thrombosis after abdominal, thoracic, or pelvic surgeries or total hip replacement and IM or SC to treat orthostatic hypotension.

CONTRAINDICATIONS

Breast-feeding, coronary artery disease, hepatic or renal disease, hypersensitivity, uncontrolled hypertension, peripheral vascular disease, pregnancy or women who may become pregnant, sepsis. ▪ Coadministration with potent CYP3A4 inhibitors, including protease inhibitors and macrolide antibiotics, is contraindicated; see Drug/Lab Interactions.

PRECAUTIONS

IM or SC use is preferred but may be given IV to obtain a more rapid effect. ▪ Coadministration with potent CYP3A4 inhibitors, including protease inhibitors and macrolide antibiotics, increases the risk of vasospasm, leading to cerebral ischemia and/or ischemia of the extremities (peripheral). May be serious and/or life threatening; see Contraindications and Drug/Lab Interactions. ▪ Use only when a clear diagnosis of migraine has been established. Do not exceed dosing guidelines or use for chronic daily administration; see Usual Dose.

Monitor: Monitor vital signs; observe closely. ▪ See Drug/Lab Interactions.

Patient Education: Consider birth control options. ▪ Take only as directed. ▪ Report ineffectiveness or an increase in frequency or severity of headaches. ▪ Report chest pain, increased HR, itching, muscle pain or weakness of arms or legs, numbness or tingling of extremities, or swelling.

Maternal/Child: Category X: avoid pregnancy. See Contraindications. ▪ Safety for use in pediatric patients not established. Severe side effects (e.g., extrapyramidal reactions may occur). Pretreatment with an antiemetic may be helpful. Limit pediatric use to patients who have not responded to less toxic treatment.

Elderly: Increased risk of hypothermia and ischemic complications (e.g., cardiac, peripheral). ▪ Consider age-related renal impairment.

DRUG/LAB INTERACTIONS

Contraindicated with potent CYP3A4 inhibitors, including **antifungals** (e.g., itraconazole [Sporanox], ketoconazole [Nizoral]), **protease inhibitors** (e.g., ritonavir [Norvir], nelfinavir [Viracept], and indinavir [Crixivan]), **and macrolide antibiotics** (e.g., clarithromycin [Biaxin], erythromycin, and troleandomycin [TAO]); see Contraindications and Precautions. ▪ Administer less potent CYP3A4 inhibitors with caution as vasospasm may occur. **Less potent inhibitors** include, but are not limited to, saquinavir (Invirase), nefazodone, fluconazole (Diflucan), grapefruit juice, fluoxetine (Prozac), fluvoxamine (Luvox), zileuton (Zyflo), and clotrimazole (Gyne-Lotrimin, Mycelex). ▪ Opposes vasodilating effects of **nitrates** (e.g., nitroglycerin), decreasing their effectiveness. ▪ May cause hypertensive crisis in combination with other **vasopressors** (e.g., epinephrine). ▪ May cause peripheral vasoconstriction with ischemia and/or cyanosis with **beta-adrenergic blockers** (e.g., propranolol [Inderal]) and **nicotine.**

SIDE EFFECTS

Rare in therapeutic doses, but may include angina pectoris, blindness, gangrene, muscle pains, muscle weakness, nausea, numbness and tingling of the fingers and toes, pleural and retroperitoneal fibrosis, thirst, uterine bleeding, and vomiting.

ANTIDOTE

Discontinue the drug and notify the physician of any side effects. Another drug will probably be chosen if further treatment is indicated. Vasodilators (nitroprusside sodium) and CNS stimulants (e.g., caffeine and sodium benzoate) are indicated as an antidote. Heparin and low-molecular-weight dextran may be used to reduce thrombosis due to excessive vasoconstriction. Hemodialysis may be indicated. Resuscitate as necessary.

DILTIAZEM HYDROCHLORIDE
(dill-**TYE**-a-zem hy-droh-**KLOR**-eyed)

Cardizem

Calcium channel blocker
Antiarrhythmic

pH 3.7 to 4.1

USUAL DOSE
0.25 mg/kg of body weight initially (20 mg for the average patient). Some patients may respond to an initial dose of 0.15 mg/kg. A second dose of 0.35 mg/kg may be given in 15 minutes if needed to achieve HR reduction (25 mg for the average patient). Any additional bolus doses used to achieve an appropriate response must be individualized to each patient. Patients with PSVT will probably respond to bolus doses and may not require an infusion, but to maintain reduction in HR in patients with atrial fibrillation or atrial flutter, immediately follow with an intravenous infusion at an initial rate of 10 mg/hr. May only be used for up to 24 hours. Some patients may maintain response with an initial rate of 5 mg/hr. Infusion may be increased by 5 mg/hr increments to a maximum dose of 15 mg/hr. Discontinue infusion within 24 hours. Oral antiarrhythmic agents (e.g., digoxin, quinidine, procainamide, calcium channel blockers [e.g., diltiazem, verapamil], beta blockers [e.g., atenolol, metoprolol, propranolol]) to maintain reduced HR are usually started within 3 hours of initial bolus of diltiazem.

DOSE ADJUSTMENTS
Specific mg/kg dose must be used for patients with low body weights. ▪ Reduced dose may be indicated in impaired hepatic or renal function. ▪ Dose selection should be cautious in the elderly. Reduced doses may be indicated based on potential for decreased organ function and concomitant disease or drug therapy. ▪ See Drug/Lab Interactions.

DILUTION
Available as a solution in 25- or 50-mg vials (5 mg/mL), as a powder with supplied diluent (Lyo-ject syringe 25 mg [5 mg/mL]), and in a piggyback monovial containing 100 mg (with transfer needle set to facilitate preparation of an infusion). Dilute according to the following charts.

Cardizem Injectable or Cardizem Lyo-Ject Syringe				
	Quantity of Cardizem (Diltiazem) Injection	Final Concentration	Administration	
Diluent Volume			Dose	Infusion Rate
100 mL	125 mg (25 mL)	1 mg/mL	5 mg/hr 10 mg/hr 15 mg/hr	5 mL/hr 10 mL/hr 15 mL/hr
250 mL	250 mg (50 mL)	0.83 mg/mL	5 mg/hr 10 mg/hr 15 mg/hr	6 mL/hr 12 mL/hr 18 mL/hr
500 mL	250 mg (50 mL)	0.45 mg/mL	5 mg/hr 10 mg/hr 15 mg/hr	11 mL/hr 22 mL/hr 33 mL/hr
100 mL	100 mg (1 monovial)	1 mg/mL	5 mg/hr 10 mg/hr 15 mg/hr	5 mL/hr 10 mL/hr 15 mL/hr
250 mL	200 mg (2 monovials)	0.8 mg/mL	5 mg/hr 10 mg/hr 15 mg/hr	6.25 mL/hr 12.5 mL/hr 18.8 mL/hr
500 mL	200 mg (2 monovials)	0.4 mg/mL	5 mg/hr 10 mg/hr 15 mg/hr	12.5 mL/hr 25 mL/hr 37.5 mL/hr

IV injection: May be given undiluted through Y-tube or three-way stopcock of tubing containing NS, D5W, or D5/$\frac{1}{2}$NS.

Infusion: May be further diluted for infusion in any of the above solutions.

Filters: No data available from manufacturer.

Storage: Vials may be stored at room temperature for up to 1 month, then discarded. Refrigeration before and after dilution preferred. Use within 24 hours of dilution. Discard unused medication and/or solution. Do not freeze.

COMPATIBILITY   (Underline Indicates Conflicting Compatibility Information)

Consider any drug NOT listed as compatible to be INCOMPATIBLE until consulting a pharmacist; specific conditions may apply.

Manufacturer recommends that **all formulations** not be mixed with any other drugs in the same container and, if possible, that they not be co-infused in the same IV line.

Cardizem Lyo-Ject Syringe is listed by the manufacturer as **incompatible** at the **Y-site** with acetazolamide (Diamox), acyclovir (Zovirax), aminophylline, ampicillin, ampicillin/sulbactam (Unasyn), diazepam (Valium), furosemide (Lasix), hydrocortisone sodium succinate (Solu-Cortef), methylprednisolone (Solu-Medrol), mezlocillin (Mezlin), nafcillin (Nallpen), phenytoin (Dilantin), rifampin (Rifadin), sodium bicarbonate. **Cardizem** is listed as **incompatible** with all of the above and insulin (regular).

Cardizem Monovial is listed by the manufacturer as **incompatible** at the **Y-site** with acetazolamide (Diamox), acyclovir (Zovirax), diazepam (Valium), furosemide (Lasix), phenytoin (Dilantin), rifampin (Rifadin).

Manufacturer lists **Cardizem Lyo-Ject Syringe** as **compatible** at the **Y-site** with insulin (regular) and lists the **Cardizem Monovial** (1 mg/mL) in NS as **compatible** at the **Y-site** with aminophylline, ampicillin, ampicillin/sulbactam (Unasyn), hydrocortisone sodium succinate (Solu-Cortef), insulin (regular), methylprednisolone (Solu-Medrol), mezlocillin (Mezlin), nafcillin (Nallpen), sodium bicarbonate.

One source lists the following **compatibilities** but does not differentiate formulations:

Y-site: Acetazolamide (Diamox), acyclovir (Zovirax), albumin, amikacin, aminophylline, amphotericin B (conventional), ampicillin, ampicillin/sulbactam (Unasyn), argatroban, aztreonam (Azactam), bivalirudin (Angiomax), bumetanide, caspofungin (Cancidas), cefazolin (Ancef), cefotaxime (Claforan), cefotetan, cefoxitin (Mefoxin), ceftaroline (Teflaro), ceftazidime (Fortaz), ceftriaxone (Rocephin), cefuroxime (Zinacef), ciprofloxacin (Cipro IV), clindamycin (Cleocin), dexmedetomidine (Precedex), digoxin (Lanoxin), dobutamine, dopamine, doripenem (Doribax), doxycycline, epinephrine (Adrenalin), erythromycin (Erythrocin), esmolol (Brevibloc), fenoldopam (Corlopam), fentanyl, fluconazole (Diflucan), gentamicin, heparin, hetastarch in electrolytes (Hextend), hetastarch in NS (Hespan), hydrocortisone sodium succinate (Solu-Cortef), hydromorphone (Dilaudid), imipenem-cilastatin (Primaxin), labetalol, lidocaine, lorazepam (Ativan), meperidine (Demerol), methylprednisolone (Solu-Medrol), metoclopramide (Reglan), metoprolol (Lopressor), metronidazole (Flagyl IV), midazolam (Versed), milrinone (Primacor), morphine, multivitamins (M.V.I.), nafcillin (Nallpen), nesiritide (Natrecor), nicardipine (Cardene IV), nitroglycerin IV, nitroprusside sodium, norepinephrine (Levophed), oxacillin (Bactocill), penicillin G potassium, pentamidine, potassium chloride (KCl), potassium phosphates, procainamide (Pronestyl), ranitidine (Zantac), sodium bicarbonate, sulfamethoxazole/trimethoprim, telavancin (Vibativ), theophylline, ticarcillin/clavulanate (Timentin), tobramycin, vancomycin, vasopressin, vecuronium.

RATE OF ADMINISTRATION

IV injection: Each single dose equally distributed over 2 minutes.

Infusion: 5 mg to 15 mg/hr based on patient response. See charts under Dilution for diluent, dose, and infusion rate information. Use of a metriset (60 gtt/min) required; volumetric infusion pump preferred.

ACTIONS

Directly inhibits the influx of calcium ions through slow channels during membrane depolarization of cardiac and vascular smooth muscle. Effective in supraventricular tachycardias because it slows conduction through the AV node, prolongs the effective refractory period, reduces ventricular rates, and helps to prevent embolic complications. Also slows conduction through the SA node. Prevents re-entry phenomena through the AV node. Reduces HR (10% with a single dose, 20% at peak effectiveness), systolic and diastolic BP, systemic vascular resistance, pulmonary artery systolic and diastolic BPs, and coronary vascular resistance with no significant effect on contractility, left ventricular end diastolic pressure, right atrial pressure, or pulmonary capillary wedge pressure. Increases cardiac output and stroke volume. Has little or no effect on normal AV nodal conduction at normal HRs. Produces less myocardial depression than verapamil. Effective within 3 minutes; maximum effect should occur within 2 to 7 minutes and last for 1 to 3 hours. 70% to 80% bound to plasma proteins. Metabolized in the liver. Half-life is approximately 3.4 hours following a bolus injection and increases to 4.1 to 4.9 hours with continuous infusion. Excreted in urine and bile. Secreted in breast milk.

INDICATIONS AND USES
Temporary control of rapid ventricular rate in atrial fibrillation or atrial flutter unless associated with an accessory bypass tract (e.g., Wolff-Parkinson-White syndrome or short PR syndrome). ▪ Rapid conversion of paroxysmal supraventricular tachycardia (PSVT) to normal sinus rhythm including AV nodal re-entrant tachycardias and reciprocating tachycardias associated with an extranodal accessory pathway (e.g., Wolff-Parkinson-White syndrome or short PR syndrome).

CONTRAINDICATIONS
Atrial fibrillation or flutter when associated with an accessory bypass tract (e.g., Wolff-Parkinson-White or short PR syndrome), cardiogenic shock, congestive heart failure (severe) unless secondary to supraventricular tachyarrhythmia treatable with diltiazem, known sensitivity to diltiazem, second- or third-degree AV block or sick sinus syndrome (unless functioning ventricular pacemaker in place), severe hypotension, patients receiving IV beta-adrenergic blocking agents (e.g., atenolol [Tenormin], propranolol [Inderal]) within 2 to 4 hours, ventricular tachycardia. Not recommended for wide QRS tachycardias of uncertain origin or for tachycardias induced by drugs or poisons.

PRECAUTIONS
For short-term use only. ▪ Initial administration of IV diltiazem should take place in a facility with adequate personnel, equipment, and supplies to monitor the patient and respond to any medical emergency. ▪ While diltiazem will effectively decrease HR, cardioversion will probably be required to convert atrial fibrillation or atrial flutter to a normal sinus rhythm. ▪ Valsalva maneuver recommended before use of diltiazem in all paroxysmal supraventricular tachycardias if clinically appropriate. ▪ Use IV diltiazem with caution in patients with pre-existing impaired ventricular function (e.g., congestive heart failure, acute myocardial infarction, or pulmonary congestion documented by x-ray); may exacerbate disease. Use of oral diltiazem in these patients is contraindicated. ▪ May cause second- or third-degree AV block in sinus rhythm; discontinue diltiazem if AV block occurs. ▪ Can cause life-threatening tachycardia with severe hypotension in atrial fibrillation or flutter in patients with an accessory bypass tract and periods of asystole in patients with sick sinus syndrome. ▪ Use with caution in impaired renal or hepatic function. ▪ Ventricular premature beats (VPBs) may occur on conversion of PSVT to sinus rhythm; considered to have no clinical significance. ▪ Continue regular dosing on day of OR and thereafter unless otherwise specified by physician. If discontinued, may cause severe angina or MI.

Monitor: Accurate pretreatment diagnosis differentiating wide-complex QRS tachycardia of supraventricular origin from ventricular origin is imperative. ▪ ECG monitoring during administration preferred; must be available. ▪ Monitor BP and HR closely. ▪ Emergency resuscitation drugs and equipment must always be available. ▪ See Drug/Lab Interactions.

Maternal/Child: Category C: large doses (5 to 10 times mg/kg dose) have resulted in embryo and fetal death and skeletal abnormalities in animals. ▪ Discontinue breastfeeding. ▪ Safety and effectiveness for use in pediatric patients not established.
Elderly: See Dose Adjustments. ▪ Half-life may be prolonged. ▪ May cause tinnitus.

DRUG/LAB INTERACTIONS

Do not give concomitantly (within a few hours) with IV **beta-adrenergic blocking agents** (e.g., atenolol [Tenormin], propranolol [Inderal]); see Contraindications. May result in bradycardia, AV block, and/or depression of contractility. Use extreme caution if these drugs are administered orally or if patient has received before admission; usually tolerated. ▪ May result in additive effects with **any agent known to affect cardiac contractility and/or SA or AV node conduction** (e.g., digoxin [Lanoxin], disopyramide [Norpace], procainamide [Pronestyl], beta-blockers [e.g., propranolol], quinidine). ▪ Is used with **digoxin,** but monitor for excessive slowing of HR and/or AV block. ▪ Coadministration with **amiodarone** (Nexterone) may result in bradycardia and decreased cardiac output. Monitor closely. ▪ May increase effects of certain **benzodiazepines** (e.g., midazolam [Versed], triazolam [Halcion]), **buspirone** (BuSpar), **methylprednisolone** (Solu-Medrol). ▪ May increase serum concentrations of **digoxin, HMG-CoA reductase inhibitors** (e.g., atorvastatin [Lipitor], simvastatin [Zocor]), **imipramine** (Tofranil), **sirolimus** (Rapamune), **and tacrolimus** (Prograf). Monitor serum levels and/or monitor for S/S of toxicity. ▪ May potentiate **anesthetics;** titrate both drugs carefully. ▪ May decrease metabolism and increase serum concentrations and toxicity of **drugs metabolized by the cytochrome P$_{450}$ enzyme system** (e.g., amlodipine [Norvasc], carbamazepine [Tegretol], cyclosporine [Sandimmune], quinidine, theophylline, valproate [Depacon]). ▪ Metabolism may be decreased and serum concentrations increased by **cimetidine** (Tagamet) **and ranitidine** (Zantac). ▪ Metabolism may be increased and serum concentrations decreased by **rifampin** (Rifadin). Adjust dose as needed. ▪ May increase **moricizine** (Ethmozine) serum concentrations. Moricizine may decrease diltiazem concentrations. ▪ May increase **nifedipine** (Procardia) serum concentrations; nifedipine may increase diltiazem serum concentrations. ▪ Variable effects when administered with **lithium.** Has caused decreased effectiveness of lithium and may cause neurotoxicity. ▪ **Any drug metabolized in the liver** may cause competitive inhibition of metabolism (e.g., insulin).

SIDE EFFECTS

Arrhythmia (junctional rhythm or isorhythmic dissociation), flushing, hypotension (asymptomatic and symptomatic), and injection site reactions (burning, itching) occurred most frequently and were most often mild and transient but could have serious potential. Amblyopia, asthenia, atrial flutter, AV block (first- or second-degree), bradycardia, chest pain, congestive heart failure, constipation, dizziness, dry mouth, dyspnea, edema, elevated alkaline phosphatase and AST, headache, hyperuricemia, nausea, paresthesia, pruritus, sinus node dysfunction, sinus pause, skin eruptions (including rare reports of exfoliative dermatitis or Stevens-Johnson syndrome), sweating, syncope, ventricular arrhythmias, ventricular fibrillation, ventricular tachycardia, and vomiting have occurred.

ANTIDOTE

Discontinue diltiazem if a high-degree AV block occurs in sinus rhythm. Notify physician promptly of all side effects. Treatment will depend on clinical situation; maintain IV fluids as indicated. Rapid ventricular response in atrial flutter/fibrillation should respond to cardioversion, procainamide, and/or lidocaine. Treat bradycardia, AV block, and asystole with standard AHA protocol (atropine, isoproterenol, pacing). Treat cardiac failure with inotropic agents (isoproterenol, dopamine, or dobutamine) and diuretics. Calcium chloride will reverse effects of verapamil; may be useful with diltiazem. Dopamine or norepinephrine (levarterenol) and Trendelenburg position should reverse hypotension. Treat hypersensitivity reactions or resuscitate as necessary. Not removed by hemodialysis.

DINUTUXIMAB BBW
(dye-new-**TUX**-ih-mab)

Unituxin

Antineoplastic
(monoclonal antibody)

pH 6.8

USUAL DOSE
Verify adequate hematologic, respiratory, hepatic, and renal function *before initiating each course of dinutuximab*; see Monitor.

Administer required premedication and hydration *before initiation of each dinutuximab infusion.*

Hydration: Administer NS 10 mL/kg as an IV infusion over 1 hour just before initiating each dinutuximab infusion.

Premedication: *Analgesics:* Immediately before initiating dinutuximab infusion, administer morphine sulfate 50 mcg/kg IV. Follow with a morphine sulfate drip at an infusion rate of 20 to 50 mcg/kg/hr during and for 2 hours after completion of dinutuximab. Additional 25 to 50 mcg/kg IV doses of morphine may be administered as needed for pain up to once every 2 hours followed by an increase in the morphine infusion rate in clinically stable patients. Consider using fentanyl or hydromorphone (Dilaudid) if morphine is not tolerated. If pain is not managed adequately with opioids, consider use of gabapentin (Neurotin) or lidocaine in conjunction with IV morphine.

Antihistamines: 20 minutes before initiating dinutuximab infusion, administer an antihistamine such as diphenhydramine (Benadryl) 0.5 to 1 mg/kg (maximum dose of 50 mg) IV over 10 to 15 minutes. Repeat every 4 to 6 hours as tolerated during the dinutuximab infusion.

Antipyretics: 20 minutes before initiating dinutuximab infusion, administer acetaminophen 10 to 15 mg/kg (maximum dose 650 mg). Repeat every 4 to 6 hours as needed for fever or pain. Administer ibuprofen 5 to 10 mg/kg every 6 hours as needed for control of persistent fever or pain.

Dinutuximab: 17.5 mg/M^2/day as an IV infusion over 10 to 20 hours for 4 consecutive days for a maximum of 5 cycles. See Rate of Administration.

Schedule of Dinutuximab Administration for Cycles 1, 3, and 5						
Cycle Day	1 through 3	4	5	6	7	8 through 24*
Dinutuximab		X	X	X	X	

*Cycles 1, 3, and 5 are 24 days in duration.

Schedule of Dinutuximab Administration for Cycles 2 and 4						
Cycle Day	1 through 7	8	9	10	11	12 through 32*
Dinutuximab		X	X	X	X	

*Cycles 2 and 4 are 32 days in duration.

DOSE ADJUSTMENTS
Manage adverse reactions by infusion interruption, infusion rate reduction, dose reduction, or permanent discontinuation of dinutuximab as outlined in the following charts; see Rate of Administration, Monitor, and Antidote.

Continued

Dinutuximab Dose Modification for Infusion-Related Reactions

Mild to moderate adverse reactions (e.g., transient rash, fever, chills, localized urticaria) that respond promptly to symptomatic treatment	Onset of reaction	Reduce dinutuximab infusion rate to 50% of the previous rate and monitor closely.
	After resolution	Gradually increase infusion rate up to a maximum rate of 1.75 mg/M^2/hr.
Prolonged or severe adverse reactions (e.g., mild bronchospasm without other symptoms, angioedema that does not affect the airway)	Onset of reaction	Immediately interrupt dinutuximab.
	After resolution	If S/S resolve rapidly, resume dinutuximab infusion at 50% of the previous rate and monitor closely.
	First recurrence	Discontinue dinutuximab until the following day. If symptoms resolve and continued treatment is warranted, premedicate with hydrocortisone 1 mg/kg IV (maximum dose 50 mg) and administer dinutuximab at a rate of 0.875 mg/M^2/hr in an intensive care unit.
	Second recurrence	Permanently discontinue dinutuximab.

Dinutuximab Dose Modification for Capillary Leak Syndrome

Moderate to severe but not life-threatening capillary leak syndrome	Onset of reaction	Immediately interrupt dinutuximab.
	After resolution	Resume dinutuximab infusion at 50% of the previous rate.
Life-threatening capillary leak syndrome	Onset of reaction	Discontinue dinutuximab for the current cycle.
	After resolution	In subsequent cycles, administer dinutuximab at 50% of the previous rate.
	First recurrence	Permanently discontinue dinutuximab.

Dinutuximab Dose Modification for Hypotension Requiring Medical Intervention

Symptomatic hypotension, systolic blood pressure (SBP) less than lower limit of normal for age, or SBP decreased by more than 15% compared to baseline	Onset of reaction	Interrupt dinutuximab infusion.
	After resolution	Resume dinutuximab infusion at 50% of the previous rate. If blood pressure remains stable for at least 2 hours, increase the infusion rate as tolerated up to a maximum rate of 1.75 mg/M^2/hr.

Dinutuximab Dose Modification for Severe Systemic Infection or Sepsis

Infections such as severe Grade 3 or 4 bacteremia requiring IV antibiotics or other urgent intervention.	Onset of reaction	Discontinue dinutuximab until resolution of infection, and then proceed with subsequent cycles of therapy.

Dinutuximab Dose Modification for Neurologic Disorders of the Eye

Disorders such as blurred vision, dilated pupil with sluggish light reflex, eyelid ptosis, fixed or unequal pupils, mydriasis, papilledema, optic nerve disorder, or other visual disturbances that do not cause vision loss.	Onset of reaction	Discontinue dinutuximab infusion until resolution.
	After resolution	Reduce dinutuximab dose by 50%.
	First recurrence or if accompanied by visual impairment	Permanently discontinue dinutuximab.

Dinutuximab Dose Modification for Severe Pain	
Severe pain	Decrease dinutuximab infusion rate to 0.875 mg/M^2/hr. Discontinue dinutuximab if pain is not adequately controlled despite infusion rate reduction and institution of maximum supportive measures. See Premedication, Analgesics.

DILUTION

Available in a single-use vial containing 17.5 mg/5 mL (3.5 mg/mL). Do not use if solution is cloudy, has pronounced discoloration, or contains particulate matter. Aseptically withdraw the required volume of dinutuximab and inject into a 100-mL bag of NS. Mix by gentle inversion. *Do not shake.*

Filters: Specific information not available.

Storage: Before use, store in refrigerator at 2° to 8° C (36° to 46° F) in outer carton to protect from light. Do not freeze or shake vials. Diluted solution may be refrigerated, but the infusion must begin within 4 hours of preparation. Discard diluted solution 24 hours after preparation. Discard unused contents of vial.

COMPATIBILITY

Specific information not available; consult pharmacist.

RATE OF ADMINISTRATION

For use as a diluted IV infusion only. Do not administer as an IV push or bolus. Initiate at an infusion rate of 0.875 mg/M^2/hr for 30 minutes. Gradually increase as tolerated to a maximum rate of 1.75 mg/M^2/hr. Manage adverse reactions by infusion interruption, infusion rate reduction, dose reduction, or permanent discontinuation of dinutuximab; see Dose Adjustments.

ACTIONS

Dinutuximab is a chimeric monoclonal antibody produced in the murine myeloma cell line SP2/0. It binds to the glycolipid GD2. This glycolipid is expressed on neuroblastoma cells and on normal cells of neuroectodermal origin, including the central nervous system and peripheral nerves. Dinutuximab binds to cell surface GD2 and induces cell lysis of GD2-expressing cells through antibody-dependent, cell-mediated cytotoxicity (ADCC) and complement-dependent cytotoxicity (CDC). Terminal half-life is approximately10 days.

INDICATIONS AND USES

Treatment of pediatric patients with high-risk neuroblastoma who achieve at least a partial response to prior first-line, multiagent, multimodality therapy. Used in combination with granulocyte-macrophage colony-stimulating factor (GM-CSF), interleukin-2 (IL-2), and 13-*cis*-retinoic acid (RA).

CONTRAINDICATIONS

History of anaphylaxis with dinutuximab.

PRECAUTIONS

For use as a diluted IV infusion only. Do not administer as an IV push or bolus. ▪ Administered under the direction of a physician knowledgeable in its use in a facility with adequate diagnostic and treatment facilities to monitor the patient and respond to any medical emergency. ▪ Serious and potentially life-threatening infusion reactions requiring urgent intervention, including blood pressure support, bronchodilator therapy, corticosteroids, infusion rate reduction, infusion interruption, or permanent discontinuation of dinutuximab, have occurred. ▪ Pain was reported in the majority of patients despite pretreatment with analgesics. Pain was most commonly described as abdominal, back, extremity, or musculoskeletal pain; chest pain; generalized pain; neuralgia; and arthralgia. ▪ Dinutuximab causes severe neuropathic pain. Both peripheral and motor neuropathy have been reported. Neuropathic effects appear more severe in adult patients compared with pediatric patients. Severe motor neuropathy was observed in adults. ▪ Capillary leak syndrome was reported. ▪ Severe hypotension was reported. Prehydration is required; see Usual Dose. ▪ Severe bacteremia requiring IV antibiotics or other urgent intervention has occurred. ▪ Neurologic disorders of the eye have been reported. ▪ Bone marrow suppression (e.g., severe anemia, febrile neutropenia, neutropenia, and thrombocytopenia) was reported. ▪ Electrolyte abnormalities (e.g., hypocalcemia, hypokalemia, and hyponatremia) occur in at least 25% of patients, and some developed inappropriate antidiuretic hormone secretion resulting in severe hyponatremia. ▪ Hemolytic-uremic syndrome has been reported. ▪ Has not been studied in patients with hepatic or renal impairment. ▪ A protein substance; has a potential for immunogenicity. ▪ See Dose Adjustments, Monitor, Maternal/Child, and Antidote.

Monitor: Verify that patients have adequate hematologic, respiratory, hepatic, and renal function before initiating each course of dinutuximab therapy. ▪ Administer required IV hydration and premedication with antihistamines, analgesics, and antipyretics before each dose. ▪ Obtain baseline CBC and platelets and monitor closely during therapy. ▪ Obtain baseline serum electrolytes and monitor daily during therapy. ▪ Monitor for S/S of an infusion reaction during and for at least 4 hours after completion of each infusion (e.g., bronchospasm, dyspnea, facial and upper airway edema, hypotension, stridor, urticaria). Infusion reaction generally occurred during or within 24 hours of completing an infusion. Because of an overlap in S/S, it is difficult to distinguish between infusion reactions and hypersensitivity reactions. ▪ Assess pain frequently; see Usual Dose, Dose Adjustments, and Antidote. ▪ Monitor for S/S of peripheral sensory or motor neuropathy (e.g., burning, numbness, tingling, or weakness). ▪ Monitor for S/S of capillary leak syndrome (e.g., edema, fatigue, hemoconcentration, hypotension, light-headedness, nausea, weakness). Interrupt or discontinue dinutuximab. ▪ Monitor blood pressure closely. For symptomatic hypotension, interrupt or discontinue dinutuximab and provide supportive management. ▪ Monitor for S/S of infection and temporarily discontinue dinutuximab until resolution of the infection. ▪ Monitor for S/S of eye disorders (e.g., dilated pupil with sluggish light reflex or other visual disturbances that do not cause vision loss). Interrupt dinutuximab infusion until resolution. ▪ Monitor for S/S of hemolytic-uremic syndrome (e.g., anemia, decreased urine output, dizziness, edema, fatigue, hematuria, pallor, renal insufficiency). If symptoms appear, discontinue dinutuximab. ▪ See Dose Adjustments, Precautions, Maternal/Child, and Antidote.

Patient Education: Review manufacturer's medication guide. ▪ Effective contraception required during treatment with dinutuximab and for at least 2 months following the last dose of dinutuximab. ▪ Promptly report a known or suspected pregnancy. ▪ Some side effects may require extensive supportive treatment and interruption or discontinuation of dinutuximab. ▪ Promptly report S/S of an infusion reaction (e.g., difficulty breathing, dizziness, facial or lip swelling, light-headedness, urticaria) that occur during or within 24 hours following the infusion. ▪ Promptly report severe or worsening pain and S/S of neuropathy such as burning, numbness, tingling, or weakness. ▪ Promptly report edema, fatigue, light-headedness, or nausea. ▪ Promptly report blurred vision, diplopia, photophobia, ptosis, or unequal pupil size. ▪ Promptly report bruising or fatigue. ▪ Promptly report heart palpitations, muscle cramping, or seizures. ▪ Promptly report decreased urine output, edema, fainting, hematuria, or pallor.

Maternal/Child: Avoid pregnancy. Based on its mechanism of action, dinutuximab can cause fetal harm when administered to a pregnant woman. ▪ Discontinue breastfeeding. ▪ Safety and effectiveness for use in pediatric patients as part of a multiagent, multimodality therapy have been established; see Indications.

Elderly: Safety and effectiveness for use in the elderly have not been established.

DRUG/LAB INTERACTIONS

No drug-drug interaction studies have been conducted with dinutuximab.

SIDE EFFECTS

The most common side effects reported in 25% or more of patients are anemia, capillary leak syndrome, diarrhea, fever, hypoalbuminemia, hypocalcemia, hypokalemia, hyponatremia, hypotension, increased ALT and AST, infusion reactions, lymphopenia, neutropenia, pain, thrombocytopenia, urticaria, and vomiting. The most common serious side effects reported in 5% or more of patients include capillary leak syndrome, fever, hypokalemia, hypotension, infections, infusion reactions, and pain. Decreased appetite, device-related infections, edema, hemorrhage, hyperglycemia, hypertension, hypertriglyceridemia, hypomagnesemia, hypophosphatemia, hypoxia, increased serum creatinine, nausea, peripheral neuropathy, proteinuria, tachycardia, and weight increase have also been reported.

ANTIDOTE
Keep physician informed of all side effects. May constitute a medical emergency or will be treated symptomatically as indicated. Permanently discontinue dinutuximab in patients with any of the following: (1) Grade 3 or 4 anaphylaxis (life-threatening infusion reactions), (2) Grade 3 or 4 serum sickness, (3) Grade 3 pain unresponsive to maximum supportive measures, (4) Grade 4 sensory neuropathy or Grade 3 sensory neuropathy that interferes with daily activities for more than 2 weeks, (5) Grade 2 peripheral motor neuropathy, (6) subtotal or total vision loss, (7) Grade 4 hyponatremia despite appropriate fluid management. Interrupt or discontinue dinutuximab and provide supportive management in (1) severe or prolonged infusion reactions, (2) symptomatic or severe capillary leak syndrome, (3) systemic infection, (4) symptomatic hypotension, and (5) patients with a dilated pupil and a sluggish light reflex or other visual disturbances that do not cause vision loss. Permanently discontinue dinutuximab and provide supportive management for signs of hemolytic-uremic syndrome. Treat these side effects aggressively; see Dose Adjustments, Precautions, and Monitor.

DIPHENHYDRAMINE HYDROCHLORIDE

(dye-fen-**HY**-drah-meen
hy-droh-**KLOR**-eyed)

Antihistamine
Antidyskinetic/antiparkinsonism
Antiemetic
Antivertigo agent
Sedative-hypnotic

Benadryl, Benadryl PF, Diphenhydramine PF

pH 5 to 6

USUAL DOSE
10 to 50 mg. Up to 100 mg may be given. Individualize dose based on patient symptoms and response. Total dosage should not exceed 400 mg/24 hr.

PEDIATRIC DOSE
See Contraindications and Maternal/Child.

Pediatric patients after neonatal period: 1.25 mg/kg/dose every 6 hours as needed or 150 mg/M^2/24 hr in equally divided doses given every 6 hours (37.5 mg/M^2 every 6 hours). Never exceed a total dosage of 300 mg/24 hr.

Anaphylaxis or phenothiazine overdose: 1 to 2 mg/kg IV slowly.

DOSE ADJUSTMENTS
Reduce dose for the elderly or debilitated. ▪ See Drug/Lab Interactions.

DILUTION
May be given undiluted.

Filters: No data available from manufacturer.

Storage: Store below 40° C (104° F), preferably between 15° and 30° C (59° and 86° F). Protect from light and freezing.

COMPATIBILITY
(Underline Indicates Conflicting Compatibility Information)
Consider any drug NOT listed as compatible to be INCOMPATIBLE until consulting a pharmacist; specific conditions may apply.

One source suggests the following **compatibilities:**

Additive: Amikacin, aminophylline, ascorbic acid, bleomycin (Blenoxane), colistimethate (Coly-Mycin M), erythromycin (Erythrocin), fat emulsion IV, lidocaine, methyldopa, nafcillin (Nallpen), penicillin G potassium and sodium.

Y-site: Abciximab (ReoPro), acetaminophen (Ofirmev), acyclovir (Zovirax), aldesleukin (Proleukin), amifostine (Ethyol), argatroban, azithromycin (Zithromax), aztreonam (Azactam), bivalirudin (Angiomax), caspofungin (Cancidas), ceftaroline (Teflaro), ciprofloxacin (Cipro IV), cisatracurium (Nimbex), cladribine (Leustatin), dexmedetomidine (Precedex), docetaxel (Taxotere), doripenem (Doribax), doxorubicin liposomal (Doxil), etoposide phosphate (Etopophos), famotidine (Pepcid IV), fenoldopam (Corlopam), fentanyl, filgrastim (Neupogen), fluconazole (Diflucan), fludarabine (Fludara), gallium nitrate (Ganite), gemcitabine (Gemzar), granisetron (Kytril), heparin, hetastarch in electrolytes (Hextend), hydrocortisone sodium succinate (Solu-Cortef), hydromorphone (Dilaudid), idarubicin (Idamycin), linezolid (Zyvox), melphalan (Alkeran), meperidine (Demerol), meropenem (Merrem IV), methadone (Dolophine), morphine, ondansetron (Zofran), oxaliplatin (Eloxatin), paclitaxel (Taxol), pemetrexed (Alimta), piperacillin/tazobactam (Zosyn), potassium chloride (KCl), propofol (Diprivan), remifentanil (Ultiva), sargramostim (Leukine), tacrolimus (Prograf), teniposide (Vumon), thiotepa, vinorelbine (Navelbine).

RATE OF ADMINISTRATION
25 mg or fraction thereof over 1 minute. Extend injection time in nonemergency situations and pediatric patients. See Maternal/Child.

ACTIONS
A potent antihistamine, it is capable of blocking the effects of histamine at various receptor sites, either eliminating a hypersensitivity reaction or greatly modifying it. It also has anticholinergic (antispasmodic), antiemetic, antivertigo, and sedative effects. It has rapid onset of action and is widely distributed throughout the body, including the CNS. A portion of this drug is metabolized in the liver; the rest is excreted unchanged in the urine. Half-life is 1 to 4 hours. Some secretion may occur in breast milk.

INDICATIONS AND USES
Allergic reactions to blood or plasma. ▪ Supplemental therapy to epinephrine in anaphylaxis and other uncomplicated allergic/hypersensitivity reactions requiring prompt treatment (e.g., angioedema, pruritus, urticaria). ▪ Preoperative or generalized sedation. ▪ Management of parkinsonism, including drug-induced (e.g., phenothiazines [e.g., prochlorperazine (Compazine)]). ▪ Severe nausea and vomiting. ▪ Motion sickness. ▪ To replace oral therapy when it is impractical or contraindicated.

CONTRAINDICATIONS
Breast-feeding, hypersensitivity to antihistamines, newborn or premature infants.

PRECAUTIONS
IV route used only in emergency situations. ▪ Avoid SC or perivascular injection. ▪ Use with extreme caution in infants, children, elderly or debilitated individuals, asthmatic attack, bladder neck obstruction, narrow-angle glaucoma, lower respiratory tract infections, prostatic hypertrophy, pyloroduodenal obstruction, and stenosing peptic ulcer.
Monitor: Will induce drowsiness. ▪ Monitor vital signs; observe closely. ▪ See Drug/Lab Interactions.
Patient Education: Do not drive or operate hazardous equipment until effects wear off. ▪ May cause drowsiness and dizziness; request help to ambulate. ▪ Avoid alcohol and other CNS depressants (e.g., diazepam [Valium], narcotics).
Maternal/Child: See Contraindications, Precautions, Monitor, and Side Effects. ▪ Category B: use only when clearly needed. May increase risk of abnormalities during the first trimester. ▪ Not recommended during breast-feeding. Small amounts may be distributed into breast milk, causing irritability or excitement in infants. ▪ Use extreme caution in infants and children; may cause hallucinations, convulsions, or death. May also reduce mental alertness and cause paradoxical excitation.
Elderly: See Dose Adjustments, Precautions, Monitor, and Side Effects. ▪ May cause confusion, dizziness, hyperexcitability, hypotension, and/or sedation. ▪ Sensitivity to anticholinergic effects is increased (e.g., blurred vision, constipation, dry mouth, urinary retention).

DRUG/LAB INTERACTIONS

Increases effectiveness of **epinephrine** and is often used in conjunction with it. ▪ Additive central nervous system effects with **alcohol, other CNS depressants** (e.g., hypnotics, sedatives, and tranquilizers), and **procarbazine** (Matulane). Reduced dose of potentiated drug may be indicated. ▪ **MAO inhibitors** (e.g., selegiline [Eldepryl]) prolong and intensify the anticholinergic (drying) effects of antihistamines. Concurrent use not recommended. ▪ Effectiveness of many drugs is reduced in combination with diphenhydramine because of increased metabolism. ▪ May inhibit the wheal and flare reaction to **antigen skin tests.**

SIDE EFFECTS

Rare when used as indicated: anaphylaxis; blurring of vision; confusion; constipation; diarrhea; difficulty in urination; diplopia; drowsiness; drug rash; dryness of mouth, nose, and throat; epigastric distress; headache; hemolytic anemia; hypotension; insomnia; nasal stuffiness; nausea; nervousness; palpitations; photosensitivity; rapid pulse; restlessness; thickening of bronchial secretions; tightness of the chest and wheezing; tingling, heaviness, weakness of hands; urticaria; vertigo; vomiting. Overdose may cause convulsions, hallucinations, and death in pediatric patients.

ANTIDOTE

For exaggerated drowsiness or other disturbing side effects, discontinue the drug and notify the physician. Side effects will usually subside within a few hours or may be treated symptomatically. Treat hypotension promptly; may lead to cardiovascular collapse. Use dopamine, norepinephrine, or phenylephrine. Epinephrine is contraindicated for hypotension; further hypotension will occur. Propranolol (Inderal) is the drug of choice for ventricular arrhythmias. Treat convulsions with diazepam (Valium) 0.1 mg/kg IV slowly. Some central anticholinergic effects may require physostigmine. Avoid analeptics (e.g., caffeine); may cause convulsions. Epinephrine must be available to treat anaphylaxis. Resuscitate as necessary.

DIPYRIDAMOLE
(dye-peer-**ID**-ah-mohl)

Coronary vasodilator
Diagnostic agent
Antiplatelet agent

Persantine

pH 2.2 to 3.2

USUAL DOSE
Myocardial perfusion imaging: 0.57 mg/kg of body weight equally distributed over 4 minutes (0.142 mg/kg/min). A 70-kg adult would receive a total dose of 39.9 mg (10 mg/min). Maximum dose is 60 mg. Thallium should be injected within 5 minutes following the 4-minute infusion of dipyridamole.

Antiplatelet agent (unlabeled): 250 mg/24 hr as an infusion.

DILUTION
Each 1 mL (5 mg) must be diluted with a minimum of 2 mL D5W, D5/^{1}/$_2$NS, or D5NS. Total volume should range from a minimum of 20 mL to 50 mL (39.9 mg [8 mL] would be diluted in a minimum of 16 mL for a total infusion of 24 mL; additional diluent can be used to facilitate titration). May not be given undiluted; will cause local irritation.

Antiplatelet agent: Each 250-mg dose should be diluted with 250 mL D5W (1 mg/mL). Concentration may be increased if larger doses required.

Storage: Undiluted drug should be stored at CRT and protected from direct light; avoid freezing.

COMPATIBILITY
Specific information not available. Consider specific use; consult pharmacist.

RATE OF ADMINISTRATION
A single dose must be equally distributed over 4 minutes (0.142 mg/kg/min).

Antiplatelet agent: 10 mg/hr as a continuous infusion. Use of a microdrip (60 gtt/mL) or infusion pump recommended.

ACTIONS
A coronary vasodilator that will cause an increase in coronary blood flow velocity of from 3.8 to 7 times greater than resting velocity. Action may result from the inhibition of adenosine uptake. Peak velocity is reached in 2.5 to 8.7 minutes. Will cause a 20% increase in HR and a mild but significant decrease in systolic and diastolic BP in the supine position. Vital signs may take up to 30 minutes to return to baseline measurements. Used in combination with thallium, visualization shows dilation with sustained enhanced flow of intact vessels, leaving reduced pressure and flow across areas of hemodynamically important coronary vascular constriction. Results achieved are comparable to exercise-induced thallium imaging. Metabolized in the liver. Excreted in bile. Secreted in breast milk.

INDICATIONS AND USES
An alternative to exercise in thallium myocardial perfusion imaging for the evaluation of coronary artery disease in patients who cannot exercise adequately.

Unlabeled uses: Prophylactic inhibition of platelet aggregation in thromboembolism and myocardial infarction.

CONTRAINDICATIONS
Hypersensitivity to dipyridamole.

PRECAUTIONS
Administered by or under the direction of the cardiologist. ▪ Full facilities for treatment of any airway problem, cardiac emergency, or hypersensitivity, including laboratory analysis, must be available. ▪ Theophylline (Aminophylline) and other emergency drugs must be immediately available. ▪ Patients with a history of unstable angina or a history of asthma may be at greater risk; use extreme caution. ▪ This drug has caused two fatal myocardial infarctions as well as other serious side effects in a small percentage of patients; clinical information to be gained must be weighed against risk to the patient.

Monitor: An IV line with a Y-tube or three-way stopcock must be in place. ▪ Monitor vital signs continuously during infusion and for at least 15 minutes after or until return to baseline. ▪ ECG monitoring using at least 1 chest lead should be continuous. ▪ Patient is usually in a supine position, but tests have been conducted in a sitting position. Lower to supine with head tilted down (Trendelenburg) if hypotension occurs.

Maternal/Child: Category B: safety for use during pregnancy not established. Use only if clearly needed. ▪ Temporarily discontinue breast-feeding. ▪ Safety for use in pediatric patients not established.

DRUG/LAB INTERACTIONS

Theophylline bronchodilators (e.g., aminophylline, oxtriphylline [Choledyl], theophylline) reverse the effect of dipyridamole on myocardial blood flow. Interferes with dipyridamole-assisted **myocardial perfusion studies.** Withhold bronchodilators for 36 hours before testing.

SIDE EFFECTS

BP lability, chest pain/angina pectoris, dizziness, dyspnea, ECG abnormalities (e.g., extrasystoles, ST-T changes, tachycardia), fatigue, flushing, headache, hypertension, hypotension, nausea, pain (unspecified), paresthesia. Numerous other side effects occur in less than 1% of patients.

Major: Bronchospasm, cerebral ischemia (transient), fatal and nonfatal myocardial infarction, ventricular fibrillation, ventricular tachycardia (symptomatic) occurred in 0.3% of patients.

ANTIDOTE

Physician will be present throughout test administration. Theophylline (Aminophylline) is an adenosine receptor antagonist and will reverse the adenosine-mediated effects of dipyridamole (e.g., angina pectoris, bronchospasm, severe hypotension, ventricular arrhythmias). If bronchospasm or chest pain occurs, administer 50 to 250 mg of theophylline at a rate not to exceed 50 mg over 30 seconds. If symptoms are not relieved by 250 mg of theophylline, sublingual nitroglycerin may be helpful. Persistent chest pain may indicate impending potentially fatal myocardial infarction. If patient condition permits, thallium may be injected and allowed to circulate for 1 minute before injection of theophylline; this will permit initial thallium perfusion imaging before reversal of vasodilatory effects of dipyridamole on coronary circulation. Use head-down supine position for hypotension before administering theophylline. After reversal of vasodilatory action, treat arrhythmias as indicated. Resuscitate as necessary.

DOBUTAMINE HYDROCHLORIDE
(doh-**BYOU**-tah-meen hy-droh-**KLOR**-eyed)

Inotropic agent
Cardiac stimulant

pH 2.5 to 5.5

USUAL DOSE
0.5 to 1 mcg/kg/min initially in patients likely to respond to minimum treatment. The usual effective initial dose ranges from 2.5 to 15 mcg/kg of body weight/min. AHA guidelines suggest 2 to 20 mcg/kg/min. Gradually adjust rate at 2- to 10-minute intervals to effect desired response. AHA guidelines recommend titrating so HR does not increase by more than 10% of baseline. Up to 40 mcg/kg/min has been used in some instances; increases potential for toxicity (e.g., myocardial ischemia). U.S. experience in controlled trials does not extend beyond 48 hours of therapy.

PEDIATRIC DOSE
2 to 20 mcg/kg/min. Initial dose usually 5 to 10 mcg/kg/min. Adjust rate to effect desired response; see Maternal/Child.

DOSE ADJUSTMENTS
Lower-end initial doses may be appropriate in the elderly based on potential for decreased organ function, concomitant disease, or other drug therapy. See Drug/Lab Interactions.

DILUTION
Available prediluted in D5W, or each 250-mg (20-mL) vial must be further diluted to at least 50 mL. Any amount of infusion solution desired above 50 mL may be used (250 mg in 1 L equals 250 mcg/mL; 250 mg in 500 mL equals 500 mcg/mL; 250 mg in 250 mL equals 1,000 mcg/mL). Adjust to fluid requirements of the patient. **Compatible** with D5W, D10W, D5/½NS, D5NS, D5/Isolyte M, LR, D5LR, Normosol-M in D5W, 20% Osmitrol in water, NS, or sodium lactate.

Filters: No data available from manufacturer. Another source suggests no significant drug loss through a 0.22-micron cellulose ester membrane filter.

Storage: When mixed in infusion solution, use within 24 hours. Pink coloring of solution does not affect potency; will crystallize if frozen.

COMPATIBILITY
(Underline Indicates Conflicting Compatibility Information)

Consider any drug NOT listed as compatible to be INCOMPATIBLE until consulting a pharmacist; specific conditions may apply.

Manufacturer states, "Do not add to sodium bicarbonate or any other strongly alkaline solution" (e.g., aminophylline, barbiturates [e.g., phenobarbital (Luminal)]). Manufacturer recommends not using other drugs as additives, not using in conjunction with other agents, and not using with diluents containing both sodium bisulfate and ethanol.

One source suggests the following **compatibilities:**

Additive: *Not recommended by manufacturer.* Amiodarone (Nexterone), atracurium (Tracrium), atropine, calcium chloride, ciprofloxacin (Cipro IV), dopamine, enalaprilat (Vasotec IV), epinephrine (Adrenalin), flumazenil (Romazicon), heparin, hydralazine, isoproterenol (Isuprel), lidocaine, meperidine (Demerol), meropenem (Merrem IV), morphine, nitroglycerin IV, norepinephrine (Levophed), phentolamine (Regitine), phenylephrine (Neo-Synephrine), potassium chloride (KCl), procainamide (Pronestyl), propranolol (Inderal), ranitidine (Zantac), verapamil, zidovudine (AZT, Retrovir).

Y-site: *Not recommended by manufacturer.* Alprostadil, amifostine (Ethyol), amiodarone (Nexterone), anidulafungin (Eraxis), argatroban, atracurium (Tracrium), aztreonam (Azactam), bivalirudin (Angiomax), calcium chloride, calcium gluconate, caspofungin (Cancidas), cefepime (Maxipime), ceftaroline (Teflaro), ceftazidime (Fortaz), ciprofloxacin (Cipro IV), cisatracurium (Nimbex), cladribine (Leustatin), dexmedetomidine (Precedex), diazepam (Valium), diltiazem (Cardizem), docetaxel (Taxotere), dopamine, doripenem (Doribax), doxorubicin liposomal (Doxil), enalaprilat (Vasotec IV), epinephrine (Adrenalin), etoposide phosphate (Etopophos), famotidine (Pepcid IV), fenoldopam (Corlopam), fentanyl, fluconazole (Diflucan), furosemide (Lasix), gemcitabine (Gemzar), granisetron (Kytril), heparin, hetastarch in electrolytes (Hextend), hydromorphone (Dilaudid), 6% hydroxyethyl starch (Voluven), insulin (regular), labetalol, levofloxacin (Levaquin), lidocaine, linezolid (Zyvox), lorazepam (Ativan), magnesium sulfate, meperidine (Demerol), midazolam (Versed), milrinone (Primacor), morphine, nicardipine (Cardene IV), nitroglycerin IV, nitroprusside sodium, norepinephrine (Levophed), oxaliplatin (Eloxatin), pancuronium, potassium chloride (KCl), propofol (Diprivan), ranitidine (Zantac), remifentanil (Ultiva), tacrolimus (Prograf), telavancin (Vibativ), theophylline, thiotepa, tigecycline (Tygacil), tirofiban (Aggrastat), vasopressin, vecuronium, verapamil, zidovudine (AZT, Retrovir).

RATE OF ADMINISTRATION

Begin with recommended dose for body weight and seriousness of condition. Gradually increase to effect desired response. May take up to 10 minutes to achieve peak effect of a specific dose. Maintain at correct therapeutic level with microdrip (60 gtt/mL) or infusion pump. Half-life of dobutamine is only about 2 minutes. See Maternal/Child.

Infusion Rate (mL/hr) for Dobutamine 500 mcg/mL											
	Patient's Weight (kg)										
Drug Delivery Rate (mcg/kg/min)	5	10	20	30	40	50	60	70	80	90	100	110
0.5	0.3	0.6	1.2	1.8	2.4	3	3.6	4.2	4.8	5.4	6	6.6
1	0.6	1.2	2.4	3.6	4.8	6	7.2	8.4	9.6	11	12	13
2.5	1.5	3	6	9	12	15	18	21	24	27	30	33
5	3	6	12	18	24	30	36	42	48	54	60	66
7.5	4.5	9	18	27	36	45	54	63	72	81	90	99
10	6	12	24	36	48	60	72	84	96	108	120	132
12.5	7.5	15	30	45	60	75	90	105	120	135	150	165
15	9	18	36	54	72	90	108	126	144	162	180	198
17.5	11	21	42	63	84	105	126	147	168	189	210	231
20	12	24	48	72	96	120	144	168	192	216	240	264

Infusion Rate (mL/hr) for Dobutamine 1,000 mcg/mL												
	Patient's Weight (kg)											
Drug Delivery Rate (mcg/kg/min)	5	10	20	30	40	50	60	70	80	90	100	110
0.5	0.15	0.3	0.6	0.9	1.2	1.5	1.8	2.1	2.4	2.7	3	3.3
1	0.3	0.6	1.2	1.8	2.4	3	3.6	4.2	4.8	5.4	6	6.6
2.5	0.75	1.5	3	4.5	6	7.5	9	11	12	14	15	17
5	1.5	3	6	9	12	15	18	21	24	27	30	33
7.5	2.3	4.5	9	14	18	23	27	32	36	41	45	50
10	3	6	12	18	24	30	36	42	48	54	60	66
12.5	3.8	7.5	15	23	30	38	45	53	60	68	75	83
15	4.5	9	18	27	36	45	54	63	72	81	90	99
17.5	5.3	11	21	32	42	53	63	74	84	95	105	116
20	6	12	24	36	48	60	72	84	96	108	120	132

Infusion Rate (mL/hr) for Dobutamine 2,000 mcg/mL												
	Patient's Weight (kg)											
Drug Delivery Rate (mcg/kg/min)	5	10	20	30	40	50	60	70	80	90	100	110
0.5	0.08	0.15	0.3	0.45	0.6	0.75	0.9	1.1	1.2	1.4	1.5	1.7
1	0.15	0.3	0.6	0.9	1.2	1.5	1.8	2.1	2.4	2.7	3	3.3
2.5	0.38	0.75	1.5	2.3	3	3.8	4.5	5.3	6	6.8	7.5	8.3
5	0.75	1.5	3	4.5	6	7.5	9	11	12	14	15	17
7.5	1.1	2.3	4.5	6.8	9	11	14	16	18	20	23	25
10	1.5	3	6	9	12	15	18	21	24	27	30	33
12.5	1.9	3.8	7.5	11	15	19	23	26	30	34	38	41
15	2.3	4.5	9	14	18	23	27	32	37	41	45	50
17.5	2.6	5.3	11	16	21	26	32	37	42	47	53	58
20	3	6	12	18	24	30	36	42	48	54	60	66

ACTIONS

A synthetic catecholamine chemically related to dopamine, it is a direct-acting inotropic agent possessing beta-stimulator activity. Induces short-term increases in cardiac output by improving stroke volume with minimum increases in rate and BP, minimum rhythm disturbances, and decreased peripheral vascular resistance. Usually most effective for only a few hours. May improve atrioventricular conduction. Peak effect obtained in 2 to 10 minutes. Has a very short duration of action. Half-life is 2 minutes; may be up to 5 minutes in preterm infants. Metabolized in the liver and other tissues. Metabolites are primarily excreted in the urine.

INDICATIONS AND USES

Short-term inotropic support in cardiac decompensation resulting from depressed contractility (organic heart disease or cardiac surgical procedures).

Unlabeled uses: Increase cardiac output in pediatric patients with congenital heart disease undergoing cardiac catheterization.

CONTRAINDICATIONS
Hypersensitivity to any components (contains sulfites), idiopathic hypertrophic subaortic stenosis, shock without adequate fluid replacement.

PRECAUTIONS
Use extreme caution in myocardial infarction; increases in HR of more than 10% may increase myocardial ischemia and size of infarction. ▪ Contains sulfites; use caution in patients with allergies. ▪ Precipitous hypotension occurs rarely; usually reverses with a decrease in rate of administration; see Antidote. ▪ Ineffective if marked mechanical obstruction (e.g., severe valvular aortic stenosis) is present. ▪ Use for long-term treatment of CHF has been associated with increased risks of hospitalization and death.
Monitor: Correct hypovolemia and acidosis as indicated before initiating treatment. ▪ Observe patient's response continuously; monitor HR, ectopic activity, BP, and urine flow. Measure pulmonary wedge pressure, central venous pressure, and cardiac output if possible. ▪ May cause significant increase in BP or HR, especially systolic pressure. Patients with pre-existing hypertension may be at increased risk of developing an increased pressor response. ▪ Monitor for changes in fluid balance, electrolytes, and acid-base balance. ▪ Use digoxin preparation before starting dobutamine in patients with atrial fibrillation with rapid ventricular response. ▪ See Drug/Lab Interactions.
Maternal/Child: Category B: use only if benefits outweigh risks. Safety for use in pregnancy, breast-feeding, and pediatric patients not established. ▪ Increases cardiac output and systemic BP in pediatric patients of every age-group, usually at infusion rates that are lower than those that cause significant tachycardia. Less effective than dopamine in premature neonates.
Elderly: Lower-end initial doses may be indicated; see Dose Adjustments. ▪ Differences in response compared to younger adults not identified, but greater sensitivity of some elderly cannot be ruled out.

DRUG/LAB INTERACTIONS
May be ineffective if **beta-blocking drugs** (e.g., propranolol [Inderal]) have been given. ▪ Produces higher cardiac output and lower pulmonary wedge pressure when given concomitantly with **nitroprusside sodium.** ▪ May cause serious arrhythmias in presence of **cyclopropane or halogen anesthetics,** severe hypertension with **oxytocic drugs, or guanethidine** (Ismelin). ▪ Pressor response increased with **tricyclic antidepressants** (e.g., amitriptyline [Elavil], imipramine [Tofranil]) and **rauwolfia alkaloids** (e.g., reserpine); may cause hypertension. ▪ Has been given concurrently without evidence of drug interaction with acetaminophen (Tylenol), atropine, digoxin preparations, folic acid, furosemide, glyceryl trinitrate (nitroglycerin), heparin, isosorbide dinitrate (Iso-Bid), lidocaine, morphine, potassium chloride, protamine, and spironolactone (Aldactone).

SIDE EFFECTS
Anginal pain, chest pain, headache, hypertension, hypokalemia, increased ventricular ectopic activity, myocardial ischemia, nausea, palpitations, shortness of breath, tachycardia. Hypersensitivity reactions (e.g., bronchospasm, eosinophilia, fever, skin rash) have been reported. Local inflammatory changes may occur with infiltration.
Overdose: In addition to all of the above, overdose may cause anorexia, anxiety, excessive hypertension or hypotension, myocardial ischemia, tremor, ventricular tachycardia, and/or fibrillation.

ANTIDOTE
Notify physician of all side effects. Decrease infusion rate and notify physician immediately if number of PVCs increases or there is a marked increase in pulse rate (30 or more beats) or BP (50 or more mm Hg systolic). For accidental overdose, reduce rate or temporarily discontinue until condition stabilizes. Maintain a patent airway with adequate oxygenation and ventilation. Treat ventricular tachyarrhythmias with propranolol (Inderal) or lidocaine. Hypertension usually responds to a reduced rate or temporarily discontinuing dobutamine. Reduce rate or discontinue dobutamine if hypotension occurs. May require treatment with vasopressors (e.g., dopamine, norepinephrine). See Precautions.

DOCETAXEL BBW

(doh-seh-**TAX**-ell)

Docefrez, Taxotere

Antineoplastic agent
(taxane)

USUAL DOSE

Premedication for all patients except those with hormone-refractory prostate cancer: Must be pretreated with oral corticosteroids to reduce the incidence and severity of fluid retention and hypersensitivity reactions. Usual regimen is dexamethasone (Decadron) 8 mg PO twice a day for 3 days. Begin 1 day before each docetaxel infusion.

Premedication for hormone-refractory prostate cancer: Administer oral dexamethasone 8 mg at 12 hours, 3 hours, and 1 hour before each docetaxel infusion (another steroid, prednisone, is part of the combination therapy).

Breast cancer: 60 to 100 mg/M^2 as an infusion. Repeat every 3 weeks.

Combination therapy for adjuvant treatment of operable node-positive breast cancer: 75 mg/M^2 as an infusion. Administer 1 hour after doxorubicin 50 mg/M^2 and cyclophosphamide 500 mg/M^2. Repeat every 3 weeks for 6 cycles. Prophylactic G-CSF (e.g., filgrastim [Neupogen]) may be used to mitigate the risk of hematologic toxicity. See doxorubicin and cyclophosphamide monographs.

Prostate cancer (hormone refractory): 75 mg/M^2 as an infusion. Repeat every 3 weeks. Prednisone 5 mg PO twice daily is administered continuously throughout treatment. See Premedication.

First-line treatment of non–small-cell lung cancer (NSCLC): 75 mg/M^2 as an infusion over 1 hour. Follow immediately with cisplatin 75 mg/M^2 as an infusion over 30 to 60 minutes. Repeat regimen every 3 weeks. *Premedicate* with antiemetics and hydration as required for cisplatin administration; see cisplatin monograph.

NSCLC after failure of prior chemotherapy: 75 mg/M^2 as an infusion. Repeat every 3 weeks. Larger doses increased toxicity, infection, and treatment-related mortality.

Gastric adenocarcinoma: 75 mg/M^2 as an infusion over 1 hour. Follow immediately with cisplatin 75 mg/M^2 as an infusion over 1 to 3 hours (both on Day 1 only). *Premedicate* with antiemetics and hydration as required for cisplatin administration; see cisplatin and fluorouracil monographs. Follow the cisplatin infusion with fluorouracil 750 mg/M^2 as an infusion equally distributed over 24 hours. Repeat fluorouracil dose for 4 more 24-hour infusions (total of 5 days). Repeat regimen every 3 weeks. In the study, G-CSF (filgrastim [Neupogen]) was recommended during the second and/or subsequent cycles to prevent or attenuate febrile neutropenia, documented infection with neutropenia, or neutropenia lasting more than 7 days.

Induction chemotherapy followed by radiotherapy for treatment of inoperable, locally advanced squamous cell cancer of the head and neck (SCCHN): 75 mg/M^2 as an infusion over 1 hour. Follow immediately with cisplatin 75 mg/M^2 as an infusion over 1 hour (both on Day 1 only). *Premedicate* with antiemetics and hydration as required for cisplatin administration; see cisplatin monograph. Follow the cisplatin infusion with fluorouracil 750 mg/M^2 as an infusion equally distributed over 24 hours. Repeat fluorouracil for four more 24-hour infusions (total of 5 days). See fluorouracil monograph. Repeat regimen every 3 weeks for a total of four cycles. Prophylactic antibiotics were used in clinical studies. Following chemotherapy, patients should receive radiotherapy.

Induction chemotherapy followed by chemoradiotherapy for treatment of locally advanced (un-resectable, low surgical cure, or organ preservation) SCCHN: 75 mg/M^2 as an infusion over 1 hour. Follow with cisplatin 100 mg/M^2 as a 30-minute to 3-hour infusion (both on Day 1 only). *Premedicate* with antiemetics and hydration as required for cisplatin administration; see cisplatin monograph. Follow the cisplatin infusion with fluorouracil 1,000 mg/M^2 as an infusion equally distributed over 24 hours. Repeat fluorouracil for three more 24-hour infusions (total of 4 days). See fluorouracil monograph. Repeat regimen every 3 weeks for 3 cycles. Prophylactic antibiotics were used in clinical studies. Following chemotherapy, patients should receive chemoradiotherapy.

Treatment of ovarian cancer (unlabeled): 60 to 75 mg/M^2 as an infusion in combination with carboplatin. Repeat every 3 weeks.

Metastatic bladder cancer (unlabeled): 100 mg/M^2 every 3 weeks as a single agent or 35 mg/M^2 on Days 1 and 8 of a 21-day cycle in combination with gemcitabine and cisplatin. Administer for at least 6 cycles or until disease progression or unacceptable toxicity.

Treatment of esophageal cancer (unlabeled): 75 mg/M^2 as a 1-hour infusion every 21 days used in combination with fluorouracil and cisplatin.

DOSE ADJUSTMENTS

All diagnoses: Withhold therapy if neutrophils below 1,500/mm^3 or platelets below 100,000 cells/mm^3. A 25% reduction in the dose of docetaxel is recommended during subsequent cycles following severe neutropenia (less than 500/mm^3) lasting 7 days or more, febrile neutropenia, or a Grade 4 infection. ▪ Withhold therapy if bilirubin is greater than the ULN or if AST and/or ALT is greater than 1.5 times the ULN concomitant with alkaline phosphatase greater than 2.5 times the ULN. ▪ Discontinue therapy in patients who develop Grade 3 or higher peripheral neuropathy. ▪ Dose selection should be cautious in the elderly. Reduced doses may be indicated based on the potential for decreased organ function and concomitant disease or drug therapy. ▪ Consider additional dose adjustments when docetaxel is given in combination with other chemotherapeutic agents. ▪ See Precautions and Drug/Lab Interactions.

Breast cancer: Reduce dose to 75 mg/M^2 for patients initially dosed at 100 mg/M^2 who experience febrile neutropenia, severe neutropenia (neutrophils below 500/mm^3 for more than 1 week), severe or cumulative cutaneous reaction, or severe peripheral neuropathy. Further reduce to 55 mg/M^2 or discontinue docetaxel if any of the previously listed reactions persist. ▪ Patients receiving the lower dose of docetaxel (60 mg/M^2) may have the dose increased gradually if lower dose was well tolerated. ▪ Discontinue therapy in patients who develop Grade 3 or greater peripheral neuropathy.

Combination therapy for adjuvant treatment of operable node-positive breast cancer: Patients who experience febrile neutropenia should receive G-CSF (e.g., filgrastim [Neupogen]) in all subsequent cycles. Patients who continue to experience this reaction should remain on G-CSF and have their docetaxel dose decreased to 60 mg/M^2. ▪ Reduce docetaxel dose to 60 mg/M^2 in patients who experience Grade 3 or 4 stomatitis. ▪ Reduce docetaxel dose from 75 to 60 mg/M^2 in patients who experience severe or cumulative cutaneous reactions or moderate neurosensory signs and/or symptoms. If side effects persist at the lower dose, discontinue therapy.

Prostate cancer: Reduce Taxotere dose from 75 to 60 mg/M^2 in patients who experience dose-limiting toxicities (e.g., febrile neutropenia, neutrophils less than 500 cells/mm^3 for more than 1 week, severe or cumulative cutaneous reactions, or moderate neurosensory signs and/or symptoms). If side effects persist at the lower dose, discontinue therapy.

Non–small-cell lung cancer after failure of prior chemotherapy: In NSCLC patients who experience either febrile neutropenia, neutrophils less than 500 cells/mm^3 for more than 1 week, severe or cumulative cutaneous reactions, or other Grade 3 or 4 nonhematologic toxicities, withhold docetaxel until resolution of toxicity, then resume at 55 mg/M^2. ▪ Discontinue therapy in patients who develop Grade 3 or greater peripheral neuropathy.

First-line treatment of NSCLC: Reduce dose to 65 mg/M^2 in patients whose nadir of platelet count during the previous course of therapy was less than 25,000 cells/mm^3, in patients who experienced febrile neutropenia, and in patients with serious nonhematologic toxicities. Dose may be further reduced to 50 mg/M^2 as indicated. See cisplatin monograph for cisplatin dose adjustments.

Gastric adenocarcinoma and head and neck cancer: Patients who experience febrile neutropenia, documented infection with neutropenia, or neutropenia lasting more than 7 days

Continued

should receive G-CSF (e.g., filgrastim [Neupogen]) in all subsequent cycles. Patients who continue to experience this reaction should remain on G-CSF and have their Taxotere dose decreased to 60 mg/M^2. Reduce dose further to 45 mg/M^2 if subsequent episodes of complicated neutropenia occur. ▪ Reduce Taxotere dose from 75 to 60 mg/M^2 in patients who experience Grade 4 thrombocytopenia. ▪ If the previously mentioned toxicities persist, discontinue therapy. ▪ Additional dose adjustments are outlined in the following chart.

Additional Recommended Dose Adjustments for Toxicities in Gastric Adenocarcinoma or Head and Neck Cancer Patients Treated with Docetaxel in Combination with Cisplatin and Fluorouracil	
Toxicity	Dose Adjustment
Diarrhea Grade 3	**First episode:** Reduce 5-FU dose by 20%. **Second episode:** Reduce docetaxel dose by 20%.
Diarrhea Grade 4	**First episode:** Reduce docetaxel and 5-FU doses by 20%. **Second episode:** Discontinue treatment.
Stomatitis Grade 3	**First episode:** Reduce 5-FU dose by 20%. **Second episode:** Stop 5-FU only at all subsequent cycles. **Third episode:** Reduce docetaxel dose by 20%.
Stomatitis Grade 4	**First episode:** Stop 5-FU only at all subsequent cycles. **Second episode:** Reduce docetaxel dose by 20%.
AST/ALT >2.5 to ≤5 × ULN and AP ≤2.5 × ULN, or AST/ALT >1.5 to ≤5 × ULN and AP >2.5 to ≤5 × ULN	Reduce docetaxel dose by 20%.
AST/ALT >5 × ULN and/or AP >5 × ULN	Discontinue docetaxel.
Peripheral neuropathy Grade 2	Reduce cisplatin dose by 20%.
Peripheral neuropathy Grade 3	Discontinue cisplatin treatment.
Ototoxicity Grade 3	Discontinue cisplatin treatment.
Rise in SCr ≥ Grade 2 (>1.5 × normal value) despite adequate rehydration	Determine CrCl before each subsequent cycle and consider the following dose reductions as outlined below.
CrCl ≥60 mL/min	Full dose of cisplatin given. Repeat CrCl before each treatment cycle.
CrCl >40 and <60 mL/min	Reduce dose of cisplatin by 50% at subsequent cycle. If CrCl was >60 mL/min at end of cycle, give full dose at the next cycle. If no recovery observed, omit cisplatin from the next treatment cycle.
CrCl <40 mL/min	Omit dose of cisplatin for **that treatment cycle only.** Discontinue cisplatin if CrCl remains at <40 mL/min. Reduce cisplatin dose by 50% if CrCl was >40 and <60 mL/min at end of cycle. Give full cisplatin dose if CrCl is >60 mL/min at end of cycle.
Plantar-palmar toxicity Grade 2 or greater	Discontinue fluorouracil until recovery, then reduce fluorouracil dose by 20%.
Other greater than Grade 3 toxicities except alopecia and anemia	Delay 5-FU chemotherapy (for a maximum of 2 weeks from the planned date of infusion) until resolution to ≤Grade 1. If medically appropriate, resume treatment.

DILUTION
Specific techniques required; see Precautions. If Taxotere or diluted solution comes into contact with skin, immediately and thoroughly wash with soap and water. If Taxotere or diluted solution comes into contact with mucosa, immediately and thoroughly wash with water.

Available in multiple formulations and in *several concentrations; read label carefully.* Formulations are *NOT* interchangeable in a dose. *Do not use the two-vial formulation (injection concentrate and diluent [contains 13% ethanol in water for injection]) with the one-vial formulation. Read prescribing information carefully for product-specific dilution, storage, and stability information.* Recently approved in a nonalcohol formula in a single-dose vial; specific product information not available at time of printing.

Single-bottle formulations (generic and Taxotere): Available in 10 mg/mL and 20 mg/mL concentrations in multiple sizes. Manually rotate to mix thoroughly. Requires no initial dilution and is ready to add to an infusion solution; *read label carefully* to avoid overdose. Allow required number of vials to stand at room temperature for 5 minutes if refrigerated. Using a 21-gauge needle, withdraw required amount of concentrate and inject into a 250-mL infusion bag or bottle of NS or D5W; *see all formulations below.* Manually rotate to mix thoroughly.

Two-vial formulation (generic): Available in 20 mg/0.5 mL or in 80 mg/2 mL vials *(concentration is 4 times greater than the single-bottle formulation; read label carefully).* Allow required number of vials to stand at room temperature for 5 minutes if refrigerated. Reconstitute the appropriate vial (20 or 80 mg) with the entire contents of the diluent vial. Resulting concentration is 10 mg/mL. Mix well by repeated inversions for at least 45 seconds. *Do not shake.* Allow to stand until most of the foam dissipates. After this initial reconstitution, withdraw the required amount of 10 mg/mL concentrate and inject into a 250-mL bag or bottle of NS or D5W; *see all formulations below.*

Docefrez (lyophilized powder): Available as 20 mg/vial and 80 mg/vial with diluent (35.4% ethanol in polysorbate 80) provided by manufacturer. Allow required number of vials to stand at room temperature for 5 minutes. Using a syringe with an 18- to 21-gauge, 1½-inch needle, withdraw the required amount of diluent. Reconstitute the 20-mg vial with 1 mL from its diluent vial (concentration is 25 mg/mL or 20 mg/0.8 mL), and reconstitute the 80-mg vial with 4 mL from its diluent vial (concentration is 24 mg/mL). *These concentrations differ from other formulations; read label carefully.* Shake reconstituted vial well to completely dissolve the powder. Solution should be clear but may have some air bubbles due to the polysorbate 80. Allow reconstituted solution to stand for a few minutes to allow any air bubbles to dissipate. Reconstituted solution may be used immediately or stored at RT or in the refrigerator for a maximum of 8 hours. Reconstituted solution is supersaturated and therefore may crystallize over time. If crystals appear, the solution must not be used and should be discarded. After this initial reconstitution, withdraw the required dose and inject into a 250-mL bag or bottle of NS or D5W; *see all formulations below.*

All formulations: Final dilution should be in glass or polypropylene bottles or polypropylene or polyolefin plastic bags for infusion. Thoroughly mix the infusion by manual rotation. Should be administered through polyethylene-lined administration sets. Desired concentration should be between 0.3 and 0.74 mg/mL (100 mg in 250 mL = 0.4 mg/mL). If a dose greater than 200 mg is required, use a larger volume of NS or D5W so that a final concentration of 0.74 mg/mL is not exceeded. Solution should be clear.

Filters: Not required. Manufacturer indicates that studies show no loss of potency with in-line filtration through a 0.22-micron filter.

Storage: *Storage requirements and stability are brand specific; check prescribing information.* Storage requirements are manufacturer dependent. Some products may be stored at RT. Others require refrigeration.

Most formulations: Most formulations when fully diluted in NS or D5W should be used within 4 hours (including the 1-hour infusion time). **Taxotere** (one-vial formulation) and **Docefrez** are stable for 6 hours (including the 1-hour infusion time). At least one generic product is available as a multiple-dose vial that is stable for 28 days when refrigerated.

COMPATIBILITY

Consider any drug NOT listed as compatible to be INCOMPATIBLE until consulting a pharmacist; specific conditions may apply.

Leaches out plasticizers, including DEHP, from PVC infusion bags and administration sets. Use glass or polypropylene bottles or plastic (polypropylene or polyolefin) bags and polyethylene-lined administration sets to minimize patient exposure to leached DEHP. Do not allow concentrate to come into contact with plasticized PVC equipment or devices used to prepare solutions.

One source suggests the following **compatibilities:**

Y-site: Acyclovir (Zovirax), amifostine (Ethyol), amikacin, aminophylline, ampicillin, ampicillin/sulbactam (Unasyn), anidulafungin (Eraxis), aztreonam (Azactam), bumetanide, buprenorphine (Buprenex), butorphanol (Stadol), calcium gluconate, cefazolin (Ancef), cefepime (Maxipime), cefotaxime (Claforan), cefotetan, cefoxitin (Mefoxin), ceftazidime (Fortaz), ceftriaxone (Rocephin), cefuroxime (Zinacef), chlorpromazine (Thorazine), ciprofloxacin (Cipro IV), clindamycin (Cleocin), dexamethasone (Decadron), diphenhydramine (Benadryl), dobutamine, dopamine, doripenem (Doribax), doxycycline, droperidol (Inapsine), enalaprilat (Vasotec IV), famotidine (Pepcid IV), fluconazole (Diflucan), furosemide (Lasix), ganciclovir (Cytovene IV), gemcitabine (Gemzar), gentamicin, granisetron (Kytril), heparin, hydrocortisone sodium succinate (Solu-Cortef), hydromorphone (Dilaudid), imipenem-cilastatin (Primaxin), leucovorin calcium, lorazepam (Ativan), magnesium sulfate, mannitol, meperidine (Demerol), meropenem (Merrem IV), mesna (Mesnex), metoclopramide (Reglan), metronidazole (Flagyl IV), morphine, ondansetron (Zofran), oxaliplatin (Eloxatin), palonosetron (Aloxi), pemetrexed (Alimta), piperacillin/tazobactam (Zosyn), potassium chloride (KCl), prochlorperazine (Compazine), promethazine (Phenergan), ranitidine (Zantac), sodium bicarbonate, sulfamethoxazole/trimethoprim, ticarcillin/clavulanate (Timentin), tobramycin, vancomycin, zidovudine (AZT, Retrovir).

RATE OF ADMINISTRATION
A single dose, properly diluted, equally distributed over 1 hour. Room temperature should be cool and lighting should be low.

ACTIONS
An antineoplastic. A novel, semisynthetic, antimicrotubule agent derived from the needles of the yew plant. It inhibits cancer cell division. Microtubules assemble and disassemble during the cell cycle. Docetaxel promotes assembly and blocks disassembly of microtubules, preventing the cancer cells from dividing. The end result is cancer cell death. Highly protein bound. Probably metabolized in the liver by CYP3A4, an isoenzyme of the P_{450} family. Half-life is 11.1 hours. Eliminated primarily through feces and, to a lesser extent, urine and bile.

INDICATIONS AND USES
Treatment of locally advanced or metastatic breast cancer after failure of prior chemotherapy. ▪ In combination with doxorubicin and cyclophosphamide for adjuvant treatment of operable node-positive breast cancer. ▪ As a single agent in the treatment of locally advanced or metastatic NSCLC after failure of platinum-based chemotherapy (e.g., cisplatin). ▪ In combination with cisplatin for treatment of patients with unresectable, locally advanced, or metastatic NSCLC who have not previously received chemotherapy for this condition. ▪ In combination with prednisone for the treatment of androgen-independent (hormone refractory) metastatic prostate cancer. ▪ In combination with cisplatin and fluorouracil for the treatment of advanced gastric adenocarcinoma, including adenocarcinoma of the gastroesophageal junction, in patients who have not received prior chemotherapy for advanced disease. ▪ In combination with cisplatin and fluorouracil for induction therapy of locally advanced SCCHN. Following chemotherapy, patients should receive radiotherapy.

Unlabeled uses: Treatment of metastatic bladder cancer, esophageal cancer, ovarian cancer, soft tissue sarcomas, and adenocarcinomas of unknown primary site; consult literature.

CONTRAINDICATIONS

Baseline neutropenia less than 1,500 cells/mm³, history of hypersensitivity reactions to docetaxel or other drugs formulated with polysorbate 80, severe impaired liver function. In the United States, docetaxel is not recommended for patients with a bilirubin above the ULN or in patients with ALT and/or AST greater than 1.5 times the ULN range and increases in alkaline phosphatase greater than 2.5 times the ULN range; see Precautions.

PRECAUTIONS

Follow guidelines for handling cytotoxic agents. See Appendix A, p. 1331. ▪ Usually administered by or under the direction of the physician specialist. ▪ Adequate diagnostic and treatment facilities must be readily available. ▪ Reversible myelosuppression is the major dose-limiting toxicity of docetaxel. The median time to nadir was 7 days, and the median duration of severe neutropenia (<500 cells/mm³) was 7 days. Myelosuppression may be more frequent and more severe in patients who have received prior cytotoxic drug therapy or radiation therapy. ▪ Incidence of febrile neutropenia and/or neutropenic infection increased in patients receiving docetaxel (Taxotere) in combination with cisplatin and fluorouracil (5-FU). ▪ Incidence of mortality increased in patients with abnormal liver function, in patients receiving higher doses, and in patients with NSCLC and a history of prior treatment with platinum-based chemotherapy who receive docetaxel as a single agent at a dose of 100 mg/M². ▪ Patients with elevations of bilirubin or abnormalities of transaminase concurrent with alkaline phosphatase are at increased risk for the development of Grade 4 neutropenia, febrile neutropenia, infections, severe thrombocytopenia, severe stomatitis, severe skin toxicity, and toxic death. ▪ Not recommended for patients with hepatic impairment; see Contraindications. Risk of toxicity and death is significant. Patients with isolated elevations of transaminases greater than 1.5 times the ULN have a higher rate of adverse events but not of death. Alcohol content should be considered if given to patients with hepatic impairment. ▪ Severe hypersensitivity reactions characterized by generalized rash/erythema, hypotension and/or bronchospasm or, rarely, fatal anaphylaxis have been reported. ▪ In addition to myelosuppression and hypersensitivity reactions, localized erythema of the extremities with edema followed by desquamation, severe fluid retention, severe neurosensory symptoms (e.g., dysesthesia, pain, paresthesia), and severe asthenia (usually in metastatic breast cancer patients) has been reported. ▪ Severe fluid retention may occur despite premedication with dexamethasone. ▪ Use with caution in patients with pleural effusion; may be exacerbated by docetaxel-induced fluid retention. ▪ Treatment-related acute myeloid leukemia (AML) or myelodysplasia has occurred in patients given docetaxel in combination with other chemotherapy agents and/or radiotherapy. ▪ Cystoid macular edema (CME) has been reported; see Monitor. ▪ Cases of intoxication have been reported with some formulations of docetaxel due to the alcohol content. Alcohol content may affect the CNS and should be considered in patients in whom alcohol intake should be avoided or minimized. May affect ability to drive or use machinery immediately after the infusion. ▪ When administering combination therapy, consult all appropriate drug monographs for relevant information. ▪ See Drug/Lab Interactions.

Monitor: Obtain baseline CBC with differential and platelets; monitor frequently during therapy and before each dose. See Dose Adjustments. ▪ Obtain baseline bilirubin, AST, ALT, and alkaline phosphatase; monitor as indicated during therapy (recommended before each dose). ▪ Determine absolute patency of vein. A stinging or burning sensation indicates extravasation; discontinue injection; use another vein. ▪ Obtain baseline vital signs; monitor during and after infusion. ▪ Monitor for hypersensitivity reactions, especially during the first and second infusions; may occur within minutes. Discontinue docetaxel if reaction is severe. Hypersensitivity reactions may occur even in patients premedicated with dexamethasone. ▪ Monitor for localized erythema of the palms of the hands and soles of the feet with or without desquamation. Skin eruptions generally occur within 1 week after docetaxel infusion, resolve before the next infusion, and are not disabling. However, severe reactions have been reported. A reduced dose may be indicated if severe. ▪ Monitor for fluid retention. Severe salt restriction and treatment with oral diuretics may be indicated. S/S of severe fluid retention include abdominal distension (severe), cardiac tamponade, dyspnea at rest, peripheral or generalized edema, pleural effusion. ▪ Observe for signs of peripheral neurotoxicity (e.g., neurosensory symptoms such as dysesthesia, pain, paresthesia, and peripheral motor neuropathy manifested primarily as distal extremity weakness); docetaxel may need to be discontinued; see Dose Adjustments. In patients with gastric adenocarcinoma or SCCHN, a baseline neurologic exam is recommended. Repeat every 2 cycles and at the end of treatment; see Dose Adjustments. ▪ Observe for signs of infection. Use of prophylactic antibiotics may be indicated pending C/S in a febrile, neutropenic patient. Monitor patients receiving docetaxel (Taxotere), cisplatin, fluorouracil (5-FU) combination therapy closely for febrile neutropenia and/or neutropenic infection. ▪ Monitor for thrombocytopenia (platelet count less than 50,000/mm^3); see Dose Adjustments. Initiate precautions to prevent excessive bleeding (e.g., inspect IV sites, skin, and mucous membranes; use extreme care during invasive procedures; test urine, emesis, stool, and secretions for occult blood). ▪ Monitor for signs of existing or developing impaired vision. A prompt comprehensive ophthalmologic exam is indicated. If CME is diagnosed, discontinue docetaxel. ▪ Hematologic follow-up required due to risk of delayed myelodysplasia or myeloid leukemia.

Patient Education: Avoid pregnancy; nonhormonal birth control recommended. ▪ Review of monitoring requirements (e.g., CBCs, liver function tests) and adverse events before therapy imperative. ▪ Pretreatment with dexamethasone as prescribed is imperative. ▪ Report pain or burning at injection site and any unusual or unexpected symptoms or side effects as soon as possible (e.g., constipation, fever, hypersensitivity reaction [e.g., difficulty breathing, itching, rash], nausea and vomiting, shortness of breath, swelling of feet and legs, weight gain, change in vision). ▪ Review all medications (prescription and nonprescription) with nurse and/or physician. ▪ Medication contains alcohol. May affect ability to drive or operate machinery immediately after infusion. ▪ See Appendix D, p. 1333. ▪ Obtain name and telephone number of a contact person for emergencies, questions, or problems. ▪ Seek resources for counseling or supportive therapy. ▪ Risk of delayed myelodysplasia or myeloid leukemia requires hematologic follow-up. Changes in blood counts due to leukemia and other blood disorders may occur years after treatment.

Maternal/Child: Category D: avoid pregnancy; may cause fetal harm. ▪ Discontinue breast-feeding. ▪ Efficacy in pediatric patients as monotherapy or in combination has not been established. The overall safety profile in pediatric patients receiving monotherapy or combination therapy with cisplatin and 5-fluorouracil was consistent with the known safety profile in adults. The alcohol content of docetaxel should be taken into account when given to pediatric patients.

Elderly: Dose selection should be cautious; see Dose Adjustments. ▪ May be at increased risk for developing side effects such as anemia, anorexia, diarrhea, dizziness, febrile neutropenia, infections, lethargy, nail changes, peripheral edema, stomatitis, and weight loss. ▪ Monitor hepatic function carefully.

DRUG/LAB INTERACTIONS
A substrate of CYP3A4. Metabolism may be modified by concomitant administration of other medications that induce, inhibit, or are metabolized by CYP3A4. Metabolism inhibited and serum levels increased with **strong CYP3A4 inhibitors** (e.g., imidazole antifungals [e.g., itraconazole (Sporanox), ketoconazole (Nizoral), voriconazole (VFEND)], protease inhibitors [e.g., atazanavir (Reyataz), indinavir (Crixivan), nelfinavir (Viracept), ritonavir (Norvir), saquinavir (Invirase)], clarithromycin [Biaxin], nefazodone, and telithromycin [Ketek]). Avoid use. A pharmacokinetic study suggests considering a 50% dose reduction of docetaxel if coadministration of a strong CYP3A4 inhibitor is required; monitor closely for toxicity. ▪ Docetaxel clearance is not affected by coadministration of **prednisone** or **cisplatin.** ▪ Metabolism of docetaxel may be modified by **other agents that induce, inhibit, or are metabolized by CYP3A4** (e.g., cyclosporine [Sandimmune], phenytoin [Dilantin], phenobarbital [Luminal], tacrolimus [Prograf], and many others). ▪ Additive bone marrow suppression may occur with **radiation therapy and/or other bone marrow–suppressing agents** (e.g., azathioprine, chloramphenicol, melphalan [Alkeran]). Dose reduction may be required. ▪ Leukopenic and/or thrombocytopenic effects may be

increased with **drugs that cause blood dyscrasias** (e.g., anticonvulsants [e.g., carbamazepine (Tegretol), phenytoin (Dilantin)], NSAIDs [e.g., ibuprofen (Advil, Motrin), naproxen (Aleve, Naprosyn)]). Adjust dose based on differential and platelet count. ▪ Risk of infection is increased with concurrent use of **other immunosuppressants** (e.g., azathioprine, chlorambucil [Leukeran], cyclophosphamide [Cytoxan], cyclosporine [Sandimmune], glucocorticoid corticosteroids [e.g., dexamethasone], muromonab CD-3 [Orthoclone], tacrolimus [Prograf]). ▪ Do not administer **live virus vaccines** to patients receiving antineoplastic agents.

SIDE EFFECTS

Generally reversible but can be fatal. Most common side effects across all indications are alopecia, anemia, anorexia, asthenia, constipation, diarrhea, dysgeusia, dyspnea, febrile neutropenia, fluid retention (e.g., ascites, edema, pericardial effusion, pleural effusion), hypersensitivity reactions (e.g., back pain, chest tightness, chills, drug fever, dyspnea, flushing, hypotension, pruritus, rash), infection, mucositis, myalgia, nail disorders, nausea, neuropathy, neutropenia, pain, skin reactions, thrombocytopenia, and vomiting. Increased incidence of bone marrow suppression (anemia, leukopenia, neutropenia, thrombocytopenia) and/or severity of side effects is dose dependent and can be dose limiting. Abdominal pain; acute myeloid leukemia and myelodysplastic syndrome; acute pulmonary edema; acute respiratory distress syndrome; alcohol intoxication; altered hearing; amenorrhea; arthralgia; bleeding episodes; cardiac arrhythmias; CHF; colitis; confusion; conjunctivitis; cough; cutaneous reactions (e.g., localized rash on hands, feet, arms, face, thorax; erythema multiforme; severe hand and foot syndrome; Stevens-Johnson syndrome; toxic epidermal necrolysis); diarrhea; DIC (often in association with sepsis or multiorgan failure); dizziness; enteritis; esophagitis/dysphagia/odynophagia; eye disorders (e.g., CME); fatigue; fever with or without infection; gastrointestinal pain and cramping; heartburn; hepatitis (sometimes fatal, primarily in patients with pre-existing liver disease); hypotension; increased ALT, AST, and bilirubin; infusion site reactions; interstitial pneumonia; lethargy; lymphedema; myocardial ischemia; neurosensory symptoms (e.g., dysesthesia, pain, paresthesia); neutropenic infection; paresthesias (e.g., pain, burning sensation); perforation of the large intestine; renal insufficiency; seizures or transient loss of consciousness; stomatitis; taste perversion; tearing; vasodilation.

Overdose: Bone marrow suppression, mucositis, peripheral neurotoxicity.

Post-Marketing: Acute pulmonary edema, acute respiratory distress syndrome/pneumonitis, alopecia (permanent), cystoid macular edema, deep vein thrombosis, dehydration, duodenal ulcer, dyspnea, esophagitis, GI hemorrhage, hyponatremia, ileus, interstitial lung disease, interstitial pneumonia, intestinal obstruction, ischemic colitis, MI, neutropenic enterocolitis, pneumonitis, pulmonary embolism, pulmonary fibrosis, radiation pneumonitis, radiation recall phenomenon, renal failure (most commonly associated with concomitant nephrotoxic drugs), respiratory failure, scleroderma-like changes (usually preceded by peripheral lymphedema), thrombophlebitis, transient visual disturbances.

ANTIDOTE

Keep physician informed of all side effects. Most will be treated symptomatically as indicated. Most hypersensitivity reactions will subside with temporary discontinuation of docetaxel, and incidence seems to decrease with subsequent doses. Discontinue docetaxel if a severe hypersensitivity reaction occurs. Severe reactions may require epinephrine (Adrenalin), antihistamines (e.g., diphenhydramine [Benadryl]), corticosteroids (e.g., dexamethasone [Decadron]), or bronchodilators (e.g., albuterol, theophylline [Aminophylline]). Patients with a history of a severe hypersensitivity reaction should not be rechallenged. If CME is diagnosed, discontinue docetaxel and initiate appropriate treatment. Consider alternative non-taxane cancer treatment. Neutropenia can be profound, and the nadir usually occurs about Day 8. Recovery is generally rapid and spontaneous but may be treated with filgrastim (Neupogen, Zarxio) or pegfilgrastim (Neulasta). Severe thrombocytopenia may require platelet transfusions. Severe anemia (less than 8 Gm/dL) may require packed cell transfusions. Hypotension and bradycardia do not usually occur at the same time except in hypersensitivity. Treat only if symptomatic. Treat any serious or symptomatic arrhythmia (e.g., conduction abnormalities, ventricular tachycardia) promptly and monitor continuously during subsequent doses. Serious cutaneous reactions with desquamation (rare), serious fluid retention (more frequent with cumulative doses of 1,300 mg/M^2), persistent febrile neutropenia, severe peripheral neuropathy, or severe liver impairment may require discontinuation of docetaxel. There is no specific antidote for overdose. Supportive therapy will help sustain the patient in toxicity. Resuscitate if indicated.

DOLASETRON MESYLATE

(dohl-**AH**-seh-tron **MES**-ih-layt)

Antiemetic

(5HT$_3$ receptor antagonist)

Anzemet

pH 3.2 to 3.8

USUAL DOSE

Prevention of postoperative nausea and/or vomiting: 12.5 mg as a single dose 15 minutes before cessation of anesthesia. If prophylaxis fails, a repeat dose should **NOT** be administered as rescue therapy.

Treatment of postoperative nausea and/or vomiting: 12.5 mg as a single dose as soon as nausea or vomiting presents.

PEDIATRIC DOSE

Doses are those recommended for *pediatric patients 2 to 16 years of age.* Safety and effectiveness in pediatric patients under 2 years of age not established; see Contraindications and Maternal/Child. Dolasetron solution for injection may be mixed with apple or applegrape juice for oral administration to pediatric patients. See prescribing information for oral doses.

Prevention of postoperative nausea and/or vomiting: 0.35 mg/kg up to a maximum dose of 12.5 mg as a single dose 15 minutes before cessation of anesthesia. If prophylaxis fails, a repeat dose should **NOT** be administered as rescue therapy.

Treatment of postoperative nausea and/or vomiting: 0.35 mg/kg up to a maximum dose of 12.5 mg as a single dose as soon as nausea or vomiting presents.

DOSE ADJUSTMENTS

No dose adjustments required for the elderly, renal failure, or impaired hepatic function; however, caution and lower-end dosing are suggested in elderly patients. Consider decreased organ function and concomitant disease or drug therapy.

DILUTION

IV injection: A single dose may be given undiluted.

IV infusion: A single dose may be further diluted up to 50 mL in NS, D5W, D5/^{1}/$_2$NS, D5LR, LR, or 10% mannitol.

Storage: Store vials at CRT; protect from light. Stable after dilution at CRT for 24 hours or 48 hours if refrigerated.

COMPATIBILITY

(Underline Indicates Conflicting Compatibility Information)

Consider any drug NOT listed as compatible to be INCOMPATIBLE until consulting a pharmacist; specific conditions may apply.

Manufacturer states, "Should not be mixed with other drugs. Flush the infusion line with a **compatible** IV solution before and after administration."

One source suggests the following **compatibilities:**

Y-site: Acetaminophen (Ofirmev), azithromycin (Zithromax), caspofungin (Cancidas), dexmedetomidine (Precedex), fenoldopam (Corlopam), hetastarch in electrolytes (Hextend), and oxaliplatin (Eloxatin).

RATE OF ADMINISTRATION

Flush infusion line before and after administration. May cause bradycardia, severe hypotension, and syncope during or shortly after administration.

IV injection: A single dose over 30 seconds.

IV infusion: Administer a single dose over 15 minutes.

ACTIONS

An antinauseant and antiemetic agent. A selective antagonist of specific serotonin ($5\text{-}HT_3$) receptors, similar to granisetron and ondansetron. 5-HT3 receptors are located on the nerve terminals of the vagus in the periphery and centrally in the chemoreceptor trigger zone. By antagonizing these receptors, nausea and vomiting are prevented. Rapidly and completely metabolized to its active metabolite, hydrodolasetron. Maximum concentration of hydrodolasetron occurs 0.6 hours after injection or infusion. Widely distributed in the body, 69% to 77% bound to plasma protein. Eliminated by multiple routes. Hydrodolasetron is partially metabolized. Average half-life is 7.3 hours. Excreted in urine and feces as unchanged drug and metabolites. Not known if dolasetron is secreted in breast milk.

INDICATIONS AND USES

Prevention of postoperative nausea and vomiting in adults and pediatric patients 2 years of age and older when indicated. When prophylaxis has failed, a repeat dose should not be initiated as rescue therapy. ▪ Treatment of postoperative nausea and/or vomiting in adults and pediatric patients 2 years of age and older.

CONTRAINDICATIONS

Known hypersensitivity to dolasetron. ▪ Contraindicated in adult and pediatric patients for the prevention of nausea and vomiting associated with initial and repeat courses of emetogenic cancer chemotherapy because of risk for dose-dependent QTc prolongation.

PRECAUTIONS

Prolongs the QT interval in a dose-dependent fashion. Torsades de pointes has been reported. Avoid use in patients with congenital long QT syndrome, hypokalemia, or hypomagnesemia. ▪ Has been shown to cause dose-dependent prolongation of the PR and QRS interval. Second- or third-degree atrioventricular block, cardiac arrest, and serious ventricular arrhythmias, including fatalities in both adult and pediatric patients, have been reported. At particular risk are patients with underlying structural heart disease, pre-existing conduction system abnormalities, sick sinus syndrome, atrial fibrillation with slow ventricular response, or myocardial ischemia; elderly patients; or patients receiving drugs known to prolong the PR interval (such as verapamil) and QRS interval (e.g., flecainide [Tambocor] or quinidine). Use with caution and monitor ECG. Avoid use in patients with or at risk for complete heart block unless they have an implanted pacemaker. ▪ Use with caution in patients who have or may develop prolongation of cardiac conduction intervals, particularly QT intervals (e.g., patients with hypokalemia, hypomagnesemia, congenital QT syndrome, cumulative high-dose anthracycline therapy [e.g., doxorubicin (Adriamycin)], patients taking diuretics with potential for inducing electrolyte abnormalities [e.g., furosemide (Lasix), hydrochlorothiazide] or antiarrhythmic drugs or other drugs that lead to QT prolongation [amiodarone (Nexterone), procainamide (Pronestyl), quinidine]). ▪ Serotonin syndrome has been reported with $5\text{-}HT_3$ receptor antagonists. Most reports were associated with concomitant use of serotonergic drugs (e.g., selective serotonin reuptake inhibitors [e.g., paroxetine (Paxil), escitalopram (Lexapro)], serotonin and norepinephrine reuptake inhibitors [e.g., duloxetine (Cymbalta), venlafaxine (Effexor XR)], monoamine oxidase inhibitors [e.g., selegiline (Eldepryl)], mirtazapine [Remeron], fentanyl, lithium, tramadol [Ultram], and intravenous methylene blue). Some cases were fatal. ▪ Cross-sensitivity has been reported in patients who received other selective 5HT₃-receptor agonists (e.g., granisetron [Kytril], ondansetron [Zofran]). These reactions have not been seen with dolasetron. ▪ See Contraindications, Maternal/Child, Drug/Lab Interactions, and Side Effects.

Monitor: Observe closely. Monitor VS. Any patient found to have a second-degree or higher AV conduction block should be monitored continuously. ▪ Correct hypokalemia and hypomagnesemia before administration of dolasetron. Monitor after administration as clinically indicated. ▪ Monitor ECG in patients with CHF, bradycardia, or renal impairment; in the elderly; and in all patients at risk for prolongation of the PR and QRS interval; see Precautions. ▪ Monitor for serotonin syndrome, especially when dolasetron is used concurrently with other serotonergic drugs. Symptoms associated with serotonin syndrome may include the following combination of S/S: mental status changes (e.g., agitation, coma, delirium, hallucinations), autonomic instability (e.g., diaphoresis, dizziness, flushing, hyperthermia, labile blood pressure, tachycardia), neuromuscular symptoms (e.g., hyperreflexia, incoordination, myoclonus, rigidity, tremor), seizures, with or without GI symptoms (e.g., diarrhea, nausea, vomiting). ▪ Ambulate slowly to avoid orthostatic hypotension.

Patient Education: Request assistance for ambulation. ▪ May cause serious cardiac arrhythmias; discuss medical history with physician and promptly report a perceived change in heart rate, fainting, or light-headedness. ▪ Report promptly if nausea persists. ▪ Maintain adequate hydration. ▪ Review prescription medications with health care provider. ▪ Promptly report S/S of serotonin syndrome (e.g., altered mental status, autonomic instability, and neuromuscular symptoms); see Precautions.

Maternal/Child: Category B: no evidence of impaired fertility or harm to fetus. Use during pregnancy only if clearly needed. ▪ Use caution if required during breast-feeding. ▪ See Contraindications. ▪ Safety and effectiveness for use in pediatric patients under 2 years of age not established. ▪ Plasma clearance increased and half-life reduced in pediatric patients.

Elderly: Use with caution and continuous ECG monitoring in the elderly; they are at particular risk for prolongation of the PR, QRS, and QT interval. ▪ See Dose Adjustments and Contraindications.

DRUG/LAB INTERACTIONS

Does not induce or inhibit the cytochrome P_{450} drug metabolizing system, but metabolism of its active metabolite, hydrodolasetron, is mediated by enzymes in the P_{450} system. Plasma levels increased when given concurrently with **cimetidine** (Tagamet [inhibitor of cytochrome P_{450}]), and decreased when given concurrently with **rifampin** (Rifadin [inducer of cytochrome P_{450}]); clinical significance not known. ▪ Clearance decreased when given concurrently with **atenolol.** ▪ See Precautions and use extreme caution with **diuretics** with potential for inducing electrolyte abnormalities (e.g., furosemide [Lasix], hydrochlorothiazide) **or antiarrhythmic drugs or other drugs that lead to prolonged QT intervals** (e.g., amiodarone [Nexterone], procainamide [Pronestyl], quinidine). ▪ Serotonin syndrome (including altered mental status, autonomic instability, and neuromuscular symptoms) has been reported following the concomitant use of 5-HT$_3$ receptor antagonists and other serotonergic drugs, including selective serotonin reuptake inhibitors (SSRIs) and serotonin and norepinephrine reuptake inhibitors (SNRIs); see Precautions. ▪ Clearance not affected by **ACE inhibitors** (e.g., enalapril), **diltiazem** (Cardizem), **furosemide** (Lasix), **glyburide** (DiaBeta), **nifedipine** (Procardia), **propranolol** (Inderal), and **verapamil.** ▪ Does not influence anesthesia recovery time.

SIDE EFFECTS

Dizziness, drowsiness, headache, pain, and urinary retention are most common. Sinus arrhythmia, hypotension, orthostatic hypotension, and numerous other side effects may occur in fewer than 2% of patients. May cause bradycardia, severe hypotension, and syncope during or shortly after administration. Can cause ECG interval changes (PR, QT, JT prolongation, and QRS widening). These changes may lead to cardiovascular consequences (e.g., cardiac arrhythmias, heart block). Usually self-limiting with declining blood levels, but may last as long as 24 hours.

Overdose: Severe hypotension and dizziness.

Post-Marketing: Wide complex tachycardia, VT, VF, and cardiac arrest have been reported rarely. Serotonin syndrome has been reported as a 5-HT$_3$ class reaction.

ANTIDOTE
Most side effects will be treated symptomatically. Keep physician informed. Overdose in one patient was treated with plasma expanders (e.g., albumin, dextran), dopamine, atropine, and continuous BP and ECG monitoring. Epinephrine, atropine, and/or cardiac pacing may be required to treat ECG interval changes. Prolonged QT interval may lead to VT or other ventricular arrhythmias; telemetry monitoring may be indicated. If symptoms of serotonin syndrome occur, discontinue dolasetron and initiate supportive care. There is no specific antidote. Treat anaphylaxis and resuscitate as necessary. Not known if dolasetron is removed by hemodialysis.

DOPAMINE HYDROCHLORIDE BBW
(**DOH**-pah-meen hy-droh-**KLOR**-eyed)

Inotropic agent
Cardiac stimulant
Vasopressor

pH 2.5 to 5

USUAL DOSE
Where appropriate, restoration of blood volume with a suitable plasma expander or whole blood should be instituted or completed before administration of dopamine; the goal is a central venous pressure of 10 to 15 cm H_2O or a pulmonary wedge pressure of 14 to 18 mm Hg.

Adults: 2 to 5 mcg/kg of body weight/min initially in patients likely to respond to minimum treatment. 5 to 10 mcg/kg/min may be required initially to correct hypotension in the seriously ill patient. Gradually increase by 5 to 10 mcg/kg/min at 10- to 30-minute intervals until optimum response occurs. Average dose is 20 mcg/kg/min; over 50 mcg/kg/min has been required in some instances but is not recommended. If more than 20 mcg/kg/min is required to maintain BP, consider use of norepinephrine (Levophed) in addition. Doses over 20 mcg/kg/min decrease renal perfusion.

Bradycardia: AHA guidelines recommend dopamine infusion 2 to 10 mcg/kg/min. Titrate to desired effect; taper slowly. Indicated if atropine is ineffective. Alternately, transcutaneous pacing or epinephrine infusion 2 to 10 mcg/min may be used.

PEDIATRIC DOSE
See Maternal/Child. Note comments in Usual Dose. Usual starting dose is 1 to 5 mcg/kg/min. Dose increments range from 2.5 to 5 mcg/kg/min. Usual maximum dose is 15 to 20 mcg/kg/min. Doses up to 50 mcg/kg/min have been administered. Titrate dose gradually to desired effect.

DOSE ADJUSTMENTS
Reduce dose to one tenth of the calculated amount for individuals who have been treated with MAO inhibitors (e.g., selegiline [Eldepryl]) within 2 to 3 weeks of administration of dopamine. ▪ Lower-end initial doses may be appropriate in the elderly based on potential for decreased organ function and concomitant disease or drug therapy. ▪ See Drug/Lab Interactions.

DILUTION
Each 200-mg, 400-mg, or 800-mg ampule must be diluted in 250 to 500 mL of the following IV solutions and given as an infusion: NS, D5W, D5NS, D5/$\frac{1}{2}$NS, D5LR, $\frac{1}{6}$ M sodium lactate, or LR injection. See the following chart.

Final Dopamine Concentration (mcg/mL) When Dopamine 40 mg/mL or 80 mg/mL Is Mixed with Various Volumes of Infusion Solution			
Concentration of Dopamine	40 mg/mL		80 mg/mL
Volume of Dopamine	5 mL (200 mg)	10 mL (400 mg)	10 mL (800 mg)
250 mL diluent	800 mcg/mL	1,600 mcg/mL	3,200 mcg/mL
500 mL diluent	400 mcg/mL	800 mcg/mL	1,600 mcg/mL
1,000 mL diluent	200 mcg/mL	400 mcg/mL	800 mcg/mL

Also available prediluted in 250 mL or 500 mL of D5W. Dopamine concentration varies. More concentrated solutions may be used if absolutely necessary to reduce fluid volume. **Storage:** Store at CRT. Protect from freezing. Discard diluted solution after 24 hours. Do not use if solution is darker than slightly yellow.

COMPATIBILITY   (Underline Indicates Conflicting Compatibility Information)
Consider any drug NOT listed as compatible to be INCOMPATIBLE until consulting a pharmacist; specific conditions may apply.
Manufacturer states, "Do not add to sodium bicarbonate or any other strongly alkaline solution (e.g., aminophylline, barbiturates [e.g., phenobarbital (Luminal)]), oxidizing agents, or iron salts. Dopamine is inactivated in alkaline solution." Do not mix with alteplase or amphotericin B.

One source suggests the following **compatibilities:**
Additive: Aminophylline, atracurium (Tracrium), calcium chloride, chloramphenicol (Chloromycetin), ciprofloxacin (Cipro IV), dobutamine, enalaprilat (Vasotec IV), flumazenil (Romazicon), gentamicin, heparin, hydrocortisone sodium succinate (Solu-Cortef), lidocaine, mannitol (Osmitrol), meropenem (Merrem IV), methylprednisolone (Solu-Medrol), nitroglycerin IV, oxacillin (Bactocill), potassium chloride (KCl), ranitidine (Zantac), verapamil.
Y-site: Aldesleukin (Proleukin), alprostadil, amifostine (Ethyol), amiodarone (Nexterone), anidulafungin (Eraxis), argatroban, atracurium (Tracrium), aztreonam (Azactam), bivalirudin (Angiomax), caffeine citrate (Cafcit), caspofungin (Cancidas), cefepime (Maxipime), ceftaroline (Telflaro), ceftazidime (Fortaz), ciprofloxacin (Cipro IV), cisatracurium (Nimbex), cladribine (Leustatin), daptomycin (Cubicin), dexmedetomidine (Precedex), diltiazem (Cardizem), dobutamine, docetaxel (Taxotere), doripenem (Doribax), doxorubicin liposomal (Doxil), enalaprilat (Vasotec IV), epinephrine (Adrenalin), esmolol (Brevibloc), etoposide phosphate (Etopophos), famotidine (Pepcid IV), fenoldopam (Corlopam), fentanyl, fluconazole (Diflucan), foscarnet (Foscavir), furosemide (Lasix), gemcitabine (Gemzar), granisetron (Kytril), heparin, hetastarch in electrolytes (Hextend), hydrocortisone sodium succinate (Solu-Cortef), hydromorphone (Dilaudid), 6% hydroxyethyl starch (Voluven), labetalol, levofloxacin (Levaquin), lidocaine, linezolid (Zyvox), lorazepam (Ativan), meperidine (Demerol), methylprednisolone (Solu-Medrol), metronidazole (Flagyl IV), micafungin (Mycamine), midazolam (Versed), milrinone (Primacor), morphine, mycophenolate (CellCept IV), nicardipine (Cardene IV), nitroglycerin IV, nitroprusside sodium, norepinephrine (Levophed), ondansetron (Zofran), oxaliplatin (Eloxatin), pancuronium, pantoprazole (Protonix IV), pemetrexed (Alimta), piperacillin/tazobactam (Zosyn), potassium chloride (KCl), propofol (Diprivan), ranitidine (Zantac), remifentanil (Ultiva), sargramostim (Leukine), tacrolimus (Prograf), telavancin (Vibativ), theophylline, thiotepa, tigecycline (Tygacil), tirofiban (Aggrastat), vasopressin, vecuronium, verapamil, warfarin (Coumadin), zidovudine (AZT, Retrovir).

RATE OF ADMINISTRATION
Begin with recommended dose for body weight and seriousness of condition. Gradually increase by 5 to 10 mcg/kg/min to produce desired response. Titrate to desired hemodynamic or renal response. When titrating to the desired increase in systolic BP, the opti-

mum dosage rate for renal response may be exceeded and may necessitate a rate reduction after the hemodynamic condition is stabilized. Use of a volumetric infusion pump is recommended for accuracy. Optimum urine flow determines correct evaluation of dosage. Decrease dose gradually; may cause marked hypotension if discontinued suddenly. Expansion of blood volume with IV fluids may be indicated.

Dopamine Infusion Rate (mL/hr): 400 mcg/mL Concentration						
Desired Dose	Weight in Kilograms					
	50 kg	60 kg	70 kg	80 kg	90 kg	100 kg
	(mL/hr)	(mL/hr)	(mL/hr)	(mL/hr)	(mL/hr)	(mL/hr)
5 mcg/kg/min	37.5	45	52.5	60	67.5	75
10 mcg/kg/min	75	90	105	120	135	150
20 mcg/kg/min	150	180	210	240	270	300
30 mcg/kg/min	225	270	315	360	405	450
40 mcg/kg/min	300	360	420	480	540	600

Dopamine Infusion Rate (mL/hr): 800 mcg/mL Concentration						
Desired Dose	Weight in Kilograms					
	50 kg	60 kg	70 kg	80 kg	90 kg	100 kg
	(mL/hr)	(mL/hr)	(mL/hr)	(mL/hr)	(mL/hr)	(mL/hr)
5 mcg/kg/min	18.75	22.5	26.25	30	33.75	37.5
10 mcg/kg/min	37.5	45	52.5	60	67.5	75
20 mcg/kg/min	75	90	105	120	135	150
30 mcg/kg/min	112.5	135	157.5	180	202.5	225
40 mcg/kg/min	150	180	210	240	270	300

ACTIONS

Dopamine is a naturally occurring catecholamine that possesses alpha, beta, and dopaminergic receptor–stimulating actions. The effects of dopamine are dose-related. At low doses (0.5 to 2 mcg/kg/min), dopamine causes vasodilation in the renal, mesenteric, coronary, and intracerebral vascular beds, thereby increasing glomerular filtration rate, renal blood flow, sodium excretion, and urine flow. At medium doses (2 to 10 mcg/kg/min), beta-adrenoceptors are stimulated, resulting in improved myocardial contractility, increased sinoatrial rate, and enhanced impulse conduction in the heart. Systolic and pulse pressure may increase, but there is little, if any, effect on diastolic pressure at these doses. At higher doses (10 to 20 mcg/kg/min), alpha-adrenoceptors are stimulated, resulting in vasoconstriction and an increase in blood pressure. At doses above 20 mcg/kg/min, alpha effects predominate and vasoconstriction may compromise circulation in the limbs and override the dopaminergic effects of dopamine, reversing renal dilation and natriuresis. Dopamine is widely distributed. It has an onset of action of 5 minutes, a duration of action of 10 minutes, and a plasma half-life of 2 minutes. Metabolized in the liver, kidney, and plasma by monoamine oxidase (MAO) and catechol O-methyltransferase (COMT), with about 25% of the dose being converted to norepinephrine. Primarily excreted in urine.

INDICATIONS AND USES

To correct hemodynamic imbalances, including hypotension resulting from shock syndrome of myocardial infarction, trauma, endotoxic septicemia, open heart surgery, renal failure, and chronic cardiac decompensation. ■ Drug of choice for hypotension and shock. ■ AHA guidelines recommend dopamine as the second drug of choice after atropine to treat symptomatic bradycardia.

Unlabeled uses: Chronic obstructive pulmonary disease, congestive heart failure, infant respiratory distress syndrome, symptomatic bradycardia, calcium channel blocker overdose, beta-blocker overdose, and drug-induced hypovolemic shock; consult literature.

CONTRAINDICATIONS

Hypersensitivity to any components (contains sulfites), pheochromocytoma, uncorrected tachyarrhythmias, ventricular fibrillation.

PRECAUTIONS

Some preparations contain sulfites; use caution in patients with allergies. ▪ Avoid hypovolemia. ▪ Presence of hypoxia, hypercapnia, or acidosis may reduce the effectiveness of dopamine and/or increase the incidence of dopamine-induced adverse events. ▪ Use caution in patients with a history of occlusive vascular disease (e.g., atherosclerosis, arterial embolism, Raynaud's disease).

Monitor: Recognition of signs and symptoms of hemodynamic imbalance and prompt treatment with dopamine will improve prognosis. ▪ Close monitoring of BP, cardiac output, cardiac rhythm, and urine output required. Avoid hypertension. If possible, check central venous pressure or pulmonary wedge pressure before administration and as ordered thereafter. ▪ Use larger veins (antecubital fossa) and avoid extravasation; may cause necrosis and sloughing of tissue. Central vein preferred for continuous infusions; see Antidote. ▪ If possible, correct hypovolemia with IV fluids, whole blood or plasma as indicated; correct acidosis if present. ▪ Monitor for decreased urine output, increased tachycardia, or new arrhythmias. ▪ With high-dose administration, palpate pulses and monitor extremities for signs of peripheral vasoconstriction (e.g., coldness, paresthesias). ▪ Therapy may be continued until the patient can maintain hemodynamic and renal functions. ▪ See Maternal/Child and Drug/Lab Interactions.

Maternal/Child: Category C: safety for use in pregnancy and breast-feeding not established. If used, benefits must outweigh risks. ▪ Safety for use in pediatric patients not established. Has been used, but experience is limited. ▪ Do not administer into an umbilical arterial catheter. Vasospastic events have been reported when dopamine is infused through the umbilical artery.

Elderly: Lower-end initial doses may be appropriate; see Dose Adjustments. ▪ Differences in response compared to younger adults not identified.

DRUG/LAB INTERACTIONS

Alkaline solutions, including sodium bicarbonate, inactivate dopamine. ▪ May cause serious arrhythmias in presence of **cyclopropane or halogen anesthetics.** ▪ May cause severe hypertension with **oxytocic drugs** (e.g., methylergonovine [Methergine] or oxytocin). ▪ **MAO inhibitors** (e.g., selegiline [Eldepryl]) prolong and potentiate the effect of dopamine. Concurrent use may cause hypertensive crisis. ▪ Concurrent administration of low-dose dopamine and diuretic agents may produce an additive or potentiating effect on urine flow. ▪ Antagonizes effects of **guanethidine** (Ismelin). ▪ Cardiac effects may be antagonized by **alpha- or beta-blocking agents** (e.g., metoprolol [Lopressor], propranolol [Inderal]). ▪ **Tricyclic antidepressants** (e.g., amitriptyline [Elavil]) may potentiate the cardiovascular effects of dopamine. ▪ May cause severe bradycardia and hypotension with **phenytoin** (Dilantin). ▪ **Alpha-adrenergic blocking agents** (e.g., doxazosin [Cardura], tamsulosin [Flomax]) antagonize the peripheral vasoconstriction caused by high-dose dopamine. ▪ **Butyrophenones** (e.g., haloperidol [Haldol]) and **phenothiazines** (e.g., chlorpromazine [Thorazine], prochlorperazine [Compazine]) can suppress the dopaminergic renal and mesenteric vasodilation induced with low-dose dopamine. ▪ See Dose Adjustments.

SIDE EFFECTS

Aberrant conduction/arrhythmias (e.g., atrial fibrillation, ectopic beats, widened QRS complex, ventricular arrhythmias), anginal pain, anxiety, azotemia, bradycardia, dyspnea, headache, hypertension, hypotension, nausea, palpitation, piloerection, tachycardia, vasoconstriction, vomiting. Gangrene of the extremities has occurred with high doses administered for prolonged periods and in patients with occlusive vascular disease receiving a low dose of dopamine.

ANTIDOTE

Notify the physician of all side effects. Decrease infusion rate and notify the physician immediately for decrease in established urine flow rate, disproportionate rise in diastolic BP (i.e., a marked decrease in pulse pressure), increasing tachycardia, or new arrhythmias. For accidental overdosage with hypertension, reduce rate or temporarily discontinue until condition stabilizes. Phentolamine, an alpha-adrenergic blocker, may be useful in an overdose situation that does not respond to discontinuation of dopamine. To prevent sloughing and necrosis in areas where extravasation has occurred, use a fine hypodermic needle to inject 5 to 10 mg of phentolamine (Regitine) diluted in 10 to 15 mL normal saline liberally throughout the tissue in the extravasated area. Begin as soon as extravasation is recognized.

# DORIPENEM (**DOR**-i-**PEN**-em)	**Antibacterial** **(carbapenem)**
Doribax	**pH 4.5 to 5.5**

USUAL DOSE

18 years of age and older: 500 mg every 8 hours. Duration of therapy is based on diagnosis as listed in the following chart.

Doripenem Dosing Guidelines			
Infection	Dosage	Frequency	Duration
Complicated intra-abdominal infection	500 mg	q 8 hr	5-14 days*
Complicated UTI, including pyelonephritis	500 mg	q 8 hr	10 days†

*Duration includes a possible switch to an appropriate oral therapy after at least 3 days of parenteral therapy and once clinical improvement has been demonstrated.
†Duration can be extended up to 14 days for patients with concurrent bacteremia.

DOSE ADJUSTMENTS

Reduced doses are indicated based on degree of renal insufficiency as noted in the following chart.

Dosage of Doripenem in Patients with Renal Impairment	
Estimated CrCl (mL/min)	Recommended Dosage Regimen
>50 mL/min	No dosage adjustment necessary
≥30 to ≤50 mL/min	250 mg q 8 hr
>10 to <30 mL/min	250 mg q 12 hr

No dose adjustment indicated based on age, gender, race, or impaired hepatic function. ▪ Dosing should be cautious in the elderly, and reduced doses may be indicated based on the potential for decreased renal function. ▪ There is insufficient information to make dose adjustment recommendations for patients undergoing hemodialysis.

DILUTION

Available in vials containing 250 mg or 500 mg.
250-mg vial: Reconstitute the 250-mg vial with 10 mL of SWFI or NS. Shake gently to form a suspension. Resulting concentration is 25 mg/mL. **Caution: The constituted suspen-**

sion is not for direct injection. Withdraw the suspension using a syringe with a 21-gauge needle, and add it to an infusion bag containing 50 or 100 mL of NS or D5W. Shake gently until clear. The final infusion solution concentration is approximately 4.2 mg/mL (50-mL infusion bag) or 2.3 mg/mL (100-mL infusion bag). Infusions range from clear and colorless to clear and slightly yellow.

500-mg vial: Reconstitute a 500-mg vial with 10 mL of SWFI or NS. Shake gently to form a suspension with a resultant concentration of 50 mg/mL. **Caution: The reconstituted suspension is not for direct injection.** Withdraw the suspension using a syringe with a 21-gauge needle and add it to an infusion bag containing 100 mL of NS or D5W. Shake gently until clear. The final infusion solution concentration is 4.5 mg/mL. Infusions range from clear and colorless to clear and slightly yellow.

To prepare a 250-mg dose from a 500-mg vial, follow the directions above for the 500-mg vial dilution. Remove 55 mL from the infusion bag that contains the 500-mg dose of doripenem diluted in NS or D5W and discard. The remaining solution will contain 250 mg of doripenem at a concentration of 4.5 mg/mL. Alternately to prevent waste, you could prepare 2 doses (one for immediate use and one for use in 8 hours) by dividing the 10 mL of reconstituted solution in half and adding each 5 mL of reconstituted solution to 50 mL of NS or D5W. Refrigerate the unused dose; see Storage.

Storage: Store unopened vial at CRT. Reconstituted vials are stable for 1 hour prior to transfer to an infusion bag. Infusion solutions diluted in NS are stable for 12 hours at RT and 72 hours refrigerated. Infusion solutions diluted in D5W are stable for 4 hours at RT and 24 hours refrigerated. (Times noted above reflect storage and infusion time.) Do not freeze infusion solutions.

COMPATIBILITY   (Underline Indicates Conflicting Compatibility Information)
Consider any drug NOT listed as compatible to be INCOMPATIBLE until consulting a pharmacist; specific conditions may apply.
Manufacturer states, "Should not be mixed with or physically added to solutions containing other drugs."

One source suggests the following **compatibilities:**
Y-site: Acyclovir (Zovirax), amikacin, aminophylline, amiodarone (Nexterone), amphotericin B (conventional), amphotericin B cholesteryl (Amphotec), amphotericin B lipid complex (Abelcet), amphotericin B liposomal (AmBisone), anidulafungin (Eraxis), atropine, azithromycin (Zithromax), bumetanide, calcium gluconate, carboplatin (Paraplatin), caspofungin (Cancidas), ceftaroline (Teflaro), ciprofloxacin (Cipro IV), cisplatin, cyclophosphamide (Cytoxan), cyclosporine (Sandimmune), daptomycin (Cubicin), dexamethasone (Decadron), digoxin (Lanoxin), diltiazem (Cardizem), diphenhydramine (Benadryl), dobutamine, docetaxel (Taxotere), dopamine, doxorubicin (Adriamycin), enalprilat (Vasotec IV), esmolol (Brevibloc), esomeprazole (Nexium IV), etoposide phosphate (Etopophos), famotidine (Pepcid IV), fentanyl, fluconazole (Diflucan), fluorouracil (5-FU), foscarnet (Foscavir), furosemide (Lasix), gemcitabine (Gemzar), gentamicin, granisetron (Kytril), heparin, hydrocortisone sodium succinate (Solu-Cortef), hydromorphone (Dilaudid), ifosfamide (Ifex), insulin, labetalol, levofloxacin (Levaquin), linezolid (Zyvox), lorazepam (Ativan), magnesium sulfate, mannitol (Osmitrol), meperidine (Demerol), methotrexate, methylprednisolone (Solu-Medrol), metoclopramide (Reglan), metronidazole (Flagyl IV), micafungin (Mycamine), midazolam (Versed), milrinone (Primacor), morphine, moxifloxacin (Avelox), norepinephrine (Levophed), ondansetron (Zofran), paclitaxel (Taxol), pantoprazole (Protonix IV), phenobarbital (Luminal), phenylephrine (Neo-Synephrine), potassium chloride, ranitidine (Zantac), sodium bicarbonate, sodium phosphate, tacrolimus (Prograf), telavancin (Vibativ), tigecycline (Tygacil), tobramycin, vancomycin, voriconazole (VFEND IV), zidovudine (AZT, Retrovir).

RATE OF ADMINISTRATION
A single dose as an infusion equally distributed over 1 hour.

ACTIONS

A synthetic, broad-spectrum, carbapenem antibiotic. Bactericidal to selected aerobic and anaerobic gram-positive and gram-negative bacteria. Bactericidal activity results from the inhibition of bacterial cell wall synthesis. Stable to hydrolysis by most beta-lactamases, including penicillinases and cephalosporinases produced by gram-positive and gram-negative bacteria, with the exception of carbapenem-hydrolyzing beta-lactamases. Less than 10% bound to plasma proteins. Penetrates into several body fluids and tissues, including those at the site of infection for the approved indications. Metabolized via dehydropeptidase-I. Elimination half-life is approximately 1 hour. Primarily eliminated unchanged by the kidneys.

INDICATIONS AND USES

As a single agent for treatment of complicated intra-abdominal infections and complicated urinary tract infections, including pyelonephritis caused by susceptible strains of microorganisms in patients 18 years of age or older.

Limitation of use: Doripenem is not approved for the treatment of ventilator-associated bacterial pneumonia.

CONTRAINDICATIONS

Known hypersensitivity to doripenem or to other carbapenems (e.g., ertapenem [Invanz], imipenem-cilastatin [Primaxin]). ■ Anaphylactic reactions to beta-lactams (e.g., penicillins and cephalosporins); see Precautions.

PRECAUTIONS

To reduce the development of drug-resistant bacteria and maintain its effectiveness, doripenem should be used to treat only those infections proven or strongly suspected to be caused by bacteria. ■ Culture and sensitivity studies are indicated to determine susceptibility of the causative organism to doripenem. ■ Serious and occasionally fatal hypersensitivity reactions have been reported in patients receiving therapy with beta-lactams. More likely in patients with a history of sensitivity to multiple allergens; obtain a careful history. Cross-sensitivity among beta-lactam antibiotics is possible. ■ Increased mortality and lower clinical response rates were reported in patients with ventilator-associated bacterial pneumonia in a clinical trial; see Limitation of use. ■ Seizures have been reported. Risk may be increased in patients with a history of CNS disorders (e.g., stroke or a history of seizures), in patients with compromised renal function, and in patients given doses greater than 500 mg every 8 hours. ■ Prolonged use may cause superinfection because of overgrowth of nonsusceptible organisms. ■ *Clostridium difficile*–associated diarrhea (CDAD) has been reported. May range from mild diarrhea to fatal colitis. Consider in patients who present with diarrhea during or after treatment with doripenem. ■ Although cross-resistance may occur, some isolates resistant to other carbapenems may be susceptible to doripenem. ■ Pneumonitis has been reported when doripenem was used investigationally via inhalation. Do not administer doripenem by this route. ■ See Drug/Lab Interactions.

Monitor: Baseline and periodic monitoring of renal function and CBC with differential may be beneficial. ■ Monitor for early symptoms or hypersensitivity reactions. Emergency equipment must be readily available. ■ Monitor for onset of CNS symptoms and/or seizures. ■ Monitor IV site carefully and rotate as indicated. ■ See Drug/Lab Interactions.

Patient Education: Promptly report S/S of hypersensitivity reaction or pain at injection site. ■ Promptly report diarrhea or bloody stools that occur during treatment or up to several months after an antibiotic has been discontinued; may indicate CDAD and require treatment. ■ Review history of any CNS disorder (e.g., stroke, history of seizures); may be at increased risk for seizures. ■ Patients with a history of seizures should review medication profile with physician before taking doripenem; see Drug/Lab Interactions.

Maternal/Child: Category B: should be used during pregnancy and breast-feeding only if clearly needed. ■ Safety and effectiveness for use in pediatric patients not established.

Elderly: Response similar to that seen in younger patients, but greater sensitivity of some older individuals cannot be ruled out (e.g., increased plasma concentrations). ■ Dosing should be cautious in the elderly; see Dose Adjustments. ▪ Monitoring of renal function may be indicated.

DRUG/LAB INTERACTIONS

Carbapenems may reduce serum **valproic acid** concentrations to subtherapeutic levels, resulting in loss of seizure control. Monitor valproic acid levels. Consider alternative antibacterial therapy. If administration of doripenem is necessary, supplemental anticonvulsant therapy should be considered. ▪ Concurrent use with **probenecid** results in elevated doripenem plasma concentrations. Concurrent use is not recommended. ▪ Does not appear to induce or inhibit the major cytochrome P_{450} isoenzymes, so it should not affect the clearance of drugs that are metabolized by these pathways.

SIDE EFFECTS

The most common adverse reactions are diarrhea, headache, nausea, phlebitis, and rash (allergic rash, bullous dermatitis, erythema, erythema multiforme, macular/papular eruptions, urticaria). Other reactions may include anemia, CDAD, hepatic enzyme elevations, hypersensitivity reactions (including anaphylaxis), oral candidiasis, pruritus, and vulvomycotic infection.

Post-Marketing: Anaphylaxis, interstitial pneumonia, leukopenia, neutropenia, renal impairment/failure, seizures, Stevens-Johnson syndrome, thrombocytopenia, and toxic epidermal necrolysis.

ANTIDOTE

Keep physician informed of all side effects. Most minor side effects will be treated symptomatically. Discontinue doripenem at the first sign of hypersensitivity. Treat hypersensitivity reactions as indicated; may require epinephrine, airway management, oxygen, IV fluids, antihistamines (e.g., diphenhydramine [Benadryl]), corticosteroids (e.g., hydrocortisone sodium succinate [Solu-Cortef]), and pressor amines (e.g., dopamine). Treat CDAD with fluids, electrolytes, protein supplements, and oral vancomycin (Vancocin) or metronidazole (Flagyl) as indicated. In severe cases, surgical evaluation may be indicated. Doripenem is partially removed by hemodialysis.

DOXERCALCIFEROL

(**DOX**-err-kal-**sif**-er-ol)

Hectorol Injection

USUAL DOSE

Optimal dose of doxercalciferol must be individualized. The dose is adjusted in an attempt to achieve intact parathyroid hormone (iPTH) levels within a targeted range of 150 to 300 pg/mL. See Precautions and Monitor. Recommended initial dose for a patient with an iPTH level greater than 400 pg/mL is 4 mcg administered as a bolus dose three times weekly at the end of dialysis (approximately every other day). Total weekly dose is 12 mcg/week. Maximum dose was limited to 18 mcg/week in clinical studies.

DOSE ADJUSTMENTS

Adjust dosing based on patient response in order to lower blood iPTH into the range of 150 to 300 pg/mL. The following chart is a suggested approach to dose titration. Doses higher than 18 mcg weekly have not been studied. During titration monitor iPTH, serum calcium, phophorus, and calcium $\times$ phosphorus product (Ca $\times$ P) weekly. Maximize iPTH suppression while maintaining serum calcium and phosphorous levels in prescribed ranges; see Monitor. ▪ Immediately suspend dosing if hypercalcemia, hyperphosphatemia, or a Ca $\times$ P product of greater than 55 mg^2/dL^2 is noted. Reinitiate therapy at a dose that is 1 mcg lower when parameters have normalized. ▪ Patients with impaired hepatic function may not metabolize doxercalciferol appropriately; see Precautions.

Suggested Dose Adjustment Guidelines for Doxercalciferol	
iPTH Level	**Doxercalciferol Dose Guidelines**
Decreased by <50% and above 300 pg/mL	Increase by 1 to 2 mcg at 8-week intervals as necessary
Decreased by >50% and above 300 pg/mL	Maintain
150-300 pg/mL	Maintain
<100 pg/mL	Suspend for 1 week, then resume at a dose that is at least 1 mcg lower

DILUTION

May be given undiluted. Available as 2 mcg/mL solution in 2-mL vials.

Storage: Store unopened vials at 25° C (77° F); range: 15° to 30° C (59° to 86° F). Protect from light. Discard unused portion.

COMPATIBILITY

Specific information not available. Consider specific use; consult pharmacist.

RATE OF ADMINISTRATION

Administer as a bolus dose at the end of dialysis.

ACTIONS

A synthetic vitamin D analog. Metabolizes to a naturally occurring, biologically active form of vitamin D_2 that regulates blood calcium at levels required for essential body functions (i.e., intestinal absorption of dietary calcium, tubular reabsorption of calcium by the kidney and, in conjunction with the parathyroid hormone [PTH], the mobilization of calcium from the skeleton). Acts directly on bone cells (osteoblasts) to stimulate skeletal growth and on the parathyroid glands to suppress PTH synthesis and secretion. In uremic patients, deficient production of biologically active vitamin D metabolites leads to secondary hyperparathyroidism, which contributes to the development of metabolic bone disease. Doxercalciferol is activated in the liver. Peak blood levels are reached in 2.1 to 13.9 hours. Mean half-life range is 32 to 96 hours.

INDICATIONS AND USES

Reduction of elevated iPTH levels in the management of secondary hyperparathyroidism in patients undergoing chronic renal dialysis.

CONTRAINDICATIONS

Evidence of vitamin D toxicity, hypercalcemia, hyperphosphatemia, or known hypersensitivity to any ingredient in this product; see Precautions.

PRECAUTIONS

Overdose of any form of vitamin D, including doxercalciferol, is dangerous. Progressive hypercalcemia due to overdose of vitamin D and its metabolites may require emergency attention. Acute hypercalcemia may exacerbate tendencies for cardiac arrhythmias and seizures and may potentiate the action of digoxin drugs. Chronic administration may place patient at risk of hypercalcemia, elevated Ca $\times$ P product, and generalized vascular and other soft-tissue calcification. If clinically significant hypercalcemia develops, dose should be reduced or held. Do not allow the Ca $\times$ P product to exceed 55 mg^2/dL^2. See Side Effects and Antidote. ▪ To avoid possible additive effects and hypercalcemia, phosphate or vitamin D-related compounds should not be taken concomitantly with doxercalciferol. ▪ Oversuppression of iPTH levels may lead to adynamic bone syndrome. ▪ Hyperphosphatemia can exacerbate hyperparathyroidism. ▪ Use caution in patients with impaired hepatic function. More frequent monitoring of iPTH, calcium, and phosphorus levels is recommended. ▪ Patients with higher pretreatment serum levels of calcium (more than 10.5 mg/dL) or phosphorus (more than 6.9 mg/dL) may be more likely to experience hypercalcemia or hyperphosphatemia; see Contraindications.

Monitor: During initiation of therapy, obtain baseline serum iPTH, calcium, and phosphorus levels, and determine levels weekly during the early phase of treatment (i.e., first 12 weeks). For dialysis patients, serum or plasma iPTH and serum calcium, phosphorus, and alkaline phosphatase should be determined periodically. See Dose Adjustments. ▪ Calculate Ca $\times$ P (should be less than 55 mg^2/dL^2). ▪ Monitor serum calcium levels weekly after all dose changes and during subsequent dose titration. ▪ Monitor for signs and symptoms of hypercalcemia. See Side Effects. Radiographic evaluation of suspect anatomical regions may be useful in the early detection of generalized vascular or other soft-tissue calcification. ▪ Oral calcium-based or other non–aluminum-containing phosphate binders and a low phosphate diet are indicated to control serum phosphorus levels in dialysis patients. Hyperphosphatemia can lessen the effectiveness of doxercalciferol in reducing blood PTH levels. After initiating doxercalciferol therapy, the dose of calcium-containing phosphate binders should be decreased to correct persistent mild hypercalcemia (10.6 to 11.2 mg/dL for 3 consecutive determinations), or increased to correct persistent mild hyperphosphatemia (7 to 8 mg/dL for 3 consecutive determinations). ▪ Persistent or markedly elevated serum calcium levels may be corrected by dialysis against a reduced calcium or calcium-free dialysate. ▪ See Precautions and Drug/Lab Interactions.

Patient Education: Report symptoms of hypercalcemia promptly. Dose adjustment or treatment may be required. Strict adherence to dietary supplementation of calcium and restriction of phosphorus is required to ensure optimal effectiveness of therapy. Phosphate-binding compounds (e.g., calcium acetate [Phos-lo]) may be needed to control serum phosphorus levels in patients with CRF, but excessive use of aluminum-containing products (e.g., aluminum hydroxide gel [Alternagel]) should be avoided. ▪ Review all nonprescription drugs with physician.

Maternal/Child: Category B: safety for use in pregnancy not established; use only if clearly needed. ▪ Discontinue breast-feeding. ▪ Safety and effectiveness for use in pediatric patients not established.

Elderly: No overall differences in effectiveness or safety observed.

DRUG/LAB INTERACTIONS

Specific interaction studies have not been performed. ▪ **Digoxin** toxicity is potentiated by hypercalcemia. Use caution when doxercalciferol is prescribed concomitantly with digoxin compounds. ▪ **Phosphate or vitamin D**–related compounds should not be taken concomitantly with doxercalciferol. ▪ May reduce serum total **alkaline phosphatase levels.** ▪ **Magnesium-containing antacids** may cause hypermagnesemia; concomitant use is not recommended. ▪ Concomitant use with **cytochrome P₄₅₀ enzyme inducers** (e.g., glutethimide, phenobarbital [Luminal], phenytoin [Dilantin], rifampin [Rifadin]) may affect hydroxylation of doxercalciferol and require dose adjustments. ▪ Concomitant use with **cytochrome P₄₅₀ enzyme inhibitors** (e.g., erythromycin, ketoconazole [Nizoral]) may inhibit metabolism of the active form of vitamin D, decreasing effectiveness.

SIDE EFFECTS

Dose-limiting side effects are hypercalcemia, hyperphosphatemia, and oversuppression of iPTH (less than 150 pg/mL). Overdose or chronic administration may lead to hypercalcemia. Signs and symptoms of vitamin D intoxication associated with hypercalcemia include: *Early:* anorexia, bone pain, constipation, dry mouth, headache, metallic taste, muscle pain, nausea, somnolence, vomiting, and weakness. *Late:* albuminuria, anorexia, apathy, arrested growth, cardiac arrhythmias, conjunctivitis (calcific), death, decreased libido, dehydration, ectopic calcification, elevated AST and ALT, elevated BUN, hypercholesterolemia, hypertension, hyperthermia, nocturia, overt psychosis (rare), pancreatitis, photophobia, polydipsia, polyuria, pruritus, rhinorrhea, sensory disturbances, somnolence, urinary tract infections, and weight loss.

Overdose: Hypercalcemia, hypercalciuria, hyperphosphatemia, and oversuppression of PTH secretion leading in certain cases to adynamic bone disease. High intake of calcium and phosphate concomitant with doxercalciferol may lead to similar abnormalities. High levels of calcium in the dialysate bath may contribute to hypercalcemia.

ANTIDOTE

Notify physician of any side effects. Treatment of patients with clinically significant hypercalcemia (more than 1 mg/dL above the upper limit of normal range) consists of immediate dose reduction or interruption of the therapy and includes a low-calcium diet, withdrawal of calcium supplements, patient mobilization, attention to fluid and electrolyte imbalances, assessment of electrocardiographic abnormalities (critical in patients receiving digoxin), forced diuresis, and hemodialysis or peritoneal dialysis against a calcium-free dialysate, as warranted. Monitor serum calcium levels frequently until calcium levels return to within normal limits. Not removed from blood during hemodialysis. When serum calcium levels return to within normal limits (usually 2 to 7 days), therapy may be restarted at a dose that is at least 1 mcg lower than prior therapy.

DOXORUBICIN HYDROCHLORIDE `BBW` ▪
DOXORUBICIN HYDROCHLORIDE
LIPOSOMAL INJECTION `BBW`

Antineoplastic
(anthracycline antibiotic)

(dox-oh-**ROO**-bih-sin hy-droh-**KLOR**-eyed)
(dox-oh-**ROO**-bih-sin hy-droh-**KLOR**-eyed **LIP**-oh-sohm-ul)

ADR, Adriamycin ▪ Doxil

pH 3.8 to 6.5 ▪ pH 6.5

USUAL DOSE

Assessment required before dosing; see Precautions and Monitor.

CONVENTIONAL DOXORUBICIN

60 to 75 mg/M^2 once every 21 days as a *single agent.* When used in *combination* with other agents, the most common dose of doxorubicin is 40 to 75 mg/M^2 every 21 to 28 days.

Breast cancer with lymph node involvement after resection: Doxorubicin 60 mg/M^2 in combination with cyclophosphamide 600 mg/M^2 given IV sequentially on Day 1 of each 21-day treatment cycle. Four cycles have been administered.

Adjuvant treatment of operable node-positive breast cancer: Treatment protocol includes doxorubicin, cyclophosphamide, and docetaxel. Administer doxorubicin 50 mg/M^2 and cyclophosphamide 500 mg/M^2. One hour later, give docetaxel 75 mg/M^2. Repeat every 3 weeks for 6 cycles. See docetaxel and cyclophosphamide monographs.

DOXIL (LIPOSOMAL DOXORUBICIN)

Do not substitute Doxil for conventional doxorubicin.

AIDS-related Kaposi's sarcoma: 20 mg/M^2 as an IV infusion over 60 minutes every 21 days until disease progression or unacceptable toxicity.

Ovarian cancer: 50 mg/M^2 as an IV infusion over 60 minutes every 28 days until disease progression or unacceptable toxicity.

Multiple myeloma: Given in combination with bortezomib (Velcade).

Bortezomib: Administer 1.3 mg/M^2 as an IV bolus on Days 1, 4, 8, and 11 of each 21-day cycle; see bortezomib monograph.

Doxil: Administer 30 mg/M^2 as an IV infusion over 60 minutes on Day 4 of each 21-day cycle following bortezomib. Continue regimen for 8 cycles or until disease progression or the occurrence of unacceptable toxicity.

Breast cancer (unlabeled): 50 mg/M^2 as an IV infusion over 60 minutes every 4 weeks. Other combination protocols are in use.

PEDIATRIC DOSE

CONVENTIONAL DOXORUBICIN: In combination with other chemotherapeutic agents as first-line treatment, 30 to 60 mg/M^2 every 21 to 42 days. See Maternal/Child.

DOXIL: Safety for use in pediatric patients not established.

DOSE ADJUSTMENTS

ALL DOXORUBICINS: *Elevated serum bilirubin:* Give 50% of above doses for serum bilirubin from 1.2 to 3 mg/mL and 25% for serum bilirubin above 3 mg/mL. Discontinue therapy for serum bilirubin greater than 5 mg/dL (doxorubicin prescribing information). ▪ Reduce dose in patients with impaired hepatic function. ▪ See Precautions.

CONVENTIONAL DOXORUBICIN: Consider lower-end doses or longer intervals between cycles for heavily pretreated patients, elderly patients, or obese patients.

Breast cancer with lymph node involvement after resection: Reduce dose to 75% of the starting dose for neutropenic fever/infection. If necessary, delay the next cycle of treatment until the ANC is 1,000 cells/mm^3 or more and the platelet count is 100,000 cells/mm^3 or more and nonhematologic toxicities have resolved.

DOXIL: Dose adjustments are required in hematologic toxicity (see the following chart) and in patients with stomatitis or hand-foot syndrome (HFS) (see product literature for guidelines). Adjust or delay a dose as described in the product literature at the first sign of a Grade 2 or higher adverse event. Do not increase Doxil dose after a dose reduction for toxicity.

Doxil Dosing Based on Hematologic Toxicity (Neutropenia or Thrombocytopenia)	
Grade	Modification
1	Resume treatment with no dose reduction.
2	Delay until ANC ≥1,500 and platelets ≥75,000; resume treatment at previous dose.
3	Delay until ANC ≥1,500 and platelets ≥75,000; resume treatment at previous dose.
4	Delay until ANC ≥1,500 and platelets ≥75,000; resume at 25% dose reduction or continue previous dose with prophylactic granulocyte growth factor.

Dose adjustments for Doxil in combination therapy with bortezomib for treatment of multiple myeloma are listed in the following chart. See bortezomib monograph for bortezomib dose adjustments.

Dose Adjustments for Doxil in Combination Therapy with Bortezomib	
Patient Status	Doxil
Fever ≥38° C and ANC <1,000/mm³	Withhold dose for this cycle if before Day 4. Decrease dose by 25% if after Day 4 of previous cycle.
On any day of drug administration after Day 1 of each cycle: Platelet count <25,000/mm³ Hemoglobin <8 Gm/dL ANC <500/mm³	Withhold dose for this cycle if before Day 4. Decrease dose by 25% if after Day 4 of previous cycle AND if bortezomib is reduced for hematologic toxicity.
Grade 3 or 4 nonhematologic drug-related toxicity	Do not dose until recovered to Grade <2, then reduce dose by 25%.
Neuropathic pain or peripheral neuropathy	No dose adjustments.

DILUTION
Specific techniques required; see Precautions.
CONVENTIONAL DOXORUBICIN: Each 10 mg must be diluted with 5 mL of NS to obtain a final concentration of 2 mg/mL. Do not use bacteriostatic diluent. Shake gently to dissolve completely. Also available in preservative-free solutions. May be further diluted in 50 mL or more D5W or NS and given as a continuous infusion through a central venous line.

DOXIL: Doses up to 90 mg must be diluted in 250 mL D5W. Not a clear solution, but a translucent red liposomal dispersion. Do not use filters. Doses over 90 mg should be diluted in 500 mL D5W. See Compatibility.

Filters: *Conventional doxorubicin:* Data not available from manufacturer; however, one source indicates no evidence of drug loss when administered through a 0.2-micron in-line nylon filter, and another source indicates no significant drug loss using various types of 0.2-micron filters.

Doxil: Do not use filters during preparation or administration.

Storage: *Conventional doxorubicin:* Retain vials in carton until time of use. Refrigerate unopened vials containing solution. Refrigeration can result in the formation of a gelled product. If this occurs, place vial at RT for 2 to 4 hours to return the product to a slightly viscous mobile solution. Vials containing lyophilized powder may be stored at CRT. All forms should be protected from light.

Doxil: Refrigerate unopened vials at 2° to 8° C (36° to 46° F). Do not freeze. Refrigerate diluted solution and use within 24 hours.

COMPATIBILITY   (Underline Indicates Conflicting Compatibility Information)
Consider any drug NOT listed as compatible to be INCOMPATIBLE until consulting a pharmacist; specific conditions may apply.

CONVENTIONAL DOXORUBICIN

Manufacturer lists fluorouracil and heparin as **incompatible** and states mixing with other drugs is not recommended unless specific **compatibility** data available. Avoid contact with alkaline solutions; can lead to hydrolysis of doxorubicin.

One source suggests the following **compatibilities:**

Additive: Bleomycin (Blenoxane), cyclophosphamide (Cytoxan), dacarbazine (DTIC), ondansetron (Zofran), paclitaxel (Taxol), vinblastine, vincristine.

Y-site: Amifostine (Ethyol), anidulafungin (Eraxis), aztreonam (Azactam), bleomycin (Blenoxane), caspofungin (Cancidas), cisplatin, cladribine (Leustatin), cyclophosphamide (Cytoxan), doripenem (Doribax), droperidol (Inapsine), etoposide phosphate (Etopophos), filgrastim (Neupogen), fludarabine (Fludara), fluorouracil (5-FU), gemcitabine (Gemzar), granisetron (Kytril), leucovorin calcium, linezolid (Zyvox), melphalan (Alkeran), methotrexate, metoclopramide (Reglan), mitomycin (Mutamycin), ondansetron (Zofran), oxaliplatin (Eloxatin), paclitaxel (Taxol), sargramostim (Leukine), sodium bicarbonate, teniposide (Vumon), thiotepa, topotecan (Hycamtin), vinblastine, vincristine, vinorelbine (Navelbine).

DOXIL

Specific information not available. Manufacturer states, "Do not mix Doxil with other drugs. Do not use any other diluent (use D5W only). Do not use any bacteriostatic agents (e.g., benzyl alcohol)."

One source suggests the following **compatibilities:**

Y-site: *Not recommended by manufacturer.* Acyclovir (Zovirax), allopurinol (Aloprim), aminophylline, ampicillin, aztreonam (Azactam), bleomycin (Blenoxane), butorphanol (Stadol), calcium gluconate, carboplatin (Paraplatin), cefazolin (Ancef), cefepime (Maxipime), cefoxitin (Mefoxin), ceftriaxone (Rocephin), chlorpromazine (Thorazine), ciprofloxacin (Cipro IV), cisplatin, clindamycin (Cleocin), cyclophosphamide (Cytoxan), cytarabine (ARA-C), dacarbazine (DTIC), dexamethasone (Decadron), diphenhydramine (Benadryl), dobutamine, dopamine, droperidol (Inapsine), enalaprilat (Vasotec IV), etoposide (VePesid), famotidine (Pepcid IV), fluconazole (Diflucan), fluorouracil (5-FU), furosemide (Lasix), ganciclovir (Cytovene IV), gentamicin, granisetron (Kytril), heparin, hydrocortisone sodium succinate (Solu-Cortef), hydromorphone (Dilaudid), ifosfamide (Ifex), leucovorin calcium, lorazepam (Ativan), magnesium sulfate, mesna (Mesnex), methotrexate, methylprednisolone (Solu-Medrol), metronidazole (Flagyl IV), ondansetron (Zofran), potassium chloride (KCl), prochlorperazine (Compazine), ranitidine (Zantac), sulfamethoxazole/trimethoprim, ticarcillin/clavulanate (Timentin), tobramycin, vancomycin, vinblastine, vincristine, vinorelbine (Navelbine), zidovudine (AZT, Retrovir).

RATE OF ADMINISTRATION

CONVENTIONAL DOXORUBICIN

IV injection: A single dose of properly diluted medication over a minimum of 3 to 10 minutes. Should be given through a central line or a secure and free-flowing peripheral venous line containing NS, 1/2NS, or D5W. Slow injection rate further for erythematous streaking along the vein or facial flushing.

Continuous infusion: Central venous line required. Equally distributed over time interval outlined in given protocol.

DOXIL

Do not administer as an undiluted suspension or as an IV bolus. For IV infusion only. Rapid infusion may increase risk of acute infusion-related reactions. Primarily occurs during the first infusion; may resolve with a reduced rate or may take up to a day after infusion completed to resolve.

Begin with an initial rate of 1 mg/min to minimize the risk of infusion reactions. If no adverse infusion-related effects, the rate may be increased from the initial rate of 1 mg/min to evenly distribute and complete infusion over 1 hour. Avoid rapid flushing of the infusion line.

ACTIONS

CONVENTIONAL DOXORUBICIN: A highly cytotoxic anthracycline topoisomerase II inhibitor that is cell-cycle specific for the S phase. Widely distributed and rapidly cleared from plasma, it interferes with cell division by binding with DNA to slow production of nucleic acid synthesis. Metabolized in the liver. Elimination half-life is 20 to 48 hours. Does not cross blood-brain barrier. Slowly excreted in bile and urine. Secreted in breast milk. **DOXIL:** Doxorubicin encapsulated in long-circulating STEALTH liposomes (phospholipids). The small size of these liposomes and their persistence in the circulation enable them to evade immune system detection and penetrate the often altered and/or compromised vasculature of tumors. Once distributed to tumor tissue, the doxorubicin is released by an unknown mechanism. It differs from conventional doxorubicin because it mostly confines itself to vascular fluid volume. Metabolized and eliminated renally. Plasma clearance is slower. Half-life is extended to 55 hours. Concentration in Kaposi's sarcoma lesions is much higher than in normal skin (range is 3 to 53 times higher).

INDICATIONS AND USES

CONVENTIONAL DOXORUBICIN: Adjuvant therapy in women with evidence of axillary lymph node involvement following resection of primary breast cancer. ▪ Treatment of acute lymphoblastic leukemia, acute myeloblastic leukemia, Hodgkin's lymphoma, non-Hodgkin's lymphoma, metastatic breast cancer, metastatic Wilms' tumor, metastatic neuroblastoma, metastatic soft tissue sarcoma, metastatic bone sarcoma, metastatic ovarian carcinoma, metastatic transitional cell bladder carcinoma, metastatic thyroid carcinoma, metastatic gastric carcinoma, metastatic bronchogenic carcinoma. **DOXIL:** Treatment of AIDS-related Kaposi's sarcoma in patients whose disease has progressed on prior combination chemotherapy or who are intolerant to combination chemotherapy. ▪ Treatment of metastatic carcinoma of the ovary in patients with disease that is refractory to platinum-based chemotherapy regimens (e.g., cisplatin, carboplatin [Paraplatin]). ▪ Treatment of multiple myeloma in combination with bortezomib (Velcade) in patients who have received one prior therapy but have not previously received bortezomib.

Unlabeled uses: *Doxil:* Treatment of refractory metastatic breast cancer.

CONTRAINDICATIONS

CONVENTIONAL DOXORUBICIN: Severe myocardial insufficiency, recent myocardial infarction (occurring within the last 4 to 6 weeks), severe persistent drug-induced myelosuppression, severe hepatic impairment (Child-Pugh Class C or serum bilirubin level greater than 5 mg/dL). **ALL DOXORUBICINS:** History of hypersensitivity to conventional or liposomal formulations of doxorubicin or to their components.

PRECAUTIONS

ALL DOXORUBICINS: Follow guidelines for handling cytotoxic agents and patient excreta. Precautions recommended for up to 5 days after a dose. See Appendix A, p. 1331. ▪ Usually administered by or under the direction of a physician specialist, with facilities for monitoring the patient and responding to any medical emergency. ▪ For IV use only. Do not give IM or SC. ▪ *Do Not Substitute* Doxil for conventional doxorubicin. Severe side effects have resulted. Differences in liposomal products as well as conventional products can substantially affect the functional properties of these agents; do not substitute one agent for another. ▪ Use extreme caution in pre-existing drug-induced bone marrow suppression, existing heart disease, hepatic impairment, previous treatment with other anthracyclines (e.g., daunorubicin), other cardiotoxic agents (e.g., bleomycin), concurrent cyclophosphamide therapy, or radiation therapy encompassing the heart; risk of cardiotoxicity increased and may occur at lower doses. ▪ All forms of doxorubicin may cause cardiotoxicity. May be manifest by acute (e.g., arrhythmias, including life-threatening arrhythmias, ECG abnormalities) or delayed (e.g., reduction in LVEF, CHF) events. Life-threatening or fatal congestive heart failure may occur during therapy or months after therapy is completed. Cardiotoxicity occurs with increasing frequency as cumulative doses increase above 300 mg/M². The risk of developing CHF increases rapidly with increasing total cumulative doses above 400 mg/M²; see Antidote. Prior use of other anthracyclines or anthracenediones should be included in calculations of total cumulative dose. Patients with active or dormant cardiovascular disease or patients who have received radiotherapy to the mediastinal area or concomitant therapy with other anthracyclines (e.g., daunorubicin, idarubicin), anthracenediones, or other cardiotoxic agents (e.g., bleomycin, cyclophosphamide, mitoxantrone, mitomycin C, trastuzumab) may be at greater risk. Consider the use of dexrazoxane to reduce the incidence and severity of cardiomyopathy due to doxorubicin in patients who have received a cumulative dose of 300 mg/M² and who will continue to receive doxorubicin. ▪ May cause severe myelosuppression resulting in serious infection, septic shock, required transfusions, hospitalization, hemorrhage, and death. ▪ See Maternal/Child and Side Effects.

CONVENTIONAL DOXORUBICIN: In addition to cardiomyopathy, pericarditis and myocarditis have been reported during or after therapy with doxorubicin. ▪ Secondary acute myelogenous leukemia (AML) and myelodysplastic syndrome (MDS) have been reported and generally occur within 1 to 3 years of treatment. ▪ Tumor lysis syndrome may occur; see Monitor.

DOXIL: Benefits must outweigh risks if Doxil is used in patients with a history of cardiovascular disease. ▪ Acute infusion-related reactions and serious, sometimes life-threatening or fatal hypersensitivity/anaphylactoid-like reactions have been reported; see Monitor. ▪ Has caused hand-foot syndrome (HFS). Incidence may be increased with higher doses or increased frequency. Generally seen after 2 or 3 cycles, but may occur earlier. May be severe and require a dose adjustment or discontinuation of Doxil. ▪ Secondary oral cancers, primarily squamous cell carcinoma, have been reported in patients who have received Doxil for a year or longer. Malignancies have been diagnosed both during treatment and up to 6 years after completion of therapy. ▪ Severe, additive myelosuppression may occur in Kaposi's sarcoma patients and may be dose limiting.

Monitor: ALL DOXORUBICINS: Monitoring of CBC including differential and platelet count, uric acid levels, electrolytes, liver function (AST, ALT, alkaline phosphatase, and bilirubin), kidney function, ECG, chest x-ray, echocardiogram, and left ventricular ejection fraction (LVEF) is necessary before and during therapy. At a minimum, CBC with platelets should be monitored before each dose. Testing for renal and hepatic function may also be indicated; see Dose Adjustments. ▪ Observe for S/S of cardiotoxicity (e.g., fast or irregular HR, shortness of breath, swelling of the feet or lower legs). Endomyocardial biopsy or gated radionuclide scans have been used to monitor potential cardiac toxicity. Increase frequency of assessment as cumulative dose exceeds 300 mg/M². Use same method of assessment of LVEF at all time points. ▪ Be alert for signs of bone marrow suppression, bleeding, or infection. ▪ Monitor for thrombocytopenia (platelet count less than 50,000/mm³). Initiate precautions to prevent excessive bleeding (e.g., inspect IV sites, skin, and mucous membranes; use extreme care during invasive procedures; test urine, emesis, stool, and secretions for occult blood). ▪ Use of prophylactic antibiotics may be indicated pending C/S in a febrile, neutropenic patient. Sepsis in a neutropenic patient has resulted in discontinuation of treatment and, in rare cases, death. ▪ Prophylactic antiemetics are indicated. ▪ See Drug/Lab Interactions.

CONVENTIONAL DOXORUBICIN: Monitor for tumor lysis syndrome. S/S include hyperkalemia, hyperphosphatemia, hyperuricemia, hypocalcemia, metabolic acidosis, urate crystalluria, and renal failure. Prevent or alleviate tumor lysis syndrome with appropriate supportive and pharmacologic measures. ▪ Maintain adequate hydration and urine alkalinization. ▪ Allopurinol may prevent formation of uric acid crystals. ▪ Use only large veins. Avoid veins over joints or in extremities with compromised venous or lymphatic drainage. Determine absolute patency of vein. A stinging or burning sensation indicates extravasation; severe cellulitis and tissue necrosis will result. *Extravasation may occur with or without stinging or* *burning and even if blood returns well on aspiration of infusion needle.* Observe and touch site frequently to feel air and/or liquid under the skin. If extravasation occurs, discontinue injection; use another vein; see Antidote.

DOXIL: Monitor for S/S of acute infusion reactions and/or hypersensitivity (e.g., apnea, asthma, back pain, bronchospasm, chills, cyanosis, facial swelling, fever, flushing, headache, hypotension, pruritus, rash, shortness of breath, syncope, tachycardia, tightness in the chest or throat). The majority of infusion-related reactions occur during the first infusion. ■ Monitor for HFS (skin eruptions characterized by swelling, pain, erythema, and possible desquamation of the skin on the hands and feet). ■ Monitor for the presence of oral ulceration or oral discomfort that may be indicative of secondary oral cancer. ■ Extravasation may cause irritation at infusion site. Discontinue and use another vein.

Patient Education: ALL DOXORUBICINS: Urine and other body fluids will be reddish for several days (from dye, not hematuria). ■ Effective birth control required for both women and men during and for 6 months after treatment. May cause infertility in both men and women. ■ Effects may be additive with current medications. Review all medications (prescription and nonprescription) with nurse and/or physician. ■ Promptly report cough, fast heartbeat, shortness of breath, and/or swelling of the feet or lower legs. ■ Report S/S of infection (e.g., chills, fever, painful urination), stomatitis, bothersome side effects, or any unusual bleeding (e.g., bruising, tarry stools). ■ Report IV site burning, stinging, puffiness, or the feeling of liquid under the skin and any other side effects promptly. ■ Report tingling, burning, redness, flaking, swelling, blisters or small sores on the palms of hands or soles of feet. ■ See Precautions. ■ See Appendix D, p. 1333.

Maternal/Child: ALL DOXORUBICINS: Category D: avoid pregnancy; can cause fetal harm. ■ Has been used only when benefits outweigh risks. ■ Discontinue breast-feeding.

CONVENTIONAL DOXORUBICIN: Treatment during childhood may result in abnormal cardiac function. ■ Infants and children are at increased risk for developing delayed cardiotoxicity; follow-up cardiac evaluation is recommended; see Precautions. ■ In infants under 2 years of age, doxorubicin clearance is similar to adults, but clearance may be increased in pediatric patients over 2 years of age. ■ May contribute to prepubertal growth failure and/or gonadal impairment (which is usually temporary). ■ See Precautions, extended recommendations for handling patient excreta.

DOXIL: Safety for use in pediatric patients not established.

Elderly: ALL DOXORUBICINS: Response similar to that seen in younger adults, but greater sensitivity of some older individuals cannot be ruled out. ■ Cardiotoxicity and myelotoxicity may be more severe in patients over 70 years of age. ■ Consider age-related organ impairment and concomitant disease and/or drug therapy; see Dose Adjustments.

DRUG/LAB INTERACTIONS

Studies not yet completed for Doxil; interactions may be similar to conventional doxorubicins. ■ Doxorubicin is a major substrate for cytochrome P_{450} CYP3A4 and CYP2D6 and P-glycoprotein. Clinically significant interactions have been reported with inhibitors of CYP3A4 and CYP2D6 and P-glycoprotein (e.g., **verapamil**), resulting in increased concentrations and clinical effects of doxorubicin. Inducers of CYP3A4 (e.g., **phenobarbital, phenytoin, St. John's wort**) and P-glycoprotein may decrease the concentration of doxorubicin. Avoid concurrent use with **inhibitors or inducers of CYP3A4 and CYP2D6 and P-glycoprotein.** ■ Avoid concurrent administration of doxorubicin (Adriamycin) and **trastuzumab** (Herceptin); results in an increased risk of cardiac dysfunction. ■ May exacerbate **cyclophosphamide**-induced hemorrhagic cystitis or increase hepatotoxicity of **6-mercaptopurine.** ■ May increase bone marrow toxicity of **other chemotherapeutic agents and radiation.** ■ **Barbiturates** increase clearance and decrease effects. ■ May decrease serum levels of **digoxin.** ■ May decrease serum levels of **anticonvulsants** (e.g., phenytoin [Dilantin], carbamazepine [Tegretol], valproate [Depacon]). ■ Risk of cardiotoxicity increased in patients previously treated with **other anthracyclines** (e.g., idarubicin [Idamycin]) **and/or radiation encompassing the heart.** ■ **Cyclosporine** (Sandimmune) **and streptozocin** (Zanosar) may decrease clearance and increase toxicity of doxorubicin. ■ **Paclitaxel** (Taxol) appears to decrease the clearance of doxorubicin. Administration of doxorubicin before paclitaxel is recommended to prevent increased toxicity. ■ Coadministration with high-dose **progesterone** may increase doxorubicin toxicity. ■ Many drug interactions possible; observe patient closely. ■ Do not administer **live virus vaccines** to patients receiving antineoplastic drugs. ■ Increased toxicity to mucosa, myocardium, skin (including redness and exfoliative changes), and liver possible when given concurrently **with or after radiation.** ■ **Dexrazoxane** is given with doxorubicin to reduce cardiotoxic effects. May also decrease antitumor effectiveness if given before a cumulative dose of doxorubicin 300 mg/M^2 is reached or other chemotherapeutic agents are included in the protocol (e.g., fluorouracil). ■ See Precautions.

SIDE EFFECTS

ALL DOXORUBICINS: Abdominal pain; alopecia (complete); anorexia; asthenia; bone marrow suppression (e.g., anemia, hypochromic anemia, leukopenia, neutropenia [ANC less than 1,000/mm^3], thrombocytopenia may be dose-limiting); cardiac toxicity (e.g., CHF); constipation; decreased serum calcium; depressed QRS voltage; diarrhea; dry skin; esophagitis; fatigue; fever; gonadal suppression; headache; hyperpigmentation of nail beds and dermal creases; hypersensitivity reactions (including life-threatening or fatal anaphylaxis); hyperuricemia; increase in alkaline phosphatase, ALT, AST, bilirubin, BUN, glucose, SCr; infection; mucositis; nausea; oral moniliasis; paresthesia; prolonged PT; rash; recall of skin reactions due to prior radiotherapy; stomatitis; weakness; vomiting.

DOXIL: In addition to all of the above, acute infusion reactions, hand-foot syndrome, secondary oral cancer. *Kaposi's sarcoma* patients may be taking numerous other drugs that may confuse the overall side effect picture (e.g., didanosine [ddI], stavudine [D4T], sulfamethoxazole/trimethoprim, zalcitabine [ddC], zidovudine [AZT, Retrovir]).

Post-Marketing: Muscle spasms, myelogenous leukemia, pulmonary embolism, and skin and subcutaneous tissue disorders (e.g., erythema multiforme, Stevens-Johnson syndrome, and toxic epidermal necrolysis).

Overdose: ALL DOXORUBICINS: Increase in bone marrow suppression and mucositis.

ANTIDOTE

ALL DOXORUBICINS: Most side effects will either be tolerated or treated symptomatically. Keep the physician informed. Bone marrow toxicity may require cessation of therapy. Administration of whole blood products (e.g., packed RBCs, platelets, leukocytes) and/or blood modifiers (e.g., darbepoetin alfa [Aranesp], epoetin alfa [Epogen], filgrastim [Neupogen, Zarxio], pegfilgrastim [Neulasta], sargramostim [Leukine]) may be indicated to treat bone marrow toxicity. Acute cardiac failure occurs suddenly (most common when total cumulative dosage approaches 550 mg/M^2) and frequently does not respond to currently available treatment (digoxin, diuretics [e.g., furosemide (Lasix)], ACE inhibitors [e.g., enalapril]). Close monitoring of accumulated dosage, bone marrow, ECG, chest x-ray, echocardiography, and systolic ejection fraction may prevent most serious and potentially fatal cardiac side effects. There is no specific antidote. Supportive therapy as indicated will help sustain the patient in toxicity. Treat hypersensitivity reactions as required; discontinue therapy if severe.

CONVENTIONAL DOXORUBICIN: Discontinue doxorubicin in patients who develop signs or symptoms of cardiomyopathy. For extravasation, attempt to aspirate extravasated fluid before removing needle. Do not flush line or apply pressure to site. Elevate the extremity and apply ice for 15 minutes four times a day for 3 days. If appropriate, administer dexrazoxane at the site of extravasation as soon as possible and within the first 6 hours after extravasation. Site should be observed promptly by a reconstructive surgeon.

DOXIL: In addition to all of the above, treatment may have to be interrupted or discontinued for severe hand-foot syndrome or acute infusion reactions. Infusion reactions may resolve with slowing of infusion rate. May be able to control hand-foot syndrome by allowing it to resolve and by increasing intervals between subsequent cycles. For extravasation, discontinue infusion and apply ice over site for 30 minutes to alleviate local reaction.

DOXYCYCLINE HYCLATE
(dox-ih-**SYE**-kleen **HI**-klayt)

Antibacterial
(tetracycline)
Antiprotozoal
Antimalarial

Doxy 100, Doxy 200, Vibramycin

pH 1.8 to 3.3

USUAL DOSE
Parenteral therapy is indicated only when oral therapy is not indicated. Transfer to oral therapy as soon as practical.

ADULTS AND PEDIATRIC PATIENTS OVER 45 KG
200 mg the first day in one or two infusions followed by 100 to 200 mg/24 hr on subsequent days with 200 mg administered in one or two infusions. Depends on severity of the infection.

Primary and secondary syphilis: 300 mg daily for at least 10 days.

Acute pelvic inflammatory disease: 100 mg every 12 hours. Used in combination with cefoxitin 2 Gm every 6 hours.

Prevention and/or treatment of anthrax postexposure: 100 mg every 12 hours. Continue therapy for 60 days.

PEDIATRIC DOSE

PEDIATRIC PATIENTS 45 KG OR LESS (BUT OVER 8 YEARS)
2 mg/lb (4.4 mg/kg) of body weight on the first day of treatment, administered in one or two infusions followed by 1 to 2 mg/lb (2.2 to 4.4 mg/kg) of body weight/day on subsequent days given as one or two infusions. Dose depends on severity of infection. Transfer to oral therapy as soon as practical. Do not exceed adult dose. See Maternal/Child.

Prevention and/or treatment of anthrax postexposure: 1 mg/lb (2.2 mg/kg) of body weight every 12 hours in children weighing less than 45 kg. Do not exceed adult dose. Continue therapy for 60 days.

DOSE ADJUSTMENTS
See Drug/Lab Interactions.

DILUTION
Check expiration date. Outdated ampules may cause nephrotoxicity. Each 100 mg or fraction thereof is diluted with 10 mL of SWFI or NS (may also be reconstituted with any of the **compatible** solutions listed for further dilution). Further dilute each 100 mg (10 mL) with 100 to 1,000 mL of a **compatible** infusion solution such as NS, D5W, R, LR, D5LR, 10% invert sugar in water, Normosol-M or Normosol-R in 5% dextrose in water, or other **compatible** solutions (see literature). Recommended concentrations 0.1 to 1 mg/mL. 100 mg in 1,000 mL of solution equals 0.1 mg/mL, 100 mg in 100 mL equals 1 mg/mL.

Storage: Store vials at CRT in carton; protect from light. Stable for 48 hours when diluted with NS or D5W to concentrations between 0.1 and 1 mg/mL and stored at 25° C (77° F). Protect from direct sunlight during storage and infusion. These dilutions may be stored for 72 hours if refrigerated and protected from sunlight *and* artificial light. Infusion must be completed within 12 hours. Solutions must be used within these time periods or discarded. See manufacturer's prescribing information for stability data when mixed with other solutions.

COMPATIBILITY
(Underline Indicates Conflicting Compatibility Information)

Consider any drug NOT listed as compatible to be INCOMPATIBLE until consulting a pharmacist; specific conditions may apply.

One source suggests the following **compatibilities:**

Additive: <u>Meropenem (Merrem IV)</u>, ranitidine (Zantac).

Y-site: Acyclovir (Zovirax), amifostine (Ethyol), amiodarone (Nexterone), aztreonam (Azactam), bivalirudin (Angiomax), cisatracurium (Nimbex), cyclophosphamide (Cytoxan), dexmedetomidine (Precedex), diltiazem (Cardizem), docetaxel (Taxotere), etoposide phosphate (Etopophos), fenoldopam (Corlopam), filgrastim (Neupogen), fludarabine (Fludara), gemcitabine (Gemzar), granisetron (Kytril), hetastarch in electrolytes (Hextend), hetastarch in NS (Hespan), hydromorphone (Dilaudid), linezolid (Zyvox), magnesium sulfate, melphalan (Alkeran), meperidine (Demerol), meropenem (Merrem IV), morphine, ondansetron (Zofran), propofol (Diprivan), remifentanil (Ultiva), sargramostim (Leukine), tacrolimus (Prograf), telavancin (Vibativ), teniposide (Vumon), theophylline, thiotepa, vinorelbine (Navelbine).

RATE OF ADMINISTRATION

Avoid rapid administration. Duration of infusion may vary with dose but is usually 1 to 4 hours. The recommended minimum infusion time for 100 mg of a 0.5 mg/mL solution is 1 hour.

ACTIONS

A broad-spectrum tetracycline antibiotic, bacteriostatic against many microorganisms, including gram-positive, gram-negative, anaerobic, atypical, and parasitic organisms. Thought to interfere with the protein synthesis of microorganisms. Doxycycline is well distributed in most body tissues and is highly bound to plasma protein. Half-life is 18 to 22 hours. Concentrated by the liver in the bile and excreted in urine and feces. Crosses the placental barrier. Secreted in breast milk.

INDICATIONS AND USES

Infections caused by susceptible strains of several microorganisms, including many gram-positive, gram-negative, anaerobic, atypical bacteria (e.g., *Rickettsia, Chlamydia, Chlamydophila, Mycoplasma*) or parasites (e.g., *Balantidium coli, Entamoeba* species). Types of infections treated may include GU infections, including those caused by *Chlamydia trachomatis* and *Neisseria gonorrhoeae;* respiratory tract infections, including mycoplasma pneumonia; skin and soft tissue infections; syphilis; and others. ■ To substitute for contraindicated penicillin or sulfonamide therapy. ■ Adjunct to amebicides in acute intestinal amebiasis. ■ Prevention and/or treatment of anthrax in all its forms, including cutaneous and inhalation anthrax postexposure.

CONTRAINDICATIONS

Known hypersensitivity to tetracyclines. Not recommended in pediatric patients under 8 years or in pregnancy or breast-feeding.

PRECAUTIONS

Sensitivity studies indicated to determine susceptibility of the causative organism to doxycycline. ■ To reduce the development of drug-resistant bacteria and maintain its effectiveness, doxycycline should be used to treat or prevent only those infections proven or strongly suspected to be caused by bacteria. ■ Continue for at least 2 to 3 days after all symptoms of infection subside. ■ Avoid prolonged use of drug; superinfection caused by overgrowth of nonsusceptible organisms may result. ■ *Clostridium difficile*–associated diarrhea (CDAD) has been reported. May range from mild to life threatening. Consider in patients who present with diarrhea during or after treatment with doxycycline. ■ Initiate oral therapy as soon as possible. ■ Cross-resistance with other tetracyclines is common. ■ Intracranial hypertension (IH, pseudotumor cerebri) has been associated with the use of tetracyclines, including doxycycline. Clinical manifestations include headache, blurred vision, diplopia, vision loss, and papilledema. Women of childbearing age who are overweight or have a history of IH are at greater risk for developing tetracycline-associated IH. ■ In venereal diseases in which coexistent syphilis is suspected, perform a dark-field examination before initiating tetracyclines. Repeat blood serology monthly for at least 4 months. ■ The antianabolic action of tetracyclines may cause an increase in BUN. Studies to date indicate that this does not occur with the use of doxycycline in patients with impaired renal function. ■ All infections due to group A beta-hemolytic streptococci should be treated for at least 10 days.

Monitor: Determine absolute patency of vein and avoid extravasation; thrombophlebitis may occur. ▪ Monitor for S/S of intracranial hypertension. If visual symptoms develop during treatment with doxycycline, prompt ophthalmologic evaluation is warranted. Intracranial pressure can remain elevated for weeks after drug cessation. Continue ophthalmologic monitoring until patient stabilizes. Permanent vision loss can occur. ▪ Monitor hematopoietic, renal, and hepatic studies periodically in long-term therapy. ▪ Monitor for S/S of hypersensitivity reactions. ▪ See Drug/Lab Interactions.

Patient Education: Report severe diarrhea, S/S of hypersensitivity reactions, or S/S of IH promptly. ▪ Alert patient to photosensitive skin reaction. ▪ Consider birth control options.

Maternal/Child: Category D: avoid pregnancy; see Contraindications. ▪ May cause skeletal retardation in the fetus and infants. ▪ Exposure during last half of pregnancy, infancy, and childhood to the age of 8 years may cause permanent discoloration of the teeth. Avoid exposure in this age-group unless treating anthrax or unless other drugs are contraindicated or are not likely to be effective. ▪ Discontinue breast-feeding.

DRUG/LAB INTERACTIONS

Inhibits **oral contraceptives;** may result in pregnancy or breakthrough bleeding. ▪ Interferes with bactericidal action of **all penicillins** (e.g., ampicillin, oxacillin). Avoid concomitant use. ▪ Serum levels decreased by **barbiturates, carbamazepine** (Tegretol), **hydantoins** (e.g., phenytoin), and others. ▪ May depress **plasma prothrombin activity;** a reduction in **anticoagulant** dose may be indicated. ▪ Avoid concomitant use with **isotretinoin** (Amnesteem, Claravis, Sotret); both agents can cause pseudotumor cerebri.

SIDE EFFECTS

Relatively nontoxic in average doses. More toxic in large doses or if given too rapidly. Anogenital lesions, anorexia, blood dyscrasias (eosinophilia, neutropenia, thrombocytopenia), diarrhea, dysphagia, elevated BUN, enterocolitis, nausea, skin rashes, vomiting.

Major: Hypersensitivity reactions (including anaphylaxis), angioneurotic edema, CDAD, drug rash with eosinophilia and systemic symptoms (DRESS), intracranial hypertension (may be caused by pseudotumor cerebri [blurred vision, diplopia, headache, papilledema, vision loss]), bulging fontanels in infants, exfoliative dermatitis, hepatotoxicity, pancreatitis, photosensitivity, systemic candidiasis, thrombophlebitis.

ANTIDOTE

Notify the physician of all side effects. If minor side effects are progressive or any major side effect occurs, discontinue the drug, treat hypersensitivity reactions as indicated, or resuscitate as necessary. Mild cases of CDAD may respond to discontinuation of doxycycline. Treat antibiotic-related pseudomembranous colitis with fluid, electrolytes, protein supplements, and oral vancomycin (Vancocin) or metronidazole (Flagyl). Not removed by hemodialysis.

DROPERIDOL BBW
(droh-**PER**-ih-dohl)

Inapsine

Antiemetic
Anesthesia adjunct

pH 3 to 3.8

USUAL DOSE

May cause serious proarrhythmic effects and death; reserve use to patients for whom other treatments are ineffective or inappropriate. Dose should be individualized and initiated at a low dose. Adjust upward, with caution, to achieve the desired effect. Consider age, body weight, physical status, underlying pathologic conditions, use of other drugs, type of anesthesia to be used, and surgical procedure involved; see Precautions. Maximum recommended initial dose is 2.5 mg. Additional 1.25-mg doses may be given to achieve the desired effect but should be used only if the potential benefit outweighs the potential risk.

Prevention of perioperative nausea and vomiting: Dose should be individualized; maximum initial dose is 2.5 mg by slow IV injection. Additional 1.25-mg doses may be given with caution to achieve desired effect only if benefits outweigh potential risk. 0.625 to 1.25 mg has been shown to have an effect similar to ondansetron (Zofran) 4 mg.

PEDIATRIC DOSE

Prevention of perioperative nausea and vomiting, pediatric patients 2 to 12 years: The maximum recommended dose is 0.1 mg/kg (100 mcg/kg). Another source suggests 0.03 to 0.07 mg/kg/dose (30 to 70 mcg/kg/dose) over 2 minutes or up to 0.1 mg/kg/dose with caution to achieve desired effect only if benefits outweigh potential risk and total dose does not exceed 2.5 mg. May be given IM or IV. See Maternal/Child.

DOSE ADJUSTMENTS

Initiate at a low dose and adjust upward with caution to achieve the desired effect. ■ Reduce dose of narcotics and all CNS depressants to one fourth or one third of usual dose before, during, and for 24 hours after injection of droperidol. ■ If other CNS depressants (e.g., narcotics) have been given previously, reduce dose of droperidol. ■ Reduce dose for elderly, debilitated, and poor-risk patients and those with impaired kidney or liver function.

DILUTION

May be given undiluted. Give through Y-tube or three-way stopcock of the infusion set. May be added to a convenient volume of selected infusion solutions (D5W, NS, or LR).

Filters: No data available from manufacturer.

Storage: Store vials at CRT; protect from light. Diluted solutions stable at CRT for at least 48 hours (up to 7 days in selected solutions; see literature).

COMPATIBILITY
(Underline Indicates Conflicting Compatibility Information)

Consider any drug NOT listed as compatible to be INCOMPATIBLE until consulting a pharmacist; specific conditions may apply.

Manufacturer states, "Will precipitate if mixed with barbiturates" (e.g., phenobarbital [Luminal]).

One source suggests the following **compatibilities:**

Y-site: Acyclovir (Zovirax), amifostine (Ethyol), azithromycin (Zithromax), aztreonam (Azactam), bivalirudin (Angiomax), bleomycin (Blenoxane), cisatracurium (Nimbex), cisplatin, cladribine (Leustatin), cyclophosphamide (Cytoxan), dexmedetomidine (Precedex), docetaxel (Taxotere), doxorubicin (Adriamycin), doxorubicin liposomal (Doxil), etoposide phosphate (Etopophos), famotidine (Pepcid IV), fenoldopam (Corlopam), filgrastim (Neupogen), fluconazole (Diflucan), fludarabine (Fludara), gemcitabine (Gemzar), granisetron (Kytril), heparin, hetastarch in electrolytes (Hextend), hydrocortisone sodium succinate (Solu-Cortef), idarubicin (Idamycin), linezolid (Zyvox), melphalan (Alkeran), meperidine (Demerol), metoclopramide (Reglan), mitomycin (Mutamycin), ondansetron (Zofran), oxaliplatin (Eloxatin), paclitaxel (Taxol), potassium chloride

(KCl), propofol (Diprivan), remifentanil (Ultiva), sargramostim (Leukine), teniposide (Vumon), thiotepa, vinblastine, vincristine, vinorelbine (Navelbine).

RATE OF ADMINISTRATION

IV injection: *Adults:* 2.5 mg or fraction thereof over 1 to 2 minutes. *Pediatric patients:* A single dose or fraction thereof over a minimum of 2 minutes.

Infusion: Titrate by dose and desired patient response. Do not exceed rate for IV injection.

ACTIONS

An antianxiety agent that produces marked tranquilization and sedation. Has an antiemetic action also. It produces mild alpha-adrenergic blockade and produces peripheral vascular dilation. May decrease an abnormally high pulmonary arterial pressure. A dose-dependent and significant QT prolongation at all dose levels (0.1, 0.175, and 0.25 mg/kg) has been observed within 10 minutes of administration in patients without known cardiac disease. Effective in 3 to 10 minutes with maximum results in 30 minutes. Lasts 2 to 4 hours. Some effects persist for 12 hours. Metabolized in the liver. Excreted in urine and feces. Crosses placental barrier very slowly. Secreted in breast milk.

INDICATIONS AND USES

To reduce the incidence of nausea and vomiting associated with surgical and diagnostic procedures.

Unlabeled uses: Antiemetic in cancer chemotherapy including potent emetic agents (e.g., cisplatin). ▪ Treatment of acute psychotic episodes manifested by severe agitation and combativeness. ▪ Adjunct to local or general anesthesia.

CONTRAINDICATIONS

Known hypersensitivity to droperidol or other butyrophenones (e.g., haloperidol [Haldol]) and patients with known or suspected QT prolongation, including those with congenital long QT syndrome.

PRECAUTIONS

Use of agents other than droperidol is recommended. ▪ QT prolongation and torsades de pointes have been reported with doses at or below those recommended. Some cases have occurred in patients with no known risk factors for QT prolongation, and some cases have been fatal. ▪ Use with extreme caution in patients who may be at risk for development of prolonged QT syndrome (e.g., clinically significant bradycardia [less than 50 bpm]; CHF or any clinically significant cardiac disease; use of a diuretic; treatment with Class Ia antiarrhythmics and/or Class III antiarrhythmics; treatment with MAO inhibitors [e.g., selegiline (Eldepryl)]; concomitant treatment with other drug products known to prolong the QT interval; electrolyte imbalance, in particular hypokalemia or hypomagnesemia; alcoholism; or concomitant treatment with drugs that may cause electrolyte imbalance or hypovolemia). See Drug Interactions. ▪ Other risk factors may include patients over 65 years of age, alcohol abuse, pheochromocytoma, and the use of agents such as benzodiazepines, volatile anesthetics, and IV opiates. ▪ Correct hypokalemia and/or hypomagnesemia before administration. ▪ When used without a general anesthetic, topical anesthesia is still required when appropriate (e.g., bronchoscopy). ▪ May worsen symptoms of Parkinson's disease.

Monitor: A potent drug. Obtain a baseline ECG on all patients. Do not administer droperidol if a prolonged QT interval exists (QTc greater than 440 msec for males or 450 msec for females). ▪ Monitor VS and ECG closely. Monitor for palpitations, syncope, and/or other symptoms of irregular cardiac rhythm and evaluate promptly. ▪ Resuscitation equipment, a narcotic antagonist (if a narcotic has been used concurrently), IV infusion line, IV fluids, and equipment and drugs to manage emergency situations must be readily available. ▪ In patients for whom the benefit is believed to outweigh the risks of potentially serious arrhythmias, monitor for arrhythmias during the treatment and for 2 to 3 hours after treatment. ▪ Orthostatic hypotension is common; move and position patients with care. ▪ EEG pattern may be slow in returning to normal postoperatively. See Precautions.

Patient Education: Avoid activities that require alertness for 24 hours after receiving droperidol. ▪ Do not drink alcoholic beverages or take other CNS depressants (e.g., antihistamines, pain medications, sleeping pills) for 24 hours after receiving droperidol.

Maternal/Child: Category C: safety for use during pregnancy not established; is rarely used. An exception is selected use during cesarean section; it has also been used to treat hyperemesis gravidarum (no longer recommended). ▪ Is secreted in breast milk; avoid breast-feeding. ▪ Pediatric patients may be more susceptible to extrapyramidal side effects, especially acute dystonic reactions. ▪ Safety for use in pediatric patients under 2 years not established.

Elderly: See Dose Adjustments. ▪ More likely to experience hypotension, excessive sedation, and prolonged QT syndrome.

DRUG/LAB INTERACTIONS

Concurrent use with **fentanyl** may cause hypotension and decrease pulmonary arterial pressure. ▪ May cause precipitous hypotension with **epinephrine.** ▪ Use caution with **other CNS depressant drugs** (e.g., barbiturates, tranquilizers, opioids, and general anesthetics); may have additive or potentiating effects **with droperidol;** see Dose Adjustments. ▪ Increased risk of QT prolongation and torsades de pointes with **other drugs known to increase the QT interval** (e.g., **Class Ia antiarrhythmics** [e.g., disopyramide (Norpace), procainamide (Pronestyl), quinidine] **and/or Class III antiarrhythmics** [e.g., amiodarone (Nexterone), dofetilide (Tikosyn), ibutilide (Corvert), sotalol (Betapace)], **anticonvulsants** [e.g., fosphenytoin (Cerebyx)], **antidepressants** [e.g., amitriptyline (Elavil), imipramine (Tofranil)], **antihistamines** [e.g., diphenhydramine (Benadryl)], **antimalarials** [e.g., chloroquine], **antineoplastics** [e.g., doxorubicin (Adriamycin)], **azole antifungal agents** [e.g., itraconazole (Sporanox)], **calcium channel blockers** [e.g., nicardipine (Cardene)], **fluoroquinolones, other neuroleptics** [e.g., haloperidol, lithium], **and many others**); see Precautions. ▪ Concurrent administration with **volatile anesthetics, benzodiazepines** (e.g., diazepam [Valium], midazolam [Versed]), or **IV opiates** (e.g., morphine) may produce prolonged QT syndrome. Initiate therapy at a low dose and adjust with caution. ▪ Concomitant treatment with **diuretics** (e.g., furosemide [Lasix)]), **laxatives, steroids with mineralocorticoid potential** (e.g., hydrocortisone) may cause electrolyte imbalance, hypovolemia, and/or induce hypokalemia or hypomagnesemia. ▪ Concurrent use with **other agents that produce hypotension** may cause orthostatic hypotension; risk is increased with **agents that produce vasodilation** (e.g., amiodarone (Nexterone), milrinone [Primacor], nitroprusside sodium [Nitropress], nicardipine [Cardene]). ▪ See Dose Adjustments and Precautions.

SIDE EFFECTS

Common: Abnormal EEG, chills, dizziness, hallucinations, hypotension, restlessness, shivering, tachycardia.

Major/overdose: Apnea; cardiac arrest; extrapyramidal symptoms; hypotension (severe); neuroleptic malignant syndrome (altered consciousness, muscle rigidity, and autonomic instability); palpitations, syncope, or other symptoms of irregular cardiac rhythm; QT prolongation and torsades de pointes; respiratory depression; ventricular tachycardia; death.

ANTIDOTE

Notify the physician of any side effect. Minor side effects will probably be transient; for major side effects discontinue the drug, treat symptomatically, and notify the physician. Treat hypotension with fluid therapy (rule out hypovolemia) and vasopressors such as dopamine or levarterenol (Levophed). Phenylephrine may help to counteract the alpha-blocking effects of droperidol. Epinephrine is contraindicated for hypotension. Further hypotension will occur. Treat extrapyramidal symptoms with benztropine mesylate (Cogentin) or diphenhydramine (Benadryl). Treat cardiac arrhythmias as indicated (e.g., magnesium sulfate for torsades de pointes, lidocaine for ventricular tachycardia). An increase in temperature, HR, or CO_2 production may be symptoms of neuroleptic malignant syndrome or malignant hyperpyrexia. Consider prompt treatment with dantrolene (Dantrium). Resuscitate as necessary.

ECULIZUMAB BBW

(eck-you-**LIZ**-you-mab)

Soliris

pH 7

USUAL DOSE

A meningococcal vaccine must be administered at least 2 weeks before initial dosing with eculizumab to all patients who have not been previously vaccinated. A booster dose may be required for patients previously vaccinated. Revaccinate according to current medical guidelines. Quadrivalent, conjugated meningococcal vaccines are strongly recommended.

Paroxysmal nocturnal hemoglobinuria (PNH): Administer 600 mg as an infusion weekly for the first 4 weeks, followed by 900 mg for the fifth dose 1 week later, then 900 mg every 2 weeks thereafter.

Atypical hemolytic uremic syndrome (aHUS) in patients 18 years of age or older: Administer 900 mg as an infusion weekly for the first 4 weeks, followed by 1,200 mg for the fifth dose 1 week later, then 1,200 mg every 2 weeks thereafter.

PEDIATRIC DOSE

See general comments under Usual Dose.

Atypical hemolytic uremic syndrome (aHUS) in patients less than 18 years of age: Administer eculizumab based on body weight as outlined in the following chart.

Atypical Hemolytic Uremic Syndrome (aHUS) Dose in Patients Less Than 18 Years of Age		
Patient Body Weight	Induction	Maintenance
40 kg and over	900 mg weekly × 4 doses	1,200 mg at week 5; then 1,200 mg every 2 weeks
30 kg to less than 40 kg	600 mg weekly × 2 doses	900 mg at week 3; then 900 mg every 2 weeks
20 kg to less than 30 kg	600 mg weekly × 2 doses	600 mg at week 3; then 600 mg every 2 weeks
10 kg to less than 20 kg	600 mg × 1 dose	300 mg at week 2; then 300 mg every 2 weeks
5 kg to less than 10 kg	300 mg × 1 dose	300 mg at week 2; then 300 mg every 2 weeks

DOSE ADJUSTMENTS

A variance of 1 to 2 days in the scheduled administration time points is allowed if indicated. ▪ Age, gender, race, and renal function do not appear to influence the pharmacokinetics of eculizumab. ▪ Supplemental dosing of eculizumab is required in the setting of concomitant support with PE/PI (plasmapheresis or plasma exchange, or fresh frozen plasma infusion). See the following chart for supplemental dosing based on the type of intervention.

Continued

Supplemental Dose of Eculizumab After PE/PI			
Type of Intervention	Most Recent Eculizumab Dose	Supplemental Eculizumab Dose with Each PE/PI Intervention	Timing of Supplemental Dose
Plasmapheresis or plasma exchange	300 mg	300 mg per each plasmapheresis or plasma exchange session	Within 60 minutes after each plasmapheresis or plasma exchange
Plasmapheresis or plasma exchange	600 mg or more	600 mg per each plasmapheresis or plasma exchange session	Within 60 minutes after each plasmapheresis or plasma exchange
Fresh frozen plasma (FFP) infusion	300 mg or more	300 mg per each infusion of fresh frozen plasma	60 minutes before each infusion of fresh frozen plasma

DILUTION

Available in 300 mg/30 mL single-use vials (10 mg/mL). Withdraw the required dose of eculizumab (2 vials are required for the 600-mg dose, 3 vials are required for the 900-mg dose, and 4 vials are required for the 1,200-mg dose) and transfer it to an infusion bag. Must be further diluted to a 5 mg/mL concentration by adding an amount of NS, ½NS, D5W, or Ringer's lactate to the infusion bag equal to the total volume of the eculizumab.

Preparation and Reconstitution of Eculizumab		
Eculizumab Dose	Diluent Volume	Final Volume
300 mg	30 mL	60 mL
600 mg	60 mL	120 mL
900 mg	90 mL	180 mL
1,200 mg	120 mL	240 mL

Invert gently to ensure thorough mixing. Allow the diluted solution to reach room temperature before infusion. Do not use an artificial heat source (e.g., microwave). Discard unused portions; contains no preservatives.

Filters: Specific information not available.

Storage: Refrigerate vials in original carton at 2° to 8° C (36° to 46° F) and protect from light. Do not use beyond the expiration date on the vial. Diluted solution is stable for 24 hours refrigerated or at CRT. Do not freeze or shake.

COMPATIBILITY

Specific information not available.

RATE OF ADMINISTRATION

Do not administer as an IV push or a bolus injection. For infusion via gravity feed, syringe-type pump, or infusion pump.

Adults: A single dose as an infusion over 35 minutes. If infusion is slowed or stopped for any reason, the total infusion time should not exceed 2 hours.

Pediatric patients: A single dose as an infusion over 1 to 4 hours.

ACTIONS

A recombinant, DNA-derived, humanized IgG monoclonal antibody. A genetic mutation in patients with paroxysmal nocturnal hemoglobinuria (PNH) leads to the generation of abnormal RBCs (known as PNH cells) that are deficient in terminal complement inhibitors; this deficiency makes these RBCs sensitive to persistent terminal complement-mediated destruction. Ongoing destruction of these RBCs is called hemolysis. Eculizumab, a complement inhibitor, specifically binds to the complement protein C5 and prevents complement-mediated intravascular hemolysis. It improves the lives of patients suffering from this disease by directly targeting the underlying disease process and markedly decreasing the ongoing RBC destruction that causes the hemolysis responsible for the S/S of PNH. In aHUS, impairment in the regulation of complement activity leads to uncontrolled terminal complement activation, resulting in platelet activation, endothelial cell damage, and thrombotic microangiopathy. Eculizumab inhibits the complement-mediated thrombotic microangiopathy (TMA) in patients with aHUS. Half-life is 190 to 354 hours.

INDICATIONS AND USES
A complement inhibitor for the treatment of patients with paroxysmal nocturnal hemoglobinuria (PNH) to reduce hemolysis. PNH is a rare, disabling, and life-threatening genetic mutation blood disorder defined by chronic RBC destruction (hemolysis). Symptoms may include anemia; disabling fatigue; dysphagia; dyspnea; erectile dysfunction; hemoglobinuria; jaundice; recurrent pain in the abdomen, back, or head; renal dysfunction; and thromboses. Average age of onset is the early 30s. ▪ Treatment of patients with atypical hemolytic uremic syndrome (aHUS) to inhibit complement-mediated thrombotic microangiography.

Limitation of use: Eculizumab is NOT indicated for treatment of patients with Shiga toxin *E. coli*–related hemolytic uremic syndrome (STEC-HUS).

CONTRAINDICATIONS
Do not use in patients with unresolved serious *Neisseria meningitidis* infection or in patients not currently vaccinated against *N. meningitidis* unless the risk of delaying eculizumab therapy outweighs the risk of developing meningococcal infection.

PRECAUTIONS
For IV infusion only; do not administer by IV push or bolus injection.
▪ Susceptibility to serious meningococcal infections (septicemia and/or meningitis) is increased. Meningococcal infections may become rapidly life threatening or fatal if not recognized and treated early. ▪ Comply with the most current Advisory Committee on Immunization Practices (ACIP) recommendations for meningococcal vaccination in patients with complement deficiencies. Revaccinate according to current medical guidelines, considering the duration of eculizumab therapy. ▪ A meningococcal vaccine must be administered at least 2 weeks before initial dosing with eculizumab to all patients who have not been previously vaccinated unless the risks of delaying eculizumab therapy outweigh the risks of developing meningococcal infection. If urgent eculizumab therapy is indicated in an unvaccinated patient, administer the meningococcal vaccine as soon as possible. In clinical studies, such patients received antibiotics for prophylaxis of meningococcal infection until at least 2 weeks after vaccination. Benefits and risks of antibiotic prophylaxis not established. Vaccination reduces, but does not eliminate, the risk of meningococcal infections. ▪ Use caution in patients with any systemic infection. ▪ Eculizumab blocks terminal complement activation. Patients have increased susceptibility to infections, especially with encapsulated bacteria. *Aspergillus* infections have occurred in immunocompromised and neutropenic patients. Pediatric patients may be at increased risk of developing serious infections due to *Streptococcus pneumoniae* or *Haemophilus influenzae* type B (Hib). Administer vaccinations for prevention of these infections according to medical guidelines. ▪ Serious hemolysis may occur in patients who discontinue eculizumab therapy; see Monitor. ▪ A protein product; infusion reactions may occur. Hypersensitivity reactions, including anaphylaxis, are possible; however, infusion reactions severe enough to discontinue eculizumab did not occur during clinical trials. ▪ Has a potential for immunogenicity. Low titers of antibodies to eculizumab have been detected but did not appear to correlate to clinical response. ▪ Continue established anticoagulant therapy during eculizumab treatment; the effect of withdrawal of anticoagulant therapy during eculizumab therapy has not been established. ▪ Eculizumab is available through a restricted program under a Risk Evaluation and Mitigation Strategy (REMS). Prescribers must be enrolled in the program. Contact manufacturer for further information.

Monitor: Obtain baseline CBC with differential and platelets, lactic dehydrogenase (LDH), SCr, and bilirubin. ▪ LDH levels increase during hemolysis and with TMA. Monitoring may assist in determining the effectiveness of eculizumab therapy. ▪ Monitor for early S/S of meningococcal infections (moderate to severe headache with nausea or vomiting, fever, or a stiff neck or stiff back; fever of 103° F [39.4° C] or higher; fever and a rash; confusion; and/or severe muscle aches with flu-like symptoms and light sensitivity). Evaluate immediately and treat with antibiotics if indicated. Discontinue eculizumab during treatment of serious meningococcal infections. ▪ Monitor for other types of infections. ▪ Monitor for S/S of an infusion or hypersensitivity reaction (e.g., chills, dyspnea, pruritus) during infusion and for at least 1 hour postinfusion. Slow or temporarily discontinue the infusion as indicated. ▪ Monitor patients with PNH who discontinue eculizumab for a minimum of 8 weeks to detect serious hemolysis and other reactions (e.g., blood clots; chest pain; confusion; decreased hemoglobin, hematocrit, and haptoglobin; difficulty breathing; elevated LDH, bilirubin, or SCr; free serum hemoglobin; and hemoglobinuria with pink/red urine). ▪ Monitor patients with aHUS who discontinue eculizumab for S/S of TMA complications for a minimum of 12 weeks. Clinical S/S of TMA may include angina, dyspnea, mental status changes, seizures, or thrombosis. Changes in laboratory parameters that may indicate TMA include a decrease in platelet count or an increased SCr and LDH.

Patient Education: Read the patient medication guide before initiating eculizumab and before each dose. ▪ Meningococcal vaccination is required before initiating therapy. Previously vaccinated individuals may require a booster dose. Vaccination may not prevent meningococcal infection. Important to receive and stay up-to-date on all recommended immunizations. Discuss immunization status with physician. ▪ Eculizumab affects the immune system and can lower the ability to fight infections. Immediately report S/S of a meningococcal infection (moderate to severe headache with nausea or vomiting, fever, or a stiff neck or stiff back; fever of 103° F [39.4° C] or higher; fever and a rash; confusion; and/or severe muscle aches with flu-like symptoms and light sensitivity). Manufacturer supplies a patient safety card that lists these symptoms. Card should be carried at all times during treatment and for 3 months after the last dose of eculizumab is administered. Share card with all health care providers treating you. ▪ Promptly report other S/S of an infection. ▪ Promptly report chills, dyspnea, and/or itching during or soon after an infusion. ▪ Report a suspected pregnancy and/or tell your doctor if you are breast-feeding. ▪ Stopping the infusions may have serious side effects and requires prolonged monitoring for development of hemolysis or TMA. Increased risk of meningococcal infection continues for several weeks after eculizumab is discontinued.

Maternal/Child: Category C: use during pregnancy only if the benefits justify the potential risk to the fetus. Eculizumab is a recombinant IgG moleculte that is expected to cross the placenta. Pregnant women with PNH and their fetuses have high rates of morbidity and mortality during pregnancy and postpartum. Treatment with eculizumab may increase fetal survival and decrease maternal complications. ▪ Use caution if breast-feeding; IgG is secreted in breast milk, but antibodies may not enter the neonatal and infant circulation in substantial amounts. Consider risks to infant versus benefits of breast-feeding. ▪ Safety and effectiveness for treatment of PNH in pediatric patients less than 18 years of age not established. ▪ Safety and effectiveness for treatment of aHUS appear similar in pediatric and adult patients. Follow medical guidelines for vaccinations for prevention of infections due to *Neisseria meningitidis, Streptococcus pneumoniae,* and Hib.

Elderly: Limited experience did not identify age-related differences in safety and effectiveness.

DRUG/LAB INTERACTIONS

Formal drug interaction studies have not been completed. ▪ Continue established anticoagulant therapy during eculizumab treatment; the effect of withdrawal of anticoagulant therapy during eculizumab therapy has not been established.

SIDE EFFECTS

Meningococcal infections (meningitis and/or septicemia) and the progression of PNH are the most serious side effects reported; may be life threatening and may occur in patients who have been vaccinated. The most commonly reported side effects in patients with **PNH** are back pain, headache, nasopharyngitis, and nausea. Other reported side effects include constipation, cough, fatigue, herpes simplex infections, influenza-like illness, myalgia, pain in extremity, respiratory tract infection, and sinusitis. The most commonly reported side effects in patients with **aHUS** are abdominal pain, anemia, cough, diarrhea, fever, headache, hypertension, nasopharyngitis, nausea, peripheral edema, upper respiratory infection, UTI, and vomiting. Other reported side effects include arthralgia, asthenia, back pain, bronchitis, fatigue, gastroenteritis, hypokalemia, hypotension, insomnia, leukopenia, neoplasms (benign, malignant, and unspecified), proteinuria, pruritus, rash, and renal impairment.

Post-Marketing: Cases of serious or fatal meningococcal infections have been reported.

ANTIDOTE

Keep physician informed of all side effects. Some will be treated symptomatically. Potential meningococcal infections must be evaluated immediately and treated with antibiotics promptly; may be life threatening. Treat hypersensitivity or infusion reactions as indicated; may respond to slowing or temporarily discontinuing the infusion or may require the use of epinephrine, corticosteroids, diphenhydramine bronchodilators (e.g., albuterol, aminophylline), IV saline, oxygen, and/or acetaminophen. Total infusion time should not exceed 2 hours. If TMA complications occur after eculizumab is discontinued, consider reinstitution of treatment, plasma therapy (plasma exchange or FFP infusion), or appropriate organ-specific supportive measures. Resuscitate as necessary.

EDETATE CALCIUM DISODIUM BBW

(ED-eh-tayt KAL-see-um DYE-so-dee-um)

Calcium Disodium Edetate, Calcium Disodium Versenate, Calcium EDTA

Antidote
Chelating agent
Lead mobilization

pH 6.5 to 8

USUAL DOSE

Specific fluid requirements indicated; see Monitor and Maternal/Child. Do not exceed recommended daily dose.

Asymptomatic adults and pediatric patients with blood lead levels over 20 mcg/dL but under 70 mcg/dL: 1,000 mg/M^2/24 hr (50 mg/kg/24 hr) for 3 to 5 days. After a rest period of 2 to 4 days (preferably up to 2 weeks) to allow for redistribution of lead, repeat the process, if indicated, based on severity of lead toxicity and patient tolerance.

Symptomatic adults and pediatric patients with blood levels over 70 mcg/dL: Dimercaprol (BAL) will be given IM in divided doses every 4 hours for a minimum of 3 or up to 5 days. 4 hours after the first dose of BAL, begin edetate calcium disodium 1,000 mg/M^2/24 hr or 25 to 50 mg/kg/24 hr for 5 days. If blood lead concentrations rebound to above 45 mcg/dL within 5 to 7 days after the initial course, repeat the edetate calcium disodium. Do not repeat the dimercaprol regimen.

DOSE ADJUSTMENTS

Reduce dose in pre-existing renal disease and/or adults with lead nephropathy. In adults with lead nephropathy dose is based on serum creatinine levels and repeated monthly until lead excretion is reduced toward normal according to the following chart.

Dose Adjustments in Impaired Renal Function and/or Adults with Lead Nephropathy	
Serum Creatinine Level	Dose
<2 mg/dL	1,000 mg/M^2/24 hr for 5 days
2-3 mg/dL	500 mg/M^2/24 hr for 5 days
3-4 mg/dL	500 mg/M^2/48 hr for 3 doses
>4 mg/dL	500 mg/M^2/week

DILUTION
Add total daily dose to 250 to 500 mL of D5W or NS for infusion.
Storage: Before use, store at CRT.

COMPATIBILITY
Consider any drug NOT listed as compatible to be INCOMPATIBLE until consulting a pharmacist; specific conditions may apply.
Manufacturer lists amphotericin B (conventional), hydralazine, D10W, 10% invert sugar in NS, LR, Ringer's solution, $1/6$ M lactate as **incompatible.** Must be diluted in specific IV solutions; see Dilution.

RATE OF ADMINISTRATION
References vary greatly. Manufacturer recommends the total daily dose be evenly distributed over 8 to 12 hours. May cause an increase in intracranial pressure with too-rapid injection in patients with lead encephalopathy and cerebral edema.

ACTIONS
A chelating agent. Helps to remove metals, especially lead, from the body. Will form a stable chelate with metals that have the ability to displace calcium from the molecule (e.g., lead, zinc, cadmium). Distributed primarily in the extracellular fluid. Half-life is 20 to 60 minutes. Chelated compounds are excreted in urine; up to 50% in 1 hour and 95% in 24 hours. The primary source of lead chelated by edetate calcium disodium is from bone. Following administration, urinary lead output increases and blood lead concentration decreases, but brain lead is significantly increased due to internal redistribution of lead.

INDICATIONS AND USES
Reduction of blood levels and depot stores of lead in lead poisoning (acute and chronic) and lead encephalopathy in both pediatric and adult patients.
Unlabeled uses: Treatment of poisoning by radioactive and nuclear fission products such as plutonium, thorium, uranium, and yttrium. ▪ Treatment of poisoning from other heavy metals such as chromium, manganese, nickel, zinc, and possibly vanadium.

CONTRAINDICATIONS
Anuria, active renal disease, or hepatitis.

PRECAUTIONS
Do not confuse with edetate disodium, which does not chelate lead but actually removes calcium from the body and can be very dangerous. ▪ Patients with lead encephalopathy and cerebral edema may have a lethal increase in intracranial pressure with IV infusion; IM injection preferred; see Maternal/Child. ▪ Equally effective with IM or IV administration. IM route is used for all patients with overt lead encephalopathy and has been suggested as the preferred route by some for young pediatric patients. ▪ Usually given IM in pediatric patients, unless given concurrently with BAL (insufficient IM injection sites); see Maternal/Child. ▪ May produce toxic and fatal effects. ▪ Produces the same renal damage as lead poisoning (e.g., proteinuria and microscopic hematuria). ▪ Nephrotoxicity is dose dependent and may be reduced by ensuring adequate diuresis before treatment begins. ▪ Use with caution in mild renal disease; see Dose Adjustments. ▪ Patients must be removed from the source of contamination promptly. ▪ Use for diagnosis of lead poisoning as a lead mobilization test is controversial; see literature. Edetate calcium disodium mobilization test should not be used in symptomatic patients or in patients with blood levels above 55 mcg/dL for whom appropriate therapy is indicated. ▪ Not effective in mercury, gold, or arsenic poisoning.
Monitor: Urine flow must be established before dimercaprol (BAL) or edetate calcium disodium is administered. IV fluids may be used. Avoid excessive fluid in patients with cerebral edema or lead encephalopathy. Once urine flow is established, further IV fluid is restricted in all patients to basal water and electrolyte requirements. ▪ Monitor urinalysis, urine sediment, renal and hepatic function, and electrolyte levels before treatment; repeat daily in serious cases and on the second and fifth day in less serious cases. Daily urine specimens are recommended to determine status of renal function. ▪ Monitor ECG and vital signs. ▪ Elevated erythrocyte protoporphyrin levels (greater than

35 mcg/dL) indicate the need to perform a venous blood lead determination. ▪ An elevation of urinary coproporphyrin (greater than 250 mcg/day in adults and greater than 75 mcg/day in pediatric patients under 80 lbs) and an elevation of urinary delta-aminolevulinic acid (greater than 4 mg/day in adults and greater than 3 mg/M^2/day in pediatric patients) are associated with blood lead levels greater than 40 mcg/dL. ▪ Excretion of calcium is not increased, but excretion of zinc and other essential metals is; monitor and replace as indicated. ▪ Obtain specific fluid orders from the physician.

Patient Education: If no urine output for 12 hours, report immediately.

Maternal/Child: Category B: safety for use during pregnancy not established; benefits must outweigh risks. ▪ Use caution in nursing mothers. ▪ Lead poisoning is often more severe in pediatric patients compared with adult patients. Lead encephalopathy occurs more often in pediatric patients. May be incipient and thus overlooked. Mortality rate in pediatric patients has been high; see Precautions. ▪ IV injection has been associated with fatality in some young children, and IM injection is considered to be the preferred route by some clinicians.

Elderly: Consider age-related organ damage.

DRUG/LAB INTERACTIONS

Steroids will increase renal toxicity. ▪ Inhibits the action of **zinc insulin** preparations by chelating the zinc.

SIDE EFFECTS

Acute renal tubular necrosis, anemia, anorexia, arthralgia, cardiac rhythm irregularities, chills, excessive thirst, fatigue, fever, headache, hematuria, hypercalcemia, hypersensitivity (e.g., sneezing, nasal congestion), hypotension, increases in liver function tests (mild), leg and other muscle cramps, malaise, myalgia, nausea, numbness, proteinuria, tetany, tingling, transient bone marrow suppression, tremors, vomiting, weakness, zinc deficiency.

ANTIDOTE

Notify the physician of any side effects. Most will improve with a decrease in rate of the infusion or will be treated symptomatically. Discontinue if urine flow stops to avoid high tissue levels of the drug. Discontinue at the first sign of renal toxicity (e.g., presence of large renal epithelial cells or increasing numbers of RBCs). Treat cerebral edema with repeated doses of mannitol. Not known if edetate calcium disodium is dialyzable.

EDETATE DISODIUM BBW
(**ED**-eh-tayt **DYE**-so-dee-um)

Antihypercalcemic agent
Calcium chelating agent

EDTA Disodium, Endrate

pH 6.5 to 7.5

USUAL DOSE
50 mg/kg of body weight/24 hr or in equally divided doses every 12 hours (25 mg/kg every 12 hours). Total dose should not exceed 3 Gm/24 hr. Usually given for 5 days, held for 2 days. Regimen may be repeated to a total of 15 doses.

PEDIATRIC DOSE
40 mg/kg of body weight/24 hr in equally divided doses every 6 to 12 hours (20 mg/kg every 12 hours, 10 mg/kg every 6 hours). Do not exceed 70 mg/kg/24 hr or adult dose, whichever is less. See instructions in Usual Dose.

DOSE ADJUSTMENTS
Dose selection should be cautious in the elderly. Reduced doses may be indicated based on potential for decreased organ function and concomitant disease or drug therapy.

DILUTION
Recommended dose must be diluted in 500 mL D5W or NS and given as an infusion. A 0.5% solution will reduce the risk of thrombophlebitis. Do not exceed cardiac reserve in any patient. Use less diluent if necessary in pediatric patients. Must be diluted to at least a 3% solution.

Storage: Store at room temperature.

COMPATIBILITY
Specific information not available. Consider specific use; consult pharmacist.

RATE OF ADMINISTRATION
Must not exceed more than 15 mg of actual medication over 1 minute. Total dose usually given over 3 to 4 hours. Rapid IV infusion may cause a sudden drop in serum calcium, resulting in tetany, convulsions, arrhythmias, and death. Reduce rate and further dilute solution for pain at injection site.

ACTIONS
A calcium-chelating agent. Also forms chelates with other polyvalent metals (e.g., magnesium, zinc). Attracts calcium ions immediately on injection and becomes calcium disodium edetate. Capable of severely depleting the body of calcium stores. Exerts a negative inotropic effect on the heart. It is well distributed in extracellular fluids and rapidly excreted in the urine.

INDICATIONS AND USES
Treatment of cardiac arrhythmias (atrial and ventricular, especially when caused by digoxin toxicity). ▪ Hypercalcemia.

CONTRAINDICATIONS
Anuria, known sensitivity to edetate disodium, renal disease.

PRECAUTIONS
Read label carefully. Deaths have been caused when edetate disodium was administered mistakenly for edetate calcium disodium. ▪ Used only when the severity of disease indicates necessity. ▪ May produce hypocalcemia quickly, especially if used for purposes other than chelating calcium. ▪ Use repeatedly with caution because of potential for nephrotoxicity and mobilization of extracirculatory calcium stores. ▪ Use caution in cardiac disease (may adversely affect myocardial contractility), diabetes (lower blood sugar may require less insulin), severe renal disease, liver disease, congestive heart failure (1 Gm of sodium in each 5 Gm), limited cardiac reserve, and patients with a history of seizures or intracranial lesions.

Monitor: Monitor vital signs and ECG before and during therapy. ▪ Confirm patency of vein, avoid extravasation; can cause tissue necrosis. ▪ Routine electrolyte panel (potassium deficiency) and urine specimens for casts and cells necessary during therapy. Magnesium, zinc, and other trace element deficiencies can occur. ▪ Keep patient in supine position during and after administration (15 to 30 minutes) to avoid postural hypotension. ▪ Obtain blood for serum calcium levels just before beginning a new infusion; specific lab methods required. ▪ Inhibits coagulation of blood (transient). Liver function tests may be indicated. ▪ See Drug/Lab Interactions.

Maternal/Child: Category C: safety for use in pregnancy or breast-feeding not established. Use with extreme caution and only if clearly needed.

Elderly: Reduced doses may be indicated; see Dose Adjustments. Monitoring of renal function is suggested.

DRUG/LAB INTERACTIONS

Inhibits **mannitol.** ▪ Potentiates **neuromuscular blocking antibiotics** (e.g., gentamicin). ▪ Inhibits coagulation of **blood** (transient). ▪ A sudden drop in calcium levels may decrease effects of **digoxin.** ▪ Obtain blood for **serum calcium levels** just before beginning a new infusion. Specific laboratory methods must be used for accurate evaluation.

SIDE EFFECTS

Anorexia, arthralgia, circumoral paresthesias, diarrhea, fatigue, fever, glycosuria, headache, hyperuricemia, hypotension, malaise, nasal congestion, nausea, numbness, sneezing, tearing, thirst, thrombophlebitis, urinary urgency, vomiting.

Major: Anaphylaxis, anemia, cardiac arrhythmias, dermatitis, hemorrhage, hypocalcemic tetany, prolonged QT interval, renal tubular destruction (reversible), seizures, death.

ANTIDOTE

Notify the physician of any side effect. For progression of minor side effects or any major side effect, discontinue drug immediately and notify the physician. Calcium gluconate is the antidote of choice and should be available for infusion at all times (use extreme caution if patient is digitalized). Treat mild hypotension by maintaining in supine position until recovery. Additional hydration indicated with S/S of nephrotoxicity. Treat anaphylaxis and resuscitate as necessary.

EDROPHONIUM CHLORIDE
(ed-roh-**FOH**-nee-um **KLOR**-eyed)

Cholinergic
Cholinesterase inhibitor
Antidote
Diagnostic agent

Enlon, Tensilon, Tensilon PF

pH 5.4

USUAL DOSE
1 to 10 mg (0.1 to 1 mL) at specified intervals depending on usage. Maximum dose should never exceed 40 mg (4 doses of 10 mg each).

Myasthenia gravis diagnosis: 10 mg (1 mL) in tuberculin syringe. Give 2 mg (0.2 mL). If no reaction occurs in 45 seconds, give remaining 8 mg (0.8 mL). Test may be repeated after 30 minutes.

Myasthenia treatment evaluation: 1 to 2 mg (0.1 to 0.2 mL) 1 hour after oral intake of drug being used for treatment. Package insert has a chart differentiating myasthenic and non-myasthenic responses.

Myasthenia crisis evaluation: 2 mg (0.2 mL) in tuberculin syringe. Give 1 mg (0.1 mL). If the patient's condition does not deteriorate, give 1 mg (0.1 mL) after 60 seconds. Improvement in cardiac status and respiration should occur.

Antagonist to curare and other nondepolarizing muscle relaxants: 10 mg (1 mL). May be repeated as necessary up to 4 doses. (Available in combination with atropine [Enlon-Plus] for use in reversal of nondepolarizing muscle relaxants.)

Terminate paroxysmal atrial tachycardia (unlabeled): 5 to 10 mg as a bolus injection. See Dose Adjustments. Repeat once in 10 minutes if necessary.

Slow supraventricular tachycardias (unlabeled): 2 mg as a test dose. Repeat 2 mg every 1 minute until arrhythmia controlled or total dose of 10 mg is given. If HR decreases, may begin an infusion of 0.25 mg/min. May be increased to 2 mg/min if necessary.

PEDIATRIC DOSE
May be given IM if the IV route is not available; however, doses are different; check literature. See Maternal/Child.

Myasthenia gravis diagnosis: Neonates: 0.1 mg (0.01 mL). **Infants:** 0.5 mg (0.05 mL).

Pediatric patients less than 34 kg: 1 mg (0.1 mL); if no response in 30 to 45 seconds, give 1 mg (0.1 mL) every 30 to 45 seconds up to 5 mg (0.5 mL). **34 kg or more,** give 2 mg (0.2 mL); if no response in 30 to 45 seconds, give 1 mg (0.1 mL) every 30 to 45 seconds up to 10 mg. Another source has the same dose for neonates but recommends 0.2 mg/kg/dose (0.02 mL/kg/dose) for **infants and other pediatric patients** with 20% of a dose given as a test dose slowly. If no response in 1 minute, give in 1-mg increments to a maximum calculated dose or 10 mg, whichever is less.

DOSE ADJUSTMENTS
Reduce antiarrhythmic dose to 5 to 7 mg in the elderly.

DILUTION
May be given undiluted. In the treatment of myasthenia crisis, this drug may be diluted in D5W or NS and given as a continuous IV. Use an infusion pump or microdrip (60 gtt/mL).

Filters: No data available from manufacturer.

COMPATIBILITY
Consider any drug NOT listed as compatible to be INCOMPATIBLE until consulting a pharmacist; specific conditions may apply.

One source suggests the following **compatibilities:**

Y-site: Heparin, hydrocortisone sodium succinate (Solu-Cortef), potassium chloride (KCl).

RATE OF ADMINISTRATION

2 mg (0.2 mL) or fraction thereof over 15 to 30 seconds.
Curare antagonist: A single dose over 30 to 45 seconds.
Antiarrhythmic: See Usual Dose.

ACTIONS

An anticholinesterase and antagonist of nondepolarizing neuromuscular-blocking agents. Inhibits the enzyme acetylcholinesterase, allowing acetylcholine to accumulate at the myoneural junction. Restores normal transmission of nerve impulses. Acts within 30 to 60 seconds and has an extremely short duration of action, seldom exceeding 10 minutes. Produces vagal stimulation, shortens refractory period of atrial muscle, and slows conduction through the AV node.

INDICATIONS AND USES

Diagnosis of myasthenia gravis. ▪ Evaluation of adequate treatment of myasthenia gravis. ▪ Evaluation of emergency treatment of myasthenia crisis. ▪ An antagonist to nondepolarizing muscle relaxants (e.g., atracurium [Tracrium]). ▪ Adjunct in treatment of respiratory depression caused by curare overdosage.
Unlabeled uses: Termination of supraventricular tachycardia unresponsive to cardiac glycosides. Adenosine is the drug of choice. ▪ Diagnosis of supraventricular tachycardia. ▪ Evaluate function of a demand pacemaker.

CONTRAINDICATIONS

Apnea, known hypersensitivity to anticholinesterase agents, intestinal and urinary obstructions of mechanical type.

PRECAUTIONS

A physician should be present when this drug is used. ▪ The term *crisis* is used when severe respiratory distress with ventilatory inadequacy occurs. The crisis may be secondary to a sudden increase in severity of myasthenia gravis (myasthenic crisis) or to overtreatment with anticholinesterase drugs (cholinergic crisis). If apnea is present, controlled ventilation must be secured before any testing with edrophonium. ▪ Use caution when administering to patients being treated with anticholinesterase drugs (e.g., neostigmine). S/S of cholinergic crisis may mimic those of myasthenic weakness, and the patient's condition may worsen with administration of edrophonium. ▪ Use caution in patients with bronchial asthma, cardiac arrhythmias, or myasthenia gravis treated with anticholinesterase drugs. ▪ Isolated cases of respiratory or cardiac arrests have been reported. ▪ Contains sulfites; use caution in patients with allergies.
Monitor: Atropine 1 mg must be available and ready for injection at all times. ▪ Continuously observe patient reactions. ▪ Anticholinesterase insensitivity may develop; withhold drugs and support respiration as necessary. ▪ See Drug/Lab Interactions.
Maternal/Child: Safety for use during pregnancy and breast-feeding not established. Use during pregnancy only if benefit justifies potential risk to mother and fetus. ▪ Discontinue breast-feeding. ▪ Safety and effectiveness in reversing neuromuscular blockade in pediatric patients not established. However, doses of 0.1 to 1.43 mg/kg have been used; effects (antagonism) were more rapid than in adults.

DRUG/LAB INTERACTIONS

Muscarinic effects antagonized by **atropine;** see Antidote. ▪ May be inhibited by **corticosteroids and magnesium.** ▪ May cause bradycardia with **digoxin glycosides.** ▪ Briefly antagonizes the effects of **nondepolarizing neuromuscular blocking agents** (e.g., atracurium, pancuronium, vecuronium). ▪ Prolongs muscle relaxant effect of **succinylcholine.**

SIDE EFFECTS

Abdominal cramps, anorexia, anxiety, bradycardia, bronchiolar spasm, cardiac arrhythmias and arrest, cold moist skin, contraction of the pupils, convulsions, diarrhea, dysphagia, fainting, increased lacrimation, increased pulmonary secretion, increased salivation, insomnia, irritability, laryngospasm, muscle weakness, nausea, perspiration, ptosis, respiratory arrest (either muscular or central), urinary frequency and incontinence, vomiting.

ANTIDOTE

If side effects occur, discontinue the drug and notify the physician. Atropine sulfate in doses of 0.4 to 0.5 mg IV will counteract most side effects and may be repeated every 3 to 10 minutes. Endotracheal intubation or tracheostomy is considered prophylactic in anesthesia or crises. Artificial ventilation, oxygen therapy, cardiac monitoring, adequate suctioning, and treatment of shock or convulsions must be instituted and maintained as necessary. Treat hypersensitivity reactions as indicated.

ELOTUZUMAB
(**EL**-oh-**TOOZ**-ue-mab)

Monoclonal antibody
Antineoplastic

Empliciti

USUAL DOSE

Premedication: To reduce the risk of infusion reactions, premedicate with the following. **Dexamethasone:** Divide into an oral and an IV dose. Administer 28 mg as an oral dose between 3 and 24 hours before elotuzumab infusion. Then 45 to 90 minutes before elotuzumab infusion, administer *dexamethasone* 8 mg IV, an *H₁ blocker* (*diphenhydramine* [25 to 50 mg orally or IV] or equivalent), an *H₂ blocker* (*ranitidine* [50 mg IV or 150 mg orally] or equivalent), and *acetaminophen* (650 to 1,000 mg orally).

Elotuzumab: 10 mg/kg as an infusion every week for the first 2 cycles and every 2 weeks thereafter in conjunction with the recommended dosing of lenalidomide (Revlimid) and dexamethasone as described in the following chart. Continue treatment until disease progression or unacceptable toxicity. Refer to the prescribing information for dexamethasone and lenalidomide and other premedications as appropriate.

Recommended Dosing Schedule of Elotuzumab in Combination with Lenalidomide and Dexamethasone								
Cycle	28-Day Cycles 1 and 2				28-Day Cycles 3+			
Day of Cycle	1	8	15	22	1	8	15	22
Premedication*	✓	✓	✓	✓	✓	—	✓	—
Dexamethasone (mg) orally†	28 mg	28 mg	28 mg	28 mg	28 mg	40 mg	28 mg	40 mg
Dexamethasone (mg) IV*	8 mg	8 mg	8 mg	8 mg	8 mg	—	8 mg	—
Elotuzumab (mg/kg) IV	10 mg/kg	10 mg/kg	10 mg/kg	10 mg/kg	10 mg/kg	—	10 mg/kg	—
Lenalidomide (mg)	Days 1 to 21 (25 mg orally)				Days 1 to 21 (25 mg orally)			

*Premedicate 45 to 90 minutes before elotuzumab infusion with medications described under Premedication in Usual Dose (dexamethasone IV, an H₁ blocker [diphenhydramine IV or PO or equivalent], an H₂ blocker [ranitidine IV or PO or equivalent], and acetaminophen PO).

†Give 28 mg of dexamethasone orally between 3 and 24 hours before elotuzumab infusion and 40 mg of dexamethasone orally on days when elotuzumab is NOT administered.

DOSE ADJUSTMENTS

If the dose of one drug in the regimen is delayed, interrupted, or discontinued, treatment with the other drugs may continue as scheduled. However, if dexamethasone is delayed or discontinued, base the decision regarding whether to administer elotuzumab on clinical judgment (i.e., risk of hypersensitivity). ■ Interrupt the elotuzumab infusion if a

Grade 2 or higher infusion reaction occurs. Upon resolution to Grade 1 or lower, restart elotuzumab infusion at 0.5 mL/min and gradually increase at a rate of 0.5 mL/min every 30 minutes as tolerated to the rate at which the infusion reaction occurred. Resume the escalation regimen if there is no recurrence of the infusion reaction; see Rate of Administration and Antidote. ▪ If the infusion reaction recurs, stop the elotuzumab infusion and do not restart on that day. ▪ A severe infusion reaction may require permanent discontinuation of elotuzumab. ▪ Dose delays and modifications for dexamethasone and lenalidomide should be performed as recommended in their Prescribing Information.

DILUTION

Available as a 300-mg or 400-mg single-dose vial. Calculate the dose (mg) based on patient weight, total volume (mL) of elotuzumab solution required, and the number of vials required using the following calculations:

$$(\text{Weight in kg} \times \text{dose/kg}) \div 300\ (400)\ \text{mg/vial} = \#\ \text{of vials required}$$

For a 60-kg patient: [(60 kg) × (10 mg/kg)] ÷ 300 (400) mg/vial = 2 vials of the 300-mg/vial solution or 1.5 vials of the 400-mg/vial solution. After patient is weighed and appropriate dose is calculated, remove sufficient vials from the refrigerator. Aseptic technique imperative. Reconstitute the 300-mg vial with 13 mL of SWFI and the 400-mg vial with 17 mL SWFI to obtain a solution with a final concentration of 25 mg/mL. Some back pressure may be experienced and is normal. To dissolve the lyophilized cake, hold vial upright and swirl the solution by rotating the vial. Gently invert the vial a few times to dissolve all the powder. Avoid vigorous agitation. *Do Not Shake;* should dissolve in less than 10 minutes. Allow the reconstituted solution to stand for 5 to 10 minutes. Solution should be colorless to slightly yellow. Do not use if opaque particles, discoloration, or other foreign particles are present. Vials contain overfill. Withdraw the calculated dose and further dilute in 230 mL of NS or D5W. The volume of NS or D5W can be adjusted so as not to exceed 5 mL/kg of patient weight at any given dose of elotuzumab. Gently invert the infusion bag to mix the solution. Infusion bags must be made of polyvinylchloride (PVC) or polyolefin.

Filters: Must be administered through an infusion set with an in-line, sterile, nonpyrogenic, low–protein binding filter (pore size 0.2 to 1.2 micrometers).

Storage: Refrigerate at 2° to 8° C (36° to 46° F) in original carton to protect from light until time of use. Do not freeze or shake. The diluted product may be stored for up to 24 hours if refrigerated and protected from light (a maximum of 8 of the 24 hours can be at RT and room light). Bring to room temperature before infusion and use immediately. Infusion should be completed within 24 hours of reconstitution. Discard any unused product remaining in vials.

COMPATIBILITY

Manufacturer states, "Do not mix elotuzumab with, or administer as an infusion with, other medicinal products." **Compatible** only with IV bags/containers made of polyvinylchloride (PVC) or polyolefin.

RATE OF ADMINISTRATION

For IV infusion only. Use of an infusion pump recommended. Initiate the infusion rate at 0.5 mL/min. Increase in a stepwise fashion (see the following chart) if no infusion reactions develop. Interrupt elotuzumab for Grade 2 or higher infusion reactions.

Recommended Infusion Rates for Elotuzumab		
Cycle 1, Dose 1	Cycle 1, Dose 2	Cycle 1, Doses 3 and 4, and All Subsequent Cycles
Time Interval Rate	Time Interval Rate	Rate
0 to 30 min: 0.5 mL/min	0 to 30 min: 1 mL/min	2 mL/min
30 to 60 min: 1 mL/min	30 min or more: 2 mL/min	2 mL/min
60 min or more: 2 mL/min	—	2 mL/min

Adjust the infusion rate following a Grade 2 or higher infusion reaction; see Dose Adjustments. The maximum infusion rate should not exceed 2 mL/min; however, in patients who have received 4 cycles of elotuzumab, the infusion rate may be increased to a maximum of 5 mL/min.

ACTIONS

Elotuzumab is a humanized recombinant IgG1 monoclonal antibody that specifically targets the SLAMF7 (signaling lymphocytic activation molecule family member 7) protein. SLAMF7 is expressed on myeloma cells independent of cytogenetic abnormalities. It is also expressed on natural killer cells, plasma cells, and some specific immune cell subsets of differentiated cells within the hematopoietic lineage. Elotuzumab targets SLAMF7 on myeloma cells and facilitates the interaction with natural killer cells to mediate the killing of myeloma cells through antibody-dependent cellular cytotoxicity (ADCC). In preclinical models, the combination of elotuzumab and lenalidomide resulted in enhanced activation of natural killer cells. When given in combination with lenalidomide/dexamethasone, approximately 97% of the maximum steady-state concentration is predicted to be eliminated with a geometric mean (CV%) of 82.4 days.

INDICATIONS AND USES

Treatment of patients with multiple myeloma who have received one to three prior therapies. Used in combination with lenalidomide and dexamethasone.

CONTRAINDICATIONS

Manufacturer states, "None." Manufacturer recommends consulting the prescribing information for lenalidomide and dexamethasone before starting therapy.

PRECAUTIONS

For IV infusion only. ▪ Administered under the direction of a physician knowledgeable in its use in a facility with adequate diagnostic and treatment facilities to monitor the patient and respond to any medical emergency. ▪ Can cause infusion reactions. Reports of infusion reactions during clinical trials were Grade 3 or lower, and most occurred during the first dose; see Monitor. ▪ Infections, including opportunistic infections, have occurred; some resulted in discontinuation of therapy or fatalities. ▪ Second primary malignancies, including hematologic malignancies, solid tumors, and skin cancers, have been reported. ▪ Hepatotoxicity (elevations in liver enzymes [ALT, AST] greater than 3 times the ULN, total bilirubin greater than 2 times the ULN, and alkaline phosphatase less than 2 times the ULN) has been reported. ▪ Can affect the determination of complete response and of disease progression in some patients with IgG kappa myeloma protein; see Drug/Lab Interactions. ▪ Clinically significant differences in the pharmacokinetics of elotuzumab were not observed based on age, gender, race, baseline LDH, albumin, renal impairment ranging from mild to severe (including ESRD with or without dialysis), and mild hepatic impairment. Pharmacokinetics of elotuzumab in patients with moderate to severe hepatic impairment is unknown. ▪ A therapeutic protein; has the potential for immunogenicity.

Monitor: Premedication required; see Usual Dose. ▪ Obtain baseline CBC and differential and monitor as indicated during therapy. ▪ Obtain baseline liver enzymes (e.g., ALT, AST, bilirubin, and alkaline phosphatase) and monitor periodically. ▪ Stop elotuzumab if Grade 3 or higher liver enzyme elevation occurs. Continuation of treatment may be considered after return to baseline values. ▪ Monitor vital signs. ▪ Monitor for S/S of infusion reactions; bradycardia, chills, fever, hypertension, and hypotension were most common. In patients who experience an infusion reaction, monitor vital signs every 30 minutes for 2 hours after the end of the elotuzumab infusion. ▪ Immediately interrupt the infusion for infusion reactions of Grade 2 or higher; see Dose Adjustments and Antidote. ▪ Monitor for S/S of infection. ▪ Monitor for S/S of second primary malignancies.

Patient Education: Review manufacturer's medication guide. ▪ Because of the combination use with lenalidomide, pregnancy must be avoided. Effective contraception is required during treatment for men and women of reproductive potential. Consult with a health professional for specific information. ▪ Premedication required to reduce the risk of infusion reactions. ▪ Immediately report any S/S of infusion-related reactions (e.g., chills, difficulty breathing, fever, rash); may occur within 24 hours of an infusion. ▪ Elotuzumab can affect the results of some tests, including testing for complete response, and additional testing may be indicated. ▪ Second primary malignancies, including skin cancer, may occur; monitoring is required. Report unusual symptoms. ▪ Report S/S of hepatotoxicity (abdominal pain, bruising, fatigue, itching, jaundice).

Maternal/Child: Combination drug regimen can cause fetal harm; avoid pregnancy; see Patient Education. ▪ Discontinue breast-feeding. Safety for use during breast-feeding is unknown. Combination drug regimen may have serious effects in a breast-feeding infant. ▪ Safety and effectiveness for use in pediatric patients not established.

Elderly: No overall differences in safety or efficacy have been reported between elderly patients and younger adults.

DRUG/LAB INTERACTIONS
No drug interaction studies have been performed. ▪ Elotuzumab may be detected on both the serum protein electrophoreses (SPEP) and immunofixation (IFE) assays used for the clinical monitoring of endogenous M protein and can interfere with correct response classification. This interference can affect the determination of complete response and possibly cause a relapse from complete response in patients with IgG kappa myeloma protein.

SIDE EFFECTS
The most frequently reported side effects include constipation, cough, decreased appetite, diarrhea, fatigue, fever, infusion reactions, nasopharyngitis, peripheral neuropathy, pneumonia, and upper respiratory tract infections. Altered mood, bradycardia, cataracts, chest pain, headache, hepatotoxicity, hypersensitivity/infusion reactions, hypertension, hypoesthesia, hypotension, infections, night sweats, oropharyngeal pain, pain in extremities, second primary malignancies, tachycardia, weight loss, and vomiting have also been reported. Reported laboratory abnormalities included elevated alkaline phosphatase, hyperglycemia, hyperkalemia, hypoalbuminemia, hypocalcemia, leukopenia, lymphopenia, low bicarbonate, and thrombocytopenia.

ANTIDOTE
Notify physician of any side effects; most will be treated symptomatically. If a Grade 2 or higher infusion reaction occurs, interrupt elotuzumab infusion and institute appropriate medical and supportive measures. Severe infusion reactions may require permanent discontinuation of elotuzumab therapy. Stop elotuzumab upon Grade 3 or higher elevation of liver enzymes. After return to baseline values, continuation of therapy may be considered. Discontinue administration at the first sign of a serious hypersensitivity reaction and treat as indicated (e.g., oxygen, diphenhydramine, epinephrine, corticosteroids, vasopressors, and/or fluids). Resuscitate as necessary. Does not appear to be removed by dialysis.

ENALAPRILAT BBW
(en-**AL**-ah-prill-at)

ACE inhibitor
Antihypertensive
Vasodilator

pH 6.5 to 7.5

USUAL DOSE
1.25 mg every 6 hours. Doses up to 5 mg every 6 hours have been tolerated for up to 36 hours, but clinical studies have not shown a need for dosage over 1.25 mg. Additional doses of 1.25 mg may be given every 6 hours except in dialysis patients. Dosage is the same when converting from oral to IV therapy. Resume oral therapy as soon as tolerated. See Precautions.

PEDIATRIC DOSE
0.625 to 1.25 mg every 6 hours. See Maternal/Child.

DOSE ADJUSTMENTS
Reduce initial dose to 0.625 mg in patients taking diuretics, patients with CHF, hyponatremia, severe volume or salt depletion, a CrCl less than 30 mL/min, and dialysis patients; see Rate of Administration. If the 0.625 dose is not clinically effective after 1 hour, it may be repeated. ▪ Blood levels markedly increased in the elderly; dose selection should be cautious. Consider decreased cardiac, hepatic, and renal function; concomitant disease; or other drug therapy. ▪ See Drug/Lab Interactions and Precautions.

DILUTION
May be given undiluted through the port of a free-flowing infusion of NS, D5W, D5NS, D5LR, or Isolyte E. May also be diluted in up to 50 mL of any of the same solutions and given as an infusion.

Storage: Store at CRT. Stable for up to 24 hours after dilution.

COMPATIBILITY   (Underline Indicates Conflicting Compatibility Information)
Consider any drug NOT listed as compatible to be INCOMPATIBLE until consulting a pharmacist; specific conditions may apply.
One source suggests the following **compatibilities:**
Additive: Dextran 40, dobutamine, dopamine, heparin, hetastarch in NS (Hespan), meropenem (Merrem IV), nitroglycerin IV, nitroprusside sodium, potassium chloride (KCl).
Y-site: Allopurinol (Aloprim), amifostine (Ethyol), amikacin, aminophylline, ampicillin, ampicillin/sulbactam (Unasyn), aztreonam (Azactam), bivalirudin (Angiomax), butorphanol (Stadol), calcium gluconate, cefazolin (Ancef), ceftaroline (Teflaro), ceftazidime (Fortaz), chloramphenicol (Chloromycetin), cisatracurium (Nimbex), cladribine (Leustatin), clindamycin (Cleocin), dexmedetomidine (Precedex), dextran 40, dobutamine, docetaxel (Taxotere), dopamine, doripenem (Doribax), doxorubicin liposomal (Doxil), erythromycin (Erythrocin), esmolol (Brevibloc), etoposide phosphate (Etopophos), famotidine (Pepcid IV), fenoldopam (Corlopam), fentanyl, filgrastim (Neupogen), ganciclovir (Cytovene IV), gemcitabine (Gemzar), gentamicin, granisetron (Kytril), heparin, hetastarch in electrolytes (Hextend), hetastarch in NS (Hespan), hydrocortisone sodium succinate (Solu-Cortef), labetalol, lidocaine, linezolid (Zyvox), magnesium sulfate, melphalan (Alkeran), meropenem (Merrem IV), methylprednisolone (Solu-Medrol), metronidazole (Flagyl IV), morphine, nafcillin (Nallpen), nicardipine (Cardene IV), nitroprusside sodium, oxaliplatin (Eloxatin), pemetrexed (Alimta), penicillin G potassium, phenobarbital (Luminal), piperacillin/tazobactam (Zosyn), potassium chloride (KCl), potassium phosphates, propofol (Diprivan), ranitidine (Zantac), remifentanil (Ultiva), sodium acetate, sulfamethoxazole/trimethoprim, teniposide (Vumon), thiotepa, tobramycin, vancomycin, vinorelbine (Navelbine).

RATE OF ADMINISTRATION
A single dose must be evenly distributed over 5 minutes. Extend rate of infusion up to 1 hour in patients at risk for severe hypotension (e.g., heart failure, hyponatremia, high-dose diuretic therapy, recent intensive diuresis or increase in diuretic dose, renal dialysis, or severe volume and/or salt depletion of any etiology).

ACTIONS
An antihypertensive agent. An angiotensin-converting enzyme inhibitor that prevents conversion of angiotensin I to angiotensin II. Peripheral arterial resistance is reduced in hypertensive patients. In patients with heart failure, significant reduction in pulmonary capillary wedge pressure (preload), peripheral vascular resistance (afterload), BP, and heart size occurs, as well as an increase in cardiac output (stroke index) and exercise tolerance time. Initial response may take 15 minutes to 1 hour. Peak BP reduction occurs in 1 to 4 hours, and effects last up to 6 hours. Peak effects of subsequent doses may be greater than the initial dose. Excreted in urine. Crosses placental barrier. Secreted in breast milk.

INDICATIONS AND USES
Treatment of hypertension when oral therapy is not practical. ▪ Heart failure not adequately responsive to diuretics and digoxin. Enalaprilat is used in addition to digoxin and diuretics. ▪ Hypertensive emergencies (effects are variable).
Unlabeled uses: Treatment of hypertension or renal crisis in scleroderma.

CONTRAINDICATIONS
Hypersensitivity to enalaprilat or its components, a history of angioedema related to previous treatment with an ACE inhibitor, or hereditary or idiopathic angioedema.

PRECAUTIONS
Has been used IV for up to 7 days. ▪ Use caution in patients with a history of angioedema (see Contraindications), aortic stenosis, or hypertrophic cardiomyopathy. ▪ Use caution in patients with collagen vascular disease and renal disease; neutropenia and/or agranulocytosis have been reported. Monitoring of WBC may be indicated. ▪ Use caution in surgery, with anesthesia, or with agents that produce hypotension. ▪ May rarely cause a syndrome that starts with cholestatic jaundice, progresses to hepatic necrosis, and may progress to death. Discontinue in patients who develop elevated liver enzymes or jaundice. ▪ ACE inhibitors often cause a persistent, nonproductive cough, which should resolve when drug is discontinued. ▪ Average dose for conversion to oral therapy is 5 mg/day as a single dose. When a reduced dose of enalaprilat IV has been indicated (e.g., diuretics, impaired renal function, dialysis), reduce initial oral dose to 2.5 mg/day as a single dose. Adjust either by patient response. ▪ Patients sensitive to one ACE inhibitor may be sensitive to another. ▪ See Monitor and Drug/Lab Interactions.
Monitor: Monitor vital signs very frequently. May cause precipitous drop in BP following the first dose. ▪ Use extreme caution in fluid-depleted patients. Patients with congestive heart failure may become hypotensive at any time. Arrhythmias or conduction defects may occur. ▪ Monitor BUN and SCr. An increase in either may require a decrease in dose of enalaprilat or discontinuation of a diuretic. ▪ Diuretics given concomitantly may cause a precipitous drop in BP within the first hour of the initial dose; observe the patient closely. Severe dietary salt restriction or dialysis will aggravate this effect. ▪ May cause oliguria or progressive azotemia in patients with severe congestive heart failure whose renal function is dependent on the activity of the renin-angiotensin-aldosterone system. Acute renal failure and death are possible. ▪ May cause hyperkalemia. May cause a significant increase in serum potassium with potassium-sparing diuretics or potassium supplements. Use with caution and only in documented hypokalemia. Use salt substitutes with caution. Monitor serum potassium levels. ▪ Monitoring of WBC may be indicated in patients with collagen vascular disease or renal disease. ▪ See Drug/Lab Interactions.
Patient Education: Consider birth control options. ▪ May cause dizziness; avoid sudden changes in posture and request assistance for ambulation if necessary.

Maternal/Child: Avoid pregnancy; Category C (first trimester) and Category D (second and third trimester). Can cause fetal and neonatal morbidity and death. Infants exposed to ACE inhibitors during the first trimester of pregnancy may have an increased risk of major congenital malformations. If pregnancy occurs, discontinue immediately; many alternate antihypertensive agents. ▪ Observe any infant with in utero exposure for hypotension, oliguria, and hyperkalemia. ▪ Has caused reversible acute renal failure in a premature infant whose mother received enalaprilat. ▪ Safety for use in breast-feeding not established. ▪ Safety for use in pediatric patients not established but has been used. ▪ May contain benzyl alcohol, which has been associated with a fatal "gasping syndrome" in neonates.

Elderly: Dose selection should be cautious; see Dose Adjustments and Precautions/Monitor. ▪ May be less sensitive to effects due to a decrease in plasma renin activity or more sensitive to hypotensive effects due to increased blood levels (decreased renal excretion).

DRUG/LAB INTERACTIONS
Use caution in surgery, with **anesthesia,** or with any **agents that produce hypotension.** ▪ May be used concomitantly with other **antihypertensive agents** (e.g., thiazide diuretics [chlorothiazide (Diuril)]). Effects are additive. ▪ **Diuretics** given concomitantly may cause a precipitous drop in BP. ▪ May cause hyperkalemia with **potassium-sparing diuretics** (e.g., spironolactone [Aldactone], triamterene [Dyrenium], amiloride [Midamor]), **potassium supplements, potassium-containing salt substitutes, or low-salt milk.** ▪ Use caution and consider lower doses when administering **nitroglycerin, nitroprusside sodium, other nitrates, or other vasodilators** (e.g., hydralazine). ▪ In patients with compromised renal function, concurrent use with **NSAIDs** (e.g., ibuprofen [Advil, Motrin], naproxen [Aleve, Naprosyn]) may result in further deterioration of renal function. ▪ Concurrent use with **NSAIDs** may also decrease the hypotensive effects of enalaprilat by inhibiting the renal prostaglandin synthesis and/or by causing sodium and fluid retention. ▪ May increase **lithium** concentration, resulting in lithium toxicity. ▪ Interac-

tion with some **imaging agents** (e.g., iodohippurate, technetium) may render diagnostic renal function tests inconclusive. ▪ May decrease **hemoglobin and hematocrit** slightly. ▪ See Precautions and Monitor.

SIDE EFFECTS

Abdominal pain, angioedema, anosmia (absence of sense of smell), atrial fibrillation, bradycardia, chest pain, conjunctivitis, cough (persistent, dry), diarrhea, dizziness, dry eyes, dyspnea, eosinophilic pneumonitis, fatigue, flank pain, gynecomastia, headache, hepatotoxicity, herpes zoster, hoarseness, hyperkalemia, hypotension (severe), impotence, insomnia, muscle cramps, nausea, palpitations, paresthesias, photosensitivity, pneumonia, pruritus, pulmonary edema, pulmonary embolism and infarction, pulmonary infiltrates, rash, Raynaud's phenomenon, renal failure (reversible), rhinorrhea, somnolence, sore throat, taste disturbances, tearing, toxic epidermal necrolysis, vomiting. Anaphylaxis has been reported.

ANTIDOTE

For minor side effects, notify the physician. Most will be tolerated or treated symptomatically. If symptoms progress or any major side effect occurs (angioedema, precipitous hypotension, hyperkalemia), discontinue drug and notify the physician immediately. Hypotension should respond to IV fluids if the patient's condition allows their use. Other drugs in the regimen may need to be discontinued or the dosage reduced. Epinephrine, diphenhydramine (Benadryl), and hydrocortisone may be used to treat angioedema. Maintain the patient as indicated. If cardiac arrhythmias occur, treat appropriately. Hemodialysis may be useful in toxicity.

EPINEPHRINE HYDROCHLORIDE

(ep-ih-**NEF**-rin hy-droh-**KLOR**-eyed)

Cardiac stimulant
Bronchodilator
Antiallergic
Vasopressor

Adrenalin Chloride

pH 2.5 to 5

USUAL DOSE

Hypersensitivity reactions or bronchospasm: 0.1 to 0.25 mg (1 to 2.5 mL of a 0.1 mg/mL concentration). Start with a small dose, giving only as much as required to alleviate undesirable symptoms, and repeat as necessary (usually every 20 to 30 minutes), gradually increasing dose depending on need. Another source suggests 0.2 to 0.5 mg of 0.1 mg/mL concentration. May be repeated as necessary.

Bradycardia: AHA guidelines recommend epinephrine infusion 2 to 10 mcg/min; titrate to desired effect. Indicated if atropine is ineffective. Alternately, transcutaneous pacing or dopamine infusion 2 to 10 mcg/kg/min may be used.

Cardiac arrest: AHA guidelines recommend 1 mg (10 mL of a 0.1 mg/mL concentration) IV; may repeat every 3 to 5 minutes. Follow each dose with a 20-mL IV flush to ensure delivery to systemic circulation. See Compatibility. Doses up to 0.2 mg/kg have been used for specific indications (beta-blocker or calcium channel blocker overdose). May also be given as a continuous infusion by adding 1 mg of epinephrine (1 mL of a 1 mg/mL solution) to 500 mL NS or D5W. Begin with an infusion rate of 0.1 to 0.5 mcg/kg/min and titrate to response. The dose for a 70-kg patient would be 7 to 35 mcg/min. Higher doses of epinephrine are controversial.

Endotracheal: A diluted solution may be given through the endotracheal tube before an IV is established. AHA guidelines recommend 2 to 2.5 mg (of a 1 mg/mL solution) diluted in 10 mL NS. Another source suggests administering the IV dose through the endotracheal tube if an IV line has not been established.

Vasopressor or maintenance dose: 1 to 10 mcg/min titrated to desired response. AHA guidelines recommend that epinephrine be used to treat symptomatic bradycardia after atropine as an alternative infusion to dopamine or to treat severe hypotension when atropine and transcutaneous pacing fail, when hypotension accompanies bradycardia, or with a phosphodiesterase enzyme inhibitor. For profound bradycardia or hypotension, 2 to 10 mcg/min may be given as an infusion (1 mg of 1 mg/mL concentration in 500 mL NS or D5W) at a rate of 0.1 to 0.5 mcg/kg/min titrated to response.

PEDIATRIC DOSE

See Maternal/Child.

Hypersensitivity reactions or bronchospasm in infants and children: 0.01 mg/kg (0.1 mL/kg of a 0.1 mg/mL concentration). May repeat at 20-minute to 4-hour intervals. One source suggests a maximum dose of 0.3 mg, another 0.5 mg. Usually given SC as a 1 mg/mL concentration.

Severe anaphylactic shock in infants and children: One source suggests 0.1 mg IV of a 0.01 mg/mL concentration (0.1 mL of a 1 mg/mL concentration diluted in 10 mL NS) given over 5 to 10 minutes. Another source suggests 0.01 mL/kg of a 1 mg/mL concentration SC. Maximum 0.3 mL/dose. Repeat every 15 minutes as needed.

Bradycardia in infants and children: AHA guidelines recommend 0.01 mg/kg (0.1 mL/kg of a 0.1 mg/mL concentration) to treat symptomatic bradycardia. If IV access is not readily available, AHA guidelines recommend 0.1 mg/kg (0.1 mL/kg) of a 1 mg/mL concentration via ET.

Asystolic or pulseless arrest in infants and children: AHA guidelines recommend 0.01 mg/kg (0.1 mL/kg of a 0.1 mg/mL concentration). Another source recommends 0.01 mg/kg of a 0.1 mg/mL concentration and suggests that the first dose should not exceed 1 mg (10 mL of a 0.1 mg/mL concentration). Repeat every 3 to 5 minutes during arrest. Up to 0.1 to 0.2 mg/kg may be used if initial doses are ineffective. May be given via ET (0.1 mg/kg [0.1 mL/kg of a 1 mg/mL concentration]) every 3 to 5 minutes until IV established, then begin with first IV dose. A third source suggests 0.01 to 0.03 mg/kg (0.1 to 0.3 mL/kg) of a 0.1 mg/mL concentration initially. May repeat every 3 to 5 minutes in neonates. In infants and children subsequent doses of 0.1 mg/kg every 3 to 5 minutes may be given if needed. Prepare an infusion and titrate from 0.1 to 1 mcg/kg/min to desired effect. Use upper dosing range if asystole is present. With higher dose, be aware of preservative content to avoid toxicity.

DOSE ADJUSTMENTS
See Drug/Lab Interactions. ▪ Doses larger than 1 mg may not be indicated in patients over 65 years of age and patients in ventricular fibrillation.

DILUTION
New changes in labeling eliminate the use of ratios; what was previously a 1:1,000 solution will now be referred to only as a 1 mg/mL solution, a 1:10,000 solution will now be referred to only as a 0.1 mg/mL solution, and a 1:100,000 solution will now be referred to only as a 0.01 mg/mL solution.

Check label. Not all epinephrine solutions can be given IV. The 1 mg/mL strength is for SC or IM use only. It must be further diluted with at least 10 mL of NS to prepare a 0.1 mg/mL solution before IV use.

IV Injection: Available prediluted (0.1 mg/mL) in 10-mL syringes. Available in a 30-mL vial (30 mg [1 mg/mL solution]) to facilitate larger doses or continuous infusion. Each 1 mg (1 mL) of 1 mg/mL solution must be diluted in at least 10 mL of NS to prepare a 0.1 mg/mL solution.

Infusion: For occasional use as a vasopressor or for maintenance, epinephrine may be further diluted in 250 to 500 mL D5W; see the following chart. Give through Y-tube or three-way stopcock of infusion set. See chart on inside back cover for additional **compatible** solutions.

Epinephrine HCl Infusion Rates						
Desired Dose	1 mg in 500 mL D5W (2 mcg/mL)			1 mg in 250 mL D5W 2 mg in 500 mL D5W (4 mcg/mL)		
mcg/min	mcg/hr	mL/min	mL/hr	mcg/hr	mL/min	mL/hr
1	60	0.5	30	60	0.25	15
2	120	1	60	120	0.5	30
3	180	1.5	90	180	0.75	45
4	240	2	120	240	1	60
5	300	2.5	150	300	1.25	75
6	360	3	180	360	1.5	90
7	420	3.5	210	420	1.75	105
8	480	4	240	480	2	120

In *cardiac arrest,* 1 mg is sometimes added to 500 mL of NS or D5W.
Filters: No data available from manufacturer.
Storage: Store at CRT unless otherwise specified by manufacturer. Do not use if brown or if a sediment is present. Deteriorates rapidly. Protect from light and freezing.

COMPATIBILITY   (Underline Indicates Conflicting Compatibility Information)
Consider any drug NOT listed as compatible to be INCOMPATIBLE until consulting a pharmacist; specific conditions may apply.
Manufacturer states, "Readily destroyed and precipitate forms with alkalis, alkaline solutions (e.g., sodium bicarbonate and oxidizing agents)." *If coadministration with sodium bi-*

carbonate is indicated, give at separate sites. Unstable in any solution with a pH over 5.5 (e.g., aminophylline, ampicillin, lidocaine, warfarin [Coumadin]).

One source suggests the following **compatibilities:**

Additive: Amikacin, dobutamine, furosemide (Lasix), ranitidine (Zantac), verapamil.

Y-site: Amiodarone (Nexterone), anidulafungin (Eraxis), atracurium (Tracrium), bivalirudin (Angiomax), calcium chloride, calcium gluconate, caspofungin (Cancidas), ceftazidime (Fortaz), cisatracurium (Nimbex), dexmedetomidine (Precedex), diltiazem (Cardizem), dobutamine, dopamine, famotidine (Pepcid IV), fenoldopam (Corlopam), fentanyl, furosemide (Lasix), heparin, hetastarch in electrolytes (Hextend), hydrocortisone sodium succinate (Solu-Cortef), hydromorphone (Dilaudid), labetalol, levofloxacin (Levaquin), lorazepam (Ativan), midazolam (Versed), milrinone (Primacor), morphine, nicardipine (Cardene IV), nitroglycerin IV, nitroprusside sodium, norepinephrine (Levophed), pancuronium, pantoprazole (Protonix IV), phytonadione (vitamin K$_1$), potassium chloride (KCl), propofol (Diprivan), ranitidine (Zantac), remifentanil (Ultiva), tigecycline (Tygacil), tirofiban (Aggrastat), vasopressin, vecuronium, warfarin (Coumadin).

RATE OF ADMINISTRATION

IV injection: Each 1 mg or fraction thereof over 1 minute or longer. May be given more rapidly in cardiac resuscitation; follow with 20-mL IV flush.

Infusion: Vasopressor or maintenance: 1 to 10 mcg/min titrated to desired patient response.

Cardiac arrest: Titrated to deliver a single dose over 3 to 5 minutes based on patient response. Must be delivered by central venous access. Use an infusion pump to control rate.

ACTIONS

A naturally occurring hormone secreted by the adrenal glands. A sympathomimetic drug, it imitates almost all actions of the sympathetic nervous system. Stimulates both alpha- and beta-adrenergic receptors. It is a vasoconstrictor and delays the absorption of many drugs; a potent cardiac stimulant, it strengthens the myocardial contraction (positive inotropic effect) and increases cardiac rate (positive chronotropic effect). Increases myocardial and cerebral blood flow during CPR. A potent dilator or relaxant of smooth muscle, especially bronchial muscle. Decreases blood supply to the abdomen and increases blood supply to skeletal muscles. Elevates systolic BP, lowers diastolic BP, and increases pulse pressure. Seldom used as a vasopressor because of its short duration of action. High-dose infusions (greater than 0.2 mcg/min) may produce profound vasoconstriction, compromising perfusion and possibly compromising renal and splanchnic blood flow. It is rapidly inactivated in the body by the liver and various enzymes and is excreted in changed form in the urine. Crosses placental barrier. Secreted in breast milk.

INDICATIONS AND USES

Cardiac resuscitation. First-line drug of choice when initial CPR, intubation, ventilation, and initial defibrillation have failed to achieve response in ventricular fibrillation, pulseless ventricular tachycardia, asystole, or pulseless electrical activity. ▪ Drug of choice for anaphylactic shock. ▪ Antidote of choice for histamine overdose and hypersensitivity reactions including bronchial asthma, urticaria, and angioneurotic edema. ▪ Stokes-Adams syndrome. ▪ Occasionally used as a vasopressor (e.g., symptomatic bradycardia).

CONTRAINDICATIONS

Anesthesia with halogenated hydrocarbons or cyclopropane, cerebral arteriosclerosis, hypertension, labor and delivery if maternal BP exceeds 130/80 mm Hg (may cause prolonged uterine atony with hemorrhage), hyperthyroidism, narrow-angle glaucoma, nervous instability, organic brain damage, patients receiving high doses of digoxin, shock. Do not use to treat overdosage of phenothiazines (e.g., chlorpromazine [Thorazine]); a further drop in BP will occur, and irreversible shock may result. Do not use concurrently with esmolol (Brevibloc).

PRECAUTIONS

Usual route is SC except in cardiac resuscitation or as a vasopressor infusion. ▪ Use caution in the elderly, in diabetics, in hypotension (except in anaphylactic shock), in patients receiving thyroid preparations, and in patients with cardiac disease, a history of seizures, or long-term emphysema or bronchial asthma with degenerative heart disease. ▪ Often used with corticosteroids in treatment of anaphylactic shock. ▪ Increasing BP and HR may cause myocardial ischemia, angina, and increased myocardial oxygen demand. ▪ Larger doses in cardiac arrest are based on optimal response range of epinephrine (0.045 to 0.2 mg/kg). May not improve survival or neurologic outcome and may cause postresuscitation myocardial dysfunction. ▪ Higher doses may be required to treat poison-induced shock.

Monitor: Check BP and HR every 5 minutes. ▪ Monitoring of ECG and serum potassium and glucose concentrations may be indicated. ▪ Vasoconstriction-induced tissue sloughing can occur. Avoid administering in areas of limited blood supply (e.g., fingers, toes) or if peripheral vascular disease is present. ▪ Infusion during cardiac arrest must be administered by central venous access to ensure delivery to systemic circulation and to avoid extravasation. ▪ Intracardiac injection or IV injection in cardiac arrest must be accompanied by cardiac massage to perfuse drug into the myocardium and permit effective defibrillation. ▪ Correct acidosis, hypoxemia. ▪ See Drug/Lab Interactions.

Maternal/Child: Category C: may cause anoxia in fetus. ▪ Discontinue breast-feeding. May produce tachyarrhythmias in pediatric patients. ▪ High doses in animals have caused increased hypertension with lower cardiac output. Risk of intracranial hemorrhage may be increased in infants and children (especially preterm infants) if hypotension is followed by hypertension. ▪ See Contraindications.

Elderly: May be more sensitive to the effects of beta-adrenergic receptor agonists (e.g., hypertension, hypokalemia, tachycardia, tremor). Patients with cardiac disease may be at increased risk for adverse effects. ▪ See Dose Adjustments and Precautions.

DRUG/LAB INTERACTIONS

May be used alternately with isoproterenol (Isuprel), but they may not be used together. Both are direct cardiac stimulants, and death may result. Adequate interval between doses must be maintained. ▪ Do not use concomitantly with **other sympathomimetic agents** (e.g., ephedrine, dopamine). Additive effects may cause toxicity. ▪ Simultaneous use with **oxytocics** (e.g., methylergonovine), **MAO inhibitors** (e.g., isocarboxazid [Marplan]), **furazolidone** (Furoxone), **or guanethidine** (Ismelin) may result in hypertension or cause hypertensive crisis. ▪ Pressor response increased by **tricyclic antidepressants** (e.g., amitriptyline [Elavil], imipramine [Tofranil]), **antihistamines** (e.g., diphenhydramine [Benadryl]), **rauwolfia alkaloids** (e.g., reserpine), **sodium levothyroxine, and urinary alkalizers;** may cause hypertension. ▪ May cause hypertension with **nonselective beta-adrenergic blockers** (e.g., propranolol). ▪ Inhibited by **ergot alkaloids and phenothiazines** (e.g., prochlorperazine [Compazine]). ▪ Inhibits **insulin and oral hypoglycemic agents;** increased dose may be required. ▪ **Hydrocarbon anesthetics** (e.g., enflurane, halothane) **and digoxin** may sensitize the myocardium and increase the risk of arrhythmias. ▪ Use with **theophylline** may increase cardiac, CNS, or GI side effects. ▪ Concurrent use with **alpha-adrenergic blocking agents** (e.g., doxazosin [Cardura], labetalol, prazosin [Minipress], terazosin [Hytrin]) may antagonize the hypertensive effects of epinephrine. ▪ Interacts with many other drugs. ▪ See Contraindications for additional drug interactions.

SIDE EFFECTS

Often transitory; sometimes occur with average doses.

Anxiety, dizziness, dyspnea, glycosuria, pallor, palpitations.

Overdose (frequently caused by too-rapid injection): Bradycardia (transient followed by tachycardia), cerebrovascular hemorrhage, collapse (rapid), fibrillation, headache (severe), hypertension, hypotension (irreversible), pulmonary edema, pupillary dilation, renal failure, restlessness, tachycardia, weakness, death.

ANTIDOTE

Treatment is primarily supportive. If side effects from the average dose become progressively worse, discontinue the drug and notify the physician. IM or SC route may be preferable. For a severe reaction caused by toxicity, treat the patient for shock and administer an antihypertensive agent such as phentolamine (Regitine) or nitroprusside sodium. Treat cardiac arrhythmias with a beta-adrenergic blocker (propranolol). Resuscitate as necessary.

EPIRUBICIN HYDROCHLORIDE BBW

(ep-ee-**ROO**-bih-sin hy-droh-**KLOR**-eyed)

Ellence ▪ Pharmorubicin PFS ✤

Antineoplastic
(anthracycline antibiotic)

pH 3 ▪ pH 4 to 5.5

USUAL DOSE

ELLENCE

Recommended starting dose is 100 to 120 mg/M^2. Patients receiving the 120-mg/M^2 dose should also receive prophylactic antibiotic therapy with sulfamethoxazole/trimethoprim or a fluoroquinolone (e.g., ciprofloxacin [Cipro]). Ellence is usually given in repeated 3- to 4-week cycles. Total dose may be given on Day 1 of each cycle or equally divided and given on Days 1 and 8 of each cycle.

One regimen used is 60 mg/M^2 of epirubicin as an infusion on Days 1 and 8 given in a regimen with oral cyclophosphamide 75 mg/M^2 on Days 1 to 14 and fluorouracil 500 mg/M^2 on Days 1 and 8. Repeat every 28 days for six cycles. Another regimen used is 100 mg/M^2 of epirubicin as an infusion together with fluorouracil 500 mg/M^2 and cyclophosphamide 500 mg/M^2. All three agents are given on Day 1 and are repeated every 21 days for 6 cycles. In either regimen the total dose of epirubicin may be given on Day 1 of each cycle or equally divided and given on Days 1 and 8 of each cycle.

✤PHARMORUBICIN PFS

Metastatic breast cancer: *Single agent:* 75 to 90 mg/M^2 once every 21 days. This dose may be divided and given on Day 1 and Day 2. An alternative weekly dose schedule of 12.5 to 25 mg/M^2 has been used and has been reported to produce less clinical toxicity than higher doses given every 3 weeks. ***Combination therapy:*** 50 mg/M^2. Used in combination with cyclophosphamide and fluorouracil.

Early-stage breast cancer (Stage II-IIIA): 50 to 60 mg/M^2 given on Days 1 and 8 every 4 weeks. Used in combination with cyclophosphamide and fluorouracil.

Small-cell lung cancer: *Single agent:* 90 to 120 mg/M^2 once every 3 weeks. ***Combination therapy:*** 50 to 90 mg/M^2. Several combinations have been used (e.g., with either cisplatin or ifosfamide; with cyclophosphamide and vincristine; with cyclophosphamide and etoposide; or with cisplatin and etoposide).

Non–small-cell lung cancer: *Single agent:* 120 to 150 mg/M^2 on Day 1 every 3 to 4 weeks. ***Combination therapy:*** 90 to 120 mg/M^2 on Day 1 every 3 to 4 weeks. Used in combination with cisplatin, etoposide, mitomycin, and vinblastine.

Non-Hodgkin's lymphoma: *Single agent:* 75 to 90 mg/M^2 once every 3 weeks. ***Combination therapy:*** 60 to 75 mg/M^2. Used in combination with cyclophosphamide, prednisone, and vincristine with or without bleomycin for the treatment of newly diagnosed non-Hodgkin's lymphoma.

Hodgkin's disease: *Combination therapy:* 35 mg/M^2 once every 2 weeks or 70 mg/M^2 once every 3 to 4 weeks. Used in combination with bleomycin, dacarbazine, and vinblastine.

Ovarian cancer: *Single agent:* 50 to 90 mg/M^2 once every 3 or 4 weeks in patients who have had prior therapy. ***Combination therapy:*** 50 to 90 mg/M^2 once every 3 or 4 weeks can be added to their regimen in patients who have had prior therapy; or the same dose in combination with cisplatin and cyclophosphamide is used for initial therapy of ovarian cancer.

Locally unresectable or metastatic gastric cancer: *Single agent:* 75 to 100 mg/M^2 once every 3 weeks. ***Combination therapy:*** 80 mg/M^2 once every 3 to 4 weeks. Used in combination with fluorouracil.

DOSE ADJUSTMENTS

ALL FORMULATIONS: Reduced dose required with elevated serum bilirubin. Give 50% of a dose for serum bilirubin from 1.2 to 3 mg/dL or AST 2 to 4 times the ULN. Give 25% of a dose for serum bilirubin greater than 3 mg/mL or AST greater than 4 times the ULN.

ELLENCE: Consider reducing starting dose to 75 to 90 mg/M^2 in heavily pretreated patients, those with pre-existing bone marrow suppression, or in the presence of neoplastic bone marrow infiltration. ■ Consider reduced dose in patients with severe renal impairment (SCr greater than 5 mg/dL). ■ Base dose adjustments after the first treatment cycle on hematologic response during treatment cycle nadir and nonhematologic toxicities. In patients who received the full dose on Day 1, reduce dose to 75% of initial first dose in subsequent cycles for platelet count less than 50,000/mm^3, absolute neutrophil count (ANC) less than 250/mm^3, neutropenic fever, or Grade 3 or 4 nonhematologic toxicity. Delay dose in subsequent treatment cycles until platelet count recovers to at least 100,000/mm^3, ANC recovers to at least 1,500/mm^3, and nonhematologic toxicities have recovered to equal to or less than Grade 1. For patients receiving a divided dose, reduce the Day-8 dose to 75% of the Day-1 dose if platelet counts are 75,000 to 100,000/mm^3 and ANC is 1,000 to 1,499/mm^3. Omit the Day-8 dose if platelet counts are less than 75,000/mm^3, ANC less than 1,000/mm^3, or Grade 3 or 4 nonhematologic toxicity has occurred.

❦**PHARMORUBICIN PFS:** Use lower dose in range for patients with inadequate marrow reserves due to old age, prior therapy, or neoplastic marrow infiltration. ■ Reduced dose, delay, or suspension of epirubicin may be required based on hematologic toxicity; manufacturer provides no specific recommendations. ■ No dose adjustment required in impaired renal function.

DILUTION
Specific techniques required; see Precautions.
ELLENCE: Available as 2 mg/mL in 25-mL and 100-mL vials. A ready-to-use, preservative-free solution; further dilution not required. Must be given through Y-tube or three-way stopcock of a free-flowing infusion of NS or D5W.

❦**PHARMORUBICIN PFS:** Available as 2 mg/mL in 5-mL, 25-mL, and 100-mL vials. Use of the 100-mL vial should be restricted to a pharmacy admixture program using a sterile transfer or dispensing device. Enter any vial only once and withdraw desired dose into a syringe. No further dilution is required.

Filters: Manufacturer indicates that studies show some initial potency loss in the first few minutes with the use of cellulose ester membrane or nylon filters; however, the total amount of drug loss is negligible. A second source has a similar statement.

Storage: *Ellence:* Refrigerate vials at 2° to 8° C (34° to 46° F); protect from light. Do not freeze. Refrigeration may result in a gel-formed product; will return to a slightly viscous to mobile solution within 2 to 4 hours. Must be used within 24 hours of removal from refrigeration. Discard unused solution.

❦*Pharmorubicin:* Store unopened PFS vials in refrigerator; keep in original cartons to protect from light. Use any filled syringe within 24 hours if stored at room temperature and within 48 hours if refrigerated. Syringes prepared from the pharmacy bulk vial must be used within 24 or 48 hours of the initial puncture of that vial based on method of storage. Once the transfer set has been inserted in the bulk vial, any remaining undispensed drug must be discarded in 8 hours.

COMPATIBILITY
Consider any drug NOT listed as compatible to be INCOMPATIBLE until consulting a pharmacist; specific conditions may apply.
Manufacturers recommend not mixing with other drugs in the same syringe. Avoid prolonged contact with alkaline solutions; will result in hydrolysis of all forms of epirubicin. Do not mix with heparin or fluorouracil (5-FU); may precipitate. **Incompatible** with ifosfamide (Ifex) when combined in syringe or solution with mesna (Mesnex).

One source suggests the following **compatibilities:**
Additive: Ifosfamide (Ifex).
Y-site: Oxaliplatin (Eloxatin).

RATE OF ADMINISTRATION

IV injection: *All formulations:* An initial starting dose of 100 to 120 mg/M^2 should be infused over 15 to 20 minutes. Lower starting doses or modified doses may be administered over a minimum of 3 minutes and up to 20 minutes. Must be given through Y-tube or three-way stopcock of a free-flowing infusion of NS or D5W. Slow injection rate further for erythematous streaking along the vein or facial flushing.

ACTIONS

A semi-synthetic, anthracycline, antineoplastic antibiotic agent. Exact method of action is unknown. Rapidly and widely distributed into tissue. Inhibits DNA, RNA, and protein synthesis and interferes with replication and transcription. Free radicals cause further cytotoxic activity. Metabolized in the liver and by other organs and cells, including RBCs. WBC nadir is reached in 10 to 14 days and should return to normal by Day 21. Elimination half-life is 30 to 40 hours. Does not cross blood-brain barrier. Primarily excreted in bile; some excretion in urine.

INDICATIONS AND USES

ELLENCE: A component of adjuvant therapy in patients with evidence of axillary-node tumor involvement following resection in primary breast cancer.

✤PHARMORUBICIN: Treatment of metastatic as well as early-stage breast cancer, small-cell lung cancer (both limited and extensive disease), advanced non–small-cell lung cancer, non-Hodgkin's lymphoma, Hodgkin's disease, Stage III and IV ovarian cancer, and metastatic and locally unresectable gastric cancers. May be used as a single agent or in combination with other chemotherapeutic agents.

Unlabeled uses: ALL FORMULATIONS: Treatment of soft-tissue sarcomas in combination with other agents. Treatment of esophageal and esophagogastric junction cancers in combination with other agents. Ellence has been used in place of Pharmorubicin for various indications.

CONTRAINDICATIONS

Patients with cardiomyopathy and/or heart failure, recent myocardial infarction, or severe arrhythmias. ▪ Baseline neutrophil count less than 1,500 cells/mm^3. ▪ Contraindicated in patients who have received previous treatment with maximum recommended cumulative doses of epirubicin, other anthracyclines, or anthracenediones (e.g., daunorubicin [Cerubidine], doxorubicin [Adriamycin], idarubicin [Idamycin], mitoxantrone [Novantrone], or mitomycin C). ▪ Hypersensitivity to epirubicin, other anthracyclines, or anthracenediones. ▪ Has not been evaluated in patients with severe hepatic impairment. Do not use in this patient population.

PRECAUTIONS

Follow guidelines for handling cytotoxic agents. See Appendix A, p. 1331. In addition to standard precautions, treat spills or leakage with 1% sodium hypochlorite. For accidental contact with eyes or skin, flush with copious amounts of water, soap and water, or sodium bicarbonate. ▪ Administered by or under the direction of the physician specialist, with facilities for monitoring the patient and responding to any medical emergency. ▪ For IV use only. Do not give IM or SC. ▪ May cause severe myelosuppression, which is usually the dose-limiting toxicity. ▪ May cause serious, irreversible myocardial toxicity with congestive heart failure and/or cardiomyopathy as the cumulative dose approaches 900 mg/M^2. Cardiotoxicity may be acute or delayed, occurring months to years after treatment. Exceeding 900 mg/M^2 is not recommended; the maximum cumulative dose used in clinical trials was 720 mg/M^2. ▪ Cardiotoxicity may occur at lower cumulative doses whether or not cardiac risk factors are present. ▪ Use extreme caution in pre-existing drug-induced bone marrow suppression, existing heart disease, previous treatment with other anthracyclines (e.g., daunorubicin, doxorubicin, idarubicin), other cardiotoxic agents (e.g., bleomycin, trastuzumab [Herceptin]), or radiation therapy encompassing the heart; toxicity may occur at lower cumulative doses and may be additive; see Drug/Lab Interactions. ▪ Administration of epirubicin after previous radiation therapy may induce an inflammatory recall reaction at the irradiation site. ▪ Incidence of secondary leukemia may be increased. Risk of developing acute myelogenous leukemia and/or myelodysplastic syndrome (AML/MDS) increases when epirubicin is given in combination with DNA-damaging antineoplastic agents, when patients have been heavily pretreated with cyto-toxic drugs, or when doses of anthracyclines have been escalated. The cumulative probability of developing AML/MDS is particularly increased in patients who have received more than 720 mg/M^2 of epirubicin or more than 6,300 mg/M^2 of cyclophosphamide. ▪ Thrombophlebitis and thromboembolic events, including pulmonary embolism, have been reported.

Monitor: Before beginning treatment with epirubicin, patients should recover from acute toxicities (e.g., stomatitis, neutropenia, thrombocytopenia, and infections) resulting from previous chemotherapy. ▪ Obtain baseline CBC, including differential and platelet count; serum calcium, phosphate, and potassium; SCr; uric acid level; liver function tests (AST, ALT, alkaline phosphatase, and serum bilirubin). ▪ Obtain baseline cardiac evaluations with an ECG and a MUGA scan or an echocardiogram to evaluate left ventricular ejection fraction (LVEF). ▪ Monitor lab values during therapy, especially before each dose. ▪ Monitor ECG, chest x-ray, echocardiogram, and/or radionuclide angiography in patients who have had mediastinal radiation, other anthracycline or anthracene therapy, those with pre-existing cardiac disease or S/S of impending heart disease, or those who have received prior epirubicin cumulative doses exceeding 550 mg/M^2. ▪ Monitor for signs of cardiac toxicity (e.g., rapid or irregular HR, shortness of breath, swelling of abdomen, feet, and lower legs); early signs usually include sinus tachycardia and nonspecific ST-T wave changes in the ECG. ▪ Use only large veins. Avoid veins over joints or in extremities with compromised venous or lymphatic drainage. Determine absolute patency of vein. Extravasation may occur with or without stinging or burning along the injection site even if blood returns well on aspiration of the infusion needle. Observe site frequently. Extravasation can result in severe cellulitis and tissue necrosis; if it occurs, discontinue injection; use another vein. ▪ Prevention and treatment of hyperuricemia due to tumor lysis syndrome may be accomplished with adequate hydration and, if necessary, allopurinol and alkalinization of urine. ▪ Be alert for signs of bone marrow suppression, bleeding, or infection. ▪ Use of prophylactic antibiotics may be indicated pending C/S in a febrile neutropenic patient. ▪ Monitor for thrombocytopenia (platelet count less than 50,000/mm^3). Initiate precautions to prevent excessive bleeding (e.g., inspect IV sites, skin, and mucous membranes; use extreme care during invasive procedures; test urine, emesis, stool, and secretions for occult blood). ▪ Prophylactic antiemetics are indicated. ▪ See Drug/Lab Interactions.

Patient Education: Urine will be reddish for several days (from drug, not hematuria). ▪ Effective contraception methods required for both men and women; avoid pregnancy. May damage testicular tissue and spermatozoa. ▪ Report IV site burning, stinging, or puffiness promptly. ▪ Report rapid or irregular HR, shortness of breath, and swelling of the abdomen, feet, or lower legs. ▪ Report vomiting, dehydration, fever, or other evidence of infection. ▪ Review side effects; may be severe (e.g., nausea and vomiting, cardiotoxicity). ▪ See Appendix D, p. 1333.

Maternal/Child: Category D: can cause fetal harm. Avoid pregnancy. In males, possible sperm DNA damage raises concerns about genetic abnormalities in fetuses. Duration of this effect is unknown. ▪ Discontinue breast-feeding. ▪ Information on safety for use in pediatric patients not available. Some studies suggest that pediatric patients may be at greater risk for anthracycline-induced acute cardiotoxicity and/or chronic CHF.

Elderly: Cardiotoxicity and myelotoxicity may be more severe; monitor closely for dose-related toxicities. ▪ See Dose Adjustments. ▪ There is a major decrease in plasma clearance of epirubicin in women over 70 years of age; monitor closely for signs of toxicity. ▪ See Dose Adjustments.

DRUG/LAB INTERACTIONS
May increase bone marrow and GI toxicity of other **chemotherapeutic agents.** ▪ Increased toxicity including skin redness and exfoliative changes possible when given concurrently with or after **radiation.** ▪ Monitoring of cardiac function may be indicated in patients taking **medications that may cause heart failure** (e.g., calcium channel blockers such as

verapamil), beta-blockers (e.g., propranolol). ▪ Plasma clearance decreased and serum levels increased by **cimetidine** (Tagamet); discontinue cimetidine. ▪ Epirubicin is extensively metabolized in the liver; **changes in hepatic function induced by concomitant therapies** may affect epirubicin metabolism, pharmacokinetics, effectiveness, and toxicity. ▪ Risk of cardiotoxicity increased in patients previously treated with maximum cumulative doses of **other anthracyclines** (e.g., doxorubicin [Adriamycin], idarubicin [Idamycin]) **and/ or radiation encompassing the heart.** ▪ Risk of cardiotoxicity is also increased when epirubicin is administered with **other cardiotoxic agents;** if possible, epirubicin-based therapy should be delayed until other cardiotoxic agents have been cleared from the circulation. Careful cardiac monitoring is required if delay is not feasible. ▪ Concomitant administration with other cytotoxic drugs may produce additive toxicity, especially hematologic and GI effects. ▪ Leukopenic and/or thrombocytopenic effects may be increased with **drugs that cause blood dyscrasias** (e.g., anticonvulsants [e.g., carbamazepine (Tegretol), phenytoin (Dilantin)], NSAIDs [e.g., ibuprofen (Advil, Motrin), naproxen (Aleve, Naprosyn)]). ▪ Administration of epirubicin immediately before or after **paclitaxel** increased the systemic exposure (AUC) of epirubicin. The mean AUC of epirubicin's metabolites increased when paclitaxel was administered immediately after epirubicin. Epirubicin had no effect on the exposure of paclitaxel. ▪ Administration of epirubicin immediately before or after **docetaxel** had no effect on the systemic exposure of epirubicin. However, the mean AUC of epirubicin's metabolites increased when docetaxel was administered immediately after epirubicin. Epirubicin had no effect on the AUC of docetaxel. ▪ Do not administer **live virus vaccines** to patients receiving antineoplastic agents. Killed or inactivated vaccines may be administered; however, the response to these vaccines may be diminished. ▪ See Precautions.

SIDE EFFECTS

Acute adverse events occurring in 10% or more of patients included alopecia, amenorrhea, conjunctivitis/keratitis, diarrhea, hematologic toxicity (anemia, leukopenia, neutropenia, thrombocytopenia), infection, lethargy, local toxicity, mucositis, nausea/vomiting, and rash/itch. Dose-limiting toxicities are infection, myelosuppression, and cardiotoxicity (usually delayed, manifested by reduced LVEF and/or S/S of CHF [e.g., ascites, dependent edema, dyspnea, gallop rhythm, hepatomegaly, pleural effusion, pulmonary edema, tachycardia]). Other serious cardiovascular adverse reactions that have occurred include AV block, bradycardia, bundle branch block, thromboembolism, and ventricular tachycardia. Severe cellulitis, vesication, local pain, and tissue necrosis can occur with extravasation. Venous sclerosis may result from injection into small veins or repeated injection into the same vein. Other side effects are anorexia, febrile neutropenia, fever, hot flashes, malaise, mucositis (esophagitis, stomatitis), phlebitis, recall of skin reaction associated with prior radiation. Hypersensitivity reactions have been reported.

Overdose: May cause an acute myocardial dysfunction within 24 hours. Bone marrow aplasia, gastrointestinal bleeding, Grade 4 mucositis, hyperthermia, lactic acidosis, multiple organ failure, and death have been reported following significant overdoses.

Post-Marketing: Anaphylaxis; chills; dehydration; erythema; flushing; GI disorders (e.g., bleeding, burning, pain, ulceration); hyperpigmentation of the skin, nails, and oral mucosa; hyperuricemia; pneumonia; pulmonary embolism; sepsis; urticaria; and vascular disorders (arterial embolism, hemorrhage, phlebitis, shock, and thrombophlebitis).

ANTIDOTE

Most side effects will either be tolerated or treated symptomatically. Keep the physician informed. Hematopoietic toxicity (leukopenia, thrombocytopenia) may require dose reduction or cessation of therapy, antibiotics, platelet and granulocyte transfusions, darbepoetin alfa (Aranesp), epoetin alfa (Epogen), filgrastim (Neupogen, Zarxio), pegfilgrastim (Neulasta), or sargramostim (Leukine). Acute cardiac failure occurs suddenly (most common when total cumulative doses approach 900 mg/M^2) and frequently does not respond to currently available treatment. Close monitoring of accumulated dose, bone marrow, ECG, chest x-ray, echocardiography, and systolic ejection fraction may prevent most serious and potentially fatal cardiac side effects. There is no specific antidote. Supportive therapy as indicated will help sustain the patient in toxicity. Dexrazoxane is currently available to prevent cardiotoxicity of doxorubicin in specific situations; in the future it may be considered with epirubicin. If extravasation occurs, attempt aspiration of the infiltrated epirubicin. Elevate the extremity and apply local intermittent ice compresses for up to 3 days. Observe the site frequently. Should be seen by a reconstructive surgeon if local pain persists or skin changes progress after 3 to 4 days. Ulceration may require early wide excision of the involved area. Treat hypersensitivity reactions as indicated.

EPOETIN ALFA BBW
(ee-**POH**-ee-tin **AL**-fah)

Recombinant human erythropoietin
Antianemic agent

EPO, Epogen, Eprex✦, Erythropoietin, Procrit

pH 5.8 to 7.2

USUAL DOSE
In all situations, rate of hematocrit increase is dose dependent and varies among patients. Availability of iron stores, baseline hematocrit, and concurrent medical problems affect the rate and extent of response. In controlled clinical trials, patients experienced greater risks for death, serious adverse cardiovascular reactions, and stroke when administered erythropoiesis-stimulating agents (ESAs) to target a hemoglobin level of greater than 11 Gm/dL. Use the lowest dose for each patient that will gradually increase the hemoglobin concentration to avoid the need for RBC transfusion; see Precautions and Monitor.

Anemia associated with chronic kidney disease (CKD) for patients on dialysis: Initiate epoetin when the hemoglobin level is less than 10 Gm/dL. *Starting dose:* 50 to 100 units/kg of body weight three times a week. May be given by IV or SC injection or into the venous line at the end of a dialysis session. The IV route is recommended in patients on hemodialysis; see Precautions. A 55-kg (120-lb) individual would receive 2,750 units at 50 units/kg, 4,125 units at 75 units/kg, and 5,500 units at 100 units/kg. Entire contents of a vial (2,000, 3,000, or 4,000 units) have been used instead of an exact calculated dose.

Anemia associated with chronic kidney disease (CKD) for patients NOT on dialysis: Consider initiating epoetin only when the hemoglobin level is less than 10 Gm/dL and the following two considerations apply: (1) the rate of hemoglobin decline indicates the likelihood of requiring a RBC transfusion, and (2) reducing the risk of alloimmunization and/or other RBC transfusion-related risks is a goal. *Starting dose:* 50 to 100 units/kg of body weight three times a week.

Anemia in zidovudine-treated, HIV-infected patients: May be given IV or SC. 100 units/kg 3 times a week. Obtain endogenous serum erythropoietin level (before transfusion) before initiating therapy; see Monitor. Serum erythropoietin levels in adults should be equal to or less than 500 mUnits/mL, and the zidovudine dose should be equal to or less than 4,200 mg/week.

Anemia associated with cancer patients on chemotherapy: SC injection recommended. ESAs shortened overall survival and/or increased the risk of tumor progression or recurrence in clinical studies of patients with certain types of cancer; see Precautions. Initiate epoetin in patients on cancer chemotherapy only if the hemoglobin is less than 10 Gm/dL and there is a minimum of 2 additional months of planned chemotherapy. Use the lowest dose necessary to avoid RBC transfusions. *Starting dose:* 150 units/kg of body weight 3 times a week until completion of chemotherapy course. An alternative schedule is 40,000 units weekly until completion of chemotherapy course.

Reduction of allogeneic blood transfusions in surgery patients: SC injection recommended. Obtain hemoglobin before initiating therapy. Should be greater than 10 Gm/dL but less than or equal to 13 Gm/dL. 300 units/kg/day for 10 days before surgery, on the day of surgery, and for 4 days after surgery. An alternate regimen is 600 units/kg once each week on Days 21, 14, and 7 before surgery and again on the day of surgery. Deep venous thrombosis prophylaxis is recommended during epoetin therapy (e.g., enoxaparin [Lovenox]); see Precautions.

PEDIATRIC DOSE
May be given by IV or SC injection. The IV route is recommended in patients on hemodialysis; see Precautions. Use the lowest dose for each patient that will gradually increase the hemoglobin concentration to avoid the need for RBC transfusion; see Precautions and Monitor.

Anemia of CKD requiring dialysis in pediatric patients 1 month to 16 years of age: *Initial:* 50 units/kg of body weight 3 times a week. The IV route is recommended for patients on hemodialysis. May also be given into the venous line at the end of the dialysis session. Safety and effectiveness for use in infants under 1 month of age not established.

Anemia in zidovudine-treated, HIV-infected pediatric patients 8 months to 17 years (unlabeled): Doses of 50 to 400 units/kg 2 to 3 times a week have been reported. See all comments under the similar section in Usual Dose. Adjust dose to achieve and maintain the lowest hemoglobin level sufficient to avoid the need for RBC transfusion; see Dose Adjustments.

Anemia associated with pediatric cancer patients on chemotherapy, ages 5 to 18 years: 600 units/kg IV weekly until completion of chemotherapy course. Do not exceed 40,000 units. Increase dose to 900 units/kg weekly if hemoglobin increases by less than 1 Gm/dL and remains below 10 Gm/dL after the initial 4 weeks of therapy. Do not exceed a dose of 60,000 units.

NEONATAL DOSE

Anemia of prematurity (unlabeled): 25 to 100 units/kg/dose SC 3 times a week or 200 to 400 units/kg/dose IV/SC 3 to 5 times a week for 2 to 6 weeks. Total dose per week is 600 to 1,400 units/kg. Use the lowest dose that will gradually increase the hemoglobin concentration to avoid the need for RBC transfusion; see Precautions, Monitor, and Dose Adjustments.

DOSE ADJUSTMENTS

Dose adjustment is based on hemoglobin. Adjust dose to achieve and maintain the lowest hemoglobin level sufficient to avoid the need for RBC transfusion.

All adult and pediatric patients with CKD: When adjusting therapy, consider hemoglobin rate of rise, hemoglobin rate of decline, ESA responsiveness, and hemoglobin variability. A single hemoglobin excursion may not require a dose adjustment. Dose should be started slowly and adjusted for each patient to achieve and maintain the lowest hemoglobin level sufficient to avoid the need for RBC transfusion. Allow sufficient time before adjusting a dose; increased hemoglobin levels may not be observed for 2 to 6 weeks. ▪ Do not increase the dose more frequently than once every 4 weeks. Decreases in dose can occur more frequently. ▪ If the hemoglobin rises rapidly (e.g., more than 1 Gm/dL in any 2-week period), reduce the dose by 25% or more as needed to reduce rapid responses. ▪ For patients who do not respond adequately after 4 weeks of therapy (e.g., the hemoglobin has not increased by more than 1 Gm/dL), increase the dose by 25%. ▪ For patients who do not respond adequately over a 12-week escalation period, increasing the dose further is unlikely to improve response and may increase risks. Discontinue epoetin if responsiveness does not improve.

Patients with CKD on dialysis: If the hemoglobin level approaches or exceeds 11 Gm/dL, reduce or interrupt the dose of epoetin.

Patients with CKD NOT on dialysis: If the hemoglobin level exceeds 10 Gm/dL, reduce or interrupt the dose of epoetin.

Zidovudine-treated, HIV-infected patients and cancer patients on chemotherapy: If hemoglobin does not increase after 8 weeks of therapy, increase dose by 50 to 100 units/kg. May increase dose at 4- to 8-week intervals until hemoglobin reaches a level needed to avoid RBC transfusions or dose reaches 300 units/kg. ▪ Withhold dose if the hemoglobin exceeds 12 Gm/dL. Restart dose at 25% below previous dose when hemoglobin falls to less than 11 Gm/dL. ▪ Discontinue epoetin if increase in hemoglobin is not achieved at a dose of 300 units/kg for 8 weeks.

Cancer patients on chemotherapy: *Reduce dose* by 25% when the hemoglobin reaches a level needed to avoid transfusion or increases more than 1 Gm/dL in any 2-week period. *Withhold dose* if the hemoglobin exceeds a level needed to avoid transfusion, and restart at 25% below the previous dose when the hemoglobin approaches a level at which transfusions may be required. ▪ Increase adult dose to 300 units/kg three times a week or 60,000 units weekly if hemoglobin increases by less than 1 Gm/dL and remains below 10 Gm/dL after the initial 4 weeks of therapy. ▪ Discontinue epoetin after 8 weeks if no response as measured by hemoglobin levels or by continued need for RBC transfusions.

DILUTION

Available in numerous concentrations; check dose on vial carefully. May be given undiluted as an IV injection. Do not shake during preparation; will render it biologically inactive. Single-dose vial contains no preservatives. Use only 1 dose per vial, then discard. Never re-enter vial. Now available in multidose vial with preservative; sterile technique imperative.

Storage: Refrigerate single and multidose vials before use, multidose vial after initial use. Discard in 21 days. Do not freeze or shake. Protect from light.

Filters: Not required; however, it was filtered during manufacturing with 0.2-micron millipore filters. No significant loss of potency expected with the use of non–protein binding filters of a similar size or larger.

COMPATIBILITY

Manufacturers state, "Do not dilute or administer in conjunction with other drug solutions." One source indicates there may be protein loss from adsorption to PVC containers and tubing. Manufacturer suggests it may be mixed 1-to-1 with bacteriostatic NS in a syringe when prepared from a single-dose vial for SC injection; see literature.

RATE OF ADMINISTRATION

A single dose over at least 1 minute.

ACTIONS

An amino acid glycoprotein manufactured by recombinant DNA technology. Has the same biologic effects as erythropoietin produced naturally by the kidneys. Stimulates bone marrow to produce RBCs, increasing the reticulocyte count within 10 days and the red cell count, hemoglobin, and hematocrit within 2 to 6 weeks. Normal iron stores are necessary because it steps up RBC production to a rate above what the body usually makes. New cells need iron, which is quickly depleted. Half-life is 4 to 13 hours. Continued therapy will maintain improved RBC levels and decrease need for transfusions.

INDICATIONS AND USES

Treatment of anemia associated with chronic kidney disease in adults and pediatric patients, including patients on dialysis and not on dialysis, to decrease the need for red blood cell (RBC) transfusion. ▪ Treatment of anemias related to zidovudine (AZT, Retrovir) therapy in HIV-infected patients. ▪ To reduce the need for allogeneic blood transfusions among patients with perioperative hemoglobin greater than 10 to less than or equal to 13 Gm/dL who are at high risk for perioperative blood loss from elective, noncardiac, nonvascular surgery. ▪ Treatment of chemotherapy-induced anemia in adult cancer patients who have nonmyeloid malignancies in which anemia is due to the effect of concomitant myelosuppressive chemotherapy and who, upon initiation of therapy, have a minimum of 2 additional months of planned chemotherapy.

Limitations of use: Not indicated for use in patients receiving hormonal agents, therapeutic biologic products, or radiotherapy unless receiving concomitant myelosuppressive chemotherapy. ▪ Not indicated for patients receiving myelosuppressive therapy when the anticipated outcome is cure; see Precautions. ▪ Has not been shown to improve quality of life, fatigue, or patient well-being. ▪ Not indicated in patients scheduled for surgery who are willing to donate autologous blood. ▪ Not indicated in patients undergoing cardiac or vascular surgery. ▪ Not indicated as a substitute for a RBC transfusion in patients who require immediate correction of anemia.

Unlabeled uses: Anemia of prematurity.

CONTRAINDICATIONS

Known hypersensitivity to epoetin alfa, uncontrolled hypertension, pure red cell aplasia (PRCA). Epoetin alfa from multidose vials containing benzyl alcohol is contraindicated in neonates, infants, pregnant women, and nursing mothers.

PRECAUTIONS

All patients: May be given IV or SC in patients not receiving dialysis. May be given to dialysis patients into the venous line at the end of the dialysis procedure to eliminate additional venous access. Erythropoiesis-stimulating agents (ESAs) increase the risk of death, MI, stroke, venous thromboembolism, and thrombosis of vascular access. Patients experienced greater risks of these adverse events when ESAs were administered to target a hemoglobin of greater than 11 Gm/dL. No trial has identified a hemoglobin target level, an epoetin alfa dose, or a dosing strategy that does not increase these risks. Use the lowest epoetin alfa dose sufficient to reduce the need for RBC transfusions. ■ Use with caution in patients with coexistent cardiovascular disease and stroke. Patients with CKD who have an insufficient hemoglobin response to ESA therapy may be at even greater risk for cardiovascular reactions and mortality than other patients. ■ In clinical trials, ESAs increased the risk of death in patients undergoing CABG surgery and the risk of deep venous thrombosis in patients undergoing orthopedic procedures. ■ Increases in hemoglobin of greater than 1 Gm/dL during any 2-week period have been associated with an increased incidence of cardiac arrest, exacerbations of hypertension, congestive heart failure (CHF), vascular thrombosis/ischemia/infarction, acute MI, deep vein thrombosis (DVT), pulmonary embolus, and fluid overload/edema and may be associated with neurologic events (e.g., seizures, stroke). See Dose Adjustments. ■ In addition to low baseline hematocrit and inadequate iron stores, delayed or diminished response may result from concurrent medical problems (infections, inflammatory or malignant processes, occult blood loss, underlying hematologic disease, folic acid or vitamin B_{12} deficiency, hemolysis, aluminum intoxication, osteitis fibrosa cystica, pure red cell aplasia [PRCA], anti-erythropoietin antibody–associated anemia). Correct or exclude other causes of anemia before initiating therapy. ■ Not intended for use in anemias caused by iron or folate deficiencies, hemolysis, or GI bleeding or for use in treating symptoms of anemia, including dizziness, fatigue, low energy, poor quality of life, or shortness of breath. ■ Not a substitute for emergency transfusion in patients requiring immediate correction of severe anemia. ■ Administration of erythropoiesis-stimulating agents (ESAs) to cancer patients shortened the overall survival time and/or increased the risk of tumor progression or recurrence in clinical studies of some patients with breast, cervical, head and neck, lymphoid, and non–small-cell lung malignancies. The risks of shortened survival time and tumor progression have not been excluded when ESAs are dosed to achieve a hemoglobin of less than 12 Gm/dL. To minimize these risks, as well as the risks of serious cardiovascular and thrombovascular events, use the lowest dose needed to avoid a red blood cell transfusion. Use only to treat anemia due to concomitant myelosuppressive chemotherapy, and discontinue after completion of a chemotherapy course. Prescribers and hospitals are now required to enroll in and comply with the ESA APPRISE Oncology Program to prescribe and/or dispense ESAs to patients with cancer. See prescribing information Black Box Warning. ■ BP may increase during therapy with epoetin. Hypertensive encephalopathy and seizures have been observed. ■ Patients with uncontrolled hypertension should not be treated with epoetin until BP has been adequately controlled. ■ Pure red cell aplasia (PRCA) and severe anemia, with or without other cytopenias, in association with neutralizing antibodies to native erythropoietin have been observed. Most often reported in CKD patients receiving epoetin alfa by SC injection. Any patient who develops a sudden loss of response to epoetin alfa accompanied by severe anemia and low reticulocyte count should be evaluated. Physicians may contact manufacturer (Amgen) for help with the evaluation of these patients. ■ Epoetin increases the risk of seizures in patients with CKD. Use with caution in patients with a seizure disorder. ■ Safety and efficacy not established in patients with a known history of underlying hematologic disorders (e.g., sickle cell anemia, myelodysplastic syndrome, or hypercoagulable disorders). ■ Serious hypersensitivity reactions, including anaphylaxis, have been reported. ■ The formulation containing albumin carries a risk for transmission of viral diseases or Creutzfeldt-Jakob disease. However, donor screening and manufacturing processes make this risk extremely remote.

Monitor: Monitor hemoglobin weekly in patients who are initiating therapy. Continue until stable and the maintenance dose has been established, then monitor at regular intervals. ■ Monitor hemoglobin weekly for at least 4 weeks following adjustment of therapy. Once stabilized, continue to monitor at regular intervals. ■ A biologic product. Monitor for S/S of hypersensitivity reactions. ■ Monitor BP routinely; initiation or intensification of antihypertensive therapy and dietary restrictions may be necessary. If BP is difficult to control by pharmacologic or dietary measures, the dose of epoetin should be reduced or withheld. ■ Normal iron stores required to support epoetin-stimulated erythropoiesis. Transferrin saturation should be at least 20% and ferritin at least 100 ng/mL. Monitor before and during therapy. Supplemental iron is usually required to increase and maintain transferrin saturation. Administration of IV parenteral iron may be necessary in some patients. ▪ Monitor for the presence of premonitory neurologic symptoms during initiation of therapy or when dose is adjusted. Seizures have been reported; see Precautions. ▪ Monitor patients with pre-existing vascular disease carefully (especially those with CKD); increase in hematocrit may precipitate a cerebrovascular accident, transient ischemic attack, or myocardial infarction. ▪ Dialysis patients may require additional anticoagulation with heparin to prevent clotting of artificial kidney or clotting of the vascular access (AV shunt) and to maintain efficiency of the dialysis procedure.

Patient Education: Risk of seizures, especially during first 90 days of therapy. Do not drive or operate heavy equipment. ▪ Menses may resume; possibility of pregnancy. Contraception may be indicated. ▪ Additional instruction (e.g., equipment, techniques) will be required in patients who will self-administer (manufacturer supplies brochure). ▪ Stress importance of compliance with diet, iron, and vitamin (e.g., folic acid, B_{12}) supplementation and BP control. Close monitoring of BP and Hgb is imperative. ▪ Promptly report S/S of hypersensitivity reaction, pain or swelling in legs, SOB, increase in BP, dizziness, or loss of consciousness. ▪ Increased risk of mortality, serious cardiovascular events, thromboembolic events, and tumor progression or recurrence. ▪ Read Medication Guide carefully. All patients should discuss the risks of using an ESA with a health care professional. ▪ Cancer patients must sign a patient–health care provider acknowledgment form through the APPRISE Oncology Program before initiating therapy; see Precautions.

Maternal/Child: Category C: may present risk to fetus; benefits must justify risk. ▪ Some formulations contain benzyl alcohol; see Contraindications. ▪ Use caution in nursing mothers. ▪ Indicated in pediatric patients ages 1 month to 16 years of age for the treatment of anemia associated with CKD requiring dialysis. ▪ Indicated in pediatric cancer patients ages 5 to 18 years for the treatment of anemia due to myelosuppressive chemotherapy. ▪ Has been used in zidovudine-treated and anemic pediatric patients ages 8 months to 17 years. Data limited. ▪ Pharmacokinetics (absorption, distribution, metabolism, and excretion) in children and adolescents similar to adults. ▪ Limited data available for use in neonates. Clearance may be increased compared to adults.

Elderly: Response similar to that found in younger patients; however, elderly patients may have a greater sensitivity to its effects. ▪ Monitor blood chemistry and BP carefully due to increased risk of renal and/or cardiovascular complications.

DRUG/LAB INTERACTIONS
Specific information not available.

SIDE EFFECTS
Generally well tolerated. Occur most frequently in patients with chronic renal failure. Increased hypertension is common, and hypertensive encephalopathy and seizures can occur. Clotted vascular access (AV shunt) and clotting of the artificial kidney may occur during dialysis. Allergic reactions have been reported. Other reported side effects are those common to the underlying disease and not necessarily attributable to epoetin and include arthralgias, asthenia, bone marrow fibrosis, cerebrovascular accident or transient ischemic attack (CVA/TIA), chest pain, cough, diarrhea, dizziness, edema, fatigue, fever, headache, hyperkalemia, myocardial infarction, nausea, polycythemia, rash, respiratory congestion, shortness of breath, tachycardia, and vomiting. PRCA and severe anemia, with or without other cytopenias, in association with neutralizing antibodies have been reported; see Precautions.

ANTIDOTE
Notify physician of all side effects; most will be treated symptomatically. Excessive hypertension may require discontinuation of epoetin until BP is controlled or may respond to reduction in dose of epoetin or to an increase in antihypertensive therapy. Reduce dose of epoetin in patients with an increase in hemoglobin over 1 Gm/dL in any 2-week period. Consider phlebotomy in toxicity. Additional heparin may be required

during dialysis to prevent clotting. If overdose or polycythemia does occur, monitor closely for cardiovascular events and hematologic abnormalities. When resuming therapy, monitor closely for evidence of rapid increases in hemoglobin concentration (greater than 1 Gm/dL within 14 days) and reduce dose as indicated. Permanently discontinue therapy in patients with antibody-mediated anemia. Patients should not be switched to other erythropoietic proteins because antibodies may cross-react. Treat minor hypersensitivity reactions symptomatically. Discontinue drug and treat anaphylaxis as indicated; resuscitate as necessary.

EPOPROSTENOL SODIUM
(eh-poh-**PROST**-en-ohl **SO**-dee-um)

Flolan, Veletri

Vasodilating agent
Antihypertensive
(pulmonary)

pH 10.2 to 10.8

USUAL DOSE

Acute dose initiation and chronic continuous infusion: May be given through a peripheral line on a temporary basis until a central venous line is established. A central venous catheter should be put in place as soon as possible and must be used for continuous long-term 24-hour administration with an ambulatory infusion pump. Begin infusion at 2 ng/kg/min. Increase in increments of 2 ng/kg/min every 15 minutes or longer until dose-limiting pharmacologic effects occur or until a tolerance limit to the drug is established and further increases in the infusion rate are not clinically warranted; see Dose Adjustments. Most common S/S of dose-limiting effects include abdominal pain, flushing, headache, hypotension, nausea, respiratory disorders, sepsis, and vomiting. If dose-limiting pharmacologic effects occur, decrease infusion rate slowly until pharmacologic effects are tolerated; see Dose Adjustments. If the initial dose of 2 ng/kg/min is not tolerated, use a lower dose. During the first 7 days of treatment in clinical trials, the dose was increased daily to a mean dose of 4.1 ng/kg/min on Day 7 of treatment. At the end of Week 12, the mean dose was 11.2 ng/kg/min. The mean incremental increase was 2 to 3 ng/kg/min every 3 weeks. May be given concomitantly with anticoagulant therapy in selected patients; see Monitor.

DOSE ADJUSTMENTS

Changes in the chronic infusion rate are to be expected. If symptoms of primary pulmonary hypertension (PPH) persist, recur, or worsen, increase infusion rate promptly by 1 to 2 ng/kg/min. Wait at least 15 minutes to assess clinical response. Observe patient for several hours to confirm patient tolerance, and take BP and HR in supine and standing positions. In trials most patients progressed to a dose a little less than their acute dose-initiation intolerable dose within 12 weeks. ■ Occurrence of dose-related side effects that do not resolve may require a decrease in the chronic infusion rate. Reduce dose gradually in 2-ng/kg/min increments and wait at least 15 minutes to assess clinical response. Use extreme caution if decreasing the dose; abrupt withdrawal or sudden large reductions may cause a rapid return of PPH symptoms and may precipitate death. ■ In patients receiving lung transplants, doses were tapered after the initiation of cardiopulmonary bypass. ■ Dose selection for the elderly should be cautious. ■ Asymptomatic increases in pulmonary artery pressure with increases in cardiac output may occur during acute dose initiation; consider dose adjustment. ■ See Precautions.

DILUTION

Infusion pump required. It must be small and lightweight; able to adjust infusion rates in increments of 2 ng/kg/min; have occlusion, end of infusion, and low battery alarms; be accurate to ±6% of the programmed rate; be positive-pressure driven (continuous or pulsatile) with intervals between pulses not exceeding 3 minutes at rates required to deliver drug; and have a disposable reservoir cassette made of polyvinyl chloride, polypropylene, or glass with a capacity of at least 100 mL. Pumps used during trials were manufactured by Pharmacia Deltec, Medfusion, Inc., and Baxter Health Care. The infusion pump used in the most recent clinical trials was the CADD-1 HFX 5100 (SIMS Deltec).

Flolan and Generic: Sterile diluent for epoprostenol is provided by the manufacturer. Do not use any other diluent. Concentration will be determined by desired dose/kg/min and parameters of ambulatory infusion pump to be used. See Rate of Administration. Two vials of provided sterile diluent will be required to prepare each 24-hour dose in each of the concentrations in the following chart.

| Guidelines for Dilution of Epoprostenol (Flolan and Generic) to Various Concentrations ||
To Make 100 mL of Solution with Final Concentration (ng/mL) of:	Directions
3,000 ng/mL	Dissolve contents of one 0.5-mg vial with 5 mL of STERILE DILUENT for epoprostenol. Withdraw 3 mL and add to sufficient STERILE DILUENT for epoprostenol to make a total of 100 mL.
5,000 ng/mL	Dissolve contents of one 0.5-mg vial with 5 mL of STERILE DILUENT for epoprostenol. Withdraw entire vial contents and add sufficient STERILE DILUENT for epoprostenol to make a total of 100 mL.
10,000 ng/mL	Dissolve contents of two 0.5-mg vials each with 5 mL of STERILE DILUENT for epoprostenol. Withdraw entire vial contents and add sufficient STERILE DILUENT for epoprostenol to make a total of 100 mL.
15,000 ng/mL	Dissolve contents of one 1.5-mg vial with 5 mL of STERILE DILUENT for epoprostenol. Withdraw entire vial contents and add sufficient STERILE DILUENT for epoprostenol to make a total of 100 mL.

Acute dose initiation may require more than one solution strength. 3,000 ng/mL and 10,000 ng/mL concentrations should be satisfactory to deliver between 2 and 16 ng/kg/min in adults. A maximum 2-day supply can be diluted at one time (200 mL). For use at room temperature, withdraw 33.3 mL and deposit in pump reservoir cassette or sterile infusion bag for each 8-hour period. If used with cold pouches and frozen gel packs, 100 mL can be placed in the pump reservoir cassette or a 100-mL sterile infusion bag for each 24-hour period. Frozen gel packs must be changed every 12 hours. Reservoir cassettes are disposable. Most patients prepare a 24-hour dose in a new reservoir cassette before a new dose is required and use cold pouches to maintain temperature.

Veletri: Stable only when reconstituted as directed using SWFI or NS. Do not use any other diluent. A single reservoir or diluted solution prepared as directed can be administered at room temperature for up to 24 hours. If lower concentrations are chosen, pump reservoirs should be changed every 12 hours. See prescribing information for additional concentrations.

| Guidelines for Dilution of Veletri to Various Concentrations ||
To Make 100 mL of Solution with Final Concentration (ng/mL) of:	Directions
15,000 ng/mL*	Dissolve contents of one 1.5-mg vial with 5 mL of SWFI or NS. Withdraw entire vial contents and add sufficient volume of the IDENTICAL DILUENT to make a total of 100 mL.
30,000 ng/mL*	Dissolve contents of two 1.5-mg vials each with 5 mL of SWFI or NS. Withdraw entire vial contents and add sufficient volume of the IDENTICAL DILUENT to make a total of 100 mL.

*Higher concentrations may be prepared for patients who receive epoprostenol long-term.

Filters: An in-line 0.22-micron filter was used during clinical trials.

Storage: *Flolan:* Unopened vials of epoprostenol may be stored at 15° to 25° C (59° to 77° F [*generic* at CRT]) in the carton to protect from light. Diluent may be stored at 15° to 25° C (59° to 77° F [*generic* at CRT]). Protection from light not required. See expiration dates on both. Before use, reconstituted solutions *(Flolan and generic)* must be refrigerated and protected from light. Do not freeze. Reconstituted solution must be discarded after 48 hours or if accidentally frozen. While in use, must not be exposed to direct sunlight or temperatures above 25° C (77° F) or below 0° C (32° F). Stable in pump reservoir for only 8 hours at RT. Use of cold pouches with frozen gel packs can extend reservoir life to 24 hours. Time stored in refrigerator and in reservoir of pump must be included in maximum 48-hour time frame.

Veletri: Unopened vials may be stored at 20° to 25° C (68° to 77° F). Vials reconstituted with 5 mL of SWFI or NS must be protected from light and can be refrigerated at 2° to 8° C (36° to 46° F) for as long as 5 days or held at up to 20° to 25° C (68° to 77° F) for up to 48 hours. Do not freeze reconstituted solutions. Discard any reconstituted solution that has been frozen or refrigerated for more than 5 days or held at room temperature for more than 48 hours. See prescribing information for maximum duration of administration (hours) of fully diluted solutions in drug delivery reservoir.

COMPATIBILITY

Manufacturer states, "Stable only when reconstituted with the provided or recommended diluent. Must not be reconstituted or mixed with any other parenteral medications or solutions prior to or during administration." One source suggests **compatibility** at the **Y-site** with bivalirudin (Angiomax).

RATE OF ADMINISTRATION

Administered by a continuous IV infusion through a central venous catheter. Peripheral access may be used temporarily until a central line can be placed. Titrate dose as outlined in Usual Dose and Dose Adjustments. Flow must not be interrupted for longer than 2 to 3 minutes. Time to completion of administration must never exceed more than 8 hours at room temperature, more than 24 hours with use of cold pouches and changing frozen gel packs every 12 hours, or more than 48 hours from time of initial reconstitution. If dose-limiting pharmacologic effects occur, decrease infusion rate slowly until pharmacologic effects are tolerated; see Dose Adjustments. The infusion rate may be calculated using the following formula:

$$\text{Infusion rate (mL/hr)} = \frac{\text{Dose (ng/kg/min)} \times \text{Weight in kg} \times 60 \text{ min/hr}}{\text{Final concentration (ng/mL)}}$$

The following charts may be used for infusion rates at a final concentration of 3,000 ng mL or 15,000 ng/mL. See package insert for charts at additional concentrations.

Infusion Rates for Epoprostenol at a Concentration of 3,000 ng/mL							
	Dose or Drug Delivery Rate (ng/kg/min)						
Patient Weight	2	4	6	8	10	12	14	16
	Infusion Delivery Rate (mL/hr)						
10 kg	—	—	1.2	1.6	2	2.4	2.8	3.2
20 kg	—	1.6	2.4	3.2	4	4.8	5.6	6.4
30 kg	1.2	2.4	3.6	4.8	6	7.2	8.4	9.6
40 kg	1.6	3.2	4.8	6.4	8	9.6	11.2	12.8
50 kg	2	4	6	8	10	12	14	16
60 kg	2.4	4.8	7.2	9.6	12	14.4	16.8	19.2
70 kg	2.8	5.6	8.4	11.2	14	16.8	19.6	22.4
80 kg	3.2	6.4	9.6	12.8	16	19.2	22.4	25.6
90 kg	3.6	7.2	10.8	14.4	18	21.6	25.2	28.8
100 kg	4	8	12	16	20	24	28	32

Infusion Rates for Epoprostenol at a Concentration of 15,000 ng/mL							
	Dose or Drug Delivery Rate (ng/kg/min)						
Patient Weight	4	6	8	10	12	14	16
	Infusion Delivery Rate (mL/hr)						
20 kg	—	—	—	—	1	1.1	1.3
30 kg	—	—	1	1.2	1.4	1.7	1.9
40 kg	—	1	1.3	1.6	1.9	2.2	2.6
50 kg	—	1.2	1.6	2	2.4	2.8	3.2
60 kg	1	1.4	1.9	2.4	2.9	3.4	3.8
70 kg	1.1	1.7	2.2	2.8	3.4	3.9	4.5
80 kg	1.3	1.9	2.6	3.2	3.8	4.5	5.1
90 kg	1.4	2.2	2.9	3.6	4.3	5	5.8
100 kg	1.6	2.4	3.2	4	4.8	5.6	6.4

ACTIONS

A naturally occurring prostaglandin. It directly vasodilates pulmonary and systemic arterial vascular beds and inhibits platelet aggregation. Right and left ventricle afterload is reduced, and cardiac output and stroke volume are increased. Effect on HR is dose related. Produces dose-related increases in cardiac index and stroke volume and dose-related decreases in pulmonary vascular resistance, total pulmonary resistance, and mean systemic arterial pressure. Has been shown to increase exercise capacity, improve hemodynamic status, and extend survival. Onset of action is immediate. Half-life is approximately 6 minutes at body pH of 7.4. Metabolized to two primary metabolites by rapid hydrolyzation and enzymatic degradation.

INDICATIONS AND USES

Treatment of pulmonary arterial hypertension (PAH [WHO Group 1]) to improve exercise capacity. Effectiveness established predominantly in patients with NYHA Functional Class III-IV symptoms and etiologies of idiopathic or heritable PAH or PAH associated with connective tissue diseases.

CONTRAINDICATIONS
Congestive heart failure due to severe left ventricular systolic dysfunction, known hypersensitivity to epoprostenol or related compounds (e.g., alprostadil [prostaglandin E_1, Prostin VR Pediatric]), or patients who develop pulmonary edema during dose initiation.

PRECAUTIONS
Administered by or under the direction of the physician specialist. ▪ During dose initiation, facilities for monitoring the patient and responding to any medical emergency must be available. ▪ Causes of secondary pulmonary hypertension should be eliminated and diagnosis of PPH carefully established. ▪ Abrupt withdrawal, interruptions in drug delivery, or sudden large reductions in dose may result in rebound pulmonary hypertension, including dyspnea, dizziness, and weakness. Death of one patient was attributed to these causes. Backup medication and equipment must always be available. ▪ Use of a multilumen catheter should be considered if other IV therapy is used. ▪ Not recommended for patients who develop pulmonary edema during acute dose initiation; may develop pulmonary veno-occlusive disease; see Contraindications. ▪ Asymptomatic increases in pulmonary artery pressure with increases in cardiac output may occur during acute dose initiation; consider dose adjustment. ▪ Cardiac catheterization is used during trials for acute dose initiation but is not necessary; consider benefit versus risk. In patients undergoing lung transplants, it is recommended that the dose of epoprostenol be tapered after initiation of cardiopulmonary bypass. ▪ A potent inhibitor of platelet aggregation; an increased risk for hemorrhagic complications may occur, particularly in patients with other risk factors for bleeding. ▪ See Monitor, Patient Education, Drug/Lab Interactions.

Monitor: ECG monitoring and frequent monitoring of vital signs recommended during acute dose initiation. ▪ Observe for dose-limiting side effects. ▪ To reduce the risk of pulmonary thromboembolism or systemic embolism through a patent foramen ovale, anticoagulant therapy is recommended concomitantly unless contraindicated. ▪ Therapy may be required for months or years; consideration must be given to the ability of the patient and family to manage this care. ▪ Monitor standing and supine HR and BP for several hours after any adjustment. ▪ Thorough patient teaching and continued support services are imperative to facilitate a good clinical outcome. ▪ See Precautions, Patient Education, Drug/Lab Interactions.

Patient Education: After initial dose titration and training, this is a self-administered drug. Must assume responsibility for drug reconstitution, drug administration, and care of the permanent central venous catheter. ▪ Aseptic technique during reconstitution and with routine care of permanent indwelling central venous catheter is imperative to prevent infection. ▪ Report fever or any sign of infection at catheter site (e.g., redness, warmth). ▪ Delivery of medication cannot be interrupted. Interruption will cause a rapid return of PPH symptoms. ▪ Should have access to a backup infusion pump and intravenous infusion sets to avoid potential interruption in drug delivery. ▪ Dose adjustments should be made only under the direction of the physician except in an emergency situation (e.g., unconsciousness, collapse).

Maternal/Child: Category B: use only if clearly needed. No evidence of fetal harm in animal studies to date. ▪ Safety for use during labor and delivery not established. ▪ Use caution in nursing mothers; safety not established. ▪ Safety for use in pediatric patients not established.

Elderly: See Dose Adjustments. Decreased organ function (cardiac, hepatic, renal), concomitant disease, and other drug therapy may cause concern. Response of younger patients versus the elderly not documented.

DRUG/LAB INTERACTIONS
Has been used with digoxin, diuretics, anticoagulants, oral vasodilators, and oxygen. ▪ Hypotension may be increased with **diuretics, antihypertensive agents, or other vasodilators.** ▪ Risk of bleeding may be increased with **antiplatelet agents, anticoagulants, or**

NSAIDs (e.g., ibuprofen [Advil, Motrin], naproxen [Aleve, Naprosyn]). ■ May decrease clearance of **furosemide** (Lasix) and **digoxin;** monitor digoxin levels.

SIDE EFFECTS

Acute dose initiation: Most common S/S of dose-limiting effects include flushing, headache, hypotension, nausea, and vomiting. Abdominal pain, agitation, anxiety/nervousness, back pain, bradycardia, chest pain, constipation, dizziness, dyspepsia, dyspnea, hyperesthesia, musculoskeletal pain, paresthesia, respiratory disorders, sepsis, sweating, tachycardia, and many other side effects may occur.

Chronic continuous infusion: Any of the above and arthralgia, bleeding at various sites, chills, diarrhea, fatigue, fever, flu-like symptoms, infection (may be local at site of catheter insertion), jaw pain, pallor, pulmonary edema, rash, sepsis, thrombocytopenia.

Overdose: Hypotension, hypoxemia, respiratory arrest, and death may occur.

Post-Marketing: Anemia, hypersplenism, hyperthyroidism, pancytopenia, splenomegaly.

ANTIDOTE

Continuous maintenance of drug flow imperative. Keep physician informed of all side effects. Most will be treated with dose reduction; some may require symptomatic treatment. Call 1-800-9-FLOLAN for drug or pump problems with Flolan.

EPTIFIBATIDE

(**ep**-tih-**FY**-beh-tide)

Antiplatelet agent

Integrilin

pH 5.35

USUAL DOSE

Used in combination with heparin and aspirin. A calculated CrCl greater than or equal to 50 mL/min is required in patients receiving the following doses. Use of the Cockroft-Gault equation is recommended for calculating CrCl. Discontinue eptifibatide infusion before CABG surgery and in patients requiring thrombolytic therapy.

ACUTE CORONARY SYNDROME

Eptifibatide: 180 mcg/kg as an IV bolus as soon as possible following diagnosis. Follow with a continuous infusion of 2 mcg/kg/min until hospital discharge or initiation of coronary artery bypass graft (CABG) surgery for up to 72 hours. Alternately, if a patient is to undergo a percutaneous coronary intervention (PCI) while receiving eptifibatide, the infusion should be continued up to hospital discharge or for 18 to 24 hours after the procedure, whichever comes first. Patient may receive up to 96 hours of therapy. See Dosing Chart by Weight on the following page and Dose Adjustments. Dose in patients with a calculated CrCl greater than or equal to 50 mL/min weighing more than 121 kg should not exceed a bolus of 22.6 mg or an infusion rate of 15 mg/hr.

Aspirin: 160 to 325 mg PO initially and daily thereafter.

Heparin: *Medical management:* Suggested heparin dose to achieve the target aPTT of 50 to 70 seconds during medical management is *Weight 70 kg or more,* 5,000 units as an IV bolus followed by an infusion of 1,000 units/hr. *Weight less than 70 kg,* 60 units/kg as an IV bolus followed by an infusion of 12 units/kg/hr.

Patients undergoing PCI: Target ACT is 200 to 300 seconds during PCI. If heparin is initiated before PCI, give additional boluses during PCI as needed to keep ACT in range. Heparin infusion after PCI is discouraged.

PERCUTANEOUS CORONARY INTERVENTION (PCI)

Eptifibatide: 180 mcg/kg as an IV bolus immediately before initiation of PCI followed by a continuous infusion of 2 mcg/kg/min. Repeat bolus of 180 mcg/kg 10 minutes after the first bolus. Continue infusion until hospital discharge or for up to 18 to 24 hours, whichever comes first. A minimum of 12 hours of infusion is recommended. See the following chart and Dose Adjustments. Dose in patients with a calculated CrCl greater than or equal to 50 mL/min weighing more than 121 kg should not exceed a bolus of 22.6 mg or an infusion rate of 15 mg/hr.

Aspirin: 160 to 325 mg PO 1 to 24 hours before PCI and daily thereafter.

Heparin: Target ACT is 200 to 300 seconds during PCI. In patients not treated with heparin within 6 hours of PCI, give 60 units/kg as a bolus. Give additional boluses as needed during PCI to keep ACT in range. Heparin infusion is discouraged after PCI.

FOR BOTH INDICATIONS

Refer to the following Eptifibatide Dosing Chart by Weight.

	Eptifibatide Dosing Chart by Weight				
Patient Weight	180 mcg/kg Bolus Volume	2 mcg/kg/min Infusion Rate		1 mcg/kg/min Infusion Rate	
	From 2 mg/mL Vial	From 2 mg/mL 100-mL Vial	From 0.75 mg/mL 100-mL Vial	From 2 mg/mL 100-mL Vial	From 0.75 mg/mL 100-mL Vial
37-41 kg	3.4 mL	2 mL/hr	6 mL/hr	1 mL/hr	3 mL/hr
42-46 kg	4 mL	2.5 mL/hr	7 mL/hr	1.3 mL/hr	3.5 mL/hr
47-53 kg	4.5 mL	3 mL/hr	8 mL/hr	1.5 mL/hr	4 mL/hr
54-59 kg	5 mL	3.5 mL/hr	9 mL/hr	1.8 mL/hr	4.5 mL/hr
60-65 kg	5.6 mL	3.8 mL/hr	10 mL/hr	1.9 mL/hr	5 mL/hr
66-71 kg	6.2 mL	4 mL/hr	11 mL/hr	2 mL/hr	5.5 mL/hr
72-78 kg	6.8 mL	4.5 mL/hr	12 mL/hr	2.3 mL/hr	6 mL/hr
79-84 kg	7.3 mL	5 mL/hr	13 mL/hr	2.5 mL/hr	6.5 mL/hr
85-90 kg	7.9 mL	5.3 mL/hr	14 mL/hr	2.7 mL/hr	7 mL/hr
91-96 kg	8.5 mL	5.6 mL/hr	15 mL/hr	2.8 mL/hr	7.5 mL/hr
97-103 kg	9 mL	6 mL/hr	16 mL/hr	3 mL/hr	8 mL/hr
104-109 kg	9.5 mL	6.4 mL/hr	17 mL/hr	3.2 mL/hr	8.5 mL/hr
110-115 kg	10.2 mL	6.8 mL/hr	18 mL/hr	3.4 mL/hr	9 mL/hr
116-121 kg	10.7 mL	7 mL/hr	19 mL/hr	3.5 mL/hr	9.5 mL/hr
>121 kg	11.3 mL	7.5 mL/hr	20 mL/hr	3.7 mL/hr	10 mL/hr

DOSE ADJUSTMENTS

ACUTE CORONARY SYNDROME

In patients with a calculated CrCl less than 50 mL/min, give a bolus of 180 mcg/kg. Decrease rate of the continuous infusion to 1 mcg/kg/min. In patients with a calculated CrCl less than 50 mL/min or a SCr greater than 2 mg/dL and weighing more than 121 kg, a maximum bolus of 22.6 mg followed by a maximum infusion rate of 7.5 mg/hr should be administered.

PCI

In patients with a calculated CrCl less than 50 mL/min, give a bolus of 180 mcg/kg. Decrease rate of the continuous infusion to 1 mcg/kg/min. Repeat bolus of 180 mcg/kg 10 minutes after the first bolus. In patients with a calculated CrCl less than 50 mL/min or a SCr greater than 2 mg/dL and weighing more than 121 kg, a maximum bolus of 22.6 mg followed by a maximum infusion rate of 7.5 mg/hr should be administered.

ALL DIAGNOSES

Dose reduction may be indicated in patients over 75 years of age weighing less than 50 kg. ■ See Dosing Chart by Weight in Usual Dose. ■ See Contraindications.

DILUTION

The 10-mL vial contains 20 mg of eptifibatide; the 100-mL vials contain 75 mg or 200 mg of eptifibatide.

IV bolus: Given undiluted. Withdraw total bolus dose (usually from the 10-mL vial) into a syringe.

Infusion: Usually given undiluted directly from the 75 mg/100 mL (0.75 mg/mL) or the 200 mg/100 mL (2 mg/mL) vials using an IV infusion pump. The 100-mL vial should be spiked with a vented infusion set. Center the spike within the circle on the stopper top. May be diluted with NS or D5NS. Use of a metriset or infusion pump appropriate.

Storage: Refrigerate vials at 2° to 8° C (36° to 46° F) or they may be kept at CRT for up to 2 months. Protect from light until administration. Do not use beyond the expiration or discard date. Discard any unused portion left in the vial.

COMPATIBILITY   (Underline Indicates Conflicting Compatibility Information)

Consider any drug NOT listed as compatible to be INCOMPATIBLE until consulting a pharmacist; specific conditions may apply.

Manufacturer lists furosemide (Lasix) as **incompatible** and states "is **incompatible** with any solution or drug not specifically listed as **compatible.**"

Manufacturer lists as **compatible** at **Y-site** with NS or D5NS with or without up to 60 mEq/L of potassium chloride as well as with alteplase (t-PA), atropine sulfate, dobutamine, heparin, lidocaine, meperidine (Demerol), metoprolol (Lopressor), midazolam (Versed), morphine, nitroglycerin IV, verapamil.

Another source adds the following **compatibilities:**

Y-site: Amiodarone (Nexterone), argatroban, bivalirudin (Angiomax), metoprolol (Lopressor), and <u>micafungin (Mycamine)</u>.

RATE OF ADMINISTRATION

IV bolus: A single dose IV push over 1 to 2 minutes.

Infusion: See Dosing Charts by Weight under Usual Dose.

ACTIONS

A cyclic heptapeptide (amino acid) that reversibly binds to the platelet receptor glycoprotein GP IIb/IIIa of human platelets and inhibits platelet aggregation by preventing the binding of fibrinogen, von Willebrand factor, and other adhesive ligands to GP IIb/IIIa. Inhibits platelet aggregation in a dose- and concentration-dependent manner. Recovery of platelet function after termination of the eptifibatide infusion is rapid. Administered alone, eptifibatide has no measurable effect on PT or aPTT. Does not exert a pharmacologic effect on other integrins. Recommended regimens of a bolus followed by an infusion produce immediate inhibition of platelet aggregation and an early peak level, followed by a small decline, with steady state achieved within 4 to 6 hours. This decline can be prevented by administering a second bolus. Plasma elimination half-life is approximately 2.5 hours. 50% cleared from plasma by the kidneys. Balance of clearance is by nonrenal mechanisms. Has been shown to reduce clinical events (e.g., acute MI, need for urgent intervention) in patients undergoing PCI during drug administration and in those receiving medical management alone.

INDICATIONS AND USES

Used in combination with heparin, aspirin and, in selected situations, a thienopyridine (e.g., clopidogrel [Plavix], prasugrel [Effient]). ▪ Treatment of patients with acute coronary syndrome (unstable angina or non–ST-segment elevation MI), including those who are to be managed medically and those undergoing PCI. In this setting, has been shown to decrease the rate of a combined endpoint of death or new MI. ▪ Treatment of patients undergoing PCI, including those undergoing intracoronary stenting. In this setting has been shown to decrease the rate of a combined endpoint of death, new MI, or need for urgent intervention.

CONTRAINDICATIONS

Known hypersensitivity to any component of the product. ▪ Current or planned administration of another parenteral glycoprotein GPIIb/IIIa inhibitor (e.g., abciximab [ReoPro], tirofiban [Aggrastat]). ▪ Dependency on renal dialysis. ▪ History of bleeding diathesis or evidence of active abnormal bleeding within the previous 30 days. ▪ History of stroke within 30 days or any history of hemorrhagic stroke. ▪ Major surgery within the preceding 6 weeks. ▪ Severe hypertension (systolic BP greater than 200 mm Hg or diastolic BP greater than 110 mm Hg) not adequately controlled on antihypertensive therapy.

PRECAUTIONS

Use caution when given with drugs that affect hemostasis (e.g., NSAIDs [e.g., ibuprofen (Advil, Motrin), naproxen (Aleve, Naprosyn)], clopidogrel [Plavix], dipyridamole [Persantine], ticlopidine [Ticlid], warfarin [Coumadin]). Limited data on the use of eptifibatide in patients receiving thrombolytic agents (e.g., alteplase [t-PA, Activase]), reteplase [Retavase], streptokinase [Streptase]) do not allow an estimate of the bleeding risk associated with concomitant use. Systemic thrombolytic therapy should be used with caution in patients who have received eptifibatide. See Drug/Lab Interactions. ▪ Use with caution in patients with renal insufficiency; clearance is reduced and plasma levels are elevated; see Dose Adjustments. There is no experience in patients dependent on dialysis. ▪ Bleeding is the most common complication encountered during therapy. ▪ Risk of major bleeding increased inversely with patient weight, especially for patients weighing less than 70 kg. ▪ Most major bleeding occurs at the arterial access site for cardiac catheterization or from the GI or GU tracts. ▪ Acute profound thrombocytopenia has been reported; see Monitor. ▪ Because eptifibatide is readily reversible, procedures such as emergency CABG may be performed safely shortly after discontinuation of an infusion without the need for platelet transfusions. ▪ Development of antibodies to eptifibatide and immune-mediated thrombocytopenia have been reported; may be associated with hypotension and/or other signs of hypersensitivity. ▪ No clinical experience in patients with a baseline platelet count less than 100,000/mm^3. Monitor closely if use is indicated.

Monitor: Before therapy obtain platelet count, hemoglobin or hematocrit, SCr, and PT/aPTT. Obtain ACT in patients undergoing PCI. ▪ Maintain target aPTT between 50 and 70 seconds unless PCI is to be performed. During PCI, the ACT should be maintained between 200 and 300 seconds. ▪ The aPTT or ACT should be checked before sheath removal. The sheath should not be removed unless the aPTT is less than 45 seconds or the ACT is less than 150 seconds. In patients treated with heparin, bleeding can be minimized by close monitoring of the aPTT. ▪ If acute profound thrombocytopenia occurs or the platelet count drops to less than 100,000/mm^3, heparin and eptifibatide should be discontinued. Monitor serial platelet counts, assess the presence of drug-dependent antibodies, and initiate appropriate therapy as indicated. ▪ Monitor the patient for signs of bleeding; take vital signs (avoiding automatic BP cuffs); observe any invaded sites at least every 15 minutes (e.g., sheaths, IV sites, cutdowns, punctures, Foleys, NGs); watch for hematuria, hematemesis, bloody stool, petechiae, hematoma, flank pain, muscle weakness. Perform neuro checks frequently. If during therapy bleeding cannot be controlled with pressure, heparin and eptifibatide should be discontinued. ▪ Use care in handling patient; minimize use of urinary catheters, nasotracheal intubation, and nasogastric tubes. Avoid arterial puncture, venipuncture, and IM injection. Use extreme precautionary methods and only compressible sites if these procedures are absolutely necessary (i.e., avoid subclavian or jugular veins). Apply pressure for 30 minutes to any invaded site and then apply pressure dressings. Saline or heparin locks suggested to facilitate blood draws. ▪ See Precautions.

Additional monitoring for patients receiving PCI: After PCI, eptifibatide should be continued until hospital discharge or for up to 18 to 24 hours, whichever comes first. See suggested time frames under each dose. Heparin use is discouraged after the PCI procedure. The femoral artery sheath may be removed during eptifibatide infusion, but only after heparin has been discontinued and its effects largely reversed. Heparin should be discontinued 3 to 4 hours before pulling the sheath, and an aPTT less than 45 seconds or an ACT of less than 150 seconds should be documented. ▪ Care should be taken to obtain proper hemostasis after removal of the sheath using standard compressive techniques followed by close observation. Sheath hemostasis should be achieved at least 2 to 4 hours before hospital discharge.

Patient Education: Compliance with all measures to minimize bleeding (e.g., strict bed rest, positioning) is imperative. ▪ Avoid use of razors, toothbrushes, and other sharp items. ▪ Use caution while moving to avoid excessive bumping. ▪ Report all episodes of bleeding and apply local pressure if indicated. ▪ Expect oozing from IV sites.

Maternal/Child: Category B: safety for use in pregnancy not established; use only if clearly needed. ▪ It is not known whether eptifibatide is excreted in breast milk; use caution if administered to a nursing mother. ▪ Safety and effectiveness for use in pediatric patients not established.

Elderly: Dose adjusted by weight; see Dosing Charts by Weight in Usual Dose. ▪ Clearance decreased and plasma levels increased in older patients; incidence of bleeding complications was higher and eptifibatide-associated bleeding was greater in the elderly during studies. ▪ No apparent difference in effectiveness between older and younger patients.

DRUG/LAB INTERACTIONS

All studies with eptifibatide included the use of **aspirin and heparin.** In the ESPRIT study, **clopidogrel** (Plavix) **or ticlopidine** (Ticlid) were administered routinely, starting the day of PCI. Concomitant use, although indicated, increases the risk of bleeding. ▪ Use caution when given with **drugs that affect hemostasis** such as **thrombolytics** (e.g., alteplase [t-PA, Activase], reteplase [Retavase], streptokinase [Streptase]), **oral anticoagulants** (e.g., warfarin [Coumadin]), **NSAIDs** (e.g., ibuprofen [Advil, Motrin], naproxen [Aleve, Naprosyn]), **dipyridamole** (Persantine), **ticlopidine** (Ticlid), **clopidogrel** (Plavix), **selected antibiotics** (e.g., cefotetan). ▪ Avoid concomitant treatment with **other inhibitors of platelet receptor glycoprotein GPIIb/IIIa** (e.g., abciximab [ReoPro], tirofiban [Aggrastat]; may have potentially serious additive effects. See Contraindications. ▪ **Enoxaparin** (Lovenox) 1 mg/kg SC every 12 hours for 4 doses has been administered without altering the effects of eptifibatide.

SIDE EFFECTS

Bleeding is the most frequent adverse event; may occur more frequently in patients undergoing CABG or PCI, or in the elderly or those weighing less than 70 kg. Bleeding is usually reported as mild oozing, but major bleeding (e.g., GI bleeding, pulmonary hemorrhage, intracranial hemorrhage, and stroke) may occur. Fatal bleeding events have been reported. Laboratory findings related to bleeding include decrease in hemoglobin, hematocrit, and platelet count and occult blood in urine and feces. Other side effects that have been reported include hypersensitivity reactions, hypotension, and thrombocytopenia (acute and profound). Incidence in studies similar to that seen with placebo.

Acute toxicity: Specific information not available for humans, but decreased muscle tone, dyspnea, loss of righting reflex, petechial hemorrhages in the femoral and abdominal areas, and ptosis occurred in animals.

Post-Marketing: Immune-mediated thrombocytopenia.

ANTIDOTE

Keep physician informed of laboratory values and side effects. Discontinue the infusion of eptifibatide and heparin if any serious bleeding not controllable with pressure occurs, if CABG surgery is initiated, and/or if patient requires thrombolytic therapy. If acute profound thrombocytopenia occurs or the platelet count drops to less than 100,000/mm^3, heparin and eptifibatide should be discontinued. Monitor serial platelet counts, assess the presence of drug-dependent antibodies, and initiate appropriate therapy as indicated. Monitor closely; platelet transfusion may be required. If a hypersensitivity reaction should occur, discontinue the infusion and treat as indicated by severity (e.g., epinephrine, dopamine, theophylline, antihistamines such as diphenhydramine [Benadryl], and/or corticosteroids as necessary). No specific antidote is available. Platelet inhibition reverses rapidly when infusion is discontinued. Hemodialysis may be useful in an overdose situation.

ERIBULIN MESYLATE
(**ER**-ih-**BUE**-lin **MES**-ih-late)

Antineoplastic
(antimicrotubular)

Halaven

USUAL DOSE
1.4 mg/M^2 IV over 2 to 5 minutes on Days 1 and 8 of a 21-day cycle.

DOSE ADJUSTMENTS
Dose adjustment not required based on age, gender, or race. ▪ Reduce dose in patients with mild hepatic impairment (Child-Pugh Class A) to 1.1 mg/M^2 IV. ▪ Patients with moderate hepatic impairment (Child-Pugh Class B) should receive 0.7 mg/M^2 IV. ▪ Patients with moderate or severe renal impairment (CrCl 15 to 49 mL/min) should receive 1.1 mg/M^2 IV. ▪ Do not administer dose on Day 1 or Day 8 in patients with an ANC less than 1,000/mm^3, platelets less than 75,000/mm^3, or Grade 3 or 4 nonhematologic toxicities. ▪ The Day 8 dose may be delayed for a maximum of 1 week. If toxicities do not resolve or improve to Grade 2 or less by Day 15, omit the dose. If toxicities resolve or improve to Grade 2 or less by Day 15, administer at a reduced dose as outlined in the following chart and initiate the next cycle no sooner than 2 weeks later. ▪ If a dose has been delayed for toxicity and the toxicities have recovered to Grade 2 severity or less, resume eribulin as outlined in the following chart. ▪ Do not re-escalate eribulin dose after it has been reduced.

Recommended Dose Reductions for Eribulin Mesylate	
Event Description	Recommended Eribulin Dose
Permanently reduce the 1.4 mg/M^2 eribulin dose for any of the following: • ANC <500/mm^3 for >7 days • ANC <1,000/mm^3 with fever or infection • Platelets <25,000/mm^3 • Platelets <50,000/mm^3 requiring transfusion • Nonhematologic Grade 3 or 4 toxicities* • Omission or delay of Day 8 eribulin dose in previous cycle for toxicity	1.1 mg/M^2
Occurrence of any event requiring permanent dose reduction while receiving 1.1 mg/M^2	0.7 mg/M^2
Occurrence of any event requiring permanent dose reduction while receiving 0.7 mg/M^2	Discontinue eribulin

*Toxicities graded in accordance with National Cancer Institute (NCI) Common Terminology Criteria for Adverse Events (CTCAE), Version 3.0.

DILUTION
Specific techniques required; see Precautions. Available in a single-use vial containing 1 mg/2 mL (0.5 mg/mL). Withdraw calculated dose and administer undiluted or may dilute in 100 mL NS.

Filter: Information not available.

Storage: Store unopened vials in carton at CRT. Do not freeze. Store undiluted solution drawn up into a syringe for up to 4 hours at RT or 24 hours under refrigeration (4° C [40° F]). Store diluted solution for up to 4 hours at RT or 24 hours under refrigeration (4° C [40° F]). Discard unused portion of vial.

COMPATIBILITY
Manufacturer states, "Do not dilute in or administer through an IV line containing solutions with dextrose. Do not administer in the same intravenous line concurrent with other medicinal products."

RATE OF ADMINISTRATION
An IV injection evenly distributed over 2 to 5 minutes.

ACTIONS
A synthetic analog of halichondrin B, a product isolated from a marine sponge. Eribulin is a non-taxane microtubule inhibitor. Inhibits the growth phase of microtubules without affecting the shortening phase and sequesters tubulin into nonproductive aggregates. Exerts its effects via a tubulin-based antimitotic mechanism leading to G_2/M cell-cycle block, disruption of mitotic spindles and, ultimately, apoptotic cell death after prolonged mitotic blockage. Plasma protein binding is 49% to 65%. Mean elimination half-life is approximately 40 hours. There are no major human metabolites. Is eliminated primarily in feces unchanged. Small amount excreted as unchanged drug in urine.

INDICATIONS AND USES
Treatment of patients with metastatic breast cancer who have previously received at least two chemotherapeutic regimens for the treatment of metastatic disease. Prior therapy should have included an anthracycline and a taxane in either the adjuvant or metastatic setting. ▪ Treatment of patients with unresectable or metastatic liposarcoma who have received a prior anthracycline-containing regimen.

CONTRAINDICATIONS
Manufacturer states, "None." ▪ Do not administer in patients with an ANC less than 1,000/mm³, platelets less than 75,000/mm³, or Grade 3 or 4 nonhematologic toxicities. ▪ Should be avoided in patients with congenital long QT syndrome.

PRECAUTIONS
Follow guidelines for handling cytotoxic agents. See Appendix A, p. 1331. ▪ May cause severe neutropenia (ANC less than 500/mm³) lasting more than 1 week. Higher incidence of Grade 4 neutropenia and febrile neutropenia seen in patients with ALT or AST greater than 3 times the ULN and in patients with a bilirubin greater than 1.5 times the ULN. Deaths from complications of febrile neutropenia and neutropenic sepsis have been reported. In clinical trials, the mean time to nadir was 13 days, and the mean time to recovery from severe neutropenia was 8 days. ▪ Grades 3 and 4 peripheral neuropathy have been reported. Peripheral neuropathy was the most common toxicity leading to discontinuation of therapy. Neuropathy may not be reversible. ▪ QT prolongation, independent of eribulin concentration, was observed on Day 8 in an uncontrolled, open-label ECG study. ▪ Has not been studied in patients with severe hepatic impairment (Child-Pugh Class C). ▪ See Dose Adjustments.

Monitor: Obtain baseline CBC with platelets, bilirubin, liver function tests, SCr, and electrolytes. ▪ Obtain CBC with platelets before each dose. Increase frequency of hematologic monitoring in patients who develop severe cytopenias (Grade 3 or 4); see Dose Adjustments. ▪ Assess for peripheral motor and sensory neuropathy before each dose; see Dose Adjustments. ▪ ECG monitoring is recommended in patients with CHF or bradyarrhythmias; in patients taking drugs that prolong the QT interval, such as Class Ia and III antiarrhythmics (e.g., amiodarone [Nexterone], disopyramide [Norpace], dofetilide [Tikosyn], ibutilide [Corvert], N-acetylprocainamide, procainamide [Pronestyl], quinidine, sotalol [Betapace]); and in patients with electrolyte abnormalities. Correct hypokalemia or hypomagnesemia before initiating therapy, and monitor electrolytes periodically during therapy. ▪ Monitor for nausea and vomiting. Use prophylactic antiemetics to reduce nausea and vomiting and increase patient comfort. ▪ Observe closely for signs of infection. Prophylactic antibiotics may be indicated pending results of C/S in a febrile neutropenic patient. ▪ In patients with thrombocytopenia (platelet count less than 50,000/mm³), initiate precautions to prevent excessive bleeding (e.g., inspect IV sites, skin, and mucous membranes; use extreme care during invasive procedures; test urine, emesis, stool, and secretions for occult blood).

Patient Education: Avoid pregnancy. Women should use effective contraception during treatment with eribulin and for 2 weeks following the final dose. Males with female partners of reproductive potential should use effective contraception during treatment and for 3.5 months following the final dose. ▪ May result in damage to male reproductive tissues, leading to impaired fertility of unknown duration. ▪ Promptly report S/S of infection (e.g., fever, chills, cough, burning or pain on urination). ▪ Report symptoms of peripheral neuropathy (e.g., numbness, tingling, or burning in hands or feet).

Maternal/Child: Category D: can cause fetal harm. ▪ Discontinue breast-feeding. ▪ Safety and effectiveness for use in pediatric patients not established.

Elderly: No overall differences in safety were observed between older and younger patients. ▪ Consider age-related cardiac, hepatic, or renal dysfunction.

DRUG/LAB INTERACTIONS

No drug-drug interactions are expected with CYP3A4 inhibitors, CYP3A4 inducers, or P-glycoprotein (P-gp) inhibitors. No clinically relevant interaction observed with the strong CYP3A4 inhibitor and a P-gp inhibitor, ketoconazole (Nizoral). No clinically relevant interaction observed with the CYP3A4 inducer rifampin (Rifadin). ▪ Does not inhibit CYP1A2, CYP2C9, CYP2C19, CYP2D6, CYP2E1, or CYP3A4 enzymes or induce CYP1A2, CYP2C9, CYP2C19, or CYP3A4 enzymes at relevant clinical concentrations, and it is not expected to alter the plasma concentrations of drugs that are substrates of these enzymes. ▪ A substrate and a weak inhibitor of the drug efflux transporter P-gp in vitro.

SIDE EFFECTS

The most common side effects were abdominal pain, alopecia, anemia, asthenia, constipation, fatigue, fever, nausea, neutropenia, and peripheral neuropathy. The most common serious side effects were febrile neutropenia and neutropenia. The most common side effects resulting in discontinuation of eribulin were fatigue, peripheral neuropathy, and thrombocytopenia. Grade 3 or 4 laboratory abnormalities included hypocalcemia, hypokalemia, and neutropenia. Other reported side effects included anorexia, arthralgia, cough, diarrhea, dyspnea, fever, headache, liver function test abnormalities, mucosal inflammation, myalgia, pain (back, bone, extremity), UTI, vomiting, and weight loss. Less frequently reported side effects included abdominal pain, anemia, anxiety, back pain, depression, dizziness, dry mouth, dysgeusia, dyspepsia, hyperglycemia, hypophosphatemia, hypotension, increased lacrimation, insomnia, muscle spasm or weakness, oropharyngeal pain, peripheral edema, rash, stomatitis, thrombocytopenia, and upper respiratory tract infection.

Post-Marketing: Dehydration, hepatotoxicity, hypersensitivity, hypomagnesemia, interstitial lung disease, lymphopenia, neutropenic sepsis, pancreatitis, pneumonia, pruritus, sepsis, Stevens-Johnson syndrome, and toxic epidermal necrolysis.

ANTIDOTE

Keep physician informed of all side effects. Most will be treated symptomatically as indicated. Neutropenia can be profound. Colony-stimulating factors (G-CSF [filgrastim], GM-CSF [sargramostim]) have been administered to aid in neutrophil recovery. Severe peripheral neuropathies may necessitate discontinuation of eribulin. There is no specific antidote for overdose. Supportive therapy will help sustain the patient in toxicity. Resuscitate if indicated.

ERTAPENEM
(er-tah-**PEN**-em)

Antibacterial
(carbapenem)

Invanz

pH 7.5

USUAL DOSE
Duration of therapy is based on diagnosis as listed in the following chart. May be given IV for up to 14 days or IM for up to 7 days.

Ertapenem Dosing Guidelines			
Infection*	Daily Dose (IV or IM) in Adults and Pediatric Patients 13 Years of Age and Older	Daily Dose (IV or IM) in Pediatric Patients 3 Months to 12 Years of Age	Duration
Complicated intra-abdominal infections	1 Gm	15 mg/kg q 12 hr†	5-14 days
Complicated skin and skin structure infections, including diabetic foot infections‡	1 Gm	15 mg/kg q 12 hr†	7-14 days§
Community-acquired pneumonia	1 Gm	15 mg/kg q 12 hr†	10-14 days‖
Complicated urinary tract infections, including pyelonephritis	1 Gm	15 mg/kg q 12 hr†	10-14 days‖
Acute pelvic infections, including postpartum endomyometritis, septic abortion, and post-surgical gynecologic infections.	1 Gm	15 mg/kg q 12 hr†	3-10 days
Prophylaxis of surgical site infection in adults for elective colorectal surgery	1 Gm		Single intravenous dose given 1 hour before surgical incision

*Due to designated pathogens.
†Not to exceed 1 Gm/24 hr.
‡Has not been studied in diabetic foot infections with concomitant osteomyelitis.
§Adult patients with diabetic foot infections received up to 28 days of treatment (parenteral or parenteral plus oral switch therapy).
‖Duration includes a possible switch to an appropriate oral therapy, after at least 3 days of parenteral therapy, once clinical improvement has been demonstrated.

DOSE ADJUSTMENTS
Reduce dose to 0.5 Gm (500 mg) daily in adults with a CrCl at or less than 30 mL/min/1.73 M^2, including adults with end-stage renal insufficiency (CrCl ≤10 mL/min/1.73 M^2). No dose adjustment indicated in adults with a CrCl at or more than 31 mL/min/1.73 M^2. Give a supplementary dose of 150 mg to patients who received the daily dose within 6 hours of a dialysis session. No data are available for pediatric patients with renal insufficiency or pediatric patients on hemodialysis. No data on patients undergoing peritoneal dialysis or hemofiltration. ▪ No dose adjustment indicated based on age, gender, or impaired hepatic function. ▪ Dosing should be cautious in the elderly, and reduced doses may be indicated based on potential for decreased organ function.

DILUTION
Reconstitute each 1-Gm vial of ertapenem with 10 mL SWFI, NS, BWFI. Shake well to dissolve, and dilute immediately as outlined below.
Adults and pediatric patients 13 years of age and older: Further dilute in 50 mL of NS.
Pediatric patients 3 months to 12 years of age: Withdraw the volume equal to the 15 mg/kg dose and dilute in NS to a final concentration of 20 mg/mL or less.

Also supplied in single-dose ADD-Vantage vials containing 1 Gm of ertapenem. Reconstitute as directed with 50 mL or 100 mL of NS; see prescribing information for directions.

Storage: Store unopened vials at or below 25° C (77° F). Dilute reconstituted solution immediately. Use diluted solution within 6 hours when stored at RT. May refrigerate for up to 24 hours and use within 4 hours after removal. Do not freeze.

COMPATIBILITY (Underline Indicates Conflicting Compatibility Information)

Consider any drug NOT listed as compatible to be INCOMPATIBLE until consulting a pharmacist; specific conditions may apply.

Manufacturer states, "Do not mix or co-infuse ertapenem with other medications. Do not use diluents containing dextrose."

One source suggests the following **compatibilities:**

Y-site: Heparin, hetastarch in NS (Hespan), potassium chloride (KCl), telavancin (Vibativ), tigecycline (Tygacil).

RATE OF ADMINISTRATION

A single dose as an infusion equally distributed over 30 minutes.

ACTIONS

A unique, synthetic 1-beta-methyl-carbapenem structurally related to beta-lactam antibiotics. Effective against gram-positive and gram-negative aerobic and anaerobic bacteria. May effectively replace some combination therapies. Does not cover *Pseudomonas* and *Acinetobacter* species. Bactericidal activity results from inhibition of bacterial cell wall synthesis. Stable against hydrolysis by a variety of beta-lactamases, including penicillinases, cephalosporinases, and extended-spectrum beta-lactamases. Hydrolyzed by metallo-beta-lactamases. Widely distributed throughout the body into many body tissues and fluids. Highly protein bound. Average half-life is 4 hours. Primarily excreted in urine (some as unchanged drug). Some excretion in feces. May cross the placental barrier. Secreted in breast milk.

INDICATIONS AND USES

Treatment of adult and pediatric patients with moderate to severe infections caused by susceptible strains of microorganisms in conditions that include complicated intra-abdominal infections; complicated skin and skin structure infections, including diabetic foot infections **without** osteomyelitis; community-acquired pneumonia; complicated urinary tract infections, including pyelonephritis; and acute pelvic infections, including postpartum endomyometritis, septic abortion, and postsurgical gynecologic infections. ▪ Prophylaxis of surgical site infections in adults following elective colorectal surgery. ▪ Not recommended for use in the treatment of meningitis in pediatric patients (lack of sufficient CSF penetration).

CONTRAINDICATIONS

Known hypersensitivity to any component of ertapenem or other drugs in the same class (e.g., imipenem-cilastatin), or in patients who have had anaphylactic reactions to beta-lactams (e.g., penicillins and cephalosporins); see Precautions.

PRECAUTIONS

To reduce the development of drug-resistant bacteria and maintain its effectiveness, ertapenem should be used to treat or prevent only those infections proven or strongly suspected to be caused by bacteria. ▪ Culture and sensitivity studies indicated to determine susceptibility of the causative organism to ertapenem. ▪ Serious and occasionally fatal hypersensitivity reactions have been reported in patients receiving therapy with beta-lactams. More likely in patients with a history of sensitivity to multiple allergens; obtain a careful history and watch for early symptoms of hypersensitivity reactions. Emergency equipment must be readily available; cross-sensitivity is possible. ▪ Prolonged use may cause superinfection because of overgrowth of nonsusceptible organisms. ▪ CNS stimulation and seizures have been reported. Use with caution in patients with CNS disorders (e.g., brain lesions or history of seizures) and/or compromised renal function. ▪ *Clostridium difficile*–associated diarrhea (CDAD) has been reported. May range from mild diarrhea to fatal colitis. Consider in patients who present with diarrhea during or after treatment with ertapenem. ▪ See Monitor and Drug/Lab Interactions.

Monitor: Monitor closely for S/S of hypersensitivity reactions (e.g., difficulty breathing, itching, rash, swelling of eyelids, lips, or face). ▪ Obtain baseline CBC with differential and platelets, and baseline kidney and liver studies (e.g., CrCl, serum creatinine, ALT, AST, serum bilirubin). Monitor periodically during prolonged therapy. ▪ Monitor patients who are at risk for CNS stimulation or are receiving anticonvulsant therapy. If focal tremors, myoclonus, or seizures occur, neurologic evaluation and dose reduction or discontinuation of ertapenem may be indicated. ▪ Monitor IV site carefully and rotate as indicated. ▪ See Precautions.

Patient Education: Promptly report S/S of hypersensitivity reaction (e.g., rash, shortness of breath, hives), fever, sore throat, unusual bleeding or bruising, severe stomach cramps, seizures, and pain or discomfort at the injection site. ▪ Promptly report diarrhea or bloody stools that occur during treatment or up to several months after an antibiotic has been discontinued; may indicate CDAD and require treatment. ▪ Patients with a history of seizures should review medication profile with physician before taking ertapenem; see Drug/Lab Interactions.

Maternal/Child: Category B: use during pregnancy only if clearly needed. ▪ Safety for use during breast-feeding not established; is found in breast milk. Benefits must outweigh risks to infant (e.g., diarrhea, candidiasis, or allergic response). Undetectable in breast milk 5 days after ertapenem is discontinued. ▪ Following a 1-Gm daily IV dose, plasma concentrations and half-life of ertapenem in pediatric patients 13 to 17 years of age are comparable to those in adults. ▪ Compared to plasma clearance in adults, plasma clearance (mL/min/kg) in pediatric patients 3 months to 12 years of age is approximately twofold higher. 30 mg/kg/24 hr (15 mg/kg every 12 hours) is comparable to a 1-Gm dose daily in adults. Half-life in pediatric patients 3 months to 12 years of age is 2.5 hours compared to 4 hours for adults and pediatric patients 13 years of age or older. ▪ Not recommended for use in infants under 3 months; no data available; see Indications and Uses.

Elderly: Dosing should be cautious in the elderly; see Dose Adjustments. ▪ Response similar to that seen in younger patients, but may be more sensitive to side effects. ▪ Monitoring of renal function may be indicated.

DRUG/LAB INTERACTIONS

Carbapenems may reduce serum **valproic acid** concentrations to subtherapeutic levels, resulting in a loss of seizure control. Monitor valproic acid levels. Consider alternative antibacterial therapy. If administration of ertapenem is necessary, supplemental anticonvulsant therapy should be considered. ▪ **Probenecid** reduces the renal clearance of ertapenem, resulting in increased plasma concentrations. Coadministration is not recommended. ▪ In vitro studies indicate that ertapenem does not inhibit metabolism mediated by any of the following cytochrome P_{450} (CYP) isoforms: 1A2, 2C9, 2C19, 2D6, 2E1, and 3A4. ▪ In vitro studies indicate that ertapenem does not inhibit P-glycoprotein–mediated transport of digoxin or vinblastine and that ertapenem is not a substrate for P-glycoprotein–mediated transport. ▪ No other drug interaction studies have been conducted.

SIDE EFFECTS

Adults: Diarrhea, headache, infusion site reactions, nausea, and vaginitis in females were most common and described as mild to moderate. Other side effects that were reported in greater than 2% of patients included abdominal pain, altered mental status, constipation, dizziness, fever, and vomiting. The most commonly reported laboratory abnormalities were elevated ALT, AST, and alkaline phosphatase and increased platelets and eosinophils. Numerous other side effects occurred in fewer than 1% of patients.

Pediatric patients: Side effects similar to adults. Diarrhea, infusion site pain, erythema, and vomiting were most common.

Major: CDAD, CNS stimulation (e.g., anxiety, confusion, depression, insomnia, nightmares, paranoia, restlessness, seizures, tremor), hypersensitivity reactions (e.g., anaphylaxis, cardiovascular collapse, death, dyspnea, edema [facial, laryngeal, or pharyngeal], hypotension, itching, rash, shock, urticaria), and pseudomembranous colitis.

Post-Marketing: Abnormal coordination, altered mental status (including aggression, delirium, and hallucinations), anaphylaxis, depressed level of consciousness, drug rash with eosinophilia and systemic symptoms (DRESS syndrome), dyskinesia, gait disturbance, muscular weakness, myoclonus, teeth staining, tremor.

ANTIDOTE

Keep physician informed of all side effects. Most minor side effects will be treated symptomatically. Discontinue ertapenem at the first sign of hypersensitivity (e.g., skin rash). Treat hypersensitivity reactions as indicated; may require epinephrine, airway management, oxygen, IV fluids, antihistamines (e.g., diphenhydramine [Benadryl]), corticosteroids (e.g., hydrocortisone sodium succinate [Solu-Cortef]), and pressor amines (e.g., dopamine). Treat CNS symptoms as indicated; may require dose reduction and/or anticonvulsants (e.g., phenytoin [Dilantin], diazepam [Valium]) for seizures. Mild cases of CDAD may respond to discontinuation of the drug. Treat CDAD with fluids, electrolytes, protein supplements, and oral vancomycin (Vancocin) or metronidazole (Flagyl) as indicated. In severe cases, surgical evaluation may be indicated. Ertapenem is partially removed by hemodialysis.

ERYTHROMYCIN LACTOBIONATE

(eh-**rih**-throw-**MY**-sin **LAK**-to-**bye**-oh-nayt)

Erythrocin

**Antibacterial
(macrolide)**

pH 6.5 to 7.7

USUAL DOSE

IV formulation used when oral administration is not possible or when the severity of the infection requires immediate high serum levels of erythromycin. Begin oral therapy as soon as practical.

Antibacterial: 15 to 20 mg/kg of body weight/24 hr in equally divided doses every 6 hours (3.75 to 5 mg/kg every 6 hours). Range is 350 to 500 mg every 6 hours. Continuous infusion over 24 hours is preferred. Up to 4 Gm/24 hr has been given for severe infections. See Elderly.

Legionnaires' disease: 1 to 4 Gm/day in divided doses (250 mg to 1 Gm every 6 hours). Optimum doses not established.

Pelvic inflammatory disease: 500 mg every 6 hours for 3 days. Follow with oral erythromycin 250 mg every 6 hours for 7 days.

Diabetic gastroparesis (unlabeled): 200 mg immediately before each meal. When practical, continue treatment with oral erythromycin 3 times daily, 30 minutes before meals, for 4 weeks.

PEDIATRIC DOSE

15 to 20 mg/kg of body weight/24 hr in equally divided doses every 6 hours is recommended (3.75 to 5 mg/kg every 6 hours). Another source recommends 20 to 50 mg/kg/24 hr in equally divided doses every 6 hours (5 to 12.5 mg/kg every 6 hours). See Maternal/Child.

DOSE ADJUSTMENTS

Reduced dose may be required in impaired liver function.

DILUTION

Each 500 mg or fraction thereof must be reconstituted with 10 mL of SWFI without preservatives to avoid precipitation. Forms a 5% solution. Shake well to ensure dilution. May be further diluted with NS, Normosol, or LR. If a dextrose solution is used, add sodium bicarbonate (Neut) 1 mL for each 100 mL of solution.

Continuous infusion (preferred): Further dilute to a 1 mg/mL solution (e.g., each 1 Gm in 1,000 mL of NS, Normosol, or LR).

Intermittent infusion: Dilute to a final concentration of 1 to 5 mg/mL. No less than 100 mL of IV diluent should be used (1 Gm in 1,000 mL equals 1 mg/mL; 1 Gm in 200 mL equals 5 mg/mL). Available in ADD-Vantage vials for use with ADD-Vantage infusion containers.

Storage: Store unopened vials at CRT. Solutions diluted from *lyophilized powder vials* are stable for 8 hours at CRT. *ADD-Vantage vials:* Solutions diluted in NS must be completely administered within 8 hours; solutions diluted in D5W must be completely administered within 2 hours.

COMPATIBILITY   (Underline Indicates Conflicting Compatibility Information)

Consider any drug NOT listed as compatible to be INCOMPATIBLE until consulting a pharmacist; specific conditions may apply.

One source suggests the following **compatibilities:**

Additive: Aminophylline, ampicillin, ascorbic acid, diphenhydramine (Benadryl), hydrocortisone sodium succinate (Solu-Cortef), lidocaine, penicillin G potassium and sodium, pentobarbital (Nembutal), potassium chloride (KCl), prochlorperazine (Compazine), ranitidine (Zantac), sodium bicarbonate, verapamil.

Y-site: Acyclovir (Zovirax), amiodarone (Nexterone), anidulafungin (Eraxis), bivalirudin (Angiomax), cyclophosphamide (Cytoxan), dexmedetomidine (Precedex), diltiazem (Cardizem), doxapram (Dopram), enalaprilat (Vasotec IV), esmolol (Brevibloc), famotidine (Pepcid IV), fenoldopam (Corlopam), foscarnet (Foscavir), heparin, hetastarch in electrolytes (Hextend), hydromorphone (Dilaudid), idarubicin (Idamycin), labetalol, lorazepam (Ativan), magnesium sulfate, meperidine (Demerol), midazolam (Versed), morphine, multivitamins (M.V.I.), nicardipine (Cardene IV), tacrolimus (Prograf), theophylline, zidovudine (AZT, Retrovir).

RATE OF ADMINISTRATION

Administer with a volume control set. A slow infusion rate is recommended to reduce pain along the injection site.

Continuous infusion (preferred): A 0.1% to 0.2% solution equally distributed over 6 to 24 hours.

Intermittent infusion: 1 Gm or fraction thereof in at least 100 mL over 20 to 60 minutes.

Diabetic gastroparesis (unlabeled): 1 to 3 mg/kg/hr, usually approximately over 15 minutes.

ACTIONS

Macrolide antibiotic, bactericidal and bacteriostatic. Effective against a number of gram-positive and some gram-negative organisms as well as *Mycoplasma pneumoniae*. Inhibits protein synthesis by binding to ribosomal subunits of susceptible organisms. Diffuses readily into most bodily fluids. Metabolized by the liver and excreted in urine and bile. Crosses placental barrier. Secreted in breast milk.

INDICATIONS AND USES

Treatment of mild to moderate infections of the upper and lower respiratory tract, skin and skin structures, and gynecologic infections caused by susceptible organisms. ▪ Alternative treatment in several sexually transmitted diseases in females with a history of penicillin sensitivity. ▪ Legionnaires' disease. ▪ Additional indications listed for oral formulation.

Unlabeled uses: Diabetic gastroparesis.

CONTRAINDICATIONS

Known erythromycin sensitivity. See Drug/Lab Interactions. ▪ Coadministration with ritonavir (Norvir) and cisapride is contraindicated. Contraindicated with astemizole and terfenadine (both have been removed from the market).

PRECAUTIONS

IV formulation used when oral administration is not possible or when the severity of the infection requires immediate high serum levels of erythromycin. Switch to oral therapy when appropriate. ▪ Sensitivity studies indicated to determine susceptibility of the causative organism to erythromycin. ▪ To reduce the development of drug-resistant bacteria and maintain its effectiveness, erythromycin should be used to treat or prevent only those infections proven or strongly suspected to be caused by bacteria. ▪ Superinfection may occur from overgrowth of nonsusceptible organisms. ▪ Use caution in impaired liver function. ▪ Hepatic dysfunction, with or without jaundice, has been reported in patients taking oral erythromycin. ▪ Use caution in patients with a history of cardiac disease (may induce torsades de pointes). ▪ Use caution in patients with myasthenia gravis; weakness may be aggravated. ▪ *Clostridium difficile*–associated diarrhea (CDAD) has been reported. May range from mild diarrhea to fatal colitis. Consider in patients who present with diarrhea during or after treatment with erythromycin.

Monitor: Monitor vital signs. ▪ Monitor IV site for redness and inflammation. ▪ See Drug/Lab Interactions.

Patient Education: Promptly report diarrhea or bloody stools that occur during treatment or up to several months after an antibiotic has been discontinued; may indicate CDAD and require treatment.

Maternal/Child: Category B: use only if clearly needed. ▪ Considered safe for use in breast-feeding; use caution. ▪ Some products contain benzyl alcohol; not recommended for use in neonates.

Elderly: When doses of 4 Gm/day or higher are used, the risk of developing erythromycin-induced hearing loss is increased in elderly patients, particularly those with impaired renal or hepatic function. ▪ May be more susceptible to development of torsades de pointes. ▪ May experience increased effects of oral anticoagulation; see Drug/Lab Interactions.

DRUG/LAB INTERACTIONS

Contraindicated with **ritonavir**. ▪ Antibacterial activity is antagonized by coadministration of **clindamycin, lincomycin, and chloramphenicol.** ▪ May inhibit **penicillins.** ▪ Will increase serum levels and potentiate the effects of **alfentanil, anticoagulants** (e.g., warfarin [Coumadin]), **astemizole** (see Contraindications), **bromocriptine** (Parlodel), **carbamazepine** (Tegretol), **cisapride** (Propulsid), **cyclosporine** (Sandimmune), **digoxin, disopyramide** (Norpace), **ergot alkaloids** (e.g., Hydergine), **lovastatin** (Mevacor), **methylprednisolone, midazolam** (Versed), **phenytoin** (Dilantin), **terfenadine** (see Contraindications), **theophyllines, triazolam** (Halcion), **and valproate;** serious toxicity may result. ▪ Concomitant administration with **cisapride** is contraindicated. May cause serious cardiotoxicity. ▪ Plasma concentrations of erythromycin may be increased by **antifungal agents** metabolized by CYP3A4 isoenzymes (e.g., fluconazole [Diflucan], ketoconazole [Nizoral], itraconazole [Sporanox]). May result in an increase in QT prolongation and ventricular arrhythmias. ▪ Severe **vinblastine** toxicity has been reported in conjunction with erythromycin. ▪ May increase serum levels of **sildenafil** (Viagra). ▪ Coadministration with **HMG-CoA reductase inhibitors** (e.g., simvastatin [Zocor]) results in increased serum levels of the antihyperlipidemic agent and increases the risk of severe myopathy and rhabdomyolysis. ▪ Concurrent use with **theophylline** (aminophylline) may decrease plasma levels of erythromycin. ▪ Serotonin syndrome has been reported with coadministration of erythromycin and **serotonin-uptake inhibitors** (e.g., sertraline [Zoloft], fluoxetine [Prozac]). ▪ May interfere with fluorometric determination of **urinary catecholamines.**

SIDE EFFECTS

Relatively free from side effects when given as directed. Nausea and vomiting, urticaria, and mild local venous discomfort. Increased incidence of usually reversible ototoxicity with larger doses. CDAD has been reported. Torsades de pointes has been reported; see Elderly. Anaphylaxis may occur.

ANTIDOTE

Notify the physician of early or mild symptoms. For severe symptoms, discontinue the drug, treat hypersensitivity reactions, or resuscitate as necessary and notify physician. Treat CDAD with fluids, electrolytes, protein supplements, and oral vancomycin (Vancocin) or metronidazole (Flagyl) as indicated. In severe cases, surgical evaluation may be indicated. Not removed by peritoneal dialysis or hemodialysis.

ESMOLOL HYDROCHLORIDE
(**EZ**-moh-lohl hy-droh-**KLOR**-eyed)

Beta-adrenergic blocking agent
Antiarrhythmic

Brevibloc

pH 4.5 to 5.5

USUAL DOSE

Supraventricular tachycardia (SVT) or noncompensatory sinus tachycardia: Administer by continuous IV infusion with or without a loading dose. Additional loading doses and/or titration of the maintenance infusion (stepwise dosing) may be necessary based on desired ventricular response.

Esmolol Stepwise Dosing for Supraventricular Tachycardia or Noncompensatory Sinus Tachycardia	
Step	Action
1	Optional loading dose (500 mcg/kg over 1 minute), then 50 mcg/kg/min for 4 min
2	Optional loading dose if necessary, then 100 mcg/kg/min for 4 min
3	Optional loading dose if necessary, then 150 mcg/kg/min for 4 min
4	If necessary, increase dose to 200 mcg/kg/min

In the absence of loading doses, continuous infusion of a single concentration of esmolol reaches a pharmacokinetic and pharmacodynamic steady-state in about 30 minutes. Effective maintenance dose for continuous and stepwise dosing is 50 to 200 mcg/kg/min, although doses as low as 25 mcg/kg/min have been adequate. Doses greater than 200 mcg/kg/min provide little additional lowering of heart rate, and the rate of adverse reactions increases. Maintenance infusions may be continued for up to 48 hours. See Precautions/Monitor.

Intraoperative and postoperative tachycardia and/or hypertension: *Immediate control:* 1 mg/kg over 30 seconds. Follow with an infusion of 150 mcg/kg/min (0.15 mg/kg/min) if necessary. Adjust as required to maintain desired HR and/or BP.

Gradual control: Use procedure listed for SVT.

Immediate and gradual control: Higher doses (250 to 300 mcg/kg/min [0.25 to 0.3 mg/kg/min]) may be required to control hypertension. Maintenance infusion doses greater than 200 mcg/kg/min are not recommended for the treatment of tachycardia. They provide little additional lowering of heart rate, and the rate of adverse reactions increases.

Transition to alternative drugs: After control of HR and BP is achieved and clinical status is stable,

1. Administer the first dose of the alternative drug. In 30 minutes, reduce the esmolol infusion rate by one half (50%).
2. After administration of the second dose of the alternative drug, monitor patient response carefully. If control is satisfactory and is maintained for 1 hour, discontinue the esmolol infusion.

PEDIATRIC DOSE

See Maternal/Child.

Antiarrhythmic (unlabeled): *Pediatric patients 1 to 12 years of age:* A loading dose of 100 to 500 mcg/kg (0.1 to 0.5 mg/kg) administered over 1 minute. Follow with a maintenance infusion of 25 to 100 mcg/kg/min (0.025 to 0.1 mg/kg/min). Titrate doses upward to response by 50 to 100 mcg/kg/min (0.05 to 0.1 mg/kg/min) at 5- to 10-minute intervals as needed. Dose requirements may be higher than in adults. Doses as high as 1,000 mcg/kg/min have been administered to pediatric patients 1 to 12 years of age.

Antihypertensive (postoperative [unlabeled]): *Pediatric patients 1 to 12 years of age:* A loading dose of 500 mcg/kg (0.5 mg/kg) administered over 1 minute. Follow with a maintenance infusion of 50 to 250 mcg/kg/min (0.05 to 0.25 mg/kg/min). Titrate doses upward 50 to 100 mcg/kg/min (0.05 to 0.1 mg/kg/min) as needed. Titrate to individual desired response. Dose requirements may be higher than in adults. Doses as high as 1,000 mcg/kg/min have been administered to pediatric patients 1 to 12 years of age.

DOSE ADJUSTMENTS

Reduced dose may be required in impaired renal function. No dose adjustment required if the maintenance infusion does not exceed 150 mcg/kg/min for more than 4 hours; no data available for higher doses or longer duration. ▪ No dose adjustment indicated in impaired hepatic function. ▪ Reduction required with transfer to alternate agent; see Monitor. ▪ See Drug/Lab Interactions.

DILUTION

Available premixed as 10 mg/mL in 100 mL NS or as 20 mg/mL in 100 mL NS (double strength). Single-dose vials are available as 100 mg/10 mL and may be given by IV injection without further dilution or may be further diluted in D5W, D5R, D5LR, D5NS, D5/¹/₂NS, NS, LR, ¹/₂NS, or D5W with KCl 40 mEq/L. Premixed solutions have a delivery port and a medication port (for withdrawing the initial bolus only). Ready-to-use vials may be used to administer initial and subsequent boluses.

Storage: Store vials and premix at CRT; protect from freezing and avoid excessive heat. Diluted solution stable at room temperature for 24 hours. If a bolus has been removed from the premixed bag, the bag should be used within 24 hours.

COMPATIBILITY
(Underline Indicates Conflicting Compatibility Information)

Consider any drug NOT listed as compatible to be INCOMPATIBLE until consulting a pharmacist; specific conditions may apply.

Manufacturer lists as **incompatible** with sodium bicarbonate and furosemide and states, "Do not add any additional medications to the bag" (premixed injection).

One source suggests the following **compatibilities:**

Additive: *Not recommended by manufacturer.* Aminophylline, atracurium (Tracrium), heparin, sodium bicarbonate.

Y-site: Amikacin, aminophylline, amiodarone (Nexterone), ampicillin, atracurium (Tracrium), bivalirudin (Angiomax), butorphanol (Stadol), calcium chloride, cefazolin (Ancef), ceftazidime (Fortaz), chloramphenicol (Chloromycetin), cisatracurium (Nimbex), clindamycin (Cleocin), dexmedetomidine (Precedex), diltiazem (Cardizem), dopamine, doripenem (Doribax), enalaprilat (Vasotec IV), erythromycin (Erythrocin), famotidine (Pepcid IV), fenoldopam (Corlopam), fentanyl, gentamicin, heparin, hetastarch in electrolytes (Hextend), hydrocortisone sodium succinate (Solu-Cortef), 6% hydroxyethyl starch (Voluven), insulin (regular), labetalol, linezolid (Zyvox), magnesium sulfate, methyldopate, metronidazole (Flagyl IV), micafungin (Mycamine), midazolam (Versed), morphine, nafcillin (Nallpen), nicardipine (Cardene IV), nitroglycerin IV, nitroprusside sodium, norepinephrine (Levophed), pancuronium, penicillin G potassium, phenytoin (Dilantin), potassium chloride (KCl), potassium phosphates, propofol (Diprivan), ranitidine (Zantac), remifentanil (Ultiva), sodium acetate, streptomycin, sulfamethoxazole/trimethoprim, tacrolimus (Prograf), tobramycin, vancomycin, vecuronium.

RATE OF ADMINISTRATION

IV injection: See Usual Dose.

Infusion: Titrate infusion according to procedure outlined in Usual Dose.

ACTIONS

A short-acting, B₁-selective adrenergic blocking agent with antiarrhythmic effects. Decreases HR and BP in a dose-related titratable manner. Hemodynamically similar to propranolol, but vascular resistance is not increased. Onset of action occurs within 1 to 2 minutes. Half-life is approximately 9 minutes, and the effects last about 20 to 30 minutes. Metabolized via esterases in RBCs and excreted in urine.

INDICATIONS AND USES

Management of supraventricular tachycardia (atrial fibrillation or atrial flutter) in situations requiring short-term control of ventricular rate with a short-acting agent (perioperative, postoperative, or other emergent circumstances). ▪ Management of noncompensatory tachycardia when HR requires specific intervention. ▪ Management of intraoperative and postoperative tachycardia and/or hypertension.

Limitation of use: Intended only for short-term use.

CONTRAINDICATIONS

Cardiogenic shock. ▪ Decompensated heart failure. ▪ Heart block greater than first degree. ▪ Hypersensitivity reactions, including anaphylaxis, to esmolol or any of its inactive ingredients (cross-sensitivity between beta-blockers is possible). ▪ IV administration of cardiodepressant calcium-channel antagonists (e.g., verapamil) and esmolol in close proximity (i.e., while the cardiac effects of the other drug are still present). ▪ Pulmonary hypertension. ▪ Severe sinus bradycardia. ▪ Sick sinus syndrome.

PRECAUTIONS

For IV use only. ▪ May cause hypotension at any dose but is dose related; risk is increased in patients with hemodynamic compromise, in patients receiving interacting medications, and with doses above 200 mcg/kg/min. Severe reactions may include loss of consciousness, cardiac arrest, and death. ▪ Use caution in patients with first-degree AV block, sinus node dysfunction, or conduction disorders. May be at increased risk for bradycardia. Sinus pause, heart block, severe bradycardia, and cardiac arrest have occurred. ▪ May further depress cardiac contractility and precipitate heart failure and cardiogenic shock. ▪ Use caution in patients whose BP is primarily driven by vasoconstriction associated with hypothermia (e.g., intraoperative and postoperative tachycardia and hypertension). ▪ Use with extreme caution in patients with reactive airway disease (e.g., asthma), diabetes mellitus and/or hypoglycemia, Prinzmetal's angina, pheochromocytoma, hypovolemia, peripheral circulatory disorders (Raynaud's disease, peripheral occlusive vascular disease), coronary artery disease, impaired renal function, metabolic acidosis, and hyperthyroidism. ▪ In general, patients with reactive airway disease (e.g., asthma) should not receive beta-blockers. Titrate to the lowest possible effective dose. ▪ In patients with hypoglycemia or diabetes who are receiving insulin or hypoglycemic agents, beta-blockers may mask tachycardia of hypoglycemia, but other manifestations of hypoglycemia such as dizziness and sweating may still be observed. ▪ May exacerbate angina attacks in patients with Prinzmetal's angina; do not use nonselective beta-blockers (e.g., propranolol). ▪ A paradoxical increase in BP may occur if beta-blockers are administered to patients with pheochromocytoma. If use is necessary, administer an alpha-blocker (e.g., phentolamine) before the beta-blocker. ▪ Can worsen reflex tachycardia and increase the risk of hypotension in hypovolemic patients. ▪ May increase serum potassium levels, causing hyperkalemia. Risk is increased in patients with renal impairment and is potentially life threatening in hemodialysis patients. ▪ Use caution in patients with metabolic acidosis; hyperkalemic renal tubular acidosis has been reported. ▪ Beta-adrenergic blockade may mask the clinical signs of hyperthyroidism (e.g., tachycardia). Abrupt withdrawal may precipitate thyroid storm. ▪ Patients at risk for hypersensitivity reactions may be more reactive to allergen exposure when receiving beta-blockers and may be unresponsive to the usual doses of epinephrine used to treat anaphylactic or anaphylactoid reactions; see Drug/Lab Interactions. ▪ Infusion site reactions, including irritation, inflammation, and severe reactions (e.g., thrombophlebitis, necrosis, and blistering), have occurred; avoid infusion into small veins or through a butterfly catheter. ▪ Although it has not been a problem with esmolol, it is recommended that the dose of beta-adrenergic blockers be reduced gradually to avoid rebound angina, MI, or ventricular arrhythmias. Use caution, especially in patients with coronary artery disease. ▪ Intended for short-term use only. Transfer to an alternative antiarrhythmic agent (e.g., digoxin [Lanoxin], verapamil) is required after stable clinical status and HR control are obtained; see Usual Dose. ▪ See Drug/Lab Interactions, Monitor, and Antidote.

Monitor: Continuous observation of the patient and ECG and BP monitoring are mandatory during administration. Hypotension should reverse within 30 minutes after decreasing the infusion rate or discontinuing the drug. ▪ Avoid infusion into small veins or through a butterfly catheter. Well tolerated if administered through a central vein. Monitor for infusion site reaction and prevent extravasation. Restart at an alternate infusion site. ▪ Titrate BP slowly in patients whose BP is primarily driven by vasoconstriction associated with hypothermia (e.g., intraoperative and postoperative tachycardia and hypertension). ▪ May mask symptoms of hypoglycemia; monitor blood glucose in patients with diabetes. ▪ Monitor electrolyes as indicated. Monitor patients with increased risk factors very closely; see Precautions. ▪ See Drug/Lab Interactions and Contraindications.

Maternal/Child: Category C: safety for use in pregnancy not established. Use only when clearly indicated. ▪ Discontinue breast-feeding. ▪ Safety and effectiveness for use in pediatric patients not established.

Elderly: Numbers in clinical studies are insufficient to determine if the elderly respond differently from younger subjects. Consider age-related organ impairment (e.g., bone marrow reserve, renal, hepatic); monitor and reduce dose if indicated.

DRUG/LAB INTERACTIONS

The effects of esmolol on BP, contractility, and impulse propagation can be increased with concomitant use of other drugs that can lower BP, reduce myocardial contractility, or interfere with sinus node function or electrical impulse propagation in the myocardium. May result in severe hypotension, cardiac failure, severe bradycardia, sinus pause, sinoatrial block, atrioventricular block, and/or cardiac arrest. ▪ **Sympathomimetic drugs having beta-adrenergic agonist activity** (e.g., epinephrine [Adrenalin], norepinephrine [Levophed]) will counteract the effects of esmolol. ▪ Use with **calcium channel blockers** (e.g., verapamil) may potentiate both drugs and result in severe depression of myocardium and AV conduction, severe hypotension, and fatal cardiac arrest. ▪ Increases **digoxin** blood levels, synergistic with digoxin; both drugs slow AV conduction. Concomitant use increases the risk of bradycardia. ▪ Esmolol should not be used in patients receiving **vasoconstrictive or inotropic drugs** (e.g., norepinephrine [Levophed], digoxin) because of the potential for reduced cardiac contractility when the systemic vascular resistance is high. ▪ Concomitant use with certain **antihypertensive agents** (e.g., clonidine [Catapres], guanfacine [Intuniv]) may precipitate increased withdrawal effects (withdrawal rebound hypertension). If antihypertensive therapy is to be interrupted or discontinued, discontinue the beta-blocker first and then gradually discontinue the antihypertensive agent. ▪ Concomitant use with **catecholamine-depleting drugs** (e.g., reserpine) may produce additive effects. Monitor for hypotension and bradycardia. ▪ May prolong neuromuscular blockade produced by **succinylcholine** and moderately prolong neuromuscular blockade producd by **mivacurium** (Mivacron). ▪ May mask S/S of developing hypoglycemia in patients on **insulin or oral antidiabetic agents.** ▪ Concurrent use with **xanthines** (e.g., aminophylline, theophyllines) may result in mutual inhibition of therapeutic effects. ▪ Patients taking **beta-blockers** who are exposed to a potential allergen may be unresponsive to the usual dose of epinephrine used to treat a hypersensitivity reaction.

SIDE EFFECTS

Symptomatic hypotension (dizziness, excessive sweating) and asymptomatic hypotension are most common. Inflammation or induration of the infusion site, nausea, and somnolence are also fairly common. Abdominal discomfort, abnormal thinking, agitation, anxiety, confusional state, constipation, convulsions (with one death), depression, dry mouth, dyspepsia, flushing, headache, light-headedness, pallor, paresthesia, peripheral ischemia, speech disorders, syncope, urinary retention, and vomiting have occurred.

Overdose: Cardiac effects (e.g., atrioventricular block [first-, second-, third-degree], bradycardia, cardiac failure [including cardiogenic shock], decreased cardiac contractility, hypotension, intraventricular conduction delays, junctional rhythms, cardiac arrest/asystole, and pulseless electrical activity); CNS effects (e.g., fatigue, lethargy, respiratory depression, seizures, sleep and mood disturbances, and coma). In addition, bronchospasm, hyperkalemia, hypoglycemia (especially in children), mesenteric ischemia, and peripheral cyanosis may occur.

Post-Marketing: Angioedema, cardiac arrest, coronary arteriospasm, psoriasis, urticaria.

ANTIDOTE

Notify the physician of all side effects. Decrease rate or discontinue drug if hypotension occurs. Hypotension should reverse within 30 minutes. Trendelenburg position may be appropriate. May require treatment with IV fluids or vasopressors (e.g., dopamine, norepinephrine [Levophed]), but protracted severe hypotension may result. Unresponsive hypotension and bradycardia may be reversed by glucagon 5 to 10 mg over 30 seconds followed by a continuous infusion of 5 mg/hr. Reduce rate as condition improves. Decrease rate of or discontinue esmolol if severe bradycardia develops. Treat with an anticholinergic drug (e.g., atropine) or cardiac pacing. Discontinue esmolol at the first S/S of cardiac failure and start supportive treatment (e.g., digoxin and diuretics). In shock resulting from inadequate cardiac contractility, consider IV dobutamine or dopamine. Glucagon may be useful. Discontinue the infusion if bronchospasm occurs. Administer a beta$_2$-stimulating agent (e.g., epinephrine, albuterol) and/or a theophylline derivative and monitor ventricular rate. Treat other side effects symptomatically and resuscitate as necessary.

ESOMEPRAZOLE SODIUM
(es-oh-**MEP**-rah-zohl **SO**-dee-um)

Proton pump inhibitor
(gastric acid inhibitor) (PPI)

Nexium IV

pH 9 to 11

USUAL DOSE

GERD with erosive esophagitis: Given as an alternative to oral therapy. Resume oral therapy as soon as practical. Safety and efficacy of IV use for more than 10 days not established. Dose and serum levels similar by IV or oral route.

Adults: 20 or 40 mg as an IV injection or infusion once daily for up to 10 days.

Risk reduction for rebleeding of gastric or duodenal ulcers following therapeutic endoscopy in adults: 80 mg as an IV infusion over 30 minutes followed by a continuous infusion of 8 mg/hr for 71.5 hours (a total treatment duration of 72 hours). Therapy is for management of the acute initial bleeding of gastric or duodenal ulcers and does not constitute full treatment. Follow with oral acid-suppressive therapy.

PEDIATRIC DOSE

GERD with erosive esophagitis: Administered as an infusion over 10 to 30 minutes. See comments under Usual Dose.

1 to 17 years of age: WEIGHT LESS THAN 55 KG: 10 mg. WEIGHT 55 KG OR MORE: 20 mg.

1 month to less than 1 year of age: 0.5 mg/kg.

DOSE ADJUSTMENTS

GERD with erosive esophagitis: No dose adjustment is required based on age or gender, in the elderly, in patients with renal insufficiency, or in patients with mild to moderate liver impairment (Child-Pugh Classes A and B). ■ Do not exceed a dose of 20 mg in patients with severe liver impairment (Child-Pugh Class C [10 or over]).

Risk reduction for rebleeding of gastric or duodenal ulcers following therapeutic endoscopy in adults: No adjustment of the initial 80-mg dose is required. Reduce the continuous infusion rate to a maximum of 6 mg/hr for patients with mild to moderate liver impairment (Child-Pugh Classes A and B) and to a maximum of 4 mg/hr for patients with severe liver impairment (Child-Pugh Class C). Do not exceed these maximum doses.

DILUTION
GERD with erosive esophagitis:
Injection (adults): Each 20- or 40-mg dose must be reconstituted with 5 mL of NS. A single dose equals 5 mL. Mix gently until powder is dissolved.

Infusion (adult and pediatric patients 1 month to less than 1 year of age): To determine the vial size needed for patients 1 month to less than 1 year of age, first calculate the dose (0.5 mg/kg). Reconstitute a 20- or 40-mg vial with 5 mL of NS, D5W, or LR. Further dilute to a final volume of 50 mL with NS. Withdraw desired dose to administer as an infusion.

40-MG VIAL: Concentration is 0.8 mg/mL; withdraw 25 mL for a 20-mg dose and 12.5 mL for a 10-mg dose. **20-MG VIAL:** Concentration is 0.4 mg/mL. For a 20-mg dose, administer 50 mL as an infusion. For a 10-mg dose, withdraw 25 mL and administer as an infusion. Adjust infusion amount as needed to provide the correct dose (0.5 mg/kg) for pediatric patients 1 month to less than 1 year of age.

Risk reduction for rebleeding of gastric or duodenal ulcers following therapeutic endoscopy in adults:
30-minute infusion: Two 40-mg vials required for the 80-mg dose. Reconstitute each 40-mg vial with 5 mL of NS and add contents of both vials to 100 mL of NS.
Continuous infusion: Two 40-mg vials required. Reconstitute each 40-mg vial with 5 mL of NS and add contents of both vials to 100 mL of NS. Administer at a rate of 8 mg/hr for 71.5 hours; see Dose Adjustments.

Filters: Not required or recommended; no additional data available from manufacturer.
Storage: Before use, store in carton at CRT and protect from light. Reconstituted and diluted solutions may be stored at CRT. Administer reconstituted solutions within 12 hours of reconstitution. Administer diluted solutions within 6 hours if diluted in D5W and within 12 hours if diluted in NS or LR. Discard any unused solution.

COMPATIBILITY
Consider any drug NOT listed as compatible to be INCOMPATIBLE until consulting a pharmacist; specific conditions may apply.
Manufacturer states, "Should not be administered concomitantly with any other medications through the same IV site and/or tubing." Flush the IV line with a **compatible** IV solution (NS, LR, or D5W) before and after administration of esomeprazole.

One source suggests the following **compatibilities** *(not recommended by manufacturer):*
Y-site: Ceftaroline (Teflaro), doripenem (Doribax).

RATE OF ADMINISTRATION
Flush the IV line with a **compatible** IV solution (NS, LR, or D5W) before and after administration of esomeprazole.

GERD with erosive esophagitis: *Injection (adults):* A single 20- or 40-mg dose evenly distributed over no less than 3 minutes.
Infusion (adults and pediatric patients): A single dose properly diluted as an infusion and evenly distributed over 10 to 30 minutes.
Risk reduction for rebleeding of gastric or duodenal ulcers following therapeutic endoscopy in adults: *Initial dose:* A single 80-mg dose evenly distributed over 30 minutes.
Continuous infusion: Administer at a rate of 8 mg/hr over 71.5 hours; see Dose Adjustments.

ACTIONS
A proton pump inhibitor. It suppresses gastric acid secretion by specific inhibition of the H^+/K^+-ATPase in the gastric parietal cell. It blocks the final step in acid production, thus reducing gastric acidity. Effect is dose-related. Highly bound to serum protein. Extensively metabolized in the liver by the cytochrome P_{450} isoenzyme system (CYP2C19 and CYP3A4 isozymes). Half-life is 1.1 to 1.4 hours and is prolonged with increasing doses. Primarily excreted as metabolites in urine with some excretion in feces. Secreted in breast milk.

INDICATIONS AND USES

Short-term treatment of GERD with erosive esophagitis in adults and pediatric patients 1 month to 17 years of age. Used as an alternative to oral therapy when oral esomeprazole is not possible or appropriate. ▪ Risk reduction for rebleeding in patients following therapeutic endoscopy for acute bleeding of gastric or duodenal ulcers in adults.

CONTRAINDICATIONS

Known hypersensitivity to esomeprazole (Nexium) or other substituted benzimidazoles (e.g., omeprazole [Prilosec], pantoprazole [Protonix]) or to any component of the formulation.

PRECAUTIONS

For IV use only; do not give IM or SC. ▪ Gastric malignancy may be present even though patient's symptoms improve. ▪ Discontinue as soon as the patient is able to resume oral therapy. ▪ Atrophic gastritis has been reported with long-term treatment of omeprazole, an enantiomer (a compound with a mirror image molecular structure) of esomeprazole. ▪ Decreased gastric acidity may increase bacterial count in GI tract. Risk of GI infections (e.g., *Salmonella* and *Campylobacter* and, in hospitalized patients, *Clostridium difficile*) may be slightly increased. ▪ May be associated with an increased risk for osteoporosis-related fractures of the hip, wrist, or spine. Risk increased in patients receiving high-dose (multiple daily doses) and long-term therapy (a year or longer). Use lowest dose and shortest duration of therapy appropriate for the condition being treated. ▪ Hypomagnesemia, both symptomatic and asymptomatic, has been reported rarely (usually with the use of PPIs for 3 months to more than a year). Arrhythmias, seizures, and tetany have occurred. Magnesium replacement and discontinuation of esomeprazole may be required. ▪ May be associated with an increased risk of *Clostridium difficile*–associated diarrhea (CDAD). Consider in patients who develop diarrhea that does not improve. ▪ Acute interstitial nephritis has been observed, is generally attributed to an idiopathic hypersensitivity reaction, and may occur at any time during therapy. Discontinue esomeprazole if it occurs. ▪ Use caution in transplant patients receiving mycophenolate mofetil (CellCept). ▪ See Drug/Lab Interactions.

Monitor: Observe for S/S of a hypersensitivity reaction (e.g., anaphylaxis, anaphylactic shock, angioedema, bronchospasm, acute interstitial nephritis, urticaria). ▪ Monitor vital signs, pain levels, and injection site. ▪ Consider obtaining baseline and periodic magnesium levels if prolonged therapy is indicated or in patients taking digoxin or medications that may cause hypomagnesemia (e.g., diuretics).

Patient Education: Review prescription and nonprescription drugs with physician. ▪ Oral route preferred. ▪ Promptly report cardiovascular or neurologic symptoms, including dizziness, palpitations, seizures, or tetany; may be signs of hypomagnesemia.

Maternal/Child: Category C: use during pregnancy only if the potential benefit justifies the potential risk to the fetus. ▪ Esomeprazole may be secreted in human milk; use with caution during breast-feeding. May have serious reactions in the infant and has a potential for tumorigenicity. ▪ Safety and effectiveness for use of IV formulation in pediatric patients established for ages 1 month to 17 years. Safety and effectiveness for use in neonates (0 to 1 month of age) not established.

Elderly: Safety and effectiveness similar to that seen in younger adults. ▪ Consider potential for impaired liver function; see Dose Adjustments.

DRUG/LAB INTERACTIONS

Extensively metabolized by CYP2C19 and CYP3A4. ▪ Because of profound and long-lasting inhibition of gastric acid secretion, esomeprazole may interfere with the absorption of drugs in which gastric pH is an important determinant of their bioavailability. Absorption of **atazanavir** (Reyataz), **erlotinib** (Tarceva), **iron salts** (ferrous sulfate), **ketoconazole** (Nizoral), and **mycophenolate mofetil** (CellCept) can decrease; other drugs (e.g., digoxin [Lanoxin]) can increase. Coadministration of **mycophenolate mofetil** (MMF) and **omeprazole** (Prilosec) in transplant patients receiving MMF reduces the exposure to MMF's active metabolite, mycophenolic acid; see Precautions. ▪ Increases in INR and PT have been reported when administered concurrently with **warfarin;** monitoring of INR and PT indicated. ▪ Concurrent use with **selected protease inhibitors** such as atazanavir (Reyataz) and nelfinavir (Viracept) is not recommended. Coadministration of proton pump inhibitors (e.g., esomeprazole [Nexium], pantoprazole [Protonix]) results in a significant reduction in plasma concentrations of atazanavir and nelfinavir, thus inhibiting their therapeutic effect. In contrast, elevated plasma concentrations have been reported with **other protease inhibitors** (e.g., saquinavir [Invirase]); monitoring of serum levels is recommended to avoid toxicity of the antiviral agent, and dose reduction should be considered. Unchanged serum levels have been reported with some other antiretroviral drugs. ▪ The metabolism of **diazepam** (Valium) may be decreased and serum levels increased by esomeprazole; not considered clinically significant. ▪ Administration with a **combined inhibitor of CYP2C19 and CYP3A4** (e.g., voriconazole [VFEND]) may more than double the exposure (concentration) of esomeprazole. With recommended doses of esomeprazole, a dose adjustment is not normally required; however, it may be indicated in patients who require higher doses. ▪ Concurrent administration of **oral contraceptives, diazepam, phenytoin, or quinidine** did not change the pharmacokinetic profile of esomeprazole. ▪ Drugs that **induce CYP2C19 or CYP3A4** (e.g., rifampin [Rifadin], St. John's wort) can substantially decrease esomeprazole concentrations. Avoid concomitant use. ▪ Concomitant administration of esomeprazole and **tacrolimus** may increase serum levels of tacrolimus. ▪ Concurrent administration with **naproxen** (Aleve) did not appear to alter pharmacokinetics in either drug. ▪ Studies suggest no clinically significant interactions with other drugs metabolized by the cytochrome P_{450} system (e.g., amoxicillin, clarithromycin [Biaxin], phenytoin [Dilantin], quinidine). ▪ Avoid concurrent use with **clopidogrel** (Plavix); esomeprazole may interfere with the conversion of clopidogrel into its active form and decrease its effectiveness. ▪ Coadministration with **cilostazol** (Pletal) may increase concentrations of cilostazol and its metabolite. Consider a dose reduction of cilostazol from 100 mg to 50 mg twice daily. ▪ Concomitant use of proton pump inhibitors with high-dose **methotrexate** may elevate and prolong serum levels of methotrexate and/or its metabolite. May lead to methotrexate toxicity; consider withdrawal of esomeprazole. ▪ Serum chromogranin A (CgA) levels increase secondary to drug-induced decreases in gastric acidity. Increased CgA levels may cause a false-positive result in diagnostic tests for neuroendocrine tumors. Temporarily discontinue esomeprazole at least 14 days before assessing CgA levels, and consider repeating the test (using the same commercial laboratory) if the initial CgA level is high.

SIDE EFFECTS
GERD with erosive esophagitis: Generally well tolerated. Most commonly reported side effects include abdominal pain, constipation, diarrhea, dizziness, dry mouth, flatulence, headache, injection site pain or reaction, nausea, and pruritus. Numerous other side effects may occur in fewer than 1% of patients.
Risk reduction for rebleeding of gastric or duodenal ulcers following therapeutic endoscopy in adults: In addition to the side effects listed under GERD, cough, duodenal ulcer hemorrhage, fever, and injection site reaction, including erythema, phlebitis, superficial phlebitis, swelling, and thrombophlebitis, have been reported.
Post-Marketing: Agranulocytosis, alopecia, anaphylaxis (rare), blurred vision, bone fracture, CDAD, depression, hypomagnesemia, microscopic colitis, myalgia, pancreatitis, pancytopenia, hepatitis with or without jaundice (rare), serious dermatologic reactions (including erythema multiforme, Stevens-Johnson syndrome, and toxic epidermal necrolysis [some fatal]), and shock.
Overdose: Ataxia, changes in respiratory frequency, decreased motor activity, intermittent clonic convulsions. Consider possibility of multiple drug ingestion.

ANTIDOTE
Keep physician informed of all side effects. May be treated symptomatically. If hypomagnesemia develops, magnesium replacement and discontinuation of esomeprazole may be required. Discontinue esomeprazole if acute interstitial nephritis occurs. Discontinue and initiate appropriate treatment if hypersensitivity reactions, S/S associated with post-marketing reports, or overdose occur; see Side Effects. Not removed by hemodialysis.

ETOMIDATE
(eh-**TOM**-ih-dayt)

Amidate

USUAL DOSE

Rapid sequence intubation and/or induction of anesthesia: Dose must be individualized. 0.3 mg/kg IV (range: 0.2 to 0.6 mg/kg). Titrate to effect. Smaller, incremental doses may be administered to adult patients during short operative procedures to supplement subpotent anesthetic agents, such as nitrous oxide.

Anesthesia induction for short outpatient or ER procedures (unlabeled): 0.1 mg/kg has been used effectively. If analgesia is required, concurrent administration of fentanyl may be used.

PEDIATRIC DOSE

Rapid sequence intubation and/or induction of anesthesia: *Pediatric patients up to 10 years of age:* Safety and effectiveness have not been established.

Pediatric patients 10 years of age and older: See Usual Dose.

Anesthesia induction for short outpatient or emergency department procedures (unlabeled): 0.1 mg/kg. 0.2 mg/kg has been used in pediatric patients for fractures or major joint reduction. If analgesia is required, concurrent administration of fentanyl may be used.

DOSE ADJUSTMENTS

Dose must be individualized for each patient. ▪ Caution and lower-end dosing suggested in the elderly; consider decreased organ function and concomitant disease or drug therapy. ▪ See Drug/Lab Interactions.

DILUTION

May be given undiluted. Solution must be clear.

Filters: No data available from manufacturer.

Storage: Store at CRT. Discard unused portion.

COMPATIBILITY

Consider any drug NOT listed as compatible to be INCOMPATIBLE until consulting a pharmacist; specific conditions may apply.

One source suggests the following **compatibilities:**

Y-site: Alfentanil, atracurium (Tracrium), atropine, dexmedetomidine (Precedex), ephedrine, fentanyl, lidocaine, lorazepam (Ativan), midazolam (Versed), morphine, pancuronium, phenylephrine (Neo-Synephrine), succinylcholine, sufentanil (Sufenta).

RATE OF ADMINISTRATION

A single dose equally distributed over 30 to 60 seconds. More-rapid injections may produce hypotension.

ACTIONS

A short-acting, nonbarbiturate hypnotic without analgesic activity. Depending on the dose administered, it can produce all levels of CNS depression, from light sleep to coma. Anesthetic doses can induce loss of consciousness within 60 seconds. Does not cause significant cardiovascular or respiratory depression. Incidence of respiratory depression may be less than with propofol (Diprivan) or barbiturates (e.g., thiopental [Pentothal]). Has little or no effect on myocardial metabolism, cardiac output, peripheral circulation, or pulmonary circulation. Produces a slight increase in $Paco_2$. Does not elevate plasma histamine or cause signs of histamine release. Decreases cerebral blood flow and lowers intracranial pressure. Usually lowers intraocular pressure moderately. Onset of action is within 1 minute. Duration of action is dose dependent, usually 3 to 5 minutes at a dose of 0.3 mg/kg. Metabolized in the liver and excreted primarily in the urine. Half-life is approximately 75 minutes.

INDICATIONS AND USES

Induction of general anesthesia. Useful for short outpatient, dental, and short diagnostic procedures and in high-risk patients. Usefulness of its hemodynamic properties should be weighed against the high frequency of transient skeletal muscle movements. (May be beneficial in patients with cardiopulmonary impairment because of minimal depressant effects and lack of histamine release.) One source suggests it is the intubation agent of choice in trauma and CHF. ▪ Supplementation of subpotent anesthetic agents (such as nitrous oxide in oxygen) during maintenance of anesthesia for short operative procedures such as dilation and curettage or cervical conization.

Unlabeled uses: Emergency department treatment of painful procedures such as abscess drainage, cardioversion, chest tube replacement, dislocation reduction, fracture reduction, foreign body removal.

CONTRAINDICATIONS

Hypersensitivity to etomidate. ▪ Not recommended for use during labor and delivery.

PRECAUTIONS

For IV use only. ▪ Should be administered by or under the direct supervision of persons trained in the administration of general anesthetics and in the management of complications encountered during general anesthesia (e.g., anesthesiologists, emergency department physicians) in a facility with adequate diagnostic and treatment facilities to monitor the patient and respond to any medical emergency. ▪ Induction doses of etomidate have been associated with the reduction of plasma cortisol and aldosterone concentrations that may last for 6 to 8 hours. Because of the hazards of prolonged suppression, etomidate is not intended for administration by prolonged infusion. Exogenous replacement (e.g., methylprednisolone [Solu-Medrol]) should be considered if concern exists for patients undergoing severe stress or for patients undergoing chronic oral corticosteroid therapy (e.g., prednisone).

Monitor: Monitor airway and vital signs. ▪ Monitor injection site. Use of larger, more proximal arm veins is recommended to lessen incidence and severity of pain on injection. Avoid use of wrist or hand veins if possible. ▪ See Precautions and Drug/Lab Interactions.

Patient Education: Avoid alcohol or other CNS depressants (e.g., antihistamines, benzodiazepines) for 24 hours following administration. ▪ Do not perform tasks requiring mental alertness (e.g., driving, operating hazardous machinery) for 24 hours following administration.

Maternal/Child: Category C: safety for use in pregnancy not established; benefit must justify potential risks to fetus; see Contraindications. ▪ Safety for use during breast-feeding not established; effects unknown. Use caution. ▪ Safety and effectiveness for use in pediatric patients under 10 years of age not established.

Elderly: See Dose Adjustments. ▪ May be more sensitive to effects (e.g., decreases in heart rate, cardiac index, and mean arterial BP).

DRUG/LAB INTERACTIONS

Administration of **fentanyl** 0.1 mg before induction with etomidate may shorten immediate recovery period. ▪ May have additive effects with concomitant **anesthetics, sedatives, hypnotics, and/or opiates** (e.g., fentanyl); reduced doses of etomidate may be indicated. ▪ Does not significantly alter the usual dosage requirements of **neuromuscular blocking agents** (e.g., vecuronium, pancuronium). ▪ Administration of **fentanyl or diazepam** before induction with etomidate may help decrease transient skeletal muscle movements. ▪ Succinylcholine-induced arrhythmias may still occur if **succinylcholine** is used in combination with etomidate.

SIDE EFFECTS

The most common adverse reactions are transient venous pain on injection and transient skeletal muscle movements, including myoclonus, averting movements, and eye movements. Less frequently reported side effects include apnea of short duration (5 to 90 seconds with spontaneous recovery), arrhythmia, bradycardia, hiccups and/or snoring (may indicate partial airway obstruction), hypertension, hyperventilation, hypotension, hypoventilation, laryngospasm, postoperative nausea and vomiting, and tachycardia.

ANTIDOTE

Discontinue drug if significant side effects or overdose occur. Support patient. Establish and maintain an airway; administer oxygen with assisted ventilation if needed. Resuscitate as necessary.

ETOPOSIDE BBW

(eh-**TOH**-poh-syd)

Antineoplastic
(mitotic inhibitor)

Etopophos PF, Etoposide Phosphate, VePesid, VP-16-213

pH 2.9 to 4

USUAL DOSE

Testicular cancer: 50 to 100 mg/M^2 daily for 5 days or 100 mg/M^2/day on Days 1, 3, and 5. Repeat at 3- to 4-week intervals. Used in combination with other chemotherapy agents.

Small-cell lung cancer: 35 mg/M^2/day for 4 days to 50 mg/M^2/day for 5 days. Repeat at 3- to 4-week intervals. Used in combination with other chemotherapy agents.

Hematopoietic stem cell transplantation conditioning regimen (unlabeled): 60 mg/kg as a single dose. Used in combination with other agents.

DOSE ADJUSTMENTS

Modify dose if indicated based on myelosuppressive effects of other drugs administered in combination and any previous radiation therapy or chemotherapy (compromised bone marrow reserve). Frequently given in combination with cisplatin, bleomycin, and doxorubicin. ■ Withhold dose if platelets less than 50,000/mm^3 or absolute neutrophil count less than 500/mm^3. Do not restart until adequate recovery. ■ Dose selection should be cautious in the elderly. Reduced doses may be indicated based on potential for decreased organ function and concomitant disease or drug therapy; see Elderly. ■ Reduce dose by 25% if CrCl is 15 to 50 mL/min. Further reduction may be indicated if the CrCl is less than 15 mL/min. One source recommends decreasing dose by 50% if CrCl is less than 10 mL/min. ■ Dose reduction may be required in impaired hepatic function. One source recommends a dose reduction of 50% with a bilirubin of 1.5 to 3 or an AST greater than 3 times the ULN. Use in severe hepatic impairment is contraindicated in the Canadian product labeling.

DILUTION

Specific techniques required; see Precautions.

NONPHOSPHATE PRODUCTS (E.G., VEPESID): Each 100 mg (5 mL) must be diluted in at least 250 mL of D5W or NS and given as an infusion (0.4 mg/mL). 500 mL of solution will yield 0.2 mg/mL. Maximum concentration to prevent precipitation is 0.4 mg/mL. Monitor closely for precipitation from dilution to completion of infusion. Undiluted etoposide has caused acrylic or ABS plastic devices to crack and leak; handle carefully during dilution process.

PHOSPHATE PRODUCT (E.G., ETOPOPHOS): Reconstitute each 100-mg vial with 5 or 10 mL of SWFI, D5W, or NS (with or without benzyl alcohol). 5 mL of diluent will yield 20 mg/mL, 10 mL will yield 10 mg/mL. Further dilute to concentrations as low as 0.1 mg/mL with D5W or NS for administration. A 1-mg/mL solution has a pH of 2.9. The water solubility of Etopophos decreases the potential for precipitation following dilution and during administration.

Storage: *Nonphosphate Products (e.g., VePesid):* May be stored at CRT before dilution. Stable after dilution at CRT for 96 hours (0.2 mg/mL solution) or 24 hours (0.4 mg/mL) in D5W or NS. *Phosphate Products (e.g., Etopophos):* Refrigerate in carton until use. Store reconstituted solutions in glass or plastic containers under refrigeration at 2° to 8° C (36° to 46° F) for 7 days. Solutions reconstituted with nonbacteriostatic diluents may be stored at CRT for up to 24 hours. Solutions reconstituted with bacteriostatic diluents may be stored at CRT for up to 48 hours. Store fully diluted solutions under refrigeration or at CRT for up to 24 hours.

COMPATIBILITY   (Underline Indicates Conflicting Compatibility Information)
Consider any drug NOT listed as compatible to be INCOMPATIBLE until consulting a pharmacist; specific conditions may apply.

NONPHOSPHATE PRODUCTS (E.G., VEPESID)
Hydrolysis may occur in alkaline solutions.
    One source suggests the following **compatibilities:**
Additive: Carboplatin (Paraplatin), cisplatin, fluorouracil (5-FU), ifosfamide (Ifex), mitoxantrone (Novantrone), ondansetron (Zofran); another source adds mesna (Mesnex).
Y-site: Allopurinol (Aloprim), amifostine (Ethyol), aztreonam (Azactam), cladribine (Leustatin), doxorubicin liposomal (Doxil), fludarabine (Fludara), gemcitabine (Gemzar), granisetron (Kytril), melphalan (Alkeran), methotrexate, micafungin (Mycamine), mitoxantrone (Novantrone), ondansetron (Zofran), paclitaxel (Taxol), piperacillin/tazobactam (Zosyn), sargramostim (Leukine), sodium bicarbonate, teniposide (Vumon), thiotepa, topotecan (Hycamtin), vinorelbine (Navelbine).

PHOSPHATE PRODUCTS (E.G., ETOPOPHOS)
One source suggests the following **compatibilities:**
Y-site: Acyclovir (Zovirax), amikacin, aminophylline, ampicillin, ampicillin/sulbactam (Unasyn), anidulafungin (Eraxis), aztreonam (Azactam), bleomycin (Blenoxane), bumetanide, buprenorphine (Buprenex), butorphanol (Stadol), calcium gluconate, carboplatin (Paraplatin), carmustine (BiCNU), caspofungin (Cancidas), cefazolin (Ancef), cefotaxime (Claforan), cefotetan (Cefotan), cefoxitin (Mefoxin), ceftazidime (Fortaz), ceftriaxone (Rocephin), cefuroxime (Zinacef), ciprofloxacin (Cipro IV), cisplatin, clindamycin (Cleocin), cyclophosphamide (Cytoxan), cytarabine (ARA-C), dacarbazine (DTIC), dactinomycin (Cosmegen), daunorubicin (Cerubidine), dexamethasone (Decadron), diphenhydramine (Benadryl), dobutamine, dopamine, doripenem (Doribax), doxorubicin (Adriamycin), doxycycline, droperidol (Inapsine), enalaprilat (Vasotec IV), famotidine (Pepcid IV), fluconazole (Diflucan), fludarabine (Fludara), fluorouracil (5-FU), furosemide (Lasix), ganciclovir (Cytovene IV), gemcitabine (Gemzar), gentamicin, granisetron (Kytril), heparin, hydrocortisone sodium succinate (Solu-Cortef), hydromorphone (Dilaudid), idarubicin (Idamycin), ifosfamide (Ifex), leucovorin calcium, linezolid (Zyvox), lorazepam (Ativan), magnesium sulfate, mannitol, meperidine (Demerol), mesna (Mesnex), methotrexate, metoclopramide (Reglan), metronidazole (Flagyl IV), mitoxantrone (Novantrone), morphine, nalbuphine, ondansetron (Zofran), oxaliplatin (Eloxatin), paclitaxel (Taxol), piperacillin/tazobactam (Zosyn), potassium chloride (KCl), promethazine (Phenergan), ranitidine (Zantac), sodium bicarbonate, streptozocin (Zanosar), sulfamethoxazole/trimethoprim, teniposide (Vumon), thiotepa, ticarcillin/clavulanate (Timentin), tobramycin, vancomycin, vinblastine, vincristine, zidovudine (AZT, Retrovir).

RATE OF ADMINISTRATION
NONPHOSPHATE PRODUCTS (E.G., VEPESID): Total desired dose, properly diluted (0.2 to 0.4 mg/mL) and evenly distributed over at least 30 to 60 minutes. Rapid infusion may cause marked hypotension. May be extended if fluid volume is a concern.
PHOSPHATE PRODUCTS (E.G., ETOPOPHOS): Total desired dose, properly reconstituted and diluted, may be given evenly distributed over as little as 5 minutes or up to 210 minutes. Do not give as a bolus injection.

ACTIONS
A semi-synthetic derivative of podophyllotoxin. A topoisomerase II inhibitor that is cell cycle–specific for the G_2 phase. At high concentrations, it causes lysis of cells entering mitosis. At lower concentrations, cells are inhibited from entering prophase. Appears to

cause DNA strand breaks. Etopophos (phosphate) is a water-soluble ester of etoposide that promptly converts to etoposide in plasma. The pharmacokinetics and pharmacodynamics of etoposide are similar after administration of either the phosphate or non-phosphate products. Half-life is from 4 to 11 hours (average is 7 hours). Highly protein-bound to albumin. Metabolized in the liver. Primarily excreted as unchanged drug or metabolites through urine and bile (feces).

INDICATIONS AND USES

Treatment of refractory testicular tumors (used in combination with other agents after previous surgery, chemotherapy, and radiotherapy). ▪ Treatment of small-cell lung cancer (used in combination with other chemotherapeutic agents as first-line treatment).

Unlabeled uses: Conditioning regimen for hematopoietic cell transplantation. Treatment of acute lymphocytic leukemias (ALL), Hodgkin's lymphoma, non-Hodgkin's lymphomas, carcinoma of the breast, neuroblastoma, Wilms' tumor, and many malignancies. Used alone or in combination with other agents.

CONTRAINDICATIONS

Hypersensitivity to etoposide, etoposide phosphate, or any other component of the formulations.

PRECAUTIONS

Follow guidelines for handling cytotoxic agents. See Appendix A, p. 1331. Always wear impervious gloves when handling vials containing etoposide. If a solution of etoposide contacts the skin, wash the skin immediately and thoroughly with soap and water. If there is contact with mucous membranes, flush thoroughly with water. ▪ For IV infusion only; do not give as a bolus injection. ▪ Usually administered by or under the direction of the physician specialist. ▪ Severe myelosuppression with resulting infection or bleeding may occur. Deaths have been reported. ▪ A low serum albumin may result in an increase of free (active) etoposide, resulting in an increased risk of toxicity. Occurs more frequently in pediatric patients. ▪ Hypersensitivity reactions have been reported. Higher-than-recommended concentration, the presence of polysorbate 80, and a rapid rate of infusion may contribute to the development of these reactions. ▪ A potential carcinogen; acute leukemia with or without a preleukemic phase has been rarely reported. ▪ Use with caution in hepatic or renal impairment; see Dose Adjustments. ▪ Oral dose of nonphosphate product (e.g., etoposide) is usually twice the IV dose.

Monitor: Determine absolute patency and quality of vein and adequate circulation of extremity. Avoid extravasation; may result in cellulitis, pain, swelling, and necrosis. ▪ Obtain baseline CBC with differential and platelets. Monitor before each dose and between courses. See Dose Adjustments. ▪ Monitor vital signs during infusion. ▪ Examine patient's mouth for ulceration before each dose. ▪ Monitor hepatic and renal function before and during therapy. ▪ Bone marrow recovery from a course is usually complete within 21 days. No cumulative toxicity has been reported as yet. ▪ Be alert for signs of bone marrow suppression or infection. ▪ Monitor for S/S of hypersensitivity reactions (e.g., bronchospasm, chills, dyspnea, fever, hypotension, pruritus, rash, tachycardia, urticaria). ▪ Monitor for thrombocytopenia (platelet count less than $50,000/mm^3$). Initiate precautions to prevent excessive bleeding (e.g., inspect IV sites, skin, and mucous membranes; use extreme care during invasive procedures; test urine, emesis, stool, and secretions for occult blood). ▪ Prophylactic antibiotics may be indicated pending results of C/S in a febrile neutropenic patient. ▪ Maintain adequate hydration. ▪ Prophylactic antiemetics may increase patient comfort.

Patient Education: Female patients should use effective contraception during treatment and for at least 6 months after the final dose. Males with female sexual partners of reproductive potential should use condoms during treatment and for at least 4 months after the final dose. ▪ Report IV site burning or stinging promptly. ▪ Report chills, difficult breathing, fever, and rapid heartbeat promptly. See Appendix D, p. 1333.

Maternal/Child: Category D: avoid pregnancy. Can cause fetal harm. ▪ May cause infertility. In male patients, may result in oligospermia, azoospermia, and permanent loss of fertility. May damage spermatozoa and testicular tissue, resulting in possible genetic fetal abnormalities. In female patients, may cause infertility and result in amenorrhea and premature menopause; see Patient Education. ▪ Discontinue breast-feeding. ▪ Has been used in pediatric patients, but safety and effectiveness not established. Anaphylactic reactions have been reported. Higher rates of anaphylactic-like reactions have occurred in pediatric patients who have received infusions of etoposide at higher-than-recommended concentrations. See Precautions. ▪ Depending on the preparation, VePesid may contain benzyl alcohol or polysorbate 80.

Elderly: Monitor renal, hepatic, and hematologic function closely. ▪ See Dose Adjustments. ▪ Incidence of anorexia, asthenia, dehydration, elevated BUN levels, granulocytopenia, leukopenia (Grade III or IV), mucositis, and somnolence occur more frequently in the elderly. ▪ May also be more sensitive to expected side effects (e.g., alopecia, gastrointestinal effects, infectious complications, and myelosuppression). Potential for greater sensitivity increased if renal function impaired.

DRUG/LAB INTERACTIONS

All products: Concurrent or consecutive use with other **bone marrow suppressants** (e.g., bleomycin, cisplatin, doxorubicin) **and/or radiation therapy** may produce additive bone marrow suppression. See Dose Adjustments. ▪ Do not administer **live virus vaccines** to patients receiving antineoplastic drugs. ▪ Clearance decreased and toxicity increased by **cyclosporine.** ▪ May potentiate **warfarin;** monitor PT/INR. ▪ Concomitant use of **antiepileptic medications**, including phenytoin, phenobarbital, carbamazepine, and valproic acid, is associated with increased clearance and reduced efficacy of etoposide.

PHOSPHATE PRODUCT (E.G., ETOPOPHOS): Use caution with drugs that are **known to inhibit phosphatase activities** (e.g., levamisole [Ergamisol]).

SIDE EFFECTS

Bone marrow toxicity (e.g., leukopenia, neutropenia, thrombocytopenia) can be severe, is dose related, and may be dose limiting. Side effects are usually reversible: abdominal pain, alopecia, anaphylactic-like reactions (bronchospasm, chills, diaphoresis, dyspnea, facial flushing, fever, hypertension or hypotension, pruritus, rash, tachycardia), anemia, anorexia, asthenia, back pain, constipation, coughing, cyanosis, diarrhea, dizziness, elevated liver function tests (e.g., AST, ALT), facial/tongue swelling, hepatic toxicity, hypertension, hypotension, interstitial pneumonitis/pulmonary fibrosis, laryngospasm, local soft tissue toxicity following extravasation, malaise, mucositis, nausea, neuritic pain, paralytic ileus, peripheral neurotoxicity, radiation recall dermatitis, seizures, Stevens-Johnson syndrome, stomatitis, taste alteration, thrombophlebitis, toxic epidermal necrolysis, urticaria, vomiting. Hepatic toxicity and metabolic acidosis have occurred with higher-than-recommended doses.

ANTIDOTE

Notify the physician of all side effects; symptomatic treatment is often indicated, and dose reduction or discontinuation may be necessary. For extravasation, discontinue the drug immediately and administer into another vein. No specific treatment for extravasation is recommended. Hypotension is usually due to a rapid infusion rate. Discontinue infusion. Trendelenburg position and IV fluids should reverse the hypotension; vasopressors (e.g., dopamine) may be required. After recovery, restart at slower rate. Administration of whole blood products (e.g., packed RBCs, platelets, leukocytes) and/or blood modifiers (e.g., darbepoetin alfa [Aranesp], epoetin alfa [Epogen], filgrastim [Neupogen, Zarxio], pegfilgrastim [Neulasta], sargramostim [Leukine]) may be indicated to treat bone marrow toxicity. Discontinue infusion at the first sign of a hypersensitivity reaction; antihistamines, corticosteroids, pressor agents, or volume expanders may be indicated. Resuscitate as necessary.

FACTOR IX (HUMAN) ▪ FACTOR IX COMPLEX (HUMAN)

Antihemorrhagic

(**FAK**-tor 9)

AlphaNine SD, Mononine ▪ **Bebulin VH, Profilnine SD**

pH 7 to 7.4 ▪ pH 7 to 7.4

USUAL DOSE

(International units [IU])

ALL FORMULATIONS

Completely individualized based on patient's circumstances, condition, degree of deficiency, and desired blood level percentage. Specific products may be indicated or preferred in some situations; see Indications and Uses. Range is 10 to 75 international units (IU)/kg of body weight. May be repeated every 12 hours in some situations, required only every 2 or 3 days in others. Actual number of international units contained shown on each bottle or vial. Units required to raise blood level percentages can be calculated as follows:

Body weight (kg) × Desired increase (% of normal) × 1 Unit/kg

(70 kg × 40% increase × 1 IU/kg = 2,800 IU). To maintain levels above 25%, calculate each dose to raise level to 40% to 60% of normal.

Minor hemorrhage: A single injection calculated to increase plasma level to 20% to 30%. May be repeated in 24 hours if indicated.

Major trauma or surgery: Increase plasma level to 25% to 50% and maintain at that level for a minimum of 1 week or as indicated. May require daily injections (every 18 to 30 hours).

Dental extraction: Increase plasma level to 50% before procedure; repeat if indicated.

Prophylaxis: 10 to 20 IU/kg once or twice a week or increase plasma level to 20% to 30%.

FACTOR IX COMPLEX

Reversal of coumarin effect: 15 IU/kg.

DILUTION

Diluent usually provided. Some preparations also supply double-ended needles for dilution and filter needle for aspiration into a syringe. Sterile technique imperative. Confirm expiration date. Use plastic syringes to prevent binding to glass surfaces. Factor IX and diluent should be at room temperature. Direct diluent from above to side of vial to gently moisten all contents. Swirl gently to dissolve; avoid foaming. Do not shake. May take 1 to 5 minutes. Should be clear and colorless. Must be used within 3 hours to avoid bacterial contamination. The addition of 2 to 3 units of heparin/mL factor IX complex may reduce the incidence of thrombosis. May be given through an IV administration set (often provided) if multiple vials are required. Discard any unused contents. Discard all administration equipment after single use; do not attempt to resterilize.

AlphaNine SD: Follow general directions above. After diluent is drawn through double-ended needle, remove diluent bottle first; then remove double-ended needle. *Do not invert concentrate vial until ready to withdraw contents!* Air from syringe into vial required to withdraw contents. Withdraw through filter.

Mononine: Follow general directions listed previously. After diluent is drawn through double-ended needle, remove diluent bottle first; then remove double-ended needle. *Use only the provided self-venting filter spike to transfer Mononine to a syringe! Do not inject any air into Mononine vial; could cause product loss.* Discard filter and use only provided wing needle and micropore tubing to administer.

Filters: Usually supplied by manufacturer. If more than one vial is required for a dose, multiple vials may be drawn into the same syringe; however, a new filter needle must be used to withdraw the contents of each vial of factor IX and/or factor IX complex (Human). Manufacturers of **AlphaNine SD** and **Mononine** provide a filter needle, which is to be used to withdraw reconstituted solution into a syringe. Discard filter needle after aspiration into the syringe. No further filtering is required for administration.

Storage: Store lyophilized powder at 2° to 8° C (36° to 46° F); do not freeze. Do not refrigerate after dilution. **Mononine** may be stored at room temperature before dilution for up to 30 days.

COMPATIBILITY
Specific information not available. Consider specific use; consult pharmacist.

RATE OF ADMINISTRATION
Average rate is 2 to 3 mL or 100 units/min. Completely individualized according to patient's condition. Decrease rate of administration for side effects such as burning or pain at injection site, chills, fever, flushing, headache, tingling, or changes in BP or pulse. Never exceed 10 mL/min.

ACTIONS
A lyophilized concentrate of human coagulation factors: IX (plasma thromboplastin and antihemophilic factor B), II (prothrombin), VII (proconvertin), and X (Stuart-Prower factor). In contrast to other products, AlphaNine SD and Mononine are highly purified factor IX and contain only minimal amounts of the other factors. All products are obtained from fresh human plasma and prepared, irradiated, and dried by specific processes. Additional processes are used to prepare AlphaNine SD and Mononine that markedly reduce the possibility of viral contamination. Concentration of 25 units/mL is 25 times greater than normal plasma. Preparations contain varying amounts of total protein in each vial. Half-life is approximately 24 hours (range 18 to 36 hours).

INDICATIONS AND USES
All factor IX products: Prevention/control of bleeding in patients with factor IX deficiency due to hemophilia B. Indicated to correct or prevent a dangerous bleeding episode or to perform surgery. ■ Prophylaxis to prevent spontaneous bleeding in patients with proven specific congenital deficiency (hemophilia B).

Factor IX (human): Preferred for surgical coverage; treatment of crush injuries and/or large IM hemorrhages requiring several days of replacement therapy; and treatment in neonates, individuals with severe hepatocellular dysfunction, or those with a history of thrombotic complications associated with factor IX complex.

Factor IX complex: Prevention/control of bleeding in patients with hemophilia A who have inhibitors to factor VIII. ■ Reversal of coumarin effect (fresh-frozen plasma preferred unless risk of hepatitis transfer would be life threatening). ■ Hemorrhage caused by hepatitis-induced lack of production of liver-dependent coagulation factors. ■ Proplex T is used for prevention or control of bleeding episodes in patients with factor VII deficiency.

CONTRAINDICATIONS
Factor IX complex: Known liver disease with suspicion of intravascular coagulation or fibrinolysis. ■ Factor VII deficiency except for Proplex T.

Mononine: Known hypersensitivity to mouse protein. ■ No other known contraindications for **AlphaNine SD** or **Bebulin VH**. ■ **AlphaNine SD, Bebulin VH,** and **Mononine** are not indicated for replacement of any other coagulation factors.

PRECAUTIONS
Used when plasma infusions would result in hypervolemia and/or proteinemia or when blood volume or RBC replacement is not indicated. ■ Use extreme caution in newborns, infants, postoperative patients, and patients with liver disease. Factor IX (human) (e.g., AlphaNine SD, Mononine) would be preferred because studies show no incidence of thrombin generation. ■ Fresh-frozen plasma may be required in addition to factor IX complex when prompt reversal is required. ■ Danger of thromboembolic episodes (DIC, myocardial infarction, pulmonary embolism, venous thrombosis) increases with plasma levels over 50%. ■ Large or frequently repeated doses of factor IX complex may cause intravascular hemolysis in patients with type A, B, or AB blood.

Monitor: Monitor the patient's levels of coagulation factors before, after, and between administrations. *Do not overdose;* see Side Effects. ▪ AIDS or hepatitis is possible for the recipient. Health care professionals should exercise caution in handling. Possibility markedly reduced with additional preparation process of AlphaNine SD and Mononine. ▪ Observe for signs and symptoms of postoperative thrombosis or disseminated intravascular coagulation (DIC). Risk multiplies with repeated administrations except for AlphaNine, AlphaNine SD, and Mononine.

Patient Education: Alert to possible risk of HIV virus and hepatitis. ▪ Report early signs of hypersensitivity promptly (burning or pain along injection site, hives, rash, tightness of chest, wheezing). ▪ Notify physician if medication seems less effective. May be developing antibodies to factor IX. ▪ Carry identification card. ▪ Proper preparation and administration imperative if given in home.

Maternal/Child: Category C: safety for use during pregnancy not established; use only if clearly indicated; see Precautions. ▪ Use extreme caution in neonates with hepatitis; high rate of morbidity.

DRUG/LAB INTERACTIONS
Concurrent use of **aminocaproic acid** (Amicar) may increase risk of thrombosis.

SIDE EFFECTS
Burning or pain along injection site, changes in BP, chills, fever, flushing, headache, nausea, tingling, urticaria, vomiting.

Major: Anaphylaxis, DIC, hepatitis, myocardial infarction, postoperative thrombosis (rare with pure factor IX [Human] products), pulmonary embolism. Consider risk potential of contracting AIDS and hepatitis; markedly reduced with pure factor IX (Human) products (AlphaNine, AlphaNine SD, and Mononine).

ANTIDOTE
Temporarily discontinue or decrease rate of administration for minor side effects. For major symptoms, discontinue, and notify physician. Treat hypersensitivity reactions as indicated; a different lot may not cause reaction. For thrombosis or DIC, anticoagulation with heparin may be indicated.

FACTOR IX (RECOMBINANT)

(**FAK**-tor 9 [re-**KOM**-be-nant])

Alprolix, BeneFIX, IDELVION, IXINITY, RIXUBIS

USUAL DOSE (International units [IU])

Available recombinant factor IX products include:

Alprolix (recombinant): A coagulation factor IX Fc fusion protein consisting of the human coagulation factor IX sequence covalently linked to the Fc domain of human immunoglobulin G_1 (IgG_1). Does not contain proteins derived from animal or human sources.

BeneFIX (recombinant), IXINITY (recombinant), RIXUBIS (recombinant): Coagulation factor IX proteins produced by a genetically engineered mammalian cell line derived from Chinese hamster ovary (CHO) cells. No human or animal proteins are added during any stage of manufacturing.

IDELVION (recombinant): A coagulation factor IX, albumin fusion protein (rIX-FP) comprising genetically fused recombinant coagulation factor IX and recombinant albumin. Does not contain proteins derived from animal or human sources.

Adults and pediatric patients: Completely individualized based on the degree of deficiency, the location and extent of bleeding, the patient's clinical condition and age, and the pharmacokinetic parameters of factor IX, such as incremental recovery and half-life. Base dose and frequency on individual clinical response. Units required to raise blood level percentages are somewhat increased with recombinant products compared with other factor IX products and can be calculated using the following formulas:

$$\text{Number of factor IX IU required} = \text{Body weight (in kg)} \times \text{Desired factor IX increase}$$
$$(\% \text{ of normal or IU/dL}) \times \text{Reciprocal of observed recovery (IU/kg per IU/dL)}$$

The observed recovery for the various products is as follows:

Alprolix: One IU of recombinant product/kg of body weight increases the circulating level of factor IX by 1% (IU/dL).

BeneFIX: One IU of recombinant product/kg of body weight increases the circulating level of factor IX by 0.8% (IU/dL) for adults and by 0.7% (IU/dL) in pediatric patients under 15 years of age.

IDELVION: One IU of recombinant product/kg of body weight is expected to increase the circulating level of factor IX by 1.3% (IU/dL) in patients 12 years of age or older and by 1% (IU/dL) in pediatric patients less than 12 years of age.

IXINITY: One IU of recombinant product/kg of body weight increases the circulating level of factor IX by 0.98% (IU/dL).

RIXUBIS: One IU of recombinant product/kg of body weight increases the circulating level of factor IX by 0.9% (IU/dL) for patients 12 years of age or older and by 0.7% (IU/dL) in pediatric patients under 12 years of age.

In the presence of an inhibitor, higher doses may be required. See examples of dose calculation in prescribing information.

The following chart may be used to guide dosing in the prevention of bleeding episodes.

Continued

Factor IX (Recombinant) Dosing Guidelines for Prevention and Control of Bleeding in Adults and Pediatric Patients			
Type of Bleeding Episodes	Circulating Factor IX Activity Required (% of normal or IU/dL)	Dosing Interval (hours)	Duration of Therapy (days)
Minor Uncomplicated or early bleeds: hemarthroses, superficial muscle (except iliopsoas) with no neurovascular compromise, other soft tissue or oral bleeding	**Alprolix** 30 to 60	48 hours	Repeat every 48 hours if there is further evidence of bleeding
	BeneFIX 20 to 30	12 to 24 hours	1 to 2 days
	IDELVION* 30 to 60	48 to 72 hours	At least 1 day until bleeding stops and healing is achieved A single dose should be sufficient for the majority of bleeds
	IXINITY 30 to 60	24 hours	1 to 3 days until healing is achieved
	RIXUBIS 20 to 30	12 to 24 hours	At least 1 day until healing is achieved
Moderate Intramusclar or soft tissue with dissection, mucous membranes, dental extractions, hematuria, hemarthrosis of longer duration, recurrent hemarthrosis, deep lacerations	**Alprolix** 30 to 60	48 hours	Repeat every 48 hours if there is further evidence of bleeding
	BeneFIX and RIXUBIS 25 to 50	12 to 24 hours	Treat until bleeding stops and healing begins, about 2 to 7 days
	IDELVION* 30 to 60	48 to 72 hours	At least 1 day until bleeding stops and healing is achieved A single dose should be sufficient for the majority of bleeds
	IXINITY 40 to 60	24 hours	2 to 7 days until healing is achieved
Major Life-threatening or limb-threatening hemorrhage, iliopsoas and deep muscle with neurovascular injury or substantial blood loss, pharyngeal, retropharyngeal, retroperitoneal, CNS	**Alprolix** 80 to 100	Consider a repeat dose after 6 to 10 hours and then every 24 hours for the first 3 days	Due to the long half-life of Alprolix, the dose may be reduced and frequency may be extended after Day 3 to every 48 hours or longer until bleeding stops and healing is achieved
	BeneFIX and RIXUBIS 50 to 100	12 to 24 hours	7 to 10 days until bleeding stops and healing is achieved
	IDELVION* 60 to 100	48 to 72 hours	7 to 14 days until bleeding stops and healing is achieved Maintenance dose weekly
	IXINITY 60 to 100	12 to 24 hours	2 to 14 days until healing is achieved

Source: Roberts and Eberst and Srivastava et al. 2013.
*Adapted from the WFH Guidelines for the Management of Hemophilia.

Dosing for perioperative management is provided in the following chart.

Factor IX (Recombinant) Dosing for Perioperative Management in Adults and Pediatric Patients			
Type of Surgery	Circulating Factor IX Level Required (% or IU/dL)	Dosing Interval (hours)	Duration of Therapy (days)
Minor (e.g., tooth extraction)	**Alprolix** 50 to 80	A single infusion may be sufficient	Repeat as needed after 24 to 48 hours until bleeding stops and healing is achieved
	BeneFIX 20 to 30	12 to 24 hours	1 to 2 days until bleeding stops and healing is achieved
	IDELVION* 50 to 80	48 to 72 hours	At least 1 day or until healing is achieved A single dose should be sufficient for the majority of minor surgeries
	IXINITY **Preoperative:** 50 to 80 **Postoperative:** 30 to 80	24 hours	1 to 5 days depending on type of procedure
	RIXUBIS 30 to 60	24 hours	At least 1 day until healing is achieved
Major (e.g., intracranial, intra-abdominal, intrathoracic, joint replacement, pharyngeal, retropharyngeal, retroperitoneal)	**Alprolix** 60 to 100 (initial level)	Consider a repeat dose after 6 to 10 hours and then every 24 hours for the first 3 days	Due to the long half-life of Alprolix, the dose may be reduced and frequency in the postsurgical setting may be extended after Day 3 to every 48 hours or longer until bleeding stops and healing is achieved
	BeneFIX 50 to 100	12 to 24 hours	7 to 10 days until bleeding stops and healing is achieved
	IDELVION* 60 to 100 (initial level)	48 to 72 hours	7 to 14 days or until bleeding stops and healing is achieved Repeat dose every 48 to 72 hours for the first week or until healing is achieved Maintenance dose 1 to 2 times per week
	IXINITY **Preoperative:** 60 to 80 **Postoperative:** 40 to 60 **Postoperative:** 30 to 50 **Postoperative:** 20 to 40	8 to 24 hours	 1 to 3 days 4 to 6 days 7 to 14 days
	RIXUBIS 80 to 100	8 to 24 hours	7 to 10 days until bleeding stops and healing is achieved

*Adapted from the WFH Guidlines for the Management of Hemophilia.

Routine prophylaxis dosing is as follows:

Alprolix dosing for routine prophylaxis in adults and pediatric patients: Routine starting regimens are either 50 IU/kg once weekly or 100 IU/kg once every 10 days. Adjust dose based on patient response.

IDELVION dosing for routine prophylaxis in patients 12 years of age or older: Recommended dose is 25 to 40 IU/kg every 7 days. Patients who are well-controlled on this regimen may be switched to a 14-day interval at 50 to 75 IU/kg.

IDELVION dosing for routine prophylaxis in pediatric patients less than 12 years of age: Recommended dose is 40 to 55 IU/kg every 7 days.

Continued

RIXUBIS dosing for routine prophylaxis in adults: Dose for previously treated patients is 40 to 60 IU/kg twice weekly for patients 12 years of age and older and 60 to 80 IU/kg twice weekly for patients under 12 years of age. Dose titration may be necessary based on individual patient's age, bleeding pattern, and physical activity.

DOSE ADJUSTMENTS

Adjust dose and frequency of repeated infusions by using factor IX activity and pharmacokinetic parameters such as half-life and incremental recovery, as well as by taking the clinical situation into consideration. ▪ Patients at the lower end of the observed factor IX recovery range may require upward dose adjustment; see Monitor. ▪ Dose adjustment may be necessary in pediatric patients under 12 years of age; see Maternal/Child.

DILUTION

Actual number of international units contained is shown on each bottle or vial. **Alprolix** is supplied in a kit that includes single-use vials containing 500, 1,000, 2,000, or 3,000 IU/vial. **BeneFIX** is supplied in a kit that includes single-use vials containing 250, 500, 1,000, 2,000, or 3,000 IU/vial. **IDELVION** is available in a kit that includes single-use vials containing 250, 500, 1,000, or 2,000 IU/vial. **IXINITY** is available in single-use vials containing 500, 1,000, or 1,500 IU/vial. **RIXUBIS** is available in single-use vials containing 250, 500, 1,000, 2,000, or 3,000 IU/vial. Sterile technique imperative. Confirm expiration date. Plastic syringes may be indicated to prevent binding to glass surfaces. Factor IX and diluent should be at room temperature. Provided diluent, dilution, and transfer equipment are specific to each product; consult manufacturer's detailed preparation and reconstitution process in prescribing information. When diluted, solution should be clear and colorless. (**IDELVION** may be yellow to colorless.) Multiple vials may be drawn in the same larger syringe per manufacturer's specific directions. Most products must be used within 3 hours of reconstitution. **IDELVION** must be used within 4 hours of reconstitution.
Filters: Supplied by manufacturer if indicated. If more than one vial is required for a dose, multiple vials may be drawn into the same syringe; see Dilution.
Storage: *Alprolix:* Refrigerate kit at 2° to 8° C (36° to 46° F). Store in original package and protect from light. *Do not refrigerate after reconstitution.*
BeneFIX: If product is labeled for RT storage, it may be stored at CRT or refrigerated at 2° to 8° C (36° to 46° F). If product is labeled for refrigeration, store at 2° to 8° C (36° to 46° F).
IDELVION: Store in original carton to protect from light in the refrigerator or at RT (2° to 25° C [36° to 77° F]). Do not freeze. *Do not refrigerate after reconstitution.*
IXINITY: Store at 2° to 25° C (36° to 77° F) in original carton to protect from light. *Do not refrigerate after reconstitution.*
RIXUBIS: Refrigerate at 2° to 8° C (36° to 46° F) for up to 24 months.
All products: Avoid freezing. Do not use after the expiration date. Discard unused product.
All products except IDELVION: Must be used within 3 hours of reconstitution. **IDELVION** must be used within 4 hours of reconstitution. **Alprolix, BeneFIX,** and **RIXUBIS** may be stored at room temperature not exceeding 30° C (86° F) for up to 6 months (12 months for RIXUBIS) before expiration (mark date removed from refrigerator on carton). Do not return to the refrigerator.

COMPATIBILITY

Alprolix, IXINITY: Manufacturer states, "Do not administer in the same tubing or container with other medications."
BeneFIX: Do not administer in the same tubing or container with other medicinal products. Do not allow blood to enter the syringe; if red blood cell agglutination is observed, discard everything and start over with new product and supplies.
IDELVION: Manufacturer states, "Do not mix or administer in the same tubing or container with other medicinal products."
RIXUBIS: Specific information not available. Consider specific use; consult pharmacist and note **compatibility** under BeneFIX.

RATE OF ADMINISTRATION

Alprolix, IDELVION, IXINITY, RIXUBIS: Administer as an IV bolus infusion. Rate of administration should be determined by patient's comfort level and no faster than 10 mL/min.

BeneFIX: Administer over a period of several minutes. Adapt to the comfort level of each individual patient.

All products: Record the name and batch number of the product in the patient record.

ACTIONS

An antihemorrhagic. A purified protein produced by recombinant DNA technology for use in the treatment of factor IX deficiency. Its primary amino acid sequence is identical to a form of plasma-derived factor IX, and it has structural and functional characteristics similar to those of endogenous factor IX. Inherently free from the risk of transmission of human bloodborne pathogens such as HIV, hepatitis viruses, and parvovirus. Factor IX is the specific clotting factor deficient in patients with hemophilia B and in patients with acquired factor IX deficiencies. Factor IX (recombinant) increases plasma levels of factor IX and can temporarily correct the coagulation defect in these patients, restoring hemostasis. Normalizes aPTT. Average half-life of *Alprolix* is 86 hours. Half-life of *BeneFIX* ranges from 11 to 36 hours. The fusion of the recombinant coagulation factor IX with recombinant albumin extends the half-life of factor IX with *IDELVION*. The half-life of *IDELVION* ranges from 104 to 118 hours in adults and from 87 to 93 hours in pediatric patients less than 18 years of age (depending on dose). *IXINITY* half-life ranges from 17 to 31 hours. *RIXUBIS* half-life ranges from 16 to 42 hours.

INDICATIONS AND USES

All Products: Control and prevention of bleeding episodes in adult and pediatric patients with hemophilia B (congenital factor IX deficiency or Christmas disease). ▪ Perioperative management in adult and pediatric patients with hemophilia B. **IXINITY** use is limited to patients 12 years of age or older.

Alprolix, IDELVION, RIXUBIS: Routine prophylaxis to prevent or reduce the frequency of bleeding episodes in adults and pediatric patients with hemophilia B.

Limitations of use: *All Products:* Not indicated for induction of immune tolerance in patients with hemophilia B; see Precautions.

BeneFIX: Not indicated for treatment of other factor deficiencies (e.g., factors II, VII, VIII, and X), hemophilia A patients with inhibitors to factor VIII, reversal of coumarin-induced anticoagulation, or bleeding due to low levels of liver-dependent coagulation factors.

CONTRAINDICATIONS

Alprolix: Known history of hypersensitivity reactions (including anaphylaxis) to the product or its excipients.

BeneFIX, IDELVION, IXINITY, RIXUBIS: Known history of hypersensitivity to the products or their excipients, including hamster protein.

RIXUBIS: Disseminated intravascular coagulation (DIC) and/or signs of fibrinolysis.

PRECAUTIONS

All Products: For IV bolus infusion only; see Rate of Administration. Safety and effectiveness of continuous infusion have not been established. ▪ Usually administered under the supervision of a physician experienced in the treatment of hemophilia B. ▪ Hypersensitivity reactions, including anaphylaxis, have been reported. Risk may be highest during the early phases of initial exposure in previously untreated patients. An association between the occurrence of factor IX inhibitor and allergic reactions has been reported. ▪ Thromboembolic episodes (e.g., disseminated intravascular coagulation [DIC], myocardial infarction, pulmonary embolism, arterial or venous thrombosis) have been reported with factor IX concentrates. Most have been reported in patients receiving factor IX complex concentrates or factor IX via continuous infusions. ▪ Because of potential thromboembolic problems, use caution in patients with liver disease, patients with signs of fibrinolysis, patients in the perioperative or postoperative period, neonates, or patients at risk for thromboembolic phenomena or DIC. Benefit must be weighed against risk.

- Factor IX inhibitors may develop; see Monitor. ■ Nephrotic syndrome has been reported following attempted immune tolerance induction in hemophilia B patients with factor IX inhibitors. Safety for use in immune tolerance induction not established.

Monitor: *All Products:* To ensure desired factor IX activity levels are achieved and maintained, precise monitoring using the one-stage factor IX activity assay is recommended, especially during surgical intervention. Adjust dose and frequency as required. *Do not overdose;* see Side Effects. ■ Monitor vital signs. ■ Monitor for S/S of hypersensitivity reaction (e.g., angioedema, chest pain, dizziness, dyspnea, fever, flushing, hypotension, nausea, pruritus, rash, rigors, urticaria, wheezing). ■ Monitor for early signs of thrombotic events and consumptive coagulopathy; see Precautions. ■ Monitor for development of factor IX inhibitors. Failure to attain the expected factor IX activity plasma levels or to control bleeding with an appropriate dose may indicate development of factor IX inhibitors. Assays used to determine if factor IX inhibitor is present should be titered in Bethesda units (BUs). ■ Patients dosed with high-purity factor IX products who develop inhibitors are at increased risk for anaphylaxis with repeat doses. Evaluate patients who experience a hypersensitivity reaction for the presence of an inhibitor.

Patient Education: *All Products:* Read manufacturer-supplied patient product information. ■ Hypersensitivity reactions can occur. Promptly report difficulty breathing, hives, itching, tightness of the chest, and/or wheezing. If self-administering, discontinue use and contact physician immediately. ■ Contact provider for lack of clinical response. May indicate development of inhibitors.

Maternal/Child: *All Products:* Use during pregnancy only if clearly indicated and/or the potential benefit justifies the potential risk. ■ Use caution during breast-feeding. ■ Pediatric patients may have higher factor IX body weight–adjusted clearance, shorter half-life, and lower recovery. Higher dose per kilogram of body weight or more frequent dosing may be needed. ■ Safety and effectiveness of IXINITY for use in pediatric patients less than 12 years of age not established.

Elderly: *All Products:* Numbers in clinical studies insufficient to determine whether the elderly respond differently than do younger subjects.

DRUG/LAB INTERACTIONS

Specific information not available. Factor IX activity measurements in the clinical lab may be affected by the type of activated partial thromboplastin time (aPTT) reagent or laboratory standard used.

SIDE EFFECTS

Alprolix: Headache and oral paresthesia were most common. Breath odor, dizziness, dysgeusia, fatigue, hypotension, infusion site pain, obstructive uropathy, and palpitations have been reported. No inhibitors were detected and no events of anaphylaxis were reported during clinical studies.

BeneFIX: Dizziness, headache, injection site pain, injection site reaction, nausea, and rash were most common. Blurred vision, cellulitis at IV site, chest tightness, drowsiness, dry cough, factor IX inhibition, fever, flushing, hives, hypoxia, phlebitis at IV site, renal infarct, shaking, taste perversion, and vomiting have been reported. Hypersensitivity reactions (including bronchospastic reactions and/or hypotension and anaphylaxis) and the development of high-titer inhibitors requiring alternate treatments to factor IX therapy are the most serious.

IDELVION: Most commonly reported reaction is headache. Dizziness, eczema, hypersensitivity reactions, and rash have been reported.

IXINITY: Most commonly reported reaction is headache. Apathy, asthenia, depression, dysgeusia, influenza, injection site discomfort, lethargy, and pruritic rash have been reported.

RIXUBIS: Dysgeusia, pain in extremity, and positive furin antibody test were most common during clinical studies.

All Products: Anaphylaxis, angioedema, dyspnea, hypotension, inadequate factor IX recovery, inhibitor development, and thrombosis may occur.

Post-Marketing: *BeneFIX:* Anaphylaxis, angioedema, dyspnea, hypotension, and thrombosis. *RIXUBIS:* Hypersensitivity (including dyspnea, pruritus), rash, and urticaria.

ANTIDOTE

Temporarily discontinue or decrease rate of administration for minor side effects. If any major symptoms appear, discontinue drug, notify physician, and consider alternative hemostatic measures. Treat hypersensitivity reactions as indicated. For thrombosis or DIC, anticoagulation with heparin may be indicated.

FACTOR XIII CONCENTRATE (HUMAN) Antihemorrhagic
(**FAK**-tor **THIR**-teen **HUE**-man)

Corifact

USUAL DOSE (International units [IU])

Dose must be individualized based on body weight, laboratory values, and patient's clinical condition.

Initial dose in adult and pediatric patients: 40 international units/kg.

Subsequent doses in adult and pediatric patients: Should be guided by the most recent trough factor XIII (coagulation factor XIII) activity level. Dose every 28 days (4 weeks) to maintain a trough factor XIII activity level of approximately 5% to 20%. Recommended dosing adjustments of ±5 units/kg should be based on trough factor XIII activity levels as shown in the chart in Dose Adjustments and on the patient's clinical condition.

DOSE ADJUSTMENTS

Guide dose adjustments based on a specific assay used to determine factor XIII levels (e.g., Berichrom Activity Assay).

Dose Adjustment of Factor XIII Concentrate Using the Berichrom Activity Assay	
Factor XIII Activity Trough Level (%)	Dosage Change
One trough level of <5%	Increase by 5 units/kg
Trough level of 5% to 20%	No change
Two trough levels of >20%	Decrease by 5 units/kg
One trough level of >25%	Decrease by 5 units/kg

DILUTION

Available as a single-use vial containing 1,000 to 1,600 units of factor XIII as a lyophilized concentrate. Actual units of potency stated on vial label. Sterile diluent and Mix2Vial filter transfer set provided. Sterile technique imperative. Confirm expiration date. Record the batch number of the product in the patient's medical record with each infusion. Bring factor XIII concentrate and diluent to RT. Place vial, diluent, and Mix2Vial transfer set on a flat surface. Remove flip caps on vial and diluent, and wipe stoppers with provided alcohol swab; allow to dry. Peel away the lid on the Mix2Vial transfer set, but leave it in the clear package. Hold the diluent vial tightly on a flat surface and pick up the Mix2Vial transfer set by its clear package. Push the plastic spike at the blue end of the Mix2Vial transfer set through the center of the diluent vial stopper. Carefully remove only the clear packaging from the transfer set. Invert the diluent vial with the Mix2Vial transfer set attached, and push the plastic spike of the transparent adapter firmly through the center of the factor XIII concentrate. Diluent will automatically transfer into the vial. With all parts still attached, gently swirl to fully dissolve. ***Do not shake.*** Solution should be colorless to slightly yellowish and slightly opalescent. Grasp the factor XIII side with one hand and the diluent side with the other and unscrew the set into 2 pieces. Draw air into an empty 20-mL sterile syringe. With the factor XIII vial upright, screw the syringe to the Mix2Vial transfer set. Inject air into the factor XIII vial. Keep the syringe plunger pressed, and invert the system upside down to draw the concentrate into the syringe by pulling the plunger back slowly. Keep the plunger facing down and remove syringe from transfer set. Attach the syringe to a suitable IV administration set. If the same patient is to receive more than one vial, contents of multiple vials may be pooled. Use a separate, unused Mix2Vial transfer set for each vial. Must be used within 4 hours of reconstitution.

Filters: Mix2Vial filter transfer set provided.

Storage: Protect from light; refrigerate vials and diluent in carton at 2° to 8° C (36° to 46° F). Do not freeze. Stable for 24 months up to the expiration date on the carton under refrigeration. May be stored at RT not to exceed 25° C (77° F) for up to 6 months; however, it cannot be returned to refrigeration. Mark date removed from refrigeration. Do not use beyond expiration date on carton and vial labels or beyond end of RT storage, whichever comes first. Must be used within 4 hours of reconstitution. Do not refrigerate or freeze the reconstituted solution. Contains no preservatives; a single-use vial; discard partially used vials.

COMPATIBILITY

Manufacturer states, "Do not mix with other medicinal products, and administer through a separate infusion line."

RATE OF ADMINISTRATION

Initial dose: Do not exceed 4 mL/min.

ACTIONS

A heat-treated, lyophilized factor XIII (coagulation factor XIII) concentrate made from pooled human plasma. Several manufacturing steps are used to inactivate or remove both enveloped and nonenveloped viruses. Factor XIII circulates in blood and is present in platelets, monocytes, and macrophages. Activated factor XIII (factor XIIIa) promotes cross-linking of fibrin during coagulation and is essential to the physiologic protection of the clot against fibrinolysis. Cross-linked fibrin is the end result of the coagulation cascade and provides tensile strength to a primary hemostatic platelet plug. Half-life is approximately 6.6 ± 2.29 days. The increase in plasma levels of factor XIII after administration lasts approximately 28 days.

INDICATIONS AND USES

Routine prophylactic treatment of congenital factor XIII deficiency in adult and pediatric patients. To be effective, a trough factor XIII activity level of approximately 5% to 20% should be maintained.

Limitation of use: There are no controlled trials demonstrating a direct benefit on treatment of bleeding episodes.

CONTRAINDICATIONS

Known anaphylactic or severe hypersensitivity reactions to human plasma–derived products or to any components of the product.

PRECAUTIONS

For IV use only. ▪ Hypersensitivity reactions have occurred; emergency equipment, medications, and supplies must be available. ▪ Neutralizing inhibitory antibodies against factor XIII have been detected in patients receiving factor XIII. ▪ Thromboembolic complications have been reported. Assess benefit versus risk in pregnant women because of their hypercoagulable state and potential for increased risk of thromboembolic events. ▪ Made from human plasma and may contain infectious agents (e.g., HIV, Creutzfeldt-Jakob disease, hepatitis B, or hepatitis C). Numerous steps in the manufacturing process are used to reduce the potential for infection. ▪ Consider appropriate vaccination against hepatitis A and B.

Monitor: Monitor trough factor XIII activity levels as outlined in Usual Dose and Dose Adjustments. ▪ Monitor for S/S of hypersensitivity reactions (e.g., chest pain, dizziness, dyspnea, fever, flushing, hypotension, nausea, pruritus, rash, rigors, urticaria). ▪ Monitor for possible development of inhibitory antibodies (e.g., response to treatment is inadequate, expected plasma factor XIII activity levels are not attained, or breakthrough bleeding occurs). ▪ Monitor for thromboembolic complications (e.g., chest pain, dyspnea, edema, hemoptysis, leg pain, or positive Homans' sign). ▪ Monitor for S/S of viral infection (e.g., chills, drowsiness, fever, runny nose followed by joint pain and rash or abdominal pain, dark urine, jaundice, nausea, vomiting).

Patient Education: Manufactured from pooled human plasma. Possibility of viral transmission exists. Promptly report S/S of viral infections (e.g., chills, drowsiness, fever, runny nose followed by joint pain and rash or abdominal pain, dark urine, jaundice, nausea, vomiting). ▪ Promptly report difficulty breathing, pruritus, or rash. ▪ Promptly report breakthrough bleeding.

Maternal/Child: Category C: use only if clearly needed; see Precautions. ▪ Use only if clearly needed in breast-feeding women. ▪ No apparent differences in the safety profile in pediatric patients compared with adults. Pediatric patients less than 16 years of age had a shorter half-life and faster clearance compared with adults.

Elderly: Numbers in clinical studies insufficient to determine whether elderly patients respond differently than younger subjects.

DRUG/LAB INTERACTIONS
Specific information not available.

SIDE EFFECTS
The most commonly reported side effects included arthralgia, chills, elevated thrombin-antithrombin levels, fever, headache, hypersensitivity reactions (including allergy, erythema, pruritus, and rash), and increased hepatic enzymes. Other reported side effects included abdominal pain, diarrhea, epistaxis, flu-like syndrome, hematoma, URT infection, and vomiting.

Post-Marketing: Hypersensitivity reactions (including anaphylaxis), factor XIII inhibition (neutralizing antibodies), thrombotic events (e.g., embolism, thrombosis), viral infection (possible).

ANTIDOTE
Keep physician informed of side effects; most will be treated symptomatically. Discontinue administration and treat hypersensitivity reactions as indicated. A different lot may not cause a reaction. For thrombosis, anticoagulation may be indicated. Resuscitate as necessary.

FAMOTIDINE
(fah-**MOH**-tih-deen)

Antiulcer agent
(H$_2$ antagonist)
Gastric acid inhibitor

Famotidine PF, Pepcid

pH 5.7 to 6.4

USUAL DOSE
20 mg (2 mL) every 12 hours. Increase frequency of dose, not amount, if necessary for pain relief. In hypersecretory states (e.g., Zollinger-Ellison syndrome), higher doses may be required. Adjust dose to individual patient needs.

PEDIATRIC DOSE
Age 1 to 16 years: Starting dose is 0.25 mg/kg every 12 hours. Treatment duration and dose must be individualized based on clinical response, pH determination, and/or endoscopy. Doses up to 0.5 mg/kg every 12 hours may be required for gastric acid suppression. Another source suggests 0.6 to 0.8 mg/kg/24 hr (0.3 to 0.4 mg/kg every 12 hours or 0.2 to 0.27 mg/kg every 8 hours). May need to reduce interval to every 8 hours because of increased elimination. Maximum dose is 40 to 80 mg/24 hr based on diagnosis.
Neonate (unlabeled): 0.5 mg/kg/dose/24 hr.

DOSE ADJUSTMENTS
Reduce dose by one-half or increase the dosing interval to 36 to 48 hours in patients with moderate or severe renal dysfunction (CrCl less than 50 mL/min). Adjust based on patient response. Half-life may exceed 20 hours if CrCl less than 10 mL/min.

DILUTION
IV injection: Available in vials containing 10 mg/mL and as premixed solution 20 mg/50 mL. Each 20-mg vial must be diluted with 5 to 10 mL of NS or other **compatible** infusion solutions for injection (e.g., D5W, D10W, LR, SWFI).
Intermittent infusion: Each 20 mg may be diluted in 100 mL of D5W or other **compatible** infusion solution and given piggyback.
Storage: Refrigerate vials before dilution. Manufacturer recommends use of diluted solutions within 48 hours. However, studies suggest diluted solutions are physically and chemically stable at RT for 7 days. Store premixed Galaxy containers at CRT; avoid excessive heat. If solution freezes, bring to RT; allow sufficient time to solubilize.

COMPATIBILITY
(Underline Indicates Conflicting Compatibility Information)
Consider any drug NOT listed as compatible to be INCOMPATIBLE until consulting a pharmacist; specific conditions may apply.
May form a precipitate with sodium bicarbonate in concentrations greater than 0.2 mg/mL.
One source suggests the following **compatibilities:**
Solutions: Selected TNA and TPN solutions and fat emulsion IV.
Additive: Cefazolin (Ancef), fat emulsion IV, flumazenil (Romazicon), vancomycin.
Y-site: Acyclovir (Zovirax), allopurinol (Aloprim), amifostine (Ethyol), aminophylline, amiodarone (Nexterone), ampicillin, ampicillin/sulbactam (Unasyn), anidulafungin (Eraxis), atropine, aztreonam (Azactam), bivalirudin (Angiomax), calcium gluconate, caspofungin (Cancidas), cefazolin (Ancef), cefotaxime (Claforan), cefotetan (Cefotan), cefoxitin (Mefoxin), ceftaroline (Teflaro), ceftazidime (Fortaz), ceftriaxone (Rocephin), cefuroxime (Zinacef), chlorpromazine (Thorazine), cisatracurium (Nimbex), cladribine (Leustatin), dexamethasone (Decadron), dexmedetomidine (Precedex), dextran 40, digoxin (Lanoxin), diphenhydramine (Benadryl), dobutamine, docetaxel (Taxotere), dopamine, doripenem (Doribax), doxorubicin (Adriamycin), doxorubicin liposomal (Doxil), droperidol (Inapsine), enalaprilat (Vasotec IV), epinephrine (Adrenalin), erythromycin (Erythrocin), esmolol (Brevibloc), etoposide phosphate (Etopophos), fenoldopam (Corlopam), filgrastim (Neupogen), fluconazole (Diflucan), fludarabine (Fludara), folic acid,

furosemide (Lasix), gemcitabine (Gemzar), gentamicin, granisetron (Kytril), heparin, hetastarch in electrolytes (Hextend), hydrocortisone sodium succinate (Solu-Cortef), hydromorphone (Dilaudid), imipenem-cilastatin (Primaxin), insulin (regular), isoproterenol (Isuprel), labetalol, lidocaine, linezolid (Zyvox), lorazepam (Ativan), magnesium sulfate, melphalan (Alkeran), meperidine (Demerol), methylprednisolone (Solu-Medrol), metoclopramide (Reglan), midazolam (Versed), morphine, nafcillin (Nallpen), nicardipine (Cardene IV), nitroglycerin IV, nitroprusside sodium, norepinephrine (Levophed), ondansetron (Zofran), oxacillin (Bactocill), oxaliplatin (Eloxatin), paclitaxel (Taxol), palonosetron (Aloxi), pemetrexed (Alimta), phenylephrine (Neo-Synephrine), phenytoin (Dilantin), phytonadione (vitamin K_1), potassium chloride (KCl), potassium phosphates, procainamide (Pronestyl), propofol (Diprivan), remifentanil (Ultiva), sargramostim (Leukine), sodium bicarbonate, telavancin (Vibativ), teniposide (Vumon), theophylline, thiamine (vitamin B_1), thiotepa, ticarcillin/clavulanate (Timentin), tirofiban (Aggrastat), verapamil, vinorelbine (Navelbine).

RATE OF ADMINISTRATION
IV injection: Each 20 mg or fraction thereof over at least 2 minutes.
Intermittent infusion: Each 20-mg dose over 15 to 30 minutes.

ACTIONS
A histamine H_2 antagonist, it inhibits both daytime and nocturnal basal gastric acid secretion. It also inhibits gastric acid secretion stimulated by food and pentagastrin. Onset of action occurs within 30 minutes and lasts for 10 to 12 hours. No cumulative effect with repeated doses. 30 to 60 times more potent than cimetidine. Elimination half-life is 2.5 to 3.5 hours. Eliminated by renal and other metabolic routes. Crosses placental barrier. Secreted in breast milk.

INDICATIONS AND USES
Short-term treatment of active duodenal ulcers, benign gastric ulcers, and pathologic hypersecretory conditions in hospitalized patients or in patients unable to take oral medication. ■ Used orally for short-term treatment of gastroesophageal reflux disease (GERD), including erosive or ulcerative esophagitis.
Unlabeled uses: GI bleeding. ■ Stress ulcer prophylaxis.

CONTRAINDICATIONS
Known hypersensitivity to H_2 receptor antagonists (e.g., cimetidine [Tagamet], famotidine [Pepcid IV], ranitidine [Zantac]) or their components; cross-sensitivity has occurred.

PRECAUTIONS
Use with caution in patients with moderate or severe renal dysfunction; see Dose Adjustments. ■ CNS adverse effects have been reported in patients with impaired renal function. ■ Gastric malignancy may be present even though patient is asymptomatic. ■ Effects maintained with oral dosage. Total treatment usually discontinued after 4 to 8 weeks.
Monitor: Use antacids concomitantly to relieve pain. ■ See Precautions.
Patient Education: Stop smoking or at least avoid smoking after last dose of the day. ■ Gastric pain and ulceration may recur after medication is stopped.
Maternal/Child: Category B: use during pregnancy only when clearly needed. ■ Advisable to discontinue breast-feeding. ■ Plasma clearance is reduced and half-life is increased in pediatric patients under 3 months of age compared to older pediatric patients with pharmacokinetic parameters similar to adults.
Elderly: Response similar to that seen in younger patients; however, greater sensitivity in the elderly cannot be ruled out. ■ Consider risk of renal dysfunction; reduced doses and monitoring of renal function may be indicated; see Dose Adjustments.

DRUG/LAB INTERACTIONS
May inhibit gastric absorption of **ketoconazole** (Nizoral). ■ May decrease **cyclosporine** serum levels when famotidine is given concurrently with ketoconazole and cyclosporine.

SIDE EFFECTS

Constipation, diarrhea, dizziness, and headache are the most common side effects. Hypersensitivity reactions (bronchospasm, fever, pruritus, rash, eosinophilia) can occur. Abdominal discomfort, agitation, alopecia, anorexia, anxiety, arthralgias, confusion, decreased libido, depression, dry mouth, dry skin, elevated ALT, flushing, grand mal seizure, hallucinations, insomnia, interstitial pneumonia, malaise, muscular pain, nausea and vomiting, orbital edema, palpitations, paresthesias, somnolence, taste disorder, thrombocytopenia, tinnitus, and toxic epidermal necrolysis/Stevens-Johnson syndrome (very rare) have been reported. Convulsions in patients with impaired renal function have been reported rarely.

ANTIDOTE

Notify physician of all side effects. May be treated symptomatically or may respond to decrease in frequency of dosage. Resuscitate as necessary for overdosage.

FAT EMULSION, INTRAVENOUS BBW*

Clinolipid 20%, Intralipid 10%, 20%, & 30%, Liposyn II 10% & 20%, Liposyn III 10%, 20%, & 30%

Nutritional supplement
(fatty acid)

pH 6 to 9

*This drug is on the Black Box Warning list; however, a BBW is not provided in the parenteral prescribing information.

USUAL DOSE

Dose depends on energy expenditure and on patient's clinical status, body weight, tolerance, and ability to metabolize. Some solutions may contain aluminum; see Precautions.
Total parenteral nutrition component: *Intralipid and Liposyn:* 500 mL of 10% or 20% on the first day. Increase dose gradually each day. *Clinolipid* suggests a dose of 1 to 1.5 Gm/kg/day (equal to 5 to 7.5 mL/kg/day). Do not exceed 60% of the patient's total caloric intake or 2.5 Gm/kg/day *(Clinolipid and Intralipid)* or 3 Gm/kg/day *(Liposyn).* Amino acids and carbohydrates should account for the remaining caloric input.
Prevention of fatty acid deficiency: *Intralipid and Liposyn:* 500 mL of 10% or 250 mL of 20% twice a week should supply the recommended 4% of caloric intake as linoleate. 8% to 10% of the caloric input should supply adequate amounts of essential fatty acids (EFA); see Dose Adjustments.

PEDIATRIC DOSE

Some solutions may contain aluminum; see Precautions.
Total parenteral nutrition component: *Intralipid and Liposyn:* 0.5 to 1 Gm/kg of body weight. Increase dose gradually each day. Do not exceed 60% of total caloric intake. Amino acids and carbohydrates should account for the remaining caloric input. Maximum dose recommended by the American Academy of Pediatrics is 3 Gm fat/kg/24 hr. Another source suggests maximum may be as high as 4 Gm fat/kg/24 hr.
Premature infants: *Intralipid and Liposyn:* Treatment of premature and low-birth-weight infants must be based on careful benefit-risk assessment. Strict adherence to the recommended total daily dose is mandatory. Hourly infusion rate should be as slow as possible. Never exceed 1 Gm/kg in 4 hours. Begin with 0.5 Gm fat/kg/24 hr (5 mL/kg/24 hr of 10% solution). May be increased based on infant's ability to eliminate fat. See comments under Pediatric Dose, Rate of Administration, Precautions, and Maternal/Child.
Prevention of fatty acid deficiency: *Intralipid and Liposyn:* 5 to 10 mL/kg/day of a 10% solution or 2.5 to 5 mL/kg/day of a 20% solution. 8% to 10% of caloric input should be supplied by IV fat emulsion. Essential fatty acid deficiency accompanied by stress may require an increased dose to correct the deficiency.

DOSE ADJUSTMENTS

Lower initial starting doses and smaller incremental advances are suggested in patients with elevated triglyceride levels. Checking of triglycerides is recommended before each incremental advance. ■ If essential fatty acid deficiency occurs together with stress, dose may need to be increased. ■ Reduce dose in patients who develop serum triglyceride concentrations above 400 mg/dL to prevent consequences associated with hypertriglyceridemia.

DILUTION

Follow manufacturer's specific instructions for preparation of each individual brand. Must be given as prepared by manufacturer; check labels for aluminum content; see Precautions. Use only freshly opened solutions; discard remainder of partial dose. Do not use if there appears to be an oiling out of the emulsion. **Intralipid 30% is not to be given by direct IV infusion.** Packaged for bulk use in a pharmacy admixture program. Must be specifically combined with dextrose solutions and amino acids (TPN) so total fat content does not exceed 20%. When combined with dextrose, check mixture closely for the presence of precipitates. Prepared for an individual patient in the pharmacy.

Filters: Do not use filters of less than 1.2 microns with lipid emulsions. *Clinolipid:* Use of a 1.2-micron inline filter during administration (alone or as part of an admixture) is recommended. *Intralipid and Liposyn:* A 1.2-micron inline filter may be used during administration (alone or as part of an admixture). FDA suggests the use of a 1.2-micron filter for admixtures containing lipids (e.g., 3 in 1).

Storage: Must be stored at temperatures not exceeding 25° C (77° F). Specific storage conditions required (see literature). Do not freeze. Manufacturer recommends admixtures (3 in 1) be refrigerated for no more than 24 hours after mixing and completely infused within 24 hours after removal from refrigeration.

COMPATIBILITY

Consider any drug NOT listed as compatible to be INCOMPATIBLE until consulting a pharmacist; specific conditions may apply.

Lipids may extract phthalates from phthalate-plasticized PVC (DEHP). Non-phthalate infusion sets recommended; available with most commercial products.

Manufacturer recommends not mixing with any electrolyte or other nutrient solution. Infuse separately; do not disturb emulsion; no additives or medications are to be placed in bottle or tubing with the exception of heparin 1 to 2 units/mL (may be added before administration [activates lipoprotein lipase]). In actual practice, carbohydrates, amino acids, and fat emulsion are mixed in specific percentages and in a specific order to meet individual total parenteral nutritional needs but should be prepared in the pharmacy. Any addition of supplemental vitamins, minerals, or electrolytes (e.g., calcium, magnesium, phosphates) may cause a precipitate unless a specific order is followed. Precipitates are difficult to detect in lipids.

RATE OF ADMINISTRATION

Lipids may extract phthalates from phthalate-plasticized PVC (DEHP). Non-phthalate infusion sets recommended; available with most commercial products.

May be administered via a Y-tube or three-way stopcock near the infusion site. Rates of both solutions (fat emulsion and amino acid products) should be controlled by infusion pumps. Keep fat emulsion line higher than all other lines (has low specific gravity and could run up into other lines).

Do not hang flexible plastic containers in series connection, do not pressurize to increase flow rates without first fully evacuating residual air from the container, and do not use vented IV administration sets. All may result in air embolism.

Adult: 10%: 1 mL/min or 0.1 Gm fat/min for the first 15 to 30 minutes. If no untoward effects, the dose may be increased to 2 mL/min. The daily dose should not exceed 2.5 Gm fat/kg (25 mL of 10% solution per kg) *(Clinolipid, Intralipid)* or 3 Gm fat/kg *(Liposyn)*. On the first day of therapy, a maximum of 500 mL of 10% solution is recommended.

20%: 0.5 mL/min or 0.1 Gm fat/min for the first 15 to 30 minutes. If no untoward effects, the rate may be increased to 1 mL/min. The daily dose should not exceed 2.5 Gm fat/kg

(12.5 mL of 20% solution per kg) *(Clinolipid, Intralipid)* or 3 Gm fat/kg *(Liposyn)*. On the first day of therapy, a maximum of 500 mL of 20% solution is recommended.

Premature infants: *Intralipid and Liposyn:* 0.5 Gm fat/kg/24 hr (5 mL of 10% or 2.5 mL of 20% per 24 hours). Hourly infusion rate should be as slow as possible. Adjust rate and/or increase amount based on the infant's ability to eliminate fat. Never exceed 1 Gm/kg in 4 hours. See comments under Usual Dose and Maternal/Child.

Pediatric: *Intralipid and Liposyn:* **10%:** 0.1 mL/min for the first 10 to 15 minutes. Reduce initial rate to 0.05 mL/min for a *20%* solution. If no untoward effects, rate may be increased to administer 1 mL/kg/hr of *10%* solution or 0.5 mL/kg/hr of *20%*. One source suggests a maximum rate of 0.17 Gm/kg/hr. An infusion pump is recommended. Do not exceed a rate of 50 mL/hr (20%) or 100 mL/hr (10%).

ACTIONS

An isotonic nutrient that serves as an important substrate for energy production. Used as a source of calories and essential fatty acids. Fatty acids are important for membrane structure and function as precursors for bioactive molecules (e.g., prostaglandins) and as regulators of gene expression. Total caloric value (fat, phospholipid, and glycerol) is 1.1 cal/mL for the 10% emulsion and 2 cal/mL for the 20% emulsion. Various formulations contain various components (e.g., *Intralipid:* soybean oil, egg yolk phospholipids, glycerin, and water; *Liposyn:* safflower oil, soybean oil, various linoleic acid components and glycerin; *Clinolipid:* refined olive oil, refined soybean oil, linoleic acid, and phospholipids. The fatty acids, phospholipids, and glycerol found in lipid emulsions are metabolized by cells to carbon dioxide and water. This metabolism results in the generation of energy. Increases heat production and oxygen consumption. Decreases respiratory quotient. Some lipids are excreted through the biliary system.

INDICATIONS AND USES

To provide additional calories and essential fatty acids for patients requiring parenteral nutrition whose caloric requirements cannot be met by glucose or who will be receiving parenteral nutrition over extended periods (over 5 days usually). ■ To prevent essential fatty acid deficiency.

Limitation of use: *Clinolipid* is not indicated for use in pediatric patients.

CONTRAINDICATIONS

Severe disorders of fat metabolism, such as pathologic hyperlipemia, lipoid nephrosis, and acute pancreatitis with hyperlipemia. ■ Severe egg allergies. *Clinolipid:* Known hypersensitivity to egg or soybean proteins or any ingredients; hyperlipidemia concentrations above 1,000 mg/dL.

PRECAUTIONS

Isotonic; may be administered by a peripheral vein or central venous infusion; when administered with dextrose and amino acids, choice of peripheral or central vein is based on osmolarity of the final infusate. ■ Fatty acids displace bilirubin bound to albumin. Use caution in jaundiced or premature infants. ■ Deaths in preterm infants have been reported; see Maternal/Child. ■ Use caution in pulmonary disease, liver disease, anemia, or blood coagulation disorders or when there is any danger of fat embolism. ■ Patients requiring parenteral nutrition may be at higher risk for infection. ■ Hypersensitivity reactions are possible. ■ Fat overload syndrome has been reported (rare); see Monitor. ■ Parenteral nutrition–associated liver disease has been reported with use for extended periods of time, especially in preterm infants. May present as cholestasis or steatohepatitis. ■ Some solutions may contain aluminum. In impaired kidney function, aluminum may reach toxic levels. Premature neonates are particularly at risk because of their immature kidneys and requirement for calcium and phosphate, which also contain aluminum. Research indicates that patients with impaired renal function who receive more than 4 to 5 mcg/kg/day of parenteral aluminum are at risk for developing CNS or bone toxicity associated with aluminum accumulation. ■ See Maternal/Child.

Monitor: Monitor lipids routinely; lipemia should clear daily. ■ Correct severe water and electrolyte disorders, severe fluid overload states, and severe metabolic disorders before administration. ■ Obtain baseline values and monitor blood glucose, fluid and electrolyte status, hemogram, blood coagulation, liver and kidney function, triglycerides, CBC and platelet count, and serum osmolarity as indicated, especially in neonates. Discontinue use for significant abnormality. ▪ Monitor for S/S of hypersensitivy (e.g., bronchospasm, chills, dyspnea, fever, hypotension, rash). ▪ Monitor for S/S of infection. ▪ Monitor for S/S of fat overload syndrome. Reduced or limited ability to metabolize and clear lipids may result in a sudden deterioration of patient condition accompanied by anemia, coagulation disorders, deteriorating liver function, fever, hepatomegaly, hyperlipidemia, leukopenia, thrombocytopenia, and CNS manifestations (e.g., coma). ▪ Monitor for S/S of essential fatty acid deficiency. ▪ See Maternal/Child.

Maternal/Child: Category C: use in pregnancy only when clearly needed; safety not established. ▪ Use caution if emulsion is administered to a woman who is breast-feeding. ▪ Use extreme caution in neonates; death from intravascular fat accumulation in the lungs has occurred. Strict adherence to dose and rate of administration is imperative. Premature and small-for-gestational-age infants have poor clearance. Administration of less than the maximum recommended dose should be considered in these patients to decrease the likelihood of intravenous fat overload. Monitor serum triglycerides and/or plasma free fatty acid levels to assess infant's ability to eliminate infused fat from the circulation; must clear between daily infusions. Frequent, even daily, platelet counts are recommended in neonatal patients receiving TPN with IV fat emulsion. *Clinolipid:* Safety and effectiveness for use in pediatric patients, including preterm infants, has not been established. Use in pediatric patients is not recommended.

Elderly: *Clinolipid:* No overall differences in safety and/or effectiveness.

DRUG/LAB INTERACTIONS

Intralipid and Liposyn: No specific information available; see Dilution. *Clinolipid:* Drug interaction studies not performed. ▪ Olive and soybean oils contain vitamin K_1. May decrease the anticoagulant activity of **coumarin derivatives** (e.g., warfarin). ▪ May interfere with certain **lab tests** if samples are taken before the lipids are eliminated from the serum (5 to 6 hours).

SIDE EFFECTS

Intralipid and Liposyn: Back pain, chest pain, cyanosis, dizziness, dyspnea, flushing, headache, hypercoagulability, hyperlipemia, hypersensitivity reactions, hyperthermia, nausea and vomiting, sepsis (from contamination of IV catheter), sleepiness, sweating, thrombophlebitis (from concurrent hyperalimentation fluids), thrombocytopenia in neonates (rare), and transient increase in liver enzymes may occur.

Clinolipid: Abnormal liver function tests, hyperglycemia, hyperlipidemia, hypoproteinemia, nausea, and vomiting were most common. Hypersensitivity and infectious complications (e.g., fever of unknown origin, septicemia, UTI) have been reported.

All formulations with long-term therapy: Abnormal liver function tests, hepatomegaly, jaundice due to central lobular cholestasis, leukopenia, overloading syndrome, splenomegaly, thrombocytopenia, and deposition of brown pigment in the reticuloendothelial tissue of the liver may occur.

Post-Marketing: Diarrhea, pruritus.

ANTIDOTE

Notify physician of all side effects. Many will be treated symptomatically. Treat hypersensitivity reactions promptly and resuscitate as necessary. For accidental overdose, stop the infusion. Obtain blood sample for inspection of plasma, triglyceride concentration, or measurement of plasma light-scattering activity by nephelometry. Repeat blood samples until the lipid has cleared. Stop infusion immediately for any signs of acute respiratory distress. May represent pulmonary embolus or interstitial pneumonitis, which may be caused by an unseen precipitate of electrolytes (e.g., calcium and phosphates) in the solution. Lipids administered and fatty acids produced are not dialyzable.

FENOLDOPAM MESYLATE

(feh-**NOL**-doh-pam **MES**-ih-layt)

Corlopam

Antihypertensive
Vasodilator

USUAL DOSE

Initiate dosing at 0.01 to 0.3 mcg/kg/min as a continuous infusion. Titrate in increments of 0.05 to 0.1 mcg/kg/min every 15 minutes or longer until target blood pressure is reached. The maximum infusion rate reported in clinical studies was 1.6 mcg/kg/min. Doses lower than 0.1 mcg/kg/min and slow up-titration have been associated with less reflex tachycardia. Maintenance infusions may be continued for up to 48 hours. Transition to oral therapy with another agent can begin any time after blood pressure is stable during fenoldopam infusion. Avoid hypotension and rapid decreases in BP.

PEDIATRIC DOSE

Initiate dosing at 0.2 mcg/kg/min as a continuous infusion. Titrate dose by 0.3 to 0.5 mcg/kg/min every 20 to 30 minutes to a maximum dose of 0.8 mcg/kg/min. Higher doses generally produced no further decreases in mean arterial pressure (MAP) but did worsen tachycardia. See Maternal/Child.

DOSE ADJUSTMENTS

Dose adjustment is not required in end-stage renal disease; in patients on continuous ambulatory peritoneal dialysis (CAPD); in severe hepatic failure; or by age, gender, or race. Effects of hemodialysis have not been evaluated. ■ Caution and lower-end dosing suggested in elderly patients. Consider decreased organ function and concomitant disease or drug therapy.

DILUTION

Each 10 mg (1 mL) must be diluted with 250 mL of NS or D5W and given as a continuous infusion. (10 mg in 250 mL, 20 mg in 500 mL, or 40 mg in 1,000 mL all yield 40 mcg/mL.) Use of an infusion pump is recommended.

Pediatric dilution: Mix to yield a final concentration of 60 mcg/mL (6 mg in 100 mL, 15 mg in 250 mL, or 30 mg in 500 mL of D5W or NS). Use of an infusion pump capable of delivering low infusion rates is required.

Storage: Store unopened ampules or vials at 2° to 30° C (35.6° to 86° F). Discard diluted solution if not being administered to a patient after 4 hours at RT or after 24 hours refrigerated.

COMPATIBILITY

(Underline Indicates Conflicting Compatibility Information)

Consider any drug NOT listed as compatible to be INCOMPATIBLE until consulting a pharmacist; specific conditions may apply. Consider specific use and need for continuous adjustment.

One source suggests the following **compatibilities**:

Y-site: Alfentanil, amikacin, aminocaproic acid (Amicar), amiodarone (Nexterone), ampicillin/sulbactam (Unasyn), argatroban, atracurium (Tracrium), atropine, aztreonam (Azactam), butorphanol (Stadol), calcium gluconate, cefazolin (Ancef), cefepime (Maxipime), cefotaxime (Claforan), cefotetan (Cefotan), ceftazidime (Fortaz), ceftriaxone (Rocephin), cefuroxime (Zinacef), chlorpromazine (Thorazine), ciprofloxacin (Cipro IV), cisatracurium (Nimbex), clindamycin (Cleocin), dexmedetomidine (Precedex), digoxin (Lanoxin), diltiazem (Cardizem), diphenhydramine (Benadryl), dobutamine, dolasetron (Anzemet), dopamine, doxycycline, droperidol (Inapsine), enalaprilat (Vasotec IV), ephedrine, epinephrine (Adrenalin), erythromycin (Erythrocin), esmolol (Brevibloc), famotidine (Pepcid IV), fentanyl, fluconazole (Diflucan), gentamicin, granisetron (Kytril), heparin, hetastarch in electrolytes (Hextend), hydrocortisone sodium succinate (Solu-Cortef), hydromorphone (Dilaudid), isoproterenol (Isuprel), labetalol, levofloxacin (Levaquin), lidocaine, linezolid (Zyvox), lorazepam (Ativan), magnesium, mannitol (Osmitrol), meperidine (Demerol), metoclopramide (Reglan), metronidazole (Flagyl IV), micafungin (Mycamine), midazolam (Versed), milrinone (Primacor), morphine, nalbuphine, naloxone, nicardipine (Cardene IV), nitroglycerin IV, norepinephrine (Levophed), ondansetron (Zofran), pancuronium, phenylephrine (Neo-Synephrine), piperacillin/tazobactam (Zosyn), potassium chloride, procainamide (Pronestyl), promethazine (Phenergan), propofol (Diprivan), propranolol, quinupristin/dalfopristin (Synercid), ranitidine (Zantac), remifentanil (Ultiva), rocuronium (Zemuron), sufentanil (Sufenta), sulfamethoxazole/trimethoprim, theophylline, ticarcillin/clavulanate (Timentin), tobramycin, vancomycin, vecuronium, verapamil.

RATE OF ADMINISTRATION
Do not give as a bolus injection; must be given as an infusion. See Usual Dose and Pediatric Dose for recommended initial infusion rate, titration, and maximum recommended infusion rate. Use of an infusion pump is recommended. To calculate the infusion rate in mL/hr, use the following formula:

$$\text{Infusion rate (mL/hr)} = \frac{[\text{Dose (mcg/kg/min)} \times \text{Weight (kg)} \times 60 \text{ min/hr}]}{\text{Concentration (mcg/mL)}}$$

Example: For a 60-kg patient at an initial dose of 0.01 mcg/kg/min using the 40 mcg/mL concentration, the infusion rate would be:

$$\text{Infusion rate (mL/hr)} = \frac{[0.01 \text{ mcg/kg/min} \times 60 \text{ kg} \times 60 \text{ min/hr}]}{40 \text{ mcg/mL}} = 0.9 \text{ mL/hr}$$

Avoid hypotension and rapid decreases in BP. Manufacturer's prescribing information contains charts of infusion rates per hour for a range of doses and a range of weights for both adult and pediatric patients.

ACTIONS
A peripherally acting rapid-acting vasodilator. Is an agonist at the D_1 receptor and binds with moderate affinity to the $alpha_2$ adrenoreceptor. Causes a dose-dependent fall in systolic and diastolic BP. May cause a reflex increase in HR. Decreases peripheral vascular resistance. Increases renal blood flow, diuresis, and natriuresis. Onset of action begins within 5 minutes, and with continuous infusion, steady-state concentrations (peak effects) are reached in 15 to 20 minutes. Elimination half-life is about 5 minutes. Metabolized in the liver primarily by conjugation (without cytochrome P_{450} enzymes). Primarily eliminated in urine; some excretion in feces.

INDICATIONS AND USES
Adult patients: In-hospital, short-term (up to 48 hours) management of severe hypertension when rapid, but quickly reversible, emergency reduction of BP is indicated, including malignant hypertension with deteriorating end-organ function.
Pediatric patients: In-hospital, short-term (up to 4 hours) for reduction in BP.
Unlabeled uses: Renal protection before study with contrast dye.

CONTRAINDICATIONS
Manufacturer states, "None known."

PRECAUTIONS
Use limited to the hospital. Adequate personnel and appropriate equipment must be available for continuous monitoring. ▪ Use extreme caution in patients with open-angle glaucoma or intraocular hypertension. Has caused a dose-dependent increase in intraocular pressure. Upon discontinuation of fenoldopam, intraocular pressure returned to baseline values within 2 hours. ▪ Causes a dose-related tachycardia with infusion rates above 0.1 mcg/kg/min in adults. May diminish over time in adults but is consistent at higher doses. Has not been reported but could lead to ischemic cardiac events or worsened heart failure. ▪ Tachycardia occurred in pediatric patients at doses greater than or equal to 0.8 mcg/kg/min. ▪ Rapidly decreases serum potassium leading to hypokalemia; see Monitor. ▪ Use caution; contains sulfites. Sulfite sensitivity is seen more frequently in asthmatic individuals. ▪ See Drug/Lab Interactions.

Monitor: Determine patency of vein; avoid extravasation. ▪ Monitor BP and HR frequently, especially during titration. Avoid hypotension. ▪ Monitor serum electrolytes frequently; hypokalemia has been observed after less than 6 hours of fenoldopam infusion. Oral or intravenous supplements may be required. ▪ Transfer to oral antihypertensive agents when BP is stable. May be added during fenoldopam infusion or following its discontinuation; monitor effects carefully. ▪ See Precautions and Drug/Lab Interactions.

Patient Education: Report IV site burning or stinging promptly. ▪ Request assistance with ambulation.

Maternal/Child: Category B: use only if clearly needed. ▪ Discontinue breast-feeding; not known if fenoldopam is secreted in breast milk (is secreted in milk of rats). ▪ Antihypertensive effects have been studied in pediatric patients under 1 month of age (at least 2 kg or full term) to 12 years of age. Pharmacokinetics are independent of age when corrected for body weight. Clinical studies did not include adolescents (12 to 16 years of age). Dose selection for this group should consider clinical condition and concomitant drug therapy.

Elderly: Dose selection should be cautious; see Dose Adjustments. ▪ Response similar to other age-groups.

DRUG/LAB INTERACTIONS

No specific drug interaction studies have been conducted. ▪ Concurrent use not recommended with **beta-adrenergic blocking agents** (e.g., atenolol [Tenormin], esmolol [Brevibloc], metoprolol [Lopressor], propranolol). May cause unexpected hypotension from beta-blocker inhibition of the reflex response to fenoldopam (e.g., tachycardia). Monitor BP frequently if concurrent use is required.

SIDE EFFECTS

Dose-dependent side effects may include hypotension with resulting tachycardia, flushing, headache, and nausea. Additional side effects unrelated to dose include abdominal pain or fullness; angina; anxiety; cardiac failure; chest pain; diaphoresis; diarrhea; dizziness; ECG T-wave inversion; extrasystoles; fever; hypokalemia; increased BUN, SCr, glucose, transaminases, and lactate dehydrogenase; injection site reaction; insomnia; ischemic heart disease; muscle spasm; MI; nasal congestion; nervousness; oliguria; palpitations; postural hypotension; urinary infection; and vomiting.

Post-Marketing: Abdominal distension, cardiogenic shock, decreased oxygen saturation, ECG ST-segment depression, hypotension.

ANTIDOTE

Keep physician informed of all side effects. Most will be treated symptomatically. Use oral and/or intravenous potassium to treat hypokalemia. Reduce dose gradually as desired BP is reached. Discontinue fenoldopam immediately for excessive hypotension. Half-life is short. Recovery should begin within 5 to 15 minutes; support patient as indicated (e.g., Trendelenburg position, IV fluids if appropriate). With short half-life the need for vasopressors is unlikely. Discontinue fenoldopam and treat life-threatening arrhythmias as indicated.

FENTANYL CITRATE
(**FEN**-tah-nil **SIT**-rayt)

Opioid analgesic
(agonist)
Anesthesia adjunct

Fentanyl, Fentanyl Citrate PF

pH 4 to 7.5

USUAL DOSE
Dose should be individualized, taking into account factors such as age, body weight, concomitant drugs or diseases, and the type of surgery or procedure to be performed. In all situations, use smallest effective dose at maximum intervals.

Adjunct to regional anesthesia: 50 to 100 mcg (0.05 to 0.1 mg).

Adjunct to general anesthesia: *Low dose:* 2 mcg/kg of body weight.

Moderate dose: 2 to 20 mcg/kg of body weight. Additional doses of 25 to 100 mcg may be administered as needed.

High dose: 20 to 50 mcg/kg of body weight. Additional doses of 25 mcg to one half the initial loading dose may be administered as needed.

General anesthetic: 50 to 100 mcg/kg of body weight administered with oxygen and a muscle relaxant.

Pain management (unlabeled): An initial dose of 25 to 100 mcg (0.025 to 0.1 mg). Titrate to effect.

PEDIATRIC DOSE
Adjunct to general anesthesia in pediatric patients over 2 years of age: 1 to 3 mcg/kg/dose over 3 to 5 minutes. May repeat in 30 to 60 minutes. To give as an infusion, begin with 1 mcg/kg/hr and titrate to effect. Maximum dose is 3 mcg/kg/hr. See Maternal/Child.

Pain management (unlabeled): 0.5 to 2 mcg/kg/dose every 1 to 2 hours as needed. Titrate to effect.

DOSE ADJUSTMENTS
Reduce dose in patients receiving other CNS depressants, such as general anesthetics, alcohol, anticholinergics, antihistamines, barbiturates, cimetidine (Tagamet), hypnotics, sedatives, psychotropic agents, and narcotic analgesics. When concurrent administration is required, consider reducing the initial opioid dose to one fourth to one third of normal. ▪ Reduce dose or increase intervals for elderly, debilitated, and poor-risk patients or those with impaired pulmonary, hepatic, or renal function. ▪ See Drug/Lab Interactions.

DILUTION
Small volumes may be given undiluted (usually by the anesthesiologist). Further dilution with at least 5 mL of SWFI or NS for injection to facilitate titration is appropriate. Other IV solutions may be used. May be given through Y-tube or three-way stopcock of infusion set.

Storage: Store at room temperature and protect from light before dilution. Use promptly.

COMPATIBILITY
(Underline Indicates Conflicting Compatibility Information)

Consider any drug NOT listed as compatible to be INCOMPATIBLE until consulting a pharmacist; specific conditions may apply.

One source suggests the following **compatibilities:**

Y-site: Abciximab (ReoPro), acetaminophen (Ofirmev), acyclovir (Zovirax), alprostadil, amiodarone (Nexterone), amphotericin B cholesteryl (Amphotec), anidulafungin (Eraxis), argatroban, atracurium (Tracrium), atropine, bivalirudin (Angiomax), caffeine citrate, caspofungin (Cancidas), ceftaroline (Teflaro), cisatracurium (Nimbex), dexamethasone (Decadron), dexmedetomidine (Precedex), diazepam (Valium), diltiazem (Cardizem), diphenhydramine (Benadryl), dobutamine, dopamine, doripenem (Doribax), doxapram (Dopram), enalaprilat (Vasotec IV), epinephrine (Adrenalin), esmolol (Brevibloc), etomidate (Amidate), fenoldopam (Corlopam), furosemide (Lasix), heparin, heta-starch in electrolytes (Hextend), hydrocortisone sodium succinate (Solu-Cortef), hydro-morphone (Dilaudid), 6% hydroxyethyl starch (Voluven), ketorolac (Toradol), labetalol, levofloxacin (Levaquin), linezolid (Zyvox), lorazepam (Ativan), metoclopramide (Reglan), midazolam (Versed), milrinone (Primacor), morphine, nafcillin (Nallpen), ne-siritide (Natrecor), nicardipine (Cardene IV), nitroglycerin IV, norepinephrine (Levo-phed), oxaliplatin (Eloxatin), palonosetron (Aloxi), pancuronium, phenobarbital (Lumi-nal), potassium chloride (KCl), propofol (Diprivan), ranitidine (Zantac), remifentanil (Ultiva), sargramostim (Leukine), vecuronium.

RATE OF ADMINISTRATION
Administer over 1 to 5 minutes. Too-rapid administration may result in apnea or respira-tory paralysis. Rate must be titrated by desired dose and patient response.

ACTIONS
A potent opioid agonist. An opioid analgesic that is approximately 100 times more potent than morphine milligram for milligram (100 **mcg** of fentanyl is approximately equivalent to 10 **mg** of morphine). It has definite respiratory-depressant actions that outlast its anal-gesic effect. Duration and degree of respiratory depression are dose related. May slow respiratory rate and diminish sensitivity to CO_2 stimulation. Peak respiratory depressant effect of a single IV dose is noted 5 to 15 minutes following injection. In healthy indi-viduals, respiratory rate returns to normal more quickly than with other opiates. Has less emetic activity than morphine or meperidine. Histamine release rarely occurs and cardiac stability is preserved. Onset of action is almost immediate; however, the maximal anal-gesic and respiratory depressant effect may not be noted for several minutes. The usual duration of action of analgesic effect is 30 to 60 minutes after a single IV dose of up to 100 mcg. Effects are cumulative with repeat doses. Half-life is approximately 3.6 hours. Metabolized in the liver and excreted in the urine. Crosses the placental barrier. May be secreted in breast milk.

INDICATIONS AND USES
Adjunct to general and regional anesthesia. ▪ Short-term analgesia during perioperative period. ▪ For administration with a neuroleptic such as droperidol as an anesthetic pre-medication, for the induction of anesthesia, and as an adjunct in the maintenance of general and regional anesthesia. ▪ For use as an anesthetic agent with oxygen in selected high-risk patients, such as those undergoing open heart surgery or certain complicated neurologic or orthopedic procedures. ▪ Useful in short-duration minor surgery in out-patients and in diagnostic procedures or treatments that require the patient to be awake or very lightly anesthetized (e.g., bronchoscopy, radiologic studies, burn dressings, cystoscopy).

Unlabeled use: Treatment of severe pain. Has been administered as an intermittent injec-tion, as an epidural injection or infusion, and as patient-controlled analgesia (PCA).

CONTRAINDICATIONS
Patients with known intolerance to fentanyl and other opioid agonists.

PRECAUTIONS
Primarily used by or under the direct observation of the anesthesiologist. ▪ Adequate facilities should be available for monitoring and ventilation. An opioid antagonist (e.g., naloxone), resuscitative equipment, and oxygen should be readily available. ▪ Schedule II opioid agonists, including hydromorphone, morphine, oxymorphone, oxycodone, fen-tanyl, and methadone, have the highest potential for abuse and risk of producing respira-tory depression. Alcohol, CNS depressants, and other opioids potentiate the respiratory depressant effects of fentanyl, increasing the risk for respiratory depression that might result in death; see Drug/Lab Interactions. ▪ May cause muscle rigidity, particularly with muscles of respiration. May occur or recur infrequently in the extended postopera-tive period, usually following increased doses. Respiratory depression secondary to chest wall rigidity has been reported in the postoperative period. Intraoperative hyperventila-

tion may further alter postoperative response to CO_2. ▪ Respiratory depression may cause an increased PCO_2, cerebral vasodilation, and increased intracranial pressure. Clinical course of head injury may be obscured. ▪ Use extreme caution in craniotomy, head injury, and increased intracranial pressure. ▪ Use caution in debilitated patients, in the elderly, in patients with impaired hepatic or renal function, and in patients with pulmonary disease; reduced dose may be indicated. ▪ Use caution when administered with a neuroleptic agent (e.g., droperidol [Inapsine]). Neuroleptics have been associated with QT prolongation, torsades de pointes, and cardiac arrest. Use extreme caution in patients at risk for prolonged QT syndrome, such as patients with clinically significant bradycardia (less than 50 bpm) or clinically significant cardiac disease (including baseline-prolonged QT interval), patients treated with Class I (e.g., disopyramide [Norpace], quinidine) and Class III antiarrhythmics (e.g., amiodarone [Nexterone], ibutilide [Corvert], sotalol [Betapace]), patients treated with MAO inhibitors, patients undergoing concomitant treatment with other agents known to prolong the QT interval, patients with electrolyte imbalance (particularly hypokalemia and hypomagnesemia), or patients treated with concomitant agents (e.g., diuretics) that may cause electrolyte imbalance. Cardiac dysrhythmias, cardiac arrest, and death have been reported. ▪ Symptoms of acute abdominal conditions may be masked. ▪ Use caution in patients with bradyarrhythmias. ▪ Cough reflex is suppressed. ▪ Use caution in patients with a possible hypersensitivity to opiates and in premature infants or labor and delivery of premature infants.

Monitor: Oxygen, controlled respiratory equipment, naloxone, and neuromuscular blocking agents (e.g., succinylcholine) must always be available. May cause rigidity of respiratory muscles; may require a muscle relaxant to permit artificial ventilation. ▪ Observe patient frequently; monitor vital signs and oxygenation. Patient will appear to be asleep and may forget to breathe unless commanded to do so. ▪ Keep patient supine; orthostatic hypotension and fainting may occur. ▪ ECG monitoring indicated when a neuroleptic drug is administered with fentanyl. ▪ See Precautions.

Patient Education: Avoid alcohol or other CNS depressants (e.g., antihistamines, diazepam [Valium]). ▪ Blurred vision, dizziness, drowsiness, or light-headedness may occur; request assistance with ambulation. ▪ Review all medications for interactions.

Maternal/Child: Category C: safety for use in pregnancy and labor and delivery not established; has impaired fertility and had embryocidal effects in rats. ▪ Use caution with breast-feeding. ▪ Safety for use in pediatric patients under 2 years of age not established; has caused chest wall rigidity in neonates and may be associated with methemoglobinemia and hypotension in premature neonates; see Precautions.

Elderly: See Dose Adjustments and Precautions. ▪ May markedly decrease pulmonary ventilation. ▪ May be more sensitive to effects (e.g., respiratory depression, urinary retention, constipation). ▪ Lower doses may provide effective analgesia. ▪ Consider age-related organ impairment; may delay postoperative recovery.

DRUG/LAB INTERACTIONS

Other CNS depressant drugs (e.g., barbiturates, tranquilizers, opioids, and general anesthetics) will have additive effects with fentanyl. CNS toxicity may also be increased by other centrally acting medications such as **antidepressants** (e.g., amitriptyline [Elavil], imipramine [Tofranil], nortriptyline [Aventyl]), **MAO inhibitors** (e.g., selegiline [Eldepryl]), **neuromuscular blocking agents** (e.g., atracurium [Tracrium]), **and phenothiazines** (e.g., chlorpromazine [Thorazine]). Reduced dose of both drugs may be indicated. ▪ May enhance the serotonergic effect of **MAO inhibitors**. This could result in serotonin syndrome (hypertension, hyperthermia, shivering). ▪ Cardiovascular depression may result from concurrent use of **diazepam** (Valium) or **nitrous oxide and high-dose fentanyl.** ▪ Monitor closely for S/S of respiratory depression and CNS depression with concurrent use of **protease inhibitors** (e.g., saquinavir [Invirase], ritonavir [Norvir]). ▪ Concurrent use with neuroleptic agents (e.g., **droperidol**) may cause hypotension and decrease pulmonary arterial pressure; see Precautions. ■ CNS and cardiovascular effects may be additive with concurrent use of tranquilizing agents (**antianxiety agents** [e.g., diazepam (Valium), midazolam (Versed)]), **phenothiazines** (e.g., chlorpromazine [Thorazine]). Consider differences in the duration of action of each drug and use caution.

SIDE EFFECTS

Apnea, bradycardia, respiratory depression, and respiratory muscle rigidity are most common. Untreated, they may lead to respiratory arrest, circulatory depression, and cardiac arrest. Bronchoconstriction, diaphoresis, dizziness, hypersensitivity reactions (e.g., anaphylaxis, laryngospasm, pruritus, urticaria), hypertension, hypotension, nausea, respiratory depression (slight), and vomiting have been reported.

ANTIDOTE

With increasing severity of any side effect or onset of symptoms of overdose, discontinue the drug and notify the physician. Naloxone will reverse serious respiratory depression. A patent airway, artificial ventilation, oxygen therapy, and other symptomatic treatment must be instituted promptly. Treat hypotension with a Trendelenburg position and IV fluids or vasopressors (e.g., dopamine, norepinephrine [Levophed]) as needed. Avoid epinephrine if a neuroleptic agent has also been administered. May paradoxically decrease BP when given with neuroleptics that block alpha-adrenergic activity. A fast-acting muscle relaxant (e.g., succinylcholine) may be required to facilitate ventilation. Use atropine to treat bradycardia. Muscle rigidity during anesthesia induction or surgery must be controlled with neuromuscular blocking agents (e.g., atracurium [Tracrium], vecuronium) and controlled ventilation with oxygen. Use a neuromuscular blocking agent prophylactically to prevent muscle rigidity or to induce muscle relaxation after rigidity occurs. Resuscitate as necessary.

FERRIC CARBOXYMALTOSE INJECTION

(**FER**-ik kar-box-ee **MAWL**-tose)

Hematinic
Iron supplement
Antianemic

Injectafer

pH 5 to 7

USUAL DOSE
Dose is expressed in terms of mg of elemental iron. Each course consists of 2 doses given at least 7 days apart. Treatment may be repeated if iron deficiency recurs.

Patients weighing 50 kg or more: Give in 2 doses separated by at least 7 days. Give each dose as 750 mg for a total cumulative dose not to exceed 1,500 mg of iron per course.

Patients weighing less than 50 kg: Give in 2 doses separated by at least 7 days. Give each dose as 15 mg/kg body weight for a total cumulative dose not to exceed 1,500 mg of iron per course.

DILUTION
Available in a 750 mg/15 mL (50 mg/mL) single-use vial. May be given undiluted as a slow intravenous push or further diluted in NS and given as an infusion. When administering as an infusion, dilute dose in no more than 250 mL of NS. Do not dilute to concentrations below 2 mg/mL.

Filters: No data available from manufacturer.

Storage: Store unopened vials at CRT. Do not freeze. Solutions diluted with NS to a concentration of 2 to 4 mg/mL are stable for 72 hours at RT. Vials are single use. Discard any unused product.

COMPATIBILITY
Specific information not available.

RATE OF ADMINISTRATION
Slow IV push: A single undiluted dose at a rate of 100 mg/min (7.5 minutes for a 750-mg dose).

Infusion: Administer over at least 15 minutes.

ACTIONS
A colloidal iron (III) hydroxide in complex with carboxymaltose, a carbohydrate polymer that releases iron. Used to replenish the total body iron stores in patients with iron deficiency. Iron is critical for normal hemoglobin synthesis to maintain oxygen transport and necessary for metabolism and synthesis of DNA and various other processes. Rapidly cleared from the plasma following administration. Iron distributes into liver, spleen, and bone marrow. Because the disappearance of iron from serum depends on the need for iron in the iron stores and iron-utilizing tissues of the body, serum clearance of iron is expected to be more rapid in patients with iron deficiency as compared with healthy individuals. Terminal half-life is 7 to 12 hours. Renal elimination of iron is negligible. Excreted in breast milk.

INDICATIONS AND USES
Treatment of iron deficiency anemia in adult patients who have intolerance to oral iron or have had an unsatisfactory response to oral iron and in adult patients who have non–dialysis dependent chronic kidney disease.

CONTRAINDICATIONS
Known hypersensitivity to ferric carboxymaltose or any of its components.

PRECAUTIONS
Serious hypersensitivity reactions, including anaphylactic-type reactions, some of which have been life-threatening and fatal, have been reported. Patients may present with shock, hypotension, loss of consciousness, and/or collapse. Other serious reactions potentially associated with hypersensitivity have included pruritus, rash, urticaria, and wheezing. ■ Administer in a facility with adequate diagnostic and treatment facilities to

monitor the patient and respond to any medical emergency. ▪ Transient elevations in systolic blood pressure, sometimes occurring with dizziness, facial flushing, or nausea, have been reported. ▪ Avoid extravasation. Brown discoloration of extravasation site may be long lasting.

Monitor: Confirm IV placement. If extravasation occurs, discontinue administration at that site. Monitor for S/S of hypersensitivity reactions during and after administration for at least 30 minutes and until clinically stable; see Precautions. ▪ Monitor vital signs and monitor for S/S of hypertension following administration. ▪ Periodic monitoring of hematologic and hematinic parameters (hemoglobin, hematocrit, serum ferritin, and transferrin saturation) is indicated during parenteral iron replacement therapy; see Drug/Lab Interactions.

Patient Education: Review any possible reactions to past parenteral iron therapy. ▪ Report S/S of a hypersensitivity reaction promptly.

Maternal/Child: Category C: use in pregnancy only if clearly needed and if potential benefit justifies the potential risk to the fetus. ▪ Safety for use during breast-feeding not established. Mean breast milk iron levels were higher in lactating women receiving ferric carboxymaltose than in lactating women receiving oral ferrous sulfate. ▪ Safety and effectiveness for use in pediatric patients not established.

Elderly: Differences in response between elderly and younger patients have not been identified, but greater sensitivity of some older individuals cannot be ruled out.

DRUG/LAB INTERACTIONS

Drug interactions involving ferric carboxymaltose have not been studied. ▪ In the 24 hours following administration of ferric carboxymaltose, laboratory assays may overestimate serum iron and transferrin-bound iron by also measuring the iron in ferric carboxymaltose.

SIDE EFFECTS

The most common side effects are dizziness, flushing, hypertension, hypophosphatemia, and nausea. Less frequently reported side effects include abdominal pain, constipation, diarrhea, dysgeusia, elevated ALT and gamma glutamyl transferase, headache, hypersensitivity reactions, hypertension, hypotension, injection site discoloration and pain, paresthesia, rash, sneezing, and vomiting.

Overdose: Hemosiderosis.

Post-Marketing: Angioedema, arthralgia, back pain, chest discomfort, chills, dyspnea, erythema, fever, pruritus, syncope, tachycardia, urticaria.

ANTIDOTE

Keep physician informed of all side effects. Discontinue drug if severe hypersensitivity reactions occur. Treat hypersensitivity reactions as indicated; may require epinephrine, airway management, oxygen, IV fluids, antihistamines (e.g., diphenhydramine [Benadryl]), corticosteroids (e.g., hydrocortisone sodium succinate [Solu-Cortef]), and pressor amines (e.g., dopamine). Treat hypertension as indicated. Resuscitate as needed.

FERUMOXYTOL BBW

(**FER**-ue-**MOX**-i-tol)

Feraheme

Antianemic
Iron supplement

pH 6 to 8

USUAL DOSE

An initial IV dose of 510 mg followed by a second IV dose of 510 mg 3 to 8 days later. Administer as an IV infusion over at least 15 minutes. After 1 month and an evaluation of the hematologic response, the recommended dose may be repeated in patients with persistent or recurrent iron deficiency anemia. Administer to hemodialysis patients at least 1 hour into dialysis session, after blood pressure has stabilized. Patient should receive infusion in a reclined or semi-reclined position; see Monitor. See Drug/Lab Interactions.

DOSE ADJUSTMENTS

No dose adjustment is required and no gender differences have been observed.

DILUTION

Available in a single-use vial containing 510 mg of elemental iron in 17 mL (30 mg/mL of elemental iron). Black to reddish brown in color. This single dose must be further diluted in 50 to 200 mL of NS or D5W for administration as an IV infusion.

Filters: Specific information not available.

Storage: Store unopened vials at CRT. When added to D5W or NS at concentrations of 2 to 8 mg of elemental iron/mL, may be stored at RT for up to 4 hours. However, immediate use is preferred.

COMPATIBILITY

Specific information not available. Given as an IV injection. Consider flushing the IV line with NS before and after injection.

RATE OF ADMINISTRATION

Administer as an IV infusion over at least 15 minutes.

ACTIONS

An iron-replacement product. A superparamagnetic iron oxide that is coated with a carbohydrate shell. The shell helps to isolate the bioactive iron from plasma components until the iron-carbohydrate complex enters the reticuloendothelial system macrophages of the liver, spleen, and bone marrow. The iron is released from the complex within the macrophages and then either enters the intracellular storage iron pool (e.g., ferritin) or is transferred to plasma transferrin for transport to erythroid precursor cells for incorporation into hemoglobin. Exhibits dose-dependent, capacity-limited elimination from plasma with a half-life of approximately 15 hours.

INDICATIONS AND USES

Treatment of iron deficiency anemia in adult patients with chronic kidney disease (CKD).

CONTRAINDICATIONS

Known hypersensitivity to ferumoxytol or any of its components. ■ History of allergic reaction to any intravenous iron product. ■ Should not be used in patients with evidence of iron overload or in patients with anemia not caused by iron deficiency.

PRECAUTIONS

Fatal and serious hypersensitivity reactions, including anaphylaxis, have been reported. Reactions have occurred after the first dose or subsequent doses of ferumoxytol in patients in whom a previous dose was tolerated. Patients with a history of multiple drug allergies may have a greater risk of anaphylaxis. Consider risk versus benefit of administration. ■ Facilities for monitoring the patient and responding to any medical emergency must be available. ■ Use only when truly indicated. Excessive therapy with parenteral iron can lead to excess storage of iron with the possibility of iatrogenic hemosiderosis. One source recommends discontinuing oral iron before administering parenteral iron. ■ Clinically significant hypotension may occur following injection. ■ May transiently affect the diagnostic ability of MRI studies.

Anticipated MRI studies should be conducted before administration of ferumoxytol. Alteration of MRI studies may last for up to 3 months. See manufacturer's prescribing information if MRI studies must be obtained after ferumoxytol administration. Ferumoxytol does not interfere with x-ray, computed tomography (CT), positron emission tomography (PET), single photon emission computed tomography (SPECT), ultrasound, or nuclear medicine imaging.

Monitor: Patient should be in a reclined or semi-reclined position during and after administration to prevent postural hypotension. ▪ BP should be stable in patients receiving hemodialysis before dose is administered. ▪ Monitor BP and HR during and after dose administration. ▪ Observe for hypersensitivity reactions (e.g., anaphylaxis, cardiac or cardiopulmonary arrest, clinically significant hypotension, pruritus, rash, syncope, unresponsiveness, urticaria, or wheezing) during and for at least 30 minutes and until clinically stable after administration. ▪ Evaluate hematologic response (hemoglobin, hematocrit, ferritin, iron, and transferrin saturation) at least 1 month after the second dose. Regularly monitor response during parenteral iron therapy. Avoid evaluation of therapy immediately after therapy. In the 24 hours following administration, laboratory assays may overestimate serum iron and transferrin-bound iron by also measuring the iron in the ferumoxytol complex.

Patient Education: Review FDA-approved patient package insert. ▪ Review any possible reactions to past parenteral iron therapy. ▪ Promptly report S/S of a hypersensitivity reaction (e.g., hives, itching, rash, shortness of breath, wheezing).

Maternal/Child: Category C: use during pregnancy only if potential benefit to the mother justifies the potential risk to the fetus. ▪ Discontinue breast-feeding. ▪ Safety and effectiveness for use in pediatric patients not established.

Elderly: No overall differences in safety and efficacy were observed between older and younger patients. However, greater sensitivity of older patients cannot be ruled out. Elderly patients with multiple or serious comorbidities who experience hypersensitivity reactions and/or hypotension after administration of ferumoxytol may have more severe outcomes. Consider risk versus benefit of administration.

DRUG/LAB INTERACTIONS

Drug-drug interaction studies have not been conducted. ▪ May reduce the absorption of concomitantly administered **oral iron** preparations. ▪ Allow at least 30 minutes between administration of ferumoxytol and administration of other medications that could potentially cause serious hypersensitivity reactions and/or hypotension (e.g., chemotherapeutic agents or monoclonal antibodies.)

SIDE EFFECTS

The most common side effects are constipation, diarrhea, dizziness, hypotension, nausea, and peripheral edema. Serious side effects may include hypersensitivity reactions (e.g., anaphylaxis, pruritus, rash, urticaria, or wheezing) and hypotension. Other reported side effects are abdominal pain, back pain, chest pain, cough, dyspnea, ecchymosis, edema, fever, headache, infusion site swelling, muscle spasm, vomiting.

Post-Marketing: Anaphylactic/anaphylactoid reactions (fatal, life-threatening, or serious), angioedema, cardiac/cardiopulmonary arrest, CHF, cyanosis, hypotension (clinically significant), ischemic myocardial events, loss of consciousness, syncope, tachycardia/rhythm abnormalities, and unresponsiveness.

ANTIDOTE

Notify the physician of significant side effects. Treat hypersensitivity reactions, or resuscitate as necessary. Epinephrine (Adrenalin) and diphenhydramine (Benadryl) should always be available. In overdose, monitor CBC, iron studies, vital signs, blood gases, glucose, and electrolytes. Maintain fluid and electrolyte balance. Correct acidosis with sodium bicarbonate. Deferoxamine is an iron chelating agent and may be useful in iron toxicity or overdose. Dialysis will not remove iron alone but will remove the iron deferoxamine complex and is indicated if oliguria or anuria is present.

FIBRINOGEN CONCENTRATE (HUMAN)

Coagulation factor I

(fi-**BRIN**-oh-gen **KON**-sen-trayt)

RiaSTAP

USUAL DOSE

Individualize dosing, duration of dosing, and frequency of administration based on the extent of bleeding, laboratory values, and clinical condition. A target fibrinogen level of 100 mg/dL should be maintained until hemostasis is obtained.

Dose when baseline fibrinogen level IS known: Calculate individually for each patient based on the target plasma fibrinogen level, which is based on the type of bleeding, actual measured plasma fibrinogen level, and body weight using the following formula:

$$\text{Dose (mg/kg)} = \frac{(\text{Target level [mg/dL]} - \text{Measured level [mg/dL]})}{1.7 \text{ (mg/dL per mg/kg body weight)}}$$

Dose when baseline fibrinogen level IS NOT known: 70 mg/kg.

DILUTION

Available as a single-use vial containing 900 to 1,300 mg lyophilized fibrinogen concentrate powder. Fibrinogen potency for each lot is printed on the vial label and carton. Bring fibrinogen concentrate to room temperature. Reconstitute with 50 mL SWFI. Gently swirl until the powder is completely dissolved. Solution should be colorless and may be clear or slightly opalescent. Do not shake. Administer within 24 hours of reconstitution.

Filters: Specific information not available.

Storage: Store in carton between 2° and 25° C (36° and 77° F). Protect from light. Do not freeze in powder or reconstituted form. Do not use beyond expiration date on vial. Reconstituted solution is stable for 24 hours at CRT. Discard partially used vials.

COMPATIBILITY

Manufacturer states, "Do not mix with other medicinal products or intravenous solutions, and should be administered through a separate injection site."

RATE OF ADMINISTRATION

A single dose is to be given at a rate not to exceed 5 mL/min.

ACTIONS

Fibrinogen (factor I) is a soluble plasma glycoprotein made from cryoprecipitate derived from pooled human plasma. It is a physiologic substrate of three enzymes—thrombin, factor XIIIa, and plasmin—and is an essential part of the coagulation cascade required for forming blood clots and preventing bleeding. In patients with congenital fibrinogen deficiency, it replaces the missing or low coagulation factor (normal levels range from 200 to 400 mg/dL). Less than 100 mg/dL can be associated with spontaneous bleeding; without treatment, these patients are at risk for potentially life-threatening bleeding. Half-life is 78.7 ± 18.13 hours (range 55.73 to 117.26 hours).

INDICATIONS AND USES

Treatment of acute bleeding episodes in patients with congenital fibrinogen deficiency, including afibrinogenemia and hypofibrinogenemia. ▪ Not indicated for use in dysfibrinogenemia (malfunction of fibrinogen in the blood).

CONTRAINDICATIONS

Known hypersensitivity to fibrinogen concentrate or its components.

PRECAUTIONS

For IV use only. ▪ Administration under the supervision of a physician is recommended. ▪ Severe hypersensitivity reactions, including anaphylaxis, may occur. Administer in a facility capable of monitoring the patient and responding to any medical emergency. Epinephrine (Adrenalin) should be immediately available. ▪ Thrombotic events (e.g., myocardial infarction, pulmonary embolism, arterial thrombosis, deep vein thrombosis) have occurred in patients with congenital fibrinogen deficiency with or without the use of fibrinogen concentrate therapy. Consider benefit versus risk. ▪ Made from human plasma and may contain infectious agents (e.g., HIV, Creutzfeldt-Jakob disease, hepatitis B, or hepatitis C). Numerous steps in the manufacturing process are used to reduce the potential for infection.

Monitor: Monitor fibrinogen levels during treatment. A target fibrinogen level of 100 mg/dL should be maintained until hemostasis is obtained. ▪ Observe for symptoms of a hypersensitivity reaction (e.g., chest pain, dizziness, dyspnea, fever, flushing, hypotension, nausea, pruritus, rash, rigors, urticaria). ▪ Monitor patients for S/S of thrombotic events.

Patient Education: Inform patient of risks for infectious agent transmission and of safety precautions taken during the manufacturing process. ▪ Promptly report symptoms of a hypersensitivity reaction (e.g., difficulty breathing, feeling faint, hives, itching, tightness in the chest, wheezing). ▪ Promptly report symptoms of a possible thrombosis (e.g., altered consciousness or speech; loss of sensation or motor power; new-onset swelling and pain in abdomen, chest, or limbs; shortness of breath).

Maternal/Child: Category C: safety and effectiveness for use during pregnancy, labor and delivery, and breast-feeding not studied; use only if clearly needed. ▪ Clinical studies included 5 patients between 8 and 16 years of age; a shorter half-life and faster clearance were noted in these patients.

Elderly: Numbers in clinical studies are insufficient to determine if the elderly respond differently than younger subjects.

DRUG/LAB INTERACTIONS
No drug interaction studies have been conducted.

SIDE EFFECTS
The most common side effects reported include chills, fever, headache, hypersensitivity reactions, nausea, and vomiting. The most serious side effects include hypersensitivity reactions (e.g., anaphylaxis, dyspnea, hives, hypotension, rash, tightness of the chest, urticaria, and wheezing) and thrombotic events (e.g., myocardial infarction, pulmonary embolism, arterial thrombosis, deep vein thrombosis).

ANTIDOTE
Keep the physician informed of all side effects. Interrupt or discontinue injection, if indicated, until symptoms subside; then resume at a tolerated rate. ▪ Discontinue fibrinogen concentrate if anaphylaxis or thrombotic events occur. Treat thrombotic events as indicated. Treat anaphylaxis with oxygen, epinephrine (Adrenalin), antihistamines (e.g., diphenhydramine [Benadryl]), vasopressors (e.g., dopamine), corticosteroids, albuterol, IV fluids, and ventilation equipment as indicated. Resuscitate as necessary.

FILGRASTIM ▪ FILGRASTIM-sndz*
(fill-**GRASS**-tim)

**G-CSF, Human Granulocyte
Colony-Stimulating Factor, Neupogen ▪ Zarxio***

Colony-stimulating factor
Antineutropenic

pH 4

USUAL DOSE
Neupogen and Zarxio: Do not use 24 hours before to 24 hours after the administration of cytotoxic chemotherapy because of the potential sensitivity of rapidly dividing myeloid cells to cytotoxic chemotherapy. Safety and effectiveness for use with concurrent radiation therapy have not been evaluated; simultaneous use should be avoided.

Cancer patients receiving myelosuppressive chemotherapy or induction and/or consolidation chemotherapy for acute myeloid leukemia (AML): The recommended starting dose is 5 mcg/kg/24 hr administered as a single daily injection by subcutaneous injection, short intravenous infusion, or continuous intravenous infusion. Administer daily for up to 2 weeks or until the ANC has reached 10,000/mm^3 following the expected chemotherapy-induced neutrophil nadir. Duration of therapy needed may be dependent on the myelosuppressive potential of the chemotherapy regimen employed. Expect a transient increase in neutrophil counts 1 to 2 days after initiation of therapy. In clinical trials, efficacy was observed at doses of 4 to 8 mcg/kg/day. See Monitor.

Bone marrow transplant (BMT): 10 mcg/kg/24 hr as an IV infusion over 4 or 24 hours. Give the first dose at least 24 hours after cytotoxic chemotherapy and 24 hours after bone marrow infusion.

Zarxio: Direct administration of less than 0.3 mL (180 mcg) is not recommended due to the potential for dosing errors. The spring mechanism of the BD UltraSafe Passive™ Needle Guard apparatus interferes with the visibility of the graduated markings corresponding to 0.1 mL and 0.2 mL.

DOSE ADJUSTMENTS
Neupogen and Zarxio: Consider dose escalation in increments of 5 mcg/kg for each chemotherapy cycle, according to the duration and severity of the ANC nadir. Discontinue filgrastim if the ANC surpasses 10,000/mm^3 after the chemotherapy-induced ANC nadir has occurred. ▪ During neutrophil recovery after BMT, titrate the daily dose against the neutrophil response as shown in the following chart.

Filgrastim Dose Adjustments (Neupogen and Zarxio) During Neutrophil Recovery Following a Bone Marrow Transplant (BMT)	
Absolute Neutrophil Count (ANC)	**Filgrastim Dose**
When ANC >1,000/mm^3 for 3 consecutive days	Reduce to 5 mcg/kg/day*
Then: If ANC remains >1,000/mm^3 for 3 more consecutive days	Discontinue filgrastim*
Then: If ANC decreases to <1,000/mm^3	Resume at 5 mcg/kg/day

*If ANC decreases to less than 1,000/mm^3 at any time during the 5 mcg/kg/day administration, increase filgrastim to 10 mcg/kg/day; the above steps should then be followed.

▪ Consider dose reduction and/or interruption of therapy in patients who develop glomerulonephritis or cutaneous vasculitis thought to be related to filgrastim therapy; see Antidote.

*A biosimilar product. Biosimilars are biological products that are licensed (approved) by the FDA because they are highly similar to an already FDA-approved biological product (known as the reference product [e.g., filgrastim (Neupogen)]) but have allowable differences because they are made from living organisms. Biosimilars also have no clinically meaningful differences in terms of safety, purity, and potency from the reference product.

DILUTION
Neupogen: Available as a single-dose vial with either 300 mcg/mL or 480 mcg/1.6 mL and as a prefilled syringe with an UltraSafe Needle Guard® as 300 mcg/0.5 mL or 480 mcg/0.8 mL.

Zarxio: Available as a prefilled syringe with an UltraSafe Passive™ Needle Guard as 300 mcg/0.5 mL or 480 mcg/0.8mL.

Neupogen and Zarxio: Remove from refrigerator to allow to warm to room temperature for a minimum of 30 minutes and a maximum of 24 hours.

Neupogen (vials): Confirm expiration date to ensure valid product. Avoid shaking. Contains no preservatives; use sterile technique, entering vial only once to withdraw a single dose. Dilute with D5W to concentrations of 5 to 300 mcg/mL. With concentrations from 5 to 15 mcg/mL, filgrastim must be combined with albumin to a final concentration of 2 mg/mL to prevent adsorption to plastic (e.g., add 2 mL of 5% albumin to each 50 mL of D5W). Discard any unused portion. Should be clear and colorless. Do not dilute to less than 5 mcg/mL.

Neupogen and Zarxio (prefilled syringes): Primarily used for SC administration; however, **Zarxio** syringes may be diluted for IV use in D5W to concentrations between 5 and 15 mcg/mL. With concentrations from 5 to 15 mcg/mL, Zarxio also must be combined with albumin to a final concentration of 2 mg/mL to prevent adsorption to plastic (e.g., add 2 mL of 5% albumin to each 50 mL of D5W). Do not dilute to less than 5 mcg/mL.

Storage: *Neupogen and Zarxio:* Before use, store in refrigerator in original packaging to protect from light. Avoid freezing; if frozen, thaw in the refrigerator before administration. Discard if frozen more than once. Do not expose to direct sunlight. Avoid shaking. Discard any vial, diluted solution, or prefilled syringe left at RT for more than 24 hours, including administration time.

COMPATIBILITY   (Underline Indicates Conflicting Compatibility Information)
Consider any drug NOT listed as compatible to be INCOMPATIBLE until consulting a pharmacist; specific conditions may apply.

Neupogen and Zarxio: Manufacturer states, "Do not dilute with saline at any time; product may precipitate." **Incompatible** with saline.

Neupogen: One source suggests the following **compatibilities:**

Solution: Diluted in D5W or D5W plus Albumin (human), filgrastim is **compatible** with glass bottles, PVC and polyolefin IV bags, and polypropylene syringes; see Dilution.

Y-site: Acyclovir (Zovirax), allopurinol (Aloprim), amikacin, aminophylline, ampicillin, ampicillin/sulbactam (Unasyn), aztreonam (Azactam), bleomycin (Blenoxane), bumetanide, buprenorphine (Buprenex), butorphanol (Stadol), calcium gluconate, carboplatin (Paraplatin), carmustine (BiCNU), cefazolin (Ancef), cefotetan (Cefotan), ceftazidime (Fortaz), chlorpromazine (Thorazine), cisplatin, cyclophosphamide (Cytoxan), cytarabine (ARA-C), dacarbazine (DTIC), daunorubicin (Cerubidine), dexamethasone (Decadron), diphenhydramine (Benadryl), doxorubicin (Adriamycin), doxycycline, droperidol (Inapsine), enalaprilat (Vasotec IV), famotidine (Pepcid IV), fluconazole (Diflucan), fludarabine (Fludara), gallium nitrate (Ganite), ganciclovir (Cytovene IV), <u>gentamicin</u>, granisetron (Kytril), hydrocortisone sodium succinate (Solu-Cortef), hydromorphone (Dilaudid), idarubicin (Idamycin), ifosfamide (Ifex), <u>imipenem-cilastatin (Primaxin)</u>, leucovorin calcium, lorazepam (Ativan), mechlorethamine (nitrogen mustard), melphalan (Alkeran), meperidine (Demerol), mesna (Mesnex), methotrexate, metoclopramide (Reglan), mitoxantrone (Novantrone), morphine, nalbuphine, ondansetron (Zofran), potassium chloride (KCl), promethazine (Phenergan), ranitidine (Zantac), sodium bicarbonate, streptozocin (Zanosar), sulfamethoxazole/trimethoprim, ticarcillin/clavulanate (Timentin), tobramycin, vancomycin, vinblastine, vincristine, vinorelbine (Navelbine), zidovudine (AZT, Retrovir).

RATE OF ADMINISTRATION
Neupogen and Zarxio: *Intermittent infusion:* A single dose over 15 to 30 minutes.

Continuous infusion: A single dose over 4 or 24 hours. In all situations, flush IV line with D5W before and after administration.

ACTIONS

Neupogen and Zarxio: A human granulocyte colony-stimulating factor (G-CSF). Colony-stimulating factors are glycoproteins that bind to specific hematopoietic cell surface receptors and stimulate proliferation, differentiation commitment, and some end-cell functional activation. Endogenous granulocyte colony-stimulating factor is produced by monocytes, fibroblasts, and endothelial cells. G-CSF is lineage-specific with selectivity for the neutrophil lineage. Using DNA recombinant technology, filgrastim and filgrastim-sndz are produced by inserting the human granulocyte colony-stimulating factor gene into specifically prepared *Escherichia coli* bacteria. It regulates the production of neutrophils within the bone marrow and affects neutrophil progenitor proliferation, differentiation, and selected end-cell functional activation. In studies, administration of filgrastim and filgrastim-sndz resulted in a dose-dependent increase in circulating neutrophil counts. Absolute monocyte counts also increased in a dose-dependent manner; however, the percentage of monocytes in the differential count remained within the normal range. Increases in lymphocyte counts were also reported in some individuals. With discontinuation of therapy, neutrophil counts returned to baseline in most cases within 4 days. The elimination half-life is approximately 3.5 hours. Filgrastim and filgrastim-sndz have been shown to be safe and effective in accelerating the recovery of neutrophil counts following a variety of chemotherapy regimens. In studies, benefits to therapy were shown to be prevention of infection as manifested by febrile neutropenia, decreased hospitalization, and decreased IV antibiotic usage. The incidence, severity, and duration of severe neutropenia (absolute neutrophil count [ANC] less than 500/mm^3) following chemotherapy were all significantly reduced.

INDICATIONS AND USES

Neupogen and Zarxio: Decrease the incidence of infection (febrile neutropenia) in patients with nonmyeloid malignancies receiving myelosuppressive anticancer drugs associated with a significant incidence of severe neutropenia with fever. ▪ Reduce the time to neutrophil recovery and the duration of fever, following induction or consolidation chemotherapy treatment of adults with AML. ▪ Decrease duration of neutropenia and related clinical problems (e.g., febrile neutropenia) in patients with nonmyeloid malignancies receiving myeloablative chemotherapy followed by BMT. ▪ Used SC to treat severe chronic neutropenia (e.g., congenital, cyclic, or idiopathic) after all diseases associated with neutropenia have been ruled out. Administered chronically to reduce the incidence and duration of sequelae of neutropenia (e.g., fever, infections, oropharyngeal ulcers) in symptomatic patients. ▪ Used SC or as a 24-hour SC infusion to mobilize hematopoietic progenitor cells into the peripheral blood for collection by leukapheresis with transplantation after myeloablative chemotherapy.

Neupogen: Used SC to increase survival in patients acutely exposed to myelosuppressive doses of radiation. (Efficacy studies could not be conducted in humans with acute radiation syndrome for ethical and feasibility reasons. Approval of this indication was based on efficacy studies conducted in animals and on data supporting the use of filgrastim for other approved indications.)

CONTRAINDICATIONS

Neupogen and Zarxio: Serious hypersensitivity reaction to human granulocyte colony-stimulating factors such as filgrastim or pegfilgrastim.

PRECAUTIONS

Neupogen and Zarxio: Should be administered under the direction of a physician knowledgeable about appropriate use for each indication (e.g., expert in bone marrow transplantation). ▪ Frequently given by SC injection. ▪ Use extreme caution in any malignancy with myeloid characteristics. The possibility that filgrastim can act as a growth factor for any tumor type, particularly myeloid malignancies, cannot be excluded. Safety in chronic myeloid leukemia (CML) and myelodysplasia has not been established. ▪ When filgrastim is used to mobilize peripheral blood progenitor cells (PBPCs), tumor cells may be released from the marrow and subsequently collected in the leukapheresis product. The effect of reinfusion of tumor cells has not been well studied. Data are inconclusive. ▪ Acute respiratory distress syndrome (ARDS) has been reported. Evaluate for ARDS if fever, lung infiltrates, or respiratory distress develop. ▪ Hypersensitivity reactions have been reported. Majority have occurred with initial exposure. Allergic reactions, including anaphylaxis, can recur within days after the discontinuation of initial anti-allergic treatment; see Monitor. ▪ Splenic rupture has been reported; fatalities have occurred. ▪ Glomerulonephritis has occurred in patients receiving filgrastim. ▪ Severe sickle cell crises have been reported with the use of filgrastim in patients with sickle cell trait or sickle cell disease. Fatalities have occurred. Consider risk versus benefit. ▪ Capillary leak syndrome (CLS) has been reported. Episodes vary in frequency and severity and may be life threatening if treatment is delayed. ▪ Use caution in patients with congenital severe chronic neutropenia (SCN); risk of developing cytogenetic abnormalities, myelodysplastic syndromes (MDS), and acute myelogenous leukemia (AML) may be increased. If a patient with SCN develops abnormal cytogenetics or myelodysplasia, the risk versus benefit of continuing filgrastim therapy should be considered. ▪ Alveolar hemorrhage manifesting as pulmonary infiltrates and hemoptysis and requiring hospitalization has been reported in healthy donors undergoing peripheral blood progenitor cell (PBPC) mobilization. Hemoptysis resolved when filgrastim was discontinued. Use of filgrastim for PBPC mobilization in healthy donors is not an approved indication. ▪ Moderate to severe cutaneous vasculitis has been reported in patients treated with filgrastim. Most reports involved patients with SCN receiving long-term filgrastim therapy. ▪ As with any therapeutic protein, potential for immunogenicity exists. ▪ Thrombocytopenia has been reported; see Monitor. ▪ Removable needle cap of prefilled syringes contains latex. Safe use in latex-sensitive individuals has not been studied.

Monitor: *Neupogen and Zarxio:* Obtain a CBC and platelet count before chemotherapy begins and twice weekly thereafter to monitor the neutrophil count and to avoid leukocytosis. ▪ Increase frequency of monitoring of CBC and platelet count after bone marrow infusion. ▪ Because higher doses of chemotherapy may be tolerated, side effects associated with the chemotherapeutic drug may be more pronounced; observe carefully. ▪ Observe for S/S of hypersensitivity reactions (e.g., hypotension, rash, tightness of the chest, urticaria, wheezing). ▪ Evaluate patients complaining of left upper abdominal pain and/or shoulder pain for an enlarged spleen or splenic rupture. ▪ Monitor respiratory status. ▪ Monitor for S/S of CLS (e.g., edema, hypoalbuminemia, hypotension, and hemoconcentration). ▪ Monitor for glomerulonephritis. Has been diagnosed based on the development of azotemia, hematuria, and proteinuria and with renal biopsy. ▪ See Precautions.

Patient Education: *Neupogen and Zarxio:* Promptly report any symptoms of infection (e.g., fever), abdominal or left shoulder pain, bruising, hypersensitivity reaction (itching, redness, swelling at the injection site) or dyspnea, with or without fever. ▪ Promptly report symptoms of glomerulonephritis (e.g., swelling of face or ankles, dark-colored urine or blood in the urine, decrease in urine production) or cutaneous vasculitis (e.g., purpura, erythema). ▪ May be self-injected SC by the patient at home; requires instruction. Literature includes a patient handout.

Maternal/Child: *Neupogen and Zarxio:* Category C: safety for use during pregnancy not established. Use only if benefit justifies the potential risk to the fetus. ▪ Secretion through breast milk not established; use caution during breast-feeding. ▪ Safety and effectiveness for use in pediatric patients with severe chronic neutropenia (SCN) have been established. Experience in pediatric patients similar to adult population in patients with cancer. May cause bone pain, fever, or rash. ▪ The relationship is unclear; however, pediatric patients with congenital neutropenia have developed cytogenetic abnormalities and have undergone transformation to MDS and AML while receiving chronic filgrastim therapy.

Elderly: *Neupogen and Zarxio:* Age-related differences in safety and efficacy have not been observed.

DRUG/LAB INTERACTIONS

Neupogen and Zarxio: Interaction with other drugs has not been evaluated. ▪ Use with caution **any drug that may potentiate the release of neutrophils** (e.g., lithium). ▪ Increased hematopoietic activity of the bone marrow in response to growth factor therapy has been associated with transient positive bone-imaging changes. Consider when interpreting **bone-imaging results.** ▪ Increases in **LDH, serum alkaline phosphatase, and serum uric acid** have been seen.

SIDE EFFECTS

Neupogen and Zarxio: *Cancer patients receiving myelosuppressive chemotherapy:* Most common adverse reactions were cough, dyspnea, fever, pain, and rash.

Patients with acute myeloid leukemia (AML) receiving induction or consolidation chemotherapy: Most common adverse reactions were epistaxis, pain, and rash.

Bone marrow transplant (BMT): Most common adverse reaction was rash.

Other reported reactions included arthralgia, back pain, bone pain, chest pain, dizziness, fatigue, headache, increased alkaline phosphatase and lactate dehydrogenase, nausea, pain in an extremity, and thrombocytopenia. Hypersensitivity reactions (itching, redness, swelling at the injection site) have occurred; anaphylaxis is possible. Complaints of dose-related bone pain are common and may require analgesics. Serious side effects include acute respiratory distress syndrome (ARDS), alveolar hemorrhage and hemoptysis, capillary leak syndrome, cutaneous vasculitis, glomerulonephritis, leukocytosis, sickle cell disorders, splenic rupture, and thrombocytopenia.

Post-Marketing: Acute respiratory distress syndrome (ARDS), alveolar hemorrhage and hemoptysis, anaphylaxis, capillary leak syndrome, cutaneous vasculitis, glomerulonephritis, leukocytosis, sickle cell disorders, splenic rupture, splenomegaly, Sweet's syndrome (acute febrile neutrophilic dermatosis), and thrombocytopenia. Decreased bone density and osteoporosis have been reported in pediatric patients with severe chronic neutropenia (SCN) receiving chronic therapy.

ANTIDOTE

Neupogen and Zarxio: Notify physician promptly if any signs of infection (fever) or other potential side effects occur. Monitor potential leukocytosis with twice-weekly CBCs. Discontinue therapy after ANC surpasses 10,000/mm^3 and the chemotherapy nadir has occurred. Discontinue filgrastim and notify physician immediately if a generalized hypersensitivity reaction should occur. Treat hypersensitivity reactions as indicated. Withhold or discontinue for other side effects (e.g., ARDS, hemoptysis). Patients who experience CLS should receive standard symptomatic treatment, which may include the need for intensive care. Hold filgrastim therapy in patients with cutaneous vasculitis. May restart at reduced dose when symptoms resolve and ANC has decreased. Consider dose reduction and/or interruption of therapy in patients who develop glomerulonephritis. Discontinue filgrastim if leukocyte count rises to greater than 100,000/mm^3 during administration of filgrastim for PBPC mobilization.

FLUCONAZOLE
(flew-**KON**-ah-zohl)

Diflucan

Antifungal
(azole derivative)

pH 3.5 to 8

USUAL DOSE
Daily dose should be based on the infecting organism and the patient's response to therapy. Treatment should be continued until clinical parameters or laboratory tests indicate that active fungal infection has subsided. IV dose has been used for a maximum of 14 days. Plasma levels are similar with IV or oral, so oral dose can replace IV dose at any time. See Monitor.

Oropharyngeal candidiasis: Initial dose of 200 mg followed by 100 mg/day for a minimum of 14 days. PO maintenance therapy usually required in AIDS patients to prevent relapse.

Esophageal candidiasis: Initial dose of 200 mg followed by 100 mg/day for a minimum of 21 days and for at least 2 weeks after symptoms subside. Up to 400 mg/24 hr may be used.

Urinary tract or peritoneal candidiasis: 50 to 200 mg/day has been used.

Systemic candidiasis: Optimum therapeutic dose and duration of therapy not established. Doses up to 400 mg/day have been used.

Treatment of acute cryptococcal meningitis: Initial dose of 400 mg followed by 200 mg/day for a minimum of 10 to 12 weeks after CSF culture becomes negative.

Suppression of cryptococcal meningitis: 200 mg/day. Usually required in patients with AIDS to prevent relapse.

Prevention of candidiasis in bone marrow transplant: 400 mg/day. If severe neutropenia (less than $500/mm^3$) is expected, begin fluconazole prophylaxis several days ahead of expected neutropenia. Continue for 7 days after neutrophils reach $1,000/mm^3$.

PEDIATRIC DOSE
Experience with pediatric patients is limited; see Maternal/Child.

In pediatric patients, 3 mg/kg is equivalent to an adult dose of 100 mg, 6 mg/kg to 200 mg, and 12 mg/kg to 400 mg. Some older pediatric patients may have clearance similar to an adult. Do not exceed 600 mg/day.

Oropharyngeal candidiasis: Initial dose of 6 mg/kg of body weight followed by 3 mg/kg/day for a minimum of 14 days.

Esophageal candidiasis: Initial dose of 6 mg/kg of body weight followed by 3 mg/kg/day for a minimum of 21 days and for at least 2 weeks after symptoms subside. Up to 12 mg/kg has been used.

Systemic candidiasis: 6 to 12 mg/kg/day. See Comments in Adult Dose.

Treatment of acute cryptococcal meningitis: Initial dose of 12 mg/kg of body weight followed by 6 mg/kg/day for a minimum of 10 to 12 weeks after CSF culture becomes negative. Up to 12 mg/kg/day has been used.

Suppression of cryptococcal meningitis: 6 mg/kg/day.

NEONATAL DOSE
Experience is limited to pharmacokinetic studies in premature newborns; see Maternal/Child.

Birth to 2 weeks of age in premature neonates: Manufacturer suggests using pediatric doses and extending the intervals to once every 72 hours. Prolonged half-life is seen in premature newborns (gestational age 26 to 29 weeks). After 2 weeks, dose may be given every 24 hours.

DOSE ADJUSTMENTS
In all adult situations the infecting organism and response to therapy may justify increased doses up to 400 mg daily. ▪ After the initial loading dose, reduce each dose by 50% in patients with a CrCl at or less than 50 mL/min. ▪ Give 100% of the recommended dose after each dialysis in patients receiving regular dialysis. ▪ Dose reduction

in children with renal insufficiency should parallel that recommended for adults.   ■ See Drug/Lab Interactions.

DILUTION

Packaged prediluted and ready for use as an iso-osmotic solution containing 2 mg/mL in both glass bottles and Viaflex Plus plastic containers. Do not remove moisture barrier overwrap of plastic container until ready for use. Tear overwrap down side at slit to open, and remove sterile inner bag. Plastic may appear somewhat opaque due to sterilization process but will clear. Squeeze inner bag firmly to check for leaks. Discard if leakage noted; sterility is impaired. Do not use if cloudy or precipitated.

Storage: Store glass bottles between 5° C (41° F) and 30° C (86° F); store plastic containers between 5° C (41° F) and 25° C (77° F). Protect both from freezing.

COMPATIBILITY   (Underline Indicates Conflicting Compatibility Information)

Consider any drug NOT listed as compatible to be INCOMPATIBLE until consulting a pharmacist; specific conditions may apply.

Manufacturer states, "Do not add supplementary medication."

One source suggests the following **compatibilities** *(not recommended by manufacturer)*:

Additive: Acyclovir (Zovirax), amikacin, amphotericin B (conventional), cefazolin (Ancef), <u>ceftazidime (Fortaz)</u>, ciprofloxacin (Cipro IV), clindamycin (Cleocin), gentamicin, heparin, meropenem (Merrem IV), metronidazole (Flagyl IV), morphine, potassium chloride (KCl), theophylline.

Y-site: Acyclovir (Zovirax), aldesleukin (Proleukin), allopurinol (Aloprim), amifostine (Ethyol), amikacin, aminophylline, amiodarone (Nexterone), ampicillin/sulbactam (Unasyn), <u>anidulafungin (Eraxis)</u>, aztreonam (Azactam), benztropine (Cogentin), bivalirudin (Angiomax), <u>caspofungin (Cancidas)</u>, cefazolin (Ancef), cefepime (Maxipime), cefotetan (Cefotan), cefoxitin (Mefoxin), ceftaroline (Teflaro), <u>ceftazidime (Fortaz)</u>, chlorpromazine (Thorazine), cisatracurium (Nimbex), daptomycin (Cubicin), dexamethasone (Decadron), dexmedetomidine (Precedex), diltiazem (Cardizem), dimenhydrinate, diphenhydramine (Benadryl), dobutamine, docetaxel (Taxotere), dopamine, doripenem (Doribax), doxorubicin liposomal (Doxil), droperidol (Inapsine), etoposide phosphate (Etopophos), famotidine (Pepcid IV), fenoldopam (Corlopam), filgrastim (Neupogen), fludarabine (Fludara), foscarnet (Foscavir), gallium nitrate (Ganite), ganciclovir (Cytovene IV), gemcitabine (Gemzar), gentamicin, granisetron (Kytril), heparin, hetastarch in electrolytes (Hextend), immune globulin intravenous (Gamunex-C), leucovorin calcium, linezolid (Zyvox), lorazepam (Ativan), melphalan (Alkeran), meperidine (Demerol), meropenem (Merrem IV), metoclopramide (Reglan), metronidazole (Flagyl IV), midazolam (Versed), morphine, nafcillin (Nallpen), nitroglycerin IV, ondansetron (Zofran), oxacillin (Bactocill), paclitaxel (Taxol), pancuronium, pemetrexed (Alimta), penicillin G potassium, <u>phenytoin (Dilantin)</u>, piperacillin/tazobactam (Zosyn), prochlorperazine (Compazine), promethazine (Phenergan), propofol (Diprivan), quinupristin/dalfopristin (Synercid 2 mg/mL), ranitidine (Zantac), remifentanil (Ultiva), sargramostim (Leukine), tacrolimus (Prograf), <u>telavancin (Vibativ)</u>, teniposide (Vumon), theophylline, thiotepa, ticarcillin/clavulanate (Timentin), tigecycline (Tygacil), tobramycin, vancomycin, vasopressin, vecuronium, vinorelbine (Navelbine), zidovudine (AZT, Retrovir).

RATE OF ADMINISTRATION

A single dose as a continuous infusion at a rate not to exceed 200 mg/hr. Do not use plastic containers in series connections; air embolism could result.

ACTIONS

A synthetic, broad-spectrum, bis-Triazole antifungal agent. Inhibits fungal growth of *Candida* and *Cryptococcus neoformans* by acting on a key enzyme and depriving the fungus of ergosterol; the cell membrane becomes unstable and can no longer function normally. Human sterol synthesis is not affected. Peak plasma concentrations achieved in 1 to 2 hours; half-life extends for 30 hours (range 20 to 50 hours). Administration of a loading dose (on day 1) of twice the usual daily dose results in a plasma concentration close to steady state by Day 2 when given IV or PO. Penetrates into all body fluids studied (see prescribing information) in similar and effective concentrations and remains constant with daily single-dose administration. 80% excreted as unchanged drug and about 11% excreted as metabolites in the urine. Secreted in breast milk.

INDICATIONS AND USES

Oropharyngeal and esophageal candidiasis. ▪ Serious candidal infections, including GU tract infections, peritonitis, and systemic Candida infections including candidemia, disseminate candidiasis, and pneumonia. May be an appropriate and less toxic alternative to amphotericin B. ▪ Cryptococcal meningitis, including suppressive therapy to prevent relapse. ▪ Prevention of candidiasis in bone marrow transplant patients. ▪ Used orally for additional indications (e.g., candidiasis prophylaxis).

Unlabeled uses: Has been used in many other fungal or parasitic infections.

CONTRAINDICATIONS

Hypersensitivity to fluconazole or any of its components. Use caution in patients hypersensitive to other azoles (e.g., ketoconazole). ▪ Coadministration with drugs known to prolong the QT interval that are metabolized via the enzyme CYP3A4, such as astemizole (removed from market), cisapride (Propulsid), erythromycin, pimozide (Orap), and quinidine.

PRECAUTIONS

For IV use only; do not give IM. ▪ Specimens for fungal culture and serologic and histopathologic testing should be obtained before therapy to isolate and identify causative organisms. Therapy may begin as soon as all specimens are obtained and before results are known. ▪ Inadequate treatment may lead to a recurrence of active infection; continue treatment until clinical parameters or laboratory tests indicate that active fungal infection has subsided. See specific recommendations in Usual Dose. ▪ Use caution in patients with pre-existing liver disease. ▪ Serious hepatotoxicity may occur. Causal relationship uncertain, but many patients are taking hepatotoxic drugs for treatment of malignancies and AIDS. Note any abnormal liver function tests (e.g., AST). If any clinical signs and symptoms consistent with liver disease develop, discontinue drug. Has caused deaths. ▪ Associated with prolongation of the QT interval. Rare cases of torsades de pointes have been reported. More common in seriously ill patients with multiple confounding factors, such as heart disease, electrolyte abnormalities, and concomitant medications that may have been contributory (e.g., Class IA antiarrhythmic agents [e.g., quinidine, procainamide (Pronestyl)] and Class III antiarrhythmic agents [e.g., amiodarone (Nexterone), sotalol]). ▪ Exfoliative skin disorders have been reported. Fatalities have occurred in patients with serious underlying diseases. ▪ Use with caution in patients with renal dysfunction; see Dose Adjustment. ▪ Anaphylaxis has been reported rarely. ▪ See Drug/Lab Interactions.

Monitor: Obtain baseline liver function tests and SCr; monitor periodically during treatment. ▪ Observe for S/S of hypersensitivity or skin reactions. Closely monitor patients with deep-seated fungal infections who develop rashes; discontinue fluconazole if lesions progress; see Antidote. ▪ Consider ECG monitoring in patients at risk for QT prolongation. ▪ See Drug/Lab Interactions.

Patient Education: May cause serious problems with selected medications; review prescription and nonprescription drugs with physician or pharmacist. ▪ May cause dizziness or seizures. Do not drive or operate hazardous machinery until effects of fluconazole are known.

Maternal/Child: Category D: safety for use in pregnancy and breast-feeding not established. There have been rare cases of distinct congenital anomalies in infants exposed in utero to high-dose maternal fluconazole during most or all of the first trimester. ▪ Use caution if administered to nursing mothers. ▪ Safety profile has been studied in pediatric patients ages 1 day to 17 years. Efficacy in pediatric patients under 6 months of age has not been established. However, a small number of patients ranging from age 1 day to 6 months have been treated safely (unlabeled).

Elderly: Differences in response compared to younger adults not identified; however, may be at increased risk for side effects (e.g., acute renal failure, anemia, diarrhea, rash, and vomiting). ▪ Use caution; consider decreased cardiac, hepatic, or renal function and effects of concomitant disease or other drug therapy. ▪ See Dose Adjustments and Drug/Lab Interactions.

DRUG/LAB INTERACTIONS

A potent CYP2C9 inhibitor and a moderate CYP3A4 inhibitor. Closely monitor patients who are treated concomitantly with **drugs with a narrow therapeutic index metabolized by CYP2C9 or CYP3A4.** The enzyme-inhibiting effect of fluconazole can last for 4 to 5 days after it is discontinued. ▪ Avoid concurrent use with **erythromycin**; may increase the risk of cardiotoxicity (prolonged QT interval, torsades de pointes) and, consequently, sudden death. ▪ Potentiated by **hydrochlorothiazide**; decreases renal clearance of fluconazole. ▪ Inhibits metabolism and increases serum levels of **phenytoin, sirolimus** (Rapamune), **oral tacrolimus** (Prograf), **and theophyllines;** careful monitoring of their plasma levels is required; nephrotoxicity has been reported with tacrolimus. ▪ Inhibits metabolism and increases serum levels of **cyclosporine**. Monitor levels and SCr. Cyclosporine dose reduction may be indicated with concomitant use. ▪ Potentiates **coumarin-type anticoagulants** (e.g., warfarin); monitor PT and INR frequently. ▪ Potentiates **sulfonylureas** (oral hypoglycemic agents [e.g., glimepiride (Amaryl), glipizide (Glucotrol XL), glyburide (DiaBeta), tolbutamide]); monitor blood glucose levels. Adjust the dose of the oral hypoglycemic agent as indicated. ▪ **Rifampin** increases metabolism; fluconazole dose may need to be increased. One source recommends avoiding concurrent use. ▪ Increases serum levels of **zidovudine** (AZT, Retrovir). Dose reduction may be necessary. ▪ Increases serum levels of **rifabutin** (Mycobutin). Uveitis has been reported in patients receiving rifabutin and fluconazole concomitantly. Monitoring is recommended. ▪ Risk of cardiac arrhythmias increased with **cisapride** (Propulsid), **erythromycin, pimozide** (Orap), and **quinidine**; concurrent use not recommended; see Contraindications. ▪ Fluconazole may inhibit metabolism and increase plasma concentrations of **carbamazepine** (Tegretol); monitor carbamazepine concentrations. ▪ Avoid concomitant use with **voriconazole** (VFEND). Potential for voriconazole toxicity remains if voriconazole is initiated within 24 hours of the last dose of fluconazole. ▪ May decrease metabolism and increase serum concentrations of **celecoxib** (Celebrex) and other **NSAIDs** (e.g., diclofenac [Arthrotec], naproxen [Aleve, Naprosyn]). Monitor for toxicity related to NSAIDs and adjust dose as needed. ▪ May decrease metabolism and increase serum concentrations of **selected benzodiazepines** that are metabolized by the cytochrome P_{450} system (e.g., midazolam [Versed], triazolam [Halcion]); a decrease in benzodiazepine dose should be considered. ▪ May increase serum concentrations and adverse effects of **alfentanil, buspirone** (BuSpar), **calcium channel blockers** (e.g., amlodipine [Norvasc], felodipine [Plendil], isradipine [Dynacirc CR], nifedipine [Procardia XL]), **corticosteroids, fentanyl, haloperidol** (Haldol), **methadone** (Dolophine), **nisoldipine** (Sular), **tolterodine** (Detrol), **tricyclic antidepressants** (e.g., amitriptyline [Elavil], imipramine [Tofranil]), **and vinca alkaloids** (e.g., vincristine). Reduce doses of the above drugs as indicated to avoid toxicity. Dose may need to be increased when fluconazole is discontinued. **Tolterodine** dose should be limited to no more than 1 mg twice daily when coadministered with fluconazole. ▪ Inhibits metabolism of **losartan** (Cozaar) to its active metabolite. Monitor BP closely. ▪ Coadministration may increase plasma levels of some **protease inhibitors** (e.g., nelfinavir [Viracept], saquinavir [Invirase]), increasing the risk of toxicity. ▪ Increases serum levels of **HMG-CoA reductase inhibitors** (e.g., atorvastatin [Lipitor], lovastatin [Mevacor], simvastatin [Zocor]); rhabdomyolysis has been reported. If coadministration is necessary, reduced doses of the HMG-CoA reductase inhibitor are indicated. **Pravastatin** (Pravachol) levels may be the least affected. ▪ Increases systemic exposure to **tofacitinib** (Xeljanz). Dose reduction required with coadministration; see tofacitinib prescribing information. ▪ May increase the plasma concentrations and therapeutic effects of **zolpidem**

(Ambien). ▪ An increase in serum bilirubin and creatinine have been observed with concurrent use of **cyclophosphamide** (Cytoxan) and fluconazole (Diflucan). Use caution and monitor if combined use is required. ▪ No significant pharmacokinetic interaction between fluconazole and **azithromycin** (Zithromax) has been observed. ▪ May **elevate liver function tests** (e.g., ALT, AST, alkaline phosphatase, and bilirubin).

SIDE EFFECTS

Abdominal pain, diarrhea, dizziness, dry mouth, dyspepsia, exfoliative skin disorders, headache, hepatic reactions, hypercholesterolemia, hypersensitivity reactions (including anaphylaxis with angioedema, face edema, and pruritus), hypertriglyceridemia, hypokalemia, increased appetite, increased sweating, leukopenia (including neutropenia and agranulocytosis), nausea, pallor, QT prolongation, rash, seizures, taste perversion, thrombocytopenia, torsades de pointes, tremor, vomiting.

Overdose: Cyanosis, decreased motility, decreased respirations, hallucinations, lacrimation, loss of balance, salivation, urinary incontinence. Clonic convulsions preceded death in experimental animals. Changes in renal and hematologic function test results and hepatic abnormalities have been seen in some patients, particularly those with serious underlying diseases such as AIDS and cancer. Clinical significance and relationship to treatment are unclear.

Post-Marketing: Asthenia, cholestasis, fatigue, fever, hepatocellular damage, insomnia, malaise, myalgia, paresthesia, somnolence.

ANTIDOTE

Notify physician of all side effects; most will be treated symptomatically. Discontinue drug and notify physician of abnormal liver function tests progressing to clinical signs and symptoms of liver disease. Rash may be the first sign of an exfoliative skin disorder in immunocompromised patients; discontinue drug and notify physician. In overdose a 3-hour dialysis session will decrease plasma levels by 50%. Treat anaphylaxis or resuscitate if indicated.

FLUDARABINE PHOSPHATE BBW

(floo-**DAIR**-ah-bean **FOS**-fayt)

Fludara

Antineoplastic
(antimetabolite)

pH 7.2 to 8.2 (lyophilized)
pH 7.3 to 7.7 (liquid)

USUAL DOSE
25 mg/M^2/day for 5 consecutive days. Repeat every 4 weeks. Optimum duration of treatment not established. If there is no major toxicity, treat until maximum response achieved, then administer three additional complete cycles.

PEDIATRIC DOSE
Safety and effectiveness for use in pediatric patients not established; see Maternal/Child.
Pediatric acute lymphocytic leukemia (ALL) patients (unlabeled): Give an initial loading bolus of 10.5 mg/M^2 on Day 1 followed by a continuous infusion of 30.5 mg/M^2/day on Days 1 through 5.
Pediatric patients with solid tumors (unlabeled): Dose-limiting myelosuppression was observed with a loading dose of 8 mg/M^2 on Day 1 followed by a continuous infusion of 23.5 mg/M^2/day on Days 1 through 5. Maximum tolerated dose in solid tumor pediatric patients was a loading dose of 7 mg/M^2/day followed by a continuous infusion of 20 mg/M^2/day for 5 days.

DOSE ADJUSTMENTS
Decrease or delay dose based on evidence of hematologic or nonhematologic toxicity. Increased toxicity may occur in the elderly and in patients with renal insufficiency or bone marrow impairment. Monitor closely and adjust dose as indicated. ▪ Adjust initial starting doses for patients with renal impairment as indicated in the following chart.

Fluarabine Starting Dose Adjustment for Renal Impairment	
Creatinine Clearance	Starting Dose
≥80 mL/min	25 mg/M^2 (full dose)
50-79 mL/min	20 mg/M^2
30-49 mL/min	15 mg/M^2
<30 mL/min	Do not administer

DILUTION
Specific techniques required; see Precautions. Available as a sterile solution 50 mg/2 mL (25 mg/mL) or as a lyophilized solid cake (50 mg) requiring reconstitution with 2 mL of SWFI (25 mg/mL). Should dissolve within 15 seconds. In clinical studies, each single dose was further diluted in 100 to 125 mL of NS or D5W and given as an infusion over 30 minutes.
Filters: Specific information from studies not available; contact manufacturer for further information.
Storage: Refrigerate between 2° and 8° C (36° to 46° F) before dilution. No preservative; use within 8 hours of dilution.

COMPATIBILITY
Consider any drug NOT listed as compatible to be INCOMPATIBLE until consulting a pharmacist; specific conditions may apply.
Manufacturer states, "Should not be mixed with other drugs."
One source suggests the following **compatibilities** *(not recommended by manufacturer):*
Y-site: Allopurinol (Aloprim), amifostine (Ethyol), amikacin, aminophylline, ampicillin, ampicillin/sulbactam (Unasyn), aztreonam (Azactam), bleomycin (Blenoxane), butorphanol (Stadol), carboplatin (Paraplatin), carmustine (BiCNU), cefazolin (Ancef), cefo-

taxime (Claforan), cefotetan (Cefotan), ceftazidime (Fortaz), ceftriaxone (Rocephin), cefuroxime (Zinacef), cisplatin, clindamycin (Cleocin), cyclophosphamide (Cytoxan), cytarabine (ARA-C), dacarbazine (DTIC), dactinomycin (Cosmegen), dexamethasone (Decadron), diphenhydramine (Benadryl), doxorubicin (Adriamycin), doxycycline, droperidol (Inapsine), etoposide (VePesid), etoposide phosphate (Etopophos), famotidine (Pepcid IV), filgrastim (Neupogen), fluconazole (Diflucan), fluorouracil (5-FU), furosemide (Lasix), gemcitabine (Gemzar), gentamicin, granisetron (Kytril), heparin, hydrocortisone sodium succinate (Solu-Cortef), hydromorphone (Dilaudid), ifosfamide (Ifex), imipenem-cilastatin (Primaxin), lorazepam (Ativan), magnesium sulfate, mannitol, mechlorethamine (nitrogen mustard), melphalan (Alkeran), meperidine (Demerol), mesna (Mesnex), methotrexate, methylprednisolone (Solu-Medrol), metoclopramide (Reglan), mitoxantrone (Novantrone), morphine, multivitamins (M.V.I.), nalbuphine, ondansetron (Zofran), pentostatin (Nipent), piperacillin/tazobactam (Zosyn), potassium chloride (KCl), promethazine (Phenergan), ranitidine (Zantac), sodium bicarbonate, sulfamethoxazole/trimethoprim, teniposide (Vumon), thiotepa, ticarcillin/clavulanate (Timentin), tobramycin, vancomycin, vinblastine, vincristine, vinorelbine (Navelbine), zidovudine (AZT, Retrovir).

RATE OF ADMINISTRATION
Single daily dose properly diluted for infusion over 30 minutes.

ACTIONS
A potent antineoplastic agent. A fluorinated nucleotide analog of the antiviral agent vidarabine. Rapidly converts to the active metabolite 2-fluoro-ara-ATP and interferes with the synthesis of DNA. Actual mechanism of action unknown and may be multifaceted. Median time to response in studies of patients with refractory chronic lymphocytic leukemia (CLL) was 7 to 21 weeks (range 1 to 68 weeks). Elimination half-life is approximately 20 hours. Total body clearance of the active metabolite is correlated with the CrCl, indicating the importance of renal excretion for drug elimination.

INDICATIONS AND USES
Treatment of patients with B-cell CLL who have not responded to or progressed during treatment with at least one standard alkylating agent–containing regimen. ▪ Safety and effectiveness in previously untreated or nonrefractory patients with CLL not established. **Unlabeled uses:** Treatment of non-Hodgkin's lymphoma, acute lymphocytic leukemia, acute myeloid leukemia, prolymphocytic leukemia or prolymphocytoid variant of CLL, mycosis fungoides, hairy-cell leukemia, and Waldenström's macroglobulinemia. Dose and/or efficacy not established.

CONTRAINDICATIONS
Hypersensitivity to fludarabine or its components (e.g., mannitol and sodium hydroxide). ▪ Not recommended for use in patients with severely impaired renal function (CrCl less than 30 mL/min). ▪ Not recommended for use in combination with pentostatin (Nipent); see Drug/Lab Interactions.

PRECAUTIONS
Follow guidelines for handling cytotoxic agents. See Appendix A, p. 1331. ▪ Administered by or under the direction of the physician specialist. ▪ Use with caution in advanced age, renal insufficiency, or bone marrow impairment, or in patients with immunodeficiency or a history of opportunistic infection. ▪ Severe myelosuppression (anemia, neutropenia, and thrombocytopenia) is common. Median time to nadir counts was 13 days for granulocytes and 16 days for platelets. ▪ Most patients have hematologic impairment at baseline because of disease or prior myelosuppressive therapy. Myelosuppression may be severe and cumulative. ▪ Several instances of trilineage bone marrow hypoplasia or aplasia resulting in pancytopenia, sometimes resulting in death, have been reported. Clinically significant cytopenias lasted from 2 months to 1 year and occurred in untreated and previously treated patients. ▪ Use of irradiated blood product is recommended for patients requiring transfusions during fludarabine therapy because transfusion-associated graft-versus-host disease has been reported. ▪ Use caution in patients with large tumor burdens; may cause tumor lysis syndrome. Response can occur within 1 week. ▪

Life-threatening and sometimes fatal cases of autoimmune phenomena, such as hemolytic anemia, autoimmune thrombocytopenia/thrombocytopenic purpura (ITP), Evans syndrome, and acquired hemophilia, have been reported; see Antidote. ▪ Serious, sometimes fatal infections, including opportunistic infections and reactivations of latent viral infections (e.g., varicella zoster virus [VZV], Epstein-Barr virus, and JC virus [progressive multifocal leukoencephalopathy]), as well as disease progression and transformation (e.g., Richter's syndrome) have been reported. ▪ Severe neurotoxicity characterized by delayed blindness, coma, and death has been reported in patients who received doses that were approximately 4 times greater than the recommended dose. Significant neurotoxicity has also been reported in patients receiving doses in the recommended range. Symptoms may appear 7 to 225 days after the last dose. ▪ Do not administer **live virus vaccines** during or after treatment with fludarabine. ▪ See Side Effects.
Monitor: Observe closely for signs of toxicity, both hematologic and nonhematologic. ▪ Obtain baseline CBC, including differential and platelet count. Repeat regularly to monitor hematopoietic suppression (especially neutrophils and platelets) and hemolysis. ▪ Obtain baseline CrCl. ▪ Observe closely for all signs of infection and any fever of unknown origin. ▪ Prophylactic antibiotics may be indicated pending results of C/S in a febrile neutropenic patient. ▪ Consider prophylactic therapy in patients at risk for developing opportunistic infections. ▪ Nausea and vomiting usually less severe than with many other antineoplastics; prophylactic administration of antiemetics may be indicated. ▪ Monitor for early signs of tumor lysis syndrome (e.g., flank pain, hematuria). Prevention and treatment of hyperuricemia due to tumor lysis syndrome may be accomplished with adequate hydration and, if necessary, allopurinol (Aloprim) and alkalinization of urine. ▪ Monitor for evidence of hemolysis. ▪ Monitor for S/S of neurotoxicity (e.g., agitation, coma, confusion, seizures). ▪ Monitor for thrombocytopenia (platelet count less than 50,000/mm^3). Initiate precautions to prevent excessive bleeding (e.g., inspect IV sites, skin, and mucous membranes; use extreme care during invasive procedures; test urine, emesis, stool, and secretions for occult blood).
Patient Education: Avoid pregnancy; birth control recommended for both males and females during therapy and for at least 6 months after fludarabine regimen has been completed. ▪ Use caution while driving or operating machinery. Agitation, confusion, fatigue, seizures, visual disturbances, and weakness have been reported. ▪ Adherence to periodic blood count monitoring is imperative. ▪ See Appendix D, p. 1333.
Maternal/Child: Category D: both males and females should use contraception and avoid pregnancy; may cause fetal harm; see Patient Education. ▪ Discontinue breast-feeding. ▪ Safety and effectiveness for use in pediatric patients not established; however, data have been submitted to the FDA using the doses described under Pediatric Dose. In pediatric patients, platelet counts appeared to be more sensitive than hemoglobin and WBCs to the effects of fludarabine.
Elderly: See Precautions and Dose Adjustments.

DRUG/LAB INTERACTIONS
Do not use with **pentostatin** (Nipent); may increase risk of fatal pulmonary toxicity. ▪ Do not administer **live virus vaccines** during or after treatment with fludarabine.

SIDE EFFECTS
Are frequent, may be dose limiting, and may cause death. Most common side effects include myelosuppression (anemia, neutropenia, thrombocytopenia), chills, cough, diarrhea, fatigue, fever, infection (including opportunistic and pneumonia), mucositis, nausea and vomiting, and weakness. The most serious side effects include CNS toxicity, hemolytic anemia, pulmonary toxicity, and severe bone marrow suppression. Other reported side effects include agitation, anorexia, arrhythmia, bone marrow aplasia or hypoplasia (may result in pancytopenia), cerebral hemorrhage, coma, confusion, dyspnea, dysuria, edema, elevated hepatic enzymes, esophagitis, GI bleeding/hemorrhage, headache, heart failure, hemorrhagic cystitis, infection, malaise, myalgia, pain, paresthesia, peripheral neuropathy, pulmonary toxicity (ARDS, dyspnea, interstitial pulmonary infiltrate, pulmonary fibrosis, pulmonary hemorrhage, respiratory distress and failure), rashes, seizures, sinusitis, stomatitis, visual disturbances. Onset of flank pain and hematuria may indicate

tumor lysis syndrome (hyperkalemia, hyperphosphatemia, hyperuricemia, hypocalcemia, metabolic acidosis, urate crystalluria, and renal failure); one reported.

Overdose: Severe bone marrow suppression (neutropenia and thrombocytopenia). Severe neurologic toxicity including delayed blindness, coma, and death occurred from 21 to 60 days after the last dose in 36% of patients treated with doses only 4 times greater than the recommended dose. Has occurred (in no more than 0.2% of patients) with average doses.

Post-Marketing: Erythema multiforme, Stevens-Johnson syndrome, toxic epidermal necrolysis, and pemphigus (some with fatal outcomes); rare cases of myelodysplastic syndrome and acute myeloid leukemia associated with prior, concomitant, or subsequent treatment with alkylating agents, topoisomerase inhibitors (e.g., irinotecan [Camptosar]), or irradiation; progressive multifocal leukoencephalopathy (PML) within a few weeks to a year (most with a fatal outcome; some patients had prior and/or concurrent chemo-therapy); trilineage bone marrow hypoplasia or aplasia resulting in pancytopenia and death; and worsening or flare-up of pre-existing skin cancer lesions and/or new onset of skin cancer during or after treatment with fludarabine.

ANTIDOTE

Notify physician of all side effects. Most will be treated symptomatically. Some toxicity is necessary to produce remission. Delay or discontinue the drug for serious hematologic depression. Administration of whole blood products (e.g., packed RBCs, platelets, leu-kocytes) and/or blood modifiers (e.g., darbepoetin alfa [Aranesp], epoetin alfa [Epogen], filgrastim [Neupogen, Zarxio], pegfilgrastim [Neulasta], sargramostim [Leukine]) may be indicated to treat bone marrow toxicity. Restart as soon as signs of bone marrow re-covery occur. Delay or discontinue if neurotoxicity occurs. There is no specific antidote; supportive therapy as indicated will help sustain the patient in toxicity. Symptoms of pulmonary toxicity may improve with the use of corticosteroids; rule out an infectious origin before use. Steroids may or may not be useful in controlling hemolytic episodes.

FLUMAZENIL BBW
(floo-**MAZ**-eh-nill)

Benzodiazepine antagonist
Antidote

Romazicon

pH 4

USUAL DOSE
Reversal of conscious sedation or in general anesthesia: 0.2 mg (2 mL) as an initial dose. Assess level of consciousness. May be repeated at 1-minute intervals, assessing level of consciousness between each dose, until desired level of consciousness achieved or a total cumulative dose of 1 mg (10 mL) has been given (average dose to awakening is 0.6 mg to 1 mg). If resedation occurs (may occur if flumazenil wears off before the benzodiazepine), the above process may be repeated at 20-minute intervals as indicated. Do not give more than a cumulative dose of 1 mg in a 20-minute period or 3 mg in any 1 hour.
Management of suspected benzodiazepine overdose: 0.2 mg (2 mL) as an initial dose. Assess level of consciousness. If results inadequate, give an additional dose of 0.3 mg (3 mL) in 1 minute. If results are still inadequate, 0.5 mg (5 mL) may be repeated at 1-minute intervals. Assess level of consciousness between each dose until desired level of consciousness achieved or a total cumulative dose of 3 mg (30 mL) has been given (average dose to awakening is 1 mg to 3 mg). If a partial response is achieved with 3 mg, continue dosing in 0.5-mg increments until awakening or a cumulative dose of 5 mg is reached (rarely required). If patient has not responded to a cumulative dose of 5 mg within 5 minutes, benzodiazepines are not the major cause of sedation; discontinue use. If desired results are achieved and resedation occurs (expected), no more than 1 mg given in 0.5-mg increments may be given in any 20-minute period and no more than a cumulative total dose of 3 mg in any 1 hour.

PEDIATRIC DOSE
Reversal of conscious sedation: 0.01 mg/kg (up to 0.2 mg). Assess level of consciousness. May repeat at 1-minute intervals, assessing level of consciousness between each dose until desired level of consciousness achieved or a maximum total dose of 0.05 mg/kg (or 1 mg) has been given. Mean total dose administered in trials was 0.65 mg. See Maternal/Child.

DOSE ADJUSTMENTS
Not required for the elderly. ▪ Reduce dose and extend intervals after the initial dose in impaired liver function. ▪ Individualize dose in high-risk patients. Administer the smallest amount that is effective and wait for peak effect (6 to 10 minutes). Slower titration rates and lower total doses may be especially important in these patients (see Precautions) to reduce emergent confusion and agitation, to prevent seizures, and to evaluate effect.

DILUTION
May be given undiluted through a free-flowing IV into a large vein (to minimize pain at injection site). **Compatible** with D5W, D2½W, LR, ½NS, and NS if further dilution required by a specific situation.
Storage: Store unopened vials at CRT. Discard in 24 hours if drawn undiluted into a syringe or diluted in any solution.

COMPATIBILITY
Consider any drug NOT listed as compatible to be INCOMPATIBLE until consulting a pharmacist; specific conditions may apply.
One source suggests the following **compatibilities:**
Additive: Aminophylline, dobutamine, dopamine, famotidine (Pepcid IV), heparin, lidocaine, procainamide (Pronestyl), ranitidine (Zantac).

RATE OF ADMINISTRATION
Series of small injections allows control of the reversal of sedation to desired endpoint, avoids abrupt awakening, and minimizes the possibility of adverse effects. Rapid

injection may cause withdrawal symptoms in patients with long-term exposure to benzodiazepines.

Reversal of conscious sedation or in general anesthesia: Each single dose over 15 seconds. **Management of suspected benzodiazepine overdose:** Each single dose (0.2 mg [2 mL], 0.3 mg [3 mL], 0.5 mg [5 mL], respectively) is given over 30 seconds.

ACTIONS

A benzodiazepine antagonist. Competes with benzodiazepines, inhibiting their effect at benzodiazepine receptor sites. Action is very specific and reverses the effects of benzodiazepines only. Antagonizes (reverses) the sedation, impairment of recall, psychomotor impairment, and ventilatory depression produced by benzodiazepines. Duration and degree of reversal are related to dose and plasma concentration (both for amount of benzodiazepine and amount of flumazenil). Onset of action usually occurs within 1 to 2 minutes of reaching the appropriate dose, with peak effect at 6 to 10 minutes. Enables the physician to control the duration of action of benzodiazepines and to evaluate the patient's postoperative condition earlier and may facilitate the postprocedural course. In overdose, it allows the physician to communicate sooner with patients who have taken an excessive dose. Extensively metabolized in the liver. Half-life is 40 to 80 minutes. Excreted in changed form in urine and to a small extent in feces.

INDICATIONS AND USES

Adults: Complete or partial reversal of the effects of general anesthesia induced and/or maintained with benzodiazepines (e.g., diazepam [Valium], midazolam [Versed]). ▪ Complete or partial reversal of the sedative effects of benzodiazepines used to produce and/or maintain conscious sedation (e.g., diagnostic and therapeutic procedures). ▪ Adjunct to conventional treatment in managing benzodiazepine overdose (e.g., chlordiazepoxide [Librium], diazepam [Valium], lorazepam [Ativan], midazolam [Versed]).

Pediatric patients 1 to 17 years of age: Reversal of conscious sedation induced with benzodiazepines; see Maternal/Child. ▪ Not approved for other indications but has been used at doses similar to those used for reversal of conscious sedation; see Maternal/Child.

CONTRAINDICATIONS

Known hypersensitivity to flumazenil or any benzodiazepine, patients who are on benzodiazepine therapy for control of potentially life-threatening conditions (e.g., control of intracranial pressure, status epilepticus), and patients showing signs of serious cyclic antidepressant overdose. ▪ Use in treatment of benzodiazepine dependence is not recommended.

PRECAUTIONS

Excess administration increases risk of side effects and decreases desired therapeutics of benzodiazepines. ▪ Will not reverse the central nervous system (CNS) effects of drugs such as alcohol, analgesics, antidepressants, barbiturates, and narcotics. In overdose, will bring the patient to a conscious state only if a benzodiazepine is responsible for the sedation. Has reversed benzodiazepine-induced hypotension and bradycardia unresponsive to other measures (e.g., IV fluids, atropine, dopamine). ▪ Convulsions may occur, especially in patients who rely on benzodiazepines to control seizures or are physically dependent on benzodiazepines for long-term sedation, in overdose cases in which patients are showing signs of serious cyclic antidepressant overdose (some clinicians recommend a diagnostic ECG or quantitative analytical testing before use—see Contraindications), or in ICU patients who may have an unrecognized dependence on benzodiazepines because of frequent use as a sedative (can occur with only 3 to 5 days of benzodiazepine administration). Intubation with ventilatory and circulatory support may be the treatment of choice for these high-risk patients; see Dose Adjustments. ▪ Risk of adverse reactions increased in patients with a history of alcohol, benzodiazepine, or sedative use (increased frequency of benzodiazepine tolerance and dependence). Can precipitate benzodiazepine withdrawal (also high-risk; see Dose Adjustments). ▪ Use extreme caution in head injury (may alter cerebral blood flow or cause convulsions). ▪ Do not use until effects of neuromuscular blockade have been fully reversed. ▪ May cause panic attacks in patients with a history of panic disorder. ▪ Flumazenil may not completely reverse respiratory depression due to benzodiazepines in patients with serious lung disease. Additional ventilatory support may be required. ▪ Half-life prolonged based on amount of hepatic impairment. ▪ Ingestion of food increases clearance of flumazenil.

Monitor: Confirm secure airway, ventilation, and IV access before administration as indicated. ▪ Monitor BP, HR, and respirations closely. ECG monitoring and oxygenation determination by pulse oximetry is recommended. ▪ Emergency equipment and supplies, including drugs for seizure control (see Antidote), must always be available. ▪ Observe continuously for resedation, respiratory depression, preseizure activity, or other residual benzodiazepine effects for an appropriate period (2 or more hours). ▪ Extend observation time for larger doses, in presence of long-acting benzodiazepines (e.g., diazepam [Valium]), or large doses of short-acting benzodiazepines (e.g., more than 10 mg of midazolam [Versed]). ▪ Observe ambulatory patients for a minimum of 2 hours after a 1-mg dose; resedation after 2 hours is unlikely. Extend observation time as above. ▪ Awake patients may require pain medication sooner than those without benzodiazepine reversal. ▪ All postprocedural instructions must be given to the patient verbally and in writing; does not reverse benzodiazepine amnesia. ▪ See Drug/Lab Interactions.

Patient Education: Review medication use, especially benzodiazepine, alcohol, and sedative use prior to surgery or procedure. ▪ Effects of benzodiazepines may recur; for 24 to 48 hours memory and judgment may be impaired. ▪ All instructions should be in writing. ▪ Do not drive, operate hazardous machinery, or engage in activities that require alertness. ▪ Do not take alcohol, other CNS depressants (e.g., antihistamines, barbiturates), or nonprescription drugs for 24 hours.

Maternal/Child: Category C: use only if benefit justifies risk. ▪ Not recommended during labor and delivery because effect on newborn unknown. ▪ Safety for use in breastfeeding not established. ▪ Safety and effectiveness for reversal of conscious sedation induced with benzodiazepines have been established in pediatric patients 1 to 17 years of age. Resedation may occur, especially in pediatric patients 1 to 5 years of age. Safety and effectiveness of repeated flumazenil doses in pediatric patients experiencing resedation have not been established. ▪ Safety and effectiveness for other uses listed under adult indications have not been established. However, published anecdotal reports have cited safety profiles and dosing guidelines similar to those used in reversal of conscious sedation. ▪ Half-life appears to be shorter and more variable in pediatric patients.

Elderly: See Dose Adjustments. Age-related differences in safety and effectiveness have not been observed; however, a greater sensitivity of some older patients cannot be ruled out. ▪ Monitor carefully; benzodiazepine-induced sedation may be deeper and more prolonged.

DRUG/LAB INTERACTIONS
May cause cardiac arrhythmias or convulsions in cases of mixed drug overdose. These toxic effects may emerge (especially with **cyclic antidepressants** [e.g., amitriptyline (Elavil), imipramine (Tofranil)]) with reversal of benzodiazepine effect; see Precautions. May reverse sedative and anticonvulsant effects. ▪ May precipitate withdrawal symptoms if given to chronic **benzodiazepine** users. ▪ No specific deleterious interactions noted when flumazenil administered after **narcotics, inhalational anesthetics, muscle relaxants, and muscle relaxant antagonists** administered in conjunction with sedation or anesthesia. ▪ Not recommended for use in **epileptic patients** who have been receiving benzodiazepines for a prolonged period. ▪ Lab test interactions have not been evaluated.

SIDE EFFECTS
Most common at doses above 1 mg and/or with abrupt reversal.

Abnormal vision, agitation, anxiety, dizziness, dry mouth, dyspnea, emotional lability, fatigue, flushing, headache, hot flashes, hypertension, hyperventilation, insomnia, involuntary movements, irritability, muscle tension, nausea, pain or reaction (rash, thrombophlebitis) at the injection site, palpitations, panic, paresthesia, sweating, tachycardia, tinnitus, tremors, and vomiting. Convulsions, fear, and panic attacks may occur; see Precautions. Deaths have been reported. Risk increased in patients with serious underlying disease or in patients who overdose on nonbenzodiazepine drugs (usually cyclic antidepressants).

Overdose: Agitation, anxiety, arrhythmias, convulsions, hyperesthesia, increased muscle tone.

ANTIDOTE

Notify the physician of any side effect. Treat symptoms of benzodiazepine withdrawal (agitation, confusion, dizziness, emotional lability, or sensory distortions) with a barbiturate, benzodiazepine, or other sedative. Larger doses may be required because of presence of flumazenil. Treat convulsions from overdose with barbiturates, benzodiazepines, and phenytoin (Dilantin). Maintain an adequate airway, adequate ventilation, and IV access at all times. Hemodialysis not effective in overdose if 1 hour has passed since administration.

FLUOROURACIL BBW

(flew-roh-**YOUR**-ah-sill)

Adrucil, 5-Fluorouracil, 5-FU

Antineoplastic
(antimetabolite)

pH 9.2

USUAL DOSE

Many dosing regimens are in use. May be given as an injection or as a continuous infusion. Manufacturer recommends 12 mg/kg of body weight/24 hr for 4 days. Total dose should not exceed 800 mg/24 hr. If no toxicity is observed, one-half dose (6 mg/kg) is given on Days 6, 8, 10, and 12 unless toxicity occurs. No medication is given on Days 5, 7, 9, or 11. Discontinue therapy on Day 12, even if no toxicity is apparent. See Precautions/Monitor. The most common form of maintenance therapy is to repeat the entire course of therapy beginning 30 days after the previous course is completed and any toxicity has subsided or to give a single dose of 10 to 15 mg/kg/week, not to exceed 1 Gm/week. Dose adjustments of subsequent doses are made depending on side effects and tolerance.

Advanced colorectal cancer (unlabeled dose): Various protocols have been used. Examples are leucovorin calcium 20 mg/M^2 followed by fluorouracil 425 mg/M^2, or leucovorin calcium 200 mg/M^2 followed by fluorouracil 370 mg/M^2 daily for 5 days. Repeat at 4-week intervals twice, then repeat every 28 to 35 days based on complete recovery from toxic effects. Do not initiate or continue in any patient with GI toxicity until completely subsided. Reduce fluorouracil dose based on tolerance to previous course; reduce 20% for moderate hematologic or GI toxicity, 30% for severe toxicity. Increase fluorouracil dose 10% if no toxicity. Leucovorin calcium dose is not adjusted. Alternatively, fluorouracil may also be used in combination with levoleucovorin; dose is different; see levoleucovorin monograph. Fluorouracil and leucovorin calcium are also used in combination with irinotecan (Camptosar); see irinotecan monograph.

Breast cancer (unlabeled dose): Various protocols have been used. An example is fluorouracil 600 mg/M^2 on Days 1 and 8 of each cycle combined with cyclophosphamide (Cytoxan) 100 mg/M^2 on Days 1 through 14 of each cycle and methotrexate 40 mg/M^2 on Days 1 and 8 of each cycle. Repeat cycles monthly (allowing a 2-week rest between cycles). Repeat for 6 to 12 cycles (6 to 12 months). Doxorubicin (Adriamycin) has also been included in this regimen. In patients older than 60 years, reduce the fluorouracil dose to 400 mg/M^2 and the initial methotrexate dose to 30 mg/M^2.

DOSE ADJUSTMENTS

For poor-risk patients or those in a poor nutritional state, either reduce dose by one half or more throughout a course of therapy or give 6 mg/kg/day for 3 days. If no toxicity observed, give 3 mg/kg on Days 5, 7, and 9. Give nothing on Days 4, 6, or 8. Do not exceed 400 mg/day. ▪ Dose based on ideal body weight in presence of edema, ascites, or obesity. ▪ Reduce dose in patients who have received high-dose pelvic irradiation or other cytotoxic drug therapy with alkylating agents (e.g., cisplatin, ifosfamide [Ifex]). ▪ One source recommends a dose adjustment in patients with impaired hepatic function. Give the full dose if the bilirubin is 5 or less on the day of administration; omit the dose if the bilirubin is greater than 5. ▪ Used with other antineoplastic drugs in reduced doses to achieve tumor remission. ▪ See Usual Dose.

DILUTION

Specific techniques required; see Precautions. May be slightly discolored without affecting safety and potency. Dissolve any precipitate by heating to 60° C (140° F) and shaking vigorously. Let cool to body temperature before using.

IV injection: May be given undiluted. May inject through Y-tube or three-way stopcock of a free-flowing infusion.

Infusion: May be further diluted with D5W or NS and given as an infusion. Doses up to 2 Gm are being given with extreme caution under the specific supervision of experienced specialists. Leucovorin calcium has been mixed into the solution with fluorouracil.

Storage: Store at room temperature; protect from light.

COMPATIBILITY   (Underline Indicates Conflicting Compatibility Information)

Consider any drug NOT listed as compatible to be INCOMPATIBLE until consulting a pharmacist; specific conditions may apply.

One source suggests the following **compatibilities:**

Additive: Bleomycin (Blenoxane), cyclophosphamide (Cytoxan), etoposide (VePesid), hydromorphone (Dilaudid), ifosfamide (Ifex), methotrexate, mitoxantrone (Novantrone), vincristine.

Y-site: Allopurinol (Aloprim), amifostine (Ethyol), anidulafungin (Eraxis), aztreonam (Azactam), bleomycin (Blenoxane), cisplatin, cyclophosphamide (Cytoxan), doripenem (Doribax), doxorubicin (Adriamycin), doxorubicin liposomal (Doxil), etoposide phosphate (Etopophos), fludarabine (Fludara), furosemide (Lasix), gemcitabine (Gemzar), granisetron (Kytril), heparin, hydrocortisone sodium succinate (Solu-Cortef), leucovorin calcium, linezolid (Zyvox), mannitol, melphalan (Alkeran), methotrexate, metoclopramide (Reglan), mitomycin (Mutamycin), ondansetron (Zofran), paclitaxel (Taxol), palonosetron (Aloxi), pemetrexed (Alimta), piperacillin/tazobactam (Zosyn), potassium chloride (KCl), propofol (Diprivan), sargramostim (Leukine), teniposide (Vumon), thiotepa, vinblastine, vincristine.

RATE OF ADMINISTRATION

IV injection: A single dose over 1 to 15 minutes.

Infusion: A single dose is usually administered over 24 hours. Toxicity may be lessened by extended administration.

ACTIONS

An antimetabolite. A fluorinated pyrimidine antagonist, cell cycle specific, that interferes with the synthesis of DNA and RNA. Through various chemical processes this deprivation acts more quickly on rapidly growing cells and causes their death. Distributes into tumors, intestinal mucosa, bone marrow, liver, and readily crosses the blood-brain barrier into cerebrospinal fluid and brain tissue. Metabolized by the liver within 3 hours. Half-life is approximately 16 minutes. Excretion is through the urine and as respiratory CO_2.

INDICATIONS AND USES

To suppress or slow neoplastic growth. Palliative treatment of cancers of the breast, colon, pancreas, rectum, and stomach. May be used alone or in combination with other agents.

Unlabeled uses: Has been used for the treatment of bladder, cervical, endometrial, esophageal, head and neck, ovarian, prostatic, skin (topical), and other cancers. Consult oncology literature for protocols in use.

CONTRAINDICATIONS

Potentially serious infections, depressed bone marrow function, poor nutritional state, hypersensitivity, major surgery within the previous month.

PRECAUTIONS

Follow guidelines for handling cytotoxic agents. See Appendix A, p. 1331. ▪ Administered by or under the direction of the physician specialist with facilities for monitoring the patient and responding to any medical emergency. Hospitalization, at least during the initial course of therapy, is recommended. ▪ Use caution in patients who have had high-dose pelvic irradiation, previous alkylating agents (e.g., cisplatin), other antimetabolic drugs (e.g., methotrexate), metastatic tumor involvement of the bone marrow, impaired hepatic or renal function, or dihydropyrimidine dehydrogenase deficiency. ▪ Pseudomembranous colitis has been reported. May range from mild to life threatening. Consider in patients that present with diarrhea during or after treatment with fluorouracil.

Monitor: Confirm patency of vein. Avoid extravasation. Change peripheral injection site every 48 hours. ▪ Obtain a CBC with differential and platelet count before each dose. When given with leucovorin calcium, repeat weekly the first two courses and then at the time of anticipated WBC nadir in following courses. Electrolytes and liver function tests should be done before the first three courses, then every other course. ▪ Be alert for signs of bone marrow suppression or infection. Prophylactic antibiotics may be indicated pending results of C/S in a febrile neutropenic patient. ▪ Examine mouth and lips daily for sores or other signs of stomatitis. ▪ Prophylactic antiemetics may reduce nausea and vomiting and increase patient comfort. ▪ Toxicity increased by any form of therapy that adds to stress, poor nutrition, and bone marrow suppression. ▪ Monitor for thrombocytopenia (platelet count less than 50,000/mm^3). Initiate precautions to prevent excessive bleeding (e.g., inspect IV sites, skin, and mucous membranes; use extreme care during invasive procedures; test urine, emesis, stool, and secretions for occult blood). ▪ See Drug/Lab Interactions.

Patient Education: Nonhormonal birth control recommended. ▪ See Appendix D, p. 1333. ▪ Report IV site burning and stinging promptly. ▪ Drink at least 2 liters of fluid each day.

Maternal/Child: Category D: avoid pregnancy; can cause fetal harm. ▪ Discontinue breastfeeding. ▪ Safety for use in pediatric patients not established.

Elderly: May be more sensitive to toxic effects of the drug. Consider age-related organ impairment. ▪ See Dose Adjustments.

DRUG/LAB INTERACTIONS

Potentiates **anticoagulants**. ▪ Do not administer **live virus vaccines** to patients receiving antineoplastic drugs. ▪ **Cimetidine** (Tagamet), **interferon alfa, and leucovorin calcium** may increase toxicity. ▪ Additive bone marrow suppression may occur with **radiation therapy, other bone marrow–suppressing agents** (e.g., azathioprine, chloramphenicol, irinotecan [Camptosar], melphalan [Alkeran], vinorelbine [Navelbine]), **and/or agents that cause blood dyscrasias** (e.g., metronidazole [Flagyl IV]). ▪ **Thiazide diuretics** (e.g., chlorothiazide [Diuril]) may prolong antineoplastic-induced leukopenia. ▪ May decrease metabolism and increase serum levels of **phenytoin** (Dilantin).

SIDE EFFECTS

Abnormal bromsulphalein (BSP), prothrombin, total protein, sedimentation rate; alopecia (reversible), anaphylaxis, bleeding, bone marrow suppression (agranulocytosis, anemia, leukopenia, pancytopenia, thrombocytopenia), cerebellar syndrome, cramps, dermatitis, diarrhea, disorientation, dry lips, erythema, esophagopharyngitis and stomatitis (may lead to sloughing and ulceration), euphoria, frequent stools, GI ulceration and bleeding, headache, hemorrhage from any site, increased skin pigmentation, infection, lacrimal duct stenosis, mouth soreness and ulceration, myocardial ischemia, nail changes, nausea, palmar-plantar erythrodysesthesia syndrome (tingling of hands and feet followed by pain, redness, and swelling), photophobia, photosensitivity, pneumopathy (cough, shortness of breath), thrombophlebitis, visual changes, vomiting (intractable). Diarrhea and stomatitis are most common and may be more severe with a prolonged duration in patients on combination therapy. Pseudomembranous colitis has been reported.

ANTIDOTE

Keep physician informed of any side effects. Discontinue the drug and notify physician promptly at the first sign of toxicity (e.g., bleeding, diarrhea, esophagopharyngitis, gastritis, intractable vomiting, rapidly falling white count, sores in or around the lips or mouth, stomatitis). Nadir of leukocyte count occurs around days 9 to 14. Recovery should be by day 30. Discontinue the drug if the WBC count is less than 3,500/mm^3 or platelets are less than 100,000/mm^3; should reach 4,000/mm^3 and 130,000/mm^3 respectively in 2 weeks; if they do not, discontinue treatment. Administration of whole blood products (e.g., packed RBCs, platelets, leukocytes, and/or blood modifiers (e.g., darbepoetin alfa [Aranesp], epoetin alfa [Epogen], filgrastim [Neupogen, Zarxio], pegfilgrastim [Neulasta], sargramostim [Leukine]) may be indicated to treat bone marrow toxicity. Continue to monitor for 4 weeks. Palmar-plantar erythrodysesthesia syndrome has been treated with oral pyridoxine (vitamin B$_6$), 100 to 150 mg daily. Death may occur from the progression of many side effects. There is no specific antidote; supportive therapy as indicated will help sustain the patient in toxicity.

FOLIC ACID
(**FOH**-lik **AS**-id)

Nutritional supplement
(vitamin)
Antianemic

pH 8 to 11

USUAL DOSE

Therapeutic dose: 0.1 to 1 mg daily (never give less than 0.1 mg). Larger doses may be required.

Maintenance dose: 0.4 mg daily. *Pregnant or lactating females:* 0.8 mg daily.

PEDIATRIC DOSE

See Maternal/Child.

Therapeutic dose: 0.1 to 1 mg daily (never give less than 0.1 mg).

Maintenance dose: *Infants:* 0.1 mg daily. *Under 4 years:* Up to 0.3 mg daily. *Over 4 years:* Same as adult.

DOSE ADJUSTMENTS

Increased initial and maintenance doses may be required in alcoholism, hemolytic anemia, anticonvulsant therapy, or chronic infection.

DILUTION

Each dose (up to 5 mg) should be diluted in at least 50 mL of SWFI, D5W, or NS. May be added to most IV solutions and given as an infusion.

Storage: Protect from light and freezing.

COMPATIBILITY

Consider any drug NOT listed as compatible to be INCOMPATIBLE until consulting a pharmacist; specific conditions may apply.

Manufacturer lists as **incompatible** with calcium gluconate (even though a precipitate cannot be seen), doxapram (Dopram), heavy metal ions, iron sulfate, oxidizing agents, reducing agents, solutions with a pH less than 5.

One source suggests the following **compatibilities:**

Y-site: Famotidine (Pepcid IV).

RATE OF ADMINISTRATION

5 mg or fraction thereof over a minimum of 1 minute; usually given over 30 minutes or more in an infusion.

ACTIONS

Folic acid (pteroylglutamic acid) is part of the vitamin B complex. In humans, exogenous folate is required for nucleoprotein synthesis and the maintenance of normal erythropoiesis. It is the precursor of tetrahydrofolic acid, an important cofactor involved in the synthesis of amino acids and DNA. Stimulates the production of RBCs, WBCs, and platelets. Metabolized in the liver and excreted in the urine. Crosses the placental barrier. Secreted in breast milk.

INDICATIONS AND USES

For prevention and treatment of folic acid deficiency. Megaloblastic anemias resulting from folic acid deficiency may be seen in sprue; anemias of malnutrition, pregnancy, infancy, and childhood; developmental or surgical anomalies of the GI tract; and other conditions.

CONTRAINDICATIONS

Pernicious anemia unless used in combination with diagnostic testing.

PRECAUTIONS

Folic acid is not commonly administered by the IV route. Oral or IM administration provides adequate absorption in most cases. ▪ Obscures the peripheral blood picture and prevents the diagnosis of pernicious anemia. May actually aggravate the neurologic symptoms.
Monitor: Obtain CBC before and during therapy.
Maternal/Child: Category A: an important vitamin before and during pregnancy. Folate-deficient mothers have a higher incidence of fetal anomalies and complications of pregnancy. ▪ Safe for use during breast-feeding; infant may require supplementation if mother is folate deficient. ▪ Some products contain benzyl alcohol as a preservative. Avoid use in neonates.
Elderly: More likely to have folate deficiency.

DRUG/LAB INTERACTIONS

Toxic effects of antineoplastic folic acid antagonists are blocked by **folinic acid** (leucovorin calcium) but not by folic acid IV. ▪ Increases **hydantoin** metabolism (e.g., phenytoin [Dilantin]); seizures may result. ▪ Inhibited by **dihydrofolate reductase inhibitors** (e.g., methotrexate, trimethoprim), **pyrimethamine, and triamterene** and by depressed **hematopoiesis, alcoholism,** and deficiencies of **vitamins B$_6$, B$_{12}$, C, and E.** ▪ **Aminosalicylic acid** (Pamisyl) or **sulfasalazine** (Azulfidine) may decrease serum folate levels. ▪ **Oral contraceptives** may inhibit folate metabolism.

SIDE EFFECTS

Almost nonexistent. Confusion, some slight flushing or feeling of warmth, nausea; anaphylaxis can occur.

ANTIDOTE

If anaphylaxis occurs, discontinue drug, treat anaphylaxis, and notify physician. Resuscitate as necessary.

FOMEPIZOLE INJECTION

(foh-**MEP**-ih-zoll in-**JEK**-shun)

Antidote

Antizol

USUAL DOSE

Ethylene glycol is the main component of antifreeze and coolants. Methanol is the main component of windshield washer fluid and a component of products such as Sternol (for fondue pots), Heet (gasoline antifreeze), and various paint products. Begin fomepizole treatment immediately upon suspicion of ethylene glycol or methanol ingestion based on patient history and/or anion gap metabolic acidosis, increased osmolar gap, visual disturbances, or oxalate crystals in the urine, or a documented serum ethylene glycol or methanol concentration greater than 20 mg/dL.

Adults with blood concentrations over 20 mg/dL but less than 50 mg/dL: Administer a loading dose of 15 mg/kg as a slow intravenous infusion. Follow with 10 mg/kg every 12 hours times 4 doses, then 15 mg/kg every 12 hours until ethylene glycol or methanol concentrations are undetectable or have been reduced below 20 mg/dL and the patient is asymptomatic with normal pH.

Adults with blood concentrations of 50 mg/dL or higher, renal failure, or significant or worsening metabolic acidosis: In addition to dosing as above, dialysis should be considered to correct metabolic abnormalities and to lower the ethylene glycol or methanol concentrations below 50 mg/dL.

Dosage with renal dialysis: Amount of loading dose and following doses (mg/kg) remains the same, but fomepizole is dialyzable and the frequency of dosing should be increased to every 4 hours during hemodialysis. Base frequency on the following chart.

Fomepizole Dosing in Patients Requiring Dialysis	
DOSE AT THE BEGINNING OF HEMODIALYSIS	
If <6 hours since last fomepizole dose Do not administer dose	If ≥6 hours since last fomepizole dose Administer next scheduled dose
DOSING DURING HEMODIALYSIS	
Dose every 4 hours	
DOSING AT THE TIME HEMODIALYSIS IS COMPLETED	
Time between last dose and the end of the hemodialysis	
<1 hour	Do not administer dose at the end of hemodialysis
1-3 hours	Administer 1/2 of next scheduled dose
>3 hours	Administer next scheduled dose
MAINTENANCE DOSING OFF HEMODIALYSIS	
Give next scheduled dose 12 hours from last dose administered	

DOSE ADJUSTMENTS

Fomepizole has not been studied sufficiently to determine whether the pharmacokinetics differ for the elderly (see Elderly), pediatric patients, between genders, in renal insufficiency (excreted renally), or in hepatic insufficiency (metabolized by the liver).

DILUTION

Fomepizole solidifies at temperatures less than 25° C (77° F). If it is solidified, liquefy by running the vial under warm water or by holding in the hand. Solidification does not affect the efficacy, safety, or stability. Withdraw the appropriate dose. Each single dose **must be diluted** in at least 100 mL of NS or D5W and given as an infusion. Mix well. **Storage:** Store vials at CRT 20° to 25° C (68° to 77° F). Diluted solutions are stable refrigerated or at CRT for 48 hours; however, manufacturer states should be used within 24 hours of dilution.

COMPATIBILITY

Specific information not available. Consider specific use; consult pharmacist.

RATE OF ADMINISTRATION

Each single dose must be given as a slow intravenous infusion equally distributed over 30 minutes. **Do not give undiluted or by bolus injection;** has caused serious venous irritation and phlebosclerosis.

ACTIONS

A synthetic competitive alcohol dehydrogenase inhibitor. Effectively blocks formation of toxic metabolites (glycolic and oxalic acids [ethylene glycol] and formic acid [methanol]). These toxins can induce metabolic acidosis, nausea and vomiting, seizures, stupor, coma, calcium oxaluria, acute tubular necrosis, blindness, and death. Has shown minimal CNS depressant effects. Plasma half-life varies with dose and has not been calculated. Rapidly distributes into total body water. Metabolized in the liver by the P_{450} mixed-function oxidase system. Significant increases in the elimination rate occur after 30 to 40 hours. Excreted in urine.

INDICATIONS AND USES

An antidote for ethylene glycol (antifreeze) or methanol (windshield wiper fluid) poisoning, or for use in suspected ethylene glycol or methanol ingestion either alone or in combination with hemodialysis.

CONTRAINDICATIONS

Known serious hypersensitivity to fomepizole or other pyrazoles (e.g., sulfinpyrazone [Anturane]).

PRECAUTIONS

Acute ethylene glycol or methanol poisoning is a medical emergency that is characterized by a syndrome that can include CNS depression, severe metabolic acidosis, renal failure, and coma. Can be lethal if left untreated or when treatment is delayed due to delayed diagnosis. The lethal dose of ethylene glycol is approximately 1.4 mL/kg. The lethal dose of methanol is approximately 1.2 mL/kg. ▪ If ethylene glycol or methanol poisoning is left untreated, the natural progression of the poisoning leads to accumulation of toxic metabolites, including glycolic and oxalic acids (ethylene glycol) and formic acid (methanol). These metabolites can induce metabolic acidosis, nausea and vomiting, seizures, stupor, coma, calcium oxaluria, acute tubular necrosis, and death. ▪ The diagnosis of these poisonings may be difficult because ethylene glycol and methanol levels diminish in the blood as they are metabolized. ▪ The ethylene glycol or methanol concentrations and the acid-base balance, as determined by serum electrolyte (anion gap) and/or arterial blood gas analysis, should be frequently monitored and used to guide treatment. ▪ Fomepizole has caused minor hypersensitivity reactions (mild rash, eosinophilia).

Monitor: Maintain a patent airway and support ventilation as indicated; CNS and respiratory distress may occur suddenly. ▪ Gastric lavage may be indicated if performed soon after ingestion or in patients who are comatose or at risk for seizures. ▪ Patients must be managed for metabolic acidosis, acute renal failure (ethylene glycol), adult respiratory distress syndrome, visual disturbances (methanol), and hypocalcemia (may result in tetany). Sodium bicarbonate may be required to treat metabolic acidosis. Correct electrolyte imbalance and maintain adequate urine output with IV fluids. A decrease in the amount of fluids will be required in impending renal failure to prevent fluid overload; monitor closely. ▪ Potassium supplementation and oxygen administration are usually necessary. ▪ Administer IV calcium to patients with seizures or tetany that may be caused by decreased calcium, but do not attempt to correct hypocalcemia itself (may increase precipitation of calcium oxalate crystals in the tissues). ▪ Hemodialysis is necessary in the anuric patient and should be considered in patients with severe metabolic acidosis or azotemia and in any patient with high ethylene glycol or methanol concentrations (equal to or greater than 50 mg/dL). ▪ ECG should be continuous to monitor for cardiac irregularities. ▪ EEG may be required in the comatose patient. ▪ The effective inhibition of alcohol dehydrogenase requires fomepizole plasma concentrations in the range of 100 to 300 micromol/L (8.6 to 24.6 mg/L). ▪ To assess treatment success, obtain baseline and frequently monitor measurements of blood gases, pH, electrolytes, BUN, creatinine, and urinalysis in addition to other laboratory tests as indicated by each patient's condition. ▪ To assess the status of ethylene glycol or methanol and their respective metabolite clearances, obtain baseline ethylene glycol or methanol plasma and urine concentrations and presence of urinary oxalate crystals (ethylene glycol) and monitor frequently. ▪ Obtain baseline and monitor hepatic enzymes and WBC counts during treatment; transient increases in serum transaminase levels and eosinophilia have been noted with repeated fomepizole dosing. ▪ Monitor for signs of hypersensitivity reactions; see Precautions.

Patient Education: Monitoring of urine output imperative. ▪ Cooperation with adequate hydration and frequent laboratory analysis required. ▪ Request assistance with ambulation.

Maternal/Child: Category C: use during pregnancy only if clearly needed. ▪ Decreased testicular mass in rats. ▪ Use caution during breast-feeding; not known if fomepizole is secreted in breast milk. ▪ Safety and effectiveness for use in pediatric patients not established.

Elderly: Risk of toxic reactions may be greater in patients with impaired renal function; consider age-related renal impairment.

DRUG/LAB INTERACTIONS

Has not been studied, but reciprocal interactions (increasing or decreasing clearance, effects, or toxicity) may occur with concomitant use of **drugs that induce or inhibit the cytochrome P$_{450}$ system** (e.g., carbamazepine [Tegretol], cimetidine [Tagamet], ketoconazole [Nizoral], phenytoin [Dilantin]). Oral fomepizole significantly reduced the rate of elimination of **ethanol** (by 40%) in healthy subjects. Ethanol decreased the rate of elimination of fomepizole (by 50%).

SIDE EFFECTS

Most common side effects are dizziness, headache, and nausea. Abdominal pain, abnormal smell, anemia, anorexia, arrhythmias (bradycardia, tachycardia), back pain (lower), blurred vision, decreased awareness of surroundings, diarrhea, DIC, feeling of drunkenness, fever, hangover, heartburn, hiccups, hypersensitivity reactions (e.g., mild rash, eosinophilia), hypotension, injection site reaction, light-headedness, lymphangitis, multisystem organ failure, nystagmus, pharyngitis, phlebitis, phlebosclerosis, seizure, shock, slurred speech, somnolence, taste changes (bad or metallic), vertigo, visual problems, vomiting occurred in up to 6% of patients.

Overdose: Dizziness, nausea, and vertigo occurred in healthy volunteers given 3 to 6 times the recommended dose.

ANTIDOTE

Keep physician informed of all side effects, laboratory results, and concurrent medical problems. Dialysis may be indicated for changes in patient condition (e.g., renal failure, significant or worsening metabolic acidosis, or a measured ethylene glycol or methanol concentration of greater than 50 mg/dL) or in the treatment of overdose. Treat side effects symptomatically as indicated. Resuscitate as necessary.

FOSAPREPITANT DIMEGLUMINE
(fos-ap-**RE**-pi-tant dye-**MEG**-loo-meen)

Emend

Antiemetic
Substance P/NK$_1$
receptor antagonist

USUAL DOSE
150 mg as IV infusion over 20 to 30 minutes approximately 30 minutes before chemotherapy. Given in combination with dexamethasone and a 5-HT$_3$ antagonist as outlined in the following charts.

Recommended Dosing for the Prevention of Nausea and Vomiting Associated with Highly Emetogenic Cancer Chemotherapy (HEC)				
	Day 1	Day 2	Day 3	Day 4
Fosaprepitant IV*	150 mg IV	None	None	None
Dexamethasone†	12 mg PO	8 mg PO	8 mg PO twice daily	8 mg PO twice daily
5-HT$_3$ antagonist (e.g., granisetron [Kytril], ondansetron [Zofran])	Consult prescribing information for the selected 5-HT$_3$ antagonist for dosing information	None	None	None

*Administer fosaprepitant 30 minutes before chemotherapy.
†Administer dexamethasone (Decadron) 30 minutes before chemotherapy on Day 1, in the morning on Day 2, and in the mornings and evenings on Days 3 and 4. The dose was chosen to account for the drug interaction.

Recommended Dosing Regimen for the Prevention of Nausea and Vomiting Associated with Moderately Emetogenic Cancer Chemotherapy (MEC)	
	Day 1
Fosaprepitant IV*	150 mg IV
Dexamethasone†	12 mg PO
5-HT$_3$ antagonist (e.g., granisetron [Kytril], ondansetron [Zofran])	Consult prescribing information for the selected 5-HT$_3$ antagonist for dosing information

*Administer fosaprepitant 30 minutes before chemotherapy.
†Administer dexamethasone (Decadron) 30 minutes before chemotherapy on Day 1. The dose was chosen to account for the drug interaction.

DOSE ADJUSTMENTS
No dose adjustment indicated based on age, race, gender, body mass index (BMI), renal status (including patients with ESRD on dialysis), or mild to moderate hepatic insufficiency. Data in patients with severe hepatic insufficiency (Child-Pugh score >9) not available.

DILUTION
Reconstitute each 150-mg vial with 5 mL of NS. Direct stream of NS to side of vial to avoid foaming. Swirl gently; do not shake. Prepare an infusion bag with 145 mL of NS. Withdraw entire volume of reconstituted vial and transfer it into the infusion bag. Gently invert the bag 2 to 3 times. Final concentration is 1 mg/mL.
Storage: Store unopened vials at 2° to 8° C (36° to 46° F). Diluted solution is stable for 24 hours at RT.

COMPATIBILITY
Manufacturer states, "Should not be mixed or reconstituted with solutions for which physical and chemical **compatibility** have not been established. Fosaprepitant (Emend) for

injection is **incompatible** with any solutions containing divalent cations (e.g., calcium or magnesium), including lactated Ringer's solution and Hartmann's solution."

RATE OF ADMINISTRATION
A single dose as an infusion equally distributed over 20 to 30 minutes.

ACTIONS
A prodrug of aprepitant, a substance P/neurokinin$_1$ (NK$_1$) receptor antagonist. Has little or no affinity for 5HT$_3$, dopamine, and corticosteroid receptors. Fosaprepitant is rapidly converted to aprepitant following IV administration. Aprepitant inhibits emesis induced by cytotoxic chemotherapeutic agents, such as cisplatin, via central actions. Crosses the blood-brain barrier and occupies brain NK$_1$ receptors. Augments the antiemetic activity of the 5HT$_3$-receptor antagonist ondansetron and the corticosteroid dexamethasone and inhibits both the acute and delayed phases of cisplatin-induced emesis. Highly protein bound. Undergoes extensive metabolism, primarily by CYP3A4 and to a lesser extent by CYP1A2 and CYP2C19. Eliminated primarily by metabolism; not renally excreted. Half-life is approximately 9 to 13 hours.

INDICATIONS AND USES
Given in combination with other antiemetics for the prevention of acute and delayed nausea and vomiting associated with initial and repeat courses of highly emetogenic cancer chemotherapy, including high-dose cisplatin. ▪ In combination with other antiemetics for the prevention of delayed nausea and vomiting associated with initial and repeat courses of moderately emetogenic cancer chemotherapy.
Limitation of use: Has not been studied for treatment of established nausea and vomiting.

CONTRAINDICATIONS
Hypersensitivity to fosaprepitant or any components of the product. ▪ Concurrent use with pimozide (Orap); see Drug Interactions.

PRECAUTIONS
Fosaprepitant is rapidly converted to aprepitant, which is a substrate, inhibitor, and inducer of CYP3A4. Use with caution in patients receiving concomitant medications that are primarily metabolized through CYP3A4; see Drug Interactions. ▪ Use with caution in patients with severe hepatic insufficiency (Child-Pugh score >9); see Dose Adjustments. ▪ Hypersensitivity reactions have been observed; see Monitor.
Monitor: Monitor for S/S of a hypersensitivity reaction during the infusion (e.g., anaphylaxis, dyspnea, erythema, flushing). ▪ Monitor IV site. ▪ See Drug/Lab Interactions.
Patient Education: Read manufacturer-supplied patient package insert before starting therapy. ▪ Discontinue use of fosaprepitant and promptly report S/S of a hypersensitivity reaction (e.g., difficulty breathing or swallowing, hives, itching, rash). ▪ Efficacy of hormonal contraceptives may be reduced during and for 28 days following administration of the last dose of fosaprepitant; includes birth control pills, skin patches, implants, and certain IUDs. Alternative or backup methods of contraception should be used during treatment and for 1 month following the last dose of fosaprepitant. ▪ Numerous drug interactions possible. A complete review of all prescription, nonprescription, and herbal products is required before each dose. ▪ Patients on chronic warfarin therapy should have their INR checked in the 2-week period, particularly at 7 to 10 days, following initiation of regimen. ▪ Report infusion site reactions.
Maternal/Child: Should be used during pregnancy only if clearly needed. ▪ Information on use during breast-feeding not available. Use caution. ▪ Safety and effectiveness for use in pediatric patients not established.
Elderly: Response similar to that seen in younger patients, but greater sensitivity of some older individuals cannot be ruled out.

DRUG/LAB INTERACTIONS
Fosaprepitant is rapidly converted to aprepitant. When given as a single 150-mg dose, it is a **weak inhibitor of CYP3A4,** and the weak inhibition of CYP3A4 continues for 2 days after the single dose. Single-dose fosaprepitant does not induce CYP3A4. **Aprepitant is a substrate, inhibitor, and inducer of CYP3A4. It is also an inducer of CYP2C9.** ▪ Efficacy of

hormonal contraceptives may be reduced during and for 28 days following administration of the last dose of fosaprepitant or aprepitant; see Patient Education. ▪ Patients on chronic warfarin therapy should be closely monitored over a 2-week period, particularly at 7 to 10 days following initiation of fosaprepitant with each chemotherapy cycle. Co-administration may result in a clinically significant decrease in INR. ▪ Concurrent use with pimozide (Orap) is contraindicated. Inhibition of CYP3A4 by fosaprepitant or aprepitant could result in elevated plasma concentrations of pimozide, potentially causing serious or life-threatening reactions; see Contraindications. ▪ Fosaprepitant/aprepitant can increase plasma concentrations of dexamethasone (Decadron) and methylprednisolone (Solu-Medrol). When given concurrently with fosaprepitant or aprepitant, reduce the dexamethasone and methylprednisolone PO doses by approximately 50% and the methylprednisolone IV dose by approximately 25%. (Dexamethasone doses listed in Usual Dose take drug interaction into account.) ▪ Coadministration of fosaprepitant or aprepitant with chemotherapy agents metabolized by CYP3A4 (e.g., irinotecan [Camptosar], ifosfamide [Ifex], imatinib [Gleevec], vinblastine, and vincristine) should be done with caution and careful monitoring. In clinical studies, the oral aprepitant regimen was commonly administered with etoposide, vinorelbine, paclitaxel, and docetaxel. Dose adjustments were not required. ▪ May increase plasma levels of benzodiazepines (e.g., alprazolam [Xanax], midazolam [Versed], triazolam [Halcion]). Monitor for sedation. ▪ Aprepitant is a CYP2C9 inducer. Has been shown to induce metabolism of CYP2C9 substrates (e.g., phenytoin [Dilantin], tolbutamide, warfarin [Coumadin]), thus decreasing plasma concentrations. Monitor patients receiving CYP2C9 substrates as indicated (e.g., plasma drug concentrations, therapeutic effect/efficacy, blood sugar control). ▪ Concurrent use with CYP3A4 inhibitors (e.g., clarithromycin [Biaxin], diltiazem [Cardizem], itraconazole [Sporanox], ketoconazole [Nizoral], nefazodone, nelfinavir [Viracept], ritonavir [Norvir], troleandomycin [TAO]) may increase aprepitant or fosaprepitant plasma concentrations. Use caution. ▪ Coadministration with CYP3A4 inducers (e.g., carbamazepine [Tegretol], phenytoin [Dilantin], rifampin [Rifadin]) may decrease fosaprepitant or aprepitant plasma concentrations and decrease efficacy. ▪ Aprepitant is a moderate inhibitor of CYP3A4. Use with caution in patients receiving concomitant medications that are primarily metabolized through CYP3A4. ▪ Has been given with dolasetron (Anzemet), granisetron (Kytril), and ondansetron (Zofran). Clinically significant drug interactions were not observed. ▪ Fosaprepitant or aprepitant is unlikely to interact with drugs that are substrates for the P-glycoprotein transporter.

SIDE EFFECTS
The most common side effects reported include anemia, asthenia, diarrhea, dyspepsia, fatigue, leukopenia, pain in extremity, peripheral neuropathy, and urinary tract infections. Other reported side effects include infusion site reactions (e.g., erythema, induration, pain, pruritus), infusion site thrombophlebitis, and neutropenia.

Post-Marketing: Hypersensitivity reactions (including anaphylaxis), pruritus, rash, Stevens-Johnson syndrome, toxic epidermal necrolysis, and urticaria have been reported. Events of ifosfamide-induced neurotoxicity after fosaprepitant and ifosfamide coadministration have also been reported.

ANTIDOTE
Keep physician informed of all side effects. Most minor side effects will be treated symptomatically. Discontinue fosaprepitant at the first sign of hypersensitivity. Treat hypersensitivity reactions as indicated; may require epinephrine, airway management, oxygen, IV fluids, antihistamines (e.g., diphenhydramine [Benadryl]), corticosteroids (e.g., hydrocortisone sodium succinate [Solu-Cortef]), and pressor amines (e.g., dopamine). Fosaprepitant is not removed by hemodialysis.

FOSCARNET SODIUM BBW

Antiviral

(fos-**KAR**-net **SO**-dee-um)

Foscavir

pH 7.4

USUAL DOSE

An individualized dose should be calculated based on body weight (mg/kg), renal function, indication of use, and dosing frequency. To reduce the risk of nephrotoxicity, creatinine clearance (mL/min/kg) should be calculated even if SCr is within the normal range. Adequate hydration and other specific testing required; see Monitor.

CMV retinitis: 90 mg/kg every 12 hours or 60 mg/kg every 8 hours for 14 to 21 days. Length of induction treatment based on clinical response. Begin a maintenance dose of 90 mg/kg/day the next day (Day 15 to 22). If retinitis progresses during the maintenance regimen, re-treat with the induction and maintenance regimens. Maintenance dose may be increased to 120 mg/kg/day in patients who show excellent tolerance to foscarnet or those who require early re-induction because of retinitis progression. Normal renal function required. For patients who have relapsed after induction and re-induction monotherapy with either foscarnet or ganciclovir, practitioners may consider combination therapy, which adds the alternate drug to the regimen. See the Clinical Trials section of the foscarnet sodium prescribing information.

Acyclovir-resistant HSV patients: 40 mg/kg every 8 or 12 hours for 2 to 3 weeks or until healed.

DOSE ADJUSTMENTS

Must be reduced and individualized according to patient's renal function. Safety and efficacy data for patients with baseline SCr greater than 2.8 mg/dL or measured 24-hour CrCl less than 50 mL/min are limited. Dose adjustment may be required during treatment even if patient had normal renal function initially. Specific calculation and testing are required for both induction and maintenance dose. Specific calculation for induction is shown in the following chart.

	Foscarnet Dose Adjustment Guide for Induction			
	Acyclovir-Resistant HSV		CMV Retinitis	
CrCl (mL/min/kg)	Dose of 40 mg/kg q 12 hr	Dose of 40 mg/kg q 8 hr	Dose of 60 mg/kg q 8 hr	Dose of 90 mg/kg q 12 hr
>1.4 mL/min/kg	40 mg/kg q 12 hr	40 mg/kg q 8 hr	60 mg/kg q 8 hr	90 mg/kg q 12 hr
>1-1.4 mL/min/kg	30 mg/kg q 12 hr	30 mg/kg q 8 hr	45 mg/kg q 8 hr	70 mg/kg q 12 hr
>0.8-1 mL/min/kg	20 mg/kg q 12 hr	35 mg/kg q 12 hr	50 mg/kg q 12 hr	50 mg/kg q 12 hr
>0.6-0.8 mL/min/kg	35 mg/kg q 24 hr	25 mg/kg q 12 hr	40 mg/kg q 12 hr	80 mg/kg q 24 hr
>0.5-0.6 mL/min/kg	25 mg/kg q 24 hr	40 mg/kg q 24 hr	60 mg/kg q 24 hr	60 mg/kg q 24 hr
≥0.4-0.5 mL/min/kg	20 mg/kg q 24 hr	35 mg/kg q 24 hr	50 mg/kg q 24 hr	50 mg/kg q 24 hr
<0.4 mL/min/kg	Not recommended	Not recommended	Not recommended	Not recommended

Specific calculation for maintenance dose is shown in the following chart.

Continued

Foscarnet Dose Adjustment Guide for Maintenance in CMV Retinitis		
CrCl (mL/min/kg)	90 mg/kg/day (once daily)	120 mg/kg/day (once daily)
>1.4 mL/min/kg	90 mg/kg q 24 hr	120 mg/kg q 24 hr
>1-1.4 mL/min/kg	70 mg/kg q 24 hr	90 mg/kg q 24 hr
>0.8-1 mL/min/kg	50 mg/kg q 24 hr	65 mg/kg q 24 hr
>0.6-0.8 mL/min/kg	80 mg/kg q 48 hr	105 mg/kg q 48 hr
>0.5-0.6 mL/min/kg	60 mg/kg q 48 hr	80 mg/kg q 48 hr
≥0.4-0.5 mL/min/kg	50 mg/kg q 48 hr	65 mg/kg q 48 hr
<0.4 mL/min/kg	Not recommended	Not recommended

Foscarnet is not recommended in patients undergoing hemodialysis because dosage guidelines have not been established.

DILUTION

An individualized dose at the required concentration (24 mg/mL or 12 mg/mL) for the route administration (central line or peripheral line) must be aseptically prepared before dispensing. Remove any excess quantity of medication from the infusion bottle using aseptic technique. To avoid any possibility of overdose, only the calculated dose should be in the infusion bottle. Discard any excess before administration.

Central line: Standard 24-mg/mL solution may be given undiluted.

Peripheral line: Each 1 mL of a calculated dose must be diluted with 1 mL of D5W or NS (yields a 12-mg/mL solution).

Storage: Store at CRT. Avoid excessive heat and freezing. Use only if vacuum is present and solution is clear and colorless. Use solution within 24 hours of entry into bottle.

COMPATIBILITY   (Underline Indicates Conflicting Compatibility Information)

Consider any drug NOT listed as compatible to be INCOMPATIBLE until consulting a pharmacist; specific conditions may apply.

Manufacturer states, "Administer only with NS or D5W solutions; no other drug or supplement should be administered concurrently via the same catheter." Because of chelating properties, a precipitate can occur. Manufacturer specifically lists as **incompatible** with 30% dextrose, solutions containing calcium (e.g., LR, TPN), acyclovir (Zovirax), amphotericin B (conventional), diazepam (Valium), digoxin (Lanoxin), *ganciclovir (Cytovene IV)*, leucovorin calcium, midazolam (Versed), pentamidine, phenytoin (Dilantin), prochlorperazine (Compazine), sulfamethoxazole/trimethoprim, vancomycin.

One source suggests the following **compatibilities:**

Additive: *Not recommended by manufacturer.* Potassium chloride (KCl).

Y-site: *Not recommended by manufacturer.* Aldesleukin (Proleukin), amikacin, aminophylline, ampicillin, aztreonam (Azactam), cefazolin (Ancef), cefoxitin (Mefoxin), ceftazidime (Fortaz), ceftriaxone (Rocephin), cefuroxime (Zinacef), chloramphenicol (Chloromycetin), clindamycin (Cleocin), dexamethasone (Decadron), dopamine, doripenem (Doribax), erythromycin (Erythrocin), fluconazole (Diflucan), furosemide (Lasix), gentamicin, heparin, hydrocortisone sodium succinate (Solu-Cortef), hydromorphone (Dilaudid), imipenem-cilastatin (Primaxin), lorazepam (Ativan), metoclopramide (Reglan), metronidazole (Flagyl IV), morphine, nafcillin (Nallpen), oxacillin (Bactocill), penicillin G potassium, ranitidine (Zantac), sulfamethoxazole/trimethoprim, ticarcillin/clavulanate (Timentin), tobramycin, vancomycin.

RATE OF ADMINISTRATION

Infusion pump required to deliver accurate dose evenly distributed over specific time frame. Excessive plasma levels and toxicity (including hypocalcemia) will occur with too-rapid rate of infusion. Advisable to clear tubing with NS if possible before and after administration through Y-tube or three-way stopcock. Never exceed 1 mg/kg/min.

CMV retinitis: *Induction doses:* Each 60-mg/kg dose equally distributed over a minimum of 1 hour. Increase to 1½ to 2 hours for 90-mg/kg dose.
Maintenance dose: Each dose equally distributed over a minimum of 2 hours.
Acyclovir-resistant HSV: Each dose equally distributed over a minimum of 1 hour.

ACTIONS

An antiviral agent capable of inhibiting replication of herpesviruses, including cytomegalovirus (CMV), herpes simplex virus types 1 and 2 (HSV-1, HSV-2), and varicella-zoster virus (VZV [unlabeled]). Does not destroy existing viruses but stops them from reproducing and invading healthy cells. Also capable of chelating metal ions (e.g., calcium, magnesium). CMV strains resistant to ganciclovir and HSV strains resistant to acyclovir may be sensitive to foscarnet. Some penetration into bone and cerebrospinal fluid. Plasma half-life ranges from 2 to 6 hours and increases markedly with renal impairment. Terminal half-life determined by urinary excretion was 87.5 +/− 41.8 hours, possibly due to release of foscarnet from bone. Excreted unchanged in urine.

INDICATIONS AND USES

Treatment of CMV retinitis in patients with AIDS. Most frequently used in patients who do not tolerate or are resistant to ganciclovir. Combination therapy with ganciclovir is indicated for patients who have relapsed after monotherapy with either drug. ■ Treatment of acyclovir-resistant mucocutaneous HSV infections in immunocompromised patients.

CONTRAINDICATIONS

Hypersensitivity to foscarnet.

PRECAUTIONS

For IV use only. ■ Safety and efficacy of foscarnet have not been established for treatment of other CMV infections (e.g., pneumonitis, gastroenteritis), congenital or neonatal CMV disease, other HSV infections (e.g., retinitis, encephalitis), congenital or neonatal HSV disease, or CMV or HSV in nonimmunocompromised individuals. Use should be limited to treatment of conditions listed in Indications and Uses above. ■ May cause potentially life-threatening changes in renal function with cumulative exposure. Careful monitoring of renal function and dose adjustment is imperative. Changes can occur at any time, most likely during second week of therapy. Elevations in SCr are usually reversible following dose adjustment or discontinuation of therapy. ■ Confirm diagnosis of CMV retinitis by indirect ophthalmoscopy. Diagnosis may be supported by cultures of CMV from the throat and body fluids such as urine and blood; negative culture does not rule out CMV retinitis. ■ Use caution in patients with a history of impaired renal function, altered calcium or other electrolyte levels, neurologic or cardiac abnormalities, a low baseline absolute neutrophil count (ANC), and those receiving other drugs known to influence minerals and electrolytes; see Drug/Lab Interactions. Has caused hyperphosphatemia, hypocalcemia, hypokalemia, hypomagnesemia, and hypophosphatemia, resulting in cardiac disturbances, seizures, and tetany. ■ Seizures related to alterations in plasma minerals and electrolytes have been reported. Several cases were associated with death. Risk factors for seizures included impaired baseline renal function, low total serum calcium, and underlying CNS conditions. ■ Contains 5.5 mg sodium/mL. Avoid use in patients who may not tolerate a large amount of sodium or water (e.g., patients with cardiomyopathy) or in patients on a controlled-sodium diet. ■ Anemia has been reported in 33% of patients receiving foscarnet. ■ Resistance has been reported to develop. May be higher in patients treated for a prolonged period. Consider the possibility of resistance in patients who show poor clinical response or who experience persistent viral excretion during treatment. ■ Amino acid substitutions conferring foscarnet resistance with cross-resistance to ganciclovir, cidofovir, and acyclovir have been identified. ■ Sensitivity testing of the viral isolate is recommended before repeat treatment and/or to evaluate sensitivity versus development of resistance.

Monitor: Baseline 24-hour CrCl verified by creatinine index; baseline SCr, calcium, magnesium, potassium, phosphorus, and electrolytes required before treatment begins. Correct any deficiencies. ■ Repeat entire testing process 2 to 3 times a week during induction therapy and weekly during maintenance therapy. Foscarnet dose must be adjusted as indicated by test results. More frequent testing may be indicated in specific patients. Supplementation of minerals and electrolytes may be required during treatment. ▪ To minimize renal toxicity, hydration adequate to establish diuresis is recommended before and during treatment. Clinically dehydrated patients should be adequately hydrated before initiating therapy. Give 750 to 1,000 mL NS or D5W before the first foscarnet infusion to establish diuresis. With subsequent infusions, give 750 to 1,000 mL concurrently with 90 to 120 mg/kg foscarnet and a minimum of 500 mL concurrently with 40 to 60 mg/kg. Oral rehydration may be considered in certain patients. Hydration fluid may need to be decreased if clinically warranted. ▪ Discontinue foscarnet if CrCl drops below 0.4 mL/min/kg. Monitor patient daily until resolution of renal impairment is ensured. Safety for use in these patients has not been studied. ▪ Anemia may be severe enough to require transfusion. ▪ Phlebitis or pain may occur at site of infusion; confirm patency of vein and use large veins to ensure adequate blood flow for rapid dilution and distribution. ▪ See Drug/Lab Interactions.

Patient Education: Not a cure. Retinitis may recur during maintenance or after treatment; regular ophthalmologic exams imperative. ▪ Complete healing of HSV infections may occur, but most relapse. ▪ Perioral tingling, numbness in the extremities or paresthesias indicate electrolyte abnormalities; report immediately. ▪ Close monitoring of renal function and electrolyte balance during treatment is imperative. ▪ Cases of male and female genital irritation/ulceration have been reported. Adequate hydration and increased personal hygiene may minimize some side effects. ▪ May cause CNS side effects (e.g., dizziness, seizures, somnolence) that could result in impairment. Use caution when driving or operating machinery. ▪ Dose modification or discontinuation may be required for major side effects.

Maternal/Child: Category C: use only if clearly needed; has caused skeletal anomalies in animals. ▪ Discontinue breast-feeding. ▪ Safety for use in pediatric patients not established; deposited in teeth and bones, and deposition greater in young animals. Use only if benefits outweigh risks.

Elderly: Safety and effectiveness not established; however, foscarnet has been used in patients over 65 years of age. Side effects seen are similar to other age-groups. Consider age-related renal impairment in dose selection, and monitor renal function; see Dose Adjustments.

DRUG/LAB INTERACTIONS
Because of physical **incompatibilities,** foscarnet sodium and **ganciclovir sodium** must never be mixed. ▪ Has caused hypocalcemia with parenteral **pentamidine;** deaths have been reported. ▪ Capable of causing calcium or electrolyte disorders. Use particular caution when administering **any drug known to influence serum calcium concentrations, other minerals, or electrolytes** (e.g., hypocalcemic agents [gallium nitrate (Ganite)], diuretics [furosemide (Lasix), mannitol], adrenocortical steroids). ▪ Elimination of foscarnet may be impaired and toxicity increased by **drugs that inhibit renal tubular secretion.** When **diuretics** are indicated, **thiazides** (e.g., hydrochlorothiazide) are recommended over **loop diuretics** (e.g., furosemide [Lasix]) because the latter inhibit renal tubular secretion. ▪ Avoid concomitant use with other **nephrotoxic drugs** (e.g., acyclovir [Zovirax], aminoglycosides [e.g., gentamicin], amphotericin B [conventional], cyclosporine [Sandimmune], methotrexate, pentamidine, tacrolimus [Prograf]) unless benefits outweigh risks. ▪ Use with **fluoroquinolones** (e.g., ciprofloxacin [Cipro]) may increase the risk of seizures; monitor patient carefully. ▪ Abnormal renal function has been reported in patients receiving foscarnet and **ritonavir** (Norvir) or foscarnet and **ritonavir and saquinavir** (Invirase). ▪ There is no clinically significant interaction with zidovudine (AZT) or probenecid. ▪ The combination antiviral activity of foscarnet and **ganciclovir** or **acyclovir** is not antagonistic in cell culture.

SIDE EFFECTS
Impaired renal function, alterations in plasma minerals and electrolytes, and seizures are major side effects and are dose limiting. Abnormal renal function, including acute renal failure, decreased CrCl, and increased SCr; anemia; bone marrow suppression; diarrhea; fatigue;

fever; headache; hyperphosphatemia; hypocalcemia (perioral tingling, numbness in extremities, paresthesias, tetany); hypokalemia; hypomagnesemia; hypophosphatemia; irritation at injection site; irritation and ulcerations of penile and vaginal epithelium; nausea; rigors; seizure; vomiting; and death have occurred. All deaths could not be directly related to foscarnet. Abdominal pain, anorexia, anxiety, asthenia, confusion, coughing, depression, dizziness, dyspnea, granulocytopenia, hypoesthesia, infection, involuntary muscle contractions, leukopenia, malaise, neuropathy, pain, rash, sweating, and vision abnormalities have occurred in 5% of patients. Numerous other side effects have occurred in fewer than 5% of patients.

Post-Marketing: Crystal-induced nephropathy, esophageal ulcerations, renal tubular acidosis, renal tubular necrosis, muscle disorders (e.g., myopathy, myositis, muscle weakness, rhabdomyolysis), vesiculobullous eruptions (e.g., erythema multiforme, toxic epidermal necrolysis, Stevens-Johnson syndrome).

ANTIDOTE

There is no specific antidote. Keep physician informed. Adequate hydration and careful monitoring will help reduce potential for renal impairment and may minimize other side effects. Elevations in SCr are usually reversible (within 1 week) with dose adjustment or discontinuation but have caused death. Discontinue foscarnet if CrCl falls below 0.4 mL/min/kg. Monitor daily until resolution of renal impairment is ensured. Discontinue foscarnet if perioral tingling, numbness in the extremities, or paresthesias occur during or after infusion; evaluate calcium and electrolyte levels (decrease in ionized serum calcium may not be reflected in total serum calcium); notify physician. Administration of foscarnet can be resumed following seizures or cardiac disturbances after treatment of underlying disease, electrolyte disturbance, or after dose adjustment. Overdose can occur with too-rapid rate of infusion. Hemodialysis and hydration may be useful in overdose. Treat anaphylaxis and resuscitate as indicated.

FOSPHENYTOIN SODIUM BBW

(FOS-fen-ih-toyn SO-dee-um)

Cerebyx

Anticonvulsant
(hydantoin)

pH 8.6 to 9

USUAL DOSE

1.5 mg of fosphenytoin sodium is equivalent to 1 mg phenytoin sodium and is referred to as 1 mg phenytoin sodium equivalents (PE). The amount and concentration of fosphenytoin is always expressed in terms of mg PE. Fosphenytoin 15 to 20 mg PE/kg is equivalent to phenytoin 15 to 20 mg/kg, or a 1,000-mg PE dose of fosphenytoin is equivalent to a 1,000-mg dose of phenytoin. Because of the risk of hypotension and cardiac arrhythmias, fosphenytoin should be administered no faster than 150 mg PE/min; see Rate of Administration, Precautions, and Monitor.

Status epilepticus: *Adult loading dose:* 15 to 20 mg PE/kg. Full effect is not immediate; concomitant administration of an IV benzodiazepine (e.g., diazepam [Valium]) is usually necessary to control status epilepticus. If seizures are not controlled, consider other anticonvulsants and other measures as needed (e.g., barbiturates or anesthesia).

Maintenance dose: 4 to 6 mg PE/kg/24 hr in divided doses.

Another source adds: *Elderly loading dose:* 14 mg PE/kg. See all comments under Usual Dose. See Elderly.

Nonemergent indications: *Loading dose:* 10 to 20 mg PE/kg. *Maintenance dose:* 4 to 6 mg PE/kg/24 hr in divided doses. Because of the risk of cardiac and local toxicity associated with IV fosphenytoin, oral phenytoin should be administered whenever possible.

Substitute for oral phenytoin: May be substituted at the same total daily phenytoin sodium equivalents (PE) dose (due to a 10% increase in bioavailability [IV/IM to oral], plasma levels with the IV/IM product may be increased slightly).

PEDIATRIC DOSE

See comments in Usual Dose.

Status epilepticus loading dose (unlabeled): 15 to 20 mg PE/kg at a rate of 3 mg PE/kg/min; do not exceed 150 mg PE/min.

Nonemergent loading dose: 10 to 20 mg PE/kg.

Maintenance dose: 4 to 6 mg PE/kg/24 hr initially; may be given as a single dose or divided into 2 doses. Safety for use in pediatric patients not established. Limited data available; no significant differences apparent to this date; see Maternal/Child.

DOSE ADJUSTMENTS

Reduced doses may be required in the elderly (see Usual Dose), in impaired renal or hepatic function, or in patients with hypoalbuminemia. ▪ See Precautions, Monitor, Drug/Lab Interactions, and Antidote.

DILUTION

Use only clear solutions. Should be diluted in D5W or NS to a concentration of 1.5 to 25 mg PE/mL. Supplied solution is 50 mg PE/mL. *Do not confuse the amount of drug to be given in PE with the concentration of the drug in the vial; serious errors have occurred.* Dilute each milliliter of fosphenytoin with 1 mL of diluent to equal 25 mg PE/mL. Dilute a 1,000-mg PE dose in 100 mL diluent to equal 10 mg PE/mL.

Storage: Keep refrigerated; do not store at room temperature for more than 48 hours. For single use only. Discard any unused product after opening.

COMPATIBILITY

Consider any drug NOT listed as compatible to be INCOMPATIBLE until consulting a pharmacist; specific conditions may apply.

One source suggests the following **compatibilities:**

Additive: Hetastarch in NS (Hespan), mannitol, potassium chloride (KCl).

Y-site: Lorazepam (Ativan), phenobarbital (Luminal).

RATE OF ADMINISTRATION

Each 100 to 150 mg PE or fraction thereof over a minimum of 1 minute. Do not exceed a rate of 150 mg PE/min. Risk of severe hypotension and cardiac arrhythmias increased. Slow or temporarily stop rate of infusion for cardiovascular side effects or for burning, itching, numbness, or pain along injection site.

Pediatric rate: Manufacturer recommends 1 to 3 mg PE/kg/min for pediatric patients. Another source suggests a rate of 1.6 mg PE/kg/min.

ACTIONS

A water-soluble prodrug of phenytoin. Converts to phenytoin, phosphate, and formaldehyde within 15 minutes of IV/IM administration. An anticonvulsant, chemically related to barbiturates. Selectively stabilizes seizure threshold and depresses seizure activity in the motor cortex. Modulation of voltage-dependent sodium channels of neurons thought to be the primary cellular mechanism responsible for anticonvulsant activity. Also exerts a depressant effect on the myocardium by selectively elevating the excitability threshold of the cell, reducing the cell's response to stimuli. Peak levels of fosphenytoin are achieved by the end of an infusion, but conversion to therapeutic serum levels of phenytoin takes longer. The conversion half-life of fosphenytoin to phenytoin is approximately 15 minutes. Extensively bound to protein, fosphenytoin displaces phenytoin from protein binding sites and increases free phenytoin (dose and rate dependent). Phenytoin's half-life is 12 to 28.9 hours. It is metabolized in the liver by hepatic cytochrome P_{450} enzymes (CYP2C9 and CYP2C19) and excreted in urine. Crosses the placental barrier. Secreted in breast milk.

INDICATIONS AND USES

Treatment and control of generalized tonic-clonic status epilepticus. ▪ Treatment or prophylaxis of seizures in neurosurgical patients. ▪ Substitute for oral phenytoin when oral administration is not feasible or prompt increases in antiepileptic drug levels are needed. *Cerebyx must not be given orally.*

CONTRAINDICATIONS

Hypersensitivity to fosphenytoin, any of its components, phenytoin, or other hydantoins. ▪ Sinus bradycardia, sinoatrial block, second- and third-degree AV block, and Adams-Stokes syndrome. ▪ Coadministration with delavirdine (Rescriptor).

PRECAUTIONS

Doses of fosphenytoin are expressed in terms of milligrams of phenytoin equivalents (mg PE) to avoid the need to perform molecular weight–based adjustments when substituting fosphenytoin for phenytoin or vice versa; no adjustment required when substituting fosphenytoin or vice versa. Labeling of fosphenytoin has been updated by the manufacturer to reduce the incidence of dosing errors. To ensure accuracy, confirm actual dose and volume to be administered with a pharmacist or another RN. ▪ Advantages of fosphenytoin over present phenytoin products include solubility in IV solutions, improved infusion site tolerance, more rapid rate of administration, and well-tolerated IM option. ▪ IV route indicated in emergency situations (e.g., status epilepticus). May be given IM in nonemergency situations. ▪ Oral phenytoin is preferred in nonemergency situations because of the risks of cardiac and local toxicity associated with IV fosphenytoin. Adverse cardiovascular reactions have occurred during and after infusions and have been reported with infusion rates above the recommended rate as well as with infusion rates at or below the recommended rate. ▪ May cause severe cardiovascular reactions (e.g., hypotension, bradycardia, various degrees of AV block, QT interval prolongation) that have resulted in asystole, cardiac arrest, and death; use extreme caution in elderly or seriously ill patients and in patients with hypotension or severe myocardial insufficiency. Risk of hypotension and cardiac arrhythmias increased by higher IV doses and/or rapid administration. ▪ Intended for short-term parenteral use (up to 5 days). ▪ Transfer to oral phenytoin therapy as soon as feasible. ▪ Abrupt withdrawal may cause increased seizure activity. Gradually reduce dose, discontinue, or substitute alternative antiepileptic agents. ▪ Discontinue immediately for hypersensitivity reactions; with caution substitute a nonhydantoin anticonvulsant. ▪ In patients who have experienced phenytoin hypersensitivity, alternatives to structurally similar drugs such as carboxamides (e.g., carbamazepine [Tegretol]), barbiturates, succinimides, and oxazolidinediones (e.g., trimethadione) should be considered. ▪ May exacerbate porphyria. ▪ Drug reaction with eosinophilia and systemic symptoms (DRESS), also known as multiorgan hypersensitivity, has been reported. DRESS usually presents with fever, rash, and/or lymphadenopathy in association with other organ system involvement such as hepatitis, nephritis, hematologic abnormalities, myocarditis, or myositis. Eosinophilia is often present. Deaths have been reported. ▪ May cause acute phenytoin hepatotoxicity, which may manifest as elevated liver function tests, jaundice, hepatomegaly, leukocytosis, eosinophilia, and/or acute hepatic failure. These events may be part of the spectrum of DRESS or may occur in isolation. Discontinue immediately and substitute alternate anticonvulsant therapy. ▪ Has caused lymphadenopathy and hemopoietic complications (e.g., agranulocytosis, granulocytopenia, leukopenia, thrombocytopenia, or pancytopenia with or without bone marrow suppression). Lymph node involvement may occur with or without S/S resembling DRESS. If lymphadenopathy occurs, substitute alternate anticonvulsant therapy. ▪ Sensory disturbances, including severe burning, itching, and paresthesia, have been reported; more common with higher doses and/or rates. ▪ Purple glove syndrome (edema, discoloration, and pain distal to the injection site) has occurred and may or may not be associated with extravasation. The syndrome may not develop for several days. ▪ Serious dermatologic reactions have been reported, including toxic epidermal necrolysis (TEN) and Stevens-Johnson syndrome (SJS). Usually occurs within 28 days but may occur later. If a rash develops, the patient should be evaluated for S/S of DRESS. ▪ Use caution with low serum albumin levels, and adjust dose as indicated. Phenytoin is highly bound to serum protein, and a reduced albumin causes an increase in free drug availability and may increase toxicity. ▪ Not effective for absence seizures; combined therapy required if both conditions present. ▪ Not indicated for seizures due to hypoglycemia or other metabolic causes. ▪ Inhibits insulin release and may increase serum glucose; monitoring indicated in diabetics. ▪ May lower serum folate levels. ▪ Antiepileptic drugs (AEDs) increase the risk of suicidal thoughts or behavior in patients taking these drugs for any indication. Patients treated with any AED for any indication should be monitored for the emergence or worsening of depression, suicidal thoughts or behavior, and/or any unusual changes in mood or behavior. Some psychotic symptoms and/or behavioral changes resolved without intervention. Others required dose reduction or discontinuation of the antiepileptic agent. ▪ Confusional states referred to as delirium, psychosis, encephalopathy or, rarely, irreversible cerebellar dysfunction have been reported when plasma phenytoin concentrations are sustained above the optimum range. At the first sign of acute toxicity, determination of plasma phenytoin concentration is recommended.

Monitor: Monitor ECG, BP, and respirations continuously during loading dose and for at least 10 to 20 minutes after infusion is complete. ▪ Allow fosphenytoin time to convert to phenytoin; accurate serum levels are not available until 2 hours after the end of an IV infusion or 4 hours after IM injection. Narrow margin of error between therapeutic and toxic dose. Plasma levels above 10 mcg/mL usually control seizure activity. The acceptable range is 5 to 20 mcg/mL (unbound phenytoin concentration of 1 to 2 mcg/mL). Toxicity begins with nystagmus at levels exceeding 20 mcg/mL. ▪ Monitoring of unbound phenytoin concentrations may be more useful in patients with renal or hepatic impairment or in patients with hypoalbuminemia. ▪ Observe for rash and discontinue if one appears. If rash is mild, fosphenytoin may be resumed when the rash has completely disappeared. Discontinue fosphenytoin if the mild rash occurs again, if the initial rash is serious in nature (e.g., exfoliative, purpuric, bullous), or if Stevens-Johnson syndrome or toxic epidermal necrolysis is suspected. Do not resume; consider alternative therapy. ▪ Phosphate is produced as a metabolite; monitor in patients who require phosphate restriction (e.g., renal impairment). ▪ Monitor patients who are gravely ill, have impaired liver or renal function or hypoalbuminemia, or are elderly. May show early signs of toxicity. ▪

Determine absolute patency of vein; avoid extravasation. Not as alkaline as phenytoin. ▪ Observe patient closely for signs of CNS side effects; see Precautions.
Patient Education: Report burning, itching, numbness, pain, or rash. ▪ Consider birth control options; nonhormonal birth control recommended. ▪ May increase the risk of suicidal thoughts and behavior. Promptly report emergence or worsening of the S/S of depression, any unusual changes in mood or behavior, or thoughts about self-harm. ▪ Women who are pregnant or who become pregnant should be encouraged to enroll in the North American Antiepileptic Drug (NAAED) Pregnancy Registry.
Maternal/Child: Category D: avoid pregnancy. Prenatal exposure to phenytoin may increase the risk of congenital malformations and other adverse developmental outcomes. Consider risk versus benefit. ▪ An increase in seizure frequency may occur during pregnancy; if phenytoin is required, monitoring of plasma phenytoin levels may be helpful. ▪ Newborns whose mothers received phenytoin during pregnancy may develop a life-threatening bleeding disorder that can be prevented by giving vitamin K to the mother before delivery and to the neonate after birth. ▪ Discontinue breast-feeding. ▪ Safety and effectiveness for use in pediatric patients not established. ▪ See Patient Education.
Elderly: See Dose Adjustments. ▪ Sensitivity and/or toxicity may be increased because serum concentrations may be elevated due to reduced clearance, or low serum albumin may cause a decrease in protein binding and an increase in free phenytoin.

DRUG/LAB INTERACTIONS
No drugs are known to interfere with the conversion of fosphenytoin to phenytoin, although phosphatase activity may have an impact. ▪ *Capable of innumerable catastrophic drug interactions; review of drug profile by pharmacist imperative.* In all situations, monitoring of phenytoin serum levels may be indicated. ▪ Coadministration with **delavirdine** (Rescriptor) is contraindicated. Has the potential for loss of virologic response and possible resistance to delavirdine or to the class of nonnucleoside reverse transcriptase inhibitors. ▪ Serum levels and toxicity of phenytoin may be increased by **alcohol (acute intake), amiodarone** (Nexterone), **antiepileptic agents** (e.g., felbamate [Felbatol], topiramate [Topamax], oxcarbazepine [Trileptal]), **azoles** (e.g., fluconazole [Diflucan], itraconazole [Sporanox], ketoconazole (Nizoral], miconazole [Oravig], voriconazole [VFEND]), **capecitabine** (Xeloda), **chloramphenicol, chlordiazepoxide** (Librium), **disulfiram** (Antabuse), **estrogens, fluorouracil, fluoxetine** (Prozac), **fluvastatin** (Lescol), **fluvoxamine** (Luvox), **H₂ antagonists** (e.g., cimetidine [Tagamet]), **halothane, isoniazid** (INH), **methylphenidate** (Ritalin), **omeprazole** (Prilosec), **phenothiazines** (e.g., prochlorperazine [Compazine]), **salicylates** (aspirin), **sertraline** (Zoloft), **succinimides** (e.g., ethosuximide [Zarontin]), **sulfonamides** (e.g., sulfamethizole, sulfaphenazole, sulfadiazine, sulfamethoxazole/trimethoprim [Bactrim]), **ticlopidine** (Ticlid), **tolbutamide, trazodone** (Deseryl), **and warfarin** (Coumadin). ▪ Serum levels and effectiveness of phenytoin may be decreased by **anticancer drugs** usually in combination (e.g., bleomycin [Blenoxane], carboplatin [Paraplatin], cisplatin, doxorubicin [Adriamycin], methotrexate), **carbamazepine** (Tegretol), **chronic alcohol abuse, diazepam** (Valium), **diazoxide** (Proglycem), **folic acid, fosamprenavir** (Lexiva), **nelfinavir** (Viracept), **reserpine, rifampin** (Rifadin), **ritonavir** (Norvir), **St. John's wort, theophylline, and vigabatrin** (Sabril). ▪ Serum levels of phenytoin may be increased or decreased by **phenobarbital** (Luminal), **valproate sodium** (Depacon), **valproic acid** (Depakene). Similarly, phenytoin may unpredictably affect the levels and efficacy of these drugs. ▪ Phenytoin will inhibit the effects of **azoles** (e.g., fluconazole [Diflucan], itraconazole [Sporanox], ketoconazole [Nizoral], posaconazole [Noxafil], voriconazole [VFEND]), **corticosteroids, doxycycline, estrogens, furosemide** (Lasix), **irinotecan** (Camptosar), **oral contraceptives, paclitaxel** (Taxol), **paroxetine** (Paxil), **quinidine, rifampin** (Rifadin), **sertraline** (Zoloft), **teniposide** (Vumon), **theophylline, and vitamin D.** Dose adjustment of these agents may be indicated. ▪ Decreases plasma concentrations of **active metabolites of albendazole** (Albenza), **antiepileptic agents** (e.g., carbamazepine [Tegretol], felbamate [Felbatol], lamotrigine [Lamictal], oxcarbazepine [Trileptal], topiramate [Topamax]), **atorvastatin** (Lipitor), certain **HIV antivirals** (e.g., efavirenz [Sustiva], lopinavir/

ritonavir [Kaletra], indinavir [Crixivan], nelfinavir [Viracept], ritonavir [Norvir], saquinavir [Invirase]), **chlorpropamide** (Diabinese), **clozapine** (Clozaril), **cyclosporine** (Sandimmune), **digoxin** (Lanoxin), **fluvastatin** (Lescol), **folic acid, methadone** (Dolophine), **mexiletine, nifedipine** (Procardia), **nimodipine, nisoldipine** (Sular), **praziquantel** (Biltricide), **quetiapine** [Seroquel], **simvastatin** (Zocor), and **verapamil**. Adjust doses of these agents as indicated. ▪ May increase or decrease PT/INR responses when coadministered with **warfarin** (Coumadin). ▪ When given with **fosamprenavir** (Lexiva) alone, phenytoin may decrease the concentration of **amprenavir** (Agenerase), the active metabolite. When given in combination with **fosamprenavir and ritonavir** (Norvir), phenytoin may increase the concentration of **amprenavir**. ▪ Resistance to the neuromuscular blocking action of the **nondepolarizing neuromuscular blocking agents** pancuronium, vecuronium, rocuronium (Zemuron), and cisatracurium (Nimbex) has occurred in patients receiving long-term administration of phenytoin. Monitor for more rapid than expected recovery from neuromuscular blockade. ▪ Alters some **clinical laboratory tests** (e.g., may decrease T_4, increase glucose, alkaline phosphatase, and GGT; may produce low results in dexamethasone or metyrapone tests).

SIDE EFFECTS
Transient ataxia, dizziness, headache, nystagmus, paresthesia, pruritus, and somnolence are the most common side effects and are dose- and rate-related. Risks of side effects increased with upper-end doses given at upper-end rates. The more important adverse clinical events caused by IV use of fosphenytoin are cardiovascular collapse and/or CNS depression. Coma, hyperreflexia, hypotension, lethargy, nausea, slurred speech, tremor, and vomiting are also signs of increased toxicity. Confusional states (e.g., delirium, encephalopathy, psychosis) and, rarely, irreversible cerebellar dysfunction can occur with high plasma concentrations. Fosphenytoin breaks down into formate and phosphate metabolites that may cause formate and phosphate toxicity in overdose situations (hypocalcemia, metabolic acidosis, muscle spasms, paresthesia, and seizures). Psychotic symptoms, including aggression, agitation, anger, anxiety, apathy, depersonalization, depression, emotional lability, hallucinations, hostility, irritability, and suicidal tendencies, have occurred with antiepileptic agents.

Major/overdose: Arrhythmias (e.g., asystole, bradycardia, cardiac arrest, tachycardia), ataxia, coma, dysarthria, hyperreflexia, hypocalcemia, hypotension, lethargy, metabolic acidosis, nausea, nystagmus, respiratory depression, slurred speech, syncope, tremor, and vomiting. Deaths have been reported.

Post-Marketing: Anaphylactoid reactions, including anaphylaxis.

ANTIDOTE
Notify physician of any side effects. Obtain serum plasma levels at first signs of toxicity; reduce dose. If symptoms persist or major side effects appear, discontinue fosphenytoin and notify physician. Treat symptomatically, maintain a patent airway, and resuscitate as necessary. Discontinue fosphenytoin at the first sign of a rash unless the rash is clearly not drug related. If TEN or SJS is suspected, do not rechallenge; consider alternate therapy. Evaluate for multiorgan hypersensitivity reactions (DRESS). Cardiovascular toxicity, including hypotension or cardiac arrhythmias, may respond to a decrease in infusion rate. One source says hemodialysis may be helpful in overdose. Another source says hemodialysis, peritoneal dialysis, forced fluid diuresis, exchange transfusions, and plasmapheresis are ineffective. In overdose, measure ionized free calcium levels to guide treatment in phosphate toxicity.

FUROSEMIDE BBW
(fur-**OH**-seh-myd)

Diuretic (loop)

Lasix

pH 8 to 9.3

USUAL DOSE
Adjust dose and dose schedule to individual patient needs. Reserve parenteral therapy for emergent situations or for patients unable to take oral therapy. Switch to oral therapy as soon as practical.

Edema: 20 to 40 mg. May be repeated in 2 hours. If necessary, increase dosage by 20-mg increments (under close medical supervision and no sooner than 2 hours after previous dose) until desired diuresis is obtained. After the initial diuresis the minimum effective dose may be given once or twice every 24 hours as required for maintenance.

New-onset pulmonary edema: 40 mg. Dose may be increased to 80 mg after 1 hour if satisfactory response is not obtained. AHA guidelines recommend less than 0.5 mg/kg. Additional therapy (e.g., digoxin, oxygen) may be administered concurrently as needed.

Hypertensive crisis: AHA guidelines recommend 0.5 to 1 mg/kg over 1 to 2 minutes. If no response, increase dose to 2 mg/kg.

Acute pulmonary edema or post–cardiac arrest cerebral edema: AHA guidelines recommend 0.5 to 1 mg/kg over 1 to 2 minutes. If no response, increase dose to 2 mg/kg.

PEDIATRIC DOSE
See Maternal/Child.

Diuretic: 1 to 2 mg/kg of body weight. After 2 hours increase by 1-mg/kg increments to effect desired response. Effective dose may be given every 6 to 12 hours. Another source suggests 1 to 2 mg/kg/dose every 6 to 12 hours. Do not exceed 6 mg/kg/dose.

NEONATAL DOSE
Diuretic: 0.5 to 1 mg/kg/dose every 8 to 24 hours. Maximum dose is 2 mg/kg/dose. Literature reports suggest that the maximum dose for premature infants should not exceed 1 mg/kg/day. See Maternal/Child.

DOSE ADJUSTMENTS
Higher doses may be required in renal insufficiency and acute or chronic renal failure. ▪ Reduced dose or extended intervals may be appropriate in the elderly. ▪ Extend dosing intervals in neonates because half-life is prolonged. ▪ See Drug/Lab Interactions.

DILUTION
May be given undiluted. May be given through Y-tube or three-way stopcock of infusion set. Not usually added to IV solutions, but large doses may be added to NS, LR, D5W, D5NS and given as an infusion. pH of solution must be over 5.5. Some sources recommend protecting diluted solutions from light to prevent photodegradation (minimized at pH 7).

Filters: One source found no significant drug loss when filtered through a 0.22-micron filter.

Storage: Store vials at CRT. Protect from light. If diluted for infusion, discard after 24 hours.

COMPATIBILITY
(Underline Indicates Conflicting Compatibility Information)

Consider any drug NOT listed as compatible to be INCOMPATIBLE until consulting a pharmacist; specific conditions may apply.

Furosemide may precipitate at a pH below 7. Manufacturer states, "Acid solutions, including other parenteral medications (e.g., amrinone, ciprofloxacin, labetalol, milrinone) must not be administered concurrently in the same infusion." Additionally, "Furosemide should not be added to an IV line containing any of these acidic products."

One source suggests the following **compatibilities:**

Additive: <u>Amikacin</u>, aminophylline, <u>amiodarone (Nexterone)</u>, ampicillin, atropine, bumetanide, calcium gluconate, cefuroxime (Zinacef), dexamethasone (Decadron), digoxin (Lanoxin), <u>epinephrine (Adrenalin)</u>, <u>gentamicin</u>, heparin, <u>hydrocortisone sodium succinate (Solu-Cortef)</u>, lidocaine, mannitol (Osmitrol), meropenem (Merrem IV), midazolam (Versed), morphine, nitroglycerin IV, potassium chloride (KCl), ranitidine (Zantac), sodium bicarbonate, theophylline, <u>tobramycin</u>, <u>verapamil</u>.

Y-site: Allopurinol (Aloprim), amifostine (Ethyol), amikacin, <u>amiodarone (Nexterone)</u>, amphotericin B cholesteryl (Amphotec), <u>anidulafungin (Eraxis)</u>, argatroban, aztreonam (Azactam), bivalirudin (Angiomax), bleomycin (Blenoxane), cefepime (Maxipime), ceftaroline (Teflaro), ceftazidime (Fortaz), <u>cisatracurium (Nimbex)</u>, cisplatin, cladribine (Leustatin), cyclophosphamide (Cytoxan), dexmedetomidine (Precedex), <u>dobutamine</u>, docetaxel (Taxotere), <u>dopamine</u>, doripenem (Doribax), doxorubicin liposomal (Doxil), <u>epinephrine (Adrenalin)</u>, etoposide phosphate (Etopophos), <u>famotidine (Pepcid IV)</u>, fentanyl, fludarabine (Fludara), fluorouracil (5-FU), foscarnet (Foscavir), gallium nitrate (Ganite), granisetron (Kytril), heparin, hetastarch in electrolytes (Hextend), hydrocortisone sodium succinate (Solu-Cortef), hydromorphone (Dilaudid), 6% hydroxyethyl starch (Voluven), indomethacin (Indocin IV), leucovorin calcium, linezolid (Zyvox), lorazepam (Ativan), melphalan (Alkeran), <u>meperidine (Demerol)</u>, meropenem (Merrem IV), methotrexate, metoprolol (Lopressor), <u>micafungin (Mycamine)</u>, mitomycin (Mutamycin), <u>morphine</u>, <u>nitroglycerin IV</u>, nitroprusside sodium, norepinephrine (Levophed), oxaliplatin (Eloxatin), paclitaxel (Taxol), <u>pantoprazole (Protonix IV)</u>, piperacillin/tazobactam (Zosyn), potassium chloride (KCl), propofol (Diprivan), ranitidine (Zantac), remifentanil (Ultiva), sargramostim (Leukine), tacrolimus (Prograf), teniposide (Vumon), thiotepa, tirofiban (Aggrastat), tobramycin.

RATE OF ADMINISTRATION

IV injection: Each 40 mg or fraction thereof should be given over 1 to 2 minutes.

Infusion: *Adults:* 0.1 mg/kg/hr. *Pediatric patients:* 0.05 mg/kg/hr. Titrate to effect. High-dose therapy in an infusion should not exceed a rate of 4 mg/min.

ACTIONS

A potent loop diuretic, structurally related to sulfonamides. Onset of action is prompt, usually within 5 minutes. Duration of action and half-life are approximately 2 hours. Inhibits the reabsorption of sodium and chloride in the proximal and distal tubules and in the loop of Henle, causing increased excretion of water, sodium, chloride, magnesium, and calcium. Highly protein bound. Metabolized and excreted in the urine. Crosses the placental barrier. Secreted in breast milk.

INDICATIONS AND USES

Parenteral therapy should be reserved for patients unable to take oral medications or for emergency clinical situations. ▪ Edema associated with congestive heart failure, cirrhosis of the liver with ascites, and renal disease including the nephrotic syndrome. Particularly useful when an agent with a greater diuretic potential is required. ▪ Adjunctive therapy in acute pulmonary edema. Indicated when rapid onset of diuresis is necessary (e.g., acute pulmonary edema).

CONTRAINDICATIONS

Anuria, hypersensitivity to furosemide.

PRECAUTIONS

A potent diuretic; may precipitate excessive diuresis with water and electrolyte depletion. Careful medical supervision is required. ▪ Use caution and improve basic condition first in hepatic coma, electrolyte depletion, and advanced cirrhosis of the liver. ▪ May be used concurrently with aldosterone antagonists (e.g., spironolactone [Aldactone]) for more effective diuresis and to prevent excessive potassium loss. ▪ If increasing azotemia and oliguria develop during treatment of severe progressive renal disease, furosemide should be discontinued. ▪ Use extreme caution in known sulfonamide sensitivity. ▪ Risk of ototoxicity (tinnitus, reversible or irreversible hearing impairment and deafness) increases with higher doses, rapid injection, severe renal dysfunction, hypoproteinemia, or concurrent use with other ototoxic drugs; see Drug/Lab Interactions. ▪ May activate or exacerbate systemic lupus erythematosus. ▪ Use caution in patients with severe symptoms of urinary retention (because of bladder emptying disorders, prostatic hypertrophy, urethral narrowing). May experience acute urinary retention related to increased production and retention of urine.

Monitor: Monitor BP frequently, especially during initial therapy. ▪ May precipitate excessive diuresis with water and electrolyte depletion. Routine checks on electrolyte panel, CO_2, and BUN are necessary during therapy. Electrolyte replacement may be required. ▪ May increase blood glucose and has precipitated diabetes mellitus. ▪ Monitor for other S/S of fluid or electrolyte imbalance, which may include dryness of the mouth, drowsiness, lethargy, muscle cramps or fatigue, nausea or vomiting, oliguria, tachycardia, thirst, and weakness. ▪ May lower serum calcium level; may cause tetany. ▪ Hyperuricemia can occur. Rarely precipitates acute gout attack. ▪ See Drug/Lab Interactions.

Patient Education: Hypotension may cause dizziness; request assistance with ambulation. ▪ Report cramps, dizziness, muscle weakness, or nausea promptly. ▪ May cause a decrease in potassium levels and require a supplement. ▪ Skin may become photosensitive; avoid unprotected exposure to sun. ▪ Therapy for diabetes may require adjustment; monitoring of serum glucose required.

Maternal/Child: Category C: use during pregnancy only when clearly needed and benefits outweigh potential risks to fetus. Treatment during pregnancy requires monitoring of fetal growth because of the potential for higher fetal birth weights. ▪ Use caution in breast-feeding; may inhibit lactation. ▪ Safety for use in pediatric patients not established. ▪ Prolonged use in premature infants may result in nephrocalcinosis and nephrolithiasis. Has also been observed in pediatric patients under 4 years of age who have been treated chronically with furosemide. ▪ May increase risk of persistent patent ductus arteriosus in preterm infants with respiratory distress syndrome. ▪ Premature infants receiving doses exceeding 1 mg/kg/day may develop plasma levels that could be associated with toxicity, including ototoxicity. Hearing loss in neonates has been associated with the use of furosemide.

Elderly: Protein binding and clearance is decreased in the elderly. ▪ Consider increased sensitivity to hypotensive and electrolyte effects. Dose selection should be cautious, starting at the lower end of the dosing range. ▪ May be more susceptible to dehydration; observe carefully. ▪ Avoid rapid contraction of plasma volume and hemoconcentration. May cause thromboembolic episodes (e.g., CVA, pulmonary emboli). ▪ The initial diuretic effect in older patients is decreased relative to younger patients.

DRUG/LAB INTERACTIONS

Causes excessive potassium depletion with **corticosteroids, thiazide diuretics** (e.g., hydrochlorothiazide), **amphotericin B** (all formulations). ▪ Potentiates **antihypertensive drugs** (e.g., angiotensin-converting enzyme [ACE] inhibitors [e.g., enalapril (Vasotec), enalaprilat (Vasotec IV), lisinopril (Zestril)], angiotensin II receptor blockers [e.g., losartan (Cozaar)], nitroglycerin, nitroprusside sodium); reduced dose of the antihypertensive agent or both drugs may be indicated. ▪ May cause transient or permanent deafness with doses exceeding the usual or when given in conjunction with **other ototoxic drugs** (e.g., aminoglycosides [e.g., gentamicin], cisplatin). ▪ **Amphotericin B** (all formulations) may increase potential for ototoxicity and nephrotoxicity; avoid concurrent use. ▪ Nephrotoxicity increased by **other nephrotoxic agents** (e.g., aminoglycosides, cephalosporins [e.g., ciprofloxacin (Cipro)], cisplatin, cyclosporine [Sandimmune], radiocontrast agents, vancomycin); avoid concurrent use. ▪ May increase serum levels of **lithium** (may cause toxicity). ▪ May cause cardiac arrhythmias with **amiodarone** (Nexterone) **or digoxin** (potassium depletion). ▪ May enhance or inhibit actions of **nondepolarizing muscle relaxants** (e.g., atracurium [Tracrium]). ▪ May potentiate the action of **succinylcholine.** ▪ Effects line. ▪ Effects may be inhibited by **NSAIDs** (e.g., ibuprofen [Motrin]) **or probene-cid.** ▪ May cause profound diuresis and serious electrolyte abnormalities with **thiazide diuretics** (e.g., chlorothiazide [Diuril]) because of synergistic effects. ▪ May be inhibited by **phenytoin** (Dilantin). ▪ Do not use concomitantly with **ethacrynic acid** (Edecrin); risk of ototoxicity markedly increased. ▪ **Salicylates** may decrease the diuretic effect of furosemide. ▪ **Furosemide** may increase serum levels of salicylates, increasing the risk of toxicity. ▪ May decrease arterial responsiveness to **norepinephrine.** Dose adjustment may be required. ▪ May enhance adverse effects of **chloral hydrate.** Concomitant use not recommended. ▪ **Methotrexate** and other drugs that undergo significant renal tubular secretion may decrease the effectiveness of furosemide. ▪ Furosemide may decrease renal elimination of other drugs that undergo tubular secretion. High-dose treatment of both furosemide and these other drugs may result in elevated serum levels and may potentiate toxicity. ▪ Concomitant use of **cyclosporine** and furosemide has been associated with increased risk of gouty arthritis secondary to furosemide-induced hyperuricemia and cyclosporine impairment of renal urate excretion. ▪ See Precautions.

SIDE EFFECTS
Usually occur in prolonged therapy, seriously ill patients, or following large doses.

Anemia, anorexia, blurring of vision, deafness (reversible), diarrhea, dizziness, elevated hepatic enzymes, eosinophilia, headache, hyperglycemia, hyperuricemia, hypokalemia, increases in serum cholesterol and triglyceride levels, leg cramps, lethargy, leukopenia, mental confusion, nausea, paresthesia, postural hypotension, pruritus, rash, tinnitus, urinary frequency, urticaria, vomiting, weakness.

Major: Anaphylactic shock, blood volume reduction, circulatory collapse, dehydration, excessive diuresis, hepatic encephalopathy in patients with hepatic insufficiency, hypokalemia, metabolic acidosis, Stevens-Johnson syndrome, toxic epidermal necrolysis, vascular thrombosis and embolism.

Overdose: Blood volume reduction, dehydration, electrolyte imbalances, hypochloremic alkalosis, and hypotension.

ANTIDOTE
If minor side effects are noted, discontinue the drug and notify the physician, who may treat the side effects symptomatically and continue the drug. If side effects are progressive or any major side effect occurs, discontinue the drug immediately and notify the physician. Treatment of major side effects is symptomatic and aggressive. Monitor serum electrolytes, carbon dioxide level, and BP frequently, and replace excessive fluid and electrolyte losses as needed. Hemodialysis does not accelerate furosemide elimination. Resuscitate as necessary.

GANCICLOVIR SODIUM BBW
(gan-**SYE**-kloh-veer **SO**-dee-um)

Antiviral

Cytovene IV

pH 9 to 11

USUAL DOSE
Adequate hydration and specific testing required; see Monitor.

CMV retinitis: 5 mg/kg of body weight every 12 hours for 14 to 21 days. Begin a maintenance dose the next day (Day 15 to 22) of 5 mg/kg daily for 7 days each week or 6 mg/kg daily for 5 days each week. See Precautions/Monitor. After IV induction and when retinitis is stable, Cytovene capsules may be used for maintenance therapy; see Precautions. If retinitis progresses during the maintenance regimen, initiate the twice-daily program again. Do not exceed recommended dose or infusion rate. Larger doses or increased rates of infusion have resulted in increased toxicity. For patients who have relapsed after induction and reinduction monotherapy with either ganciclovir or foscarnet, practitioners may consider an unlabeled combination therapy, which adds the alternate drug to the regimen. Information on this combination regimen is available from Roche and in the Clinical Trials section of the foscarnet sodium prescribing information.

Prevention of CMV disease in transplant recipients: 5 mg/kg every 12 hours for 7 to 14 days. Follow with maintenance regimen as outlined in CMV retinitis. Length of treatment based on immunosuppression degree and duration; 3 to 4 months or longer is common. CMV disease may occur if treatment is stopped prematurely.

Prevention of CMV disease in HIV-infected adolescents and adults (unlabeled): 5 to 6 mg/kg/dose for 5 to 7 days each week. Cytovene capsules may be used.

PEDIATRIC DOSE

Safety for use in pediatric patients under 12 years of age not established. ▪ Use extreme caution; long-term carcinogenicity and reproductive toxicity are probable. Benefit must outweigh risks. See Indications and Maternal/Child.

CMV retinitis in pediatric patients over 3 months of age (unlabeled): 2.5 mg/kg every 8 hours for 14 to 21 days followed by a maintenance dose of 6 to 6.5 mg/kg/day was used during clinical trials. When retinitis progressed, the adult dosing regimen for induction and maintenance was followed. Another source suggests the adult dose regimen listed in Usual Dose.

Prevention of CMV disease in transplant recipients (unlabeled): Same as adults; see Usual Dose.

Prevention of CMV disease in HIV-infected individuals (unlabeled): 5 mg/kg/dose IV daily.

DOSE ADJUSTMENTS

Dose selection should be cautious in the elderly. Reduced doses may be indicated based on the potential for decreased organ function and concomitant disease or drug therapy. Assess renal function before administration to elderly patients and adjust dose appropriately; see Elderly. ▪ Withhold dose if absolute neutrophil count (ANC) less than 500 cells/mm^3 or platelets less than 25,000 cells/mm^3. ▪ See Drug/Lab Interactions. ▪ With impaired renal function, reduce dose according to the following chart.

Ganciclovir Induction and Maintenance Dose Guidelines in Impaired Renal Function				
Creatinine Clearance (mL/min)	Ganciclovir IV Induction Dose (mg/kg)	Dosing Interval (hours)	Ganciclovir Maintenance Dose (mg/kg)	Dosing Interval (hours)
≥70	5 mg/kg	12 hours	5 mg/kg	24 hours
50-69	2.5 mg/kg	12 hours	2.5 mg/kg	24 hours
25-49	2.5 mg/kg	24 hours	1.25 mg/kg	24 hours
10-24	1.25 mg/kg	24 hours	0.625 mg/kg	24 hours
<10	1.25 mg/kg	3 times per week following hemodialysis	0.625 mg/kg	3 times per week following hemodialysis

DILUTION

Specific techniques required; see Precautions. Initially dissolve the 500-mg vial with 10 mL SWFI (50 mg/mL). Do not use bacteriostatic water containing parabens; will cause precipitation. Shake well to dissolve completely. Discard if particulate matter or discoloration observed. Withdraw desired dose and further dilute with NS, D5W, Ringer's, or LR to provide a concentration less than 10 mg/mL (70-kg adult at 5 mg/kg equals 350 mg; dissolved in 100 mL of solution equals 3.5 mg/mL).

Filters: Use not required by manufacturer; however, use of a filter would not have an adverse effect.

Storage: Store unopened vials below 40° C (104° F). Reconstituted solution in vial stable at CRT for 12 hours. Do not refrigerate. Solution fully diluted for administration must be refrigerated and used within 24 hours to reduce incidence of bacterial contamination.

Stable for 14 days refrigerated at 5° C (41° F) if prepared in PVC bags and reconstituted with SWFI and further diluted with NS.

COMPATIBILITY   (Underline Indicates Conflicting Compatibility Information)

Consider any drug NOT listed as compatible to be INCOMPATIBLE until consulting a pharmacist; specific conditions may apply.

Because of physical **incompatibilities,** ganciclovir sodium and *foscarnet sodium* must never be mixed.

One source suggests the following **compatibilities:**

Y-site: Allopurinol (Aloprim), amphotericin B cholesteryl (Amphotec), anidulafungin (Eraxis), caspofungin (Cancidas), cisatracurium (Nimbex), docetaxel (Taxotere), doxorubicin liposomal (Doxil), enalaprilat (Vasotec IV), etoposide phosphate (Etopophos), filgrastim (Neupogen), fluconazole (Diflucan), granisetron (Kytril), linezolid (Zyvox), melphalan (Alkeran), paclitaxel (Taxol), pemetrexed (Alimta), propofol (Diprivan), remifentanil (Ultiva), teniposide (Vumon), thiotepa.

RATE OF ADMINISTRATION

A single dose must be administered at a constant rate over 1 hour as an infusion. Use of an infusion pump or microdrip (60 gtt/mL) recommended. *Do not give by rapid or bolus IV injection.* Excessive plasma levels and toxicity will occur with too-rapid rate of injection. Advisable to clear tubing with NS before and after administration through Y-tube or three-way stopcock.

ACTIONS

An antiviral agent that inhibits DNA synthesis and stops cytomegalovirus (CMV) from multiplying. Does not destroy existing viruses but stops them from reproducing and invading healthy cells. May allow a weakened immune system to defend the body against the CMV infection. May also be inhibitory against herpes simplex virus 1 and 2, Epstein-Barr virus, and varicella zoster virus, but clinical studies have not been done. Onset of action is prompt, and therapeutic levels are maintained for 3 to 6 hours with some drug remaining 11 hours after infusion. Widely distributed in tissues and body fluids. Half-life is 2.6 to 4.4 hours. Crosses the placental barrier. Suspected to be secreted in breast milk. Approximately 90% excreted unchanged in urine in patients with normal renal function.

INDICATIONS AND USES

Treatment of CMV retinitis in immunocompromised individuals, including patients with AIDS. ▪ CMV disease prevention in at-risk transplant patients. ▪ Safety and effectiveness for use in congenital or neonatal CMV disease, treatment of established CMV disease other than retinitis, or nonimmunocompromised individuals not established. Use should be limited to treatment of conditions listed above. ▪ Now available as an ophthalmic surgical aid (intravitreal implant) to treat CMV retinitis. ▪ Ganciclovir (Cytovene) capsules are used for prevention of CMV retinitis in at-risk patients with advanced HIV infection and in the prevention of CMV disease in solid-organ transplant recipients; see Precautions. Valganciclovir (Valcyte) is an oral drug recently approved for the treatment of CMV retinitis, and it is also being used for maintenance.

Unlabeled uses: Treatment of other CMV infections (e.g., gastroenteritis, hepatitis, pneumonitis) in immunocompromised patients. ▪ Treatment of polyradiculopathy caused by CMV infections. ▪ Combination therapy (ganciclovir and foscarnet) to treat progressive retinitis refractory to single therapy.

CONTRAINDICATIONS

Hypersensitivity to ganciclovir or acyclovir; patients with a neutrophil count less than 500 cells/mm^3 or a platelet count less than 25,000 cells/mm^3; patients receiving zidovudine (AZT, Retrovir) because both drugs cause granulocytopenia.

PRECAUTIONS

A nucleoside analog; follow guidelines for handling and disposal of cytotoxic agents. See Appendix A, p. 1331. ▪ For IV use only; IM or SC administration will cause severe tissue irritation. ▪ Hematologic toxicity (anemia, granulocytopenia, thrombocytopenia) is common; see Monitor. ▪ Use with caution in patients with pre-existing cytopenias or a history of cytopenic reactions to other drugs, chemicals, or irradiation. ▪ Ganciclovir is not a cure for CMV infections. Maintenance therapy is almost always necessary to prevent relapse in patients with AIDS. ▪ Resistance has been reported to develop. May be higher in patients treated for a prolonged period. ▪ Cidofovir is also an agent for treatment of CMV retinitis. ▪ Risk of a more rapid rate of disease progression is increased with oral ganciclovir. Use in maintenance recommended only if benefits of avoiding daily IV infusions outweigh risk.

Monitor: Confirm diagnosis of CMV retinitis by indirect ophthalmoscopy. Diagnosis may be supported by cultures of CMV (e.g., urine, blood, throat); negative culture does not rule out CMV retinitis. ▪ Continue ophthalmologic exams during induction and maintenance treatment to monitor CMV status. ▪ CBC with differential and platelet counts, SCr, and CrCl are required before treatment is initiated. Monitor CBC and platelet counts frequently, especially in patients with previous leukopenia from ganciclovir or other nucleoside analogs or those with neutrophils less than 1,000 cells/mm³ at beginning of treatment and in patients undergoing hemodialysis. Withhold dose if absolute neutrophil count (ANC) less than 500 cells/mm³ or platelets less than 25,000 cells/mm³. Monitor SCr or CrCl every 2 weeks. ▪ Maintain adequate hydration and urine flow before and during infusion. ▪ Phlebitis or pain may occur at site of infusion; confirm patency of vein and use small needles and large veins to ensure adequate blood flow for rapid dilution and distribution. ▪ Granulocytopenia usually occurs within 14 days but may occur at any time; recovery should begin within 3 to 7 days of discontinuing ganciclovir. ▪ Consider the possibility of viral resistance if retinitis does not show significant improvement with treatment. ▪ See Drug/Lab Interactions.

Patient Education: Must use effective birth control throughout treatment. Men should continue barrier contraception for at least 90 days. ▪ Not a cure; retinitis may still progress. Frequent ophthalmoscopic examinations important. ▪ Cooperation for close monitoring of blood cell counts is imperative to control side effects (e.g., anemia, neutropenia, thrombocytopenia). ▪ Report any unexpected side effects promptly (e.g., chills, fever, unusual bleeding or bruising). ▪ Patients with AIDS receiving zidovudine (AZT, Retrovir) may not tolerate ganciclovir. ▪ High frequency of impaired renal function increased with concomitant use of nephrotoxic agents (e.g., cyclosporine, amphotericin); high risk for transplant recipients.

Maternal/Child: Category C: avoid pregnancy. A potential carcinogen. Teratogenic and embryotoxic; has caused aspermatogenesis and will cause birth defects. Do not use during pregnancy unless risk is justified. May cause temporary or permanent infertility in men and women. ▪ Discontinue nursing during treatment; minimum interval required before resuming breast-feeding is unknown. ▪ Use extreme caution in pediatric patients under 12 years of age. Long-term carcinogenicity and reproductive toxicity are probable. Benefit must outweigh risks.

Elderly: Dose selection should be cautious; see Dose Adjustments. Monitor renal function during therapy and adjust dose as indicated.

DRUG/LAB INTERACTIONS

Because of physical **incompatibilities,** ganciclovir and **foscarnet** must never be mixed. ▪ Additive toxicity may occur with concomitant use of **other drugs that inhibit replication of rapidly dividing cell populations** (e.g., dapsone, pentamidine, flucytosine [Ancobon], vincristine, vinblastine, doxorubicin [Adriamycin], amphotericin B [conventional], sulfamethoxazole/trimethoprim [Bactrim]). ▪ May cause severe anemia and neutropenia with **zidovudine** (AZT, Retrovir). Combination used in patients with AIDS is rarely tolerated. ▪ Concurrent treatment with **didanosine** (Videx) may cause increased didanosine levels. ▪ May cause seizures with **imipenem-cilastatin** (Primaxin). ▪ Potentiated by **probenecid and other drugs that may reduce renal clearance;** will increase toxicity. ▪ Impaired renal function may be markedly increased with other **nephrotoxic agents** (e.g., cyclosporine, amphotericin B). ▪ Concurrent or consecutive use with **other bone marrow suppressants** (e.g., antineoplastics, amphotericin B, zidovudine and/or radiation therapy) may produce additive bone marrow suppression. ▪ Drug interaction studies with drugs commonly used in transplant recipients have not been conducted. ▪ See Contraindications.

SIDE EFFECTS

Anemia, leukopenia, and thrombocytopenia are most common and are generally reversible if treatment is discontinued. Abdominal pain; anorexia; chills; diarrhea; fever; infection; nausea; neuropathy; pain, infection, and sepsis at injection site; phlebitis; pruritus; rash; retinal detachment; sepsis; sweating; and vomiting occur in some patients. Abnormal kidney function and/or failure, abnormal vision, alopecia, anxiety, arthralgia, asthenia, chest pain, confusion, constipation, cough, decreased CrCl, depression, dizziness, dry mouth, dry skin, dyspepsia, dyspnea, edema, eructation, headache, hypertension, increased ALT and AST, increased creatinine, insomnia, leg cramps, malaise, myalgia, myasthenia, pancytopenia, seizures, somnolence, stomatitis, taste perversion, tinnitus, tremor, and weight loss have occurred. Gastrointestinal perforation, multiple organ failure, pancreatitis, and sepsis have occurred and may be fatal. Numerous additional side effects may occur.

Overdose: Acute renal failure, hematuria, hepatitis, irreversible pancytopenia, persistent bone marrow suppression, and seizures have occurred.

ANTIDOTE

Notify physician of all side effects; most will be treated symptomatically. Filgrastim (Neupogen, Zarxio) 1 to 10 mcg/kg/day has been used to maintain the neutrophil count. Discontinue drug if neutrophils fall below 500 cells/mm^3 or platelets fall below 25,000 cells/mm^3. Hydration and hemodialysis (up to 50% removal) are useful in overdose. Treat anaphylaxis and resuscitate as necessary.

GEMCITABINE HYDROCHLORIDE

(jem-**SIGHT**-ah-been hy-droh-**KLOR**-eyed)

Gemzar

Antineoplastic
(miscellaneous)

pH 2.7 to 3.3

USUAL DOSE

Pancreatic cancer: 1,000 mg/M^2 as outlined in the following treatment schedule:

Weeks 1-8: Weekly dosing for the first 7 weeks followed by 1 week of rest.

After Week 8: Weekly dosing on Days 1, 8, and 15 of 28-day cycles.

Non–small-cell lung cancer (NSCLC): 1,000 mg/M^2 as an infusion on Days 1, 8, and 15 of each 28-day cycle. Given in combination with cisplatin. Administer cisplatin 100 mg/M^2 IV on Day 1 after the infusion of gemcitabine. An alternate schedule is gemcitabine 1,250 mg/M^2 on Days 1 and 8 of each 21-day cycle. Administer cisplatin 100 mg/M^2 IV on Day 1 after the infusion of gemcitabine. See cisplatin monograph for administration and hydration guidelines.

Breast cancer: 1,250 mg/M^2 as an infusion on Days 1 and 8 of each 21-day cycle. Given in combination with paclitaxel (Taxol). On Day 1, administer paclitaxel 175 mg/M^2 as a 3-hour infusion before the gemcitabine infusion. Premedication required; see paclitaxel monograph.

Ovarian cancer: 1,000 mg/M^2 as an infusion on Days 1 and 8 of a 21-day cycle. Given in combination with carboplatin (Paraplatin). On Day 1, administer carboplatin at AUC 4 after gemcitabine administration.

Bladder cancer (unlabeled): 1,000 mg/M^2 on Days 1, 8, and 15. Repeat cycle every 28 days. Given in conjunction with cisplatin.

Hodgkin's lymphoma (relapsed) or non-Hodgkin's lymphoma (refractory) (unlabeled): 1,000 mg/M^2 on Days 1 and 8 of a 21-day cycle.

Adenocarcinoma of the pancreas: Given in combination with Abraxane; see paclitaxel protein-bound particles for injectable suspension (Abraxane) monograph.

DOSE ADJUSTMENTS

Clearance decreased in women and the elderly. May be less likely to progress to subsequent cycles; see Precautions and Elderly.

Treatment of pancreatic cancer and NSCLC: Reduce dose based on the degree of hematologic toxicity according to the following chart.

Gemcitabine Dose Reduction Guidelines Indicated for Dose Reduction in Pancreatic Cancer and NSCLC			
Absolute Granulocyte Count (cells/mm³)		Platelet Count (cells/mm³)	% of Full Dose to Be Administered
≥1,000	and	≥100,000	100%
500-999	or	50,000-99,999	75%
<500	or	<50,000	Hold

Treatment of breast cancer (combination with paclitaxel): Reduce dose based on degree of hematologic toxicity according to the following chart.

Dose Reduction Guidelines for Gemcitabine in Combination with Paclitaxel for Myelosuppression on Day of Treatment in Breast Cancer				
Treatment Day	Absolute Granulocyte Count (cells/mm³)		Platelet Count (cells/mm³)	% of Full Dose
Day 1	≥1,500	and	≥100,000	100%
	<1,500	or	<100,000	Hold
Day 8	≥1,200	and	>75,000	100%
	1,000–1,199	or	50,000–75,000	75%
	700–999	and	≥50,000	50%
	<700	or	<50,000	Hold

See paclitaxel monograph for additional dose adjustment guidelines.

Treatment of ovarian cancer in combination with carboplatin: Reduce dose based on the degree of hematologic toxicity according to the following charts.

Dose Reduction Guidelines for Gemcitabine in Combination with Carboplatin for Myelosuppression on Day of Treatment in Ovarian Cancer				
Treatment Day	Absolute Granulocyte Count (cells/mm³)		Platelet Count (cells/mm³)	% of Full Dose
Day 1	≥1,500	and	≥100,000	100%
	<1,500	or	<100,000	Delay treatment cycle
Day 8	≥1,500	and	≥100,000	100%
	1,000–1,499	or	75,000–99,999	50%
	<1,000	or	<75,000	Hold

Gemcitabine dose modification for myelosuppression in previous cycle in ovarian cancer: Reduce dose based on myelosuppression occurrence according to the chart on the following page.

Continued

Gemcitabine Dose Modification for Myelosuppression in Previous Cycle in Ovarian Cancer		
Occurrence	Myelosuppression During Treatment Cycle	Dose Modification
Initial occurrence	• Absolute granulocyte count <500 cells/mm³ for more than 5 days • Absolute granulocyte count <100 cells/mm³ for more than 3 days • Febrile neutropenia • Platelets <25,000 cells/mm³ • Cycle delay of more than 1 week due to toxicity	Permanently reduce dose to 800 mg/M² on Day 1 and Day 8
Subsequent occurrence	Occurrence of any of the above toxicities after the initial dose reduction	Permanently reduce dose to 800 mg/M² on Day 1 only

See carboplatin monograph for additional dosing guidelines.

Gemcitabine Dose Modifications for Nonhematologic Adverse Reactions
Permanently discontinue gemcitabine for any of the following:
• Unexplained dyspnea or other evidence of severe pulmonary toxicity • Severe hepatic toxicity • Hemolytic-uremic syndrome (HUS) • Capillary leak syndrome (CLS) • Posterior reversible encephalopathy syndrome (PRES) • Withhold gemcitabine or reduce dose by 50% for other severe (Grade 3 or 4) nonhematologic toxicity until resolved. No dose modifications are recommended for alopecia, nausea, or vomiting.

DILUTION

Specific techniques required; see Precautions. Each 200 mg must be reconstituted with 5 mL NS without preservatives (25 mL NS for 1 Gm). Yields 38 mg/mL. Shake to dissolve. Do not use less solution to reconstitute; dissolution will be incomplete. The appropriate dose ***must*** be further diluted with NS to concentrations as low as 0.1 mg/mL. 1,500 mg diluted in 250 mL yields 6 mg/mL. 750 mg in 100 mL yields 7.5 mg/mL.

Filters: Reconstituted solution may be filtered through a 0.22- or 0.45-micron pre-filter.

Storage: Store unopened vials at CRT. Reconstituted or diluted solutions are stable at CRT for 24 hours. Do not refrigerate in any form; may crystallize. Discard unused portion.

COMPATIBILITY   (Underline Indicates Conflicting Compatibility Information)

Consider any drug NOT listed as compatible to be INCOMPATIBLE until consulting a pharmacist; specific conditions may apply.

Manufacturer states, "**Compatibilities** with other drugs have not been studied. No **incompatibilities** observed with IV bottles or PVC bags and administration sets."

One source suggests the following **compatibilities:**

Y-site: Amifostine (Ethyol), amikacin, aminophylline, ampicillin, ampicillin/sulbactam (Unasyn), anidulafungin (Eraxis), aztreonam (Azactam), bleomycin (Blenoxane), bumetanide, buprenorphine (Buprenex), butorphanol (Stadol), calcium gluconate, carboplatin (Paraplatin), carmustine (BiCNU), cefazolin (Ancef), cefotetan (Cefotan), cefoxitin (Mefoxin), ceftazidime (Fortaz), ceftriaxone (Rocephin), cefuroxime (Zinacef), chlorpromazine (Thorazine), ciprofloxacin (Cipro IV), cisplatin, clindamycin (Cleocin), cyclophosphamide (Cytoxan), cytarabine (ARA-C), dactinomycin (Cosmegen), daunorubicin (Cerubidine), dexamethasone (Decadron), dexrazoxane (Zinecard), diphenhydramine (Benadryl), dobutamine, docetaxel (Taxotere), dopamine, doripenem (Doribax), doxorubicin (Adriamycin), doxycycline, droperidol (Inapsine), enalaprilat (Vasotec IV), etoposide (VePesid), etoposide phosphate (Etopophos), famotidine (Pepcid IV), fluconazole (Diflucan), fludarabine (Fludara), fluorouracil (5-FU), gentamicin, granisetron (Kytril), heparin, hydrocortisone sodium succinate (Solu-Cortef), hydromorphone (Dilaudid), idarubicin (Idamycin), ifosfamide (Ifex), leucovorin calcium, linezolid (Zyvox), lorazepam (Ativan), mannitol, meperidine (Demerol), mesna (Mesnex), metoclopramide (Reglan), metronidazole (Flagyl IV), mitoxantrone (Novantrone), morphine, nalbuphine, ondansetron (Zofran), oxaliplatin (Eloxatin), paclitaxel (Taxol), palonosetron (Aloxi), potassium chloride (KCl), promethazine (Phenergan), ranitidine (Zantac), sodium bicarbonate, streptozocin (Zanosar), sulfamethoxazole/trimethoprim, teniposide (Vumon), thiotepa, ticarcillin/clavulanate (Timentin), tobramycin, topotecan (Hycamtin), vancomycin, vinblastine, vincristine, vinorelbine (Navelbine), zidovudine (AZT, Retrovir).

RATE OF ADMINISTRATION
A single dose as an infusion equally distributed over 30 minutes. Do not extend infusion time beyond 60 minutes; will increase toxicity.

ACTIONS
A nucleoside metabolic inhibitor with antineoplastic activity. Metabolized intracellularly to two active nucleosides. Cell phase specific, these nucleosides induce internucleosomal DNA fragmentation, primarily killing cells undergoing DNA synthesis (S-phase) and also blocking the progression of cells through the G_1/S-phase boundary. Very little is bound to plasma protein. Volume of distribution is increased by infusion length. Half-life is shorter (42 to 94 minutes) with a short infusion (less than 70 minutes), and longer (245 to 638 minutes) with a long infusion (more than 70 minutes). Half-life is slightly longer and rate of clearance is lower in women and in the elderly, resulting in higher concentrations for any given dose. Primarily excreted in urine.

INDICATIONS AND USES
First-line treatment for patients with locally advanced (nonresectable Stage II or Stage III) or metastatic (Stage IV) adenocarcinoma of the pancreas in patients previously treated with fluorouracil. ▪ First-line treatment in combination with cisplatin for the treatment of inoperable, locally advanced (Stage IIIA or IIIB) or metastatic (Stage IV) non–small-cell lung cancer. ▪ First-line treatment in combination with paclitaxil for treatment of metastatic breast cancer after failure of previous anthracycline chemotherapy unless anthracyclines (e.g., doxorubicin [Adriamycin], idarubicin [Idamycin]) were clinically contraindicated. ▪ Treatment in combination with carboplatin for patients with advanced ovarian cancer that has relapsed at least 6 months after completion of platinum-based therapy.
Unlabeled uses: Treatment of metastatic bladder cancer. ▪ Treatment of testicular cancer. ▪ Treatment of cancer of the head and neck.

CONTRAINDICATIONS
Hypersensitivity to gemcitabine or any of its components.

PRECAUTIONS
Follow guidelines for handling cytotoxic agents. See Appendix A, p. 1331. ▪ Administered by or under the direction of the physician specialist. ▪ Adequate diagnostic and treatment facilities must be available. ▪ For IV use only. May be administered on an outpatient basis. ▪ Prolongation of the infusion time beyond 60 minutes and more frequent than weekly dosing have been shown to increase toxicity (e.g., clinically significant hypotension, severe flu-like symptoms, myelosuppression, and asthenia). ▪ Myelosuppression (e.g., anemia, neutropenia, and thrombocytopenia) is the dose-limiting toxicity. Occurs with gemcitabine as a single agent, and the risk increases when it is combined with other cytotoxic drugs; see Dose Adjustments. ▪ Clearance in women and the elderly is reduced; women, especially older women, were more likely not to proceed to a subsequent cycle and to experience Grade 3 or 4 neutropenia and thrombocytopenia. No age or gender dose adjustments recommended. ▪ Use with caution in impaired renal or hepatic function. Clear dose recommendations are not available; data from clinical

studies insufficient. ▪ Hepatotoxicity, including liver failure and death, has been reported. Use in patients with concurrent liver metastases or a history of alcoholism, hepatitis, or liver cirrhosis may lead to exacerbation of the underlying hepatic insufficiency. ▪ Hemolytic-uremic syndrome (HUS) and/or renal toxicity, including renal failure leading to death or requiring dialysis, has been reported. ▪ Gemcitabine is a potent radiosensitizer. Depending on the site being radiated, concurrent use with gemcitabine may cause severe, life-threatening esophagitis and pneumonitis. Data suggest that gemcitabine can be started after the acute effects of radiation have resolved or at least 1 week after radiation is completed. Radiation recall has been reported in patients who receive gemcitabine after prior radiation. ▪ Pulmonary toxicity (e.g., adult respiratory distress syndrome [ARDS], interstitial pneumonitis, pulmonary edema, pulmonary fibrosis) has been reported. Fatalities have occurred. Onset of pulmonary symptoms may occur up to 2 weeks after the last dose of gemcitabine. Discontinue gemcitabine in patients who develop unexplained dyspnea, with or without bronchospasm, or who have any evidence of pulmonary toxicity. ▪ Capillary leak syndrome (CLS) and posterior reversible encephalopathy syndrome (PRES) have been reported. ▪ Use caution in patients who have had previous cytotoxic chemotherapy or radiation therapy.

Monitor: Monitor for bone marrow suppression. ▪ Obtain a CBC, including differential and platelet count, before each dose; see Dose Adjustments. ▪ Obtain baseline renal function (e.g., SCr) and liver function tests (e.g., AST, ALT) and repeat periodically. ▪ Monitor serum calcium, magnesium, potassium, and SCr during combination therapy with cisplatin. ▪ Monitor vital signs. ▪ Maintain adequate hydration. ▪ Nausea and vomiting are frequent and were severe in 15% of patients; prophylactic administration of antiemetics will increase patient comfort. ▪ Observe closely for S/S of infection. May cause fever in the absence of infection, or prophylactic antibiotics may be indicated pending results of C/S in a febrile or nonfebrile patient. ▪ Monitor for thrombocytopenia (platelet count less than 50,000/mm^3). Initiate precautions to prevent excessive bleeding (e.g., inspect IV sites, skin, and mucous membranes; use extreme care during invasive procedures; test urine, emesis, stool, and secretions for occult blood). ▪ Consider a diagnosis of HUS if anemia with evidence of microangiopathic hemolysis, elevation of bilirubin or LDH, reticulocytosis, severe thrombocytopenia, and/or evidence of renal failure (elevation of SCr or BUN) develops; discontinue gemcitabine. ▪ Monitor for S/S of CLS (sudden edema, rapid drop in blood pressure, shock, hemoconcentration, hypoalbuminemia). ▪ Monitor for S/S of PRES (blindness, confusion, headache, hypertension, lethargy, seizure, or other visual or neurologic disturbances). Confirm diagnosis of PRES with MRI. ▪ Not a vesicant, but monitor injection site for inflammation and/or extravasation.

Patient Education: Nonhormonal birth control recommended. ▪ See Appendix D, p. 1333. ▪ Report any unusual or unexpected symptoms or side effects (e.g., shortness of breath, cough, blood in stool or urine, change in color or volume of urine, S/S of infection, jaundice, unusual bruising or bleeding) as soon as possible.

Maternal/Child: Category D: avoid pregnancy. May cause fetal harm. ▪ Discontinue breast-feeding. ▪ Safety and effectiveness for use in pediatric patients not established.

Elderly: Clearance reduced in the elderly; hematologic toxicity requiring reduction, delay, or omission of subsequent doses is higher than in younger adults; however, incidence of nonhematologic toxicity is similar. Elderly men and women are more likely to experience Grade 3 or 4 thrombocytopenia. Elderly women are also more likely to experience Grade 3 or 4 neutropenia. Usual dose adjustments based on toxicity are considered appropriate. Age-related impaired renal function may further reduce clearance and increase toxicity.

DRUG/LAB INTERACTIONS
Interaction of gemcitabine with other drugs has not been adequately studied. ▪ Additive bone marrow suppression may occur with **radiation therapy, other bone marrow–suppressing agents** (e.g., amphotericin B [traditional and lipid], azathioprine, chloramphenicol, melphelan [Alkeran]), and/or **immunosuppressants** (e.g., chlorambucil [Leukeran], cyclo-

phosphamide [Cytoxan], cyclosporine [Sandimmune], glucocorticoid corticosteroids [e.g., dexamethasone], muromonab-CD3 [Orthoclone], tacrolimus [Prograf]); dose reduction may be required. ▪ Do not administer **live virus vaccines** to patients receiving antineoplastic agents.

SIDE EFFECTS

The most common side effects are anemia, dyspnea, fever, hematuria, hepatic transaminitis, increased alkaline phosphatase, nausea, neutropenia, peripheral edema, proteinuria, rash, thrombocytopenia, and vomiting. Less frequently reported side effects include alopecia, anorexia, arrhythmias, arthralgia, bone marrow toxicity (e.g., anemia, leukopenia, neutropenia, thrombocytopenia), bone pain, bronchospasm, capillary leak syndrome, cerebrovascular accident, CHF, constipation, diarrhea, edema, elevated lab tests (e.g., BUN, creatinine, hematuria, proteinuria), fatigue, febrile neutropenia, flu syndrome (e.g., anorexia, chills, cough, headache, myalgia, weakness), hemolytic-uremic syndrome, hemorrhage, hepatotoxicity, hypertension, increased liver function tests (e.g., ALT, AST, GGT, alkaline phosphatase, and bilirubin), infection, injection site reaction, myalgia, myocardial infarction, neuropathy (motor and sensory), pain, paresthesias, peripheral vasculitis and gangrene, posterior reversible encephalopathy syndrome (PRES), pruritus, pulmonary toxicity (including pulmonary edema, pulmonary fibrosis, interstitial pneumonitis, ARDS, respiratory failure), radiation recall reactions, severe skin reactions (e.g., desquamation and bullous skin eruptions), somnolence, and stomatitis. Anaphylaxis and hemolytic-uremic syndrome have been reported.

ANTIDOTE

Keep physician informed of all side effects. Symptomatic and supportive treatment is indicated. Permanently discontinue gemcitabine if any of the following occur: unexplained dyspnea or other evidence of severe pulmonary toxicity, severe hepatic toxicity, hemolytic-uremic syndrome, capillary leak syndrome, or posterior reversible encephalopathy syndrome (PRES). Reduce dose or withhold gemcitabine until myelosuppression improves to specific criteria; see Dose Adjustments. If gemcitabine-induced pneumonitis or esophagitis is confirmed or suspected, discontinue permanently (in one study severe stomatitis and pharyngeal damage required patients to be fed by feeding tube for up to 12 months after receiving doses of 300 mg/M^2 [25% of the usual dose]). Anemia may require RBC transfusions. Other whole blood products (e.g., platelets, leukocytes) and/or blood modifiers (e.g., darbepoetin alfa [Aranesp], epoetin alfa [Epogen], filgrastim [Neupogen, Zarxio], pegfilgrastim [Neulasta], sargramostim [Leukine]) may be indicated to treat bone marrow toxicity. Most side effects are reversible with dose reduction or temporary withholding of gemcitabine. No known antidote for overdose. If hemolytic-uremic syndrome occurs, discontinue gemcitabine; renal failure may not be reversible even with discontinuation of therapy, and dialysis may be required. Treat hypersensitivity reactions as indicated; may require epinephrine, airway management, oxygen, IV fluids, antihistamines (e.g., diphenhydramine [Benadryl]), corticosteroids (e.g., hydrocortisone sodium succinate [Solu-Cortef]), and pressor amines (e.g., dopamine).

G-H

GENTAMICIN SULFATE BBW
(jen-tah-**MY**-sin **SUL**-fayt)

Antibacterial
(aminoglycoside)

pH 3 to 5.5

USUAL DOSE

3 mg/kg of body weight/24 hr equally divided into 3 doses (1 mg/kg every 8 hours). Up to 5 mg/kg/24 hr may be given if indicated. Reduce to usual dose as soon as feasible. Another source suggests 1 to 2.5 mg/kg/dose every 8 to 12 hours. A loading dose of 2 mg/kg is commonly used. **Dosage based on ideal body weight.** Studies suggest that in certain populations a single daily dose of 4 to 7 mg/kg (instead of divided into 2 to 3 doses) may provide higher peak levels and enhance drug effectiveness while actually reducing or having no adverse effects on risk of toxicity. Various procedures for monitoring blood levels are in use. Some health facilities are monitoring with trough levels; others may draw levels at predetermined times and plot the concentration on nomograms. Depending on the protocol in place, doses or intervals may be adjusted. See Dose Adjustments and Precautions/Monitor.

Prevention of bacterial endocarditis in dental, respiratory tract, GI or GU tract surgery or instrumentation: 1.5 mg/kg 30 minutes before procedure. Do not exceed 80 mg. Repeat in 8 hours. Given concurrently with ampicillin, vancomycin, or amoxicillin.

Pelvic inflammatory disease: 2 mg/kg as an initial dose. Follow with 1.5 mg/kg every 8 hours for 4 days or 48 hours after patient improves. Given concurrently with clindamycin.

PEDIATRIC DOSE

See Maternal/Child.

6 to 7.5 mg/kg of body weight/24 hr (2 to 2.5 mg/kg every 8 hours). A single daily dose is also being used in pediatric patients. See comments under Usual Dose. 10 mg/mL product available for pediatric use.

Prevention of bacterial endocarditis in dental, respiratory tract, GI or GU tract surgery or instrumentation: 2 mg/kg. See Adult Dose for instructions.

NEONATAL DOSE

See Maternal/Child.

2.5 mg/kg. Intervals adjusted based on age as follows:

0 to 7 days of age; less than 28 weeks' gestation: Every 24 hours.

28 to 34 weeks' gestation: Every 18 hours.

Over 34 weeks' gestation: Every 12 hours.

Over 7 days of age; less than 28 weeks' gestation: Every 18 hours.

28 to 34 weeks' gestation: Every 12 hours.

Over 34 weeks' gestation: Every 8 hours.

Another source suggests that higher doses (4 to 5 mg/kg/dose) at extended intervals (24 to 48 hours) may be used.

DOSE ADJUSTMENTS

Reduce daily dose commensurate with amount of renal impairment according to the following chart. Other protocols are in use; see literature. ▪ Once-daily dosing is not usually used for patients with ascites, burns covering more than 20% of the total body surface area, CrCl less than 40 mL/min (including patients requiring dialysis), CrCl greater than 120 mL/min, cystic fibrosis, endocarditis, mycobacterium infections, or in infants or during pregnancy. ▪ Reduced dose or extended intervals may be indicated in elderly adults. ▪ See Monitor and Drug/Lab Interactions.

Gentamicin Dosing Guidelines for Impaired Renal Function (Dose at 8-Hour Intervals After the Initial Dose)		
Serum Creatinine (mg%)	Approximate Creatinine Clearance Rate (mL/min/1.73 M²)	Percent of Usual Dose to Be Administered q 8 hr
<1	>100	100%
1.1-1.3	71-100	80%
1.4-1.6	56-70	65%
1.7-1.9	46-55	55%
2-2.2	41-45	50%
2.3-2.5	36-40	40%
2.6-3	31-35	35%
3.1-3.5	26-30	30%
3.6-4	21-25	25%
4.1-5.1	16-20	20%
5.2-6.6	11-15	15%
6.7-8	≤10	10%

The recommended dose at the end of each dialysis period is 1 to 1.7 mg/kg depending on the severity of the infection. 2 mg/kg may be administered to pediatric patients. The amount of gentamicin removed by dialysis may vary; however, an 8-hour dialysis session may reduce serum concentrations by 50%. Another source suggests the following dose guidelines for impaired renal function.

Conventional Gentamicin Dosing Guidelines for Impaired Renal Function	
Approximate Creatinine Clearance Rate (mL/min/1.73 M²)	Administer Conventional Dose at the Following Intervals
>60 mL/min	Every 8 hours
40 to 60 mL/min	Every 12 hours
20 to 40 mL/min	Every 24 hours
<20 mL/min	Loading dose, then monitor levels

High-dose therapy: Interval may be extended (e.g., every 48 hours) in patients with moderate renal impairment (CrCl 30 to 59 mL/min) and/or adjusted based on serum level determinations.

DILUTION
Available premixed in several concentrations. Vials equal 10 or 40 mg/mL. Further dilute each single dose in 50 to 200 mL of IV NS or D5W. Decrease volume of diluent for pediatric patients. Commercially diluted solutions available.

COMPATIBILITY   (Underline Indicates Conflicting Compatibility Information)
Consider any drug NOT listed as compatible to be INCOMPATIBLE until consulting a pharmacist; specific conditions may apply.
Manufacturer states, "Do not physically premix with other drugs; administer separately." Inactivated in solution with beta-lactam antibiotics (e.g., cephalosporins, penicillins) and

vancomycin. Do not mix in the same solution. Appropriate spacing required because of physical **incompatibilities.** See Drug/Lab Interactions.

One source suggests the following **compatibilities:**

Additive: *Not recommended by manufacturer.* Atracurium (Tracrium), aztreonam (Azactam), bleomycin (Blenoxane), cefotaxime (Claforan), cefoxitin (Mefoxin), ceftriaxone (Rocephin), cefuroxime (Zinacef), ciprofloxacin (Cipro IV), clindamycin (Cleocin), cytarabine (ARA-C), dextran 40, dopamine, fluconazole (Diflucan), furosemide (Lasix), linezolid (Zyvox), mannitol (Osmitrol), meropenem (Merrem IV), metronidazole (Flagyl IV), midazolam (Versed), penicillin G sodium, ranitidine (Zantac), verapamil.

Y-site: Acyclovir (Zovirax), alprostadil, amifostine (Ethyol), amiodarone (Nexterone), anidulafungin (Eraxis), atracurium (Tracrium), aztreonam (Azactam), bivalirudin (Angiomax), caspofungin (Cancidas), cefepime (Maxipime), ceftaroline (Teflaro), ceftazidime (Fortaz), ciprofloxacin (Cipro IV), cisatracurium (Nimbex), cyclophosphamide (Cytoxan), cytarabine (ARA-C), daptomycin (Cubicin), dexmedetomidine (Precedex), diltiazem (Cardizem), docetaxel (Taxotere), doripenem (Doribax), doxapram (Dopram), doxorubicin liposomal (Doxil), enalaprilat (Vasotec IV), esmolol (Brevibloc), etoposide phosphate (Etopophos), famotidine (Pepcid IV), fenoldopam (Corlopam), filgrastim (Neupogen), fluconazole (Diflucan), fludarabine (Fludara), foscarnet (Foscavir), gemcitabine (Gemzar), granisetron (Kytril), hetastarch in electrolytes (Hextend), hydromorphone (Dilaudid), 6% hydroxyethyl starch (Voluven), insulin (regular), labetalol, levofloxacin (Levaquin), linezolid (Zyvox), lorazepam (Ativan), magnesium sulfate, melphalan (Alkeran), meperidine (Demerol), meropenem (Merrem IV), midazolam (Versed), milrinone (Primacor), morphine, multivitamins (M.V.I.), nicardipine (Cardene IV), ondansetron (Zofran), paclitaxel (Taxol), palonosetron (Aloxi), pancuronium, potassium chloride (KCl), remifentanil (Ultiva), sargramostim (Leukine), tacrolimus (Prograf), telavancin (Vibativ), teniposide (Vumon), theophylline, thiotepa, tigecycline (Tygacil), vasopressin, vecuronium, vinorelbine (Navelbine), zidovudine (AZT, Retrovir).

RATE OF ADMINISTRATION

Each single dose, properly diluted, over 30 to 60 minutes, up to 2 hours in pediatric patients. Studies suggest bolus dosing (versus infusion over 30 minutes) may produce an earlier bactericidal effect, which is sustained. No dose, dilution, or rate recommendations are available at this time.

ACTIONS

Aminoglycoside antibiotic with neuromuscular blocking action. Bactericidal against specific gram-negative bacilli, including *Escherichia coli, Klebsiella, Proteus,* and *Pseudomonas.* Not effective for fungi or viral infections. Well distributed throughout all body fluids; serum and urine levels remain adequate for 6 to 12 hours. Usual half-life is 2 hours. Half-life prolonged in infants, postpartum females, fever, liver disease and ascites, spinal cord injury, cystic fibrosis, and the elderly; shorter in severe burns. Crosses placental barrier. Excreted through kidneys.

INDICATIONS AND USES

Treatment of serious infections of the GI (peritonitis), respiratory, and urinary tracts; CNS (meningitis); skin; bone; soft tissue (burns); septicemia; and bacterial neonatal sepsis. ▪ Primarily used when penicillin and other less toxic antibiotics are ineffective or contraindicated. ▪ Prevention of bacterial endocarditis in dental, respiratory tract, GI, or GU surgery or instrumentation. ▪ Used concurrently with clindamycin to treat pelvic inflammatory disease. ▪ Considered initial therapy after culture and sensitivity is drawn in suspected or confirmed gram-negative infections or other serious infections. ▪ Treat suspected infection in the immunosuppressed patient. ▪ May be used synergistically in gram-positive infections. ▪ Used concurrently with penicillin for endocarditis and neonatal sepsis.

CONTRAINDICATIONS

Known gentamicin or aminoglycoside sensitivity, renal failure. Sulfite sensitivity may be a contraindication.

PRECAUTIONS

Sensitivity studies indicated to determine susceptibility of the causative organism to gentamicin. ▪ Use extreme caution if therapy is required over 7 to 10 days. ▪ Superinfection may occur from overgrowth of nonsusceptible organisms. ▪ Use caution in infants, children, and the elderly. ▪ Advanced age and dehydration may increase risk of toxicity. ▪ May contain sulfites; use caution in patients with asthma. ▪ Aminoglycosides are nephrotoxic; risk for nephrotoxicity is increased in patients with impaired renal function and in patients who receive high doses or prolonged therapy. ▪ Use extreme caution in patients with end-stage renal disease. ▪ Single daily dosing has been used effectively in abdominal, pelvic inflammatory, and GU infections in patients with normal renal function. Not recommended in bacteremia caused by *Pseudomonas aeruginosa,* endocarditis, meningitis, during pregnancy, or in patients less than 6 weeks postpartum. Limited data available for use in all other situations (e.g., burns, cystic fibrosis, elderly, pediatrics, renal impairment). ▪ Potentially nephrotoxic, ototoxic, and neurotoxic. Risk of neurotoxicity (e.g., auditory and vestibular ototoxicity) is increased in patients with pre-existing renal damage or in normal renal function with prolonged use. Partial or total irreversible deafness may continue to develop after gentamicin is discontinued. ▪ *Clostridium difficile*–associated diarrhea (CDAD) has been reported. May range from mild diarrhea to fatal colitis. Consider in patients who present with diarrhea during or after treatment with gentamicin.

Monitor: Narrow range between toxic and therapeutic levels. Periodically monitor peak and trough concentrations. Therapeutic level is between 4 and 8 mcg/mL. Avoid trough levels above 2 mcg/mL and prolonged peak levels above 12 mcg/mL; adjust dose as indicated. Risk of renal and eighth cranial nerve toxicity increased. Monitor frequently in patients with impaired renal function. ▪ Watch for decrease in urine output and rising BUN and SCr. May require decreased dose. ▪ Routine gentamicin serum levels and evaluation of hearing are recommended. ▪ Closely monitor renal and eighth cranial nerve function, especially in patients with known or suspected reduced renal function at onset of therapy and in patients who develop signs of renal dysfunction during therapy. Monitor urine for decreased specific gravity, increased protein, and the presence of cells or casts. Serial audiograms are recommended, particularly in high-risk patients. ▪ Maintain good hydration. ▪ Monitor serum calcium, magnesium, sodium, and potassium; levels may decline. Depressed levels have caused mental confusion, paresthesia, positive Chvostek and Trousseau signs (provoked spasm of facial muscles and other muscles; occurs in tetany), and tetany in adults; muscle weakness and tetany in infants. ▪ Closely monitor patients with impaired renal function for nephrotoxicity and neurotoxicity (e.g., auditory and vestibular ototoxicity, convulsions, muscle twitching, numbness, tingling); nephrotoxicity may be reversible. ▪ In extended treatment, daily monitoring of serum levels, electrolytes, and renal, auditory, and vestibular functions is recommended. ▪ See Drug/Lab Interactions.

Patient Education: Report promptly: dizziness, hearing loss, weakness, or any changes in balance. ▪ Promptly report diarrhea or bloody stools that occur during treatment or up to several months after an antibiotic has been discontinued; may indicate CDAD and require treatment. ▪ Consider birth control options.

Maternal/Child: Category D: avoid pregnancy. Potential hazard to fetus. ▪ Safety for use during breast-feeding not established; use extreme caution. ▪ Peak concentrations are generally lower in infants and young children.

Elderly: Consider less toxic alternatives. Half-life prolonged. Longer intervals between doses may be more important than reduced doses. ▪ Advanced age and dehydration may increase risk for toxicity. ▪ Monitor renal function and drug levels carefully. Measurement of CrCl more useful than BUN or SCr to assess renal function. ▪ See Precautions.

DRUG/LAB INTERACTIONS

Inactivated in solution with **penicillins** but is synergistic when used in combination with **beta-lactam antibiotics** (e.g., sulbactam sodium, clavulanate potassium, cephalosporins, penicillins) and **vancomycin.** Do not mix in the same solution. Dose adjustment and appropriate spacing required because of physical **incompatibilities** and interactions. Synergism may be inconsistent; measure aminoglycoside levels. ▪ Concurrent and/or sequential use topically or systemically with any other **neurotoxic or nephrotoxic agent** should be avoided (e.g.,

G-H

amikacin, cephaloridine, cisplatin, colistin [Coly-Mycin S], kanamycin, neomycin, polymyxin B, paromomycin [Humatin], streptomycin, tobramycin, vancomycin). ▪ May have dangerous additive effects with **anesthetics** (e.g., enflurane), **other neuromuscular blocking antibiotics** (e.g., kanamycin, streptomycin), **beta-lactam antibiotics** (e.g., cephalosporins), **diuretics** (e.g., furosemide [Lasix]), **vancomycin,** and many others. ▪ **Neuromuscular blocking muscle relaxants** (e.g., atracurium [Tracrium], succinylcholine) are potentiated by aminoglycosides. *Apnea can occur.* ▪ Aminoglycosides are also potentiated by **anticholinesterases** (e.g., edrophonium), **antineoplastics** (e.g., nitrogen mustard, cisplatin). ▪ May be antagonized by **bacteriostatic antibiotics** (e.g., chloramphenicol, erythromycin, tetracyclines); bactericidal action may be impacted.

SIDE EFFECTS

Occur more frequently with impaired renal function, higher doses, or prolonged administration, in dehydrated or elderly patients, and in patients receiving other ototoxic or nephrotoxic drugs.

Anorexia, burning, dizziness, fever, headache, hypertension, hypotension, itching, lethargy, muscle twitching, nausea, numbness, rash, roaring in ears, seizures, tingling sensation, tinnitus, urticaria, vomiting, weight loss.

Major: Acute organic brain syndrome; blood dyscrasias; CDAD; convulsions; elevated bilirubin, BUN, SCr, AST, and ALT; hearing loss; laryngeal edema; neuromuscular blockade; oliguria; respiratory depression or arrest.

ANTIDOTE

Notify the physician of all side effects. If minor side effects persist or any major symptom appears, notify the physician; may require dose adjustment or discontinuation of gentamicin. Treatment is symptomatic. In overdose or toxic reactions, hemodialysis may be indicated. Rate of gentamicin removal is lower with peritoneal dialysis. Monitor fluid balance, CrCl, and plasma levels carefully. Complexation with ticarcillin may be as effective as hemodialysis. Consider exchange transfusion in the newborn. Calcium salts or neostigmine may reverse neuromuscular blockade. Treat CDAD with fluids, electrolytes, protein supplements, and oral vancomycin (Vancocin) or metronidazole (Flagyl) as indicated. In severe cases, surgical evaluation may be indicated. Resuscitate as necessary.

GLUCAGON (rDNA ORIGIN)
(**GLOO**-kah-gon)

Antihypoglycemic
Diagnostic agent
Antidote

GlucaGen, Glucagon for Injection   pH 2.5 to 3.5

USUAL DOSE
Hypoglycemia in adults and pediatric patients weighing more than 20 kg (Glucagon [44 lb]) to 25 kg (GlucaGen [55 lb]): 1 mg. May be given IV, IM, or SC. May be repeated if needed. For severe hypoglycemia or when patient fails to respond to glucagon, IV dextrose should be administered. After patient responds to treatment, give fast-acting and long-acting oral carbohydrates to restore liver glycogen and prevent the recurrence of hypoglycemia.

Diagnostic aid: stomach, duodenal bulb, duodenum, and small bowel: 0.2 to 0.5 mg IV or 1 mg IM before procedure begins. When diagnostic procedure is over, administer oral carbohydrates to patients who have been fasting if this is compatible with the diagnostic procedure.

Diagnostic aid: colon: 0.5 to 0.75 mg IV or 1 to 2 mg IM before procedure begins. When diagnostic procedure is over, administer oral carbohydrates to patients who have been fasting if this is compatible with the diagnostic procedure.

Management of cardiac effects of beta-blocker or calcium channel blocker overdose (unlabeled): 3 to 10 mg (0.05 to 0.15 mg/kg) over 3 to 5 minutes. May be followed by an infusion of 3 to 5 mg/hr (0.05 to 0.1 mg/kg/hr). Titrate to patient response.

PEDIATRIC DOSE
Hypoglycemia in infants and children weighing less than 20 kg (Glucagon [44 lb]) to 25 kg (GlucaGen [55 lb]): 20 to 30 mcg/kg or 0.5 mg. See comments under Usual Dose. If the weight is unknown, use 0.5 mg for pediatric patients younger than 6 years of age and 1 mg for those 6 years of age and older.

DOSE ADJUSTMENTS
For uses other than hypoglycemia, lower-end doses may be indicated in the elderly; consider impaired organ function and concurrent disease or other drug therapy.

DILUTION
Dilute 1 unit (1 mg) with 1 mL SWFI (may be supplied) to achieve a final concentration of approximately 1 mg/mL. Shake vial gently until completely dissolved. Concentrations greater than 1 mg/mL are not recommended. Do not add to IV solutions. May be given through Y-tube or three-way stopcock of infusion set if a dextrose solution is infusing.

Reverse effects of beta blockade: Reconstitute each 1 unit (1 mg) with 1 mL SWFI. For *continuous infusion* this reconstituted solution may be further diluted in D5W to deliver 1 to 5 mg/hr.

Storage: Use immediately after reconstitution. Discard any unused portion. Before reconstitution, may be stored at RT for up to 24 months in original package to protect from light. Do not freeze. If solution shows any sign of gel formation or particles after reconstitution, it should be discarded.

COMPATIBILITY
May form a precipitate with saline solutions and solutions with a pH of 3 to 9.5. Consider specific use; consult pharmacist.

RATE OF ADMINISTRATION
Too-rapid rate of injection or doses over 1 mg may increase incidence of side effects (e.g., nausea and vomiting).

1 unit (1 mg) or fraction thereof over 1 minute.

G-H

ACTIONS

An antihypoglycemic agent and a gastrointestinal motility inhibitor. A polypeptide hormone identical to naturally occurring human glucagon produced by recombinant DNA technology. Induces liver glycogen breakdown, releasing glucose from the liver. Glucagon acts only on liver glycogen; hepatic stores of glycogen are necessary for glucagon to produce an antihypoglycemic effect. Blood glucose is raised within 10 minutes. Maximum glucose concentrations are seen about 30 minutes after administration. Duration of antihypoglycemic effect is 60 to 90 minutes. Extrahepatic effect produces relaxation of the smooth muscle of the stomach, duodenum, small bowel, and colon, inhibiting GI motility. Onset of smooth muscle relaxation is less than 1 minute. Duration of smooth muscle relaxation is dose-dependent and ranges from 9 to 25 minutes. Has a half-life of 8 to 18 minutes. Degraded in the liver, kidney, and plasma. Does not cross the placental barrier.

INDICATIONS AND USES

Treatment of severe hypoglycemia (e.g., during insulin therapy in the management of diabetes mellitus). ▪ As a diagnostic aid in the radiologic examination of the stomach, duodenum, small bowel, and colon when diminished intestinal motility would be advantageous.

Unlabeled uses: May be helpful in reversing adverse beta-blockade of beta-adrenergic blocking agents (e.g., propranolol) in overdose situations. ▪ If conventional therapy is ineffective, may be helpful in reversing myocardial depression of calcium channel blockers (e.g., diltiazem [Cardizem]).

CONTRAINDICATIONS

Glucagon for injection: Known hypersensitivity to glucagon or its components, patients with known pheochromocytoma, insulinoma, or glucagonoma. **GlucaGen:** Known hypersensitivity to GlucaGen, lactose, or any of its components; patients with pheochromocytoma or insulinoma.

PRECAUTIONS

Easily absorbed IM or SC. ▪ If glucagon and glucose do not awaken patient, coma is probably caused by a condition other than hypoglycemia. ▪ Use caution in patients with a history suggestive of glucagonoma; secondary hypoglycemia may occur. Treat with adequate carbohydrate intake; see Contraindications and Monitor. ▪ May cause the release of catecholamines in patients with pheochromocytoma. Use is contraindicated; see Antidote. ▪ Should not be administered to patients suspected of having insulinoma; see Contraindications. Administration may produce an initial increase in blood glucose; however, it may directly or indirectly stimulate exaggerated insulin release from the insulinoma, producing hypoglycemia. Administer IV or oral glucose to a patient who develops symptoms of hypoglycemia. ▪ Treatment with glucagon in patients with diabetes mellitus may cause hyperglycemia. ▪ Evaluation by a physician is recommended for all patients who experience severe hypoglycemia. ▪ Use caution in patients with conditions that result in low levels of releasable glucose (e.g., adrenal insufficiency, chronic hypoglycemia, prolonged fasting, starvation). Insufficient glucose stores will result in inadequate reversal of hypoglycemia. Treatment with dextrose is recommended. ▪ Use caution; hypersensitivity reactions have occurred, usually in association with endoscopic examination during which other agents are administered (e.g., contrast media, local anesthetics). ▪ When used to inhibit gastrointestinal motility, use caution in patients with known cardiac disease. Glucagon exerts positive inotropic and chronotropic effects and may cause tachycardia and hypertension. ▪ Hypotension has been reported for up to 2 hours after use as premedication for upper GI endoscopy procedures. ▪ Not all products are packaged with the syringe and diluent necessary for rapid preparation and administration during an emergency outside of a health care facility. Ensure that correct product is prescribed and dispensed for outpatient use. ▪ See Drug/Lab Interactions.

Monitor: Prolonged hypoglycemia may result in damage to the central nervous system. Monitor blood glucose levels and mentation. Repeat dose and supplement with IV dextrose (50%) if needed. ▪ Monitor BP and HR. In patients with cardiac disease, cardiac monitoring may be indicated. ■ Test patients suspected of having glucagonoma for glucagon levels before treatment, and monitor for changes in blood glucose levels during treatment. ■ Emesis on awakening is common. Prevent aspiration by turning patient face down. ■ Depletes glycogen stores, especially in children and adolescents; supplement with fast-acting and long-acting oral carbohydrates on awakening to replenish liver glycogen and to prevent recurrence of hypoglycemia. ■ Monitor for S/S of hypersensitivity (e.g., dizziness, dyspnea, fever, flushing, hypotension, nausea, pruritus, rash, rigors, urticaria). ■ In patients with diabetes mellitus, monitor for hyperglycemia. Administration of insulin may be indicated.

Patient Education: Eat some form of sugar if hypoglycemia recurs. ■ Report episodes of hypoglycemia and glucagon use at home. Dose adjustment of diabetes medications may be indicated. ■ Hypoglycemia may impair ability to concentrate or react. Do not drive or operate machinery until oral carbohydrates have been consumed and hypoglycemic episode has resolved. ■ Teach patient and family proper storage and preparation of glucagon from kits. Include signs of hypoglycemia and procedures to be followed after administration to an unconscious patient.

Maternal/Child: Category B: use during pregnancy only if clearly needed. Use caution during breast-feeding. Not absorbed through the GI tract; it would be unlikely to have any effect on the infant. ■ Does not cross the placental barrier. ■ Safety and effectiveness for treatment of hypoglycemia in pediatric patients have been demonstrated; however, safety and effectiveness for use in pediatric patients as a diagnostic aid have not been established.

Elderly: Cautious dosing may be indicated in the elderly; see Dose Adjustments. ■ Differences in response compared to younger adults not identified. ■ If used to inhibit gastrointestinal motility, use caution in elderly patients with known cardiac disease.

DRUG/LAB INTERACTIONS

Beta-blockers (e.g., metoprolol [Lopressor], sotalol) may cause a temporary increase in BP and pulse; treatment may be required in patients with cardiac disease or pheochromocytoma. ■ Concurrent use with **indomethacin** (Indocin) may cause glucagon to lose its ability to raise blood glucose and may even produce hypoglycemia. ■ Coadministration with **anticholinergic** agents (e.g., atropine) is not recommended due to increased GI side effects. ■ May increase the anticoagulant effects of **warfarin** (Coumadin). ■ **Insulin** reacts antagonistically toward glucagon; use caution when glucagon is used as a diagnostic aid in patients with diabetes.

SIDE EFFECTS

Rare in recommended doses: hyperglycemia (in diabetic patients), hypersensitivity reactions (e.g., anaphylaxis, dyspnea, hypotension, rash), hypoglycemia, hypoglycemic coma, hypotension, increased BP, increased HR, nausea, vomiting. Increases in BP and HR may be greater in patients taking beta-blockers.

Overdose: Nausea and vomiting, increase in BP and HR, inhibition of GI tract motility, hypokalemia.

ANTIDOTE

Nausea and vomiting are tolerable and do occur in hypoglycemia. Antiemetics are indicated when larger doses are given. Increased BP and HR may require treatment in patients with coronary heart disease or pheochromocytoma. Treat sudden increases in BP with phentolamine 5 to 10 mg IV. In overdose situations, glucagon may decrease serum potassium levels; supplemental potassium may be indicated. For any other side effects, discontinue the drug and notify the physician. Treat hypersensitivity reactions and resuscitate as necessary. Insulin administration may be indicated in acute overdose. Effects of dialysis unknown; unlikely to provide benefit because of the short half-life of glucagon and the nature of the symptoms of overdose.

GLUCARPIDASE

(gloo-**KAR**-pi-dase)

Voraxaze

USUAL DOSE

50 units/kg as a single intravenous injection over 5 minutes.

PEDIATRIC DOSE

See Usual Dose.

DOSE ADJUSTMENTS

No dose adjustment is recommended in patients with renal impairment. ▪ Has not been studied in patients with hepatic impairment.

DILUTION

Available in a vial containing 1,000 units of lyophilized powder. Reconstitute with 1 mL of NS to provide a solution containing 1,000 units/vial. Roll and tilt vial gently to mix. *Do not shake.* Solution should be clear and colorless. Withdraw calculated dose from vial for administration as a bolus injection.

Storage: Refrigerate unopened vials at 2° to 8° C (36° to 46° F). Do not freeze. Do not use beyond expiration date on vial. Use reconstituted solution immediately or store under refrigeration for up to 4 hours. Discard any unused product.

COMPATIBILITY

Specific information not available. Consider specific use and potential for hypersensitivity reactions.

RATE OF ADMINISTRATION

Administer as an injection evenly distributed over 5 minutes. Flush IV line before and after administration.

ACTIONS

A carboxypeptidase enzyme produced by recombinant DNA technology. Hydrolyzes the carboxyl-terminal glutamate residue from folic acid and classic antifolates such as methotrexate. Converts methotrexate to its inactive metabolite, 4-deoxy-4-amino-N10-methylpteroic acid (DAMPA) and glutamate. Glucarpidase provides an alternate nonrenal pathway for methotrexate elimination in patients with renal dysfunction during high-dose methotrexate treatment. The desired end point of therapy is a rapid and sustained clinically important reduction (RSCIR) in methotrexate concentration, which is defined as attaining a plasma methotrexate concentration less than or equal to 1 μmol/L at 15 minutes and sustaining it for up to 8 days after administration of glucarpidase. The likelihood of attaining a RSCIR correlates with the pre-glucarpidase methotrexate concentration. However, even patients with methotrexate concentrations greater than 50 μmol/L were able to achieve greater than 95% reduction in methotrexate concentrations for up to 8 days following glucarpidase administration. Glucarpidase distribution is restricted to the plasma volume. Mean elimination half-life is 5.6 hours.

INDICATIONS AND USES

Treatment of toxic plasma methotrexate concentrations (greater than 1 μmol/L) in patients with delayed methotrexate clearance due to impaired renal function. **Limitation of use:** Not indicated for use in patients who exhibit the expected clearance of methotrexate (plasma methotrexate concentrations within 2 standard deviations of the mean methotrexate excretion curve specific for the dose of methotrexate administered) or in patients with normal or mildly impaired renal function because of the potential risk of subtherapeutic exposure to methotrexate.

CONTRAINDICATIONS

Manufacturer states, "None."

PRECAUTIONS

Serious hypersensitivity reactions, including anaphylaxis, have been reported. ▪ Efficacy of a second dose of glucarpidase in patients with markedly elevated pre-glucarpidase methotrexate concentrations was not demonstrated in studies. ▪ Continue hydration, alkalinization of the urine, and leucovorin rescue as indicated; see Monitor and methotrexate and leucovorin monographs. ▪ A protein substance, it has the potential to produce immunogenicity. Anti-glucarpidase antibodies have been detected in a small number of patients treated with glucarpidase.

Monitor: Obtain baseline and periodic renal function tests (e.g., SCr and BUN). ▪ Watch for early S/S of hypersensitivity or infusion reactions (e.g., chills, dyspnea, fever, flushing, headache, hives, itching, numbness, rash, throat tightness). ▪ Monitor methotrexate concentrations. During the first 48 hours after glucarpidase administration, methotrexate concentrations can be reliably measured only by a chromatographic method. During this period, DAMPA (the inactive metabolite of methotrexate) interferes with the measurement of methotrexate concentration using immunoassays. ▪ Continue to administer leucovorin after glucarpidase. Do not administer leucovorin within 2 hours before or after a dose of glucarpidase; see Drug/Lab Interactions. ▪ For 48 hours after glucarpidase administration, determine the leucovorin dose based on the patient's pre-glucarpidase methotrexate concentration. Beyond 48 hours, administer leucovorin based on the measured methotrexate concentration. Continue therapy with leucovorin until the methotrexate concentration has been maintained below the leucovorin treatment threshold for a minimum of 3 days; see leucovorin monograph. Monitor for S/S of potential methotrexate toxicity (e.g., abdominal distress, chills, dizziness, fever, leukopenia, malaise, nausea, stomatitis, undue fatigue).

Patient Education: Promptly report any S/S of a hypersensitivity reaction or an infusion reaction (e.g., chills, feeling hot, fever, flushing, headache, hives, itching, numbness, rash, throat tightness or breathing problems, tingling). ▪ Continued monitoring of methotrexate levels and renal status is imperative.

Maternal/Child: Category C: no human or animal data. Safety for use during pregnancy and breast-feeding not established. Use only if clearly needed. ▪ Effectiveness in pediatric patients has been established in clinical studies. No overall differences in safety were observed between pediatric patients (age 1 month to 17 years of age) and adult patients.

Elderly: No overall differences in safety or effectiveness were observed between elderly patients and younger patients.

DRUG/LAB INTERACTIONS

Leucovorin is a substrate for glucarpidase. Do not administer leucovorin within 2 hours before or after a dose of glucarpidase. ▪ Other potential exogenous substrates of glucarpidase include **reduced folates and folate antimetabolites.**

SIDE EFFECTS

The most commonly reported side effects included flushing, headache, hypotension, nausea, paraesthesia, and vomiting. Other reported adverse reactions included blurred vision, diarrhea, hypersensitivity reactions (including anaphylaxis), hypertension, rash, throat irritation or tightness, and tremor.

ANTIDOTE

Notify the physician of any side effects. Discontinue the drug if indicated. Treat hypersensitivity reactions as indicated (airway, oxygen, IV fluids, antihistamines [e.g., diphenhydramine (Benadryl)], corticosteroids [e.g., hydrocortisone sodium succinate (Solu-Cortef)], epinephrine, pressor amines [e.g., dopamine]) and resuscitate as necessary.

G-H

GLYCOPYRROLATE

(**GLYE**-koh-**pye**-roh-layt)

Robinul

Anticholinergic
Antidote

pH 2 to 3

USUAL DOSE

Dose equivalents in mL are based on the 0.2 mg/mL concentration. Check vial for correct concentration.

Preanesthetic medication: 0.004 mg/kg (0.02 mL/kg) of body weight IM 30 to 60 minutes before anesthesia induction. Usually given at the same time as the preanesthetic narcotic and/or sedative.

Intraoperative medication: 0.1 mg (0.5 mL) IV. Repeat as needed at 2- to 3-minute intervals to counteract drug-induced or vagal traction reflexes and associated arrhythmias (e.g., bradycardia). Attempt to determine the etiology of arrhythmia and the procedures required to correct parasympathetic imbalance.

Reversal of neuromuscular blockade: 0.2 mg (1 mL) IV for each 1 mg of neostigmine or 5 mg of pyridostigmine (Regonol); to minimize the bradycardia and excessive secretions caused by these agents used to reverse the neuromuscular blockade of nondepolarizing muscle relaxants. May be administered simultaneously and may be mixed in the same syringe.

Peptic ulcer: 0.1 mg (0.5 mL) at 4-hour intervals 3 to 4 times/day. May be given IV or IM. Adjust frequency of administration based on patient response. Some may require only a single dose. If a more profound effect is required, dose may be increased to 0.2 mg (1 mL).

Respiratory antisecretory: 0.1 to 0.2 mg/dose (0.5 to 1 mL/dose) every 4 to 8 hours. Maximum dose suggested is 0.2 mg/dose or 0.8 mg/24 hr.

PEDIATRIC DOSE

See Maternal/Child.

Preanesthetic medication: Same as Usual Dose. *Infants 1 month to 2 years of age:* May require up to 0.009 mg/kg (0.045 mL/kg) of body weight.

Intraoperative medication: Rarely needed in pediatric patients because of the long duration of action from the preanesthetic dose. If required, administer 0.004 mg/kg (0.02 mL/kg) of body weight IV. Do not exceed 0.1 mg (0.5 mL) in a single dose. Repeat as needed at 2- to 3-minute intervals to counteract drug-induced or vagal traction reflexes and associated arrhythmias (e.g., bradycardia). Attempt to determine the etiology of arrhythmia and the procedures required to correct parasympathetic imbalance.

Reversal of neuromuscular blockade: Same as Usual Dose.

Peptic ulcer: Not recommended for treatment of peptic ulcer in pediatric patients; see Maternal/Child.

Respiratory antisecretory: 0.004 to 0.01 mg/kg/dose (0.02 to 0.05 mL/kg/dose) every 4 to 8 hours. Maximum dose suggested is 0.2 mg/dose or 0.8 mg/24 hr.

DOSE ADJUSTMENTS

Caution and lower-end dosing suggested for elderly patients based on potential for decreased organ function and concomitant disease or drug therapy. ▪ Elimination prolonged in patients with renal failure. Dose adjustment not provided; see Precautions. ▪ See Drug/Lab Interactions.

DILUTION

May be given undiluted. Administer through Y-tube or three-way stopcock of infusion tubing containing D5 or D10 in water or saline, D5/½NS, NS, or Ringer's. May be further diluted with D5 or D10 in water or saline.

Filters: No data available from manufacturer.

Storage: Store at CRT.

COMPATIBILITY

Consider any drug NOT listed as compatible to be INCOMPATIBLE until consulting a pharmacist; specific conditions may apply.

Manufacturer lists as **incompatible** with lactated Ringer's and states, "Stability is questionable above a pH of 6. May form a precipitate or a gas with chloramphenicol (Chloromycetin), diazepam (Valium), dimenhydrinate, methohexitol (Brevital), pentazocine (Talwin), pentobarbital (Nembutal), sodium bicarbonate; do not combine in the same syringe." Dexamethasone (Decadron) will result in a pH above 6.

One source suggests the following **compatibilities:**

Y-site: Dexmedetomidine (Precedex), palonosetron (Aloxi), propofol (Diprivan).

RATE OF ADMINISTRATION

0.2 mg or fraction thereof over 1 to 2 minutes.

ACTIONS

A synthetic anticholinergic agent. It inhibits the action of acetylcholine. It reduces the volume and free acidity of gastric secretions and controls excessive pharyngeal, tracheal, and bronchial secretions. Antagonizes muscarinic symptoms (e.g., bronchorrhea, bronchospasm, bradycardia, and intestinal hypermotility) induced by cholinergic drugs. Onset of action is within 1 minute. Vagal blocking effects last 2 to 3 hours, and antisialagogic (inhibited saliva flow) effects last up to 7 hours. Metabolism has not been studied. Half-life is 0.7 to 0.96 hours. Excreted primarily in urine and to a small extent in bile. Does not effectively cross the blood-brain barrier. Crosses the placental barrier in very small amounts.

INDICATIONS AND USES

Adjunctive therapy in peptic ulcer. ▪ Protection against the peripheral muscarinic effects (e.g., bradycardia and excessive secretions) of cholinergic agents such as neostigmine and pyridostigmine (Regonol) given to reverse the neuromuscular blockade due to nondepolarizing muscle relaxants (e.g., atracurium [Tracrium]). ▪ Reduction of salivary, tracheobronchial, and pharyngeal secretions preoperatively. ▪ Reduction of volume and free acidity of gastric secretions. ▪ Other intraoperative uses controlled by the anesthesiologist (counteract drug-induced or vagal traction reflexes and associated arrhythmias, prevent aspiration pneumonitis).

CONTRAINDICATIONS

Known hypersensitivity to glycopyrrolate. May be contraindicated in patients with glaucoma, obstructive uropathy, obstructive disease of the GI tract, paralytic ileus, intestinal atony of the elderly or debilitated, unstable cardiovascular status in acute hemorrhage, severe ulcerative colitis, toxic megacolon, and myasthenia gravis when used for treatment of peptic ulcer disease because of long duration of therapy. ▪ Do not use in neonates.

PRECAUTIONS

Use IV only when immediate drug effect is essential. ▪ Use extreme caution in autonomic neuropathy, asthma, glaucoma, pregnancy, breast-feeding, cardiac arrhythmias, congestive heart failure, coronary artery disease, hepatic or renal disease, hiatal hernia, hypertension, hyperthyroidism, incomplete intestinal obstruction (diarrhea may be an early symptom), ulcerative colitis, and prostatic hypertrophy. Anticholinergic drugs may aggravate these conditions. ▪ Obtain cardiac history before administration of glycopyrrolate; may exacerbate pre-existing tachycardia. ▪ Heat prostration can occur with the use of anticholinergic agents in the presence of fever or high environmental temperatures. Pediatric patients and the elderly are at increased risk.

Monitor: Urinary retention can be avoided if the patient voids just before each dose. ▪ See Drug/Lab Interactions.

Patient Education: Use caution if a task requires alertness; may cause blurred vision, dizziness, or drowsiness. ▪ Report constipation, difficulty urinating, dry mouth, flushing, increased light sensitivity, or skin rash promptly. ▪ Use caution during exercise or hot weather. Increased heat sensitivity may result in heatstroke.

G-H

Maternal/Child: Category B: safety for use in pregnancy not established. ▪ It is not known whether this drug is secreted in breast milk; may suppress lactation; use caution. ▪ Safety and effectiveness for use in pediatric patients under 16 years of age not established for management of peptic ulcer. ▪ Dysrhythmias have been observed in pediatric patients. ▪ Pediatric patients may have an increased response to anticholinergics and be at increased risk for side effects (e.g., paradoxical hyperexcitability). Infants and young children, patients with Down syndrome, and pediatric patients with spastic paralysis or brain damage are especially susceptible to this increased response. ▪ *Contains benzyl alcohol; do not use in neonates;* see Contraindications.

Elderly: Differences in response compared to younger adults not observed. ▪ Dosing should be cautious; see Dose Adjustments. ▪ May produce excitement, agitation, confusion, or drowsiness in the elderly. ▪ May precipitate undiagnosed glaucoma. ▪ Risk of urinary retention and constipation increased. ▪ May increase memory impairment.

DRUG/LAB INTERACTIONS

Potentiated by other drugs with **anticholinergic activity** (e.g., amantadine [Symmetrel], **antiparkinson drugs** [e.g., levodopa (Larodopa, Dopar)], **atropine, phenothiazines** [e.g., prochlorperazine (Compazine)], **tricyclic antidepressants** [e.g., amitriptyline (Elavil), imipramine (Tofranil)]). Reduced dose of either or both drugs may be indicated. ▪ Concomitant administration with **KCl** in a wax matrix may increase the risk and severity of KCl-induced GI lesions (due to slower GI transit time). ▪ May decrease antipsychotic effects of **phenothiazines.** Dose adjustment may be required. ▪ Risk of ventricular arrhythmias increased when given in presence of **cyclopropane.** Risk is less than with atropine and when given in doses of 0.1 mg or less. ▪ Potentiates **atenolol** (Tenormin) and **digoxin.**

SIDE EFFECTS

Anaphylaxis, anticholinergic psychosis, arrhythmias, blurred vision, cardiac arrest, confusion, constipation, decreased sweating, dizziness, drowsiness, dry mouth, headache, heat prostration, hypertension, hypotension, impotence, increased ocular tension, injection site reactions, insomnia, loss of taste, malignant hyperthermia, muscular weakness, nausea and vomiting, nervousness, palpitation, paralysis, photophobia, pruritus, respiratory arrest, seizures, suppression of lactation, tachycardia, urinary hesitancy and retention, urticaria, weakness.

Overdose: A curare-like action may occur (i.e., neuromuscular blockade leading to muscular weakness and possible paralysis).

ANTIDOTE

Notify physician of all side effects. May be treated symptomatically or drug may be discontinued. Treat hypotension with IV fluids and/or pressor agents (e.g., dopamine). Initiate artificial respiration if overdose with paralysis of respiratory muscles occurs. Neostigmine, in 0.25-mg increments, may be used to counteract peripheral anticholinergic effects. May repeat every 5 to 10 minutes to a maximum dose of 2.5 mg. Need for repetitive doses of neostigmine should be based on close monitoring of the decrease in HR and the return of bowel sounds. Physostigmine, in increments of 0.5 to 2 mg, may be used to counteract CNS effects. May repeat as needed to a maximum dose of 5 mg. Proportionately smaller doses should be used in pediatric patients. Resuscitate as necessary.

GOLIMUMAB BBW
(goe-**LIM**-ue-mab)

Monoclonal antibody
Antirheumatic agent
TNF-blocker

Simponi Aria pH 5.5

USUAL DOSE
Preliminary patient evaluation required; see Monitor.

Begin with an initial dose of 2 mg/kg as an infusion over 30 minutes. Repeat at Week 4 and then every 8 weeks thereafter. Given in combination with methotrexate. See methotrexate monograph. Patients may continue taking other nonbiologic disease-modifying antirheumatic drugs (DMARDs), corticosteroids, NSAIDs, and/or analgesics.

The efficacy and safety of switching between IV and SC formulations and routes of administration of golimumab has not been established.

DILUTION
Available as a 50 mg/4 mL concentrated solution for infusion (12.5 mg/mL). Determine the number of vials required using the following calculations:

$$(\text{Weight in kg} \times \text{dose/kg}) \div 50 \text{ mg} = \# \text{ of vials required}$$

For a 60-kg patient: [(60 kg) × (2 mg/kg)] ÷ 50 mg/vial = 2.4 vials. After patient is weighed and appropriate dose is calculated, remove sufficient vials from the refrigerator. Aseptic technique imperative. Solution should be colorless to light yellow and may develop a few translucent particles because golimumab is a protein. Do not use if opaque particles, discoloration, or other foreign particles are present. Withdraw the calculated dose (9.6 mL in above example) from the required number of vials. This calculated dose must be further diluted in NS to a final total volume of 100 mL. Withdraw and discard a volume of NS equal to the calculated volume of golimumab from a 100-mL bottle or bag of NS and slowly add golimumab solution. Mix gently.

Filters: Must be administered through an infusion set with an in-line, sterile, nonpyrogenic, low–protein binding filter (pore size 0.22 micrometer or less).

Storage: Refrigerate at 2° C to 8° C (36° F to 46° F) in original carton to protect from light. Do not freeze or shake. The diluted product may be stored at RT for up to 4 hours, including infusion time. Do not use beyond expiration date. Discard any unused product remaining in vials.

COMPATIBILITY
Manufacturer recommends not infusing concomitantly in the same IV line with other agents. No **compatibility** studies have been conducted.

RATE OF ADMINISTRATION
Use of an infusion set with an in-line, sterile, nonpyrogenic, low–protein binding filter (pore size 0.22 micrometer or less) is required. Use of an infusion pump is helpful. Administer a single dose as an infusion over 30 minutes. Flush the IV line with NS at the end of the infusion to ensure the total dose is received.

ACTIONS
A human monoclonal antibody that binds to both the soluble and transmembrane bioactive forms of human tumor necrosis factor alpha (TNFα). This interaction prevents the binding of TNFα to its receptors, thereby inhibiting the biological activity of TNFα (a cytokine protein). There has been no evidence of the golimumab antibody binding to other TNF superfamily ligands. Elevated TNFα levels in the blood, synovium, and joints have been implicated in the pathophysiology of rheumatoid arthritis (RA). Golimumab is thought to be distributed primarily in the circulatory system with limited extravascular distribution. Elimination pathways have not been characterized. Mean terminal half-life

G-H

is estimated to be 9 to 15 days in healthy subjects and 10 to 18 days in patients with RA. Crosses the placental barrier.

INDICATIONS AND USES
Treatment of adult patients with moderate to severely active rheumatoid arthritis. Used in combination with methotrexate.

CONTRAINDICATIONS
Manufacturer states, "None."

PRECAUTIONS
TNFα mediates inflammation and modulates cellular immune response. Anti-TNF therapies, including golimumab, may affect normal immune responses. ▪ Administered under the direction of a physician knowledgeable in its use in a facility with adequate diagnostic and treatment facilities to monitor the patient and respond to any medical emergency. ▪ Patients treated with golimumab are at increased risk for developing serious infection that may lead to hospitalization or death. Most patients who developed these infections were taking concomitant immunosuppressant therapy (e.g., methotrexate, corticosteroids) that, in addition to their underlying disease, may predispose them to infection. Treatment with golimumab should not be initiated in patients with an active infection, including clinically important localized infections. ▪ Discontinue golimumab if a patient develops a serious infection. Reported infections with TNF-blockers include active tuberculosis, including reactivation of latent tuberculosis; invasive fungal infections (e.g., histoplasmosis, coccidioidomycosis, candidiasis, aspergillosis, blastomycosis, and pneumocytosis); and bacterial, viral, and other infections due to opportunistic pathogens, including *Legionella* and *Listeria*. ▪ Patients with TB have frequently presented with disseminated or extrapulmonary disease. ▪ Patients with histoplasmosis or other invasive fungal infections may present with disseminated, rather than localized, disease. Antigen and antibody testing for histoplasmosis may be negative. ▪ Consider the risks and benefits of golimumab treatment before initiating therapy in patients with chronic or recurrent infection, patients who have been exposed to TB, patients with a history of an opportunistic infection, patients who have resided or traveled in areas of endemic tuberculosis or endemic mycoses (e.g., histoplasmosis, coccidioidomycosis, or blastomycosis), or patients with underlying conditions that may predispose them to infection. ▪ Has been associated with the reactivation of hepatitis B virus (HBV) in patients who are chronic hepatitis B carriers (i.e., surface antigen–positive). Fatalities have been reported. ▪ Lymphoma and other malignancies, some fatal, have been reported in pediatric and adolescent patients treated with TNF-blockers; most of these patients were receiving concomitant immunosuppressants. ▪ Rare post-marketing cases of hepatosplenic T-cell lymphoma (HSTCL) have been reported in patients treated with TNF-blocking agents. This rare type of T-cell lymphoma has a very aggressive disease course and is usually fatal. Nearly all cases have occurred in adolescents and young adult males with Crohn's disease or ulcerative colitis who have been treated with azathioprine or 6-mercaptopurine concomitantly with a TNF-blocker at or before diagnosis. ▪ Consider risk versus benefit in adult patients with a known malignancy other than a successfully treated nonmelanoma skin cancer (NMSC) or when considering continuing a TNF-blocker in patients who develop a malignancy. ▪ In controlled trials, more cases of lymphoma were seen in patients receiving anti-TNF treatment compared with the control group. Patients with RA and other chronic inflammatory diseases, particularly patients with highly active disease and/or chronic exposure to immunosuppressant therapies, may be at higher risk than the general population for developing lymphoma and other malignancies. Melanoma and Merkel cell carcinoma have also been reported in patients treated with TNF-blocking agents. ▪ Concurrent use with abatacept (Orencia) or anakinra (Kineret) is not recommended; see Drug/Lab Interactions. ▪ Cases of worsening CHF and new-onset CHF have been reported with TNF-blockers, including golimumab. Some incidents have resulted in hospitalization and increased mortality. Use with caution in patients with a history of CHF. ▪ TNF-blockers have been associated with rare cases of new onset or exacerbation of CNS demyelinating disorders, including multiple sclerosis and peripheral demyelinating disorders such as Guillain-Barré syndrome. Use with caution if indicated in these patients. ▪ Treatment with TNF-blockers, including golimumab, may re-

sult in the formation of antinuclear antibodies. Rarely, treatment with TNF-blockers may result in a lupus-like syndrome. If symptoms suggestive of a lupus-like syndrome develop, discontinue golimumab. ▪ Use caution if switching from one biologic product to another (e.g., abatacept [Orencia], adalimumab [Humira], infliximab [Remicade], golimumab [Simponi], rituximab [Rituxan]); overlapping biological activity may further increase the risk of infection. ▪ Use caution in patients who have or have had significant cytopenias; aplastic anemia, leukopenia, neutropenia, thrombocytopenia, and pancytopenia have been reported. ▪ May receive vaccinations, except for live virus vaccines; see Drug/Lab Interactions. ▪ Hypersensitivity reactions have been reported. ▪ Has not been studied in patients with impaired hepatic or renal function.

Monitor: Before initiating TNF-blocker therapy, including golimumab therapy, patients should be tested for HBV infection. If the test is positive, consultation with a physician with expertise in the treatment of hepatitis B is recommended before beginning treatment. Consider risk versus benefit in patients who are carriers of HBV. ▪ In patients who are carriers of HBV and require treatment with TNF-blockers, closely monitor for clinical and laboratory signs of active HBV throughout treatment and for several months after completion of treatment. If HBV reactivation occurs, discontinue golimumab; see Antidote. ▪ Evaluate patients for active and latent TB before and throughout therapy. Initiate treatment for latent TB before therapy with golimumab. ▪ Anti-tuberculosis treatment of patients with a reactive TB skin test may reduce the risk of TB reactivation in patients receiving golimumab. Consider antituberculosis therapy for patients with a history of latent or active TB (if an adequate course of treatment cannot be confirmed) and for patients with a negative TB test who have risk factors for TB infection. Consultation with a physician with expertise in the treatment of TB is recommended. ▪ Consider a diagnosis of TB in patients who develop a new infection during treatment. ▪ Monitor for S/S of infection during and after treatment with golimumab, including the possible development of TB in patients who tested negative for latent TB before initiating therapy. Discontinue if a serious infection, an opportunistic infection, or sepsis occurs; see Precautions and Antidote. ▪ A prompt and complete diagnostic workup appropriate for an immunocompromised patient is indicated for patients who develop a new infection during treatment. Monitor closely and initiate appropriate antimicrobial therapy. Consider empiric antifungal therapy in patients at risk for invasive fungal infections who develop severe systemic illness. ▪ Monitor patients for S/S of malignancy. Periodic skin examination is recommended for all patients, particularly those with risk factors for skin cancer. ▪ Closely monitor patients with S/S of CHF. ▪ Monitor for S/S of a hypersensitivity reaction (e.g., anaphylaxis, dyspnea, hives, nausea, and pruritus). Most hypersensitivity reactions occurred during or within 1 hour of the infusion. Some reactions occurred after the first administration of golimumab.

Patient Education: Read the manufacturer's medication guide before each treatment with golimumab. ▪ Tell health care professionals about heart conditions, previous or current infections, and recent or past exposure to TB or histoplasmosis. ▪ Review all medicines and disease history with pharmacist or physician before initiating treatment. ▪ Promptly report S/S of infection (e.g., burning on urination; chills; cough; diarrhea; fever; stomach pain; warm, red, or painful skin; or sores on body). ▪ Promptly report new or worsening conditions such as heart failure (e.g., shortness of breath, swelling feet), demyelinating disorders, autoimmune diseases, liver disease, cytopenias, or psoriasis. ▪ Report S/S of hypersensitivity reactions (e.g., itching, rash, swelling in the throat). ▪ Report changes of growths on your skin during or after golimumab treatment. ▪ Promptly report possible symptoms of lupus (e.g., excessive tiredness, new joint or muscle pain, rash on cheeks, sun sensitivity). ▪ Report recently receiving or being scheduled to receive a live virus vaccine or treatment with weakened bacteria (such as BCG for bladder cancer) to your physician. ▪ Consider potential benefit and risks of golimumab. ▪ See Appendix D, p. 1333.

Maternal/Child: Category B: use during pregnancy only if clearly needed. ▪ Discontinue breast-feeding. ▪ Safety and effectiveness for use in pediatric patients less than 18 years of age not established. ▪ Infants exposed to golimumab in utero and infants born to mothers treated with golimumab during pregnancy may be at increased risk for infection for up to 6 months, and administration of live virus vaccines is not recommended for 6 months after the last dose of golimumab to the mother.

Elderly: Numbers in clinical studies insufficient to determine if the elderly respond differently than younger subjects. ▪ Patients over 65 years of age and those with comorbid conditions may also be at increased risk for infections.

DRUG/LAB INTERACTIONS

Golimumab should be used with **methotrexate**. Following IV administration, concomitant administration of methotrexate decreased golimumab clearance by reducing the development of anti-golimumab antibodies. ▪ Concurrent administration with **other biologic products,** including **anakinra** (Kineret) or **abatacept** (Orencia) may be associated with an increased risk of serious infections without any increase in benefit. Anakinra is also associated with an increased risk of neutropenia. Concurrent administration of TNF-blocking agents (e.g., golimumab) with other biologics approved to treat RA, including anakinra or abatacept, is not recommended. ▪ Concomitant use of **NSAIDs** (e.g., ibuprofen [Advil, Motrin], naproxen [Aleve, Naprosyn]), **oral corticosteroids** (e.g., prednisone), or **sulfasalazine** did not influence golimumab SC clearance. ▪ **Live virus vaccines** and **therapeutic infectious agents** (e.g., BCG bladder instillation for treatment of cancer) should not be given concurrently with golimumab. Could result in clinical infection, including disseminated infections. In addition, for infants who had in utero exposure to infliximab, it is recommended that live vaccines not be given for at least 6 months after birth; see Precautions and Maternal/Child. ▪ Cytochrome P_{450} enzymes may be suppressed by increased levels of cytokines during chronic inflammation. Golimumab antagonizes cytokine activity, and the formation of the CYP_{450} enzyme may be normalized. When initiating or discontinuing golimumab in patients treated with **CYP_{450} substrates with a narrow therapeutic index,** monitoring of the effect (e.g., **warfarin** [Coumadin]) or drug concentrations (e.g., **cyclosporine** [Sandimmune] or **theophylline**) is recommended. Dose adjustment may be necessary.

SIDE EFFECTS

The most common side effects are bronchitis, hypertension, rash, upper respiratory tract infections, and viral infections. The most serious were malignancies (e.g., lymphoma, nonmelanoma skin cancer) and serious infections (e.g., abscess, cellulitis, invasive fungal infections, opportunistic infections, pneumonia, sepsis, and tuberculosis). Other less common side effects include bullous skin reactions, constipation, dizziness, increased liver function tests (e.g., ALT, AST), lower respiratory tract infection (pneumonia), decreased neutrophil count, paresthesia, pyelonephritis, sinusitis, and superficial fungal infections.

Post-Marketing: No post-marketing experience is available for golimumab. The adverse reactions listed have been identified during postapproval use of the subcutaneous formulation of golimumab. Hypersensitivity/infusion-related reactions, interstitial lung disease, melanoma, sarcoidosis, serious systemic hypersensitivity reactions (including anaphylactic reactions), and skin exfoliation. Rare cases of hepatosplenic T-cell lymphoma have been reported with TNF-blockers.

ANTIDOTE

Notify physician of any side effects; most will be treated symptomatically. Discontinue golimumab if patient experiences a serious infection, new or worsening S/S of heart failure, or a hypersensitivity reaction. Treat a hypersensitivity reaction with oxygen, epinephrine (Adrenalin), antihistamines (e.g., diphenhydramine [Benadryl]), vasopressors (e.g., dopamine), corticosteroids, albuterol, IV fluids, and ventilation equipment as indicated. Discontinue golimumab in patients who develop HBV reactivation, and initiate antiviral therapy with appropriate supportive treatment. Safety of resuming therapy after HBV is controlled is not known; use caution if resumption of therapy is considered and monitor closely. Discontinue if demyelinating disorders or S/S of lupus occur.

GRANISETRON HYDROCHLORIDE
(gran-**ISS**-eh-tron hy-droh-**KLOR**-eyed)

Antiemetic
(5-HT$_3$ receptor antagonist)

Kytril

pH 4 to 6

USUAL DOSE
Chemotherapy-induced nausea and vomiting (prophylaxis): A single dose of 10 mcg/kg of body weight as an injection or as an infusion. Begin within 30 minutes before giving emetogenic cancer chemotherapy (e.g., cisplatin, carboplatin) and only on the day(s) chemotherapy is given. Clinical trials used doses up to 40 mcg/kg with effects similar to the recommended 10-mcg/kg dose. Some studies question the effectiveness of a 10-mcg/kg dose. Repeat doses are frequently required to prevent nausea with chemotherapy. Oral granisetron is available.

Prevention and treatment of postoperative nausea and vomiting: 1 mg before induction of anesthesia, immediately before reversal of anesthesia, or postoperatively.

PEDIATRIC DOSE
Chemotherapy-induced nausea and vomiting (prophylaxis) in pediatric patients 2 to 16 years of age: Identical to adult dose. See Maternal/Child.

DOSE ADJUSTMENTS
No dose adjustment required for the elderly or in renal failure or impaired hepatic function.

DILUTION
Read label carefully. Available in two concentrations (0.1 mg/mL and 1 mg/mL). The 0.1-mg/mL vial contains no preservatives. The 1-mg/mL single-dose and multidose vials contain benzyl alcohol. Sterile technique imperative when withdrawing a single dose from the multidose vial; see Storage.

A single dose may be given undiluted by IV injection or further diluted to a total volume of 20 to 50 mL with NS or D5W and given as an infusion.

Storage: Store vials at CRT or below. Do not freeze; protect from light. Should be administered after dilution (preservative free) but is stable up to 24 hours at room temperature. Discard multidose vial within 30 days of initial penetration.

COMPATIBILITY
(Underline Indicates Conflicting Compatibility Information)
Consider any drug NOT listed as compatible to be INCOMPATIBLE until consulting a pharmacist; specific conditions may apply.
Manufacturer recommends not mixing in solution with other drugs as a general precaution.

One source suggests the following **compatibilities:**
Additive: *Not recommended by manufacturer.* Dexamethasone (Decadron), methylprednisolone (Solu-Medrol).

Y-site: Acetaminophen (Ofirmev), acyclovir (Zovirax), allopurinol (Aloprim), amifostine (Ethyol), amikacin, aminophylline, amphotericin B cholesteryl (Amphotec), ampicillin, ampicillin/sulbactam (Unasyn), aztreonam (Azactam), bleomycin (Blenoxane), bumetanide, buprenorphine (Buprenex), butorphanol (Stadol), calcium gluconate, carboplatin (Paraplatin), carmustine (BiCNU), cefazolin (Ancef), cefepime (Maxipime), cefotaxime (Claforan), cefotetan (Cefotan), cefoxitin (Mefoxin), ceftaroline (Teflaro), ceftazidime (Fortaz), ceftriaxone (Rocephin), cefuroxime (Zinacef), chlorpromazine (Thorazine), ciprofloxacin (Cipro IV), cisplatin, cladribine (Leustatin), clindamycin (Cleocin), cyclophosphamide (Cytoxan), cytarabine (ARA-C), dacarbazine (DTIC), dactinomycin (Cosmegen), daunorubicin (Cerubidine), dexamethasone (Decadron), dexmedetomidine (Precedex), diphenhydramine (Benadryl), dobutamine, docetaxel (Taxotere), dopamine, doripenem (Doribax), doxorubicin (Adriamycin), doxorubicin liposomal (Doxil), doxycycline, droperidol (Inapsine), enalaprilat (Vasotec IV), etoposide (VePesid), etoposide phosphate (Etopophos), famotidine (Pepcid IV), fenoldopam (Corlopam), filgrastim (Neupogen), fluconazole (Diflucan), fludarabine (Fludara), fluorouracil (5-FU), furosemide (Lasix), gallium nitrate (Ganite), ganciclovir (Cytovene IV), gemcitabine (Gemzar), gentamicin, heparin, hetastarch in electrolytes (Hextend), hydrocortisone sodium succinate (Solu-Cortef), hydromorphone (Dilaudid), idarubicin (Idamycin), ifosfamide (Ifex), imipenem-cilastatin (Primaxin), leucovorin calcium, linezolid (Zyvox), lorazepam (Ativan), magnesium sulfate, mechlorethamine (nitrogen mustard), melphalan (Alkeran), meperidine (Demerol), mesna (Mesnex), methotrexate, methylprednisolone (Solu-Medrol), metoclopramide (Reglan), metronidazole (Flagyl IV), mitomycin (Mutamycin), mitoxantrone (Novantrone), morphine, nalbuphine, oxaliplatin (Eloxatin), paclitaxel (Taxol), pemetrexed (Alimta), piperacillin/tazobactam (Zosyn), potassium chloride (KCl), prochlorperazine (Compazine), promethazine (Phenergan), propofol (Diprivan), ranitidine (Zantac), sargramostim (Leukine), sodium bicarbonate, streptozocin (Zanosar), sulfamethoxazole/trimethoprim, teniposide (Vumon), thiotepa, ticarcillin/clavulanate (Timentin), tobramycin, topotecan (Hycamtin), vancomycin, vinblastine, vincristine, vinorelbine (Navelbine), zidovudine (AZT, Retrovir).

RATE OF ADMINISTRATION
IV injection: A single dose over 30 seconds.
Intermittent infusion: A single dose equally distributed over 5 minutes.

ACTIONS
An antinauseant and antiemetic agent. A selective antagonist of specific serotonin (5-HT_3) receptors. Chemotherapeutic agents such as cisplatin increase the release of serotonin from specific cells in the GI tract, causing emesis. By antagonizing these receptors, chemotherapy-induced nausea and vomiting are prevented. Has little effect on BP, HR, ECG, plasma prolactin, or aldosterone concentrations. Moderately bound to protein (65%). Distributes freely between plasma and RBCs. Metabolized in the liver by hepatic cytochrome P_{450} enzymes. Mean half-life is approximately 9 hours. Excreted in urine and feces.

INDICATIONS AND USES
Prevention of nausea and vomiting associated with initial and repeat courses of emetogenic cancer therapy, including high-dose cisplatin. Has been shown to be effective with most emetogenic antineoplastic agents. ▪ Prevention and treatment of postoperative nausea and vomiting in adults.
Unlabeled uses: Prevention of nausea and vomiting associated with total body radiation or fractional abdominal radiation.

CONTRAINDICATIONS
Known hypersensitivity to granisetron.

PRECAUTIONS
Stool softeners or laxatives may be required to prevent constipation. ▪ See Drug/Lab Interactions. ▪ Hypersensitivity reactions have been reported. Use caution in patients who have exhibited hypersensitivity to other selective 5-HT_3 receptor antagonists. Cross-sensitivity has been reported between dolasetron (Anzemet) and other agents in this class (e.g., granisetron, ondansetron). ▪ The use in patients following abdominal surgery or in patients with chemotherapy-induced nausea and vomiting may mask a progressive ileus and/or gastric distension. ▪ Does not stimulate GI motility and should not be used instead of NG suction. ▪ QT prolongation has been reported. Use with caution in patients with pre-existing arrhythmias, cardiac conduction disorders, or electrolyte abnormalities or in patients who are taking other medications that can prolong the QT interval; see Drug/Lab Interactions. ▪ Serotonin syndrome has been reported with 5-HT_3 receptor antagonists. Most reports were associated with concomitant use of serotonergic drugs (e.g., selective serotonin reuptake inhibitors [e.g., paroxetine (Paxil), escitalopram (Lexapro)], serotonin and norepinephrine reuptake inhibitors [e.g., duloxetine (Cymbalta), venlafaxine (Effexor)], monoamine oxidase inhibitors [e.g., selegiline (Eldepryl)], mir-

tazapine (Remeron), fentanyl, lithium, tramadol (Ultram), and intravenous methylene blue). Some cases were fatal. ▪ Not recommended if nausea and vomiting are not expected postoperatively unless nausea and vomiting must be avoided during the postoperative period.

Monitor: Ambulate slowly to avoid orthostatic hypotension. ▪ Monitor for S/S of hypersensitivity (e.g., anaphylaxis, hypotension, shortness of breath, urticaria). ▪ Monitor ECG in patients at risk for prolongation of the PR and QRS interval; see Precautions. ▪ Monitor for serotonin syndrome, especially when dolasetron is used concurrently with other serotonergic drugs. Symptoms associated with serotonin syndrome may include the following combination of S/S: mental status changes (e.g., agitation, coma, delirium, hallucinations), autonomic instability (e.g., diaphoresis, dizziness, flushing, hyperthermia, labile blood pressure, tachycardia), neuromuscular symptoms (e.g., hyperreflexia, incoordination, myoclonus, rigidity, tremor), seizures, with or without GI symptoms (e.g., diarrhea, nausea, vomiting).

Patient Education: Request assistance for ambulation. ▪ Report promptly if nausea persists for more than 10 minutes. ▪ Maintain adequate hydration. ▪ Stool softeners may be required to avoid constipation. ▪ Promptly report S/S of serotonin syndrome (e.g., altered mental status, autonomic instability, and neuromuscular symptoms); see Precautions.

Maternal/Child: Category B: no evidence of impaired fertility or harm to fetus. Benzyl alcohol may cross the placenta; see Dilution. Use during pregnancy only if benefits justify risks. ▪ Use caution if required during breast-feeding. ▪ Safety and effectiveness for use in the treatment of chemotherapy-induced nausea and vomiting in pediatric patients under 2 years of age have not been established. ▪ Not recommended for prevention and treatment of postoperative nausea and vomiting in pediatric patients due to a lack of efficacy and QT prolongation observed in a clinical trial.

Elderly: Response similar to other age-groups. ▪ Clearance lower and half-life prolonged but has no clinical significance.

DRUG/LAB INTERACTIONS

Metabolism may be inhibited by **ketoconazole** (Nizoral). Clinical significance unknown. ▪ Does not induce or inhibit the cytochrome P_{450} drug metabolizing system, but definitive interaction studies have not been done. Its clearance and half-life may be affected by **inducers of these enzymes** such as anticonvulsants (e.g., carbamazepine [Tegretol], phenobarbital [Luminal], phenytoin [Dilantin]) or rifampin (Rifadin) or by **inhibitors of these enzymes** (e.g., cimetidine [Tagamet], calcium channel blockers [e.g., diltiazem (Cardizem), verapamil], antiviral agents [e.g., indinavir (Crixivan), ritonavir [Norvir], saquinavir [Invirase]). ▪ Has been safely administered with **benzodiazepines** (e.g., lorazepam [Ativan], midazolam [Versed]), **neuroleptics** (e.g., chlordiazepoxide [Librium]), and **antiulcer drugs** (e.g., ranitidine [Zantac]) commonly prescribed with antiemetic treatment. ▪ Does not appear to interact with emetogenic cancer chemotherapies. ▪ Concurrent use with **drugs known to prolong the QT interval** (e.g., amiodarone [Nexterone], antihistamines, azole antifungals [e.g., itraconazole (Sporanox)], disopyramide [Norpace], fluoroquinolones [e.g., levofloxacin (Levaquin)], ibutilide [Corvert], mexiletine, phenothiazines [e.g., thioridazine (Mellaril)], procainamide [Pronestyl], quinidine, and tricyclic antidepressants [e.g., amitriptyline (Elavil), imipramine (Tofranil)]) may result in clinical consequences. ▪ Serotonin syndrome (including altered mental status, autonomic instability, and neuromuscular symptoms) has been reported following the concomitant use of 5-HT$_3$ receptor antagonists and other serotonergic drugs, including selective serotonin reuptake inhibitors (SSRIs) and serotonin and norepinephrine reuptake inhibitors (SNRIs); see Precautions.

SIDE EFFECTS

Asthenia (5%), constipation (3%), diarrhea (4%), headache (14%), somnolence (4%), and weakness (5%) occur most frequently. Hypersensitivity reactions, including anaphylaxis (rare), have occurred. Transient elevation of AST or ALT may occur. Other side effects include abdominal pain, anemia, anxiety, bradycardia, coughing, dizziness, dyspepsia, fever, hypertension, hypotension, infection, insomnia, leukocytosis, oliguria, pain. Other side effects have occurred in fewer than 2% of patients but could not be clearly associated with granisetron.

Post-Marketing: QT prolongation. Serotonin syndrome has been reported as a 5-HT$_3$ class reaction.

ANTIDOTE
Most side effects will be treated symptomatically. Keep physician informed as indicated. There is no specific antidote. If symptoms of serotonin syndrome occur, discontinue granisetron and initiate supportive care. Treat anaphylaxis and resuscitate as necessary.

HEMIN BBW
(**HEE**-men)

Porphyrin inhibitor

Panhematin

USUAL DOSE
A single dose of 1 to 4 mg/kg of body weight/24 hr of hematin for 3 to 14 days. This dose could be repeated in 12 hours for severe cases. Never exceed a total dose of 6 mg/kg/24 hr. Length of treatment dependent on severity of symptoms and clinical response. See Precautions.

DILUTION
Each vial containing 313 mg of hemin must be diluted with 43 mL of SWFI (provides 301 mg of hematin). Shake well for 2 to 3 minutes to ensure dissolution. Each 1 mL contains 7 mg hematin. Each 0.14 mL contains 1 mg hematin. May be given directly from vial as an infusion or through Y-tube or three-way stopcock of infusion set.

Filters: Use of a 0.45-micron or smaller in-line filter recommended.

Storage: Store in refrigerator at 2° to 8° C (36° to 46° F). Contains no preservative, decomposes rapidly; discard unused solution.

COMPATIBILITY
Undergoes rapid chemical decomposition in solution. Manufacturer states, "No drug or chemical agent should be added unless its effect on the chemical and physical stability has been determined." Specific information not available; consult pharmacist.

RATE OF ADMINISTRATION
A single dose evenly distributed over 10 to 15 minutes.

ACTIONS
An iron-containing metalloporphyrin enzyme inhibitor extracted from RBCs. Inhibits rate of porphyria/heme biosynthesis in the liver and bone marrow by an unknown mechanism. Induces remission of symptoms only; not curative. Some excretion occurs in urine and feces.

INDICATIONS AND USES
To control symptoms of recurrent attacks of acute intermittent porphyria in selected patients (often related to the menstrual cycle in susceptible women).

CONTRAINDICATIONS
Hypersensitivity to hemin; porphyria cutanea tarda.

PRECAUTIONS
Confirm diagnosis of acute porphyria before use (positive Watson-Schwartz or Hoechst test). Administered by or under the supervision of a physician experienced in the treatment of porphyrias and in facilities equipped to monitor the patient and respond to any medical emergency. ▪ Alternate therapy of 400 Gm glucose/24 hr for 1 to 2 days should be tried before use of hemin is initiated. ▪ Give as early as possible with onset of attack to achieve the most benefit. ▪ Must

be given before irreversible neuronal damage of porphyria has begun. ▪ See Drug/Lab Interactions.

Monitor: Use of a large arm vein or central venous catheter recommended to avoid phlebitis. ▪ Effectiveness monitored by decrease in urine concentration of S-aminolevulinic acid (ALA), uroporphyrinogen (UPG), or porphobilinogen (PBG).

Maternal/Child: Category C: safety for use during pregnancy, breast-feeding, and in pediatric patients not established.

DRUG/LAB INTERACTIONS

Action inhibited by **estrogens, barbiturates, and steroid metabolites.** Avoid concurrent use. ▪ Has mild anticoagulant effects. Avoid concurrent use with **anticoagulants** (e.g., heparin, warfarin [Coumadin]).

SIDE EFFECTS

Almost nonexistent with usual dosage and appropriate technique; fever, phlebitis. Reversible renal shutdown has been reported with excessive doses.

ANTIDOTE

Discontinue temporarily if known or questionable side effect appears, and notify physician. Renal shutdown of overdose has responded to ethacrynic acid (Edecrin) and mannitol. Treat anaphylaxis (antihistamines, epinephrine, corticosteroids) and resuscitate as necessary.

HEPARIN SODIUM   Anticoagulant
(**HEP**-ah-rin **SO**-dee-um)

Hepalean♦, Heparin Lock-Flush, Heparin Sodium PF, Hep-Flush 10, Hep-Lock, Hep-Lock U/P   pH 5 to 7.5

USUAL DOSE

Confirm choice of the correct heparin product; see Precautions.

As of 2009 USP heparin has a new reference standard and a new test method for manufacturers to use in determining accurate potency. The adjustment in reference standard results in approximately a 10% reduction in the potency of heparin and makes it commensurate with the World Health Organization International Standard unit dose. In most situations this new reference standard will not require a dose adjustment; however, dose adjustments and more frequent monitoring may be indicated in selected clinical situations.

Intermittent injection for therapeutic anticoagulation (based on a 68-kg [150-lb] patient): 10,000 units initially. Dosage is repeated every 4 to 6 hours and adjusted according to coagulation test results. Usually 5,000 to 10,000 units. Initial and repeat doses may be given undiluted or may be diluted in 50 to 100 mL of NS.

IV infusion for therapeutic anticoagulation (based on a 68-kg [150-lb] patient): An initial bolus dose of 5,000 units is required. 20,000 to 40,000 units/24 hr in NS or other **compatible** infusion solution. Adjust dose according to coagulation test results.

Treatment of venous thromboembolism (VTE): American College of Chest Physicians recommends an initial bolus of 80 units/kg (alternately 5,000 units) followed by an initial continuous infusion of 18 units/kg/hr (alternately 1,000 units/hr) for VTE. An initial bolus of 70 units/kg followed by an initial infusion of 15 units/kg/hr has been recommended for cardiac or stroke patients.

Adjuvant therapy in treatment of AMI: AHA guidelines recommend an initial bolus dose of 60 units/kg of body weight (maximum dose 4,000 units). Follow with an infusion of 12 units/kg/hr. The initial maximum recommended infusion rate is 1,000 units/hr. Adjust to maintain aPTT at 1.5 to 2 times control. Other protocols are in use.

Continued

Adjuvant therapy during treatment with thrombolytic agents (e.g., alteplase, reteplase, streptokinase) and glycoprotein GPIIb/IIIa receptor antagonists (e.g., abciximab, eptifibitide, tirofiban): See individual monographs for suggested doses.

Open heart surgery: 150 to 400 units/kg of body weight during surgical procedure, depending on duration of procedure. Frequently, a dose of 300 units/kg is administered for procedures estimated to last less than 60 minutes. 400 units/kg may be given for procedures estimated to last longer than 60 minutes.

Disseminated intravascular coagulation: Use and dose of heparin is based on severity of DIC and underlying cause and extent of thrombosis. Several dosing regimens have been used; see literature.

Maintain patency of indwelling venipuncture devices (e.g., heparin-lock, catheter, or implanted port) intended for intermittent use: Consult device manufacturer's instructions for specific requirements regarding its use. 10 unit/mL concentration is commonly used for younger infants (less than 10 kg). Higher concentration of 100 units/1 mL is used in older infants, pediatric patients, and adults. Volume of heparin flush solution should be similar to volume of catheter. May be used after initial placement of the device in the vein, after each medication injection, after withdrawal of blood for laboratory tests, or every 8 to 24 hours to maintain patency of device. Confirm patency by aspirating before each injection. Flush with SWFI or NS before and after any medication **incompatible** with heparin. Reinstill heparin after second flush. If additional medications are not needed, each single dose of heparin will prevent clotting within the lumen of indwelling venipuncture devices for up to 24 hours.

Blood transfusion: 400 to 600 units/100 mL whole blood.

Converting to an oral anticoagulant: When converting from heparin to **warfarin** (Coumadin), begin warfarin on the first or second day of heparin therapy at the usual initial dose and determine PT/INR at the usual intervals. To ensure continuous anticoagulation, continue full heparin therapy for several days until the PT/INR has reached a therapeutic range (INR of 2 or greater) for at least 24 hours. Once target PT/INR has been achieved and maintained, heparin therapy can be discontinued without tapering. When initiating oral therapy with **dabigatran (Pradaxa)**, stop the heparin infusion immediately after the first dose of oral dabigatran. For intermittent IV administration of heparin, start dabigatran 0 to 2 hours before the time that the next dose of intermittent heparin was to have been administered.

PEDIATRIC DOSE

Read label carefully. Comes in many strengths. Confirm use of the correct strength. Fatal hemorrhages have occurred in pediatric patients, including neonates, as a result of medication errors in which heparin sodium injection vials have been confused with heparin-lock flush vials.

Do not use products containing benzyl alcohol in neonates or infants. Preservative-free solution is required for neonates and infants. See Maternal/Child.

Full-dose continuous IV infusion: A *loading dose* of 75 to 100 units/kg administered over 10 minutes and a *maintenance dose* (to maintain an aPTT of approximately 60 to 85 seconds or a range corresponding to an anti-factor Xa level of 0.35 to 0.7) based on age as follows:

Infants less than 2 months: (Have the highest requirements) Average 28 units/kg/hr.

Infants 2 months to 1 year of age: 25 to 30 units/kg/hr.

Over 1 year of age: 18 to 20 units/kg/hr.

Older pediatric patients: May require less heparin, similar to the weight-adjusted dose in adults (18 units/kg/hr).

Another source suggests a *loading dose* of 50 units/kg followed by a *maintenance dose* of 25 units/kg/hr or up to 20,000 units/M^2 equally distributed over 24 hours. All doses should be adjusted to coagulation tests.

Disseminated intravascular coagulation: Use and dose of heparin are based on severity of DIC and underlying cause and extent of thrombosis. Several dosing regimens have been used; see literature.

Patency of indwelling venipuncture devices: See Maternal/Child. Safety and effectiveness of the 100-USP units/mL heparin-lock flush solution for pediatric patients not established. Patency for peripheral devices (e.g., single- and double-lumen central catheters) is usually accomplished with 10 units/mL heparin solution in younger infants (e.g., less than 10 kg) and with 100 units/mL for older infants, children, and adults. Avoid approaching therapeutic unit/kg dose. Follow catheter manufacturer's guidelines. See all comments under similar section in Usual Dose.

DOSE ADJUSTMENTS

Reduction of initial dose indicated in low-birth-weight infants and may be indicated in patients 60 years of age and older (especially women). Adjust dose based on coagulation tests; see Monitor. ■ Increased dose may be required in smokers (half-life shortened and elimination rate increased).

DILUTION

May be given undiluted or diluted in any given amount of NS, dextrose, or Ringer's solution for infusion and given by IV injection, as an intermittent IV, or continuous IV infusion. When added to an infusion solution for continuous IV administration, invert container a minimum of 6 times to ensure adequate mixing and to prevent pooling of heparin in the solution. Available in several strengths for administration or dilution as well as in several premixed concentrations and volumes. Unit-dose heparin flush syringes are not for multiple use; discard unused portions.

Intermittent injection or infusion: Usually given undiluted or may be diluted in 50 to 100 mL of NS or D5W.

Continuous infusion: Available in several manufacturer-supplied concentrations. If prepared, may be diluted in 250 to 1,000 mL of **compatible** solution to provide a 24-hour dose. See chart on inside back cover.

Blood transfusion: Add 7,500 units heparin to 100 mL NS. Add 6 to 8 mL of this sterile solution to each 100 mL of whole blood.

Filters: No significant reduction in potency when 10,000 units diluted in D5W or NS was filtered through a 0.22-micron cellulose ester membrane filter.

Storage: Store at CRT. Do not freeze. Do not use if solution is discolored or contains a precipitate. Storage of prepared (diluted) heparin infusion solutions should not exceed 4 hours at RT or 24 hours refrigerated.

COMPATIBILITY
(Underline Indicates Conflicting Compatibility Information)

Consider any drug NOT listed as compatible to be INCOMPATIBLE until consulting a pharmacist; specific conditions may apply.

Several sources recommend not mixing or administering through the same IV line with other drugs until **compatibility** confirmed. To avoid precipitation with heparin, they also caution to flush with SWFI or NS before and after any acidic or **incompatible** medication or solution. Manufacturer lists as **incompatible** in solution with alteplase (Activase, Cathflo), amikacin, atracurium (Tracrium), ciprofloxacin (Cipro IV), cytarabine (ARA-C), daunorubicin (Cerubidine), droperidol (Inapsine), erythromycin (Erythrocin), gentamicin, idarubicin (Idamycin), kanamycin, mitoxantrone (Novantrone), polymyxin B, promethazine (Phenergan), streptomycin, and tobramycin.

One source suggests the following **compatibilities:**

Additive: Aminophylline, amphotericin B (conventional), ampicillin, anti-thymocyte globulin (rabbit) (Thymoglobulin), ascorbic acid, bleomycin (Blenoxane), calcium gluconate, cefepime (Maxipime), ceftazidime (Fortaz), chloramphenicol (Chloromycetin), clindamycin (Cleocin), colistimethate (Coly-Mycin M), dimenhydrinate, dobutamine, dopamine, enalaprilat (Vasotec IV), esmolol (Brevibloc), fluconazole (Diflucan), flumazenil (Romazicon), furosemide (Lasix), hydrocortisone sodium succinate (Solu-Cortef), hydromorphone (Dilaudid), isoproterenol (Isuprel), lidocaine, lincomycin (Lincocin), magnesium sulfate, meropenem (Merrem IV), methyldopate, methylprednisolone (Solu-Medrol), mitomycin (Mutamycin), nafcillin (Nallpen), norepinephrine (Levophed), octreotide (Sandostatin), penicillin G potassium and sodium, potassium chloride, ranitidine (Zantac), sodium bicarbonate, vancomycin, verapamil.

Y-site: Acetaminophen (Ofirmev), acyclovir (Zovirax), <u>aldesleukin (Proleukin)</u>, allopurinol (Aloprim), amifostine (Ethyol), aminophylline, ampicillin, ampicillin/sulbactam (Unasyn), <u>anidulafungin (Eraxis)</u>, <u>anti-thymocyte globulin (rabbit) (Thymoglobulin)</u>, atracurium (Tracrium), atropine, aztreonam (Azactam), bivalirudin (Angiomax), bleomycin (Blenoxane), caffeine citrate, calcium gluconate, cefazolin (Ancef), cefotetan (Cefotan), ceftaroline (Teflaro), ceftazidime (Fortaz), ceftriaxone (Rocephin), chlorpromazine (Thorazine), <u>cisatracurium (Nimbex)</u>, cisplatin, cladribine (Leustatin), clindamycin (Cleocin), cyclophosphamide (Cytoxan), <u>dacarbazine (DTIC)</u>, daptomycin (Cubicin), dexamethasone (Decadron), dexmedetomidine (Precedex), digoxin (Lanoxin), <u>diltiazem (Cardizem)</u>, diphenhydramine (Benadryl), <u>dobutamine</u>, docetaxel (Taxotere), dopamine, doripenem (Doribax), doxapram (Dopram), doxorubicin liposomal (Doxil), <u>droperidol (Inapsine)</u>, edrophonium (Enlon), enalaprilat (Vasotec IV), epinephrine (Adrenalin), ertapenem (Invanz), erythromycin (Erythrocin), esmolol (Brevibloc), estrogens, conjugated (Premarin), ethacrynic acid (Edecrin), etoposide phosphate (Etopophos), famotidine (Pepcid IV), fenoldopam (Corlopam), fentanyl, fluconazole (Diflucan), fludarabine (Fludara), fluorouracil (5-FU), foscarnet (Foscavir), furosemide (Lasix), gallium nitrate (Ganite), gemcitabine (Gemzar), granisetron (Kytril), hetastarch in electrolytes (Hextend), hydralazine, hydrocortisone sodium succinate (Solu-Cortef), hydromorphone (Dilaudid), 6% hydroxyethyl starch (Voluven), insulin (regular), isoproterenol (Isuprel), <u>labetalol</u>, leucovorin calcium, lidocaine, linezolid (Zyvox), lorazepam (Ativan), magnesium sulfate, melphalan (Alkeran), meperidine (Demerol), meropenem (Merrem IV), methotrexate, methyldopate, methylergonovine (Methergine), <u>methylprednisolone (Solu-Medrol)</u>, metoclopramide (Reglan), metoprolol (Lopressor), metronidazole (Flagyl IV), <u>micafungin (Mycamine)</u>, midazolam (Versed), milrinone (Primacor), mitomycin (Mutamycin), morphine, nafcillin (Nallpen), neostigmine, <u>nicardipine (Cardene IV)</u>, nitroglycerin IV, nitroprusside sodium, norepinephrine (Levophed), ondansetron (Zofran), oxacillin (Bactocill), oxaliplatin (Eloxatin), oxytocin (Pitocin), paclitaxel (Taxol), <u>palonosetron (Aloxi)</u>, pancuronium, pemetrexed (Alimta), penicillin G potassium, pentazocine (Talwin), phytonadione (vitamin K_1), piperacillin/tazobactam (Zosyn), potassium chloride (KCl), procainamide (Pronestyl), prochlorperazine (Compazine), <u>promethazine (Phenergan)</u>, propofol (Diprivan), propranolol, <u>quinidine gluconate</u>, ranitidine (Zantac), remifentanil (Ultiva), sargramostim (Leukine), sodium bicarbonate, succinylcholine, tacrolimus (Prograf), <u>telavancin (Vibativ)</u>, theophylline, thiotepa, ticarcillin/clavulanate (Timentin), tigecycline (Tygacil), tirofiban (Aggrastat), tranexamic acid (Cyklokapron), <u>vancomycin</u>, vasopressin, vecuronium, vinblastine, vincristine, <u>vinorelbine (Navelbine)</u>, warfarin (Coumadin), zidovudine (AZT, Retrovir).

RATE OF ADMINISTRATION

A single injection (5,000 units or fraction thereof) may be given over 1 minute. A continuous IV infusion may be given over 4 to 24 hours, depending on specific dosage of heparin required, amount of heparin added, and amount of infusion fluid used as a diluent. Continuous IV infusion is the preferred method of administration. Use an infusion pump for accuracy.

ACTIONS

An anticoagulant with immediate and predictable effects on the blood. Inhibits reactions that lead to clotting of blood and the formation of fibrin clots. Heparin combines with other factors in the blood to inhibit the conversion of prothrombin to thrombin and fibrinogen to fibrin. Adhesiveness of platelets is reduced. Well-established clots are not dissolved, but growth is prevented and newer clots may be dissolved. Duration of action is short, about 4 to 6 hours. Average plasma half-life is 30 to 180 minutes. The half-life of the anticoagulant effect of heparin is approximately 1.5 hours and does not increase with dose. Metabolic fate not fully determined. May be partially metabolized in the liver and the reticuloendothelial system. Small amount excreted as unchanged drug in the urine.

INDICATIONS AND USES

Prevention and/or treatment of all types of thromboses and emboli, including deep vein thrombosis (DVT), pulmonary emboli (PE), thromboembolic complications associated with atrial fibrillation (AF), and peripheral arterial embolism. ■ Treatment of disseminated intravascular coagulation (DIC). ■ Prevention of clotting in arterial and cardiac surgery and during blood transfusion, extracorporeal circulation, and dialysis procedures. ■ Maintain patency of an indwelling venipuncture device designed for intermittent injection or infusion therapy or blood sampling (e.g., heparin-lock, catheter, or implanted port).

Unlabeled uses: Adjunct in treatment of coronary occlusion with acute myocardial infarction (MI). ■ Adjunct to use of glycoprotein GP IIb/IIIa receptor antagonists in percutaneous coronary intervention (PCI). ■ ST-elevation MI, as an adjunct to thrombolysis.

CONTRAINDICATIONS

History of heparin-induced thrombocytopenia (HIT) and heparin-induced thrombocytopenia and thrombosis (HITT). ■ Severe thrombocytopenia. ■ Patients receiving full-dose heparin unless blood coagulation tests can be performed at appropriate intervals. ■ Hypersensitivity to heparin (or any of its components [may contain sulfites]) or pork products. ■ Uncontrolled bleeding except in DIC. ■ Do not administer heparin preparations preserved with benzyl alcohol to neonates, infants, pregnant women, or breast-feeding mothers.

PRECAUTIONS

Read label carefully. Comes in many strengths. Confirm use of the correct strength. Fatal hemorrhages have occurred in pediatric patients, including neonates, as a result of medication errors in which heparin sodium injection vials have been confused with heparin-lock flush vials. ■ For IV or SC use only; avoid IM administration (may cause hematomas). ■ Derived from animal protein (pork). ■ Avoid using heparin in the presence of major bleeding, except when the benefits of heparin therapy outweigh the potential risks. ■ Use extreme caution in any disease state or clinical condition in which risk of hemorrhage may be increased, such as subacute bacterial endocarditis; severe hypertension; during or following spinal tap, spinal anesthesia, or major surgery (especially major surgery involving the brain, spinal cord, or eye); hemophilia; thrombocytopenia; gastrointestinal ulcerative lesions; vascular purpuras; continuous tube drainage of the stomach or small intestine; menstruation; severe liver disease with impaired hemostasis; severe renal disease; or in patients with indwelling catheters. ■ Resistance to heparin increased in cancer, fever, infections with thrombosing tendencies, MI, postsurgical patients, thrombophlebitis, and thrombosis. ■ May cause thrombocytopenia; monitor closely. ■ May develop heparin-induced thrombocytopenia (HIT), an antibody-mediated reaction resulting from irreversible aggregation of platelets. HIT may progress to heparin-induced thrombocytopenia and thrombosis (HITT), which involves the development of venous and arterial thromboses. HIT and HITT may occur during heparin treatment or may be delayed for up to several weeks after heparin treatment is discontinued; see Monitor. ■ See Elderly for additional precautions. ■ Repeated flushing of an indwelling venipuncture device with heparin may result in a systemic anticoagulant effect. ■ Heparin-lock flush solution is intended for maintenance of patency of intravenous injection devices only and is not to be used for anticoagulant therapy. ■ See Maternal/Child.

Monitor: Obtain baseline coagulation studies (e.g., whole blood clotting time [WBCT], activated coagulation time [ACT], activated partial thromboplastin time [aPTT], and INR) and a baseline CBC with platelets. ■ Dose is considered adequate when the aPTT is 1.5 to 2 times normal or when the WBCT is elevated approximately 2.5 to 3 times the control value. Confirm desired control level with physician. ■ During the early stages of treatment, coagulation tests are often done before each intermittent injection or every 4 hours with a continuous infusion. Once the patient is adequately anticoagulated and stable, monitoring may be decreased to daily. Reinstitute more frequent monitoring with any dose adjustment, change in patient condition, or change in therapy that might affect anticoagulation status. Notify the physician if aPTT, ACT, or WBCT is above therapeutic level. ■ Monitor platelet count periodically. Discontinue heparin if it falls below 100,000 or a thrombosis forms. May develop HIT or HITT. Immune-mediated HIT is diagnosed based on clinical findings supplemented by laboratory tests confirming the presence of antibodies to heparin or platelet activation induced by heparin. Thrombotic events may be the initial presentation for HITT and may include DVT, cerebral vein thrombosis, limb ischemia, mesenteric thrombosis, thrombus formation on a prosthetic cardiac valve, or renal artery thrombosis; skin necrosis; gangrene of the extremities that may lead to amputation; MI; pulmonary embolism; stroke; or death. HIT and HITT may occur during heparin therapy or may be delayed. Evaluate patients for HIT and HITT if they present with thrombocytopenia or thrombosis after heparin is discontinued. Can occur up to several weeks after heparin is discontinued. ■ Also monitor hematocrit and occult blood in stool. ■ Hemorrhage can occur at any site and is the primary complication. Monitor closely. Consider the possibility of a hemorrhagic event with an unexplained fall in hematocrit, a fall in BP, or any other unexplained symptom. GI or urinary tract bleeding may indicate an underlying lesion. Certain hemorrhagic complications may be difficult to detect and can be very serious (e.g., adrenal [with resultant adrenal insufficiency], ovarian [corpus luteum], and retroperitoneal hemorrhage). ■ Use extensive precautionary methods to prevent bleeding if patient requires IM injection, arterial puncture, or venipuncture. ■ Monitor coagulation tests closely in patients who develop resistance to heparin. Adjustment of heparin doses based on anti-Factor Xa levels may be warranted; see Precautions.

Patency of indwelling venipuncture devices: Obtain a baseline aPTT prior to insertion of an indwelling venipuncture device. Repeated heparin injections can alter aPTT. ■ To avoid precipitation, irrigate indwelling venipuncture devices with NS before and after injecting acidic or **incompatible** solutions. ■ Heparin and/or NS may interfere with blood samples drawn from these devices, especially if drawn on a frequent basis. Clear the heparin flush solution by aspirating and discarding a volume of solution equal to that of the indwelling venipuncture device before the desired blood sample is drawn.

Patient Education: Report all episodes of bleeding and apply local pressure if indicated. ■ Report tarry stools. ■ Compliance with all measures to minimize bleeding is very important (e.g., avoid use of razors, toothbrushes, other sharp items). ■ Use caution while moving to avoid excess bumping. ■ Promptly report S/S of any other side effects (e.g., hypersensitivity reaction, HIT, HITT).

Maternal/Child: Category C: preferred anticoagulant in pregnancy but must be used with caution. Hemorrhage most likely to occur during the last trimester or postpartum. Has caused stillbirths and prematurity. ■ Not secreted in breast milk. ■ Some preparations may contain benzyl alcohol; do not use in neonates, infants, pregnant women, or breastfeeding mothers; see Contraindications. ■ Use to maintain patency of umbilical artery catheters has been associated with an increased risk of intraventricular hemorrhage in low-birth-weight infants. ■ Use heparin-lock flush with caution in infants with diseases with an increased risk of hemorrhage. The 100 units/mL concentration should not be used in neonates or infants who weigh less than 10 kg because of the risk of systemic anticoagulation. Use caution when using the 10 units/mL concentration in premature infants who weigh less than 1 kg and are receiving frequent flushes, because a therapeutic heparin dose may be given in a 24-hour period. Use minimal doses and preservative-free preparations, and monitor carefully. ■ See Dose Adjustments and Precautions.

Elderly: Higher plasma levels of heparin and longer aPTTs may occur in patients over 60 years of age. Higher incidence of bleeding in patients 60 years of age and older (especially women). Lower doses of heparin may be indicated; see Dose Adjustments.

DRUG/LAB INTERACTIONS

Increased risk of bleeding with **drugs that can interfere with platelet aggregation and/or increase the risk of bleeding** (e.g., **systemic salicylates** [aspirin], **NSAIDs** including celecoxib [Celebrex] and ibuprofen [Motrin], **platelet aggregation inhibitors** [e.g., clopidogrel (Plavix), prasugrel (Effient), ticagrelor (Brilinta)], **glycoprotein GPIIb/IIIa receptor antago-**

nists [e.g., abciximab (ReoPro), eptifibatide (Integrilin), tirofiban (Aggrastat)], **some cephalosporins** [e.g., cefotetan], **dextran, or other thrombolytic agents** [e.g., alteplase, streptokinase]); use heparin with caution in patients receiving such agents. ▪ Anticoagulant effect of heparin is enhanced by concurrent treatment with **antithrombin III (human)** (Thrombate III). ▪ Resistance to heparin anticoagulation may occur following administration of **streptokinase** as a systemic thrombolytic agent; adjust dose of heparin based on more frequent aPTTs. ▪ Inhibited by **antihistamines, digoxin, nicotine, nitrates, tetracyclines, and others;** may counteract anticoagulant action of heparin. ▪ Potentiates **oral anticoagulants** (e.g., apixaban [Eliquis], dabigatran [Pradaxa], rivaroxaban [Xarelto], warfarin [Coumadin]). ▪ See Precautions/Monitor. ▪ Use caution when administered with or around **other anticoagulants.** Lab data may not provide an accurate baseline. ▪ Numerous **lab values** (e.g., aminotransferase levels [AST, ALT], PT) may be altered. Notify lab of heparin use. Diagnostic results may not be attainable. See Monitor. ▪ When heparin is given concomitantly with warfarin (Coumadin), the PT may be prolonged. Wait at least 5 hours after IV bolus heparin dose before drawing PT. If heparin is being administered as a continuous infusion, may draw PT at any time.

SIDE EFFECTS
The most common side effects are elevations of aminotransferase levels and general hypersensitivity reactions, usually chills, fever, and urticaria (anaphylactoid reactions, including shock, asthma, headache, itching and burning on plantar side of feet, lacrimation, nausea and vomiting, and rhinitis may occur less frequently); hemorrhage (bruising, epistaxis, hematuria, tarry stools [adrenal hemorrhage (with resultant acute adrenal insufficiency), ovarian hemorrhage (corpus luteum hemorrhage that may be fatal), and/or retroperitoneal hemorrhage may be difficult to detect]); HIT and HITTS (including delayed-onset cases); injection site irritation; and thrombocytopenia.

ANTIDOTE
Discontinue drug and notify physician of any side effects. Protamine sulfate is a heparin antagonist and specifically indicated in overdose or desired heparin reversal. Each milligram of protamine neutralizes approximately 100 units heparin. No more than 50 mg should be administered, very slowly, in any 10-minute period. Administration of protamine can cause severe hypotension and anaphylactoid reactions. Use with caution and have emergency equipment and medications readily available. If HIT (with or without thrombosis) is diagnosed or strongly suspected, discontinue all sources of heparin, including heparin flushes. Use an alternative anticoagulant. Any future use of heparin should be avoided, especially within 3 to 6 months after the diagnosis of HIT or HITT and while patients test positive for HIT antibodies. Whole blood transfusion may be indicated. If heparin-induced thrombocytopenia or white clot syndrome occurs, discontinue heparin and administer a non-heparin anticoagulant (e.g., argatroban, bivalirudin [Angiomax]) as an alternate form of anticoagulation. Follow-up with oral anticoagulation (e.g., warfarin [Coumadin]) may also be indicated. Avoid use of heparin for at least 3 to 6 months or for as long as the patient tests positive for HIT antibodies.

G-H

HEPATITIS B IMMUNE GLOBULIN INTRAVENOUS (HUMAN)

Immunizing agent
(passive)

(hep-ah-**TY**-tiss ih-**MUNE GLAW-**byoo-lin IV)

HepaGam B

pH 5.6

USUAL DOSE

(International units [IU])

Prevention of hepatitis B recurrence following liver transplantation: Administered by a set dosing regimen designed to attain serum levels of antibodies to hepatitis B surface antigen (anti-HBs) greater than 500 IU/L. Each dose should contain 20,000 IU calculated from the measured potency as stamped on the vial label. Administer the first dose of 20,000 IU concurrently with grafting of the transplanted liver (the anhepatic phase). Administer each subsequent dose of 20,000 IU as recommended in the following chart.

Hepatitis B IGIV Dosing Regimen			
Anhepatic Phase	Week 1 Postoperative	Weeks 2-12 Postoperative	Month 4 Onward
First dose of 20,000 IU	20,000 IU daily from Day 1 through Day 7; see Dose Adjustments	20,000 IU every 2 weeks from Day 14 (Week 2) through Week 12	20,000 IU monthly

DOSE ADJUSTMENTS

(International units [IU])

Increased doses may be required in patients who fail to reach anti-HBs levels of 500 IU/L within the first week after liver transplantation. Particularly susceptible to an extensive decrease of circulated anti-HBs are patients who have surgical bleeding or abdominal fluid drainage (greater than 500 mL) or those who undergo plasmapheresis. If the desired anti-HBs levels are not reached, increase the dosing regimen to a half-dose (10,000 IU [calculated from the measured potency as stamped on the vial label]) and administer IV every 6 hours until the target anti-HBs level is reached.

DILUTION

A ready-to-use liquid preparation; should be clear to opalescent. Multiple vials will be required. *Do not shake vials; avoid foaming.* Bring to room temperature before administration. Administer through a separate IV line using an IV administration set and an infusion pump.

Filters: No data available from manufacturer.

Storage: Store between 2° and 8° C (36° and 46° F). Do not freeze. Do not use after expiration date. Use within 6 hours of opening the vial, and discard partially used vials.

COMPATIBILITY

Manufacturer states, "Administer through a separate IV line using an IV administration set via infusion pump."

RATE OF ADMINISTRATION

Set infusion pump rate at 2 mL/min. Decrease to 1 mL/min or slower for patient discomfort, infusion-related adverse events, or concern about the speed of infusion.

ACTIONS

A solvent/detergent-treated sterile solution of purified gamma globulin containing anti-HBs. Prepared from plasma donated by healthy, screened donors with high titers of anti-HBs. Purified by an anion-exchange column chromatography manufacturing method. It provides passive immunization for individuals exposed to the hepatitis B virus by binding to the surface antigen and reducing the rate of hepatitis B infection. Following liver transplantation, hepatitis B virus re-infection can occur immediately at the time of liver reperfusion due to a circulating virus or later from a virus retained in extrahepatic sites.

Provides an immediate immune response to the hepatitis B virus. Mechanism of action is not known but may occur through several pathways (e.g., through blockage of a putative HBV receptor, neutralization of circulating virions through immune precipitation and immune complex formation, triggering of an antibody-dependent cell-mediated cytotoxicity response that results in target cell lysis, or binding to hepatocytes and interaction with HBsAg within cells). Clinical effectiveness is dependent on dose, length of administration, and viral replication status of the patient at the time of transplant. Bioavailability is complete and immediate and is distributed quickly between plasma and extravascular fluid. Immune globulins are metabolized by being broken down in the reticuloendothelial system. IM injection results in mean peak concentrations within 4 to 5 days of administration and an elimination half-life of 22 to 25 days. A slightly decreased half-life is expected following IV administration.

INDICATIONS AND USES

Prevention of hepatitis B recurrence following liver transplantation in HBsAg-positive liver transplant patients. Recommended for use in patients who have no or low levels of viral replication at the time of liver transplantation. ▪ Used IM for postexposure prophylaxis in the following settings: acute exposure to blood containing HBsAg, perinatal exposure of infants born to HBsAg-positive mothers, sexual exposure to HBsAg-positive persons, and household exposure to persons with acute HBV infection.

CONTRAINDICATIONS

History of anaphylactic or severe systemic reactions to human globulins. ▪ Weigh benefits versus risk of hypersensitivity reactions in IgA-deficient individuals; see Precautions.

PRECAUTIONS

Administer in a facility with adequate equipment and supplies to monitor the patient and respond to any medical emergency. ▪ Hypersensitivity and/or infusion reactions may occur. ▪ Individuals deficient in IgA may have the potential to develop IgA antibodies and have an anaphylactoid reaction. ▪ Contains maltose, which can interfere with select blood glucose monitoring systems (those based on the glucose dehydrogenase pyrroloquinequinone [GDH-PQQ] method). May cause falsely elevated glucose readings, result in inappropriate insulin administration, and cause life-threatening hypoglycemia. In contrast, cases of true hypoglycemia may go untreated if the hypoglycemic state is masked by falsely elevated results. ▪ Derived from human plasma. Despite screening and purification processes, may have the potential risk of transmitting infectious agents (e.g., viruses [e.g., HIV, hepatitis]) or the Creutzfeldt-Jakob disease agent. ▪ Has not been evaluated in combination with antiviral therapy posttransplantation. ▪ See Patient Education and Drug/Lab Interactions.

Monitor: Hepatitis B IGIV is most effective in patients with no or low levels of HBV replication at the time of transplantation. Monitor serum HBsAg and levels of anti-HBs antibody regularly and pre-infusion to track treatment response and adjust dose when indicated. ▪ Infusion reactions may occur; usually related to rate of infusion. Monitor closely during and following an infusion. ▪ Use caution and observe diabetic patients closely; see Precautions. Only glucose-specific testing systems can be used in patients receiving hepatitis IGIV. Review product information of the blood glucose testing system to confirm that it can be used with maltose-containing parenteral products. ▪ Monitor for S/S of a hypersensitivity reaction.

Patient Education: Regular monitoring of serum HBsAg and anti-HBs antibody levels imperative. ▪ Vaccination with live virus vaccines should be deferred until approximately 3 months after administration of hepatitis B IGIV. Revaccination may be required if the previous vaccination occurred within 2 weeks of the initial hepatitis IGIV dose.

Maternal/Child: Category C: use during pregnancy only if clearly indicated. ▪ Use caution during breast-feeding. ▪ Safety and effectiveness for use in pediatric patients under 18 years of age not established.

Elderly: Safety and effectiveness not established.

DRUG/LAB INTERACTIONS

May reduce the effectiveness of **live virus vaccines** (e.g., measles, mumps, rubella, varicella). Vaccination with live virus vaccines should be deferred until approximately 3 months after administration of hepatitis B IGIV. ▪ Contains **maltose**, which can interfere with select blood glucose monitoring systems (those based on the glucose dehydrogenase pyrroloquinequinone [GDH-PQQ] method). May cause falsely elevated glucose readings. Use only glucose-specific testing systems in patients receiving hepatitis B IGIV. ▪ Passively transferred antibodies may cause a misleading positive result in **serologic testing** (e.g., Coombs' test). ▪ No data available on drug interactions with other medications.

SIDE EFFECTS

Arthralgia, chills, fever, headaches, hypersensitivity reactions, moderate or low back pain, nausea, and vomiting are the most common. Other reported side effects include agitation, amnesia, aphthous stomatitis, diarrhea, dyspepsia, edema, fatigue, gingival hyperplasia, hepatobiliary disease, hyperglycemia, hypertension, hypotension, infectious diarrhea, liver transplant rejection, nocturia, pleural effusion, pneumonia, presbyopia, pruritus, rash, sepsis, splenomegaly, tremors.

ANTIDOTE

Reduce rate of infusion for patient discomfort, infusion-related side effects, or other concerns. Discontinue the drug immediately for any signs of a hypersensitivity reaction. Notify the physician. Antihistamines (e.g., diphenhydramine [Benadryl]) or analgesic agents may be indicated for symptoms related to immune complex formation. Resume infusion at a slower rate if symptoms subside. Treat anaphylaxis immediately. Epinephrine, diphenhydramine (Benadryl), corticosteroids, and ventilation equipment must always be available.

HETASTARCH BBW

(**HET**-ah-starch)

Hespan, Hextend

Plasma volume expander

pH 5.5 to 5.9

USUAL DOSE

HESPAN, HEXTEND

Plasma volume expansion: Variable. Total dosage and rate of administration depend on amount of fluid loss and resultant hemoconcentration. Age, weight, and clinical condition of the patient are also considered. Usually 500 to 1,000 mL. Total dose usually does not exceed 1,500 mL/24 hr for the typical 70-kg patient (approximately 20 mL/kg of body weight). Higher doses, usually in conjunction with blood and/or blood products, have been used in postoperative and trauma patients who have had severe blood loss.

HESPAN

Leukapheresis: 250 to 700 mL with citrate anticoagulant in continuous flow centrifugation procedures. Do not use Hextend for leukapheresis.

DOSE ADJUSTMENTS

Avoid use in patients with pre-existing renal impairment. Information on dose adjustment in hepatic impairment is not available.

DILUTION

HESPAN: Available as a 6% solution in 500-mL containers properly diluted in NS and ready for use. Calculated osmolarity is approximately 310 mOsm/L.

HEXTEND: Available as a 6% solution in 500-mL containers properly diluted in lactated electrolyte solution and ready for use. Lactated electrolyte solution contains dextrose, normal physiologic levels of calcium and sodium, and slightly lower than normal physiologic levels of potassium and magnesium.

Storage: Store at CRT. Avoid excessive heat. Do not freeze. Do not use if color is a turbid deep brown or a crystalline precipitate is visible. Discard unused portions.

COMPATIBILITY (Underline Indicates Conflicting Compatibility Information)
Consider any drug NOT listed as compatible to be INCOMPATIBLE until consulting a pharmacist; specific conditions may apply.

HESPAN

One source suggests the following **compatibilities:**
Additive: Enalaprilat (Vasotec IV), fosphenytoin (Cerebyx), oxacillin (Bactocill).
Y-site: Ampicillin, cefazolin (Ancef), diltiazem (Cardizem), doxycycline, enalaprilat (Vasotec IV), ertapenem (Invanz), nicardipine (Cardene IV).

HEXTEND

Safety and **compatibility** of other additives not established. Contains calcium; do not administer simultaneously through the same administration set as blood; coagulation likely.

One source suggests the following **compatibilities:**
Y-site: Alfentanil, amikacin, aminophylline, amiodarone (Nexterone), ampicillin, ampicillin/sulbactam (Unasyn), atracurium (Tracrium), azithromycin (Zithromax), aztreonam (Azactam), bumetanide, butorphanol (Stadol), calcium gluconate, cefazolin (Ancef), cefepime (Maxipime), cefotaxime (Claforan), cefotetan (Cefotan), cefoxitin (Mefoxin), ceftazidime (Fortaz), cefuroxime (Zinacef), chlorpromazine (Thorazine), ciprofloxacin (Cipro IV), cisatracurium (Nimbex), clindamycin (Cleocin), dexamethasone (Decadron), digoxin (Lanoxin), diltiazem (Cardizem), diphenhydramine (Benadryl), dobutamine, dolasetron (Anzemet), dopamine, doxycycline, droperidol (Inapsine), enalaprilat (Vasotec IV), ephedrine, epinephrine (Adrenalin), erythromycin (Erythrocin), esmolol (Brevibloc), famotidine (Pepcid IV), fenoldopam (Corlopam), fentanyl, fluconazole (Diflucan), furosemide (Lasix), gentamicin, granisetron (Kytril), heparin, hydrocortisone sodium succinate (Solu-Cortef), hydromorphone (Dilaudid), isoproterenol (Isuprel), ketorolac (Toradol), labetalol, levofloxacin (Levaquin), lidocaine, lorazepam (Ativan), magnesium sulfate, mannitol, meperidine (Demerol), methylprednisolone (Solu-Medrol), metoclopramide (Reglan), metronidazole (Flagyl IV), midazolam (Versed), milrinone (Primacor), morphine, nalbuphine, nitroglycerin IV, nitroprusside sodium, norepinephrine (Levophed), ondansetron (Zofran), palonosetron (Aloxi), pancuronium, phenylephrine (Neo-Synephrine), piperacillin/tazobactam (Zosyn), potassium chloride (KCl), procainamide (Pronestyl), prochlorperazine (Compazine), promethazine (Phenergan), ranitidine (Zantac), rocuronium (Zemuron), succinylcholine, sufentanil (Sufenta), sulfamethoxazole/trimethoprim, theophylline, ticarcillin/clavulanate (Timentin), tobramycin, vancomycin, vecuronium, verapamil.

RATE OF ADMINISTRATION

Variable, depending on indication, present blood volume, and patient response. Initial 500 mL may be given at rates approaching 20 mL/kg of body weight per hour. If additional hydroxyethyl starch is required, reduce flow to lowest rate possible to maintain hemodynamic status. If pressure infusion is used (flexible containers), withdraw all air through medication port before infusing. If a pumping device is used for administration, discontinue pumping action before the container runs dry or air embolism may result.

Leukapheresis: Usually infused at a constant ratio to venous whole blood (i.e., 1:8).

ACTIONS

A synthetic colloid solution. Pharmacologically classified as a plasma volume expander. The amount of plasma volume expansion produced approximates that of 5% albumin and decreases over the succeeding 24 to 36 hours. **Hextend** supports oncotic pressure and provides electrolytes. Its electrolyte content resembles that of normal plasma. **Hespan** supports oncotic pressure and increases erythrocyte sedimentation rate. Improves the efficiency of granulocyte collection by centrifugal means. Hetastarch molecules are rapidly eliminated by renal excretion.

G-H

INDICATIONS AND USES

HESPAN AND HEXTEND: Treatment of hypovolemia when plasma volume expansion is desired.

HESPAN: Adjunct in leukapheresis to improve harvesting and increase yield of granulocytes.

CONTRAINDICATIONS

Do not use in critically ill adult patients, including patients with sepsis. ▪ Severe liver disease. ▪ Hypersensitivity to hetastarch. ▪ Clinical conditions in which volume overload is a potential problem (such as CHF or renal disease with oliguria or anuria not related to hypovolemia). ▪ Pre-existing coagulation or bleeding disorders. ▪ **Hextend** contains lactate; not for use in leukapheresis or in the treatment of lactic acidosis.

PRECAUTIONS

HESPAN AND HEXTEND: For IV infusion only. ▪ Not a substitute for whole blood or plasma proteins. ▪ In critically ill adult patients, including patients with sepsis, the use of hydroxyethyl starch (HES) products, including Hespan and Hextend, increases the risk of mortality and renal replacement therapy. ▪ Avoid use in patients with pre-existing renal dysfunction. ▪ Discontinue use at the first sign of renal injury. ▪ Use caution in heart disease, congestive heart failure, pulmonary edema, and liver disease. ▪ Anaphylactic reactions have occurred, even after solutions containing hetastarch have been discontinued. Patients allergic to corn may also be allergic to hetastarch. ▪ Administration of large volumes may transiently alter the coagulation mechanism due to hemodilution and a mild direct inhibitory action on factor VIII. Hemodilution by isotonic solutions containing 6% hetastarch may also result in a 24-hour decline of total protein, albumin, and fibrinogen levels and in transient prolongation of prothrombin, activated partial thromboplastin, clotting, and bleeding times. Volumes greater than 25% of blood volume within 24 hours may cause significant hemodilution (decreased hematocrit and plasma proteins). Administration of packed RBCs, platelets, or fresh frozen plasma may be indicated. ▪ When used over a period of days, hetastarch has been associated with coagulation abnormalities in conjunction with an acquired reversible von Willebrand's–like syndrome and/or factor VIII deficiency. If a severe factor VIII deficiency is identified, replacement therapy may be indicated. If coagulopathy develops, it may take days to resolve. ▪ Not recommended for use as a cardiac bypass pump prime, while the patient is undergoing cardiopulmonary bypass, or in the immediate period after the pump has been discontinued. Risk of coagulopathies and bleeding increased.

HEXTEND: Use extreme caution in patients with metabolic or respiratory alkalosis; contains lactate ions. Excessive lactate may result in metabolic alkalosis. ▪ Contains electrolytes; use caution in patient populations in which sodium or potassium administration or retention could pose a problem (e.g., renal insufficiency, CHF, hyperkalemia, edema). Use caution in patients receiving corticosteroids and in renal or cardiac disease, particularly in digitalized patients. ▪ Contains dextrose; use caution in patients with overt diabetes.

Monitor: *Hespan and Hextend:* Monitor vital signs, hemoglobin, hematocrit, platelet count, prothrombin time, partial thromboplastin time, and renal and liver function tests. ▪ Acid-base balance, electrolytes, and serum protein evaluation are also necessary during therapy. ▪ Monitor renal function in hospitalized patients for at least 90 days because the use of renal replacement therapy has been reported up to 90 days after administration of hydroxyethyl starch solutions. ▪ May reduce coagulability of the circulating blood. Observe patient for increased bleeding and/or circulatory overload. Risk increased with higher doses.

Hespan: Monitor donors undergoing repeated leukapheresis procedures; may have a slight decline in platelet count and hemoglobin levels resulting from hemodilution by hetastarch and saline and the collection of platelets and erythrocytes. Temporary declines in total protein, albumin, calcium, and fibrinogen may also be present. Regular and frequent clinical evaluation and complete blood counts are necessary for proper monitoring of Hespan use during leukapheresis. If frequency of leukapheresis is to exceed the guidelines for whole blood donation, additional testing may be indicated; see manufacturer's prescribing information.

Maternal/Child: Category C: embryocidal to rabbits. Use only if benefit justifies the potential risk to the fetus. ▪ Use caution during breast-feeding. ▪ Safety and effectiveness for use in pediatric patients not established, but has been used. Increased prothrombin time noted in pediatric patients who received more than 20 mL/kg/24 hr.

Elderly: Differences in response between elderly and younger patients not identified. Risk of toxic reactions may be greater in patients with impaired renal function. Monitoring of renal function suggested in the elderly.

DRUG/LAB INTERACTIONS

Use with caution in patients receiving other drugs that affect coagulation (e.g., **anticoagulants** [e.g., argatroban, bivalirudin (Angiomax), heparin, warfarin (Coumadin)], **platelet aggregation inhibitors** [e.g., clopidogrel (Plavix), dipyridamole (Persantine), ticlopidine (Ticlid)], **glycoprotein GPIIb/IIIa receptor antagonists** [e.g., abciximab (ReoPro), eptifibatide (Integrilin), tirofiban (Aggrastat)], **plicamycin** [Mithracin], **valproic acid** [Depacon]). Close monitoring of aPTT and PT indicated. ▪ May increase **indirect bilirubin** levels. Total bilirubin remained normal. ▪ Elevated serum amylase levels have been observed, although no association with pancreatitis has been demonstrated.

SIDE EFFECTS

The most common adverse reactions are circulatory overload, coagulopathy, hemodilution, hypersensitivity (including anaphylaxis), and metabolic acidosis. Anemia and/or bleeding due to hemodilution and/or factor VIII deficiency, acquired von Willebrand's–like syndrome, and other coagulopathies, including DIC; chills; congestive heart failure; elevated serum amylase; fever; headache; increased urine specific gravity; intracranial bleeding; itching; muscle pains; peripheral edema; pulmonary edema; submaxillary and parotid glandular enlargement; urticaria; and vomiting have been reported.

Post-Marketing: Death, renal failure requiring renal replacement therapy.

ANTIDOTE

Notify the physician of any side effect. Discontinue the drug immediately at the first sign of a hypersensitivity reaction, provided other means of sustaining the circulation are available. Antihistamines such as diphenhydramine (Benadryl) are helpful. Epinephrine (Adrenalin) may also be indicated. Not eliminated by dialysis. Many side effects can result in medical emergencies. Deaths from severe hypersensitivity reactions have occurred. Treat as indicated and resuscitate as necessary.

HYDRALAZINE HYDROCHLORIDE
(hy-**DRAL**-ah-zeen hy-droh-**KLOR**-eyed)

Antihypertensive
Vasodilator

pH 3.4 to 4

USUAL DOSE
10 to 40 mg. Begin with a low dose. Increase gradually as indicated. Repeat every 3 to 6 hours as necessary. Maximum dose is 300 to 400 mg/24 hr.

Eclampsia: 5 to 10 mg every 20 minutes. If no effect after a total dose of 20 mg, use another agent.

PEDIATRIC DOSE
See Maternal/Child (unlabeled).

0.1 to 0.5 mg/kg/dose every 4 to 6 hours. Initial dose should not exceed 20 mg. Maximum IV dose is 0.2 to 0.8 mg/kg/dose up to 40 mg. Another source suggests 0.1 to 0.2 mg/kg/dose (not to exceed 20 mg) every 4 to 6 hours as needed. Up to 1.7 to 3.5 mg/kg/day divided in 4 to 6 doses.

DOSE ADJUSTMENTS
Reduced dose may be required with advanced renal disease and in the elderly. ▪ See Drug/Lab Interactions.

DILUTION
May be given undiluted. Do not add to IV solutions. May be given through Y-tube or three-way stopcock of infusion set. Color changes occur in most 10% dextrose solutions and after drawing through a metal filter. Use immediately after drawing up solution.

Filters: See Dilution.

COMPATIBILITY
(Underline Indicates Conflicting Compatibility Information)

Consider any drug NOT listed as compatible to be INCOMPATIBLE until consulting a pharmacist; specific conditions may apply.

One source suggests the following **compatibilities:**

Additive: Dobutamine.

Y-site: <u>Caspofungin (Cancidas)</u>, heparin, hydrocortisone sodium succinate (Solu-Cortef), <u>nitroglycerin IV</u>, potassium chloride, verapamil.

RATE OF ADMINISTRATION
Adults: A single dose over 1 minute.

Pediatric patients: A single dose over 3 to 5 minutes.

ACTIONS
A potent antihypertensive drug. It lowers BP by direct relaxation of smooth muscle of arteries and arterioles. Peripheral vasodilation and decreased peripheral vascular resistance result. HR, cardiac output, and stroke volume are all increased. Renal blood flow increased in some cases, while cerebral blood flow maintained. Onset of action is 5 to 20 minutes. Average duration of action is 2 to 6 hours. Metabolized by the liver and excreted in urine. Crosses placental barrier. Secreted in breast milk.

INDICATIONS AND USES
Severe essential hypertension. ▪ Vasodilation in cardiogenic shock. ▪ Drug of choice for pregnancy-induced hypertension (eclampsia).

CONTRAINDICATIONS
Hypersensitivity to hydralazine, coronary artery disease, mitral valvular rheumatic heart disease.

PRECAUTIONS
IV use recommended only when the oral route is not feasible. ▪ Rarely the drug of choice for hypertension unless used in combination (effectiveness increased and side effects decreased) with spironolactone (Aldactone), reserpine, guanethidine (Ismelin), and thiazide diuretics. ▪ Tolerance is easily developed but subsides about 7 days after the drug is discontinued. ▪ Use caution in advanced renal disease, cerebrovascular

accidents, congestive heart failure, coronary insufficiency, headache, increased intracranial pressure, and tachycardia. ▪ Use in pregnancy should be limited to treatment of eclampsia.

Monitor: Check BP every 5 minutes until stabilized at the desired level. Check every 15 minutes thereafter throughout crisis. Average maximum decrease occurs in 10 to 80 minutes. ▪ Withdraw drug gradually to avoid rebound hypertension.

Patient Education: Report chest pain, fatigue, fever, joint or muscle pain promptly.

Maternal/Child: Category C: can cause fetal abnormalities; see Indications and Precautions. ▪ Safety for use in pediatric patients not established. ▪ May be used in breast-feeding women.

Elderly: Increased risk of hypotension. ▪ Consider age-related renal impairment.

DRUG/LAB INTERACTIONS

Sometimes used with a **beta-adrenergic blocking drug** (e.g., propranolol) **or diuretics** (e.g., hydrochlorothiazide [Aldactazide]); use caution; may potentiate effects. ▪ Potentiated by **anesthetics, MAO inhibitors** (e.g., selegiline [Eldepryl]), **and other antihypertensive agents.** ▪ Inhibits **epinephrine, levarterenol** (Levophed). ▪ Use with **diazoxide** can cause profound hypotension. ▪ **NSAIDs** (e.g., ibuprofen [Motrin]) may decrease antihypotensive effect.

SIDE EFFECTS

May often be minimized by initiating therapy with a small dose and increasing the dose gradually.

Anxiety, depression, dry mouth, flushing, headache, nausea, numbness, palpitations, paresthesia, postural hypotension, tachycardia, tingling, unpleasant taste, vomiting.

Major: Angina, blood dyscrasias, chills, coronary insufficiency, delirium, dependent edema, fever, ileus, lupus erythematosus (simulated), myocardial ischemia and infarction, rheumatoid syndrome (simulated), toxic psychosis.

ANTIDOTE

If minor side effects occur, notify the physician, who will probably treat them symptomatically. Beta-adrenergic blocking agents (e.g., propranolol) will control tachycardia. Pyridoxine will relieve numbness, tingling, and paresthesia. Antihistamines, barbiturates, and salicylates may be required. Treat hypotension with a vasopressor that is least likely to precipitate cardiac arrhythmias. If side effects are progressive or any major side effects occur, discontinue the drug immediately and notify the physician. Treatment is symptomatic. Resuscitate as necessary. Occasionally methyldopa (Aldomet) will be used as a substitute because it is effective for the same indications but has fewer side effects.

G-H

HYDROCORTISONE SODIUM SUCCINATE

(hy-droh-**KOR**-tih-zohn **SO**-dee-um **SUK**-sih-nayt)

Hormone (corticosteroid)
Anti-inflammatory
Antiemetic

A-Hydrocort, Solu-Cortef

pH 7 to 8

USUAL DOSE

The IV route is usually used in an emergency situation or when oral dosing is not feasible. The lowest possible dose should be used to control condition. When reduction in dosage is possible, reduction should be gradual. Larger doses may be justified by patient condition. Repeat until adequate response, then decrease dose as indicated. Doses must be individualized and are not always reduced for pediatric patients. High dose treatment is utilized until patient condition stabilizes, usually no longer than 48 to 72 hours. Complications secondary to treatment with corticosteroids are dependent on the size of dose and duration of therapy.

Average dose range is 100 to 500 mg repeated as necessary every 2, 4, or 6 hours. For severe shock, doses up to 2 Gm or more every 2 to 10 hours have been given. Maximum dose is 8 Gm/24 hr. A minimum dose of no less than 25 mg/24 hr is recommended. Increased doses are indicated in patients undergoing corticosteroid therapy who are subjected to any unusual stressful situation (e.g., illness, surgery).

Other sources recommend:

Acute asthma: 1 to 2 mg/kg/dose every 6 hours for 24 hours. Follow with 0.5 to 1 mg/kg every 6 hours.

Anti-inflammatory or immunosuppressive: 15 to 240 mg every 12 hours.

Life-threatening shock: 50 mg/kg initially. Repeat in 4 hours and/or every 24 hours as needed *or*

0.5 to 2 Gm initially. Repeat every 2 to 6 hours as needed.

Adrenal insufficiency (acute): 100 mg as an IV bolus. Follow with 300 mg/day in divided doses every 8 hours or as a continuous infusion for 48 hours. Change to oral dosing when patient is stable.

Physiologic replacement: 20 to 30 mg/day (usually given PO).

PEDIATRIC DOSE

See Maternal/Child.

Average dose range in pediatric patients is 0.56 to 8 mg/kg/day in 3 to 4 divided doses (0.19 to 2.67 mg/kg every 8 hours or 0.14 to 2 mg/kg every 6 hours).

Other sources recommend:

Acute asthma: 1 to 2 mg/kg/dose every 6 hours for 24 hours; then 2 to 4 mg/kg/24 hr in equally divided doses every 6 hours (0.5 to 1 mg/kg every 6 hours). For status asthmaticus, another source suggests a *loading dose (optional)* of 4 to 8 mg/kg up to a maximum dose of 250 mg.

Maintenance dose: 8 mg/kg/24 hr in equally divided doses every 6 hours (2 mg/kg every 6 hours).

Anti-inflammatory: 1 to 5 mg/kg/24 hr, or 0.5 to 2.5 mg/kg every 12 hours, or 30 to 150 mg/M²/24 hr, or 15 to 75 mg/M² every 12 hours.

Adrenal insufficiency (acute): 1 to 2 mg/kg/dose bolus, then 25 to 150 mg/day in divided doses every 6 to 8 hours (8.33 to 50 mg every 8 hours or 6.25 to 37.5 mg every 6 hours) in infants and young children. In older children the bolus dose is the same, followed by 150 to 250 mg/day in divided doses every 6 to 8 hours (50 to 83.33 mg every 8 hours or 37.5 to 62.5 mg every 6 hours).

Physiologic replacement: 0.5 to 0.75 mg/kg/day given every 8 hours (usually given PO).

DOSE ADJUSTMENTS

Reduced dose may be required in the elderly. ▪ See Drug/Lab Interactions.

DILUTION

Available in Act-O-Vials and Univials, which are reconstituted by removing the protective cap, turning the rubber stopper a quarter turn, and pressing down, allowing the diluent into the lower chamber. Agitate gently. Using sterile techniques, a needle can be easily inserted through the center of the rubber stopper to withdraw the solution. Also available in flip-top vials. For these other preparations, reconstitute each 250 mg or fraction thereof with 2 mL bacteriostatic water for injection. Agitate gently to mix solution. May be given by IV injection, or each 100 mg (250 mg, 500 mg, or more) may be further diluted in at least 100 mL (250 mL, 500 mL, or more) but not more than 1,000 mL of D5W, NS, or D5NS.

Storage: Store vials and solutions at RT (20° to 25° C [68° to 77° F]). Protect solution from light. Discard unused solutions after 3 days. If fluid restriction is necessary, 100 to 3,000 mg may be added in 50 mL of **compatible** solution. Resultant solution is stable for 4 hours.

COMPATIBILITY   (Underline Indicates Conflicting Compatibility Information)

Consider any drug NOT listed as compatible to be INCOMPATIBLE until consulting a pharmacist; specific conditions may apply.

Manufacturer states, "Should not be diluted or mixed with other solutions."

One source suggests the following **compatibilities:**

Solution: Most commonly used IV solutions, fat emulsion 10% IV.

Additive: Amikacin, aminophylline, amphotericin B (conventional), ampicillin, anti-thymocyte globulin (rabbit) (Thymoglobulin), calcium chloride, calcium gluconate, chloramphenicol (Chloromycetin), clindamycin (Cleocin), cytarabine (ARA-C), daunorubicin (Cerubidine), dimenhydrinate, dopamine, erythromycin (Erythrocin), furosemide (Lasix), heparin, lidocaine, magnesium sulfate, metronidazole (Flagyl IV), mitomycin (Mutamycin), mitoxantrone (Novantrone), norepinephrine (Levophed), penicillin G potassium and sodium, potassium chloride (KCl), vancomycin, verapamil.

Y-site: Acetaminophen (Ofirmev), acyclovir (Zovirax), allopurinol (Aloprim), amifostine (Ethyol), aminophylline, amphotericin B cholesteryl (Amphotec), ampicillin, anidulafungin (Eraxis), anti-thymocyte globulin (rabbit) (Thymoglobulin), argatroban, atracurium (Tracrium), atropine, aztreonam (Azactam), bivalirudin (Angiomax), calcium gluconate, caspofungin (Cancidas), ceftaroline (Teflaro), chlorpromazine (Thorazine), cisatracurium (Nimbex), cladribine (Leustatin), cytarabine (ARA-C), dexamethasone (Decadron), digoxin (Lanoxin), diltiazem (Cardizem), diphenhydramine (Benadryl), docetaxel (Taxotere), dopamine, doripenem (Doribax), doxorubicin liposomal (Doxil), droperidol (Inapsine), edrophonium (Enlon), enalaprilat (Vasotec IV), epinephrine (Adrenalin), esmolol (Brevibloc), estrogens, conjugated (Premarin), ethacrynic acid (Edecrin), etoposide phosphate (Etopophos), famotidine (Pepcid IV), fenoldopam (Corlopam), fentanyl, filgrastim (Neupogen), fludarabine (Fludara), fluorouracil (5-FU), foscarnet (Foscavir), furosemide (Lasix), gallium nitrate (Ganite), gemcitabine (Gemzar), granisetron (Kytril), heparin, hetastarch in electrolytes (Hextend), hydralazine, isoproterenol (Isuprel), lidocaine, linezolid (Zyvox), lorazepam (Ativan), magnesium sulfate, melphalan (Alkeran), meperidine (Demerol), methylergonovine (Methergine), morphine, neostigmine, nicardipine (Cardene IV), norepinephrine (Levophed), ondansetron (Zofran), oxacillin (Bactocill), oxaliplatin (Eloxatin), oxytocin (Pitocin), paclitaxel (Taxol), pancuronium, penicillin G potassium, pentazocine (Talwin), phytonadione (vitamin K$_1$), piperacillin/tazobactam (Zosyn), procainamide (Pronestyl), prochlorperazine (Compazine), promethazine (Phenergan), propofol (Diprivan), propranolol, remifentanil (Ultiva), sodium bicarbonate, succinylcholine, tacrolimus (Prograf), telavancin (Vibativ), teniposide (Vumon), theophylline, thiotepa, vecuronium, vinorelbine (Navelbine).

RATE OF ADMINISTRATION

Each 100 mg or fraction thereof over 30 seconds to 1 minute. Extend to 10 minutes for larger doses (500 mg or more). IV injection is usually the route of choice and eliminates the possibility of overloading the patient with IV fluids. At the discretion of the physician, a continuous infusion may be given, properly diluted over the specified time desired.

ACTIONS

Contains the principal hormone secreted by the adrenal cortex and has both glucocorticoid and mineralocorticoid properties. Has potent metabolic, anti-inflammatory, and innumerable other effects. Peak plasma levels achieved promptly. Metabolized in the liver and excreted as inactive metabolites in the urine. Elimination half-life is 1 to 2 hours. Crosses placental barrier. Secreted in breast milk.

INDICATIONS AND USES

Agents of choice for adrenocortical insufficiency; total, relative, and operative. ▪ Agents of choice for acute exacerbation of disease for patients on steroid therapy. ▪ Occasionally used for asthma or shock, but nonmineralocorticoid steroids are preferred (e.g., dexamethasone, methylprednisolone).

CONTRAINDICATIONS

Absolute contraindications except in life-threatening situations: Hypersensitivity to any product component, including sulfites; systemic fungal infections. ▪ Administration of live or live-attenuated vaccines in patients receiving an immunosuppressive dose of corticosteroids.

Relative contraindications: Active or latent peptic ulcer, active or latent tuberculosis, chickenpox, diverticulitis, fresh intestinal anastomoses, measles, myasthenia gravis, ocular herpes simplex, pregnancy, thromboembolic tendencies, vaccinia.

PRECAUTIONS

To avoid relative adrenocortical insufficiency, do not stop therapy abruptly. Taper off. Patient is observed carefully, especially under stress, for up to 2 years. The exception is very short-term therapy. ▪ Anaphylactoid reactions have occurred (incidence is rare). ▪ Increased doses are indicated in patients undergoing corticosteroid therapy who are subjected to any unusual stressful situation (e.g., illness, surgery). ▪ Should not be used for treatment of traumatic brain injury. May increase mortality. ▪ Use with caution in patients who have had a recent MI. May be associated with left ventricular free wall rupture. ▪ Kaposi's sarcoma has been reported in patients receiving corticosteroid therapy, most often for chronic conditions. Clinical improvement may occur if therapy is discontinued. ▪ Use with caution in patients with CHF, hypertension, or renal insufficiency; see Monitor. ▪ Use with caution in patients with active or latent peptic ulcer disease, diverticulitis, fresh intestinal anastomoses, and nonspecific ulcerative colitis; may increase risk of perforation. Prophylactic antacids may prevent peptic ulcer complications. ▪ May induce psychological side effects (e.g., euphoria, insomnia, mood swings, depression, psychosis) or may aggravate existing emotional instability or psychotic tendencies.

Monitor: Monitor electrolytes. May cause sodium retention and potassium and calcium excretion. Dietary salt restriction and potassium supplementation may be necessary. May cause hypertension secondary to fluid and electrolyte disturbances. ▪ May increase susceptibility to infection, reactivate latent infectious diseases, or mask signs of infection. ▪ Monitor blood glucose. May increase insulin needs in diabetes. ▪ Administer before 9 AM to reduce suppression of individual's own adrenocortical activity. ▪ Periodic ophthalmic exams may be necessary with prolonged treatment. ▪ See Drug/Lab Interactions.

Patient Education: Do not discontinue abruptly. ▪ Advise all medical personnel of current or past corticosteroid use. ▪ Report edema, tarry stools, or weight gain promptly. Anorexia, diarrhea, dizziness, fatigue, low blood sugar, nausea, weakness, weight loss, and vomiting may indicate adrenal insufficiency after dose reduction or discontinuation of therapy; report any of these symptoms. ▪ May mask signs of infection and/or decrease resistance. ▪ Patients with diabetes may have an increased requirement for insulin or oral hypoglycemics. ▪ Avoid immunization with live virus vaccines. ▪ Carry ID stating steroid dependent if receiving prolonged therapy.

Maternal/Child: Category C: could produce fetal abnormalities. ▪ Discontinue breast-feeding. ▪ Observe newborn for hypoadrenalism if mother has received large doses. ▪ Observe growth and development in long-term use in pediatric patients.

Elderly: Reduced muscle mass and plasma volume may require a reduced dose. ▪ Monitor BP, blood glucose, and electrolytes carefully; increased risk of hypertension. ▪ Higher risk of glucocorticoid-induced osteoporosis.

DRUG/LAB INTERACTIONS
Aminoglutethimide (Cytadren) may increase the metabolism of hydrocortisone, thereby decreasing therapeutic effects. Monitor carefully if concurrent use is necessary. ▪ Metabolism increased and effects reduced by **hepatic enzyme–inducing agents** (e.g., alcohol, barbiturates [e.g., phenobarbital], hydantoins [e.g., phenytoin (Dilantin)], and rifampin [Rifadin]); dose adjustment may be required when adding or deleting from drug profile. ▪ Risk of hypokalemia increased with **amphotericin B or potassium-depleting diuretics** (e.g., thiazides, furosemide, ethacrynic acid). Monitor potassium levels and cardiac function. Increased risk of **digoxin** toxicity secondary to hypokalemia. ▪ May also decrease effectiveness of **potassium supplements;** monitor serum potassium. ▪ **Diuretics** decrease sodium and fluid retention effects of corticosteroids; corticosteroids decrease sodium excretion and diuretic effects of diuretics. ▪ May antagonize effects of **anticholinesterases** (e.g., neostigmine), **isoniazid** (INH), **salicylates, and somatrem;** dose adjustments may be required. ▪ Clearance decreased and effects increased with **estrogens, oral contraceptives, macrolide antibiotics** (e.g., azithromycin [Zithromax]), **and ketoconazole** (Nizoral). ▪ May interact with **anticoagulants, nondepolarizing muscle relaxants** (e.g., atracurium [Tracrium]), **or theophyllines;** may inhibit or potentiate action. ▪ Monitor patients receiving **insulin or thyroid hormones** carefully; dose adjustments of either or both agents may be required. ▪ Increased activity of both **hydrocortisone and cyclosporine** may occur with concurrent use. Therapeutic use is beneficial for organ transplants; however, toxicity may also be increased, and convulsions have been reported. ▪ Concurrent use with **aspirin or NSAIDs** (e.g., ibuprofen [Motrin], naproxen [Aleve, Naprosyn]) may increase the risk of GI side effects. ▪ Administration of **live or live-attenuated vaccines** is contraindicated in patients receiving immunosuppressive dose of corticosteroids. Inactivated vaccines may be administered; however, the response to these vaccines cannot be predicted. ▪ Altered **protein-binding capacity** will impact effectiveness of this drug. ▪ **Corticosteroids** may suppress reactions to skin tests. ▪ See Dose Adjustments.

SIDE EFFECTS
Do occur but are usually reversible: alteration of glucose metabolism including hyperglycemia and glycosuria; Cushing's syndrome (e.g., moon face, fat pads); electrolyte and calcium imbalance; euphoria or other psychic disturbances; hypersensitivity reactions including anaphylaxis; increased BP; increased intracranial pressure; masking of infection; menstrual irregularities; perforation and hemorrhage from aggravation of peptic ulcer; protein catabolism with negative nitrogen balance; spontaneous fractures; sweating, headache, or weakness; thromboembolism; transitory burning or tingling; and many others.

ANTIDOTE
Notify the physician of any side effect. Will probably treat the side effect if necessary. Resuscitate as necessary for anaphylaxis and notify physician. Keep epinephrine immediately available.

G-H

HYDROMORPHONE HYDROCHLORIDE BBW

(hy-droh-**MOR**-fohn hy-droh-**KLOR**-eyed)

Opioid analgesic
(agonist)

Dilaudid, Dilaudid HP

pH 3.5 to 5.5, 4.5 to 6.5

USUAL DOSE

Individualize dose based on age; general condition and medical status; degree of opioid tolerance; daily dose, potency, and specifics of previous opioids prescribed; concurrent medications; type and severity of pain; risk factors for abuse or addiction (e.g., previous or current abuse problem, family history of abuse, history of mental illness or depression); balance between pain control and adverse reactions.

Dispense with caution; dosing errors due to confusion between different concentrations and between mg and mL could result in accidental overdose and death. Oral and IV doses of hydromorphone and IV doses with doses of other opioids are *NOT* equivalent; see prescribing information for a discussion on opioid conversion and equianalgesic potency for conversion to hydromorphone injection.

IV injection: Usual starting dose is 0.2 to 1 mg every 2 to 3 hours as needed for pain. Titrate dose to achieve acceptable pain management and tolerable adverse events.

Infusion: Used postoperatively with a patient-controlled analgesic device (PCA) and in selected terminally ill cancer patients. One source suggests a concentration of 0.2 mg/mL, with a starting patient-controlled dose of 0.1 to 0.2 mg (range 0.05 to 0.4 mg) that can be activated at prescribed intervals. Must be administered through a controlled infusion device that may be patient activated. The initial loading dose, the continuous background infusion (if prescribed), additional patient-activated doses with a specific time interval, additional health care professional–provided boluses with a specific time interval, and the total dose allowed per hour must be determined by the physician specialist and individualized for each patient.

PEDIATRIC DOSE

Individualized on the basis of age and weight (unlabeled). One source suggests 0.015 mg/kg/dose every 4 to 6 hours as needed in pediatric patients; see Contraindications and Maternal/Child.

DOSE ADJUSTMENTS

Dose selection should be cautious in the elderly and debilitated. Reduced initial doses may be indicated based on the potential for increased sensitivity, decreased organ function, and concomitant disease or drug therapy. ▪ Depending on the degree of impairment, one-fourth to one-half the usual starting dose is recommended in patients with impaired renal or hepatic function. ▪ Use lower initial doses in opiate-naïve patients. ▪ Doses appropriate for the general population may cause serious respiratory depression in vulnerable patients. ▪ Increase doses as required if analgesia is inadequate, tolerance develops, or pain severity increases. The first sign of tolerance is usually a reduced duration of effect. ▪ Decrease dose if excessive side effects are observed early in the dosing interval. If this results in breakthrough pain at the end of the dosing interval, the dosing interval may be shortened. ▪ See Drug/Lab Interactions.

DILUTION

Available in more than one concentration (1 mg/mL, 2 mg/mL, and 4 mg/mL) and hydromorphone-HP (a high-potency [10 mg/mL]) formulation. Do not confuse hydromorphone-HP with standard formulations of hydromorphone or other opioids; overdose and death could result. Hydromorphone-HP is usually reserved for compounding in the pharmacy or for use in opioid-tolerant patients. Verify concentration to avoid overdose and/or death.

IV injection: May be given undiluted; further dilution with 5 mL NS to facilitate titration is appropriate. May give through Y-tube or three-way stopcock of infusion set.

Infusion: Each 0.1 to 1 mg is usually diluted in 1 mL NS to provide 0.1 to 1 mg/mL for use in a narcotic syringe infusor system. Dilaudid is available in 1-, 2-, or 4-mg/mL clear ampules. Dilaudid-HP is available in 10-mg/mL amber ampules and as lyophilized powder that must be reconstituted with 25 mL SWFI for a concentration of 10 mg/mL. Generic hydromorphone is available in similar concentrations; check mg/mL carefully. Use concentrated preparations for larger doses. May be diluted in larger amounts of D5W, D5NS, D5/^{1}/$_2$NS, or NS for infusion and given through a standard infusion pump (requires very close titration).

Storage: Store at CRT and protect from light and freezing. Stable for 24 hours at 25 C° (77° F), protected from light, in most common large-volume parenteral solutions.

COMPATIBILITY   (Underline Indicates Conflicting Compatibility Information)
   Consider any drug NOT listed as compatible to be INCOMPATIBLE until consulting a pharmacist; specific conditions may apply.
   One source suggests the following **compatibilities:**
   Additive: Fluorouracil (5-FU), heparin, midazolam (Versed), ondansetron (Zofran), potassium chloride (KCl), promethazine (Phenergan), verapamil.
   Y-site: Acetaminophen (Ofirmev), acyclovir (Zovirax), allopurinol (Aloprim), amifostine (Ethyol), amikacin, ampicillin, atropine, aztreonam (Azactam), bivalirudin (Angiomax), caspofungin (Cancidas), cefazolin (Ancef), cefotaxime (Claforan), cefoxitin (Mefoxin), ceftaroline (Teflaro), ceftazidime (Fortaz), cefuroxime (Zinacef), chloramphenicol (Chloromycetin), cisatracurium (Nimbex), cladribine (Leustatin), clindamycin (Cleocin), dexamethasone (Decadron), dexmedetomidine (Precedex), diazepam (Valium), diltiazem (Cardizem), diphenhydramine (Benadryl), dobutamine, docetaxel (Taxotere), dopamine, doripenem (Doribax), doxorubicin liposomal (Doxil), doxycycline, epinephrine (Adrenalin), erythromycin (Erythrocin), etoposide phosphate (Etopophos), famotidine (Pepcid IV), fenoldopam (Corlopam), fentanyl, filgrastim (Neupogen), fludarabine (Fludara), foscarnet (Foscavir), furosemide (Lasix), gemcitabine (Gemzar), gentamicin, granisetron (Kytril), heparin, hetastarch in electrolytes (Hextend), 6% hydroxyethyl starch (Voluven), ketorolac (Toradol), labetalol, levofloxacin (Levaquin), linezolid (Zyvox), lorazepam (Ativan), magnesium sulfate, melphalan (Alkeran), metoclopramide (Reglan), metronidazole (Flagyl IV), micafungin (Mycamine), midazolam (Versed), milrinone (Primacor), morphine, nafcillin (Nallpen), nicardipine (Cardene IV), nitroglycerin IV, norepinephrine (Levophed), ondansetron (Zofran), oxacillin (Bactocill), oxaliplatin (Eloxatin), paclitaxel (Taxol), palonosetron (Aloxi), pemetrexed (Alimta), penicillin G potassium, phenobarbital (Luminal), piperacillin/tazobactam (Zosyn), propofol (Diprivan), ranitidine (Zantac), remifentanil (Ultiva), sulfamethoxazole/trimethoprim, tacrolimus (Prograf), teniposide (Vumon), thiotepa, tobramycin, vancomycin, vecuronium, vinorelbine (Navelbine).

RATE OF ADMINISTRATION
   Rapid IV administration increases the possibility of hypotension and respiratory depression.
   IV injection: Administer a single dose over a minimum of 2 to 3 minutes. Frequently titrated according to symptom relief and respiratory rate.
   Infusion: All parameters (outlined in Usual Dose) should be ordered by the physician. Any dose requiring a controlled infusion device requires accurate titration and close monitoring.

ACTIONS
   A mu-opioid receptor agonist closely related to morphine. Precise mode of action unknown, but opioids are believed to combine with specific CNS opiate receptors. Pharmacologic effects include analgesia, anxiolysis, cough suppression, euphoria, and feelings of relaxation. Seven times more potent than morphine milligram for milligram. Produces respiratory depression by direct effect on brainstem respiratory centers and reduces the responsiveness to increases in carbon dioxide. Causes a reduction of motility in the GI tract. May produce hypotension due to either peripheral vasodilation, release of histamine, or both. Onset of action is prompt, and half-life is about 2.3 hours. Hydromor-

G-H

phone is metabolized in the liver and excreted in the urine. Crosses placental barrier. Secreted in breast milk.

INDICATIONS AND USES

Hydromorphone (1 mg/mL, 2 mg/mL, or 4 mg/mL): Management of pain in patients for whom an opioid analgesic is appropriate.

High-potency hydromorphone (10 mg/mL): Management of moderate-to-severe pain in opioid-tolerant patients who require larger-than-usual doses of opioids to provide adequate pain relief. Patients considered opioid-tolerant are those who are taking at least 60 mg oral morphine/day, 25 mcg transdermal fentanyl/hr, 30 mg oral oxycodone/day, 8 mg hydromorphone/day, 25 mg oral oxymorphone/day, or an equianalgesic dose of another opioid for 1 week or longer.

CONTRAINDICATIONS

Hypersensitivity to hydromorphone, any of its components, or sulfite-containing medications. ▪ Acute or severe bronchial asthma, respiratory depression in the absence of resuscitation equipment or in unmonitored settings. ▪ In patients with, or at risk for developing, GI obstruction, especially paralytic ileus. ▪ Hydromorphone-HP is contraindicated in patients who are not opioid tolerant.

PRECAUTIONS

Hydromorphone-HP is for use in opioid-tolerant patients only. ▪ Use of hydromorphone and hydromorphone-HP carries the risk of respiratory depression, abuse, and medication errors. Do not confuse hydromorphone-HP formulations with standard formulations of hydromorphone or with other opioids; overdose and death could result. ▪ Schedule II opioid agonists, including hydromorphone, morphine, oxymorphone, oxycodone, fentanyl, and methadone, have the highest potential for abuse and a risk of producing fatal overdose due to respiratory depression. Alcohol, CNS depressants, and other opioids potentiate the respiratory depressant effects of hydromorphone, increasing the risk for respiratory depression that might result in death; see Drug/Lab Interactions. ▪ Use caution in elderly or debilitated patients and in patients with conditions accompanied by hypoxia or hypercapnia or upper airway obstruction. In these patients, even moderate therapeutic doses may dangerously decrease pulmonary ventilation. ▪ Use with extreme caution in patients with COPD, cor pulmonale, a substantially decreased respiratory reserve, hypoxia, hypercapnia, or pre-existing respiratory depression. Usual therapeutic doses may decrease respiratory drive while simultaneously increasing airway resistance to the point of apnea. Consider using nonopioid analgesics, or administer under careful medical supervision at the lowest effective dose in these patients. ▪ Use with alcohol and other CNS depressants increases the risk of respiratory depression, hypotension, or profound sedation and could result in coma or death; see Drug/Lab Interactions. ▪ Use with caution and reduce initial doses in elderly or debilitated patients; in patients with severe impairment of hepatic, pulmonary, or renal function; and in patients with myxedema or hypothyroidism, adrenocortical insufficiency (e.g., Addison's disease), CNS depression or coma, toxic psychoses, prostatic hypertrophy or urethral stricture, acute alcoholism, delirium tremens, or kyphoscoliosis associated with respiratory depression. ▪ The respiratory depressant effects of hydromorphone promote carbon dioxide retention, resulting in increased intracranial pressure (ICP). This increase in ICP may be markedly exaggerated in the presence of head injury, intracranial lesions, or other conditions that predispose patients to ICP. The effects on pupillary response and consciousness can obscure the clinical course and neurologic signs of further pressure increases in patients with head injuries. ▪ May cause severe hypotension in patients whose ability to maintain blood pressure is compromised by a depleted blood volume or a concurrent administration of drugs such as general anesthetics, phenothiazines, or other agents that compromise vasomotor tone; see Drug/Lab Interactions. ▪ Use with caution in patients in circulatory shock. Vasodilation caused by the drug may further reduce cardiac output and BP. ▪ May produce orthostatic hypotension in ambulatory patients. ▪ Avoid administration in patients with GI obstruction. Use with caution in patients who are at risk for developing ileus. Diminishes peristalsis and may prolong obstruction. ▪ Symptoms of acute abdominal conditions may be masked. Use with caution in patients with biliary tract disease, including acute pancreatitis; may cause spasm of the sphincter of Oddi and diminish biliary and pancreatic secretions. ▪ Cough reflex may be suppressed. ▪ Seizures and myoclonus have been reported in patients administered high parenteral doses. May also aggravate pre-existing seizures in patients with a convulsive disorder and may induce or aggravate seizures in some clinical settings. ▪ Tolerance (the need to increase doses to maintain a defined effect such as analgesia) to the different effects of hydromorphone may develop to varying degrees and at varying rates. ▪ A Schedule II controlled substance. Physical dependence can develop but is not a factor in the presence of chronic cancer and noncancer pain. Physical dependence is manifest by withdrawal symptoms after abrupt discontinuation of a drug or upon administration of an antagonist. ▪ Abuse and addiction are separate and distinct from physical dependence and tolerance. Abuse poses a hazard of overdose and death. Use with caution in patients with alcoholism and other drug dependencies. See prescribing information for further discussion regarding abuse, addiction, physical dependence, and tolerance. ▪ Some products may use a latex stopper and some may contain sulfites; may cause a hypersensitivity reaction in susceptible patients. ▪ See Maternal/Child.

Monitor: Oxygen, naloxone, and equipment to establish and maintain an airway must be available. ▪ Assess baseline pain, reassess after administration of hydromorphone, and adjust dose or interval as required. ▪ Monitor vital signs and observe patient frequently to continuously based on dose administered. ▪ Keep patient supine; orthostatic hypotension and fainting may occur; less likely with continuous low doses, but observe closely during ambulation. ▪ Uncontrolled pain causes sleep deprivation, decreases pain threshold, and increases pain. When pain is finally controlled, expect the patient to sleep more until recovery from sleep deprivation. ▪ Laxatives with or without stool softeners will be required to avoid constipation and fecal impaction, especially with increased doses and extended use. Maintain adequate hydration.

Patient Education: Avoid alcohol or other CNS depressants (e.g., barbiturates, benzodiazepines [e.g., diazepam (Valium)]). ▪ May cause blurred vision, drowsiness, or dizziness; use caution in tasks that require alertness. ▪ Request assistance with ambulation. ▪ May be habit forming. ▪ Take only as directed. ▪ Report unrelieved pain or unacceptable side effects promptly.

Maternal/Child: Category C: use during pregnancy only if the potential benefit justifies the risk to the fetus. ▪ Use during labor and delivery may produce respiratory depression and a physiologic effect in neonates. May also prolong labor by reducing the strength, duration, and frequency of contractions. ▪ Not recommended for use in breast-feeding mothers. ▪ Infants born to mothers physically dependent on opioids will also be physically dependent and may exhibit respiratory difficulties and withdrawal symptoms (e.g., excessive crying, fever, hyperactive reflexes, increased respiratory rate, increased stools, sneezing, tremors, vomiting, yawning). Neonatal opioid withdrawal syndrome may be life threatening and should be treated according to established protocols. ▪ Safety and effectiveness for use in pediatric patients not established. ▪ Pediatric patients may be more sensitive to effects (e.g., respiratory depression).

Elderly: See Dose Adjustments and Precautions. ▪ May be more susceptible to effects (e.g., respiratory depression, urinary retention, constipation). ▪ Lower doses may provide effective analgesia.

DRUG/LAB INTERACTIONS

Potentiated by **phenothiazines and other CNS depressants** such as opioid analgesics, alcohol, anticholinergics, antihistamines, barbiturates, centrally acting antiemetics, general anesthetics, hypnotics, sedatives, MAO inhibitors (e.g., selegiline [Eldepryl]), psychotropic agents (e.g., antidepressants, antianxiety agents), and skeletal muscle relaxants (e.g., cyclobenzaprine [Flexeril]). Side effects (e.g., CNS or respiratory depression, constipation, hypotension) may be additive. Reduced dosages of both drugs may be indicated. Hydromorphone may enhance the action of neuromuscular blocking agents (e.g., atracurium [Tracrium]) and produce an increased degree of respiratory depression. ▪ Do not initiate treatment with hydromorphone within 14 days of use of a **MAO inhibitor.** ▪ Administration of **agonist/antagonist analgesics** (e.g., butorphanol [Stadol], buprenorphine [Buprenex]) to an opiate-dependent patient receiving a pure opiate may precipitate withdrawal symptoms. ▪ Concurrent use with **anticholinergics** (e.g., dimenhydrinate) or **drugs with anticholinergic activity** may cause urinary retention, severe constipation, and paralytic ileus. ▪ Plasma **amylase and lipase determinations** may be unreliable for 24 hours following opioid administration.

SIDE EFFECTS

Most frequently occurring side effects include dizziness, dry mouth, dysphoria, euphoria, flushing, light-headedness, nausea, pruritus, sedation, sweating, and vomiting. Other side effects may include abnormal dreams; agitation; alteration of moods; anorexia; antidiuretic effects; anxiety; arrhythmias (e.g., bradycardia, palpitations, tachycardia); biliary colic; blurred or impaired vision; bronchospasm; chills; depression; disorientation and hallucination; drug abuse, addiction, and dependence; GI effects (e.g., abdominal pain, constipation, diarrhea, ileus) and effects in sphincter of Oddi; headache; hypotension; increased intracranial pressure; injection site pain and urticaria; insomnia; laryngospasm; miosis; muscle rigidity; nervousness; nystagmus; paresthesia; rash; seizures; shock; taste alteration; tremor; urinary retention or hesitancy; weakness.

Overdose: Apnea, atypical snoring, bradycardia, cardiac arrest, circulatory depression or collapse, cold and clammy skin, constricted pupils, hypotension (severe), partial or complete airway obstruction, respiratory depression or arrest, skeletal muscle flaccidity, somnolence progressing to stupor or coma, and death.

Post-Marketing: Anaphylactic reactions, confused state, convulsions, dyskinesia, dyspnea, erectile dysfunction, increased hepatic enzymes, hyperalgesia, hypersensitivity reactions, injection site reactions, myoclonus, oropharyngeal swelling, peripheral edema, and somnolence.

ANTIDOTE

Notify the physician of any side effect. If minor side effects progress or any major side effect occurs, including the onset of symptoms of overdose, discontinue the drug and notify the physician. Naloxone will reverse serious cardiovascular, CNS, and respiratory reactions. Naloxone use should be reserved for situations in which clinically significant respiratory or circulatory depression is present. Titrate naloxone dose carefully to avoid precipitating an acute abstinence syndrome or uncontrolled pain. The duration of action of hydromorphone may exceed the duration of action of naloxone. Monitor patient carefully. Repeat doses of naloxone may be required. A patent airway, artificial ventilation, oxygen therapy, and other symptomatic treatment must be instituted promptly. Treat anaphylaxis as indicated or resuscitate as necessary.

HYDROXOCOBALAMIN

Antidote

(hy-**DROX**-oh-koh-**BAL**-ah-min)

Cyanokit

pH 3.5 to 6

USUAL DOSE

Manufacturer provides a quick-use reference guide in carton to facilitate immediate administration. It covers reconstitution, mixing, infusion rate, common S/S of cyanide poisoning with or without smoke inhalation, **incompatibilities,** and alternate diluents.

Initial dose: 5 Gm administered by IV infusion over 15 minutes. Based on severity of poisoning and clinical response, a second 5-Gm dose may be administered for a total dose of 10 Gm.

PEDIATRIC DOSE

Safety and effectiveness for use in pediatric patients not established but has been used outside the United States.

Initial dose (unlabeled): 70 mg/kg.

DOSE ADJUSTMENTS

No dose adjustments required in the elderly. ▪ Potential need for dose adjustment in patients with impaired hepatic or renal function has not been studied.

DILUTION

Each kit contains one 5-Gm, 250-mL glass vial of lyophilized hydroxocobalamin, a sterile transfer spike, a sterile vented infusion tubing, a quick-use reference guide, and a package insert. The glass vial is marked with a fill line for diluent. Using a sterile spike, transfer 200 mL of NS diluent into the glass vial (to the fill line [25 mg/mL]). If NS is not available, LR or D5W may be used. **Do Not Shake!** Invert or rock vial for at least 60 seconds to mix. Solution should be clear and dark red. Attach infusion tubing and begin infusion of the first vial; see Rate of Administration.

Filters: Specific information not available.

Storage: Store kit at CRT. See package insert for allowable storage temperatures for kit transport in extreme weather conditions. Reconstituted product may be held at a temperature not to exceed 40° C (104° F) for up to 6 hours. Do not freeze. Discard any unused portion after 6 hours.

COMPATIBILITY

Manufacturer lists as **incompatible** with ascorbic acid, blood products (whole blood, packed red cells, platelet concentrate, and/or fresh frozen plasma), diazepam (Valium), dobutamine, dopamine, fentanyl, nitroglycerin IV, pentobarbital (Nembutal), propofol (Diprivan), sodium nitrite, sodium thiosulfate. Do not administer simultaneously through the same IV line. Use of a separate line on the opposing extremity is recommended.

RATE OF ADMINISTRATION

Each 5-Gm dose properly diluted and evenly distributed over 15 minutes. The rate of infusion for the second 5-Gm dose may range from 15 minutes (for a patient in extremis) to 2 hours based on patient condition.

ACTIONS

A high dose of cyanide can result in death within minutes by inhibiting the cells' ability to use oxygen (inhibition of cytochrome oxidase results in arrest of cellular respiration). Specifically, cyanide binds with a component of cytochrome oxidase (cytochrome a3), prevents the cell from using oxygen, and forces anaerobic metabolism; this results in lactate production, cellular hypoxia, and metabolic acidosis. Each molecule of hydroxocobalamin can bind one cyanide ion to form cyanocobalamin (vitamin B_{12}) and reverse the toxic process. Cyanocobalamin is then excreted in urine.

INDICATIONS AND USES

Treatment of known or suspected cyanide poisoning. Administer without delay if clinical suspicion of cyanide poisoning is high. Symptoms of cyanide poisoning include chest tightness, confusion, dyspnea, headache, nausea. Signs of cyanide poisoning include altered mental status (e.g., confusion, disorientation), seizures or coma, mydriasis (excessive dilation of the pupil of the eye), abnormally rapid or deep breathing (early), abnormally slow breathing or apnea (late), hypertension (early), hypotension (late), cardiovascular collapse, vomiting, plasma lactate concentration equal to or greater than 8 mmol/L. Smoke inhalation victims with cyanide poisoning have usually been exposed to fire and smoke in an enclosed area and may present with soot around mouth, nose, and/ or oropharynx or an altered mental status. They may have a plasma lactate concentration equal to or greater than 10 mmol/L.

CONTRAINDICATIONS

Manufacturer states, "None"; see Precautions.

PRECAUTIONS

For IV use only. ▪ In addition to treatment with hydroxocobalamin, immediate confirmation of airway patency, adequacy of oxygenation and hydration, cardiovascular support (may be hypotensive or hypertensive), and management of seizure activity is required. Decontamination measures may also be indicated. ▪ Use caution in patients with known hypersensitivity to hydroxocobalamin or cyanocobalamin (vitamin B_{12}). Consider alternative treatments if available (e.g., sodium nitrite and sodium thiosulfate). ▪ Collection of a pretreatment blood sample would be useful in confirming a diagnosis of cyanide poisoning but should not delay treatment. ▪ May cause photosensitivity. ▪ Use in patients with impaired hepatic or renal function has not been studied. ▪ See Drug/Lab Interactions.

Monitor: Immediately confirm airway patency, adequacy of oxygenation, and adequate hydration. ▪ If feasible, draw a pretreatment blood sample; see Precautions. ▪ Monitor BP (may be hypotensive or hypertensive [BP equal to or greater than 180 mm Hg systolic or equal to or greater than 110 mm Hg diastolic has been reported with this treatment]). Hypertension may occur at the beginning of the infusion, is usually at a maximum by the end of the infusion, and should return to baseline within 4 hours. Note Compatibility if treatment is required. ▪ Monitor for seizures. Note Compatibility if treatment is required. ▪ Monitor for S/S of hypersensitivity reactions (e.g., anaphylaxis, angioneurotic edema, chest tightness, dyspnea, edema, pruritus, rash, urticaria).

Patient Education: Skin redness may last up to 2 weeks. Avoid sun exposure while skin is red. ▪ Urine redness may last up to 5 weeks. ▪ An acne-like rash may appear 7 to 28 days after treatment. Has usually resolved without treatment. ▪ Discontinue breastfeeding; talk with your physician to see when and if you can resume. ▪ Report any side effect that is troublesome or doesn't go away.

Maternal/Child: Category C: has caused skeletal and visceral abnormalities in animal studies. Because cyanide readily crosses the placenta, maternal cyanide poisoning results in fetal cyanide poisoning that can be life threatening to the mother and fetus. Consider benefit versus risk before use in pregnancy and labor and delivery. ▪ Discontinue breastfeeding until cleared with physician. ▪ Safety and effectiveness for use in pediatric patients not established but has been used outside the United States.

Elderly: Safety and effectiveness similar to that seen in younger adults.

DRUG/LAB INTERACTIONS

Formal drug interaction studies have not been conducted. ▪ **Sodium nitrite and sodium thiosulfate** are also used to treat cyanide poisoning. They are **incompatible** with hydroxocobalamin and must be administered in a separate IV line if used concurrently. Safety of coadministration has not been established. ▪ Because of its deep red color, hydroxocobalamin **interferes with numerous clinical laboratory tests.** Effects persist for varying lengths of time depending on test. See package insert for specifics. ▪ Deep red color may cause hemodialysis machines to shut down (an erroneous detection of a "blood leak"). Consider before hemodialysis is initiated in patients treated with hydroxocobalamin.

SIDE EFFECTS

Most common side effects include chromaturia, decreased lymphocytes, erythema, headache, hypertension, injection site reactions, nausea, and rash. Hypersensitivity reactions and hypertension are the most serious side effects associated with hydroxocobalamin. Other reactions that may occur include abdominal discomfort, chest discomfort, diarrhea, dizziness, dry throat, dyspepsia, dysphagia, dyspnea, hematochezia (blood in stool), hot flashes, impaired memory, irritation, peripheral edema, pruritus, redness and swelling of the eyes, restlessness, throat tightness, urticaria, and vomiting.

ANTIDOTE
Keep physician informed of all side effects; will be treated symptomatically. Note Compatibility before treating hypertension or seizures; use an alternate IV line if indicated. Severe hypersensitivity reactions may require epinephrine (Adrenalin), antihistamines (e.g., diphenhydramine [Benadryl]), corticosteroids (e.g., hydrocortisone), or bronchodilators (e.g., albuterol, theophylline). Data on overdose not available; manage symptomatically. Hemodialysis may be effective and is indicated for significant hydroxocobalamin toxicity. Cardiac and/or respiratory arrest may occur before treatment has an effect; resuscitate as indicated.

6% HYDROXYETHYL STARCH 130/0.4 IN 0.9% SODIUM CHLORIDE INJECTION BBW
Plasma volume substitute

(hy-**DROX**-ee-eth-ihl starch)

Voluven pH 4 to 5.5

USUAL DOSE
Variable depending on patient's blood loss, maintenance or restoration of hemodynamics, and hemodilution (dilution effect). Daily dose may be administered repetitively over several days. Titrate to individual colloid needs, hydration status, and hemodynamics.
Initial infusion: Administer initial 10 to 20 mL of infusion slowly. Observe patient continuously for S/S of a possible hypersensitivity reaction.
Daily dose: Up to 50 mL/kg of body weight per day (equivalent to 3 Gm hydroxyethyl starch and 7.7 mEq sodium/kg body weight). This dose is equivalent to 3,500 mL for a 70-kg patient.

PEDIATRIC DOSE
See Usual Dose. Pediatric dose should be adjusted to the individual patient's colloid needs, taking into account the patient's underlying disease state and hemodynamic and hydration status. Doses used in clinical trials are listed in the following chart.

Pediatric Dosing of 6% Hydroxyethyl Starch 130/0.4 in 0.9% Sodium Chloride in Clinical Trials		
Pediatric Age-Groups	Recommended Daily Dose	Mean Daily Dose ± SD* in Clinical Trials
<2 years	Up to 50 mL/kg body weight in all age-groups	16 ± 9 mL/kg body weight
2 to 12 years		36 ± 11 mL/kg body weight
>12 years		Same as adult dose

*SD, Standard deviation

DOSE ADJUSTMENTS
Use caution in patients with cardiac or renal dysfunction and in the elderly. Avoid fluid overload. Volume status, infusion rate, and urine output should be closely monitored. Lower-end initial dosing may be appropriate. Titrate to effect.

DILUTION

Available as a 6% solution in a ready-to-use 500-mL flexible plastic intravenous solution container. Remove overwrap immediately before administration. See manufacturer instructions for use of free/flex IV container. Administer through a nonvented standard infusion set. Air inlet of infusion set must be closed.

Storage: Store at 15° to 25° C (59° to 77° F). Do not freeze. Use immediately after insertion of administration set. Manufacturer recommends changing administration set at least once every 24 hours. For single use only. Discard any unused portion.

COMPATIBILITY

Consider any drug NOT listed as compatible to be INCOMPATIBLE until consulting a pharmacist; specific conditions may apply.

Manufacturer states the safety and **compatibility** of additives have not been established.

One source suggests the following **compatibilities**:

Y-site: Ampicillin, calcium chloride, calcium gluconate, cefazolin (Ancef), ceftriaxone (Rocephin), ciprofloxacin (Cipro IV), clindamycin (Cleocin), dimenhydrinate, dobutamine, dopamine, esmolol (Brevibloc), fentanyl, furosemide (Lasix), gentamicin, heparin, hydromorphone (Dilaudid), insulin, labetalol, levofloxacin (Levaquin), magnesium sulfate, meperidine (Demerol), methylprednisolone (Solu-Medrol), metronidazole (Flagyl IV), midazolam (Versed), morphine, moxifloxacin (Avelox), multivitamins (M.V.I.), nitroglycerin IV, norepinephrine (Levophed), octreotide (Sandostatin), potassium chloride, potassium phosphates, propofol (Diprivan), sodium bicarbonate, vasopressin.

RATE OF ADMINISTRATION

Variable depending on indication, present blood volume, and patient response. Initial 10 to 20 mL should be infused slowly, keeping the patient under close observation because of possible anaphylactoid reactions. Do not hang flexible plastic containers in series connection, do not pressurize to increase flow rates without first fully evacuating residual air from the container, and do not use vented IV administration sets. All may result in air embolism.

ACTIONS

A synthetic colloid for use in plasma volume expansion. Contains hydroxyethyl starch in a colloidal solution that expands plasma volume when administered intravenously. After isovolemic exchange of blood with 500 mL of Voluven in healthy volunteers, blood volume is maintained for at least 6 hours. Elimination half-life is 12 hours, and approximately 62% is excreted as hydroxyethyl starch molecules in urine within 72 hours.

INDICATIONS AND USES

Treatment and prophylaxis of hypovolemia in adults and children. It is not a substitute for red blood cells or coagulation factors in plasma.

CONTRAINDICATIONS

Do not use in critically ill adult patients, including patients with sepsis. ▪ Known hypersensitivity to hydroxyethyl starch. ▪ Clinical conditions with fluid overload (e.g., pulmonary edema, congestive heart failure). ▪ Renal failure with oliguria or anuria not related to hypovolemia. ▪ Patients receiving dialysis. ▪ Severe hypernatremia or severe hyperchloremia. ▪ Intracranial bleeding. ▪ Pre-existing coagulation or bleeding disorders. ▪ Severe liver disease.

PRECAUTIONS

For IV use only. ▪ Hypersensitivity reactions, including anaphylaxis, have been reported with solutions containing hydroxyethyl starch. ▪ Use caution in patients with cardiac insufficiency. ▪ In critically ill adult patients, including patients with sepsis, the use of hydroxyethyl starch (HES) products, including Voluven, increases the risk of mortality and renal replacement therapy. ▪ Avoid use in patients with pre-existing renal dysfunction. ▪ Discontinue at the first sign of renal injury. ▪ Avoid fluid overload; see Dose Adjustments. ▪ In cases of severe dehydration, a crystalloid solution should be administered first. In general, sufficient fluid should be administered to avoid dehydration. ▪ At high dosages, the dilutional effects may result in decreased levels of coagulation factors and other plasma proteins and a decrease in hematocrit.

Monitor: Monitor for S/S of hypersensitivity reactions (e.g., mild influenza-like symptoms, bradycardia, tachycardia, bronchospasm, hypotension, noncardiac pulmonary edema, anaphylaxis); see Rate of Administration. ▪ Clinical evaluation and periodic laboratory determinations are necessary to monitor fluid balance, electrolyte concentrations, kidney function, acid-base balance, and coagulation parameters during prolonged parenteral therapy or whenever the patient's condition warrants such evaluation. ▪ Monitor coagulation status of patients undergoing open heart surgery with CABG. Excess bleeding has been reported. ▪ Monitor BP, HR, and urine output. ▪ Monitor fluid status and rate of administration closely, especially in patients with cardiac or renal insufficiency. ▪ Continue to monitor renal function in hospitalized patients for at least 90 days because use of renal replacement therapy (RRT) has been reported up to 90 days after administration. ▪ Monitor liver function and coagulation parameters. ▪ Maintain adequate hydration of patient with additional IV fluids.

Maternal/Child: Category C: benefit must justify potential risk to the fetus. Embryocidal to rabbits. ▪ Information on use during labor and delivery unknown. Use only if clearly needed. ▪ Use caution during breast-feeding. ▪ See Pediatric Dose.

Elderly: Differences in response between elderly and younger patients not identified, but greater sensitivity of some older individuals cannot be ruled out. Risk of adverse reactions may be greater in patients with impaired renal function. Monitoring of renal function suggested in the elderly.

DRUG/LAB INTERACTIONS
No interactions with other drugs or nutritional products are known. ▪ Elevated serum amylase levels may be observed temporarily following administration. May interfere with diagnosis of pancreatitis. ▪ Dilutional effects may result in decreased levels of coagulation factors and other plasma proteins and a decrease in hematocrit.

SIDE EFFECTS
Most common side effects include elevated serum amylase, hemodilution (resulting in a dilution of blood components [e.g., coagulation factors and other plasma proteins and a decrease in hematocrit]), and pruritus. Anaphylactoid/hypersensitivity reactions and disturbances in blood coagulation beyond dilution effects have occurred rarely. Increased mortality and need for renal replacement therapy in critically ill patients, including sepsis, were most serious.

Overdose: May lead to overloading of circulatory system (e.g., pulmonary edema).

Post-Marketing: Anaphylactic/anaphylactoid/hypersensitivity reactions and hypotension/shock/circulatory collapse, mortality, need for renal replacement therapy.

ANTIDOTE
Notify the physician of any side effect. Discontinue the drug immediately at the first sign of a hypersensitivity reaction and treat reaction as indicated. Antihistamines (diphenhydramine [Benadryl]) and epinephrine (Adrenalin) may be indicated. Discontinue infusion immediately in the event of circulatory overload. A diuretic (furosemide [Lasix]) may be administered if necessary. Discontinue at the first sign of renal injury or coagulopathy. Treat side effects as indicated and resuscitate as necessary.

IBANDRONATE SODIUM

(i-**BAN**-dro-nate **SO**-dee-um)

Boniva

Bone resorption inhibitor
Bisphosphonate

USUAL DOSE

3 mg as an IV injection over 15 to 30 seconds every 3 months. Supplemental calcium and vitamin D may be required. See Precautions. Do not administer more frequently than every 3 months; if a dose is missed, administer it as soon as it can be rescheduled, and schedule the next injection for 3 months from that date.

DOSE ADJUSTMENTS

No dose adjustment is indicated based on age, gender, or impaired hepatic function. ▪ No dose adjustment is indicated for impaired kidney function in patients with a CrCl equal to or greater than 30 mL/min; see Contraindications.

DILUTION

May be given undiluted. Available in a prefilled syringe with a 25-gauge needle and a needle-stick protection device. Administer only with the provided 25-gauge needle.

Storage: Store at CRT. Syringes are for single use only; discard unused drug.

COMPATIBILITY

Manufacturer states, "Must not be mixed with calcium-containing solutions or other intravenously administered drugs."

RATE OF ADMINISTRATION

A single dose as an IV injection over 15 to 30 seconds.

ACTIONS

A nitrogen-containing bisphosphonate. Action is based on its affinity for hydroxyapatite, which is part of the mineral matrix of bone. Ibandronate inhibits osteoclast activity and reduces bone resorption and turnover. In postmenopausal women with osteoporosis, it increases bone mineral density and reduces the incidence of vertebral fractures. Either rapidly binds to bone (40% to 50% of a dose) or is excreted unchanged in urine (50% to 60%). No evidence that it is metabolized in humans. Terminal half-life is dose dependent and ranged from 4.6 to 25.5 hours in studies in which 2 and 4 mg of ibandronate were administered. Renal clearance is related to CrCl. Patients with a CrCl less than 30 mL/min have a more than twofold increase in exposure (AUC) than do patients with a CrCl greater than 80 mL/min.

INDICATIONS AND USES

Treatment of osteoporosis in postmenopausal women.

Limitation of use: Safety and effectiveness based on clinical data of 1-year duration; optimal duration of use has not been determined. Re-evaluate on a periodic basis. Consider discontinuing ibandronate after 3 to 5 years of use in patients at low risk for fracture, and re-evaluate risk for fracture periodically in patients who discontinue ibandronate.

CONTRAINDICATIONS

Hypersensitivity to ibandronate or its excipients, uncorrected hypocalcemia, severe impaired renal function (CrCl less than 30 mL/min or SCr greater than 2.3 mg/dL).

PRECAUTIONS

For IV injection only. Confirm patency of vein. Intra-arterial or paravenous administration could lead to tissue damage. ▪ Anaphylaxis, including fatal events, has been reported. Administer in a facility equipped to monitor the patient and respond to any medical emergency. ▪ Disturbances of bone and mineral metabolism (e.g., hypocalcemia, hypovitaminosis D) must be treated before administration of ibandronate. ▪ Bisphosphonates have been associated with a deterioration in renal function (e.g., increased SCr, acute renal failure [rare]). Use caution in patients who have concomitant diseases or are taking concomitant medications that may have adverse effects on the kidney. ▪ Osteonecrosis of the jaw (ONJ) has been reported in patients receiving bisphosphonates. The majority of cases have been in cancer patients undergoing dental procedures. Risk factors include cancer, concomitant therapy (e.g., chemotherapy, angiogenesis inhibitors, radiotherapy, corticosteroids), and comorbid conditions (e.g., anemia, coagulopathies, infection, pre-existing oral disease). Risk may increase with duration of exposure to bisphosphonates. Consider dental exam and appropriate preventive dentistry before beginning therapy with bisphosphonates. Avoid invasive dental procedures during bisphosphonate therapy. Dental surgery may exacerbate ONJ in patients who develop ONJ while on bisphosphonate therapy. ▪ Severe and occasionally incapacitating bone, joint, and muscle pain has been reported rarely. Symptoms may occur from one day to several months after initiation of treatment. In most cases, pain resolves when ibandronate is discontinued; in some patients, however, symptoms resolved slowly or persisted. ▪ Atypical, low-energy, or low-trauma fractures of the femoral shaft have been reported in bisphosphonate-treated patients. May be bilateral. Many patients report prodromal pain in the affected area, which usually presents as dull, aching thigh pain weeks to months before a complete fracture occurs. Patients presenting with thigh or groin pain should be evaluated to rule out an incomplete femur fracture. Patients presenting with an atypical fracture should also be assessed for S/S of fracture in the contralateral limb.

Monitor: Obtain baseline measurements of serum calcium, magnesium, phosphate, and serum creatinine; see Precautions. Perform a routine oral examination before administration. ▪ May cause a transient decrease in serum calcium values. ▪ Daily supplements of calcium and vitamin D may be required during therapy with ibandronate if dietary intake is inadequate. ▪ Monitor SCr before each dose. Nephropathy has been reported; see Precautions. Withhold treatment for renal deterioration. ▪ Monitor for S/S of a hypersensitivity reaction (e.g., chest pain, dizziness, dyspnea, fever, flushing, hypotension, nausea, pruritus, rash, rigors, urticaria). ▪ Influenza-like side effects (e.g., bone, muscle, or joint pains; chills; fever; fatigue) consistent with an acute-phase reaction have been reported. Incidence is higher with IV administration. Usually occurs within 3 to 7 days of injection. Symptoms generally subside within 24 to 48 hours, and treatment other than acetaminophen has not been required.

Patient Education: Read manufacturer's patient information sheet before each infusion. ▪ Daily supplements of calcium and vitamin D may be required during therapy with ibandronate. ▪ Avoid pregnancy; report a suspected pregnancy immediately. ▪ Discuss your health history (e.g., kidney problems, diabetes, high blood pressure, heart disease, planned tooth extraction) and prescription and nonprescription medications with health care providers, including your dentist. ▪ Promptly report jaw problems. ▪ Promptly report chills and/or fever and other S/S of a hypersensitivity reaction (e.g., chest pain, dizziness, feeling faint, flushing, hives, itching, nausea, pruritus, rash, shortness of breath). ▪ Report development of bone, joint, or muscle pain promptly. Onset of pain is variable. ▪ Promptly report thigh or groin pain. ▪ Do not administer more frequently than every 3 months; if a dose is missed, administer it as soon as it can be rescheduled, and schedule the next injection for 3 months from that date. ▪ Laboratory monitoring of renal function required before each dose.

Maternal/Child: Category C: use during pregnancy only if benefits justify risks to the mother and fetus. Bisphosphonates do cause fetal harm in animals. ▪ Found in milk of lactating animals; safety for use during breast-feeding not established. ▪ Safety and effectiveness for use in pediatric patients not established.

Elderly: Response similar to that seen in younger patients; however, greater sensitivity cannot be ruled out. ▪ Monitor renal function. Consider impaired renal function and concomitant disease or drug therapy.

DRUG/LAB INTERACTIONS

Does not inhibit cytochrome P_{450} isoenzymes. ▪ Secretory pathway does not appear to include known acidic or basic transport systems involved in the excretion of other drugs. ▪ Limited studies show no interaction between ibandronate and melphalan (Alkeran), oral prednisolone, or tamoxifen (Nolvadex). ▪ Bisphosphonates are known to interfere with the use of **bone-imaging agents;** ibandronate has not been studied.

SIDE EFFECTS

Abdominal pain, arthralgia, and back pain are the most common side effects. Other commonly reported side effects include headache, increased SCr, influenza-like illness (bone, muscle, or joint pains; chills; fever; fatigue), and injection site reactions (redness or swelling). Less frequent side effects include bronchitis, constipation, cystitis, depression, diarrhea, dizziness, dyspepsia, extremity pain, gastritis, gastroenteritis, hypertension, hypocalcemia, insomnia, localized osteoarthritis, myalgia, nasopharyngitis, nausea, rash, upper respiratory infection, urinary tract infection.

Overdose: Hypocalcemia, hypomagnesemia, and hypophosphatemia.

Post-Marketing: Acute renal failure; atypical, low-energy, or low-trauma fractures of the femoral shaft; hypersensitivity reactions, including anaphylaxis (with fatalities), angioedema, asthma exacerbation, bronchospasm, dermatitis bullous, erythema multiforme, rash, and Stevens-Johnson syndrome; severe or incapacitating musculoskeletal pain.

ANTIDOTE

Keep physician informed of side effects. Most will respond to symptomatic treatment. Withhold treatment for renal deterioration. Treat clinically relevant reductions in serum levels of calcium, magnesium, and phosphorus with IV administration of calcium gluconate, magnesium sulfate, and/or potassium or sodium phosphate as indicated. Discontinue ibandronate if severe bone, joint, or muscle pain develops. To be beneficial, dialysis must be administered within 2 hours of overdose. Treat anaphylaxis and/or resuscitate as indicated.

IBUPROFEN BBW

(**EYE**-bue-**PROE**-fen)

Caldolor

NSAID

pH 7.4

USUAL DOSE

Use the lowest effective dose for the shortest duration of time based on individual needs and response. Re-evaluate after the initial dose. Adjust dose and frequency as indicated. Total daily dose should not exceed 3,200 mg. Adequate hydration and correction of hypovolemia required before administration to reduce the risk of adverse renal reactions.

Analgesia: 400 to 800 mg every 6 hours as necessary.

Antipyretic: 400 mg every 4 to 6 hours or 100 to 200 mg every 4 hours as necessary.

PEDIATRIC DOSE

Pediatric Dosing of Ibuprofen for Fever and Pain			
Age-Group	Dose	Dosing Interval	Maximum Daily Dose*
6 months to less than 12 years	10 mg/kg up to 400 mg max	Every 4 to 6 hr as needed	40 mg/kg or 2,400 mg
12 to 17 years	400 mg	Every 4 to 6 hr as needed	2,400 mg

*Maximum daily dose is 40 mg/kg or 2,400 mg, whichever is less.

See comments under Usual Dose and Maternal/Child.

DOSE ADJUSTMENTS

To minimize the potential risk for an adverse cardiovascular (CV) event, use the lowest effective dose for the shortest duration possible. ■ Lower-end initial and reduced doses may be indicated in the elderly and/or debilitated. Consider potential for decreased organ function and concomitant disease or drug therapy.

DILUTION
Must be diluted to a final concentration of 4 mg/mL or less for both adult and weight-based pediatric dosing. Infusion without dilution can cause hemolysis. Further dilute in NS, D5W, or LR.
Filters: Specific information not available; consult pharmacist.
Storage: Store vials at CRT. Diluted solutions stable for up to 24 hours at 20° to 25° C (68° to 77° F) and with ambient room lighting.

COMPATIBILITY
Specific information not available; consult pharmacist.

RATE OF ADMINISTRATION
Adult: A single dose as an infusion over no less than 30 minutes.
Pediatric: A single dose as an infusion over no less than 10 minutes.

ACTIONS
A nonsteroidal anti-inflammatory drug (NSAID) that has anti-inflammatory, analgesic, and antipyretic activity. Mechanism of action is not completely understood but involves inhibition of cyclooxygenase (COX-1 and COX-2). Ibuprofen is a mixture of two isomers: [-]R- and [+]S-. The [+]S- isomer is responsible for the activity of ibuprofen. The [-]R- isomer slowly converts to the active [+]S- isomer to maintain levels of the active drug in the circulation. Highly protein bound; the mean half-life of a 400-mg dose is 2.2 hours, and the mean half-life of an 800-mg dose is 2.44 hours. Metabolized in the liver via oxidation and excreted in the urine.

INDICATIONS AND USES
Management of mild to moderate pain. ▪ Management of moderate to severe pain as an adjunct to opioid analgesics. ▪ Reduction of fever.

CONTRAINDICATIONS
Known hypersensitivity (anaphylactoid reactions, serious skin reactions) to ibuprofen or other NSAIDs. ▪ Known history of asthma, urticaria, or allergic-type reactions after taking aspirin or other NSAIDs. ▪ In the setting of coronary artery bypass graft (CABG) surgery. ▪ See Maternal/Child.

PRECAUTIONS
For IV infusion only. ▪ NSAIDs increase the risk for serious cardiovascular (CV) thrombotic events, including MI and stroke, which can be fatal. This risk may occur early in treatment and may increase with duration of use. The increase in CV thrombotic risk has been observed most consistently at higher doses. ▪ Avoid the use of ibuprofen in patients with a recent MI or in patients with heart failure unless the benefits are expected to outweigh the risks. Studies have shown these patients to be at increased risk for reinfarction, CV-related death, and all-cause mortality. ▪ NSAIDs increase the risk for serious GI ulceration, bleeding, and/or perforation. Can occur at any time, with or without warning symptoms, and can be fatal. Use extreme caution in patients with a prior history of peptic ulcer disease or GI bleeding. Risk is also increased in elderly or debilitated patients, in patients with advanced liver disease, and with concomitant use of aspirin, oral corticosteroids, anticoagulants, alcohol, selective serotonin reuptake inhibitors (SSRIs), or smoking. ▪ May cause elevations of liver function tests (e.g., ALT, AST). Rare cases of serious, sometimes fatal, hepatic injury (fulminant hepatitis, liver necrosis, hepatic failure) have occurred. ▪ May cause fluid retention and edema; use caution in patients with CHF or edema; see Drug/Lab Interactions. ▪ May precipitate hypertension or worsen pre-existing hypertension; see Drug/Lab Interactions. ▪ In addition to the usual caution in patients with reduced hepatic or renal function, NSAIDs may cause a dose-dependent reduction in renal prostaglandin formation and, secondarily, in renal blood flow, which can precipitate renal failure. Patients with impaired renal function, heart failure, liver dysfunction, dehydration, or hypovolemia; elderly patients; and patients receiving ACE inhibitors (e.g., enalapril [Vasotec], lisinopril [Zestril]), angiotensin receptor blockers (ARBs) (e.g., losartan [Cozaar], valsartan [Diovan]), or diuretics are at greatest risk. ▪ Avoid ibuprofen use in patients with advanced renal disease unless the benefits are expected to outweigh the risk. ▪ Increases in serum potassium, including hyperkalemia, have been reported. ▪ Anaphylactic reac-

tions have occurred in patients with and without known hypersensitivity to ibuprofen and in patients with aspirin-sensitive asthma. Cross-reactivity between aspirin and other NSAIDs has been reported in aspirin-sensitive patients; see Contraindications. Use caution in patients with pre-existing asthma (without known aspirin sensitivity), and monitor for changes in S/S of asthma. ▪ May cause serious skin reactions (e.g., exfoliative dermatitis, Stevens-Johnson syndrome, toxic epidermal necrolysis) without warning; some have been fatal. ▪ Anti-inflammatory and antipyretic effects may reduce the utility of these diagnostic signs in detecting infections. ▪ May cause anemia. Anemia may be due to occult or gross GI blood loss, fluid retention, or an incompletely described effect on erythropoiesis. ▪ NSAIDs inhibit platelet aggregation and may increase the risk of bleeding; see Drug/Lab Interactions. ▪ Aseptic meningitis and ophthalmologic effects (e.g., blurred or diminished vision, changes in color vision) have been reported with oral ibuprofen. ▪ See Maternal/Child.

Monitor: Correct hypovolemia before administration and maintain adequate hydration. ▪ Obtain baseline vital signs and monitor frequently during therapy. CBC, electrolytes, liver function tests, and SCr or CrCl may be indicated for a baseline or as needed as symptoms develop. ▪ Monitor patients with or without a previous history of CV disease for S/S of CV events (e.g., chest pain, dyspnea, edema, hypertension, limb or facial paralysis). ▪ Monitor for edema or signs of worsening heart failure. ▪ Observe for S/S of GI ulceration or bleeding and/or liver dysfunction. ▪ Monitor renal function, especially in patients with impaired renal function. ▪ Monitor for S/S of hypersensitivity reactions (e.g., anaphylaxis, pruritus, rash, urticaria, or wheezing). ▪ Monitor patients who may be adversely affected by alterations in platelet function (e.g., patients with coagulation disorders or patients receiving anticoagulants).

Patient Education: Side effects have resulted in extended hospitalization and could be fatal. ▪ Promptly report any S/S of CV thrombotic events (e.g., chest pain, shortness of breath, slurred speech, weakness), GI adverse events (e.g., dyspepsia, epigastric pain, hematemesis, melena), hepatotoxicity (e.g., diarrhea, fatigue, flu-like symptoms, jaundice, lethargy, nausea, right upper quadrant tenderness), heart failure (e.g., edema, shortness of breath, weight gain), and/or a hypersensitivity reaction (e.g., difficulty breathing, swelling of the face or throat) or any type or rash. ▪ Avoid use of concomitant NSAIDs (e.g., naproxen [Aleve, Naprosyn], celecoxib [Celebrex]). Over-the-counter medications for the treatment of fever, cold, and insomnia may contain NSAIDs. Consult pharmacist before use. ▪ Discuss use of low-dose aspirin for cardiac prophylaxis with health care provider before initiating concomitant therapy; see Maternal/Child.

Maternal/Child: Avoid use starting at 30 weeks' gestation; premature closure of the ductus arteriosus in the fetus may occur. Use before 30 weeks' gestation only if the potential benefit justifies the potential risk to the fetus. ▪ Effects during labor and delivery unknown. ▪ Use with caution during breast-feeding. ▪ Safety and effectiveness for use in pediatric patients under 6 months of age not established.

Elderly: Increased risk for serious NSAID-associated GI, cardiovascular, and/or renal adverse events. ▪ Dosing should be cautious; see Dose Adjustments.

DRUG/LAB INTERACTIONS

Concurrent use with **aspirin** or other **salicylates** (e.g., diflunisal, salsalate) is not recommended; may increase the risk of toxicity and serious GI events. ▪ Synergistic effect on bleeding with **anticoagulants** (e.g., heparin, warfarin [Coumadin]), **antiplatelet agents** (e.g., aspirin), **SSRIs** (e.g., fluoxetine [Prozac], paroxetine [Paxil], sertraline [Zoloft]), and **serotonin-norepinephrine reuptake inhibitors (SNRIs)** (e.g., duloxetine [Cymbalta], venlafaxine [Effexor]); risk of bleeding increased. Monitor patients closely if concomitant use indicated. ▪ NSAIDs may decrease the effectiveness of **ACE inhibitors** (e.g., enalapril [Vasotec], lisinopril [Zestril]), **angiotensin receptor blockers (ARBs)** (e.g., losartan [Cozaar], valsartan [Diovan]), and **beta-blockers** (e.g., metoprolol [Lopressor], propranolol [Inderal]); monitor BP. ▪ Coadministration with an **ACE inhibitor** or **ARB** may result in deterioration of renal function in at-risk patients; monitor renal function. ▪ Ibuprofen can reduce the natriuretic effects of **loop diuretics** (e.g., furosemide [Lasix]) and **thiazide** diuretics (e.g., hydrochlorothiazide); observe for signs of worsening renal function and ensure diuretic/therapeutic effectiveness. ▪ May increase **digoxin** serum concentration and prolong half-life of digoxin; monitor digoxin levels with concomitant use. ▪ Concurrent use of **lithium** with NSAIDs may decrease lithium clearance, increasing plasma levels of lithium; observe for signs of lithium toxicity. ▪ Concurrent use of NSAIDs with **methotrexate** may enhance methotrexate toxicity (e.g., neutropenia, thrombocytopenia, renal dysfunction); monitor for signs of methotrexate toxicity. ▪ Concomitant use with **cyclosporine** (Sandimmune) may increase cyclosporine's nephrotoxicity; monitor renal function. ▪ Concomitant use with **pemetrexed** (Alimta) may increase the risk of pemetrexed-associated myelosuppression and renal and GI toxicity; avoid concomitant use for 2 to 5 days before pemetrexed administration and for 2 days following administration in patients with mild to moderate renal impairment (CrCl 45 to 79 mL/min). See pemetrexed monograph.

SIDE EFFECTS
Adults: The most common side effects are dizziness, flatulence, headache, hemorrhage, and nausea and vomiting. Other side effects include abdominal discomfort, anemia, bacteremia, bacterial pneumonia, cough, diarrhea, dyspepsia, eosinophilia, hyperkalemia, hypernatremia, hypertension, hypoalbuminemia, hypokalemia, hypoproteinemia, hypotension, increased blood urea, increased lactic dehydrogenase (LDH), neutropenia, peripheral edema, thrombocytosis, urinary retention, wound hemorrhage. See Precautions for potential major side effects.

Pediatric patients: The most common side effects are anemia, headache, infusion site pain, nausea, and vomiting.

Overdose: Acute renal failure, coma, drowsiness, epigastric pain, GI bleeding, hypertension, lethargy, nausea, respiratory depression, and vomiting.

ANTIDOTE
Keep the physician informed of significant side effects. With increasing severity or onset of symptoms of any major side effect (e.g., CHF; edema; hypersensitivity reactions; GI bleeding, ulceration, or perforation; hepatic or renal effects; hypertension; skin reactions; thrombotic events), discontinue the drug and notify the physician. A patent airway, artificial ventilation, oxygen therapy, and other symptomatic treatment must be instituted promptly if indicated. Treat anaphylaxis with epinephrine (Adrenalin), diphenhydramine (Benadryl), and corticosteroids as indicated. No known antidote. Forced diuresis, alkalinization of urine, hemodialysis, or hemoperfusion may not be useful due to high protein binding.

IBUPROFEN LYSINE
(eye-byou-**PROH**-fen **LIE**-seen)

NSAID
(patent ductus arteriosus adjunct)

NeoProfen

pH 7

NEONATAL DOSE
All doses are based on birth weight. A course of therapy is three doses given at 24-hour intervals.

Initial dose: 10 mg/kg. Follow with a dose of 5 mg/kg in 24 hours and repeat at 48 hours; see Dose Adjustments.

After completion of the first course, no further doses are indicated if the ductus arteriosus closes or is significantly reduced in size. If the ductus arteriosus fails to close or reopens, a second course, alternative pharmacologic therapy, or surgery may be necessary.

DOSE ADJUSTMENTS
If urine output is less than 0.6 mL/kg/hr at any time a dose is to be given, withhold dose until lab studies confirm a return to normal renal function.

DILUTION
Each single dose must be diluted to an appropriate volume for administration as an infusion over 15 minutes with dextrose or saline. Prepare for infusion and begin administration within 30 minutes of preparation. A fresh solution should be prepared just before each administration. Contains no preservatives; discard any unused portion.

Filters: Specific information not available.

Storage: Store vials in cartons at CRT and protect from light until use. Use reconstituted solution within 30 minutes of preparation.

COMPATIBILITY
Manufacturer states, "Should not be simultaneously administered in the same IV line with Total Parenteral Nutrition" (TPN). If required, interrupt TPN for 15 minutes before and after ibuprofen administration. Maintain IV line patency with dextrose or saline infusion.

RATE OF ADMINISTRATION
Administer via the IV port nearest the insertion site.

A single dose, properly diluted, and infused continuously over 15 minutes.

ACTIONS
A nonsteroidal anti-inflammatory drug (NSAID). Mechanism of action by which it causes closure of a patent ductus arteriosus (PDA) is unknown; however, in adults it is an inhibitor of prostaglandin synthesis. By closing the patent ductus arteriosus, the need for surgical intervention is eliminated. Half-life varies inversely with postnatal age, but in general the half-life in infants is more than 10 times longer than in adults. In lower-birth-weight premature infants, half-life may range from 20 to 51 hours. Metabolism and excretion have not been studied in premature infants. In adults, it is metabolized in the liver and excreted in the urine and feces.

INDICATIONS AND USES
Closure of a clinically significant patent ductus arteriosus in premature infants weighing between 500 and 1,500 Gm who are no more than 32 weeks' gestational age when usual medical management (e.g., fluid restriction, diuretics, respiratory support) is not effective. Consequences beyond 8 weeks after treatment have not been evaluated.

CONTRAINDICATIONS
Bleeding (especially active intracranial hemorrhage or GI bleeding), coagulation defects, suspected necrotizing enterocolitis, infants with congenital heart disease (e.g., pulmonary atresia, severe coarctation of the aorta, severe tetralogy of Fallot) who require pa-

tency of the ductus arteriosus for satisfactory pulmonary or systemic blood flow, proven or suspected untreated infection, significant renal impairment, thrombocytopenia.

PRECAUTIONS

For IV use only; see Monitor. ▪ Reserve for infants with clear evidence of a clinically significant PDA. ▪ For use only in a highly supervised setting such as an intensive care nursery. ▪ No long-term evaluations available. Effects of ibuprofen on neurodevelopmental outcome and growth and on disease processes associated with prematurity (e.g., retinopathy of prematurity, chronic lung disease) have not been assessed. ▪ May alter the usual signs of infection. Use with extreme caution in the presence of an existing controlled infection and in infants at risk for infection. ▪ Can inhibit platelet aggregation. ▪ Can prolong bleeding time in adults; use caution in infants with underlying hemostatic defects; see Contraindications. ▪ Can displace bilirubin from albumin-binding sites; use with caution in infants with elevated total bilirubin.

Monitor: Confirm absolute patency of vein. Avoid extravasation; will irritate tissue. Administration via an umbilical arterial line has not been studied. ▪ Obtain baseline and monitor vital signs, oxygenation, acid-base status, fluid and electrolyte balance, and kidney function (SCr, BUN, urine output). ▪ Can cause a reduction in urine output, increased BUN and SCr, and a decreased CrCl; may progress to oliguria or renal failure. Monitor all infants closely, especially those with some degree of renal impairment. ▪ May inhibit platelet aggregation; monitor for signs of bleeding. ▪ Monitor for signs of infection.

DRUG/LAB INTERACTIONS

Drug interactions have not been studied.

SIDE EFFECTS

The most commonly reported side effects include adrenal insufficiency, anemia, apnea, atelectasis, decreased urine output, edema, GI disorders (including nonnecrotizing enterocolitis), hematuria, hypernatremia, hypocalcemia, hypoglycemia, increased BUN and SCr, intraventricular hemorrhage and other bleeding, renal failure, renal insufficiency, respiratory failure, respiratory infection, sepsis, skin lesion or irritation, and urinary tract infection. Other side effects of unknown association include abdominal distension, cardiac failure, cholestasis, convulsions, feeding problems, gastritis, gastroesophageal reflux, hypotension, ileus, infections, inguinal hernia, injection site reactions, jaundice, lab abnormalities (e.g., hyperglycemia, neutropenia, thrombocytopenia), and tachycardia.

Post-Marketing: GI perforation, necrotizing enterocolitis, and pulmonary hypertension.

Overdose: Breathing difficulties, coma, drowsiness, hypotension, irregular heartbeat, kidney failure, seizures, and vomiting have occurred in individuals (not necessarily in premature infants) following overdose of oral ibuprofen.

ANTIDOTE

Discontinue the drug and notify the physician of all side effects. Based on severity, side effects may be treated symptomatically or drug will be completely discontinued in favor of surgical intervention. In case of overdose, there is no specific antidote. Treat symptomatically and follow for several days after apparent recovery; GI ulceration and hemorrhage may occur. Resuscitate as necessary.

IBUTILIDE FUMARATE BBW

(ih-**BYOU**-tih-lyd **FU**-mar-ayt)

Antiarrhythmic

Corvert

pH 4.6

USUAL DOSE

Guidelines for Ibutilide Dosing		
Patient Weight	Initial Infusion (over 10 minutes)	Second Infusion
60 kg (132 lb) or more	1 mg ibutilide fumarate (one vial [10 mL])	If the arrhythmia does not terminate within 10 minutes after the end of the initial infusion, a second 10-minute infusion of equal strength may be administered 10 minutes after completion of the first infusion.
Less than 60 kg (132 lb)	0.01 mg/kg ibutilide fumarate (0.1 mL/kg)	

Discontinue infusion promptly when the presenting arrhythmia is terminated (desired effect). Must also be discontinued immediately if sustained or nonsustained ventricular tachycardia or marked prolongation of QT or QTc occurs (adverse effects). Postconversion treatment with appropriate antiarrhythmics (e.g., digoxin, verapamil, or propranolol) is usually required.

DOSE ADJUSTMENTS

Dose selection should be cautious in the elderly. Reduced doses may be indicated based on the potential for decreased organ function and concomitant disease or drug therapy. ▪ No adjustments required in patients with impaired hepatic or renal function; see Monitor. Lower doses may be indicated in post–cardiac surgery patients. In recent studies one or two infusions of 0.5 mg in patients weighing 60 kg or more or 0.005 mg/kg/dose for patients under 60 kg was effective in terminating atrial fibrillation and/or flutter.

DILUTION

May be given undiluted or may be diluted in 50 mL of NS or D5W and given as an infusion. 1 mg (10 mL of a 0.1-mg/mL solution) of ibutilide in 50 mL diluent yields 0.017 mg/mL.

Storage: Store at CRT in carton until use. Stable after dilution for 24 hours at room temperature, 48 hours if refrigerated.

COMPATIBILITY

Manufacturer lists as **compatible** with NS and D5W packaged in glass, polyvinyl chloride, or polyolefin infusion containers. Additional information not available; consult pharmacist.

RATE OF ADMINISTRATION

A single dose by injection or infusion over 10 minutes.

ACTIONS

A Class III antiarrhythmic agent that produces mild slowing of the sinus rate and atrioventricular conduction. Delays repolarization by activation of a slow inward current (sodium) rather than blocking outward potassium currents. Prolonged atrial and ventricular action potential duration and refractoriness result. Produces dose-related prolongation of the QT interval (may result from dose of ibutilide or rate of injection). Conversion of atrial flutter/fibrillation usually occurs within 30 minutes but may take up to 90 minutes after the start of the infusion. Most patients remain in normal sinus rhythm (NSR) for 24 hours. At recommended doses, ibutilide has no clinically significant effects on cardiac output, mean pulmonary arterial pressure, or pulmonary capillary wedge pressure. Rapidly distributed and metabolized. Elimination half-life is 6 hours (range 2 to 12 hours). Primarily excreted in urine (7% as unchanged drug). Excreted in small amounts in feces.

INDICATIONS AND USES

Rapid conversion of recent-onset atrial fibrillation or atrial flutter to sinus rhythm. Patients with more recent onset of arrhythmia have a higher rate of conversion. Effectiveness was less in those with a longer-duration arrhythmia.

CONTRAINDICATIONS

Known hypersensitivity to ibutilide or any of its components. ▪ Not recommended in patients who have had a previous polymorphic ventricular tachycardia (e.g., torsades de pointes). ▪ See Drug/Lab Interactions.

PRECAUTIONS

For IV infusion only. ▪ Usually administered by or under the direction of the physician specialist. ▪ Skilled personnel and proper equipment (e.g., cardiac monitors, intracardiac pacing facilities, cardioverter/defibrillator, emergency drugs) must be immediately available. ▪ May cause life-threatening arrhythmias (e.g., torsades de pointes) with or without documented QT prolongation. ▪ Correct hypokalemia and hypomagnesemia before use; may exaggerate a prolonged QT and cause arrhythmias. ▪ Adequate anticoagulation (usually at least 2 weeks) is required for any patient with atrial fibrillation of more than 2 to 3 days' duration. ▪ Select patients carefully; benefits (potential for maintaining sinus rhythm) must outweigh risks. Patients with chronic atrial fibrillation are more likely to revert back to atrial fibrillation after conversion to sinus rhythm. Patients with a QTc interval greater than 440 msec or a serum potassium less than 4.0 mEq/L are at very high risk to develop life-threatening arrhythmias. ▪ Patients with a history of CHF may be more susceptible to sustained polymorphic VT. ▪ Slightly more effective in atrial flutter than atrial fibrillation. ▪ See Drug/Lab Interactions.

Monitor: Obtain weight, baseline vital signs, and ECG before administration. Continuous ECG monitoring during and after infusion indicated to observe for arrhythmias. Watch for QT or QTc prolongation; may cause arrhythmia (torsades de pointes) with or without QT prolongation. ▪ Monitor BP and HR. Bradycardia, a varying HR, and/or hypokalemia may increase risk of arrhythmia. ▪ Arrhythmia occurs most frequently within 40 minutes of completion of infusion but may occur for up to 3 hours after infusion. Monitor ECG for a minimum of 4 hours or until QTc has returned to baseline. Monitor longer if there are any episodes of arrhythmias or if the patient has impaired liver function.

Patient Education: Report promptly any feeling of faintness, difficulty breathing, or pain or stinging along injection site.

Maternal/Child: Category C: benefits must outweigh risks. Caused birth defects and was embryocidal in rats. ▪ Temporarily discontinue breast-feeding. ▪ Safety and effectiveness for use in pediatric patients under 18 years of age not established.

Elderly: No age-related differences observed. Median age in clinical trials was 65 years. ▪ Lower-end initial doses may be indicated; see Dose Adjustments.

DRUG/LAB INTERACTIONS

Should not be given concurrently with **Class Ia antiarrhythmics** (e.g., disopyramide [Norpace], procainamide [Pronestyl], quinidine) **or other Class III antiarrhythmics** (e.g., amiodarone [Nexterone], sotalol [Betapace]). Withhold any of these agents for at least 5 half-lives before ibutilide infusion and for 4 hours after. ▪ Incidence of arrhythmia may be increased with **other drugs that prolong the QT interval** (e.g., phenothiazines [e.g., promethazine (Phenergan)], tricyclic antidepressants [e.g., amitriptyline (Elavil)], tetracyclic antidepressants [e.g., maprotiline (Ludiomil)]). ▪ Monitor **serum digoxin levels** to avoid digoxin toxicity. ▪ Use with **digoxin, beta-blockers, or calcium channel blockers** does not alter safety or effectiveness of ibutilide. However, **sotalol** is a beta-blocker, and its use with ibutilide is restricted because it has Class III antiarrhythmic activity; see first sentence above.

SIDE EFFECTS

Sustained polymorphic VT (1.7%) and nonsustained polymorphic VT (2.7%) can deteriorate into ventricular fibrillation and be fatal. May cause many other arrhythmias (e.g., first-, second-, or third-degree AV block [1.5%], bradycardia [1.2%], bundle branch block [1.9%], nonsustained monomorphic VT [4.9%], prolonged QT segment [1.2%], PVCs [5.1%], tachycardia [2.7%]), CHF (0.5%), headache (3.6%), hypertension (1.2%), hypotension (2%), nausea (1.9%), palpitation (1%).

Overdose: Side effects exaggerated with overdose in humans. Acute overdose in animals resulted in CNS depression, rapid gasping breathing, convulsions.

ANTIDOTE

If proarrhythmias occur, discontinue ibutilide; correct electrolyte abnormalities (e.g., potassium and magnesium). Overdrive cardiac pacing, electrical cardioversion, or defibrillation may be required. Infusions of magnesium sulfate may be helpful. Avoid treatment with antiarrhythmic agents. VT that deteriorates to VF will require immediate defibrillation.

IDARUBICIN HYDROCHLORIDE BBW
(eye-dah-**ROOB**-ih-sin hy-droh-**KLOR**-eyed)

Idamycin PFS, Idarubicin PFS, IDR

Antineoplastic
(anthracycline antibiotic)

pH 5 to 7

USUAL DOSE

Adult acute myeloid leukemia (AML) induction therapy:

Induction: Idarubicin 12 mg/M^2/day for 3 days. Used in combination with cytarabine (Ara-C). Cytarabine 100 mg/M^2/day may be given as a continuous infusion on Days 1 to 7 (daily for 7 days), or alternately the cytarabine may be given as an IV injection of 25 mg/M^2 followed immediately by a continuous infusion of cytarabine 200 mg/M^2/day on Days 1 to 5 (daily for 5 days). See Precautions/Monitor. If unequivocal evidence of leukemia remains after the first course, a second course may be given; see Dose Adjustments. The benefit of an aggressive consolidation and maintenance program in prolonging the duration of remissions and survival has not been proven. See prescribing information for regimens used in clinical trials.

DOSE ADJUSTMENTS

Delay second course until full recovery if severe mucositis has occurred and reduce dose by 25%. ▪ Consider dose reductions in impaired liver and kidney function based on bilirubin and/or creatinine levels above the normal range. Do not administer if bilirubin is above 5 mg/dL. In one Phase III clinical trial, patients with bilirubin levels between 2.6 and 5 mg/dL received a 50% reduction in dose.

DILUTION

Specific techniques required (see Precautions). Idamycin PFS is a liquid formulation; each 5 mg of powdered idamycin must be reconstituted with 5 mL of nonbacteriostatic NS for injection (1 mg/mL). Use extreme caution inserting the needle; vial contents are under negative pressure. Avoid any possibility of inhalation from aerosol or any skin contamination.

Filters: No data available from manufacturer.

Storage: PFS product must be refrigerated. Reconstituted idamycin is stable for 7 days under refrigeration (2° to 8° C [36° to 46° F]) or 3 days (72 hours) at room temperature (15° to 30° C [59° to 86° F]). Discard unused solution appropriately.

COMPATIBILITY

Consider any drug NOT listed as compatible to be INCOMPATIBLE until consulting a pharmacist; specific conditions may apply.

Manufacturer states, "Should not be mixed with other drugs unless specific **compatibility** data are available," and lists as **incompatible** with heparin. Prolonged contact with solutions of an alkaline pH (e.g., sodium lactate, sodium bicarbonate) will result in degradation of idarubicin.

One source suggests the following **compatibilities:**

Y-site: Amifostine (Ethyol), amikacin, aztreonam (Azactam), cladribine (Leustatin), cyclophosphamide (Cytoxan), cytarabine (ARA-C), diphenhydramine (Benadryl), droperidol (Inapsine), erythromycin (Erythrocin), etoposide phosphate (Etopophos), filgrastim (Neupogen), gemcitabine (Gemzar), granisetron (Kytril), imipenem-cilastatin (Primaxin), magnesium sulfate, mannitol, melphalan (Alkeran), metoclopramide (Reglan), potassium chloride (KCl), ranitidine (Zantac), sargramostim (Leukine), thiotepa, vinorelbine (Navelbine).

RATE OF ADMINISTRATION

A single dose of properly diluted medication over 10 to 15 minutes through Y-tube or three-way stopcock of a free-flowing infusion of D5W or NS.

ACTIONS

A highly toxic, synthetic, antibiotic, antineoplastic agent. An analog of daunorubicin. Rapidly distributed; has an increased rate of cellular uptake compared to other anthracyclines. It inhibits synthesis of DNA and interacts with the enzyme topoisomerase II. Results in a greater number of remissions and longer survival than previous protocols (daunorubicin and cytarabine). It is severely immunosuppressive. Extensive extrahepatic metabolism. Half-life averages 20 to 22 hours. Slowly excreted in bile and urine.

INDICATIONS AND USES

Treatment of acute myeloid leukemia (AML) in adults in combination with other approved antileukemic drugs.

Unlabeled uses: Treatment of acute lymphoblastic leukemia in pediatric patients; see Maternal/Child.

CONTRAINDICATIONS

Not absolute; pre-existing bone marrow suppression, impaired cardiac function, pre-existing infection; see Precautions/Monitor. ▪ Do not administer if bilirubin above 5 mg/dL.

PRECAUTIONS

Follow guidelines for handling cytotoxic agents. See Appendix A, p. 1331. ▪ Administered by or under the direction of the physician specialist, with facilities for monitoring the patient and responding to any medical emergency. ▪ For IV use only. Do not give IM or SC. ▪ Use extreme caution in pre-existing drug-induced bone marrow suppression, existing heart disease, previous treatment with other anthracyclines (e.g., daunorubicin), other cardiotoxic agents (e.g., bleomycin), or radiation therapy encompassing the heart. ▪ Myocardial toxicity may cause potentially fatal acute congestive heart failure, acute life-threatening arrhythmias, or other cardiomyopathies. Cardiac toxicity is more common in patients who have received prior anthracyclines (e.g., doxorubicin) or who have pre-existing cardiac disease. ▪ May cause severe myelosuppression. ▪ Use with caution in patients with hepatic or renal dysfunction. Metabolism and excretion of idarubicin may be impaired; see Dose Adjustments.

Monitor: Determine absolute patency of vein. A stinging or burning sensation indicates extravasation, but extravasation may occur without stinging or burning; severe cellulitis and tissue necrosis can occur with extravasation. Discontinue injection; use another vein. ▪ Monitoring of WBCs, RBCs, platelet count, liver function, kidney function, ECG, chest x-ray, echocardiography, and systolic ejection fraction indicated before and during therapy. ▪ Severe myelosuppression occurs with effective therapeutic doses. Observe closely for all signs of infection or bleeding. ▪ Monitor for thrombocytopenia (platelet count less than 50,000/mm^3). Initiate precautions to prevent excessive bleeding (e.g., inspect IV sites, skin, and mucous membranes; use extreme care during invasive procedures; test urine, emesis, stool, and secretions for occult blood). ▪ Prophylactic antibiotics may be indicated pending results of C/S in a febrile neutropenic patient. ▪ Prophylactic antiemetics may reduce nausea and vomiting and increase patient comfort. ▪ Monitor uric acid levels; maintain hydration; allopurinol and urine alkalinization may be indicated. ▪ See Precautions.

Patient Education: Nonhormonal birth control recommended. ▪ Report IV site burning or stinging promptly. ▪ See Appendix D, p. 1333.

Maternal/Child: Category D: avoid pregnancy. May produce teratogenic effects on the fetus. Contraceptive measures indicated during childbearing years. ▪ Discontinue breast-feeding before taking idarubicin. ▪ Safety and efficacy for use in pediatric patients not established but has been used; consult literature.

Elderly: Cardiotoxicity or myelotoxicity may be more severe. Patients over 60 years of age who were undergoing induction experienced CHF, serious arrhythmias, chest pain, myocardial infarction, and asymptomatic declines in left ventricular ejection fraction more frequently than younger patients. ▪ Monitor renal, hepatic, and hematologic functions closely.

DRUG/LAB INTERACTIONS
Bone marrow toxicity is additive with **other chemotherapeutic agents.** ▪ Risk of cardiotoxicity increased in patients previously treated with maximum cumulative doses of **other anthracyclines** (e.g., doxorubicin [Adriamycin], mitoxantrone [Novantrone]) **and/or radiation encompassing the heart.** ▪ Leukopenic and/or thrombocytopenic effects may be increased with **drugs that cause blood dyscrasias** (e.g., anticonvulsants [e.g., carbamazepine (Tegretol), phenytoin (Dilantin)], NSAIDs [e.g., ibuprofen (Advil, Motrin), naproxen (Aleve, Naprosyn)]). Adjust dose based on differential and platelet count. ▪ Do not administer **live virus vaccines** to patients receiving antineoplastic drugs. ▪ See Precautions/Monitor.

SIDE EFFECTS
Acute congestive heart failure, alopecia (reversible), arrhythmias, bone marrow suppression (marked with average doses), cramping, decrease in systolic ejection fraction, depressed QRS voltage, diarrhea, erythema and tissue necrosis (if extravasation occurs), fever, headache, hemorrhage (severe), hepatic function changes, infection, mucositis, myocarditis, nausea, pericarditis, renal function changes, seizures, skin rash, urticaria (local), vomiting.

ANTIDOTE
Most side effects will be tolerated or treated symptomatically. Keep physician informed. Close monitoring of bone marrow, ECG, chest x-ray, echocardiography, and systolic ejection fraction may prevent most serious and potentially fatal side effects. There is no specific antidote, but adequate supportive care including platelet transfusions, antibiotics, and symptomatic treatment of mucositis is required. For extravasation, elevate the extremity and apply intermittent ice packs over the area immediately and 4 times a day for $1/2$ hour. Continue for 3 days. Consider aspiration of as much infiltrated drug as possible, flooding of the site with NS, and injection of hydrocortisone sodium succinate (Solu-Cortef) throughout extravasated tissue. Use a 27- or 25-gauge needle. Site should be observed promptly by a reconstructive surgeon. If ulceration begins or there is severe persistent pain at the site, early wide excision of the involved area will be considered. Hemodialysis or peritoneal dialysis probably not effective in overdose.

IDARUCIZUMAB
(**EYE**-da-roo-**KIZ**-ue-mab)

Antidote
Monoclonal antibody

Praxbind

pH 5.3 to 5.7

USUAL DOSE
5 Gm provided as two separate vials, each containing 2.5 Gm/50 mL. There are limited data to support administration of an additional 5-Gm dose of idarucizumab; see Precautions.

DOSE ADJUSTMENTS
No dose adjustment is required in renally impaired patients. ▪ Formal studies in patients with hepatic impairment have not been conducted.

DILUTION
A colorless to slightly yellow, clear to slightly opalescent solution available as a 2.5 Gm/50 mL injection in a single-use vial. Administer undiluted by withdrawing and injecting the contents of 2 vials with a syringe or by hanging and infusing the contents of 2 vials.

Filter: Specific information not available.

Storage: Store unopened vials in the refrigerator at 2° to 8° C (36° to 46° F). Do not freeze. Do not shake. Before use, the unopened vial may be kept at RT 25° C (77° F) for up to 48 hours if stored in the original package to protect from light, or up to 6 hours when exposed to light. Once solution has been removed from the vial, administration should begin promptly or within 1 hour.

COMPATIBILITY
Manufacturer states, "Do not mix with other medicinal products. A pre-existing IV line may be used for administration. The line must be flushed with NS prior to infusion. No other infusion should be administered in parallel via the same IV access."

RATE OF ADMINISTRATION
Administer by bolus injection by injecting both vials consecutively one after another via syringe. Alternatively, may administer as two rapid consecutive infusions by hanging and infusing each vial one after another. Flush IV line with NS before administration of idarucizumab.

ACTIONS
A recombinant humanized monoclonal antibody fragment (Fab); it is derived from an IgG1 isotype molecule whose target is the direct thrombin inhibitor dabigatran. Idaruciz-umab is a specific reversal agent for dabigatran. It binds to dabigatran and its acyl gluc-uronide metabolites with a higher affinity than the binding affinity of dabigatran to thrombin, thereby neutralizing their anticoagulant effect. In studies, the plasma concentrations of unbound dabigatran were reduced to below the lower limit of quantification immediately after the administration of 5 Gm idarucizumab. Subjects' diluted thrombin time (dTT), ecarin clotting time (ECT), activated partial thromboplastin time (aPTT), thrombin time (TT), and activated clotting time (ACT) parameters returned to baseline levels. Idarucizumab is rapidly eliminated with an initial half-life of 47 minutes and a terminal half-life of 10.3 hours. Some drug is recovered in the urine. The remaining part of the dose is assumed to be eliminated via protein catabolism, mainly in the kidney. Idarucizumab is thought to be metabolized via pathways that involve the biodegradation of the antibody to smaller peptides or amino acids, which are then reabsorbed and incorporated in the general protein synthesis.

INDICATIONS AND USES
Reversal of the anticoagulant effects of dabigatran (Pradaxa) when reversal is needed for emergency surgery/urgent procedures or in life-threatening or uncontrolled bleeding.

Limitations of use: This indication is approved under accelerated approval based on a reduction in unbound dabigatran and normalization of coagulation parameters in healthy volunteers. Continued approval for this indication may be contingent on the results of an ongoing cohort case series study.

CONTRAINDICATIONS
Manufacturer states, "None."

PRECAUTIONS
For IV use only. ▪ Idarucizumab treatment should be used in conjunction with standard supportive measures. ▪ Reversing dabigatran therapy exposes patients to the thrombotic risk of their underlying disease. To reduce this risk, resumption of anticoagulant therapy should be considered as soon as medically appropriate. Dabigatran treatment can be initiated 24 hours after administration of idarucizumab. No changes in the pharmacokinetics or pharmacodynamics of dabigatran were noted upon re-initiation 24 hours after administration of idarucizumab. ▪ Elevated coagulation parameters (e.g., activated partial thromboplastin time [aPPT], ecarin clotting time [ECT]) have been observed 12 and 24 hours after administration of a 5-Gm dose of idarucizumab in a limited number of patients. Administration of an additional 5-Gm dose of idarucizumab may be considered if the reappearance of clinically relevant bleeding together with elevated coagulation parameters is observed after administration of the initial dose. Similarly, patients who require a second emergency surgery/urgent procedure and have elevated coagulation parameters may receive an additional 5-Gm dose of idarucizumab. The safety and effectiveness of repeat treatment with idarucizumab have not been established. ▪ Adverse events possibly indicative of hypersensitivity reactions have been reported. The risk of using idarucizumab in a patient with known hypersensitivity to idarucizumab (e.g., anaphylactic reaction) or to any of its excipients needs to be weighed cautiously against the potential benefit of such an emergency treatment. If an anaphylactic reaction or other serious reaction occurs, immediately discontinue administration of idarucizumab. ▪ The recommended dose of idarucizumab contains 4 Gm of sorbitol as an excipient. Patients with the condition of hereditary fructose intolerance (HFI) have experienced serious adverse reactions (e.g., acute liver failure, hypoglycemia, hypophosphatemia, increase in uric acid, metabolic acidosis) after receiving parenteral administration of sorbitol. When prescribing idarucizumab to patients with HFI, consider the combined daily metabolic load of sorbitol/fructose from all sources, including idarucizumab and other drugs containing sorbitol. The minimum amount of sorbitol at which serious adverse reactions may occur in these patients is not known. ▪ Idarucizumab is a specific reversal agent for dabigatran, with no impact on the effect of other anticoagulant or antithrombotic therapies. ▪ As with all proteins, there is a potential for immunogenicity with idarucizumab. Pre-existing antibodies with cross-reactivity to idarucizumab were detected in some subjects. No impact on the pharmacokinetics or the reversal effect of idarucizumab or on hypersensitivity reactions was observed in these subjects.

Monitor: Monitor coagulation parameters (e.g., aPPT and ECT [if available]). ▪ Monitor for S/S of clinically relevant bleeding and thromboembolic events. ▪ Monitor for S/S of hypersensitivity reactions (e.g., bronchospasm, fever, pruritus, rash).

Patient Education: Increased thromboembolic risk with reversal of dabigatran. Resume anticoagulant therapy as directed when deemed stable. ▪ Seek immediate medical attention for any S/S of bleeding. ▪ Seek immediate medical attention for S/S of a hypersensitivity reaction (e.g., rash, wheezing). Reactions may occur during or after administration of idarucizumab. ▪ Inform patients with HFI that idarucizumab contains sorbitol. Adverse reactions related to the parenteral administration of sorbitol may occur during or after administration and should be promptly reported.

Maternal/Child: Risk to fetus unknown. Administer during pregnancy only if clearly needed. ▪ Safety and effectiveness during labor and delivery have not been studied. ▪ Use caution during breast-feeding; risk to infant unknown. ▪ Safety and effectiveness have not been established in pediatric patients.

Elderly: No overall differences in safety or effectiveness have been observed between elderly patients and younger patients.

DRUG/LAB INTERACTIONS

Formal drug interaction studies have not been conducted. ▪ In vitro data suggest that the inhibition of dabigatran by idarucizumab is not affected by coagulation factor concentrates (3-factor or 4-factor prothrombin complex concentrates [PCCs], activated PCC, or recombinant factor VIIa).

SIDE EFFECTS

The most frequently reported adverse reactions were constipation, delirium, fever, headache, hypokalemia, and pneumonia. Hypersensitivity reactions (e.g., bronchospasm, fever, hyperventilation, pruritus, and rash) and thromboembolic events have been reported.

ANTIDOTE

Notify physician of any side effects; most will be treated symptomatically. Discontinue administration at the first sign of a serious hypersensitivity reaction and treat as indicated (e.g., oxygen, diphenhydramine, epinephrine, corticosteroids, vasopressors, and/or fluids). Resuscitate as necessary.

IFOSFAMIDE BBW

(eye-**FOS**-fah-myd)

Antineoplastic
(alkylating agent/
nitrogen mustard)

Ifex, Ifosfamide/Mesna Kit

pH 6

USUAL DOSE

Specific testing recommended before each dose; see Monitor.

1.2 Gm/M^2/day for 5 consecutive days. Repeat every 3 weeks as hematologic recovery permits. To prevent hemorrhagic cystitis, ifosfamide should be given with extensive hydration (e.g., at least 2 liters of oral or IV fluid/day), and mesna should be administered with every dose. Ifosfamide dose has been mixed with the initial mesna dose each day in the same solution. Appears to be **compatible.**

DOSE ADJUSTMENTS

Reduced dose may be required in renal or hepatic impairment. Adequate data not available. ▪ Dosing should be cautious in the elderly. Consider decrease in cardiac, hepatic, and renal function; concomitant disease; or other drug therapy. See Elderly. ▪ Severe myelosuppression is frequent, especially when ifosfamide is given with other chemotherapeutic agents. Dose adjustments of all agents may be required. Adjustment of dose interval may be required. Unless clinically essential, the dose should be held for WBCs less than 2,000/mm^3 and/or platelets less than 50,000/mm^3. See Monitor and Drug/Lab Interactions.

DILUTION

Specific techniques required; see Precautions. Each 1 Gm must be diluted with 20 mL SWFI or bacteriostatic water for injection (parabens or benzyl alcohol preserved only). Shake solution to dissolve. May be further diluted with D5W, NS, LR, or SWFI to a final concentration of 0.6 to 20 mg/mL. Further dilution with D2½W, ½NS, and D5NS is also acceptable for larger volumes. 1 Gm in 20 mL or 3 Gm in 60 mL equals 50 mg/mL; 1 Gm in 50 mL equals 20 mg/mL; 1 Gm in 200 mL equals 5 mg/mL. Generic product available in a kit containing ifosfamide and mesna.

Filters: Studies measured potency of ifosfamide in combination with mesna through a 5-micron filter. No significant drug loss for ifosfamide; mesna was not measured.

Storage: Store at CRT 20° to 25° C (68° to 77° F). Protect from temperatures above 30° C (86° F). Reconstituted and further diluted solution should be refrigerated and used within 24 hours. Solutions containing benzyl alcohol can reduce stability.

COMPATIBILITY

(Underline Indicates Conflicting Compatibility Information)

Consider any drug NOT listed as compatible to be INCOMPATIBLE until consulting a pharmacist; specific conditions may apply.

One source suggests the following **compatibilities:**

Additive: Carboplatin (Paraplatin), cisplatin, epirubicin (Ellence), etoposide (VePesid), fluorouracil (5-FU), mesna (Mesnex).

Y-site: Allopurinol (Aloprim), amifostine (Ethyol), amphotericin B cholesteryl (Amphotec), anidulafungin (Eraxis), aztreonam (Azactam), caspofungin (Cancidas), doripenem (Doribax), doxorubicin liposomal (Doxil), etoposide phosphate (Etopophos), filgrastim (Neupogen), fludarabine (Fludara), gallium nitrate (Ganite), gemcitabine (Gemzar), granisetron (Kytril), linezolid (Zyvox), melphalan (Alkeran), ondansetron (Zofran), oxaliplatin (Eloxatin), paclitaxel (Taxol), palonosetron (Aloxi), pemetrexed (Alimta), piperacillin/tazobactam (Zosyn), propofol (Diprivan), sargramostim (Leukine), sodium bicarbonate, teniposide (Vumon), thiotepa, topotecan (Hycamtin), vinorelbine (Navelbine).

RATE OF ADMINISTRATION

A single dose over a minimum of 30 minutes as an infusion. Extend administration time based on amount of diluent and patient condition.

ACTIONS

An alkylating agent. Chemically related to the nitrogen mustards and a synthetic analog of cyclophosphamide. A prodrug that requires activation by hepatic cytochrome P_{450} isoenzymes to exert its cytotoxic activity. Exact mechanism of action not determined, but its cytotoxic action is primarily through DNA cross-links caused by alkylation by iso-phosphoramide mustard at guanine N7 positions. The formation of inter- and intra-strand cross-links in the DNA results in cell death. Distribution takes place with minimal tissue binding and little plasma protein binding. Extensively bound by red blood cells. Extensively metabolized in the liver by cytochrome P_{450} isoenzymes (considerable individual variation). Elimination half-life for a usual dose is about 7 hours. Half-life is extended with larger doses. Ifosfamide and its metabolites are excreted in urine. Secreted in breast milk.

INDICATIONS AND USES

Used in combination with other specific antineoplastic agents for third-line chemo-therapy of germ cell testicular cancer. Should be used in combination with mesna for prophylaxis of hemorrhagic cystitis.

Unlabeled uses: Bladder, cervical, and ovarian cancers; Ewing's sarcoma; Hodgkin's and non-Hodgkin's lymphoma; small-cell lung cancer; osteosarcoma; soft tissue sarcomas.

CONTRAINDICATIONS

Hypersensitivity to ifosfamide; urinary outflow obstruction.

PRECAUTIONS

Follow guidelines for handling cytotoxic agents. See Appendix A, p. 1331. ▪ Usually administered by or under the direction of the physician specialist. ▪ Exclude or correct any urinary tract obstructions; see Contraindications. ▪ Administer cautiously, if at all, to patients with an infection (including an active urinary tract infection), severe immuno-suppression, or compromised bone marrow reserve as indicated by leukopenia, granulo-cytopenia, extensive bone marrow metastases, prior radiation therapy, or prior treatment with other cytotoxic agents. ▪ Myelosuppression can be severe and lead to fatal infections. Deaths have been reported. Risk of myelosuppression is dose-dependent and is increased in patients with reduced renal function and when ifosfamide is administered as a single high dose compared to fractionated doses. Severe myelosuppression is often observed when ifosfamide is used in combination with other chemotherapeutic/hematotoxic agents and/or radiation therapy. ▪ CNS toxicities can be severe and result in encephalopathy and death. ▪ Nephrotoxic and urotoxic. Acute tubular necrosis, acute renal failure, and chronic renal failure have been reported, and deaths have occurred. Benefits must outweigh risks if ifos-famide is used in patients with pre-existing renal impairment or reduced nephron reserve. Glomerular and tubular disorders of renal function are common and may become appar-ent during therapy or months and years after stopping treatment. They may resolve, re-main stable, or progress even after completion of treatment. Hemorrhagic cystitis can be se-vere and may require blood transfusions. Urotoxic effects can be reduced by the prophylactic use of mesna. Risk of hemorrhagic cystitis is dose-dependent and increases with the administra-tion of single high doses compared to fractionated administration. Past or concomitant radiation of the bladder or busulfan therapy may also increase risk. ▪ Use caution in patients with risk factors for cardiotoxicity or pre-existing cardiac disease. Cardiotoxicity (e.g., supraventricular or ventricular arrhythmias, decreased QRS voltage and ST-segment or T-wave changes, toxic cardiomyopathy leading to heart failure with conges-tion and hypotension, pericardial effusion, fibrinous pericarditis, epicardial fibrosis), sometimes with fatal outcomes, has been reported. Risk is dose dependent and is in-creased with prior or concomitant treatment with other cardiotoxic agents or radiation of the cardiac region and, possibly, renal impairment. ▪ Pulmonary toxicity (e.g., intersti-tial pneumonitis, pulmonary fibrosis, and other forms of pulmonary toxicity) has been reported, sometimes with fatal outcomes. ▪ Hypersensitivity reactions, including ana-phylaxis, have been reported. Cross-sensitivity between oxazaphosphorine cytotoxic agents (e.g., cyclophosphamide [Cytoxan]) has been reported. ▪ May interfere with normal wound healing. ▪ Risk of secondary malignancies has been reported. ▪ Veno-

occlusive liver disease has been reported. ▪ Studies in patients with hepatic or renal impairment have not been conducted. Use with caution.
Monitor: Monitor blood counts prior to and at intervals after each treatment cycle. CBC with differential and platelet count and hemoglobin are recommended before each daily dose and as clinically indicated. Unless clinically essential, WBC count should be above 2,000/mm³ and platelet count above 50,000/mm³. ▪ Evaluate glomerular and tubular kidney function before, during, and after treatment. ▪ Monitor urinary sediment regularly for erythrocytes and other signs of urotoxicity/nephrotoxicity. ▪ Urinalysis before each dose recommended. Withhold drug if RBCs in urine exceed 10 per high-powered field. Reinstitute after complete resolution with vigorous oral or parenteral hydration. Mesna given concurrently should prevent hemorrhagic cystitis. ▪ Monitor serum and urine chemistries, including phosphorus and potassium, regularly; administer replacement as indicated. ▪ Monitor for S/S of renal dysfunction (e.g., decreased glomerular filtration rate, increased SCr, aminoaciduria, cylindruria, enzymuria, glycosuria, phosphaturia, proteinuria, and tubular acidosis). ▪ Adequate hydration required; encourage fluid intake (minimum of 2 L/day) and frequent voiding to prevent cystitis. ▪ Nadir of the leukocyte count tends to be reached during the second week after administration. ▪ Monitor for S/S of hypersensitivity (e.g., chest pain, dizziness, dyspnea, fever, flushing, hypotension, nausea, pruritus, rash, rigors, urticaria). ▪ Monitor for S/S of pulmonary toxicity and treat as indicated. ▪ Pneumonias, as well as other bacterial, fungal, viral, and parasitic infections, have been reported, and latent infections can be reactivated. Observe constantly for signs of infection (e.g., fever, sore throat, tiredness) or unusual bleeding or bruising. Antimicrobial prophylaxis may be indicated in certain cases of neutropenia. Antibiotics and/or antimycotics must be given if neutropenic fever occurs. ▪ Monitor for thrombocytopenia (platelet count less than 50,000/mm³). Initiate precautions to prevent excessive bleeding (e.g., inspect IV sites, skin, and mucous membranes; use extreme care during invasive procedures; test urine, emesis, stool, and secretions for occult blood). ▪ Monitor for CNS toxicity. Blurred vision, coma, confusion, extrapyramidal symptoms, hallucinations, peripheral neuropathy, psychotic behavior, seizures, somnolence, and urinary incontinence have been reported. Neurotoxicity may appear within a few hours to a few days after the first administration and usually resolves within 48 to 72 hours of discontinuing ifosfamide, although symptoms may persist. Recurrence after several uneventful treatment courses has occurred. Discontinue treatment if encephalopathy occurs. ▪ Prophylactic administration of antiemetics recommended. ▪ See Drug/Lab Interactions.
Patient Education: Nonhormonal birth control recommended. Females should avoid pregnancy and males should not father a child during therapy and for up to 6 months after the end of therapy; see Maternal/Child. ▪ CNS toxicity may impair the ability to operate an automobile or other heavy machinery. ▪ Side effects are numerous and may be fatal; review all potential side effects with your health care professional before treatment. ▪ See Appendix D, p. 1333.
Maternal/Child: Category D: can cause fetal harm. Females should avoid pregnancy and males should not father a child during therapy and for up to 6 months after the end of therapy. May cause amenorrhea in females and oligospermia or azoospermia in males. Sterility has been reported. ▪ Discontinue breast-feeding. ▪ Safety and effectiveness for use in pediatric patients not established. Fanconi syndrome, renal rickets, and growth retardation have been reported in pediatric patients. Prepubescent females may become sterile or are at risk for developing premature menopause. Prepubescent males may not develop secondary sexual characteristics normally and may have oligospermia or azoospermia.
Elderly: Consider age-related organ impairment. Dose selection should be cautious; see Dose Adjustments. Monitor renal, hepatic, and hematologic functions closely.

DRUG/LAB INTERACTIONS

See Dose Adjustments. ▪ A substrate for both CYP3A4 and CYP2B6. **CYP3A4 inducers** (e.g., carbamazepine [Tegretol], fosphenytoin [Cerebyx], phenytoin [Dilantin], phenobarbital [Luminal], rifampin [Rifadin], and St. John's wort) may increase the metabolism of ifosfamide to its active alkylating metabolites and increase the formation of the neurotoxic/nephrotoxic metabolite chloroacetaldehyde. Monitor closely for signs of toxicity; consider dose adjustment. **CYP3A4 inhibitors** (e.g., aprepitant [Emend], fosaprepitant [Emend for injection], fluconazole [Diflucan], grapefruit and grapefruit juice, itraconazole [Sporanox], ketoconazole [Nizoral], sorafenib [Nexavar]) may decrease the metabolism of ifosfamide to its active alkylating metabolites, perhaps decreasing the effectiveness of treatment. ▪ May have additive effects with **other drugs that act on the CNS** (e.g., antihistamines, antiemetics, narcotics, or sedatives). Use with caution or discontinue if encephalopathy occurs. ▪ Do not administer **live virus vaccines** to patients receiving antineoplastic drugs.

SIDE EFFECTS

Hematuria, hemorrhagic cystitis, and bone marrow suppression are dose-limiting side effects. The most common side effects included alopecia, anemia, CNS toxicity, hematuria, infection, leukopenia, nausea, and vomiting. Other commonly reported side effects were anorexia, confusion, constipation, depressive psychosis with hallucinations, diarrhea, and somnolence. Cardiotoxicity, coagulopathy, coma, cranial nerve dysfunction, dermatitis, disorientation, dizziness, fatigue, fever of unknown origin, hypersensitivity reactions, hypertension, hypotension, liver dysfunction, malaise, neutropenia, osteomalacia, phlebitis, polyneuropathy, pulmonary symptoms, thrombocytopenia, or seizures may occur.

Overdose: Manifestations of dose-dependent toxicities such as CNS toxicity, mucositis, myelosuppression, nephrotoxicity.

Post-Marketing: Anaphylaxis; angioedema; benign and malignant neoplasms; hematotoxicity (e.g., agranulocytosis, bone marrow failure, DIC, febrile bone marrow aplasia, hemolytic anemia, hemolytic uremic syndrome, methemoglobinemia, neonatal anemia); infections, including reactivation of latent infections (e.g., herpes zoster, *Pneumocystis jiroveci*, progressive multifocal leukoencephalopathy [PML], *Strongyloides*, viral hepatitis, and other viral and fungal infections); pneumonia; sepsis and septic shock (including fatal outcomes); psychiatric disorders; syndrome of inappropriate antidiuretic hormone secretion (SIADH); tumor lysis syndrome; and numerous other serious side effects have been reported.

ANTIDOTE

Minor side effects will be treated symptomatically if necessary. Discontinue ifosfamide and notify physician immediately if hematuria, hemorrhagic cystitis, confusion, coma, WBC below 2,000 mm³, or platelets below 50,000/mm³ occur. Administration of whole blood products (e.g., packed RBCs, platelets, leukocytes) and/or blood modifiers (e.g., darbepoetin alfa [Aranesp], epoetin alfa [Epogen], filgrastim [Neupogen, Zarxio], pegfilgrastim [Neulasta], sargramostim [Leukine]) may be indicated to treat bone marrow suppression. Maintain supportive therapy for CNS symptoms until complete resolution; occasionally, recovery has been incomplete. Discontinue treatment if encephalopathy occurs. There is no specific antidote. Supportive therapy as indicated will help sustain the patient in toxicity. Cystitis prophylaxis with mesna may prevent or limit urotoxic effects. Ifosfamide and its metabolites are dialyzable.

IMIPENEM-CILASTATIN

(em-ee-**PEN**-em sigh-lah-**STAT**-in)

Primaxin

Antibacterial
(carbapenem)

pH 6.5 to 8.5

USUAL DOSE

Range is from 250 mg to 1 Gm every 6 to 8 hours. Dose based on severity of disease, susceptibility of pathogens, condition of the patient, age, weight, and CrCl. Adult doses in the following chart are limited to patients with a CrCl equal to or greater than 71 mL/min/1.73 M^2 and a body weight equal to or greater than 70 kg; see Dose Adjustments. Because of high antimicrobial activity, do not exceed the lower of 50 mg/kg/24 hr or 4 Gm/24 hr in adult or pediatric patients. Continue for at least 2 days after all symptoms of infection subside.

Imipenem-Cilastatin Dosing Guidelines				
Type or Severity of Infection	Fully Susceptible Organisms	Total Daily Dose	Moderately Susceptible Organisms	Total Daily Dose
Mild	250 mg q 6 hr	1 Gm	500 mg q 6 hr	2 Gm
Moderate	500 mg q 8 hr or 500 mg q 6 hr	1.5 Gm 2 Gm	500 mg q 6 hr or 1 Gm q 8 hr	2 Gm 3 Gm
Severe/life-threatening	500 mg q 6 hr	2 Gm	1 Gm q 8 hr or 1 Gm q 6 hr	3 Gm 4 Gm
Uncomplicated UTI	250 mg q 6 hr	1 Gm	250 mg q 6 hr	1 Gm
Complicated UTI	500 mg q 6 hr	2 Gm	500 mg q 6 hr	2 Gm

Adult and pediatric patients over 12 years of age with cystic fibrosis and normal renal function: Higher doses up to 90 mg/kg/day have been used. Do not exceed 4 Gm/24 hr.

PEDIATRIC DOSE

Not recommended for use in pediatric patients with CNS infections because of the risk of seizures, or in pediatric patients weighing less than 30 kg with impaired renal function (no data available). Because of high antimicrobial activity, do not exceed the lower of 50 mg/kg/24 hr or 4 Gm/24 hr in adult or pediatric patients.

Infants 3 months of age or less, weighing 1,500 Gm or more: For non-CNS infections:

Less than 1 week of age: 25 mg/kg every 12 hours.

1 to 4 weeks of age: 25 mg/kg every 8 hours.

4 weeks to 3 months of age: 25 mg/kg every 6 hours.

Premature infants weighing from 670 to 1,890 Gm in the first week of life were given 20 mg/kg every 12 hours in one study (see package insert).

Infants and other pediatric patients over 3 months of age: For non-CNS infections: 15 to 25 mg/kg/dose every 6 hours. See statements in Usual Dose. Maximum dose is 2 Gm/day for treatment of infections caused by fully susceptible organisms and 4 Gm/day for moderately susceptible organisms.

DOSE ADJUSTMENTS

Dose adjustments are extensive and required for all patients weighing less than 70 kg, as well as all patients with a CrCl less than 71 mL/min/1.73 M^2. Dose adjustments also vary based on total daily dose required (e.g., 1, 1.5, 2, 3, or 4 Gm). See charts in package insert. ■ Reduced doses may be required in the elderly based on weight and/or decreased renal function. ■ Cleared by hemodialysis; administer after hemodialysis and at 12-hour intervals thereafter. ■ See Precautions/Monitor and Drug/Lab Interactions.

DILUTION

Reconstitute each single dose with 10 mL of **compatible** infusion solutions (e.g., D5W, D10W, NS [see chart on inside back cover or literature]); also **compatible** in D5W with 0.15% KCl and mannitol 5% and 10%. Shake well and transfer the resulting suspension to 100 mL of the same infusion solution. Rinse vial with an additional 10 mL of infusion solution to ensure complete transfer of vial contents to the infusion solution. Agitate until clear. Also available in ADD-Vantage vials for use with ADD-Vantage infusion containers.

Neonatal dilution: Use preservative-free solutions for reconstitution of neonatal doses.

Filters: Manufacturer's data limited; indicates that use of a filter system when withdrawing the suspension from the vial would probably result in filter clogging and decrease the available antibiotic. An in-house study documented **compatibility** of the final diluted solution with a 0.22-micron in-line filter.

Storage: Store dry powder below 25° C (77° F). Diluted solutions are stable at room temperature for 4 hours after preparation or 24 hours if refrigerated. Do not freeze.

COMPATIBILITY   (Underline Indicates Conflicting Compatibility Information)

Consider any drug NOT listed as compatible to be INCOMPATIBLE until consulting a pharmacist; specific conditions may apply.

Manufacturer states, "Should not be mixed with or physically added to other antibiotics." See Drug/Lab Interactions.

One source suggests the following **compatibilities:**

Y-site: Acyclovir (Zovirax), amifostine (Ethyol), anidulafungin (Eraxis), aztreonam (Azactam), caspofungin (Cancidas), cisatracurium (Nimbex), diltiazem (Cardizem), docetaxel (Taxotere), famotidine (Pepcid IV), filgrastim (Neupogen), fludarabine (Fludara), foscarnet (Foscavir), granisetron (Kytril), idarubicin (Idamycin), insulin (regular), linezolid (Zyvox), melphalan (Alkeran), methotrexate, ondansetron (Zofran), propofol (Diprivan), remifentanil (Ultiva), tacrolimus (Prograf), telavancin (Vibativ), teniposide (Vumon), thiotepa, tigecycline (Tygacil), vasopressin, vinorelbine (Navelbine), zidovudine (AZT, Retrovir).

RATE OF ADMINISTRATION

Intermittent IV: Each 500 mg or fraction thereof over 20 to 30 minutes. Doses greater than 500 mg should be infused over 40 to 60 minutes. Slow infusion rate if patient develops nausea and vomiting, dizziness, hypotension, or sweating. May be given through Y-tube or three-way stopcock of infusion set.

ACTIONS

A potent broad-spectrum antibacterial agent. Imipenem is a carbapenem antibiotic; cilastatin inhibits the kidney enzyme responsible for the metabolism of imipenem. Both components are present in equal amounts. Bactericidal to many gram-negative, gram-positive, and anaerobic organisms. Bactericidal activity results from the inhibition of bacterial wall synthesis. Effective against many otherwise resistant organisms. Has a high degree of stability in the presence of beta-lactamases produced by gram-negative and gram-positive bacteria. Rapidly and widely distributed into many body fluids and tissues. Metabolized in the kidneys. Half-life is approximately 1 hour. Excreted in the urine. May cross the placental barrier.

INDICATIONS AND USES

Treatment of serious lower respiratory tract, urinary tract, skin and skin structure, bone and joint, gynecologic, intra-abdominal, and polymicrobic infections; bacterial septicemia; and endocarditis. Most effective against specific organisms (see literature).

Unlabeled uses: Treatment of febrile neutropenia and melioidosis (a rare infection in humans and animals).

CONTRAINDICATIONS

Known sensitivity to any component of this product. ▪ See Maternal/Child and Precautions.

PRECAUTIONS

Specific sensitivity studies are indicated to determine susceptibility of the causative organism to imipenem-cilastatin. ■ To reduce the development of drug-resistant bacteria and maintain its effectiveness, imipenem-cilastatin should be used to treat or prevent only those infections proven or strongly suspected to be caused by bacteria. ■ Serious and occasionally fatal hypersensitivity reactions have been reported in patients receiving therapy with beta-lactams (e.g., carbapenems, cephalosporins, penicillins). More likely in patients with a history of sensitivity to multiple allergens; obtain a careful history. Cross-sensitivity is possible. ■ Avoid prolonged use of drug; superinfection caused by overgrowth of nonsusceptible organisms may result. ■ CNS adverse effects, including confusional states, myoclonic activity, and seizures, have been reported. Incidence increases with higher doses, compromised renal function, or pre-existing CNS disorders. ■ Not recommended in patients with a CrCl less than 5 mL/min/1.73 M^2 unless hemodialysis is instituted within 48 hours. ■ For patients on hemodialysis, benefits of use must outweigh risk of seizures. ■ *Clostridium difficile*–associated diarrhea (CDAD) has been reported. May range from mild diarrhea to fatal colitis. Consider in patients who present with diarrhea during or after treatment with imipenem-cilastatin. ■ Safety and effectiveness for use in meningitis not established. ■ Clinical improvement has been observed in patients with cystic fibrosis, COPD, and lower respiratory tract infections caused by *Pseudomonas aeruginosa;* however, effective bacterial eradication may not occur. ■ See Maternal/Child and Drug/Lab Interactions.

Monitor: May cause thrombophlebitis. Use small needles and large veins, and rotate infusion sites. ■ Electrolyte imbalance and cardiac irregularities resulting from sodium content are possible. Contains 3.2 mEq of sodium/Gm. ■ Monitor renal, hepatic, and hemopoietic systems in prolonged therapy. ■ Some strains of *Pseudomonas aeruginosa* may develop resistance fairly rapidly during treatment. Periodic susceptibility testing should be done when clinically indicated. ■ See Drug/Lab Interactions.

Patient Education: Promptly report diarrhea or bloody stools that occur during treatment or up to several months after an antibiotic has been discontinued; may indicate CDAD and require treatment. ■ Patients with a history of seizures should review medication profile with physician before taking imipenem; see Drug/Lab Interactions.

Maternal/Child: Category C: use only if potential benefit outweighs potential risk during pregnancy and breast-feeding.

Elderly: Consider weight and age-related renal impairment. See Dose Adjustments. ■ Response similar to that seen in younger patients; however, greater sensitivity in the elderly cannot be ruled out.

DRUG/LAB INTERACTIONS

Carbapenems may reduce serum **valproic acid** concentrations to subtherapeutic levels, resulting in loss of seizure control. Monitor valproic acid levels. Consider alternative antibacterial therapy. If administration of imipenem is necessary, supplemental anticonvulsant therapy should be considered. ■ May be used concomitantly with **aminoglycosides and other antibiotics,** but these drugs must never be mixed in the same infusion or given concurrently. ■ Use with **ganciclovir** (Cytovene) may cause generalized seizures. Use only if benefit outweighs risk. ■ Half-life and plasma levels slightly increased by **probenecid.** Avoid concurrent use. ■ Concurrent use with **cyclosporine** (Sandimmune) may decrease cyclosporine metabolism. Elevated cyclosporine levels and neurotoxicity (e.g., agitation, confusion, tremor) have been reported.

SIDE EFFECTS

Full scope of hypersensitivity reactions including anaphylaxis, pruritus, rash, and urticaria. Abdominal pain; abnormal clotting time; agitation; altered CBC and electrolytes; anuria; burning, discomfort, and pain at injection site; CDAD; confusion; diarrhea; dizziness; dyskinesia; dyspnea; elevated alkaline phosphatase, AST, ALT, bilirubin, creatinine, BUN, LDH; fever; gastroenteritis; glossitis; headache; heartburn; hemorrhagic colitis; hepatic failure; hepatitis (including fulminant hepatitis); hyperventilation; hypotension; increased salivation; myoclonus; nausea and vomiting; paresthesia; pharyngeal pain; polyarthralgia; polyuria; positive direct Coombs' test; presence of WBCs or RBCs, protein casts, bilirubin, or urobilinogen in urine; seizures; somnolence; thrombophlebitis; tinnitus; tongue papillar hypertrophy; transient hearing loss in the hearing impaired; vertigo; and many others.

ANTIDOTE
Notify physician of any side effects. Discontinue the drug if indicated. Treat hypersensitivity reactions as indicated; may require epinephrine, airway management, oxygen, IV fluids, antihistamines (e.g., diphenhydramine [Benadryl]), corticosteroids (e.g., hydrocortisone sodium succinate [Solu-Cortef]), and pressor amines (e.g., dopamine). Resuscitate as necessary. Begin anticonvulsants if focal tremors, myoclonus, or seizures occur. If symptoms continue, decrease dose or discontinue the drug. Infusion rate reactions (e.g., dizziness, hypotension, N/V, and sweating) may respond to a decrease in rate of infusion. Mild cases of CDAD may respond to discontinuation of the drug. Treat CDAD with fluids, electrolytes, protein supplements, and oral vancomycin (Vancocin) or metronidazole (Flagyl) as indicated. In severe cases, surgical evaluation may be indicated. Hemodialysis may be useful in overdose.

IMMUNE GLOBULIN INTRAVENOUS BBW

Immunizing agent (passive)

(im-**MUNE GLAW**-byoo-lin IV)

Bivigam, Carimune NF, Flebogamma, Gammagard Liquid, Gammagard S/D, Gammaked, Gammaplex, Gamunex-C, IGIV, Octagam, Privigen

pH 4 to 7.2

USUAL DOSE
For all indications, ensure adequate hydration before administration.

PRIMARY IMMUNODEFICIENCY (PID) DISEASES
Bivigam and Gammuplex: 300 to 800 mg/kg as a single-dose IV infusion every 3 to 4 weeks. Monitor clinical response and trough levels to adjust dose as appropriate. Desired trough level of total IgG concentrations is a minimum of 500 mg/dL (target is 600 mg/dL).

Carimune NF: 400 to 800 mg/kg as a single-dose IV infusion. Administer once every 3 to 4 weeks. Use of a 3% solution is recommended for the first infusion in previously untreated agammaglobulinemic or hypogammaglobulinemic patients. Subsequent infusions may be administered at a higher concentration based on patient tolerance.

Flebogamma, Gammagard Liquid, Gammagard S/D, Gammaked, Gamunex-C, and Octagam 5%: 300 to 600 mg/kg as a single-dose IV infusion every 3 to 4 weeks. Individualize dose and interval based on clinical response. If a patient receiving *Gammaked, Gamunex-C,* or *Octagam* is routinely receiving a dose of less than 400 mg/kg and is at risk for measles exposure (i.e., traveling to a measles endemic area), administer a dose of at least 400 mg/kg just before the expected measles exposure. If a patient is exposed to measles, administer a dose of 400 mg/kg as soon as possible after exposure.

Privigen: 200 to 800 mg/kg as a single-dose IV infusion every 3 to 4 weeks. Adjust dose to achieve desired serum trough levels and clinical response.

IDIOPATHIC THROMBOCYTOPENIC PURPURA (ITP)
All products must be given by IV infusion for ITP patients. Do not administer SC due to a potential risk of hematoma.

Carimune NF: 400 mg/kg/day for 2 to 5 consecutive days based on platelet count and clinical response. A 6% solution is recommended for use in ITP; see chart in Rate of Administration. May be discontinued in acute ITP of childhood if an initial platelet count

Continued

response to the first 2 doses is adequate (30,000 to 50,000/mm³). After induction, if clinically significant bleeding occurs and/or the platelet count falls below 30,000/mm³, a maintenance dose of 400 mg/kg may be given as a single infusion. If response inadequate, increase to 800 to 1,000 mg/kg. May be given intermittently to maintain platelet count.

Flebogamma 10%: 1 Gm/kg/day for 2 consecutive days.

Gammagard S/D: 1 Gm/kg. Up to 3 doses can be given on alternate days based on clinical response and platelet count.

Gammaked and Gamunex-C: 1 Gm/kg/day (10 mL/kg/day) for 2 consecutive days for a total dose of 2 Gm/kg. May withhold the second 1 Gm/kg dose if an adequate platelet response is seen within 24 hours. Alternately, the 2 Gm/kg total dose can be administered as 400 mg/kg/day (4 mL/kg/day) for 5 consecutive days. The high-dose regimen (1 Gm/kg/day for 1 to 2 days) is not recommended for individuals with expanded fluid volumes or when fluid volume may be a concern.

Gammaplex, Octagam 10%, and Privigen: *Chronic ITP:* 1 Gm/kg/day for 2 consecutive days for a total dose of 2 Gm/kg.

B-Cell Chronic Lymphocytic Leukemia (CLL)

Gammagard S/D: 400 mg/kg every 3 to 4 weeks.

Chronic Inflammatory Demyelinating Polyneuropathy (CIDP)

Gamunex-C and Gammaked: *Loading dose:* 1 Gm/kg/day (10 mL/kg/day) for 2 consecutive days or 0.5 Gm/kg/day (5 mL/kg/day) for 4 consecutive days. With either regimen the total dose is 2 Gm/kg. Follow with *maintenance dose* of 1 Gm/kg every 3 weeks. The maintenance dose may be given as a total dose of 1 Gm/kg (10 mL/kg) on Day 1 or divided into 2 doses of 500 mg/kg/day given over 2 consecutive days.

Multifocal Motor Neuropathy (MMN)

Gammagard Liquid: Dose range is 0.5 to 2.4 Gm/kg/month based on clinical response.

PEDIATRIC DOSE

Kawasaki Syndrome

Gammagard S/D: A single dose of 1 Gm/kg as an IV infusion. Alternately, 400 mg/kg/day may be administered for 4 consecutive days. Begin within 7 days of onset of fever. Concomitant administration of aspirin 80 to 100 mg/kg/day in 4 divided doses is indicated.

Other Indications

See specific product manufacturer prescribing information for age restrictions for other indications.

See mg/kg or Gm/kg dose recommendations under Usual Dose. Begin with the lowest recommended dose. With most brands, clinical studies suggested that no difference in dosing is necessary and no special precautions are indicated. According to the manufacturers, infants and neonates were not included in clinical studies for primary immunodeficiency diseases or Kawasaki disease. All age-groups were represented in clinical studies for idiopathic thrombocytopenic purpura. See Maternal/Child.

DOSE ADJUSTMENTS

Adjust dose according to IgG levels and clinical response. Frequency and dose will vary from patient to patient. No controlled clinical trials are available to determine optimum trough serum IgG level.

DILUTION

Requirements for dilution of liquid and lyophilized powder preparations are brand specific and vary considerably; see manufacturer's package insert. Some may be further diluted only with D5W or with D5W and/or NS; others cannot be diluted. Some require D5W or NS to flush the infusion line.

All formulations: Do not mix with IGIV products from other manufacturers. Do not mix with other medicinal products. Administer through a separate infusion line or flush line before and after administration. Do not use if solution is cloudy, turbid, or contains particulate matter. Do not freeze. Do not use if previously frozen. Do not use beyond expiration date. For single use only; use promptly or discard unused product. Bring to room temperature before reconstitution (if required) or administration.

Most formulations: *Do not shake.* If large doses are to be administered, several vials may be pooled using aseptic technique (time limits or specific processes may apply); see specific product.

Bivigam, Flebogamma, Gamunex-C, Gammagard Liquid, Gammaked, Gammaplex, Octagam, and ***Privigen*** are liquid preparations and are ready to use.

Carimune NF is a lyophilized product, ***and Gammagard S/D*** is a freeze-dried product. Both require reconstitution. Absolute sterile technique is required at all steps of the reconstitution process. Filtration may be required as drawn into a syringe for administration or as administered through IV tubing. Check both brands for specific equipment and specific dilution requirements.

Bivigam: A ready-to-use 10% sterile solution; do not dilute. Available as 5 Gm in 50 mL or 10 Gm in 100 mL. Does not contain sucrose. Warm to room temperature before use and maintain at room temperature during administration. *Do not shake.* Several vials may be pooled using aseptic technique into sterile infusion bags and infused. pH 4 to 4.6.

Carimune NF: Contains sucrose; see Precautions. Available as a lyophilized powder in 3-, 6-, and 12-Gm vials. Reconstitute with NS, D5W, or SWFI. Package insert has a chart with dilution requirements for all concentrations. *Do not shake.* Immediate use is recommended unless reconstituted under a sterile laminar flow hood; then it may be refrigerated and administration must begin within 24 hours. Several reconstituted vials of identical concentration and diluent may be pooled in an empty sterile glass or plastic IV infusion container using aseptic technique. pH 6.4 to 6.8. A 6% solution of *Carimune NF* is recommended for use in ITP.

Flebogamma: Contains sorbitol; does not contain sucrose. A ready-to-use 5% (50 mg/mL) sterile solution; available as 0.5 Gm in 10 mL, 2.5 Gm in 50 mL, 5 Gm in 100 mL, 10 Gm in 200 mL, and 20 Gm in 400 mL. Also available as a ready-to-use 10% (100 mg/mL) sterile solution of 5 Gm in 50 mL, 10 Gm in 100 mL, and 20 Gm in 200 mL concentrations. Further dilution with other solutions not recommended. Using aseptic technique, several vials may be pooled into an empty sterile solution container. See Filters. pH 5 to 6.

Gammagard Liquid: Does not contain sucrose. A ready-to-use 10% solution available as 1 Gm in 10 mL, 2.5 Gm in 25 mL, 5 Gm in 50 mL, 10 Gm in 100 mL, and 20 Gm in 200 mL. Warm to room temperature before use. *Do not shake.* May be further diluted only with D5W. See Filters. pH 4.6 to 5.1.

Gammagard S/D: Does not contain sucrose. A freeze-dried preparation. Must be warmed to room temperature before reconstitution if refrigerated. Diluent (SWFI), transfer device, administration set with integral airway, and filter provided with each single-use vial. Available in 2.5-, 5-, and 10-Gm single-dose vials with diluent. Use full amount of diluent (50, 96, 192 mL) to prepare a 5% solution (50 mg/mL), or remove one half the amount of diluent (25, 48, 96 mL) to prepare a 10% solution (100 mg/mL). *Do not shake.* Must be used within 2 hours of dilution if prepared outside a laminar flow hood. Administer within 24 hours if prepared aseptically inside a sterile laminar flow hood and stored in the original glass container or pooled into ViaFlex bags under constant refrigeration. Record date and time of reconstitution/pooling. pH 6.4 to 7.2.

Gammaked: Does not contain sucrose. A ready-to-use 10% solution. Available as 1 Gm in 10 mL, 2.5 Gm in 25 mL, 5 Gm in 50 mL, 10 Gm in 100 mL, and 20 Gm in 200 mL. Bring to room temperature before administration if refrigerated. Use an 18-gauge needle or dispensing pin to penetrate the stopper of the 10-mL vial. Use 16-gauge needles or dispensing pins for the 25 mL and larger sizes. May be further diluted with D5W if required. Do not use any other diluent. *Do not shake.* Content of vials may be pooled under aseptic conditions into sterile infusion bags but must be infused within 8 hours of pooling. pH is 4 to 4.5.

Gammaplex: Does not contain sucrose but does contain fructose; see Contraindications. A ready-to-use 5% sterile solution. Available as 2.5 Gm in 50 mL, 5 Gm in 100 mL, and 10 Gm in 200 mL. *Do not shake.* Begin infusion within 2 hours if multiple vials are pooled under aseptic conditions. Bring to room temperature before administration if refrigerated. pH 4.8 to 5.1.

Gamunex-C: Does not contain sucrose. A ready-to-use 10% sterile solution. Available in 1-, 2.5-, 5-, 10-, and 20-Gm single-dose vials. Bring to room temperature before administration if refrigerated. Use an 18-gauge needle to penetrate the stopper of the 1-Gm size. Use a 16-gauge needle to penetrate the stopper of the 2.5- to 20-Gm sizes. Penetration of the stopper in the center of the raised ring and perpendicular to it is recommended. May be further diluted with D5W if required. Do not use any other diluent. Filtration during administration is not required. Use within 8 hours if multiple vials are pooled under aseptic conditions. pH 4 to 4.5.

Octagam: Does not contain sucrose but does contain maltose; see Contraindications. A ready-to-use 5% or 10% sterile solution. The 5% solution is available as 1-, 2.5-, 5-, 10-, and 25-Gm single-dose vials. The 10% solution is available as 2- 5-, 10-, and 20-Gm single-dose vials. *Do not shake.* Use within 8 hours if multiple vials are pooled under aseptic conditions. Bring to room temperature before administration if refrigerated. pH 5.1 to 6 (5%); pH 4.5 to 5 (10%).

Privigen: Does not contain sucrose but does contain L-proline; see Contraindications. A ready-to-use 10% sterile solution. Available in 5-, 10-, 20-, and 40-Gm single-dose vials. *Do not shake.* May be further diluted with D5W if required. Do not use any other diluent. Filtration during administration is not required. Content of vials may be pooled under aseptic conditions into sterile infusion bags but infusion should begin within 8 hours of pooling; contains no preservatives. pH 4.6 to 5.

Filters: Filter or filter needle is provided by most manufacturers. *Carimune NF and Flebogamma* may be filtered with a larger pore filter size but is not required by manufacturers (filters greater than or equal to 15 microns will be less likely to slow infusion [0.2-micron antibacterial filters may be used with *Carimune NF, Flebogamma, and Octagam*]). *Carimune NF* is nano-filtered. Filtration of *Gamunex-C* during administration is not required; however, use of a non–protein-binding, 0.22-micron filter is permissible. Use of an in-line filter is optional with *Gammagard Liquid and Octagam.*

Storage: Storage requirements are brand specific and vary considerably from refrigeration only to continuous or partial storage at RT not exceeding 30° C (77° F); see manufacturer's package insert. Do not use after expiration date. Discard partially used vials. Do not use if solution is turbid or has been frozen. Some specifically state, "Do not heat or microwave."

COMPATIBILITY

Consider any drug NOT listed as compatible to be INCOMPATIBLE until consulting a pharmacist; specific conditions may apply.

Manufacturers recommend administration through a separate IV line without admixture with other drugs and state, "Do not combine one IGIV product with an IGIV product from another manufacturer." *Gammagard Liquid, Gammaked, Gamunex-C, and Privigen* are **compatible** only with D5W and are **incompatible** with NS. *Flebogamma and Octagam* should not be further diluted with any solution.

Most preparations may be infused sequentially into a primary IV of D5W or NS, or the tubing may be flushed with D5W or NS before and after administration.

One source suggests the following **compatibilities:** *Not recommended by manufacturers.*
Y-site: Fluconazole (Diflucan), sargramostim (Leukine).

RATE OF ADMINISTRATION

All formulations: Too-rapid infusion may cause a precipitous hypotensive reaction. Decrease rate of infusion at onset of patient discomfort or any adverse reactions; see Antidote. Decrease rate in patients at risk for neuromuscular disorders. See Precautions and individual products for suggested decrease in rates for patients at risk for thrombosis or developing renal dysfunction. Administer via separate IV tubing with filter or filter needle (provided by most manufacturers if required). Do not mix with IGIV products from other manufacturers or with other drugs or IV solutions. An infusion pump will facilitate an accurate rate of administration.

Bivigam: Does not contain sucrose. 0.5 mg/kg/min for the first 10 minutes. If no discomfort or adverse effects, may be increased every 20 minutes by 0.8 mg/kg/min up to 6 mg/kg/min. In patients at risk for thrombosis or developing renal dysfunction, administer at the minimum dose and rate of infusion that is practicable.

Carimune NF: Contains sucrose; see Precautions. An initial infusion rate of 0.5 mg/kg/min for 30 minutes. May then be increased to 1 mg/kg/min for the next 30 minutes. May be gradually increased in steps up to a maximum of 3 mg/kg/min as tolerated. The first dose in previously untreated agammaglobulinemic or hypogammaglobulinemic patients must be a 3% solution. After the first dose, subsequent infusions may be administered at a higher concentration as tolerated; see Precautions. In patients at risk for thrombosis or developing renal dysfunction, administer at the minimum dose; the maximum rate of infusion should not exceed 2 mg/kg/min.

Flebogamma: Does not contain sucrose. In patients at risk for thrombosis or developing renal dysfunction, administer at the minimum dose and rate of infusion that is practicable.

Primary immunodeficiency (PI): Initiate 5% solution at 0.01 mL/kg/min (0.5 mg/kg/min) for the first 30 minutes. If no discomfort or adverse effects, may be gradually increased to a maximum rate of 0.1 mL/kg/min (5 mg/kg/min).

Primary immunodeficiency (PI) and idiopathic thrombocytopenic purpura (ITP): Initiate 10% solution at 0.01 mL/kg/min (1 mg/kg/min) for the first 30 minutes. If no discomfort or adverse effects, may be gradually increased to a maximum rate of 0.08 mL/kg/min (8 mg/kg/min).

Gammagard Liquid: Does not contain sucrose. In patients at risk for developing renal dysfunction or thrombotic episodes, the maximum infusion rate should be less than 3.3 mg/kg/min (less than 2 mL/kg/hr).

Primary immunodeficiency (PI): 0.5 mL/kg/hr (0.8 mg/kg/min) for the first 30 minutes. If no discomfort or adverse effects, may be gradually increased every 30 minutes to a maximum rate of 5 mL/kg/hr (8 mg/kg/min).

Multifocal motor neuropathy (MMN): 0.5 mL/kg/hr. (0.8 mg/kg/min) for the first 30 minutes. If no discomfort or adverse effects, may be gradually increased every 30 minutes to a maximum rate of 5.4 mL/kg/hr (9 mg/kg/min).

Gammagard S/D: Dose not contain sucrose. 5% solution 0.5 mL/kg/hr. May be gradually increased to a maximum rate of 4 mL/kg/hr if no discomfort or adverse effects. If 5% solution well tolerated at 4 mL/kg/hr, a 10% solution can be used. Begin with 0.5 mL/kg/hr. If no adverse effects, gradually increase up to a maximum of 8 mL/kg/hr. In patients at risk for developing renal dysfunction, the concentration and infusion rate should be less than 3.3 mg/kg/min (less than 2 mL/kg/hr of 10% or less than 4 mL/kg/hr of 5%).

Gammaked: Does not contain sucrose. In patients at risk for thrombosis or developing renal dysfunction, administer at the minimum dose and rate of infusion that is practicable.

Primary immunodeficiency (PI) and idiopathic thrombocytopenic purpura (ITP): 1 mg/kg/min (0.01 mL/kg/min). If the infusion is well tolerated, the rate may be gradually increased to a maximum of 8 mg/kg/min (0.08 mL/kg/min).

Chronic inflammatory demyelinating polyneuropathy (CDIP): 2 mg/kg/min (0.02 mL/kg/min). If the infusion is well tolerated, the rate may be gradually increased to a maximum of 8 mg/kg/min (0.08 mL/kg/min).

Gammaplex: Does not contain sucrose. 0.5 mg/kg/min (0.01 mL/kg/min) for the first 15 minutes. If no discomfort or adverse effects, may be gradually increased every 15 minutes to 4 mg/kg/min (0.08 mL/kg/min). In patients at risk for thrombosis or developing renal dysfunction, administer at the minimum dose and rate of infusion that is practicable.

Gamunex-C: Does not contain sucrose. In patients at risk for thrombosis or developing renal dysfunction, administer at the minimum dose and rate of infusion that is practicable.

Primary immunodeficiency (PI) and idiopathic thrombocytopenic purpura (ITP): 1 mg/kg/min (0.01 mL/kg/min) for the first 30 minutes. If no discomfort or adverse effects, may be gradually increased to a maximum rate of 8 mg/kg/min (0.08 mL/kg/min).

Chronic inflammatory demyelinating polyneuropathy (CIDP): 2 mg/kg/min (0.02 mL/kg/min). If no discomfort or adverse effects, may be gradually increased to a maximum rate of 8 mg/kg/min (0.08 mL/kg/min).

Octagam: Does not contain sucrose; does contain maltose. In patients at risk for thrombosis or developing renal dysfunction, administer at the minimum dose and rate of infusion that is practicable.

Primary immunodeficiency (PI): Initiate 5% solution at 0.5 mg/kg/min for the first 30 minutes. If no discomfort or adverse effects, may increase gradually in 30-minute increments to a maximum rate of 3.33 mg/kg/min.

Idiopathic thrombocytopenic purpura (ITP): Initiate 10% solution at 1 mg/kg/min for the first 30 minutes. If no discomfort or adverse effects, may increase gradually in 30-minute increments to a maximum rate of 12 mg/kg/min.

Privigen: Does not contain sucrose. IV line may be flushed with D5W or NS. In patients at risk for thrombosis or developing renal dysfunction, administer at the minimum dose and rate of infusion that is practicable.

Primary immunodeficiency: 0.5 mg/kg/min (0.005 mL/kg/min) initially. If no discomfort or adverse effects, may be gradually increased to a maximum rate of 8 mg/kg/min (0.08 mL/kg/min).

Chronic immune thrombocytopenic purpura: 0.005 mL/kg/min (0.5 mg/kg/min) initially. If no discomfort or adverse effects, may be gradually increased to a maximum rate of 0.04 mL/kg/min (4 mg/kg/min).

ACTIONS

A preparation of concentrated human immunoglobulin G (IgG) antibodies. Obtained, purified, and standardized from human plasma. Specific methods during the manufacturing process (e.g., cold ethanol fractionation, detergents, solvents, nanofiltration) inactivate blood-borne viruses (e.g., hepatitis, HIV). Used as replacement therapy in primary and secondary immunodeficiencies. Active against bacterial, viral, parasitic, and mycoplasma antigens. Capable of both opsonization and neutralization of microbes and toxins. Also contains antibodies capable of interacting with and altering the activity of the immune system as well as antibodies capable of reacting with cells such as erythrocytes. (The role of these antibodies and the mechanisms of action of IgG have not been fully clarified.) Provides immediate antibody levels following infusion. The immediate peak in serum IgG is followed by a rapid decay due to equilibration between the plasma and extravascular fluid compartments. Half-life is variable (approximately 3 to 6 weeks) but may be decreased by fever or infection (increased catabolism or consumption). Crosses the placenta.

INDICATIONS AND USES

Selected products are approved for different uses; see Usual Dose. All provide rapid-onset, short-term passive immunization. Labeled uses include: *Primary immunodeficiency diseases:* Replacement therapy in adults, adolescents, and other pediatric patients unable to produce adequate amounts of IgG antibodies, especially in the following situations: need for immediate increase in intravascular immunoglobulin levels, small muscle mass or bleeding tendencies that contraindicate IM injection, and selected disease states (e.g., congenital agammaglobulinemia, common variable immunodeficiency [CVID], combined immunodeficiency, X-linked agammaglobulinemia, Wiskott-Aldrich syndrome). ■ *Treatment of acute and chronic idiopathic thrombocytopenic purpura (also called immune thrombocytopenic purpura or primary immune thrombocytopenia):* Temporary increase in platelet counts in patients with idiopathic thrombocytopenic purpura and with thrombocytopenia associated with bone marrow transplant. ■ *Treatment of chronic inflammatory demyelinating polyneuropathy (CIDP):* Improvement of neuromuscular disability and impairment and maintenance therapy to prevent relapse. ■ *Adjunct in chronic lymphocytic leukemia:* Prevention of bacterial infections in patients with hypogammaglobulinemia or recurrent bacterial infection associated with B-cell CLL. ■ *Multifocal motor neuropathy (MMN):* To improve muscle strength and disability in adult patients. ■ *Kawasaki syndrome:* Prevention of coronary artery aneurysms associated with Kawasaki syndrome. ■ Safety and effectiveness of *Gammagard S/D, Gammaplex, and Octagam 10%* in pediatric patients with chronic ITP have not been established; see Maternal/Child for additional limitations with other products. ▪ Several formulations are approved for SC use in specific diagnoses; consult prescribing information.

Unlabeled uses: There are numerous unlabeled uses; consult literature.

CONTRAINDICATIONS

Individuals known to have anaphylactic or severe hypersensitivity responses to the administration of human immune globulin. ▪ IgA-deficient patients with pre-existing anti-IgA antibodies and a history of hypersensitivity. ▪ *Gammaplex* is contraindicated in patients with hereditary intolerance to fructose; also contraindicated in infants and neonates for whom sucrose or fructose tolerance has not been established. ▪ *Octagam* is contraindicated in patients with acute hypersensitivity to corn (contains maltose, which is derived from corn). ▪ *Privigen* is contraindicated in patients with hyperprolinemia because it contains L-proline as a stabilizer.

PRECAUTIONS

Check label; must state, "For IV use." ▪ Some formulations may be given SC; however, all products must be given by IV infusion for ITP patients. Do not administer SC due to a potential risk for hematoma. ▪ Hypersensitivity reactions have occurred; administer in a facility with adequate equipment and supplies to monitor the patient and respond to any medical emergency. ▪ Use extreme caution in individuals with a history of prior systemic hypersensitivity reactions. Incidence of anaphylaxis may be increased, especially with repeated injections. IgA-deficient patients, especially those with antibodies against IgA, are at greater risk for developing severe hypersensitivity reactions. ▪ Some packaging of these products may contain latex; use caution in sensitive individuals. ▪ IGIV products have been associated with renal dysfunction, acute renal failure, osmotic nephrosis, and death. Use extreme caution in patients with any degree of renal insufficiency; in patients age 65 years and older; in patients with diabetes mellitus, paraproteinemia, sepsis, or volume depletion; and/or in patients receiving known nephrotoxic drugs. If used, should be administered at the minimum dose and rate of infusion practicable. *Products containing sucrose as a stabilizer (e.g., Carimune NF) have demonstrated an increased risk for renal dysfunction.* Consider benefit versus risk before use. ▪ Increases in SCr and/or BUN may progress to oliguria and anuria requiring dialysis; however, some patients improve spontaneously with discontinuation of IGIV. ▪ May cause aseptic meningitis syndrome (AMS), especially with high doses (greater than 1 Gm/kg) and/or rapid infusion. May begin from 2 hours to 2 days after treatment. Symptoms are drowsiness, fever, headache (severe), nausea and vomiting, nuchal rigidity, painful eye movements, and photophobia. Cerebrospinal fluid (CSF) studies are often positive with pleocytosis, predominantly from the granulocyte series and elevated protein levels. ▪ Hyperproteinemia, with resultant changes in serum viscosity, and electrolyte imbalances (e.g., hyponatremia) may occur. Distinguish true hyponatremia from pseudohyponatremia to determine correct treatment. Decreasing serum-free water in patients with pseudohyponatremia may lead to volume depletion with a further increase in serum viscosity, which may predispose to thromboembolic events. ▪ IGIV products have been associated with thrombotic events. Risk factors may include advanced age, prolonged immobilization, hypercoagulable conditions, history of venous or arterial thrombosis, use of estrogens, indwelling vascular catheter, hyperviscosity, and cardiovascular risk factors (e.g., cerebrovascular disease, coronary artery disease, diabetes, hypertension). Thrombosis may occur in the absence of known risk factors. If used, should be administered at the minimum dose and rate of infusion practicable. Ensure adequate hydration before administration. ▪ Baseline assessment of blood viscosity should be made in patients at risk for hyperviscosity, including those with cryoglobins, fasting chylomicronemia, markedly high triglycerides, or monoclonal gammopathies. ▪ May rarely cause hemolysis, which can result in hemolytic anemia due to enhanced RBC sequestration. High doses (greater than 2 Gm/kg) and non-O blood group may be risk factors for hemolysis. Cases of severe hemolysis-related renal dysfunction/failure or DIC have occurred following infusion; see Monitor. ▪ Consider risk/benefit before use of high-dose regimens (greater than 1 Gm/kg) in chronic ITP patients at increased risk for acute kidney injury, hemolysis, thrombosis, or volume overload. ▪ Noncardiogenic pulmonary edema (transfusion-related acute lung injury [TRALI]) has been reported; see Monitor. ▪ Derived from human blood. Despite purification processes, may carry risk of transmitting infectious agents (e.g., viruses [e.g., HIV, hepatitis] or Creutzfeldt-Jakob disease [CJD] agent). ▪ Patients with gammaglobulinemia or extreme hypogamma-globulinemia who have never before received immunoglobulin substitution treatment or patients whose time from the last treatment is greater than 8 weeks may be at risk for developing inflammatory reactions (e.g., chills, fever, nausea, vomiting) on rapid infusion. Initiate slowly and increase rate as tolerated.

Monitor: Use of larger veins recommended to reduce infusion-site discomfort, especially with 10% solutions. ▪ Correct volume depletion before administration in all patients, especially patients with pre-existing renal insufficiency. ▪ Recording of lot number on vials is recommended. ▪ Monitor vital signs and observe patient continuously during infusion. A precipitous drop in BP or anaphylaxis can occur at any time. Emergency equipment and supplies must be at bedside. ▪ Monitor renal function (e.g., BUN, SCr) and urine output in patients at increased risk for renal failure. Obtain baseline studies, monitor at intervals, and discontinue IGIV if renal function deteriorates. See Precautions. ▪ Monitor for hyperproteinemia with resultant changes in serum viscosity and electrolyte imbalances. ▪ Monitor for S/S of thrombosis and assess blood viscosity in patients at risk for hyperviscosity. ▪ Monitor for S/S of hemolysis (e.g., lysis of red blood cells, liberation of hemoglobin), significant drop in hemoglobin or hematocrit, and hemolytic anemia. ▪ Monitor for S/S of TRALI (e.g., fever, hypoxemia, normal left ventricular function, pulmonary edema, severe respiratory distress). Usually occurs within 1 to 6 hours after completion of the infusion. Manage with oxygen and adequate ventilatory support. If TRALI is suspected, both the product and the patient serum should be tested for the presence of antineutrophil antibodies. ▪ Monitor for volume overload.

Patient Education: Report a burning sensation in the head, chills, cyanosis, diaphoresis, dyspnea, faintness or light-headedness, fatigue, fever, hives, itching or rash, neck pain or difficulty moving neck, tachycardia, wheezing. ▪ Report chest pain or tightness, pain and/or swelling of an arm or a leg with warmth over the affected area, difficulty passing urine, decreased urine output, fluid retention, edema, shortness of breath, or sudden weight gain. ▪ Remote risk of viral or CJD infection; consider risk versus benefit of therapy. See Drug/Lab Interactions.

Maternal/Child: Category C: use with caution in pregnancy; no adverse effects documented, but adequate studies are not available. ▪ Safety for use in breast-feeding not established. ▪ Response in pediatric patients usually exceeds response in adults. ▪ Safety and effectiveness of *Gammagard S/D* in pediatric patients with chronic ITP have not been established. ▪ Safety and effectiveness of *Gammagard S/D* in Kawasaki disease have been established. ▪ Use of *Privigen* to treat primary immunodeficiency in pediatric patients under 3 years of age or to treat chronic immune thrombocytopenic purpura in pediatric patients under 15 years of age not established. ▪ Safety and effectiveness of *Bivigam* not established for use in pediatric patients under 6 years of age. ▪ Safety and effectiveness of *Flebogamma 5% and 10% and Gammaplex* in pediatric patients under 2 years of age have not been established. ▪ Safety and effectiveness of *Octagam 10%* in pediatric patients have not been established. ▪ Safety and effectiveness of *Gammagard Liquid* for treatment of PI in pediatric patients under 2 years of age have not been established. ▪ Safety and effectiveness for use in pediatric patients with MMN have not been established. ▪ Safety and effectiveness of *Gammaked* and *Gamunex-C* for use in pediatric patients with CIDP have not been established.

Elderly: Use with extreme caution. Incidence of renal insufficiency, thrombosis, and other side effects increased due to age, potential for decreased organ function, and pre-existing medical conditions. Do not exceed recommended dose and infuse at the minimum infusion rate practicable; see Precautions.

DRUG/LAB INTERACTIONS

Do not administer **live virus vaccines** from 2 weeks before to at least 3 months after immune globulin IV. Passive transfer of antibodies may transiently interfere with the response to live virus vaccines, such as measles, mumps, rubella, and varicella; see prescribing information if there is a risk of measles exposure or if accidental exposure has occurred. ▪ Provides immediate antibody levels that last for about 3 weeks. In selected patients, may have an immune-modulating effect that may alter their response to **corticosteroids or antineoplastic agents.** ▪ Concurrent use with **nephrotoxic drugs** (e.g., aminoglycosides [e.g., gentamicin], amphotericin B [Amphotec, conventional], cidofovir [Vistide], rifampin [Rifadin]) may increase risk of renal insufficiency. ▪ Products that contain **maltose** *(Octagam)* may interfere with blood and urine glucose tests. ▪ Various antibody titers may be raised temporarily, resulting in **false-positive serologic testing.** ▪ May cause a positive **direct or indirect antiglobulin (Coombs') test.**

SIDE EFFECTS
Arthralgia, asthenia, back pain, chills, diarrhea, dizziness, fatigue, fever, flushing, headache, hyperhidrosis, hypertension, infusion site pain/reactions, lethargy, nausea and vomiting, pharyngitis, rash, sinusitis, upper abdominal pain, and urticaria were reported most commonly. Full range of hypersensitivity symptoms, including anaphylaxis, is possible. Angioedema, erythema, fever, and urticaria are most frequently observed. Anxiety, chest tightness, cough, decreased diastolic BP, difficulty breathing, elevated ALT and AST (temporary), hemolytic anemia (reversible), increased BUN and SCr (may occur as soon as 1 to 2 days following infusion), leg cramps, light-headedness, malaise, migraine, myalgia, pharyngolaryngeal pain, and tachycardia have been reported. Severe reactions (e.g., circulatory collapse, fever, loss of consciousness, nausea and vomiting, sudden onset of dyspnea) have occurred and are more common in patients with antibody deficiencies. Noncardiogenic pulmonary edema (transfusion-related acute lung injury [TRALI]) has been reported. Acute renal failure, acute tubular necrosis, osmotic nephrosis, and proximal tubular nephropathy have been reported; may result in death. Is made from human plasma; process attempts to eliminate risk of hepatitis or HIV infection. A precipitous hypotensive reaction can occur and is most frequently associated with too-rapid rate of injection. Aseptic meningitis syndrome and hemolysis occur infrequently. See Precautions.

Post-Marketing: Abdominal pain, apnea, ARDS, back pain, bronchospasm, bullous dermatitis, cardiac arrest, coma, cyanosis, dyspnea, epidermolysis, erythema multiforme, hepatic dysfunction, hypotension, hypoxemia, leukopenia, loss of consciousness, pancytopenia, positive direct antiglobulin (Coombs') test, pulmonary edema, seizures, Stevens-Johnson syndrome, thromboembolism, and tremor have been reported with IGIV products.

ANTIDOTE
Reduce rate for patient discomfort, for any sign of adverse reaction, and in patients at risk for renal insufficiency or thrombosis. If symptoms subside promptly, the infusion may be resumed at a lower rate. Decreasing the volume of subsequent infusions may also prevent or decrease the incidence of adverse reactions. Loop diuretics (e.g., furosemide [Lasix]) may be helpful in the management of fluid overload. Patients who continue to experience adverse reactions after rate and/or volume have been reduced may be premedicated with hydrocortisone 1 to 2 mg/kg 30 minutes before the immune globulin infusion. Pretreatment with acetaminophen (Tylenol) and diphenhydramine (Benadryl) or trying a different brand of immune globulin may also be useful. Discontinue the drug immediately for any signs of a hypersensitivity reaction, thrombotic event, or renal insufficiency. Notify the physician. May be treated symptomatically and infusion resumed at slower rate if symptoms subside. Treat anaphylaxis immediately. Epinephrine (Adrenalin), diphenhydramine (Benadryl), oxygen, vasopressors (e.g., dopamine), corticosteroids, and ventilation equipment must always be available. Manage TRALI with oxygen and ventilatory support. Resuscitate as necessary.

INDOMETHACIN SODIUM
(in-doh-**METH**-ah-sin **SO**-dee-um)

Prostaglandin inhibitor
(patent ductus arteriosus adjunct)

Indocin IV

pH 6 to 7.5

USUAL DOSE
Neonates: Three IV doses, specific to age at first dose, given at 12- to 24-hour intervals constitute a course of therapy.
Less than 48 hours of age: First dose (0.2 mg/kg of body weight), second dose (0.1 mg/kg), third dose (0.1 mg/kg).
2 to 7 days of age: 0.2 mg/kg for each of 3 doses.
Over 7 days of age: First dose (0.2 mg/kg), then 0.25 mg/kg for the next 2 doses.

If ductus arteriosus reopens, a second course of 1 to 3 doses as described for each neonate age may be repeated one time given at 12- to 24-hour intervals. If neonate remains unresponsive to indomethacin therapy after 2 courses, surgery may be required for closure of the ductus arteriosus.

DOSE ADJUSTMENTS
If urine output is less than 0.6 mL/kg/hr at any time a dose is to be given, withhold dose until lab studies confirm normal renal function.

DILUTION
Each 1 mg must be diluted with at least 1 mL NS or SWFI without preservatives (0.1 mg/0.1 mL); may be diluted with 2 mL diluent (0.05 mg/0.1 mL). The preservative benzyl alcohol is toxic in neonates. A fresh solution should be prepared just before each administration. Discard any unused portion.
Filters: No data available from manufacturer.
Storage: Store unopened vials in carton at CRT. Protect from light. Use reconstituted solution immediately.

COMPATIBILITY
Consider any drug NOT listed as compatible to be INCOMPATIBLE until consulting a pharmacist; specific conditions may apply.
Manufacturer states, "Prepare only with preservative-free NS or SWFI"; further dilution with IV solutions is not recommended and may precipitate with solutions with a pH below 6.

One source suggests the following **compatibilities:**
Y-site: Dextrose 2.5% and 5%, furosemide (Lasix), insulin (regular), potassium chloride (KCl), sodium bicarbonate, nitroprusside sodium.

RATE OF ADMINISTRATION
A single dose, properly diluted, by IV injection over 20 to 30 minutes.

ACTIONS
A potent inhibitor of prostaglandin synthesis. Through an unconfirmed method of action (thought to be inhibition of prostaglandin synthesis), it causes closure of a patent ductus arteriosus 75% to 80% of the time, eliminating the need for surgical intervention. Plasma half-life varies inversely with postnatal age and weight and ranges from 12 to 20 hours. Metabolized in the liver and eventually excreted in urine and bile.

INDICATIONS AND USES
Closure of a hemodynamically significant patent ductus arteriosus in premature infants weighing between 500 and 1,750 Gm if usual medical management (e.g., fluid restriction, diuretics, digoxin, respiratory support) has not been effective after 48 hours.

CONTRAINDICATIONS
Bleeding, especially active intracranial hemorrhage or GI bleeding; coagulation defects; necrotizing enterocolitis; infants with congenital heart disease (e.g., pulmonary atresia, severe coarctation of the aorta, severe tetralogy of Fallot) who require patency of the

ductus arteriosus for satisfactory pulmonary or systemic blood flow; proven or suspected untreated infection; significant renal impairment; thrombocytopenia.

PRECAUTIONS

Clinical evidence of a hemodynamically significant patent ductus arteriosus (respiratory distress, a continuous murmur, a hyperactive precordium, cardiomegaly and pulmonary plethora on chest x-ray) should be present before use is considered. ▪ For use only in a highly supervised setting such as an intensive care nursery. ▪ May increase potential for GI or intraventricular bleeding. ▪ Use caution in presence of existing controlled infection; may mask signs and symptoms of exacerbation. ▪ May suppress water excretion to a greater extent than sodium excretion. Hyponatremia may result. ▪ For IV use only. ▪ Surgery indicated if condition is not responsive to two courses of therapy.

Monitor: Vital signs, oxygenation, acid-base status, fluid and electrolyte balance, and kidney function (SCr, BUN, urine output) must be monitored and maintained. ▪ Can cause marked reduction in urine output (over 50%), increase BUN and SCr, and reduce glomerular filtration rate and CrCl. These symptoms usually disappear when therapy completed but may cause acute renal failure, especially in infants with impaired renal function from other causes. ▪ May inhibit platelet aggregation; monitor for signs of bleeding. ▪ Discontinue drug if signs of impaired liver function appear. ▪ Confirm absolute patency of vein. Avoid extravasation; will irritate tissue. ▪ See Drug/Lab Interactions.

DRUG/LAB INTERACTIONS

May reduce elimination and increase serum concentrations of **drugs that are renally excreted** (e.g., aminoglycosides [e.g., gentamicin], digoxin [Lanoxin]). Monitor drug levels and adjust doses as needed to avoid toxicity. ▪ Observe neonate closely for signs of **digoxin toxicity;** frequent monitoring of ECG and digoxin serum levels is indicated. ▪ Use with **furosemide** (Lasix) may help to maintain renal function. ▪ Concomitant use with **anticoagulants** may increase risk of bleeding; monitoring of PT suggested. ▪ Coadministration with **ACE inhibitors** (e.g., enalapril [Vasotec]) may result in deterioration of renal function, including renal failure.

SIDE EFFECTS

Abdominal distension; acidosis; alkalosis; apnea; bleeding into the GI tract (gross or microscopic); bradycardia; DIC; elevated BUN or creatinine; exacerbation of pre-existing pulmonary infection; fluid retention; gastric perforation; hyperkalemia; hypoglycemia; hyponatremia; intracranial bleeding; necrotizing enterocolitis; oliguria; oozing from needle puncture sites; pulmonary hemorrhage; pulmonary hypertension; reduced urine sodium, chloride, potassium, urine osmolality, free water clearance, or glomerular filtration rate; renal failure; retrolental fibroplasia; thrombocytopenia; transient ileus; uremia; vomiting.

ANTIDOTE

Discontinue the drug and notify the physician of all side effects. Based on severity, side effects may be treated symptomatically or drug will be completely discontinued in favor of surgical intervention. Resuscitate as necessary.

INFLIXIMAB BBW • INFLIXIMAB-dyyb BBW*
(in-**FLIX**-ih-mab)

Monoclonal antibody
Inflammatory bowel disease agent
Antirheumatic agent
TNF-blocking agent

Remicade, Inflectra*　　　　　　　　　　　　　　　　　　　pH 7.2

USUAL DOSE
Preliminary patient evaluation required; see Monitor.

Inflectra and Remicade: *Premedication:* Administer at the physician's discretion. May include antihistamines (e.g., diphenhydramine [Benadryl]), H_2 blockers (e.g., famotidine [Pepcid IV]), acetaminophen, and/or corticosteroids (e.g., hydrocortisone).

Crohn's disease and fistulizing Crohn's disease: Begin with an initial dose of 5 mg/kg as an infusion. Repeat at 2 and 6 weeks and every 8 weeks thereafter. For patients who respond and then lose their response, consideration may be given to treatment with 10 mg/kg. If there is no response by Week 14, response with continued dosing is unlikely; consider discontinuing infliximab. See Precautions.

Rheumatoid arthritis: 3 mg/kg as an infusion. Repeat dose at 2 and 6 weeks, then every 8 weeks thereafter. Given in combination with methotrexate at a minimum dose of 12.5 mg/week (median dose of 15 mg/week). See methotrexate monograph. If response to infliximab is incomplete, dose may be adjusted up to 10 mg/kg or interval decreased to every 4 weeks. Risk of infection may be increased at higher doses.

Ankylosing spondylitis: 5 mg/kg as an infusion. Repeat at 2 and 6 weeks, then every 6 weeks thereafter.

Psoriatic arthritis: 5 mg/kg as an infusion. Repeat dose at 2 and 6 weeks, then every 8 weeks thereafter. May be used with or without methotrexate.

Ulcerative colitis and plaque psoriasis: 5 mg/kg as an infusion. Repeat dose at 2 and 6 weeks, then every 8 weeks thereafter.

PEDIATRIC DOSE
Preliminary patient evaluation required; see Monitor. See Maternal/Child.

Crohn's disease *(Inflectra and Remicade)* **and ulcerative colitis†** *(Remicade):* 5 mg/kg as an infusion. Repeat at 2 and 6 weeks. Follow with a maintenance regimen of 5 mg/kg every 8 weeks.

DOSE ADJUSTMENTS
Inflectra and Remicade: Do not exceed a dose of 5 mg/kg in patients with moderate to severe CHF (NYHA Class III/IV); see Contraindications.

DILUTION
Inflectra and Remicade: Each vial contains 100 mg of infliximab. When reconstituted as directed below, each milliliter of solution contains 10 mg of infliximab. Calculate the dose and the number of vials required and the total volume of reconstituted infliximab solution required. Reconstitute each 100-mg vial with 10 mL of SWFI, using a syringe equipped with a 21-gauge or smaller needle. Direct the stream of SWFI to side of vial. Swirl gently; do not shake. Allow reconstituted solution to stand for 5 minutes. Solution should be colorless to light yellow and opalescent and may develop a few translucent particles as infliximab is a protein. Do not use if opaque particles, discoloration, or other

---

*A biosimilar product. Biosimilars are biological products that are licensed (approved) by the FDA because they are highly similar to an already FDA-approved biological product (known as the reference product [e.g., infliximab (Remicade)]) but have allowable differences because they are made from living organisms. Biosimilars also have no clinically meaningful differences from the reference product in terms of safety, purity, and potency.

†*Inflectra* is not approved for ulcerative colitis in pediatric patients due to marketing exclusivity for Remicade.

foreign particles are present. The total dose of reconstituted solution must be further diluted with NS to a final volume of 250 mL. (May withdraw a volume of NS equal to the calculated volume of reconstituted infliximab from a 250-mL bottle or bag of NS and slowly add reconstituted solution.) Do not dilute the reconstituted infliximab solution with any other diluent. Mix gently. Infusion concentration should range between 0.4 mg/mL and 4 mg/mL. The infusion should begin within 3 hours of reconstitution and dilution.

Filters: *Inflectra and Remicade:* Must be administered through an infusion set with an in-line, sterile, nonpyrogenic, low–protein binding filter (pore size equal to or less than 1.2 microns). Flush and prime tubing/filter system with NS before administration of infusion.

Storage: *Inflectra and Remicade:* Refrigerate unopened vials at 2° to 8° C (36° to 46° F). Discard any unused portion. Do not use beyond expiration date on vials.

COMPATIBILITY

Inflectra and Remicade: Manufacturer recommends not infusing concomitantly in the same IV line with other agents until specific **compatibility** data are available.

RATE OF ADMINISTRATION

Inflectra and Remicade: Begin the infusion within 3 hours of reconstitution and dilution. Flush and prime tubing/filter system with NS before administration. A single dose should be given over a period of not less than 2 hours. Upon completion of infusion, IV line should be flushed thoroughly with 15 to 20 mL of NS to ensure all active drug is delivered to the patient. Patients experiencing a mild to moderate infusion-related reaction may be able to continue therapy at a reduced rate; see Antidote.

ACTIONS

Inflectra and Remicade: A chimeric IgG1 monoclonal antibody that binds specifically to human tumor necrosis factor alpha (TNFα). Is composed of human constant and murine variable regions. Neutralizes the biologic activity of TNFα by binding with high affinity to the soluble and transmembrane forms of TNFα and inhibiting binding of TNFα with its receptors. Infliximab does not neutralize TNFβ. Biologic activities attributed to TNFα include induction of pro-inflammatory cytokines such as IL-1 and IL-6, enhancement of leukocyte migration by increasing endothelial layer permeability and expression of adhesion molecules by endothelial cells and leukocytes, activation of neutrophil and eosinophil functional activity, and induction of acute phase reactants and other liver proteins, as well as tissue-degrading enzymes produced by synoviocytes and/or chondrocytes. Elevated concentrations of TNFα have been found in involved tissues and fluids of patients with Crohn's disease, rheumatoid arthritis, ankylosing spondylitis, ulcerative colitis, psoriatic arthritis, and plaque psoriasis. These elevated concentrations correlate with elevated disease activity. Treatment with infliximab blocks the biological activities attributed to TNFα. After treatment, patients have decreased levels of serum IL-6 and C-reactive protein compared to baseline. Infliximab is distributed predominantly within the vascular space. Has a prolonged terminal half-life of 7.7 to 9.5 days. Produced by a recombinant cell line cultured by continuous perfusion and is purified by a series of steps that include measures to inactivate and remove viruses.

INDICATIONS AND USES

Adult and pediatric patients 6 years of age and older: Reduce the S/S and induce and maintain clinical remission in patients with moderately to severely active Crohn's disease who have had an inadequate response to conventional therapy (*Inflectra* and *Remicade*). ■ Reduce the S/S and induce and maintain clinical remission and mucosal healing in patients with moderately to severely active ulcerative colitis who have had an inadequate response to conventional therapy. (*Inflectra* and *Remicade* may be used in adults; however, use in pediatric patients is limited to Remicade due to marketing exclusivity for Remicade.) In addition, *Inflectra* and *Remicade* are indicated to help eliminate corticosteroid use in adult patients with ulcerative colitis.

Adult patients: *Inflectra and Remicade:* Reduce the number of draining enterocutaneous and rectovaginal fistula(s) and maintain fistula closure in fistulizing Crohn's disease. ■ Given in combination with methotrexate to improve physical function, inhibit progression of structural damage, and reduce S/S in patients with moderately to severely active rheumatoid arthritis. ▪ Reduce S/S in active ankylosing spondylitis. ▪ Reduce the S/S of active arthritis, inhibit progression of structural damage, and improve physical function in psoriatic arthritis. ▪ Used for treatment of patients with chronic severe (i.e., extensive and/or disabling) plaque psoriasis who are candidates for systemic treatment and when other systemic treatments are less appropriate.

CONTRAINDICATIONS
Inflectra and Remicade: Known hypersensitivity to infliximab, murine proteins, or other components of the product. ▪ Administration of doses exceeding 5 mg/kg in patients with moderate to severe (NYHA Class III/IV) CHF.

PRECAUTIONS
Inflectra and Remicade: Administer in a facility that is equipped to monitor the patient and respond to any medical emergency. ▪ TNFα mediates inflammation and modulates cellular immune response. Anti-TNF therapies, including infliximab, may affect normal immune responses. ▪ Patients treated with infliximab are at increased risk for developing serious infections that may lead to hospitalization or death. Many of the serious infections have occurred in patients undergoing concomitant immunosuppressive therapy (e.g., methotrexate, corticosteroids) that, in addition to their underlying disease, may predispose them to infections; see Drug/Lab Interactions. Discontinue infliximab if patient experiences a serious infection or sepsis. Reported infections with TNF-blockers include active tuberculosis, including reactivation of latent tuberculosis; invasive fungal infections (e.g., histoplasmosis, coccidioidomycosis, candidiasis, aspergillosis, blastomycosis, and pneumocytosis); and bacterial, viral, and other infections due to opportunistic pathogens, including *Legionella* and *Listeria*. ▪ Patients with TB have frequently presented with disseminated or extrapulmonary disease. ▪ Cases of tuberculosis reactivation or new tuberculosis infections have been observed in patients receiving infliximab, including patients who have previously received treatment for latent or active tuberculosis. Cases of active tuberculosis have also occurred in patients being treated with infliximab during treatment for latent tuberculosis. ▪ Antituberculosis treatment of patients with a reactive TB skin test reduces the risk of TB reactivation in patients receiving infliximab. ▪ Patients with histoplasmosis or other invasive fungal infections may present with disseminated rather than localized disease. Antigen and antibody testing for histoplasmosis may be negative. ▪ Treatment with infliximab should not be initiated in patients with an active infection, including clinically important localized infections. Consider the risks and benefits of infliximab treatment before initiating therapy in patients with chronic or recurrent infection, patients who have been exposed to TB, patients with a history of an opportunistic infection, patients who have resided in or traveled to areas of endemic tuberculosis or endemic mycoses (e.g., histoplasmosis, coccidioidomycosis, or blastomycosis), or patients with underlying conditions that may predispose them to infection. ▪ Has been associated with the reactivation of hepatitis B virus (HBV) in patients who are chronic hepatitis B carriers (i.e., surface antigen–positive). Fatalities have been reported. ▪ Infliximab therapy has been associated with adverse outcomes in patients with heart failure and should be used in these patients only after consideration of other treatment options. A higher incidence of worsening CHF, increased mortality, and a higher rate of cardiovascular adverse events have been seen in patients with moderate to severe CHF. Occurs more frequently in patients receiving a 10 mg/kg dose. Do not use doses greater than 5 mg/kg in patients with moderate to severe CHF; see Contraindications. Discontinue for new-onset CHF or for worsening CHF, and consider discontinuing in patients with CHF who have not had a significant response to infliximab. Use with caution in patients with mild CHF (NYHA Class I/II); monitor closely. ▪ Hypersensitivity reactions characterized by urticaria, dyspnea, and/or hypotension have occurred in association with infliximab infusion. Most occur during or within 2 hours of the infusion. Discontinue infusion if severe reaction occurs. Medications for management of hypersensitivity reaction (e.g., acetaminophen [Tylenol], diphenhydramine [Benadryl], corticosteroids [e.g., hydrocortisone] and/or epinephrine) should be readily available. ▪ Se-

rum sickness–like reactions (dysphagia, fever, hand and facial edema, headache, myalgias, polyarthralgias, sore throat) have been reported and have occurred as early as after the second dose and when infliximab was interrupted and then re-initiated after an extended period. These reactions are associated with a marked increase in antibodies to infliximab, a loss of detectable serum concentrations of infliximab, and a possible loss of drug efficacy. ▪ Readministration of infliximab after a period of no treatment resulted in a higher incidence of infusion reactions relative to regular maintenance treatment in clinical trials. Evaluate risk versus benefit of readministration after a period of no treatment, especially if considering a re-induction regimen given at 0, 2, and 6 weeks. For cases in which maintenance therapy for psoriasis has been interrupted, infliximab should be re-initiated with a single dose followed by maintenance therapy. ▪ Infliximab therapy may result in formation of autoimmune antibodies and, rarely, in the development of a lupus-like syndrome. Discontinue therapy if this occurs. In clinical studies, symptoms resolved with discontinuation of therapy. ▪ Lymphoma and other malignancies, some fatal, have been reported in children and adolescent patients treated with TNF blockers, including infliximab. Most of the affected patients were receiving concomitant immunosuppressants. ▪ Cases of hepato-splenic T-cell lymphoma have been reported. The majority of reported cases have occurred in adolescents and young adult males being treated with infliximab for Crohn's disease or ulcerative colitis. This type of lymphoma has a very aggressive disease course and is usually fatal. Almost all affected patients received concomitant treatment with a TNF-blocker and azathioprine or 6-mercaptopurine (Purinethol) at or before diagnosis. When treating patients with inflammatory bowel disease, particularly adolescents and young adults, the decision whether to use infliximab alone or in combination with other immunosuppressants should consider the possibility that there is a higher risk of developing hepatosplenic T-cell lymphoma (HSTCL) with combination therapy versus an observed increased risk of immunogenicity and hypersensitivity reactions with infliximab monotherapy. ▪ Use caution in patients with moderate to severe COPD; may have an increased risk of malignancy, especially of the lungs and head or neck. ▪ The potential role of TNF-blocking therapy in the development of lymphoma, leukemia, melanoma, Merkel cell carcinoma, and other malignancies is not known. Patients with Crohn's disease, ulcerative colitis, rheumatoid arthritis, or plaque psoriasis, particularly with highly active disease and/or exposure to immunosuppressant therapies, may be at higher risk (up to several-fold) than the general population for the development of lymphoma, leukemia, and other malignancies, even in the absence of TNF-blocking therapy. Use caution when considering infliximab therapy in patients with a history of malignancy or when continuing treatment in patients who develop a malignancy while receiving infliximab. ▪ In clinical trials, nonmelanoma skin cancers were more common in psoriasis patients with previous phototherapy. ▪ Rare cases with CNS manifestations of systemic vasculitis, seizures, and new-onset or exacerbation of clinical symptoms and/or radiographic evidence of CNS demyelinating disorders (e.g., multiple sclerosis, optic neuritis) and peripheral demyelinating disorders (e.g., Guillain-Barré syndrome) have been reported. Use with caution in patients with any of these existing neurologic disorders. Consider discontinuing therapy if any of these disorders develop. ▪ Severe hepatic reactions, including liver failure, jaundice, hepatitis, cholestasis, and autoimmune hepatitis, have been reported. Reactions have occurred anywhere from 2 weeks to more than a year after initiation of treatment and have resulted in death or the need for a liver transplant. ▪ Leukopenia, neutropenia, thrombocytopenia, and pancytopenia, some with fatal outcome, have been reported. ▪ Use caution when switching between biological disease-modifying antirheumatic drugs (e.g., **abatacept** [Orencia], **adalimumab** [Humira], **anakinra** [Kineret], **etanercept** [Enbrel]) **or other TNF-blocking agents** (e.g., golimumab [Simponi Aria]); overlapping biological activity may further increase the risk of infection; see Drug/Lab Interactions. ▪ Administration of live virus vaccines or therapeutic infectious agents (e.g., BCG bladder instillation for treatment of cancer) concurrently with infliximab is not recommended. Could result in clinical infections, including disseminated infections. ▪ See Drug/Lab Interactions and Maternal/Child.

Monitor: *Inflectra and Remicade:* Evaluate patients for tuberculosis risk factors and test for latent infection before initiating infliximab and periodically during therapy. Initiate treatment of latent TB before therapy with infliximab. Antituberculosis therapy should also be considered before initiating infliximab in patients with a history of latent or active tuberculosis for whom an adequate course of treatment cannot be confirmed and in patients with a negative test for latent tuberculosis but risk factors for tuberculosis infection. Consultation with a physician with expertise in the treatment of TB is recommended to aid in deciding whether initiating antituberculosis therapy is appropriate for a given patient. ■ During and after treatment, monitor for the development of tuberculosis in patients who tested negative for latent tuberculosis infection before initiating therapy. Tests for latent tuberculosis infection may also be falsely negative while on therapy with infliximab. Tuberculosis should be strongly considered in patients who develop a new infection during infliximab therapy, especially in patients who have previously or recently traveled to countries with a high prevalence of TB or who have had close contact with a person with active TB. ■ Before initiating TNF-blocker therapy, including infliximab, patients should be tested for HBV infection. Consultation with a physician with expertise in the treatment of hepatitis B is recommended if a patient tests positive for hepatitis B surface antigen. ■ In patients who are carriers of HBV and require treatment with TNF-blockers, closely monitor for clinical and laboratory signs of active HBV infection throughout treatment and for several months after completion of treatment. If HBV reactivation occurs, discontinue infliximab; see Antidote. ■ Monitor for S/S of infection during and after treatment; discontinue if a serious infection occurs and initiate appropriate antimicrobial treatment. Empiric antifungal therapy may be appropriate pending results of a diagnostic workup in patients at risk for invasive fungal infections; see Precautions. ■ Monitor cardiac status closely for new-onset or worsening CHF; see Precautions. ■ Patients may develop antibodies to infliximab. In clinical trials, patients who were antibody-positive were more likely to have higher rates of clearance and reduced efficacy and to experience an infusion reaction than were patients who were antibody-negative. The incidence of antibody development was lower among patients receiving immunosuppressant therapies (e.g., 6-mercaptopurine, azathioprine, corticosteroids). ■ Monitor for S/S of hepatotoxicity (e.g., jaundice and/or marked liver enzyme elevations [equal to or greater than 5 times the upper limit of normal]). ■ Monitor CBC with differential and platelet count periodically. ■ Monitor for S/S of hypersensitivity or infusion reaction (e.g., anaphylaxis, chills, dyspnea, fever, flu-like symptoms, GI symptoms, headache, hypotension, rash). ■ Monitor BP and pulse every 30 minutes during infusion. If patient experiences a significant change in vital signs (e.g., drop in diastolic BP of 15 to 20 mm Hg) or exhibits any symptoms that may indicate hypersensitivity, stop infusion. Evaluate symptoms and treat appropriately. Continue to monitor patient for at least 30 minutes after completion of the infusion. ■ Monitor for S/S of malignancies such as HSTCL (e.g., abdominal pain, hepatomegaly, night sweats, persistent fever, weight loss) and lymphoma. ■ Periodic skin examination is recommended for all patients, particularly those with risk factors for skin cancer.

Patient Education: *Inflectra and Remicade:* Read manufacturer's medication guide before each treatment with infliximab. ■ Tell health care professionals of heart conditions, previous or current infections, and recent or past exposure to TB or histoplasmosis. ■ Review all medicines and disease history with pharmacist or physician before initiating treatment. ■ Promptly report abdominal pain, fever, S/S of heart failure (e.g., shortness of breath, swelling feet), infection, numbness, tingling, or visual disturbances. ■ Report S/S of hypersensitivity reactions (e.g., itching, rash, swelling in the throat). Usually occur during or immediately following the infusion but may occur from 3 to 12 days later. ■ Report changes of growths on your skin during or after infliximab treatment. ■ Report symptoms of a cytopenia such as bruising, bleeding, or persistent fever. ■ Report recently receiving or being scheduled to receive a live virus vaccine or treatment with a weakened bacteria (such as BCG for bladder cancer) to your physician.

Maternal/Child: *Inflectra and Remicade:* Category B: use during pregnancy only if clearly needed. ■ Has potential for harm to the nursing infant; discontinue breast-feeding. ■ At least a 6-month waiting period following birth is recommended before the administration of any live vaccine to infants exposed in utero to infliximab. Infliximab crosses the placental barrier and has been detected in these infants up to 6 months after the last dose of infliximab to the mother, and these infants may be at increased risk for infection. ▪ Safety and effectiveness for use in pediatric patients with ulcerative colitis and/or Crohn's disease who are less than 6 years of age not established. ▪ Safety and effectiveness for use in pediatric patients with juvenile rheumatoid arthritis was evaluated in a multicenter trial. The study failed to establish effectiveness; see prescribing information for details. ▪ Before initiating infliximab therapy in pediatric patients with Crohn's disease or ulcerative colitis, all vaccinations should be brought up-to-date. ▪ Long-term (greater than 1 year) safety and effectiveness in pediatric patients with Crohn's disease not established.

Elderly: *Inflectra and Remicade:* Specific differences in safety and effectiveness not noted; the incidence of serious side effects may be increased. An increase in the incidence of serious infections has been noted in patients 65 years and older, and because there is a higher incidence of infections in the elderly population in general, caution should be used in treating the elderly. See Precautions.

DRUG/LAB INTERACTIONS

Inflectra and Remicade: Specific interaction studies have not been performed. ▪ Concurrent administration with **anakinra** (Kineret), an interleukin-1 antagonist, **or abatacept** (Orencia), an antirheumatic agent, may be associated with an increased risk of serious infections. The added benefit of combination therapy has not been documented. Anakinra is also associated with an increased risk of neutropenia. Concurrent administration of TNF α-blocking agents (e.g., infliximab) with anakinra or abatacept is not recommended. ▪ May cause increased immunosuppression and increased risk of infection with **tocilizumab** (Actemra); concurrent use should be avoided. ▪ Concurrent use of infliximab with other biological products (**adalimumab** [Humira], **etanercept** [Enbrel], **golimumab** [Simponi Aria]) used to treat the same conditions as infliximab is not recommended; may increase risk of infection. ▪ The majority of patients with Crohn's disease, rheumatoid arthritis, or psoriatic arthritis received one or more of the following concomitant medications without evidence of any type of negative drug interaction: aminosalicylates, antibiotics, antivirals, corticosteroids, 6-mercaptopurine (Purinethol), azathioprine, folic acid, methotrexate, narcotics, NSAIDs (e.g., ibuprofen [Motrin, Advil], naproxen [Aleve, Naprosyn]), and sulfasalazine. ▪ Patients receiving **immunosuppressants** (e.g., 6-mercaptopurine, azathioprine, corticosteroids) tended to experience fewer infusion reactions as compared to patients on no immunosuppressants. ▪ Concomitant **methotrexate** use may decrease incidence of anti-infliximab antibody production and increase infliximab concentrations. ▪ **Live virus vaccines and therapeutic infectious agents** (e.g., BCG for bladder instillation for treatment of cancer) should not be given concurrently with infliximab. Could result in clinical infection, including disseminated infection. In addition, it is also recommended that live vaccines not be given to infants after in utero exposure to infliximab for at least 6 months following birth; see Precautions and Maternal/Child. ▪ Cytochrome P_{450} enzymes may be suppressed by increased levels of cytokines during inflammation. Infliximab antagonizes cytokine activity, and the formation of the CYP450 enzymes may be normalized. When initiating or discontinuing infliximab in patients treated with **CYP450 substrates with a narrow therapeutic index,** monitoring of the effect (e.g., warfarin [Coumadin]) or drug concentrations (e.g., cyclosporine [Sandimmune] or theophylline) is recommended. Dose adjustment may be necessary.

SIDE EFFECTS

Inflectra and Remicade: The most commonly reported side effects include abdominal pain, headache, infection (e.g., pharyngitis, sinusitis, upper respiratory tract, and urinary tract), and infusion-related reactions. The most common reasons for discontinuation of therapy were infusion-related reactions (e.g., dyspnea, fever, flushing, headache, rash) occurring during or within 2 hours of infusion or infections (bacterial, fungal, protozoal, and viral). See Precautions. Other less common side effects include abscess, anaphylactic-like reactions (including laryngeal/pharyngeal edema and severe bronchospasm), anemia, anxiety, arthralgia, autoantibodies/lupus-like syndrome, back pain, conjunctivitis, constipation, depression, diarrhea, dizziness, dyspepsia, dysuria, flushing, hot flashes, HACA development, hepatitis B virus reactivation, hepatotoxicity (autoimmune hepatitis, increased liver function tests, jaundice, liver failure), insomnia, intestinal obstruction, lymphoproliferative disorders, malignancies including lymphoma, moniliasis, myalgia, pain, paresthesia, peripheral edema, rash, sarcoidosis, seizures, serum sickness–like reactions, stomatitis, tachycardia, vertigo, and visual disturbances. See Precautions. Infections (bacterial, fungal, protozoal, and viral) including TB, invasive opportunistic infections (e.g., histoplasmosis, listeriosis, and pneumocystosis), new-onset or worsening CHF, CNS demyelinating disorders, and deaths have been reported.

Post-Marketing: *Inflectra and Remicade:* Cholestasis, erythema multiforme, hepatitis, hepatosplenic T-cell lymphomas, idiopathic and/or thrombotic thrombocytopenic purpura, interstitial lung disease (including pulmonary fibrosis/interstitial pneumonitis and, very rarely, rapidly progressive disease), jaundice, liver failure, melanoma and Merkel cell carcinoma, myocardial ischemia/infarction, neuropathies, neutropenia, pericardial effusion, peripheral demyelinating disorders (e.g., Guillain-Barré syndrome, chronic inflammatory demyelinating polyneuropathy, and multifocal motor neuropathy), psoriasis (including new-onset and pustular, primarily palmar/plantar), Stevens-Johnson syndrome, systemic and cutaneous vasculitis, toxic epidermal necrolysis, and transverse myelitis have been reported; fatalities have occurred.

Pediatric patients with Crohn's disease: *Inflectra and Remicade:* Anemia, bacterial infection, blood in stool, bone fracture, flushing, leukopenia, neutropenia, respiratory tract allergic reactions, and viral infections were reported more commonly in pediatric patients than in adult patients receiving similar treatment regimens. Serious side effects were infections (some fatal), including opportunistic infections and tuberculosis, infusion reactions, and hypersensitivity reactions. Malignancies (including hepatosplenic T-cell lymphomas), transient hepatic enzyme abnormalities, lupus-like syndromes, and the development of autoantibodies were less common, yet serious, reactions.

ANTIDOTE

Inflectra and Remicade: Notify physician of any side effects; most will be treated symptomatically. Discontinue infliximab if patient experiences a serious infection, significant changes in vital signs, new or worsening S/S of heart failure, hepatotoxicity, a hypersensitivity reaction, a lupus-like syndrome (fever, pleuritic pain, pleural effusion), a neurologic disorder, or significant hematologic abnormalities. Treat hypersensitivity and/or infusion reactions with acetaminophen (Tylenol), antihistamines (diphenhydramine [Benadryl]), corticosteroids, dopamine, and epinephrine as indicated. Slow or suspend infusion for a mild or moderate infusion-related reaction. Upon resolution of the reaction, re-initiation at a lower infusion rate and/or therapeutic administration of antihistamines, acetaminophen, and/or corticosteroids may be attempted with caution. If patient does not tolerate the infusion after these interventions, infliximab should be discontinued; see Usual Dose. Lupus-like syndrome usually subsides within 10 days of discontinuing infliximab. Discontinue infliximab in patients who develop HBV reactivation, and initiate antiviral therapy with appropriate supportive treatment. Safety of resuming therapy after HBV is controlled is not known; use caution if resumption of therapy is considered, and monitor closely.

INSULIN INJECTION (REGULAR) ▪
INSULIN ASPART rDNA origin ▪
INSULIN GLULISINE rDNA origin ▪
INSULIN LISPRO rDNA origin
(**IN**-sue-lin in-**JEK**-shun ▪ **IN**-sue-lin **AS**-part)

Hormone
Antidiabetic agent

Humulin R, Novolin ge Toronto ❋
▪ **NovoLog** ▪ **Apidra** ▪ **Humalog**

pH 7 to 7.8 ▪ pH 7.2 to 7.6 ▪
pH 7.3 ▪ pH 7 to 7.8

USUAL DOSE

Only regular insulin, insulin aspart, insulin glulisine, and insulin lispro may be given IV. Confirm by label or package insert that a particular insulin product is for IV use; see Precautions.

Dose varies greatly. Will be dependent on patient's condition and response. Insulin requirements may be altered during stress or major illness or with changes in exercise, meal pattern, or coadministered drugs. It is imperative that dosing is individualized and adjusted based on blood glucose determinations because of the marked loss of insulin from adsorption to glass and plastic infusion containers and tubing; see Precautions.

Low-dose treatment in ketoacidosis: The American Diabetes Association recommends 0.15 unit/kg as a loading dose (10.5 units for a 70-kg patient), followed by a continuous infusion of 0.1 unit/kg/hr (7 units/hr for a 70-kg patient). Plasma glucose should decrease at a rate of 50 to 75 mg/dL/hr. If plasma glucose concentrations do not fall by 50 mg/dL within the first hour of insulin therapy, the insulin infusion rate may be doubled every hour, provided the patient is adequately hydrated. Decrease the rate of infusion when plasma glucose reaches 250 to 300 mg/dL. Start a separate IV of D5/¹/₂NS when plasma glucose reaches 300 mg/dL. Administer insulin to maintain serum glucose concentrations between 150 and 200 mg/dL in patients with diabetic ketoacidosis. Continue until metabolic acidosis is corrected. Administer an appropriate dose of insulin SC 30 minutes before discontinuing the insulin infusion (intermediate-acting insulin recommended).

Diabetes mellitus with hyperosmolar coma, nonketotic (unlabeled): An initial bolus dose of 0.1 unit/kg followed by a continuous infusion of 0.1 unit/kg/hr until the blood glucose falls to 250 mg/dL.

Hyperkalemia (unlabeled): Insulin may be used in patients with or without diabetes mellitus to treat hyperkalemia. Must be administered with a dextrose solution in nondiabetic patients. Begin with an initial dose of 5 to 10 units of regular insulin and 50 mL of dextrose 50% as an IV bolus. Follow with a continuous infusion of 10% dextrose with regular insulin 20 units/L. Administer at 50 mL/hr to prevent fasting hyperkalemia.

Diagnosis of growth hormone deficiency (regular insulin [unlabeled use]): 0.05 to 0.15 unit/kg of body weight as a rapid, one-time injection.

PEDIATRIC DOSE

Ketoacidosis or hyperosmolar hyperglycemia: *Fluids:* Consider initial potential for dehydration and administer 10 to 20 mL/kg of NS or LR over 1 hour.

Regular insulin and insulin aspart: Administer 0.1 unit/kg/hr as a continuous infusion. Goal is to reduce glucose by 80 to 100 mg/dL/hr. When glucose reaches 250 to 300 mg/dL, or if glucose decreases more than 100 mg/dL/hr, add D5W to fluids. SC insulin may be started once pH and bicarbonate are within normal limits. Discontinue insulin infusion 1 hour after SC dose. Monitor glucose levels and serum electrolytes and continue fluid replacement as appropriate.

Continued

DOSE ADJUSTMENTS

A reduced dose of insulin may be indicated when infusions are discontinued and SC administration is indicated. As in Usual Dose, base on blood glucose determinations and patient's response to therapy. ▪ Dose requirements may be reduced in patients with renal or hepatic impairment. ▪ Dose adjustment may be indicated if it is necessary to change from one insulin product to another.

DILUTION

Regular insulin: Use only if clear. May be given undiluted either directly into the vein or through a Y-tube or three-way stopcock. Another regimen adds 100 units of insulin (1 mL) to 100 mL of NS. This solution yields 1 unit/mL and is usually given at a rate of 0.1 unit/kg of body weight/hr (70-kg adult would receive 7 units/hr).

Insulin aspart: May be diluted in NS to a final concentration of 0.05 to 1 unit/mL. Use a polypropylene infusion bag. See Precautions.

Humulin R U-100: Must be diluted with NS to achieve a final concentration of 0.1 to 1 unit/mL (100 units of insulin [1 mL] to 100 mL of NS yields 1 unit/mL). Use polyvinyl chloride (PVC) infusion bags.

Insulin glulisine: May be diluted only with NS to achieve a final concentration of 0.05 unit/mL to 1 unit/mL (e.g., dilute 100 units in 100 mL NS). Polyvinyl chloride (PVC) infusion systems, including tubing, must be used.

Insulin lispro: Must be diluted with NS to achieve a final concentration of 0.1 to 1 unit/mL (100 units of insulin [1 mL] to 100 mL of NS yields 1 unit/mL).

Storage: Vials: Store unopened vials in refrigerator. A vial that is in use may be stored at RT for 28 days *(insulin aspart, insulin glulisine, and insulin lispro)* or 31 days *(regular insulin).* Protect from sunlight and freezing.

Infusions: Some insulin will be initially adsorbed to the material of the infusion bag. *Regular insulin and insulin lispro:* Infusion bags prepared as indicated in dilution are stable for 48 hours refrigerated and then may be used at RT for up to an additional 48 hours. *Insulin glulisine:* Infusion bags prepared as indicated in dilution are stable at RT for 48 hours. *Insulin aspart:* Infusion bags prepared as indicated in dilution are stable at RT for 24 hours.

COMPATIBILITY   (Underline Indicates Conflicting Compatibility Information)

Consider any drug NOT listed as compatible to be INCOMPATIBLE until consulting a pharmacist; specific conditions may apply.

Manufacturer states, "**Insulin glulisine** is stable (**compatible**) only with NS; do not use other solutions for infusion and do not mix with other insulins for IV administration."

One source suggests the following **compatibilities:**

These compatibilities refer to regular insulin only; information on specific compatibilities for insulin aspart, insulin glulisine, and insulin lispro are not available.

Additive: Meropenem (Merrem IV).

Y-site: Amiodarone (Nexterone), ampicillin, ampicillin/sulbactam (Unasyn), aztreonam (Azactam), caspofungin (Cancidas), cefazolin (Ancef), cefepime (Maxipime), cefotetan, ceftaroline (Teflaro), ceftazidime (Fortaz), digoxin (Lanoxin), dobutamine, doripenem (Doribax), doxapram (Dopram), esmolol (Brevibloc), famotidine (Pepcid IV), gentamicin, heparin, 6% hydroxyethyl starch (Voluven), imipenem-cilastatin (Primaxin), indomethacin (Indocin IV), levofloxacin (Levaquin), magnesium sulfate, meperidine (Demerol), meropenem (Merrem IV), midazolam (Versed), milrinone (Primacor), morphine, nitroglycerin IV, nitroprusside sodium, oxytocin (Pitocin), pantoprazole (Protonix IV), pentobarbital (Nembutal), propofol (Diprivan), sodium bicarbonate, tacrolimus (Prograf), ticarcillin/clavulanate (Timentin), tobramycin, vancomycin, vasopressin.

RATE OF ADMINISTRATION

Each 50 units or fraction thereof over 1 minute. When given in an IV infusion, the rate should be ordered by the physician and will depend on insulin and fluid needs; see Dilution for example. Decrease rate when plasma glucose reaches 300 mg/dL. Manufacturer recommends that the rate of *insulin lispro* be regularly adjusted to maintain blood glucose concentrations between 100 and 160 mg/dL.

ACTIONS

A hormone produced by the pancreas that controls the storage and metabolism of carbohydrates, proteins, and fat. Responsible for regulation of glucose metabolism. Binds to insulin receptors on muscle and fat cells and lowers blood glucose by facilitating cellular uptake of glucose and inhibiting output of glucose from the liver. Also inhibits lipolysis, proteolysis, and gluconeogenesis and enhances protein synthesis and conversion of excess glucose into fat. Rapidly and widely distributed. The glucose-lowering activities of regular insulin, insulin aspart, insulin glulisine, and insulin lispro are equipotent when administered by the IV route. The average elimination half-life is dose dependent and ranges from 0.25 to 1 hour depending on dose and product.

INDICATIONS AND USES

Regular insulin: Treatment of diabetes mellitus (Type 1, Type 2, and gestational). ■ Treatment of complications associated with diabetes (e.g., diabetic coma, hyperosmolar hyperglycemia with or without coma [hyperglycemia and dehydration], ketoacidosis with or without coma [plasma glucose exceeding 250 mg/dL with arterial pH of 7 to 7.24 or less and serum bicarbonate of 10 to 15 mEq/L or less]). ■ In combination with glucose to treat hyperkalemia. ■ Add to total parenteral nutrition to control hyperglycemia.

Humulin R U-100, insulin aspart, insulin glulisine, and insulin lispro: Treatment of patients with diabetes mellitus to improve glycemic control. Usually used as part of a SC injection regimen or as a SC infusion administered via an external insulin pump. May be given IV. Proper medical supervision is required to prevent hypoglycemia and hypokalemia.

Unlabeled uses: Diagnosis of growth hormone deficiency. ■ Continuous intravenous infusions administered via a special pump have been used to treat severe brittle diabetics who have failed more conventional therapy.

CONTRAINDICATIONS

Contraindicated during episodes of hypoglycemia and in patients hypersensitive to regular human insulin, insulin aspart, insulin glulisine, insulin lispro, or one of the excipients of any of these products.

PRECAUTIONS

Only regular insulin, insulin aspart, insulin glulisine, and insulin lispro may be given IV. All insulin formulations for IV use are standardized at 100 units/mL.

Regular insulin, insulin aspart, insulin glulisine, and insulin lispro: Any change in insulin should be made cautiously and only under medical supervision. Concomitant oral antidiabetic treatment may need to be adjusted. ■ Hypoglycemia and hypokalemia are potential side effects of insulin therapy. Use caution in patients in whom these side effects may be clinically relevant (e.g., patients who are fasting, have autonomic neuropathy, are using potassium-lowering drugs [e.g., diuretics], or are taking drugs sensitive to serum potassium levels [e.g., digoxin]). ■ Severe hypoglycemia may lead to unconsciousness and/or convulsions and may result in temporary or permanent impairment of brain function or death. Early warning symptoms of hypoglycemia may be different or less pronounced under certain conditions such as long-standing diabetes, diabetic nerve disease, and the use of medications such as beta-blockers. ■ Untreated hypokalemia may cause respiratory paralysis, ventricular arrhythmia, and death. ■ Use with caution in patients with renal or hepatic impairment; see Dose Adjustments. Frequent monitoring may be required. ■ Insulin requirements may be altered during illness or stress. ■ Anti-insulin antibodies have been reported. Clinical significance of anti-insulin antibodies is unknown. ■ Systemic hypersensitivity reactions have been reported. May include hypotension, pruritus, rash, shortness of breath, sweating, tachycardia, and/or wheezing. Anaphylaxis has occurred. ■ Use with thiazolidinediones (TZDs [e.g., pioglitazone (Actos)]) may cause heart failure. See Drug/Lab Interactions.

Regular insulin: Insulin potency may be reduced by at least 20% and possibly up to 80% via the glass or plastic infusion container and plastic IV tubing before it actually reaches the venous system when given by infusion. The percentage adsorbed is inversely proportional to the concentration of insulin (the larger the dose, the less adsorption) and takes place within 30 to 60 minutes. Albumin is sometimes added to reduce this adsorption.

Other additives (e.g., electrolytes, other drugs, vitamins) may also reduce adsorption. Other methods of compensation for insulin loss include the addition of added insulin to saturate binding sites or the use of a syringe pump (instead of infusion containers) to reduce surface area for adsorption.

Monitor: Response to insulin measured by blood glucose, blood pH, acetone, BUN, sodium, potassium, chloride, and CO_2 levels. Monitor patient carefully in all situations. ▪ Glucose and potassium levels must be monitored closely during IV administration of insulin to avoid potentially fatal hypoglycemia and hypokalemia. ▪ Glycosylated hemoglobin (HgbA1c) may be measured to assess long-term glycemic control. ▪ Hypovolemia is a common complication of diabetic acidosis. ▪ See Drug/Lab Interactions. ▪ Insulin is inactivated at pH above 7.5.

Patient Education: Monitor blood glucose as directed. ▪ Adhere to consistent diet and exercise programs. ▪ Avoid alcohol. ▪ Review medications or changes in medication regimen with a health care professional. ▪ Review S/S of hypoglycemia and hyperglycemia with a health care professional. Be familiar with the treatment for each. ▪ Insulin requirements may change with onset of illness. Monitor glucose carefully and adjust insulin therapy as required.

Maternal/Child: *Regular insulin:* Category B: human insulin is drug of choice for control of diabetes in pregnancy. Additional insulin may be required to control serum glucose and avoid ketoacidosis. Monitor carefully; insulin requirements may drop immediately postpartum. Normal prepregnancy dose should be achieved within 6 weeks. Patients with gestational diabetes usually do not require insulin therapy following childbirth. ▪ Use caution in breast-feeding. ▪ Breast-feeding may decrease insulin requirements. ▪ Inadequately controlled maternal blood glucose late in pregnancy may cause increased insulin production in the fetus. Monitor and treat neonatal hypoglycemia postpartum.

Insulin aspart and insulin lispro: Category B: careful monitoring of glucose control is essential; see comments under regular insulin. ▪ Use caution during breast-feeding.

Insulin glulisine: Category C: use caution and assess risk versus benefit. Careful monitoring of glucose control is essential; see comments under regular insulin. ▪ Use caution with breast-feeding. Considered **compatible,** but women with diabetes who are lactating may require adjustments of their insulin doses. ▪ Safety and effectiveness of IV administration for use in pediatric patients not established.

DRUG/LAB INTERACTIONS

Hypoglycemic effect is potentiated by **ACE inhibitors** (e.g., enalapril [Vasotec], lisinopril [Zestril]), **anabolic steroids** (e.g., nandrolone [Durabolin]), **disopyramide** (Norpace), **fluoxetine** (Prozac), **fibrates** (e.g., fenofibrate [Tricor]), **guanethidine, MAO inhibitors** (e.g., selegiline [Eldepryl]), **oral antidiabetic agents** (e.g., glyburide [DiaBeta]), **pentoxifylline** (Trental), **salicylates, sulfonamides, and many others.** ▪ Drugs that may reduce blood glucose–lowering effect include **atypical antipsychotic medications** (e.g., olanzapine [Zyprexa], clozapine [Clozaril]), **corticosteroids, danazol** (Cyclomen), **diazoxide, diuretics** (e.g., furosemide [Lasix]), **glucagon, isoniazid** (INH), **niacin, oral contraceptives, phenothiazine derivatives** (e.g., chlorpromazine [Thorazine]), **protease inhibitors** (e.g., indinavir [Crixivan]), **somatropin** (Humatrope), **sympathomimetic agents** (e.g., dobutamine, epinephrine [Adrenalin], albuterol [Ventolin]), **thyroid preparations, and others.** ▪ **Alcohol, beta-adrenergic blockers including ophthalmics** (e.g., propranolol, metoprolol [Lopressor]), **clonidine** (Catapres), **and lithium** may either potentiate or inhibit the blood glucose–lowering effect of insulin. ▪ Hypoglycemic effects may be decreased in **smokers;** dose adjustment may be required. ▪ Will affect serum potassium levels; use caution in patients taking **digoxin.** ▪ **Octreotide** (Sandostatin) may alter insulin, glucagon, and growth hormone secretion, resulting in hypoglycemia or hyperglycemia. Monitor serum glucose and adjust insulin dose as indicated. Octreotide also markedly increases adsorption of insulin to glass and plastic and reduces availability. ▪ **Pentamidine** is toxic to the beta cells of the pancreas. Patients may develop hypoglycemia initially as insulin is released. This may be followed by hypoinsulinemia and hyperglycemia with continued pentamidine therapy. ▪ S/S of hypoglycemia may be masked in the presence of **beta-blockers,** clonidine (Catapres), **guanethidine** (Ismelin), **and reserpine.** ▪ **Thiazolidinediones** (TZDs [e.g., pioglitazone (Actos)]) can cause dose-related fluid retention, particularly when used in combination with insulin. Fluid retention may lead to or exacerbate heart failure. Patients receiving concomitant therapy should be monitored for S/S of heart failure. Dose reduction or discontinuation of the TZD may be indicated if heart failure develops.

SIDE EFFECTS

Hypoglycemia with overdose. *Mild to moderate:* Abnormal behavior; anxiety; blurred vision; depressed mood; dizziness; drowsiness; headache; hunger; inability to concentrate; irritability; light-headedness; palpitation; personality changes; restlessness; sleep disturbances; slurred speech; sweating; tingling in the hands, feet, lips, or tongue; tremors; unsteady movement.

Severe: Coma, disorientation, hypokalemia (with ECG changes), seizures, unconsciousness, and death. Hypersensitivity reactions, including anaphylaxis, may occur; death is rare. Abdominal pain, chest pain, diarrhea, headache, hyporeflexia, nausea, and sensory disturbances have also been reported.

ANTIDOTE

Discontinue the drug immediately and notify physician of adverse reactions or hypoglycemia. *Glucagon* 1 to 2 mg IM or SC is the specific antidote for insulin overdose. It may be supplemented by glucose 50% IV and/or oral carbohydrates such as glucose gel or orange juice. Oral carbohydrates may be sufficient to combat early symptoms of hypoglycemia. Correct hypokalemia as indicated. Hypersensitivity reactions usually respond to symptomatic treatment.

INTERFERON ALFA-2b, RECOMBINANT BBW

Biologic response modifier
Antineoplastic

(in-ter-**FEER**-on **AL**-fah)

Intron A   pH 6.9 to 7.5

USUAL DOSE

(International units [IU])

Pretreatment with acetaminophen may lessen flu-like side effects. To enhance tolerability, injections should be administered in the evening when possible. *Not all dosage forms and strengths are appropriate for some indications; see Dilution.*

Malignant melanoma: *Induction:* 20,000,000 IU/M² as an infusion for 5 consecutive days per week for 4 weeks. Begin therapy within 56 days of surgical resection.

Maintenance: Follow with 10,000,000 IU/M² as a SC injection three times each week for 48 weeks.

Total treatment regimen lasts for 1 year and should be completed unless there is progression of disease or the drug is discontinued because of specific side effects.

DOSE ADJUSTMENTS

Moderate to severe adverse events may require modification of the dosage regimen or, in some cases, termination of therapy. Temporarily discontinued for serious adverse reactions, if granulocytes decrease to less than 500/mm³, or ALT/AST increases to 5 to 10 times the ULN. When adverse reactions subside or improvement of granulocytes or liver function tests occurs, treatment can be restarted at 50% of the previous dose. Discontinue permanently if serious adverse reactions persist, if a severe adverse reaction recurs at a reduced dose, if granulocytes decrease to less than 250/mm³, if platelet counts decrease to less than 25,000/mm³, or if ALT/AST increases to more than 10 times the upper limit of normal. ▪ See Elderly.

DILUTION

Intron A Solution for Injection is NOT recommended for IV administration and should not be used for the induction phase of malignant melanoma. Only the sterile powder is suitable for dilution for IV use. Do not use different brands of interferon in any single treatment regimen; variations exist and may adversely affect dosage and response to treatment. Powder for Injection is available in 10, 18, and 50 million IU vials; select one most appropriate for desired dose. Allow product to come to RT before use. Reconstitute immediately before use with 1 mL of SWFI (provided). (The SWFI supplied by the manufacturer contains 5 mL. Discard remaining 4 mL.) Gently swirl to dissolve. Withdraw desired dose and inject into 100 mL of NS. Final concentration should be at least 10 million IU/100 mL. **Storage:** Unopened vials of powder for injection should be refrigerated. After reconstitution, solution should be used immediately but can be refrigerated at 2° to 8° C (36° to 46° F) for 24 hours. Single-dose vial. Discard any unused portion.

COMPATIBILITY
Specific information not available. Consider specific use; consult pharmacist. One source indicates **compatibility** with NS, LR, and R solutions and **incompatibility** with dextrose solutions.

RATE OF ADMINISTRATION
A single dose equally distributed over 20 minutes. Administration at bedtime and the use of acetaminophen may prevent or partially reduce common side effects (e.g., fever, headache, "flu-like" symptoms).

ACTIONS
A naturally occurring small protein and glycoprotein of the interferon family produced by recombinant DNA techniques. It binds to specific membrane receptors on the cell surface and initiates a complex sequence of intracellular events (e.g., induction of specific enzymes, suppression of cell proliferation, immunomodulating activities [e.g., enhancement of phagocytic activity of macrophages, augmentation of the specific cytotoxicity of lymphocytes for target cells, inhibition of virus replication in virus-infected cells]). Peak concentration achieved within 30 minutes. Half-life about 2 hours; undetectable 4 hours after infusion. The kidney may be the site of interferon catabolism. Has produced a significant increase in relapse-free and overall survival in patients with malignant melanoma.

INDICATIONS AND USES
Adjuvant to surgical treatment in patients with malignant melanoma who are free of disease but at high risk for systemic recurrence within 56 days of surgery. ▪ Used IM or SC to treat hairy cell leukemia, follicular non-Hodgkin's lymphoma, AIDS-related Kaposi's sarcoma, chronic hepatitis B, chronic hepatitis C, and intralesionally to treat condylomata acuminata.

CONTRAINDICATIONS
Hypersensitivity to interferon alfa or any of its components. ▪ Decompensated liver disease or autoimmune hepatitis.

PRECAUTIONS
May cause or aggravate life-threatening or fatal neuropsychiatric (e.g., depression, aggressive and/or suicidal behavior), autoimmune, ischemic, or infectious disorders. Close monitoring with periodic clinical and laboratory evaluations required. Discontinue therapy if S/S of any of the previous conditions are persistently severe or worsen. Symptoms resolve in most cases. ▪ Because of fever and other flu-like symptoms associated with its use, interferon alfa should be used cautiously in patients with a history of pulmonary disease (e.g., COPD), diabetes mellitus prone to ketoacidosis, coagulation disorders (e.g., thrombophlebitis, pulmonary embolism), or severe myelosuppression. ▪ Use cautiously in patients with a history of cardiovascular disease (e.g., unstable angina, recent MI, and previous or current arrhythmic disorder). Cardiovascular adverse events (e.g., arrhythmia, cardiomyopathy, hypotension, MI, tachycardia) have been reported. Supraventricular arrhythmias occurred rarely and appeared to be correlated with pre-existing conditions or prior therapy with cardiotoxic agents. ▪ Depression and suicidal behavior (including suicidal ideation, suicidal at-

tempts, and completed suicides), homicidal ideation, and aggressive behavior sometimes directed toward others have been reported; see Monitor and Maternal/Child. ▪ Use with caution in patients with a history of psychiatric disorders and in patients with substance use disorders. Drug screening and periodic health evaluation, including psychiatric symptom monitoring, may be indicated. ▪ Severe cytopenias, including rare cases of aplastic anemia, have been reported; see Monitor. ▪ Ophthalmologic disorders (e.g., decrease or loss of vision; retinopathy, including macular edema, retinal artery or vein thrombosis, retinal hemorrhage, and cotton wool spots; optic neuritis; papilledema; and serous retinal detachment) may be induced or aggravated by treatment with interferons; see Monitor. ▪ Use caution in patients with psoriasis and sarcoidosis; may exacerbate disease. ▪ Rare cases of autoimmune diseases (e.g., lupus erythematosus, Raynaud's phenomenon, rhabdomyolysis, rheumatoid arthritis, thrombocytopenia, and vasculitis) have been reported; may require discontinuation of therapy. ▪ Serum neutralizing antibodies have been detected in some patients; clinical significance unknown. ▪ Ischemic and hemorrhagic cerebrovascular events have been reported. A causal relationship between interferon therapy and these side effects is difficult to establish. ▪ Endocrine disorders (e.g., hypothyroidism, hyperthyroidism, diabetes mellitus) have developed in patients receiving interferon alfa-2b. ▪ Hepatotoxicity, including fatality, has been reported. Interferon alfa increases the risk of hepatic decompensation and death in patients with cirrhosis. ▪ Pulmonary disorders (e.g., dyspnea, pulmonary infiltrates, pneumonia, bronchiolitis obliterans, interstitial pneumonitis, pulmonary hypertension, and sarcoidosis), some resulting in respiratory failure and/or patient deaths, may be induced or aggravated by interferons. Recurrence of respiratory failure has been observed with interferon rechallenge. ▪ Acute serious hypersensitivity reactions have been reported. ▪ Elevated triglyceride levels have been observed. Hypertriglyceridemia may result in pancreatitis.

Monitor: Obtain baseline CBC including differential and platelet count, blood chemistries (electrolytes, glucose, liver function tests, and TSH), and chest x-ray. Obtain baseline eye exam for all patients and periodically for patients with pre-existing ophthalmologic disorders (e.g., diabetic or hypertensive retinopathy). Obtain baseline ECG if there is a history of cardiovascular disease and/or patient is in advanced stages of cancer. Monitor all tests periodically during therapy. Adjust or discontinue therapy as appropriate. ▪ In patients with malignant melanoma, monitor CBC with differential and platelet count and liver function tests weekly during the induction phase and monthly during maintenance. Dose adjustments will be determined by results. Discontinue therapy if neutrophil count drops below 500 cells/mm³. ▪ Hepatic function should be monitored in all patients receiving interferon. Obtain serum bilirubin, ALT, AST, alkaline phosphatase, and LDH at 2, 8, and 12 weeks following initiation of therapy and then every 6 months while on therapy. ▪ Monitor for thrombocytopenia (platelet count less than 50,000/mm³). Discontinue therapy if platelet count drops below 25,000/mm³. Initiate precautions to prevent excessive bleeding (e.g., inspect IV sites, skin, and mucous membranes; use extreme care during invasive procedures; test urine, emesis, stool, and secretions for occult blood). ▪ Monitor for S/S of a hypersensitivity reaction (e.g., anaphylaxis, angioedema, bronchoconstriction, urticaria). ▪ Closely monitor any patient with a history of cardiovascular disease (see Precautions); arrhythmias (including supraventricular arrhythmias and tachycardia), hypotension, and transient reversible cardiomyopathy have occurred. ▪ Hypotension may occur during administration or up to 2 days after therapy; monitor BP frequently. May require fluid replacement to maintain intravascular volume. ▪ Maintain adequate hydration, particularly during initial states of treatment. ▪ Monitor for signs of depression and/or aggressive or suicidal behavior. If psychiatric problems develop, patients should be carefully monitored during treatment and in the 6-month follow-up period. If psychiatric symptoms persist or worsen or if suicidal or homicidal ideation or aggressive behavior toward others is identified, treatment with interferon alpha should be discontinued. The patient should be followed closely, with psychiatric intervention as appropriate. Use of narcotics, hypnotics, or sedatives may be required to manage adverse effects; use with caution and monitor carefully. ▪ Monitor thyroid function, liver function tests, blood glucose, and triglyceride levels; abnormalities not normalized by medication may require discontinuing interferon. ▪ Determine cause of persistent fever (not thought to be due to the flu-like syndrome commonly reported in patients treated with interferon alfa). ▪ Repeat chest x-ray if cough, dyspnea, fever, or other respiratory symptoms occur. Monitor closely if pulmonary infiltrates or evidence of pulmonary function impairment is present; may require discontinuing interferon. ▪ Obtain an eye exam for any patient who complains of changes in visual acuity, visual fields, or other ophthalmologic symptoms. ▪ See Precautions.

Patient Education: Cooperation for close monitoring and prompt reporting of side effects is imperative. Side effects may include depression (including suicidal ideation), cardiovascular toxicity (e.g., chest pain), ophthalmologic toxicity (e.g., loss of or change in vision), pancreatitis (abdominal pain), cytopenias (persistently high fevers, bruising). ▪ Review manufacturer's medication guide before each dose. ▪ Home use may require extensive patient education. Review Instructions for Use provided by manufacturer. ▪ Do not change brands of interferon without medical consultation. Variations in dosage, routes of administration, and adverse reactions exist among different brands. ▪ Do not drive or operate machinery; mental alertness may be impaired. ▪ Administration at bedtime and/or use of acetaminophen may be helpful to prevent the most common flu-like side effects. Remain well hydrated. ▪ Side effects may decrease in severity as treatment continues. ▪ See Appendix D, p. 1333.

Maternal/Child: Category C: has been shown to have abortifacient effects in monkeys. Should be used only if benefits justify risks. ▪ Discontinue breast-feeding. ▪ Safety for use in pediatric patients under 18 years of age for indications other than chronic hepatitis B or C has not been established. ▪ Suicidal ideation or attempts have occurred more often among pediatric patients (primarily adolescents) compared to adult patients.

Elderly: Incidence of encephalopathy, obtundation, and coma has occurred, especially at higher doses. ▪ Cardiovascular adverse events and confusion have been reported more frequently in the elderly. ▪ Consider age-related decreases in organ function and concomitant disease and drug therapy. Careful monitoring required. Make dose adjustments based on symptoms and/or lab abnormalities.

DRUG/LAB INTERACTIONS
Specific information not available. Use caution with any **other potentially myelosuppressive agent** (e.g., cisplatin, zidovudine [AZT, Retrovir]). ▪ May increase serum levels of **theophylline;** monitoring of theophylline levels recommended. ▪ See Precautions.

SIDE EFFECTS
Occur in high percentages of patients; may be serious enough to require a decreased dose or discontinuation of drug. Usually rapidly reversible after therapy is discontinued, but may require up to 3 weeks to resolve. The most frequently reported adverse reactions were flu-like symptoms (chills, fatigue, fever, headache, and myalgia). In patients treated for malignant melanoma, the most frequently reported adverse reaction was fatigue. Adverse reactions that were reported in greater than 20% of patients included alopecia, altered taste sensation, anemia, anorexia, chills, depression, diarrhea, dizziness/vertigo, fever, headache, increased AST, myalgia, nausea/vomiting, and neutropenia. Severe adverse reactions (ECOG [Eastern Cooperative Oncology Group] Toxicity Criteria Grade 3 or 4) reported in greater than 10% of patients included chills, fatigue, fever, headache, increased AST, myalgia, and neutropenia/leukopenia. Many other side effects may occur.

Post-Marketing: Stevens-Johnson syndrome, toxic epidermal necrolysis, erythema multiforme, injection site necrosis, myositis, hearing loss, pulmonary fibrosis, and a wide variety of autoimmune and immune-mediated disorders (e.g., idiopathic thrombocytopenic purpura and thrombotic thrombocytopenic purpura) have been identified in post-marketing reports.

ANTIDOTE

Keep physician informed of all side effects. Some will be tolerated or treated symptomatically. Discontinue interferon immediately for any acute serious hypersensitivity reactions and treat as appropriate; may require epinephrine, airway management, oxygen, IV fluids, antihistamines (e.g., diphenhydramine [Benadryl]), corticosteroids (e.g., hydrocortisone sodium succinate [Solu-Cortef]), and pressor amines (e.g., dopamine). Discontinue drug for any patient who develops severe depression or other psychiatric disorder. Close patient monitoring and psychiatric intervention may be indicated. Discontinue for myelosuppression that persists after dose reduction, endocrine abnormalities or persistently elevated triglycerides associated with symptoms of potential pancreatitis (e.g., abdominal pain, nausea, vomiting) not normalized by medication, serious liver function abnormalities (Grade 3 hepatic injury or hepatic decompensation [Child-Pugh score >6 (Class B and C)]), new or worsening ophthalmologic disorders, serious pulmonary function impairment, or pulmonary infiltrates. Treatment of overdose with hemodialysis or peritoneal dialysis is not considered effective. Resuscitate as necessary.

IPILIMUMAB BBW

(ip-i-**LIM**-ue-mab)

Yervoy

Monoclonal antibody
Antineoplastic

pH 7

USUAL DOSE

Unresectable or metastatic melanoma: 3 mg/kg administered as an IV infusion over 90 minutes every 3 weeks for a total of 4 doses. In the event of toxicity, doses may be delayed, but all treatment must be administered within 16 weeks of the first dose.

Adjuvant treatment of melanoma: 10 mg/kg as an IV infusion over 90 minutes every 3 weeks for 4 doses followed by 10 mg/kg every 12 weeks for up to 3 years. In the event of toxicity, doses are omitted, not delayed.

DOSE ADJUSTMENTS

The recommended treatment modifications for immune-mediated adverse reactions to ipilimumab are outlined in the following chart.

Treatment Modifications of Ipilimumab for Immune-Mediated Adverse Reactions		
Target/Organ System	Adverse Reaction (CTCAE, v3)	Treatment Modification
Endocrine	Symptomatic endocrinopathy	Withhold ipilimumab. Resume ipilimumab in patients with complete or partial resolution of adverse reactions (Grade 0 or 1) and who are receiving less than 7.5 mg prednisone or equivalent per day.
	• Symptomatic reactions lasting 6 weeks or longer • Inability to reduce corticosteroid dose to 7.5 mg prednisone or equivalent per day	Permanently discontinue ipilimumab.
Ophthalmologic	Grade 2 through 4 reactions • Not improving to Grade 1 within 2 weeks while receiving topical therapy or • Requiring systemic treatment	Permanently discontinue ipilimumab.
All other	Grade 2	Withhold ipilimumab. Resume ipilimumab in patients with complete or partial resolution of adverse reactions (Grade 0 or 1) and who are receiving less than 7.5 mg prednisone or equivalent per day.
	• Grade 2 reactions lasting 6 weeks or longer • Inability to reduce corticosteroid dose to 7.5 mg prednisone or equivalent per day • Grade 3 or 4 reactions	Permanently discontinue ipilimumab.

■ Permanently discontinue ipilimumab for severe or life-threatening adverse reactions; see Precautions and Antidote. ■ No dose adjustment indicated in renal impairment or mild hepatic impairment.

DILUTION

Available as a 5 mg/mL solution in 50-mg and 200-mg vials. Solution may have a clear to pale yellow color and may contain translucent-to-white amorphous particles. Discard vial if solution is cloudy or if there is pronounced discoloration. ***Do not shake.*** Allow vials to stand at RT for approximately 5 minutes. Withdraw required volume of ipilimumab and transfer into an infusion bag containing NS or D5W. Final concentration of diluted solution should range from 1 to 2 mg/mL. Mix diluted solution by gentle inversion. For example, a dose for a 70-kg patient with metastatic melanoma would be 70 kg × 3 mg/kg dose = 210 mg. Withdraw 210 mg (42 mL of a 5 mg/mL solution) and transfer to a 100-mL bag of NS or D5W. Final concentration = 210 mg ÷ 142 mL = 1.5 mg/mL.

Filters: Administer through a line equipped with a sterile, nonpyrogenic, low–protein binding, in-line filter.

Storage: Refrigerate vials at 2° to 8° C (36° to 46° F). Do not freeze. Protect from light. Store diluted solution for no more than 24 hours under refrigeration (2° to 8° C [36° to 46° F]) or at RT. Discard partially used vials.

COMPATIBILITY
Manufacturer states, "Do not mix with, or administer as an infusion with, other medicinal products." Flush IV line with NS or D5W after each dose.

RATE OF ADMINISTRATION
A single dose equally distributed as an infusion over 90 minutes. Administer through a line equipped with a low–protein binding in-line filter. Flush line with NS or D5W after each dose; see Filters.

ACTIONS
An IgG1 kappa immunoglobulin. A recombinant, human monoclonal antibody that binds to the cytotoxic, T-lymphocyte–associated antigen 4 (CTLA-4). CTLA-4 is a negative regulator of T-cell activity. Ipilimumab binds to CTLA-4 and blocks the interaction of CTLA-4 with its ligands, CD80/CD86. Blockade has been shown to augment T-cell activation and proliferation, including the activation and proliferation of tumor-infiltrating T-effector cells. Inhibition of CTLA-4 signaling can also reduce T-regulatory cell function, which may contribute to a general increase in T-cell responsiveness, including the antitumor immune response. Terminal half-life is 15.4 days. Renal impairment and mild hepatic impairment did not have a clinically important effect on the pharmacokinetics of ipilimumab.

INDICATIONS AND USES
Treatment of unresectable or metastatic melanoma. ▪ Adjuvant treatment of patients with cutaneous melanoma with pathologic involvement of regional lymph nodes of more than 1 mm who have undergone complete resection, including total lymphadenectomy.

CONTRAINDICATIONS
Manufacturer states, "None."

PRECAUTIONS
May result in severe and fatal immune-mediated adverse reactions. Reactions may involve any organ system; however, the most common severe immune-mediated adverse reactions are enterocolitis, hepatitis, dermatitis (including toxic epidermal necrolysis), neuropathy, and endocrinopathy. Most reactions are manifested during treatment; however, a minority occurred weeks to months after discontinuation of ipilimumab. See manufacturer's literature for clinical trial information outlining the different clinical courses observed for each of the immune-mediated reactions. Most, but not all, patients experienced partial or complete resolution of reactions following treatment; see Antidote. ▪ Severe, life-threatening, or fatal immune-mediated enterocolitis, hepatotoxicity, and dermatitis have been reported. ▪ Severe, life-threatening, or fatal motor or sensory neuropathy, Guillain-Barré syndrome, or myasthenia gravis have been reported. ▪ Severe to life-threatening immune-mediated endocrinopathies that require hospitalization or urgent medical intervention or that interfere with activities of daily living have been reported. Endocrinopathies have included hypophysitis, hypopituitarism, adrenal insufficiency, hypogonadism, hypothyroidism, hyperthyroidism, and Cushing's syndrome. ▪ Severe immune-mediated reactions involving other organ systems (e.g., hemolytic anemia, meningitis, myocarditis, nephritis, pancreatitis, pericarditis, pneumonitis, uveitis, iritis) have been reported rarely. ▪ A small number of patients have tested positive for binding antibodies against ipilimumab. Infusion-related or peri-infusional reactions consistent with hypersensitivity or anaphylaxis were not reported

in these patients, and neutralizing antibodies against ipilimumab were not detected. ■ Immune-mediated ocular disease unresponsive to topical immunosuppressive therapy has been reported. ■ Has not been studied in patients with moderate to severe hepatic impairment. ■ See Drug Interactions.

Monitor: Obtain baseline clinical chemistries, including liver function tests, adrenocorticotropic (ACTH) level, and thyroid function tests. Repeat before each dose and as indicated based on symptoms. ■ Assess patients for signs and symptoms of enterocolitis (diarrhea [greater than 6 to 7 stools/day above baseline], abdominal pain, mucus or blood in stool, with or without fever) and of GI perforation (peritoneal signs and ileus). In symptomatic patients, rule out infectious etiologies or malignant causes and consider endoscopic evaluation for persistent or severe symptoms. ■ Monitor for immune-mediated hepatitis (moderate hepatotoxicity: AST or ALT elevations of 2.5 to 5 times the ULN or total bilirubin elevation of more than 1.5 to 3 times the ULN; severe hepatotoxicity: AST or ALT elevations of more than 5 times the ULN or total bilirubin elevations more than 3 times the ULN). In patients with hepatotoxicity, rule out infectious or malignant causes and increase the frequency of liver function test monitoring until resolution of symptoms. ■ Monitor for immune-mediated dermatitis (e.g., pruritus, rash, Stevens-Johnson syndrome, toxic epidermal necrolysis, rash complicated by full-thickness dermal ulceration, or necrotic, bullous, or hemorrhagic manifestations). Unless an alternate etiology has been identified, S/S of dermatitis should be considered immune mediated. ■ Monitor for symptoms of motor or sensory neuropathy (e.g., unilateral or bilateral weakness, sensory alterations, or paresthesia that interferes with daily activities). ■ Monitor for clinical S/S of endocrinopathies, including hypophysitis (inflammation of the pituitary gland), adrenal insufficiency (including adrenal crisis), and hyperthyroidism or hypothyroidism. Patients may present with fatigue, headache, mental status changes, abdominal pain, unusual bowel habits, and hypotension. Unless an alternate etiology has been identified, S/S of endocrinopathies should be considered immune mediated. ■ Monitor for clinical S/S of immune-mediated ocular disease. ■ See Precautions.

Patient Education: Review Medication Guide before each dose. Severe immune-mediated reactions have been reported. ■ Promptly report any side effects. ■ May cause fetal harm. Use effective contraception during treatment with ipilimumab and for 3 months after the last dose of ipilimumab.

Maternal/Child: Based on animal data; may cause fetal harm. Use during pregnancy only if the potential benefit justifies the potential risk to the fetus. ■ Discontinue breastfeeding. ■ Safety and effectiveness for use in pediatric patients not established.

Elderly: No overall differences in safety or efficacy were reported between elderly patients and younger patients.

DRUG/LAB INTERACTIONS

Formal drug interaction studies have not been performed. ■ Increases in transaminases with or without concomitant increases in total bilirubin have occurred with concurrent administration of ipilimumab with vemurafenib (Zelboraf).

SIDE EFFECTS

The most common side effects are colitis, diarrhea, fatigue, pruritus, and rash. In addition to these reactions, decreased appetite, fever, headache, insomnia, nausea, vomiting, and weight loss were commonly reported with the 10 mg/kg dose. 15% of patients receiving 3 mg/kg ipilimumab as monotherapy and 12% of patients receiving 3 mg/kg ipilimumab combined with an investigational gp100 peptide vaccine experienced Grade 3 to 5 immune-mediated reactions. In contrast, 41% of patients receiving 10 mg/kg ipilimumab experienced Grade 3 to 5 immune-mediated reactions. Severe to fatal immune-mediated reactions include dermatitis, endocrinopathy (adrenal insufficiency, hyperthyroidism, hypopituitarism, primary hypothyroidism), enterocolitis (including intestinal perforation), eosinophilia, hepatotoxicity, meningitis, myocarditis, nephritis, neuropathy, pericarditis, pneumonitis, and uveitis. Reported laboratory abnormalities include decreased hemoglobin and increased alkaline phosphatase, amylase, ALT, AST, bilirubin, creatinine, and lipase. Other reported side effects include acute respiratory distress syndrome, encephalitis, esophagitis, hearing loss, infusion reaction, intestinal ulcer, myositis, ocular myositis, polymyositis, renal failure, sarcoidosis, and urticaria. Other immune-mediated adverse reactions were reported in fewer than 1% of patients; see manufacturer's prescribing information.

Post-Marketing: Drug reaction with eosinophilia and systemic symptoms (DRESS syndrome)

ANTIDOTE

Keep physician informed of all side effects. Permanently discontinue ipilimumab and initiate systemic high-dose corticosteroid therapy (e.g., 1 to 2 mg/kg/day of prednisone or equivalent) for severe immune-mediated reactions (e.g., Grades 3 to 5). With improvement to Grade 1 or less, initiate corticosteroid taper and continue to taper over at least 1 month. Consider adding anti-TNF (e.g., infliximab [Remicade]) or other immunosuppressant agents for management of immune-mediated enterocolitis unresponsive to systemic corticosteroids within 3 to 5 days or recurring after symptom improvement. Withhold ipilimumab dosing for moderate enterocolitis; administer antidiarrheal treatment (e.g., loperamide [Imodium]) and, if persistent for more than 1 week, initiate systemic corticosteroids at a dose of 0.5 mg/kg/day of prednisone or the equivalent. Mycophenolate (CellCept) may be considered in patients with persistent, severe hepatitis despite high-dose corticosteroids. Withhold ipilimumab dosing in patients with moderate hepatotoxicity, dermatitis, or neuropathy (neuropathy not interfering with daily activities). For mild to moderate dermatitis, such as localized rash and pruritus, treat symptomatically with topical or systemic steroids if no improvement of symptoms within 1 week. Initiate appropriate hormone replacement therapy in patients with symptomatic endocrinopathies. Administer corticosteroid eye drops to patients who develop uveitis, iritis, or episcleritis. Resuscitate as necessary.

IRINOTECAN HYDROCHLORIDE BBW
*IRINOTECAN LIPOSOME INJECTION BBW

Antineoplastic
(topoisomerase 1 inhibitor)

(**eye**-rih-noh-**TEE**-kan hy-droh-**KLOR**-eyed)
(**eye**-rih-noh-**TEE**-kan **LIP**-oh-sohm-ul)

Camptosar, CPT-11 ▪ ONIVYDE

pH 3 to 3.8 (Camptosar)

USUAL DOSE
CONVENTIONAL IRINOTECAN

Premedication with antiemetics recommended. Dexamethasone 10 mg and a 5-HT$_3$ blocker (e.g., ondansetron [Zofran] or granisetron [Kytril]) should be given on the day of treatment. Begin at least 30 minutes before giving irinotecan. In addition, prophylactic or therapeutic atropine may be indicated in patients experiencing cholinergic symptoms. See Monitor.

First-line treatment of colorectal cancer: Premedication as described above is recommended. Initiate regimen with the dose of irinotecan over 90 minutes. Follow immediately with the dose of leucovorin calcium (see leucovorin calcium monograph). Follow the leucovorin immediately with the dose of fluorouracil (see fluorouracil monograph). Doses and modified dosing recommendations are based on the chart Combination-Agent Dosage Regimens and Dose Modifications. Doses of irinotecan and fluorouracil may require modification based on toxicity.

See the following chart, Combination-Agent Dosage Regimens and Dose Modifications, and see Dose Adjustments, combination therapy, and/or package insert.

Combination-Agent Dosage Regimens and Dose Modifications* (Irinotecan/Fluorouracil [5-FU]/Leucovorin Calcium [LV])				
Regimen 1 6-wk course with bolus 5-FU/LV (next course begins on Day 43)	irinotecan leucovorin 5-FU	125 mg/M^2 IV over 90 min, Day 1, 8, 15, 22 20 mg/M^2 IV bolus, Day 1, 8, 15, 22 500 mg/M^2 IV bolus, Day 1, 8, 15, 22		
	Starting Dose and Modified Dose Levels (mg/M^2)			
		Starting Dose	Dose Level −1	Dose Level −2
	irinotecan	125 mg/M^2	100 mg/M^2	75 mg/M^2
	leucovorin	20 mg/M^2	20 mg/M^2	20 mg/M^2
	5-FU	500 mg/M^2	400 mg/M^2	300 mg/M^2
Regimen 2 6-wk course with infusional 5-FU/LV (next course begins on Day 43)	irinotecan leucovorin 5-FU bolus 5-FU infusion†	180 mg/M^2 IV over 90 min, Day 1, 15, 29 200 mg/M^2 IV over 2 hr, Day 1, 2, 15, 16, 29, 30 400 mg/M^2 IV bolus, Day 1, 2, 15, 16, 29, 30 600 mg/M^2 IV over 22 hr, Day 1, 2, 15, 16, 29, 30		
	Starting Dose and Modified Dose Levels (mg/M^2)			
		Starting Dose	Dose Level −1	Dose Level −2
	irinotecan	180 mg/M^2	150 mg/M^2	120 mg/M^2
	leucovorin	200 mg/M^2	200 mg/M^2	200 mg/M^2
	5-FU bolus	400 mg/M^2	320 mg/M^2	240 mg/M^2
	5-FU infusion†	600 mg/M^2	480 mg/M^2	360 mg/M^2

*Dose reductions beyond dose level −2 by decrements of ~20% may be warranted for patients continuing to experience toxicity. Provided intolerable toxicity does not develop, treatment with additional courses may be continued indefinitely as long as patients continue to experience clinical benefit.
†Infusion follows bolus administration.

Treatment of colorectal cancer after failure of treatment with fluorouracil: Irinotecan: Administer as an infusion based on the following chart, Irinotecan Single-Agent Regimens and Dose Modifications. See Premedication. After adequate recovery, additional doses may be repeated in a similar cycle and continued indefinitely in patients who attain a response or in those whose disease remains stable.

Irinotecan Single-Agent Regimens and Dose Modifications		
Weekly Regimen*	125 mg/M² IV over 90 min, Day 1, 8, 15, 22 then 2-wk rest	
	Starting Dose and Modified Dose Levels (mg/M²) ‡	
	Starting Dose	Dose Level −1	Dose Level −2
	125 mg/M²	100 mg/M²	75 mg/M²
Once-Every-3-Weeks Regimen†	350 mg/M² IV over 90 min, once every 3 wks ‡	
	Starting Dose and Modified Dose Levels (mg/M²)	
	Starting Dose	Dose Level −1	Dose Level −2
	350 mg/M²	300 mg/M²	250 mg/M²

*Subsequent doses may be adjusted as high as 150 mg/M² or to as low as 50 mg/M² in 25 to 50 mg/M² decrements depending upon individual patient tolerance.
†Subsequent doses may be adjusted as low as 200 mg/M² in 50 mg/M² decrements depending upon individual patient tolerance.
‡Provided intolerable toxicity does not develop, treatment with additional courses may be continued indefinitely as long as patients continue to experience clinical benefit.

Onivyde (Liposomal Irinotecan)
Do not substitute ONIVYDE for other drugs containing irinotecan HCl.
   Administer **ONIVYDE before** administering leucovorin and fluorouracil.
Premedication: Administer a corticosteroid and an antiemetic 30 minutes before the **ONIVYDE** infusion.
Metastatic adenocarcinoma of the pancreas: 70 mg/M² as an IV infusion over 90 minutes every 2 weeks. In patients known to be homozygous for the UGT1A1*28 allele, the recommended starting dose is 50 mg/M² as an IV infusion over 90 minutes. Increase dose to 70 mg/M² as tolerated in subsequent cycles. In clinical trials doses of **ONIVYDE**, 70 mg/M² was followed by leucovorin 400 mg/M² IV over 30 minutes, followed by fluorouracil 2,400 mg/M² IV over 46 hours every 2 weeks.

DOSE ADJUSTMENTS
Conventional Irinotecan
   A reduction in the starting dose by one dose level may be required in patients with a performance status of 2, in patients who have previously received pelvic/abdominal irradiation, and in patients with increased bilirubin levels; see Elderly. Available information insufficient to recommend a dose for patients with bilirubin greater than 2 mg/dL.
▪ Consider decreasing the **starting dose** by at least one level of irinotecan when administered in combination with other agents or as a single agent to a patient known to be homozygous for the UGT1A1*28 allele (an allele is an alternative form of a gene). The precise dose reduction for this patient population is not known. Subsequent dose modification should be based on individual patient tolerance as outlined in the following charts. Heterozygous patients (patients who carry one variant allele) appear to tolerate normal starting doses. ▪ See Precautions.
Combination therapy: Decrease dose based on toxicity as described in the following chart.
Continued

Guidelines for Dose Adjustments in Combination Schedules
(Irinotecan/Fluorouracil [5-FU]/Leucovorin Calcium [LV])

Patients should return to pretreatment bowel function without requiring antidiarrhea medications for at least 24 hours before the next chemotherapy administration. A new course of therapy should also not begin until the granulocyte count has recovered to ≥1,500/mm^3 and the platelet count has recovered to ≥100,000/mm^3. Treatment should be delayed 1 to 2 weeks to allow for recovery from treatment-related toxicities. If the patient has not recovered after a 2-week delay, consideration should be given to discontinuing therapy.

Toxicity CTCAE* Grade (Value)	During a Course of Therapy	At the Start of Subsequent Courses of Therapy†
No toxicity	Maintain dose level	Maintain dose level
Neutropenia		
1 (1,500 to 1,999/mm^3)	Maintain dose level	Maintain dose level
2 (1,000 to 1,499/mm^3)	↓1 dose level	Maintain dose level
3 (500 to 999/mm^3)	Omit dose until resolved to ≤Grade 2, then ↓1 dose level	↓1 dose level
4 (<500/mm^3)	Omit dose until resolved to ≤Grade 2, then ↓2 dose levels	↓2 dose levels
Neutropenic fever	Omit dose, then ↓2 dose levels when resolved	
Other hematologic toxicities	Dose modifications for leukopenia or thrombocytopenia during a course of therapy and at the start of subsequent courses of therapy are also based on Common Terminology Criteria for Adverse Events and are the same as previously recommended for neutropenia.	
Diarrhea		
1 (2-3 stools/day >pretx‡)	Delay dose until resolved to baseline, then give same dose	Maintain dose level
2 (4-6 stools/day >pretx)	Omit dose until resolved to baseline, then ↓1 dose level	Maintain dose level
3 (7-9 stools/day >pretx)	Omit dose until resolved to baseline, then ↓1 dose level	↓1 dose level
4 (≥10 stools/day >pretx)	Omit dose until resolved to baseline, then ↓2 dose levels	↓2 dose levels
Other nonhematologic toxicities		
Grade 1	Maintain dose level	Maintain dose level
Grade 2	Omit dose until resolved to ≤Grade 1, then ↓1 dose level	Maintain dose level
Grade 3	Omit dose until resolved to ≤Grade 2, then ↓1 dose level	↓1 dose level
Grade 4	Omit dose until resolved to ≤Grade 2, then ↓2 dose levels	↓2 dose levels
	For mucositis/stomatitis decrease only 5-FU, not irinotecan	*For mucositis/stomatitis decrease only 5-FU, not irinotecan*

*Common Terminology Criteria for Adverse Events.
†Relative to the starting dose of the previous cycle.
‡Pretreatment.

Single-agent therapy: Reduce dose based on toxicity levels in the following chart, Guidelines for Irinotecan Dose Adjustments in Single-Agent Schedules. The most common reasons for dose reduction are late diarrhea, neutropenia, and leukopenia.

Guidelines for Irinotecan Dose Adjustments in Single-Agent Schedules*			
A new course of therapy should not begin until the granulocyte count has recovered to $\geq$1,500/mm³, the platelet count has recovered to $\geq$100,000/mm³, and treatment-related diarrhea is fully resolved. Treatment should be delayed 1 to 2 weeks to allow for recovery from treatment-related toxicities. If the patient has not recovered after a 2-week delay, consideration should be given to discontinuing irinotecan.			
Worst Toxicity CTCAE† Grade (Value)	During a Course of Therapy	At the Start of the Next Courses of Therapy (After Adequate Recovery). Compared with the Starting Dose in the Previous Course*	
	Weekly	Weekly	Once Every 3 Weeks
No toxicity	Maintain dose level	$\uparrow$25 mg/M² up to a maximum dose of 150 mg/M²	Maintain dose level
Neutropenia			
1 (1,500 to 1,999/mm³)	Maintain dose level	Maintain dose level	Maintain dose level
2 (1,000 to 1,499/mm³)	$\downarrow$25 mg/M²	Maintain dose level	Maintain dose level
3 (500 to 999/mm³)	Omit dose until resolved to $\leq$Grade 2, then $\downarrow$25 mg/M²	$\downarrow$25 mg/M²	$\downarrow$50 mg/M²
4 (<500/mm³)	Omit dose until resolved to $\leq$Grade 2, then $\downarrow$50 mg/M²	$\downarrow$50 mg/M²	$\downarrow$50 mg/M²
Neutropenic fever	Omit dose until resolved, then $\downarrow$50 mg/M²	$\downarrow$50 mg/M²	$\downarrow$50 mg/M²
Other hematologic toxicities	Dose modifications for leukopenia, thrombocytopenia, and anemia during a course of therapy and at the start of subsequent courses of therapy are also based on Common Terminology Criteria for Adverse Events and are the same as recommended for neutropenia above.		
Diarrhea			
1 (2-3 stools/day >pretx‡)	Maintain dose level	Maintain dose level	Maintain dose level
2 (4-6 stools/day >pretx)	$\downarrow$25 mg/M²	Maintain dose level	Maintain dose level
3 (7-9 stools/day >pretx)	Omit dose until resolved to $\leq$Grade 2, then $\downarrow$25 mg/M²	$\downarrow$25 mg/M²	$\downarrow$50 mg/M²
4 ($\geq$10 stools/day >pretx)	Omit dose until resolved to $\leq$Grade 2, then $\downarrow$50 mg/M²	$\downarrow$50 mg/M²	$\downarrow$50 mg/M²
Other nonhematologic toxicities			
Grade 1	Maintain dose level	Maintain dose level	Maintain dose level
Grade 2	$\downarrow$25 mg/M²	$\downarrow$25 mg/M²	$\downarrow$50 mg/M²
Grade 3	Omit dose until resolved to $\leq$Grade 2, then $\downarrow$25 mg/M²	$\downarrow$25 mg/M²	$\downarrow$50 mg/M²
Grade 4	Omit dose until resolved to $\leq$Grade 2, then $\downarrow$50 mg/M²	$\downarrow$50 mg/M²	$\downarrow$50 mg/M²

*All dose modifications should be based on the worst preceding toxicity.
†Common Terminology Criteria for Adverse Events.
‡Pretreatment.

Continued

ONIVYDE

There is no recommended dose of **ONIVYDE** for patients with serum bilirubin above the upper limit of normal. ▪ Withhold **ONIVYDE** for an absolute neutrophil count below 1,500/mm^3 or neutropenic fever. ▪ Withhold **ONIVYDE** for diarrhea of Grade 2 to 4 severity. ▪ See the following chart for dose modifications recommended for adverse reactions.

Recommended Dose Modifications for Adverse Reactions to ONIVYDE			
Toxicity NCI CTCAE, v 4.0*	Occurrence	ONIVYDE Adjustment in Patients Receiving 70 mg/M^2	ONIVYDE Adjustment in Patients Homozygous for UGT1A1*28 Without Previous Increase to 70 mg/M^2
Grade 3 or 4 adverse reactions	1. Withhold ONIVYDE. 2. Initiate loperamide for late-onset diarrhea of **any** severity. 3. Administer IV or SC atropine 0.25 to 1 mg (unless clinically contraindicated) for early-onset diarrhea of **any** severity. 4. Upon recovery to ≤ Grade 1, resume ONIVYDE at:		
	First	50 mg/M^2	43 mg/M^2
	Second	43 mg/M^2	35 mg/M^2
	Third	Discontinue ONIVYDE	Discontinue ONIVYDE
Interstitial lung disease	First	Discontinue ONIVYDE	Discontinue ONIVYDE
Anaphylactic reaction	First	Discontinue ONIVYDE	Discontinue ONIVYDE

*NCI CTCAE, v 4.0, National Cancer Institute Common Toxicity Criteria for Adverse Events, version 4.0.

For recommended dose modifications for fluorouracil (5-FU) and/or leucovorin (LV), refer to their monographs and/or full prescribing information.

DILUTION

Specific techniques required; see Precautions.

CONVENTIONAL IRINOTECAN: Available in single-dose vials in 2-mL, 5-mL, and 15-mL sizes with a concentration of 20 mg/mL. Must be diluted for infusion with D5W (preferred) or NS to concentrations between 0.12 and 2.8 mg/mL. Usually diluted in 250 to 500 mL D5W.

ONIVYDE: Available in a single-dose vial containing 43 mg irinotecan free base at a concentration of 4.3 mg/mL. It is a slightly yellow, opaque, liposomal dispersion. Withdraw the calculated volume from the vial and dilute in 500 mL D5W or NS. Mix by gentle inversion. Protect diluted solution from light.

Filters: *Conventional irinotecan:* Specific information not available. *ONIVYDE:* Do not use in-line filters.

Storage: *Conventional irinotecan:* Packaged in a blister pack to protect against accidental breakage and leakage. Store in carton protected from light at CRT. When mixed with D5W, is chemically and physically stable for 48 hours if refrigerated and in ambient fluorescent lighting and for 24 hours at CRT. ***Do not refrigerate if mixed with NS;*** a precipitate may form. Stable for 24 hours at CRT when mixed in NS. Because of the risk of microbial contamination, the manufacturer recommends that solutions mixed in D5W or NS be used within 4 hours if kept at RT. However, if reconstitution and dilution are performed under strict aseptic conditions (e.g., on a laminar air flow bench), the solution should be used (i.e., infusion completed) within 12 hours at RT or 24 hours (D5W) if refrigerated. Avoid freezing.

ONIVYDE: Refrigerate in carton at 2° to 8° C (36° to 46° F) to protect from light. Do not freeze. Administer diluted solution within 4 hours of preparation when stored at RT or within 24 hours if refrigerated. Allow diluted solution to come to RT before administration. Do not freeze. Discard unused portion.

COMPATIBILITY (Underline Indicates Conflicting Compatibility Information)

Consider any drug NOT listed as compatible to be INCOMPATIBLE until consulting a pharmacist; specific conditions may apply.

CONVENTIONAL IRINOTECAN

Manufacturer states, "Other drugs should not be added to the infusion solution." Consider specific use and toxicity.

One source suggests the following **compatibilities:**

Y-site: Oxaliplatin (Eloxatin) and <u>palonosetron (Aloxi)</u>.

ONIVYDE

Specific information not available. Consider specific use and toxicity; consult pharmacist.

RATE OF ADMINISTRATION

Both formulations: A single dose as an infusion equally distributed over 90 minutes.

ONIVYDE: Do not use in-line filter.

ACTIONS

CONVENTIONAL IRINOTECAN: A semi-synthetic derivative of camptothecin. An alkaloid extract from plants such as *Camptotheca acuminata*. A class of antineoplastic agent that inhibits the enzyme topoisomerase I required for DNA replication. Together with its active metabolite SN-38 it causes cell death by damaging DNA produced during the S-phase of cell synthesis. Maximum plasma SN-38 levels are reached within 1 hour of infusion end. Extensively distributed to body tissues. Terminal half-life of irinotecan is about 6 to 12 hours; SN-38 is 10 to 20 hours. Irinotecan is moderately bound to plasma proteins (30% to 68%), but SN-38 is highly bound (95%). Metabolic conversion of irinotecan to SN-38 primarily occurs in the liver. SN-38 is conjugated to a glucuronide metabolite by the enzyme UDP-glucuronosyltransferase 1A1 (UGT1A1). Approximately 25% to 50% excreted through bile and urine.

ONIVYDE: A topoisomerase 1 inhibitor encapsulated in a lipid bilayer vesicle or liposome. Topoisomerase 1 relieves torsional strain in DNA by inducing single-strand breaks. Irinotecan and its active metabolite SN-38 bind reversibly to the topoisomerase 1–DNA complex and prevent re-ligation of the single-strand breaks, leading to cell death. 95% of irinotecan remains liposome-encapsulated. Terminal elimination half-life is approximately 25.8 hours. Protein binding is less than 0.44% of the total irinotecan in ONIVYDE. Metabolism and excretion of irinotecan liposome have not been evaluated.

INDICATIONS AND USES

CONVENTIONAL IRINOTECAN: As a component of first-line therapy in combination with 5-fluorouracil (5-FU) and leucovorin (LV) for patients with metastatic carcinoma of the colon or rectum. ▪ For patients with metastatic carcinoma of the colon or rectum whose disease has recurred or progressed following initial fluorouracil-based therapy.

ONIVYDE: Treatment of patients with metastatic adenocarcinoma of the pancreas after disease progression following gemcitabine-based therapy. Used in combination with fluorouracil and leucovorin.

Limitation of use of ONIVYDE: Not indicated as a single agent for the treatment of patients with metastatic adenocarcinoma of the pancreas.

CONTRAINDICATIONS

Both formulations: History of hypersensitivity to conventional or liposomal formulations of irinotecan or any of their components.

PRECAUTIONS

Both formulations: Follow guidelines for handling cytotoxic agents. See Appendix A, p. 1331. ▪ Administered by or under the direction of the physician specialist. ▪ Adequate diagnostic and treatment facilities must be available. ▪ Can cause severe or life-threatening neutropenia and fatal neutropenic sepsis. ▪ Patients who are homozygous for the UGT1A1*28 allele have decreased UGT1A1 enzyme activity. This leads to a higher exposure to SN-38 and an increased risk for neutropenia; see Dose Adjustments. A laboratory test is available to determine the UGT1A1 status of patients. ▪ Can cause severe or life-threatening diarrhea that may be either early or late onset (see discussion under individual agents). ▪ Severe hypersensitivity reactions, including anaphylaxis, have been reported.

▪ Interstitial pulmonary disease has been reported and can be fatal. Use caution in patients with pleural effusions and/or impaired pulmonary function. Risk factors may include pre-existing lung disease or use of pneumotoxic agents (e.g., amiodarone [Nexterone]), radiation therapy, or colony-stimulating factors; see Antidote.

CONVENTIONAL IRINOTECAN: Can induce both early and late forms of diarrhea that appear to be mediated by different mechanisms. Both forms may be severe. Interrupt therapy and reduce subsequent doses if severe diarrhea occurs; see Dose Adjustments. Late diarrhea may be complicated by colitis, ulceration, bleeding, ileus, obstruction, and infection. Cases of megacolon and intestinal perforation have been reported. Patients must not be treated with irinotecan until resolution of any bowel obstruction. ▪ Hepatic dysfunction may impair the metabolism of both irinotecan and SN-38. Patients with a bilirubin of 1 to 2 mg/dL are at increased risk for developing Grade 3 or 4 neutropenia. The manufacturer does not recommend a dose for patients with a bilirubin greater than 2 mg/dL and states that insufficient information is available. ▪ May cause severe myelosuppression. Deaths due to sepsis following severe neutropenia have been reported. ▪ Use with caution in patients with renal impairment. Has not been studied. Not recommended for use in patients on dialysis. ▪ Use caution in the elderly (may have an increased incidence and severity of diarrhea) and in patients who have had previous cytotoxic therapy or previous pelvic/abdominal irradiation (likely to have an increased incidence and severity of myelosuppression). Monitor closely. ▪ Use caution in patients with poor performance status. Patients with a baseline performance status of 2 had higher rates of hospitalization, neutropenic fever, thromboembolism, first-cycle treatment discontinuation, and early deaths than patients with a performance status of 0 or 1. ▪ Contains sorbitol. Do not use in patients with hereditary fructose intolerance. ▪ The Mayo Clinic regimen of 5-FU/LV (administered for 4 to 5 days every 28 days) should not be used in combination with irinotecan outside a carefully controlled, well-designed clinical study. Regimen has caused increased toxicity and death. ▪ See Monitor.

ONIVYDE: Severe or life-threatening neutropenia, neutropenic fever or sepsis, and fatal neutropenic sepsis have occurred. The incidence of Grade 3 or 4 neutropenia was higher among Asian patients compared with Caucasian patients in clinical trials. Withhold ONIVYDE for absolute neutrophil count below 1,500/mm³ or neutropenic fever; see Monitor. ▪ Severe diarrhea has occurred in patients receiving liposomal irinotecan in combination with fluorouracil and leucovorin. Withhold ONIVYDE for diarrhea of Grade 2 to 4 severity. An individual patient may experience both early- and late-onset diarrhea; see Monitor. ▪ Do not administer ONIVYDE to patients with bowel obstruction. ▪ Not studied in patients with hepatic impairment. ▪ No pharmacokinetic effects noted in patients with mild to moderate renal impairment. Data for severe renal impairment are insufficient.

Monitor: BOTH FORMULATIONS: Prophylactic antiemetics are recommended; see Usual Dose. To reduce nausea and vomiting and increase patient comfort after initial dosing, additional antiemetics should be available (e.g., prochlorperazine [Compazine], ondansetron [Zofran], granisetron [Kytril]). ▪ Monitor vital signs. ▪ Obtain an accurate bowel history to evaluate changes in bowel habits after administration of irinotecan. ▪ Monitor for "early" diarrhea. Occurs during or within 24 hours of irinotecan administration and is cholinergic in nature. Usually transient and only infrequently is severe. May be accompanied by other cholinergic symptoms (e.g., abdominal cramping, bradycardia, diaphoresis, flushing, increased salivation, lacrimation, miosis, rhinitis). Patients who have a cholinergic reaction to irinotecan will probably have similar reactions to subsequent doses. Atropine 0.25 to 1 mg IV or SC may be considered for treatment or for prophylactic use unless clinically contraindicated. ▪ Monitor for "late" diarrhea (more than 24 hours after irinotecan administration), which probably results from cytotoxic effects on GI epithelium. May be prolonged; may cause dehydration, electrolyte imbalances, or sepsis; and can be life threatening. At first onset, give loperamide (Imodium) 4 mg; give 2 mg every 2 hours (4 mg every 4 hours during the night) until diarrhea-free for a minimum of 12 hours. Monitor carefully; replace fluids and electrolytes as needed; see Patient Education. ▪ Maintain adequate hydration. Orthostatic hypotension or dizziness may indicate dehydration. ▪ Initiate antibiotic therapy in patients who develop ileus, fever, or severe neutropenia. ▪ Be alert for signs of bone marrow suppression or infection. Prophylactic antibiotics may be indicated pending results of C/S in a febrile or nonfebrile neutropenic patient. ▪ Monitor for thrombocytopenia (platelet count less than 50,000/mm^3). Initiate precautions to prevent excessive bleeding (e.g., inspect IV sites, skin, and mucous membranes; use extreme care during invasive procedures; test urine, emesis, stool, and secretions for occult blood). ▪ Monitor for S/S of a hypersensitivity reaction (e.g., chest pain, chills, dizziness, dyspnea, fever, flushing, hypotension, nausea, pruritus, rash, urticaria) or an infusion reaction (e.g., asthenia, chills, fatigue, fever, vomiting). ▪ Monitor for S/S of interstitial lung disease. Withhold therapy in patients with new or progressive cough, dyspnea, and fever pending diagnostic evaluation; see Precautions and Antidote. ▪ See Dose Adjustments.

CONVENTIONAL IRINOTECAN: Obtain a WBC with differential, hemoglobin, and platelet count before each dose. Expected nadir for platelets is 14 days, and 21 days for hemoglobin, neutrophils, and leukocytes. ▪ Obtain baseline electrolytes and liver function tests. ▪ Not a vesicant, but monitor injection site for inflammation and/or extravasation. ▪ If late-onset diarrhea develops, subsequent weekly chemotherapy treatments should be delayed until pretreatment bowel function has returned for at least 24 hours without the need for antidiarrheal medication. If Grade 2, 3, or 4 late diarrhea recurs, subsequent doses of irinotecan should be decreased; see Dose Adjustments. ▪ Avoid use of diuretics and laxatives in patients with diarrhea. ▪ Monitor renal function and hydration status. Rare cases of renal impairment or acute renal failure have been reported, usually in patients who became dehydrated from vomiting and/or diarrhea.

ONIVYDE (LIPOSOMAL IRINOTECAN): Prophylactic antiemetics and corticosteroids are recommended 30 minutes before ONIVYDE infusion. ▪ Monitor CBC on Days 1 and 8 of every cycle and more frequently if clinically indicated. Withhold ONIVYDE if the absolute neutrophil count (ANC) is below 1,500/mm^3 or if neutropenic fever occurs. Resume when the ANC is 1,500 mm^3 or above; see Dose Adjustments. ▪ Monitor for infusion reactions occurring on the day of administration. S/S have included periorbital edema, pruritus, rash, and urticaria.

Patient Education: *Both formulations:* Review manufacturer's medication guide. ▪ Report any unusual or unexpected symptoms or side effects as soon as possible. ▪ Report black or bloody stools, diarrhea not under control within 24 hours, dry mouth, fever or chills, inability to retain oral fluids due to nausea and vomiting, infections, symptoms of dehydration (e.g., light-headedness, dizziness, fainting), urine changes, or vomiting immediately; each must be treated promptly. Have loperamide (Imodium) available. Dose of loperamide prescribed for late diarrhea is higher than the usual dose recommendation. Limit use at this dose to 48 hours to avoid risk of paralytic ileus. ▪ May cause dizziness or visual disturbances (usually within 24 hours of administration); use caution in tasks that require alertness. ▪ Compliance with regimen imperative (e.g., taking temperature, obtaining lab work, adequate rest, nourishment, and fluids). ▪ Effective birth control required for both women and men; see Maternal/Child. ▪ Inform health care professionals of any problems with previous treatments. ▪ See Appendix D, p. 1333.

Maternal/Child: *Both formulations:* Safety and effectiveness for use in pediatric patients not established.

Conventional irinotecan: Category D: avoid pregnancy. May cause fetal harm. ▪ Discontinue breast-feeding.

ONIVYDE: Can cause fetal harm; avoid pregnancy. Advise females of reproductive potential to use effective contraception during treatment and for 1 month after the final dose. Advise males with female partners of reproductive potential to use condoms during treatment and for 4 months after the final dose. ▪ Discontinue breast-feeding during treatment and for 1 month after the final dose.

Elderly: *Conventional irinotecan:* Half-life slightly extended. ▪ Reduce starting dose by one dose level to 300 mg/M^2 in patients 70 years and older in the single-agent, once-every-3-weeks regimen. No change in the starting dose is recommended for elderly patients receiving the weekly dose schedule of irinotecan. See Usual Dose and Dose Adjustments. ▪ Risk of early and late diarrhea increased in the elderly. ▪ Monitor carefully;

may dehydrate more quickly from diarrhea. Begin loperamide therapy promptly. Avoid laxatives.

ONIVYDE: No overall differences in safety and effectiveness observed between the elderly and younger patients.

DRUG/LAB INTERACTIONS

Interaction of **conventional irinotecan** and/or **ONIVYDE** with other drugs has not been adequately studied.

Both formulations: Concomitant use with **CYP3A4 enzyme–inducing anticonvulsants and strong CYP3A4 inducers** may increase the metabolism of irinotecan, which decreases concentrations and effectiveness. Avoid use of **strong CYP3A4 inducers** (e.g., carbamazepine [Tegretol], oxcarbazepine [Trileptal], phenobarbital [Luminal], phenytoin [Dilantin], rifampin [Rifadin], rifabutin [Micobutin], St. John's wort) if possible. Substitute non–enzyme inducing therapies at least 2 weeks before initiation of irinotecan therapy. ▪ **CYP3A4 inhibitors** (e.g., clarithromycin [Biaxin], indinavir [Crixivan], itraconazole [Sporanox], ketoconazole [Nizoral], lopinavir/ritonavir [Kaletra], nefazodone, nelfinavir [Viracept], ritonavir [Norvir], saquinavir [Invirase], teleprevir [Incivek], voriconazole [VFEND]) **and UGT1A1 inhibitors** (e.g., atazanavir [Reyataz], gemfibrozil [Lopid], indinavir [Crixivan], ketoconazole [Nizoral]) may decrease metabolism, which increases serum concentrations and the risk of toxicity. Avoid the use of **strong CYP3A4 or UGT1A1 inhibitors** if possible. Discontinue at least 1 week before starting irinotecan therapy. ▪ Do not administer **live virus vaccines** to patients receiving antineoplastic drugs.

Conventional irinotecan: Additive bone marrow suppression may occur with **radiation therapy and/or other bone marrow–suppressing agents** (e.g., azathioprine, chloramphenicol, melphalan [Alkeran]). Dose reduction may be required. ▪ Concurrent administration with **irradiation** is not recommended. ▪ Use caution or withhold **diuretics** (e.g., furosemide [Lasix]) **and laxatives** during treatment; may increase risk of dehydration secondary to vomiting and/or diarrhea.

SIDE EFFECTS

Conventional irinotecan: Myelosuppression (anemia, leukopenia, neutropenia) and diarrhea ("early" [e.g., abdominal cramping or pain, diaphoresis] or "late") occur in patients and are the most common dose-limiting toxicities with irinotecan administration.

Combination therapy: Common adverse reactions (greater than 30%) observed in combination therapy are abdominal pain, abnormal bilirubin, alopecia, anemia, anorexia, asthenia, constipation, diarrhea, fever, infection, leukopenia (including lymphocytopenia), mucositis, nausea, neutropenia, pain, thrombocytopenia, and vomiting.

Single-agent therapy: Common adverse reactions (greater than 30%) observed in single-agent therapy are abdominal pain, alopecia, anemia, anorexia, asthenia, constipation, diarrhea, fever, leukopenia (including lymphocytopenia), nausea, neutropenia, weight loss, and vomiting.

Other reported side effects with irinotecan include abdominal bloating, back pain, chills, confusion, coughing, dehydration, dizziness, dyspepsia, dyspnea, edema, exfoliative dermatitis, flatulence, flushing, headache, hypersensitivity reactions (including anaphylaxis), hyponatremia, hypotension, increased alkaline phosphatase and AST, increased bilirubin, insomnia, interstitial pulmonary disease, muscular contractions or cramps, myocardial infarction, neutropenic fever, neutropenic infection, paresthesia, pneumonia, pulmonary embolism, rash, rhinitis, somnolence, stomatitis, thrombophlebitis, and weight loss may occur. In addition, ileus without preceding colitis has occurred. Renal impairment or failure has occurred, usually in patients who became volume depleted from severe vomiting and/or diarrhea.

ONIVYDE: Asthenia, decreased appetite, diarrhea, fatigue, fever, lymphopenia, nausea, neutropenia, stomatitis, and vomiting are most common. The most common serious side effects were acute renal failure, dehydration, diarrhea, fever, nausea, neutropenic fever or neutropenic sepsis, pneumonia, sepsis, septic shock, thrombocytopenia, and vomiting. Diarrhea, vomiting, and sepsis were the most common reasons for discontinuing therapy.

Anemia, diarrhea, nausea, and neutropenia were the most common reasons for dose reduction.

Post-Marketing: Asymptomatic elevated pancreatic enzymes (e.g., amylase, lipase), dysarthria (transient), ischemic or ulcerative colitis, megacolon, myocardial ischemic events, pancreatitis.

ANTIDOTE

Keep physician informed of all side effects and monitor carefully. Adjust or omit dose as indicated for toxicity; see Dose Adjustments. Treat diarrhea immediately; see Monitor. In the event of an acute onset of new or progressive, unexplained pulmonary symptoms (e.g., cough, dyspnea, fever), interrupt irinotecan and other coprescribed chemotherapeutic agents pending diagnostic evaluation. If interstitial pulmonary disease is diagnosed, discontinue irinotecan and other chemotherapy and initiate appropriate treatment as needed. Administration of whole blood products (e.g., packed RBCs, platelets, leukocytes) and/or blood modifiers (e.g., darbepoetin alfa [Aranesp], epoetin alfa [Epogen], filgrastim [Neupogen, Zarxio], pegfilgrastim [Neulasta], sargramostim [Leukine]) may be indicated to treat bone marrow toxicity. Death may occur from the progression of many side effects. No known antidote for overdose. Maximum supportive care (e.g., to prevent dehydration due to diarrhea and to treat any infectious complications) will help sustain patient in toxicity. If extravasation occurs, flush site with SWFI, elevate the extremity, and apply ice.

IRON DEXTRAN INJECTION BBW

(EYE-ern DEKS-tran in-JEK-shun)

Hematinic
Antianemic
Iron supplement

DexFerrum, DexIron✚, InFeD, Infufer✚, Proferdex

pH 4.5 to 7

USUAL DOSE

Iron-deficiency anemia: A test dose is required on the first day. The maximum daily dose is 100 mg/day.

Test dose: 0.5 mL (25 mg) on the first day as a test dose. Wait 1 hour. If no adverse reactions, administer the remainder of the initial therapeutic dose of 1.5 mL (75 mg).

Therapeutic dose: Repeat the total dose of 2 mL (100 mg)/24 hr daily until results achieved or maximum calculated dosage reached (see dosage charts in literature or formula below). A total calculated dose has been given as an infusion. Though not FDA approved, this method is preferred by some to multiple small-dose infusions or injections. To calculate the total amount of iron dextran (mL) required to restore hemoglobin and to replenish iron stores in adults and pediatric patients weighing over 15 kg (lean body weight [LBW]):

Dose (mL) = 0.0442 (Desired Hb − Observed Hb) × LBW in kg + (0.26 × LBW in kg)

If actual weight is less than LBW or in pediatric patients between 5 and 15 kg, use actual weight in kg. Calculated dose is in **mL.**

Iron replacement for blood loss: Dose should represent the equivalent amount of iron represented in blood loss. Begin with a test dose of 0.5 mL (25 mg). Wait 1 hour. If no adverse reactions, calculate the desired dose with the following formula and administer the balance of the replacement dose over 2 to 3 daily doses:

Amount of replacement iron **(mg)** = Blood loss **(mL)** × Hematocrit

Calculated dose is in **mg;** convert to **mL** before administration.

Formula is based on the approximation that 1 mL of normocytic, normochromic red cells contains 1 mg of elemental iron.

PEDIATRIC DOSE

Injectable iron not normally used in infants less than 4 months of age. See Maternal/Child.

Iron-deficiency anemia: Test dose: 0.5 mL (25 mg) for pediatric patients or 0.25 mL (12.5 mg) for infants over at least 5 minutes on the first day. Wait 1 hour. If no adverse reactions, may give remainder of daily dose. Direct IV push is not recommended; diluting with NS for infusion may lower the incidence of phlebitis. If actual weight is less than LBW or for pediatric patients between 5 and 15 kg, use actual weight in kg. The following daily doses have been recommended for IM injection by one source: *less than 5 kg,* 25 mg; *5 to 10 kg,* 50 mg; *more than 10 kg,* 100 mg. Repeat daily until results achieved or maximum calculated dosage reached (see dosage charts in literature or the formula listed earlier).

Iron replacement for blood loss: Calculate dose by formula used for adult dose. Dose should represent the equivalent amount of iron represented in blood loss. Begin with a test dose of 0.5 mL (25 mg) for pediatric patients or 0.25 mL (12.5 mg) for infants over at least 5 minutes on the first day. Wait 1 hour. If no adverse reactions, administer the balance of the replacement dose over 2 to 3 daily doses.

DILUTION

Given undiluted, or up to the total desired dose may be further diluted in 50 to 1,000 mL NS for infusion. D5W may cause additional local pain and phlebitis.

Filters: No data available from manufacturer.

Storage: Store unopened vials at CRT, protect from freezing.

COMPATIBILITY

Manufacturer states, "Do not mix with other medications or add to parenteral nutrition solutions."

RATE OF ADMINISTRATION

Test dose: 25 mg over 5 minutes (DexFerrum) or over 30 seconds (InFeD). Specific rates of test dose infusions not available for other manufacturers.

IV injection: If no adverse reactions to the test dose, administer 1 mL (50 mg) or a fraction thereof over 1 minute or more. Extend injection time in pediatric patients.

Infusion: If no adverse reactions to the test dose, infuse remaining dose over 1 to 8 hours (based on amount of dose, amount of diluent, and patient comfort).

ACTIONS

Iron dextran is removed from the plasma by cells of the reticuloendothelial system, which split the complex into its components of iron and dextran. Iron is immediately bound to protein moieties to form hemosiderin or ferritin, the physiologic forms of iron, or to a lesser extent to transferrin. This iron replenishes hemoglobin and depleted iron stores. Serum ferritin peaks approximately 7 to 9 days after iron dextran administration and slowly returns to baseline after about 3 weeks. Dextran is metabolized or excreted. Negligible amounts of iron are lost via the urinary or alimentary pathways after administration of iron dextran. Some placental transfer of iron dextran may occur. Trace amounts of unmetabolized iron dextran are excreted in breast milk.

INDICATIONS AND USES

Iron deficiency anemia in patients for whom oral administration is unsatisfactory or impossible; identify and treat the cause of the anemia.

Unlabeled uses: Iron supplementation for patients taking epoetin alfa (Epogen).

CONTRAINDICATIONS

Manifestation of hypersensitivity reactions; any anemia other than iron deficiency.

PRECAUTIONS

Anaphylactic-type reactions, including fatalities, have been reported. Fatal reactions have occurred both after the test dose and in situations in which the test dose was tolerated. Administer in facilities equipped to monitor the patient and respond to any medical emergency. Patients with a history of drug allergy or multiple drug allergies may be at increased risk for anaphylactic-type reactions. Concomitant use of angiotensin-converting enzyme inhibitors (e.g., enalapril [Vasotec], lisinopril [Zestril]) may also increase the risk of reactions. Facilities for monitoring the patient and responding to any medical emergency must be readily available. ▪ Iron dextran products are not clinically interchangeable. They differ in chemical characteristics and may differ in clinical and adverse effects. ▪ Large IV doses have been associated with an increased incidence of side effects, including arthralgia, backache, chills, dizziness, fever, headache, malaise, myalgia, nausea, and vomiting. The onset of these side effects is often delayed (1 to 2 days) and symptoms generally subside within 3 to 4 days. Maximum daily recommended dose is 100 mg (2 mL) of undiluted iron dextran. ▪ Use with caution in patients with severe liver impairment, cardiovascular disease, or a history of significant allergies and/or asthma. ▪ Do not administer during the acute phase of infectious kidney disease. ▪ Patients with rheumatoid arthritis may experience increased joint pain and swelling after administration of iron dextran. ▪ Administration of parenteral iron therapy should be limited to patients in whom clinical and laboratory investigations have established an iron-deficient state. Unwarranted therapy may cause excess storage of iron and possible exogenous hemosiderosis.

Monitor: Keep patient lying down after injection to prevent postural hypotension. ▪ Observe continuously for a hypersensitivity reaction during an infusion. Monitor vital signs. ▪ Monitor hemoglobin, hematocrit, reticulocyte count, total iron-binding capacity (TIBC), and percent of saturation of transferrin as indicated to monitor therapy and iron status. May take up to 3 weeks to see response. ▪ Monitor serum ferritin assays in prolonged therapy. Consider possibility of false results for months after injection caused by delayed

utilization. ▪ In patients undergoing chronic renal dialysis who are receiving iron dextran complex, the correlation of body iron stores and serum ferritin may not be valid.
Patient Education: Promptly report S/S of hypersensitivity (e.g., rash, itching, SOB). ▪ Promptly report any other side effects, immediate or delayed.
Maternal/Child: Category C: use only if absolutely necessary in pregnancy, breast-feeding, or childbearing years. ▪ Injectable iron not normally used in infants younger than 4 months of age.

DRUG/LAB INTERACTIONS

Inhibited by **chloramphenicol.** ▪ Concurrent administration of medicinal iron with **dimercaprol** (BAL in Oil) will result in the formation of a toxic complex. Either postpone iron therapy or treat severe iron deficiency with transfusions. ▪ Effectiveness negated by **deferoxamine** (Desferal), an iron chelating agent. May be affected by **other chelating agents** (e.g., edetate disodium). Give iron dextran at least 2 hours after a chelating agent. ▪ May cause **false serum iron values** within 1 to 2 weeks of large doses of iron dextran. ▪ May cause a **false elevated bilirubin, false decreased calcium, or affect numerous other tests or scans.** ▪ See Monitor.

SIDE EFFECTS

Backache, dizziness, headache, itching, local phlebitis at injection site, malaise, nausea, rash, shivering, transitory paresthesias.
Major: Anaphylaxis (fatalities have occurred); arthritic reactivation; dyspnea; febrile episodes; hypotension; leukocytosis; local phlebitis; lymphadenopathy; peripheral vascular flushing, especially with too-rapid injection; tachycardia; urticaria; shock (severe iron toxicity increases vasodilation and venous pooling and decreases circulating blood volume. Results in decreased cardiac output, hypotension, increased peripheral vascular resistance, and shock).
Overdose: Serum iron levels greater than 300 mcg/dL may indicate iron poisoning. Overdose with iron dextran is unlikely. May result in hemosiderosis, and excess iron may increase susceptibility to infection. If acute toxicity is seen, it may present as:
> *Early:* Abdominal pain, diarrhea, vomiting.
> *Late:* Bluish-colored lips, fingernails, and palms of hands; acidosis, drowsiness, shallow and rapid breathing, clammy skin, weak and fast heartbeat, hypotension, hypoglycemia, cardiovascular collapse.

ANTIDOTE

Discontinue the drug and notify the physician of early symptoms. For severe symptoms, discontinue drug, treat hypersensitivity reactions, or resuscitate as necessary, and notify physician. Epinephrine (Adrenalin) and diphenhydramine (Benadryl) should always be available. In overdose, monitor CBC, iron studies, vital signs, blood gases, and glucose and electrolytes. Maintain fluid and electrolyte balance. Correct acidosis with sodium bicarbonate. Deferoxamine is an iron chelating agent and may be useful in iron toxicity or overdose. Dialysis will not remove iron alone but will remove the iron deferoxamine complex and is indicated if oliguria or anuria is present.

IRON SUCROSE
(**EYE**-ern **SOO**-kros)

Hematinic
Iron supplement
Antianemic

Venofer   pH 10.5 to 11.1

USUAL DOSE
Dose is expressed in terms of mg of elemental iron. The usual total treatment course of iron sucrose is 1,000 mg. Treatment may be repeated if iron deficiency recurs.

Test dose (optional): 50 mg. Test dose is not required but was administered in some of the clinical trials. May be given at the physician's discretion.

Adult patients with hemodialysis-dependent chronic kidney disease (HDD-CKD): 100 mg as a slow IV injection or as a 15-minute infusion during consecutive hemodialysis sessions. Administered early during the dialysis session. Repeat as needed to maintain target levels of hemoglobin, hematocrit, and laboratory parameters of iron stores within acceptable limits. Frequency of dosing should be no more than three times weekly.

Adult patients with non–dialysis dependent chronic kidney disease (NDD-CKD): 200 mg as a slow IV injection over 2 to 5 minutes or as an infusion of 200 mg in a maximum of 100 mL of NS over 15 minutes. Administer on 5 different days within a 14-day period to a total cumulative dose of 1,000 mg. Alternately, there is limited experience with administering a 500-mg dose on Day 1 and Day 14 as a 3.5- to 4-hour infusion in a maximum of 250 mL of NS.

Adult patients with peritoneal dialysis–dependent chronic kidney disease (PDD-CKD): 300 mg as an infusion on Day 1 and Day 14. Follow with 400 mg as an infusion on Day 28. A total cumulative dose of 1,000 mg given in 3 doses over 28 days. Each infusion is diluted in a maximum of 250 mL NS and administered over 1.5 to 2.5 hours; see Rate of Administration.

PEDIATRIC DOSE
Pediatric patients (2 years of age and older) with hemodialysis-dependent chronic kidney disease (HDD-CKD) for iron maintenance treatment: The dosing for iron replacement treatment in pediatric patients with HDD-CKD has not been established.

Iron maintenance treatment: 0.5 mg/kg. Do not exceed 100 mg/dose. Administer every 2 weeks for 12 weeks; given undiluted by slow IV injection over 5 minutes or diluted in 25 mL of NS and administered over 5 to 60 minutes. Regimen may be repeated if necessary.

Pediatric patients (2 years of age and older) with non–dialysis dependent chronic kidney disease (NDD-CKD) or peritoneal dialysis–dependent chronic kidney disease (PDD-CKD) who are undergoing erythropoietin therapy for iron maintenance treatment: The dosing for iron replacement treatment in pediatric patients with NDD-CKD or PDD-CKD has not been established.

Iron maintenance treatment: 0.5 mg/kg. Do not exceed 100 mg/dose. Administer every 4 weeks for 12 weeks; given undiluted by slow IV injection over 5 minutes or diluted in 25 mL of NS and administered over 5 to 60 minutes. Regimen may be repeated if necessary.

DOSE ADJUSTMENTS
Begin at the low end of the dosing range in elderly patients. Consider the potential for decreased organ function and concomitant disease or drug therapy. ■ Withhold in patients with evidence of tissue iron overload; see Monitor.

DILUTION
Available in several sizes of single-dose vials. Check vial carefully and select the size that is closest to the desired dose. All contain 20 mg/mL of elemental iron. May be given undiluted or further diluted in NS. Do not dilute to concentrations below 1 mg/mL.

Test dose (optional): 50 mg should be diluted in 50 mL of NS.

Adult patients with hemodialysis-dependent chronic kidney disease (HDD-CKD): 100-mg dose may be given undiluted or may be further diluted in a maximum of 100 mL of NS and given as an infusion.

Adult patients with non–dialysis dependent chronic kidney disease (NDD-CKD): 200-mg dose may be given undiluted or may be further diluted in a maximum of 100 mL of NS. The 500-mg dose may be further diluted in a maximum of 250 mL of NS and given as an infusion.

Adult patients with peritoneal dialysis–dependent chronic kidney disease (PDD-CKD): Each 300- or 400-mg dose must be diluted in a maximum of 250 mL NS and given as an infusion.

Pediatric patients receiving iron maintenance treatment: A single dose may be given undiluted or diluted in 25 mL of NS and given as an infusion; see Usual Dose.

Filters: No data available from manufacturer.

Storage: Store unopened vials in original carton at CRT. Do not freeze. Diluted iron infusions should be used immediately after preparation. Discard any unused portion. When diluted with NS to a concentration of 1 to 2 mg/mL in PVC or non-PVC infusion bags, iron sucrose is stable for 7 days at CRT. When undiluted (20 mg/mL) or diluted with NS to a concentration of 2 to 10 mg/mL and stored in a plastic syringe, iron sucrose is stable for 7 days at CRT or refrigerated.

COMPATIBILITY

Manufacturer states, "Do not mix with other medications or add to parenteral nutrition solutions."

RATE OF ADMINISTRATION

Too-rapid administration may cause hypotension or symptoms of overdose; see Side Effects.

Test dose (optional): A single dose over 3 to 10 minutes.

Slow IV injection in adults: A single undiluted dose over 2 to 5 minutes. In dialysis patients, administer into the dialysis line during the dialysis session.

Infusion in adults: This method of administration may reduce the risk of hypotensive episodes.

Adult hemodialysis-dependent chronic kidney disease patients (HDD-CKD): A single 100-mg dose given as a slow IV injection over 2 to 5 minutes. Alternately may be given as an infusion equally distributed over at least 15 minutes.

Adult non–dialysis dependent chronic kidney disease patients (NDD-CKD): A single 200-mg dose as a slow IV injection over 2 to 5 minutes or as an infusion equally distributed over 15 minutes. Has also been administered as an infusion in a 500-mg dose equally distributed over 3.5 to 4 hours.

Adult peritoneal dialysis–dependent chronic kidney disease patients (PDD-CKD): A single 300-mg dose equally distributed over 1.5 hours or a single 400-mg dose equally distributed over 2.5 hours.

Pediatric patients receiving iron maintenance treatment: A single dose as a slow IV injection over 5 minutes or diluted with 25 mL NS and administered as an infusion over 5 to 60 minutes; see Usual Dose.

ACTIONS

An aqueous complex of polynuclear iron (III)-hydroxide in sucrose. Used to replenish the total body iron stores in patients with iron deficiency. Iron is critical for normal hemoglobin synthesis to maintain oxygen transport and necessary for metabolism and synthesis of DNA and various other processes. Following intravenous administration, iron sucrose is dissociated by the reticuloendothelial system into iron and sucrose. Iron distributes into liver, spleen, and bone marrow. Because iron disappearance from serum depends on the need for iron in the iron stores and iron-utilizing tissues of the body, serum clearance of iron is expected to be more rapid in iron-deficient patients as compared to healthy individuals. Half-life of the iron component is 6 hours. The sucrose component is eliminated mainly by urinary excretion. Most iron is stored in the body in hemoglobin, bone marrow, spleen, liver, and ferritin. Small amounts are eliminated in the urine. Significant increases in serum iron and ferritin and significant decreases in total iron-binding capacity occur within 4 weeks of beginning iron sucrose treatment.

INDICATIONS AND USES
Treatment of iron deficiency anemia in patients with chronic kidney disease (CKD).

CONTRAINDICATIONS
Known hypersensitivity to iron sucrose or any of its inactive components. Should not be used in patients with evidence of iron overload or in patients with anemia not caused by iron deficiency.

PRECAUTIONS
Use only when truly indicated to avoid excess storage of iron. Not recommended for use in patients with iron overload. ▪ Potentially fatal hypersensitivity reactions characterized by anaphylactic shock, loss of consciousness, collapse, hypotension, dyspnea, or convulsions have been reported. Medications and equipment for resuscitation must be readily available. ▪ Hypotension has been reported frequently and may be related to rate of administration and/or total dose administered. Follow guidelines for dosing and administration. See Usual Dose and Rate of Administration.

Monitor: Confirm IV placement and avoid extravasation; injection site discoloration has been reported following extravasation. ▪ Monitor vital signs during and immediately following administration. Recumbent position during and after administration may help to prevent postural hypotension. Hypotensive effects may be additive to transient hypotension during dialysis and/or from too-rapid rate of administration. ▪ Monitor for S/S of hypersensitivity reactions during and after administration for at least 30 minutes and until clinically stable; see Precautions. Reactions may occur after the first dose or subsequent doses of iron sucrose. ▪ Periodic monitoring of hematologic and hematinic parameters (hemoglobin, hematocrit, serum ferritin and transferrin saturation) is indicated during parenteral iron replacement therapy. Takes about 4 weeks of treatment to see increased serum iron and ferritin and decreased TIBC (total iron-binding capacity). Transferrin saturation values increase rapidly after IV adminstration of iron sucrose; thus serum iron values may be reliably obtained 48 hours after the last IV dose.

Patient Education: Review any possible reactions to past parenteral iron therapy. ▪ Report S/S of a hypersensitivity reaction promptly.

Maternal/Child: Category B: use in pregnancy only if clearly needed. ▪ Safety for use during breast-feeding not established. ▪ Safety and effectiveness for iron replacement treatment in pediatric patients have not been established. Safety and effectiveness for iron maintenance treatment have been established for pediatric patients 2 years of age and older. ▪ Necrotizing enterocolitis in 5 premature infants (weight less than 1,250 Gm) with 2 deaths has been reported in one country in which iron sucrose is approved for use in pediatric patients. No causal relationship to drugs could be established; it may be a complication of prematurity in very-low-birth-weight infants.

Elderly: Differences in response between elderly and younger patients have not been identified. Lower-end initial doses may be appropriate in the elderly; see Dose Adjustments.

DRUG/LAB INTERACTIONS
Drug interactions involving iron sucrose have not been studied. May reduce the absorption of concomitantly administered **oral iron preparations;** concurrent use not recommended.

SIDE EFFECTS
Adult patients: Arthralgia, back pain, chest pain, diarrhea, dizziness, headache, hypotension, injection site burning or pain, muscle cramps, nausea, pain in extremity, peripheral edema, pruritus, and vomiting are most common. Other side effects varied according to the type of chronic kidney disease patient who was receiving iron sucrose (e.g., hemodialysis dependent, peritoneal dialysis–dependent, non–dialysis dependent) and included abdominal pain, altered taste, asthenia, catheter site infection, conjunctivitis, cough, dyspnea, ear pain, fecal occult blood positive, feeling abnormal, fever, fluid overload, gout, graft complications, hyperglycemia, hypersensitivity reactions, hypertension, hy-

poesthesia, hypoglycemia, injection site extravasation, myalgia, nasal congestion, nasopharyngitis, peritoneal infection, pharyngitis, sinusitis, upper respiratory infection.

Pediatric patients: Arteriovenous fistula thrombosis, cough, dizziness, fever, headache, hypertension, hypotension, nausea, peritonitis, renal transplant, respiratory tract viral infection, and vomiting occurred.

Overdose: Serum iron levels greater than 300 mcg/dL may indicate iron poisoning. May result in hemosiderosis. Excess iron may increase susceptibility to infection. If acute toxicity is seen, it may present as abdominal and muscle pain, cardiovascular collapse, dizziness, dyspnea, edema, headache, hemosiderosis, hypotension, joint aches, nausea, pale eyes, paresthesia, sedation, vomiting.

Post-Marketing: Life-threatening hypersensitivity reactions (e.g., anaphylactic shock, angioedema, bronchospasm, collapse, convulsions, dyspnea, loss of consciousness, pruritus, rash, shock, wheezing), bradycardia, chromaturia, confusion, CHF, light-headedness, sweating, swelling of joints.

ANTIDOTE

Reduce rate of infusion for hypotension or other symptoms. Most symptoms are successfully treated with IV fluids, hydrocortisone sodium succinate (Solu-Cortef), and/or antihistamines (e.g., diphenhydramine [Benadryl]). Volume expanders (e.g., albumin, dextran, hetastarch [Hespan]) may be indicated. Keep physician informed of all side effects. Discontinue drug if severe hypersensitivity reactions occur. Treat hypersensitivity reactions as indicated; may require epinephrine, airway management, oxygen, IV fluids, antihistamines (e.g., diphenhydramine [Benadryl]), corticosteroids (e.g., hydrocortisone sodium succinate [Solu-Cortef]), and pressor amines (e.g., dopamine). Resuscitate as needed. Not removed by dialysis.

ISAVUCONAZONIUM SULFATE
(eye-sah-vew-koh-nah-**ZOH**-nee-um **SUL**-fayt)

Antifungal
(azole derivative)

Cresemba

USUAL DOSE
Obtain specimens for fungal culture and other relevant lab studies (including histopathology) to isolate and identify causative organism(s) before initiating therapy. Institute antifungal therapy and adjust based on results of culture and lab studies.

Loading dose: 372 mg (1 vial) as an infusion every 8 hours for 6 doses.

Maintenance dose: 372 mg (1 vial) as an infusion once daily. Initiate 12 to 24 hours after the last loading dose. Oral formulation (2 capsules = 372 mg) may be substituted when appropriate.

DOSE ADJUSTMENTS
No dose adjustment is required based on age, gender, or race or in patients with mild, moderate, or severe renal impairment, including ESRD. ▪ No dose adjustment is required with mild to moderate hepatic impairment.

DILUTION
Available as a lyophilized powder containing 372 mg isavuconazonium sulfate (equivalent to 200 mg isavuconazole). Reconstitute 1 vial with 5 mL of SWFI. Gently shake to dissolve the powder completely. Solution should be clear and free of particulates. Withdraw 5 mL from the reconstituted vial and inject into a 250-mL bag of NS or D5W. Final concentration is approximately 1.5 mg/mL. Diluted solution may have visible translucent to white particulates, which will be removed by in-line filtration. Use gentle mixing or roll bag to minimize the formation of particulates. Avoid unnecessary vibration or vigorous shaking of the solution. Do not use a pneumatic transport system.

Filters: Must be administered using an infusion set that contains a sterile, nonpyrogenic, in-line filter (pore size of 0.2 to 1.2 micrometers).

Storage: Before use, refrigerate at 2° to 8° C (36° to 46° F). Reconstituted solution should be further diluted and used immediately but may be stored below 25° C for a maximum of 1 hour before further dilution. Diluted solution must be used within 6 hours if kept at RT or may be immediately refrigerated. Complete the infusion within 24 hours. Do not freeze.

COMPATIBILITY
Manufacturer states, "Do not infuse isavuconazonium with other intravenous medications." **Compatible** only with NS or D5W.

RATE OF ADMINISTRATION
Do not administer as an IV bolus; for use as a diluted IV infusion only. Administer a single dose as an infusion equally distributed over a minimum of 60 minutes. Flush the IV line before and after each isavuconazonium infusion with NS or D5W. Administer through an infusion set that contains a sterile, nonpyrogenic, in-line filter (pore size of 0.2 to 1.2 micrometers).

ACTIONS
Isavuconazonium is a prodrug of isavuconazole, an azole antifungal drug. Acts by inhibiting the synthesis of ergosterol, a key component of fungal cell membranes. Rapidly hydrolyzed in blood to isavuconazole by esterases, predominantly by butylcholinesterase. Extensively distributed and highly protein bound, predominantly to albumin. Following IV administration, maximum plasma concentrations of the prodrug and inactive products were detectable during infusion and declined rapidly following the end of administration. Mean plasma half-life is 130 hours. CYP3A4, CYP3A5 and, subsequently, uridine diphosphate-glucuronosyltransferase (UGT) are involved in the metabolism of isavuconazole. Primarily excreted as metabolites in urine and feces.

INDICATIONS AND USES

Treatment of invasive aspergillosis and invasive mucormycosis in patients 18 years of age and older.

CONTRAINDICATIONS

Known hypersensitivity to isavuconazole. ▪ Coadministration of strong CYP3A4 inhibitors such as ketoconazole (Nizoral) or high-dose ritonavir (Norvir [400 mg every 12 hours]). ▪ Coadministration of strong CYP3A4 inducers such as rifampin (Rifadin), carbamazepine (Tegretol), St. John's wort, or long-acting barbiturates (e.g., phenobarbital [Luminal]). ▪ Patients with familial short QT syndrome. ▪ See Drug/Lab Interactions.

PRECAUTIONS

Do not administer as an IV bolus; for use as a diluted IV infusion only. ▪ Elevations in liver function tests (e.g., ALT, AST, alkaline phosphatase, total bilirubin) have been reported, were generally reversible, and did not require discontinuation of isavuconazonium. ▪ Severe hepatic reactions (e.g., cholestasis, hepatitis, or hepatic failure, including death) have been reported in patients with serious underlying medical conditions (e.g., hematologic malignancy) during treatment with azole antifungal agents, including isavuconazonium. ▪ Has not been studied in patients with severe hepatic impairment (Child-Pugh Class C); use in these patients only when benefits outweigh risks. ▪ Infusion-related reactions have been reported. ▪ Serious hypersensitivity and severe skin reactions, such as anaphylaxis or Stevens-Johnson syndrome, have been reported with other azole antifungal agents. There is no information regarding cross-sensitivity between isavuconazole and other azole antifungal agents. Use caution in patients with hypersensitivity to other azoles. ▪ In vitro and animal studies suggest cross-resistance between isavuconazole and other azoles. Relevance of cross-resistance to clinical outcome has not been fully characterized. Patients failing prior azole therapy may require alternative antifungal therapy. ▪ See Drug/Lab Interactions.

Monitor: Obtain specimens for fungal culture and other relevant lab studies (including histopathology) to isolate and identify causative organism(s) before initiating therapy. Institute antifungal therapy and adjust based on results of culture and lab studies. ▪ Obtain baseline liver function tests and repeat as necessary. Monitor more frequently in patients who develop abnormal liver function tests and when treating patients with severe hepatic impairment. ▪ Monitor for infusion-related reactions (e.g., chills, dizziness, dyspnea, hypoesthesia, hypotension, and paresthesia). ▪ Monitor for S/S of hypersensitivity reactions (e.g., hypotension, rash, tightness of the chest, urticaria, wheezing). ▪ Monitor for S/S of skin reactions (e.g., rash, blisters).

Patient Education: Review manufacturer's medication guide. ▪ Review of health history and medication profile is imperative. ▪ Avoid pregnancy; nonhormonal birth control recommended; see Drug/Lab Interactions. Should pregnancy occur, notify physician and discuss potential hazards. ▪ Promptly report S/S of a hypersensitivity/infusion reaction (e.g., itching, hives, shortness of breath, or a serious skin reaction [e.g., rash]).

Maternal/Child: Category C: may cause fetal harm. Use during pregnancy only if the potential benefit to the patient outweighs the risk to the fetus. Report a suspected pregnancy. ▪ Discontinue breast-feeding. ▪ Safety and effectiveness for use in patients under 18 years of age have not been established.

Elderly: Response similar to that seen in younger adults.

DRUG/LAB INTERACTIONS

Isavuconazole is a sensitive substrate of CYP3A4. CYP3A4 inhibitors or inducers may alter the plasma concentrations of isavuconazole. Isavuconazole is a moderate inhibitor of CYP3A4, a mild inhibitor of P-glycoprotein (P-gp), and an organic cation transporter 2 (OCT2). ▪ Coadministration of isavuconazonium with **strong CYP3A4 inhibitors** such as ketoconazole (Nizoral) or high-dose ritonavir (Norvir [400 mg every 12 hours]) is *contraindicated*. Strong CYP3A4 inhibitors can significantly increase the plasma concentration of isavuconazole. ▪ Coadministration of isavuconazonium with **strong CYP3A4 inducers** such as rifampin (Rifadin), carbamazepine (Tegretol), St. John's wort, or long-acting barbiturates (e.g., phenobarbital [Luminal]) is **_contraindicated._** Strong CYP3A4 inducers can significantly decrease the plasma concentration of isavuconazole. ▪ Coadministration with **lopinavir/ritonavir** (Kaletra) can significantly increase the plasma concentration of isavuconazole, and **isavuconazole** may decrease the antiviral effectiveness of lopinavir/ritonavir. ▪ Coadministration with **atorvastatin** (Lipitor) may increase atorvastatin exposure and toxicity. ▪ Coadministration with **cyclosporine** (Sandimmune), **mycophenolate** (CellCept), **sirolimus** (Rapamune), and **tacrolimus** (Prograf) may increase exposure of these drugs. Monitor drug concentrations of these drugs and/or drug-related toxicities and adjust doses as needed. ▪ May increase exposure of **midazolam** (Versed). Consider dose reduction of midazolam with concomitant administration. ▪ May decrease exposure of **bupropion** (Wellbutrin, Zyban). Dose increase of bupropion may be necessary with coadministration; do not exceed the maximum recommended dose. ▪ Concomitant administration with **digoxin** increases digoxin exposure. Monitor serum digoxin concentrations and adjust dose as necessary.

SIDE EFFECTS
The most commonly reported side effects include back pain; constipation; cough; diarrhea; dyspnea; elevated ALT, AST, alkaline phosphatase, total bilirubin, and GGT; headache; hypokalemia; nausea and vomiting; and peripheral edema. Hepatic adverse drug reactions, infusion-related or hypersensitivity reactions, and embryo-fetal toxicity are considered the most serious. Abdominal pain, acute respiratory failure, anxiety, chest pain, decreased appetite, delirium, dyspepsia, fatigue, hypomagnesemia, hypotension, injection site reaction, insomnia, pruritus, rash, and renal failure have also been reported.

ANTIDOTE
Notify physician of all side effects; most will be treated symptomatically. If a hypersensitivity reaction, infusion reaction, or severe cutaneous reaction occurs, discontinue the infusion and treat as indicated. Discontinue isavuconazonium if clinical S/S consistent with liver disease develop that may be attributable to isavuconazonium. No known specific antidote. Not removed by hemodialysis.

ISOPROTERENOL HYDROCHLORIDE
(**eye**-so-**PROH**-ter-ih-nohl hy-droh-**KLOR**-eyed)

Isuprel

Cardiac stimulant
(inotropic/chronotropic)
Bronchodilator
Antiarrhythmic

pH 3.5 to 4.5

USUAL DOSE
In all situations, adjust the rate of infusion based on HR, CVP, BP, respiratory rate, and urine output.

Recommended Isoproterenol Dose for Adults with Atropine-Resistant Hemodynamically Significant Bradycardia, Heart Block, Adams-Stokes Attacks, and Cardiac Arrest			
Route of Administration	Preparation of Dilution	Initial Dose	Subsequent Dose Range*
Bolus intravenous injection	Dilute 1 mL (0.2 mg) to 10 mL with NS or D5W	0.02 to 0.06 mg (1 to 3 mL of diluted solution)	0.01 to 0.2 mg (0.5 to 10 mL of diluted solution)
Intravenous infusion	Dilute 10 mL (2 mg) in 500 mL D5W (4 mcg/mL)	5 mcg/min (1.25 mL of diluted solution per minute)	
Intracardiac	Use solution 0.2 mg/mL undiluted	0.02 mg (0.1 mL)	

*Subsequent dose depends on the ventricular rate and the rapidity with which the cardiac pacemaker can take over when the drug is gradually withdrawn.
AHA recommendation is 2 to 10 mcg/min if an external pacemaker is not available.

Recommended Isoproterenol Dose for Adults with Shock (Cardiogenic, CHF, Hypoperfusion [Low Cardiac Output], Hypovolemic, Septic)		
Route of Administration	Preparation of Dilution*	Infusion Rate†
Intravenous infusion	Dilute 5 mL (1 mg) in 500 mL of D5W (2 mcg/mL)	0.5 to 5 mcg/min (0.25 to 2.5 mL of diluted solution)

*Concentrations up to 10 times greater have been used when limitation of volume is essential.
†Rates over 30 mcg/min have been used in advanced stages of shock. Adjust infusion rate based on HR, CVP, BP, and urine flow. If HR exceeds 110 beats/min, consider decreasing rate or temporarily discontinue the infusion.

Recommended Isoproterenol Dose for Adults with Bronchospasm Occurring During Anesthesia			
Route of Administration	Preparation of Dilution	Initial Dose	Subsequent Dose
Bolus intravenous injection	Dilute 1 mL (0.2 mg) to 10 mL with NS or D5W	0.01 to 0.02 mg (0.5 to 1 mL of diluted solution)	Repeat initial dose as necessary

Complete heart block following closure of ventricular septal defects: 0.04 to 0.06 mg (2 to 3 mL of a 0.02 mg/mL dilution) as a bolus injection. May maintain a sinus rhythm with a HR above 90 to 100 beats/min or may relapse into complete heart block again.
Diagnosis of mitral regurgitation (unlabeled): 4 mcg/min as an infusion (1 mL/min of a 4 mcg/mL dilution).
Diagnosis of coronary artery disease or lesions (unlabeled): 1 to 3 mcg/min as an infusion (0.25 to 0.75 mL/min of a 4 mcg/mL dilution).
Refractory torsades de pointes, bradycardia in heart transplant patients, beta-adrenergic blocker poisoning: AHA recommends 2 to 10 mcg/min (0.5 to 2.5 mL/min of a 4 mcg/mL dilu-

tion). Titrate to adequate heart rate. In torsades de pointes titrate to increase heart rate until VT is suppressed.

PEDIATRIC DOSE
See Dilution and Maternal/Child.
0.05 to 2 mcg/kg/min. Begin with 0.1 mcg/kg/min as an infusion. Increase by 0.1 mcg/kg/min until desired effect. Titrate to patient response and monitor cardiac status carefully. Maximum dose is 2 mcg/kg/min. Another source suggests a maximum dose of 1 mcg/kg/min.
Complete heart block after closure of ventricular septal defects in infants: 0.01 to 0.03 mg (0.5 to 1.5 mL of a 0.02 mg/mL solution) as a bolus injection. See comments in Usual Dose.

DOSE ADJUSTMENTS
Lower-end initial doses may be appropriate in the elderly; consider the potential for decreased organ function and concomitant disease or drug therapy.

DILUTION
IV injection: Available in a 0.2 mg/mL solution. Dilute 1 mL of a 0.2 mg/mL solution with 10 mL NS or D5W to provide a concentration of 0.02 mg/mL.
Infusion: *Atropine-resistant, hemodynamically significant bradycardia, heart block, Adams-Stokes attacks, and cardiac arrest:* Dilute 10 mL (2 mg of a 0.2 mg/mL solution) in 500 mL D5W (4 mcg/mL). *Shock:* Dilute 5 mL (1 mg of a 0.2 mg/mL solution) in 500 mL D5W (2 mcg/mL). Use an infusion pump or microdrip (60 gtts equals 1 mL) to administer. Less diluent may be used to reduce fluid intake.
Filters: No data available from manufacturer. Another source cites no significant loss in drug potency in several studies using various types and sizes of filters from 0.22 to 5 microns in size.
Storage: Store between 8° and 15° C (46° to 59° F) unless otherwise specified by manufacturer. Do not use if pink or brown in color or contains a precipitate.

COMPATIBILITY
Consider any drug NOT listed as compatible to be INCOMPATIBLE until consulting a pharmacist; specific conditions may apply.
One source suggests the following **compatibilities:**
Additive: Atracurium (Tracrium), calcium chloride, dobutamine, heparin, magnesium sulfate, multivitamins (M.V.I.), potassium chloride (KCl), ranitidine (Zantac), succinylcholine, verapamil.
Y-site: Amiodarone (Nexterone), atracurium (Tracrium), bivalirudin (Angiomax), cisatracurium (Nimbex), dexmedetomidine (Precedex), famotidine (Pepcid IV), fenoldopam (Corlopam), heparin, hetastarch in electrolytes (Hextend), hydrocortisone sodium succinate (Solu-Cortef), levofloxacin (Levaquin), milrinone (Primacor), nitroprusside sodium, pancuronium, potassium chloride (KCl), propofol (Diprivan), remifentanil (Ultiva), tacrolimus (Prograf), vecuronium.

RATE OF ADMINISTRATION
IV injection: Each 1 mL of a 0.02 mg/mL solution or fraction thereof over 1 minute. Follow with a 20-mL flush of NS if indicated to ensure distribution to circulation.
Infusion: Titrate to desired dose, HR, and rhythm; see the following infusion rate chart. Decrease rate of infusion as necessary. Ventricular rate generally should not exceed 110 beats/min.

Isoproterenol (Isuprel) Infusion Rates						
Desired Dose	1 mg in 500 mL D5W (2 mcg/mL)			1 mg in 250 mL D5W 2 mg in 500 mL D5W (4 mcg/mL)		
mcg/min	mcg/hr	mL/min	mL/hr	mcg/hr	mL/min	mL/hr
2	120	1	60	120	0.5	30
5	300	2.5	150	300	1.25	75
10	600	5	300	600	2.5	150
15	900	7.5	450	900	3.75	225
20	1,200	10	600	1,200	5	300
25	1,500	12.5	750	1,500	6.25	375
30	1,800	15	900	1,800	7.5	450

ACTIONS

A nonselective synthetic cardiac beta receptor stimulant (sympathomimetic amine) similar to epinephrine and norepinephrine. Has positive inotropic and chronotropic actions more potent than those of epinephrine. It increases cardiac output, cardiac work, coronary flow, and venous return. Improves atrioventricular conduction. Stimulates only the higher ventricular foci, allowing a more normal cardiac pacemaker to take over, thus suppressing ectopic pacemaker activity. Decreases peripheral vascular resistance by relaxing arterial smooth muscle and is a most effective bronchial smooth muscle relaxant. Onset of action is immediate and lasts 1 to 2 hours. Metabolized by the liver and inactivated by various enzyme systems. Excreted in the urine.

INDICATIONS AND USES

Treatment of mild or transient episodes of heart block that do not require cardioversion or pacemaker therapy. ▪ Treatment of serious episodes of heart block and Adams-Stokes attacks (except when caused by VT or VF). ▪ May be used in cardiac arrest until defibrillation or pacemaker (the treatments of choice) is available. ▪ Bronchospasm during anesthesia. ▪ Management of shock (cardiogenic, CHF, hypoperfusion [low cardiac output], hypovolemic, septic). Adequate fluid and electrolyte replacement required. ▪ AHA recommends cautious use in symptomatic bradycardia if a pacemaker is not available, treatment of refractory torsades de pointes unresponsive to magnesium sulfate, temporary control of bradycardia in heart transplant patients (denervated heart unresponsive to atropine), and treatment of poisoning from beta-adrenergic blockers (e.g., metoprolol [Lopressor]).

Unlabeled uses: Aid in diagnosis of the etiology of mitral regurgitation. ▪ Aid in diagnosis of coronary artery disease or lesions. ▪ Pulmonary embolism to increase pulmonary blood volume and decrease pulmonary arterial pressure and vascular resistance.

CONTRAINDICATIONS

Tachyarrhythmias, patients with tachycardia or heart block caused by digoxin intoxication, angina pectoris, ventricular arrhythmias that require inotropic therapy.

PRECAUTIONS

IV injection in cardiac standstill must be accompanied by cardiac massage to perfuse drug into the myocardium. Current JAMA recommendations do not include isoproterenol in the treatment of cardiac arrest or hypotension. ▪ Fourth-line agent for bradycardia; considered possibly helpful but may be harmful. ▪ Can cause a severe drop in BP and can be very harmful in bradycardia. ▪ Use extreme caution when inhalant anesthetics (e.g., cyclopropane) are being administered and supplementary to digoxin administration. ▪ Use caution in coronary insufficiency, diabetes, hyperthyroidism, known sensitivity to sympathomimetic amines, history of seizures, hypertension, and pre-existing cardiac arrhythmias with tachycardia. ▪ Increased cardiac output and work can increase ischemia and worsen arrhythmias. ▪ Contains sulfites; use caution in allergic patients.

Monitor: Decrease rate of infusion as necessary. Ventricular rate generally should not exceed 110 beats/min. Maintain adequate blood volume and correct acidosis. ▪ Continuous cardiac monitoring, central venous pressure readings, BP, respiratory rate, and urine flow measurements are advisable during therapy with isoproterenol. ▪ Monitoring of serum glucose, magnesium, and potassium may be indicated. ▪ See Drug/Lab Interactions and Maternal/Child.

Maternal/Child: Category C: safety for use in pregnancy or breast-feeding not established. Benefits must outweigh risks. ▪ Safety and effectiveness in pediatric patients not established. ▪ In asthmatic pediatric patients, IV infusion of isoproterenol has caused clinical deterioration, myocardial necrosis, CHF, and death. Risks of cardiac toxicity may be increased by other factors such as acidosis, hypoxemia, coadministration of corticosteroids or methylxanthines (e.g., aminophylline). Continuous assessment of VS, frequent ECGs, and daily measurement of cardiac enzymes (e.g., CPK, MB) is suggested if isoproterenol infusion is required.

Elderly: Difference in response from younger adults not known. May be more sensitive to the effects of beta-adrenergic agents (e.g., hypertension, hypokalemia, tachycardia, tremor). Patients with cardiac disease may be at increased risk for cardiac effects. ▪ Lower-end initial doses may be appropriate; see Dose Adjustments.

DRUG/LAB INTERACTIONS

May be used alternately with epinephrine (Adrenalin), but they may not be used together. Both are direct cardiac stimulants; serious arrhythmias and death may result. An adequate interval between doses must be maintained. ▪ Do not use concomitantly with other **sympathomimetic agents** (e.g., ephedrine, dopamine). Additive effects may cause toxicity. May be used after effects of previous drug have subsided. ▪ Simultaneous use with **oxytoxics** may cause hypertensive crisis. ▪ May cause hypertension with **guanethidine** (Ismelin). ▪ **Digoxin, quinidine, and halogenated hydrocarbon anesthetics** (e.g., halothane) may sensitize myocardium and cause serious arrhythmias. ▪ Antagonized by **propranolol.** May be used to treat tachycardia caused by isoproterenol, but tachycardia and hypotension secondary to peripheral vasodilation may occur. ▪ Potentiated by **tricyclic antidepressants** (e.g., imipramine [Tofranil]). ▪ Concomitant use with **theophylline** increases the risk of cardiotoxicity. ▪ See Contraindications.

SIDE EFFECTS

Anginal pain, cardiac arrhythmias, flushing, headache, hyperglycemia, hypokalemia, nausea, nervousness, palpitations, sweating, tachycardia, vomiting. Cardiac dilation, marked hypotension, pulmonary edema, and death may occur with prolonged use or overdose. Adams-Stokes attacks have been reported.

ANTIDOTE

Notify the physician of any side effect. Treatment will probably be symptomatic. For ventricular rate over 110 beats/min, PVCs, or ECG changes, decrease rate of infusion or discontinue drug. Vasodilators (e.g., nitrates) may be useful for treatment of hypertension. For accidental overdose, discontinue drug immediately, resuscitate and sustain patient, and notify physician.

IXABEPILONE BBW

(ix-ab-**EP**-i-lone)

Ixempra Kit

Antineoplastic
(microtubule inhibitor)

USUAL DOSE

Premedication: An H_1 antagonist (e.g., diphenhydramine [Benadryl]) and an H_2 antagonist (e.g., ranitidine [Zantac], famotidine [Pepcid]) should be administered orally 60 minutes prior to ixabepilone to minimize the chance of a hypersensitivity reaction. Patients who experience a hypersensitivity reaction require premedication with a corticosteroid (e.g., dexamethasone 20 mg IV 30 minutes before infusion or orally 60 minutes before infusion) in addition to pretreatment with the H_1 and H_2 antagonists.

Ixabepilone: 40 mg/M^2 as an infusion over 3 hours every 3 weeks. Doses for patients with a body surface area (BSA) greater than 2.2 M^2 should be calculated based on 2.2 M^2. Administered alone or in combination with capecitabine (Xeloda) 1,000 mg/M^2 twice daily for 2 weeks followed by 1 week of rest.

DOSE ADJUSTMENTS

If toxicities are present, therapy should be delayed to allow recovery. ▪ Dosing adjustment guidelines for monotherapy and combination therapy are listed in the following chart. *If toxicities recur, an additional 20% dose reduction should be made.*

Dose Adjustments Guidelines	
Ixabepilone (Monotherapy or Combination Therapy)	**Ixabepilone Dose Modification**
NONHEMATOLOGIC	
Grade 2 neuropathy (moderate) lasting ≥7 days	Decrease the dose by 20%
Grade 3 neuropathy (severe) lasting <7 days	Decrease the dose by 20%
Grade 3 neuropathy (severe) lasting ≥7 days or disabling neuropathy	Discontinue treatment
Any Grade 3 toxicity (severe) other than neuropathy	Decrease the dose by 20%
Transient Grade 3 arthralgia/myalgia or fatigue	No change in dose required
Grade 3 hand-foot syndrome (palmar-plantar erythrodysesthesia)	No change in dose required
Any Grade 4 toxicity (disabling)	Discontinue treatment
HEMATOLOGIC	
Neutrophils <500 cells/mm³ for ≥7 days	Decrease the dose by 20%
Febrile neutropenia	Decrease the dose by 20%
Platelets <25,000/mm³ or platelets <50,000/mm³ with bleeding	Decrease the dose by 20%
Capecitabine **(When Used in Combination with Ixabepilone)**	**Capecitabine** **Dose Modification**
NONHEMATOLOGIC	Follow capecitabine prescribing information
HEMATOLOGIC	
Platelets <25,000/mm³ or platelets <50,000/mm³ with bleeding	Hold for concurrent diarrhea or stomatitis until platelet count >50,000/mm³, then continue at same dose
Neutrophils <500 cells/mm³ for ≥7 days or febrile neutropenia	Hold for concurrent diarrhea or stomatitis until neutrophil count >1,000/mm³, then continue at same dose

Dose adjustments at the start of a cycle should be based on nonhematologic toxicity or blood counts from the preceding cycle following the previous guidelines. Patients should not begin a new cycle unless the neutrophil count is at least 1,500 cells/mm³, the platelet count is at least 100,000 cells/mm³, and nonhematologic toxicities have improved to Grade 1 (mild) or have resolved. ■ Combined use with capecitabine is contraindicated in patients who have AST or ALT >2.5 times the ULN or bilirubin >1 times the ULN; see Contraindications and Precautions. ■ Patients with hepatic impairment who are receiving monotherapy should be dosed according to the guidelines listed in the following chart.

Dose Adjustments for Ixabepilone as Monotherapy in Patients with Hepatic Impairment				
	Transaminase Levels		Bilirubin Levels*	Ixabepilone Dose† (mg/M²)
Mild	AST and ALT ≤2.5 × ULN	and	≤1 × ULN	40
	AST or ALT ≤10 × ULN	and	≤1.5 × ULN	32
Moderate	AST and ALT ≤10 × ULN	and	>1.5 × ULN to ≤3 × ULN	20-30
Severe	AST or ALT >10 × ULN	or	>3 × ULN	Not recommended

*Excluding patients whose total bilirubin is elevated due to Gilbert's disease.
†Dosage recommendations are for the first course of therapy; further decreases in subsequent courses should be based on individual tolerance.

Patients with moderate hepatic impairment should start with 20 mg/M². The dose in subsequent cycles may be increased up to, but should not exceed, 30 mg/M² if tolerated. ■ Reduce dose to 20 mg/M² when coadministered with a strong CYP3A4 inhibitor; see Drug Interactions. If the strong inhibitor is discontinued, wait for at least 1 week before adjusting the ixabepilone dose upward to the indicated dose. ■ If coadministration of a strong CYP3A4 inducer is required and alternatives are not feasible (e.g., the patient has been maintained on a strong CYP3A4 inducer), the dose may be gradually increased from 40 mg/M² to 60 mg/M² if tolerated; see Drug Interactions. Increase infusion duration of 60 mg/M² dose to 4 hours and monitor patient closely for toxicity. If CYP3A4 inducer is discontinued, return to original dose. ■ No dose adjustment indicated based on age, race, and gender. ■ Minimally excreted by the kidney; no studies conducted in patients with renal impairment.

DILUTION
Specific techniques required; see Precautions. Available as a 15-mg or 45-mg Ixempra Kit that contains two vials; one vial contains the indicated amount of ixabepilone, and the other contains a manufacturer-supplied diluent. Only the manufacturer-supplied diluent may be used for reconstitution. Calculate dose and remove required number of kits from refrigerator. Let stand at RT for approximately 30 minutes. A white precipitate may appear in the diluent vial. This will dissolve as the vial warms to RT. Withdraw diluent and slowly inject it into the ixabepilone vial. (The 15-mg vial is reconstituted with 8 mL of diluent, and the 45-mg vial is reconstituted with 23.5 mL.) Gently swirl and invert until completely dissolved. Concentration of reconstituted solution is 2 mg/mL. Must be further diluted to a final concentration of 0.2 to 0.6 mg/mL with LR, Plasma-Lyte A Injection pH 7.4, or NS 250 to 500 mL (the pH of the NS must be adjusted to between 6 and 9 by adding 2 mEq [i.e., 2 mL of an 8.4% w/v solution or 4 mL of a 4.2% w/v solution] of sodium bicarbonate injection before adding the ixabepilone). A 250-mL bag will be sufficient for most doses. Withdraw the calculated dose from the ixabepilone vials and transfer to a DEHP-free IV bag containing an appropriate volume of infusion solution to achieve the final desired concentration. Thoroughly mix by manual rotation. Should be administered through a DEHP-free, polyethylene-lined administration set.
Filter: Must be administered through an in-line filter with a microporous membrane of 0.2 to 1.2 microns.

Storage: Store unopened vials at 2° to 8° C (36° to 46° F) in original carton. Protect from light. Reconstituted solution may be stored in vial for 1 hour at RT and room light. Once diluted, solution is stable for a maximum of 6 hours at RT. Administration must be completed within this 6-hour period.

COMPATIBILITY

Manufacturer states, "DEHP-free infusion containers and administration sets must be used." Must be reconstituted with manufacturer-supplied diluent only and further diluted with the infusion solutions noted in Dilution. Indicated solutions have a pH between 6 to 9, which is required for ixabepilone stability.

RATE OF ADMINISTRATION

A single dose as an infusion equally distributed over 3 hours. In patients who experience a hypersensitivity reaction, increase duration of infusion and premedicate with corticosteroids and H_1 and H_2 antagonists; see Usual Dose. Increase duration of infusion to 4 hours in patients receiving 60 mg/M^2 dose; see Dose Adjustments.

ACTIONS

A microtubule inhibitor belonging to a class of antineoplastic agents, the epothilones. A semi-synthetic analog of epothilone B. Binds directly to β-tubulin subunits on microtubules, leading to suppression of microtubule dynamics. Blocks cells in the mitotic phase of the cell division cycle, leading to cell death. Has antitumor activity against multiple human tumor xenografts and is active in xenografts that are resistant to multiple agents, including taxanes, anthracyclines, and vinca alkaloids. Has demonstrated synergistic antitumor activity in combination with capecitabine. In addition to direct antitumor activity, ixabepilone has antiangiogenic activity. 67% to 77% bound to plasma proteins. Extensively metabolized in the liver, primarily by CYP3A4. Eliminated primarily as metabolized drug in feces and urine. Half-life is approximately 52 hours.

INDICATIONS AND USES

In combination with capecitabine (Xeloda) for the treatment of patients with metastatic or locally advanced breast cancer resistant to treatment with an anthracycline and a taxane or for patients whose cancer is taxane resistant and for whom further anthracycline therapy is contraindicated. Anthracycline resistance is defined as progression while on therapy or within 6 months in the adjuvant setting or 3 months in the metastatic setting. Taxane resistance is defined as progression while on therapy or within 12 months in the adjuvant setting or 4 months in the metastatic setting. ▪ As monotherapy for the treatment of metastatic or locally advanced breast cancer in patients whose tumors are resistant or refractory to anthracyclines, taxanes, and capecitabine.

CONTRAINDICATIONS

History of severe (CTCAE Grade 3 or 4) hypersensitivity reaction to agents containing Cremophor® EL or its derivatives. ▪ Neutrophil count less than 1,500 cells/mm^3 or platelet count less than 100,000 cells/mm^3. ▪ In combination with capecitabine in patients with AST or ALT greater than 2.5 times the ULN or bilirubin greater than 1 times the ULN.

PRECAUTIONS

Follow guidelines for handling cytotoxic agents. See Appendix A, p. 1331. ▪ Should be administered by or under the direction of the physician specialist in facilities equipped to monitor the patient and respond to any medical emergency. ▪ Ixabepilone in combination with capecitabine is contraindicated in patients with significant hepatic insufficiency due to increased risk of toxicity and neutropenia-related death; see Contraindications. ▪ Use caution in patients with hepatic insufficiency receiving monotherapy. Risk of toxicity is increased and data are limited; see Dose Adjustments. ▪ Premedication is required to minimize the chance of a hypersensitivity reaction; see Usual Dose. ▪ Peripheral neuropathy is a common side effect and was the most common cause of treatment discontinuation in clinical studies. It is cumulative and generally reversible. May require dose reduction or delay in therapy; see Dose Adjustments. Use caution in patients with diabetes mellitus or pre-existing peripheral neuropathy. Risk of severe neuropathy may be increased. ▪ Myelosuppression is dose dependent and primarily manifested as neutropenia. Hold therapy in patients with a neutrophil count less than 1,500 cells/mm^3; see Dose Adjustments and Contraindications. ▪ Use caution in patients with a history of cardiac disease. Adverse cardiac events (e.g., myocardial ischemia, ventricular dysfunction, and supraventricular arrhythmias) have been reported. ▪ Not studied in patients with renal impairment.

Monitor: Obtain baseline and periodic CBC with differential and platelet count. ▪ Obtain baseline and periodic bilirubin, AST, and ALT. ▪ Monitor for S/S of a hypersensitivity reaction (e.g., bronchospasm, dyspnea, flushing, rash). ▪ Monitor for S/S of peripheral neuropathy (primarily sensory [e.g., burning sensation, discomfort, hyperesthesia, hypoesthesia, neuropathic pain or paresthesia]). Most cases of new-onset or worsening neuropathy occurred during the first 3 cycles. ▪ Monitor for thrombocytopenia (platelet count less than 50,000/mm^3); see Dose Adjustments and Contraindications. Initiate precautions to prevent excessive bleeding (e.g., inspect IV sites, skin, and mucous membranes; use extreme care during invasive procedures; test urine, emesis, stool, and secretions for occult blood).

Patient Education: Promptly report any numbness or tingling of feet, S/S of infection (fever, chills cough), or S/S of a hypersensitivity reaction (chest tightness, dyspnea, flushing, pruritus, rash, urticaria). ▪ Avoid pregnancy. Use of nonhormonal birth control is required. ▪ Promptly report chest pain, difficulty breathing, palpitations, or unusual weight gain; these may be signs of adverse cardiac events.

Maternal/Child: Category D: avoid pregnancy; may cause fetal harm. ▪ Discontinue breast-feeding. ▪ Effectiveness for use in pediatric patients not established. Evaluation in two clinical studies suggests that pediatric patients have a safety profile consistent with that seen in adults.

Elderly: The incidence of Grade 3 and 4 adverse reactions was higher when used in combination with capecitabine in clinical studies. As monotherapy, no overall difference in safety was seen in the elderly compared with younger adults.

DRUG/LAB INTERACTIONS

Use of concomitant strong **CYP3A4 inhibitors** (e.g., amprenavir [Agenerase], atazanavir [Reyataz], clarithromycin [Biaxin], delavirdine [Rescriptor], indinavir [Crixivan], itraconazole [Sporanox], ketoconazole [Nizoral], nefazodone, nelfinavir [Viracept], ritonavir [Norvir], saquinavir [Invirase], telithromycin [Ketek], or voriconazole [VFEND]) may increase plasma concentrations of ixabepilone. Avoid concomitant use if possible. If required, decrease dose of ixabepilone to 20 mg/M^2 and monitor closely for acute toxicity. If strong inhibitor is discontinued, wait for at least 1 week before adjusting ixabepilone dose upward to indicated dose. ▪ **Grapefruit juice** may increase plasma concentrations of ixabepilone and should be avoided. ▪ **Rifampin** (Rifadin), a potent CYP3A4 inducer, decreases ixabepilone plasma concentrations. Other strong **CYP3A4 inducers** (e.g., carbamazepine [Tegretol], dexamethasone [Decadron], phenobarbital [Luminal], phenytoin [Dilantin], rifabutin [Mycobutin]) may also decrease ixabepilone plasma concentrations, decreasing effectiveness. Avoid use if possible; see Dose Adjustments. ▪ **St. John's wort** may decrease ixabepilone plasma concentrations, decreasing effectiveness. Avoid use. ▪ Ixabepilone does not inhibit CYP enzymes and is not expected to alter plasma concentrations of other drugs.

SIDE EFFECTS

The most common side effects in patients receiving monotherapy included alopecia, anemia, arthralgia, asthenia, diarrhea, fatigue, leukopenia, mucositis, musculoskeletal pain, myalgia, nausea, neutropenia, peripheral sensory neuropathy, stomatitis, thrombocytopenia, and vomiting. In combination therapy, the following additional side effects were commonly reported: abdominal pain, anorexia, constipation, nail disorder, and hand-foot syndrome (palmar-plantar erythrodysesthesia). Other less commonly reported side effects included chest pain, cough, dehydration, dizziness, dyspnea, edema, febrile neutropenia, fever, gastroesophageal reflux disease, headache, hot flush, hypersensitivity reactions (including anaphylaxis), increased lacrimation, infection, insomnia, pain, pruritus, rash, skin exfoliation, skin hyperpigmentation, taste disorder.

Overdose: Fatigue, GI symptoms (e.g., abdominal pain, anorexia, diarrhea, nausea, stomatitis), musculoskeletal pain/myalgia, and peripheral neuropathy.

Post-Marketing: Radiation recall has been reported.

ANTIDOTE

Keep physician informed of all side effects. Most minor side effects will be treated symptomatically. Monitor patient closely. Discontinuation should be considered in patients who develop cardiac ischemia or impaired cardiac function. Discontinue ixabepilone at the first sign of a severe hypersensitivity reaction. Treat hypersensitivity reactions as indicated; may require epinephrine, airway management, oxygen, IV fluids, antihistamines (e.g., diphenhydramine [Benadryl]), corticosteroids, (e.g., hydrocortisone sodium succinate [Solu-Cortef]), and pressor amines (e.g., dopamine). Patients who experience a hypersensitivity reaction may be able to continue therapy. Rate reduction and additional pretreatment with corticosteroids may be attempted in subsequent cycles; see Usual Dose.

KETOROLAC TROMETHAMINE BBW   NSAID
(kee-toh-**ROH**-lack tro-**METH**-ah-meen)

Toradol   pH 6.9 to 7.9

USUAL DOSE

Adults under 65 years: 30 mg. May repeat every 6 hours. Maximum dose is 120 mg/24 hr. Do not increase the dose or frequency for breakthrough pain. Consider alternating with low doses of opioids (e.g., morphine or meperidine). Ketorolac oral may be used only as continuation therapy to parenteral dosing. Maximum oral dose is 40 mg/24 hr. Do not administer for longer than 5 days (IV/IM alone or combined use with oral).

Adults over 65 years, patients with impaired renal function, and/or patients under 50 kg (110 lb): 15 mg. May repeat every 6 hours. Maximum dose is 60 mg in 24 hours. Note all restrictions for adults under 65 years outlined above.

PEDIATRIC DOSE

See Maternal/Child.

Pediatric patients 2 to 16 years of age: One dose of 0.5 mg/kg up to a maximum dose of 15 mg. 0.5 mg/kg IV every 6 hours has been administered in a limited number of patients (unlabeled).

Short-term postoperative pain management (unlabeled): 1 mg/kg alone or as an adjunct.

DOSE ADJUSTMENTS

Required for patients under 50 kg (110 lb), patients over 65 years of age, and patients with reduced renal function (moderately elevated SCr); see Usual Dose. Further dose reductions may be required with high-dose salicylates; see Drug/Lab Interactions.

DILUTION

Confirm IV use. Some 2-mL tubex syringes are for IM use only. May be given undiluted through Y-tube or three-way stopcock of infusion set. Administration through a free-flowing IV is preferred.

Storage: Store at CRT; protect from light.

COMPATIBILITY   (Underline Indicates Conflicting Compatibility Information)

Consider any drug NOT listed as compatible to be INCOMPATIBLE until consulting a pharmacist; specific conditions may apply.

May form a precipitate if admixed with drugs with a low pH (e.g., meperidine [Demerol], morphine, promethazine [Phenergan]).

One source suggests the following **compatibilities:**
Solution: D5W, NS, D5NS, LR, R.
Y-site: Acetaminophen (Ofirmev), cisatracurium (Nimbex), dexmedetomidine (Precedex), fentanyl, hetastarch in electrolytes (Hextend), hydromorphone (Dilaudid), methadone (Dolophine), morphine, remifentanil (Ultiva).

RATE OF ADMINISTRATION
A single dose over a minimum of 15 seconds; evenly distributed over 1 to 2 minutes is preferred.

ACTIONS
A nonsteroidal anti-inflammatory drug (NSAID) with peripheral analgesic, anti-inflammatory, and antipyretic actions. Inhibits prostaglandin synthesis. 30 to 60 mg produces analgesia similar to morphine 12 mg or Demerol 100 mg. Studies reflect less drowsiness, nausea, and vomiting. Not a narcotic agonist or antagonist. Cardiac and hemodynamic parameters are not altered. Onset of action is 30 to 60 minutes. Half-life varies from 3.8 to 8.6 hours based on age and clinical status. Relief in some patients may last 6 to 8 hours. Excreted primarily in urine. Secreted in breast milk.

INDICATIONS AND USES
Short-term management of moderately severe, acute pain (no longer than 5 days). ▪ NOT indicated for minor or chronic painful conditions.
Unlabeled uses: Postoperative short-term pain management in pediatric patients.

CONTRAINDICATIONS
Hypersensitivity to ketorolac, its components, or to acetylsalicylic acid (ASA) or other NSAIDs; labor and delivery; breast-feeding; preoperative or intraoperative medication when hemostasis is critical due to increased risk of bleeding; patients currently receiving ASA or NSAIDs (e.g., ibuprofen [Advil, Motrin], naproxen [Aleve, Naprosyn]); active peptic ulcer disease; recent GI bleeding or perforation; patients with a history of peptic ulcer disease or GI bleeding; suspected or confirmed cerebrovascular bleeding; hemorrhagic diathesis; incomplete hemostasis; high risk of bleeding; advanced renal impairment; or patients at risk for renal failure because of volume depletion. Do not use for epidural or intrathecal administration; contains alcohol. See Drug/Lab Interactions.

PRECAUTIONS
Use only recommended doses; increased doses will not be more effective and will increase the risk of serious adverse events. ▪ Hypersensitivity reactions, including anaphylaxis, have been reported. Administer in a facility with adequate diagnostic and treatment facilities to monitor the patient and respond to any medical emergency. ▪ Inhibits platelet aggregation and may prolong bleeding time. ▪ May cause serious GI ulceration and bleeding without warning. ▪ In addition to the usual caution in patients with reduced hepatic or renal function, ketorolac may also cause a dose-dependent reduction in renal prostaglandin formation. Can precipitate renal failure in patients with impaired renal function, heart failure, or liver dysfunction; in the elderly; or in patients receiving diuretics. ▪ Use caution in patients with cardiac decompensation, hypertension, or similar conditions; may cause fluid retention and edema. ▪ Use caution in patients with pre-existing asthma, especially aspirin-sensitive asthma. Severe bronchospasm has been reported.
Monitor: Correct hypovolemia before giving ketorolac and maintain adequate hydration. ▪ Observe patient frequently, especially for heartburn or signs and symptoms of GI upset or bleeding, and monitor vital signs. ▪ Monitor BUN, SCr, liver enzymes, occult blood loss, urinalysis, urine output, and signs of pain relief (e.g., increased appetite and activity). ▪ Observe closely during ambulation. ▪ Low doses of narcotics may be required to treat breakthrough pain.
Patient Education: Side effects have resulted in extended hospitalization and could be fatal. ▪ Discard any remaining oral ketorolac at end of 5-day total cumulative maximum time for use.
Maternal/Child: See Contraindications. ▪ Category C: safety for use not established. Use only if other alternatives are not available. ▪ Discontinue breast-feeding. ▪ Multiple dose treatment in pediatric patients has not been studied; limited data available.

Elderly: See Dose Adjustments and Precautions. ▪ More sensitive to side effects. ▪ Incidence of GI bleeding and acute renal failure increases with age.

DRUG/LAB INTERACTIONS

Probenecid inhibits clearance and may triple plasma levels of ketorolac. Concomitant use is contraindicated. ▪ Potentiated by **salicylates** (especially high-dose regimens). May double plasma levels of ketorolac. Reduce dose of ketorolac by half. ▪ May decrease clearance and increase toxicity of **methotrexate.** ▪ Additive if used with other **NSAIDs** (see Contraindications); side effects may increase markedly. ▪ May potentiate **lithium** levels. ▪ May increase risk of bleeding, especially from the GI tract, when given concomitantly with **anticoagulants** (e.g., warfarin [Coumadin], heparin) or **thrombolytic agents** (e.g., alteplase [tPA]). ▪ May increase risk of bleeding when given with **agents that may cause thrombocytopenia or inhibit or interfere with platelet aggregation** (e.g., clopidogrel [Plavix], valproic acid [Depacon]) and **serotonin reuptake inhibitors** (e.g., paroxetine [Paxil]). ▪ Can precipitate renal failure concomitantly with **diuretics** (e.g., furosemide [Lasix]); see Precautions. ▪ Can reduce response to **furosemide** (Lasix) **or other diuretics** in normovolemic healthy individuals. ▪ May increase risk of renal impairment with **ACE inhibitors** (e.g., enalapril [Vasotec]). ▪ Nephrotoxicity of both agents may be increased with **other nephrotoxic agents** (e.g., aminoglycosides [e.g., gentamicin], cyclosporine [Sandimmune]). ▪ May potentiate **nondepolarizing muscle relaxants** (e.g., atracurium [Tracrium]). ▪ Has caused seizures in a few patients taking **antiepileptics** (e.g., phenytoin [Dilantin], carbamazepine [Tegretol]). ▪ May cause hallucinations with **antipsychotics** (e.g., thiothixene [Navane]), **antidepressants** (e.g., fluoxetine [Prozac]). ▪ May cause **elevations of liver function tests** AST and ALT.

SIDE EFFECTS

Average dose: Diarrhea, dizziness, dyspepsia, drowsiness, edema, GI bleeding, GI pain, headache, injection site pain, nausea, and sweating are most common. Capable of all side effects of other NSAIDs, especially with extended use: abnormal taste, abnormal vision, asthenia, asthma, confusion, constipation, depression, dry mouth, dypsnea, euphoria, excessive thirst, flatulence, inability to concentrate, insomnia, liver function abnormalities, melena, myalgia, nervousness, oliguria, pallor, paresthesia, peptic ulcer, rectal bleeding, stimulation, stomatitis, pruritus, purpura, urinary frequency, urticaria, vasodilation, vertigo, vomiting.

Overdose: Abdominal pain, diarrhea, labored breathing, metabolic acidosis, pallor, peptic ulcer, rales, vomiting.

ANTIDOTE

With increasing severity of any side effect or onset of symptoms of overdose, discontinue the drug and notify the physician. A patent airway, artificial ventilation, oxygen therapy, and other symptomatic treatment must be instituted promptly if indicated. Treat anaphylaxis with epinephrine (Adrenalin), diphenhydramine (Benadryl), and corticosteroids as indicated. Not significantly cleared by dialysis.

LABETALOL HYDROCHLORIDE
(lah-**BET**-ah-lohl hy-droh-**KLOR**-eyed)

Alpha/beta-adrenergic
blocking agent
Antihypertensive

pH 3 to 4

USUAL DOSE
Dose must be individualized based on degree of hypertension and patient response.

20 mg as an initial dose by IV injection. May repeat with injections of 40 to 80 mg at 10-minute intervals until desired BP is achieved, or may be diluted and given as a continuous infusion. Usually effective with 50 to 200 mg. Do not exceed a total dose of 300 mg. Initiate oral labetalol after desired BP has been achieved and the supine diastolic pressure starts to rise. See literature for dose regimen. AHA recommends 10 mg IV over 1 to 2 minutes. May repeat or double dose every 10 minutes to a maximum dose of 150 mg. Or initial dose may be given by IV injection followed by an infusion of 2 to 8 mg/min. Titrate slowly to achieve desired results without exceeding maximum dose.

DOSE ADJUSTMENTS
See Precautions and Drug/Lab Interactions.

DILUTION
IV injection: May be given undiluted in a 5 mg/mL concentration.

Continuous infusion: May be diluted in most commonly used IV solutions (see chart on inside back cover). Addition of 200 mg (40 mL) to 160-mL solution yields 1 mg/mL, 300 mg (60 mL) to 240 mL yields 1 mg/mL, or 200 mg (40 mL) to 250 mL yields 2 mg/3 mL. Amount of solution may be decreased if required by fluid restrictions of the patient.

Storage: Store unopened vial between 2° and 30° C (36° and 86° F). Do not freeze. Protect from light. Stable after dilution for 24 hours at room temperature or refrigerated.

COMPATIBILITY
(Underline Indicates Conflicting Compatibility Information)

Consider any drug NOT listed as compatible to be INCOMPATIBLE until consulting a pharmacist; specific conditions may apply.

Manufacturer lists 5% sodium bicarbonate as **incompatible** and indicates to use care when administering alkaline drugs, including furosemide (Lasix).

One source suggests the following **compatibilities:**

Y-site: Amikacin, aminophylline, amiodarone (Nexterone), ampicillin, bivalirudin (Angiomax), butorphanol (Stadol), calcium gluconate, cefazolin (Ancef), ceftazidime (Fortaz), chloramphenicol (Chloromycetin), clindamycin (Cleocin), dexmedetomidine (Precedex), diltiazem (Cardizem), dobutamine, dopamine, doripenem (Doribax), enalaprilat (Vasotec IV), epinephrine (Adrenalin), erythromycin (Erythrocin), esmolol (Brevibloc), famotidine (Pepcid IV), fenoldopam (Corlopam), fentanyl, gentamicin, heparin, hetastarch in electrolytes (Hextend), hydromorphone (Dilaudid), 6% hydroxyethyl starch (Voluven), lidocaine, linezolid (Zyvox), lorazepam (Ativan), magnesium sulfate, meperidine (Demerol), metronidazole (Flagyl IV), midazolam (Versed), milrinone (Primacor), morphine, nicardipine (Cardene IV), nitroglycerin IV, nitroprusside sodium, norepinephrine (Levophed), oxacillin (Bactocill), penicillin G potassium, potassium chloride (KCl), potassium phosphates, propofol (Diprivan), ranitidine (Zantac), sodium acetate, sulfamethoxazole/trimethoprim, telavancin (Vibativ), tobramycin, vancomycin, vecuronium.

RATE OF ADMINISTRATION
IV injection: Each 20 mg or fraction thereof over at least 2 minutes.

Continuous infusion: Begin at 2 mg/min. Adjust according to orders of physician and BP response. Another source suggests 0.5 to 2 mg/min. Use of a microdrip (60 gtt/mL) or an infusion pump may be helpful.

ACTIONS

An adrenergic receptor blocking agent with both selective alpha-1-adrenergic and nonselective beta-adrenergic receptor blocking activity. Causes dose-related falls in BP without reflex tachycardia or significant reduction in HR. Maximum effect of each dose is reached in 5 minutes. Half-life is 5.5 hours, but some effects last up to 16 hours. Metabolized and excreted as metabolites in urine and through bile to feces. Crosses the placental barrier. Present in small amounts in breast milk.

INDICATIONS AND USES

Control of BP in severe hypertension.

Unlabeled uses: Treatment of clonidine withdrawal hypertension. ▪ Decrease BP and relieve symptoms in patients with pheochromocytoma.

CONTRAINDICATIONS

Obstructive airway disease including asthma, cardiogenic shock, greater than first-degree heart block, overt cardiac failure, severe bradycardia, other conditions associated with severe and prolonged hypotension, and hypersensitivity to labetalol or its components.

PRECAUTIONS

Use caution in impaired liver function. ▪ Hepatic injury has been reported. Has occurred after both short-term and long-term treatment. Usually reversible, but hepatic necrosis and death have been reported. ▪ Use extreme caution in patients with any degree of cardiac failure; may further depress myocardial contractility. Does not alter effectiveness of digoxin on heart muscle. ▪ Effective in lowering BP in pheochromocytoma but has caused a paradoxical hypertensive response in some patients. ▪ Use with extreme caution in diabetics or patients with a history of hypoglycemia. May mask the symptoms of hypoglycemia and reduce the release of insulin in response to hyperglycemia. ▪ Routine withdrawal of chronic beta-blocker therapy before surgery is not recommended. However, the effect of the alpha-adrenergic activity of labetalol has not been evaluated in the surgical setting. Deaths have occurred when labetalol has been used during surgery. ▪ Intraoperative floppy iris syndrome has been observed during cataract surgery in some patients treated with alpha-1 blockers. Characterized by a combination of a flaccid iris, progressive miosis despite preoperative dilation with standard mydriatic drugs, and potential prolapse of the iris. Modification of the surgical technique may be required. ▪ See Drug/Lab Interactions.

Monitor: Keep patient supine. Postural hypotension can occur for up to 3 hours after administration. Ambulate with care and assistance. ▪ Monitor BP before and 5 and 10 minutes after each direct IV injection. Monitor at least every 5 minutes during infusion. Avoid rapid or excessive falls in either systolic or diastolic BP. When severely elevated BP drops too rapidly, catastrophic reactions can occur (e.g., cerebral infarction, optic nerve infarction, angina, ischemic ECG changes). ▪ Monitor for S/S of CHF. ▪ Although rebound angina, myocardial infarction, or ventricular arrhythmias have not been a problem with labetalol, it is recommended that the dose of beta-adrenergic blockers be reduced gradually to avoid these conditions. ▪ See Drug/Lab Interactions.

Patient Education: Report cough, dizziness, irregular pulse, or shortness of breath promptly. ▪ May cause dizziness or fainting; request assistance with ambulation.

Maternal/Child: Category C: use in pregnancy only when clearly indicated and benefit outweighs risk. Hypotension, bradycardia, hypoglycemia, and respiratory depression have been reported in infants of mothers who were treated with labetalol for hypertension during pregnancy. Has been used during labor and delivery. ▪ Use caution during breastfeeding. ▪ Safety and effectiveness for use in pediatric patients not established.

Elderly: Use with caution in age-related peripheral vascular disease; risk of hypothermia increased. ▪ May exacerbate mental impairment.

DRUG/LAB INTERACTIONS

Amiodarone (Nexterone) may enhance the bradycardic effect of beta-blockers. ▪ Inhibits **beta-agonist bronchodilators** (e.g., albuterol [Ventolin]); increased doses may be required, especially in asthmatics. ▪ Synergistic with **halothane anesthesia.** High concentrations of halothane (3% or above) should not be used. The degree of hypotension will be increased, and the possibility of a large reduction in cardiac output and an increase in central venous pressure exists. Notify anesthesiologist that patient is receiving labetalol. ▪ Potentiated by **cimetidine** (Tagamet). May blunt the reflex tachycardia produced by **nitroglycerin.** May cause further hypotension with **nitroglycerin.** ▪ The use of labetalol with **calcium channel blockers** (e.g., diltiazem [Cardizem], verapamil) may potentiate both drugs and result in severe depression of myocardium, AV conduction, and severe hypotension. ▪ May mask the hypoglycemic effects of **insulin and other antidiabetic agents.** May inhibit the mobilization of glucose from hepatic stores. Monitor glucose carefully in diabetic patients. ▪ Patients receiving beta-blockers who have a history of severe anaphylactic reaction to a variety of allergens may be unresponsive to the usual doses of **epinephrine** used to treat an allergic reaction. ▪ May interfere with lab tests in the **diagnosis of pheochromocytoma.** ▪ May cause a **false-positive urine test** for amphetamine use.

SIDE EFFECTS
Diaphoresis, dizziness, flushing, moderate hypotension, numbness, severe postural hypotension, nausea, somnolence, tingling of scalp, and ventricular dysrhythmias (e.g., intensified atrioventricular block) occur most frequently.

ANTIDOTE
Notify the physician of all side effects. Decrease rate or discontinue drug if hypotension occurs. Notify physician immediately. Trendelenburg position may be appropriate. May require treatment with IV fluids or vasopressors (e.g., norepinephrine [levarterenol], dopamine). Use atropine or epinephrine for severe bradycardia; digoxin, diuretics, dopamine, or dobutamine for cardiac failure; norepinephrine (Levophed) for hypotension; epinephrine (Adrenalin) and/or albuterol for bronchospasm; and diazepam (Valium) for seizures. Unresponsive hypotension and bradycardia may be reversed by glucagon 5 to 10 mg over 30 seconds followed by a continuous infusion of 5 mg/hr. Reduce rate as condition improves. Treat other side effects symptomatically and resuscitate as necessary. Hemodialysis is not effective.

J–L

LACOSAMIDE
(la-**KOE**-sa-mide)

Anticonvulsant

Vimpat

pH 3.5 to 5

USUAL DOSE

Serum levels similar by oral or IV route; no dose or frequency adjustment is necessary. Transfer to oral therapy as soon as practical. Twice-daily IV infusions have been used for up to 5 days.

Monotherapy: Begin with an initial dose of 100 mg twice daily (200 mg/day); dose should be increased by 50 mg twice daily (100 mg/day) every week up to a recommended maintenance dose of 150 to 200 mg twice daily (300 to 400 mg/day). Alternatively, lacosamide may be initiated with a single loading dose of 200 mg* followed approximately 12 hours later by 100 mg twice daily (200 mg/day); this dose regimen should be continued for 1 week. Based on individual response and tolerability, the dose can be increased at weekly intervals by 50 mg twice daily (100 mg/day) until the recommended maintenance dose of 150 to 200 mg twice daily (300 to 400 mg/day) is achieved. For patients who are already on a single antiepileptic and are converting to lacosamide monotherapy, the therapeutic dose of 150 to 200 mg twice daily should be maintained for at least 3 days before initiating withdrawal of the concomitant antiepileptic drug. A gradual withdrawal of the concomitant antiepileptic drug over at least 6 weeks is recommended.

Adjuvant therapy: Begin with an initial dose of 50 mg twice daily (100 mg/day). Based on individual patient response and tolerability, the dose may be increased at weekly intervals by 50 mg twice daily (100 mg/day). The recommended maintenance dose is 100 to 200 mg twice daily (200 to 400 mg/day). Alternatively, lacosamide may be initiated with a single loading dose of 200 mg* followed approximately 12 hours later by 100 mg twice daily (200 mg/day); this dose regimen should be continued for 1 week. Based on individual response and tolerability, the dose can be increased at weekly intervals by 50 mg twice daily (100 mg/day) as needed until the maximum recommended maintenance dose of 200 mg twice daily (400 mg/day) is achieved.

*Monotherapy and adjuvant therapy: The loading dose should be administered with medical supervision because of the increased incidence of CNS adverse reactions. There is no evidence that doses greater than 400 mg/day offer additional benefit, and they have been associated with a higher incidence of side effects.

Transfer from an IV dose to an oral dose: Transfer at the equivalent daily dose and frequency of the IV dose.

DOSE ADJUSTMENTS

Titrate dose with caution in patients with renal or hepatic impairment and in the elderly.
■ No dose adjustment is indicated for patients with mild to moderate renal impairment.
■ 300 mg is the maximum recommended dose for patients with severe renal impairment (a CrCl equal to or less than 30 mL/min) and for patients with end-stage renal disease. A supplemental dose of up to 50% should be considered after a 4-hour hemodialysis treatment. ■ A maximum dose of 300 mg/day is recommended for patients with mild or moderate hepatic impairment. ■ Not recommended for patients with severe hepatic impairment. ■ Patients with renal or hepatic impairment who are taking strong inhibitors of CYP3A4 and CYP2C9 may have a significant increase in exposure of lacosamide. Consult with pharmacist. Dose reduction may be required. ■ Dose adjustment not required based on gender or race or in the elderly; see Elderly.

DILUTION

Available as a 200 mg/20 mL (10 mg/mL) solution for injection.
May be given undiluted or may be further diluted with NS, D5W, or LR. See Rate of Administration.

Filters: Specific information not available.

Storage: Store unopened vials at CRT. Do not freeze. Diluted solutions should not be stored for more than 4 hours at RT. Discard unused portions of vial.

COMPATIBILITY

Solutions: Compatible with NS, D5W, and LR. Additional information not available.

RATE OF ADMINISTRATION

A single dose as an infusion over 30 to 60 minutes is preferred. When medically necessary, may be infused over 15 minutes. Incidence of CNS side effects (e.g., dizziness, paresthesia, and somnolence) may be higher with the 15-minute infusion.

ACTIONS

An antiepileptic (anticonvulsant) drug. The precise mechanism of action is unknown. In vitro studies have shown that it selectively enhances the slow inactivation of voltage-gated sodium channels, resulting in stabilization of hyperexcitable neuronal membranes and inhibition of repetitive neuronal firing. Some effects are reached at the end of infusion. Steady-state plasma concentrations are achieved after 3 days of administration. Doses above 400 mg/day do not appear to have additional benefit. Less than 15% bound to plasma proteins. Partially metabolized. Half-life is approximately 13 hours. Excreted as metabolites and as unchanged drug in urine.

INDICATIONS AND USES

Monotherapy or adjunctive therapy in the treatment of partial-onset seizures in adult patients (17 years of age and older) with epilepsy. IV injection is used as a temporary alternative to oral therapy. May be used alone or in combination with other antiepileptic drugs (AEDs).

CONTRAINDICATIONS

Manufacturer indicates none; see Precautions.

PRECAUTIONS

For IV use only. ▪ Antiepileptic drugs (AEDs) increase the risk of suicidal thoughts or behavior in patients taking these drugs for any indication. Patients treated with any AED for any indication should be monitored for the emergence or worsening of depression, suicidal thoughts or behavior, and/or any unusual changes in mood or behavior. In an analysis of AED clinical trials, symptoms occurred as early as 1 week after starting AEDs and persisted for the duration of treatment. May require a dose reduction or discontinuation of lacosamide. Many illnesses for which AEDs are prescribed, including epilepsy, are associated with morbidity and mortality and an increased risk of suicidal thoughts and behavior. Consider that these symptoms may also be related to the illness being treated. ▪ May cause dizziness and ataxia. Dizziness was the adverse event most frequently leading to discontinuation of therapy. Onset of symptoms commonly observed during titration. ▪ Dose-dependent prolongations in PR intervals have been observed. First- and second-degree AV heart block, complete AV heart block, and bradycardia have been reported. Use caution in patients with known conduction problems (e.g., marked first-degree AV block, second-degree or higher AV block, and sick sinus syndrome without a pacemaker), sodium channelopathies (e.g., Brugada syndrome), or severe cardiac disease such as myocardial ischemia or heart failure. ▪ May cause atrial arrhythmias (atrial fibrillation or atrial flutter), especially in patients with diabetic neuropathy or cardiovascular disease. ▪ Syncope or loss of consciousness was reported. Often associated with changes in orthostatic hypotension, atrial flutter/fibrillation (and associated tachycardia), or bradycardia. Most commonly seen in patients with a history of risk factors for cardiac disease, in patients receiving medications that slow AV conduction, and in patients with diabetic neuropathy. Most cases were associated with doses above the recommended 400 mg/day. ▪ A delayed multiorgan hypersensitivity reaction (also known as Drug Reaction with Eosinophilia and Systemic Symptoms, or DRESS) occurred in one patient and manifested as symptomatic hepatitis and nephritis, which resolved over time. DRESS has been reported with other AEDs and typically presents with a fever and rash associated with other organ involvement, such as eosinophilia, hepatitis, nephritis, lymphadenopathy, and/or myocarditis. ▪ Not recommended for patients with severe hepatic impairment. ▪ To minimize the potential for increased seizure frequency, withdraw AEDs (including lacosamide) gradually (over a minimum of 1 week). ▪ Physical dependence has not been demonstrated; however, psychological dependence cannot be excluded because of the ability of lacosamide to produce a euphoria-type response.

Monitor: Baseline CBC, CrCl, bilirubin, and liver function tests indicated; monitor as needed. ▪ Monitor vital signs. ▪ Monitor for seizure activity. ▪ Monitor for the emergence or worsening of depression, suicidal thoughts or behavior, and/or any unusual changes in mood or behavior. ▪ Observe patient closely for signs of CNS side effects, prolonged PR interval, and/or symptoms of DRESS; see Precautions. ▪ Obtain a baseline ECG in patients with known conduction problems and/or severe cardiac disease. Repeat ECG after lacosamide is titrated to steady-state concentrations.

Patient Education: Read patient information guide provided by manufacturer. ▪ May cause dizziness, fainting, and somnolence; use caution performing tasks that require alertness (e.g., operating machinery, driving). ▪ Inform your health care professional if you are pregnant or breast-feeding. ▪ May increase the risk of suicidal thoughts and behavior. Promptly report emergence or worsening of S/S of depression, any unusual changes in mood or behavior, or thoughts about self-harm. ▪ Has caused atrial arrhythmias. Promptly report palpitations, rapid pulse, and/or shortness of breath. ▪ May cause various degrees of heart block. Report slow or irregular pulse, light-headedness, or fainting. ▪ Promptly report S/S of hypersensitivity (e.g., fever, rash) or liver toxicity (e.g., fatigue, jaundice, dark urine). ▪ Women who are pregnant or who become pregnant should be encouraged to enroll in the North American Antiepileptic Drug (NAAED) Pregnancy Registry. ▪ Review prescription and nonprescription drugs with your physician.

Maternal/Child: Category C: animal studies demonstrated developmental toxicity (increased embryofetal and perinatal mortality, growth deficit). Use during pregnancy only if the potential benefit justifies the potential risk to the fetus. Manufacturer has established a pregnancy registry to evaluate safety and outcomes; see manufacturer's literature and Patient Education. ▪ Effects during labor and delivery unknown. ▪ Discontinue breast-feeding. ▪ Safety and effectiveness for use in pediatric patients under 17 years of age not established.

Elderly: Higher plasma concentrations seen in the elderly may be due to differences in total body water and age-associated impaired renal function. Although dose adjustment based on age is not necessary, dose titration should be performed with caution; see Usual Dose.

DRUG/LAB INTERACTIONS

Use with caution in patients taking concomitant **medications that prolong the PR interval** (e.g., beta-blockers [e.g., metoprolol (Lopressor), propranolol] and calcium channel blockers [e.g., diltiazem (Cardizem), verapamil]). Increased risk of AV block or bradycardia. Baseline ECG and repeat ECG following titration to steady state recommended. ▪ No evidence of any relevant drug/drug interaction with **other antiepileptic drugs** (AEDs) such as carbamazepine (Tegretol), clonazepam (Klonopin), gabapentin (Neurontin), lamotrigine (Lamictal), levetiracetam (Keppra), oxcarbazepine (Trileptal), phenobarbital (Luminal), phenytoin (Dilantin), topiramate (Topamax), valproic acid (e.g., Depacon, Depakote), and zonisamide (Zonegran). ▪ Concurrent administration with **carbamazepine, phenobarbital, or phenytoin** has resulted in small reductions in lacosamide plasma concentrations. ▪ Minimal protein binding; unlikely to have interactions with drugs competing for protein-binding sites. ▪ Has been administered with **oral contraceptives** (containing ethinyl estradiol and levonorgestrel), **digoxin** (Lanoxin), **metformin** (Glucophage), **midazolam** (Versed), **omeprazole** (Prilosec), and **warfarin** (Coumadin) with no interference on the pharmacokinetics of either drug. ▪ Does not induce or inhibit the enzyme activity of many drugs metabolized by selected cytochrome P_{450} isoforms. In vitro studies suggest lacosamide has the potential to inhibit CYP2C19 at therapeutic concentrations; see prescribing information. ▪ Patients with renal or hepatic impairment who are taking **strong inhibitors of CYP3A4** (e.g., ritonavir [Norvir], clarithromycin

[Biaxin], ketoconazole [Nizoral]) **and CYP2C9** (e.g., fluconazole [Diflucan]) may have a significant increase in exposure of lacosamide. Dose reduction may be necessary.

SIDE EFFECTS

The most common side effects are diplopia, dizziness, headache, and nausea. Ataxia, blurred vision, diplopia, dizziness, nausea, vertigo, and vomiting led to discontinuation of lacosamide. Incidence of side effects increased with doses above 400 mg/day. Most side effects at recommended doses were considered mild or moderate and included anemia; asthenia; balance disorder; cerebellar syndrome; confusion; constipation; depression; diarrhea; dry mouth; dyspepsia; elevated liver function tests (e.g., ALT, AST); falls; fatigue; feeling drunk; fever; gait disturbance; hypoanesthesia; injection site pain, discomfort, irritation, or erythema; muscle spasms; nystagmus; oral hypoanesthesia; palpitations; paresthesia; pruritus; skin laceration; somnolence; tinnitus; and tremor. Psychiatric disorders, including aggression, agitation, anger, anxiety, apathy, depersonalization, depression, emotional lability, hallucinations, hostility, irritability, and suicidal tendencies, have been reported. May produce euphoria-type reactions. Other serious adverse reactions include ataxia and dizziness, cardiac rhythm and conduction abnormalities, multiorgan hypersensitivity reactions, and syncope.

Post-Marketing: Aggression, agitation, agranulocytosis, angioedema, hallucinations, insomnia, psychotic disorder, rash, Stevens-Johnson syndrome, toxic epidermal necrolysis, urticaria.

ANTIDOTE

Keep physician informed of all side effects. Some may not require intervention, and others may improve with a reduced dose or discontinuation of lacosamide; see Precautions and Side Effects. Discontinue lacosamide for symptoms of DRESS; use of an alternate treatment is recommended. Support patient as required in treatment of overdose. No specific antidote in overdose; however, hemodialysis will remove approximately 50% of a dose in 4 hours.

J-L

LEUCOVORIN CALCIUM
(loo-koh-**VOR**-in **KAL**-see-um)

Antidote
Antineoplastic adjunct

**Citrovorum Factor, Folinic Acid,
Leucovorin Calcium PF**

pH 6 to 8.1

USUAL DOSE

May be given IV/IM or PO. If GI toxicity is present, should be administered parenterally. **Delayed excretion or overdose of methotrexate (MTX):** 10 mg/M^2 every 6 hours until the serum MTX level is less than 0.05 micromolar. Milligram for milligram or greater than the dose of MTX is common. Administer within the first hour (or as soon as possible) in overdose or within 24 hours of MTX dose if there is delayed excretion. At least every 24 hours, obtain a SCr and MTX level. If SCr is more than 50% above pretreatment level, increase the leucovorin dose to 100 mg/M^2 every 3 hours until the serum MTX level is less than 0.05 micromolar.

Leucovorin rescue after high-dose MTX therapy: With high-dose methotrexate (12 to 15 Gm/M^2 as an infusion over 4 hours), begin leucovorin 15 mg (approximately 10 mg/M^2) 24 hours after MTX infusion started. Repeat every 6 hours for 10 doses. If MTX elimination is delayed, extend every-6-hour dosing until MTX level is less than 0.05 micromolar. If there is evidence of acute renal injury, increase leucovorin to 150 mg every 3 hours until MTX level is less than 1 micromolar, then 15 mg every 3 hours until MTX level is less than 0.05 micromolar. In both situations obtain SCr and MTX level at least every 24 hours. Other protocols are in use. Amount of leucovorin is dependent on MTX dose, MTX serum levels, and SCr.

Megaloblastic anemia: Up to 1 mg daily.

Advanced colorectal cancer: 200 mg/M^2 followed by fluorouracil (5-FU) 370 mg/M^2 or leucovorin 20 mg/M^2 followed by 5-FU 425 mg/M^2 daily for 5 days. Repeat at 4-week intervals twice, then repeat every 28 to 35 days based on complete recovery from toxic effects. Reduce 5-FU dose based on tolerance to previous course, 20% for moderate hematologic or GI toxicity, 30% for severe. Leucovorin doses remain the same. Increase 5-FU dose 10% if no toxicity. Other protocols are in use. Also approved for use with irinotecan and 5-FU.

Pemetrexed toxicity (unlabeled): A single dose of 100 mg/M^2. Follow with 50 mg/M^2 every 6 hours for 8 days.

DOSE ADJUSTMENTS

See adjustments in Usual Dose; larger reductions may be required in the elderly based on the potential for decreased renal function, especially in combination with fluorouracil. ▪ See Precautions/Monitor.

DILUTION

Each 50-mg, 100-mg, or 350-mg vial should be diluted to a 10 mg/mL to 20 mg/mL solution. For total doses less than 10 mg/M^2, dilute with bacteriostatic water for injection (contains benzyl alcohol as a preservative). Use SWFI without a preservative for any dose 10 mg/M^2 or greater. May be further diluted in 100 to 500 mL of D5W, D10W, NS, R, or LR. 1-mL (3-mg) ampules may be given undiluted (contain benzyl alcohol).

Storage: If prepared without a preservative, use immediately; stable up to 7 days with a preservative.

COMPATIBILITY

(Underline Indicates Conflicting Compatibility Information)

Consider any drug NOT listed as compatible to be INCOMPATIBLE until consulting a pharmacist; specific conditions may apply.

Several sources, including the manufacturer, cite **incompatibility** with fluorouracil (5-FU) as an additive; may form a precipitate.

One source suggests the following **compatibilities:**

Additive: Cisplatin.

Y-site: Amifostine (Ethyol), anidulafungin (Eraxis), aztreonam (Azactam), bleomycin (Blenoxane), cisplatin, cladribine (Leustatin), cyclophosphamide (Cytoxan), docetaxel (Taxotere), doxorubicin (Adriamycin), doxorubicin liposomal (Doxil), etoposide phosphate (Etopophos), filgrastim (Neupogen), fluconazole (Diflucan), fluorouracil (5-FU), furosemide (Lasix), gemcitabine (Gemzar), granisetron (Kytril), heparin, linezolid (Zyvox), methotrexate, metoclopramide (Reglan), mitomycin (Mutamycin), oxaliplatin (Eloxatin), pemetrexed (Alimta), piperacillin/tazobactam (Zosyn), tacrolimus (Prograf), teniposide (Vumon), thiotepa, vinblastine, vincristine.

RATE OF ADMINISTRATION

Because of calcium content, do not exceed a rate of 160 mg/min (16 mL of a 10-mg/mL or 8 mL of a 20-mg/mL solution). May be given more slowly. Large doses may be infused equally distributed over 1 to 6 hours. Never exceed above limits.

ACTIONS

Potent agent for neutralizing immediate toxic effects of methotrexate (and other folic acid antagonists) on the hematopoietic system. Preferentially rescues normal cells without reversing the oncolytic effect of methotrexate. Also enhances the therapeutic and toxic effects of fluoropyrimidines (e.g., fluorouracil [5-FU]).

INDICATIONS AND USES

Treatment of accidental folic acid antagonist (e.g., methotrexate) overdose or delayed excretion of MTX. ▪ Folinic acid rescue to prevent or decrease the toxicity of massive MTX doses used to treat resistant neoplasms. ▪ Treatment of megaloblastic anemia due to folic acid deficiency when oral therapy not appropriate. ▪ In combination with fluorouracil or fluorouracil and irinotecan (Camptosar) to treat colorectal cancer.

Unlabeled uses: Adjunct in the treatment of Ewing's sarcoma, head and neck cancer, non-Hodgkin's lymphomas, and trophoblastic tumors. ▪ Treatment of pemetrexed toxicity.

CONTRAINDICATIONS

Pernicious anemia and other megaloblastic anemias secondary to lack of vitamin B_{12}. None when used as indicated for other specific uses.

PRECAUTIONS

Usually administered in the hospital by or under the direction of the physician specialist. ▪ Permits use of massive doses of methotrexate. ▪ Do not discontinue leucovorin calcium until methotrexate serum levels fall below toxic levels. ▪ Much less effective in accidental overdose after a 1-hour delay. ▪ Delayed MTX excretion may occur from third-space fluid accumulation (ascites, pleural effusion), renal insufficiency, or inadequate hydration. ▪ All doses over 25 mg should be given IM or IV (no more than 25 mg can be absorbed orally). ▪ IM or IV dosing required in presence of GI toxicity, nausea, or vomiting. ▪ Benzyl alcohol associated with gasping syndrome in premature infants.

Monitor: Monitor serum blood levels of MTX and SCr levels at least daily until level is less than 0.05 micromolar. Death can occur in 5 to 10 days if MTX remains at toxic levels longer than 48 hours. ▪ Minimum fluid intake of 3 L/24 hr and alkalinization of urine to a pH of 7 or more with oral sodium bicarbonate recommended. Begin 12 hours before MTX dose and continue for 48 hours after final dose in each sequence. Does not reduce nephrotoxicity of MTX from drug or metabolite precipitation in the kidney. ▪ See methotrexate or fluorouracil monograph.

Maternal/Child: Category C: safety for use in pregnancy and breast-feeding not established. Benefits must outweigh risks. ▪ Contains benzyl alcohol; do not use in neonates or dilute with SWFI if indicated; see Dilution.

Elderly: Response similar to that seen in younger patients; however, use caution; may have greater sensitivity to its toxic effects (e.g., greater risk for GI toxicity and severe diarrhea in combination with fluorouracil). Monitoring of renal function suggested. ▪ See Dose Adjustments.

DRUG/LAB INTERACTIONS

May inhibit **phenytoins** (e.g., Dilantin), **phenobarbital, and primidone;** may cause increased frequency of seizures. ▪ Is used in combination with **fluorouracil;** use caution; leucovorin calcium may increase toxic as well as therapeutic effects of fluorouracil. ▪ When given with **MTX,** avoid any drug that may interfere with MTX elimination or binding to serum albumin (e.g., **NSAIDs** [e.g., ibuprofen (Advil, Motrin), indomethacin, ketoprofen, naproxen (Aleve, Naprosyn)], **probenecid, procarbazine** [Matulane], **salicylates, sulfon-amides**). Consider as a possible cause of toxicity. ▪ High doses of leucovorin may reduce the effectiveness of intrathecally administered **methotrexate.** ▪ Leucovorin may enhance the toxic effects of **capecitabine** (Xeloda); monitor closely. ▪ Concurrent use with **sulfa-methoxazole and trimethoprim** may cause treatment failure and increased morbidity in HIV patients being treated for *Pneumocystis jiroveci* pneumonia.

SIDE EFFECTS

Allergic reactions including anaphylaxis have occurred rarely. Methotrexate or fluorouracil may cause many serious and dose-limiting side effects; see individual monographs.

ANTIDOTE

Keep physician informed of patient's condition. Symptomatic treatment indicated.

LEVETIRACETAM INJECTION

Anticonvulsant

(lee-ve-tye-**RA**-se-tam in-**JEK**-shun)

Keppra

pH 5.5

USUAL DOSE

Serum levels similar by oral or IV route; no dose or frequency adjustment is necessary. Transfer to oral therapy as soon as practical.

Transfer to an IV dose from an oral dose: Administer IV levetiracetam at the same dose and frequency as the oral formulation.

All indications: Initiate treatment with a daily dose of 1,000 mg/day, given as twice-daily dosing (500 mg twice daily). Monitor for 2 weeks. Dose may be increased by 1,000 mg/day (500 mg twice daily) every 2 weeks to a maximum recommended daily dose of 3,000 mg (1,500 mg twice daily).

Partial-onset seizures in adults 16 years of age and older: There is no evidence that doses *greater* than 3,000 mg/day offer additional benefit.

Myoclonic seizures in adults and adolescents 12 years of age and older with juvenile myoclonic epilepsy and primary generalized tonic-clonic seizures in adults 16 years of age and older: The effectiveness of doses *lower* than 3,000 mg/day has not been adequately studied.

PEDIATRIC DOSE

Partial-onset seizures: *1 month to under 6 months:* Initiate treatment with a daily dose of 14 mg/kg in 2 divided doses (7 mg/kg twice daily). Increase the daily dose every 2 weeks in increments of 14 mg/kg to the recommended daily dose of 42 mg/kg (21 mg/kg twice daily). In the clinical trial, the mean daily dose was 35 mg/kg in this age-group. Effectiveness of lower doses has not been studied.

6 months to under 4 years: Initiate treatment with a daily dose of 20 mg/kg in 2 divided doses (10 mg/kg twice daily). Increase the daily dose every 2 weeks in increments of 20 mg/kg to the recommended daily dose of 50 mg/kg (25 mg/kg twice daily). If the patient cannot tolerate a daily dose of 50 mg/kg, the daily dose may be reduced. In the clinical trial, the mean daily dose was 47 mg/kg in this age-group.

4 years to under 16 years: Initiate treatment with a daily dose of 20 mg/kg in 2 divided doses (10 mg/kg twice daily). Increase the daily dose every 2 weeks in increments of 20 mg/kg to the recommended daily dose of 60 mg/kg (30 mg/kg twice daily). If the patient cannot tolerate a daily dose of 60 mg/kg, the daily dose may be reduced. In the clinical trial, the mean daily dose was 44 mg/kg in this age-group. The maximum daily dose was 3,000 mg.

Myoclonic seizures in adolescents 12 years of age and older with juvenile myoclonic epilepsy: See Usual Dose.

Primary generalized tonic-clonic seizures: *6 years to under 16 years of age:* Initiate treatment with a daily dose of 20 mg/kg in 2 divided doses (10 mg/kg twice daily). Increase the daily dose every 2 weeks in increments of 20 mg/kg (10 mg/kg twice daily) to the recommended daily dose of 60 mg/kg (30 mg/kg twice daily). The effectiveness of doses lower than 60 mg/kg/day has not been adequately studied. Maximum daily dose is 3,000 mg.

DOSE ADJUSTMENTS

No dose adjustment is required for gender, race, or impaired hepatic function. ▪ Dose adjustment may be required in the elderly based on impaired renal function. ▪ Dose adjustment for adults with impaired renal function is calculated based on CrCl adjusted for body surface area and is adjusted according to the following chart.

Levetiracetam Dose Adjustment in Adults with Impaired Renal Function		
Creatinine Clearance (mL/min/1.73 M^2)	Dose in mg	Frequency
>80 mL/min/1.73 M^2	500 to 1,500 mg	Every 12 hours
50 to 80 mL/min/1.73 M^2	500 to 1,000 mg	Every 12 hours
30 to 49 mL/min/1.73 M^2	250 to 750 mg	Every 12 hours
<30 mL/min/1.73 M^2	250 to 500 mg	Every 12 hours
ESRD patients on dialysis	500 to 1,000 mg	Every 24 hours*

*Administration of a 250- to 500-mg supplemental dose following dialysis is recommended.

▪ Information is unavailable for dosage adjustments in pediatric patients with renal impairment.

DILUTION

Adults: Each vial contains 500 mg/5 mL (100 mg/mL). A single dose (500, 1,000, or 1,500 mg [1, 2, or 3 vials]) must be diluted in 100 mL of NS, LR, or D5W for infusion. Doses of 500, 1,000, or 1,500 mg are available prediluted in 100 mL of NS.

Pediatric patients: A smaller volume of infusion solution may be required due to limitations around the total daily fluid intake of the patient. The amount of diluent should be calculated such that the final concentration of the levetiracetam solution does not exceed 15 mg/mL. For example, a 1-year-old 10-kg child beginning therapy for treatment of partial-onset seizures would initiate therapy at 20 mg/kg/day = 200 mg/day = 100 mg twice daily. 100 mg (1 mL) mixed in 24 mL of **compatible** solution will provide a final concentration of 4 mg/mL. In a fluid-restricted patient, the solution volume could be decreased to as low as 5.7 mL [100 mg ÷ (1 mL from drug + 5.7 mL of solution) = 14.9 mg/mL].

Filters: Specific information not available.

Storage: Store at CRT. Diluted solution stable for at least 24 hours at CRT stored in polyvinyl chloride (PVC) bags. Discard any unused portion of vial.

COMPATIBILITY

Consider any drug NOT listed as compatible to be INCOMPATIBLE until consulting a pharmacist; specific conditions may apply.

Manufacturer lists solutions NS, LR, and D5W and other antiepileptic drugs lorazepam (Ativan), diazepam (Valium), and valproate sodium (Depacon) as **compatible** for at least 24 hours stored in polyvinyl chloride (PVC) bags at CRT.

RATE OF ADMINISTRATION

A single dose properly diluted as an infusion over 15 minutes.

ACTIONS

An antiepileptic (anticonvulsant) drug. The precise mechanism of action is unknown. In animal studies it inhibited burst firing without affecting normal neuronal excitability, which suggests that it may selectively prevent hypersynchronization of epileptiform burst firing and propagation of seizure activity in human complex partial seizures. Less than 10% bound to plasma proteins. Not extensively metabolized in humans and not liver (cytochrome P_{450}) dependent. Undergoes enzymatic hydrolysis. Half-life is 6 to 8 hours. Primarily excreted in urine as unchanged drug and metabolites. Crossed the placental barrier in animal studies. Secreted in breast milk.

INDICATIONS AND USES

IV injection is used as a temporary alternative for patients when oral administration is temporarily not feasible. ▪ Adjunctive therapy in the treatment of partial-onset seizures in adults and pediatric patients 1 month of age and older with epilepsy. ▪ Adjunctive therapy in the treatment of myoclonic seizures in adults and adolescents 12 years of age and older with juvenile myoclonic epilepsy (JME). ▪ Adjunctive therapy in the treatment of primary generalized tonic-clonic seizures in adults and pediatric patients 6 years of age and older with idiopathic generalized epilepsy.

CONTRAINDICATIONS

Manufacturer states, "None."

PRECAUTIONS

For IV use only. ▪ Associated with CNS side effects (somnolence and fatigue, coordination difficulties [abnormal gait, ataxia, incoordination], and behavioral abnormalities [e.g., aggression, agitation, anxiety, apathy, depression, emotional lability, irritability, and psychotic symptoms, including psychosis and suicidal tendencies]). Somnolence and fatigue and coordination difficulties occurred most frequently within the first 4 weeks of treatment and resolved or improved with dose reduction or discontinuation of levetiracetam. ▪ Antiepileptic drugs (AEDs) increase the risk of suicidal thoughts or behavior in patients taking these drugs for any indication. Patients treated with any AED for any indication should be monitored for the emergence or worsening of depression, suicidal thoughts or behavior, and/or any unusual changes in mood or behavior. Some behavioral changes resolved without intervention. Others required dose reduction or discontinuation of levetiracetam. ▪ Serious dermatologic reactions, including Stevens-Johnson syndrome and toxic epidermal necrolysis, have been reported. Median time to onset is 14 to 17 days, but development up to 4 months after initiation of therapy has been reported. ▪ To minimize the potential of increased seizure frequency, withdraw antiepileptic drugs (including levetiracetam) gradually. ▪ Increase in diastolic BP has been reported in patients 1 month to under 4 years of age who are receiving the oral formulation of levetiracetam. This side effect was not observed in older children or adults.

Monitor: Baseline CBC and CrCl indicated; monitor as needed. Decreases in WBC, RBC, hemoglobin, and hematocrit have been reported, but a change or discontinuation of therapy was not required. Increases in eosinophil counts and cases of agranulocytosis have also been reported. ▪ Monitor for seizure activity. ▪ Observe patient closely for signs of CNS side effects; see Precautions. ▪ Monitor vital signs. Pediatric patients 1 month to under 4 years of age should be monitored for a possible increase in diastolic BP. ▪ Monitor for serious dermatologic reactions.

Patient Education: May cause dizziness, coordination difficulties, and somnolence; use caution when performing tasks that require alertness or coordination (e.g., operating machinery, driving). ▪ Inform your health care professional if you are pregnant or breast-feeding. ▪ May increase the risk of suicidal thoughts and behavior. Promptly report emergence or worsening of S/S of depression, any unusual changes in mood or behavior, or thoughts about self-harm. ▪ Women who are pregnant or who become pregnant should be encouraged to enroll in the North American Antiepileptic Drug (NAAED) Pregnancy Registry. ▪ May cause serious dermatologic reactions; promptly report development of a rash.

Maternal/Child: Category C: animal studies demonstrated fetal skeletal abnormalities and delayed offspring growth. Use during pregnancy only if potential benefit justifies the potential risk to the fetus. ▪ Physiologic changes during pregnancy may decrease levetiracetam concentration. Monitor carefully during pregnancy. Extend monitoring to postpartum period if dose adjustments were required during the pregnancy. ▪ Effects during labor and delivery unknown. ▪ Discontinue breast-feeding. ▪ Safety and effectiveness for use in certain pediatric populations have been established; see Indications. ▪ Pharmacokinetic analysis showed that body weight was significantly correlated to the clearance of levetiracetam in pediatric patients; clearance increased with an increase in body weight.

Elderly: Safety similar to that seen in younger adults; however, total body clearance is decreased and half-life is increased. ▪ Reduced doses may be indicated; see Dose Adjustments. Monitoring of renal function suggested.

DRUG/LAB INTERACTIONS

Manufacturer states that levetiracetam "is unlikely to produce, or be subject to, pharmacokinetic interactions." ▪ Other antiepileptic drugs (AEDs) such as carbamazepine (Tegretol), gabapentin (Neurontin), lamotrigine (Lamictal), phenobarbital (Luminal), phenytoin (Dilantin), primidone (Mysoline), and valproate (Depacon) do not influence the pharmacokinetics of levetiracetam, and it does not influence their pharmacokinetics. ▪ An increase in the clearance of levetiracetam was seen in pediatric patients when it was coadministered with **enzyme-inducing AEDs** (e.g., carbamazepine [Tegretol], phenytoin [Dilantin]). Levetiracetam had no effect on plasma concentrations of carbamazepine (Tegretol), lamotrigine (Lamictal), topiramate (Topamax), or valproate (Depacon) in pediatric patients. ▪ Not an inhibitor or a substrate of cytochrome P_{450} isoforms; unlikely to have interactions with drugs metabolized by these isoenzymes in the liver. ▪ Minimal protein binding; unlikely to have interactions with drugs requiring protein-binding sites. ▪ Has been administered with oral contraceptives, digoxin (Lanoxin), and warfarin (Coumadin) with no interference on the pharmacokinetics of either drug. ▪ **Probenecid** decreases renal clearance and increases serum concentrations of one of the metabolites of levetiracetam.

SIDE EFFECTS

Adults: Asthenia, dizziness, infection, and somnolence occurred most frequently during the first 4 weeks of treatment.

Pediatric patients: Aggression, decreased appetite, fatigue, irritability, and nasal congestion were most commonly reported.

Patients of all ages: Other side effects reported and presenting anywhere from 1 to 4 weeks included amnesia; anorexia; anxiety; ataxia; cough; decreased RBC, WBC, Hct, and Hgb; depersonalization; depression; diarrhea; diplopia; emotional lability; headache; hostility; influenza; insomnia; irritability; mood swings; neck pain; nervousness; pain; paresthesia; pharyngitis; rhinitis; seizures; sinusitis; and vertigo.

Post-Marketing: Abnormal liver function tests, agranulocytosis, choreoathetosis, drug rash with eosinophilia and systemic symptoms (DRESS), dyskinesia, erythema multiforme, hepatic failure, hepatitis, hyponatremia, leukopenia, muscle weakness, neutropenia, pancreatitis, pancytopenia (with bone marrow suppression), panic attack, Stevens-Johnson syndrome, suicidal behavior, thrombocytopenia, toxic epidermal necrolysis, and weight loss. Alopecia has been reported; recovery occurred in the majority of cases if levetiracetam was discontinued.

Overdose: Aggression, agitation, coma, depressed level of consciousness, drowsiness, respiratory depression, and somnolence.

ANTIDOTE

Keep physician informed of all side effects. Some may not require intervention, and others may improve with a reduced dose or discontinuation of levetiracetam; see Precautions and Side Effects. Discontinue at first sign of rash, unless the rash is clearly not drug related. Support patient as required in treatment of overdose. No specific antidote in overdose; however, hemodialysis will remove approximately 50% of a dose in 4 hours.

LEVOFLOXACIN BBW

(**lee**-voh-**FLOX**-ah-sin)

Levaquin

Antibacterial
(fluoroquinolone)

pH 3.8 to 5.8

USUAL DOSE

250 to 750 mg once every 24 hours.* Dose and duration of treatment are based on degree of infection and specific diagnosis. CrCl equal to or greater than 50 mL/min is required. Dose and serum levels similar by oral or IV route. Transfer to oral dose as soon as practical.

Levofloxacin Dosing Guidelines		
Type of Infection[a]	Dose Every 24 Hours[b]	Duration (Days)
Acute Bacterial Exacerbation of Chronic Bronchitis	500 mg	7 days
Nosocomial Pneumonia	750 mg	7-14 days
Community-Acquired Pneumonia	500 mg or 750 mg	7-14 days 5 days
Acute Bacterial Sinusitis	500 mg or 750 mg	10-14 days 5 days
Chronic Bacterial Prostatitis	500 mg	28 days
Complicated SSSI[c]	750 mg	7-14 days
Uncomplicated SSSI[c]	500 mg	7-10 days
Complicated UTI[d] or Acute Pyelonephritis	750 mg	5 days
Complicated UTI[d] or Acute Pyelonephritis	250 mg	10 days
Uncomplicated UTI[d]	250 mg	3 days
Inhalation Anthrax (postexposure) and plague in adults[e]	500 mg	60 days (anthrax) 10 to 14 days (plague)
Inhalation Anthrax (postexposure) and plague in pediatric patients >50 kg[e]	500 mg	60 days (anthrax) 10 to 14 days (plague)[f]
Inhalation Anthrax (postexposure) and plague in pediatric patients <50 kg and ≥6 months of age[e]	8 mg/kg q 12 hr[b] (not to exceed 250 mg/dose)	60 days (anthrax) 10 to 14 days (plague)[f]

[a]Due to the designated pathogens (see Indications and Usage).
[b]Frequency is every 12 hours (not 24 hours) for treatment of inhalation anthrax and plague in pediatric patients less than 50 kg and age 6 months or more.
[c]Skin and skin structure infections.
[d]Urinary tract infections.
[e]Begin drug administration as soon as possible after suspected or confirmed exposure to aerosolized *Bacillus anthracis* or to *Yersinia pestis.* If clinically indicated, higher doses of levofloxacin (e.g., equivalent to 750 mg) can be used for the treatment of plague.
[f]See Precautions and Maternal/Child.

*Frequency is every 12 hours (not 24 hours) for treatment of inhalation anthrax and plague in pediatric patients less than 50 kg and age 6 months or more.

DOSE ADJUSTMENTS

No dose adjustment is required specifically for age, gender, race, or in impaired hepatic function. ■ Clearance is reduced and half-life is prolonged in patients with a CrCl equal to or less than 50 mL/min. See the following chart for dosing guidelines. See Important IV Therapy Facts on p. xx for formula to convert SCr to CrCl. ■ Supplemental doses are not required after hemodialysis or peritoneal dialysis.

Levofloxacin Dosing Guidelines in Impaired Renal Function			
Dosage in Normal Renal Function Every 24 hours	Creatinine Clearance 20 to 49 mL/min	Creatinine Clearance 10 to 19 mL/min	Hemodialysis or Chronic Ambulatory Peritoneal Dialysis (CAPD)
750 mg	750 mg q 48 hr	750 mg initial dose, then 500 mg q 48 hr	750 mg initial dose, then 500 mg q 48 hr
500 mg	500 mg initial dose, then 250 mg q 24 hr	500 mg initial dose, then 250 mg q 48 hr	500 mg initial dose, then 250 mg q 48 hr
250 mg	No dose adjustment required	250 mg q 48 hr; no dose adjustment required if treating uncomplicated UTI	No information on dose adjustment available

DILUTION

Available in single-use vials and as prediluted, ready-to-use infusions.

Single-use vials: Withdraw desired dose from single-use vial (10 mL for 250 mg, 20 mL for 500 mg, 30 mL for 750 mg). Each 10 mL (250 mg) must be further diluted with a minimum of 40 mL NS, D5W, D5NS, D5LR, D5/plasma-Lyte 56, D5/$\frac{1}{2}$NS with 0.15% KCl, or $\frac{1}{6}$ M sodium lactate. Desired concentration is 5 mg/mL. No preservatives; enter vial only once. When 500-mg (20-mL) vial is used to prepare two 250-mg doses, withdraw entire contents of vial at once using a single-entry procedure. Prepare and store second dose for subsequent use.

Premix flexible containers: No further dilution necessary. Available as 250 mg in 50 mL, 500 mg in 100 mL, or 750 mg in 150 mL D5W. Instructions for access to and use of premix flexible containers are on its storage carton. Do not use flexible containers in series connections.

Filters: Not required; however, contents of both vials and premixed solutions were filtered during manufacturing with polyvinyl mixed ester cellulose filters. Size not specified by manufacturer. No significant loss of potency expected.

Storage: Store vials at CRT; protect from light. Store premix at or below 25° C (77° F); protect from freezing, light, and excessive heat. Brief exposure up to 40° C (104° F) does not adversely affect the product. Both are stable to expiration date. Solutions diluted from vials are stable at or below 25° C (77° F) for 3 days and for up to 14 days if refrigerated. May be frozen for up to 6 months. Do not force thaw (e.g., microwave or water bath) and do not refreeze. Discard any unused portion of premixed solutions and/or opened vials.

COMPATIBILITY   (Underline Indicates Conflicting Compatibility Information)

Consider any drug NOT listed as compatible to be INCOMPATIBLE until consulting a pharmacist; specific conditions may apply.

Manufacturer states, "Limited **compatibility** information available; other intravenous substances, additives, or other medications should not be added to levofloxacin or infused simultaneously through the same intravenous line." Never administer in the same IV or through the same tubing with any solution containing multivalent cations (e.g., calcium, magnesium). Flush line with a **compatible** solution before and after administration of levofloxacin and/or any other drug through the same IV line.

One source suggests the following **compatibilities:**

Y-site: Amikacin, aminophylline, ampicillin, anidulafungin (Eraxis), bivalirudin (Angiomax), caffeine citrate (Cafcit), caspofungin (Cancidas), cefotaxime (Claforan), ceftaroline (Teflaro), clindamycin (Cleocin), daptomycin (Cubicin), dexamethasone (Decadron), dexmedetomidine (Precedex), dobutamine, dopamine, doripenem (Doribax), epinephrine (Adrenalin), fenoldopam (Corlopam), fentanyl, gentamicin, hetastarch in electrolytes (Hextend), hydromorphone (Dilaudid), 6% hydroxyethyl starch (Voluven), insulin (regular), isoproterenol (Isuprel), lidocaine, linezolid (Zyvox), lorazepam (Ativan), magnesium sulfate, metoclopramide (Reglan), morphine, oxacillin (Bactocill), pancuronium, penicillin G sodium, phenobarbital (Luminal), phenylephrine (Neo-Synephrine), potassium chloride, sodium bicarbonate, vancomycin.

RATE OF ADMINISTRATION

Each 250- or 500-mg dose must be equally distributed over 60 minutes as an infusion. A 750-mg dose must be equally distributed over 90 minutes as an infusion. Too-rapid administration may cause hypotension. May be given through a Y-tube or three-way stopcock of infusion set. Temporarily discontinue other solutions infusing at the same site and flush tubing with **compatible** solutions before and after levofloxacin.

ACTIONS

A synthetic, broad-spectrum, fluoroquinolone antibacterial agent. Bactericidal to aerobic gram-negative and gram-positive organisms through interference with an enzyme (topoisomerase II) needed for synthesis of bacterial DNA. May be active against bacteria resistant to aminoglycosides, beta-lactam antibiotics, and macrolides. Onset of action is prompt, and serum levels are dose related. Mean terminal half-life is 6 to 8 hours. Steady state is achieved within 48 hours. Widely distributed into body tissues, including blister fluid and lung tissues. Moderately bound to serum protein (24% to 38%). Metabolism is minimal; primarily excreted as unchanged drug in urine. Very small amounts found in bile and feces. May cross placental barrier. May be secreted in breast milk.

INDICATIONS AND USES

Treatment of adults with mild, moderate, and severe infections caused by susceptible strains of microorganisms in conditions including acute bacterial sinusitis, acute bacterial exacerbation of chronic bronchitis, and nosocomial pneumonia. ■ Treatment of community-acquired pneumonia due to many organisms, including *Streptococcus pneumoniae* (including multidrug-resistant strains [MDRSP]). MDRSP strains are resistant to two or more of the following antibiotics: penicillin, second-generation cephalosporins (e.g., cefuroxime [Zinacef]), macrolides, tetracyclines, and sulfamethoxazole/trimethoprim. ■ Treatment of complicated skin and skin structure infections, mild to moderate uncomplicated skin and skin structure infections, complicated and uncomplicated urinary tract infections, and acute pyelonephritis (including cases with concurrent bacteremia). ■ To reduce the incidence and progression of inhalational anthrax following exposure to *Bacillus anthracis.* Begin administration as soon as possible after suspected or confirmed exposure. Transfer to oral therapy when practical. ■ Treatment of plague, including pneumonic and septicemic plague, due to *Yersinia pestis,* as well as prophylaxis for plague in adults and pediatric patients 6 months of age and older. ■ Treatment of chronic bacterial prostatitis (usually oral therapy).

CONTRAINDICATIONS

History of hypersensitivity to levofloxacin, its components, or any other quinolone antimicrobial agents (e.g., ciprofloxacin [Cipro], norfloxacin [Noroxin]).

PRECAUTIONS

For IV use only. ■ Culture and sensitivity studies indicated to determine susceptibility of the causative organism to levofloxacin. ■ *Pseudomonas aeruginosa* may develop resistance during treatment. Ongoing culture and sensitivity studies indicated. ■ The emergence of bacterial resistance to fluoroquinolones and the occurrence of cross-resistance with other fluoroquinolones have been observed and are of concern. Proper use of fluoroquinolones and other classes of antibiotics is encouraged to avoid the emergence of resistant bacteria from overuse. ■ Prolonged use may cause superinfection because of overgrowth of nonsusceptible organisms. ■ Use with caution in patients with known CNS disorders that predispose to seizures or alter seizure threshold (e.g., epilepsy, severe cerebral arteriosclerosis, concomitant drug therapy). Convulsions, toxic psychosis, increased intracranial pressure (including pseudotumor cerebri), and CNS stimulation have been reported. May cause other CNS effects, including confusion, depression, dizziness, hallucinations, tremors and, rarely, suicidal thoughts or acts. ■ Use caution in patients with impaired renal function; see Dose Adjustments. ■ May be used by patients who are allergic to penicillin or intolerant of macrolides (e.g., erythromycin). ■ Cross-resistance may occur with other fluoroquinolones, but some microorganisms resistant to other fluoroquinolones may be susceptible to levofloxacin. ■ Severe, sometimes fatal hepatotoxicity has been reported. Symptoms appeared within 6 to 14 days of initiating therapy, and most cases were not associated with hypersensitivity and occurred in patients 65 years of age or older; see Patient Education and Antidote. ■ Tendinitis and tendon rupture that required surgical repair or resulted in prolonged disability have been reported in patients of all ages receiving quinolones. Most frequently involves the Achilles tendon but has also been reported with the shoulder, hand, biceps, thumb, and other tendon sites. ■ Tendon rupture or tendinitis may occur during or up to months after fluoroquinolone therapy. Risk may be increased in patients over 60 years of age; in patients taking corticosteroids; in patients with heart, kidney, or lung transplants; with strenuous physical activity; and in patients with renal failure or previous tendon disorders such as rheumatoid arthritis. ■ Prolongation of the QT interval on ECG and infrequent cases of arrhythmia (including torsades de pointes) have been reported. The risk of arrhythmia may be reduced by avoiding the use of levofloxacin in patients with known prolongation of the QT interval, uncorrected electrolyte imbalances (e.g., hypokalemia, hypomagnesemia), significant bradycardia, cardiomyopathy, or concurrent treatment with Class Ia antiarrhythmic agents (e.g., quinidine [Quinidex], procainamide [Procanbid, Procan SR]) or Class III antiarrhythmic agents (e.g., amiodarone [Nexterone], sotalol [Betapace]) and any other drug that can prolong the QT interval; avoid coadministration; see Drug/Lab Interactions. ■ Fluoroquinolones have neuromuscular blocking activity and may exacerbate muscle weakness in persons with myasthenia gravis. Serious adverse events, including a requirement for ventilatory support and deaths, have been reported in these patients. Avoid use in patients with a known history of myasthenia gravis. ■ Rare cases of peripheral neuropathy (e.g., paresthesias, hypoesthesias, dysesthesias [impairment of sensitivity or touch], or weakness) have been reported. Symptoms may occur soon after initiation of therapy and may be irreversible; see Antidote. ■ *Clostridium difficile*–associated diarrhea (CDAD) has been reported. May range from mild diarrhea to fatal colitis. Consider in patients who present with diarrhea during or after treatment with levofloxacin. ■ Serious and occasionally fatal hypersensitivity and/or anaphylactic reactions have been reported. Often occur after the first dose. ■ Other serious events (sometimes fatal) due to hypersensitivity or uncertain etiology have been reported with fluoroquinolones, including levofloxacin; usually occur after multiple doses. Manifestations may include renal impairment/failure, hematologic toxicity, and dermatologic toxicity; see Side Effects, Post-Marketing. Discontinue levofloxacin at the first appearance of a skin rash, jaundice, or other signs of hepatotoxicity or hypersensitivity. ■ Moderate to severe photosensitivity/phototoxicity reactions have been reported in patients receiving quinolones; see Patient Education. ■ Not tested in humans for postexposure prevention of inhalation anthrax; however, plasma concentrations are considered to be in a range to produce effective results. ■ Safety for use in adults beyond 28 days or in pediatric patients beyond 14 days not studied; use only for prescribed indication; benefits must outweigh risks. An increased incidence of musculoskeletal adverse events has been observed in pediatric patients.

Monitor: Hypersensitivity reactions, including anaphylaxis with the first or succeeding doses, have been reported in patients receiving quinolones, even in those without known hypersensitivity. Emergency equipment must always be available; see Precautions. ■ Obtain baseline CBC with differential, CrCl, and blood glucose. Periodic monitoring of organ systems, including hematopoietic, hepatic, and renal, is recommended. ■ Monitor for S/S of peripheral neuropathy. Discontinue levofloxacin at the first symptoms of neuropathy (e.g., pain, burning, tingling, numbness and/or weakness) or if patient is found to have deficits in light touch, pain, temperature, position sense, vibratory sensation, and/or motor strength. ▪ Maintain adequate hydration to prevent concentrated urine throughout treatment. Crystalluria and cylindruria have been reported with quinolones. ▪ Monitor infusion site for inflammation and/or extravasation. ▪ Symptomatic hyperglycemia or hypoglycemia may occur, usually in diabetic patients receiving oral hypoglycemic agents (e.g., glyburide) or insulin. Monitor blood glucose closely. ▪ See Precautions, Drug/Lab Interactions, and Antidote.

Patient Education: A patient medication guide is available from the manufacturer. ▪ Review all medicines and disease history with pharmacist or physician before initiating treatment. ▪ Inform physician of any history of myasthenia gravis. ▪ Patients with a history of myasthenia gravis should avoid the use of levofloxacin. ▪ Drink fluids liberally. ▪ Promptly report skin rash or any other hypersensitivity reaction. ▪ Promptly report pain, burning, tingling, numbness and/or weakness in extremities. Nerve damage can be permanent. ▪ Photosensitivity has occurred in a minimal number of patients, but it is best to avoid excessive sunlight or artificial ultraviolet light. May cause severe sunburn; wear protective clothing, use sunscreen, and wear dark glasses outdoors. Report a sunburn-like reaction or skin eruption promptly. ▪ Dizziness or light-headedness may interfere with ambulation and motor coordination. Use caution in tasks that require alertness. ▪ Effects of caffeine, theophylline preparations, and/or warfarin (Coumadin) may be increased; notify your physician if you take any of these agents. If diabetic and on medication, monitor your blood glucose carefully. If a hypoglycemia reaction occurs, discontinue levofloxacin and consult physician. ▪ Promptly report S/S of liver injury (e.g., dark-colored urine, fever, itching, jaundice [yellowing of skin or whites of eyes], light-colored bowel movements, loss of appetite, nausea, right upper quadrant tenderness, tiredness, vomiting, weakness). ▪ Promptly report tendon pain or inflammation; rest and refrain from exercise. ▪ Before initiating therapy, parents should inform their child's physician if their child has a history of joint-related problems, and they should notify their child's physician of any tendon or joint-related problems that occur during or after therapy. ▪ Promptly report diarrhea or bloody stools that occur during treatment or up to several months after an antibiotic has been discontinued; may indicate CDAD and require treatment. ▪ See Precautions, Monitor, Drug/Lab Interactions, and Antidote.

Maternal/Child: Category C: safety for use in pregnancy not established; benefits must outweigh risks. ▪ Discontinue breast-feeding. ▪ Safety for use in pediatric patients under 18 years of age not established. Indicated in pediatric patients 6 months of age or older only for prevention of inhalation anthrax (postexposure) and prevention and treatment of plague. Safety for use in pediatric patients under 6 months of age not established. An increased incidence of musculoskeletal disorders (arthralgia, arthritis, tendinopathy, and gait abnormality) compared with controls has been observed in pediatric patients receiving levofloxacin.

Elderly: Half-life may be slightly extended due to age-related renal impairment. Dose reduction required only in the elderly with a CrCl of 50 mL/min or less. ▪ Safety and effectiveness similar to that in younger adults; however, they may experience an increased risk of side effects (e.g., CNS effects, hepatotoxicity, tendinitis, tendon rupture, risk of QT prolongation). Monitoring of renal function may be useful. ▪ See Dose Adjustments and Precautions.

DRUG/LAB INTERACTIONS

May cause ventricular arrhythmias or torsades de pointes with **drugs that prolong the QT interval,** such as **Class Ia antiarrhythmic agents** (e.g., quinidine, procainamide [Procanbid, Procan SR]), **Class III antiarrhythmic agents** (e.g., amiodarone [Nexterone], sotalol [Betapace]), **anticonvulsants** (e.g., fosphenytoin [Cerebyx]), **antihistamines** (e.g., diphenhydramine [Benedryl]), **phenothiazines** (e.g., chlorpromazine [Thorazine]), **serotonin reuptake inhibitors** (e.g., fluoxetine [Prozac], paroxetine [Paxil]), **tricyclic antidepressants** (e.g., imipramine [Tofranil], amitryptyline [Elavil]). Avoid coadministration. ▪ Risk of

CNS stimulation and convulsive seizures may be increased with **NSAIDs** (e.g., ibuprofen [Advil, Motrin], naproxen [Aleve, Naprosyn]). ▪ May cause hyperglycemia and hypoglycemia with concurrent administration of **antidiabetic agents** (e.g., metformin [Glucophage], insulin); monitoring of blood glucose recommended. ▪ Concomitant administration with **cimetidine or probenecid** reduces levofloxacin renal clearance by 24% and 35% respectively, but dose adjustment is not required. ▪ Interactions with **theophylline** that occur with other quinolones have not been noted, but monitoring of theophylline levels is recommended with concomitant use. ▪ Some quinolones, including levofloxacin, may enhance effects of **warfarin** (Coumadin); monitoring of PT or INR is recommended with concomitant use. ▪ No dose adjustment required for either drug when levofloxacin is administered concomitantly with **cyclosporine or digoxin**. ▪ See Precautions. ▪ May cause **false-positive when testing urine for opiates**; more specific testing methods may be indicated.

SIDE EFFECTS

The most common side effects are constipation, diarrhea, dizziness, headache, insomnia, and nausea. Abdominal pain, chest pain, crystalluria, cylindruria, dyspepsia, dyspnea, edema, injection site reaction, moniliasis, photosensitivity/phototoxicity (sun sensitivity), pruritus, rash, vaginitis, and vomiting have occurred. Abnormal dreaming, abnormal gait, abnormal hepatic function, abnormal renal function, acute renal failure, agitation, anemia, anorexia, anxiety, arthralgia, cardiac arrest, CDAD, confusion, convulsions, depression, epistaxis, esophagitis, gastritis, gastroenteritis, genital moniliasis, glossitis, granulocytopenia, hallucinations, hyperglycemia, hyperkalemia, hyperkinesia, hypersensitivity reactions, hypertonia, hypoglycemia, increased alkaline phosphatase, increased hepatic enzymes, myalgia, nightmares, palpitation, pancreatitis, paresthesia, phlebitis, pseudomembranous colitis, skeletal pain, sleep disorders, somnolence, stomatitis, syncope, tendinitis, thrombocytopenia, tremor, urticaria, ventricular arrhythmia, ventricular tachycardia, and vertigo have also been reported in fewer than 1% of patients.

Post-Marketing: Abnormal EEG; hematologic abnormalities (agranulocytosis, anemia [hemolytic and aplastic], eosinophilia, leukopenia, pancytopenia, thrombocytopenia [including thrombotic thrombocytopenic purpura]); exacerbation of myasthenia gravis; eye disorders (e.g., blurred vision, diplopia, reduced visual acuity, scotoma, uveitis); hepatic failure, including fatal cases; fever; hepatitis; hypersensitivity reactions (sometimes fatal, including angioneurotic edema, anaphylaxis); interstitial nephritis; jaundice; leukocytoclastic vasculitis; multiorgan failure; muscle injury and increased muscle enzymes; paranoia; peripheral neuropathy; photosensitivity/phototoxicity reactions; prolonged INR; prolonged PT; prolonged QT interval; pseudotumor cerebri; psychosis; rhabdomyolysis; serum sickness; severe dermatologic reactions (e.g., toxic epidermal necrolysis [Lyell's syndrome], Stevens-Johnson syndrome); tachycardia; tendon rupture; tinnitus; vasodilation; and isolated reports of allergic pneumonitis, encephalopathy, suicide attempts and suicidal ideation, and torsades de pointes.

ANTIDOTE

Keep physician informed of all side effects. Most minor side effects will be treated symptomatically; monitor closely. Discontinue levofloxacin at the first sign of any major side effect (CDAD, CNS symptoms, dermatologic reactions, hepatotoxicity, hypersensitivity, hypoglycemic reactions, phototoxicity, symptoms of neuropathy, or tendon rupture). Treat hypersensitivity reactions as indicated with epinephrine, airway management, oxygen, IV fluids, antihistamines (e.g., diphenhydramine [Benadryl]), corticosteroids (e.g., Solu-Cortef), and pressor amines (e.g., dopamine). Treat CNS symptoms as indicated; may require diazepam (Valium) for seizures. Mild cases of CDAD may respond to discontinuation of levofloxacin. Treat CDAD with fluids, electrolytes, protein supplements, and oral vancomycin (Vancocin) or metronidazole (Flagyl) as indicated. In severe cases, surgical evaluation may be indicated. Complete rest is indicated for an affected tendon until treatment is available. Maintain hydration in overdose. No specific antidote; not removed by hemodialysis or peritoneal dialysis. Maintain patient until drug is excreted and symptoms subside.

LEVOLEUCOVORIN
(lee-voh-loo-koh-**VOR**-in)

Fusilev

Folate analog
Antidote
Antineoplastic adjunct

USUAL DOSE

Dosed at one-half the usual dose of the racemic form (leucovorin calcium).

Levoleucovorin rescue after high-dose methotrexate therapy: Dose is based on a methotrexate dose of 12 Gm/M^2 infused over 4 hours; see methotrexate monograph. Obtain serum creatinine and methotrexate levels at least once daily. Additional hydration and urinary alkalinization (pH 7 or greater) is indicated and should be continued until the methotrexate level is less than 0.05 micromolar. Administer and/or adjust the levoleucovorin dose or extend rescue based on the following guidelines. See Dose Adjustments, Precautions, and Monitor.

Guidelines for Levoleucovorin Administration, Adjustment, or Extension of Rescue		
Clinical Situation	Laboratory Findings	Levoleucovorin Dose and Duration
Normal methotrexate elimination	Serum methotrexate level approximately 10 micromolar at 24 hours, 1 micromolar at 48 hours, and less than 0.2 micromolar at 72 hours after methotrexate administration.	7.5 mg IV every 6 hours for 60 hours (10 doses starting at 24 hours after start of methotrexate infusion).
Delayed late methotrexate elimination	Serum methotrexate level remains above 0.2 micromolar at 72 hours and more than 0.05 micromolar at 96 hours after methotrexate administration.	Continue 7.5 mg IV every 6 hours until methotrexate level is less than 0.05 micromolar.
Delayed early methotrexate elimination and/or evidence of acute renal injury	Serum methotrexate level of 50 micromolar or more at 24 hours or 5 micromolar or more at 48 hours after methotrexate administration. **OR** 100% or greater increase in serum creatinine level at 24 hours after methotrexate administration (e.g., an increase from 0.5 mg/dL to a level of 1 mg/dL or more).	75 mg IV every 3 hours until methotrexate level is less than 1 micromolar; then 7.5 mg IV every 3 hours until methotrexate level is less than 0.05 micromolar.

Inadvertent methotrexate overdose: 7.5 mg IV every 6 hours (approximately 5 mg/M^2) until the serum methotrexate level is less than 5×10^{-8} M (0.05 micromolar). Begin levoleucovorin rescue as soon as possible after an inadvertent methotrexate overdose and within 24 hours of methotrexate administration when there is delayed excretion. The effectiveness of levoleucovorin in counteracting toxicity may decrease as the time interval between methotrexate administration and levoleucovorin rescue increases. See Dose Adjustments and Monitor.

Colorectal cancer: Several regimens are in use. See fluorouracil (5-FU) monograph for 5-FU specific information. Administer 5-FU and levoleucovorin separately to avoid the formation of a precipitate.

Flush the IV line with NS between drugs.

Levoleucovorin 100 mg/M^2 by IV injection over a minimum of 3 minutes (see Rate of Administration) followed by *5-FU* 370 mg/M^2 by IV injection *or levoleucovorin* 10 mg/M^2 by IV injection followed by *5-FU* at 425 mg/M^2 by IV injection. Repeat either regimen daily for 5 days. This 5-day course is repeated at 4-week intervals for 2 courses and then at 4- to 5-week intervals provided that complete recovery from the toxic effects of the previous course has occurred. See Dose Adjustments.

PEDIATRIC DOSE
See Usual Dose.

DOSE ADJUSTMENTS

Levoleucovorin rescue after high-dose methotrexate therapy: Some patients may have significant but less severe abnormalities in methotrexate elimination or renal function following methotrexate administration than the abnormalities described in the preceding table. These abnormalities may or may not be associated with significant clinical toxicity. If significant clinical toxicity is observed, levoleucovorin rescue should be extended for an additional 24 hours (a total of 14 doses over 84 hours) in subsequent courses of therapy. If lab abnormalities or clinical toxicities are observed, consider the possibility that the patient is taking other medications that interact with methotrexate (e.g., medications that may interfere with methotrexate elimination or binding to serum albumin [see methotrexate monograph]). ▪ Delayed methotrexate excretion may also be caused by accumulation in a third space fluid collection (i.e., ascites, pleural effusion), inadequate hydration, or renal insufficiency. Higher doses of levoleucovorin or prolonged administration may be indicated.

Inadvertent methotrexate overdose: If the 24-hour serum creatinine has increased 50% over baseline or if the 24-hour methotrexate level is greater than 5×10^{-6} M (5 micromolar) or the 48-hour level is greater than 9×10^{-7} M (0.9 micromolar), increase the dose of levoleucovorin to 50 mg/M^2 IV every 3 hours until the methotrexate level is less than 0.05 micromolar. Hydrate with a minimum of 3 liters/day and use sodium bicarbonate for urinary alkalinization (adjust to maintain a urine pH of 7 or greater).

Colorectal cancer: In subsequent courses, adjust the dose of 5-FU based on patient tolerance of the previous treatment course. Reduce 5-FU dose by 20% for patients who experienced moderate hematologic or GI toxicity in the previous course and 30% for patients who experienced severe toxicity. 5-FU dose may be increased by 10% if no toxicity was experienced in the previous course. Levoleucovorin doses are not adjusted for toxicity.

DILUTION

Levoleucovorin for injection: Reconstitute each 50-mg vial of lyophilized powder with 5.3 mL of preservative-free NS (concentration equals 10 mg/mL). Do not use other diluents. A single dose may be further diluted immediately in NS or D5W to a concentration of 0.5 mg/mL to 5 mg/mL. Do not use if solution is cloudy or a precipitate is observed.

Levoleucovorin injection: Available in ready-to-use single-use vials containing 175 mg (17.5 mL) or 250 mg (25 mL). Concentration equals 10 mg/mL. A single dose of these solutions may be further diluted to a concentration of 0.5 mg/mL in NS or D5W.

Filters: Specific information not available.

Storage: *Levoleucovorin for injection (reconstituted lyophilized powder):* Store unopened vials in carton at CRT. Protect from light. Solutions reconstituted or further diluted in NS are stable for not more than 12 hours at RT. Reconstituted solutions further diluted in D5W are stable for not more than 4 hours at RT. *Levoleucovorin injection (ready-to-use solution):* Refrigerate unopened vials in carton at 2° to 8° C (36° to 46° F). Protect from light. Solutions diluted to 0.5 mg/mL in NS or D5W are stable for not more than 4 hours at RT.

COMPATIBILITY

Manufacturer states, "Due to the risk of precipitation, do not coadminister levoleucovorin with other agents in the same admixture." Dilute only with preservative-free NS; do not use other diluents or NS with preservatives.

RATE OF ADMINISTRATION

Because of the calcium content of the solution, do not exceed a rate of injection of 16 mL/min of reconstituted solution (160 mg of levoleucovorin). When given in combination with 5-FU, flush the IV line with NS between drugs.

ACTIONS

A folate analog. An active isomer of 5-formyl tetrahydrofolic acid, the pharmacologically active isomer of leucovorin calcium. A replacement for leucovorin calcium, which also contains the pharmacologically inactive dextro isomer. Does not require reduction by the enzyme dihydrofolate reductase. Actively and passively transported across cell membranes. Converted in vivo to the primary circulating form of active reduced folate. Levoleucovorin can counteract the therapeutic and toxic effects of folic acid antagonists such as methotrexate, which act by inhibiting dihydrofolate reductase. Terminal half-life is from 5.1 to 6.8 hours.

INDICATIONS AND USES

Levoleucovorin rescue is indicated after high-dose methotrexate therapy in patients with osteosarcoma. ▪ Also indicated to diminish the toxicity and counteract the effects of impaired methotrexate elimination and of inadvertent overdose of folic acid antagonists (e.g., methotrexate, pemetrexed [Alimta]). ▪ Indicated for use in combination chemotherapy with 5-fluorouracil (5-FU) in the palliative treatment of advanced metastatic colorectal cancer. ▪ Not indicated for the treatment of pernicious anemia and megaloblastic anemias secondary to vitamin B_{12} deficiency; improper use may cause a hematologic remission while neurologic manifestations continue to progress.

CONTRAINDICATIONS

Contraindicated in patients who have had previous hypersensitivity reactions to folic acid or folinic acid.

PRECAUTIONS

For IV use only; do not administer by any other route. ▪ Contains calcium; limit rate of administration to no more than 16 mL/min (160 mg of levoleucovorin per minute). ▪ Toxicities during combination use with 5-fluorouracil (5-FU) are similar to those observed with 5-FU alone; however, GI toxicities (particularly stomatitis and diarrhea) are observed more commonly and may be more severe or of prolonged duration. ▪ Concomitant use with sulfamethoxazole/trimethoprim for the acute treatment of *Pneumocystis jiroveci* pneumonia in patients with HIV infection may cause treatment failure and morbidity.

Monitor: *All situations with methotrexate:* Obtain baseline serum methotrexate, serum creatinine, electrolytes, and urine pH. Monitor at least daily. ▪ Adequate hydration and maintenance of a urinary pH of 7 or greater with sodium bicarbonate are indicated.

Levoleucovorin rescue after high-dose methotrexate therapy: Patients who experience delayed early methotrexate elimination are likely to develop reversible renal failure. Continuing hydration and urinary alkalinization and close monitoring of fluid and electrolyte status are required until the serum methotrexate level has fallen to below 0.05 micromolar and the renal failure has resolved.

Inadvertent methotrexate overdose: See Dose Adjustments; hydration with a minimum of 3 liters/day and the use of sodium bicarbonate for urinary alkalinization (adjust to maintain a urine pH of 7 or greater) may be indicated.

Combination with 5-FU: Monitor for S/S of GI toxicity. See the 5-fluorouracil monograph for hematologic monitoring requirements.

Maternal/Child: Category C: use during pregnancy only if clearly needed. ▪ Not known if levoleucovorin is excreted in human milk; has potential for harmful effects; discontinue breast-feeding.

Elderly: Studies of levoleucovorin in the treatment of osteosarcoma did not include adults age 65 or older. ▪ Dehydration, diarrhea, and severe enterocolitis have been reported in elderly patients receiving weekly levoleucovorin and 5-fluorouracil (5-FU).

DRUG/LAB INTERACTIONS

May ameliorate the hematologic toxicity associated with **high-dose methotrexate,** but levoleucovorin has no effect on other established toxicities of methotrexate, such as nephrotoxicity resulting from drug and/or metabolite precipitation in the kidney. ▪ Folic acid in large amounts may counteract the antiepileptic effects of **phenobarbital** (Luminal), **phenytoin** (Dilantin), **and primidone** (Mysoline). Seizure activity may be increased in susceptible patients. Levoleucovorin may or may not have the same effect due to shared metabolic pathways; use caution when administering concurrently with anticonvulsant drugs. ▪ Small amounts of systemically administered levoleucovorin may enter the cerebrospinal fluid (CSF). *Do not give levoleucovorin intrathecally;* see Precautions. ▪ Increases the toxicity of **5-fluorouracil** (5-FU); dehydration, diarrhea, and severe enterocolitis have been reported in elderly patients receiving weekly levoleucovorin and 5-fluorouracil. ▪ Concomitant use with **sulfamethoxazole/trimethoprim** for the acute treatment of *Pneumocystis jiroveci* pneumonia in patients with HIV infection may cause treatment failure and morbidity. ▪ High doses of levoleucovorin may reduce the effectiveness of intrathecally administered **methotrexate.** ▪ Levoleucovorin may enhance the toxic effects of **capecitabine** (Xeloda); monitor closely.

SIDE EFFECTS
Nausea and vomiting and stomatitis were reported most commonly. Abnormal renal function, confusion, dermatitis, diarrhea, dyspepsia, dyspnea, hypersensitivity reactions, leukopenia, neuropathy, thrombocytopenia, typhlitis (inflammation of the cecum), and taste perversion have been reported.
Combination therapy with 5-fluorouracil (5-FU): Abdominal pain, alopecia, anorexia, dermatitis, diarrhea, fatigue, nausea, stomatitis, vomiting. Hypersensitivity reactions have been reported.
Post-Marketing: Dyspnea, pruritus, rash, rigors, temperature change.

ANTIDOTE
Keep physician informed of patient's condition. Symptomatic treatment indicated.

LEVOTHYROXINE SODIUM BBW
(lee-voh-thigh-**ROX**-een **SO**-dee-um)

Hormone
(thyroid)

T$_4$, L-Thyroxine

USUAL DOSE
When oral ingestion is not practical, IV dose should be ½ of any previously established oral dose; see Indications, Limitations of Use. Adjust in small increments as indicated. Initiate oral treatment as soon as possible.
Hypothyroidism (when oral therapy is not possible): Usual IV starting dose would be 6.25 to 12.5 mcg/day. Increase in increments of 12.5 mcg every 2 to 4 weeks. Base dosing on clinical response and serum thyroid and TSH levels. Average maintenance dose is 50 to 100 mcg/day PO.
Myxedema coma: 300 to 500 mcg as an initial dose. Follow with once-daily intravenous maintenance doses between 50 and 100 mcg.

PEDIATRIC DOSE
Given orally (may be crushed in food or liquid). See Precautions. Any IV dose should be 50% to 75% of the established oral dose. See pediatric literature for dosing guidelines.

DOSE ADJUSTMENTS
Age, general condition, cardiac risk factors, and clinical severity of myxedema symptoms should be considered when determining the starting and maintenance dosages. ▪ Reduce dose in elderly, functional or ECG evidence of cardiovascular disease (including angina), long-standing thyroid disease, other endocrinopathies, and severe hypothyroidism. ▪ See Drug/Lab Interactions.

DILUTION
Available in different strengths; read label carefully. Each vial of lyophilized powder is diluted with 5 mL of NS for injection (without preservatives). Shake well to dissolve completely. Reconstituted concentrations will be 20 mcg/mL for the 100-mcg vial and 100 mcg/mL for the 500-mcg vial. Do not add to IV solutions. May be given through Y-tube or three-way stopcock of infusion set.

Storage: Store dry product at CRT and protect from light. Reconstituted solution is pre-servative-free and stable for 4 hours; any remaining solution is discarded.

COMPATIBILITY
Manufacturer states, "Do not add to other IV fluids."

RATE OF ADMINISTRATION
100 mcg or fraction thereof over 1 minute.

ACTIONS
A synthetic thyroid hormone. Effective replacement for decreased or absent thyroid hormone. Thyroid hormone synthesis and secretion is regulated by the hypothalamic-pituitary-thyroid axis. Thyroid hormones regulate multiple metabolic processes and play an essential role in normal growth and development. Actions are produced predominantly by T_3 (triiodothyronine). Approximately 80% of T_3 is derived from T_4 (levothyroxine) by deiodination in peripheral tissues. The metabolic actions of thyroid hormones include augmentation of cellular respiration and thermogenesis, as well as metabolism of proteins, carbohydrates, and lipids. Circulating thyroid hormones are greater than 99% bound to plasma proteins (thyroxine-binding globulin [TBG], thyroxine-binding prealbumin [TBPA], and albumin [TBA]). The higher affinity of both TBG and TBPA for T_4 partially explains the higher serum levels, slower metabolic clearance, and longer half-life of T_4 (6 to 8 days) compared with T_3 (less than 2 days). The major pathway of thyroid hormone metabolism is through sequential deiodination. The liver is the major site of degradation for both T_4 and T_3. Primary route of elimination is through the kidneys. Small amounts are eliminated into the bile and feces.

INDICATIONS AND USES
Treatment of myxedema coma. ▪ Specific replacement therapy for reduced or absent thyroid function due to any cause (usually given orally).
Limitations of use: The relative bioavailability between oral and intravenous levothyroxine sodium for injection has not been established but has been estimated to be between 48% and 74%. Caution should be used when switching patients from oral products to the parenteral product because adequate dosing conversions have not been studied.

CONTRAINDICATIONS
Manufacturer states, "None." ▪ Not indicated for use in treatment of obesity. Risk can outweigh benefit.

PRECAUTIONS
Excessive bolus doses (greater than 500 mcg) are associated with cardiac complications, particularly in the elderly and in patients with underlying cardiac disease; see Dose Adjustments. ▪ Patients with undiagnosed endocrine disorders (e.g., adrenal insufficiency, hypopituitarism, diabetes insipidus) may experience new or worsening symptoms of these endocrinopathies. Patients should be treated with replacement glucocorticoids before initiation of treatment with levothyroxine until adrenal function has been adequately assessed. Failure to do so may precipitate an acute adrenal crisis when thyroid hormone therapy is initiated as a result of increased metabolic clearance of glucocorticoids by thyroid hormone. Patients with myxedema coma should be monitored for previously undiagnosed diabetes insipidus. ▪ Not indicated for treatment of obesity or for weight loss. Doses within the range of daily hormonal requirements are ineffective for weight reduction. Larger doses may produce serious or even life-threatening manifestations of toxicity, particularly when given in conjunction with sympathomimetic amines, such as those used for the anorectic effects.
Monitor: Observe patient closely and monitor vital signs. ▪ Monitor thyroid function tests (e.g., free T_4 index, TSH). ▪ TSH and thyroid hormone levels should be measured a few weeks after switching from IV to oral therapy. Adjust dose according to results and clinical status. ▪ Monitor TSH every 6 to 8 weeks until normalized, every 8 to 12 weeks after dose changes, and every 6 to 12 months throughout therapy.
Maternal/Child: Category A: may be used during pregnancy. ▪ Presumed safe in breast-feeding; use caution and observe infant. ▪ Myxedema coma is a disease of the elderly.

An approved oral dosage form should be used in pediatric patients for maintaining a euthyroid state in noncomplicated hypothyroidism; see Pediatric Dose.

Elderly: See Dose Adjustments; more sensitive to effects. Atrial fibrillation is a common side effect associated with levothyroxine treatment in the elderly.

DRUG/LAB INTERACTIONS

Addition of levothyroxine to **antidiabetic or insulin** therapy may result in increased antidiabetic or insulin requirements. Monitor glucose values closely, especially when thyroid therapy is initiated, changed, or discontinued. ▪ Levothyroxine increases response to **oral anticoagulant** therapy (e.g., warfarin). Reduction in dose of oral anticoagulant may be required. Monitor PT/INR. ▪ May decrease therapeutic effects of **digoxin**, necessitating an increase in the digoxin dose. Monitor serum digoxin levels. ▪ Concurrent use of **tricyclic** (e.g., amitriptyline) or **tetracyclic** (e.g., maprotiline) **antidepressants** and levothyroxine may increase the therapeutic and toxic effects of both drugs, possibly due to increased receptor sensitivity to catecholamines. ▪ Administration of **sertraline** in patients stabilized on levothyroxine may result in increased levothyroxine requirements. ▪ Concurrent use with **ketamine** may produce marked hypertension and tachycardia. Use caution. ▪ Concurrent use with **sympathomimetics** (e.g., epinephrine, norepinephrine) may increase the effects of sympathomimetics or thyroid hormone. May increase risk of coronary insufficiency. ▪ **Carbamazepine, fosphenytoin, phenytoin, and rifampin** may decrease the serum concentration of thyroid hormones. Monitor levels closely. ▪ Levothyroxine can increase the metabolism of **theophylline**, necessitating an increase in theophylline dose. Monitor theophylline levels. ▪ Changes in TBG concentration must be considered when interpreting T_3 and T_4 values, which necessitates measurement and evaluation of unbound (free) hormone and/or determination of the free levothyroxine index. Several medications and disease states can alter TBG concentrations. See manufacturer's prescribing information.

SIDE EFFECTS

Abdominal cramps, angina, arrhythmias, chest pain, diarrhea, heart palpitations, heat intolerance, increased pulse and BP, insomnia, menstrual irregularities, muscle cramps, nervousness, sweating, tachycardia, tremors, vomiting, and weight loss.

ANTIDOTE

Notify the physician of any side effect. A reduction in dose will usually decrease symptoms. Supportive treatment should be initiated as dictated by the patient's medical status.

LIDOCAINE HYDROCHLORIDE

(**LYE**-doh-kayn hy-droh-**KLOR**-eyed)

Lidocaine PF, Xylocaine PF, Xylocard ♣

Antiarrhythmic

pH 5 to 7 (Injection),
3 to 5.5 (IV infusion)

USUAL DOSE

Ventricular arrhythmia: 50 to 100 mg as a *loading dose* (0.7 to 1.4 mg/kg). Repeat after 5 minutes if desired clinical response is not produced. Follow with an infusion of 1 to 4 mg/min (20 to 50 mcg/kg/min). Should not exceed a maximum dose of 200 to 300 mg during a 1-hour period.

Refractory ventricular fibrillation or pulseless ventricular tachycardia: 1 to 1.5 mg/kg of body weight (50 to 100 mg) as a *loading dose.* May repeat 0.5 to 0.75 mg/kg every 10 minutes to desired effect, up to a total maximum cumulative dose of 3 mg/kg/24 hr. Should not exceed 200 to 300 mg during a 1-hour period. Follow with a continuous infusion of 1 to 4 mg/min (20 to 50 mcg/kg/min).

Maintenance dose: With return of perfusion, initiate an infusion of 1 to 4 mg/min (20 to 50 mcg/kg/min) in an average 70-kg adult. *Do not exceed 4 mg/min rate.* If arrhythmias occur during an infusion, give a small bolus of 0.5 mg/kg to increase plasma concentration.

Seizures unresponsive to other therapy (unlabeled): 1 mg/kg as a loading dose. If seizure does not terminate in 2 minutes, give an additional 0.5 mg/kg; a maintenance infusion of 30 mcg/kg/min has been used to prevent recurrences.

Cardiac arrest: AHA guidelines recommend a single dose of 1 to 1.5 mg/kg. An additional dose of 0.5 to 0.75 mg/kg may be given in 5 to 10 minutes to a maximum of 3 doses or a total dose of 3 mg/kg.

Perfusing arrhythmia (stable VT, wide-complex tachycardia of uncertain type, significant ectopy): AHA guidelines recommend doses ranging from 0.5 to 0.75 mg/kg and up to 1 to 1.5 mg/kg. Repeat 0.5 to 0.75 mg/kg every 5 to 10 minutes to a maximum total dose of 3 mg/kg. Follow with a continuous infusion of 1 to 4 mg/min (20 to 50 mcg/kg/min).

PEDIATRIC DOSE

See Maternal/Child (unlabeled).

Antiarrhythmic: AHA recommends 1 mg/kg as an IV injection followed immediately by an infusion of 20 to 50 mcg/kg/min (average of 30 mcg/kg/min). If 15 minutes have elapsed since the initial bolus dose before the infusion is started, administration of an additional bolus (1 mg/kg/min) is recommended when the infusion is initiated. Another source recommends 1 mg/kg IV. May repeat in 10 to 15 minutes × 2 if indicated. Maximum total dose is 3 to 5 mg/kg within the first hour. Follow with an infusion of 20 to 50 mcg/kg/min. Intratracheal dose suggested should be 2 to 2.5 times the IV dose.

DOSE ADJUSTMENTS

Reduce loading dose in digoxin toxicity with AV block. ▪ Consider loading dose reduction (not universally recommended) in congestive heart failure, reduced cardiac output, and liver disease. ▪ Lower-end initial doses may be indicated in the elderly based on potential for decreased organ function and concomitant disease or drug therapy. ▪ Reduce maintenance dose by one half in the presence of decreased cardiac output (e.g., acute MI, congestive heart failure, or shock from any cause [one source suggests not exceeding 20 mcg/kg/min]), with impaired liver function, in the elderly (over 65), and in patients receiving drugs that may decrease clearance of lidocaine or decrease liver blood flow (e.g., beta-blockers [propranolol, cimetidine (Tagamet)]). ▪ Reduce maintenance dose after 24 hours or monitor blood levels; half-life of lidocaine increases with prolonged administration.

DILUTION

Label must state "for IV use" and be preservative free. Bolus dose may be given undiluted.

Infusion: Add 1 Gm of lidocaine to 500 or 250 mL of D5W (preferred), D5/¹/₂NS, D5NS, LR, or other **compatible** solutions; see chart on inside back cover. Solution gives 2 or 4 mg/mL of lidocaine. Available premixed in 0.4% or 0.8% solutions (4 or 8 mg/mL). Titrate to desired response.

Pediatric infusion: Add 120 mg of lidocaine to 100 mL of diluent (1,200 mcg/mL). 1 to 2.5 mL/kg/hr will deliver 20 to 50 mcg/kg/min.

Storage: Store at CRT. Discard diluted solution after 24 hours. Protect from freezing.

COMPATIBILITY (Underline Indicates Conflicting Compatibility Information)

Consider any drug NOT listed as compatible to be INCOMPATIBLE until consulting a pharmacist; specific conditions may apply.

Manufacturer states, "Because doses of lidocaine are titrated to response, additives should not be introduced into premixed solutions of lidocaine."

One source suggests the following **compatibilities:**

Additive: *Not recommended by manufacturer. Physically* **compatible** *with numerous drugs. Combination may not be practical because of extensive individualized rate adjustments of lidocaine to achieve desired effects; consult pharmacist.* Alteplase (Activase, tPA), aminophylline, amiodarone (Nexterone), atracurium (Tracrium), calcium chloride, calcium gluconate, chloramphenicol (Chloromycetin), chlorothiazide (Diuril), ciprofloxacin (Cipro IV), dexamethasone (Decadron), digoxin (Lanoxin), diphenhydramine (Benadryl), dobutamine, dopamine, ephedrine sulfate, erythromycin (Erythrocin), fentanyl, flumazenil (Romazicon), furosemide (Lasix), heparin, hydrocortisone sodium succinate (Solu-Cortef), nafcillin (Nallpen), nitroglycerin IV, penicillin G potassium, pentobarbital (Nembutal), phenylephrine (Neo-Synephrine), potassium chloride (KCl), procainamide (Pronestyl), prochlorperazine (Compazine), ranitidine (Zantac), sodium bicarbonate, sodium lactate, theophylline, verapamil.

Y-site: Acetaminophen (Ofirmev), alteplase (Activase, tPA), amiodarone (Nexterone), argatroban, bivalirudin (Angiomax), cefazolin (Ancef), ceftaroline (Teflaro), ciprofloxacin (Cipro IV), cisatracurium (Nimbex), daptomycin (Cubicin), dexmedetomidine (Precedex), diltiazem (Cardizem), dobutamine, dopamine, enalaprilat (Vasotec IV), etomidate (Amidate), famotidine (Pepcid IV), fenoldopam (Corlopam), heparin, hetastarch in electrolytes (Hextend), hydrocortisone sodium succinate (Solu-Cortef), labetalol, levofloxacin (Levaquin), linezolid (Zyvox), meperidine (Demerol), micafungin (Mycamine), morphine, nicardipine (Cardene IV), nitroglycerin IV, nitroprusside sodium, palonosetron (Aloxi), potassium chloride (KCl), propofol (Diprivan), remifentanil (Ultiva), theophylline, tigecycline (Tygacil), tirofiban (Aggrastat), vasopressin, warfarin (Coumadin).

RATE OF ADMINISTRATION

Bolus dose: 25 to 50 mg or fraction thereof over 1 minute. Too-rapid injection may cause seizures.

Infusion: Using an infusion pump delivers lidocaine in recommended doses. Adjust as indicated by progress in patient's condition. See Dose Adjustments and the Infusion Rate chart.

Lidocaine Infusion Rates						
Desired Dose	1 Gm in 500 mL Diluent (2 mg/mL)			1 Gm in 250 mL Diluent (4 mg/mL)		
mg/min	mg/hr	mL/min	mL/hr	mg/hr	mL/min	mL/hr
1	60 mg/hr	0.5 mL/min	30 mL/hr	60 mg/hr	0.25 mL/min	15 mL/hr
2	120 mg/hr	1 mL/min	60 mL/hr	120 mg/hr	0.5 mL/min	30 mL/hr
3	180 mg/hr	1.5 mL/min	90 mL/hr	180 mg/hr	0.75 mL/min	45 mL/hr
4	240 mg/hr	2 mL/min	120 mL/hr	240 mg/hr	1 mL/min	60 mL/hr
Pediatric infusion:	120 mg to 100 mL diluent = 1,200 mcg/mL					
	1 to 2.5 mL/kg/hr = 20 to 50 mcg/kg/min					

IV infusions in flexible plastic containers: *With or without a pump:* Do not hang in series connection, do not pressurize to increase flow rates without first fully evacuating residual air from the container, and do not use vented IV administration sets. All may result in air embolism.

ACTIONS

Intravenous lidocaine exerts an antiarrhythmic effect by increasing the electric stimulation threshold of the ventricle during diastole. In usual therapeutic doses, produces no change in myocardial contractility, systemic arterial pressure, or absolute refractory period. Decreases neuronal membrane permeability to sodium ions, resulting in inhibition of depolarization. Onset of action should occur within 2 minutes and last approximately 10 to 20 minutes. Terminal half-life is 1.5 to 2 hours. Elimination half-life of its major metabolites ranges from 2 to 10 hours. Primarily metabolized in the liver. Excreted in the urine with about 10% excreted unchanged and 90% excreted as metabolites. Crosses placental barrier and is secreted in breast milk.

INDICATIONS AND USES

Acute management of ventricular arrhythmias (e.g., PVCs, ventricular tachycardia [VT], ventricular fibrillation [VF]) occurring during acute myocardial infarction or during cardiac manipulations, such as cardiac surgery.

Unlabeled uses: Pediatric ventricular arrhythmias, seizures unresponsive to other therapy.

CONTRAINDICATIONS

Known sensitivity to lidocaine or any other local anesthetic of the amide type. ▪ Patients with Stokes-Adams syndrome, Wolff-Parkinson-White syndrome, or severe degrees of sinoatrial, atrioventricular, or intraventricular block. ▪ Solutions containing dextrose may be contraindicated in patients with known allergies to corn or corn products.

PRECAUTIONS

Administered by health care professionals knowledgeable in its use with access to adequate equipment and appropriate emergency drugs to monitor the patient and respond to any medical emergency. ▪ Use caution in patients with severe liver or renal disease; accumulation may occur and lead to toxicity, especially with repeated use. ▪ Use caution in hypovolemia, shock, all forms of heart block, and untreated bradycardia (see Contraindications). ▪ Systemic toxicity may result in CNS depression (sedation) or irritability (twitching). May progress to frank convulsions with respiratory depression and/or arrest. ▪ Vasopressors (e.g., dopamine) may be used if circulatory depression occurs. ▪ Has been associated with malignant hyperthermia. ▪ Hypersensitivity reactions, including anaphylaxis, have been reported. ▪ Oral antiarrhythmic drugs are preferred for maintenance.

Monitor: Monitor IV flow rate and the patient's ECG continuously. Therapeutic serum levels range from 1.5 to 5 mcg/mL; above 6 mcg/mL is usually toxic. ▪ Monitor electrolytes, fluid balance, and acid-base balance. Avoid fluid overload or disturbances of serum electrolyte concentrations; may interfere with cardiac conduction or result in CHF. ▪ Half-life increases over time. Reduce rate of continuous infusion after 24 hours and monitor blood levels. ▪ Keep patient lying down to reduce hypotensive effects. ▪ Discontinue lidocaine when patient's cardiac condition is stable or any signs of toxicity become apparent (signs of excessive depression of cardiac conductivity, such as prolongation of the PR interval, widening of the QRS interval, or appearance or aggravation of arrhythmias). ▪ Keep a bolus dose, 100 mg (5 mL), available at all times for emergency use in myocardial infarction. ▪ Monitor for S/S of hypersensitivity (e.g., large hives, rash, shortness of breath or troubled breathing, swelling of eyelids, lips, or face).

Patient Education: May cause dizziness; remain at bed rest; request assistance if ambulation permitted.

Maternal/Child: Category B: use during pregnancy only if clearly needed. ▪ Safety for use in breast-feeding and pediatric patients not established.

Elderly: Lower-end initial dosing and/or mg/kg dose may be appropriate. See Dose Adjustments. ▪ Decreased lidocaine clearance and increased sensitivity to adverse effects. ▪ Consider age-related renal and hepatic impairment.

DRUG/LAB INTERACTIONS
Administration with other **antiarrhythmic agents** (e.g., amiodarone [Nexterone], phenytoin [Dilantin], procainamide [Pronestyl], propranolol, quinidine) may result in additive or antagonistic cardiac effects, and toxic effects may be additive. ▪ **Phenytoin** may stimulate the hepatic metabolism of lidocaine; clinical significance not known. ▪ **Propranolol and cimetidine** (Tagamet) may decrease lidocaine clearance and increase lidocaine toxicity. Monitor lidocaine serum concentrations and monitor closely for signs of toxicity. ▪ Potentiates neuromuscular blockade of **muscle relaxants** (e.g., succinylcholine). ▪ Use caution in patients with **digitalis toxicity** and AV block.

SIDE EFFECTS
Apprehension; blurred or double vision; confusion; dizziness; drowsiness; euphoria; light-headedness; methemoglobinemia; sensations of heat, cold, and numbness; tinnitus; vomiting.
Major: Bradycardia, cardiac arrest, cardiovascular collapse, convulsions, hypotension, malignant hyperthermia (tachycardia, tachypnea, metabolic acidosis, fever), PR interval prolonged, QRS complex widening, respiratory depression, tremors, twitching, unconsciousness. Hypersensitivity reactions, including anaphylaxis, have been reported (infrequent). According to one source, cross-sensitivity between lidocaine and procainamide or between lidocaine and quinidine has not been reported.

ANTIDOTE
Notify the physician of any side effects. For major side effects, discontinue the drug immediately and institute appropriate measures. Ensure patency of airway and adequacy of ventilation. Treat anaphylaxis immediately with oxygen, epinephrine (Adrenalin), antihistamines (e.g., diphenhydramine [Benadryl]), vasopressors (e.g., dopamine), corticosteroids, albuterol, IV fluids, and ventilation equipment as indicated. To correct CNS stimulation use diazepam (Valium), rapid ultra-short-acting barbiturates (e.g., thiopental [Pentothal]), or if under anesthesia, muscle relaxants (e.g., succinylcholine). Use vasopresssors (e.g., dopamine) and IV fluids to correct hypotension. Maintain and support patient; resuscitate as necessary.

LINEZOLID

(lih-**NAY**-zoh-lid)

Zyvox

Antibacterial
(oxazolidinone)

USUAL DOSE

Dose and duration of therapy are based on diagnosis and designated pathogens. May be transferred to oral dosing when appropriate; no dose adjustment is necessary. See Precautions.

Recommended Linezolid Doses in Pediatric and Adult Patients			
	Dosage and Route of Administration		Recommended Duration of Treatment (Consecutive Days)
Infection*	Pediatric Patients† (Birth Through 11 Years of Age)	Adults and Adolescents (12 Years of Age and Older)	
Complicated skin and skin structure infections	10 mg/kg IV or PO‡ q 8 hr	600 mg IV or PO‡ q 12 hr	10 to 14
Community-acquired pneumonia, including concurrent bacteremia			
Nosocomial pneumonia			
Vancomycin-resistant *Enterococcus faecium* infections, including concurrent bacteremia	10 mg/kg IV or PO‡ q 8 hr	600 mg IV or PO‡ q 12 hr	14 to 28
Uncomplicated skin and skin structure infections	Less than 5 years: 10 mg/kg PO‡ q 8 hr 5-11 years: 10 mg/kg PO‡ q 12 hr	Adults: 400 mg PO‡ q 12 hr Adolescents: 600 mg PO‡ q 12 hr	10 to 14

*Due to the designated pathogens (see Indications and Uses and package insert).

†Neonates less than 7 days of age: Most preterm neonates less than 7 days of age (gestational age less than 34 weeks) have lower systemic linezolid clearance values and larger AUC values than many full-term neonates and older infants. These neonates should be initiated with a dosing regimen of 10 mg/kg q 12 hr. Consideration may be given to the use of 10 mg/kg q 8 hr regimen in neonates with a suboptimal clinical response. All neonatal patients should receive 10 mg/kg q 8 hr by 7 days of life.

‡Oral dosing using either linezolid tablets or linezolid for oral suspension.

PEDIATRIC DOSE

See Usual Dose and Maternal/Child.

DOSE ADJUSTMENTS

Dose adjustment based on age, gender, renal insufficiency, or hepatic insufficiency is not required. ▪ 30% of a dose is removed during a 3-hour dialysis session. Administer linezolid after hemodialysis.

DILUTION

Available in ready-to-use flexible plastic infusion bags in a foil laminate overwrap. Available as a 2 mg/mL solution in 200-, 400-, and 600-mg infusion bags. Before use, remove overwrap and check for leaks by squeezing the bag. Do not use flexible containers in series connections.

Storage: Store at CRT. Protect from light and freezing. Keep in overwrap until ready to use. Solution may exhibit a yellow color that can intensify with time. Will not adversely affect potency.

COMPATIBILITY
Consider any drug NOT listed as compatible to be INCOMPATIBLE until consulting a pharmacist; specific conditions may apply.
Manufacturer states, "Additives should not be added to the infusion bag." If administered through the same tubing as other medications, flush line before and after infusion of linezolid with a solution that is **compatible** with linezolid (e.g., D5W, NS, LR) and with any medications administered through the common line. Manufacturer lists as **incompatible** at the **Y-site** with amphotericin B (conventional), ceftriaxone (Rocephin), chlorpromazine (Thorazine), diazepam (Valium), erythromycin (Erythrocin), pentamidine, phenytoin (Dilantin), and sulfamethoxazole/trimethoprim.

One source suggests the following **compatibilities:**
Solutions: D5W, NS, LR.
Additive: *Not recommended by manufacturer.* Aztreonam (Azactam), cefazolin (Ancef), ceftazidime (Fortaz), ciprofloxacin (Cipro IV), gentamicin, levofloxacin (Levaquin), tobramycin.
Y-site: Acyclovir (Zovirax), alfentanil (Alfenta), amikacin, aminophylline, ampicillin, ampicillin/sulbactam (Unasyn), anidulafungin (Eraxis), aztreonam (Azactam), buprenorphine (Buprenex), butorphanol (Stadol), calcium gluconate, carboplatin (Paraplatin), caspofungin (Cancidas), cefazolin (Ancef), cefotetan, cefoxitin (Mefoxin), ceftazidime (Fortaz), ceftriaxone (Rocephin), cefuroxime (Zinacef), ciprofloxacin (Cipro IV), cisatracurium (Nimbex), cisplatin, clindamycin (Cleocin), cyclophosphamide (Cytoxan), cyclosporine (Sandimmune), cytarabine (ARA-C), dexamethasone (Decadron), dexmedetomidine (Precedex), digoxin (Lanoxin), diphenhydramine (Benadryl), dobutamine, dopamine, doripenem (Doribax), doxorubicin (Adriamycin), doxycycline, droperidol (Inapsine), enalaprilat (Vasotec IV), esmolol (Brevibloc), etoposide phosphate (Etopophos), famotidine (Pepcid IV), fenoldopam (Corlopam), fentanyl, fluconazole (Diflucan), fluorouracil (5-FU), furosemide (Lasix), ganciclovir (Cytovene IV), gemcitabine (Gemzar), gentamicin, granisetron (Kytril), heparin, hydrocortisone sodium succinate (Solu-Cortef), hydromorphone (Dilaudid), ifosfamide (Ifex), imipenem-cilastatin (Primaxin), labetalol, leucovorin calcium, levofloxacin (Levaquin), lidocaine, lorazepam (Ativan), magnesium sulfate, mannitol, meperidine (Demerol), meropenem (Merrem IV), mesna (Mesnex), methotrexate, methylprednisolone (Solu-Medrol), metoclopramide (Reglan), metronidazole (Flagyl IV), midazolam (Versed), mitoxantrone (Novantrone), morphine, nalbuphine, naloxone, nicardipine (Cardene IV), nitroglycerin IV, ondansetron (Zofran), paclitaxel (Taxol), pentobarbital (Nembutal), phenobarbital (Luminal), piperacillin/tazobactam (Zosyn), potassium chloride (KCl), prochlorperazine (Compazine), promethazine (Phenergan), propranolol, ranitidine (Zantac), remifentanil (Ultiva), sodium bicarbonate, sufentanil (Sufenta), theophylline, tigecycline (Tygacil), tobramycin, vancomycin, vasopressin, vecuronium, verapamil, vincristine, zidovudine (AZT, Retrovir).

RATE OF ADMINISTRATION
Administer as an infusion over 30 to 120 minutes. Flush line before and after administration if indicated; see Compatibility.

ACTIONS
A synthetic antibacterial agent. The first agent of a new class of antibiotics, the oxazolidinones. Clinically useful in the treatment of infections caused by aerobic gram-positive bacteria. See Indications and Uses and manufacturer's literature. Inhibits bacterial protein synthesis through a mechanism of action different from that of other antibacterial agents; therefore cross-resistance between linezolid and other classes of antibiotics is unlikely. Bacteriostatic against enterococci and staphylococci. Bactericidal against most strains of streptococci. Readily distributes into well-perfused tissues. Metabolized to two inactive metabolites. Metabolic pathway is not fully understood. Half-life is 4.8 hours. Approximately 30% of a dose is excreted in the urine as linezolid and 50% is excreted as metabolites.

INDICATIONS AND USES

Treatment of adults, adolescents, and other pediatric patients with the following infections caused by susceptible strains of the designated microorganisms: vancomycin-resistant *Enterococcus faecium* infections, including cases with concurrent bacteremia; nosocomial pneumonia caused by *Staphylococcus aureus* (methicillin-susceptible and methicillin-resistant strains) or *Streptococcus pneumoniae* (including multidrug-resistant strains [MDRSP]); complicated skin and skin-structure infections (including diabetic foot infections without concomitant osteomyelitis) caused by *Staphylococcus aureus* (methicillin-susceptible and methicillin-resistant strains), *Streptococcus pyogenes,* or *Streptococcus agalactiae;* uncomplicated skin and skin-structure infections caused by *Staphylococcus aureus* (methicillin-susceptible strains only) or *Streptococcus pyogenes;* and community-acquired pneumonia caused by *Streptococcus pneumoniae* (including multidrug-resistant strains [MDRSP] and cases with concurrent bacteremia) or *Staphylococcus aureus* (methicillin-susceptible strains only). ▪ Treatment of decubitus ulcers has not been studied. ▪ Given orally to treat uncomplicated skin and skin-structure infections. ▪ Not indicated for treatment of gram-negative infections. Critical that specific gram-negative therapy be initiated immediately if a concomitant gram-negative pathogen is documented or suspected. ▪ Not approved for and should not be used for treatment of patients with catheter-related bloodstream infections or catheter-site infections.

CONTRAINDICATIONS

History of hypersensitivity to linezolid or any of its components. ▪ Avoid use in patients taking any medicinal products that inhibit monoamine oxidase A or B (e.g., isocarboxazid [Marplan], phenelzine [Nardil]) or within 2 weeks of taking any such product. ▪ Unless closely monitored for potential increases in BP, avoid use in patients with uncontrolled hypertension, pheochromocytoma, or thyrotoxicosis and/or in patients taking any of the following types of medications: directly and indirectly acting sympathomimetic agents (e.g., pseudoephedrine [Sudafed]), vasopressive agents (e.g., epinephrine [Adrenalin], norepinephrine [Levophed]), dopaminergic agents (e.g., dobutamine, dopamine); see Precautions and Drug/Lab Interactions. ▪ Unless closely monitored for S/S of serotonin syndrome or neuroleptic malignant syndrome–like (NMS-like) reactions, avoid use in patients with carcinoid syndrome and/or in patients taking any of the following medications: serotonin reuptake inhibitors (e.g., fluoxetine [Prozac], sertraline [Zoloft]), tricyclic antidepressants (e.g., amitriptyline [Elavil]), serotonin 5-HT$_1$ receptor agonists (e.g., triptans [e.g., sumatriptan (Imitrex)]), meperidine (Demerol), or buspirone (BuSpar); see Precautions and Drug/Lab Interactions.

PRECAUTIONS

Culture and sensitivity studies are indicated to determine susceptibility of the causative organism to linezolid. ▪ To reduce the development of drug-resistant bacteria and maintain its effectiveness, linezolid should be used to treat or prevent only those infections proven or strongly suspected to be caused by bacteria. ▪ Reports of vancomycin-resistant *Enterococcus faecium* (VRE) becoming resistant to linezolid during its clinical use have been published. ▪ There has been a report of methicillin-resistant *Staphylococcus aureus* (MRSA) developing resistance to linezolid during its clinical use. ▪ Combination therapy may be clinically indicated in treatment of nosocomial pneumonia or complicated skin and skin-structure infections if the documented or presumptive pathogens include gram-negative organisms. ▪ Should not be used for treatment of patients with catheter-related bloodstream infections or catheter site infections. ▪ Myelosuppression (including anemia, leukopenia, pancytopenia, and thrombocytopenia) has been reported; see Monitor. ▪ Hypoglycemia, including symptomatic episodes, has been reported in patients with diabetes who have been treated with insulin or oral hypoglycemic agents and linezolid; see Monitor and Drug/Lab Interactions. ▪ Use with caution in patients with renal failure. Although dose adjustments are not recommended in this patient population, the metabolites may accumulate. The clinical significance of this accumulation is unknown. Dose should be given after hemodialysis. ▪ Use with caution in patients with uncontrolled hypertension, severe hepatic insufficiency, pheochromocytoma, carcinoid syndrome, or untreated hyperthyroidism; see Contraindications. Use has not been studied in these patient populations. ▪ Safety and efficacy of linezolid given for longer than 28 days have not been evaluated. ▪ Neuropathy (peripheral and optic) has been reported, primarily in patients treated for longer than the maximum recommended duration of 28 days. May occur in patients treated with linezolid for shorter periods, as well as in patients treated for more than 28 days. ▪ Superinfection, caused by the overgrowth of nonsusceptible organisms, may occur with antibiotic use. Treat as indicated. ▪ *Clostridium difficile*–associated diarrhea (CDAD) has been reported. May range from mild diarrhea to fatal colitis. Consider in patients who present with diarrhea during or after treatment with linezolid. ▪ Lactic acidosis has been reported. In most cases, patients experienced repeated episodes of N/V. ▪ Serotonin syndrome and neuroleptic malignant syndrome–like (NMS-like) reactions have been reported in patients receiving linezolid and concomitant serotonergic agents; see Contraindications, Monitor, and Drug/Lab Interactions. ▪ Convulsions have been reported; however, a history of seizures was reported in some of the cases. ▪ See Monitor, Patient Education, and Drug/Lab Interactions.

Monitor: CBC with differential and platelet count should be monitored weekly, especially in patients who receive linezolid for longer than 2 weeks; those with pre-existing myelosuppression; those receiving concomitant drugs that produce bone marrow suppression (e.g., antineoplastics [cisplatin, gemcitabine (Gemzar)], chloramphenicol, immunosuppressants [e.g., azathioprine]) or affect platelet function (e.g., aspirin, epoprostenol [Flolan], NSAIDs [e.g., ibuprofen (Advil, Motrin), naproxen (Aleve, Naprosyn)], platelet aggregation inhibitors [e.g., abciximab (ReoPro), clopidogrel (Plavix), dipyridamole (Persantine), eptifibatide (Integrilin)], selected antibiotics [e.g., piperacillin], valproic acid [Depacon, Depakene]); or those with a chronic infection who have received previous or concomitant antibiotics. Consider discontinuing therapy in patients who develop or have worsening myelosuppression. Myelosuppression appears to be reversible following discontinuation of linezolid. ▪ Monitor patients with diabetes who are receiving insulin or hypoglycemic agents for hypoglycemia; see Drug/Lab Interactions. ▪ Monitoring of visual function is recommended in patients taking linezolid for extended periods (3 months or more). Prompt ophthalmic evaluation is recommended if symptoms of visual impairment appear (e.g., blurred vision, changes in visual acuity or color vision, or visual field defect). ▪ Monitor for S/S of lactic acidosis (e.g., recurrent N/V, unexplained acidosis, or a low bicarbonate level); immediate medical evaluation is indicated. ▪ Monitor for S/S of serotonin syndrome or NMS-like reactions (autonomic instability, hyperthermia, myoclonus, rigidity, and mental status changes that include extreme agitation progressing to delirium and coma) when administered concurrently with serotonergic agents; see Drug/Lab Interactions. ▪ Monitor dietary intake of tyramine; see Patient Education. Hypertension may result from excessive tyramine intake (less than 100 mg/day). ▪ See Precautions and Drug/Lab Interactions.

Patient Education: Avoid foods or beverages high in tyramine (e.g., aged cheeses, fermented or air-dried meats, sauerkraut, soy sauce, tap beers, red wines). ▪ Inform physician of any history of hypertension or seizures. See Precautions. ▪ Inform physician if taking any medications containing pseudoephedrine or phenylpropanolamine (found in many cold or allergy preparations or diet aids), if taking serotonin reuptake inhibitors (e.g., fluoxetine [Prozac], sertraline [Zoloft], paroxetine [Paxil]) or other antidepressants, or if taking an antidiabetic agent (e.g., insulin or an oral hypoglycemic agent). ▪ Promptly report diarrhea or bloody stools that occur during treatment or up to several months after an antibiotic has been discontinued; may indicate CDAD and require treatment. ▪ Report any vision changes promptly. See Drug Interactions.

Maternal/Child: Category C: safety for use in pregnancy and breast-feeding not established; benefits must outweigh risks. ▪ Volume of distribution is similar regardless of age in pediatric patients; however, clearance varies as a function of age. With the exception of preterm neonates less than 1 week of age, clearance is most rapid in the youngest age-groups (ranging from less than 1 week old to 11 years of age), resulting in lower single-dose systemic exposure (AUC) and a shorter half-life. ▪ Most preteerm neonates less than 7 days of age (gestational age less than 34 weeks) have lower systemic linezolid clearance values and larger AUC values than many full-term neonates and older infants; see Usual Dose. ▪ AUC values in patients from birth to 11 years of age dosed every 8 hours are similar to adolescents and adults dosed every 12 hours. ▪ Therapeutic concentrations are not consistent in CSF; not indicated for empiric treatment of CNS infections in pediatric patients.

Elderly: No overall difference in safety or effectiveness has been observed between these patients and younger patients. Pharmacokinetics is not significantly altered in the elderly. See Dose Adjustments.

DRUG/LAB INTERACTIONS

Linezolid is a reversible, nonselective inhibitor of monoamine oxidase and therefore has the potential to interact with **adrenergic and serotonergic agents and with tyramine-containing foods.** ▪ A reversible enhancement of the pressor response to **indirect-acting sympathomimetic agents or vasopressor or dopaminergic agents** (e.g., pseudoephedrine [Sudafed], phenylpropanolamine, epinephrine [Adrenalin], dopamine) may be seen with concomitant use. Initial doses of adrenergic agents, such as epinephrine or dopamine, should be reduced and titrated to achieve the desired response; see Contraindications. ▪ Serotonin syndrome has been reported in patients receiving concurrent therapy with linezolid and **selective serotonin reuptake inhibitors** (SSRIs) (e.g., citalopram [Celexa], escitalopram [Lexapro], fluoxetine [Prozac], fluvoxamine [Luvox], paroxetine [Paxil], sertraline [Zoloft], and vilazodone [Viibryd]) or **serotonin norepinephrine reuptake inhibitors** (SNRIs) (e.g., duloxetine [Cymbalta], desvenlafaxine [Pristiq], venlafaxine [Effexor]). Linezolid use in patients taking serotonergic drugs should be limited to life-threatening or urgent situations in which linezolid is considered to be the drug of choice (e.g., treatment of vancomycin-resistant enterococcus [VRE] infections, serious infections such as nosocomial pneumonia, or complicated skin and skin structure infections, including cases caused by MRSA). The serotonergic agent should be stopped promptly when linezolid therapy is initiated. Patients should be monitored for the development of serotonin syndrome for 2 weeks (5 weeks if fluoxetine was taken) or until 24 hours after the last dose of linezolid, whichever comes first. If S/S of serotonin syndrome develop, consider discontinuing linezolid. Patients should also be monitored for specific symptoms due to discontinuation of the serotonergic agent; see prescribing information for the specific agent; see Contraindications and Monitor. ▪ May cause hypoglycemia with **insulin or hypoglycemic agents.** Dose reduction or discontinuation of the antidiabetic agent and/or discontinuation of linezolid may be indicated. ▪ Does not appear to induce, inhibit, or be induced by the cytochrome P_{450} system and should therefore not affect drugs metabolized by this system (e.g., warfarin [Coumadin], phenytoin [Dilantin]); however, coadministration with **rifampin** (Rifadin) led to an observed reduction in linezolid plasma concentrations. The mechanism is unclear. **Other strong inducers of hepatic enzymes** (e.g., carbamazepime [Tegretol], phenytoin [Dilantin], phenobarbital [Luminal]) may also cause a decrease in linezolid concentration. ▪ Has been coadministered with aztreonam (Azactam) and gentamicin. When linezolid was coadministered with either one of these agents, no alteration of pharmacokinetics occurred in either drug. ▪ Severe myelosuppression may occur with **bone marrow suppressants and other drugs that affect platelet function;** see Monitor.

SIDE EFFECTS
The most common side effects are anemia, diarrhea, headache, nausea, and vomiting. Other reported side effects include abdominal pain; CDAD; constipation; dizziness; dysgeusia (change in sense of taste); dyspepsia; fever; hypertension; increased AST, BUN, SCr, total bilirubin; insomnia; lactic acidosis; myelosuppression (anemia, leukopenia, neutropenia, pancytopenia, thrombocytopenia); neuropathy (peripheral and optic [optic neuropathy may progress to vision loss]); oral moniliasis; pruritus; rash; seizures; serotonin syndrome (cognitive dysfunction, hyperpyrexia, hyperreflexia, lack of coordination); tongue discoloration; vaginal moniliasis; and vomiting.

Post-Marketing: Anaphylaxis, angioedema, bullous skin disorders such as Stevens-Johnson syndrome, hypoglycemia (including symptomatic episodes), and superficial tooth and tongue discoloration.

ANTIDOTE
Keep physician informed of all side effects. Discontinue drug if indicated. If S/S of serotonin syndrome develop, consider discontinuing linezolid or the serotonergic agent. Consider discontinuing linezolid in patients who develop or have worsening myelosuppression. Mild cases of CDAD may respond to discontinuation of linezolid. Treat CDAD with fluids, electrolytes, protein supplements, and oral vancomycin (Vancocin) or metronidazole (Flagyl) as indicated. In severe cases, surgical evaluation may be indicated. In the event of an overdose, initiate supportive care and maintain glomerular filtration. Both linezolid and its metabolites are partially removed by hemodialysis.

LORAZEPAM
(lor-**AYZ**-eh-pam)

Benzodiazepine
Sedative-hypnotic
Antianxiety agent
Anticonvulsant
Amnestic
Skeletal muscle relaxant
Antiemetic

Ativan, Lorazepam PF

USUAL DOSE

Dose must be individualized, especially when used in conjunction with other medications that may cause CNS depression. See Dose Adjustments, Precautions, and Drug/Lab Interactions.

Antianxiety/amnestic: 2 mg or 0.044 mg/kg of body weight, whichever is smaller, 15 to 20 minutes before procedure. For greater lack of recall 0.05 mg/kg up to 4 mg may be given. 2 mg is usually the maximum dose for patients over 50 years of age.

Sedation: 2 mg as the initial dose (may not be necessary if patient is receiving intermittent benzodiazepines [e.g., diazepam, midazolam]). Follow with an infusion of 0.5 to 1 mg/hr (0.25 to 0.5 mg/hr if less agitated or has cardiorespiratory problems). Titrate to achieve adequate sedation. Increase in 1 mg/hr increments. Up to 5 to 10 mg/hr has been used. When sedation is adequate, reduce to lowest amount needed.

Status epilepticus: 4 mg as the initial dose. May repeat once in 10 to 15 minutes if seizures continue. One source suggests a maximum dose of 8 mg within a 12-hour period. Experience with further doses is very limited. Additional intervention (e.g., concomitant administration of phenytoin) may be required. Another source suggests 0.05 mg/kg of body weight to a total dose of 4 mg. May repeat once in 10 to 15 minutes. If still not effective, use another anticonvulsant agent (e.g., phenytoin). Do not exceed a total dose of 8 mg in 12 hours.

High-dose therapy for refractory status epilepticus (unlabeled): With continuous EEG monitoring, begin a continuous infusion of lorazepam at 1 mg/hr. Increase by 1 mg/hr at 15-minute intervals until patient is seizure free. Maintain seizure-free state with lorazepam for 24 hours. Use therapeutic doses of phenytoin and phenobarbital in addition to lorazepam. At the end of 24 hours, begin to reduce the lorazepam by 1 mg/hr at hourly intervals. Observe closely and monitor EEG for signs of recurrent seizures. Repeat process if seizures recur.

Management of emetic-inducing chemotherapy (unlabeled): 0.025 mg/kg to 0.05 mg/kg (maximum dose is 4 mg) 30 minutes before chemotherapy is begun. Supplement with oral lorazepam 1 to 2 mg/hr as needed. Another source suggests 1.5 mg/M^2 (up to a maximum of 3 mg/M^2) over 5 minutes. Administer 30 to 45 minutes before administration of antineoplastic agent. May be given in combination with other antiemetics (e.g., ondansetron [Zofran], dexamethasone). Repeat every 4 hours as needed.

PEDIATRIC DOSE

Safety for use in pediatric patients under 12 years of age has not been fully studied, but it has been used for status epilepticus in neonates, infants, and children; see Maternal/Child.

Sedation: 0.05 mg/kg up to a maximum of 2 mg/dose every 4 to 8 hours.

Status epilepticus (unlabeled): *Neonates, infants, and children:* 0.05 to 0.1 mg/kg up to a maximum of 4 mg/dose. Another source suggests a maximum dose of 2 mg/dose. May repeat 0.05 mg/kg once in 10 to 15 minutes if needed.

Antiemetic, adjunct therapy (unlabeled): 0.02 to 0.05 mg/kg/dose up to a maximum of 2 mg/dose. May repeat every 6 hours as needed.

DOSE ADJUSTMENTS

Start with a small dose in the elderly and increase gradually based on response. Consider the potential for decreased organ function and concomitant disease or drug therapy. ▪

Dose adjustments are not required with impaired liver function. ▪ Dose adjustments are not required with impaired renal function unless frequent doses are given over a short period of time. ▪ Reduced dose may be indicated in the presence of other CNS depressants. ▪ Reduce dose by 50% when given concurrently with probenecid or valproate (Depacon). ▪ See Drug/Lab Interactions.

DILUTION

IV injection: Dilute immediately before use with an equal volume of SWFI, D5W, or NS. Do not shake vigorously; will result in air entrapment. Gently invert repeatedly until completely in solution. May be given by IV injection or through Y-tube or three-way stopcock of infusion tubing.

Infusion (unlabeled): Has been further diluted in D5W or NS and given as an infusion. Best solubility is in concentrations of 0.1 mg/mL or 0.2 mg/mL.

Lorazepam Guidelines for Dilution and Infusion				
Base Concentration	2 mg/mL		4 mg/mL	
Desired Concentration	0.1 mg/mL	0.2 mg/mL	0.1 mg/mL	0.2 mg/mL
Volume of diluent required for each 1 mL lorazepam	19 mL	9 mL	39 mL	19 mL

Very viscous; mix well and observe for crystallization. Crystallization does occur and is thought to be due to propylene glycol preservative. May occur more frequently in NS than in D5W and with 4-mg/mL vials of lorazepam base than with 2-mg/mL vials. Prepare only enough to last for 12 hours. If necessary for fluid restriction, a 2-mg/mL vial has been stable for 24 hours when diluted in a 1 mg (lorazepam base) to 1 mL diluent (D5W preferred). Monitor carefully.

Storage: Refrigerate before dilution; protect from light. Use only freshly prepared solutions; discard if discolored or precipitate forms. Infusions stable at room temperature for 12 hours in plastic, 24 hours in glass.

COMPATIBILITY   (Underline Indicates Conflicting Compatibility Information)

Consider any drug NOT listed as compatible to be INCOMPATIBLE until consulting a pharmacist; specific conditions may apply.

One source suggests the following **compatibilities:**

Additive: Levetiracetam (Keppra).

Y-site: Acetaminophen (Ofirmev), acyclovir (Zovirax), albumin (Albuminar), allopurinol (Aloprim), amifostine (Ethyol), amikacin, amiodarone (Nexterone), amphotericin B cholesteryl (Amphotec), atracurium (Tracrium), bivalirudin (Angiomax), bumetanide, caspofungin (Cancidas), cefotaxime (Claforan), ceftaroline (Teflaro), ciprofloxacin (Cipro IV), cisatracurium (Nimbex), cladribine (Leustatin), dexamethasone (Decadron), dexmedetomidine (Precedex), diltiazem (Cardizem), dobutamine, docetaxel (Taxotere), dopamine, doripenem (Doribax), doxorubicin liposomal (Doxil), epinephrine (Adrenalin), erythromycin (Erythrocin), etomidate (Amidate), etoposide phosphate (Etopophos), famotidine (Pepcid IV), fenoldopam (Corlopam), fentanyl, filgrastim (Neupogen), fluconazole (Diflucan), fludarabine (Fludara), foscarnet (Foscavir), fosphenytoin (Cerebyx), furosemide (Lasix), gemcitabine (Gemzar), gentamicin, granisetron (Kytril), heparin, hetastarch in electrolytes (Hextend), hydrocortisone sodium succinate (Solu-Cortef), hydromorphone (Dilaudid), labetalol, levofloxacin (Levaquin), linezolid (Zyvox), melphalan (Alkeran), methadone (Dolophine), metronidazole (Flagyl IV), micafungin (Mycamine), midazolam (Versed), milrinone (Primacor), morphine, nicardipine (Cardene IV), nitroglycerin IV, norepinephrine (Levophed), oxaliplatin (Eloxatin), paclitaxel (Taxol), palonosetron (Aloxi), pancuronium, pemetrexed (Alimta), piperacillin/tazobactam (Zosyn), potassium chloride (KCl), propofol (Diprivan), ranitidine (Zantac), remifentanil (Ultiva), sulfamethoxazole/trimethoprim, tacrolimus (Prograf), teniposide

(Vumon), thiotepa, vancomycin, vecuronium, vinorelbine (Navelbine), zidovudine (AZT, Retrovir).

RATE OF ADMINISTRATION

IV injection: Each 2 mg or fraction thereof over 1 to 5 minutes.

Infusion: Use a microdrip or infusion pump for accuracy to deliver desired dose and/or titrate to desired level of sedation.

Pediatric rate: 2 mg/min is the maximum rate of administration.

ACTIONS

A benzodiazepine with antianxiety, sedative, and anticonvulsant effects. Inhibits ability to recall events. Interacts with the GABA-benzodiazepine receptor complex in the brain. Effective in 15 to 30 minutes. Effects last an average of 6 to 8 hours, but may last as long as 12 to 24 hours. Half-life is 9.5 to 19.5 hours. Distributed in body fluids. Metabolized by the liver to inactive metabolites; some is slowly excreted in urine. Crosses the placental barrier. Excreted in breast milk.

INDICATIONS AND USES

Preanesthetic medication for adult patients. ▪ Produce sedation, relieve anxiety, and provide anterograde amnesia. ▪ Management of status epilepticus.

Unlabeled uses: High-dose therapy for status epilepticus clinically or EEG diagnosed as refractory to high doses of phenytoin and phenobarbital. ▪ Management of emetic-inducing chemotherapy. ▪ Antipanic agent. ▪ Treatment of alcohol withdrawal. ▪ Amnestic during endoscopic procedures. ▪ Skeletal muscle relaxant adjunct. ▪ Treatment of tension headaches.

CONTRAINDICATIONS

Hypersensitivity to benzodiazepines (diazepam [Valium]) or the components (e.g., polyethylene glycol, propylene glycol, or benzyl alcohol). Patients with acute narrow-angle glaucoma, sleep apnea syndrome, or severe respiratory insufficiency (except patients requiring relief of anxiety and/or diminished recall of events while being mechanically ventilated). Intra-arterial injection.

PRECAUTIONS

Rapidly and completely absorbed IM. ▪ When given as a sedative, patient is able to respond to simple instructions. ▪ Increased risk of respiratory depression; airway support, emergency drugs, and equipment must be immediately available. ▪ Dependence is possible with prolonged use or high dose. ▪ Use with extreme caution in the elderly, the very ill, or patients with limited pulmonary reserve; risk of hypoventilation and/or hypoxic cardiac arrest is increased. ▪ Use as a premedicant before local or regional anesthesia may cause excessive drowsiness and interfere with assessment of levels of anesthesia. More likely to occur with doses greater than 0.05 mg/kg or when narcotic agents are used concomitantly. ▪ Use with caution in patients with mild to moderate renal or hepatic disease. ▪ There have been reports of possible propylene and polyethylene glycol toxicity (e.g., lactic acidosis, hyperosmolality, hypotension, acute tubular necrosis) when lorazepam has been administered at higher than recommended doses. Patients with renal impairment may be at increased risk of developing toxicity. Paradoxical reactions may occur. ▪ See Antidote (e.g., risk of seizure with flumazenil).

Monitor: To reduce incidence of thrombophlebitis, avoid smaller veins. Extravasation is hazardous; arterial administration may cause arteriospasms and gangrene and/or require amputation. ▪ Bed rest required for a minimum of 3 hours after IV injection and assistance required for up to 8 hours. ▪ Monitor and maintain patent airway. Respiratory assistance and flumazenil (Romazicon) must be available. ▪ Establish an IV and monitor vital signs. **Status epilepticus:** In addition to the above, observe for and correct any other possible cause of seizure (e.g., hypoglycemia, hyponatremia, other metabolic disorders). ▪ Sedative effects may add to the impairment of consciousness seen in the postictal state (e.g., after a seizure). ▪ Neurologic consult is suggested for any patient who fails to regain consciousness.

Patient Education: May produce drowsiness or dizziness; request assistance with ambulation and use caution when performing tasks that require alertness for 24 to 48 hours or until the effects of the drug have subsided. ▪ Avoid use of alcohol or other CNS depressants (e.g., antihistamines, barbiturates) for 24 to 48 hours or until the effects of the drug have subsided. ▪ May be habit-forming with long-term use or high-dose therapy. ▪ Has amnestic potential; may impair memory. ▪ Consider birth control options.

Maternal/Child: Category D: avoid pregnancy. May cause fetal damage. Not recommended during pregnancy, labor and delivery, breast-feeding, or in pediatric patients under 12 years of age. ▪ Has FDA approval for treatment of status epilepticus in adults over 18 years of age. Safety for use in pediatric patients has not been fully studied, but has been used for status epilepticus in neonates, infants, and children. ▪ May cause paradoxical excitement in pediatric patients. ▪ Seizure activity and myoclonus have been reported in low-birth-weight neonates. ▪ Contains benzyl alcohol, which has been associated with a fatal "gasping syndrome" in neonates. ▪ Half-life prolonged in pediatric patients.

Elderly: Dosing should be cautious in the elderly; see Dose Adjustments. ▪ More sensitive to therapeutic and adverse effects (e.g., ataxia, dizziness, oversedation). ▪ IV injection may be more likely to cause apnea, bradycardia, CNS depression, hypotension, respiratory depression, and cardiac arrest. ▪ See Precautions and Drug/Lab Interactions.

DRUG/LAB INTERACTIONS

Concurrent use with **other CNS depressants** such as alcohol, antihistamines, barbiturates, MAO inhibitors (e.g., selegiline [Eldepryl]), narcotics (e.g., morphine, meperidine [Demerol], fentanyl), phenothiazines (e.g., prochlorperazine [Compazine]), and tricyclic antidepressants (e.g., imipramine [Tofranil-PM]) may result in additive effects for up to 48 hours. Reduced dose may be indicated. ▪ Concurrent administration with **valproate** (Depacon) **or probenecid** will decrease clearance of lorazepam. Reduce dose of lorazepam by one half in patients receiving concurrent valproate or probenecid. ▪ Apnea, arrhythmia, bradycardia, cardiac arrest, coma, and death have been reported when used concurrently with **haloperidol** (Haldol). ▪ Significant hypotension, respiratory depression, and stupor have been reported (rare) with concomitant use of **loxapine** (Loxapac). ▪ May increase serum concentrations of **digoxin and phenytoin** (Dilantin); monitor digoxin and phenytoin serum levels. ▪ Use with **rifampin** (Rifadin) increases clearance and reduces effects of benzodiazepines. ▪ **Theophyllines** (Aminophylline) antagonize the sedative effects of benzodiazepines. ▪ Marked sedation, salivation, ataxia and, rarely, death have been reported with concomitant use of **clozapine** (Clozaril) and lorazepam. ▪ Estrogen-containing **oral contraceptives** increase clearance and decrease effects. ▪ Inhibits antiparkinson effectiveness of **levodopa.** ▪ Incidence of hallucinations and irrational behavior and an increased incidence of sedation have been observed with concurrent use of scopolamine.

SIDE EFFECTS

Airway obstruction, apnea, blurred vision, confusion, crying, delirium, depression, excessive drowsiness, hallucinations, hypotension, injection site reaction, respiratory depression, restlessness, somnolence.

Overdose: Ataxia, coma, hypnosis, hypotension, hypotonia and, very rarely, death.

ANTIDOTE

Notify physician of all symptoms. Reduction of dose may be required. Treat hypotension with dopamine or norepinephrine (Levophed). In overdose, flumazenil (Romazicon) will reverse all sedative effects of benzodiazepines. See flumazenil monograph (risk of seizures). A patent airway, artificial ventilation, oxygen therapy, and other symptomatic and supportive treatment must be instituted promptly. Monitor vital signs and fluid status carefully. Forced diuresis and osmotic diuretics (e.g., mannitol) may increase rate of lorazepam elimination. The value of dialysis has not been adequately determined.

LYMPHOCYTE IMMUNE GLOBULIN BBW

Immunosuppressant

(**LIM**-foh-sight ih-**MUNE GLAW**-byoo-lin)

Anti-Thymocyte Globulin [Equine], Atgam

pH 6.8

USUAL DOSE

Intradermal skin test required before administration. Use 0.1 mL of a 1:1,000 dilution in NS and a saline control. If a systemic reaction (rash, dyspnea) occurs, do not administer. If a limited reaction (10-mm wheal or erythema) occurs, proceed with extreme caution. Anaphylaxis can occur even if skin test is negative.

Range is 10 to 30 mg/kg of body weight/24 hr. Actual potency and activity may vary from lot to lot. Given concomitantly with other immunosuppressive therapy (antimetabolites such as azathioprine and corticosteroids).

Delay onset of renal allograft rejection: 15 mg/kg/24 hr for 14 days, then every other day for 7 more doses. Initial dose should be given 24 hours before or after the transplant.

Treat allograft rejection: 10 to 15 mg/kg/24 hr for 14 days, then every other day for 7 more doses (optional). Initial dose should be given when first rejection episode is diagnosed.

Aplastic anemia: 10 to 20 mg/kg/24 hr for 8 to 14 days. Additional alternate-day therapy up to a total of 21 doses may be given.

PEDIATRIC DOSE

Experience with pediatric patients is limited and unlabeled. Intradermal skin test required; see Usual Dose. Has been administered to treat aplastic anemia, to manage renal allograft rejection, and to delay onset of renal allograft rejection using mg/kg doses recommended for adults.

DILUTION

Total daily dose must be further diluted with NS, D5/^{1}/$_4$NS, or D5/^{1}/$_2$NS for infusion. Invert solution while injecting drug so contact is not made with air in infusion bottle. Gently rotate diluted solution. Do not shake. Concentration should not exceed 4 mg/mL. May be infused into a vascular shunt, AV fistula, or high-flow central vein.

Filters: Use of a 0.2- to 1-micron filter recommended.

Storage: Keep refrigerated before and after dilution. Discard diluted solution after 24 hours.

COMPATIBILITY

Manufacturer states lymphocyte immune globulin may precipitate in dextrose solutions and may be unstable with highly acidic solutions.

RATE OF ADMINISTRATION

A total daily dose equally distributed over a minimum of 4 hours.

ACTIONS

A lymphocyte-selective immunosuppressant. Reduces the number of thymus-dependent lymphocytes and contains low concentrations of antibodies against other formed elements in blood. Effective without causing severe lymphopenia. Supports an increase in the frequency of resolution of an acute rejection episode. Has a serum half-life of 5 to 8 days.

INDICATIONS AND USES

Management of allograft rejection in renal transplant patients. ▪ Adjunctive to other immunosuppressive therapy to delay onset of initial rejection episode. ▪ Treatment of moderate to severe aplastic anemia in patients who are not candidates for bone marrow transplant.

CONTRAINDICATIONS

Systemic hypersensitivity reaction to previous injection of lymphocyte immune globulin or any other equine gamma-globulin preparation.

PRECAUTIONS

Administered only under the direction of a physician experienced in immunosuppressive therapy and management of renal transplant patients in a facility with adequate laboratory and supportive medical resources. ▪ Use caution in repeated courses of therapy; observe for signs of hypersensitivity reactions.

Monitor: Will cause chemical phlebitis in peripheral veins. ▪ Monitor carefully for signs of infection, leukopenia, or thrombocytopenia. Thrombocytopenia is usually transient in renal transplant patients. Platelet transfusions may be necessary in patients with aplastic anemia. Notify physician immediately so prompt treatment can be instituted and/or drug discontinued. ▪ Prophylactic antibiotics may be indicated pending results of C/S. ▪ Masked reactions may occur as dose of corticosteroids and antimetabolites is decreased. Observe carefully. ▪ Antihistamines (e.g., diphenhydramine [Benadryl]) may be required to control itching. ▪ Anaphylaxis can occur at any time. Monitor closely for S/S of a hypersensitivity reaction. Emergency equipment and supplies must be at bedside.

Patient Education: See Appendix D, p. 1333.

Maternal/Child: Category C: no studies conducted in pregnant patients. Use caution. ▪ Safety for use in breast-feeding not established. ▪ Limited experience on use in pediatric patients; see Pediatric Dose.

DRUG/LAB INTERACTIONS

See Monitor.

SIDE EFFECTS

Full range of hypersensitivity reactions, including anaphylaxis, is possible. Arthralgia, back pain, chest pain, chills, clotted AV fistula, diarrhea, dyspnea, fever, headache, hypotension, infusion site pain, leukopenia, nausea, night sweats, pruritus, rash, stomatitis, thrombocytopenia, thrombophlebitis, urticaria, vomiting, wheal and flare. Other reactions occur in fewer than 1% of patients.

ANTIDOTE

Notify physician of all side effects. Discontinue if anaphylaxis, severe and unremitting thrombocytopenia, and/or severe and unremitting leukopenia occur; see Monitor. May be discontinued if infection or hemolysis present even if appropriately treated. Clinically significant hemolysis may require erythrocyte transfusion, IV mannitol, furosemide, sodium bicarbonate, and fluids. Prophylactic or therapeutic antihistamines (e.g., diphenhydramine [Benadryl]) or corticosteroids should control chills caused by release of endogenous leukocyte pyrogens. Treat anaphylaxis immediately. Epinephrine (Adrenalin), diphenhydramine (Benadryl), oxygen, vasopressors (e.g., dopamine), corticosteroids, and ventilation equipment must always be available. Resuscitate as necessary.

MAGNESIUM SULFATE
(mag-**NEE**-see-um **SUL**-fayt)

Electrolyte replenisher
Anticonvulsant
Antiarrhythmic
Uterine relaxant

pH 3.5 to 6.5

USUAL DOSE
Individualize dose based on patient requirement and response. Discontinue as soon as desired response is obtained.

Eclampsia: Several regimens in literature. 4 Gm (32 mEq [40 mL of a 10% solution]) over 3 to 4 minutes. Subsequent doses may be given IM every 4 hours as needed, or a continuous infusion of 1 to 2 Gm/hr may be initiated. Do not exceed 30 to 40 Gm/24 hr. Frequent monitoring required; see Dose Adjustments, Precautions, and Monitor.

Seizures associated with epilepsy, glomerulonephritis, or hypothyroidism: 1 Gm.

Hypomagnesemia (mild): 1 Gm every 6 hours for 4 doses.

Hypomagnesemia (severe): 5 Gm (40 mEq) in 1,000 mL D5W or NS as an infusion evenly distributed over 3 hours.

Hyperalimentation in adults: 8 to 24 mEq/24 hr (1 to 3 Gm).

Paroxysmal atrial tachycardia (unlabeled): 3 to 4 Gm (30 to 40 mL of a 10% solution) over 30 seconds with extreme caution. Reserve for patients in whom simpler measures have failed and in whom there is no evidence of myocardial damage.

Reduction of cerebral edema (unlabeled): 2.5 Gm (25 mL of a 10% solution).

Cardiac arrest (hypomagnesemia or torsades de pointes): AHA recommends 1 to 2 Gm (2 to 4 mL of a 50% solution) diluted in 10 mL D5W over 15 minutes.

Torsades de pointes: AHA recommends a loading dose of 1 to 2 Gm in 50 to 100 mL D5W as an infusion over 5 to 60 minutes. Follow with an infusion of 0.5 to 1 Gm/hr and titrate to control the torsades.

Barium poisoning: 1 to 2 Gm.

Alleviate bronchospasm in acute asthma (unlabeled): 2 Gm given IV over 20 minutes. Usually given concurrently with inhaled albuterol (Proventil) and IV corticosteroids.

PEDIATRIC DOSE
All pediatric doses are unlabeled; see Maternal/Child.

Hypomagnesemia or hypocalcemia: 25 to 50 mg/kg of body weight. May repeat at 4- to 6-hour intervals for 3 or 4 doses. Maximum recommended single dose is 2 Gm. Maintain with 30 to 60 mg/kg/24 hr (approximately 0.25 to 0.5 mEq/kg/24 hr). Maximum dose is 1 Gm/24 hr.

Pulseless VT with torsades de pointes: AHA recommends 25 to 50 mg/kg IV push. A 50% solution equals 500 mg/mL. Maximum recommended dose is 2 Gm.

Status asthmaticus: 25 to 50 mg/kg as an infusion over 15 to 30 minutes. A 50% solution equals 500 mg/mL. Another source recommends 25 to 75 mg/kg as an infusion over 20 minutes. Maximum recommended dose is 2 Gm.

Acute nephritis in pediatric patients: 100 to 200 mg/kg as a 1% to 3% solution (1 Gm in 100 mL = 1% solution, 3 Gm in 100 mL = 3%). One-half dose should be given slowly over 15 to 20 minutes. Complete balance of dose within 1 hour. Monitor BP closely.

Hyperalimentation: *Infants:* 2 to 10 mEq (0.25 to 1.25 Gm daily).

Other pediatric patients: 0.25 to 0.5 mEq/24 hr or 30 to 60 mg/kg/24 hr.

DOSE ADJUSTMENTS
Reduce dose of other CNS depressants (e.g., narcotics, barbiturates) when given in conjunction with magnesium sulfate. ▪ Reduce dose in impaired renal function and in the elderly. ▪ Decrease maximum daily dose to 10 Gm/24 hr in patients with severe renal insufficiency. Monitor serum magnesium levels.

DILUTION

Concentrated solutions must be diluted to a concentration of 20% (200 mg/mL) or less for IV administration. D5W and NS are the most common diluents. Available in various containers in multiple concentrations and also in multiple concentrations as a premixed solution in sterile water for injection or in 5% dextrose. See Usual Dose for specific dilutions. May be given through Y-tube or three-way stopcock of infusion set.

Storage: Store at CRT. Protect from freezing. Contains no preservative. Discard any unused solution.

COMPATIBILITY   (Underline Indicates Conflicting Compatibility Information)

Consider any drug NOT listed as compatible to be INCOMPATIBLE until consulting a pharmacist; specific conditions may apply.

Will form various precipitates with alkali carbonates and bicarbonates, alkali hydroxides, arsenates, barium, calcium, clindamycin (Cleocin), hydrocortisone sodium succinate (Solu-Cortef), lead, phosphates, salicylates, strontium, and tartrates. Use caution; consult pharmacist.

One source suggests the following **compatibilities:**

Additive: Calcium chloride, calcium gluconate, chloramphenicol (Chloromycetin), cisplatin, heparin, hydrocortisone sodium succinate (Solu-Cortef), isoproterenol (Isuprel), meropenem (Merrem IV), methyldopa, norepinephrine (Levophed), penicillin G potassium, potassium chloride (KCl), sodium bicarbonate, verapamil.

Y-site: Acyclovir (Zovirax), aldesleukin (Proleukin), amifostine (Ethyol), amikacin, amiodarone (Nexterone), ampicillin, aztreonam (Azactam), bivalirudin (Angiomax), caspofungin (Cancidas), cefazolin (Ancef), cefotaxime (Claforan), cefoxitin (Mefoxin), ceftaroline (Teflaro), chloramphenicol (Chloromycetin), ciprofloxacin (Cipro IV), cisatracurium (Nimbex), clindamycin (Cleocin), dexmedetomidine (Precedex), dobutamine, docetaxel (Taxotere), doripenem (Doribax), doxorubicin liposomal (Doxil), doxycycline, enalaprilat (Vasotec IV), erythromycin (Erythrocin), esmolol (Brevibloc), etoposide phosphate (Etopophos), famotidine (Pepcid IV), fenoldopam (Corlopam), fludarabine (Fludara), gallium nitrate (Ganite), gentamicin, granisetron (Kytril), heparin, hetastarch in electrolytes (Hextend), hydrocortisone sodium succinate (Solu-Cortef), hydromorphone (Dilaudid), 6% hydroxyethyl starch (Voluven), idarubicin (Idamycin), insulin (regular), labetalol, levofloxacin (Levaquin), linezolid (Zyvox), meperidine (Demerol), metronidazole (Flagyl IV), micafungin (Mycamine), milrinone (Primacor), morphine, nafcillin (Nallpen), nicardipine (Cardene IV), nitroprusside sodium, ondansetron (Zofran), oxacillin (Bactocill), oxaliplatin (Eloxatin), paclitaxel (Taxol), penicillin G potassium, piperacillin/tazobactam (Zosyn), potassium chloride (KCl), propofol (Diprivan), remifentanil (Ultiva), sargramostim (Leukine), sulfamethoxazole/trimethoprim, telavancin (Vibativ), thiotepa, tobramycin, vancomycin.

RATE OF ADMINISTRATION

IV injection: 150 mg/min (1.5 mL of a 10% solution or its equivalent) over at least 1 minute or as directed in Usual Dose. Too-rapid administration may cause hypermagnesemia, hypotension, and asystole.

IV infusion: As directed in Usual Dose.

ACTIONS

An important cofactor for enzymatic reactions and plays an important role in neurochemical transmission and muscular excitability. A CNS depressant. It prevents or controls seizures by blocking neuromuscular transmission and decreasing the amount of acetylcholine release. Acts peripherally to produce vasodilation and may cause a lowering of BP at higher doses. Onset of anticonvulsant action is immediate and lasts for about 30 minutes. Excreted in the urine. Secreted in breast milk. Crosses the placental barrier.

INDICATIONS AND USES

Replacement therapy in magnesium deficiency (e.g., acute hypomagnesemia accompanied by signs of tetany similar to those seen in hypocalcemia). ▪ Correction or prevention of hypomagnesemia in patients receiving TPN. ▪ Prevention and control of seizures in pre-eclampsia and eclampsia.

Unlabeled uses: Prevention and control of convulsive states (epilepsy, glomerulonephritis, hypothyroidism). ▪ Cerebral edema. ▪ Acute nephritis in pediatric patients to control hypertension, encephalopathy, and convulsions. ▪ Treatment of torsades de pointes, ventricular tachycardia, and ventricular fibrillation (VT/VF) caused by hypomagnesemia. ▪ Counteract muscle-stimulating effects of barium poisoning. ▪ Treatment of paroxysmal atrial tachycardia. ▪ Treatment of acute asthma in patients who do not respond to conventional therapy.

CONTRAINDICATIONS

Presence of heart block or myocardial damage. ▪ Within 2 hours of delivery; see Maternal/Child.

PRECAUTIONS

Continuous administration of magnesium sulfate beyond 5 to 7 days to pregnant women can lead to hypocalcemia and bone abnormalities in the developing fetus, including skeletal demineralization, osteopenia, and neonatal fracture. ▪ Use caution in impaired renal function; may result in magnesium toxicity. ▪ Some solutions may contain aluminum. In impaired kidney function, aluminum may reach toxic levels. Premature neonates are particularly at risk because of their immature kidneys and requirement for calcium and phosphate, which also contain aluminum. Research indicates that patients with impaired renal function who receive greater than 4 to 5 mcg/kg/day of parenteral aluminum are at risk for developing CNS or bone toxicity associated with aluminum accumulation. ▪ Administer with caution if flushing and sweating occur (first signs of vasodilation). ▪ See Drug/Lab Interactions.

Monitor: Discontinue IV administration when the desired therapeutic effect is obtained. ▪ Monitor magnesium levels. Normal plasma magnesium levels range from 1.5 to 2.5 mEq/L. Levels usually sufficient to control convulsions range from 2.5 to 5 mEq/L. Deep tendon reflexes decrease at plasma magnesium levels above 4 mEq/L and disappear as levels approach 10 mEq/L. Respiratory paralysis will occur at this level. Heart block may occur at or below this level. Levels above 12 mEq/L may be fatal. ▪ With each repeated dose, test patellar reflex (knee jerks) and observe respirations. If the knee jerk is absent or if respirations are less than 16/min, *do not* give additional magnesium sulfate. ▪ Equipment to maintain artificial ventilation must be available at all times. Patient must be continuously observed. ▪ Maintain minimum of 100 mL of urine output every 4 hours.

Patient Education: If magnesium is given for the treatment of preterm labor, inform the woman that the efficacy and safety of such use have not been established and that use beyond 5 to 7 days may cause fetal abnormalities.

Maternal/Child: Category D: continuous administration beyond 5 to 7 days to pregnant women can lead to hypocalcemia and bone abnormalities in the developing fetus; see Precautions. Use during pregnancy only if clearly needed. ▪ Continuous administration of magnesium is an unapproved treatment for preterm labor. Safety and efficacy have not been established. Administration of magnesium outside its approved indication in pregnant women should be by trained obstetric personnel in a hospital setting with appropriate obstetric care facilities. ▪ May cause magnesium toxicity in the newborn if given IV to the mother within 2 hours of delivery. ▪ A continuous infusion given to control convulsions in toxemic mothers before delivery (especially in the 24 hours preceding) may cause signs of magnesium toxicity in the newborn (e.g., neuromuscular or respiratory depression). ▪ Use caution during breast-feeding. ▪ Safety for use in pediatric patients not established.

Elderly: See Dose Adjustments.

DRUG/LAB INTERACTIONS

Additive CNS depressant effects when used concomitantly with **barbiturates, hypnotics, narcotics, or systemic anesthetics.** See Dose Adjustments and Monitor. ▪ Potentiates **neuromuscular blocking agents** (e.g., vecuronium, succinylcholine). ▪ If **calcium** is used to treat magnesium toxicity, use in digitalized patients may cause serious changes in cardiac conduction, resulting in heart block. Use with extreme caution.

SIDE EFFECTS

Usually the result of magnesium intoxication. Cardiac and CNS depression proceeding to respiratory paralysis; circulatory collapse; depressed or absent knee jerk reflex; flaccid paralysis; flushing; hypocalcemia with signs of tetany; hypotension; hypothermia; stupor; sweating.

ANTIDOTE

Discontinue the drug and notify the physician of the occurrence of any side effect. An intravenous calcium salt (10 to 20 mL of a 5% solution [diluted if desirable with NS]) may be used to counteract the effects of hypermagnesemia. Physostigmine 0.5 to 1 mg SC may be helpful. Treat hypotension with dopamine. Employ artificial ventilation as necessary and resuscitate as necessary. Hemodialysis is effective in overdose.

Hypermagnesemia in the newborn: May require endotracheal intubation, assisted ventilation, and IV calcium.

M

MANNITOL

(**MAN**-nih-tol)

Osmitrol

Diuretic
(osmotic)

pH 4.5 to 7

USUAL DOSE

Total dose, concentration, and rate of administration should be based on the nature and severity of the condition being treated, fluid requirements, and urine output. The usual adult dose may range from 20 to 100 Gm/24 hr. In most instances, an adequate response is achieved with doses of 50 to 100 Gm/24 hr. The rate of administration is usually adjusted to maintain a urine output of at least 30 to 50 mL/hr. See Precautions and Monitor. *A test dose may be required (e.g., patients with marked oliguria or inadequate renal function).*
Test dose: Give 200 mg/kg of body weight over 3 to 5 minutes. 30 to 50 mL of urine should be produced in 1 hour. If adequate urine is not produced, repeat once. If still ineffective, re-evaluate patient.

1 Gm equal to approximately 5.5 mOsm.

Prevention of oliguric phase of acute renal failure: 50 to 100 Gm as a 5% to 25% solution. A concentrated solution may be used initially, followed by a 5% to 10% solution.
Treatment of oliguria: 50 to 100 Gm of a 15% to 25% solution.
Management of intracranial pressure in neurologic emergencies: Manufacturer recommends 0.25 Gm/kg every 6 to 8 hours. AHA recommends 0.5 to 1 Gm/kg over 5 to 10 minutes through an in-line filter. Repeat 0.25 to 2 Gm/kg every 4 to 6 hours as needed. A third source suggests 1.5 to 2 Gm/kg of body weight as a 15% to 25% solution. An osmotic gradient between the blood and cerebrospinal fluid of approximately 10 mOsm should yield a satisfactory reduction in intracranial pressure.
Reduction of intraocular pressure: 1.5 to 2 Gm/kg of body weight as a 15% or 20% solution. To obtain maximal effect, this dose may be administered over a period as short as 30 minutes. May be used 60 to 90 minutes before surgery.
Promotion of urinary excretion of toxic substances: 50 to 200 Gm. Manufacturer recommends a 5% or 25% solution as indicated if urine output remains adequate. Numerous regimens are in use. Urine output of 100 to 500 mL/hr and a positive fluid balance of 1 to 2 L should be maintained. One regimen suggests an initial loading dose of 25 Gm followed by an infusion at a rate to maintain urine output at 100 mL/hr. Discontinue if no benefit derived from 200 Gm.
Diuretic for adjunctive treatment of ascites or edema: 100 Gm of a 10% to 20% solution over 2 to 6 hours.

PEDIATRIC DOSE

See Maternal/Child. *Test dose may be required (e.g., oliguria or anuria).*
Test dose: Give 200 mg/kg of body weight or 6 Gm/M^2 over 3 to 5 minutes. 30 to 50 mL of urine should be produced in 1 hour. If adequate urine is not produced, repeat once. If still ineffective, re-evaluate patient. Maximum test dose is 12.5 Gm.
Cerebral or ocular edema: 2 Gm/kg of body weight or 60 Gm/M^2 of body surface as a 15% to 20% solution over 30 to 60 minutes.
Promotion of urinary excretion of toxic substances: 2 Gm/kg or 60 Gm/M^2 as a 5% or 10% solution as needed if urine output remains adequate. Concentration depends on fluid requirement and urine output.
Anuria/oliguria: 0.5 to 1 Gm/kg as an initial dose. Maintain with 0.25 to 0.5 Gm/kg every 4 to 6 hours. Another source suggests 2 Gm/kg or 60 Gm/M^2 over 90 minutes to several hours.
Edema and ascites: 2 Gm/kg or 60 Gm/M^2 as a 15% to 20% solution over 2 to 6 hours.

DOSE ADJUSTMENTS

Reduce dose by one half for small or debilitated patients. ▪ Dose selection in the elderly should be cautious (usually starting at the low end of the dosing range), reflecting the

greater frequency of decreased organ function and of concomitant disease or drug therapy.
- Reduced dose may be required in oliguria or impaired renal function; see Monitor.

DILUTION
Available in concentrations of 5%, 10%, 15%, 20%, or 25%. May be in flexible IV bags or in flip-top vials. No further dilution is necessary; however, if there are any crystals present in the solution, they must be completely dissolved before administration. One manufacturer recommends: To dissolve crystals in the flexible container, warm the unit to 70° C (158° F) with agitation. Heat solution using a dry-heat cabinet with overwrap intact. Use of a water bath is not recommended. To dissolve the crystals in the flip-top vial, warm the bottle in hot water at 80° C (176° F). Shake vigorously periodically. 25% mannitol injection may be autoclaved at 121° C (250° F) for 20 minutes at 15 psi. Consult prescribing information; process may differ with specific brands. Let cool to at least body temperature before administration.

Glomerular filtration rate: See Usual Dose.

Filters: Use an in-line filter for 15%, 20%, and 25% solutions.

Storage: One manufacturer recommends storing at CRT. Protect from freezing. Consult prescribing information; may be brand specific. Discard unused portions.

COMPATIBILITY   (Underline Indicates Conflicting Compatibility Information)
Consider any drug NOT listed as compatible to be INCOMPATIBLE until consulting a pharmacist; specific conditions may apply.

Sources list as **incompatible** with strongly acidic or alkaline solutions. 20% or 25% solutions of mannitol may precipitate with potassium chloride (KCl) or sodium chloride. Concomitant administration of electrolyte-free mannitol solutions with whole blood may cause pseudoagglutination. If blood must be given simultaneously, at least 20 mEq of NaCl should be added to each liter of mannitol solution; consult pharmacist. Do not use PVC infusion bags with 25% mannitol; may form a precipitate.

One source suggests the following **compatibilities:**

Additive: Amikacin, aztreonam (Azactam), cefoxitin (Mefoxin), ceftriaxone (Rocephin), cisplatin, dopamine, fosphenytoin (Cerebyx), furosemide (Lasix), gentamicin, <u>levofloxacin (Levaquin)</u>, metoclopramide (Reglan), ondansetron (Zofran), sodium bicarbonate, tobramycin, verapamil.

Y-site: Acetaminophen (Ofirmev), allopurinol (Aloprim), amifostine (Ethyol), amphotericin B cholesteryl (Amphotec), aztreonam (Azactam), bivalirudin (Angiomax), ceftaroline (Teflaro), cisatracurium (Nimbex), cladribine (Leustatin), dexmedetomidine (Precedex), docetaxel (Taxotere), doripenem (Doribax), etoposide phosphate (Etopophos), fenoldopam (Corlopam), fludarabine (Fludara), fluorouracil (5-FU), gallium nitrate (Ganite), gemcitabine (Gemzar), hetastarch in electrolytes (Hextend), idarubicin (Idamycin), linezolid (Zyvox), melphalan (Alkeran), ondansetron (Zofran), oxaliplatin (Eloxatin), paclitaxel (Taxol), <u>palonosetron (Aloxi)</u>, pemetrexed (Alimta), piperacillin/tazobactam (Zosyn), propofol (Diprivan), remifentanil (Ultiva), sargramostim (Leukine), <u>telavancin (Vibativ)</u>, teniposide (Vumon), thiotepa, vinorelbine (Navelbine).

RATE OF ADMINISTRATION
Variable; may be adjusted to obtain a urine output of at least 30 to 50 mL/hr. A single dose should be given over 30 to 90 minutes. Up to 3 Gm/kg have been given over this time span. A test dose (see Monitor) or loading doses may be given over 3 to 5 minutes.

Oliguria: A single dose over 90 minutes to several hours.

Reduction of intracranial pressure and brain mass: A single dose over 30 to 60 minutes.

Treatment of edema or ascites: A single dose over 2 to 6 hours.

ACTIONS
A sugar alcohol and most effective osmotic diuretic. It is a stable, inert, nontoxic solution. Distribution in the body is limited to extracellular compartments. Increases osmolarity of glomerular filtrate and the extracellular space. An increase in extracellular osmolarity causes the movement of water to the extracellular and vascular spaces. This action is responsible for the ability of mannitol to decrease intracranial pressure and

edema and to reduce elevated intraocular pressure. Mannitol is not reabsorbed or secreted by the tubules of the kidneys. It is excreted almost completely in the urine along with water, sodium, and chloride. Onset of diuresis is 1 to 3 hours. Reduction in cerebrospinal and intraocular fluid occurs within 15 minutes and lasts 4 to 8 hours. Rebound may occur within 12 hours.

INDICATIONS AND USES
Promotion of diuresis in the prevention and/or treatment of the oliguric phase of acute renal failure before irreversible renal failure becomes established. ▪ Reduction of intracranial pressure and treatment of cerebral edema by reducing brain mass. ▪ Reduction of extremely high intraocular pressure. ▪ Promotion of excretion of toxic substances. ▪ Reduction of generalized edema and ascites.

CONTRAINDICATIONS
Anuria, hypersensitivity to mannitol, intracranial bleeding except during craniotomy, progressive heart failure or pulmonary congestion after initiation of mannitol therapy, severe dehydration, severe pulmonary congestion or frank pulmonary edema, severe renal impairment or progressive renal dysfunction after initiation of mannitol therapy, including increasing azotemia or oliguria.

PRECAUTIONS
For IV use only. ▪ Evaluate cardiac status to avoid fulminating congestive heart failure. Use caution in renal failure; fluid overload may result. ▪ Loss of water in excess of electrolytes can cause hypernatremia. ▪ May cause osmotic nephrosis, which may progress to severe irreversible nephrosis. ▪ Use with caution in neurosurgical patients. May increase cerebral blood flow and increase risk of postoperative bleeding. ▪ Increased cerebral blood flow may worsen intracranial hypertension in pediatric patients who develop a generalized cerebral hyperemia within 48 hours of injury.

Monitor: Test dose should be used in patients with marked oliguria or impaired renal functions; see Usual Dose. ▪ Observe urine output continuously; should exceed 30 to 50 mL/hr. Insert Foley catheter if necessary. ▪ Monitor fluid status and osmolality (not to exceed 310 mOsm/kg). ▪ May obscure signs of inadequate hydration or hypovolemia. Electrolyte depletion (especially sodium and potassium) may occur. Administration of water and electrolytes is required to maintain fluid balance due to losses of these substances from urine, sweat, and expired air. Check with laboratory studies and replace as necessary. Monitor renal, cardiac, and pulmonary function. ▪ Before attempting to reduce intracranial pressure and brain mass, evaluate circulatory and renal reserve, fluid and electrolyte balance, body weight, and total input and output before and after mannitol infusion. Support with adequate ventilation and oxygenation. Reduced cerebrospinal fluid pressure must be observed within 15 minutes after starting infusion. ▪ Observe infusion site to prevent infiltration.

Maternal/Child: Category C: safety for use in pregnancy, labor, or delivery not established. Benefits must outweigh risks. ▪ Use caution in breast-feeding. ▪ Safety and effectiveness for use in pediatric patients under 12 years of age not established; however, doses are used clinically.

Elderly: Response similar to that seen in younger patients. Lower-end initial doses may be appropriate; see Dose Adjustments.

DRUG/LAB INTERACTIONS
May increase **lithium** excretion, thereby decreasing its effectiveness. ▪ Mannitol-induced hypokalemia may increase the potential for **digoxin** toxicity.

SIDE EFFECTS
Rare when used as directed but may include acidosis, backache, blurred vision, chest pain, chills, convulsions, decreased chloride levels, decreased sodium levels, dehydration, diuresis, dizziness, dryness of mouth, edema, fever, fulminating congestive heart failure, head-

ache, hyperosmolality, hypertension, hypotension, nausea, polyuria then oliguria, pulmonary edema, rhinitis, tachycardia, thirst, thrombophlebitis, and urinary retention.

ANTIDOTE
If minor side effects persist, notify the physician. For all major side effects or if urine output is under 30 to 50 mL/hr, discontinue the drug and notify the physician. Treatment will be supportive to correct fluid and electrolyte imbalances. Hemodialysis may be used to clear mannitol and reduce serum osmolality.

MELPHALAN HYDROCHLORIDE BBW
(**MEL**-fah-lan hy-droh-**KLOR**-eyed)

Antineoplastic
(alkylating agent/nitrogen mustard)

Alkeran, Evomela   pH 6.5 to 7

USUAL DOSE
Premedication: Administration of a prophylactic antiemetic is recommended.

Multiple-myeloma palliative treatment (all products): 16 mg/M^2 as an IV infusion over 15 to 20 minutes every 2 weeks for 4 doses. After recovery from toxicity, repeat dose every 4 weeks. Prednisone is administered concurrently.

Multiple-myeloma conditioning treatment (Evomela): 100 mg/M^2/day administered as an IV infusion over 30 minutes for 2 consecutive days (Day −3 and Day −2) prior to autologous stem cell transplantation (ASCT, Day 0). For patients who weigh more than 130% of their ideal body weight, body surface area should be calculated based on adjusted ideal body weight. Other unlabeled regimens are in use.

PEDIATRIC DOSE
See Maternal/Child. All pediatric doses are unlabeled; consult literature.

DOSE ADJUSTMENTS
All products: For palliative treatment, manufacturer recommends reducing dose by 50% if BUN greater than 30 mg/dL.

Evomela: No dose adjustment is necessary for conditioning treatment. For patients who weigh more than 130% of their ideal body weight, body surface area should be calculated based on adjusted ideal body weight.

Alkeran and generic: Dose reduction based on blood counts at the nadir and on the day of treatment should be considered. In one clinical study, the following reductions based on cell count were followed: reduce dose by 25% if WBC between 3,000 and 4,000/mm^3 and platelets between 75,000 and 100,000/mm^3; by 50% if WBC between 2,000 and 3,000/mm^3 and platelets between 50,000 and 75,000/mm^3. Withhold dose for WBC below 2,000/mm^3 and platelets below 50,000/mm^3. ▪ Lower-end initial doses may be indicated in the elderly. Consider impaired organ function and concomitant disease or drug therapy.

DILUTION
Specific techniques required; see Precautions. All products are available in a 50-mg single-dose vial.

Alkeran and generic: Reconstitution to completion of administration must take place within 60 minutes due to instability of melphalan (rapid hydrolysis). Rapidly inject 10 mL of supplied diluent into vial using a sterile needle (20-gauge or larger needle diameter) and syringe. Shake vigorously until a clear solution results (5 mg/mL). Use only clear solutions. Immediately, further dilute in NS to a concentration not greater than 0.45 mg/mL. Drug is very unstable and may begin to deteriorate within 30 minutes.

Evomela: Reconstitute with 8.6 mL of NS to make a 5 mg/mL solution. The NS should be assisted or pulled into the vial by a partial vacuum. Do not use if this vacuum is not present. Calculate the required volume needed for the patient dose. Withdraw this volume from the vial and inject into the appropriate volume of NS to create a solution with a final concentration of 0.45 mg/mL.

Filters: No data available from manufacturer. Another source indicates minimal adsorption with several types of filters from 0.2 to 0.45 microns in size.

Storage: *All products:* Store at CRT in carton to protect from light. *Alkeran and generic:* Keep time between reconstitution/dilution and administration to a minimum because reconstituted and diluted solutions are unstable. Complete administration within 60 minutes of reconstitution. Reconstituted solution will precipitate if refrigerated. Do not refrigerate. *Evomela:* Reconstituted solution is stable for 1 hour at RT and 24 hours if refrigerated. Diluted solution is stable for 4 hours at RT in addition to the 1 hour following reconstitution.

COMPATIBILITY   (Underline Indicates Conflicting Compatibility Information)
Consider any drug NOT listed as compatible to be INCOMPATIBLE until consulting a pharmacist; specific conditions may apply.

Evomela: Manufacturer states that Evomela should not be mixed with other melphalan hydrochloride for injection drug products.

Alkeran and generic: One source suggests the following **compatibilities:**

Y-site: Acyclovir (Zovirax), amikacin, aminophylline, ampicillin, aztreonam (Azactam), bleomycin (Blenoxane), bumetanide, buprenorphine (Buprenex), butorphanol (Stadol), calcium gluconate, carboplatin (Paraplatin), carmustine (BiCNU), caspofungin (Cancidas), cefazolin (Ancef), cefotaxime (Claforan), cefotetan, ceftazidime (Fortaz), ceftriaxone (Rocephin), cefuroxime (Zinacef), cisplatin, clindamycin (Cleocin), cyclophosphamide (Cytoxan), cytarabine (ARA-C), dacarbazine (DTIC), dactinomycin (Cosmegen), daunorubicin (Cerubidine), dexamethasone (Decadron), diphenhydramine (Benadryl), doxorubicin (Adriamycin), doxycycline, droperidol (Inapsine), enalaprilat (Vasotec IV), etoposide (VePesid), famotidine (Pepcid IV), filgrastim (Neupogen), fluconazole (Diflucan), fludarabine (Fludara), fluorouracil (5-FU), furosemide (Lasix), gallium nitrate (Ganite), ganciclovir (Cytovene IV), gentamicin, granisetron (Kytril), heparin, hydrocortisone sodium succinate (Solu-Cortef), hydromorphone (Dilaudid), idarubicin (Idamycin), ifosfamide (Ifex), imipenem-cilastatin (Primaxin), lorazepam (Ativan), mannitol, mechlorethamine (nitrogen mustard), meperidine (Demerol), mesna (Mesnex), methotrexate, methylprednisolone (Solu-Medrol), metoclopramide (Reglan), metronidazole (Flagyl IV), mitomycin (Mutamycin), mitoxantrone (Novantrone), morphine, nalbuphine, ondansetron (Zofran), pentostatin (Nipent), potassium chloride (KCl), prochlorperazine (Compazine), promethazine (Phenergan), ranitidine (Zantac), sodium bicarbonate, streptozocin (Zanosar), sulfamethoxazole/trimethoprim, teniposide (Vumon), thiotepa, ticarcillin/clavulanate (Timentin), tobramycin, vancomycin, vinblastine, vincristine, vinorelbine (Navelbine), zidovudine (AZT, Retrovir).

RATE OF ADMINISTRATION
Do not administer directly into a peripheral vein.

Alkeran and generic: Keep the time from reconstitution to dilution to administration to a minimum. Drug is very unstable and may begin to deteriorate within 30 minutes. Complete administration within 60 minutes of reconstitution. Manufacturer recommends administration by injecting slowly into a fast-running IV solution via an injection port or via a central venous line. In cases of poor peripheral venous access, consideration should be given to use of a central venous line.

Evomela: Inject slowly into a fast-running IV infusion via a central venous access line.

Palliative treatment (all products): A single dose as an IV infusion over 15 to 20 minutes.

Conditioning treatment (Evomela): A single dose as an IV infusion over 30 minutes.

ACTIONS

A phenylalanine derivative of nitrogen mustard that is a bifunctional alkylating antineoplastic agent. Cytotoxicity is related to the extent of its interstrand cross-linking with DNA. Not dependent on cell cycle phase. Active against both resting and dividing tumor cells. Binding to plasma proteins (primarily albumin) ranges from approximately 50% to 90%. Approximately 30% is irreversibly bound to plasma proteins. Eliminated from plasma primarily by chemical hydrolysis. Half-life is approximately 75 minutes. About 10% excreted as unchanged drug in urine.

INDICATIONS AND USES

All products: Palliative treatment of patients with multiple myeloma when oral therapy is not appropriate.

Evomela: High-dose conditioning treatment prior to hematopoietic progenitor (stem) cell transplantation in patients with multiple myeloma.

Unlabeled uses: *Alkeran and generic:* Conditioning regimen before autologous hematopoietic stem cell transplantation (HSCT). ■ Component of combination therapy to treat relapsed, resistant Hodgkin's lymphomas. ■ Pediatric rhabdomyosarcoma. ■ HSCT for pediatric neuroblastoma, pediatric hematologic malignancies, and Ewing sarcoma.

CONTRAINDICATIONS

All products: History of serious hypersensitivity to melphalan.

Alkeran and generic: Patients whose disease has demonstrated prior resistance to melphalan.

PRECAUTIONS

Follow guidelines for handling cytotoxic agents. See Appendix A, p. 1331. ■ Administered by or under the direction of the physician specialist, with facilities for monitoring the patient and responding to any medical emergency. ■ Severe myelotoxicity with resulting infection or bleeding may occur. Trials comparing IV to oral melphalan have shown more myelosuppression with the IV formulation. ■ For patients receiving **Evomela** as part of a conditioning regimen, myeloablation occurs in all patients. Do not begin the conditioning regimen unless a stem cell product is available for rescue. Monitor blood counts and provide supportive care for infections, anemia, and thrombocytopenia until there is adequate hematopoietic recovery. ■ When melphalan is being administered for palliative treatment, use extreme caution in patients whose bone marrow is compromised by or recovering from previous radiation or chemotherapy. ■ GI toxicity, including nausea, vomiting, mucositis, and diarrhea, has been reported with both indications. May occur in over 50% of patients receiving the conditioning regimen. Use prophylactic antiemetic therapy and provide supportive care for GI toxicity. ■ Hepatotoxicity ranging from abnormal liver function tests to hepatitis and hepatic venoocclusive disease has been reported. ■ Hypersensitivity reactions, including anaphylaxis, have been reported. ■ Do not abandon treatment prematurely when used for palliative treatment. Improvement may continue slowly over many months with repeated courses. ■ Patients with an elevated BUN had a greater incidence of severe bone marrow suppression. ■ Produces chromosomal aberrations in vitro and in vivo. Should be considered potentially leukemogenic in humans. Secondary malignancies, including acute nonlymphocytic leukemia, myeloproliferation syndrome, and carcinoma have been reported in patients treated with alkylating agents, including melphalan. ■ See Drug/Lab Interactions.

Monitor: Determine absolute patency of vein. A stinging or burning sensation indicates extravasation; cellulitis and tissue necrosis may result. Discontinue injection; use another vein; see Rate of Administration. ■ Frequently monitor platelet count, hemoglobin, white blood cell count, and differential. For palliative treatment, monitoring is indicated before each dose as well as between doses to determine optimal dose and avoid toxicity. Nadirs occur 2 to 3 weeks after treatment; recovery should occur in 4 to 5 weeks. ■ Severe myelosuppression can occur with effective doses. Withhold further doses until blood cell counts have recovered if thrombocytopenia and/or leukopenia occur. ■ Monitor renal function before and during therapy. ▪ Monitor liver function tests. ▪ Hypersensitivity reactions may occur with initial treatment or may be delayed and occur after multiple courses. Observe closely. ▪ Observe closely for all signs of infection, bleeding, or symptomatic anemia and provide supportive care as indicated. Prophylactic antibiotics may be indicated pending results of C/S in a febrile neutropenic patient. ▪ Prophylactic antiemetics may reduce nausea and vomiting and increase patient comfort. ▪ Nutritional support and analgesics may be required in patients experiencing Grade 3 or 4 mucositis. ▪ Monitor for thrombocytopenia (platelet count less than 50,000/mm³). Initiate precautions to prevent excessive bleeding (e.g., inspect IV sites, skin, and mucous membranes; use extreme care during invasive procedures; test urine, emesis, stool, and secretions for occult blood). ▪ See Drug/Lab Interactions.

Patient Education: Avoid pregnancy. Females of reproductive potential and males with female sexual partners of reproductive potential should use effective contraception methods during and after treatment. ▪ Treatment with melphalan may result in temporary or permanent infertility. ▪ Promptly report IV site burning or stinging. ▪ Acute side effects are related to bone marrow suppression, hypersensitivity reactions, GI toxicity, and pulmonary toxicity. Promptly report S/S of a hypersensitivity reaction or any potential side effects (e.g., bleeding, cough, fever, mucositis, rash). ▪ Routine laboratory monitoring is required. ▪ Major long-term toxicities are related to infertility and secondary malignancy. Discuss risks with health care provider. ▪ See Appendix D, p. 1333.

Maternal/Child: Avoid pregnancy. Based on its mechanism of action, melphalan can cause fetal harm, including teratogenicity and/or embryo-fetal lethality. ▪ Discontinue breastfeeding. ▪ Safety and effectiveness for use in pediatric patients not established; see Unlabeled Uses.

Elderly: Response similar to that seen in younger adults. However, a greater incidence of engraftment syndrome was observed in older patients. ▪ See Dose Adjustments.

DRUG/LAB INTERACTIONS

Coadministration with **cyclosporine** (Sandimmune) may result in acute renal failure. May occur after the first dose of each drug. ▪ Renal dysfunction induced by **cisplatin** may lead to decreased clearance and increased toxicity of melphalan. ▪ Threshold for lung toxicity associated with **carmustine** (BiCNU) may be reduced with concurrent use. ▪ **Interferon alfa** may decrease serum concentrations of melphalan. ▪ Use with **nalidixic acid** (NegGram) may cause severe hemorrhagic necrotic enterocolitis in pediatric patients. ▪ Do not administer **live virus vaccines** to immunocompromised patients receiving antineoplastic agents.

SIDE EFFECTS

The most common adverse reactions (occurring in at least 50% of patients) include anemia; decreased lymphocyte count, neutrophil count, platelet count, and white blood cell count; diarrhea; fatigue; hypokalemia; nausea; and vomiting. The most common serious adverse reactions were febrile neutropenia, fever, hematochezia, and renal failure. Reversible bone marrow suppression (e.g., anemia, leukopenia, thrombocytopenia) is dose-limiting. Irreversible bone marrow failure has been reported. Abdominal pain, alopecia, constipation, decreased appetite, dizziness, elevated BUN, hemolytic anemia, hepatic toxicity (including venoocclusive disease), hypersensitivity reactions (e.g., anaphylaxis, bronchospasm, dyspnea, dysgeusia, dyspepsia, edema, hypotension, mucosal inflammation, peripheral edema, pruritus, rash, urticaria, tachycardia), hypophosphatemia, interstitial pneumonitis, pulmonary fibrosis, secondary malignancies (long-term use), skin ulceration at injection site, stomatitis, and vasculitis have occurred.

Overdose: Adult respiratory distress syndrome, bone marrow suppression (severe), cholinomimetic effects (e.g., bradycardia, increased peristalsis and salivation, incontinence), convulsions, decreased consciousness, hyponatremia (inappropriate secretion of ADH), GI toxicity (colitis, diarrhea, GI bleed, mucositis, nausea, stomatitis, and vomiting), muscular paralysis, and nephrotoxicity.

ANTIDOTE

Keep physician informed of all side effects. Close monitoring of bone marrow may prevent most serious and potentially fatal side effects. WBC and platelet count nadirs occur 2 to 3 weeks after treatment with recovery in 4 to 5 weeks. Withhold further doses until blood cell counts have recovered if leukopenia or thrombocytopenia occur. There is no specific antidote, but adequate supportive care including administration of whole blood products (e.g., packed RBCs, platelets, leukocytes) and/or blood modifiers (e.g., darbepoetin alfa [Aranesp], epoetin alfa [Epogen], filgrastim [Neupogen, Zarxio], pegfilgrastim [Neulasta], sargramostim [Leukine]) may be indicated to treat bone marrow toxicity. Appropriate antibiotics may be indicated. Monitor closely until recovery (6 weeks or more). Discontinue the infusion for severe hypersensitivity reactions and treat with antihistamines, corticosteroids, pressor agents, or volume expanders; do not readminister melphalan (IV or oral). Hemodialysis probably not effective in overdose.

MEPERIDINE HYDROCHLORIDE

(meh-**PER**-ih-deen hy-droh-**KLOR**-eyed)

Opioid analgesic
(agonist)
Anesthesia adjunct

Demerol, Demerol HCl, Meperidine HCl PF

pH 3.5 to 6

USUAL DOSE

Determination of dose should be based on severity of pain and patient response.

IV injection: 5 to 10 mg every 5 minutes as needed. Do not exceed 600 mg/24 hr. IV dosing in acute pain should be limited to 48 hours or less; see Precautions.

Supplement anesthesia: 1 to 10 mg/mL dilution is usually used. Titrate under the direct observation and control of the anesthesiologist. Dose dependent on premedication, type of anesthesia, type and duration of procedure, and patient's condition.

Treatment or prevention of shaking chills (unlabeled): 0.5 mg/kg 20 minutes before shaking chills are expected to begin or 50 mg after onset of chills. Up to 150 mg has been required within 30 minutes if administered after onset.

PEDIATRIC DOSE

1 mg/kg/dose; see Maternal/Child.

DOSE ADJUSTMENTS

Reduced dose may be required in the elderly or debilitated, in hepatic or renal disease, or in numerous other disease entities; see Precautions. ▪ Doses appropriate for the general population may cause serious respiratory depression in vulnerable patients. ▪ Increase doses as required if analgesia is inadequate, tolerance develops, or pain severity increases. The first sign of tolerance is usually a reduced duration of effect. ▪ Decrease dose by 25% to 50% when administered concomitantly with phenothiazines and other centrally acting medications (e.g., sedatives). ▪ See Drug/Lab Interactions.

DILUTION

IV injection: May be given undiluted; however, further dilution with 5 mL of SWFI, NS, or other IV solutions to facilitate titration is appropriate; see chart on inside back cover.

Filters: No data available from manufacturer.

Storage: Before use, store at CRT protected from light. Do not freeze.

COMPATIBILITY
(Underline Indicates Conflicting Compatibility Information)

Consider any drug NOT listed as compatible to be INCOMPATIBLE until consulting a pharmacist; specific conditions may apply.

One source suggests the following **compatibilities:**

Additive: Cefazolin (Ancef), dobutamine, metoclopramide (Reglan), ondansetron (Zofran), sodium bicarbonate, succinylcholine, verapamil.

Y-site: Acetaminophen (Ofirmev), <u>acyclovir (Zovirax)</u>, amifostine (Ethyol), amikacin, ampicillin, ampicillin/sulbactam (Unasyn), <u>anidulafungin (Eraxis)</u>, aztreonam (Azactam), bivalirudin (Angiomax), bumetanide, <u>caspofungin (Cancidas)</u>, cefazolin (Ancef), cefotaxime (Claforan), cefotetan, cefoxitin (Mefoxin), ceftaroline (Teflaro), ceftazidime (Fortaz), ceftriaxone (Rocephin), cefuroxime (Zinacef), chloramphenicol (Chloromycetin), cisatracurium (Nimbex), cladribine (Leustatin), clindamycin (Cleocin), dexamethasone (Decadron), dexmedetomidine (Precedex), digoxin (Lanoxin), diltiazem (Cardizem), diphenhydramine (Benadryl), dobutamine, docetaxel (Taxotere), dopamine, doripenem (Doribax), doxycycline, droperidol (Inapsine), erythromycin (Erythrocin), etoposide phosphate (Etopophos), famotidine (Pepcid IV), fenoldopam (Corlopam), filgrastim (Neupogen), fluconazole (Diflucan), fludarabine (Fludara), <u>furosemide (Lasix)</u>, gallium nitrate (Ganite), gemcitabine (Gemzar), gentamicin, granisetron (Kytril), heparin, hetastarch in electrolytes (Hextend), hydrocortisone sodium succinate (Solu-Cortef), 6% hydroxyethyl starch (Voluven), insulin (regular), labetalol, lidocaine, linezolid (Zyvox), magnesium sulfate, melphalan (Alkeran), methyldopate, methylprednisolone (Solu-Medrol), metoclopramide (Reglan), metoprolol (Lopressor), metronidazole (Flagyl IV), ondansetron (Zofran), oxacillin (Bactocill), oxaliplatin (Eloxatin), oxytocin (Pitocin), paclitaxel (Taxol), <u>palonosetron (Aloxi)</u>, pemetrexed (Alimta), penicillin G potassium, piperacillin/tazobactam (Zosyn), potassium chloride (KCl), propofol (Diprivan), propranolol, ranitidine (Zantac), remifentanil (Ultiva), sargramostim (Leukine), sulfamethoxazole/trimethoprim, teniposide (Vumon), thiotepa, ticarcillin/clavulanate (Timentin), tobramycin, vancomycin, verapamil, vinorelbine (Navelbine).

RATE OF ADMINISTRATION

IV injection: A single dose over 4 to 5 minutes. Frequently titrated according to symptom relief and respiratory rate. Rapid IV administration increases the possibility of hypotension and respiratory depression.

ACTIONS

A synthetic narcotic analgesic and descending CNS depressant, similar to morphine. Has multiple actions; the most prominent involve the CNS and organs composed of smooth muscle. Principal actions of therapeutic value are analgesia and sedation. May produce less smooth muscle spasm, constipation, and depression of the cough reflex than equianalgesic doses of morphine. A parenteral dose of meperidine 60 to 80 mg is approximately equivalent in analgesic effect to 10 mg of morphine. Onset of action occurs in about 5 minutes and lasts for about 2 to 4 hours. Readily absorbed and distributed throughout the body. Metabolized to an active, toxic metabolite (normeperidine) in the liver, its extended half-life (15 to 30 hours) may lead to cumulative effects. Excreted in the urine. Crosses the placental barrier. Secreted in breast milk.

INDICATIONS AND USES

Short-term relief of moderate to severe pain. ▪ Preoperative medication. ▪ Support of anesthesia. ▪ Obstetric analgesia.

Unlabeled uses: Treatment or prevention of shaking chills (rigors) caused by some medications (e.g., amphotericin B [all formulations], aldesleukin [Proleukin]). ▪ Treatment of postoperative shivering.

CONTRAINDICATIONS

Hypersensitivity to meperidine, patients who have received MAO inhibitors (e.g., selegiline [Eldepryl]) in the previous 14 days.

PRECAUTIONS

Use of meperidine as a first-line analgesic for pain is discouraged due to its short duration of action and the risk of accumulation of its toxic metabolite, normeperidine. Accumulation of normeperidine may increase the risk of toxicity (e.g., seizures). If its use in acute pain (in patients without renal or CNS disease) cannot be avoided, the American Pain Society and ISMP recommend limiting treatment to 48 hours or less and not exceeding 600 mg/24 hr. ▪ Use with caution in glaucoma, head injuries, increased intracranial pressure (elevates spinal fluid pressure), asthma, chronic obstructive pulmonary disease, decreased respiratory reserve or respiratory depression, supraventricular tachycardia, convulsions, acute abdominal conditions before diagnosis, the elderly and debilitated, and hepatic or renal insufficiency. ▪ Use with caution and in reduced doses in patients receiving concurrent therapy with other narcotic analgesics, general anesthetics, phenothiazines (e.g., promethazine [Phenergan], prochlorperazine [Compazine]), sedative-hypnotics (including barbiturates [e.g., phenobarbital]), tricyclic antidepressants (e.g., imipramine [Tofranil]), and other CNS depressants, including alcohol. Use may result in respiratory depression, hypotension, and profound sedation or coma. See Drug/Lab Interactions. ▪ Use with caution in patients with renal dysfunction; normeperidine may accumulate, resulting in increased CNS toxicity. ▪ May cause severe hypotension in postoperative patients or in any patient whose ability to maintain blood pressure has been compromised by depleted blood volume or concomitant administration of drugs that can cause hypotension (e.g., anesthetics, phenothiazines). ▪ Use with caution in patients with sickle cell anemia, hypothyroidism, Addison's disease, pheochromocytoma, and prostatic hypertrophy or urethral stricture. Reduced doses may be indicated; see Dose Adjustments. ▪ Cough reflex may be suppressed. ▪ Morphine is usually preferred for pain during an acute MI. ▪ IM route frequently used. Frequent IM injections may lead to severe fibrosis of muscle tissue. ▪ Do not use in patients for any long-term pain relief (e.g., cancer). ▪ Psychological and physical dependence and tolerance may develop with repeated administration.

Monitor: Oxygen, controlled respiratory equipment, and naloxone must always be available. ▪ Observe patient frequently to continuously based on amount of dose and monitor vital signs. ▪ Assess baseline pain, then assess pain with vital signs. Reassess after administration of meperidine and adjust dose or interval as required. ▪ Keep patient supine; orthostatic hypotension and fainting may occur; less likely with continuous low doses, but observe closely during ambulation. ▪ Uncontrolled pain causes sleep deprivation, decreases pain threshold, and increases pain. When pain is finally controlled, expect the patient to sleep more until recovery from sleep deprivation. ▪ With use the active metabolite normeperidine accumulates to toxic levels; will lower seizure threshold. Monitor for twitching, jerking, shaky hands, tremors; may lead to grand mal seizure. ▪ Laxatives with or without stool softeners may be required to avoid constipation and fecal impaction. Maintain adequate hydration.

Patient Education: Avoid alcohol or other CNS depressants (e.g., barbiturates, benzodiazepines [e.g., diazepam (Valium)]). ▪ May cause blurred vision, dizziness, or drowsiness; use caution in tasks that require alertness. ▪ Request assistance with ambulation. ▪ May be habit forming.

Maternal/Child: Category C: safety for use before labor not established. ▪ Use during delivery may cause depression of respiration and psychophysiologic functions in the newborn requiring resuscitation. ▪ May cause serious adverse reactions in nursing infants; discontinue breast-feeding or discontinue meperidine. ▪ Not recommended for IV use in pediatric patients but is used. Consider risk versus benefit before use in neonates or young infants. Rate of elimination is slower in neonates and young infants compared to older children or adults. May be more sensitive to effects (e.g., respiratory depression) and may cause paradoxical excitation.

Elderly: See Dose Adjustments and Precautions. ▪ Elimination rate is slower than in younger adults. ▪ May be more sensitive to effects (e.g., respiratory depression, constipation, urinary retention). ▪ Lower doses may provide effective analgesia. ▪ Consider age-related organ impairment.

DRUG/LAB INTERACTIONS

Potentiated by **acyclovir** (Zovirax), **anticholinergics, cimetidine** (Tagamet), **tricyclic antidepressants** (e.g., imipramine [Tofranil]), **isoniazid** (INH), **neostigmine, neuromuscular blocking agents** (e.g., atracurium [Tracrium]), **phenothiazines, general anesthetics, other narcotic analgesics, and CNS depressants including alcohol.** Side effects (e.g., CNS depression, constipation, hypotension) may be additive. Reduced dosage of both drugs may be indicated. ▪ Do not use with **MAO inhibitors** (e.g., selegiline [Eldepryl]); may cause cardiovascular collapse. ▪ Avoid concurrent use with **sibutramine** (Meridia); may precipitate serotonin syndrome (e.g., altered consciousness, CNS irritability, motor weakness, myoclonus, shivering). ▪ **Mixed agonists/antagonists** (e.g., pentazocine [Talwin], nalbuphine, butorphanol [Stadol]) may decrease analgesic effect of meperidine and/or precipitate withdrawal symptoms. ▪ Concurrent use with **protease inhibitors** (e.g., saquinavir [Invirase], ritonavir [Norvir]) not recommended. May increase meperidine serum concentrations and increase the risk of side effects, including seizures and cardiac arrhythmias. ▪ **Hydantoins** (e.g., phenytoin [Dilantin]) may increase metabolism and decrease the half-life of meperidine; however, increased normeperidine levels have been seen. ▪ Metabolism increased and analgesic effects may be decreased or delayed in **smokers.**

SIDE EFFECTS

Dizziness, flushing, light-headedness, nausea, postural hypotension, rash, restlessness, sedation, sweating, syncope, vomiting. Side effects associated with histamine release, convulsions, and constipation may be more common with meperidine than with most other narcotic analgesics.

Major: Apnea, cardiac arrest, cardiovascular collapse, cold and clammy skin, convulsions, dilated pupils, hypersensitivity reactions (e.g., anaphylaxis, pruritus), normeperidine toxicity (jerking, tremor, twitching, shaky hands, grand mal seizure), respiratory depression, shock, tremor.

ANTIDOTE

With increasing severity of minor side effects or onset of any major side effect, discontinue the drug and notify the physician. A patent airway, artificial respiration, oxygen therapy, and other symptomatic treatment must be instituted promptly. Naloxone hydrochloride will reverse cardiovascular, CNS, and respiratory reactions. In patients who are physically dependent on narcotics, either avoid the use of a narcotic antagonist or use extreme caution and doses as small as one-fifth to one-tenth of the usual initial dose to avoid precipitating an acute withdrawal syndrome. In all patients, adjust and titrate the dose of a narcotic antagonist to reverse side effects without reversing pain control. Avoid total reversal of pain control. Resuscitate as necessary.

MEROPENEM
(**mer**-oh-**PEN**-em)

Merrem I.V.

Antibacterial
(carbapenem)

pH 7.3 to 8.3

USUAL DOSE

Dose ranges from 500 mg to 2 Gm and depends on type and severity of infection.

Complicated skin and skin structure infections in adults and pediatric patients weighing 50 kg or more: 500 mg every 8 hours. Increase to 1 Gm every 8 hours in complicated skin and skin structure infections caused by *P. aeruginosa*.

Intra-abdominal infections in adults and pediatric patients weighing 50 kg or more: 1 Gm every 8 hours.

Febrile neutropenia in adults and pediatric patients weighing 50 kg or more (unlabeled): 1 Gm every 8 hours.

Meningitis (unlabeled in adult patients): 2 Gm every 8 hours.

Burkholderia infections (melioidosis [unlabeled]): 1 Gm every 8 hours.

Mild to moderate infection, other severe infections (unlabeled): 500 mg to 1 Gm every 8 hours.

Complicated urinary tract infections (unlabeled): 500 mg to 1 Gm every 8 hours.

PEDIATRIC DOSE

30 to 120 mg/kg/day divided (10 to 40 mg) every 8 hours depending on type and severity of infection. Maximum dose is 6 Gm/day. See Maternal/Child.

Complicated skin and skin structure infections in pediatric patients over 3 months of age: 10 mg/kg every 8 hours. Maximum single dose every 8 hours is 500 mg. Increase dose to 20 mg/kg every 8 hours in complicated skin and skin structure infections caused by *P. aeruginosa*. Maximum single dose every 8 hours is 1 Gm.

Intra-abdominal infections in pediatric patients over 3 months of age: 20 mg/kg every 8 hours. Maximum single dose every 8 hours is 1 Gm.

Intra-abdominal infections in pediatric patients under 3 months of age: Dose is based on gestational age (GA) and postnatal age (PNA).

Infants under 32 weeks GA and PNA under 2 weeks: 20 mg/kg every 12 hours.

Infants under 32 weeks GA and PNA 2 weeks and older: 20 mg/kg every 8 hours.

Infants 32 weeks and older GA and PNA under 2 weeks: 20 mg/kg every 8 hours.

Infants 32 weeks and older GA and PNA 2 weeks and older: 30 mg/kg every 8 hours.

Meningitis in pediatric patients over 3 months of age: 40 mg/kg every 8 hours. Maximum single dose every 8 hours is 2 Gm.

Febrile neutropenia in pediatric patients 3 months of age and older and less than 50 kg (unlabeled): 20 mg/kg every 8 hours.

DOSE ADJUSTMENTS

Reduced dose required if CrCl is less than 51 mL/min based on the following chart.

Meropenem Recommended IV Dosage Schedule for Adults with Impaired Renal Function		
Creatinine Clearance (mL/min)	Dose (dependent on type of infection)	Dosing Interval
26-50 mL/min	Recommended dose	Every 12 hours
10-25 mL/min	One half recommended dose	Every 12 hours
<10 mL/min	One half recommended dose	Every 24 hours

Consult package insert or front matter of this text for formula to convert SCr to CrCl. ▪ No dose adjustment necessary in impaired hepatic function. ▪ Reduced dose may be required in the elderly based on decreased renal function. ▪ Information is inadequate for use in patients on hemodialysis or peritoneal dialysis. ▪ No experience in pediatric patients with renal impairment.

DILUTION

Injection: Reconstitute each 500 mg with 10 mL SWFI (1 Gm with 20 mL). Yields 50 mg/mL. Shake to dissolve and let stand until clear. May be given as an IV injection or further diluted with **compatible** infusion solutions (see Infusion and Compatibility).

Infusion: Available as infusion vials that may be directly reconstituted with a **compatible** solution and then infused. Concentration may range from 1 to 20 mg/mL.

Storage: Store unopened vials (dry powder) at RT (20° to 25° C [68° to 77° F]). Use of freshly prepared solutions preferred. Injection vials reconstituted with SWFI for bolus administration (up to 50 mg/mL) may be stored for up to 3 hours at up to 25° C (77° F) or for 13 hours at up to 5° C (41° F). Solutions prepared for infusion with NS (concentrations ranging from 1 to 20 mg/mL) may be stored for 1 hour at up to 25° C (77° F) or for 15 hours at up to 5° C (41° F). Solutions prepared for infusion with D5W (concentrations ranging from 1 to 20 mg/mL) should be used immediately. Do not freeze.

COMPATIBILITY   (Underline Indicates Conflicting Compatibility Information)

Consider any drug NOT listed as compatible to be INCOMPATIBLE until consulting a pharmacist; specific conditions may apply.

Manufacturer states, "Meropenem should not be mixed or physically added to solutions containing other drugs; **compatibility** not established."

One source suggests the following **compatibilities:**

Solution: Compatible under specific conditions (see Storage) with NS, D5W, D10W, D5NS, D5/¼NS, KCl 0.15% in D5W, Na Bicarbonate 0.02% in D5W, D5 in Normosol-M, D5LR, D2½ in ½NS, Mannitol 2.5%, R, LR, Na Lactate ⅙ M, Na Bicarbonate 5%.

Additive: *Not recommended by manufacturer.* <u>Acyclovir (Zovirax)</u>, aminophylline, atropine, dexamethasone (Decadron), dobutamine, dopamine, <u>doxycycline</u>, enalaprilat (Vasotec IV), fluconazole (Diflucan), furosemide (Lasix), gentamicin, heparin, insulin (regular), magnesium sulfate, metoclopramide (Reglan), morphine, norepinephrine (Levophed), <u>ondansetron (Zofran)</u>, phenobarbital (Luminal), ranitidine (Zantac), vancomycin, <u>zidovudine (AZT, Retrovir)</u>.

Y-site: <u>Acyclovir (Zovirax)</u>, aminophylline, <u>anidulafungin (Eraxis)</u>, atropine, <u>calcium gluconate</u>, <u>caspofungin (Cancidas)</u>, cyclosporine (Sandimmune), dexamethasone (Decadron), digoxin (Lanoxin), diphenhydramine (Benadryl), docetaxel (Taxotere), <u>doxycycline</u>, enalaprilat (Vasotec IV), fluconazole (Diflucan), furosemide (Lasix), gentamicin, heparin, insulin (regular), linezolid (Zyvox), metoclopramide (Reglan), milrinone (Primacor), morphine, norepinephrine (Levophed), <u>ondansetron (Zofran)</u>, phenobarbital (Luminal), potassium chloride (KCl), <u>telavancin (Vibativ)</u>, vancomycin, vasopressin, <u>zidovudine (AZT, Retrovir)</u>.

RATE OF ADMINISTRATION

IV injection in adults and pediatric patients over 3 months of age: A single dose (up to 1 Gm [20 mL] after dilution) over 3 to 5 minutes.

Intermittent infusion in adults and pediatric patients over 3 months of age: A single dose over 15 to 30 minutes.

Intermittent infusion in pediatric patients under 3 months of age: A single dose over 30 minutes.

Extended infusion (unlabeled): 0.5 to 2 Gm over 3 hours every 8 hours.

ACTIONS

A synthetic, broad-spectrum, carbapenem antibiotic. Bactericidal to selected gram-negative, gram-positive, and anaerobic organisms. Bactericidal activity results from the inhibition of cell wall synthesis. Readily penetrates the cell wall of susceptible organisms to reach penicillin-binding protein targets. Has significant stability to hydrolysis by penicillinases and cephalosporinases produced by gram-positive and gram-negative bacteria. Peak plasma concentrations reached by the end of an infusion. Penetrates well into most body fluids and tissues, including cerebrospinal fluid. Peak fluid and tissue concentrations reached in 0.5 to 1.5 hours. Minimal protein binding. Elimination half-life averages 1 hour in adults, 1.5 hours in pediatric patients age 3 months to 2 years, and 2.7 hours in infants under 3 months of age. 70% recovered as unchanged drug in urine within 12 hours. Not yet known if it crosses the placental barrier. Secreted in breast milk.

INDICATIONS AND USES

Indicated as single-agent therapy for treatment of the specific infections caused by susceptible organisms. Is useful as presumptive therapy in the indicated infections before identification of the causative organism because of its broad spectrum of activity. Treatment of intra-abdominal infections (e.g., complicated appendicitis, peritonitis) in adults and pediatric patients. ■ Treatment of complicated skin and skin structure infections in adults and pediatric patients 3 months of age and older. ■ Treatment of bacterial meningitis in pediatric patients 3 months of age and older. Efficacy of meropenem as monotherapy in the treatment of meningitis caused by penicillin-nonsusceptible isolates of *Streptococcus pneumoniae* has not been established. Meropenem has been found to be effective in eliminating concurrent bacteremia in association with bacterial meningitis.

Unlabeled uses: Empiric anti-infective therapy in febrile neutropenic patients. ■ Meningitis in adults. ■ Septicemia. ■ Complicated urinary tract infections caused by susceptible bacteria. ■ Respiratory tract infections. ■ Alternate or concomitant therapy in *Acinetobacter,* anthrax, *Bacillus cereus,* melioidosis caused by *Burkholderia pseudomallei, Campylobacter fetus, Capnocytophaga canimorsus, Clostridium perfringens,* glanders caused by *Burkholderia mallei, Nocardia,* and *Rhodococcus equi* infections.

CONTRAINDICATIONS

History of hypersensitivity to meropenem, its components, any other carbapenem antibiotic (e.g., imipenem-cilastatin [Primaxin]), or patients with demonstrated anaphylaxis to beta-lactams; see Precautions.

PRECAUTIONS

Specific sensitivity studies are indicated to determine susceptibility of the causative organism to meropenem. ■ To reduce the development of drug-resistant bacteria and maintain its effectiveness, meropenem should be used to treat or prevent only those infections proven or strongly suspected to be caused by bacteria. ■ Serious and occasionally fatal hypersensitivity reactions have been reported in patients receiving therapy with beta-lactams (e.g., penicillins, cephalosporins, carbapenems). More likely in patients with a history of sensitivity to multiple allergens; obtain a careful history. Cross-sensitivity is possible. ■ Seizures and other adverse CNS reactions have been reported. Occurred most commonly in patients with a history of CNS disorders (e.g., brain lesions, history of seizures) or with bacterial meningitis and/or compromised renal function. Use extreme caution; continue administration of anticonvulsants in patients with known seizure disorders. ■ Use with caution in patients with impaired renal function; thrombocytopenia may occur and the incidence of heart failure, kidney failure, seizures, and shock may be increased; see Dose Adjustments. ■ May have cross-resistance with strains resistant to other carbapenems (e.g., imipenem-cilastatin [Primaxin]). ■ Localized clusters of infections resulting from carbapenem-resistant bacteria have been reported in some regions. ■ Has the potential for neuromotor impairment (e.g., headaches, paresthesias, seizures) that can interfere with mental alertness and/or cause motor impairment; see Patient Education. ■ Avoid prolonged use of drug; superinfection caused by overgrowth of nonsusceptible organisms may result. ■ *Clostridium difficile*–associated diarrhea (CDAD) has been reported. May range from mild diarrhea to fatal colitis. Consider in patients who present with diarrhea during or after treatment with meropenem. ■ See Drug/Lab Interactions.

Monitor: Anaphylaxis has been reported. Emergency equipment must always be available. ■ Monitor infusion site for inflammation and/or extravasation. May cause thrombophlebitis. ■ Monitor for S/S of CNS reactions (e.g., focal tremors, myoclonus, seizures). ■ Monitor renal, hepatic, and hemopoietic systems in prolonged therapy. ■ Each 1 Gm contains 3.92 mEq of sodium; monitoring of electrolytes may be indicated. ■ See Drug/Lab Interactions and Side Effects.

Patient Education: Report any itching, rash, shortness of breath, or twitching sensation immediately. ▪ Report any burning, pain, or stinging at injection site. ▪ Promptly report diarrhea or bloody stools that occur during treatment or up to several months after an antibiotic has been discontinued; may indicate CDAD and require treatment. ▪ Patients with a history of seizures should review medication profile with physician before taking meropenem; see Drug/Lab Interactions. ▪ May interfere with mental alertness and/or cause motor impairment. Do not operate machinery or drive until tolerance is established.

Maternal/Child: Category B: safety for use in pregnancy not established; use only if clearly needed. ▪ Use caution during breast-feeding. ▪ Safety and effectiveness established for pediatric patients 3 months of age and older with complicated skin and skin structure infections or bacterial meningitis and for pediatric patients of all ages with complicated intra-abdominal infections. ▪ Safety data are limited to support the administration of a 40 mg/kg (up to a maximum of 2 Gm) bolus dose.

Elderly: Consider age-related renal impairment; plasma clearance is decreased with decreased renal function; see Dose Adjustments. Monitoring of renal function is suggested. Response is similar to that seen in younger patients; however, greater sensitivity in the elderly cannot be ruled out. See Precautions.

DRUG/LAB INTERACTIONS

Carbapenems may reduce serum **valproic acid** concentrations to subtherapeutic levels, resulting in a loss of seizure control. Monitor valproic acid levels. Consider alternative antibacterial therapy. If administration of meropenem is necessary, supplemental anticonvulsant therapy should be considered. ▪ **Probenecid** inhibits renal excretion and increases serum levels of meropenem, extending its half-life and increasing systemic exposure; coadministration is not recommended. ▪ May be synergistic with **aminoglycosides** against some isolates of *Pseudomonas aeruginosa*.

SIDE EFFECTS

Toxicity rate is usually low. ***Pediatric patients:*** The types of clinical adverse effects seen in pediatric patients are similar to those seen in adults. The most commonly reported adverse effects included diarrhea, diaper area moniliasis, glossitis, oral moniliasis, rash, and vomiting. In neonates and infants under 3 months of age, additional side effects that were reported irrespective of causality were convulsions, hyperbilirubinemia, and vomiting. ***Adults:*** Anemia, constipation, diarrhea, headache, nausea and vomiting, and rash are most common. Apnea, injection site reactions (e.g., edema, inflammation, pain, phlebitis), pruritus, sepsis, and shock also occurred in more than 1% of patients. Many other side effects—including CDAD; hypersensitivity reactions (including anaphylaxis); increases or decreases in hematologic, hepatic, and renal lab tests; neuromotor impairment; seizures; and thrombocytopenia—may occur in fewer than 1% of patients.

Post-Marketing: Agranulocytosis, angioedema, erythema multiforme, hemolytic anemia, leukopenia, neutropenia, positive direct or indirect Coombs' test, Stevens-Johnson syndrome, and toxic epidermal necrolysis have been reported.

ANTIDOTE

Notify physician of all side effects. Most treated symptomatically. Discontinue immediately if a hypersensitivity reaction occurs. Treat hypersensitivity reactions as indicated; may require epinephrine, airway management, oxygen, IV fluids, antihistamines (e.g., diphenhydramine [Benadryl]), corticosteroids (e.g., hydrocortisone sodium succinate [Solu-Cortef]), and pressor amines (e.g., dopamine). If focal tremors, myoclonus, or seizures occur, evaluate neurologically, initiate anticonvulsant therapy, and decide whether to decrease or discontinue meropenem. Mild cases of CDAD may respond to discontinuation of meropenem. Treat CDAD with fluids, electrolytes, protein supplements, and oral vancomycin (Vancocin) or metronidazole (Flagyl) as indicated. In severe cases, surgical evaluation may be indicated. Readily removed by hemodialysis.

MESNA
(**MEZ**-nah)

Ifosfamide/Mesna Kit, Mesnex, Uromitexan ✤

Antidote
Antineoplastic adjunct
Prophylactic for hemorrhagic cystitis

pH 6.5 to 8.5

USUAL DOSE
Specific testing recommended before each dose of ifosfamide; see Monitor.

Intravenous dose: Total daily dose is 60% of the ifosfamide dose equally divided into 3 doses. A single dose of mesna equal to 20% of the ifosfamide dose is given at the time of the ifosfamide injection and repeated 4 hours and 8 hours later (e.g., ifosfamide 1.2 Gm/M^2 would require mesna 240 mg/M^2 with the ifosfamide, 240 mg/M^2 in 4 hours, and again at 8 hours). The initial mesna dose each day may be mixed with the ifosfamide. Appears to be **compatible.** Available combined in solution with ifosfamide and as a single agent in tablet form.

Combination of intravenous and oral doses: At the time of the ifosfamide injection, give a single IV dose of mesna equal to 20% of the ifosfamide dose. At 2 hours and at 6 hours after each dose of ifosfamide, administer mesna tablets PO in a dose equal to 40% of the ifosfamide dose. The total daily dose of mesna (IV [20%] and PO [80%] combined) is 100% of the ifosfamide dose.

DOSE ADJUSTMENTS
Dose of mesna must be repeated each day ifosfamide is administered and adjusted with each increase or decrease of the ifosfamide dose.

DILUTION
Each 100 mg (1 mL) must be diluted in a minimum of 4 mL D5W, D5NS, D5/¼NS, D5/⅓NS, D5/½NS, NS, or LR. Desired concentration is 20 mg/mL.

Filters: Manufacturer's studies measured the potency of ifosfamide in combination with mesna through a 5-micron filter. No significant drug loss for ifosfamide; mesna was not measured.

Storage: Store at CRT before use. Opened multidose vials may be stored at CRT and used for up to 8 days. Diluted solutions are stable for 24 hours at 25° C (77° F). Mesna oxidizes to disulfide dimesna when exposed to oxygen.

COMPATIBILITY
(Underline Indicates Conflicting Compatibility Information)
Consider any drug NOT listed as compatible to be INCOMPATIBLE until consulting a pharmacist; specific conditions may apply.

One source suggests the following **compatibilities:**

Additive: <u>Cyclophosphamide (Cytoxan)</u>, ifosfamide (Ifex).

Y-site: Allopurinol (Aloprim), amifostine (Ethyol), aztreonam (Azactam), cladribine (Leustatin), docetaxel (Taxotere), doxorubicin liposomal (Doxil), etoposide phosphate (Etopophos), filgrastim (Neupogen), fludarabine (Fludara), gallium nitrate (Ganite), gemcitabine (Gemzar), granisetron (Kytril), linezolid (Zyvox), melphalan (Alkeran), methotrexate, <u>micafungin (Mycamine)</u>, ondansetron (Zofran), oxaliplatin (Eloxatin), paclitaxel (Taxol), pemetrexed (Alimta), piperacillin/tazobactam (Zosyn), sargramostim (Leukine), sodium bicarbonate, teniposide (Vumon), thiotepa, vinorelbine (Navelbine).

RATE OF ADMINISTRATION
A single dose over a minimum of 1 minute given as a single agent. Administer at rate for ifosfamide if given together. Another source recommends administering as an infusion over 15 to 30 minutes or as a continuous infusion maintained for 12 to 24 hours after completion of the ifosfamide infusion.

M

ACTIONS

A detoxifying agent. Reacts chemically in the kidney with urotoxic ifosfamide metabolites to detoxify them and inhibit hemorrhagic cystitis. Remains in the intravascular compartment and much of a single dose is excreted within 4 hours in urine. Does not appear to interfere with the antitumor efficacy of ifosfamide.

INDICATIONS AND USES

A prophylactic agent used to reduce the incidence of hemorrhagic cystitis caused by ifosfamide.

Unlabeled uses: May reduce the incidence of hemorrhagic cystitis caused by cyclophosphamide.

CONTRAINDICATIONS

Hypersensitivity to mesna or other thiol compounds.

PRECAUTIONS

Repeated doses are required to maintain adequate levels of mesna in the kidneys and bladder to detoxify urotoxic ifosfamide metabolites. ▪ Hemorrhagic cystitis caused by ifosfamide is dose dependent. Mesna is most effective when ifosfamide dose is less than 1.2 Gm/M^2/24 hr. Somewhat less effective when ifosfamide dose is 2 to 4 Gm/M^2/24 hr. If hematuria develops with appropriate doses of mesna, ifosfamide dose may need to be reduced or discontinued. ▪ Does not inhibit any other side effects or toxicities caused by ifosfamide therapy. ▪ Not effective in preventing hematuria caused by other conditions (e.g., thrombocytopenia). ▪ Hypersensitivity reactions ranging from mild to anaphylaxis have been reported. Patients with autoimmune disorders who are treated with cyclophosphamide and mesna may have a higher incidence of hypersensitivity reactions.

Monitor: Before administering each dose of ifosfamide, obtain a morning specimen of urine and test for hematuria. Depending on the severity of the hematuria, dose reduction or discontinuation of ifosfamide may be required. ▪ If emesis occurs within 2 hours of taking PO mesna, either repeat the PO dose or administer an IV dose.

Patient Education: Drink at least one quart of liquid daily. ▪ Report pink or red urine immediately. ▪ Report emesis within 2 hours of taking PO mesna.

Maternal/Child: Category B: use during pregnancy only if benefits clearly outweigh risks. ▪ Discontinue breast-feeding. ▪ Multidose vial contains benzyl alcohol. Do not use in neonates or infants.

Elderly: Dosing should be cautious; however, the ratio of ifosfamide to mesna should remain the same.

DRUG/LAB INTERACTIONS

May cause a false-positive reaction for **urinary ketones.** If a red-violet color develops, glacial acetic acid returns the coloring to violet.

SIDE EFFECTS

Average dose: Anorexia, bad taste in the mouth, coughing, decreased platelets associated with hypersensitivity reactions, diarrhea, dizziness, fever, flushing, headache, hyperesthesia, hypersensitivity reactions, hypertension, hypotension, increased liver enzymes, influenza-like symptoms, injection site reactions, malaise, myalgia, nausea, pharyngitis, soft stool, somnolence, ST-segment elevation, tachycardia, tachypnea, vomiting.

Overdose: Convulsions, cyanosis, diarrhea, dyspnea, fatigue, headache, hematuria, hypersensitivity reactions, hypotension, limb pain, nausea, tremor.

ANTIDOTE

No specific antidote. Keep physician informed of all side effects. Notify promptly if signs of overdose occur. Resuscitate as necessary.

METHADONE HYDROCHLORIDE BBW

(**METH**-ah-dohn hy-droh-**KLOR**-eyed)

Opioid analgesic
(agonist)
Narcotic abstinence
syndrome suppressant

Dolophine

pH 4.5 to 6.5

USUAL DOSE

Parenteral administration permitted only under specific conditions; see Indications and Precautions.

Dosing is complex and requires extensive individualization. Extended half-life, potential for prolonged respiratory depressant effects, retention in the liver (prolonging the potential duration of action), and high interpatient variability in absorption, metabolism, and relative analgesic potency must be considered.

Treatment of pain: Consider the following factors for each patient before determining an initial dose:

- Total daily dose, potency, and specific characteristics of any previously administered opioid.
- Will it be used for acute or chronic methadone dosing?
- Patient's degree of opioid tolerance.
- Patient's age, general condition, and medical status.
- Concurrent medications; see Drug/Lab Interactions.
- Type, severity, and expected duration of patient's pain.
- Acceptable balance between pain control and adverse effects.

Initial analgesic in patients who are not being treated with other opioids and are not tolerant to other opioids: 2.5 to 10 mg every 8 to 12 hours. Titrate slowly to effect. More frequent dosing may be required to maintain adequate analgesia; use extreme caution, consider extended half-life, and avoid overdose.

Conversion from oral to parenteral methadone: Begin with a 2:1 ratio (e.g., 10 mg oral methadone to 5 mg parenteral methadone); see Precautions.

Switching from other chronic opioids to parenteral methadone: Dose conversion ratios and cross-tolerance are uncertain; deaths have occurred in opioid-tolerant patients during conversion to methadone. Individualize dose based on patient's prior opioid exposure, general medical condition, concomitant medication, and anticipated breakthrough medication use. Titrate to achieve adequate pain relief balanced against tolerability of side effects. Adjust dose and/or dosing interval as necessary. The following two charts are examples of conversions.

Conversion from Oral Morphine to IV Methadone for Chronic Administration		
Total Daily Baseline Oral Morphine Dose	Estimated Total Daily Oral Methadone Dose as a Percentage of Total Daily Morphine Dose*	Estimated Daily IV Methadone Dose as a Percentage of Total Daily Oral Morphine Dose*
<100 mg	20% to 30%	10% to 15%
100 mg to 300 mg	10% to 20%	5% to 10%
300 mg to 600 mg	8% to 12%	4% to 6%
600 mg to 1,000 mg	5% to 10%	3% to 5%
>1,000 mg	Less than 5%	Less than 3%

*Divide total daily methadone dose as necessary to achieve desired dosing schedule (e.g., divide by 3 for administration every 8 hours).

Continued

Conversion from Parenteral Morphine to IV Methadone for Chronic Administration	
Total Daily Baseline Parenteral Morphine Dose	Estimated Daily IV Methadone Dose as a Percentage of Total Daily Morphine Dose*
10 mg to 30 mg	40% to 66%
30 mg to 50 mg	27% to 66%
50 mg to 100 mg	22% to 50%
100 mg to 200 mg	15% to 34%
200 mg to 500 mg	10% to 20%

*Divide total daily methadone dose as necessary to achieve desired dosing schedule (e.g., divide by 3 for administration every 8 hours).

DOSE ADJUSTMENTS
Lower-end initial doses are indicated in the elderly; consider impaired organ function and concomitant disease or drug therapy. ▪ Reduced initial doses are indicated in debilitated patients and in those with severe impaired hepatic or renal function. ▪ Clearance may be increased and half-life decreased during pregnancy. Increased doses or shorter intervals between doses may be indicated; see Maternal/Child.

DILUTION
May be given undiluted; however, to facilitate titration, further dilution of each mL with 1 to 5 mL of NS is appropriate. May be given through Y-tube or three-way stopcock of infusion set.

Storage: A multidose vial; store in carton at CRT protected from light until contents have been used.

COMPATIBILITY   (Underline Indicates Conflicting Compatibility Information)
Consider any drug NOT listed as compatible to be INCOMPATIBLE until consulting a pharmacist; specific conditions may apply.
One source suggests the following **compatibilities:**
Y-site: Atropine, dexamethasone (Decadron), <u>diazepam (Valium),</u> diphenhydramine (Benadryl), ketorolac (Toradol), lorazepam (Ativan), metoclopramide (Reglan), midazolam (Versed), phenobarbital (Luminal).

RATE OF ADMINISTRATION
A single dose as an injection over a minimum of several minutes. Titrate according to symptom relief and respiratory rate; side effects may be increased if rate of injection is too rapid.

ACTIONS
A synthetic opioid analgesic with actions similar to those of morphine. Duration of analgesic action is from 4 to 8 hours. Respiratory depressant effects occur later and persist longer than its peak analgesic effects. With repeated dosing, methadone may be retained in the liver and then slowly released, thereby prolonging the duration of action while plasma concentrations are low. Highly protein bound (85% to 90%). Metabolized in the liver by various enzymes (including cytochrome P_{450} enzymes) to inactive metabolites. Half-life is prolonged (ranges from 8 to 59 hours). Eliminated by extensive biotransformation followed by renal and fecal elimination. Secreted in saliva, breast milk, amniotic fluid, and umbilical cord plasma.

INDICATIONS AND USES
Treatment of moderate to severe pain not responsive to nonnarcotic analgesics. ▪ Temporary treatment in opioid-dependent patients unable to take oral medication. ▪ Used PO for detoxification or maintenance in opioid addiction. ▪ Parenteral products are not approved for outpatient use.

CONTRAINDICATIONS
Known hypersensitivity to methadone or any of its components. ▪ Any situation in which opioids are contraindicated (e.g., patients with respiratory depression [where resuscitative equipment is not readily available or in unmonitored settings], patients with

acute bronchial asthma or hypercarbia). ▪ Other sources add paralytic ileus and concurrent use of selegiline (Zelapar, Eldepryl).

PRECAUTIONS

If the parenteral route is indicated, the IV route is preferred; absorption by the IM or SC routes is unpredictable and may cause local tissue reaction. ▪ Schedule II opioid agonists, including hydromorphone, morphine, oxymorphone, oxycodone, fentanyl, and methadone, have the highest potential for abuse and risk of producing respiratory depression. Alcohol, CNS depressants, and other opioids potentiate the respiratory depressant effects of hydromorphone, increasing the risk of respiratory depression that might result in death; see Drug/Lab Interactions. ▪ Deaths, cardiac and respiratory, have been reported during initiation and conversion of pain patients to methadone treatment from treatment with other opioid agonists. Close monitoring is required during these times as well as during dose titration. ▪ The peak respiratory depressant effects of methadone usually occur later and last longer than the peak analgesic effects. Iatrogenic overdose may occur with short-term use, particularly during treatment initiation and dose titration. ▪ Patients tolerant to other opioids may still be sensitive to methadone. This incomplete cross-tolerance makes dose selection difficult when converting to methadone. Deaths have been reported. A high degree of "opioid tolerance" does not eliminate the possibility of methadone toxicity. ▪ Prolongation of the QT interval and infrequent cases of arrhythmia (including torsades de pointes) have been reported. May occur with any dose but appears to be more common with higher dose treatment (greater than 200 mg/day). ▪ Use with caution in patients at risk for development of prolonged QT interval (e.g., cardiac conduction abnormalities, cardiac hypertrophy, hypokalemia, hypomagnesemia) and in patients receiving concurrent treatment with other drugs that may induce electrolyte disturbances (e.g., diuretics, laxatives and, rarely, mineralocorticoid hormones) or other drugs that may prolong the QT interval; see Drug/Lab Interactions. ▪ Initiate treatment for analgesic therapy in patients with acute or chronic pain only if benefits outweigh the increased risk of QT prolongation with high doses. ▪ Use extreme caution in patients with potential respiratory insufficiency (e.g., elderly or debilitated patients, conditions accompanied by hypoxia or hypercapnia or decreased respiratory reserve [e.g., asthma, COPD, pulmonary disease or cor pulmonale, severe obesity, sleep apnea syndrome, myxedema, kyphoscoliosis, CNS depression, or coma]). Usual doses may decrease respiratory drive and simultaneously increase airway resistance, resulting in apnea. Consider use of nonopioid analgesics. If methadone is required, administer at lowest effective dose under close medical supervision. ▪ Use caution in elderly or debilitated patients, severe impaired hepatic or renal function, Addison's disease, hypothyroidism, prostatic hypertrophy, or urethral stricture; see Dose Adjustments. ▪ Use with caution in patients with head injury, other intracranial lesions, or pre-existing increased intracranial pressure. Cerebrospinal fluid pressure may be markedly exaggerated, and the clinical course of head injuries may be obscured. ▪ May mask symptoms and make diagnosis of acute abdominal conditions difficult. ▪ May cause severe hypotension in patients whose ability to maintain normal blood pressure is compromised (e.g., severe volume depletion). ▪ Patients with impaired hepatic function may be at increased risk of accumulating methadone after multiple dosing. ▪ Because of their opioid tolerance, patients receiving maintenance doses may require increased or more frequent doses of opioids to treat physical trauma, postoperative pain, or other acute pain. ▪ Do not increase methadone dose for symptoms of anxiety. ▪ Abrupt discontinuation of methadone is not recommended; may result in withdrawal symptoms (e.g., chills, lacrimation, myalgia, mydriasis, perspiration, restlessness, rhinorrhea, yawning) and may lead to relapse of illicit drug use.

Monitor: Oxygen, controlled ventilation equipment, and naloxone must always be available. ▪ Observe patient frequently to continuously based on amount of dose, and monitor VS. ▪ Assess baseline pain, then assess pain with vital signs or more frequently if needed. Reassess after administration of methadone and adjust dose or interval as required. Keep patient supine; orthostatic hypotension and fainting may occur; monitor closely during ambulation. ▪ Uncontrolled pain causes sleep deprivation, decreases pain threshold, and increases pain. When pain is finally controlled, expect the patient to sleep more until recovered from sleep deprivation. ▪ Monitor ECG in patients who develop QT prolongation and assess for modifiable risk factors (e.g., drugs with cardiac effects, drugs that may cause electrolyte abnormalities, or drugs that may inhibit the metabolism of methadone); see Drug/Lab Interactions. Consider alternate therapies for pain management. ▪ Laxatives with or without stool softeners will be required to avoid constipation and fecal impaction, especially with increased doses and extended use. Maintain adequate hydration. ▪ See Precautions and Drug/Lab Interactions.

Patient Education: Promptly report dizziness, light-headedness, palpitations, or syncope; may indicate a need for ECG monitoring. ▪ Avoid alcohol or other CNS depressants (e.g., barbiturates, benzodiazepines [e.g., diazepam (Valium)]). ▪ May cause blurred vision, dizziness, or drowsiness; use caution in tasks that require alertness. ▪ Request assistance with ambulation. ▪ May be habit forming.

Maternal/Child: Category C: potential benefit should justify potential risk to fetus. Compare the benefit of methadone to the risk of untreated addiction to illicit drugs. ▪ Total body clearance is increased during pregnancy and half-life is decreased (during 2nd and 3rd trimesters). May lead to withdrawal symptoms. Increases in dose or dosing at more frequent intervals may be indicated. ▪ Data is insufficient; however, women treated with methadone during pregnancy had improved prenatal care and did not appear to have an increased risk of miscarriage or premature delivery. Methadone in amniotic fluid and cord plasma has similar concentrations to maternal plasma. Newborn urine concentrations are less than maternal concentrations. ▪ Infants born to women treated with methadone during pregnancy may experience respiratory depression (consider methadone's long duration of action) and may be born physically dependent. Onset of withdrawal may occur in days or be delayed for 2 to 4 weeks. Withdrawal signs include fever, hyperactive reflexes, increased respiratory rate, increased stools, irritability and excessive crying, sneezing, tremors, vomiting, and yawning. May have reduced birth weight, length, and/or head circumference and some deficits in psychometric and behavioral tests. ▪ Discontinue or do not start breast-feeding. Women who are breast-feeding should wean gradually to prevent withdrawal symptoms in their infants. ▪ Safety and effectiveness for use in pediatric patients under 18 years of age not established. ▪ See Drug/Lab Interactions.

Elderly: Dosing should be cautious; see Dose Adjustments. ▪ Differences in response compared to younger adults not identified. ▪ See Precautions.

DRUG/LAB INTERACTIONS

May have additive effects with **other CNS depressants** (e.g., alcohol, general anesthetics, hypnotics or sedatives [e.g., benzodiazepines (e.g., diazepam [Valium], midazolam [Versed]), barbiturates [e.g., phenobarbital (Luminal)], other opioid analgesics, phenothiazines [e.g., prochlorperazine (Compazine)]). Concurrent use may result in hypotension, profound sedation, respiratory depression, coma, or death. ▪ Not recommended for concurrent administration with **opioid antagonists** (e.g., naloxone, naltrexone [ReVia]), **mixed agonist/antagonists, or partial agonists** (e.g., buprenorphine [Buprenex], butorphanol [Stadol], nalbuphine, pentazocine [Talwin]); may precipitate withdrawal symptoms and/or reduce analgesic effect in patients maintained on methadone. ▪ Metabolism increased and serum concentrations decreased by **cytochrome P_{450} inducers** (e.g., carbamazepine [Tegretol], phenobarbital [Luminal], phenytoin [Dilantin], rifampin [Rifadin], St. John's wort), efavirenz (Sustiva), nevirapine (Viramune), ritonavir (Norvir), and ritonavir/lopinavir combination (Kaletra). With concurrent administration, the effects of methadone are decreased; monitor for S/S of withdrawal, and adjust methadone dose as indicated. ▪ Metabolism decreased and serum concentrations increased by **cytochrome P_{450} inhibitors** (e.g., azole antifungal agents [e.g., itraconazole (Sporanox), ketoconazole (Nizoral)], macrolide antibiotics [e.g., erythromycin], selective serotonin reuptake inhibitors (SSRIs) [e.g., fluvoxamine (Luvox), sertraline (Zoloft)]). With concurrent administration, monitor methadone serum concentrations to prevent methadone toxicity. ▪ May increase serum levels of **desipramine** (Norpramin). ▪ May increase AUC of **zidovudine** and result in zidovudine toxicity. ▪ May decrease AUC and peak levels of **didanosine** (Videx) **and stavudine** (Zerit). ▪ Use caution with **MAO inhibitors** (e.g., selegiline [Eldepryl]) administered within 14 days and test for sensitivity. MAO inhibitors have caused cardiovascular collapse with other opioids (e.g., meperidine [Demerol]), not reported with methadone; see Contraindications. ▪ Use extreme caution with other **drugs that prolong the QT interval** (e.g., Class Ia antiarrhythmic agents [e.g., quinidine, procainamide (Pronestyl)], Class III antiarrhythmic agents [e.g., amiodarone (Nexterone), sotalol (Betapace)], calcium channel blockers [e.g., diltiazem (Cardizem), verapamil], some neuroleptics [e.g., phenothiazines (e.g., chlorpromazine [Thorazine])], and tricyclic antidepressants [e.g., amitriptyline (Elavil), imipramine (Tofranil)]).

SIDE EFFECTS

Hypotension and respiratory depression are dose limiting. Respiratory arrest, shock, cardiac arrest, and death have occurred.

Dizziness, light-headedness, nausea and vomiting, sedation, and sweating occur most frequently. Other reported side effects include abdominal pain, agitation, anorexia, antidiuretic effect, arrhythmias, asthenia, biliary tract spasm, cardiomyopathy, confusion, constipation, chronic hepatitis, dry mouth, edema, euphoria, flushing, glossitis, headache, heart failure, hypokalemia, hypomagnesemia, hypotension, palpitations, phlebitis, prolonged QT interval, pulmonary edema, pruritus, seizures, skin rashes, syncope, thrombocytopenia (reversible), torsades de pointes, urinary retention or hesitancy, urticaria, visual disturbances.

Overdose: Bradycardia, cold and clammy skin, constricted pupils, hypotension, respiratory depression (decrease in respiratory rate and/or tidal volume, Cheyne-Stokes respiration, cyanosis), skeletal muscle flaccidity, somnolence progressing to stupor or coma. Apnea, circulatory collapse, cardiac arrest, and death may occur.

ANTIDOTE

Keep physician informed of all side effects; may be treated symptomatically. During prolonged administration (patients on maintenance), side effects usually decrease with time. Lower doses of methadone may be indicated for dizziness, light-headedness, nausea and vomiting, sedation, and sweating. Management of major side effects or overdose requires establishing a patent airway, instituting assisted or controlled ventilation, IV fluids, vasopressors, and other supportive measures as indicated. Do not administer opioid antagonists to physically dependent patients unless clinically significant respiratory or cardiovascular depression occurs. May precipitate an acute withdrawal syndrome. If a decision is made to treat serious respiratory or circulatory depression in a physically dependent patient, administration of the antagonist should begin with care and by titration with smaller than usual doses of the antagonist. Opioid antagonists (e.g., naloxone) have a much shorter duration of action than methadone and may need repeating for up to 48 hours. Continuous monitoring is required. Forced diuresis, peritoneal dialysis, hemodialysis, or charcoal hemoperfusion may not be useful to increase methadone or metabolite elimination; however, urine acidification has been shown to increase renal elimination of methadone.

METHOTREXATE SODIUM BBW
(meth-oh-**TREKS**-ayt **SO**-dee-um)

Antineoplastic (antimetabolite)
Antipsoriatic
Antirheumatic

Methotrexate PF, MTX

pH 8.5

USUAL DOSE
Many dose limitations based on patient condition, renal and hepatic function, and concomitant drugs or therapies; see Precautions/Monitor. Doses between 100 and 500 mg/M^2 *may require* leucovorin calcium rescue. Doses over 500 mg/M^2 *require* leucovorin calcium rescue; see leucovorin calcium or levoleucovorin (Fusilev) monograph. Part of numerous protocols that change as new advances in antileukemic therapy and other cancers are developed. Selections from those protocols are included in the following text.

Acute lymphoblastic leukemia: *Induction:* 3.3 mg/M^2 in combination with prednisone 60 mg/M^2. Give daily if tolerated, and continue for up to 8 weeks or until satisfactory response (usually 4 to 6 weeks). Usually given PO.

Maintenance: Dose individualized; 15 mg/M^2/dose administered 2 times weekly IM or PO (a total weekly dose of 30 mg/M^2) or 2.5 mg/kg IV every 14 days has been used.

Mycosis fungoides: 5 to 50 mg once weekly in the early stages of disease. Adjust dose or discontinue as indicated by patient response and hematologic monitoring. 15 to 37.5 mg twice weekly may be used in patients who respond poorly to weekly therapy. Usually given PO or IM, but combination chemotherapy regimens, including higher doses of IV methotrexate with leucovorin calcium rescue, have been used in advanced stages of the disease.

Breast cancer (unlabeled): One regimen administers methotrexate 40 mg/M^2 on Days 1 and 8 of each cycle. Given in combination with PO cyclophosphamide 100 mg/M^2 on Days 1 through 14 of each cycle and fluorouracil 600 mg/M^2 on Days 1 and 8 of each cycle. In patients over 60 years of age, reduce the initial methotrexate dose to 30 mg/M^2 and the initial fluorouracil dose to 400 mg/M^2. Repeat monthly (allows a 2-week rest period between cycles) for 6 to 12 cycles.

Psoriasis: 10 to 25 mg once a week until adequate response. Some references suggest an initial test dose of 5 to 10 mg/week before initiating therapy to detect sensitivity to adverse reactions. Sources suggest 30 mg/week as a maximum dose. Use smallest effective dose. Usually given PO or IM. May be used in combination with infliximab; see infliximab monograph.

Osteosarcoma: One regimen recommends 12 Gm/M^2 as a single dose given as an infusion over 4 hours. Begin the fourth week after surgery and repeat weekly at Weeks 5, 6, 7, 11, 12, 15, 16, 29, 30, 44, and 45. A peak serum concentration of 1,000 micromolars/L at the end of the infusion is desired. Dose may be increased to 15 Gm/M^2 if required. Must be accompanied by leucovorin calcium rescue; see leucovorin calcium or levoleucovorin (Fusilev) monograph. Leucovorin calcium may be given IV or PO; levoleucovorin is IV only. When methotrexate is given in combination with leucovorin rescue, the serum creatinine must be normal, and creatinine clearance must be greater than 60 mL/min before beginning therapy. ***Osteosarcoma also requires combination chemotherapy.*** Protocols vary but may include methotrexate in combination with doxorubicin, with cisplatin, and with the combination of bleomycin, cyclophosphamide, and dactinomycin (BCD regimen). These massive doses are highly individualized and require exacting calculations and constant patient monitoring; see Precautions/Monitor.

PEDIATRIC DOSE
Safety for use in pediatric patients is limited to chemotherapy and in polyarticular-course juvenile rheumatoid arthritis. May contain benzyl alcohol; not recommended for use in neonates. See Maternal/Child.

DOSE ADJUSTMENTS

Manufacturer does not provide information on dose adjustment in patients with impaired renal or hepatic function. However, various recommendations are available in the literature. In patients with impaired hepatic function, one source recommends administering 75% of dose if bilirubin is between 3.1 and 5 or if transaminases are greater than 3 times the ULN; if bilirubin above 5, omit dose. ▪ Reduced doses may be required in patients with impaired renal function. Suggested guidelines are to administer 50% of a dose with a CrCl of 10 to 50 mL/min, and avoid use with a CrCl of less than 10 mL/min in adult patients. In pediatric patients, administer 50% of a dose with a CrCl of 10 to 50 mL/min and 30% of a dose with a CrCl of less than 10 mL/min/1.73M^2. ▪ Reduced dose may be required in patients with ascites or pleural effusions, in the very young or very elderly, in the debilitated, and in other diseases; see Precautions. ▪ Often used with other antineoplastic drugs to achieve tumor remission. ▪ See Drug/Lab Interactions.

DILUTION

Specific techniques required; see Precautions. Available in solution or as a lyophilized powder. Reconstitute powder with D5W or NS. The 1-Gm vial should be reconstituted with 19.4 mL to a concentration of 50 mg/mL. When high-dose methotrexate is administered by IV infusion, the total dose is diluted in D5W. 25 mg/mL is the maximum suggested concentration that can be given IV. Reconstitution of each 5 mg with 2 mL of preservative-free D5W or NS is suggested. Each milliliter equals 2.5 mg of methotrexate. Available in preservative-free solution. Do not use formulations or diluents with preservatives (e.g., bacteriostatic) for high-dose therapy or intrathecal injection. 1-Gm vial available for high-dose use with appropriate dilution. Not usually added to IV solutions when given in smaller doses (less than 100 mg). Discard solution if a precipitate forms. May be given through Y-tube or three-way stopcock of a free-flowing IV.

A single dose may be further diluted with D5W or NS immediately before use as an infusion with higher (100 mg or more) methotrexate doses.

Filters: No data available from manufacturer. Another source indicates no significant drug loss filtered through a nylon 0.2-micron filter.

Storage: Store in unopened container at CRT; protect from light. If prepared without a preservative, use immediately. May be stable up to 24 hours with a preservative.

COMPATIBILITY   (Underline Indicates Conflicting Compatibility Information)

Consider any drug NOT listed as compatible to be INCOMPATIBLE until consulting a pharmacist; specific conditions may apply.

One source suggests the following **compatibilities:**

Additive: Cyclophosphamide (Cytoxan), cytarabine (ARA-C), fluorouracil (5-FU), ondansetron (Zofran), sodium bicarbonate, vincristine. Other sources add dacarbazine (DTIC), furosemide (Lasix), hydrocortisone sodium succinate (Solu-Cortef), leucovorin calcium.

Y-site: Allopurinol (Aloprim), amifostine (Ethyol), amphotericin B cholesteryl (Amphotec), asparaginase (Elspar), aztreonam (Azactam), bleomycin (Blenoxane), ceftriaxone (Rocephin), cisplatin, cyclophosphamide (Cytoxan), cytarabine (ARA-C), daunorubicin (Cerubidine), doripenem (Doribax), doxorubicin (Adriamycin), doxorubicin liposomal (Doxil), etoposide (VePesid), etoposide phosphate (Etopophos), filgrastim (Neupogen), fludarabine (Fludara), fluorouracil (5-FU), furosemide (Lasix), gallium nitrate (Ganite), granisetron (Kytril), heparin, imipenem-cilastatin (Primaxin), leucovorin calcium, linezolid (Zyvox), melphalan (Alkeran), mesna (Mesnex), methylprednisolone (Solu-Medrol), metoclopramide (Reglan), mitomycin (Mutamycin), ondansetron (Zofran), oxacillin (Bactocill), oxaliplatin (Eloxatin), paclitaxel (Taxol), piperacillin/tazobactam (Zosyn), sargramostim (Leukine), teniposide (Vumon), thiotepa, vancomycin, vinblastine, vincristine, vinorelbine (Navelbine).

RATE OF ADMINISTRATION

IV injection: Each 10 mg or fraction thereof over 1 minute.

Infusion: A single dose equally distributed over 30 minutes to 4 hours or as prescribed by protocol.

ACTIONS

An antimetabolite and folic acid antagonist. Inhibits dihydrofolic acid reductase. Cell cycle–specific for the S phase. It interferes with DNA synthesis, repair, and cellular replication. Rapidly proliferating tissues are more sensitive to this effect. Widely distributed and is approximately 50% protein bound. Undergoes some hepatic and intracellular metabolism. Half-life is dose dependent and is 3 to 10 hours in patients receiving low-dose antineoplastic therapy and 8 to 15 hours in patients receiving high-dose methotrexate therapy. 80% to 90% of the administered dose is excreted unchanged in the urine within 24 hours. Clearance rates decrease with higher doses. Does not cross blood-brain barrier. Secreted in breast milk.

INDICATIONS AND USES

Used for life-threatening neoplastic disease alone or in combination with other anticancer agents in the treatment of acute lymphocytic leukemia, breast cancer, epidermal tumors of the head and neck, small-cell and squamous cell lung cancer, non-Hodgkin's lymphoma, advanced mycosis fungoides (cutaneous T-cell lymphoma). ▪ Severe disabling psoriasis or rheumatoid arthritis unresponsive to other treatment. Diagnosis of psoriasis should be established by biopsy and/or dermatology consultation before use. ▪ To prolong relapse-free survival in patients with nonmetastatic osteosarcoma who have undergone surgical resection or amputation of the primary tumor. Given as a high-dose regimen with leucovorin rescue in combination with other chemotherapeutic agents. ▪ Given PO or IM for early-stage mycosis fungoides, trophoblastic diseases (gestation choriocarcinoma, chorioadenoma destruens, and hydatidiform mole), polyarticular-course juvenile rheumatoid arthritis, rheumatoid arthritis, and other diagnoses, and given intrathecally for treatment and prophylaxis of meningeal leukemia.

Unlabeled uses: Treatment of bladder and testicular cancer. Treatment of soft tissue sarcomas and CNS tumors. Management of Crohn's disease and ectopic pregnancy and prevention of acute graft-versus-host disease. High-dose regimens for neoplastic diseases other than osteosarcoma are investigational, and therapeutic efficacy is not established.

CONTRAINDICATIONS

Hypersensitivity to methotrexate; breast-feeding mothers. Contraindicated in pregnant females with psoriasis or rheumatoid arthritis and should be used during pregnancy for treatment of neoplastic diseases only when the potential benefit outweighs the risk to the fetus. Contraindicated in psoriasis or rheumatoid arthritis patients with immunodeficiency syndromes, pre-existing blood dyscrasias, or chronic liver disease.

PRECAUTIONS

Follow guidelines for handling cytotoxic agents. See Appendix A, p. 1331. ▪ Administered by or under the direction of the physician specialist. ▪ Methotrexate should be used only in life-threatening neoplastic diseases or in patients with psoriasis or rheumatoid arthritis with severe, recalcitrant, disabling disease that is not responsive to other forms of therapy. ▪ Deaths have been reported with methotrexate use in the treatment of malignancy, psoriasis, and rheumatoid arthritis. ▪ Methotrexate elimination is reduced in patients with impaired renal function, ascites, or pleural effusions. Careful monitoring, dose reduction and, in some cases, discontinuation of therapy are required; consider evacuating excess fluid from ascites and pleural effusions before treatment if possible. ▪ Methotrexate can suppress hematopoiesis, causing anemia, aplastic anemia, pancytopenia, leukopenia, neutropenia, and/or thrombocytopenia. ▪ Serious and sometimes fatal bone marrow suppression, aplastic anemia, and GI toxicity have been reported with concomitant use of methotrexate (usually high doses) and some NSAIDs; see Drug/Lab Interactions. ▪ Leukoencephalopathy has been reported in patients who have received both IV methotrexate and craniospinal irradiation. ▪ A transient stroke-like encephalopathy has been reported with high-dose methotrexate therapy. Symptoms may include confusion, hemiparesis, transient blindness, seizures, and coma. ▪ Methotrexate-induced lung disease, including acute or chronic interstitial pneumonitis, may occur at any time, may occur even with low doses, and has been fatal. Patients may present with fever, dry cough, dyspnea, hypoxemia, and an infiltrate on chest x-ray. May require interruption of therapy and is not always fully reversible. ▪ Severe skin reactions can occur at any time and have been fatal. ▪ Transient elevations in liver enzymes may occur early during treatment. Chronic hepatotoxicity (fibrosis and cirrhosis) occurs more frequently with prolonged use and a total dose of at least 1.5 Gm. Persistent abnormalities in liver function tests and/or depression of serum albumin may be indicators of serious liver toxicity. Has resulted in deaths; see Monitor. ▪ Use with extreme caution in patients with ascites, bone marrow suppression, folate deficiency, GI obstruction, impaired renal or liver function, infection, peptic ulcer, pleural effusion, or ulcerative colitis; in debilitated patients; and in the very young or very elderly. ▪ Diarrhea and ulcerative stomatitis will require interrupting therapy; otherwise hemorrhagic enteritis and death from intestinal perforation may occur. ▪ Tumor lysis syndrome may occur, and S/S include hyperkalemia, hyperphosphatemia, hyperuricemia, hypocalcemia, metabolic acidosis, urate crystalluria, and renal failure. Prevent or alleviate tumor lysis syndrome with appropriate supportive and pharmacologic measures; see Monitor. ▪ Potentially fatal opportunistic infections, especially *Pneumocystis jiroveci* pneumonia, may occur. ▪ Risk of soft tissue necrosis and osteonecrosis may be increased with concomitant use of methotrexate and radiotherapy. ▪ May cause renal damage that may lead to acute renal failure. Nonreversible oliguric renal failure is likely to develop in patients who experience delayed early methotrexate elimination. ▪ Malignant lymphomas have been reported. May occur in patients receiving low-dose methotrexate and may not require cytotoxic treatment; discontinue methotrexate first and initiate appropriate treatment if the lymphoma does not regress. ▪ Use caution when administering high-dose methotrexate to patients receiving proton pump inhibitors; see Drug Interactions.

Monitor: Close patient observation is mandatory. Course of therapy is not repeated until all signs of toxicity from the previous course subside. ▪ CBC with platelets, chest x-ray, and renal and liver function tests before, during, and after therapy are essential to comprehensive treatment. ▪ Monitor closely for bone marrow, liver, lung, kidney, and skin toxicities. ▪ Nadir of leukocyte and platelet count usually occurs after 7 to 10 days, with recovery 7 days later. ▪ Liver biopsy, pulmonary studies, and bone marrow studies may be indicated in high-dose or long-term therapy. ▪ Monitor renal function closely; verify by CrCl levels; see Precautions. Maintain continuing adequate hydration and urine alkalinization. ▪ Prevention and treatment of hyperuricemia due to tumor lysis syndrome may be accomplished with adequate hydration and, if necessary, allopurinol and alkalinization of urine. ▪ Monitor serum methotrexate levels. ▪ Use prophylactic antiemetics to reduce nausea and vomiting and increase patient comfort. ▪ Observe closely for signs of infection. Prophylactic antibiotics may be indicated pending results of C/S in a febrile neutropenic patient. ▪ Monitor for thrombocytopenia (platelet count less than 50,000/mm³). Initiate precautions to prevent excessive bleeding (e.g., inspect IV sites, skin, and mucous membranes; use extreme care during invasive procedures; test urine, emesis, stool, and secretions for occult blood). ▪ *Administration of high-dose methotrexate* requires the following: a WBC count greater than 1,500/mm³, neutrophil count greater than 200/mm³, platelet count greater than 75,000/mm³, serum bilirubin less than 1.2 mg/dL, alanine aminotransferase (ALT) level less than 450 units, healing of any mucositis, ascites or pleural effusion must be drained dry, normal SCr, CrCl greater than 60 mL/min, 1 L/M² of IV fluid over 6 hours before dosing and 3 L/M²/day on day of infusion and for 2 days after, alkalinization of urine with sodium bicarbonate to maintain pH above 7, and repeat serum methotrexate and SCr levels at least daily until methotrexate level is below 0.05 micromolar. ▪ See Drug/Lab Interactions.

Patient Education: Avoid pregnancy. Nonhormonal birth control recommended for both females and males. Continue for at least 3 months after treatment is complete in male patients and for at least one ovulatory cycle after therapy is complete for female patients. ▪ Avoid alcohol and take only prescribed medications. Reactions can be lethal. ▪ Side effects such as dizziness and fatigue may interfere with ability to drive or operate machinery. ▪ Review early signs and symptoms of toxicity with health care provider. ▪ Close follow-up with physician is imperative. ▪ See Appendix D, p. 1333.

Maternal/Child: Category X: avoid pregnancy. Has caused fetal death and congenital anomalies. ▪ Discontinue breast-feeding. ▪ Safety for use in pediatric patients established for cancer chemotherapy and polyarticular-course juvenile rheumatoid arthritis. ▪ Serious neurotoxicity (e.g., general or focal seizures) has been reported in patients with acute lymphoblastic leukemia who have been treated with intermediate-dose methotrexate. ■ Administration of formulations containing the preservative benzyl alcohol have been associated with fatal gasping syndrome in neonates. Use preservative-free formulation of methotrexate in neonates.

Elderly: See Dose Adjustments. Dose selection should be cautious and based on the potential for decreased organ function, decreased folate stores, and concomitant disease or drug therapy. ■ Consider monitoring CrCl and methotrexate levels. ■ Monitor for early signs of hepatic, renal, or bone marrow toxicity. ■ In chronic administration, certain toxicities may be decreased by folate supplementation. ■ Post-marketing experience suggests that the occurrence of bone marrow suppression, thrombocytopenia, and pneumonitis may increase with age.

DRUG/LAB INTERACTIONS

The following drugs may enhance methotrexate toxicity when administered concomitantly: **cyclosporine** (Sandimmune), **any hepatotoxic drug** (e.g., azathioprine, retinoids [vitamin A], sulfasalazine [Azulfidine]), **etretinate** (Tegison), **NSAIDs** (e.g., ibuprofen [Advil, Motrin], ketoprofen, naproxen [Aleve, Naprosyn]), **penicillins** (e.g., amoxicillin, nafcillin [Nallpen]), **probenecid, salicylates, sulfonamides, phenytoin** (Dilantin), **pyrimethamine, trimethoprim** (component of sulfamethoxazole/trimethoprim), **and vancomycin** (given up to 10 days prior to methotrexate); interactions may be life threatening. Monitoring serum levels and/or reduced doses of methotrexate may be indicated or a longer duration of leucovorin calcium rescue may be required. One source suggests delaying administration of aspirin, NSAIDs, and probenecid for 48 hours after larger doses of methotrexate; see Precautions. ■ **NSAIDs** are used in the treatment of rheumatoid arthritis in combination with low doses of methotrexate (e.g., 7.5 to 15 mg/week). Do not administer NSAIDs before or concomitantly with high doses of methotrexate (e.g., treatment of osteosarcoma); deaths from severe hematologic and GI toxicity have been reported. ■ Use caution if high-dose methotrexate is administered in combination with **nephrotoxic chemotherapy agents** (e.g., cisplatin). ■ Concurrent use of methotrexate (primarily at high dose) with **some proton pump inhibitors** such as esomeprazole (Nexium), omeprazole (Prilosec), and pantoprazole (Protonix) may cause prolonged elevation of serum levels of methotrexate and its metabolite, hydroxymethotrexate, leading to toxicity. Discontinue several days before methotrexate administration. Consider an H_2 antagonist (e.g., ranitidine [Zantac]). ■ **Doxycycline** may increase toxicity of methotrexate in high-dose regimens. ■ **Vitamins with folic acid** may inhibit the antifolate effects of methotrexate, decreasing effectiveness. ■ May increase serum levels of **mercaptopurine** (Purinethol); dose adjustment may be required. ■ Do not administer **live virus vaccines** to patients receiving antineoplastic drugs. ■ **Procarbazine** (Matulane) may increase nephrotoxicity of methotrexate. Allow 72 hours between last dose of procarbazine and first dose of methotrexate. ■ Monitor for signs of increased bone marrow suppression with **sulfonamides** (e.g., sulfisoxazole [Gantrisin], SMZ-TMP [Bactrim]), **bone marrow–suppressing agents** (e.g., antineoplastics), **and radiation therapy.** May also cause SMZ-TMP (Bactrim)-induced megaloblastic anemia. ■ May decrease **theophylline** clearance and increase serum levels; monitor theophylline serum levels with concurrent use. ■ **Urinary alkalinizers** increase renal excretion and may reduce effectiveness.

SIDE EFFECTS

Toxicity usually dose related. Death can occur from average doses, high doses, drug interactions (e.g., NSAIDs), bone marrow toxicity, GI toxicity, hepatic toxicity, pulmonary toxicity, and/or severe skin reactions. Abdominal distress, chills, decreased resistance to infection, dizziness, fatigue, fever, leukopenia, malaise, nausea, and ulcerative stomatitis occur most frequently. Other side effects reported include abortion (spontaneous), acne, acute hepatitis, agranulocytosis, alopecia, alveolitis, anaphylaxis, anemia, anorexia, aplastic anemia, azotemia, blurred vision, chronic fibrosis and cirrhosis, convulsions, COPD, cystitis, decreased serum albumin, defective oogenesis or spermatogenesis, diabetes, diarrhea, drowsiness, enteritis, eosinophilia, erythema multiforme, erythematous rashes, exfoliative dermatitis, fetal defects or death, furunculosis, GI ulceration and bleeding, gingivitis, gynecomastia, headache, hematemesis, hematuria, hemiparesis, hepatic failure, hepatotoxicity, hypotension, infertility, interstitial pneumonitis, liver enzyme elevations, lymphadenopathy and lymphoproliferative disorders, melena (passage of dark, tarry stools), menstrual dysfunction, nephropathy (severe), neutropenia, oligospermia (transient), opportunistic infections (e.g., cytomegalovirus infection, herpes zoster, histoplasmosis, *Pneumocystis jiroveci* pneumonia), pancreatitis, pancytopenia, paresis, pericardial effusion, pericarditis, pharyngitis, photosensitivity, pigmentary changes, proteinuria, pruritus, pseudomembranous colitis, renal failure, respiratory failure, respiratory fibrosis, skin necrosis, skin ulceration, speech impairment (aphasia, dysarthria), Stevens-Johnson syndrome, stomatitis, suppressed hematopoiesis (blood cell formation), telangiectasia, thrombocytopenia, thromboembolic events (e.g., arterial thrombosis, cerebral thrombosis, deep vein thrombosis, pulmonary embolus, retinal vein thrombosis, thrombophlebitis), toxic epidermal necrolysis, transient blindness, tumor lysis syndrome, urticaria, vaginal discharge, vomiting.

ANTIDOTE

Discontinue methotrexate and notify the physician of any side effects. **Leucovorin calcium (citrovorum factor, folinic acid)** may be given PO, IM, or IV promptly to counteract inadvertent overdose. Leucovorin calcium is also indicated as a planned rescue mechanism for large doses of methotrexate required to treat some malignancies. Doses equal to dose of methotrexate are frequently required. Should be given within 1 hour in overdose, 24 hours in rescue. See specific process for overdose and for rescue for high-dose MTX in leucovorin calcium monograph. Doses up to 150 mg or 100 mg/M² every 3 hours may be required if SCr is 50% or greater than baseline measurement before methotrexate administration. Serum methotrexate must come down to below 0.05 micromolar. Continuing hydration and urinary alkalinization are mandatory to prevent precipitation in renal tubules. Monitor fluid and electrolyte status until serum methotrexate has fallen to less than 0.05 micromolar and renal failure has resolved. Glucarpidase (Voraxaze), an antidote indicated for the treatment of toxic methotrexate concentration in patients with delayed methotrexate clearance due to impaired renal function, may also be used. If glucarpidase is used, do not administer leucovorin within 2 hours before or after a dose of glucarpidase because leucovorin is a substrate for glucarpidase; see glucarpidase monograph. Administration of whole blood products (e.g., packed RBCs, platelets, leukocytes) and/or blood modifiers (e.g., darbepoetin alfa [Aranesp], epoetin alfa [Epogen], filgrastim [Neupogen, Zarxio], pegfilgrastim [Neulasta], sargramostim [Leukine]) may be indicated to treat bone marrow toxicity. Death may occur from the progression of most of these side effects. Symptomatic and supportive therapy is indicated. Charcoal hemoperfusion may be helpful, and/or acute intermittent hemodialysis with a high-flux dialyzer may be used to counteract toxicity or inadvertent overdose.

METHYLERGONOVINE MALEATE
(meth-ill-er-**GON**-oh-veen **MAL**-ee-ayt)

Uterine stimulant
(oxytocic)

Methergine

pH 2.7 to 3.5

USUAL DOSE
1 mL (0.2 mg); repeat doses should be IM or PO.

DILUTION
Check expiration date on vial; methylergonovine deteriorates with age. May be given undiluted. Some clinicians recommend dilution with 5 mL of NS. Do not add to IV solutions. May be given through Y-tube or three-way stopcock of infusion set.

Filters: No data available from manufacturer; suggests following hospital protocol for filtering from ampules.

Storage: Store in refrigerator (2° to 8° C [36° to 46° F]); protect from light.

COMPATIBILITY
Consider any drug NOT listed as compatible to be INCOMPATIBLE until consulting a pharmacist; specific conditions may apply.

One source suggests the following **compatibilities:**

Y-site: Heparin, hydrocortisone sodium succinate (Solu-Cortef).

RATE OF ADMINISTRATION
0.2 mg or fraction thereof over 1 minute. Too-rapid injection may cause severe nausea and vomiting. See Precautions.

ACTIONS
A semi-synthetic ergot alkaloid used for prevention and control of postpartum hemorrhage. An oxytocic. It exerts a direct stimulation on the smooth muscle of the uterus. Increases tone, rate, and amplitude of rhythmic contractions. Shortens third-stage labor and reduces blood loss. In therapeutic doses the prolonged initial contraction of the uterus is followed by periods of relaxation and contraction. May also produce vasoconstriction, increase CVP and BP, and may rarely produce peripheral ischemia. Effective within minutes. Half-life approximately 3.4 hours. It is probably metabolized in the liver and excreted in feces. Secreted in breast milk.

INDICATIONS AND USES
Routine management of uterine atony, hemorrhage, and subinvolution of the uterus following delivery of the placenta. ▪ Control of uterine hemorrhage in the second stage of labor following delivery of the anterior shoulder.

CONTRAINDICATIONS
Hypersensitivity, hypertension, pregnancy before third stage of labor (delivery of the placenta) except as stated in Indications, toxemia. ▪ Contraindicated for concomitant use with potent CYP3A4 inhibitors (e.g., protease inhibitors [ritonavir (Norvir)], macrolide antibiotics [erythromycin], and azole antifungals [ketoconazole (Nizoral)]); see Drug/Lab Interactions.

PRECAUTIONS
IV administration is for emergency use only. IM or oral routes are preferred and should be used after the initial IV dose. ▪ IV use may induce hypertension and/or CVA. Give slowly and monitor BP. ▪ Use caution in presence of sepsis, obliterative vascular disease, and hepatic or renal disease. ▪ Patients with coronary artery disease or risk factors for coronary artery disease (e.g., diabetes, high cholesterol, obesity, smoking) may be more susceptible to developing myocardial ischemia and infarction associated with methylergonovine-induced vasospasm. ▪ Use with caution during the second stage of labor. The necessity for manual removal of a retained placenta should occur rarely with proper technique and adequate allowance of time for a spontaneous separation. ▪ Avoid intra-arterial or peri-arterial injection. ▪ See Contraindications.

Monitor: Monitor BP. ▪ Observe for signs of excessive bleeding. ▪ See Drug/Lab Interactions.

Maternal/Child: Category C: see Contraindications and Precautions. ▪ Avoid breast-feeding during treatment with methylergonovine. Wait at least 12 hours after administration of the last dose before initiating or resuming breast-feeding. Milk secreted during this period should be discarded. May be given orally with caution during breast-feeding for up to 1 week after delivery. ▪ Inadvertent administration of methylergonovine to newborn infants resulting in convulsions, cyanosis, oliguria, and respiratory depression has been reported. Methylergonovine should be stored separately from medications intended for neonatal administration (e.g., vitamin K, hepatitis B vaccine). ▪ Safety and effectiveness for use in pediatric patients not established.

Elderly: Difference in safety and effectiveness compared to younger adults not observed. ▪ If used in the elderly, dose selection should be cautious.

DRUG/LAB INTERACTIONS

Severe hypertension and cerebrovascular accidents can result with **ephedrine and other vasopressors.** Hydralazine IV will reduce this hypertension. ▪ *Do not administer with potent CYP3A4 inhibitors,* such as **macrolide antibiotics** (e.g., erythromycin [Erythrocin], troleandomycin [TAO], clarithromycin [Biaxin]), **HIV protease inhibitors** (e.g., indinavir [Crixivan], nelfinavir [Viracept], ritonavir [Norvir]), **reverse transcriptase inhibitors** (e.g., delavirdine [Rescriptor]), **or azole antifungals** (e.g., ketoconazole [Nizoral], voriconazole [VFEND]). Serum levels increased. Elevated levels of ergot alkaloids can cause ergotism (i.e., risk for vasospasm potentially leading to cerebral ischemia and/or ischemia of the extremities). ▪ May be used cautiously with **less potent CYP3A4 inhibitors** (e.g., saquinavir [Invirase], nefazodone, fluconazole [Diflucan], grapefruit juice, fluoxetine [Prozac], fluvoxamine [Luvox], zileuton [Zyflo], and clotrimazole [Gyne-Lotrimin, Mycelex]). ▪ **Strong CYP3A4 inducers** (e.g., rifampin [Rifadin], nevirapine [Viramune]) may decrease effectiveness of methylergonovine. ▪ **Anesthetics** (e.g., halothane, methoxyflurane) may reduce oxytocic effect of methylergonovine. ▪ Produces vasoconstriction and can be expected to reduce the effect of **antianginal drugs** (e.g., nitroglycerin). ▪ Concomitant use with **other ergot alkaloids or prostaglandins** will produce additive effects. Use caution.

SIDE EFFECTS

Rare in therapeutic doses but may include the following:

Abdominal pain (caused by uterine contractions), bradycardia, chest pain (temporary), coronary artery spasm, diaphoresis, diarrhea, dilated pupils, dizziness, dyspnea, hallucinations, headache, hematuria, hypersensitivity reactions, hypertension (transient), hypotension, leg cramps, MI, nasal congestion, nausea, palpitations, rash, seizures, tachycardia, thrombophlebitis, tinnitus, vasoconstriction, vasospasm, vomiting, water intoxication, weakness.

Overdose: Cerebrovascular accident, coma, convulsions, hypertension (followed by hypotension in severe cases), hypothermia, numbness, oliguria, palpitations, respiratory depression, severe nausea and vomiting, tachycardia, tingling of the extremities.

Post-Marketing: Angina, atrioventricular block, cerebrovascular accident, paresthesia, ventricular fibrillation, ventricular tachycardia.

ANTIDOTE

Discontinue the drug immediately at the onset of any side effect and notify the physician. Most side effects are transient unless there is severe toxicity and will be treated symptomatically. Use antiemetics (e.g., prochlorperazine [Compazine], ondansetron [Zofran]) for nausea and vomiting. Treat seizures with anticonvulsants (e.g., diazepam [Valium], phenytoin [Dilantin]). Maintain adequate pulmonary ventilation, especially if convulsions or coma develop. Correct hypotension with pressor drugs (e.g., dopamine). Apply warmth to extremities to control peripheral vasospasm.

METHYLPREDNISOLONE SODIUM SUCCINATE
(meth-ill-pred-**NISS**-oh-lohn **SO**-dee-um **SUK**-sih-nayt)

A-Methapred, Solu-Medrol

Hormone
(corticosteroid)
Anti-inflammatory

pH 7 to 8

USUAL DOSE

Use the lowest possible dose to control the condition being treated. When reduction in dose is possible, the reduction should be gradual.

Average dose range is 10 to 40 mg initially. May be repeated every 4 to 6 hours as necessary. IV methylprednisolone is usually given in an emergency situation or when oral dosing is not feasible. Larger doses may be justified by patient condition. Repeat until adequate response, then decrease dose as indicated. Total dose usually does not exceed 1.5 Gm/24 hr, but higher doses have been used in life-threatening shock. High-dose treatment is used until patient condition stabilizes, usually no longer than 48 to 72 hours.

Anti-inflammatory: 10 to 40 mg. May be repeated every 4 to 6 hours as necessary.

Acute spinal cord injury high-dose therapy (unlabeled): Spinal cord injury must be less than 8 hours old and above L-2. The earlier methylprednisolone therapy begins, the better the results. *Loading dose:* 30 mg/kg of a specifically diluted solution (see Dilution) evenly distributed over 15 minutes. Maintain IV line with standard IV fluids for 45 minutes, then begin a *maintenance dose* of 5.4 mg/kg/hr for 23 hours. Discontinue 24 hours after loading dose initiated.

Status asthmaticus: Newer asthma guidelines recommend 40 to 80 mg/day in 1 to 2 divided doses until peak expiratory flow is 70% of predicted or personal best. Another source recommends a *loading dose* of 2 mg/kg followed by 0.5 to 1 mg/kg/dose every 6 hours for up to 5 days.

Acute exacerbation of multiple sclerosis: 160 mg as a single dose each day for 7 days. Follow with 64 mg every other day for 1 month.

Pneumocystis jiroveci **pneumonia (unlabeled):** Initiate within 24 to 72 hours of initial antibiotic PCP therapy. 30 mg twice daily for 5 days. Follow with 30 mg once daily for 5 days (Days 6 to 10). Then reduce to 15 mg once daily for 11 days (Days 11 to 21) or until antibiotic regimen is complete.

Severe lupus nephritis (unlabeled): 1 Gm as an infusion over 1 hour for 3 days. Follow with long-term prednisolone oral therapy.

PEDIATRIC DOSE

See Maternal/Child. Dose may be reduced for infants and pediatric patients but should be governed more by the severity of the condition and the response of the patient than by age or size. Dose should not be less than 0.5 mg/kg every 24 hours.

Anti-inflammatory/immunosuppressive: The range of initial doses is 0.11 to 1.6 mg/kg/day (3.2 to 48 mg/M^2/day) in 3 to 4 divided doses (0.0275 to 0.4 mg/kg every 6 hours or 0.036 to 0.53 mg/kg every 8 hours, or 0.8 to 12 mg/M^2 every 6 hours or 1.06 to 16 mg/M^2 every 8 hours). Another source recommends 0.5 to 1.7 mg/kg/day or 5 to 25 mg/M^2/day in divided doses every 6 to 12 hours (0.125 to 0.425 mg/kg or 1.25 to 6.25 mg/M^2 every 6 hours, or 0.25 to 0.85 mg/kg or 2.5 to 12.5 mg/M^2 every 12 hours).

Status asthmaticus: Newer asthma guidelines recommend 0.5 to 1 mg/kg every 12 hours (maximum 60 mg/day) until peak expiratory flow is 80% of predicted or personal best. Another source recommends 2 mg/kg as a *loading* dose. *Maintain* with 0.5 to 1 mg/kg every 6 hours for up to 5 days.

Severe lupus nephritis (unlabeled): 30 mg/kg every other day for 6 doses. Follow with long-term prednisolone oral therapy.

DOSE ADJUSTMENTS

Reduced dose may be required; see Precautions and Drug/Lab Interactions. ▪ Clearance of corticosteroids is decreased in patients with hypothyroidism and increased in patients with hyperthyroidism. Dose adjustment may be required.

DILUTION

Available in Act-O-Vials containing 40 mg, 125 mg, 500 mg, and 1,000 mg. Each vial has an appropriate amount of diluent. Reconstitute by pressing down on the plastic activator, allowing the diluent into the lower chamber. Agitate gently. Remove the plastic tab covering the center of the stopper and sterilize the stopper with a suitable germicide. Using sterile technique, insert a needle through the center of the rubber stopper to withdraw diluted solution. To be diluted only with diluent supplied in Act-O-Vial. Also available in vials, including a 2,000-mg dose. Should be diluted with accompanying diluent or BWFI with benzyl alcohol. May be given as direct IV, as an infusion, or further diluted in desired amounts of D5W, D5NS, or NS.

Acute spinal cord injury loading and maintenance doses: Each 1-Gm vial must be diluted to 16 mL with bacteriostatic water to maintain potency and avoid precipitation (62.5 mg/mL). Further dilute in D5W, D5NS, or NS with an amount to facilitate dose of 5.4 mg/kg/hr. (Example for a patient weighing 50 kg: [50 kg × 5.4 mg/hr = 270 mg/hr. 270 mg/hr × 23 hours = 6,210 mg total dose]. With a total dose of 6,210 mg at 62.5 mg/mL, you will have 99.36 [100] mL of reconstituted methylprednisolone. Add an additional 100 mL diluent to achieve 31.25 mg/mL. 270 mg/hr is the desired dose for this patient. 270 mg/hr divided by 31.25 mg/mL [strength of solution] equals 8.6. Administer at 8.6 mL/hr to achieve desired dose over 23 hours.)

Storage: Protect from light. Store both unreconstituted product and solution at RT (20° to 25° C [68° to 77° F]). Use solution within 48 hours of mixing. Heat sensitive; do not autoclave.

COMPATIBILITY   (Underline Indicates Conflicting Compatibility Information)

Consider any drug NOT listed as compatible to be INCOMPATIBLE until consulting a pharmacist; specific conditions may apply.

Manufacturer states, "Because of possible physical **incompatibilities,** should not be diluted or mixed with other solutions."

One source suggests the following **compatibilities:**

Additive: <u>Aminophylline</u>, chloramphenicol (Chloromycetin), clindamycin (Cleocin), <u>cytarabine (ARA-C)</u>, dopamine, granisetron (Kytril), heparin, norepinephrine (Levophed), penicillin G potassium, ranitidine (Zantac), theophylline, verapamil.

Y-site: Acetaminophen (Ofirmev), acyclovir (Zovirax), alprostadil, amifostine (Ethyol), amiodarone (Nexterone), amphotericin B cholesteryl (Amphotec), <u>anidulafungin (Eraxis)</u>, aztreonam (Azactam), bivalirudin (Angiomax), cefepime (Maxipime), ceftaroline (Teflaro), ceftazidime (Fortaz), <u>cisatracurium (Nimbex)</u>, cladribine (Leustatin), cytarabine (ARA-C), dexmedetomidine (Precedex), <u>diltiazem (Cardizem)</u>, dopamine, doripenem (Doribax), doxorubicin liposomal (Doxil), enalaprilat (Vasotec IV), famotidine (Pepcid IV), fludarabine (Fludara), granisetron (Kytril), heparin, hetastarch in electrolytes (Hextend), 6% hydroxyethyl starch (Voluven), linezolid (Zyvox), melphalan (Alkeran), meperidine (Demerol), methotrexate, metronidazole (Flagyl IV), midazolam (Versed), milrinone (Primacor), morphine, nicardipine (Cardene IV), oxaliplatin (Eloxatin), pemetrexed (Alimta), piperacillin/tazobactam (Zosyn), <u>potassium chloride (KCl)</u>, remifentanil (Ultiva), sodium bicarbonate, tacrolimus (Prograf), <u>telavancin (Vibativ)</u>, teniposide (Vumon), theophylline, thiotepa, topotecan (Hycamtin).

RATE OF ADMINISTRATION

IV injection: A single dose of 10 to 40 mg over several minutes. When higher doses are needed, administer up to 30 mg/kg over 30 minutes or more. Too-rapid administration of high doses (greater than 500 mg administered over a period of less than 10 minutes) may precipitate hypotension, cardiac arrhythmia, and sudden death. Direct IV administration of lower doses (10 to 40 mg) is usually the route of choice and eliminates the possibility of overloading the patient with IV fluids. May be given as an *infusion* in its own diluent.

At the discretion of the physician, a continuous infusion may be given, properly diluted, over a specified time. Another source suggests the following:

A single dose of up to 1.8 mg/kg or 125 mg may be given *IV push* over 3 to 15 minutes.

A single dose of 2 mg/kg or 250 mg or more may be given as an *infusion* over 15 to 30 minutes.

A single dose of 15 mg/kg or greater than 500 mg may be given as an *infusion* over 30 minutes or more.

Acute spinal cord injury: See Usual Dose and Dilution.

ACTIONS

A glucocorticoid steroid with potent metabolic, anti-inflammatory actions and innumerable other effects. Has a greater anti-inflammatory potency than prednisolone and less tendency to cause excessive potassium and calcium excretion and sodium and water retention. Has five times the potency of hydrocortisone sodium succinate. Has minimal mineralocorticoid activity. Primarily used for anti-inflammatory and immunosuppressive effects. Demonstrable effects seen within 1 hour of administration. Primarily metabolized in the liver and excreted in the urine and feces. Dose almost completely excreted after 12 hours, which allows the use of very large doses with reasonable safety. Crosses the placental barrier. Secreted in breast milk.

INDICATIONS AND USES

Includes treatment of allergic states, dermatologic diseases, endocrine disorders, gastrointestinal diseases, hematologic disorders, neoplastic diseases, nervous system disorders, ophthalmic diseases, renal diseases, respiratory diseases, and rheumatic disorders. See prescribing information for a complete list. Used primarily as an anti-inflammatory or immunosuppressant agent. May be used in conjunction with other forms of therapy, such as epinephrine for acute hypersensitivity reactions. Oral therapy should be used when appropriate.

Unlabeled uses: High-dose therapy as an adjunct to traditional spinal cord injury management; to improve neurologic recovery in an acute (less than 8 hours old) spinal cord injury above L-2. ■ Treatment of *Pneumocystis jiroveci* pneumonia as an adjunct to antibiotics.

CONTRAINDICATIONS

Absolute contraindications in long-term therapy, except in life-threatening situations: Hypersensitivity to any product component, including sulfites; systemic fungal infections. ■ Formulations containing benzyl alcohol are contraindicated in neonates and for intrathecal administration.

Relative contraindications: Active or healed tuberculosis, amebiasis (latent or active), cerebral malaria, chickenpox, ocular herpes simplex, pregnancy.

PRECAUTIONS

Not the drug of choice to treat acute adrenocortical insufficiency. ■ May produce hypothalamic-pituitary-adrenal (HPA) axis suppression with resulting glucocorticosteroid insufficiency in patients undergoing chronic or prolonged therapy. To avoid relative adrenocortical insufficiency, do not stop therapy abruptly; taper off. Patient is observed carefully, especially under stress, for up to 2 years; exception is very short-term therapy. ■ Increased doses of rapidly acting corticosteroids are indicated when patients on corticosteroid therapy are subjected to any unusual stress (e.g., surgery, hospitalization). These increased doses should be used before, during, and after the stressful situation. ■ Formulation may contain benzyl alcohol; see Contraindications and Maternal/Child. ■ Rare instances of anaphylactoid reactions have been reported in patients receiving corticosteroid therapy. ■ In one study, an increase in mortality was seen in patients with cranial trauma who had no other clear indication for corticosteroid treatment. Should not be used for treatment of traumatic brain injury. ■ Use with caution in patients who have had a recent MI. Ventricular free wall rupture has been reported. ■ Patients taking corticosteroids may be more susceptible to infections. Latent disease may be activated. Intercurrent infections may be exacerbated; see Contraindications. ■ Use with caution in patients with CHF, hypertension, or renal insufficiency. May affect fluid and electrolyte balance. ▪ Use with caution in patients with thyroid dysfunction; see Dose Adjustments. ▪ Use with caution in patients with active or latent peptic ulcers, diverticulitis, fresh intestinal anastomoses, and nonspecific ulcerative colitis. May be at increased risk for perforation. ▪ Metabolism of corticosteroids is decreased in patients with cirrhosis; effects may be enhanced. ▪ Use with caution in patients at risk for osteoporosis. Corticosteroids decrease bone formation, increase bone resorption, and decrease protein matrix of the bone. May lead to inhibition of bone growth in pediatric patients and the development of osteoporosis at any age. ▪ An acute myopathy has been reported with the use of high doses of corticosteroids. Most often seen in patients with disorders of neuromuscular transmission (e.g., myasthenia gravis) or in patients receiving concomitant therapy with neuromuscular blocking drugs. Myopathy is generalized, may involve ocular and respiratory muscles, and may result in quadriparesis. Clinical improvement following discontinuation of corticosteroids may take weeks to years. ▪ May induce psychological changes (e.g., depression, euphoria, insomnia, mood swings, personality changes, psychosis). May aggravate existing emotional instability or psychotic tendencies. ▪ Kaposi's sarcoma has been reported in patients receiving corticosteroid therapy, most often for chronic conditions. Clinical improvement has been seen with discontinuation of the corticosteroid. ▪ Prophylactic antacids may prevent peptic ulcer complications.

Monitor: Monitor electrolytes. May cause sodium retention and potassium and calcium excretion. ▪ May cause hypertension secondary to fluid and electrolyte disturbances. Monitor BP. ▪ May mask signs of infection. ▪ May increase insulin needs in patients with diabetes. Monitor serum glucose. ▪ Administer single dose before 9 AM to reduce suppression of adrenocortical activity. ▪ During prolonged therapy, routine laboratory studies such as urinalysis, 2-hour postprandial blood sugar, BP, body weight assessment, and chest x-ray should be obtained at regular intervals. Upper GI x-rays are suggested for patients with a history of ulcers or significant dyspepsia. ▪ May increase intraocular pressure. Periodic ophthalmic exams may be necessary with prolonged treatment. ▪ See Drug/Lab Interactions.

Patient Education: Report edema, tarry stools, or weight gain promptly. Report anorexia, diarrhea, dizziness, fatigue, low blood sugar, nausea, weakness, weight loss, or vomiting; may indicate adrenal insufficiency after dose reduction or discontinuing therapy. ▪ May mask signs of infection and/or decrease resistance. ▪ Diabetics may have increased requirement for insulin or oral hypoglycemics. ▪ Avoid immunizations with live virus vaccines. ▪ Avoid exposure to measles or chickenpox. Seek immediate medical advice if exposure occurs. ▪ Carry ID stating steroid dependent if receiving prolonged therapy.

Maternal/Child: Category C: corticosteroids have been shown to be teratogenic in many species. ▪ Discontinue breast-feeding. ▪ Infants born to mothers who received corticosteroids during pregnancy should be carefully monitored for signs of hypoadrenalism. ▪ May contain benzyl alcohol, which has been associated with a fatal "gasping syndrome" in neonates. ▪ Monitor growth and development of pediatric patients receiving prolonged treatment.

Elderly: Differences in response between the elderly and younger patients have not been identified. Dose selection should be cautious based on the possibility of age-related organ impairment (e.g., bone marrow reserve, renal, hepatic). May be more sensitive to effects.

DRUG/LAB INTERACTIONS

Aminoglutethimide (Cytadren) may lead to a loss of corticosteroid-induced adrenal suppression. ▪ Metabolism increased and effects reduced by **hepatic enzyme–inducing agents** (e.g., alcohol, barbiturates [e.g., phenobarbital], hydantoins [e.g., phenytoin (Dilantin)], rifampin [Rifadin]); dose adjustments may be required when adding or deleting from drug profile. ▪ Risk of hypokalemia increased with **amphotericin B or potassium-depleting diuretics** (e.g., thiazides, furosemide, ethacrynic acid). Monitor potassium levels and cardiac function. Increased risk of **digoxin** toxicity secondary to hypokalemia. ▪ May decrease effectiveness of **potassium supplements;** monitor serum potassium. ▪ **Diuretics** decrease sodium and fluid retention effects of corticosteroids; corticosteroids decrease sodium excretion and diuretic effects of diuretics. ▪ Use with **cyclosporine** in organ transplants is therapeutic but may increase cyclosporine toxicity; seizures have been reported; use caution. ▪ Clearance decreased and effects increased with **estrogens, oral contraceptives, triazole antifungals** (e.g., itraconazole [Sporanox]), **and macrolide antibiotics** (e.g., azithromycin [Zithromax], erythromycin, troleandomycin [TAO]). ▪ Coadministration of **aprepitant** (fosaprepitant [Emend]) may increase methylprednisolone levels. Dose reduction of methylprednisolone may be indicated. ▪ May interact with **anticoagulants, nondepolarizing muscle relaxants** (e.g., atracurium [Tracrium]), **or theophyllines;** may inhibit or potentiate action; monitor carefully. ▪ Monitor patients receiving **antidiabetic agents** (e.g., insulin, glyburide) **or thyroid hormones** carefully; dose adjustments of either or both agents may be required. ▪ May antagonize effects of **isoniazid and salicylates;** dose adjustments may be required. ▪ Administration of **live virus or live-attenuated vaccines** is contraindicated in patients receiving immunosuppressive doses of corticosteroids. Inactivated vaccines may be administered, but the response to such vaccines cannot be predicted. ▪ Concomitant use with **NSAIDs** (e.g., ibuprofen [Advil, Motrin], naproxen [Aleve, Naprosyn]) may increase the risk of adverse GI effects. ▪ Concomitant use with **anticholinesterase agents** (e.g., neostigmine) may produce severe weakness in patients with myasthenia gravis. If possible, anticholinesterase agents should be withdrawn at least 24 hours before initiating corticosteroid therapy. ▪ Altered **protein-binding capacity** will impact effectiveness of this drug. ▪ Corticosteroids may **suppress reactions to skin tests.** ▪ See Dose Adjustments.

SIDE EFFECTS
Do occur but are usually reversible: Cushing's syndrome; electrolyte and calcium imbalance; euphoria; glycosuria; hyperglycemia; hypersensitivity reactions, including anaphylaxis; hypertension; increased appetite; increased intracranial pressure; menstrual irregularities; peptic ulcer perforation and hemorrhage; protein catabolism; spontaneous fractures; transitory burning or tingling, sweating, headache, or weakness; thromboembolism; and many others.

ANTIDOTE
Notify the physician of any side effect. Will probably treat the side effect if necessary. Resuscitate as necessary for anaphylaxis and notify physician. Keep epinephrine immediately available.

METOCLOPRAMIDE HYDROCHLORIDE ▪BBW▪
(meh-toe-kloh-**PRAH**-myd hy-droh-**KLOR**-eyed)

Reglan

GI stimulant
Antiemetic

pH 4.5 to 6.5

USUAL DOSE
Small bowel intubation and/or radiologic examination of the small bowel: 10 mg (2 mL) as a single dose.

Antiemetic: High-dose regimen for highly emetogenic chemotherapy is rarely used; $5HT_3$ receptor antagonists (e.g., granisetron [Kytril], ondansetron [Zofran]) preferred. 2 mg/kg of body weight 30 minutes before giving emetogenic cancer chemotherapy (e.g., cisplatin, dacarbazine). Repeat every 2 hours for 2 doses, then every 3 hours for 3 doses; see Dose Adjustments. For less emetogenic regimens, 1 mg/kg/dose may be adequate.

Diabetic gastroparesis: 10 mg immediately before each meal and at bedtime. Use IV for up to 10 days if symptoms are severe. Continue treatment PO for 2 to 8 weeks.

Prevention of postoperative nausea and vomiting: 10 mg, usually given IM toward the end of surgery. Up to 20 mg may be used.

PEDIATRIC DOSE

Small bowel intubation and/or radiologic examination of the small bowel: *6 to 14 years:* 2.5 to 5 mg. *Under 6 years:* 0.1 mg/kg of body weight.

Gastroesophageal reflux or GI dysmotility (unlabeled): 0.1 to 0.2 mg/kg/dose. May be given every 6 hours if required. Maximum dose 0.8 mg/kg/24 hr (0.2 mg/kg/dose every 6 hours).

Antiemetic (unlabeled): Rarely used. 5HT$_3$-receptor antagonists preferred. A high-dose regimen for highly emetogenic chemotherapy of 1 to 2 mg/kg/dose every 2 to 6 hours has been administered but is rarely used. Premedicate with diphenhydramine (Benadryl) to reduce extrapyramidal symptoms.

DOSE ADJUSTMENTS

Antiemetic dose may be reduced to 1 mg/kg if initial doses suppress vomiting. Initial doses may be reduced to 1 mg/kg for less emetogenic regimens. ▪ Reduce initial dose by half in any patient with a CrCl less than 40 mL/min. Adjust subsequent doses as indicated. ▪ Caution and lower-end dosing suggested in elderly patients. Consider potential for decreased organ function and concomitant disease or drug therapy. ▪ See Drug/Lab Interactions.

DILUTION

May be given undiluted if dose does not exceed 10 mg. For doses exceeding 10 mg dilute in at least 50 mL of D5W, NS, D5/¹/₂NS, R, or LR, and give as an infusion.

Storage: Light sensitive; store in carton before use. Diluted solutions stable for 24 hours in normal light, 48 hours if protected from light. Do not freeze unless diluted in NS. Discard if color or particulate matter is observed.

COMPATIBILITY   (Underline Indicates Conflicting Compatibility Information)

Consider any drug NOT listed as compatible to be INCOMPATIBLE until consulting a pharmacist; specific conditions may apply.

Manufacturer lists as **incompatible** with chloramphenicol (Chloromycetin) and sodium bicarbonate.

Sources suggest the following **compatibilities:**

Additive: Manufacturer lists ampicillin, ascorbic acid, benztropine (Cogentin), cisplatin, clindamycin (Cleocin), cyclophosphamide (Cytoxan), cytarabine (ARA-C), dexamethasone (Decadron), diphenhydramine (Benadryl), doxorubicin (Adriamycin), erythromycin (Erythrocin), heparin, insulin (regular), lidocaine, mannitol, methotrexate, multivitamins (M.V.I.), penicillin G potassium, potassium acetate, and potassium phosphates. Other sources add meperidine (Demerol), meropenem (Merrem IV), morphine, potassium chloride (KCl), verapamil.

Y-site: All drugs listed by the manufacturer as **compatible** under *Additive.* Other sources add acetaminophen (Ofirmev), acyclovir (Zovirax), aldesleukin (Proleukin), amifostine (Ethyol), aztreonam (Azactam), bivalirudin (Angiomax), bleomycin (Blenoxane), ceftaroline (Teflaro), ciprofloxacin (Cipro IV), cisatracurium (Nimbex), cisplatin, cladribine (Leustatin), cyclophosphamide (Cytoxan), dexmedetomidine (Precedex), diltiazem (Cardizem), docetaxel (Taxotere), doripenem (Doribax), doxapram (Dopram), doxorubicin (Adriamycin), droperidol (Inapsine), etoposide phosphate (Etopophos), famotidine (Pepcid IV), fenoldopam (Corlopam), fentanyl, filgrastim (Neupogen), fluconazole (Diflucan), fludarabine (Fludara), fluorouracil (5-FU), foscarnet (Foscavir), gallium nitrate (Ganite), gemcitabine (Gemzar), granisetron (Kytril), heparin, hetastarch in electrolytes (Hextend), hydromorphone (Dilaudid), idarubicin (Idamycin), leucovorin calcium, levofloxacin (Levaquin), linezolid (Zyvox), melphalan (Alkeran), meperidine (Demerol), meropenem (Merrem IV), methadone (Dolophine), methotrexate, mitomycin (Mutamycin), morphine, ondansetron (Zofran), oxaliplatin (Eloxatin), paclitaxel (Taxol), palonosetron (Aloxi), pemetrexed (Alimta), piperacillin/tazobactam (Zosyn), quinupristin/dalfopristin (Synercid), remifentanil (Ultiva), sargramostim (Leukine), tacrolimus (Prograf), telavancin (Vibativ), teniposide (Vumon), thiotepa, tigecycline (Tygacil), topotecan (Hycamtin), vinblastine, vincristine, vinorelbine (Navelbine), zidovudine (AZT, Retrovir).

M

RATE OF ADMINISTRATION

Too-rapid IV injection will cause intense anxiety, restlessness, and then drowsiness.
IV injection: 10 mg or fraction thereof over 2 minutes. Reduce rate of injection in pediatric patients.
Infusion: Administer over a minimum of 15 minutes.

ACTIONS

A dopamine antagonist. Antiemetic properties appear to be the result of antagonism of central and peripheral dopamine receptors. Blocks the stimulation of medullary chemoreceptor trigger zones by dopamine. Inhibits nausea and vomiting. Increases tone and amplitude of gastric contractions, relaxes the lower pyloric sphincter and duodenal bulb, and increases peristalsis of the duodenum and jejunum, resulting in accelerated gastric emptying. Does not stimulate gastric, biliary, or pancreatic secretions. Acts even if vagal innervation not present. Action negated by anticholinergic drugs. Distributes extensively into tissues. Onset of action occurs in 1 to 3 minutes and lasts 1 to 2 hours. Average half-life is 5 to 6 hours. Excreted in urine. Secreted in breast milk.

INDICATIONS AND USES

Facilitate small bowel intubation. ▪ Stimulate gastric and intestinal emptying of barium to permit radiologic examination of the stomach and small intestine. ▪ Prevention of nausea and vomiting associated with emetogenic cancer chemotherapy. ▪ Prophylaxis of postoperative nausea and vomiting when nasogastric suction is not indicated. ▪ Diabetic gastroparesis.

CONTRAINDICATIONS

Situations in which gastric motility is contraindicated (i.e., gastric hemorrhage, obstruction, or perforation); known hypersensitivity to metoclopramide; patients with epilepsy or patients taking drugs that may also cause extrapyramidal reactions; pheochromocytoma.

PRECAUTIONS

May produce sedation, extrapyramidal symptoms, or Parkinson-like symptoms, similar to those seen with phenothiazines. Use caution in patients with pre-existing disease. ▪ Acute dystonic reactions (a type of extrapyramidal symptom [EPS]) are usually seen during the first 24 to 48 hours of treatment and are more common in pediatric patients, in adults under 30 years of age, and at higher doses used for prophylaxis of N/V due to chemotherapy. ▪ Tardive dyskinesia may develop and is usually related to duration of treatment and total cumulative dose. Avoid use for longer than 12 weeks unless benefit outweighs risk of tardive dyskinesia. ▪ Neuroleptic malignant syndrome (NMS) has been reported rarely. Potentially fatal. Discontinue metoclopramide immediately; see Monitor. ▪ Produces a transient increase in plasma aldosterone; patients with cirrhosis or CHF may develop fluid retention and volume overload. If S/S occur, discontinue metoclopramide. ▪ Use with caution in patients with hypertension. May cause release of catecholamines, exacerbating the condition. ▪ A prolactin-elevating compound; may be carcinogenic. Risk with a single dose almost nonexistent. ▪ May cause serious depression and suicidal tendencies; use extreme caution in any patient with a history of depression. ▪ Patients with NADH-cytochrome b_5 reductase deficiency are at increased risk for developing methemoglobinemia and/or sulfhemoglobinemia. In patients with G6PD deficiency who develop methemoglobinemia, methylene blue treatment is not recommended. Can cause hemolytic anemia. ▪ See Maternal/Child.

Monitor: Monitor vital signs. ▪ Pretreatment with diphenhydramine may reduce incidence of extrapyramidal symptoms with larger doses (e.g., antiemetic). ▪ Monitor for S/S of NMS (e.g., hyperthermia, muscle rigidity, altered consciousness, and evidence of autonomic instability [irregular pulse or BP, tachycardia, diaphoresis, and arrhythmias]). ▪ Discontinue therapy in patients who develop S/S of tardive dyskinesia (syndrome of potentially irreversible involuntary movements of the tongue, face, mouth, jaw, trunk, or extremities). ▪ See Precautions and Drug/Lab Interactions.

Patient Education: Use caution performing any task that requires alertness, coordination, or physical dexterity; may produce dizziness and drowsiness. ▪ If any involuntary

movement of eyes, face, or limbs occurs, notify physician promptly. ▪ Avoid alcohol or other CNS depressants (e.g., barbiturates, benzodiazepines [e.g., diazepam (Valium)]). **Maternal/Child:** Category B: use caution in pregnancy and breast-feeding. ▪ May increase milk production (elevates prolactin). ▪ Pharmacokinetics highly variable in children and neonates. ▪ Safety and effectiveness for use in pediatric patients not established except when administered to facilitate small bowel intubation. ▪ Dystonic reactions are more common in pediatric patients. ▪ Prolonged clearance in neonates may produce excessive serum concentrations. ▪ May cause methemoglobinemia in premature and full-term neonates at doses exceeding 0.5 mg/kg/24 hr. ▪ See Precautions and Side Effects.
Elderly: May be more sensitive to therapeutic or adverse effects. ▪ Long-term use increases risk of extrapyramidal effects (e.g., parkinsonism, tardive dyskinesia). ▪ See Dose Adjustments and Precautions.

DRUG/LAB INTERACTIONS
Antagonized by **anticholinergic drugs** (e.g., atropine) **and narcotic analgesics** (e.g., morphine). ▪ May potentiate **alcohol and cyclosporine.** ▪ Drugs ingested orally may be absorbed more slowly or more rapidly depending on the absorption site (e.g., inhibits **cimetidine, digoxin**). ▪ Potentiates **MAO inhibitors** (e.g., selegiline [Eldepryl]); use extreme caution or do not use. ▪ **Insulin** reactions may result from gastric stasis, making diabetic control difficult. Dose or timing of insulin may need adjustment. ▪ Extrapyramidal effects may be potentiated with concomitant use of **phenothiazines, butyrophenones, and thioxanthines** (antipsychotic drugs). ▪ Used concurrently, metoclopramide and **levodopa** have opposite effects on dopamine receptors; metoclopramide is inhibited and levodopa is potentiated.

SIDE EFFECTS
Usually mild, transient, and reversible after metoclopramide is discontinued. Hypersensitivity reactions can occur. Acute CHF, anxiety, arrhythmias, bowel disturbances, confusion, convulsions, depression (severe, may have suicidal tendencies), dizziness, drowsiness, extrapyramidal reactions, fatigue, fluid retention, hallucinations, headache, hypertension, hypotension, insomnia, methemoglobinemia in neonates, nausea, NMS (hyperthermia, muscle rigidity, altered consciousness, and evidence of autonomic instability [irregular pulse or BP, tachycardia, diaphoresis, and arrhythmias]), restlessness, sulfhemoglobinemia in adults, tardive dyskinesia. Numerous other side effects may occur.
Overdose: Disorientation, drowsiness, and extrapyramidal reactions.

ANTIDOTE
Notify physician of all side effects. Most will respond to a reduced dose or discontinuation of metoclopramide. Treat overdose or extrapyramidal reactions with diphenhydramine (Benadryl) or benztropine (Cogentin). Symptoms should disappear within 24 hours. To manage NMS, immediately discontinue metoclopramide. Intensive symptomatic treatment and monitoring are required. Bromocriptine (Parlodel) and dantrolene (Dantrium) have been used to treat NMS, but effectiveness not established. Discontinue therapy in patients who develop S/S of tardive dyskinesia; symptoms may resolve. Treat methemoglobinemia with IV methylene blue. Hemodialysis is not likely to be useful in an overdose. Resuscitate as necessary.

METOPROLOL TARTRATE $\blacksquare$BBW$\blacksquare$
(me-toe-**PROH**-lohl **TAHR**-trayt)

Beta-adrenergic blocking agent
Antiarrhythmic (post MI)

Lopressor

pH 7.5

USUAL DOSE
Treatment of myocardial infarction: 5 mg as an IV bolus dose. Initiate as soon as the patient's hemodynamic condition has stabilized. Repeat at 2-minute intervals for 2 more doses; a total dose of 15 mg (AHA recommends 5 mg at 5-minute intervals to a total dose of 15 mg). If IV doses are well tolerated, give 50 mg PO every 6 hours for 48 hours beginning 15 minutes after the last bolus. Follow with an oral maintenance dose of 100 mg twice daily. In patients who do not tolerate the full IV dose start 25 to 50 mg PO within 15 minutes of the last IV dose. Dosage based on degree of intolerance. May have to discontinue metoprolol.

Treatment of atrial fibrillation (unlabeled): 2.5 to 5 mg as an IV injection over 2 to 5 minutes as necessary to control rate up to a total dose of 15 mg in a 10- to 15-minute period if indicated.

Treatment of ventricular rate control/hypertension (unlabeled): 1.25 to 5 mg every 6 to 12 hours. Begin with a lower initial dose and titrate to response. Up to 15 mg every 3 to 6 hours has been used.

DOSE ADJUSTMENTS
See Drug/Lab Interactions. ▪ Not required in impaired renal function. ▪ In patients with impaired hepatic function, start at a low dose and titrate upward slowly.

DILUTION
May be given undiluted.

Storage: Store at CRT. Protect from light.

COMPATIBILITY
(Underline Indicates Conflicting Compatibility Information)

Consider any drug NOT listed as compatible to be INCOMPATIBLE until consulting a pharmacist; specific conditions may apply.

One source suggests the following **compatibilities:**

Y-site: Abciximab (ReoPro), alteplase (tPA), amiodarone (Nexterone), argatroban, bivalirudin (Angiomax), ceftaroline (Teflaro), diltiazem (Cardizem), eptifibatide (Integrilin), furosemide (Lasix), heparin, meperidine (Demerol), milrinone (Primacor), morphine, nesiritide (Natrecor), nitroprusside sodium (Nitropress), procainamide (Pronestyl).

RATE OF ADMINISTRATION
A single dose over 1 minute. Monitor ECG, HR, and BP and discontinue metoprolol if adverse symptoms occur (bradycardia less than 45 beats/min, heart block greater than first degree, systolic BP less than 100 mm Hg, or moderate to severe cardiac failure).

ACTIONS
Metoprolol is a cardioselective (B_1) adrenergic receptor blocker. Its mechanism of action in patients with suspected or definite myocardial infarction is not known, but its use has been shown to reduce the 3-month mortality rate in this patient population. It reduces the incidence of recurrent myocardial infarctions and reduces the size of the infarct and the incidence of fatal arrhythmias. Reduces HR, systolic BP, and cardiac output. Well distributed throughout the body, it acts within 1 to 2 minutes and lasts about 3 to 4 hours. Maximum beta blockade is achieved in approximately 20 minutes. Metabolized in the liver by the cytochrome P_{450} enzyme system, primarily CYP2D6. Excreted as metabolites in the urine. Crosses placental barrier. Secreted in breast milk.

INDICATIONS AND USES
To reduce cardiac mortality in hemodynamically stable individuals with suspected or definite myocardial infarction (used in conjunction with oral metoprolol maintenance therapy). ▪ Treatment of hypertension, angina pectoris, and CHF in oral dosage form.

Unlabeled uses: Treatment of atrial fibrillation and unstable angina. ▪ Has been used in the perioperative period to reduce cardiac morbidity and mortality in patients at risk. ▪ Treatment of ventricular rate control and hypertension in patients who cannot take PO medications.

CONTRAINDICATIONS

HR below 45 beats/min, second- or third-degree heart block, significant first-degree heart block (PR interval equal to or greater than 0.24 second), systolic BP below 100 mm Hg, or moderate to severe cardiac failure. ▪ Hypersensitivity to metoprolol or to any of the excipients. Use caution in patients with hypersensitivity to other beta-blockers (e.g., atenolol [Tenormin], esmolol [Brevibloc], propranolol). Cross-sensitivity between beta-blockers can occur. ▪ Severe peripheral arterial circulatory disorders or sick sinus syndrome in patients with angina or hypertension.

PRECAUTIONS

Use caution in CHF. Beta blockade may depress myocardial contractility and precipitate or exacerbate heart failure and cardiogenic shock. ▪ Use caution in presence of heart failure controlled by digoxin. Both drugs slow AV conduction. Bradycardia, sinus pause, heart block, and cardiac arrest have occurred. Patients with first-degree AV block, sinus node dysfunction, or conduction disorders may be at increased risk; see Antidote. ▪ May produce significant first- (PR interval equal to or greater than 0.26 second), second-, or third-degree heart block. Acute MI can also cause heart block. ▪ Metoprolol decreases sinus heart rate. MI may also produce significant lowering of HR; see Antidote. ▪ Routine withdrawal of chronically administered beta-blockers before major surgery is not necessary; however, the risks of general anesthesia and surgical procedures may be increased by the impaired ability of the heart to respond to reflex adrenergic stimuli. ▪ Use caution in patients with a history of severe anaphylactic reactions to a variety of allergens; they may be more reactive to repeated challenge (either accidental, diagnostic, or therapeutic) and may be unresponsive to the usual doses of epinephrine used to treat hypersensitivity reactions; see Drug/Lab Interactions. ▪ May mask tachycardia occurring with hypoglycemia in diabetes and tachycardia of hyperthyroidism. ▪ In general, patients with bronchospastic disease should not receive beta-blockers, including metoprolol. Because of its relative beta selectivity, metoprolol may be used with extreme caution in these patients. Monitor pulmonary function closely; see Antidote. ▪ Use with caution in patients with impaired hepatic function; see Dose Adjustments. ▪ May cause arrhythmia, angina, MI, or death if stopped abruptly (more of an issue with chronic oral therapy); see prescribing information. ▪ May cause severe bradycardia in patients with Wolff-Parkinson-White syndrome. ▪ Contraindicated in patients known to have or suspected of having a pheochromocytoma. If metoprolol is required, it should be given in combination with an alpha-blocker (e.g., phenoxybenzamine [Dibenzyline]) and only after the alpha-blocker has been initiated. ▪ See Drug/Lab Interactions.

Monitor: Continuous ECG, HR, and BP monitoring is mandatory with use of IV metoprolol. ▪ Hemodynamic status must be closely monitored. If heart failure or hypotension occurs or persists despite appropriate treatment, metoprolol should be discontinued. Assess extent of myocardial damage. Invasive monitoring of central venous, pulmonary capillary wedge, and arterial pressure may be required. ▪ See Drug/Lab Interactions and Antidote.

Patient Education: Report any breathing difficulty promptly.

Maternal/Child: Category C: safety for use in pregnancy and breast-feeding and in pediatric patients not established. ▪ If a pregnancy occurs, women should inform their physician.

Elderly: Age-related differences in safety and effectiveness not identified; however, greater sensitivity of some elderly cannot be ruled out. Dose with caution. ▪ May exacerbate mental impairment.

DRUG/LAB INTERACTIONS

Concurrent use with **calcium channel blockers** (e.g., diltiazem, verapamil) may potentiate both drugs and result in severe depression of myocardium and AV conduction and severe hypotension. ▪ Concurrent use with **antihypertensive agents,** including **alpha-adrenergic blockers** (e.g., clonidine [Catapres], guanfacine [Tenex], methyldopa, reserpine), may result in excessive hypotension. Dose adjustment may be required. ▪ Concurrent administration with **hydralazine** may decrease metabolism and increase concentrations of metoprolol. ▪ **Potent inhibitors of the CYP2D6 enzyme** may increase plasma concentrations of metoprolol and decrease its cardioselectivity. These inhibitors include **antidepressants** (e.g., clomipramine [Anafranil], desipramine [Norpramin], fluoxetine [Prozac], fluvoxamine [Luvox], paroxetine [Paxil], sertraline [Zoloft], bupropion [Wellbutrin]), **antipsychotics** (e.g., chlorpromazine, fluphenazine, haloperidol [Haldol], thioridazine [Mellaril]), **antiarrhythmics** (e.g., quinidine, propafenone [Rythmol]), **antiretrovirals** (e.g., ritonavir [Norvir]), **antihistamines** (e.g., diphenhydramine [Benadryl]), **antimalarials** (e.g., hydroxychloroquine [Plaquenil], quinidine), **allylamine antifungals** (e.g., terbinafine [Lamisil]), and **medications for stomach ulcers** (e.g., cimetidine [Tagamet]). ▪ Concurrent use within 14 days of **MAO inhibitors** (selegiline [Eldepryl]) may cause severe hypertension. ▪ Use with **sympathomimetic agents** (e.g., epinephrine, norepinephrine, phenylephrine) **or xanthines** (e.g., aminophylline) may negate therapeutic effects of both drugs. ▪ Effects of beta-adrenergic blocking agents may be decreased by **anti-inflammatory drugs** (e.g., NSAIDs), **barbiturates, rifampin, salicylates, and others.** ▪ **Inhalation anesthetics, phenytoin** (Dilantin), **and quinolone antibiotics** (e.g., ciprofloxacin) may increase myocardial depressant effects and hypotension. ▪ Beta-adrenergic blocking agents may be continued during the perioperative period in most patients; however, use caution with **selected anesthetic agents** that may depress the myocardium. ▪ Potentiates effects of **oral antidiabetics, catecholamine-depleting drugs** (e.g., reserpine), insulin, lidocaine, and skeletal muscle relaxants; monitor carefully. Dose adjustment may be required. ▪ Concurrent use with **clonidine** may precipitate acute hypertension if one or both agents are stopped abruptly. Withdraw metoprolol first. ▪ Effects decreased when hypothyroid patient is **converted to a euthyroid state;** adjust dose as indicated. ▪ Used concurrently with **digoxin or alpha-adrenergic blockers** (e.g., phentolamine [Regitine]) as indicated. ▪ Use caution; both **digoxin** and beta-blockers (e.g., atenolol, esmolol, metoprolol, propranolol) slow AV conduction. May increase risk of bradycardia. ▪ Patients taking beta-blockers who are exposed to a potential allergen may be unresponsive to the usual dose of **epinephrine** used to treat a hypersensitivity reaction. ▪ May enhance the vasoconstrictive action of **ergot alkaloids.** ▪ In general, withhold administration of a beta-blocker before **dipyridamole** testing; monitor HR carefully following dipyridamole injection.

SIDE EFFECTS

Abdominal pain, bradyarrhythmias, bronchospasm, cardiac failure, claudication, confusion, dizziness, dyspnea, elevated liver function tests, first-degree heart block, hallucinations, headache, hepatitis, hypotension, jaundice, nausea, nightmares, pruritus, rash, reduced libido, respiratory distress, second- or third-degree heart block, sleep disturbances, syncopal attacks, tiredness, unstable diabetes, vertigo, visual disturbances.

ANTIDOTE

For any side effect, discontinue drug and notify physician immediately. Patients with myocardial infarction may be more hemodynamically unstable; treat with caution. Use atropine (0.25 to 0.5 mg) for bradycardia or heart block; use isoproterenol with caution if atropine is not effective. Glucagon 5 to 10 mg IV may be effective if atropine and isoproterenol are not (investigational use). Transvenous cardiac pacing may be needed. Treat hypotension with IV fluids if indicated or vasopressors (dopamine or norepinephrine [Levarterenol]); treat cause of hypotension (e.g., bradycardia). Use all vasopressors with extreme caution; severe hypotension can result. Use digoxin and diuretics at first sign of cardiac failure; dobutamine, isoproterenol, or glucagon may be required. Use aminophylline or isoproterenol (with extreme care) for bronchospasm, and glucagon or IV glucose for hypoglycemia. Treat other side effects symptomatically; resuscitate as necessary.

METRONIDAZOLE HYDROCHLORIDE BBW
(meh-troh-**NYE**-dah-zohl hy-droh-**KLOR**-eyed)

Antibacterial
Antiprotozoal
Amebicide

Flagyl IV, Flagyl IV RTU

pH 4.5 to 7

USUAL DOSE
May transfer to oral therapy when condition warrants (usual PO dose is 7.5 mg/kg every 6 hours).

Anaerobic infections: Begin with an initial loading dose of 15 mg/kg of body weight. Follow with 7.5 mg/kg (up to 1 Gm/dose) in 6 hours and every 6 hours thereafter for 7 to 10 days or longer if indicated. Do not exceed 4 Gm in 24 hours.

Surgical prophylaxis to prevent postoperative infection in contaminated or potentially contaminated colorectal surgery: 15 mg/kg infused over 30 to 60 minutes and completed 1 hour before surgery. Follow with 7.5 mg/kg over 30 to 60 minutes in 6 hours and in 12 hours.

PEDIATRIC DOSE
Safety for use in infants and other pediatric patients not established, but is used for anaerobic infections; see Maternal/Child.

Anaerobic infections: *Pediatric patients more than 7 days of age:* 7.5 mg/kg every 6 hours with a maximum dose of 4 Gm/24 hr.

Another source recommends age- and weight-specific doses as follows:

Less than 7 days of age weighing less than 1.2 kg: 7.5 mg/kg every 48 hours.
Less than 7 days of age weighing 1.2 to 2 kg: 7.5 mg/kg every 24 hours.
Less than 7 days of age weighing 2 or more kg: 7.5 mg/kg every 12 hours.
7 days of age or older weighing less than 1.2 kg: 7.5 mg/kg every 24 hours.
7 days of age or older weighing 1.2 to 2 kg: 7.5 mg/kg every 12 hours.
7 days of age or older weighing 2 or more kg: 15 mg/kg every 12 hours.

DOSE ADJUSTMENTS
Reduce dose by 50% in patients with severe (Child-Pugh Class C) hepatic impairment. ▪ Increase intervals in neonates; see Pediatric Dose. ▪ No dose adjustment is indicated in mild to moderate impaired renal function. Recommendations vary for patients with a CrCl of less than 10 mL/min who are not on dialysis; consider reducing dose by 50% or increasing the interval to every 12 hours. ▪ Dose adjustment not indicated in anuric patients; accumulated metabolites readily removed by dialysis. 40% to 65% of a metronidazole dose can be removed by dialysis depending on length of dialysis session and type of dialyzer membrane used. If metronidazole administration cannot be separated from dialysis session, consider supplemental dose following dialysis. ▪ Continuous NG suction may remove sufficient metronidazole in gastric aspirate to reduce serum levels. No dose adjustment is recommended.

DILUTION
All solutions are prediluted and ready to use (5 mg/mL) except Flagyl IV. The powder form (Flagyl IV) is not readily available but requires a specific dilution process. Initially add 4.4 mL SWFI or NS for injection (with or without preservative) to provide a solution with an approximate concentration of 100 mg/mL (500 mg in 5 mL). Solution must be clear. Solution will be yellow to yellow-green in color with a pH of 0.5 to 2. The desired dose of properly reconstituted solution may be further diluted with NS, D5W, or LR. Do not exceed a concentration of 8 mg/mL (500 mg in 100 mL yields a concentration of 5 mg/mL). Must be neutralized before infusion with 5 mEq of sodium bicarbonate per 500 mg metronidazole to achieve an approximate pH of 6 to 7. Mix thoroughly. CO_2 gas will be generated and may require venting. Do not use plastic containers in series connections. Risk of air embolism is present. Avoid all contact with aluminum in needles and syringes in all situations.

Storage: Store at room temperature (25° C [75° F]). Do not refrigerate. Protect from light. Do not remove premixed product from overwrap until ready for use. Reconstituted vial is stable for 96 hours when stored below 86° F (30° C) in room light. Diluted, neutralized solution must be used within 24 hours of mixing. Do not refrigerate neutralized solution; precipitation may occur.

COMPATIBILITY   (Underline Indicates Conflicting Compatibility Information)
Consider any drug NOT listed as compatible to be INCOMPATIBLE until consulting a pharmacist; specific conditions may apply.

Manufacturer recommends, "Administer separately, discontinue the primary IV during administration, and do not introduce additives into the solution." Do not use equipment containing aluminum.

One source suggests the following **compatibilities:**
Additive: *Not recommended by manufacturer.* Ampicillin, cefazolin (Ancef), <u>cefepime (Maxipime)</u>, cefotaxime (Claforan), <u>cefoxitin (Mefoxin)</u>, ceftazidime (Fortaz), ceftriaxone (Rocephin), cefuroxime (Zinacef), ciprofloxacin (Cipro IV), fluconazole (Diflucan), gentamicin, hydrocortisone sodium succinate (Solu-Cortef), midazolam (Versed), penicillin G potassium, tobramycin.

Y-site: Acyclovir (Zovirax), allopurinol (Aloprim), amifostine (Ethyol), <u>anidulafungin (Eraxis)</u>, bivalirudin (Angiomax), <u>caspofungin (Cancidas)</u>, ceftaroline (Teflaro), cisatracurium (Nimbex), cyclophosphamide (Cytoxan), dexmedetomidine (Precedex), diltiazem (Cardizem), dimenhydrinate, docetaxel (Taxotere), dopamine, doripenem (Doribax), doxapram (Dopram), doxorubicin liposomal (Doxil), enalaprilat (Vasotec IV), esmolol (Brevibloc), etoposide phosphate (Etopophos), fenoldopam (Corlopam), fluconazole (Diflucan), foscarnet (Foscavir), gemcitabine (Gemzar), granisetron (Kytril), heparin, hetastarch in electrolytes (Hextend), hydromorphone (Dilaudid), 6% hydroxyethyl starch (Voluven), labetalol, linezolid (Zyvox), lorazepam (Ativan), magnesium sulfate, melphalan (Alkeran), meperidine (Demerol), methylprednisolone (Solu-Medrol), midazolam (Versed), milrinone (Primacor), morphine, nicardipine (Cardene IV), <u>palonosetron (Aloxi)</u>, piperacillin/tazobactam (Zosyn), remifentanil (Ultiva), sargramostim (Leukine), tacrolimus (Prograf), teniposide (Vumon), theophylline, thiotepa, vasopressin, vinorelbine (Navelbine).

RATE OF ADMINISTRATION
Must be given as a slow intermittent or continuous IV infusion, each single dose evenly distributed over 1 hour. Discontinue primary IV during administration.
Surgical prophylaxis: Administer each single dose over 30 to 60 minutes.

ACTIONS
A bactericidal agent with cytotoxic effects, active against specific obligate anaerobic bacteria and protozoa. Does not possess any clinically relevant activity against facultative anaerobes or obligate aerobes. Metronidazole enters the organism by passive diffusion and is reduced. The reduced form and free radicals that are produced during the reduction reaction interact with DNA, leading to inhibition of DNA synthesis and to DNA degradation and death of bacteria. The precise mechanism of action is unclear. Metronidazole is widely distributed. Plasma concentrations are directly proportional to dose given. Onset of action is prompt. Metabolized in the liver. Half-life is 8 hours. Crosses placental and blood-brain barriers. Excreted primarily in urine, some in feces. Secreted in breast milk.

INDICATIONS AND USES
Treatment of serious infections caused by susceptible strains of anaerobic bacteria, including serious intra-abdominal, skin and skin structure, gynecologic, bone and joint, CNS, and lower respiratory tract infections, bacterial septicemia, and endocarditis. Is effective in *Bacteroides fragilis* infections resistant to clindamycin, chloramphenicol, and penicillin. ▪ Perioperative prophylaxis to reduce infection rates in contaminated or potentially contaminated colorectal surgery. ▪ Given orally for amebiasis, giardiasis, *Helicobacter pylori* eradication, and other indications.
Unlabeled uses: *Clostridium difficile*–associated diarrhea (CDAD), Crohn's disease, pelvic inflammatory disease.

CONTRAINDICATIONS
Hypersensitivity to metronidazole or other nitroimidazole derivatives; use of disulfiram within the last 2 weeks; use of alcohol or products containing propylene glycol during and for at least 3 days after therapy with metronidazole.

PRECAUTIONS
A mixed (anaerobic/aerobic) infection will require use of additional antibiotics targeted for treatment of the aerobic infection. ▪ Sensitivity studies indicated to determine susceptibility of the causative organism to metronidazole. ▪ To reduce the development of drug-resistant bacteria and maintain its effectiveness, metronidazole should be used to treat or prevent only those infections proven or strongly suspected to be caused by bacteria. ▪ Avoid prolonged use of the drug; superinfection caused by overgrowth of nonsusceptible organisms may result. ▪ Symptoms of candidiasis may be exacerbated and require treatment. ▪ Encephalopathy has been reported in association with cerebellar toxicity characterized by ataxia, dizziness, and dysarthria. CNS lesions have been seen on MRI. Generally reversible within days to weeks after metronidazole is discontinued. ▪ Optic neuropathy and peripheral neuropathy (mainly sensory with S/S of numbness or paresthesia of extremities) have been reported. ▪ May cause seizures. ▪ Aseptic meningitis has been reported. Symptoms may occur within hours of dose administration and generally resolve after metronidazole is discontinued. ▪ Use caution in patients predisposed to edema and/or taking corticosteroids, in patients with impaired cardiac function (contains 27 to 28 mEq sodium/Gm), CNS disease, hepatic or renal impairment, or a history of blood dyscrasias. ▪ *Clostridium difficile*–associated diarrhea (CDAD) has been reported. May range from mild diarrhea to fatal colitis. Consider in patients who present with diarrhea during or after treatment with metronidazole. ▪ Carcinogenic in rodents; avoid unnecessary use and restrict use to approved indications.
Monitor: Rotate IV site frequently to avoid thrombophlebitis. Avoid extravasation. ▪ Mild leukopenia has been reported. Obtain total and differential leukocyte counts before, during, and after prolonged or repeated courses of therapy. ▪ Monitor for S/S of toxicity in patients with hepatic or renal impairment and in the elderly. ▪ Monitor for neurologic S/S (e.g., ataxia, dizziness, dysarthrias, numbness, paresthesia, and seizures); see Antidote. ▪ Transfer to oral dosing as soon as practical. ▪ See Drug/Lab Interactions.
Patient Education: Avoid alcohol, alcohol-containing preparations, and disulfiram; toxic reactions will occur. ▪ Promptly report any neurologic side effects (e.g., seizures, numbness, or paresthesia of an extremity). ▪ Promptly report diarrhea or bloody stools that occur during treatment or up to several months after an antibiotic has been discontinued; may indicate CDAD and require treatment.
Maternal/Child: Category B: use during pregnancy only if clearly needed. ▪ Discontinue breast-feeding during metronidazole therapy and for 24 hours after therapy ends. ▪ Safety for use in pediatric patients and neonates not established. The elimination half-life, measured during the first 3 days of life, was inversely related to gestational age. Half-life markedly extended in newborns; adjust intervals; see Pediatric Dose.
Elderly: Pharmacokinetics altered in the elderly; monitor for metronidazole-associated adverse events and adjust dose accordingly.

DRUG/LAB INTERACTIONS
Avoid **alcohol and alcohol-containing preparations** for at least 3 days after taking any dose of metronidazole; a disulfiram-like reaction (abdominal cramps, flushing, headaches, nausea and vomiting) may occur. ▪ Avoid administration of metronidazole to patients who have taken **disulfiram** within the last 2 weeks. Psychotic reactions have been reported. ▪ Concurrent use with **drugs that induce microsomal enzyme activity** (e.g., phenobarbital, phenytoin [Dilantin]) may increase metabolism of metronidazole and decrease plasma levels. ▪ Administration with **drugs that inhibit microsomal liver enzyme activity** (e.g., cimetidine [Tagamet]) may prolong the half-life of metronidazole and increase metronidazole plasma levels. ▪ May decrease clearance and increase serum concentration of **phenytoin**. ▪ May decrease metabolism and increase anticoagulant effects of **warfarin** (Coumadin). Monitor PT/INR periodically. ▪ May increase **lithium** levels and

cause toxicity. ▪ May increase plasma concentrations of **busulfan**, increasing the risk of serious busulfan toxicity. Avoid concomitant use if possible. If concomitant administration is medically necessary, monitor busulfan plasma concentration and adjust busulfan dose accordingly. ▪ May interfere with **selected chemistry studies** (e.g., AST, ALT, LDH, triglycerides, glucose hexokinase).

SIDE EFFECTS

The most serious side effects include aseptic meningitis, convulsive seizures, encephalopathy, and optic and peripheral neuropathy. Abdominal cramping; anorexia; ataxia; CDAD; confusion; constipation; cystitis; darkened deep red urine; decreased libido; depression; diarrhea; dizziness; dryness of the mouth, vagina, or vulva; dysarthria; dysuria; epigastric distress; fever; fleeting joint pain; flushing; furry tongue; glossitis; headache; incontinence; insomnia; irritability; metallic taste (expected); nasal congestion; nausea; neutropenia (reversible); numbness; painful coitus; pancreatitis; paresthesia; pelvic pressure; polyuria; proctitis; pruritus; psychosis; rash; Stevens-Johnson syndrome; stomatitis; syncope; thrombocytopenia (reversible); thrombophlebitis; toxic epidermal necrolysis; T-wave flattening; urticaria; vomiting; and weakness have occurred.

ANTIDOTE

Notify physician of all side effects. Treatment will be symptomatic and supportive. Evaluate risk versus benefit of continuing therapy in patients who develop abnormal neurologic S/S (e.g., encephalopathy, seizures, or signs of peripheral neuropathy). Treat CDAD with fluids, electrolytes, protein supplements, and oral vancomycin (Vancocin) or metronidazole (Flagyl) as indicated. In severe cases, surgical evaluation may be indicated. Removed by hemodialysis. Treat anaphylaxis and resuscitate as necessary.

MICAFUNGIN SODIUM
(my-kah-**FUN**-gin **SO**-dee-um)

Antifungal
(echinocandin)

Mycamine

pH 5 to 7

USUAL DOSE

Treatment of candidemia, acute disseminated candidiasis, *Candida* peritonitis and abscesses: 100 mg/day as an infusion. Mean duration of treatment during clinical studies was 15 days (range 10 to 47 days).

Treatment of esophageal candidiasis: 150 mg/day as an infusion. Mean duration of treatment during clinical studies was 15 days (range 10 to 30 days).

Prophylaxis of *Candida* infections in hematopoietic stem cell transplant (HSCT) recipients: 50 mg/day as an infusion. Mean duration of treatment in patients who responded successfully during clinical studies was 19 days (range 6 to 51 days).

PEDIATRIC DOSE

Recommended doses for pediatric patients based on indication and weight are outlined in the following chart.

Micafungin Dosage in Pediatric Patients 4 Months of Age or Older		
	Pediatric Dose Given Once Daily	
Indication	30 kg or less	Greater than 30 kg
Treatment of candidemia, acute disseminated candidiasis, *Candida* peritonitis and abscesses	2 mg/kg (maximum daily dose 100 mg)	
Treatment of esophageal candidiasis	3 mg/kg	2.5 mg/kg (maximum daily dose 150 mg)
Prophylaxis of *Candida* infections in HSCT recipients	1 mg/kg (maximum daily dose 50 mg)	

DOSE ADJUSTMENTS
No dose adjustment indicated based on gender or race, in the elderly, or in patients with severe renal dysfunction or mild to moderate or severe hepatic insufficiency. ▪ Not dialyzable; a supplementary dose following hemodialysis should not be required. ▪ See Drug/Lab Interactions.

DILUTION
Each 50- or 100-mg vial must be reconstituted with 5 mL of NS (without a bacteriostatic agent) or with D5W. Following reconstitution, the 50-mg vial has a final concentration of 10 mg/mL. The 100-mg vial has a final concentration of 20 mg/mL. The use of strict aseptic technique is required. Swirl vial(s) gently to dissolve. *Do not shake.* Do not use if precipitation or foreign matter is observed. Each single adult dose (50, 100, or 150 mg) must be further diluted in 100 mL NS or D5W for infusion. For pediatric patients, calculate the dose in milligrams and withdraw the required volume from the selected concentration (10 mg/mL or 20 mg/mL). Add the withdrawn volume to an infusion bag or syringe containing NS or D5W. Final concentration of diluted solution should be between 0.5 and 4 mg/mL. Concentrations greater than 1.5 mg/mL should be infused through a central line.
Filters: No study data available; if filtering is necessary, contact manufacturer.
Storage: Store unopened vials at CRT. Reconstituted solution in original vial or diluted solution is stable up to 24 hours at 25° C (77° F). Protect diluted solution from light. Discard partially used vials.

COMPATIBILITY (Underline Indicates Conflicting Compatibility Information)
Consider any drug NOT listed as compatible to be INCOMPATIBLE until consulting a pharmacist; specific conditions may apply.
Manufacturer states, "Do not mix or co-infuse micafungin with other medications. Has been shown to precipitate when mixed directly with a number of other commonly used medications." Flush IV line with NS before and after infusion.
One source suggests the following **compatibilities:**
Y-site: Aminophylline, bumetanide, calcium chloride, calcium gluconate, carboplatin (Paraplatin), cyclosporine (Sandimmune), dopamine, doripenem (Doribax), eptifibatide (Integrilin), esmolol (Brevibloc), etoposide (VePesid), fenoldopam (Corlopam), furosemide (Lasix), heparin, hydromorphone (Dilaudid), lidocaine, lorazepam (Ativan), magnesium sulfate, mesna (Mesnex), milrinone (Primacor), nitroglycerin IV, nitroprusside (Nitropress), norepinephrine (Levophed), phenylephrine (Neo-Synephrine), potassium chloride, potassium phosphates, sodium phosphates, tacrolimus (Prograf), theophylline, vasopressin.

RATE OF ADMINISTRATION
Flush IV line with NS before and after infusion.
A single dose as an infusion equally distributed over 1 hour. Rapid infusion may result in more frequent histamine-mediated reactions (e.g., facial swelling, pruritus, rash, vasodilation). To minimize the risk of infusion reactions in pediatric patients, concentrations of greater than 1.5 mg/mL should be administered via a central catheter. Injection site reactions have been reported and occur more often in patients receiving micafungin via peripheral intravenous administration.

ACTIONS

A semi-synthetic lipopeptide and the first of a new class of antifungal agents, the echinocandins. Acts by inhibiting the synthesis of 1,3-beta-D-glucan, an integral component of the fungal cell wall not present in mammalian cells. The AUC increases as doses are increased (e.g., from 50 to 150 mg or from 3 to 8 mg/kg). Highly protein bound primarily to albumin but does not competitively displace bilirubin binding to albumin. 85% of steady-state concentration achieved after three daily doses. Metabolized in the liver. A substrate and weak inhibitor of CYP3A, but CYP3A is not a major pathway for metabolism. Half-life ranges from approximately 8 to 21 hours in adults and from 5 to 22 hours in pediatric patients. Primarily excreted in feces, with some excretion in urine.

INDICATIONS AND USES

Indicated in adult and pediatric patients 4 months of age and older for treatment of candidemia, acute disseminated candidiasis, and *Candida* peritonitis and abscesses. Has not been adequately studied in patients with endocarditis, osteomyelitis, and meningitis due to *Candida* infections. ▪ Treatment of esophageal candidiasis. ▪ Prophylaxis of *Candida* infections in patients undergoing hematopoietic stem cell transplantation. ▪ Efficacy against infections caused by fungi other than *Candida* not established.

CONTRAINDICATIONS

Hypersensitivity to micafungin, any of its components, or other echinocandins (e.g., anidulafungin [Eraxis]), caspofungin (Cancidas).

PRECAUTIONS

Do not give as an IV bolus; for IV infusion only. ▪ Isolated anaphylactoid reactions (including shock) and anaphylaxis have been reported. ▪ Abnormal liver function tests have been reported. Isolated cases of significant hepatic dysfunction, hepatitis, or worsening hepatic failure have occurred. Incidence may be increased in patients with serious underlying conditions who are receiving additional concomitant medications. Evaluate risk versus benefit of continued micafungin therapy. ▪ Elevations in BUN and creatinine have been reported. Isolated cases of significant renal dysfunction or acute renal failure have occurred. ▪ Intravascular hemolysis and hemoglobinuria have been reported. Isolated cases of significant hemolysis and hemolytic anemia have occurred. Evaluate risk versus benefit of continued micafungin therapy. ▪ Reports of clinical failures resulting from development of drug resistance have been reported. ▪ See Monitor and Antidote.

Monitor: Specimens for fungal culture, serologic testing, and histopathologic testing should be obtained before therapy to isolate and identify causative organisms. Therapy may begin as soon as all specimens are obtained and before results are known. Reassess after test results are known. ▪ Baseline CBC with differential and platelet count, BUN, SCr, and liver function tests (e.g., ALT, AST) may be indicated. ▪ Monitor for S/S of a hypersensitivity reaction (e.g., bronchospasm, dyspnea, hives, hypotension, rash, pruritus, swelling of eyelids, lips, or face); discontinue infusion if a hypersensitivity reaction occurs. ▪ Monitor for evidence of worsening hepatic function (e.g., increased ALT, AST, serum alkaline phosphatase). ▪ Monitor for evidence of worsening renal function (e.g., increased BUN, SCr). ▪ Monitor for S/S of hemolytic anemia, hemolysis, and hemoglobinuria as indicated (lysis of RBCs, liberation of hemoglobin, blood in the urine). ▪ Hematologic, hepatic, and renal effects may require discontinuation of micafungin.

Patient Education: Promptly report shortness of breath, dizziness or fainting, itching, rash, or swelling of extremities. ▪ Report S/S of liver dysfunction (anorexia, fatigue, jaundice, nausea and vomiting, dark urine, or pale stools). ▪ Report any S/S of hemoglobinuria (blood in the urine). ▪ Report S/S of renal dysfunction (decrease in urine output). ▪ Review list of current medications with physician. Drug interactions are possible; see Drug/Lab Interactions.

Maternal/Child: Pregnancy category C: use during pregnancy only if benefits justify risk to fetus. Some abnormalities, including abortion, occurred in animal studies. ▪ Use caution if required during breast-feeding. Secreted in milk of drug-treated rats; not known if micafungin is secreted in human milk. ▪ Safety and effectiveness for use in pediatric patients younger than 4 months of age not established.

Elderly: Differences in response compared to younger adults not identified; however, greater sensitivity in the elderly cannot be ruled out.

DRUG/LAB INTERACTIONS

No alteration of micafungin pharmacokinetics observed with concurrent administration of amphotericin B, cyclosporine (Sandimmune), fluconazole (Diflucan), itraconazole (Sporanox), mycophenolate (CellCept), nifedipine (ProCardia XL), prednisolone, rifampin (Rifadin), ritonavir (Norvir), sirolimus (Rapamune), tacrolimus (Prograf), or voriconazole (VFEND). ▪ Concurrent doses of micafungin did not appear to alter the pharmacokinetics of cyclosporine, mycophenolate, fluconazole, prednisolone, tacrolimus, or voriconazole. ▪ The effects of **itraconazole, nifedipine, and sirolimus** are increased with concurrent administration of micafungin. Monitor for itraconazole, nifedipine, or sirolimus toxicity and reduce their dose as indicated. ▪ Effects of micafungin on the pharmacokinetics of **rifampin and ritonavir** not available. ▪ Not expected to alter effects of drugs metabolized by the CYP3A system.

SIDE EFFECTS

Side effect profile similar in both adult and pediatric patients. Most common side effects include diarrhea, fever, headache, hypokalemia, nausea, thrombocytopenia, and vomiting. The most serious side effects that may occur regardless of indication include acute intravascular hemolysis, decreased WBC, hemoglobinuria, hemolytic anemia, histamine-mediated reactions (e.g., facial swelling, pruritus, rash, vasodilation), hypersensitivity reactions (e.g., anaphylaxis and anaphylactoid reactions [including shock]), significant hepatic dysfunction (e.g., hepatitis, hepatocellular damage, hyperbilirubinemia, or worsening hepatic failure), significant renal dysfunction, and/or acute renal failure. Abdominal pain, anemia, chills, delirium, dizziness, increased liver function tests (e.g., alkaline phosphatase, ALT, AST, BUN, transaminases), injection site reactions (including inflammation, phlebitis, and thrombophlebitis), leukopenia, lymphopenia, neutropenia, and somnolence occurred in patients treated for esophageal candidiasis. In addition, constipation, decreased appetite, dysgeusia (altered sense of taste), dyspepsia, fatigue, febrile neutropenia, flushing, hiccups, hyperbilirubinemia, hypertension, hypocalcemia, hypokalemia, hypomagnesemia, hypophosphatemia, hypotension, increased drug levels, increased SCr, and mucosal inflammation occurred in patients undergoing prophylactic use during HSCT.

Patients with esophageal candidiasis: Also reported rash and phlebitis.

Patients with candidemia and other *Candida* infections and prophylaxis of *Candida* infection in HSCT: Both reported bacteremia, hypertension, hypokalemia, hypomagnesemia, hypotension, peripheral edema, tachycardia, and thrombocytopenia.

Patients with candidemia and other *Candida* infections: Also reported aggravated anemia, atrial fibrillation, bradycardia, decubitus ulcer, hyperkalemia, hypernatremia, hypoglycemia, increased blood alkaline phosphatase, pneumonia, sepsis, septic shock, vascular disorders.

Prophylaxis of *Candida* infection in HSCT: Also reported anorexia, anxiety, constipation, cough, dizziness, dyspepsia, dyspnea, epistaxis, erythema, fatigue, febrile neutropenia, fluid overload, fluid retention, flushing, hypocalcemia, mucosal inflammation, neutropenia, pruritus, rash, and rigors.

Post-Marketing: Disseminated intravascular coagulation (DIC), Stevens-Johnson syndrome, and toxic epidermal necrolysis.

ANTIDOTE

Notify physician of all side effects; most will be treated symptomatically. If a hypersensitivity reaction occurs, discontinue micafungin and treat as indicated. Appropriate treatment may include oxygen, epinephrine, antihistamines (e.g., diphenhydramine [Benadryl]), vasopressors (e.g., dopamine), corticosteroids, IV fluids, and ventilation equipment. S/S indicative of hepatic, renal, or hematologic side effects may require evaluation of benefits versus risk of continuing micafungin therapy. Not removed by hemodialysis. Resuscitate as indicated.

MIDAZOLAM HYDROCHLORIDE BBW

(my-**DAYZ**-oh-lam hy-droh-**KLOR**-eyed)

Benzodiazepine
Sedative-hypnotic
Anesthetic adjunct
Amnestic

Midazolam HCl PF, Versed

pH 3

USUAL DOSE

Dose requirements for each patient may vary and will depend on the type and amount of premedication used. Doses given below are general guidelines. Individualize dose and titrate slowly to effect. Allow 3 to 5 minutes between each small injection to evaluate the full effect before administering additional doses.

SEDATION, ANXIOLYSIS (ANTIANXIETY), AND/OR AMNESIA FOR SHORT DIAGNOSTIC, ENDOSCOPIC, AND THERAPEUTIC PROCEDURES

The desired endpoint for conscious sedation can usually be achieved in 3 to 6 minutes. Time will depend on total dose and type or dose of narcotic premedication used concomitantly.

Healthy adults under 60 years of age: 1 to 2.5 mg immediately before the procedure. Begin with 1 mg and titrate slowly up to slurred speech or 2.5 mg. Some patients respond adequately to 1 mg. If additional medication is needed, wait a full 2 minutes, then titrate additional dosage slowly in small increments (usually no more than 1 mg). Wait a full 2 minutes between each increment. A total dose exceeding 5 mg is rarely necessary. Reduce dose by 30% in the presence of narcotic premedication or other CNS depressants. 25% of the sedating dose can be used for maintenance only when clearly indicated by clinical evaluation.

Patients over 60 years of age or debilitated or chronically ill patients: 1 to 1.5 mg. Begin with 1 mg and titrate slowly up to slurred speech or 1.5 mg. May respond adequately to 1 mg. If additional medication is needed, wait a full 2 minutes, then titrate additional dosage in small increments (no more than 1 mg). Wait a full 2 minutes between each increment. A total dose exceeding 3.5 mg is rarely necessary. Reduce dose by 50% in the presence of narcotic premedication or other CNS depressants. 25% of the sedating dose can be used for maintenance only when clearly indicated by clinical evaluation.

INDUCTION OF ANESTHESIA BEFORE ADMINISTRATION OF OTHER ANESTHETIC AGENTS AND/OR MAINTENANCE OF ANESTHESIA AS A COMPONENT OF BALANCED ANESTHESIA DURING SURGICAL PROCEDURES

In all patients (unpremedicated and premedicated), allow 2 minutes from initial dose to reach peak effect. If necessary, complete induction with 25% of initial dose or use inhalational anesthesia (e.g., halothane). Doses of any agents used after induction of anesthesia with midazolam may need to be reduced to as little as 25% of the usual initial dose. 25% of the induction dose can be repeated when indicated by lightening of anesthesia.

Unpremedicated patients under 55 years of age: 0.3 to 0.35 mg/kg as an initial dose. A total dose of up to 0.6 mg/kg has been required; recovery may be prolonged.

Unpremedicated patients over 55 years of age (ASA I or II): 0.15 to 0.3 mg/kg as an initial dose.

Unpremedicated debilitated patients or those with severe systemic disease (ASA III or IV): 0.15 to 0.25 mg/kg as an initial dose. As little as 0.15 mg/kg may be adequate.

Patients premedicated with sedatives or narcotics under 55 years of age: 0.25 mg/kg as an initial dose may be adequate. **Range is 0.15 to 0.35 mg/kg of body weight.**

Patients premedicated with sedatives or narcotics over 55 years of age (Good risk [ASA I & II]): 0.2 mg/kg as an initial dose may be adequate.

Patients premedicated with sedatives or narcotics who are debilitated or those with severe systemic disease (ASA III or IV): 0.15 mg/kg as an initial dose may be adequate.

Premedication usually includes narcotics (e.g., fentanyl 1.5 to 2 mcg/kg IV 5 minutes before induction, or morphine [up to 0.15 mg/kg IM] or meperidine [up to 1 mg/kg IM])

1 hour before induction with midazolam. Sedative premedication usually includes hydroxyzine (Vistaril) 100 mg PO or a barbiturate PO 1 hour before induction.

SEDATION FOR ANESTHESIA OR TREATMENT IN A CRITICAL CARE SETTING FOR INTUBATED AND MECHANICALLY VENTILATED PATIENTS

Continuous infusion (concentration 0.5 mg/mL): Begin with a *loading dose* of 0.01 to 0.05 mg/kg (0.5 to 4 mg for a typical adult) to rapidly initiate sedation. Infuse over several minutes. May be repeated at 10- to 15-minute intervals until adequate sedation achieved.

For maintenance of sedation: An initial infusion rate of 0.02 to 0.1 mg/kg/hr (1 to 7 mg/hr) may be used. Upper-end doses may be required, but use the lowest recommended doses in patients with residual effects from anesthetic drugs or in those concurrently receiving other sedatives or opioids. Initial infusion rate may be titrated up or down by 25% to 50% to maintain desired level of sedation. Decrease by 10% to 25% every few hours to find the minimum effective infusion rate. The lowest rate that produces the desired level of sedation is recommended. Agitation, hypertension, or tachycardia in response to stimulation in adequately sedated patients may indicate need for an opioid analgesic. Reduced rate of midazolam infusion may be indicated with the addition of an opioid analgesic. Taper dose gradually if midazolam has been used for more than a few days. Abrupt discontinuation may result in withdrawal symptoms.

REFRACTORY STATUS EPILEPTICUS (UNLABELED)

0.15 to 0.3 mg/kg (usual dose 5 to 15 mg); may repeat every 10 to 15 minutes or has been given as a continuous infusion at a rate of 0.05 to 0.6 mg/kg/hr.

PEDIATRIC DOSE

In all situations dose is based on lean body weight in obese pediatric patients. See Precautions and Maternal/Child.

SEDATION, ANXIOLYSIS (ANTIANXIETY), AND/OR AMNESIA BEFORE AND DURING PROCEDURES OR BEFORE ANESTHESIA

All increments of midazolam are on a mg/kg basis. Initial dose is age, procedure, and route dependent. Total dose will depend on patient response, type and duration of the procedure, and type and dose of concomitant medications. Titrate dose of midazolam and other concomitant medications slowly to the desired clinical effect. With concomitant medications, dose of midazolam should be reduced (usually by 25% to 30%). Before beginning a procedure or repeating a dose, wait a full 2 to 3 minutes to fully evaluate the sedative effect. If further sedation is necessary, continue to titrate with small increments at 2- to 3-minute intervals until desired level of sedation achieved. Prolonged sedation and risk of hypoventilation may be associated with higher-end doses.

Nonintubated infants under 6 months of age: Uncertain when patient transfers from neonatal physiology to pediatric physiology; manufacturer has no specific dosing recommendations. Titrate with very small increments to clinical effect and monitor very carefully for airway obstruction and hypoventilation.

Pediatric patients 6 months to 5 years of age: Begin with an initial dose of 0.05 to 0.1 mg/kg. Up to 0.6 mg/kg may be required, but a total dose of 6 mg is usually not exceeded.

Pediatric patients 6 to 12 years of age: Begin with an initial dose of 0.025 to 0.05 mg/kg. Up to 0.4 mg/kg may be required, but a total dose of 10 mg is usually not exceeded.

Pediatric patients 12 to 16 years of age: See Usual Dose. May require higher-than-recommended adult doses, but total dose usually does not exceed 10 mg.

SEDATION, ANXIOLYSIS, AMNESIA

Intubated pediatric patients in critical care settings: Begin with a loading dose of 0.05 to 0.2 mg/kg. May be allowed to breathe on own through intubation tube but assisted ventilation recommended in pediatric patients receiving other CNS depressants. In hemodynamically compromised pediatric patients, titrate the loading dose in small increments and monitor for hypotension, respiratory rate, and oxygen saturation. May be followed by a continuous IV infusion at 0.06 to 0.12 mg/kg/hr (1 to 2 mcg/kg/min). Increase or

Continued

decrease infusion in 25% increments or use supplemental IV injection to maintain desired effect.

SEDATION OF INTUBATED NEONATES IN CRITICAL CARE SETTINGS

Neonates under 32 weeks: A continuous infusion at a rate of 0.03 mg/kg/hr (0.5 mcg/kg/min).

Neonates 32 weeks or older: A continuous infusion at a rate of 0.06 mg/kg/hr (1 mcg/kg/min).

Do not use loading doses in neonates. Infusion may be run more rapidly for the first several hours to establish therapeutic plasma levels. Reassess rate carefully and frequently to use the lowest possible effective dose and reduce the potential for drug accumulation. Midazolam contains benzyl alcohol and must be used with extreme caution in neonates.

REFRACTORY STATUS EPILEPTICUS (UNLABELED)

Pediatric patients 2 months of age or older: *Loading dose:* 0.15 mg/kg followed by a continuous infusion of 1 mcg/kg/min. Titrate dose upward every 5 minutes to effect. Mean dose is 2.3 mcg/kg/min (range is 1 to 18 mcg/kg/min).

DOSE ADJUSTMENTS

Reduce dose by 30% to 50%, depending on age, in the presence of narcotic premedication or other CNS depressants; see Usual Dose. ▪ Reduce dose in congestive heart failure, chronic obstructive pulmonary disease, impaired hepatic or renal function, debilitated patients, and patients over 55 years of age. Half-life is extended and depressant effects will be potentiated; see Usual Dose. ▪ Dose based on lean body weight in obese pediatric patients. ▪ See Drug/Lab Interactions.

DILUTION

Read Label Carefully and Confirm mg Dose. Available in Two Strengths, 1 mg/mL and 5 mg/mL.
IV injection: May be diluted with D5W or NS. Dilute in a sufficient amount to permit slow titration (i.e., 1 mg in 4 mL or 5 mg in 20 mL [0.25 mg/mL]). Maximum concentration after dilution should not exceed 0.5 mg/mL.

Infusion: Dilute in either of the previously listed solutions to a maximum concentration of 0.5 mg/mL. 5 mL of a 1 mg/mL (5 mg) in 5 mL of diluent yields 0.5 mg/mL. 5 mL of a 5 mg/mL (25 mg) in 45 mL diluent is usually a 24-hour supply and also yields 0.5 mg/mL. Use a controlled infusion device or at the very least a metriset (60 gtt/mL) to facilitate titration and control flow to prevent overdose.

COMPATIBILITY   (Underline Indicates Conflicting Compatibility Information)

Consider any drug NOT listed as compatible to be INCOMPATIBLE until consulting a pharmacist; specific conditions may apply.

One source suggests the following **compatibilities:**

Additive: <u>Aminophylline</u>, cefuroxime (Zinacef), ciprofloxacin (Cipro IV), furosemide (Lasix), gentamicin, hydromorphone (Dilaudid), metronidazole (Flagyl IV), ranitidine (Zantac).

Y-site: Abciximab (ReoPro), acetaminophen (Ofirmev), amikacin, amiodarone (Nexterone), <u>anidulafungin (Eraxis)</u>, argatroban, atracurium (Tracrium), bivalirudin (Angiomax), calcium gluconate, <u>caspofungin (Cancidas)</u>, cefazolin (Ancef), cefotaxime (Claforan), ceftaroline (Teflaro), ciprofloxacin (Cipro IV), cisatracurium (Nimbex), clindamycin (Cleocin), dexmedetomidine (Precedex), digoxin (Lanoxin), diltiazem (Cardizem), <u>dobutamine</u>, dopamine, doripenem (Doribax), epinephrine (Adrenalin), erythromycin (Erythrocin), esmolol (Brevibloc), etomidate (Amidate), famotidine (Pepcid IV), fenoldopam (Corlopam), fentanyl, fluconazole (Diflucan), gentamicin, heparin, hetastarch in electrolytes (Hextend), hydromorphone (Dilaudid), 6% hydroxyethyl starch (Voluven), insulin (regular), labetalol, linezolid (Zyvox), lorazepam (Ativan), methadone (Dolophine), methylprednisolone (Solu-Medrol), metronidazole (Flagyl IV), milrinone (Primacor), morphine, nicardipine (Cardene IV), nitroglycerin IV, nitroprusside sodium, norepinephrine (Levophed), <u>palonosetron (Aloxi)</u>, pancuronium, potassium chloride (KCl), <u>propofol (Diprivan)</u>, ranitidine (Zantac), remifentanil (Ultiva), theophylline, tirofiban (Aggrastat), tobramycin, vancomycin, vecuronium.

RATE OF ADMINISTRATION

IV injection: *Sedation:* Any single increment of a total dose titrated slowly over at least 2 minutes. Stop at any point that the speech becomes slurred.

Induction of anesthesia: Any single increment of a total dose over 20 to 30 seconds. Rapid injection in any situation may cause respiratory depression or apnea.

Infusion: See Usual Dose. The American Academy of Critical Care recommends limiting the use of midazolam in the critical care setting to 24 hours because its metabolites accumulate in peripheral tissue, especially with long-term infusion.

Pediatric rate: Any single increment of a total dose over a minimum of 2 to 3 minutes. Rapid injection or infusion may cause severe hypotension or seizures in infants and neonates; incidence increased with concomitant fentanyl. See comments under Infusion.

ACTIONS

A short-acting benzodiazepine CNS depressant 3 to 4 times as potent as diazepam. Has anxiolytic, hypnotic, anticonvulsant, muscle relaxant, and anterograde amnestic effects. Depressant effects are dependent on dose, route of administration, and the presence or absence of other premedications. Can depress the ventilatory response to CO_2 stimulation. Mechanics of respiration are not adversely affected with usual doses. Mean arterial pressure, cardiac output, stroke volume, and systemic vascular resistance may be slightly decreased. May cause HRs of less than 65/min to rise and more than 85/min to fall. Produces sleepiness and relief of apprehension, and diminishes patient recall very effectively. Widely distributed. Onset of action occurs within 1.5 to 5 minutes. Half-life is approximately 2.5 hours (range is 1 to 5 hours), shorter than that of diazepam (Valium). Time to recovery is usually within 2 hours but may take as long as 6 hours. Metabolized in the liver by cytochrome P_{450} mediation and excreted as metabolites in urine. Crosses the placental barrier. Secreted in breast milk.

INDICATIONS AND USES

To produce sedation, relieve anxiety, and impair memory of perioperative events. ▪ May be used with or without narcotic sedation for conscious sedation before short diagnostic, endoscopic, or therapeutic procedures (e.g., bronchoscopy, gastroscopy, cystoscopy, coronary angiography, cardiac catheterization). ▪ Induction of anesthesia before administration of other anesthetic agents. ▪ As a component in the induction and maintenance of balanced anesthesia in short surgical procedures. ▪ Continuous infusions may be used in intubated and mechanically ventilated patients for sedation as a component of anesthesia or during treatment in a critical care setting.

Unlabeled use: Treatment of refractory status epilepticus.

CONTRAINDICATIONS

Acute narrow-angle glaucoma, known hypersensitivity to midazolam, open-angle glaucoma unless receiving appropriate treatment. Not recommended in pregnancy, childbirth, breast-feeding, shock, coma, acute alcohol intoxication with depression of vital signs. Contraindicated with ritonavir (Norvir).

PRECAUTIONS

Respiratory depression and/or respiratory arrest may occur. Should be used only in a hospital or ambulatory care setting with continuous monitoring of respiratory and cardiac function (e.g., pulse oximetry). Resuscitative drugs (including flumazenil [Romazicon]) and age- and size-appropriate equipment for bag/valve/mask ventilation and intubation must be immediately available. Personnel must be skilled in airway management. ▪ A dedicated individual with no other responsibilities should monitor deeply sedated patients throughout any procedure. ▪ A topical anesthetic agent should be used with midazolam during perioral endoscopy, and premedication with a narcotic is recommended in bronchoscopy because increased cough reflex and laryngospasm frequently occur. Premedication with a narcotic is also recommended with balanced anesthesia. ▪ For IV/IM use only. Contains benzyl alcohol. Do not use for intrathecal or epidural administration. ▪ Use caution in neonates. At recommended doses benzyl alcohol is not expected to be toxic, but excessive benzyl alcohol may result in hypotension, metabolic acidosis, and increased incidence of kernicterus, especially in small preterm infants. ▪ Use extreme caution in the elderly, in patients with chronic disease states, decreased pulmonary reserve, hepatic or renal impairment, neuromuscular disorders, and in those with uncompensated acute illness (e.g., severe fluid or electrolyte disturbances); may have increased risks of hypoventilation, airway obstruction, or apnea. Peak effect may take longer. ▪ Use with caution in obese patients and patients with CHF. Half-life is prolonged. ▪ See Pediatric Dose and Maternal/Child for additional precautions with infants and other pediatric patients. ▪ Does not protect against increased intracranial pressure or circulatory changes noted with succinylcholine or pancuronium or associated with intubation under light general anesthesia. ▪ Some clinicians prefer midazolam over diazepam because of effectiveness, minimum pain if any on injection, and miscibility with many drugs and solutions.

Monitor: Obtain a careful presedation history (e.g., medical conditions, concomitant meds), and complete a physical exam. Check for airway abnormalities. ▪ Monitor respiratory and cardiac function (e.g., BP, HR, pulse oximetry) continuously. *Has caused apnea and cardiac arrest.* Monitoring of ECG desirable. Maintain a patent airway and support adequate ventilation. Record assessments using standard assessment charts for scoring, especially in pediatric patients. Monitor for both adequate and excessive sedation. ▪ Extravasation or arterial administration hazardous. ▪ Bed rest required for a minimum of 3 hours after IV injection. ▪ See Drug/Lab Interactions.

Patient Education: Do not drive or operate hazardous machinery until the day after surgery or longer. All effects must have subsided. Avoid use of alcohol or other CNS depressants (e.g., antihistamines, barbiturates) for 24 hours after last dose. ▪ May impair memory; request written postoperative instructions. ▪ Consider birth control options.

Maternal/Child: Category D: avoid pregnancy. ▪ Not recommended during pregnancy, labor and delivery, or breast-feeding. ▪ Elimination rate is faster in infants and children. ▪ Neonate has reduced or immature organ function. Clearance is decreased and half-life is increased in critically ill neonates. May be susceptible to profound and/or prolonged respiratory effects. ▪ See Precautions and Monitor.

Elderly: See Usual Dose and Dose Adjustments. Start with a small dose and increase gradually based on response. ▪ Clearance is reduced compared to younger adults, and time to recovery may be prolonged. ▪ All elderly are more sensitive to therapeutic and adverse effects (e.g., oversedation, ataxia, dizziness). Patients over 70 years of age may be particularly sensitive. IV injection may be more likely to cause apnea, bradycardia, hypotension, and cardiac arrest. ▪ See Precautions and Drug/Lab Interactions.

DRUG/LAB INTERACTIONS
Concurrent use with **other CNS depressants** (e.g., alcohol, antihistamines, barbiturates, inhalation anesthetics [e.g., halothane], MAO inhibitors [e.g., selegiline (Eldepryl)], narcotics [e.g., morphine, meperidine (Demerol), fentanyl], phenothiazines [e.g., prochlorperazine (Compazine)], thiopental, and tricyclic antidepressants [e.g., imipramine (Tofranil)]) may result in additive effects for up to 48 hours. May produce apnea or prolonged effect, depress ventilatory response to CO_2, or cause hypotension. Reduce doses of midazolam. ▪ **Agents that inhibit cytochrome P$_{450}$ activity** (e.g., triazole antifungals [e.g., itraconazole (Sporanox), ketoconazole (Nizoral), miconazole (Monistat)], cimetidine [Tagamet], diltiazem [Cardizem], verapamil, macrolide antibiotics [e.g., erythromycin], omeprazole [Prilosec], and ranitidine [Zantac]) decrease clearance and increase effects of midazolam, resulting in prolonged sedation. ▪ Reduce doses of **inhalation anesthetics** (e.g., halothane) **and/or thiopental** when used with midazolam. ▪ **Protease inhibitors** (e.g., indinavir [Crixivan], nelfinavir [Viracept], and saquinavir [Invirase]) may increase risk of prolonged sedation and respiratory depression. Concurrent use not recommended. Half-life may double with saquinavir. *Contraindicated with ritonavir (Norvir);* may cause life-threatening increased sedation and respiratory depression. Benzodiazepines metabolized by alternate routes may be safer (e.g., lorazepam [Ativan], oxazepam [Serax], temazepam [Restoril]). ▪ May increase serum concentrations of **digoxin**; monitor digoxin serum levels. ▪ Hypotensive effects of benzodiazepines may be increased by any **agent that induces hypotension** (e.g., antihypertensives, CNS depressants, diuretics, lidocaine, pacli-

taxel). Monitor BP during and after use. ■ Use with **rifampin** (Rifadin) increases clearance and reduces effects of benzodiazepines. ■ **Theophyllines** (Aminophylline) antagonize sedative effects of benzodiazepines. ■ **Smoking** increases metabolism and clearance of midazolam, decreasing plasma levels and sedative effects.

SIDE EFFECTS

The incidence of cardiorespiratory events is higher in patients undergoing procedures involving the upper airway (e.g., upper endoscopy or dental procedures). Serious cardiorespiratory events may include airway obstruction, apnea, hypotension (especially with narcotic premedication), oxygen desaturation, respiratory arrest, and/or cardiac arrhythmias or arrest. Inadequate or excessive dosing may cause agitation, combativeness, involuntary movements (e.g., clonic, tonic, muscle tremor), and hyperactivity; may be caused by cerebral hypoxia or be true paradoxical reactions. Other common reactions are coughing, drowsiness, fluctuation in vital signs, headache, hiccups, nausea and vomiting, nystagmus (especially in pediatric patients), induration, redness, or phlebitis at injection site. Capable of numerous other side effects. Has caused death and hypoxic encephalopathy. Withdrawal may be seen in patients receiving an infusion for extended periods of time.

Overdose: Sedation, somnolence, confusion, impaired coordination, diminished reflexes, coma, and untoward effect on vital signs.

ANTIDOTE

Notify the physician of all side effects. Reduction of dosage may be required or will be treated symptomatically. Discontinue the drug for major side effects or paradoxical reactions. Flumazenil (Romazicon) will reverse all sedative effects of benzodiazepines. A patent airway, artificial ventilation, oxygen therapy and other symptomatic treatment must be instituted promptly. Treat hypotension with IV fluids, Trendelenburg position, or vasopressors (e.g., dopamine) as indicated. May cause emesis; observe closely. Treat hypersensitivity reactions and resuscitate as necessary.

MILRINONE LACTATE

(**MILL**-rih-nohn **LAK**-tayt)

Primacor

Antiarrhythmic
Inotropic agent

pH 3.2 to 4

USUAL DOSE

50 mcg/kg (0.05 mg/kg) of body weight as the initial loading dose.
Follow with a maintenance infusion according to the following chart.

Milrinone Maintenance Dose Guidelines			
	Infusion Rate (mcg/kg/min)	Total Daily Dose (24 Hours)	
Minimum	0.375 mcg/kg/min	0.59 mg/kg	Administer as a continuous IV infusion.
Standard	0.50 mcg/kg/min	0.77 mg/kg	
Maximum	0.75 mcg/kg/min	1.13 mg/kg	

Titrate the infusion dose between 0.375 mcg/kg/min to 0.75 mcg/kg/min (26 mcg/min to 52 mcg/min for a 70-kg person) based on hemodynamic and clinical response. Do not exceed a total dose of 1.13 mg/kg/24 hr. Duration of infusion usually does not exceed 48 hours.

DOSE ADJUSTMENTS

Reduced dose required in impaired renal function based on CrCl according to the following chart.

Milrinone Dose Guidelines in Impaired Renal Function	
Creatinine Clearance (mL/min/1.73 M^2)	Infusion Rate (mcg/kg/min)
5 mL/min/1.73 M^2	0.2 mcg/kg/min
10 mL/min/1.73 M^2	0.23 mcg/kg/min
20 mL/min/1.73 M^2	0.28 mcg/kg/min
30 mL/min/1.73 M^2	0.33 mcg/kg/min
40 mL/min/1.73 M^2	0.38 mcg/kg/min
50 mL/min/1.73 M^2	0.43 mcg/kg/min

DILUTION

Loading dose: May be given undiluted, or each 1 mg (1 mL) may be diluted in 1 mL NS or ½NS for injection. Alternately, the loading dose may be diluted with NS, ½NS, or D5W to a total volume of 10 or 20 mL for injection.

Infusion: Dilute with NS, ½NS, or D5W. Available prediluted as 200 mcg/mL in D5W. Amount of diluent may be increased or decreased based on patient fluid requirements. Another source suggests dilution with LR.

Guidelines for Dilution of Milrinone for Infusion			
Desired Infusion Concentration (mcg/mL)	Milrinone 1 mg/mL (mL)	Diluent (mL)	Total Volume (mL)
200 mcg/mL	10 mL	40 mL	50 mL
200 mcg/mL	20 mL	80 mL	100 mL

May be given through Y-tube or three-way stopcock of IV infusion set but should never come in contact with furosemide (Lasix). Use only freshly prepared solutions.

Filters: No data available from manufacturer.

Storage: Store at room temperature before dilution; avoid freezing.

COMPATIBILITY   (Underline Indicates Conflicting Compatibility Information)

Consider any drug NOT listed as compatible to be INCOMPATIBLE until consulting a pharmacist; specific conditions may apply.

Manufacturer states, "Do not add supplementary medications." Forms an immediate precipitate with furosemide (Lasix).

One source suggests the following **compatibilities:**

Additive: Not recommended by manufacturer. Quinidine gluconate.

Y-site: Acyclovir (Zovirax), amikacin, amiodarone (Nexterone), ampicillin, argatroban, atracurium (Tracrium), bivalirudin (Angiomax), bumetanide, calcium chloride, calcium gluconate, caspofungin (Cancidas), cefazolin (Ancef), cefepime (Maxipime), cefotaxime (Claforan), ceftaroline (Teflaro), ceftazidime (Fortaz), cefuroxime (Zinacef), ciprofloxacin (Cipro IV), clindamycin (Cleocin), dexamethasone (Decadron), dexmedetomidine (Precedex), digoxin (Lanoxin), diltiazem (Cardizem), dobutamine, dopamine, doripenem (Doribax), epinephrine (Adrenalin), fenoldopam (Corlopam), fentanyl, gentamicin, heparin, hetastarch in electrolytes (Hextend), hydromorphone (Dilaudid), insulin (regular), isoproterenol (Isuprel), labetalol, lorazepam (Ativan), magnesium sulfate, meropenem (Merrem IV), methylprednisolone (Solu-Medrol), metoprolol (Lopressor), metronidazole (Flagyl IV), micafungin (Mycamine), midazolam (Versed), morphine, nesiritide (Natrecor), nicardipine (Cardene IV), nitroglycerin IV, nitroprusside sodium, norepinephrine (Levophed), oxacillin (Bactocill), pancuronium, piperacillin/tazobactam (Zosyn), potassium chloride (KCl), propofol (Diprivan), propranolol, quinidine gluconate, ranitidine (Zantac), rocuronium (Zemuron), sodium bicarbonate, telavancin (Vibativ), theophylline, ticarcillin/clavulanate (Timentin), tobramycin, torsemide (Demadex), vancomycin, vasopressin, vecuronium, verapamil.

RATE OF ADMINISTRATION

Loading dose: A single dose evenly distributed over 10 minutes.

Infusion: Use an infusion pump to deliver milrinone in recommended doses. The following manufacturer's dose chart defines selected dose in mcg/kg/min in infusion rate of mL/hr. Adjust as indicated by physician's orders and progress in patient's condition. Reduce rate or stop infusion for excessive drop in BP.

Milrinone Infusion Rate (mL/hr) Using 200 mcg/mL Concentration										
Maintenance Dose	Patient Body Weight (kg)									
(mcg/kg/min)	30	40	50	60	70	80	90	100	110	120
0.375	3.4	4.5	5.6	6.8	7.9	9	10.1	11.3	12.4	13.5
0.4	3.6	4.8	6	7.2	8.4	9.6	10.8	12	13.2	14.4
0.5	4.5	6	7.5	9	10.5	12	13.5	15	16.5	18
0.6	5.4	7.2	9	10.8	12.6	14.4	16.2	18	19.8	21.6
0.7	6.3	8.4	10.5	12.6	14.7	16.8	18.9	21	23.1	25.2
0.75	6.8	9	11.3	13.5	15.8	18	20.3	22.5	24.8	27

ACTIONS

A class of cardiac inotropic agent different in chemical structure and mode of action from digitalis glycosides and catecholamines. Similar to inamrinone, with fewer side effects. With a loading dose, peak effect occurs within 10 minutes. Continuous administration is required to maintain serum levels. It has positive inotropic action with vasodilator activity. Reduces afterload and preload by direct relaxant effect on vascular smooth muscle. Produces slight enhancement of AV node conduction. Cardiac output is improved without significant increases in HR or myocardial oxygen consumption or changes in arteriovenous oxygen difference. Pulmonary capillary wedge pressure, total peripheral resistance, diastolic BP, and mean arterial pressure are decreased. HR generally remains the same. Mean half-life is 2.4 hours. Primary route of excretion is in urine.

INDICATIONS AND USES
Short-term management of patients with acute decompensated heart failure.

CONTRAINDICATIONS
Hypersensitivity to milrinone or inamrinone.

PRECAUTIONS
Not shown to be safe or effective for use longer than 48 hours. No improvement in symptoms and an increased risk of death have been reported. ▪ Use caution in impaired renal function; serum levels may increase considerably. ▪ May be given to digitalized patients without causing signs of digoxin toxicity; correct hypokalemia with potassium supplements. ▪ May increase ventricular response in atrial flutter/fibrillation. Consider pretreatment with digoxin. ▪ Additional fluids and electrolytes may be required to facilitate appropriate response in patients who have been vigorously diuresed and may have insufficient cardiac filling pressure. Use caution. ▪ Safety for use in the acute phase of myocardial infarction not established. ▪ Should not be used in patients with severe obstructive aortic or pulmonary valvular disease in lieu of surgical relief of the obstruction. May aggravate outflow tract obstruction in hypertrophic subaortic stenosis.

Monitor: Observe closely. Continuous ECG monitoring required to allow for prompt detection and management of cardiac events, including life-threatening ventricular arrhythmias. Emergency equipment must be readily available. ▪ Monitoring of BP, urine output, renal function, fluid and electrolyte changes (especially potassium), liver function tests, and body weight is recommended. ▪ Monitoring of cardiac index, pulmonary capillary wedge pressure, central venous pressure, and plasma concentration is very useful. ▪ Observe for orthopnea, dyspnea, and fatigue. ▪ Reduce rate or stop infusion for excessive drop in BP. ▪ As cardiac output and diuresis improve, a reduction in diuretic dose may be indicated. ▪ Possible risk of arrhythmias. Risk further increased with excessive diuresis and/or hypokalemia. Replace potassium as indicated. ▪ Infusion site reactions may occur. Monitor site carefully.

Maternal/Child: Category C: safety for use during pregnancy, breast-feeding, and in pediatric patients not established. Use during pregnancy only if potential benefit justifies potential risk.

Elderly: Consider impaired renal function; may require a reduced dose.

DRUG/LAB INTERACTIONS
Theoretical potential for interaction with **calcium channel blockers** (e.g., verapamil); no clinical evidence to date. ▪ May cause additive hypotensive effects with **any drug that produces hypotension** (e.g., alcohol, benzodiazepines [e.g., diazepam, midazolam], lidocaine, paclitaxel). ▪ No untoward drug interactions observed when used in a limited number of patients concurrently with captopril, chlorthalidone (Hygroton), diazepam (Valium), digoxin (Lanoxin), furosemide (Lasix), heparin, hydralazine, hydrochlorothiazide, insulin, isosorbide dinitrate (Sorbitrate), lidocaine, nitroglycerin, prazosin (Minipress), quinidine, spironolactone (Aldactone), warfarin (Coumadin), and potassium supplements. ▪ See Monitor.

SIDE EFFECTS
Supraventricular and ventricular arrhythmias including nonsustained ventricular tachycardia do occur; rare cases of torsades de pointes have been reported. Abnormal liver function tests, anaphylactic shock (rare), angina, bronchospasm, chest pain, headaches, hypokalemia, hypotension, infusion site reactions, rash, and tremor have been reported.

ANTIDOTE
Notify the physician of any side effect. Based on degree of severity and condition of the patient, may be treated symptomatically, and dose may remain the same, be decreased, or the milrinone may be discontinued. Reduce rate or discontinue the drug at the first sign of marked hypotension and notify the physician. May be resolved by these measures alone or vasopressors (e.g., dopamine) may be required. Treat dysrhythmias with the appropriate drug. Resuscitate as necessary.

MITOMYCIN BBW
(my-toe-**MY**-sin)

Antineoplastic
(antibiotic)

MTC, Mutamycin

pH 6 to 8

USUAL DOSE
10 to 20 mg/M^2 as a single dose. May be repeated in 6 to 8 weeks after adequate bone marrow recovery; see Dose Adjustments. Discontinue drug if no response after two courses of treatment.

DOSE ADJUSTMENTS
Subsequent doses based on posttreatment leukocyte and platelet counts. Withhold dose for leukocytes below 4,000/mm^3 or platelet count below 100,000/mm^3. Adjust subsequent doses based on nadir after the prior dose according to the following chart. ■ Lower usual dose range is indicated when used with other antineoplastic drugs and radiation.

Guide to Mitomycin Dose Adjustment		
Nadir After Prior Dose		
Leukocytes/mm^3	Platelets/mm^3	Percentage of Prior Dose to Be Given
≥4,000	≥100,000	100%
3,000 to 3,999	75,000 to 99,999	100%
2,000 to 2,999	25,000 to 74,999	70%
<2,000	<25,000	50%

DILUTION
Specific techniques required; see Precautions. Each 5 mg must be diluted with 10 mL SWFI. Allow to stand at room temperature until completely in solution. May be given through Y-tube or three-way stopcock of a free-flowing infusion of NS or D5W or further diluted in either of the same solutions or sodium lactate ⅙ M and given as an infusion.
Storage: Store unopened vial at CRT. Stable after initial reconstitution at room temperature for 7 days, up to 14 days if refrigerated. When further diluted to a concentration of 20 to 40 mcg/mL, it is stable at room temperature for 3 hours in D5W, 12 hours in NS, and 24 hours in sodium lactate ⅙ M.

COMPATIBILITY
(Underline Indicates Conflicting Compatibility Information)
Consider any drug NOT listed as compatible to be INCOMPATIBLE until consulting a pharmacist; specific conditions may apply.
Sources suggest the following **compatibilities:**
Additive: Manufacturer states that mitomycin (5 to 15 mg) and heparin (1,000 to 10,000 units) in 30 mL NS is stable at CRT for 48 hours. Other sources list dexamethasone (Decadron), heparin, hydrocortisone sodium succinate (Solu-Cortef).

Y-site: Amifostine (Ethyol), bleomycin (Blenoxane), <u>caspofungin (Cancidas)</u>, cisplatin (Platinol), cyclophosphamide (Cytoxan), doxorubicin (Adriamycin), droperidol (Inapsine), fluorouracil (5-FU), furosemide (Lasix), granisetron (Kytril), heparin, leucovorin calcium, melphalan (Alkeran), methotrexate, metoclopramide (Reglan), ondansetron (Zofran), teniposide (Vumon), thiotepa, vinblastine, vincristine.

RATE OF ADMINISTRATION
IV injection: A single dose over 5 to 10 minutes.

Infusion: Rate determined by amount and type of solution, typically 15 to 30 minutes.

ACTIONS
A highly toxic antibiotic, antineoplastic agent. Cell cycle phase–nonspecific, it is most useful in G and S phases. Interferes with cell division by binding with DNA to slow production of RNA. Rapidly distributed to body tissues and ascitic fluid. Does not cross blood-brain barrier. Metabolized primarily in the liver, but some metabolism occurs in other tissues as well. Some excreted in urine.

INDICATIONS AND USES
Treatment of disseminated adenocarcinoma of the stomach or pancreas. Used in combination with other drugs. Used intravesically in bladder cancer.

Unlabeled uses: Combination chemotherapy in anal, cervical, head and neck, metastatic breast, and non–small-cell lung cancers and in malignant mesothelioma.

CONTRAINDICATIONS
Not recommended as single-agent primary therapy. Known hypersensitivity to mitomycin, thrombocytopenia, coagulation disorders, increased bleeding from other causes, potentially serious infections, SCr greater than 1.7 mg/100 mL.

PRECAUTIONS
Follow guidelines for handling cytotoxic agents. See Appendix A, p. 1331. ▪ Administered by or under the direction of the physician specialist in a facility with adequate diagnostic and treatment facilities for monitoring the patient and responding to any medical emergency. ▪ Use extreme caution in impaired renal function; see Contraindications. ▪ Acute shortness of breath and bronchospasm have occurred within minutes to hours following administration of vinca alkaloids (e.g., vincristine) in patients who have received mitomycin previously or are receiving mitomycin simultaneously. Bronchodilators, steroids and/or oxygen may be used to treat respiratory distress. ▪ Bone marrow suppression (leukopenia and thrombocytopenia) may be severe and contribute to overwhelming infections in an already compromised patient. ▪ Hemolytic uremic syndrome (hemolytic anemia, thrombocytopenia, and irreversible renal failure) has occurred in patients receiving mitomycin as a single agent or in combination with other agents. It can occur at any time during treatment, but most cases have occurred with a cumulative dose greater than 60 mg. Administration of blood products may exacerbate the symptoms.

Monitor: Monitor WBC, RBC, platelet count, PT, bleeding time, differential, and hemoglobin before, during, and 7 to 10 weeks after therapy. ▪ Monitor all patients, especially those nearing a cumulative dose of 60 mg, for unexplained anemia with fragmented cells on peripheral blood smear, thrombocytopenia, and decreased renal function; see Precautions. ▪ Determine absolute patency of vein; use of an IV catheter is preferred because severe cellulitis and tissue necrosis will result from extravasation. If extravasation occurs, discontinue injection and use another vein. Elevate extremity and apply cold compresses to extravasated area. Delayed erythema with or without ulceration has occurred at or distant to the injection site. May occur weeks to months after mitomycin administration, even when no obvious evidence of extravasation was observed during administration. ▪ May precipitate acute respiratory distress syndrome. Oxygen can be toxic to the lungs; monitor intake carefully and use only enough to provide adequate arterial saturation. ▪ Monitor fluid balance; avoid overhydration. ▪ Be alert for signs of bone marrow suppression or infection. ▪ Monitor for thrombocytopenia (platelet count less than 50,000/mm³). Initiate precautions to prevent excessive bleeding (e.g., inspect IV sites, skin, and mucous membranes; use extreme care during invasive procedures; test urine, emesis, stool, and secretions for occult blood). ▪ Prophylactic antibiotics may be indicated pending results of C/S in a febrile neutropenic patient. ▪ Prophylactic antiemetics may reduce nausea and vomiting and increase patient comfort. ▪ See Precautions and Drug/Lab Interactions.

Patient Education: Nonhormonal birth control recommended. ▪ Report shortness of breath and IV site burning and stinging promptly. ▪ See Appendix D, p. 1333.

Maternal/Child: Avoid pregnancy; may produce teratogenic effects on the fetus. ▪ Information on safety in breast-feeding or in pediatric patients not available; discontinue breast-feeding.

Elderly: Consider diminished hepatic function; monitor for early signs of toxicity.

DRUG/LAB INTERACTIONS

Do not administer **live virus vaccines** to patients receiving antineoplastic drugs. ▪ May cause shortness of breath, severe bronchospasm, and acute pneumonitis with **vinca alkaloids** (e.g., vinblastine).

SIDE EFFECTS

Alopecia, anaphylaxis, anorexia, bleeding, blurring of vision, cellulitis at injection site, confusion, CHF (patient has usually received doxorubicin [Adriamycin, Doxil]), coughing, diarrhea, drowsiness, dyspnea with nonproductive cough, edema, elevated BUN or SCr, fatigue, fever, headache, hematemesis, hemolytic uremic syndrome (microangiopathic hemolytic anemia [hematocrit less than 25%], irreversible renal failure [SCr greater than 1.6 mg/dL], and thrombocytopenia [less than 100,000/mm^3]), hemoptysis, hypertension, leukopenia, mouth ulcers, nausea, paresthesias, pneumonia, pruritus, pulmonary edema, purple discoloration of vein, radiographic evidence of pulmonary infiltrates, rash, renal failure, respiratory distress syndrome (acute), skin toxicity, stomatitis, syncope, thrombocytopenia, thrombophlebitis, vomiting.

ANTIDOTE

Most side effects will be treated symptomatically. Keep the physician informed. All are potentially serious and many can be life threatening. Hematopoietic depression requires cessation of therapy until recovery occurs. Discontinue drug if dyspnea, nonproductive cough, or radiographic evidence of pulmonary infiltrates is present. Discontinue drug for any symptoms of hemolytic uremic syndrome. There is no specific antidote. Supportive therapy as indicated will help sustain the patient in toxicity. Administration of whole blood products (e.g., packed RBCs, platelets, leukocytes) and/or blood modifiers (e.g., darbepoetin alfa [Aranesp], epoetin alfa [Epogen], filgrastim [Neupogen, Zarxio], pegfilgrastrim [Neulasta], sargramostim [Leukine]) may be indicated to treat bone marrow toxicity; see Precautions. If extravasation has occurred, L.A. dexamethasone injected into the indurated area with a fine hypodermic needle may be helpful; elevate extremity.

MITOXANTRONE HYDROCHLORIDE BBW
(my-toe-**ZAN**-trohn hy-droh-**KLOR**-eyed)

Antineoplastic
(antibiotic)

Novantrone

pH 3 to 4.5

USUAL DOSE
Preliminary evaluations and testing required; see Monitor.

Combination initial therapy for acute nonlymphocytic leukemia (ANLL) in adults:

Induction: 12 mg/M^2/day of mitoxantrone on Days 1 through 3 and cytarabine 100 mg/M^2/day as a continuous 24-hour infusion on Days 1 through 7. Should a complete remission not be achieved, repeat mitoxantrone, 12 mg/M^2/day for only 2 days, and cytarabine 100 mg/M^2/day for 5 days after all signs or symptoms of severe or life-threatening nonhematologic toxicity have cleared.

Consolidation: After full hematologic recovery (usually 6 weeks after induction therapy), administer mitoxantrone 12 mg/M^2/day by IV infusion on Days 1 and 2 and cytarabine 100 mg/M^2/day as a continuous 24-hour infusion on Days 1 to 5. May repeat in 4 weeks. Severe myelosuppression occurred in these subsequent courses. See Monitor.

Prostate cancer: 12 to 14 mg/M^2 as a short IV infusion once every 21 days. Used concurrently with steroids.

Multiple sclerosis (MS): 12 mg/M^2 as an infusion over 5 to 15 minutes. Repeat every 3 months. May be given for up to 2 years or until a cumulative dose of 140 mg/M^2 has been administered.

DOSE ADJUSTMENTS
Adjust dose based on clinical response and development and severity of toxicity. ▪ Clearance is reduced by impaired hepatic function. Treat patients with impaired hepatic function with caution; dose adjustment may be indicated. Specific recommendations not available; see Precautions.

DILUTION
Specific techniques required; see Precautions. A single dose must be diluted with at least 50 mL of NS or D5W. May be further diluted in NS, D5W, or D5NS. Must be given through Y-tube or three-way stopcock of a free-flowing infusion of D5W or NS, or may be diluted in larger amounts of the same solutions and given as a continuous infusion.

Filters: No data available from manufacturer.

Storage: Store unopened vial at RT (15° to 25° C [59° to 77° F]). Do not freeze. Diluted solution should be used immediately. After penetration of the stopper on a multidose vial, the undiluted mitoxantrone may be stored at RT for 7 days or refrigerated for up to 14 days. Do not freeze.

COMPATIBILITY
Consider any drug NOT listed as compatible to be INCOMPATIBLE until consulting a pharmacist; specific conditions may apply.

Manufacturer recommends not mixing in the same infusion with other drugs until **compatibility** data are available and states that it may form a precipitate if mixed in the same infusion with heparin.

One source suggests the following **compatibilities:**

Additive: *Not recommended by manufacturer.* Cyclophosphamide (Cytoxan), cytarabine (ARA-C), etoposide (VePesid), fluorouracil (5-FU), hydrocortisone sodium succinate (Solu-Cortef), potassium chloride (KCl).

Y-site: Allopurinol (Aloprim), amifostine (Ethyol), cladribine (Leustatin), etoposide (VePesid), etoposide phosphate (Etopophos), filgrastim (Neupogen), fludarabine (Fludara), gemcitabine (Gemzar), granisetron (Kytril), linezolid (Zyvox), melphalan (Alkeran), ondansetron (Zofran), oxaliplatin (Eloxatin), sargramostim (Leukine), teniposide (Vumon), thiotepa, vinorelbine (Navelbine).

RATE OF ADMINISTRATION

IV injection: A single dose of properly diluted medication over at least 3 to 5 minutes. Must be given through Y-tube or three-way stopcock of a free-flowing infusion of D5W or NS.

Intermittent infusion: A single dose over 15 to 30 minutes.

Infusion: Sometimes a single dose is given as a continuous infusion over 24 hours. Is combined with cytarabine.

ACTIONS

An anthracenedione, a synthetic antibiotic antineoplastic agent. Has achieved complete remissions with a single course of combination therapy. Has a cytocidal effect on proliferating and nonproliferating cells. Probably not cell-cycle specific. Inhibits DNA and RNA synthesis. Thought to reduce the number of relapses and slow down progression of MS through its ability to suppress the activity of T-cells, B-cells, and macrophages. These cells attack the myelin sheath around nerve cells, causing the symptoms of MS. Improves the presentation of brain lesions on MRI studies. Extensive distribution to tissue occurs rapidly. Partially metabolized. Exact pathways unknown. Half-life varies from 23 to 213 hours (median 75 hours). Slowly excreted in bile, urine, and feces as either unchanged drug or as inactive metabolites.

INDICATIONS AND USES

Treatment of acute nonlymphocytic leukemia in adults; includes erythroid, monocytic, myelogenous, and promyelocytic acute leukemias. Given in combination with other approved drugs. ▪ Treatment of bone pain in patients with advanced prostate cancer resistant to hormones. Used concurrently with steroids. ▪ To reduce neurologic disability and/or the frequency of clinical relapses in patients with secondary (chronic) progressive, progressive relapsing, or worsening relapsing-remitting multiple sclerosis (i.e., patients whose neurologic status is significantly abnormal between relapses). Not indicated in the treatment of patients with primary progressive MS.

Unlabeled uses: Treatment of acute lymphocytic leukemia (ALL), breast cancer, Hodgkin's lymphoma, non-Hodgkin's lymphomas, myelodysplastic syndrome, pediatric acute leukemias, pediatric sarcoma, and part of a conditioning regimen for autologous hematopoietic stem cell transplantation (HSCT).

CONTRAINDICATIONS

Hypersensitivity to mitoxantrone or other anthracyclines. ▪ Not for intrathecal use; severe injury with permanent sequelae can result.

PRECAUTIONS

For IV use only. Do not administer SC, IM, intra-arterially, or intrathecally. ▪ Follow guidelines for handling cytotoxic agents. See Appendix A, p. 1331. ▪ Use of goggles, gloves, and protective gown recommended. Flush skin copiously with warm water should any contact occur. Irrigate eyes immediately in case of contact. Clean spills with 5.5 parts calcium hypochlorite to 13 parts by weight of water for each 1 part of mitoxantrone. ▪ Usually administered by or under the direction of the physician specialist with facilities for monitoring the patient and responding to any medical emergency. ▪ Will cause severe myelosuppression; use extreme caution in pre-existing drug-induced bone marrow suppression. ▪ Should not be given to patients with baseline neutrophil counts of less than 1,500 cells/mm^3 (except for the treatment of acute nonlymphocytic leukemia). ▪ MS patients with a baseline left ventricular ejection fraction (LVEF) below the lower limit of normal or patients who have received a cumulative dose equal to or greater than 140 mg/M^2 should not be treated with mitoxantrone. ▪ May cause severe cardiac toxicity (e.g., acute congestive heart failure) in all patients, even if cardiac risk factors are not present. May occur early during therapy or months to years after completion. Risk increased with cumulative doses (equal to or greater than 140 mg/M^2), in patients with pre-existing heart disease, and in patients previously treated with anthracyclines (see Drug/Lab Interactions), other cardiotoxic drugs, or radiation therapy encompassing the heart. ▪ Use caution in impaired liver function. Clearance is decreased; see Dose Adjustments. Patients with MS who have hepatic impairment should ordinarily not be treated with mitoxantrone. ▪ Use caution if renal function is impaired; has not been studied. ▪ Urine and sclera may turn bluish in color. ▪ Therapy with mitoxantrone increases the risk of developing secondary leukemia in patients with multiple sclerosis

M

and in patients with cancer. Most commonly reported types are acute promyelocytic leukemia and acute myelocytic leukemia. The occurrence is more common when mitoxantrone is given in combination with other cytotoxic agents and/or radiotherapy or when doses of anthracyclines (e.g., doxorubicin [Adriamycin], idarubicin [Idamycin]) have been escalated. ▪ Rapid lysis of cancer cells may cause tumor lysis syndrome. ▪ See Monitor.

Monitor: Obtain baseline CBC with differential and platelet count; repeat before each dose and if S/S of infection occur. ▪ Complete a physical exam and ECG and obtain a complete history to assess for S/S of pre-existing cardiac disease. ▪ In all patients, obtain an evaluation of left ventricular ejection fraction (LVEF) by echocardiogram or MUGA (multiple-gated acquisition) before therapy begins. ▪ Evaluation of LVEF and assessment of cardiotoxicity by history, physical exam, and ECG should be repeated before each dose in MS patients. ▪ Obtain repeat LVEF as indicated in all patients. ▪ Mitoxantrone should not ordinarily be administered to MS patients who have received a cumulative dose equal to or greater than 140 mg/M^2 or to patients who experience a drop in LVEF to below the lower limit of normal or a clinically significant reduction in LVEF. MS patients should have an annual quantitative evaluation of LVEF after discontinuing mitoxantrone therapy to monitor for late-occurring cardiotoxicity. ▪ Monitoring of liver function is indicated before and during therapy. ▪ Because of rapid lysis of cancer cells, initiate hypouricemic therapy with allopurinol or similar agents before beginning treatment. Monitor uric acid levels, maintain hydration, and alkalinize urine if necessary. ▪ Observe closely and frequently for all signs of bleeding or infection. ▪ Prophylactic antibiotics may be indicated pending results of C/S in a febrile neutropenic patient. ▪ Determine absolute patency of vein. Severe local tissue damage may occur with extravasation. Phlebitis at the infusion site has also been reported. Should extravasation or phlebitis occur, discontinue injection and use another vein. ▪ Prophylactic antiemetics may reduce nausea and vomiting and increase patient comfort. ▪ Monitor for thrombocytopenia (platelet count less than 50,000/mm^3). Initiate precautions to prevent excessive bleeding (e.g., inspect IV sites, skin, and mucous membranes; use extreme care during invasive procedures; test urine, emesis, stool, and secretions for occult blood). ▪ Monitor for S/S of acute leukemia (secondary leukemia); may include excessive bruising, bleeding, and recurrent infections. ▪ See Precautions and Drug/Lab Interactions.

Patient Education: Nonhormonal birth control recommended; see Maternal/Child. ▪ Blood and cardiac tests are imperative; keep all appointments. ▪ Report IV site burning or stinging promptly. ▪ Urine may turn blue-green for 24 hours following administration. Bluish discoloration of sclera may also occur. ▪ Medication guide available; read before beginning treatment with mitoxantrone. ▪ See Appendix D, p. 1333.

Maternal/Child: Category D: avoid pregnancy. May produce teratogenic effects on the fetus. Women with MS who are biologically capable of becoming pregnant should have a pregnancy test before each dose of mitoxantrone regardless of other methods of birth control used, including birth control pills. ▪ Secreted in breast milk. Discontinue breastfeeding. ▪ Safety for use in pediatric patients not established.

Elderly: Specific age-related differences have not been identified; consider age-related organ impairment (e.g., bone marrow reserve, renal, hepatic) and possibility of increased sensitivity.

DRUG/LAB INTERACTIONS

Additive bone marrow suppression may occur with **radiation therapy and/or other bone marrow–suppressing agents** (e.g., azathioprine, chloramphenicol, melphalan [Alkeran]). Dose reduction may be required. ▪ Risk of cardiotoxicity increased in patients previously treated with maximum cumulative doses of **other anthracyclines** (e.g., doxorubicin [Adriamycin], epirubicin [Ellence], idarubicin [Idamycin]) **and/or radiation encompassing the heart.** ▪ Do not administer **live virus vaccines** to patients receiving antineoplastic drugs.

SIDE EFFECTS

Alopecia (reversible), bladder infections, menstrual disorders, mucositis, and nausea occur frequently. Other side effects include abdominal pain, acute congestive heart failure, altered electrolytes, altered liver function tests (e.g., increased ALT, AST, BUN), arrhythmias, arthralgias, bleeding, bone marrow suppression (severe with standard doses), cardiotoxicity, conjunctivitis, cough, decrease in LVEF, diarrhea, dyspnea, erythema, fever, GI bleeding, headache, hematuria, hypersensitivity reactions (e.g., dyspnea, hypotension, rash, urticaria), infections, injection site burning, jaundice, leukemia (including secondary AML), mucositis, myalgias, nail bed changes, phlebitis, renal failure, seizures, skin discoloration, stomatitis, swelling, vomiting. Interstitial pneumonitis has been reported. Anaphylaxis has been reported rarely.

Post-Marketing: Secondary acute myelogenous leukemia (AML).

ANTIDOTE

There is no specific antidote. Notify physician of all side effects. Most will be treated symptomatically. Blood and blood products, antibiotics, and other adjunctive therapies must be available. Blood modifiers (e.g., darbepoetin alfa [Aranesp], epoetin alfa [Epogen], filgrastim [Neupogen, Zarxio], pegfilgrastim [Neulasta], sargramostim [Leukine]) may be indicated to treat bone marrow toxicity. Nadir of leukocyte count occurs within 10 days. Recovery is within 21 days. For extravasation, elevate extremity and apply ice. Monitor closely and obtain surgical consult if necessary. Overdose has resulted in death. Peritoneal dialysis or hemodialysis not effective. Supportive therapy as indicated will help sustain the patient in toxicity.

M

MORPHINE SULFATE BBW

(**MOR**-feen **SUL**-fayt)

Opioid analgesic
(agonist)
Adjunct, pulmonary edema
Anesthesia adjunct

Astramorph PF, Duramorph PF

pH 2.5 to 7

USUAL DOSE

IV injection: Manufacturer recommends an initial dose of 2 to 10 mg/70 kg of body weight. Repeat every 3 to 4 hours as necessary. Doses may range from 2 to 20 mg based on patient requirements and response. Titrate to achieve pain relief with lowest dose. Frequent, repeated doses (e.g., up to every 5 minutes if needed) in small-dose increments (e.g., 1 to 4 mg) may be associated with fewer side effects than the administration of larger, less frequent doses.

Cancer patients suffering with severe chronic pain often require higher doses because of increased tolerance (up to 150 mg/hr has been given). Very high doses (275 to 440 mg/hr) are occasionally used for short periods of time (hours to days) for extreme exacerbations of pain in these drug-tolerant individuals. 1 to 3 mg/kg over 15 to 20 minutes will induce unconsciousness.

Acute MI: 2 to 4 mg initially. May give additional doses of 2 to 8 mg at 5- to 15-minute intervals as needed (AHA guidelines).

Infusion: 1 mg/mL (range is 0.1 to 1 mg/mL) in NS or D5W per controlled infusion device (may be patient activated). *Based on a 1 mg/mL dilution,* an initial loading dose may be as high as 15 mg (15 mL). The continuous background infusion to provide a level of pain relief and maintain patency of the vein may range from 1 to 2.5 mg/hr (1 to 2.5 mL). Additional doses averaging 0.5 to 1.5 mg (0.5 to 1.5 mL) may be activated by the patient at selected intervals every 3 to 60 minutes (averaging 10 to 15 minutes). Additional boluses averaging 1 to 2 mg (1 to 2 mL) may be given by health care professionals (e.g., every 30 minutes prn). In selected cancer patients all of these doses may be considerably higher.

Open heart surgery: 0.5 to 3 mg/kg as the sole anesthetic or with an anesthetic agent. Cardiovascular function not depressed if oxygen is used and adequate ventilation maintained.

Dyspnea during end-of-life care (unlabeled): 2 to 5 mg IV every 5 to 10 minutes until relief. Patient-controlled anesthesia (PCA) is recommended in the inpatient setting. Higher doses may be needed for patients taking chronic opioids.

PEDIATRIC DOSE

Analgesic: Usual range is 0.05 to 0.1 mg/kg. Administer very slowly.

Postoperative analgesia: 0.01 to 0.04 mg/kg/hr (10 to 40 mcg/kg/hr).

Selected pediatric patients with severe chronic cancer pain: 0.025 to 2.6 mg/kg/hr (average 0.04 to 0.07 mg/kg/hr).

Selected pediatric patients with severe pain during sickle cell crisis: 0.025 to 2.6 mg/kg/hr (average 0.04 to 0.07 mg/kg/hr).

NEONATAL DOSE

Elimination is reduced in neonates, and they have an increased susceptibility to CNS side effects.

Analgesia/tetralogy (cyanotic) spells (unlabeled): 0.05 to 0.2 mg/kg/dose every 4 hours. Titrate to individual response. Another source suggests an *IV injection* of 0.05 to 0.1 mg/kg/dose every 4 to 8 hours or an *IV infusion* of 0.01 to 0.02 mg/kg/hr. Titrate to individual response.

Mechanical ventilation of neonates (unlabeled): 50 mcg/kg as an initial loading dose. Administer over 30 to 60 minutes. Follow with a continuous infusion of 10 to 30 mcg/kg/hr. Titrate to individual response.

Postoperative analgesia (unlabeled): 50 mcg/kg as an initial loading dose. Administer over 30 to 60 minutes. Follow with a continuous infusion of 15 mcg/kg/hr. Titrate to individual response.

DOSE ADJUSTMENTS
Reduced dose and/or extended intervals may be required in impaired renal or hepatic function and in the elderly. ▪ Doses appropriate for the general population may cause serious respiratory depression in vulnerable patients. ▪ Increase doses as required if analgesia is inadequate, tolerance develops, or pain severity increases. The first sign of tolerance is usually a reduced duration of effect. ▪ See Drug/Lab Interactions.

DILUTION
IV injection: May be given undiluted; however, further dilution with 5 mL of SWFI or NS for injection or other IV solutions to facilitate titration is appropriate. May be given through Y-tube or three-way stopcock of infusion set.

Infusion: Each 0.1 to 1 mg is usually diluted in 1 mL NS or D5W and administered via a controlled infusion device that may be patient activated (e.g., a narcotic syringe infuser system). Available in 60-mL ampules containing 1 to 2 mg/mL for direct transfer to syringe infuser systems. (*Astramorph PF and Duramorph* are preservative free and expensive; can be used IV, but are the only choice for epidural or intrathecal injection; see drug literature. *Duramorph* is **NOT** for use in continuous microinfusion devices. *Infumorph* is **NOT** for IV use.) Fluid restriction or high doses may require more concentrated solutions. Concentrations above 5 mg/mL are rarely exceeded. Available in vials containing 25 mg/mL, which must be further diluted before infusion. Also available in ADD-Vantage vials for use with ADD-Vantage infusion containers. Is sometimes added to larger amounts (500 mL to 1 L) of IV solution in selected situations and infused via a large volume-controlled infusion pump (requires close titration).

Storage: Store at CRT. Protect from light and freezing.

COMPATIBILITY   (Underline Indicates Conflicting Compatibility Information)
Consider any drug NOT listed as compatible to be INCOMPATIBLE until consulting a pharmacist; specific conditions may apply.
One source suggests the following **compatibilities:**

Additive: Alteplase (tPA, Activase), atracurium (Tracrium), dobutamine, fluconazole (Diflucan), furosemide (Lasix), ketamine (Ketalar), meropenem (Merrem IV), metoclopramide (Reglan), ondansetron (Zofran), succinylcholine, verapamil.

Y-site: Acetaminophen (Ofirmev), acyclovir (Zovirax), allopurinol (Aloprim), amifostine (Ethyol), amikacin, aminophylline, amiodarone (Nexterone), ampicillin, ampicillin/sulbactam (Unasyn), anidulafungin (Eraxis), argatroban, atracurium (Tracrium), atropine, aztreonam (Azactam), bivalirudin (Angiomax), bumetanide, calcium chloride, caspofungin (Cancidas), cefazolin (Ancef), cefepime (Maxipime), cefotaxime (Claforan), cefotetan, cefoxitin (Mefoxin), ceftaroline (Teflaro), ceftazidime (Fortaz), ceftriaxone (Rocephin), cefuroxime (Zinacef), chloramphenicol (Chloromycetin), cisatracurium (Nimbex), cladribine (Leustatin), clindamycin (Cleocin), dexamethasone (Decadron), dexmedetomidine (Precedex), diazepam (Valium), digoxin (Lanoxin), diltiazem (Cardizem), diphenhydramine (Benadryl), dobutamine, docetaxel (Taxotere), dopamine, doripenem (Doribax), doxycycline, enalaprilat (Vasotec IV), epinephrine (Adrenalin), erythromycin (Erythrocin), esmolol (Brevibloc), etomidate (Amidate), etoposide phosphate (Etopophos), famotidine (Pepcid IV), fenoldopam (Corlopam), fentanyl, filgrastim (Neupogen), fluconazole (Diflucan), fludarabine (Fludara), foscarnet (Foscavir), furosemide (Lasix), gemcitabine (Gemzar), gentamicin, granisetron (Kytril), heparin, hetastarch in electrolytes (Hextend), hydrocortisone sodium succinate (Solu-Cortef), hydromorphone (Dilaudid), 6% hydroxyethyl starch (Voluven), insulin (regular), ketorolac (Toradol), labetalol, levofloxacin (Levaquin), lidocaine, linezolid (Zyvox), lorazepam (Ativan), magnesium sulfate, melphalan (Alkeran), meropenem (Merrem IV), methyldopate, methylprednisolone (Solu-Medrol), metoclopramide (Reglan), metoprolol (Lopressor), metronidazole (Flagyl IV), midazolam (Versed), milrinone (Primacor), nafcillin (Nallpen), nicardipine (Cardene IV), nitroglycerin IV, nitroprusside sodium, norepinephrine (Levophed), ondansetron (Zofran), oxacillin (Bactocill), oxaliplatin (Eloxatin), oxytocin (Pitocin), paclitaxel (Taxol), palonosetron (Aloxi), pancuronium, pantoprazole (Protonix IV), pemetrexed (Alimta), penicillin G potassium, phenobarbital (Luminal), piperacillin/tazobactam (Zosyn), potassium chloride (KCl), propofol (Diprivan), propranolol, ranitidine (Zantac), remifentanil (Ultiva), sodium bicarbonate, sulfamethoxazole/trimethoprim, tacrolimus (Prograf), teniposide (Vumon), thiotepa, ticarcillin/clavulanate (Timentin), tirofiban (Aggrastat), tobramycin, vancomycin, vecuronium, vinorelbine (Navelbine), warfarin (Coumadin), zidovudine (AZT, Retrovir).

RATE OF ADMINISTRATION

Frequently titrated according to symptom relief and respiratory rate. Side effects markedly increased if rate of injection too rapid. Rapid IV administration may result in chest wall rigidity.

IV injection: 15 mg or fraction thereof over 4 to 5 minutes.

Infusion: Initial loading dose, basal rate (continuous rate of infusion), patient self-administered dose and interval, additional boluses permitted, and total dose for 1 hour should be ordered by physician. Administer initial dose and boluses at rate for IV injection. For continuous infusion and self-administered dose and interval, note range of mL/hr under Usual Dose.

ACTIONS

An opium-derivative, opioid analgesic that is a descending CNS depressant. Produces a wide spectrum of pharmacologic effects, including analgesia, diminished GI mobility, dysphoria, euphoria, physical dependence, respiratory depression, and somnolence. Pain relief is effected almost immediately and lasts up to 4 to 5 hours (mean is 2 hours). Morphine induces sleep and inhibits perception of pain by binding to opiate receptors, decreasing sodium permeability, and inhibiting transmission of pain impulses. Depresses many other senses or reflexes. Relieves pulmonary congestion, lowers myocardial oxygen requirements, and reduces anxiety. Metabolized in the liver and primarily excreted in the urine and feces. Crosses the blood-brain barrier, but plasma concentration of morphine is higher than CSF concentration. Crosses the placental barrier. Secreted in breast milk.

INDICATIONS AND USES

Relief of moderate to severe acute and chronic pain (e.g., postoperative or cancer pain). ▪ Analgesic of choice in pain associated with myocardial infarction. ▪ Treatment of acute pulmonary edema associated with left ventricular failure. ▪ Used before surgery to sedate, decrease anxiety, and facilitate induction of anesthesia. ▪ Management of neonatal opiate withdrawal.

Unlabeled uses: Treatment of dyspnea in end-of-life care. ▪ Control of pain during mechanical ventilation in neonates. ▪ Control of postoperative pain in neonates.

CONTRAINDICATIONS

Hypersensitivity to morphine sulfate or any component of the formulation, bronchial asthma (acute or severe), and upper airway obstruction. Other sources include paralytic ileus, premature infants, or labor and delivery of premature infants. Specific formulations may have additional contraindications; see prescribing information. ▪ *Duramorph* is **NOT** for use in continuous microinfusion devices.

PRECAUTIONS

Schedule II opioid agonists, including hydromorphone, morphine, oxymorphone, oxycodone, fentanyl, and methadone, have the highest potential for abuse and risk of producing respiratory depression. Alcohol, CNS depressants, and other opioids potentiate the respiratory depressant effects of hydromorphone, increasing the risk of respiratory depression that might result in death; see Drug/Lab Interactions. ▪ Use caution in the elderly, in patients with impaired hepatic or renal function, and in pulmonary disease. ▪ May cause severe hypotension in an individual whose ability to maintain BP has been compromised by a depleted blood volume or a concurrent administration of drugs such as phenothiazines or general anesthetics; see Drug/Lab Interactions. ▪ Use extreme caution in craniotomy, head injury, and increased intracranial pressure; respiratory depression and intracranial pressure may be further increased. ▪ May cause sedation and pupillary changes (miosis) that may obscure the existence, extent, and course of intracranial pathology. ▪ May cause apnea in asthmatic patients. ▪ Symptoms of acute abdominal conditions may be masked. ▪ May increase ventricular response rate in presence of supraventricular tachycardias. ▪ Cough reflex is suppressed. ▪ Tolerance as well as psychological and physical dependence can develop. Tolerance for the drug gradually increases, but abstinence for 1 to 2 weeks will restore effectiveness. Risk of using a narcotic antagonist in patients chronically receiving narcotic therapy should be considered. ▪ A marked increase in dose may precipitate seizures. Use with caution in patients with known seizure disorders.

Monitor: Oxygen, controlled respiratory equipment, and naloxone must always be available. ▪ Observe patient frequently to continuously based on amount of dose and monitor vital signs. ▪ Assess baseline pain, then assess pain with vital signs and/or more frequently if needed. Reassess after administration of morphine and adjust dose or interval as required. ▪ Keep patient supine; orthostatic hypotension and fainting may occur; less likely with continuous low doses, but observe closely during ambulation. ▪ Uncontrolled pain causes sleep deprivation, decreases pain threshold, and increases pain. When pain is finally controlled, expect the patient to sleep more until recovery from sleep deprivation. ▪ Adhere to prescribed bowel care regimen to avoid constipation and/or impaction. Maintain adequate hydration. ▪ See Drug/Lab Interactions.

Patient Education: Avoid alcohol or other CNS depressants (e.g., barbiturates, benzodiazepines [e.g., diazepam (Valium)]). ▪ May cause blurred vision, dizziness, or drowsiness; use caution in tasks that require alertness. ▪ Request assistance with ambulation. ▪ May be habit forming.

Maternal/Child: Category C: safety for use in pregnancy or breast-feeding not established. Benefits must outweigh risks. ▪ May reduce strength, duration, and frequency of uterine contractions during labor and delivery. ▪ See Contraindications. ▪ Pediatric patients may be more sensitive to effects, especially respiratory depressant effects. ▪ May cause paradoxical excitation. ▪ May cause respiratory depression in the neonate when given during labor and delivery. Have naloxone and resuscitative equipment available. ▪ Infants born to mothers who have been taking morphine chronically may exhibit withdrawal symptoms.

Elderly: See Dose Adjustments and Precautions. ▪ May be more sensitive to effects (e.g., respiratory depression, constipation, urinary retention). ▪ Lower doses may provide effective analgesia. ▪ Consider age-related organ impairment.

DRUG/LAB INTERACTIONS

Alcohol, other CNS depressants (e.g., narcotic analgesics, general anesthetics, antidepressants [e.g., amitriptyline (Elavil), imipramine (Tofranil), nortriptyline (Aventyl)], barbiturates, hypnotics, sedatives), H_2 antagonists (e.g., cimetidine [Tagamet]), and some phenothiazines (e.g., chlorpromazine [Thorazine]) may increase CNS depression, respiratory depression, and hypotension; reduced dose of one or both agents indicated. ▪ **Anticholinergics** (e.g., atropine) **and antidiarrheals** may increase risk of constipation or paralytic ileus. ▪ Hypotensive effects will be increased with **diuretics** (e.g., furosemide [Lasix]), **antihypertensive agents** (especially ganglionic blockers [e.g., guanethidine (Ismelin)]), **or hypotension-producing agents** (e.g., antidepressants, benzodiazepines [e.g., diazepam], adrenergic blocking agents [e.g., propranolol], calcium channel blocking agents [e.g., diltiazem], calcium, nitroprusside sodium, nitroglycerin). ▪ Concurrent use with **rifampin** (Rifadin) may decrease analgesic effects of morphine; an alternate analgesic may be required. ▪ Markedly reduced doses of **MAO inhibitors** (e.g., selegiline [Eldepryl]) required with opiates. ▪ Administration of **agonist/antagonist analgesics** (e.g., butorphanol [Stadol] or buprenorphine [Buprenex]) to an opiate-dependent patient receiving a pure opiate may precipitate withdrawal symptoms. ▪ May potentiate anticoagulant effect of oral **warfarin**.

M

SIDE EFFECTS

Average dose: Anxiety, bradycardia, confusion, constipation, decreased libido in men and women, delayed absorption of oral medications, depression of cough reflex, dizziness, drowsiness/sedation, euphoria, histamine-related reactions (e.g., local tissue irritation, pruritus, urticaria, wheals), hypersensitivity reactions, hypothermia, increased intracranial pressure, interference with thermal regulation, menstrual irregularities (including amenorrhea), nausea, neonatal apnea, oliguria, orthostatic hypotension, physical or psychological dependence, reduced male potency, respiratory depression (slight), skeletal muscle rigidity, tremors, urinary retention, vomiting. Side effects associated with histamine and constipation may be more common with morphine than with most other narcotic analgesics.

Higher doses: CNS excitation (convulsions), respiratory depression (severe).

Overdose: Anaphylaxis, cardiac arrest, Cheyne-Stokes respiration, circulatory collapse, coma, excitation, hypotension (severe), inverted T-wave on ECG, myocardial depression (severe), pinpoint pupils, respiratory depression or arrest, tachycardia, death.

ANTIDOTE

With increasing severity of any side effect or onset of symptoms of overdose, discontinue the drug and notify the physician. Naloxone will reverse cardiovascular, CNS, and respiratory reactions. Question the diagnosis of narcotic-induced toxicity if no response is observed after administration of 10 mg of naloxone. A patent airway, artificial ventilation, oxygen therapy, and other symptomatic treatment must be instituted promptly. Resuscitate as necessary.

MOXIFLOXACIN HYDROCHLORIDE `BBW`
(mox-ee-**FLOX**-ah-sin hy-droh-**KLOR**-eyed)

Avelox

Antibacterial
(fluoroquinolone)

pH 4.1 to 4.6

USUAL DOSE

400 mg once every 24 hours. Duration of therapy is based on diagnosis as listed in the following chart. Serum levels similar by oral or IV route. Transfer to oral therapy as soon as practical; no dose adjustment necessary. The magnitude of QT prolongation may increase with increasing serum concentrations. Do not exceed recommended dose.

Moxifloxacin Dosing Guidelines		
Infection*	Daily Dose (mg)	Duration (days)
Acute bacterial sinusitis	400 mg	10 days
Acute bacterial exacerbation of chronic bronchitis	400 mg	5 days
Community-acquired pneumonia	400 mg	7-14 days
Uncomplicated skin and skin structure infections	400 mg	7 days
Complicated skin and skin structure infections	400 mg	7-21 days
Complicated intra-abdominal infections†	400 mg	5-14 days

*Due to the designated pathogens.
†Therapy should usually be started with the IV formulation.

DOSE ADJUSTMENTS

Dose adjustment is not indicated based on age, gender, or race; in impaired renal function (including patients on hemodialysis or CAPD); or in mild, moderate, or severe impaired hepatic function (Child-Pugh Classes A, B, and C). See Precautions.

DILUTION
Available in ready-to-use latex-free plexibags containing 400 mg moxifloxacin in 0.8% saline. No further dilution is necessary. Refer to directions provided with administration set.

Filters: No data available from manufacturer.

Storage: Store at CRT. Do not refrigerate; a precipitate will form. Discard unused portions.

COMPATIBILITY
Consider any drug NOT listed as compatible to be INCOMPATIBLE until consulting a pharmacist; specific conditions may apply.

Limited **compatibility** data available. Manufacturer states, "Other IV substances, additives, or other medications should not be added to moxifloxacin or infused simultaneously through the same IV line." Flush line with a solution **compatible** to both drugs before and after administration of moxifloxacin and/or any other drug through the same IV line. May be administered through a Y-tube or three-way stopcock. Temporarily discontinue other solutions infusing at the same site.

Y-site: Manufacturer lists as **compatible** with NS, D5W, D10W, SWFI, LR at ratios from 1:10 to 10:1.

One source suggests the following **compatibilities:**

Y-site: Ceftaroline (Teflaro), doripenem (Doribax), 6% hydroxyethyl starch (Voluven), vasopressin.

RATE OF ADMINISTRATION
Single dose equally distributed over 60 minutes as an infusion. Avoid rapid or bolus IV infusion. Incidence and magnitude of QT prolongation may increase with increasing concentrations or increasing rates of infusion. Flush tubing before and after moxifloxacin with a **compatible** solution.

ACTIONS
A synthetic broad-spectrum methoxy fluoroquinolone antibacterial agent. Effective against a wide range of gram-negative and gram-positive organisms, including common respiratory pathogens such as *Streptococcus pneumoniae, Haemophilus influenzae,* and *Moraxella catarrhalis,* and atypicals such as *Chlamydophila pneumoniae* and *Mycoplasma pneumoniae.* Bactericidal action results from inhibition of topoisomerase II and IV, which are required for bacterial DNA replication, transcription, repair, and recombination. Mode of action helps minimize selection of resistant mutants of gram-positive bacteria, which cause many respiratory tract infections. Mechanism of fluoroquinolones differs from that of aminoglycosides, cephalosporins, macrolides, penicillins, and tetracyclines, and fluoroquinolones may be active against pathogens resistant to these antibiotics. There is no cross-resistance between fluoroquinolones and these other antibiotics. Widely distributed throughout the body. Concentrations in most target tissues are higher than those found in plasma. Mean half-life is approximately 10.7 to 13.3 hours. Partially metabolized in the liver by glucuronide and sulfate conjugation. Excreted as unchanged drug and metabolites in feces and urine. May be secreted in breast milk.

INDICATIONS AND USES
In May 2015, moxifloxacin was approved for the prevention and treatment of septicemic and pneumonic plague. The revised manufacturer's prescribing information outlining this indication and its corresponding dose was not available at the time this edition went to print.

Treatment of adults with infections caused by susceptible strains of microorganisms in conditions that include acute bacterial sinusitis, acute bacterial exacerbation of chronic bronchitis, complicated and uncomplicated skin and skin structure infections, and complicated intra-abdominal infections. ■ Treatment of community-acquired pneumonia caused by many organisms, including *Streptococcus pneumoniae* (including multidrug-resistant strains [MDRSP]). MDRSP strains are resistant to two or more of the following antibiotics: penicillin, second-generation cephalosporins (e.g., cefuroxime [Zinacef]), macrolides, tetracyclines, and sulfamethoxazole/trimethoprim.

CONTRAINDICATIONS

History of hypersensitivity to moxifloxacin or other quinolone antibiotics (e.g., ciprofloxacin [Cipro], levofloxacin [Levaquin], norfloxacin [Noroxin]).

PRECAUTIONS

For IV use only. ▪ C/S studies indicated to determine susceptibility of the causative organism to moxifloxacin. ▪ Prolonged use may cause superinfection because of overgrowth of nonsusceptible organisms. ▪ Cross-resistance has been observed between moxifloxacin and other fluoroquinolones against gram-negative bacteria. However, gram-positive bacteria resistant to other fluoroquinolones may still be susceptible to moxifloxacin. Observed emergence of bacterial resistance to fluoroquinolones and the occurrence of cross-resistance with other fluoroquinolones are of concern. Proper use of fluoroquinolones and other classes of antibiotics is encouraged to avoid the emergence of resistant bacteria from overuse. ▪ Prolongation of the QTc interval on ECG has been reported with moxifloxacin. Infrequent cases of arrhythmia (including torsades de pointes) have been reported with the use of other fluoroquinolones. The risk of arrhythmia may be reduced by avoiding quinolone use in patients with known prolongation of the QTc interval and in the presence of uncorrected electrolyte imbalances (e.g., hypokalemia, hypomagnesemia), significant bradycardia, acute myocardial ischemia, or concurrent treatment with Class Ia antiarrhythmic agents (e.g., quinidine [Quinidex], procainamide [Procanbid, Procan SR]) or Class III antiarrhythmic agents (e.g., amiodarone [Nexterone], sotalol [Betapace]); see Rate of Administration. ▪ Use with caution in patients receiving drugs that prolong the QTc interval (e.g., antipsychotics, cisapride [Propulsid], erythromycin, and tricyclic antidepressants). ▪ Use caution in patients with mild, moderate, or severe hepatic insufficiency; associated metabolic disturbances may lead to QT prolongation. ▪ Use with caution in patients with known or suspected CNS disorders, such as severe cerebral atherosclerosis, epilepsy, or other factors that may predispose to seizures. Convulsions, increased intracranial pressure (including pseudotumor cerebri), psychosis, and CNS stimulation have been reported; see Side Effects. CNS events, including agitation, anxiety, confusion, depression, dizziness, hallucinations, insomnia, nervousness, nightmares, paranoia, suicidal thoughts or acts, and tremors may be caused by fluoroquinolones, including moxifloxacin. ▪ Tendinitis and tendon rupture that required surgical repair or resulted in prolonged disability have been reported in patients of all ages receiving quinolones. Most frequently involves the Achilles tendon but has also been reported with the shoulder, hand, biceps, thumb, and other tendon sites. ▪ Tendinitis or tendon rupture may occur during or for up to months after fluoroquinolone therapy. Risk may be increased in patients over 60 years of age; in patients taking corticosteroids; in patients with heart, kidney, or lung transplants; with strenuous physical activity; and in patients with renal failure or previous tendon disorders such as rheumatoid arthritis. ▪ Fluoroquinolones have neuromuscular blocking activity and may exacerbate muscle weakness in persons with myasthenia gravis. Serious adverse events, including requirement for ventilatory support and deaths, have been reported in these patients. Avoid use in patients with a known history of myasthenia gravis. ▪ Rare cases of peripheral neuropathy (e.g., paresthesias, hypoesthesias, dysesthesias [impairment of sensitivity or touch], or weakness) have been reported. Symptoms may occur soon after initiation of therapy and may be irreversible; see Antidote. ▪ *Clostridium difficile*–associated diarrhea (CDAD) has been reported. May range from mild diarrhea to fatal colitis. Consider in patients who present with diarrhea during or after treatment with moxifloxacin. ▪ Serious and occasionally fatal hypersensitivity and/or anaphylactic reactions have been reported. Often occur after the first dose. ▪ Other serious events (sometimes fatal) due to hypersensitivity or uncertain etiology have been reported with fluoroquinolones, including moxifloxacin. Usually occur following multiple doses. Manifestations may include things such as renal impairment/failure, hematologic toxicity, hepatic necrosis/failure, and dermatologic toxicity; see Side Effects, Post-Marketing. Discontinue moxifloxacin at the first appearance of a skin rash, jaundice, or other signs of hepatotoxicity or hypersensitivity. ▪ Moderate to severe photosensitivity/phototoxicity reactions have been reported in patients receiving quinolones; see Patient Education. ▪ See Monitor.

Monitor: Serious and occasionally fatal hypersensitivity reactions have been reported in patients receiving quinolone therapy. May be seen with first or subsequent doses. Emergency equipment must be readily available; see Side Effects. Watch for early symptoms of a hypersensitivity reaction. ▪ Monitor for S/S of peripheral neuropathy. Discontinue moxifloxacin at first symptoms of neuropathy (e.g., pain, burning, tingling, numbness and/or weakness) or if patient has deficits in light touch, pain, temperature, position sense, vibratory sensation, and/or motor strength. ▪ Obtain baseline and periodic CBC with differential. ▪ ECG monitoring for QT prolongation may be indicated in select patients. ▪ Maintain adequate hydration to prevent concentrated urine throughout treatment. Other quinolones have formed crystals. ▪ Symptomatic hyperglycemia or hypoglycemia may occur, usually in elderly diabetic patients receiving oral hypoglycemic agents (e.g., glyburide) or insulin. Monitor blood glucose closely. ▪ See Precautions, Drug/Lab Interactions, and Antidote.

Patient Education: A patient medication guide is available from the manufacturer. ▪ Drink fluids liberally. ▪ Inform physician of any history of myasthenia gravis. ▪ Patients with a history of myasthenia gravis should avoid use of moxifloxacin. ▪ Report skin rash or any other hypersensitivity reaction promptly. ▪ Dizziness or light-headedness may interfere with ambulation or motor coordination. Use caution in tasks that require alertness. ▪ Discontinue moxifloxacin and promptly report CNS side effects such as confusion, depression, dizziness, hallucinations, seizures, suicidal thoughts, tremors, or vision loss. ▪ Report tendon pain or inflammation promptly; rest and refrain from exercise. ▪ Promptly report burning, numbness, pain, tingling, or weakness in extremities. Nerve damage can be permanent. ▪ May produce changes in ECG. Report fainting spells or palpitations promptly. ▪ Review medicines and disease states with physician or pharmacist before initiating therapy. ▪ May alter glucose control in diabetic patients on insulin or oral therapy. Monitor glucose carefully. Discontinue moxifloxacin and contact physician if hypoglycemic reaction occurs. ▪ Photosensitivity has occurred in patients receiving other quinolones and, infrequently, moxifloxacin. It is best to avoid excessive sunlight or artificial ultraviolet light. May cause severe sunburn; wear protective clothing, use sunscreen, and wear dark glasses outdoors. Report a sunburn-like reaction or skin eruption promptly. ▪ Promptly report diarrhea or bloody stools that occur during treatment or up to several months after an antibiotic has been discontinued; may indicate CDAD and require treatment. ▪ See Precautions, Monitor, Drug/Lab Interactions, and Antidote.

Maternal/Child: Category C: safety for use in pregnancy not established. Benefit must outweigh risk to fetus. ▪ Has potential for harmful effects on breast-feeding infants; either discontinue breast-feeding or choose an alternate drug. ▪ Safety and effectiveness for use in pediatric patients under 18 years of age not established. ▪ Quinolones have caused erosion of cartilage in weight-bearing joints and other signs of arthropathy in juvenile animals; however, they have been used in infants and children to treat serious infections unresponsive to other antibiotic regimens.

Elderly: Safety and effectiveness similar to that of younger adults; however, elderly may experience an increased risk of side effects (e.g., CNS effects, tendinitis, tendon rupture, risk of QT prolongation). ▪ See Precautions.

DRUG/LAB INTERACTIONS

May cause ventricular arrhythmias or torsades de pointes with **drugs that prolong the QT interval,** such as **Class Ia antiarrhythmic agents** (e.g., quinidine, procainamide [Pronestyl]), **Class III antiarrhythmic agents** (e.g., amiodarone [Nexterone], sotalol [Betapace]), **anticonvulsants** (e.g., fosphenytoin [Cerebyx]), **antihistamines** (e.g., diphenhydramine [Benedryl]), **phenothiazines** (e.g., chlorpromazine [Thorazine]), **serotonin reuptake inhibitors** (e.g., fluoxetine [Prozac], paroxetine [Paxil]), **tricyclic antidepressants** (e.g., imipramine [Tofranil], amitryptyline [Elavil]). Use with caution; see Precautions. ▪ Risk of CNS stimulation and seizures may be increased with concurrent use of **NSAIDs** (e.g., ibuprofen [Advil, Motrin], naproxen [Aleve, Naprosyn]). ▪ May cause hyperglycemia and hypoglycemia with concurrent administration of **antidiabetic agents** (e.g., metformin [Glucophage], insulin); monitoring of blood glucose recommended. ▪ Not metabolized by the cytochrome P_{450} isoenzyme system. Drug-drug interactions with atenolol (Tenormin), digoxin, glyburide (DiaBeta), itraconazole (Sporanox), oral contraceptives, theophylline, and warfarin have not been observed. ▪ Does not inhibit the P_{450} isoenzyme system. Drugs metabolized by this system (e.g., cyclosporine [Sandimmune], midazolam [Versed], theophylline, or warfarin [Coumadin]) are not affected by coadministration of moxifloxacin. ▪ Digoxin, itraconazole, morphine, probenecid, ranitidine (Zantac), theophylline, and warfarin (Coumadin) have been shown not to alter the pharmacokinetics of moxifloxacin; dose adjustments are not indicated. ▪ Some quinolones, including moxifloxacin, may enhance the effects of **warfarin** (Coumadin); monitoring of PT or INR is recommended with concomitant use. ▪ See literature for additional drug/drug interactions on transfer to oral moxifloxacin. ▪ May cause a false-positive when **testing urine for opiates;** more specific testing methods may be indicated.

SIDE EFFECTS

Diarrhea, dizziness, headache, and nausea were most common and described as mild to moderate in severity. Capable of numerous other reactions in fewer than 1% of patients. **Major:** Cardiovascular effects (e.g., cardiac arrest, palpitations, QT interval prolongation, tachycardia, torsades de pointes, vasodilation, ventricular tachyarrhythmias); CDAD; CNS stimulation (e.g., anxiety, confusion, depression, hallucinations, insomnia, nightmares, paranoia, restlessness, seizures, suicidal thoughts, tremor); hepatic failure; hepatitis and jaundice (predominantly cholestatic); hyperglycemia or hypoglycemia; hypersensitivity reactions (e.g., anaphylaxis, cardiovascular collapse, death, dyspnea, edema [facial, laryngeal, or pharyngeal], hypotension, itching, rash, shock, urticaria); hypotension; increased bilirubin; increased intracranial pressure; pain, inflammation, and ruptures of the shoulder, hand, and Achilles tendon; peripheral neuropathy (e.g., pain, burning, tingling, numbness and/or weakness [see Precautions, Monitor]); photosensitivity/ phototoxicity; prolonged PT and INR; Stevens-Johnson syndrome; syncope; and toxic psychoses; see Precautions.

Post-Marketing: Acute renal insufficiency or failure, allergic pneumonitis; arthralgia; exacerbation of myasthenia gravis; hearing impairment, including deafness (reversible in most); hematologic abnormalities (agranulocytosis, anemia [hemolytic and aplastic], leukopenia, pancytopenia, thrombocytopenia, thrombotic thrombocytopenic purpura); interstitial nephritis; jaundice; liver abnormalities (e.g., acute hepatic necrosis or failure, hepatitis, jaundice); muscle weakness; myalgia; peripheral neuropathy; polyneuropathy; rash; serum sickness; severe dermatologic reactions (e.g., toxic epidermal necrolysis [Lyell's syndrome], Stevens-Johnson syndrome); suicidal ideation/thoughts; vasculitis; vision loss (transient in most cases).

ANTIDOTE

Keep physician informed of all side effects. Most minor side effects will be treated symptomatically or will resolve with continued dosing (e.g., dizziness, light-headedness); monitor closely. Discontinue at first sign of hypersensitivity (e.g., skin rash), CDAD, CNS symptoms, dermatologic reactions, hypoglycemic reactions, phototoxicity, symptoms of neuropathy, or tendon rupture. Treat allergic reactions as indicated with epinephrine, airway management, oxygen, IV fluids, antihistamines (e.g., diphenhydramine [Benadryl]), corticosteroids (e.g., Solu-Cortef), and pressor amines (e.g., dopamine). Treat CNS symptoms as indicated; may require anticonvulsants (e.g., phenytoin [Dilantin], diazepam [Valium]) for seizures and discontinuation of moxifloxacin. Mild cases of CDAD may respond to discontinuation of drug. Treat CDAD with fluids, electrolytes, protein supplements, and oral vancomycin (Vancocin) or metronidazole (Flagyl) as indicated. In severe cases, surgical evaluation may be indicated. Complete rest is indicated for an affected tendon until treatment is available. Discontinue if photosensitivity occurs. Monitoring of the ECG and adequate hydration are indicated in overdose. No specific antidote. Less than 10% of moxifloxacin and its glucuronide metabolite are removed by CAPD or hemodialysis.

MULTIVITAMIN INFUSION
(mul-ti-**VI**-tah-min in-**FU**-zhun)

Nutritional supplement
(vitamin)

Infuvite Adult, Infuvite Pediatric, M.V.I.-12, M.V.I. Adult, M.V.I. Pediatric

USUAL DOSE
Multiples of the daily dose may be given for 2 or more days in patients (adult and pediatric patients) with multiple vitamin deficiencies or markedly increased requirements. Individual components may be indicated in specific or long-standing deficiencies. Monitor blood vitamin concentrations to ensure maintenance of adequate levels. Formulations differ in the amount of each vitamin supplied and in their content (some contain vitamin K [e.g., *M.V.I. Adult and Pediatric, Infuvite (Adult and Pediatric)*], and others do not [e.g., *M.V.I.-12*]); see Drug/Lab Interactions.
All adult formulations: One 5- to 10-mL dose every 24 hours.

PEDIATRIC DOSE
See Maternal/Child.

INFUVITE PEDIATRIC
Supplemental vitamin A may be required for low-birth-weight infants.
Less than 1 kg: 30% of the contents of vial 1 and vial 2 (1.2 mL of vial 1 and 0.3 mL of vial 2).
1 to 3 kg: 65% of the contents of vial 1 and vial 2 (2.6 mL of vial 1 and 0.65 mL of vial 2).
Over 3 kg to 11 years of age: Entire contents of vial 1 (4 mL) and entire contents of vial 2 (1 mL).

M.V.I. PEDIATRIC
Less than 1 kg: 1.5 mL/24 hr.
1 to 3 kg: 3.25 mL/24 hr.
Over 3 kg to 11 years of age: 5 mL/24 hr.

DILUTION
Various preparations. Most may be reconstituted with 5 mL of SWFI or supplied diluent. All preparations must be further diluted in at least 500 mL but preferably 1,000 mL of IV fluids. Soluble in commonly used infusion fluids, including dextrose, saline, electrolyte replacement fluids, plasma, and selected protein amino acid products. Do not use if any crystals have formed. When reconstituted as directed, *Infuvite Adult* contains no more than 70 mcg/L of aluminum. M.V.I.-12 also contains aluminum.
Pediatric dilution: *Infuvite Pediatric and M.V.I. Pediatric:* Each dose should be added to at least 100 mL of dextrose, saline, or other **compatible** infusion solution. When reconstituted as directed, *M.V.I. Pediatric* contains no more than 42 mcg/L of aluminum, and *Infuvite Pediatric* contains no more than 30 mcg/L of aluminum; see Precautions. See Maternal/Child.
Storage: Before use, refrigerate at 2° to 8° C (36° to 46° F) protected from light. Manufacturers recommend immediate use of fully diluted Infuvite Pediatric and M.V.I. Adult and Pediatric. Fully diluted M.V.I.-12 and Infuvite Adult should be refrigerated and used within 24 hours.

COMPATIBILITY
(Underline Indicates Conflicting Compatibility Information)
Consider any drug NOT listed as compatible to be INCOMPATIBLE until consulting a pharmacist; specific conditions may apply.
Compatibility may vary with preparation; consult prescribing information for specifics of a preparation. Direct addition to IV fat emulsions is not recommended. Some manufacturers suggest that admixture or **Y-site** administration with vitamin solutions should be avoided. Alkaline or moderately alkaline solutions (e.g., acetazolamide [Diamox], aminophylline, chlorothiazide [Diuril], sodium bicarbonate), as well as ampicillin and tetra-

cycline, are listed as **incompatible** by one manufacturer. Folic acid may be unstable with calcium salts. *All formulations must be diluted in infusion solutions.*

One source suggests the following **compatibilities:**

Additive: Cefoxitin (Mefoxin), <u>fat emulsion IV</u>, isoproterenol (Isuprel), methyldopate, metoclopramide (Reglan), norepinephrine (Levophed), sodium bicarbonate, verapamil.

Y-site: *All formulations must be diluted in infusion solutions before administration at the Y-site.* Acyclovir (Zovirax), <u>ampicillin,</u> cefazolin (Ancef), ceftaroline (Teflaro), clindamycin (Cleocin), diltiazem (Cardizem), erythromycin (Erythrocin), fludarabine (Fludara), gentamicin, 6% hydroxyethyl starch (Voluven), tacrolimus (Prograf).

RATE OF ADMINISTRATION
A single dose given as an infusion at prescribed rate of infusion fluids.

ACTIONS
A multiple vitamin solution containing fat-soluble and water-soluble vitamins in an aqueous solution. Provides B complex and vitamins A, D, and E. Some multivitamin preparations presently available do not contain vitamin K. *Infuvite Adult, M.V.I. Adult, Infuvite Pediatric, and M.V.I. Pediatric* do contain vitamin K. Provides daily requirements or corrects an existing deficiency.

INDICATIONS AND USES
A daily multivitamin maintenance supplement for patients receiving parenteral nutrition. Provides the necessary vitamins required to maintain the body's normal resistance and repair processes. Used in situations such as surgery, trauma, burns, severe infectious disease, and comatose states, which may provoke a stress response and alteration in the body's metabolic demands. Used when oral administration is contraindicated, not possible, or insufficient. Solutions without vitamin K are indicated for patients on warfarin anticoagulant therapy who are receiving parenteral nutrition.

CONTRAINDICATIONS
Known hypersensitivity to thiamine hydrochloride or other product components; preexisting hypervitaminosis. ▪ Contraindicated prior to blood sampling for detection of megaloblastic anemia. Folic acid and cyanocobalamin in formulation may mask serum deficits.

PRECAUTIONS
Do not wait for the development of clinical signs of vitamin deficiency before initiating vitamin therapy. ▪ Hypersensitivity reactions have occurred following IV administration of multivitamin solutions containing vitamin B_1 (thiamine) and vitamin K. ▪ Hypervitaminosis A manifested by blurred vision, dizziness, headache, and nausea and vomiting has been reported in patients with renal failure or liver disease who are receiving vitamin A supplementation. Use caution. ▪ Vitamin A may adhere to plastic, resulting in inadequate vitamin A administration in the doses recommended; see Maternal/Child. ▪ Elevated blood levels of vitamin E may result if doses larger than recommended or oral or parenteral vitamin E are administered. ▪ Solutions containing multivitamins may contain aluminum. In impaired kidney function, aluminum may reach toxic levels. Premature neonates are particularly at risk because of their immature kidneys and requirement for calcium and phosphate, which also contain aluminum. Research indicates that patients with impaired renal function who receive more than 4 to 5 mcg/kg/day of parenteral aluminum are at risk for developing CNS or bone toxicity associated with aluminum accumulation. ▪ Blood draws for the detection of folic acid and cyanocobalamin deficiencies are indicated before administration to patients with megaloblastic anemia. ▪ See Drug/Lab Interactions.

Monitor: Monitor VS. ▪ Monitor for any symptoms of a hypersensitivity reaction. ▪ Moderate increase in ALT may occur in patients with active inflammatory enterocolitis. Usually reversible following discontinuation of vitamin infusion. Monitoring of ALT levels suggested. ▪ Monitor vitamin A levels in patients with liver disease and/or high alcohol consumption. ▪ Monitor renal function, calcium, phosphorous, and vitamin A levels in patients with impaired renal function. ▪ Measure blood vitamin concentrations periodically in patients receiving parenteral nutrition to determine if vitamin deficiencies or excesses are developing. Blood levels of A, C, D, and folic acid may decline in patients receiving parenteral multivitamins as their sole source of vitamins for 4 to 6 months. ▪ See Precautions, Maternal/Child, and Drug/Lab Interactions.

Maternal/Child: Recommendations for use during pregnancy vary by product. Range is from vitamin needs may exceed those of nonpregnant women to safety for use in pregnancy not established; use only if clearly needed. ▪ Recommendations for use during breast-feeding vary by product. Range is from vitamin needs may exceed those of nonpregnant women to not known if secreted in breast milk; use caution if required during breast-feeding. ▪ Vitamin A may adhere to plastic, resulting in inadequate vitamin A administration in the doses recommended. Additional vitamin A supplementation may be necessary, especially in low-birth-weight infants. ▪ Polysorbates (a component of some multivitamins) have been associated with E-Ferol syndrome (ascites, cholestasis, hepatomegaly, hypotension, metabolic acidosis, renal dysfunction, and thrombocytopenia) in low-birth-weight infants; however, this has not been reported with the use of pediatric multivitamins. ▪ See Precautions.

Elderly: Consider age-related decreased organ function and/or medical problems.

DRUG/LAB INTERACTIONS

Folic acid may lower serum concentration of **phenytoin**, resulting in increased seizure frequency; monitor serum levels of both drugs. ▪ **Phenytoin** may decrease serum folic acid concentrations; avoid during pregnancy. ▪ Folic acid may obscure pernicious anemia and may decrease the patient's response to **methotrexate** therapy. ▪ Pyridoxine may reduce effectiveness of **levodopa.** ▪ Concomitant administration of **hydralazine or isoniazid** (INH) may increase pyridoxine requirements. ▪ Vitamin K may antagonize the anticoagulant effects of **warfarin** (Coumadin) and reduce its effectiveness; monitor INR/ PT. ▪ The hematologic response to vitamin B_{12} therapy in patients with pernicious anemia may be inhibited by concomitant administration of **chloramphenicol.** ▪ Thiamine, riboflavin, pyridoxine, niacinamide, and ascorbic acid may decrease the antibiotic activity of **erythromycin, kanamycin, streptomycin, doxycycline, and lincomycin.** ▪ **Bleomycin** is inactivated in vitro by ascorbic acid and riboflavin. ▪ Ascorbic acid in the urine may cause **false-negative urine glucose** determinations.

SIDE EFFECTS

Rare when administered as recommended: Agitation; allergic reactions including anaphylaxis, angioedema, periorbital and digital edema, shortness of breath, urticaria, and wheezing; anxiety; diplopia; dizziness; erythema; fainting; headache; pruritus; rash. Vitamin A and vitamin D hypervitaminosis (symptomatology related to hypercalcemia) may occur with prolonged use of significant doses.

ANTIDOTE

With onset of any side effect, discontinue administration immediately and notify physician. Treat anaphylaxis or resuscitate as necessary.

MYCOPHENOLATE MOFETIL HYDROCHLORIDE BBW

Immunosuppressant

(**my**-koh-**FEN**-oh-layt **MAH**-fuh-teel hy-droh-**KLOR**-eyed)

CellCept Intravenous

pH 2.4 to 4.1

USUAL DOSE

Used in combination with cyclosporine (Sandimmune) and corticosteroids. Oral form should be used as soon as tolerated by the patient. Initial dose should be given within 24 hours of transplantation. The IV preparation may be used for up to 14 days.

Kidney or liver transplant: 1 Gm as an infusion twice daily (total daily dose of 2 Gm).

Heart transplant: 1.5 Gm as an infusion twice daily (total daily dose of 3 Gm).

PEDIATRIC DOSE

Limited data available; see Indications and product insert. Safety and efficacy of IV formulation not established. Usually given orally.

DOSE ADJUSTMENTS

No dose adjustments are indicated in renal transplant patients who experience delayed graft function postoperatively. ▪ Avoid doses greater than 1 Gm twice a day in renal transplant patients with severe chronic renal impairments (GFR less than 25 mL/min/1.73 M^2) outside the immediate posttransplant period. ▪ Data not available for cardiac or hepatic transplant patients with severe chronic renal impairment; potential benefits must outweigh risks. ▪ Reduce dose or interrupt the dosing cycle if neutropenia (ANC less than 1.3×10^3 [1,300 cells/mm^3]) occurs. ▪ Dose adjustment not indicated in impaired liver function. ▪ See Precautions/Monitor.

DILUTION

Specific techniques required; see Precautions. Use caution in handling and preparation. Avoid skin contact with the solution. If skin contact occurs, wash thoroughly with soap and water; rinse eyes with plain water.

Reconstitute each 500-mg vial with 14 mL of D5W (500 mg/15 mL). Shake gently to dissolve. Discard if particulate matter or discoloration is observed or if a lack of vacuum in vial is noted when diluent is added. To achieve a final concentration of 6 mg/mL, each 500 mg must be further diluted with 70 mL of D5W (1 Gm with 140 mL; 1.5 Gm with 210 mL).

Filters: Not required by manufacturer; however, no significant loss of potency is expected with the use of a filter.

Storage: Store powder and reconstituted or diluted solutions at 15° to 30° C (59° to 86° F). Most desired storage temperature is 25° C (77° F). Reconstituted or diluted solutions are best used immediately after preparation. Keep reconstituted or diluted solutions at CRT; the infusion must begin within 4 hours of reconstitution/dilution.

COMPATIBILITY

(Underline Indicates Conflicting Compatibility Information)

Consider any drug NOT listed as compatible to be INCOMPATIBLE until consulting a pharmacist; specific conditions may apply.

Manufacturer states, "Mycophenolate is **incompatible** with other IV solutions and should not be mixed or administered concurrently via the same infusion catheter with other intravenous drugs or infusion admixtures."

One source lists the following **compatibilities:**

Y-site: <u>Anidulafungin (Eraxis)</u>, <u>caspofungin (Cancidas)</u>, cefepime (Maxipime), dopamine, norepinephrine (Levophed), tacrolimus (Prograf), vancomycin.

RATE OF ADMINISTRATION

A single dose must be given as an infusion over a minimum of 2 hours. **Must not be** administered by rapid or bolus IV injection.

ACTIONS

A hydrochloride salt of mycophenolate mofetil. A potent immunosuppressive agent, inhibiting proliferation of both B- and T-lymphocytes. Has been shown to prolong the survival of allogeneic transplants (kidney, heart, liver, intestine, limb, small bowel, pancreatic islets, and bone marrow) and to reverse ongoing acute rejection episodes in animal models. Rapidly and completely metabolized to mycophenolic acid (MPA), its active metabolite. MPA is then metabolized predominantly to its inactive metabolite, mycophenolic acid glucuronide (MPAG). Secondary peak in plasma MPA concentration is usually noted 6 to 12 hours postdose. Enterohepatic recirculation is thought to contribute to MPA concentrations. Both MPA and MPAG are highly bound to albumin. In patients with renal impairment or delayed graft function, levels of MPAG may be elevated. Binding of MPA may then be reduced as a result of competition between MPAG and MPA. Plasma concentrations of metabolites are increased in patients with renal impairment. Half-life is 11.4 to 24.4 hours. Excreted primarily as MPAG in urine. Small amount excreted in feces. May cross the placental barrier. May be secreted in breast milk.

INDICATIONS AND USES

Used as part of an immunosuppressive regimen that includes cyclosporine and corticosteroids. ▪ Prophylaxis of acute organ rejection in patients receiving allogeneic kidney, heart or liver transplants. ▪ Capsules, tablets, and oral solution approved for prevention of rejection in pediatric renal transplant patients.

CONTRAINDICATIONS

Hypersensitivity to mycophenolate mofetil, mycophenolic acid, any component of the drug product, or polysorbate 80 (TWEEN).

PRECAUTIONS

For IV use only. ▪ Use caution in handling and preparation. Avoid skin contact of the solution. If contact occurs, wash thoroughly with soap and water; rinse eyes with plain water. Follow guidelines for handling cytotoxic agents. See Appendix A, p. 1331. ▪ Usually administered by or under the direction of a physician experienced in immunosuppressive therapy and the management of organ transplant patients. Adequate laboratory and supportive medical resources must be available. ▪ Use caution; hypersensitivity reactions have been observed; emergency equipment and drugs for treatment of severe hypersensitivity reactions must be immediately available. ▪ Risk of developing lymphoproliferative diseases, lymphomas, and other malignancies, particularly of the skin, is increased. Appears to be related to the intensity and duration of immunosuppression rather than to any specific agent. ▪ Patients receiving immunosuppressants are at increased risk for developing bacterial, fungal, protozoal, and new or reactivated viral infections, including opportunistic infections. Polyomavirus-associated nephropathy (PVAN), JC virus–associated progressive multifocal leukoencephalopathy (PML), cytomegalovirus (CMV) infections, and reactivation of hepatitis B (HBV) or hepatitis C (HCV) have all been reported. Reduction in immunosuppression should be considered for patients who develop evidence of new or reactivated viral infections. Physicians should also consider the risk that reduced immunosuppression presents to the functioning allograft. ▪ The overall incidence of opportunistic infections and herpesvirus infections (herpes simplex, herpes zoster, and CMV) was higher in cardiac transplant patients treated with mycophenolate than in those receiving azathioprine. ▪ PML has been reported. PML is a serious progressive neurologic disorder caused by infection of the CNS by JC virus, a member of the papovavirus family. It typically occurs in immunocompromised patients. PML is rare but may result in irreversible neurologic deterioration and death, and there is no known effective treatment. Hemiparesis, apathy, confusion, cognitive deficiencies, and ataxia are the most commonly observed clinical signs. ▪ BKVAN has been reported. May lead to deterioration in renal function and renal graft loss. Reduction in immunosuppression may be indicated. ▪ Risk of CMV viremia and CMV disease is highest among transplant recipients who are seronegative for CMV at time of transplant and receive a graft from a CMV-seropositive donor. ▪ Severe neutropenia has been reported; see Monitor. ▪ Pure red cell aplasia (PRCA) has been reported in patients receiving mycophenolate in combination with other immunosuppressive agents. May be reversible with dose reduction or discontinuation of mycophenolate. In transplant patients, reduced immunosuppression may place the graft at risk. ▪ Has been associated with an increased incidence of GI adverse effects (e.g., GI tract ulceration, hemorrhage, and/or perforation). Use caution in patients with active serious digestive system disease. ▪ Use with caution in patients with hepatic insufficiency. Metabolism of MPA may be affected by certain types of hepatic disease. ▪ Use caution in patients with severe chronic renal impairment; see Dose Adjustments. ▪ Avoid use in patients with selected rare hereditary deficiency diseases (e.g., Lesch-Nyhan, Kelley-Seegmiller syndrome). ▪ See Monitor, Patient Education, and Maternal/Child.

Monitor: Obtain baseline CBC with differential before treatment. Repeat weekly during the first month, twice monthly for the second and third months, then monthly thereafter for the first year. ▪ Monitor for neutropenia. Has been observed most frequently in the period from 31 to 180 days posttransplant. May be due to mycophenolate, concomitant medications, viral infections, or some combination of these causes. If neutropenia develops (ANC less than 1,300 cells/mm³), mycophenolate should be interrupted or the dose reduced. Appropriate diagnostic tests and treatment should be instituted. ▪ Assess neurologic status frequently. ▪ Monitor patients infected with HBV or HCV for clinical and laboratory signs suggestive of reactivation of infection. ▪ Monitor patients with severe chronic renal impairment and patients with delayed graft function closely. See Dose Adjustments and Actions.

Patient Education: Read the manufacturer's medication guide before beginning treatment with mycophenolate. ▪ In women of childbearing age, a pregnancy test is required immediately before starting mycophenolate. Test should be repeated in 8 to 10 days. Repeat pregnancy tests should be performed during routine follow-up visits. Effective contraception must be used during therapy and for 6 weeks following cessation of therapy. Females with reproductive potential must be counseled regarding pregnancy prevention and planning. Females with reproductive potential include girls who have entered puberty and all women who have a uterus and have not passed through menopause (menopause must be confirmed). See manufacturer's prescribing information for acceptable contraceptive methods. Birth control pills alone may be ineffective. If a pregnancy occurs, do not stop mycophenolate; call your health care provider. See Maternal/Child. ▪ Alternative immunosuppressants with less potential for embryo-fetal toxicity should be considered in patients who are considering pregnancy. ▪ Promptly report any S/S of infection or bone marrow suppression (e.g., unexpected bruising, bleeding). May cause serious infections. ▪ May increase risk of lymphoproliferative disease and some other malignancies. ▪ Risk of skin cancer may be increased. Reduce exposure to sunlight and UV light. Wear protective clothing and use a sunscreen with a high protection factor. ▪ Although most vaccinations may be less effective, the manufacturer suggests that flu vaccinations may be of value. ▪ Cooperation with repeated laboratory tests imperative. ▪ Review medications with the physician responsible for mycophenolate therapy. ▪ See Appendix D, p. 1333.

Maternal/Child: Category D: avoid pregnancy. Increased risk of first-trimester pregnancy loss and increased risk of congenital malformations, especially external ear and other facial abnormalities (including cleft lip and palate) and anomalies of the distal limbs, heart, esophagus, kidney, and nervous system. See manufacturer's literature for details. A negative serum or urine pregnancy test with a sensitivity of at least 25 mIU/mL immediately before beginning therapy is indicated in all women of childbearing age. Repeat testing required. Contraception required before, during, and after use. See Patient Education. Use during pregnancy only if benefit justifies risk; should pregnancy occur during treatment, discuss the desirability of continuing the pregnancy. Women using mycophenolate at any time during pregnancy are encouraged to enroll in the National Transplantation Pregnancy Registry. Patients considering pregnancy should discuss with their physician appropriate alternative immunosuppressants with less potential for embryo-fetal toxicity. ▪ Discontinue breast-feeding. ▪ Safety and effectiveness for use in pediatric patients not established; see Indications.

Elderly: No specific recommendations. Consider age-related decreased organ function and/or additional medical problems and medications. May be at increased risk for certain adverse reactions (e.g., certain infections [including CMV tissue invasive disease] and possibly GI hemorrhage and pulmonary edema). Observe carefully.

DRUG/LAB INTERACTIONS

Because oversuppression of the immune system can increase the risk of infection, combination immunosuppressant therapy should be used with caution. ▪ **Cyclosporine** (Sandimmune) may decrease serum levels of MPA (mycophenolate). Monitor levels closely when cyclosporine is added or removed from a drug regimen containing mycophenolate. ▪ Has been administered in combination with **antithymocyte globulin** (ATGAM), **cyclosporine, corticosteroids, and muromonab-CD3** (Orthoclone). Safety for use with other agents has not been determined. ▪ Manufacturer recommends not administering concomitantly with **azathioprine.** Both agents may cause bone marrow suppression and concomitant administration has not been studied. ▪ Use caution with **drugs that interfere with enterohepatic recirculation or alter the intestinal flora** (e.g., cholestyramine [Questran]). ▪ In impaired renal function, **acyclovir** (Zovirax) **and/or ganciclovir** (Cytovene) and mycophenolate may compete for tubular secretion, further increasing the serum levels of each drug; monitor patients closely. ▪ Coadministration with **probenecid** results in an increase in the AUC of MPAG and MPA. **Other agents that undergo renal tubular secretion** (e.g., acyclovir, ganciclovir) may also result in increased serum levels of mycophenolate. ▪ MPA may slightly decrease protein binding of **phenytoin** (Dilantin) **and theophylline,** increasing the free fraction of these drugs; clinical significance unknown. ▪ **Oral contraceptives and other hormonal contraceptives** (e.g., transdermal patch, vaginal ring, injection, and implant) may be less effective; use additional barrier contraceptive measures. ▪ Not recommended for concurrent administration with a combination of **metronidazole** (Flagyl) **and norfloxacin** (Noroxin); may decrease mycophenolate levels. Interaction not observed when mycophenolate is administered with either antibiotic separately. ▪ Not recommended for concurrent use with **rifampin** (Rifadin); may decrease mycophenolate levels. ▪ Coadministration with **ciprofloxacin** (Cipro) or **amoxicillin/ clavulanic acid** (Augmentin) may cause a reduction in median MPA trough concentrations. Clinical significance unknown. ▪ Concomitant administration of telmisartan (Micardis) and mycophenolate results in a decrease in MPA concentration. ▪ Do not use **live virus vaccines** in patients receiving mycophenolate; vaccinations may be less effective. See Patient Education.

SIDE EFFECTS

Diarrhea, infection, leukopenia, phlebitis, thrombosis, and vomiting occur most frequently. Other reactions that occurred in at least 20% of patients during clinical trials included abdominal pain, anorexia, anxiety, ascites, asthenia, back pain, bone marrow suppression (e.g., anemia, hypochromic anemia, leukocytosis, leukopenia, neutropenia, thrombocytopenia), chest pain, constipation, cough, creatinine and BUN increase, dizziness, dyspepsia, dyspnea, edema, fever, GI hemorrhage, headache, hypercholesterolemia, hyperglycemia, hyperkalemia, hypertension, hypocalcemia, hypokalemia, hypomagnesemia, hypotension, infection, insomnia, lactic dehydrogenase increase, LFT abnormalities, nausea, pain, paresthesia, peripheral edema, pleural effusion, progressive multifocal leukoencephalopathy, rash, renal function abnormalities, sepsis, severe neutropenia, sinusitis, tachycardia, tremor, and UTI. In renal transplant patients, those receiving 2 Gm/day demonstrated an overall better safety profile than those receiving 3 Gm/day.

Post-Marketing: Colitis, embryo-fetal toxicity, hypogammaglobulinemia, increased incidence of first-trimester pregnancy loss, infections (e.g., atypical mycobacterial infections; endocarditis; meningitis; polyomavirus-associated neuropathy [PVAN], especially due to BK virus; TB), interstitial lung disorders (including fatal pulmonary fibrosis), pancreatitis, pure red cell aplasia, viral reactivation in patients infected with HBV or HCV).

ANTIDOTE

Notify the physician of all side effects. Most can be treated symptomatically. Drug may be decreased or discontinued or other immunosuppressive agents utilized. Some side effects (e.g., neutropenia) may require temporary reduction of dosage or withholding of treatment. Consider reducing the amount of immunosuppression in patients who develop PML, taking into account the risk this may represent to the graft. At clinically encountered concentrations, MPA and MPAG are not usually removed by hemodialysis. However, at high concentrations (greater than 100 mcg/mL) small amounts of MPAG are removed. MPA may be removed by bile acid sequestrants such as cholestyramine (Questran).

NAFCILLIN SODIUM
(naf-**SILL**-in **SO**-dee-um)

Nallpen ✦

Antibacterial
(penicillinase-resistant penicillin)

pH 6 to 8.5

USUAL DOSE

500 mg to 1 Gm every 4 hours. Up to 12 Gm in 24 hours has been used in severe infections. Continue therapy for at least 48 hours after patient is afebrile and asymptomatic and cultures are negative. Usual duration of therapy is at least 14 days for severe staphylococcal infections and longer (4 to 6 weeks) for endocarditis and osteomyelitis.

Endocarditis, meningitis, osteomyelitis, or pericarditis: 1.5 to 2 Gm every 4 to 6 hours.

PEDIATRIC DOSE

Safety and effectiveness for use in pediatric patients not established. All pediatric doses are unlabeled; see Maternal/Child. Limited clinical experience with IV route in neonates and infants. Maximum dose is 12 Gm/24 hr.

Pediatric patients less than 40 kg and over 1 month of age: *Moderate infections:* 50 to 100 mg/kg/24 hr in equally divided doses every 6 hours (12.5 to 25 mg/kg every 6 hours). *Serious infections (e.g., osteomyelitis, pericarditis, endocarditis):* 100 to 200 mg/kg/24 hr in equally divided doses every 4 to 6 hours (16.6 to 33.3 mg/kg every 4 hours or 25 to 50 mg/kg every 6 hours).

NEONATAL DOSE

Safety and effectiveness for use in neonates not established. All pediatric doses are unlabeled; see Maternal/Child. Limited clinical experience with IV route in neonates and infants.

10 to 20 mg/kg every 8 to 12 hours, or 25 mg/kg with the interval adjusted based on age and weight as follows:

0 to 7 days of age and under 2,000 Gm: Every 12 hours.
Over 7 days of age and under 1,200 Gm: Every 12 hours.
Over 7 days of age and 1,200 to 2,000 Gm: Every 8 hours.
0 to 7 days of age and over 2,000 Gm: Every 8 hours.
Over 7 days of age and over 2,000 Gm: Every 6 hours.

Increase dose to 50 mg/kg every 6, 8, or 12 hours in meningitis.

DOSE ADJUSTMENTS

Dose adjustment not required for patients with renal dysfunction, including those receiving hemodialysis. ■ Measure nafcillin serum levels and adjust dose accordingly in patients with hepatic insufficiency and renal failure.

DILUTION

Each 500-mg vial is diluted with 1.7 mL of SWFI (1-Gm vial with 3.4 mL, 2-Gm vial with 6.8 mL). Each 1 mL equals 250 mg. Further dilute each dose with a minimum of 15 to 30 mL of SWFI, NS, or ½NS, or other **compatible** IV solutions (see chart on inside back cover or literature). Concentration should be 2 to 40 mg/mL. Available prediluted and in ADD-Vantage vials for use with ADD-Vantage infusion containers. May be given through Y-tube, three-way stopcock, or with additive tubing, or may be added to larger volume of **compatible** solutions.

Filters: Not required by manufacturer. Premixed and frozen solutions are filtered during manufacturing.

Storage: Store unopened vials at CRT. Refrigerate unused medication after initial dilution and discard after 7 days. Stable in specific solutions at concentrations of 2 to 40 mg/mL for 24 hours at room temperature and 96 hours if refrigerated. Frozen, premixed solutions should be stored at $-20°$ C ($-4°$ F). Thaw at room temperature or under refrigeration. Thawed solutions are stable for 72 hours at RT or 21 days refrigerated. Do not refreeze.

COMPATIBILITY   (Underline Indicates Conflicting Compatibility Information)

Consider any drug NOT listed as compatible to be INCOMPATIBLE until consulting a pharmacist; specific conditions may apply.

Inactivated in solution with aminoglycosides (e.g., amikacin, gentamicin). Do not mix in the same solution. Appropriate spacing and/or separate sites required. See Drug/Lab Interactions.

One source suggests the following **compatibilities:**

Additive: Aminophylline, chloramphenicol (Chloromycetin), chlorothiazide (Diuril), dexamethasone (Decadron), dextran 40, diphenhydramine (Benadryl), ephedrine sulfate, heparin, lidocaine, potassium chloride (KCl), prochlorperazine (Compazine), sodium bicarbonate, sodium lactate, verapamil.

Y-site: Acyclovir (Zovirax), atropine, cyclophosphamide (Cytoxan), diazepam (Valium), diltiazem (Cardizem), enalaprilat (Vasotec IV), esmolol (Brevibloc), famotidine (Pepcid IV), fentanyl, fluconazole (Diflucan), foscarnet (Foscavir), heparin, hydromorphone (Dilaudid), magnesium sulfate, morphine, nicardipine (Cardene IV), propofol (Diprivan), theophylline, vancomycin, zidovudine (AZT, Retrovir).

RATE OF ADMINISTRATION

IV injection: Each 500 mg or fraction thereof properly diluted over 5 to 10 minutes.

Intermittent IV: Administration over 30 to 60 minutes may decrease incidence of thrombophlebitis.

Infusion: When diluted in large volumes of infusion fluids, give at rate prescribed.

ACTIONS

A semi-synthetic penicillinase-resistant penicillin, used for its bactericidal activity against gram-positive organisms, primarily penicillinase-producing staphylococci. Mode of action involves inhibition of bacterial cell wall biosynthesis. Highly resistant to inactivation by staphylococcal penicillinase. Readily distributes into most body fluids and tissues except spinal fluid. Binds to serum proteins, primarily albumin. Mainly eliminated by hepatic inactivation and excretion in bile; a small amount is excreted in urine. Half-life is 30 to 60 minutes. Crosses the placental barrier. Secreted in breast milk.

INDICATIONS AND USES

Treatment of infections caused by penicillinase-producing staphylococci.

CONTRAINDICATIONS

Known hypersensitivity to any penicillin or cephalosporin (not absolute); see Precautions. Prediluted solutions containing dextrose may be contraindicated with known allergies to corn products.

PRECAUTIONS

Sensitivity studies necessary to determine susceptibility of the causative organism to nafcillin. Nafcillin should not be used in infections caused by an organism susceptible to penicillin G or due to an organism other than a resistant staphylococcus. Modify antimicrobial treatment as indicated by C/S. ■ To reduce the development of drug-resistant bacteria and maintain its effectiveness, nafcillin should be used to treat or prevent only those infections proven or strongly suspected to be caused by bacteria. ▪ Use with caution in patients with both impaired hepatic and renal function; elevated serum concentrations may cause neurotoxic reactions. See Dose Adjustments. ▪ Hypersensitivity reactions, including fatalities, have been reported in patients receiving beta-lactam antibacterial drugs; most likely to occur in patients with a history of penicillin hypersensitivity or sensitivity to multiple allergens. There have been reports of individuals with a history of penicillin hypersensitivity experiencing severe reactions when treated with cephalosporins. Check history of previous hypersensitivity reactions to penicillins, cephalosporins, or other allergens. Actual incidence of cross-allergenicity not established but may be more common with first-generation cephalosporins. ▪ Avoid prolonged use of the drug; superinfection caused by overgrowth of nonsusceptible organisms may result. ▪ *Clostridium difficile*–associated diarrhea (CDAD) has been reported. May range from mild diarrhea to fatal colitis. Consider in patients who present with diarrhea during or after treatment with nafcillin. ▪ Manufacturer's premixed solutions contain dextrose; may be contraindicated in patients with an allergy to corn or corn products.

Monitor: Obtain baseline CBC with differential and monitor during treatment. Monitor urinalysis, SCr, BUN, ALT, and AST periodically, especially with prolonged treatment. ▪ Watch for early symptoms of a hypersensitivity reaction, especially in individuals with a history of allergic problems. ▪ May cause thrombophlebitis, especially in the elderly or with too-rapid injection. Limit IV treatment to 24 to 48 hours when possible. Change to oral therapy as soon as practical. ▪ Electrolyte imbalance and cardiac irregularities from sodium content are possible. Contains up to 3.3 mEq sodium/Gm. May aggravate CHF. Observe for hypokalemia. ▪ See Drug/Lab Interactions.

Patient Education: May require alternate birth control. ▪ Promptly report diarrhea or bloody stools that occur during treatment or up to several months after an antibiotic has been discontinued; may indicate CDAD and require treatment.

Maternal/Child: Category B: use only if clearly needed. ▪ Safety and effectiveness for use in pediatric patients not established, but it is used; see Pediatric Dose. ▪ May cause diarrhea, candidiasis, or allergic response in nursing infants. ▪ Elimination rate markedly reduced in neonates and infants due to immature hepatic and renal function.

Elderly: Response similar to that seen in younger adults. Consider age-related organ impairment and concomitant disease or drug therapy. ▪ May be at increased risk for thrombophlebitis. ▪ See Precautions/Monitor and Dose Adjustments.

DRUG/LAB INTERACTIONS

May be antagonized by **bacteriostatic antibiotics** (e.g., chloramphenicol, erythromycin, tetracyclines); may interfere with bactericidal action. ▪ Potentiated by **probenecid**; toxicity may result. ▪ Synergistic when used in combination with **aminoglycosides** (e.g., amikacin, gentamicin). Synergism may be inconsistent; see Compatibility. ▪ Concomitant use with **beta-adrenergic blockers** (e.g., propranolol) may interfere with the treatment of a hypersensitivity reaction to nafcillin. ▪ Risk of bleeding with **anticoagulants** (e.g., heparin) is increased. ▪ May decrease serum levels and effectiveness of **cyclosporine** (Sandimmune). ▪ Inhibits effectiveness of **oral contraceptives;** breakthrough bleeding or pregnancy could result. ▪ High doses (9 to 12 Gm daily) may decrease serum half-life of **warfarin** (Coumadin); monitor PT up to 30 days after nafcillin completed. ▪ May reduce effectiveness of **nifedipine** (Procardia XL) by reducing its serum plasma levels. ▪ May cause **false values in common lab tests**; see literature.

SIDE EFFECTS

Bleeding abnormalities, bone marrow suppression (e.g., agranulocytosis, neutropenia), diarrhea, hypersensitivity reactions (e.g., anaphylaxis, bronchospasm, pruritus, rash, serum sickness–like symptoms, urticaria [may be immediate or delayed]), interstitial nephritis, local reactions (e.g., pain, phlebitis, thrombophlebitis, and occasionally skin sloughing with extravasation), nausea and vomiting, and renal tubular damage have been reported. CDAD and hypersensitivity myocarditis (fever, eosinophilia, rash, sinus tachycardia, ST-T changes, and cardiomegaly) can occur. Higher-than-normal doses may cause neurologic adverse reactions, including convulsions, especially with concomitant impaired hepatic insufficiency and renal dysfunction.

ANTIDOTE

Notify physician immediately of any adverse symptoms. For severe symptoms discontinue the drug, treat hypersensitivity reaction (antihistamines, epinephrine, corticosteroids), and resuscitate as necessary. Hemodialysis or peritoneal dialysis is minimally effective in overdose. Treat CDAD with fluids, electrolytes, protein supplements, and oral vancomycin (Vancocin) or metronidazole (Flagyl) as indicated. In severe cases, surgical evaluation may be indicated. Mild cases may respond to drug discontinuation alone.

NALBUPHINE HYDROCHLORIDE
(**NAL**-byoo-feen hy-droh-**KLOR**-eyed)

Narcotic analgesic
(agonist-antagonist)
Anesthesia adjunct

pH 3.5 to 3.7

USUAL DOSE

Pain control: 10 mg/70 kg. May repeat every 3 to 6 hours. In nontolerant patients, the recommended single maximum dose is 20 mg. Maximum total daily dose is 160 mg. Adjust dose and interval according to severity of pain, physical status of patient, and other medications administered concomitantly; see Dose Adjustments.

Adjunct to balanced anesthesia: A loading dose of 300 mcg (0.3 mg) to 3 mg/kg over 10 to 15 minutes. Maintain desired level of balanced anesthesia with 250 to 500 mcg/kg (0.25 to 0.5 mg/kg) as required. Administered only under the direction of the anesthesiologist.

DOSE ADJUSTMENTS

In patients dependent on opioids, initiate a dose of nalbuphine at one fourth the usual dose if their previous medication was a narcotic. Observe for symptoms of withdrawal. Increase to effective dose gradually. ▪ Reduced dose may be required in the elderly or debilitated, in impaired liver or renal function, in patients with limited pulmonary reserve, and in the presence of other CNS depressants. ▪ See Drug/Lab Interactions.

DILUTION

May be given undiluted.

Filters: No data available from manufacturer.

Storage: Store at CRT. Avoid freezing and/or prolonged exposure to light.

COMPATIBILITY

Consider any drug NOT listed as compatible to be INCOMPATIBLE until consulting a pharmacist; specific conditions may apply.

Manufacturer lists as **incompatible** with nafcillin (Nallpen) and ketorolac (Toradol).

One source suggests the following **compatibilities:**

Solution: D5NS, D10W, LR, NS.

Y-site: Acetaminophen (Ofirmev), acyclovir (Zovirax), amifostine (Ethyol), aztreonam (Azactam), bivalirudin (Angiomax), cisatracurium (Nimbex), cladribine (Leustatin), dexmedetomidine (Precedex), etoposide phosphate (Etopophos), fenoldopam (Corlopam), filgrastim (Neupogen), fludarabine (Fludara), gemcitabine (Gemzar), granisetron (Kytril), hetastarch in electrolytes (Hextend), linezolid (Zyvox), melphalan (Alkeran), oxaliplatin (Eloxatin), paclitaxel (Taxol), propofol (Diprivan), remifentanil (Ultiva), teniposide (Vumon), thiotepa, vinorelbine (Navelbine).

RATE OF ADMINISTRATION

Pain control: Each 10 mg or fraction thereof over 3 to 5 minutes. Frequently titrated according to symptom relief and respiratory rate.

Anesthesia adjunct: See Usual Dose.

ACTIONS

A synthetic narcotic agonist-antagonist analgesic. Binds to kappa, mu, and delta receptors. Acts as an agonist at kappa receptors and as a partial antagonist at mu receptors. It equals morphine in analgesic effect. Does produce respiratory depression, but this does not increase markedly with increased doses. Onset of pain relief occurs within 2 to 3 minutes and lasts about 3 to 6 hours. Metabolized in the liver. Some excretion in urine. Crosses the placental barrier. Secreted in breast milk.

INDICATIONS AND USES

Relief of moderate to severe pain. ▪ Preoperative and postoperative analgesia. ▪ Surgical anesthesia supplement. ▪ Obstetric analgesia during labor and delivery.

Unlabeled uses: 10 mg SC to reduce pruritus from epidural morphine.

CONTRAINDICATIONS

Hypersensitivity to nalbuphine or its components.

PRECAUTIONS

May precipitate withdrawal symptoms if stopped too quickly after prolonged use or if patient has been on opiates. ▪ Use caution in patients with impaired respiration (e.g., from other medications, uremia, asthma, severe infection, cyanosis, or respiratory obstruction); see Dose Adjustments. ▪ Use caution in patients with myocardial infarction who have nausea and vomiting or compromised cardiac function; effect on heart not fully evaluated. ▪ Use caution in ambulatory patients; see Patient Education. ▪ Use caution in patients with head injuries, intracranial lesions, or pre-existing increases in intracranial pressure. Nalbuphine may elevate CSF pressure and may produce effects that can obscure the clinical course of patients with head injuries (e.g., pupillary changes, sedation). ▪ Use caution in patients with a history of drug abuse or emotional instability; close monitoring is required. ▪ Use caution in the elderly and debilitated and in patients with renal or hepatic impairment; see Dose Adjustments. ▪ Use caution in patients about to undergo surgery of the biliary tract. Can cause spasm of the sphincter of Oddi. ▪ Administration during labor has caused severe fetal bradycardia; naloxone may reverse effects; see Maternal/Child. ▪ Should be administered as a supplement to general anesthesia only by persons specifically trained in the use of IV anesthetics and in the management of the respiratory effects of potent opioids. ▪ When used with anesthesia, a high incidence of bradycardia has been reported in patients who did not receive atropine preoperatively.

Monitor: Naloxone, oxygen, and controlled respiratory equipment must be available. ▪ Observe frequently; monitor vital signs. ▪ Keep patient supine to minimize side effects; orthostatic hypotension and fainting may occur. Observe closely during ambulation. ▪ Pain control usually more effective with routinely administered doses. Determine appropriate interval through clinical assessment ▪ See Drug/Lab Interactions.

Patient Education: Avoid use of alcohol or other CNS depressants (e.g., antihistamines, diazepam [Valium]). ▪ Request assistance for ambulation. ▪ Use caution performing any task that requires alertness; may cause dizziness, euphoria, and sedation. ▪ May be habit forming. Can cause withdrawal if stopped too quickly after prolonged use or if other opioids are used.

Maternal/Child: Category B: use during pregnancy (other than labor and delivery) only if benefits justify risks. Take appropriate measures (e.g., fetal monitoring) to detect and manage potential adverse effects to the fetus. ▪ Safety for use during breast-feeding not established. ▪ Fetal and neonatal bradycardia, respiratory depression at birth, apnea, cyanosis, and hypotonia have been reported. Maternal or neonatal administration of naloxone may reverse these effects. Fetal death has been reported when mothers received nalbuphine during labor and delivery. Use during labor and delivery only if clearly indicated and if benefit outweighs risk. Newborns should be monitored for respiratory depression, apnea, bradycardia, and arrhythmias if nalbuphine has been used. ▪ Not recommended for pediatric patients under 18 years of age.

Elderly: May be more sensitive to effects (e.g., respiratory depression, constipation, dizziness, urinary retention). ▪ Analgesia should be effective with lower doses. ▪ Consider age-related organ impairment.

DRUG/LAB INTERACTIONS

Potentiated by **cimetidine** (Tagamet), **phenothiazines** (e.g., chlorpromazine [Thorazine]), by **other CNS depressants** such as narcotic analgesics, general anesthetics, alcohol, anticholinergics, antihistamines, barbiturates, hypnotics, neuromuscular blocking agents (e.g., atracurium [Tracrium]), psychotropic agents, and sedatives. Reduced doses of both drugs may be indicated. ▪ May decrease analgesic effects of **other narcotics;** avoid concurrent use. ▪ Plasma **amylase and lipase** determinations may be unreliable for 24 hours following narcotic administration. ▪ Depending on the test used, nalbuphine may interfere with enzymatic methods for the detection of **opiates.** Consult test manufacturer's literature.

SIDE EFFECTS

Abdominal pain, agitation, anaphylaxis, anxiety, blurred vision, bradycardia, clammy skin, dizziness, dry mouth, fever, headache, hypertension, hypotension, injection site reaction, nausea, psychotomimetic effect (symptoms resembling a psychosis), pulmonary edema, respiratory depression, sedation, seizures, symptoms associated with histamine release, tachycardia, tremor, urinary urgency, vertigo, vomiting.

ANTIDOTE

With increasing severity of any side effect or onset of symptoms of overdose, discontinue the drug and notify the physician. Naloxone hydrochloride will reverse severe reactions. A patent airway, artificial ventilation, oxygen therapy, and other symptomatic treatment (e.g., fluids, vasopressors) must be instituted promptly.

N-O

NALOXONE HYDROCHLORIDE
(nal-**OX**-ohn hy-droh-**KLOR**-eyed)

Antidote
Narcotic antagonist

pH 3 to 4

USUAL DOSE

Narcotic overdose: 0.4 to 2 mg. Repeat in 2 to 3 minutes if indicated. The diagnosis of narcotic overdose should be questioned if no response is observed after 10 mg of naloxone. If effective, dosage may be repeated as necessary for recurrence of symptoms.

Postoperative narcotic depression: 0.1 to 0.2 mg at 2- to 3-minute intervals to desired response. Titrate to avoid excessive reduction of narcotic analgesic action.

Challenge test for suspected opioid dependence: 0.2 mg. Observe for 30 seconds for S/S of withdrawal (e.g., abdominal cramps, diaphoresis, dysphoria, nausea and vomiting, rhinorrhea). If no evidence of withdrawal, inject 0.6 mg of naloxone and observe for an additional 20 minutes. Monitor VS and observe patient again for S/S of opiate withdrawal.

PEDIATRIC DOSE

Ampules containing 0.02 mg/mL are available, but larger doses are frequently required. Adult strength is often used to reduce amount of injection and to effect desired response, which may require increased or repeat doses. One source states, "Up to 10 times a dose has been required."

Narcotic overdose: *Less than 20 kg:* 0.01 to 0.1 mg/kg of body weight initially. Based on estimated degree of overdose and respiratory depression. May repeat every 2 to 3 minutes. May dilute with SWFI. American Academy of Pediatrics recommends 0.1 mg/kg. Manufacturer recommends 0.01 mg/kg.

Over 20 kg or over 5 years of age: 2 mg. Repeat every 2 to 3 minutes as needed. A continuous infusion may be used after initial effective dose. Add 75% to 100% of effective dose to a specific amount of IV fluid and infuse evenly distributed over 1 hour. For some overdoses (e.g., methadone), weaning in 50% increments may take up to 48 hours. For others, 6 to 12 hours is adequate. If symptoms recur, rebolus and go back to 100%.

Postoperative narcotic depression: 0.005 to 0.01 mg IV at 2- to 3-minute intervals to desired response.

NEONATAL DOSE

Neonatal opiate depression: Administration into umbilical vein is preferred. 0.01 to 0.1 mg/kg of body weight initially. Based on estimated degree of overdose and respiratory depression. May repeat every 2 to 3 minutes to achieve a satisfactory response. May dilute with SWFI. American Academy of Pediatrics recommends 0.1 mg/kg repeated every 2 to 3 minutes. Manufacturer recommends 0.01 mg/kg repeated every 2 to 3 minutes. Another source suggests an initial dose of 0.01 mg/kg. If response is not satisfactory, increase subsequent doses to 0.1 mg/kg.

DILUTION

May be given undiluted, diluted with SWFI, or further diluted in NS or D5W and given as an infusion (2 mg in 500 mL equals a concentration of 0.004 mg/mL). Discard infusions after 24 hours.

Storage: Store below 40° C. Protect from light.

COMPATIBILITY

Consider any drug NOT listed as compatible to be INCOMPATIBLE until consulting a pharmacist; specific conditions may apply.

Manufacturer lists as **incompatible** with bisulfites, sulfites, long-chain or high-molecular-weight anions, solutions with an alkaline pH.

One source suggests the following **compatibilities:**

Additive: Verapamil.

Y-site: Fenoldopam (Corlopam), linezolid (Zyvox), propofol (Diprivan).

RATE OF ADMINISTRATION
Each 0.4 mg or fraction thereof over 15 seconds. Titrate infusion to patient response.

ACTIONS
A potent narcotic antagonist. Overcomes effects of narcotic overdose including respiratory depression, sedation, and hypotension. Unlike other narcotic antagonists, it does not have any narcotic effect itself. Onset of action is within 2 minutes. Duration of action is dependent on dose and route of naloxone administration. Requirement for repeat doses is dependent on amount, type, and route of narcotic administration. Metabolized in the liver and excreted in urine.

INDICATIONS AND USES
Reversal of narcotic depression. ▪ Antidote for natural (e.g., morphine) and synthetic narcotics (e.g., butorphanol, methadone, nalbuphine, and pentazocine). ▪ Diagnosis of suspected opioid tolerance or acute opiate overdose.

Unlabeled uses: Reversal of alcoholic coma and improvement of circulation in refractory shock.

CONTRAINDICATIONS
Known hypersensitivity to naloxone. ▪ The naloxone challenge test should not be performed in patients showing S/S of withdrawal or whose urine contains opioids.

PRECAUTIONS
Does not produce respiratory depression with nonnarcotic drug overdose, a beneficial action. ▪ It is ineffective against respiratory depression caused by barbiturates, anesthetics, other nonnarcotic agents, or pathologic conditions. ▪ Will precipitate acute withdrawal symptoms in narcotic addicts; use caution, especially in newborns of narcotic-dependent mothers. ▪ Use caution in cardiac disease patients or those receiving cardiotoxic drugs.

Monitor: Symptomatic treatment with oxygen and artificial ventilation as necessary should be continued until naloxone is effective. Observe patient continuously. Duration of narcotic action may exceed that of naloxone.

Maternal/Child: Category B: use in pregnancy and breast-feeding only when clearly needed. Safety for use not established. ▪ See Precautions.

DRUG/LAB INTERACTIONS
Specific information not available.

SIDE EFFECTS
Hypertension, irritability and increased crying in the newborn, nausea and vomiting, sweating, tachycardia, tremulousness. Overdose postoperatively may result in excitement, hypertension, hypotension, pulmonary edema, reversal of analgesia, ventricular tachycardia and fibrillation.

ANTIDOTE
Notify the physician of any side effect. Treatment will probably be symptomatic. Resuscitate as necessary.

N-O

NATALIZUMAB BBW

(nah-tah-**LIZZ**-u-mab)

Tysabri

Monoclonal antibody
Immunomodulator

pH 6.1

USUAL DOSE

Multiple sclerosis (MS): 300 mg as an infusion every 4 weeks.

Crohn's disease (CD): 300 mg as an infusion every 4 weeks. Discontinue if no benefit is seen after 12 weeks of therapy. For patients with CD who initiate natalizumab therapy while on chronic corticosteroids, begin steroid tapering as soon as therapeutic benefit of natalizumab has occurred. Discontinue natalizumab if the patient cannot be tapered off steroids within 6 months. Consider discontinuing therapy in patients who require more than 3 months of steroid use (excluding the original 6-month taper) in a calendar year to control their CD. Aminosalicylates may be continued during therapy with natalizumab.

DOSE ADJUSTMENTS

None indicated. Pharmacokinetics has not been studied in patients with renal or hepatic insufficiency.

DILUTION

Available in 300 mg/15 mL single-use vials. Withdraw 15 mL of concentrate (300 mg) from the vial and inject into 100 mL of NS. Gently invert to mix completely. Do not shake. No other IV diluents may be used to prepare the solution. Solution is a colorless, clear to slightly opalescent concentrate. Do not use if particulates are present or if solution is discolored.

Filters: Use of filtration devices during administration not evaluated.

Storage: Refrigerate vials at 2° to 8° C (36° to 46° F). Do not use beyond the expiration date on the vial. Do not shake or freeze. Protect from light. Following dilution, solution should be infused immediately. However, it may be refrigerated and used within 8 hours of preparation. If refrigerated, allow to warm to room temperature before infusion.

COMPATIBILITY

Manufacturer states, "Other medications should not be injected into infusion set side ports or mixed with natalizumab." Flush line with NS before and after infusion.

RATE OF ADMINISTRATION

Do not administer as an IV push or bolus injection. Infuse over approximately 1 hour. Flush line with NS before and after infusion.

ACTIONS

A recombinant humanized IgG4κ monoclonal antibody produced in murine myeloma cells. An integrin receptor antagonist. Natalizumab is thought to bind to a subunit on the surface of all leukocytes except neutrophils and inhibit the adhesion of leukocytes to their counterreceptors. The receptors for the α4 family of integrins include vascular cell adhesion molecule-1 (VCAM-1), which is expressed on activated vascular endothelium, and mucosal addressin cell adhesion molecule-1 (MAdCAM-1), which is present on vascular endothelial cells of the GI tract. Disruption of these molecular interactions prevents transmigration of leukocytes across the endothelium into inflamed parenchymal tissue. Specific mechanisms of how natalizumab exerts its effects in MS and CD have not been fully defined. In multiple sclerosis (MS), lesions are believed to occur when activated inflammatory cells, including T-lymphocytes, cross the blood-brain barrier (BBB). Leukocyte migration across the BBB involves the interaction between adhesion molecules on inflammatory cells and their counterreceptors on the endothelial cells of the vessel wall. The clinical effect of natalizumab in MS may be secondary to blockade of the molecular interaction of α4β1 integrins expressed by inflammatory cells with VCAM-1 on vascular endothelial cells and with CS-1 and/or osteopontin expressed by parenchymal cells in the brain. In clinical trials, natalizumab reduced the rate of clinical relapse and the appearance of new or newly enlarging T2 hyperintense lesions on MRI studies. The number of gadolinium-enhancing lesions on the 1-year MRI scan follow-up was also reduced. In Crohn's disease (CD), the $\alpha 4\beta 7$ integrin with the endothelial receptor MAd-CAM-1 expression has been found to be increased at active sites of inflammation in the mucosa and to contribute to the inflammatory response characteristic of CD. It is mainly expressed on gut endothelial cells. The action of natalizumab may be secondary to block-ade of molecular interaction of the $\alpha 4\beta 7$-integrin receptor with MAdCAM-1 expressed on the venular endothelium at inflammatory foci. Distribution is limited primarily to vascular space (plasma volume). Half-life is 3 to 17 days.

INDICATIONS AND USES

Monotherapy for the treatment of patients with relapsing forms of multiple sclerosis (MS). ▪ Induction and maintenance of clinical response and remission in adults with moderately to severely active Crohn's disease with evidence of inflammation who have had an inadequate response to or are unable to tolerate conventional therapy and inhibi-tors of TNFα (e.g., infliximab [Remicade]). Should not be used in combination with immunosuppressants (e.g., 6-mercaptopurine, azathioprine, cyclosporine [Sandimmune], or methotrexate) or inhibitors of TNFα; see Precautions.

CONTRAINDICATIONS

Hypersensitivity to natalizumab or any of its components, patients who have or have had progressive multifocal leukoencephalopathy (PML).

PRECAUTIONS

Natalizumab increases the risk of progressive multifocal leukoencephalopathy (PML), a rare opportunis-tic viral infection of the brain caused by the JC virus (JCV) that usually leads to death or severe dis-ability. PML typically occurs only in patients who are immunocompromised. Risk factors for the develop-ment of PML include duration of therapy (especially beyond 2 years), prior use of immunosuppressants (e.g., azathioprine, cyclophosphamide [Cytoxan], methotrexate, mitoxantrone [Novantrone], or myco-phenolate [CellCept]), and the presence of anti-JVC antibodies. Patients who are anti–JCV anti-body positive have a higher risk of developing PML. These factors should be considered in the context of expected benefits when initiating and continuing treatment with natalizumab. ▪ There are no known interventions that can reliably prevent PML or adequately treat PML if it oc-curs. Because of the risk of PML, natalizumab is available only through a special restricted distribution program called the TOUCH™ Prescribing Program. See prescribing information, or contact the manu-facturer for specific details and requirements. ▪ Anti-JCV testing should not be used to diag-nose PML. Testing positive for anti-JCV antibodies means that a person has been ex-posed to JCV in the past. Consider testing patients before treatment or during treatment if antibody status is unknown. Patients who test negative for anti-JCV antibodies are still at risk for the development of PML because of the potential for a new JCV infection or a false-negative test result. Periodic retesting of antibody status should be considered in patients previously determined to be anti–JCV antibody negative. Anti–JCV testing should not be performed for at least 2 weeks after plasma exchange due to the removal of antibodies from the serum. ▪ PML has been reported after discontinuation of natali-zumab in patients who did not have findings suggestive of PML at the time of discon-tinuation. ▪ Patients who develop PML and have discontinued natalizumab have devel-oped immune reconstitution inflammatory syndrome (IRIS). In most cases IRIS occurred after plasma exchange was used to eliminate circulating natalizumab. This syndrome has not been seen in patients discontinuing treatment for reasons unrelated to PML. ▪ Has been associated with hypersensitivity reactions, including anaphylaxis. Reactions usually occur within 2 hours of the start of the infusion. Generally associated with antibodies to natalizumab. ▪ Anti-natalizumab antibodies have been detected in some patients. Persis-tently positive antibodies were associated with a substantial decrease in effectiveness and an increase in infusion-related reactions. Approximately 82% of patients who became persistently antibody-positive developed detectable antibodies by 12 weeks. Patients who receive therapeutic monoclonal antibodies, including natalizumab, after an extended period without treatment may be at increased risk of hypersensitivity reactions with re-exposure. Consider testing for the presence of antibodies in patients who want to resume therapy after a dose interruption. ▪ Effects on immune system may increase the risk of infection, including opportunistic infection. ▪ Liver injury has been reported; it has occurred as early as 6 days after the first dose and after multiple doses. The combination of ALT, AST, and bilirubin elevations without evidence of obstruction is generally recognized as an important predictor of severe liver injury that may lead to death or the need for liver transplantation. ▪ Risk for developing encephalitis and meningitis caused by herpes simplex and varicella zoster viruses is increased. Serious, life-threatening, and sometimes fatal cases have been reported. ▪ No data available on secondary transmission of infections by live virus vaccines.

Monitor: Obtain baseline CBC and differential. Monitor periodically during treatment. ▪ Obtain a baseline MRI before initiating treatment and periodically throughout treatment. In MS patients it may be helpful in differentiating subsequent MS symptoms from PML and assessing disease progression. In CD patients it may be helpful in distinguishing pre-existing lesions from newly developed lesions. ▪ Consider determining anti-JCV antibody status before initiating natalizumab. Reassess status periodically; see Precautions. ▪ Observe patients during the infusion and for 1 hour after the infusion is complete. Discontinue infusion at the first sign of any hypersensitivity reaction (e.g., chest pain, dizziness, dyspnea, fever, flushing, hypotension, nausea, pruritus, rash, rigors, urticaria). ▪ Antibodies detected within the first 6 months of therapy may be transient and disappear. Repeat testing in 3 months. If antibodies are persistent, consider risk versus benefit of continued therapy; see Precautions. ▪ Monitor for S/S of infection. ▪ Monitor for signs of clinical relapse. ▪ Assess neurologic status frequently. S/S associated with PML are diverse and occur over days to weeks. May include progressive weakness on one side of the body, clumsiness of limbs, disturbances of vision, or changes in thinking, memory, and orientation leading to confusion and personality changes. Progression of deficits usually leads to severe disability or death over weeks to months. Withhold natalizumab if PML is suspected. ▪ Use of a gadolinium-enhanced MRI scan of the brain is recommended for diagnosis of PML and, when indicated, CSF analysis for JC viral DNA. If clinical suspicion of PML remains after initial evaluations are negative, continue to withhold natalizumab, and repeat evaluations. Continue to monitor for S/S suggestive of PML for approximately 6 months after discontinuation of natalizumab. ▪ Monitor for S/S of IRIS; may occur within days to weeks after plasma exchange. IRIS presents as a clinical decline in condition (may occur after clinical improvement); decline may be rapid and cause serious neurologic complications or death. Associated with characteristic changes in the MRI. ▪ Monitor for S/S of meningitis and encephalitis (e.g., confusion, fever, headache). ▪ Monitor for S/S of liver injury (e.g., elevated bilirubin or liver function tests, jaundice).

Patient Education: Read medication guide carefully. ▪ Review medical conditions and medications with health care provider. ▪ Promptly report any new medical problems (e.g., new or sudden change in thinking, eyesight, balance, or strength). ▪ Report infections. ▪ Promptly report S/S of hepatotoxicity (e.g., anorexia, dark urine, fatigue, jaundice, right upper abdominal discomfort), meningitis, or encephalitis (e.g., confusion, fever, headache). ▪ Immediately report any symptoms of infusion or hypersensitivity reactions (e.g., difficulty breathing, dizziness, feeling faint, itching, nausea). ▪ Discuss potential risks and benefits of treatment (e.g., risk of PML). ▪ Your physician may order a blood test to see if you have ever been exposed to JCV. Risk of PML is greatest if you have all three known risk factors; see Precautions. ▪ Scheduled follow-up visits are required as part of the TOUCH™ Program. ▪ PML has been reported following discontinuation of natalizumab. Monitor for S/S suggestive of PML for approximately 6 months after discontinuation of therapy.

Maternal/Child: Category C: use during pregnancy only if the potential benefit justifies the potential risk to the fetus. If a woman becomes pregnant while taking natalizumab, encourage enrollment in TYSARBI Pregnancy Exposure Registry. ▪ Has been detected in breast milk. Risk of this exposure to infant is unknown. ▪ Safety and effectiveness in pediatric patients with MS or CD under 18 years of age not established.

Elderly: Studies did not include sufficient numbers of patients 65 years of age and older to determine whether they respond differently than younger patients.

DRUG/LAB INTERACTIONS

Formal studies not completed. Concurrent use with **antineoplastic, immunosuppressant, or immunomodulating agents** may further increase the risk of infection, including PML and other opportunistic infections, over the risk observed with the use of natalizumab alone. Safety and efficacy of natalizumab in combination with any of these agents not established. ▪ Concurrent use of short courses of **corticosteroids** was associated with an increase in infections in clinical trials. However, the increase in infections in both the natalizumab-treated and placebo-treated patients who received steroids was similar. Corticosteroids should be tapered in patients with CD who are initiating natalizumab therapy; see Usual Dose. ▪ No data are available on the effects of **vaccination** in patients receiving natalizumab. ▪ Increases circulating **lymphocytes, monocytes, eosinophils, basophils, and nucleated red blood cells.** A return to baseline usually occurs within 16 weeks after the last dose. Elevations of **neutrophils** are not observed. ▪ May induce mild decreases in **hemoglobin,** frequently transient.

SIDE EFFECTS

The most commonly reported adverse reactions were abdominal discomfort, arthralgia, depression, diarrhea, fatigue, gastroenteritis, headache, infections (UTI, upper and lower respiratory tract), nausea, pain in extremities, rash, and vaginitis. The most commonly reported serious adverse reactions were infections, hypersensitivity reactions (including anaphylaxis), depression (including suicidal ideation), and cholelithiasis. The most commonly reported adverse reactions resulting in clinical intervention (i.e., discontinuation of natalizumab) were urticaria and other hypersensitivity reactions. Infusion-related reactions (defined as any adverse event occurring within 2 hours of the start of an infusion) included headache, dizziness, fatigue, hypersensitivity reactions, nausea, pruritus, rigors, urticaria, and vomiting. Other reported adverse reactions included abnormal liver function tests, amenorrhea, antibody formation, chest discomfort, dermatitis, irregular menstruation/dysmenorrhea, local bleeding, muscle cramps, night sweats, pruritus, somnolence, syncope, tonsillitis, tremor, urinary urgency and frequency, and vertigo. Adverse reactions reported in persistently antibody-positive patients included anxiety, dyspnea, hypertension, myalgia, and tachycardia.

Post-Marketing: Eosinophilia (resolved with discontinuation of therapy), herpes simplex virus encephalitis and meningitis, herpes zoster virus meningitis, PML in patients treated with natalizumab monotherapy.

ANTIDOTE

Keep physician informed of all side effects. Most will be treated symptomatically. Discontinue natalizumab at the first sign of liver injury, S/S of meningitis or encephalitis, S/S suggestive of PML, or with any change in neurologic status. Discontinue infusion if any S/S of a hypersensitivity or infusion reaction occur. Treat with epinephrine, corticosteroids, diphenhydramine, bronchodilators, and oxygen as indicated. Patients who experience a hypersensitivity reaction should not be retreated with natalizumab.

N-O

NECITUMUMAB BBW

(neh-**CIT**-ue-mew-mab)

Antineoplastic
(Monoclonal antibody,
epidermal growth factor
receptor [EGFR] inhibitor)

Portrazza

pH 6

USUAL DOSE

Premedication: For patients who have experienced a previous Grade 1 or 2 infusion-related reaction (IRR), premedicate with diphenhydramine (Benadryl) or equivalent before all subsequent necitumumab infusions. For patients who have experienced a second occurrence of Grade 1or 2 IRR, premedicate before all subsequent necitumumab infusions with diphenhydramine (or equivalent), acetaminophen (or equivalent), and dexamethasone (Decadron) (or equivalent).

Necitumumab: 800 mg as an IV infusion over 60 minutes on Days 1 and 8 of each 3-week cycle. Administer before gemcitabine (Gemzar) and cisplatin infusions. Continue until disease progression or unacceptable toxicity. Refer to gemcitabine and cisplatin monographs for premedication, hydration, dose recommendations, precautions, monitoring, and other requirements before administration.

DOSE ADJUSTMENTS

Reduce the infusion rate of necitumumab by 50% for a Grade 1 IRR. ▪ Stop the infusion for a Grade 2 IRR. When signs and symptoms have resolved to Grade 0 or 1, resume necitumumab at a 50% reduced rate for all subsequent infusions. ▪ Permanently discontinue necitumumab for a Grade 3 or 4 IRR. ▪ Withhold necitumumab for Grade 3 dermatologic toxicity (e.g., rash or acneiform rash) until symptoms resolve to Grade 2 or less, then resume necitumumab at a reduced dose of 400 mg for at least 1 treatment cycle. If symptoms do not worsen, dose may be increased to 600 mg and 800 mg in subsequent cycles. ▪ Permanently discontinue necitumumab for dermatologic toxicity if (1) the Grade 3 rash or acneiform rash does not resolve to Grade 2 or less within 6 weeks, (2) reactions worsen or become intolerable at a dose of 400 mg, (3) patient experiences a Grade 3 skin induration/fibrosis, or (4) patient experiences Grade 4 dermatologic toxicity. ▪ Withhold necitumumab for Grade 3 or 4 electrolyte abnormalities. Administer subsequent cycles once electrolyte abnormalities have improved to Grade 2 or less. ▪ No dose adjustment necessary based on body weight.

DILUTION

Available as a preservative-free solution in a single-dose vial containing 800 mg/50 mL (16 mg/mL). Solution should be clear. Discard if discolored or particulate matter is present. Withdraw the desired dose and further dilute to a final volume of 250 mL with NS. Do not use solutions containing dextrose. Gently invert the container to ensure adequate mixing. ***Do not freeze or shake.***

Filters: Specific information not available.

Storage: Before use, refrigerate at 2° to 8° C (36° to 46° F) in original carton to protect from light. ***Do not freeze or shake the vial.*** Diluted solution may be stored for no more than 24 hours if refrigerated or no more than 4 hours at RT. Discard any unused portion left in the vial.

COMPATIBILITY

Manufacturer states, "Do not dilute with solutions other than NS or co-infuse with other electrolytes or medication." Use of a separate line required.

RATE OF ADMINISTRATION

Administer as an infusion over 60 minutes using an infusion pump through a separate infusion line. Flush the line with NS at the end of the infusion. Reduce rate or discontinue infusion for IRR; see Dose Adjustments.

ACTIONS

A recombinant human IgG1 monoclonal antibody that specifically binds to the human epidermal growth factor receptor (EGFR) and blocks the binding of EGFR to its ligands. Expression and activation of EGFR has been correlated with malignant progression, induction of angiogenesis, and inhibition of apoptosis. Binding of necitumumab induces EGFR internalization and degradation in vitro and also leads to antibody-dependent cellular cytotoxicity in EGFR-expressing cells. Elimination half-life is approximately 14 days. The predicted time to reach steady state is approximately 100 days.

INDICATIONS AND USES

First-line treatment of patients with metastatic squamous non–small-cell lung cancer in combination with gemcitabine and cisplatin.

Limitation of use: Not indicated for treatment of nonsquamous non–small-cell lung cancer. These patients experienced more serious and fatal toxicities, including cardiopulmonary arrest/sudden death, within 30 days when administered necitumumab in combination with pemetrexed (Alimta) and cisplatin.

CONTRAINDICATIONS

Manufacturer states, "None."

PRECAUTIONS

Administered by or under the direction of a physician specialist in a facility with adequate diagnostic and treatment facilities to monitor the patient and respond to any medical emergency. ▪ Cardiopulmonary arrest and/or sudden death has been reported with necitumumab used in combination with gemcitabine and cisplatin. Some of these deaths occurred within 30 days of the last dose of necitumumab in patients with comorbid conditions, including a history of coronary artery disease, hypomagnesemia, COPD, and/or hypertension. ▪ Hypomagnesemia occurred in most patients receiving necitumumab in combination with gemcitabine and cisplatin and was severe in 20% of patients. The median time to development of hypomagnesemia and accompanying electrolyte abnormalities was 6 weeks after initiation of necitumumab. ▪ Venous and arterial thromboembolic events (VTEs and ATEs), some fatal, have been observed. The most common VTEs were pulmonary embolism and deep vein thrombosis. The most common ATEs were cerebral stroke and ischemia and myocardial infarction. Risk is higher in patients with a reported history of VTEs or ATEs. ▪ Dermatologic toxicities, some severe, have been reported. ▪ Infusion-related reactions have been reported. Most IRRs occurred after the first or second administration of necitumumab; see Premedication and Monitor. ▪ As with all therapeutic proteins, there is a potential for immunogenicity. ▪ Renal function and mild to moderate hepatic impairment have no influence on the exposure to necitumumab based on population pharmacokinetic analysis; however, no formal studies have been conducted. No patients with severe hepatic impairment were enrolled in clinical trials.

Monitor: Obtain serum electrolytes (including serum magnesium, potassium, and calcium), before each dose of necitumumab. Closely monitor for hypomagnesemia, hypocalcemia, and hypokalemia during treatment and for at least 8 weeks after the last dose is administered, with aggressive replacement when warranted during and after administration of necitumumab. ▪ Withhold necitumumab for Grade 3 or 4 electrolyte abnormalities. ▪ Monitor for S/S of venous and arterial thromboembolic events (e.g., chest pain, limb or abdominal swelling and/or pain, shortness of breath, loss of sensation or motor power, or altered consciousness, vision, or speech). ▪ Monitor for dermatologic toxicities (e.g., acne, dermatitis acneiform, dry skin, erythema, generalized rash, maculopapular rash, rash, skin fissures). Usually develops within the first 2 weeks of therapy and resolves within 17 weeks after onset; see Dose Adjustments and Antidote. ▪ Monitor for S/S of IRRs (e.g., chills, dyspnea, fever, hypotension, rash, tightness of the chest, urticaria, wheezing) during and after infusion; see Dose Adjustments and Antidote.

Patient Education: Blood levels of magnesium, potassium, and calcium may be decreased. Take medicines to replace these electrolytes exactly as advised by the physician. ▪ Risk of venous and arterial thromboembolic events is increased. Promptly report chest pain, limb or abdominal swelling and/or pain, shortness of breath, loss of sensation or motor power, or altered consciousness, vision, or speech. ▪ To reduce the risk of dermatologic reactions, minimize sun exposure with the use of protective clothing and sunscreen during treatment. ▪ Immediately report S/S of an infusion-related reaction (e.g., breathing problems, chills, fever, rash, tightness of the chest, urticaria, wheezing). ▪ There is a potential risk to a fetus and to postnatal development. Effective contraception is required in females of reproductive potential during treatment and for 3 months after the final dose. ▪ See Maternal/Child.

Maternal/Child: Based on its mechanism of action, necitumumab can cause fetal harm or developmental anomalies. Effective contraception required; see Patient Education. ▪ Discontinue breast-feeding during treatment and for 3 months after the final dose. ▪ Safety and effectiveness for use in pediatric patients not established.

Elderly: There was a higher incidence of venous thromboembolic events, including pulmonary embolism, in patients age 70 years and over compared with younger patients.

DRUG/LAB INTERACTIONS

When used in combination with gemcitabine, the dose-normalized area under the curve (AUC) of gemcitabine was increased. Exposure to cisplatin was unchanged. Gemcitabine and cisplatin had no effect on the exposure of necitumumab.

SIDE EFFECTS

The most common adverse reactions (all grades) observed more frequently in patients treated with necitumumab than with gemcitabine and cisplatin alone were dermatitis acneiform, diarrhea, hypomagnesemia, rash, and vomiting. The most common severe (Grade 3 or higher) adverse events were thromboembolic events (including pulmonary embolism), rash, and vomiting. Acne, conjunctivitis, dry skin, electrolyte abnormalities (including hypocalcemia, hypokalemia, and hypophosphatemia), headache, hemoptysis, paronychia, pruritus, skin fissures, stomatitis, VTE, and weight decrease have been reported.

ANTIDOTE

Keep physician informed of all side effects. May constitute a medical emergency or will be treated symptomatically as indicated. Reduce the infusion rate of necitumumab by 50% for Grade 1 IRRs. Stop the infusion for Grade 2 IRRs. Treat infusion-related reactions as indicated and provide premedication (e.g., diphenhydramine [Benadryl], acetaminophen, corticosteroids) for subsequent infusions; see Usual Dose. When signs and symptoms have resolved to Grade 0 or 1, resume necitumumab at a 50% reduced rate for all subsequent infusions. Withhold necitumumab for Grade 3 or 4 electrolyte abnormalities. Permanently discontinue necitumumab for any of the following: (1) Grade 3 or 4 IRR, (2) Grade 3 rash or acneiform rash that does not resolve to Grade 2 or less within 6 weeks, (3) dermatologic reactions that worsen or become intolerable at a dose of 400 mg, (4) Grade 3 skin induration/fibrosis, or (5) Grade 4 dermatologic toxicity. See Dose Adjustments, Precautions, and Monitor.

NELARABINE BBW

(nell-ah-**RA**-ben)

Antineoplastic

Arranon

pH 5 to 7

USUAL DOSE

1,500 mg/M² administered as an infusion over 2 hours on Days 1, 3, and 5. Repeat every 21 days. The recommended duration of treatment has not been clearly established. In clinical trials, treatment was generally continued until there was evidence of disease progression or until the patient experienced unacceptable toxicity, became a candidate for bone marrow transplant, or no longer continued to benefit from treatment.

PEDIATRIC DOSE

650 mg/M² administered as an infusion over 1 hour daily for 5 consecutive days. Repeat every 21 days; see Usual Dose.

DOSE ADJUSTMENTS

Discontinue therapy for neurologic events of Common Terminology Criteria for Adverse Events (CTCAE) Grade 2 or greater. Dosage may be delayed for other toxicity, including hematologic toxicity. ▪ Has not been studied in patients with hepatic or renal impairment. Because nelarabine and ara-G are partially eliminated by the kidneys, clearance may be reduced in patients with renal insufficiency. No dose adjustment is recommended for patients with a CrCl equal to or greater than 50 mL/min. Dose recommendations are not available for patients with a CrCl less than 50 mL/min; see Precautions. ▪ Use caution in dose selection for the elderly.

DILUTION

Specific techniques required; see Precautions. Nelarabine is not diluted before administration. Available in a 250 mg/50 mL (5 mg/mL) vial. Transfer the appropriate dose into a polyvinylchloride (PVC) infusion bag or glass container and administer as an infusion. Example: An adult patient with a body surface area of 2 M² would require a dose of 3,000 mg (1,500 mg/M² × 2 M² = 3,000 mg). 3,000 mg ÷ 250 mg/vial = 12 vials.

Filters: Specific information not available.

Storage: Store unopened vials at CRT. Stable in PVC infusion bags or glass containers for up to 8 hours at up to 30° C (86° F).

COMPATIBILITY

Specific information not available. Consider specific use; consult pharmacist.

RATE OF ADMINISTRATION

Adult dose: A single dose evenly distributed over 2 hours.

Pediatric dose: A single dose evenly distributed over 1 hour.

ACTIONS

A prodrug of ara-G, a T-cell selective nucleoside metabolic inhibitor. Nelarabine is demethylated to ara-G and then converted through various metabolic processes to the active 5′-triphosphate, ara-GTP. Ara-GTP is incorporated into DNA, leading to inhibition of DNA synthesis and cell death. Nelarabine and ara-G are extensively distributed throughout the body and are rapidly eliminated from the plasma, with a mean half-life of 18 minutes and 3.2 hours, respectively. They are partially eliminated by the kidneys.

INDICATIONS AND USES

Treatment of patients with T-cell acute lymphoblastic leukemia and T-cell lymphoblastic lymphoma whose disease has not responded to treatment or has relapsed following treatment with at least two chemotherapy regimens. This use is based on the induction of complete responses. Randomized trials demonstrating increased survival or other clinical benefit have not been conducted.

CONTRAINDICATIONS

Hypersensitivity to nelarabine or any of its components.

PRECAUTIONS

Follow guidelines for handling cytotoxic agents. See Appendix A, p. 1331. ▪ For IV use only. ▪ Administered by or under the direction of a physician specialist in a facility with adequate diagnostic and treatment facilities to monitor the patient and respond to any medical emergency. ▪ Neurotoxicity is the dose-limiting toxicity. Severe neurologic events have been reported and may include altered mental states (e.g., coma, confusion, severe somnolence), central nervous system effects (e.g., ataxia, convulsions), and peripheral neuropathy ranging from numbness and paresthesias to motor weakness and paralysis. Events associated with demyelination and ascending peripheral neuropathies similar in appearance to Guillain-Barré syndrome have also been reported. Full recovery from these events has not always occurred with cessation of therapy. ▪ Patients treated previously or concurrently with intrathecal chemotherapy or previously with craniospinal irradiation may be at increased risk for neurologic adverse events. ▪ Hematologic toxicity (e.g., anemia, leukopenia, neutropenia [including febrile neutropenia], thrombocytopenia) is common. ▪ Use caution in patients with renal or hepatic impairment. Use has not been studied. Patients with a CrCl less than 50 mL/min or a bilirubin greater than 3 times the ULN may be at increased risk for toxicity. Monitor closely. ▪ May develop tumor lysis syndrome. ▪ See Drug/Lab Interactions.

Monitor: Close monitoring for neurologic events is strongly recommended; see Precautions and Antidote. ▪ Obtain a baseline CBC with platelets and monitor regularly. ▪ Monitor renal and hepatic function (BUN, SCr, bilirubin). ▪ Monitor for S/S of tumor lysis syndrome (e.g., hyperkalemia, hyperphosphatemia, hyperuricemia, hypocalcemia, metabolic acidosis, urate crystalluria, and renal failure). ▪ Adequate hydration, alkalinization of urine, and allopurinol are indicated to prevent and/or treat hyperuricemia due to tumor lysis syndrome. ▪ Monitor for S/S of infection. Prophylactic antibiotics may be indicated pending results of C/S in a febrile neutropenic patient. ▪ Monitor for thrombocytopenia (platelet count less than 50,000/mm³). Initiate precautions to prevent excessive bleeding (e.g., inspect IV sites, skin, and mucous membranes; use extreme care during invasive procedures; test urine, emesis, stool, and secretions for occult blood). ▪ Avoid administration of live virus vaccines to immunocompromised patients.

Patient Education: Avoid pregnancy; nonhormonal birth control is recommended. ▪ Use caution in tasks that require alertness. ▪ Notify physician at first sign of infection or of new or worsening neurotoxicity (e.g., numbness, tingling, difficulty with fine motor coordination, unsteadiness, weakness, seizures).

Maternal/Child: Category D: avoid pregnancy; may cause fetal harm. ▪ Discontinue breast-feeding. ▪ The mean clearance of nelarabine is about 30% higher in pediatric patients than in adult patients. Half-lives of nelarabine and ara-G are shorter than those seen in adults—13 minutes and 2 hours, respectively.

Elderly: May be at increased risk of neurologic adverse events. Clearance may be reduced in the elderly due to age-related renal impairment; see Dose Adjustments and Precautions.

DRUG/LAB INTERACTIONS

Formal drug interaction studies have not been completed. ▪ Concurrent administration with **adenosine deaminase inhibitors** (e.g., pentostatin [Nipent]) is not recommended; may decrease conversion of nelarabine to its active form and decrease its effectiveness. ▪ Nelarabine and ara-G do not appear to inhibit the activities of human hepatic cytochrome P_{450} isoenzymes. ▪ Fludarabine does not appear to affect the pharmacokinetics of nelarabine, ara-G, or ara-GTP. ▪ Do not administer **live virus vaccines** to immunocompromised patients receiving antineoplastic agents.

SIDE EFFECTS

Adults: Side effects most frequently reported were anemia, constipation, cough, diarrhea, dizziness, dyspnea, fatigue, fever, headache, hyperuricemia, hypoesthesia, nausea, neutropenia, paresthesia, peripheral neurologic disorders, somnolence, thrombocytopenia, and vomiting. Other reported side effects included abdominal distension, abdominal pain, abnormal gait, anorexia, arthralgia, asthenia, back pain, blurred vision, chest pain, chills, confusion, dehydration, depression, edema, epistaxis, exertional dyspnea, extremity pain, febrile neutropenia, hyperglycemia, hypotension, increased AST, infection, insomnia, muscular weakness, myalgia, pain, peripheral edema, petechiae, pleural effusion, pneumonia, sinusitis, sinus tachycardia, stomatitis, and wheezing. *Neurologic* side effects in adults were mostly Grade 1 or 2 and included amnesia, ataxia, balance disorder, depressed level of consciousness, headache, hypoesthesia, neuropathy (peripheral, peripheral motor, and peripheral sensory), paresthesia, sensory loss, taste alteration, and tremor. Grade 3 events included aphasia, convulsion, hemiparesis, and loss of consciousness. Cerebral hemorrhage, coma, intracranial hemorrhage, leukoencephalopathy, and metabolic encephalopathy also were reported. One patient had a cerebral hemorrhage (fatal), coma, and leukoencephalopathy.

Pediatric patients: Side effects most frequently reported were anemia, decreased blood albumin and potassium levels, headache, increased transaminase levels, leukopenia, neutropenia, peripheral neurologic disorders, thrombocytopenia, and vomiting. Other reported side effects included asthenia; decreased calcium, glucose, and magnesium levels; increased bilirubin and SCr; and infection. *Neurologic* side effects that were greater than Grade 2 included ataxia, headache, hypertonia, hypoesthesia, motor dysfunction, neuropathy (peripheral, peripheral motor, and peripheral sensory), paralysis of the third and sixth nerves, paresthesia, seizures (convulsions, grand mal convulsions, status epilepticus), somnolence, tremor.

Overdose: Myelosuppression, severe neurotoxicity (coma, paralysis), and potentially death.

Post-Marketing: Demyelination and ascending peripheral neuropathies similar in appearance to Guillain-Barré syndrome, increased blood creatine phosphokinase, opportunistic infections (fatal), rhabdomyolysis, tumor lysis syndrome.

ANTIDOTE

Notify physician of any side effects. Most will be treated symptomatically. Discontinue therapy for neurologic events of Common Terminology Criteria for Adverse Events (CTCAE) Grade 2 or greater. Dosage may be delayed for other toxicity, including hematologic toxicity. Blood and blood products, antibiotics, and other adjunctive therapies must be available. Blood modifiers (e.g., darbepoetin alfa [Aranesp], epoetin alfa [Epogen], filgrastim [Neupogen, Zarxio], pegfilgrastim [Neulasta], sargramostim [Leukine]) may be indicated to treat bone marrow toxicity. No known antidote; provide supportive care in overdose. Resuscitate as necessary.

NEOSTIGMINE METHYLSULFATE

Acetylcholinesterase
inhibitor

(nee-oh-**STIG**-meen **METH**-ill-**SUL**-fayt)

Bloxiverz

pH 5.5

USUAL DOSE

Doses should be individualized. A peripheral nerve stimulator should be used to determine when neostigmine should be initiated and if additional doses are needed. Before neostigmine administration and up until complete recovery of normal ventilation, the patient should be well ventilated and a patent airway maintained. An anticholinergic agent (e.g., atropine or glycopyrrolate) should be administered before or concomitantly with neostigmine using a separate syringe.

Atropine: 0.6 to 1.2 mg IV for each 0.5 to 2 mg of neostigmine **OR**

Glycopyrrolate: 0.2 mg IV for each 1 mg of neostigmine; see Precautions.

Neostigmine: 0.03 to 0.07 mg/kg. This dose will generally achieve a train-of-four (TOF) twitch ratio of 90% within 10 to 20 minutes of administration. The recommended maximum total dose is 0.07 mg/kg or up to a total of 5 mg, whichever is less. Dose selection should be based on the extent of spontaneous recovery that has occurred at the time of administration, the half-life of the neuromuscular blocking agent (NMBA) being reversed, and whether there is a need to rapidly reverse the NMBA.

The 0.03 mg/kg dose is recommended for:

- Reversal of NMBAs with shorter half-lives (e.g., rocuronium) **OR**
- When the first twitch response to the train-of-four (TOF) stimulus is substantially greater than 10% of baseline or when a second twitch is present.

The 0.07 mg/kg dose is recommended for:

- Reversal of NMBAs with longer half-lives (e.g., pancuronium or vecuronium) **OR**
- When the first twitch response is relatively weak (i.e., not substantially greater than 10% of baseline) **OR**
- There is need for more rapid recovery.

PEDIATRIC DOSE

See Usual Dose and Maternal/Child.

DOSE ADJUSTMENTS

Individualize dose based on extent of spontaneous recovery at time of administration, the half-life of the NMBA being reversed, and whether or not there is a need to rapidly reverse the NMBA. ▪ Use with caution and with minimum effective dose in pediatric patients and in patients with coronary artery disease, cardiac arrhythmias, recent acute coronary syndrome, or myasthenia gravis; see Maternal/Child. ▪ Reduce dose if recovery from neuromuscular blockade is nearly complete. See Precautions and Monitor.

DILUTION

Available in 0.5 mg/mL and 1 mg/mL in 10-mL multiple-dose vials. May be given undiluted through Y-tube or three-way stopcock of infusion set.

Storage: Store at CRT in carton. Protect from light.

COMPATIBILITY

(Underline Indicates Conflicting Compatibility Information)

One source suggests the following **compatibilities**:

Y-site: Heparin, hydrocortisone sodium succinate (Solu-Cortef), palonosetron (Aloxi), potassium chloride.

RATE OF ADMINISTRATION

Inject slowly over a period of at least 1 minute.

ACTIONS

A competitive cholinesterase inhibitor and antagonist of nondepolarizing neuromuscular blocking agents. Inhibits the enzyme cholinesterase. By reducing the breakdown of acetylcholine, neostigmine induces an increase in acetylcholine in the synaptic cleft. Acetylcholine competes for the same binding sites as nondepolarizing NMBAs and reverses the neuromuscular blockade. The increase in acetylcholine levels results in the potentiation of both muscarinic and nicotine cholinergic activity. Does not cross the blood-brain barrier so does not significantly affect cholinergic function in the CNS. Metabolized by microsomal enzymes in the liver. Half-life ranges from 24 to 113 minutes. Excreted primarily in urine.

INDICATIONS AND USES

Reversal of the effects of nondepolarizing neuromuscular blocking agents after surgery. **Unlabeled use:** Treatment of myasthenia gravis.

CONTRAINDICATIONS

Known hypersensitivity to neostigmine (known hypersensitivity reactions have included urticaria, angioedema, erythema multiforme, generalized rash, facial swelling, peripheral edema, fever, flushing, hypotension, bronchospasm, bradycardia, and anaphylaxis). ▪ Peritonitis or mechanical obstruction of the intestinal or urinary tract.

PRECAUTIONS

For IV administration only. ▪ Should be administered by a trained health care provider familiar with the use, actions, characteristics, and complications of neuromuscular blocking agents and neuromuscular block reversal agents. ▪ Neostigmine has been associated with bradycardia. In the presence of bradycardia, it is recommended that the anticholinergic agent (atropine or glycopyrrolate) be administered before neostigmine. ▪ Cardiovascular effects such as bradycardia, hypotension, or dysrhythmia are anticipated with acetylcholinesterase inhibitors such as neostigmine. Use with caution in patients with coronary artery disease, cardiac arrhythmias, recent acute coronary syndrome, or myasthenia gravis. Risk of blood pressure and heart rate complications may be increased in these patients. ▪ Because of the possibility of hypersensitivity, atropine and medications to treat anaphylaxis should be readily available. ▪ Large doses of neostigmine administered when neuromuscular blockade is minimal can produce neuromuscular dysfunction. The dose of neostigmine should be reduced if recovery from neuromuscular blockade is nearly complete. ▪ It is important to distinguish between myasthenic crisis and cholinergic crisis caused by overdose of neostigmine. Both result in extreme muscle weakness but require radically different treatment; see Antidote. ▪ Use with caution in patients with renal and hepatic impairment. Dose adjustment is not required, but duration of action of NMBAs that are renally or hepatically eliminated may be prolonged. Patients must be carefully monitored to ensure that the effects of the NMBA do not persist beyond those of neostigmine.

Monitor: A peripheral nerve stimulation device capable of delivering a train-of-four (TOF) stimulus is required. There must be a twitch response to the first stimulus in the TOF of at least 10% of its baseline level (i.e., the response prior to the NMBA) before administering neostigmine. ▪ TOF monitoring alone should not be relied on to determine the adequacy of reversal of neuromuscular blockade as related to a patient's ability to adequately ventilate and maintain a patent airway following tracheal extubation. Satisfactory recovery should be judged by adequacy of skeletal muscle tone and respiratory measurements in addition to the response to the peripheral nerve stimulator. ▪ Continue monitoring for adequacy of reversal for a period that will ensure full recovery based on the patient's medical condition and the pharmacokinetics of neostigmine and the NMBA used.

Maternal/Child: It is not known whether neostigmine can cause fetal harm when administered to a pregnant woman; use during pregnancy, labor, or delivery only if clearly needed. Acetylcholinesterase drugs, including neostigmine, may cause uterine irritability and induce premature labor when given to pregnant women who are near-term. ▪ The effect of neostigmine on the mother and fetus with regard to labor, delivery, the need for forceps delivery or other intervention, or resuscitation of the newborn is not known. ▪ Use caution during breast-feeding. ▪ Recovery of neuromuscular activity occurs more rapidly with smaller doses of acetylcholinesterase inhibitors in pediatric patients than in adults. However, infants and small children may be at greater risk for complications from incomplete reversal of neuromuscular blockade due to decreased respiratory reserve. The risks associated with incomplete reversal outweigh any risk from giving higher doses of neostigmine. ∎ Because blood pressure in pediatric patients, particularly infants and neonates, is sensitive to changes in heart rate, the effects of an anticholinergic agent (e.g., atropine) should be observed before administration of neostigmine to lessen the probability of bradycardia and hypotension.

Elderly: Duration of action is prolonged in the elderly. However, the elderly also experience a slower spontaneous recovery from NMBAs. Dose adjustment is not generally needed, but an extended monitoring period to ensure complete reversal may be warranted.

DRUG/LAB INTERACTIONS

Pharmacokinetic interactions between neostigmine and other drugs have not been studied. ∎ Metabolized by microsomal enzymes in the liver. Use with caution when using with other drugs that may alter the activity of metabolizing enzymes or transporters.

SIDE EFFECTS

Usually attributable to exaggerated pharmacologic effects at the muscarinic receptor. The most common side effects are bradycardia, nausea, and vomiting. Other side effects include dizziness, dry mouth, dyspnea, headache, hypotension, incision site complications, insomnia, oxygen desaturation, pharyngolaryngeal pain, postoperative shivering, procedural complications, procedural pain, prolonged neuromuscular blockade, pruritus, and tachycardia.

Overdose: Bradycardia, nausea, vomiting, diarrhea, increased bronchial and salivary secretions, muscle weakness (including muscles of respiration), sweating, death (symptoms of cholinergic crisis).

Post-Marketing: Hypersensitivity reactions, anaphylaxis, arthralgia, bowel cramps, bronchospasm, cardiac arrest, cardiac arrhythmias, convulsions, diaphoresis, diarrhea, drowsiness, dysarthria, fasciculation, flatulence, flushing, hypotension, increased peristalsis, increased secretions, loss of consciousness, miosis, muscle cramps, nonspecific ECG changes, rash, respiratory depression or arrest, spasms, syncope, urinary frequency, urticaria, visual changes, weakness.

ANTIDOTE

If side effects occur, discontinue drug and notify the physician. The use of an anticholinergic agent (atropine or glycopyrrolate) may prevent or mitigate most side effects, including cardiovascular complications (bradycardia, hypotension, or dysrhythmia). In the event of an overdose, ventilation should be supported by artificial means until adequacy of spontaneous respiration is assured, and cardiac function should be monitored. Treat anaphylaxis immediately with oxygen, epinephrine (Adrenalin), antihistamines (e.g., diphenhydramine [Benadryl]), vasopressors (e.g., dopamine), corticosteroids, albuterol, IV fluids, and ventilation equipment as indicated. Resuscitate as necessary.

NESIRITIDE
(nih-**SIR**-ih-tide)

Cardiotonic
Vasodilator

Natrecor

USUAL DOSE

Prime the IV tubing with the diluted nesiritide solution before connecting to the patient and before giving the bolus dose and infusion. *Bolus must be drawn from the prepared infusion bag.*

An initial dose of 2 mcg/kg of diluted solution is given as an IV bolus over 60 seconds. Follow immediately with the diluted solution as an infusion of 0.01 mcg/kg/min (0.1 mL/kg/hr); see Dilution and Rate of Administration. *Do not initiate nesiritide at a dose that is above the recommended dose.* Do not increase rate of titration more frequently than every 3 hours. Use central hemodynamic monitoring, and do not exceed 0.03 mcg/kg/min. Experience is limited in the use of the infusion for more than 96 hours. See Dose Adjustments and Precautions.

DOSE ADJUSTMENTS

Use of the loading dose may not be appropriate for patients with low systolic blood pressure (less than 110 mm Hg) or for patients recently treated with afterload reducers (e.g., nitroprusside [Nitropress], nitroglycerin). ▪ Reduced doses are not required in impaired renal function or based on age, gender, race, baseline endogenous human B-type natriuretic peptide (hBNP) concentration, severity of CHF, or concomitant administration of an ACE inhibitor (e.g., enalapril [Vasotec]). ▪ If hypotension occurs, reduce the dose or discontinue nesiritide. Use IV fluids or changes in body position to support BP. Discontinue nesiritide if symptomatic hypotension occurs. Hypotension may be prolonged. Observe closely; reduce dose by 30% and restart nesiritide infusion (no bolus) when patient is stabilized. ▪ See Antidote.

DILUTION

Each 1.5-mg vial must be reconstituted with 5 mL of diluent withdrawn from a prefilled, preservative-free, 250-mL plastic IV bag of D5W, NS, D5/½NS, or D5/¼NS. Do not shake. Ensure complete dilution by rotating the vial gently so all surfaces, including the stopper, are in contact with the diluent. Withdraw the entire contents of the vial and add to the 250-mL plastic IV bag used for the initial reconstitution. Invert several times to ensure complete mixing. Yields a concentration of 6 mcg/mL. *Prime the tubing and withdraw the bolus dose from this final dilution.* The IV tubing should be primed with 5 mL of the infusion solution before connecting to the IV access port and before withdrawing the bolus. Use the remaining solution for the infusion.

Filters: Manufacturer did two studies. Data indicate no loss of drug potency through a 5-micron needle filter in a 500 mcg/mL concentration. With the use of an in-line, 0.22-micron filter and concentrations of 2 and 50 mcg/mL at a rate of 9 mL/hr, drug potency was initially lower but recovered to 90% in 1 hour and 100% at 2 hours.

Storage: Vials should be stored in the carton below 25° C (77° F); protect from light; do not freeze. Reconstituted solutions may be stored at 2° to 25° C (36° to 77° F) for up to 24 hours.

COMPATIBILITY
(Underline Indicates Conflicting Compatibility Information)

Consider any drug NOT listed as compatible to be INCOMPATIBLE until consulting a pharmacist; specific conditions may apply.

Manufacturer lists as **incompatible** with bumetanide, enalaprilat (Vasotec IV), ethacrynic acid (Edecrin), furosemide (Lasix), heparin, hydralazine, insulin (regular), and any injectable drug that contains the preservative sodium metabisulfite. Manufacturer states, "Do not coadminister as infusions with nesiritide through the same IV catheter." If an **incompatible** drug has been administered, the IV catheter must be flushed with a **compatible** solution (see Dilution) before and after the administration of nesiritide. Do not

N-O

administer through a heparin-coated catheter (central or peripheral). Binds to heparin and could bind to the lining of a heparin-coated catheter and decrease the amount of nesiritide delivered to the patient.

One source suggests the following **compatibilities:**

Y-site: Amiodarone (Nexterone), argatroban, digoxin (Lanoxin), diltiazem (Cardizem), fentanyl, metoprolol (Lopressor), milrinone (Primacor), nicardipine (Cardene IV), nitroglycerin IV, nitroprusside (Nitropress), propranolol, quinidine gluconate, torsemide (Demadex), verapamil.

RATE OF ADMINISTRATION

If the IV line has been used to administer other drugs, flush it with a solution **compatible** to nesiritide before administration and then prime it with nesiritide solution. The IV tubing should be primed with 5 mL of the infusion solution before connecting to the IV access port and before withdrawing the bolus.

IV bolus: A single dose over 60 seconds through an IV port in the tubing.

IV infusion: Use a volume-controlled infusion pump and administer at a flow rate of 0.1 mL/kg/hr to deliver the desired dose of 0.01 mcg/kg/min.

Adjust bolus volumes and rates of infusion by weight according to the following chart.

Nesiritide Weight-Adjusted Bolus Volume and Infusion Flow Rate (2 mcg/kg Bolus Followed by a 0.01 mcg/kg/min Infusion)		
Patient Weight (kg)	Volume of Bolus (mL)	Rate of Infusion (mL/hr)
60 kg	20 mL	6 mL/hr
70 kg	23.3 mL	7 mL/hr
80 kg	26.7 mL	8 mL/hr
90 kg	30 mL	9 mL/hr
100 kg	33.3 mL	10 mL/hr
110 kg	36.7 mL	11 mL/hr

Alternately, the following formulas can be used to calculate the correct bolus volume and infusion rate:

$$\text{Bolus volume (mL)} = \text{Patient weight (kg)} \div 3$$

$$\text{Infusion flow rate (mL/hr)} = 0.1 \times \text{Patient weight (kg)}$$

ACTIONS

A recombinant form of human B-type natriuretic peptide (hBNP). Has the same 32–amino acid sequence as the endogenous peptide produced by the ventricular myocardium. Binds to specific receptors of vascular smooth muscle and endothelial cells, resulting in increased intracellular concentrations of cGMP and smooth muscle cell relaxation. Dilates veins and arteries. Produces dose-dependent reductions in pulmonary capillary wedge pressure (PCWP) and systemic arterial pressure in patients with heart failure. Has no effect on cardiac contractility or measures of cardiac electrophysiology (e.g., atrial and ventricular refractory times or atrioventricular node conduction) in animals. 60% of the 3-hour effect on PCWP reduction and 70% of the 3-hour effect on systolic blood pressure (SBP) reduction is achieved within 15 minutes. Half-life is approximately 18 minutes. Duration of action may be longer than predicted based on half-life and may be dose dependent. Mechanism of elimination has not been studied.

INDICATIONS AND USES

Treatment of acutely decompensated CHF in patients who have dyspnea at rest or with minimal activity. Has been shown to reduce PCWP and improve short-term symptoms of dyspnea (3 hours).

CONTRAINDICATIONS

Hypersensitivity to nesiritide or its components (a recombinant protein manufactured using *Escherichia coli*). ▪ Cardiogenic shock. ▪ Patients with a persistent systolic BP less than 100 mm Hg. ▪ Not recommended in patients for whom vasodilating agents are not appropriate (e.g., restrictive or obstructive cardiomyopathy, constrictive pericarditis, pericardial tamponade, significant valvular stenosis), for other conditions in which cardiac output is dependent on venous return, or for patients who may have or are known to have low cardiac filling pressures.

PRECAUTIONS

Safety and effectiveness for use longer than 96 hours not established. ▪ Administered by or under the supervision of a physician experienced in its use and in a facility equipped to monitor the patient and respond to any medical emergency. ▪ An *E. coli*–derived protein product; hypersensitivity reactions have been reported and may be more likely to occur in individuals with a history of sensitivity to recombinant peptides; obtain patient history. ▪ May decrease renal function; see Monitor. ▪ May cause azotemia in patients with severe CHF whose renal function may depend on the activity of the renin-angiotensin-aldosterone system. Some patients have required first-time dialysis.

Monitor: Incidence of hypotension is similar to nitroglycerin, but duration of hypotension is longer. Monitor BP closely. Reduce rate or stop infusion for excessive drop in BP; see Dose Adjustments and Antidote. ▪ Observe patient continuously; monitor urine output, renal function, fluid and electrolyte changes, and body weight. Monitor SCr during treatment and after treatment is completed until values have stabilized. Monitoring of cardiac index and PCWP useful. ▪ Observe for orthopnea, dyspnea, and fatigue. ▪ Monitor for S/S of a hypersensitivity reaction (e.g., hives, rash, shortness of breath or troubled breathing, swelling of eyelids, lips, or face). ▪ As cardiac output and diuresis improve, a reduction in diuretic dose may be indicated. ▪ See Precautions and Drug/Lab Interactions.

Patient Education: Report dizziness or faintness; request assistance for ambulation.

Maternal/Child: Category C: use during pregnancy only if potential benefit justifies possible risk to the fetus. ▪ Not known if nesiritide is secreted in breast milk; use caution in women who are breast-feeding. ▪ Safety and effectiveness for use in pediatric patients not established.

Elderly: Response similar to that found in younger patients; however, use with caution in the elderly; may have a greater sensitivity to its effects.

DRUG/LAB INTERACTIONS

Trials specifically examining potential drug interactions have not been conducted. ▪ May cause additive hypotension with **ACE inhibitors** (e.g., enalapril [Vasotec]) **and other drugs that may cause hypotension** (e.g., antidepressants [e.g., amitriptyline (Elavil)], antihypertensives, benzodiazepines [e.g., diazepam (Valium), lorazepam (Ativan)], magnesium sulfate). ▪ Has been administered with angiotensin II receptor antagonists, anticoagulants, beta-blockers (e.g., atenolol [Tenormin]), calcium channel blockers (e.g., diltiazem [Cardizem], verapamil), Class III antiarrhythmic agents (e.g., amiodarone [Nexterone], sotalol [Betapace]), digoxin, diuretics, dobutamine, dopamine, oral ACE inhibitors, oral nitrates, and statins (e.g., simvastatin [Zocor]). No specific effect on the action of nesiritide was noted, but hypotensive effects are additive. ▪ Effects of concurrent use with **other IV vasodilators** (e.g., milrinone, nitroglycerin, or nitroprusside sodium), **drugs affecting the renin-angiotensin system** (e.g., angiotensin receptor blockers [e.g., losartan (Cozaar), candesartan (Atacand)] and/or angiotensin-converting enzyme inhibitors [e.g., enalapril (Vasotec), captopril]), **and afterload reducers** (e.g., nitroprusside [Nitropress], enalapril [Vasotec], captopril) have not been studied, but hypotensive effects would be additive.

SIDE EFFECTS

Hypotension is the primary side effect; may be symptomatic and can be dose limiting; see Antidote. Back pain, dizziness, headache, increased serum creatinine (SCr), and nausea are most common. Other reported side effects include abdominal pain, amblyopia (vision impairment), anemia, angina, anxiety, apnea, arrhythmias (e.g., atrial fibrillation, AV node conduction abnormalities, bradycardia, PVCs, tachycardia, VT), catheter pain, confusion, fever, hemoptysis, increased cough, increased serum creatinine, injection site reaction, insomnia, leg cramps, paresthesia, somnolence, sweating, tremor, and vomiting. Hypersensitivity reactions and anaphylaxis may occur. A meta-analysis of seven clinical trials demonstrated that nesiritide did not increase mortality rate in patients with acute decompensated heart failure at Day 30 or Day 180.

Post-Marketing: Hypersensitivity reactions, infusion site extravasation, pruritus, rash.

ANTIDOTE

Notify the physician of any side effects. Based on degree of severity and condition of the patient; may be treated symptomatically; dose may remain the same, be decreased, or be discontinued. Reduce rate or discontinue nesiritide at the first sign of marked hypotension and notify the physician. Hypotension may respond to a Trendelenburg position and IV fluids (avoid fluid overload). Hypotension may last for hours; observation for a prolonged period may be indicated before restarting nesiritide. After hypotension is stabilized, nesiritide may be restarted; do not administer a bolus dose, and reduce the rate of infusion by 30%. Treat hypersensitivity reactions as indicated.

NICARDIPINE HYDROCHLORIDE

Calcium channel blocker
Antihypertensive

(nye-**KAR**-dih-peen hy-droh-**KLOR**-eyed)

Cardene IV

pH 3.7 to 4.7

USUAL DOSE

Must be individualized based on the severity of hypertension and the response of each patient. Blood pressure decrease is dependent on the rate of infusion and frequency of dose adjustments. Gradual reduction based on clinical situation is best. Avoid too-rapid or excessive drop in BP. See Precautions. Transfer to oral medication as soon as clinical condition permits.

To substitute for oral nicardipine therapy: 0.5 mg/hr will achieve similar plasma concentration to an oral dose of 20 mg every 8 hours; 1.2 mg/hr to an oral dose of 30 mg every 8 hours; 2.2 mg/hr to an oral dose of 40 mg every 8 hours.

Gradual reduction of BP in a drug-free patient: Initiate therapy at 5 mg/hr. May be increased by 2.5 mg/hr every 15 minutes until desired BP reduction is achieved. Do not exceed 15 mg/hr.

Rapid reduction of BP in a drug-free patient: Initiate a 5-mg/hr dose as above, but increases of 2.5 mg/hr may be given every 5 minutes until desired BP reduction is achieved (AHA guidelines recommend 5 to 15 minutes). Do not exceed 15 mg/hr.

Maintenance: When desired BP is achieved, reduce rate to 3 mg/hr. This is the average maintenance rate. Adjust as needed to maintain desired response.

Transfer to an oral antihypertensive agent: The first dose of oral nicardipine should be given 1 hour before discontinuing infusion. Initiate any other oral antihypertensive agent on discontinuation of infusion.

DOSE ADJUSTMENTS

Lower doses and slower titration suggested in heart failure and impaired hepatic or renal function; see Precautions. ▪ Lower-end initial doses may be indicated in the elderly. Consider potential for decreased organ function and concomitant disease or drug therapy.

DILUTION

Available as a premixed solution containing 0.1 mg/mL in D5W or NS or in a vial that requires further dilution. Each vial (25 mg in 10 mL) must be diluted with 240 mL of **compatible** infusion solution to equal a concentration of 0.1 mg/mL; in this 0.1 mg/mL concentration, 2.5 mg/hr equals 25 mL/hr, 3 mg/hr equals 30 mL/hr, 5 mg/hr equals 50 mL/hr, and 15 mL/hr equals 150 mL/hr. **Compatible** in ½NS, NS, D5W, D5/½NS, D5NS. Also **compatible** in D5W with 40 mEq of potassium added.

Fluid-restricted or pediatric patients: One source recommends mixing up to 50 mg in 100 mL (0.5 mg/mL). To avoid superficial phlebitis, administration via a central line is recommended for this concentration.

Filters: No data available from manufacturer.

Storage: Store vials in carton, protected from light at CRT. Has a light yellow color. Diluted solution is stable at room temperature for 24 hours. Store prediluted solutions at CRT; protect from light and excessive heat and avoid freezing.

COMPATIBILITY   (Underline Indicates Conflicting Compatibility Information)
Consider any drug NOT listed as compatible to be INCOMPATIBLE until consulting a pharmacist; specific conditions may apply.
Manufacturer states, "Do not combine with any product in the same IV line or premixed container. Do not add supplementary medication to the bag." Manufacturer lists as **incompatible** with sodium bicarbonate 5% and LR.

One source suggests the following **compatibilities:**

Additive: *Not recommended by manufacturer.* Potassium chloride (KCl).

Y-site: *Not recommended by manufacturer.* Amikacin, aminophylline, aztreonam (Azactam), butorphanol (Stadol), calcium gluconate, cefazolin (Ancef), ceftazidime (Fortaz), chloramphenicol (Chloromycetin), clindamycin (Cleocin), dextran 40 in 5% dextrose, diltiazem (Cardizem), dobutamine, dopamine, enalaprilat (Vasotec IV), epinephrine (Adrenalin), erythromycin (Erythrocin), esmolol (Brevibloc), famotidine (Pepcid IV), fenoldopam (Corlopam), fentanyl, gentamicin, heparin, hetastarch in NS (Hespan), hydrocortisone sodium succinate (Solu-Cortef), hydromorphone (Dilaudid), labetalol, lidocaine, linezolid (Zyvox), lorazepam (Ativan), magnesium sulfate, methylprednisolone (Solu-Medrol), metronidazole (Flagyl IV), midazolam (Versed), milrinone (Primacor), morphine, nafcillin (Nallpen), nesiritide (Natrecor), nitroglycerin IV, nitroprusside sodium, norepinephrine (Levophed), penicillin G potassium, potassium chloride (KCl), potassium phosphates, ranitidine (Zantac), sodium acetate, sulfamethoxazole/trimethoprim, tobramycin, vancomycin, vecuronium.

RATE OF ADMINISTRATION
Must be administered as a slow, continuous infusion. Adjust as indicated in Usual Dose and Dose Adjustments.

ACTIONS
The first dihydropyridine calcium channel blocker for IV use. Inhibits influx of calcium ions into cardiac muscle and smooth muscle without altering serum calcium. Contractile processes are dependent on calcium movement through specific channels. Effects seen are more selective to vascular smooth muscle than cardiac muscle. Causes coronary and peripheral blood vessels to dilate and relax, reducing systemic vascular resistance. Increases cardiac output, coronary blood flow, and myocardial oxygen supply without increasing cardiac oxygen demand. Reduces BP without significantly affecting cardiac conduction and usually does not depress cardiac function. Produces dose-dependent decreases in BP. Begins to reduce BP in minutes; achieves 50% of ultimate decrease in 45 minutes. When discontinued, can lose 50% of effect within 30 minutes, but gradually decreasing effects persist for up to 50 hours. Effects more prominent in hypertensive than in normotensive volunteers. Highly protein bound. Extensively metabolized in the liver. Half-life is 14.4 hours. Excreted in urine and feces. Crosses placental barrier. Minimally secreted in breast milk.

INDICATIONS AND USES
Short-term treatment of hypertension when oral therapy is not feasible or not desirable.

CONTRAINDICATIONS
Advanced aortic stenosis (reduced diastolic pressure may worsen rather than improve myocardial oxygen balance). ■ Known hypersensitivity to nicardipine.

PRECAUTIONS

Use caution in patients with coronary artery disease. May cause increase in frequency, duration, or severity of angina. ▪ Has improved left ventricle function after beta-blockade. ▪ Use caution and titrate slowly in patients with heart failure or significant left ventricular dysfunction, particularly when used in combination with a beta-blocker; possible negative inotropic effects may occur. ▪ Use caution with impaired hepatic or renal function; lower doses, slower titration, and close monitoring indicated. ▪ May produce symptomatic hypotension or tachycardia. Avoid systemic hypotension (systolic BP less than 90 mm Hg), and use with caution in patients with acute cerebral infarction or hemorrhage.

Monitor: To reduce the possibility of venous thrombosis, phlebitis, local irritation, swelling, extravasation, and/or vascular impairment, administer through a central vein or large peripheral vein rather than a small peripheral vein. Avoid intra-arterial administration. If administered via a peripheral vein, change the infusion site every 12 hours. ▪ Avoid tachycardia or too-rapid or excessive reduction in either systolic or diastolic BP. Monitor BP and HR continually during infusion and frequently after infusion. Additional monitoring of BP and HR is indicated when used in combination with a beta-blocker in patients with HF or significant left ventricular dysfunction ▪ Transfer to oral therapy as soon as clinical condition permits. ▪ See Precautions and Drug/Lab Interactions.

Patient Education: Request assistance to change position or ambulate.

Maternal/Child: Category C: use during pregnancy only if benefit justifies potential risk to the fetus. ▪ Dizziness, flushing, headache, hypotension, nausea, postpartum hemorrhage, reflex tachycardia, and tocolysis have occurred in pregnant women treated for hypertension during pregnancy. Produced hypotension in some neonates. ▪ During use in preterm labor, dyspnea, headache, hypotension, hypoxia, phlebitis at the injection site, and pulmonary edema have been reported. Neonatal side effects included acidosis (pH less than 7.25). ▪ Use caution during breast-feeding; infant exposure may occur. ▪ Safety and effectiveness for use in pediatric patients under 18 years of age not established.

Elderly: Response similar to that seen in younger adults; however, greater sensitivity in the elderly cannot be ruled out. ▪ Half-life may be prolonged. ▪ See Dose Adjustments.

DRUG/LAB INTERACTIONS

May cause possible negative inotropic effects with concurrent administration of a **beta-blocker** (e.g., atenolol [Tenormin], metoprolol [Lopressor]); see Precautions. ▪ **Cimetidine** (Tagamet) increases oral nicardipine plasma concentrations; monitor patients receiving IV nicardipine carefully. ▪ Will increase plasma levels of **cyclosporine** (Sandimmune); monitor and decrease cyclosporine dose if indicated. ▪ May potentiate the effects of **other antihypertensives.** Monitor BP closely and adjust doses as indicated. ▪ Metabolism may be increased and serum concentrations decreased by **rifampin** (Rifadin). Adjust dose as needed. ▪ Plasma protein binding of nicardipine not altered with therapeutic concentrations of furosemide (Lasix), propranolol, dipyridamole (Persantine), warfarin (Coumadin), quinidine, or naproxen (Naprosyn).

SIDE EFFECTS

Average dose: Most common side effects include headache, hypotension, nausea and vomiting, and tachycardia. Many other side effects, including ECG abnormality (e.g., angina pectoris, atrioventricular block, ST-segment depression, inverted T wave), confusion, conjunctivitis, deep vein thrombophlebitis, dyspepsia, ear disorder, fever, hypertonia, hypophosphatemia, neck pain, peripheral edema, respiratory difficulties, thrombocytopenia, tinnitus, and urinary frequency, occurred in fewer than 3% of patients. Hypersensitivity reactions (e.g., angioedema, rash, wheezing) have been reported.

Overdose: Bradycardia (following initial tachycardia), confusion, drowsiness, flushing, hypotension (marked), palpitations, slurred speech. Progressive AV block may occur with lethal overdose.

Post-Marketing: Decreased oxygen saturation (possible pulmonary shunting).

ANTIDOTE
Keep physician informed of all side effects. Headache, hypotension, and tachycardia have required a reduction in dose or discontinuation of nicardipine. When symptoms subside, nicardipine may be restarted at low doses (e.g., 3 to 5 mg/hr [30 to 50 mL/hr of a 0.1 mg/mL solution or 15 to 25 mL/hr of a 0.2 mg/mL solution]) and adjusted to maintain desired BP. In overdose, monitor BP and cardiac and respiratory functions; put patients in Trendelenburg position; use vasopressors (e.g., dopamine) for excessive hypotension. IV calcium gluconate may reverse effects of calcium entry blockade. Not removed by hemodialysis.

NITROGLYCERIN IV
(**NYE**-troe-**GLIS**-er-in)

Antianginal
Antihypertensive
Vasodilator

pH 3 to 6.5

USUAL DOSE
See Compatibility; these doses are recommended for use with non-PVC administration sets. Increased doses are required if using PVC administration sets. Effectiveness is short term; see Actions. Initiate concurrent therapy before tolerance develops (e.g., doses exceeding 200 mcg/min or administration over 12 to 24 hours).

Unstable angina, persistent ischemia, and/or congestive heart failure associated with MI: An IV bolus of 12.5 to 25 mcg followed by a continuous infusion of 10 to 20 mcg/min; increase by 5 to 10 mcg/min every 5 to 10 minutes until desired hemodynamic response. AHA recommends an IV bolus of 12.5 to 25 mcg followed by an infusion at 10 mcg/min. Increase rate by 10 mcg/min every 3 to 5 minutes until desired effect. 200 mcg/min is the usual maximum dose.

Treatment of angina in patients unresponsive to therapeutic doses of nitrates or beta-blockers: 5 mcg/min initially. Increase by 5 mcg/min increments every 3 to 5 minutes until some BP response is noted. Reduce increments and/or increase time to fine-tune to desired hemodynamic response. If no response at 20 mcg/min, 10 mcg/min increases may be used. Incremental increases of up to 20 mcg/min may be needed to achieve desired effect. No fixed optimum dose. Tolerance may develop if administered over 12 to 24 hours.

Severe hypertension or hypertensive emergency: Doses up to 100 mcg/min may be required (range is 5 to 100 mcg/min). Doses that will reduce mean arterial BP by no more than 25% over several minutes to 1 hour are suggested to prevent overaggressive therapy. If stable, follow with further reductions toward 160/100 to 110 mm Hg within the next 2 to 6 hours. When an initial response is achieved, increases in dosage increments should be reduced and/or the intervals between dose increases lengthened.

PEDIATRIC DOSE
0.25 to 0.5 mcg/kg/min initially. May increase by 0.5 to 1 mcg/kg/min increments every 3 to 5 minutes until desired response. See Maternal/Child. AHA guidelines recommend titrating by 1 mcg/kg/min every 15 to 20 minutes and state the typical dose range is 1 to 5 mcg/kg/min.

DOSE ADJUSTMENTS
Reduced dose may be required with persistent headache unrelieved by analgesics. Reduce dose gradually when weaning to prevent rebound symptoms. ■ Lower-end initial doses may be appropriate in the elderly based on potential for decreased organ function, concomitant disease, or other drug therapy.

N-O

DILUTION

Available premixed in D5W with various concentrations of nitroglycerin. All other preparations must be diluted and administered as an infusion. Use only non-PVC plastic or glass infusion bottles and specific (nonpolyvinyl chloride) infusion tubing (provided by manufacturer). Do not use filters. Dilute in a given amount of D5W or NS for infusion. Concentration dependent on initial preparation (0.5 mg/mL or 5 mg/mL) and patient fluid tolerances. 10 mL of 0.5 mg/mL in 250 mL diluent equals 20 mcg/mL (in 1,000 mL, 5 mcg/mL). 10 mL of 5 mg/mL in 250 mL diluent equals 200 mcg/mL (in 1,000 mL, 50 mcg/mL). See the following dilution chart.

Guidelines for Dilution of Nitroglycerin IV for Infusion		
Diluent Volume (mL)	Quantity of Nitroglycerin (5 mg/mL)	Approximate Final Concentration (mcg/mL)
100 mL	10 mg (2 mL)	100 mcg/mL
100 mL	20 mg (4 mL)	200 mcg/mL
100 mL	40 mg (8 mL)	400 mcg/mL
250 mL	25 mg (5 mL)	100 mcg/mL
250 mL	50 mg (10 mL)	200 mcg/mL
250 mL	100 mg (20 mL)	400 mcg/mL
500 mL	50 mg (10 mL)	100 mcg/mL
500 mL	100 mg (20 mL)	200 mcg/mL
500 mL	200 mg (40 mL)	400 mcg/mL

May be used in dilutions from 25 to 400 mcg/mL.

Pediatric dilution: 6 mg/kg nitroglycerin IV in 100 mL D5W at an infusion rate of 1 mL/hr equals 1 mcg/kg/min.

Filters: Do not use filters; see Dilution.

Storage: Protect vials from light. Solution stable for up to 24 hours.

COMPATIBILITY
(Underline Indicates Conflicting Compatibility Information)

Consider any drug NOT listed as compatible to be INCOMPATIBLE until consulting a pharmacist; specific conditions may apply.

Manufacturer states, "Do not admix with any other drug." See Dilution. Non-PVC plastic or glass infusion bottles and nonpolyvinyl chloride infusion tubing are required to deliver accurate dosing with minimal adsorption. Calculated dose will not be correct if other infusion containers or tubing are used because of excess adsorption.

One source suggests the following **compatibilities:**

Additive: *Not recommended by manufacturer.* Alteplase (tPA, Activase), aminophylline, dobutamine, dopamine, enalaprilat (Vasotec IV), furosemide (Lasix), lidocaine, verapamil.

Y-site: Amiodarone (Nexterone), amphotericin B cholesteryl (Amphotec), argatroban, atracurium (Tracrium), bivalirudin (Angiomax), cisatracurium (Nimbex), dexmedetomidine (Precedex), diltiazem (Cardizem), dobutamine, dopamine, epinephrine (Adrenalin), esmolol (Brevibloc), famotidine (Pepcid IV), fenoldopam (Corlopam), fentanyl, fluconazole (Diflucan), furosemide (Lasix), heparin, hetastarch in electrolytes (Hextend), hydralazine, hydromorphone (Dilaudid), 6% hydroxyethyl starch (Voluven), insulin (regular), labetalol, lidocaine, linezolid (Zyvox), lorazepam (Ativan), micafungin (Mycamine), midazolam (Versed), milrinone (Primacor), morphine, nesiritide (Natrecor), nicardipine (Cardene IV), nitroprusside sodium, norepinephrine (Levophed), pancuronium, pantoprazole (Protonix IV), propofol (Diprivan), ranitidine (Zantac), remifentanil (Ultiva), tacrolimus (Prograf), theophylline, tirofiban (Aggrastat), vasopressin, vecuronium, warfarin (Coumadin).

RATE OF ADMINISTRATION

Dependent on patient response and effective dose. Specific adjustments required; see Usual Dose. Use extreme caution in patients responsive to initial 5 mcg/min dose. Decrease adjustments and increase time between doses as patient begins to respond. Use of an infusion pump or microdrip (60 gtt/mL) required. Exact and constant delivery mandatory. See the following chart.

Nitroglycerin IV Guidelines for Infusion				
Concentration (mcg/mL)	50	100	200	400
Desired Dose (mcg/min)	60 Microdrops = 1 mL Flow Rate (microdrops/min = mL/hr)			
5 mcg/min	6	3	—	—
10 mcg/min	12	6	3	—
15 mcg/min	18	9	—	—
20 mcg/min	24	12	6	3
30 mcg/min	36	18	9	—
40 mcg/min	48	24	12	6
60 mcg/min	72	36	18	9
80 mcg/min	96	48	24	12
120 mcg/min	—	72	36	18
160 mcg/min	—	96	48	24
240 mcg/min	—	—	72	36
320 mcg/min	—	—	96	48
480 mcg/min	—	—	—	72
640 mcg/min	—	—	—	96

ACTIONS

A vascular smooth-muscle relaxant and vasodilator. Affects arterial and venous beds. Reduces myocardial oxygen consumption, preload, and afterload by reducing systolic, diastolic, and mean arterial blood pressure; central venous and pulmonary capillary wedge pressures; and pulmonary and systemic vascular resistance. Effective coronary perfusion is usually maintained. Low doses (30 to 40 mcg/min) produce venodilation; high doses (150 to 500 mcg/min) produce arteriolar dilation. Widely distributed throughout the body. Onset of action occurs in 1 to 2 minutes and lasts 3 to 5 minutes. Metabolized in the liver and excreted in urine.

INDICATIONS AND USES

Control of BP in perioperative hypertension (especially cardiovascular procedures). ■ Drug of choice in unstable angina or congestive heart failure associated with acute myocardial infarction. May be used in combination with dobutamine 2 to 20 mcg/kg/min to produce hemodynamic improvement while reducing risk of ischemic damage. ■ Treatment of angina pectoris if patient unresponsive to therapeutic doses of organic nitrates and/or a beta-blocker. ■ Controlled hypotension during surgical procedures.

CONTRAINDICATIONS

Anemia (severe), hypersensitivity to nitrates, hypotension or uncorrected hypovolemia, cerebral hemorrhage, closed-angle glaucoma, head trauma, increased intracranial pressure, patients taking sildenafil (Viagra), pericardial tamponade, constrictive pericarditis.

PRECAUTIONS

Special tubing causes problems with infusion pump control. Patient may still be receiving nitroglycerin IV even though pump is off or tubing clamped. Low flow rates may

N-O

actually be higher and not deliver accurate dosage. ▪ Plastic (polyvinyl chloride) tubing or containers will absorb up to 80% of diluted nitroglycerin IV. Use extreme caution and adjust dose if changing infusion equipment (e.g., IV tubing, extension tubing). Absorption greatest with slowest rate. ▪ If changing preparations from 0.8 mg/mL to 5 mg/mL, use new tubing or clear tubing with a minimum of 15 mL, adjust dose carefully, and observe effects. ▪ Use caution in patients with low left ventricular filling pressure or low pulmonary capillary wedge pressure. May have exaggerated response to low dosage. ▪ Use caution in hepatic or renal disease, pericarditis, or postural hypotension.

Monitor: Maintain adequate systemic BP and coronary perfusion pressure. HR and BP measurements mandatory; pulmonary wedge pressure recommended. ▪ Observe for tachycardia, which can decrease diastolic filling time. ▪ Observe for fall in pulmonary wedge pressure. Precedes arterial hypotension and impending shock. Reduce or discontinue drug temporarily. ▪ Headache may improve with analgesics or slightly lower dose; usually improves with time. ▪ See Drug/Lab Interactions.

Maternal/Child: Category C: safety for use in pregnancy, breast-feeding, and in pediatric patients not established.

Elderly: Hypotensive effects may be increased. ▪ Differences in response compared to younger patients not identified. ▪ Lower-end initial doses may be indicated; see Dose Adjustments.

DRUG/LAB INTERACTIONS

May cause irreversible hypotension if given within 24 to 48 hours of **impotence agents** (e.g., sildenafil citrate [Viagra, Revatio], tadalafil [Cialis], vardenafil [Levitra]). ▪ Potentiated by **alcohol** (may cause hypotension and cardiovascular collapse), **antihypertensives, aspirin, beta-adrenergic blockers** (e.g., propranolol), **other vasodilators, phenothiazines** (e.g., prochlorperazine [Compazine]), **and tricyclic antidepressants.** ▪ Inhibited by **dihydroergotamine and sympathomimetics** (e.g., vasopressors [phenylephrine], bronchodilators, decongestants, glaucoma agents, mydriatics). ▪ Inhibits **acetylcholine, histamine, norepinephrine.** ▪ Potentiates **nondepolarizing muscle relaxants** (e.g., atracurium [Tracrium]); may cause apnea. ▪ May cause marked orthostatic hypotension with **calcium channel blockers** (e.g., verapamil). ▪ May antagonize anticoagulant effects of **heparin;** monitor. ▪ Concurrent use with **alteplase** (tPA) reduces the thrombolytic effects of alteplase.

SIDE EFFECTS

Abdominal pain, angina, apprehension, dizziness, headache, hypersensitivity reactions (e.g., itching, tracheobronchitis, wheezing), hypotension, methemoglobinemia, muscle twitching, nausea, palpitations, postural hypotension, restlessness, retrosternal discomfort, tachycardia, vomiting.

Overdose: Bloody diarrhea, colic, confusion, diaphoresis, dyspnea, flushing, heart block, paralysis, tachycardia, visual disturbances. Severe hypotension may result in shock, reflex paradoxical bradycardia, inadequate cerebral circulation, constrictive pericarditis, pericardial tamponade, decreased organ perfusion, and death.

ANTIDOTE

Notify physician of all side effects. Discontinue if blurred vision or dry mouth occur. For accidental overdose with severe hypotension and reflex tachycardia and/or fall in pulmonary wedge pressure, reduce rate or temporarily discontinue until condition stabilizes. Lower head of bed (Trendelenburg position). Administer IV fluids. Use O_2 and assisted ventilation if indicated. An alpha-adrenergic agonist (e.g., phenylephrine [Neo-Synephrine]) is rarely required. Epinephrine and related compounds (dopamine) are contraindicated. Monitor levels and treat methemoglobinemia if indicated with methylene blue 0.2 mL/kg of body weight (1 to 2 mg/kg) IV and high-flow oxygen. Treat anaphylaxis and resuscitate as necessary.

NITROPRUSSIDE SODIUM BBW
(nye-troh-**PRUS**-eyed **SO**-dee-um)

Antihypertensive
Vasodilator

Nitropress

pH 3.5 to 6

USUAL DOSE
Begin with 0.25 to 0.3 mcg/kg of body weight/min. Under continuous BP monitoring, titrate upward very gradually (small increments every 2 to 3 minutes). 3 mcg/kg/min is the average effective dose; range is 0.1 to 10 mcg/kg/min. AHA guidelines recommend beginning with 0.1 mcg/kg/min. Titrate upward every 3 to 5 minutes to desired effect (up to 5 mcg/kg/min). Small adjustments can lead to major fluctuations in BP. Never exceed 10 mcg/kg/min. If 10 mcg/kg/min does not promote adequate BP reduction in 10 minutes, discontinue administration and use another antihypertensive agent. Cyanide toxicity can occur with as little as 2 mcg/kg/min and could begin to occur after 10 minutes at the maximum dose.

Acute CHF: Titrate as described previously until one of the following occurs: cardiac output is no longer increasing, perfusion of vital organs would be compromised by further reduction of BP, or maximum infusion rate (10 mcg/kg/min) is reached.

PEDIATRIC DOSE
Begin with 0.3 mcg/kg/min. Adjust slowly to individual response as in Usual Dose. AHA guidelines recommend 0.3 to 1 mcg/kg/min initially; titrate up to 8 mcg/kg/min as needed.

DOSE ADJUSTMENTS
Average effective dose may be as little as 0.5 mcg/kg/min in patients who are receiving other antihypertensive agents by any route. ▪ Reduced dose may be required in the elderly.

DILUTION
Available in a liquid formulation (25 mg/mL), or each 50 mg must be reconstituted with 2 to 3 mL of D5W or SWFI without a preservative. Must be further diluted in a minimum of 250 mL of D5W (manufacturer's recommendation). JAMA suggests NS may be used. Must be administered as an infusion. Larger amounts of solution may be used. 50 mg in 250 mL equals 200 mcg/mL. 50 mg in 500 mL equals 100 mcg/mL. Immediately after mixing, wrap infusion bottle in opaque material (e.g., aluminum foil) to protect from light. Use only freshly prepared solutions; usually discard infusion within 4 hours of mixing. (Literature now states, "Stable for 24 hours if properly protected.") ▪ Solution has a faint brownish tint; discard immediately if highly colored, blue, green, or dark red.

Pediatric dilution: Add 0.6 mg/kg to 100 mL diluent. 1 mL/hr equals 0.1 mcg/kg/min.

COMPATIBILITY   (Underline Indicates Conflicting Compatibility Information)
Consider any drug NOT listed as compatible to be INCOMPATIBLE until consulting a pharmacist; specific conditions may apply.

One source suggests the following **compatibilities:**

Additive: Enalaprilat (Vasotec IV), ranitidine (Zantac), verapamil.

Y-site: Alprostadil, <u>amiodarone (Nexterone)</u>, argatroban, atracurium (Tracrium), bivalirudin (Angiomax), calcium chloride, <u>cisatracurium (Nimbex)</u>, dexmedetomidine (Precedex), diltiazem (Cardizem), <u>dobutamine</u>, dopamine, enalaprilat (Vasotec IV), epinephrine (Adrenalin), esmolol (Brevibloc), famotidine (Pepcid IV), furosemide (Lasix), heparin, hetastarch in electrolytes (Hextend), indomethacin (Indocin IV), insulin (regular), isoproterenol (Isuprel), labetalol, lidocaine, magnesium sulfate, metoprolol (Lopressor), <u>micafungin (Mycamine)</u>, midazolam (Versed), milrinone (Primacor), morphine, nesiritide (Natrecor), <u>nicardipine (Cardene IV)</u>, nitroglycerin IV, norepinephrine (Levophed), pancuronium, potassium chloride (KCl), potassium phosphates, procainamide (Pronestyl), propofol (Diprivan), tacrolimus (Prograf), theophylline, vecuronium.

N-O

RATE OF ADMINISTRATION

Use of an infusion pump (volumetric preferred) required to regulate dose accurately. Increase mcg/kg/min rate as outlined in Usual Dose to reduce BP gradually to preset or desired levels. Do not exceed maximum dose. Response should be noted almost immediately. Manufacturer provides the following infusion rate chart in mL/hr to achieve initial (0.3 mcg/kg/min) and maximal (10 mcg/kg/min) for 50-, 100-, and 200-mcg/mL dilutions.

Nitroprusside Sodium Guidelines for Infusion							
Volume	250 mL		500 mL		1,000 mL		
Nitroprusside Sodium	50 mg		50 mg		50 mg		
Injection Concentration	200 mcg/mL		100 mcg/mL		50 mcg/mL		
Patient Weight	Infusion Rate (mL/hr)						
kg	lbs	Initial	Maximum	Initial	Maximum	Initial	Maximum
10	22	1	30	2	60	4	120
20	44	2	60	4	120	7	240
30	66	3	90	5	180	11	360
40	88	4	120	7	240	14	480
50	110	5	150	9	300	18	600
60	132	5	180	11	360	22	720
70	154	6	210	13	420	25	840
80	176	7	240	14	480	29	960
90	198	8	270	16	540	32	1,080
100	220	9	300	18	600	36	1,200

ACTIONS

A potent, rapid-acting antihypertensive agent. Produces peripheral vasodilation through direct action on smooth muscle of the blood vessels. Effective almost immediately. Will lower diastolic BP 30% to 40% or more below pretreatment levels. May increase HR and/or cardiac output slightly. Effectiveness ends when IV infusion is stopped. BP will return to pretreatment levels in 1 to 10 minutes. Rapidly converted to thiocyanate and eventually excreted in the urine.

INDICATIONS AND USES

Drug of choice for hypertensive emergencies. ▪ Cardiogenic shock. ▪ Controlled hypotension during surgery. ▪ Acute congestive heart failure.

Unlabeled uses: In combination with dopamine to reduce afterload in hypertensive patient with myocardial infarction. ▪ Treatment of left ventricular failure in combination with oxygen, morphine, and a loop diuretic.

CONTRAINDICATIONS

Compensatory hypertension (e.g., arteriovenous shunt or coarctation of the aorta); known inadequate cerebral circulation; emergency surgery on moribund patients.

PRECAUTIONS

Use only when adequate personnel and appropriate equipment are available for continuous monitoring. ▪ Precipitous decreases in BP can occur quickly. Can lead to irreversible ischemic injuries or death. ▪ Cyanide toxicity can occur with doses less than the average effective dose and will begin to occur as the maximum dose of 10 mcg/kg/min is approached. May be rapid, serious, and lethal. ▪ Methemoglobinemia may begin to occur within 16 hours if larger doses are required. ▪ Use caution in hypothyroidism, increased intracranial pressure, liver or renal impairment, and the elderly. ▪ May increase ischemia in myocardial infarction.

Monitor: Determine patency of vein; avoid extravasation. ▪ Continuous automatic BP monitoring is mandatory (intra-arterial pressure sensor preferred). Never allow systolic BP to fall below 60 mm Hg. ▪ Monitor pulmonary wedge pressure in patients with myocardial infarction or severe congestive heart failure. ▪ Monitor acid/base balance and venous oxygen concentration; may indicate cyanide toxicity. ▪ Oral antihypertensive agents may be given concomitantly to maintain ongoing BP regulation. Reduced nitroprusside sodium dose may be indicated; see Dose Adjustments. ▪ Measure blood thiocyanate levels daily if dose is 3 mcg/kg/min (1 mcg/kg/min in the anuric patient). Desired level of steady-state thiocyanate is less than 1 mmol/L. Coadministration of sodium thiosulfate in doses 5 to 10 times that of nitroprusside sodium has been used to avoid toxicity with larger doses or necessary long-term therapy. May potentiate hypotensive action; use with extreme caution. ▪ In controlled hypotension, monitor blood loss and correct hypovolemia before and during surgery. ▪ Persistent hypotension (lasting more than 1 to 10 minutes) after nitroprusside sodium is discontinued is due to another source. Monitor for sodium retention.

Patient Education: Report IV site burning or stinging promptly. ▪ Request assistance to ambulate.

Maternal/Child: Category C: safety for use in pregnancy and in pediatric patients not yet established. Has caused cyanide toxicity in fetuses of ewes, but not in humans. ▪ Discontinue breast-feeding.

Elderly: See Dose Adjustments and Precautions. ▪ Hypotensive effects may be increased. ▪ Consider age-related renal impairment.

DRUG/LAB INTERACTIONS

Potentiated by **ganglionic blocking agents** (e.g., trimethaphan [Arfonad]), **volatile liquid anesthesia** (e.g., halothane), **and circulatory depressants.** ▪ Will cause profound hypotension with **diazoxide.**

SIDE EFFECTS

Usually occur with too-rapid rate of infusion and are reversible: abdominal pain, apprehension, bradycardia, coma, decreased platelet aggregation, diaphoresis, dizziness, ECG changes, flushing, headache, hypotension (profound), ileus, increased intracranial pressure, muscle twitching, nausea, palpitations, rash, restlessness, retching, retrosternal discomfort, venous streaking. With prolonged therapy or overdose, cyanide intoxication (air hunger, bright red venous blood, confusion, elevated cyanide levels, marked clinical deterioration, metabolic acidosis, and death), hypothyroidism, or methemoglobinemia (chocolate-brown blood, impaired oxygen delivery even though cardiac output and arterial Po_2 are adequate) can occur.

ANTIDOTE

At first sign of side effects, decrease rate of administration. Never allow systolic BP to fall below 60 mm Hg. If BP begins to rise or side effects persist, notify the physician. Hemodialysis or peritoneal dialysis may be indicated for thiocyanate levels over 10 mg/dL. For massive overdose with signs of cyanide toxicity or tachyphylaxis, discontinue nitroprusside sodium. Cyanide antidote kits contain all needed medications (see sodium nitrite/sodium thiosulfate monograph on the Evolve website for complete information). Administer amyl nitrite inhalations for 15 to 30 seconds each minute until 3% sodium nitrite solution can be initiated as an IV infusion or immediately start the infusion over 2 to 4 minutes (4 to 6 mg/kg). Monitor BP carefully; may cause hypotension that will also require treatment. Next, inject sodium thiosulfate 150 to 200 mg/kg (usually about 12.5 Gm or 50 mL of the 25% solution) in 50 mL of 5% dextrose in water IV over 10 minutes. Observe patient. If signs of overdose reappear, may repeat the previously described process after 2 hours; but use one half the original dosage. Sodium nitrite provides a buffer for cyanide by converting HgB into methemoglobin; sodium thiosulfate converts cyanide into thiocyanate, which is then excreted in urine. For hypotension, slow or discontinue the IV and put the patient in Trendelenburg position. Should improve in 1 to 10 minutes. Correct hypotension with vasopressors (e.g., dopamine). Treat methemoglobinemia with methylene blue 1 to 2 mg/kg. Use with caution if considerable amounts of cyanide are bound to methemoglobin.

NIVOLUMAB
(nye-**VOL**-ue-mab)

Opdivo

Antineoplastic
(Monoclonal antibody)

pH 6

USUAL DOSE
Melanoma (single agent): 3 mg/kg administered as an IV infusion over 60 minutes every 2 weeks until disease progression or unacceptable toxicity.

Melanoma in combination with ipilimumab: 1 mg/kg as an intravenous infusion over 60 minutes, followed by ipilimumab on the same day every 3 weeks for 4 doses. The recommended subsequent dose of nivolumab as a single agent is 3 mg/kg administered as an IV infusion over 60 minutes every 2 weeks until disease progression or unacceptable toxicity; see Rate of Administration.

Classical Hodgkin lymphoma (cHL), non–small-cell lung cancer (NSCLC), and renal cell carcinoma (RCC): 3 mg/kg administered as an IV infusion over 60 minutes every 2 weeks until disease progression or unacceptable toxicity.

DOSE ADJUSTMENTS
Recommendations for dose modifications are provided in the following chart.

Recommended Dose Modifications for Nivolumab		
Adverse Reaction	Severity*	Dose Modification
Colitis	Grade 2 diarrhea or colitis	Withhold dose†
	Grade 3 diarrhea or colitis	Withhold dose† when administered as a single agent
		Permanently discontinue when administered with ipilimumab
	Grade 4 diarrhea or colitis	Permanently discontinue
Pneumonitis	Grade 2 pneumonitis	Withhold dose†
	Grade 3 or 4 pneumonitis	Permanently discontinue
Hepatitis	AST or ALT more than 3 and up to 5 times the ULN or total bilirubin more than 1.5 and up to 3 times the ULN	Withhold dose†
	AST or ALT more than 5 times the ULN or total bilirubin more than 3 times the ULN	Permanently discontinue
Hypophysitis	Grade 2 or 3 hypophysitis	Withhold dose†
	Grade 4 hypophysitis	Permanently discontinue
Adrenal insufficiency	Grade 2 adrenal insufficiency	Withhold dose†
	Grade 3 or 4 adrenal insufficiency	Permanently discontinue
Type 1 diabetes mellitus	Grade 3 hyperglycemia	Withhold dose†
	Grade 4 hyperglycemia	Permanently discontinue
Nephritis and renal dysfunction	SCr more than 1.5 and up to 6 times the ULN	Withhold dose†
	SCr more than 6 times the ULN	Permanently discontinue
Rash	Grade 3 rash	Withhold dose†
	Grade 4 rash	Permanently discontinue
Encephalitis	New-onset moderate or severe neurologic S/S	Withhold dose†
	Immune-mediated encephalitis	Permanently discontinue

Continued

Recommended Dose Modifications for Nivolumab—cont'd		
Adverse Reaction	Severity*	Dose Modification
Other	Other Grade 3 adverse reaction First occurrence Recurrence of the same Grade 3 adverse reaction	Withhold dose† Permanently discontinue
	Life-threatening or Grade 4 adverse reaction	Permanently discontinue
	Requirement of 10 mg/day or greater prednisone or equivalent for more than 12 weeks	Permanently discontinue
	Persistent Grade 2 or 3 adverse reactions lasting 12 weeks or longer	Permanently discontinue

*Toxicity graded per National Cancer Institute Common Terminology Criteria for Adverse Events, v4.0 (NCI CTCAE v4).
†Resume treatment when adverse reactions return to Grade 0 or 1.

When nivolumab is administered in combination with ipilimumab, ipilimumab should be withheld if nivolumab is withheld. ▪ No recommended dose modifications for hypothyroidism or hyperthyroidism. ▪ No dose adjustment is recommended in patients with pre-existing renal impairment or mild hepatic impairment. ▪ See Monitor and Antidote.

DILUTION
Available as a solution in single-use vials containing 40 mg/4 mL or 100 mg/10 mL (10 mg/mL). Discard the vial if the solution is cloudy, discolored, or contains extraneous particulate matter other than a few translucent-to-white, proteinaceous particles. Calculate the number of vials required for the recommended dose, and withdraw the required volume of nivolumab and transfer into an IV bag or container of NS or D5W to prepare an infusion with a final concentration ranging from 1 to 10 mg/mL. Mix diluted solution by gentle inversion. *Do not shake.* A 3-mg/kg dose for a 70-kg patient would require 210 mg of 10-mg/mL solution (21 mL). 21 mL of nivolumab added to 189 mL of NS or D5W would make a 1-mg/mL solution. Dilution of this 210-mg dose in 50 mL or 100 mL of NS would still be within the required concentration limits.

Filters: Must be administered using IV tubing that contains a sterile, nonpyrogenic, low–protein-binding, in-line filter (pore size of 0.2 to 1.2 micrometers).

Storage: Before use, refrigerate at 2° to 8° C (36° to 46° F) in original package to protect from light. Do not freeze or shake. Nivolumab does not contain a preservative. After preparation, store the prepared infusion at room temperature for no more than 4 hours or refrigerate for no more than 24 hours from the time of preparation. Administration time is included in storage time. Do not freeze. Discard partially used vials.

COMPATIBILITY
Manufacturer states, "Do not coadminister other drugs through the same intravenous line."

RATE OF ADMINISTRATION
A single dose as an infusion equally distributed over 60 minutes. Interrupt or slow rate of administration in patients with mild or moderate infusion reactions. If a common IV line is used to administer other drugs in addition to nivolumab, flush the IV line before and after each nivolumab infusion with NS or D5W. Administer through an IV tubing that contains a sterile, nonpyrogenic, low–protein-binding, in-line filter (pore size of 0.2 to 1.2 micrometers). When administered in combination with ipilimumab, infuse nivolumab first, followed by ipilimumab on the same day. Use separate infusion bags and filters for each infusion.

ACTIONS
An antineoplastic agent. Nivolumab is a human immunoglobulin G4 (IgG4) monoclonal antibody that binds to the PD-1 receptor and blocks its interaction with PD-L1 and PD-L2, thereby releasing PD-1 pathway–mediated inhibition of the immune response, including the antitumor immune response. In syngeneic mouse tumor models, blocking PD-1 activity resulted in decreased tumor growth. Mean elimination half-life is

26.7 days. Steady-state concentrations were reached by 12 weeks when administered at 3 mg/kg every 2 weeks. Clearance of nivolumab increases with increasing body weight supporting a weight-based dose. Analysis suggested that age (29 to 87 years), gender, race, baseline LDH, PD-L1 expression, tumor type, tumor size, renal impairment, and mild hepatic impairment had no effect on the clearance of nivolumab.

INDICATIONS AND USES

As a single agent for the treatment of patients with BRAF V600 wild-type unresectable or metastatic melanoma. ▪ As a single agent for the treatment of patients with BRAF V600 mutation–positive unresectable or metastatic melanoma; see Limitation of Use. ▪ In combination with ipilimumab (Yervoy) for the treatment of patients with unresectable or metastatic melanoma; see Limitation of Use. ▪ Treatment of patients with metastatic non–small-cell lung cancer (NSCLC) with progression on or after platinum-based chemotherapy. Before receiving nivolumab, patients with EGFR or ALK genomic tumor aberrations should have experienced disease progression while undergoing FDA-approved therapy for these aberrations. ▪ Treatment of patients with advanced renal cell carcinoma (RCC) who have received prior antiangiogenic therapy. ▪ Treatment of patients with classical Hodgkin lymphoma (cHL) that has relapsed or progressed after autologous hematopoietic stem cell transplantation (HSCT) and posttransplantation brentuximab vedotin (Adcetris); see Limitation of Use.

Limitation of use: Specified indications have received accelerated approval. This accelerated approval is based on progression-free survival or overall response rate. Continued approval may be contingent on verification and descriptioni of clinical benefit in the confirmatory trials.

CONTRAINDICATIONS

Manufacturer states, "None."

PRECAUTIONS

Severe pneumonitis or interstitial lung disease, including fatal cases, has occurred with nivolumab treatment. ▪ Severe diarrhea and colitis have been reported. ▪ Immune-mediated hepatitis and liver test abnormalities (elevated ALT, AST, alkaline phosphatase, total bilirubin) have occurred with nivolumab treatment. ▪ Elevated serum creatinine and immune-mediated nephritis have occurred with nivolumab treatment. ▪ Pneumonitis, colitis, hepatitis, and nephritis (renal dysfunction equal to or greater than Grade 2 increased SCr) were defined as immune-mediated when corticosteroids were required for treatment and there was no clear alternate etiology. ▪ Immune-mediated endocrinopathies, including hypophysitis, adrenal insufficiency, type 1 diabetes mellitus (with possible diabetic ketoacidosis), hypothyroidism, and hyperthyroidism, have been reported. ▪ Immune-mediated rash can occur. Rare cases of toxic epidermal necrolysis (TEN) have been reported. ▪ Immune-mediated encephalitis can occur with nivolumab treatment. ▪ Numerous other immune-mediated adverse reactions were reported in fewer than 1% of patients. ▪ Severe infusion reactions have been reported. ▪ Complications (e.g., severe or hyperacute graft-versus-host disease (GVHD), steroid-requiring febrile syndrome, hepatic veno-occlusive disease [VOD]), including fatal events, occurred in patients who received allogenic HSCT after nivolumab. ▪ See Dose Adjustments, Monitor, and Antidote for required Dose Adjustments, indicated criteria and medications for treatment, and criteria for discontinuation of nivolumab. ▪ Nivolumab has not been studied in patients with moderate or severe hepatic impairment. ▪ A protein substance; has a potential for immunogenicity.

Monitor: Obtain serum electrolytes, baseline liver function tests (e.g., ALT, AST, alkaline phosphatase, total bilirubin), serum creatinine, and thyroid function tests before initiating treatment, and monitor periodically during treatment and as indicated based on clinical evaluation. ▪ Monitor for infusion reactions; see Rate of Administration and Antidote. ▪ Monitor patients for S/S of pneumonitis (e.g., abnormal chest x-ray, chest pain, new or worsening cough, or shortness of breath). Administer corticosteroids at a dose of 1 to 2 mg/kg/day prednisone equivalents for moderate (Grade 2) or greater pneumonitis, followed by corticosteroid taper. Withhold nivolumab until resolution for moderate (Grade 2) pneumonitis; see Dose Adjustments and Antidote. ▪ Monitor patients for immune-mediated colitis. Administer corticosteroids at a dose of 1 to 2 mg/kg/day prednisone equivalents followed by corticosteroid taper for severe (Grade 3) or life-threatening (Grade 4) colitis. Administer corticosteroids at a dose of 0.5 to 1 mg/kg/day prednisone equivalents followed by corticosteroid taper for moderate (Grade 2) colitis of more than 5 days' duration; if worsening or no improvement occurs despite initiation of corticosteroids, increase dose to 1 to 2 mg/kg/day prednisone equivalents. Withhold nivolumab for moderate (Grade 2) or severe (Grade 3) immune-mediated colitis when used as a single agent or for moderate (Grade 2) colitis when used in combination with ipilimumab; see Dose Adjustments and Antidote. ▪ Monitor for S/S of hepatitis (e.g., easy bruising or bleeding, jaundice, lethargy, pain on the right side of the abdomen, severe nausea or vomiting, abnormal LFTs). Administer corticosteroids at a dose of 0.5 to 1 mg/kg/day prednisone equivalents for moderate (Grade 2) transaminase elevations, with or without concomitant elevations in total bilirubin. Administer corticosteroids at a dose of 1 to 2 mg/kg/day prednisone equivalents for severe (Grade 3) or life-threatening (Grade 4) transaminase elevations, with or without concomitant elevations in total bilirubin. Withhold nivolumab for moderate (Grade 2) immune-mediated hepatitis; see Dose Adjustments and Antidote. ▪ Monitor renal function periodically. For moderate (Grade 2) or severe (Grade 3) SCr elevation, withhold nivolumab and administer corticosteroids at a dose of 0.5 to 1 mg/kg/day prednisone equivalents followed by corticosteroid taper; if worsening or no improvement occurs, increase dose of corticosteroids to 1 to 2 mg/kg/day prednisone equivalents and permanently discontinue nivolumab. Administer corticosteroids at a dose of 1 to 2 mg/kg/day prednisone equivalents followed by corticosteroid taper for life-threatening (Grade 4) SCr elevation, and permanently discontinue nivolumab; see Dose Adjustments and Antidote. ▪ Monitor for S/S of hypophysitis (e.g., fatigue, headache, low levels of the hormones produced by the pituitary [adrenocorticotropic hormone (ACTH), thyroid-stimulating hormone (TSH), follicle-stimulating hormone (FSH), luteinizing hormone (LH), growth hormone (GH), prolactin]). Administer corticosteroids at a dose of 1 mg/kg/day prednisone equivalents for moderate (Grade 2) or higher hypophysitis. Withhold nivolumab for moderate (Grade 2) or severe (Grade 3) hypophysitis; see Dose Adjustments and Antidote. ▪ Monitor for S/S of adrenal insufficiency (e.g., fatigue, nausea, vomiting, hypotension, hyponatremia, hyperkalemia, low cortisol concentrations). Administer corticosteroids at a dose of 1 to 2 mg/kg/day prednisone equivalents for severe (Grade 3) or life-threatening (Grade 4) adrenal insufficiency. Withhold nivolumab for moderate (Grade 2) adrenal insufficiency; see Dose Adjustments and Antidote. ▪ Monitor for changes in thyroid function. Administer hormone replacement therapy for hypothyroidism. Initiate medical management for control of hyperthyroidism; see Dose Adjustments and Antidote. ▪ Monitor for hyperglycemia. Administer insulin when clinically indicated. Withhold nivolumab for severe (Grade 3) hyperglycemia until metabolic control is achieved; see Dose Adjustments and Antidote. ▪ Monitor for development of a rash. Administer corticosteroids at a dose of 1 to 2 mg/kg/day prednisone equivalents for severe (Grade 3) or life-threatening (Grade 4) rash. Withhold nivolumab for severe (Grade 3) rash; see Dose Adjustments and Antidote. ▪ Monitor for changes in neurologic status. Withhold nivolumab in patients with new-onset moderate to severe neurologic signs or symptoms. Evaluate patient to rule out infectious or other causes of moderate to severe neurologic deterioration. Evaluation may include, but is not limited to, consultation with a neurologist, brain MRI, and lumbar puncture. If other etiologies are ruled out, administer corticosteroids at a dose of 1 to 2 mg/kg/day prednisone equivalents, followed by a prednisone taper; see Dose Adjustments and Antidote. ▪ Monitor patient for any clinically significant immune-mediated adverse reactions. Immune-mediated adverse reactions may occur after nivolumab is discontinued. Examples of other immune-mediated adverse reactions that have occurred include autoimmune neuropathy, demyelination, duodenitis, facial and abducens nerve paresis, gastritis, Guillain-Barré syndrome, hypopituitarism, motor dysfunction, myasthenic syndrome, pancreatitis, polymyalgia rheumatica, sarcoidosis, systemic inflammatory response syndrome, uveitis, and vasculitis. For any suspected immune-mediated adverse reactions, exclude other causes. Based on the severity of the adverse reaction, withhold or discontinue nivolumab, administer high-dose cortico-steroids and, if appropriate, initiate hormone-replacement therapy. Upon improvement to Grade 1 or less, initiate corticosteroid taper and continue to taper over at least 1 month. Consider restarting nivolumab after completion of corticosteroid taper based on the severity of the event. ▪ Monitor for early evidence of transplant-related complications such as hyperacute GVHD, severe acute GVHD, steroid-requiring febrile syndrome, hepatic VOD, and other immune-mediated adverse reactions, and intervene promptly.

Patient Education: Review manufacturer's medication guide. ▪ Effective contraception required during treatment with nivolumab and for at least 5 months following the last dose of nivolumab. ▪ Promptly report a known or suspected pregnancy. ▪ Some side effects may require corticosteroid treatment and interruption or discontinuation of nivolumab. ▪ Promptly report S/S of pneumonitis (e.g., chest pain, new or worsening cough, or short-ness of breath). ▪ Promptly report S/S of colitis (e.g., diarrhea or severe abdominal pain). ▪ Promptly report S/S of hepatitis (e.g., easy bruising or bleeding, jaundice, lethargy, pain on the right side of the abdomen, severe nausea or vomiting). ▪ Promptly report S/S of kidney dysfunction (e.g., blood in urine, decreased urine output, loss of appetite, swelling in ankles). ▪ Promptly report S/S of hypophysitis, adrenal insufficiency, hypothyroidism, hyperthyroidism, or diabetes mellitus; see Monitor. ▪ Promptly report S/S of encephali-tis; see Monitor. ▪ Promptly report development of a rash. ▪ Keeping scheduled ap-pointments for blood work or other laboratory tests is imperative.

Maternal/Child: Avoid pregnancy. Based on mechanism of action and data from animal stud-ies, nivolumab can cause fetal harm when administered to a pregnant woman. Human IgG4 is known to cross the placental barrier, and nivolumab is an IgG4. Effects of nivolumab are likely to be greater during the second and third trimesters of pregnancy. ▪ Discontinue breast-feeding. ▪ Safety and effectiveness for use in pediatric patients not established.

Elderly: No overall differences in safety or efficacy were reported between elderly patients and younger patients.

DRUG/LAB INTERACTIONS
No formal pharmacokinetic drug-drug interaction studies conducted with nivolumab.

SIDE EFFECTS
Several immune-mediated reactions have been reported, including colitis, encephalitis, endocrinopathies, hepatitis, nephritis and renal dysfunction, pneumonitis, and rash; see Precautions, Monitor, and Antidote.

Melanoma: *Single agent:* The most common adverse reactions were diarrhea, fatigue, mus-culoskeletal pain, nausea, pruritus, and rash. ***Combination therapy:*** The most common adverse reactions were diarrhea, dyspnea, fatigue, fever, nausea, rash, and vomiting. Other reported side effects in melanoma patients included anemia, cough, dizziness, edema, erythema multiforme, exfoliative dermatitis, infusion-related reactions, intestinal perforation, iridocyclitis, lymphopenia, myopathy, neuritis, peripheral edema, peripheral and sensory neuropathy, peroneal nerve palsy, pruritus, psoriasis, Sjögren's syndrome, spondyloarthropathy, stomatitis, upper respiratory tract infection, ventricular arrhythmia, and vitiligo. Laboratory abnormalities occurring in 10% or more of nivolumab-treated patients were hyperkalemia, hypocalcemia, hyponatremia, and increased alkaline phos-phate, ALT, amylase, AST, bilirubin, creatinine, and lipase.

NSCLC: The most common adverse reactions were constipation, cough, decreased appe-tite, dyspnea, fatigue, and musculoskeletal pain. Other commonly reported or clinically significant side effects included asthenia, infection, pleural effusion, pneumonia, poly-myalgia rheumatica, pulmonary embolism, respiratory failure, and urticaria. Laboratory abnormalities occurring in 10% or more of patients were hyponatremia and increased AST, alkaline phosphatase, ALT, creatinine, and TSH.

RCC: The most common adverse reactions were arthralgia, asthenic conditions, back pain, constipation, cough, decreased appetite, diarrhea, dyspnea, headache, nausea, and rash. Other commonly reported or clinically significant side effects included abdominal pain, acute kidney injury, anemia, edema, fever, lymphopenia, musculoskeletal pain, palmar-plantar erythrodysesthesia, peripheral neuropathy, pleural effusion, pneumonia, pruritus, upper respiratory tract infection, vomiting, and weight loss. Laboratory abnormalities occurring in 15% or more of patients treated with nivolumab were hyperkalemia, hypocalcemia, hyponatremia, and increased alkaline phosphate, ALT, AST, cholesterol, creatinine, triglycerides, and TSH.

cHL: The most common adverse reactions were cough, diarrhea, fatigue, fever, and upper respiratory tract infections.

ANTIDOTE

Keep physician informed of all side effects. May constitute a medical emergency or will be treated symptomatically as indicated. Interrupt or slow the rate of administration in patients with mild or moderate infusion reactions. Discontinue in patients with a severe or life-threatening infusion reaction and treat as indicated. Permanently discontinue nivolumab in patients with any of the following: (1) any life-threatening or Grade 4 adverse reaction, (2) Grade 3 or 4 pneumonitis, (3) Grade 4 colitis or recurrent colitis upon restarting nivolumab when used as a single agent or Grade 3 or 4 colitis or recurrent colitis upon restarting nivolumab when used in combination with ipilimumab, (4) AST or ALT greater than 5 times the ULN or total bilirubin greater than 3 times the ULN, (5) Grade 3 or Grade 4 immune-mediated hepatitis, (6) creatinine greater than 6 times the ULN, (7) any severe or Grade 3 treatment-related adverse reaction that recurs, (8) Grade 3 or Grade 4 adrenal insufficiency, (9) immune-mediated encephalitis, (10) inability to reduce corticosteroid dose to 10 mg or less of prednisone or equivalent per day within 12 weeks, or (11) persistent Grade 2 or 3 treatment-related adverse reactions that do not recover to Grade 1 or resolve within 12 weeks after last dose of nivolumab. Treat these side effects aggressively; see Precautions and Monitor.

NOREPINEPHRINE BITARTRATE `BBW`   Vasopressor
(**nor**-ep-ih-**NEF**-rin by-**TAR**-trayt)

Levarterenol Bitartrate, Levophed   pH 3 to 4.5

USUAL DOSE

8 to 12 mcg/min initially. Other clinicians suggest an initial dose of 0.5 to 1 mcg/min titrated to maintain the desired BP range. Usual maintenance dose is 2 to 4 mcg/min (AHA recommendation is 0.1 to 0.5 mcg/kg/min; titrate to response). Larger doses may be given safely as long as the patient remains hypotensive and blood volume depletion is corrected. Up to 30 mcg/min may be required in patients with refractory shock. 2 mg bitartrate equals 1 mg of norepinephrine. All doses are expressed in terms of norepinephrine.

PEDIATRIC DOSE

Safety and effectiveness for use in pediatric patients not established.

Begin with an initial dose of 0.05 to 0.1 mcg/kg/min as a continuous IV infusion. Titrate to desired effect up to a maximum dose of 2 mcg/kg/min. AHA recommends 0.1 to 2 mcg/kg/min in advanced life support.

DOSE ADJUSTMENTS

Lower-end initial doses may be indicated in the elderly based on potential for decreased organ function and concomitant disease or drug therapy.

DILUTION

Must be diluted in 250 to 1,000 mL of D5W or D5NS and given as infusion. 4 mg (4 mL) in 1 L of diluent equals 4 mcg/mL. Final concentration based on fluid volume requirements of the patient. Administration in a dextrose solution reduces loss of potency resulting from oxidation. NS without dextrose is not recommended. Phentolamine (Regitine) 5 to 10 mg and/or heparin sodium to provide 100 to 200 units/hr may be added to diluent to prevent any sloughing, necrosis, and/or thrombosis from slight leakage along the vein pathway.

Storage: Before dilution, store at CRT; protect from light.

COMPATIBILITY   (Underline Indicates Conflicting Compatibility Information)

Consider any drug NOT listed as compatible to be INCOMPATIBLE until consulting a pharmacist; specific conditions may apply.

Consult pharmacist; may be inactivated by solutions with a pH above 6. **Incompatible** with whole blood; administer through **Y-site** or a separate IV line. Avoid contact with iron salts, alkalis, or oxidizing agents.

One source suggests the following **compatibilities:**

Additive: Amikacin, calcium chloride, calcium gluconate, ciprofloxacin (Cipro IV), dimenhydrinate, dobutamine, heparin, hydrocortisone sodium succinate (SoluCortef), magnesium sulfate, meropenem (Merrem IV), methylprednisolone (SoluMedrol), multivitamins (M.V.I.), potassium chloride (KCl), ranitidine (Zantac), succinylcholine, verapamil.

Y-site: Amiodarone (Nexterone), anidulafungin (Eraxis), argatroban, bivalirudin (Angiomax), caspofungin (Cancidas), ceftaroline (Teflaro), cisatracurium (Nimbex), dexmedetomidine (Precedex), diltiazem (Cardizem), dobutamine, dopamine, doripenem (Doribax), epinephrine (Adrenalin), esmolol (Brevibloc), famotidine (Pepcid IV), fenoldopam (Corlopam), fentanyl, furosemide (Lasix), heparin, hetastarch in electrolytes (Hextend), hydrocortisone sodium succinate (Solu-Cortef), hydromorphone (Dilaudid), 6% hydroxyethyl starch (Voluven), labetalol, lorazepam (Ativan), meropenem (Merrem IV), micafungin (Mycamine), midazolam (Versed), milrinone (Primacor), morphine, mycophenolate mofetil (CellCept IV), nicardipine (Cardene IV), nitroglycerin IV, nitroprusside sodium, pantoprazole (Protonix IV), potassium chloride (KCl), propofol (Diprivan), ranitidine (Zantac), remifentanil (Ultiva), telavancin (Vibativ), vasopressin, vecuronium.

RATE OF ADMINISTRATION

See Usual Dose. Use the slowest possible flow rate to correct hypotension gradually and maintain adequate or preset BP. Some response should be noted within 1 to 2 minutes of IV administration. Use of an infusion pump or microdrip (60 gtt/mL) is an aid to correct evaluation of dose. Reduce infusion rate gradually. Avoid sudden discontinuation.

Norepinephrine (Levophed) Infusion Rate						
Desired Dose	4 mg in 1,000 mL D5W or D5NS 2 mg in 500 mL D5W or D5NS 4 mcg/mL			8 mg in 1,000 mL D5W or D5NS 4 mg in 500 mL D5W or D5NS 8 mcg/mL		
mcg/min	mcg/hr	mL/min	mL/hr	mcg/hr	mL/min	mL/hr
2 mcg/min	120	0.5	30	120	0.25	15
3 mcg/min	180	0.75	45	180	0.375	22.5
4 mcg/min	240	1	60	240	0.5	30
6 mcg/min	360	1.5	90	360	0.75	45
8 mcg/min	480	2	120	480	1	60
9 mcg/min	540	2.25	135	540	1.125	67.5
10 mcg/min	600	2.5	150	600	1.25	75
11 mcg/min	660	2.75	165	660	1.375	82.5
12 mcg/min	720	3	180	720	1.5	90

ACTIONS

Levarterenol is the levo-isomer of norepinephrine. It is a sympathomimetic drug that functions as a peripheral vasoconstrictor (alpha-adrenergic action) and inotropic stimulator of the heart and dilator of coronary arteries (beta-adrenergic action). Dilates the coronary arteries more than twice as much as epinephrine can. It is rapidly inactivated in the body by various enzymes and excreted in changed form in the urine.

INDICATIONS AND USES

All hypotensive states, including those associated with spinal anesthesia, blood reactions, drug reactions, hemorrhage, myocardial infarction, pheochromocytomectomy, septicemia, surgery, sympathectomy, and trauma. ▪ Adjunct in treatment of cardiac arrest and profound hypotension.

CONTRAINDICATIONS
Do not use in hypotension from blood loss unless an emergency, in mesenteric or peripheral vascular thrombosis, or with cyclopropane or halothane (inhalant) anesthesia.

PRECAUTIONS
Whole blood or plasma should be given in a separate IV site. May be given through Y-tube connection. ▪ Use caution in the elderly and in those with peripheral vascular disease or ischemic heart disease. ▪ Use caution in previously hypertensive patients; see Monitor. ▪ Use caution in patients with allergies; some formulations contain sulfites. ▪ Therapy may be continued until the patient can maintain own BP. Decrease dosage gradually.
Monitor: Check BP every 2 minutes until stabilized at the desired level. Check every 5 minutes thereafter during therapy. Avoid hypertension. One source suggests limiting rise in BP in previously hypertensive patients to no more than 40 mm Hg below previously systolic normal. ▪ Observe for hypovolemia and replace fluids immediately. In an emergency, norepinephrine can be effective in a hypovolemic state before fluid replacement has been accomplished. ▪ Check flow rate and injection site constantly. ▪ Infusion should be through a large vein, preferably the antecubital vein, to prevent complications of prolonged peripheral vasoconstriction. Avoid veins in the hands, ankles, and legs. Use of the femoral vein may be considered. ▪ Causes severe tissue necrosis, sloughing, and gangrene. Insert a plastic IV catheter or similar intravascular device at least 6 inches long well into the large vein chosen to prevent extravasation into any surrounding tissue; see Dilution. ▪ Blanching along the vein pathway is a preliminary sign of extravasation. Change the injection site. ▪ See Drug/Lab Interactions.
Patient Education: Report IV site burning or stinging promptly. ▪ Request assistance to ambulate.
Maternal/Child: Category C: use only if clearly needed; benefits must outweigh risks. ▪ Use caution in breast-feeding.
Elderly: See Precautions. ▪ Lower-end initial doses may be indicated; see Dose Adjustments. ▪ Differences in response versus younger patients not documented.

DRUG/LAB INTERACTIONS
Pressor effects may be potentiated by **amphetamines, anesthetics, antihistamines, tricyclic antidepressants** (e.g., desipramine [Norpramin]), **rauwolfia alkaloids** (e.g., reserpine), **thyroid preparations, and methylphenidate** (Ritalin). ▪ May cause severe hypertension with **ergot alkaloids and guanethidine** (Ismelin) and severe prolonged hypertension with **MAO inhibitors** (e.g., selegiline [Eldepryl]). ▪ May cause hypotension and bradycardia with **hydantoins** (e.g., phenytoin [Dilantin]). ▪ **Halogenated hydrocarbon anesthetics** (e.g., halothane) may cause serious arrhythmias. ▪ Interacts in numerous and sometimes contradictory ways with many drugs.

SIDE EFFECTS
Rare when used as directed; anxiety, arrhythmias (e.g., bradycardia and VT), chest pain, decreased cardiac output, dyspnea, headache, ischemia, necrosis caused by extravasation, pallor, photophobia, seizures, vomiting. Persistent headache may indicate overdose and severe hypertension. Gangrene has been reported.

ANTIDOTE
To prevent sloughing and necrosis in areas where extravasation has occurred, use a fine hypodermic needle to inject 5 to 10 mg of phentolamine (Regitine) diluted in 10 to 15 mL of NS liberally throughout the tissue in the extravasated area. Phentolamine causes immediate and conspicuous local hyperemic changes if the area is infiltrated within 12 hours. Treatment should be started as soon as extravasation is recognized. Atropine may be used to counteract the bradycardia. Notify physician of any side effect. Should a sudden or uncontrolled hypertensive state occur, discontinue levarterenol, notify the physician, and if necessary, treat with an adrenergic blocking agent (e.g., phentolamine [Regitine] or phenoxybenzamine [Dibenzyline]).

OBILTOXAXIMAB BBW

(oh-bil-tox-**AX**-i-mab)

Monoclonal antibody

Anthim

pH 5.5

USUAL DOSE

Premedication: Administer diphenhydramine (Benadryl) before infusing obiltoxaximab. Although it does not prevent anaphylaxis, it may decrease the occurrence of other reported adverse reactions.

Obiltoxaximab: A single dose of 16 mg/kg administered as an infusion over 90 minutes. See chart in Pediatric Dose for adults weighing less than 40 kg.

PEDIATRIC DOSE

Premedication: See Usual Dose.

See the following chart for recommended weight-based dosing.

Recommended Dose of Obiltoxaximab for Pediatric Patients and Adults Weighing Less Than 40 kg	
Body Weight	Dose
Greater than 40 kg	16 mg/kg
Greater than 15 to 40 kg	24 mg/kg
15 kg or less	32 mg/kg

DOSE ADJUSTMENTS

Age, gender, and race have no meaningful effect on the pharmacokinetics of obiltoxaximab.

DILUTION

Available in single-dose vials containing 600 mg/6 mL (100 mg/mL). A clear to opalescent, colorless to pale yellow to pale brownish-yellow solution that may contain a few translucent-to white proteinaceous particulates. *Do not shake.* Sterile technique imperative; contains no preservatives. Obiltoxaximab solution must be diluted with NS in an appropriately sized infusion bag or syringe depending on the total volume required. Calculate the required dose:

$$\text{Suggested dose} \times \text{Patient weight (kg)} = \text{Required dose (mg)}$$

Then calculate the required volume:

$$\text{Calculated dose (mg)} \div \text{Concentration (100 mg/mL)} = \text{Required volume of obiltoxaximab (mL)}$$

Infusion bag: Withdraw a volume of solution from the infusion bag of NS equal to the calculated volume in mL of obiltoxaximab. Transfer the required volume (dose) of obiltoxaximab to the selected infusion bag. Gently invert the bag to mix the solution. *Do not shake.*

Syringe: Using an appropriately sized syringe for the total volume of infusion to be administered, withdraw the calculated volume (dose) of obiltoxaximab into the syringe, then withdraw the appropriate amount of NS into the syringe. Gently mix the solution. *Do not shake.*

See the following chart for recommended dose, total infusion volume, and infusion rate by body weight.

Obiltoxaximab Dose, Total Infusion Volume, and Infusion Rate by Body Weight		
Body Weight (Weight-Based Dosing)	Total Infusion Volume	Infusion Rate
Weight Greater Than 40 kg or Adult (16 mg/kg)		
Greater than 40 kg	250 mL	167 mL/hr
Weight Greater Than 15 kg to 40 kg (24 mg/kg)		
31 to 40 kg	250 mL	167 mL/hr
16 to 30 kg	100 mL	67 mL/hr
Weight 15 kg or Less (32 mg/kg)		
11 to 15 kg	100 mL	67 mL/hr
5 to 10 kg	50 mL	33.3 mL/hr
3.1 to 4.9 kg	25 mL	17 mL/hr
2.1 to 3 kg	20 mL	13.3 mL/hr
1.1 to 2 kg	15 mL	10 mL/hr
1 kg or less	7 mL	4.7 mL/hr

Filters: Use of a 0.22-micron in-line filter is required for administration.

Storage: Before use, refrigerate at 2° to 8° C (36° to 46° F) in original carton to protect from light. Do not freeze. Do not shake. *Infusion bag:* Prepared solution stable for 4 hours at RT or refrigerated. Discard NS withdrawn from bag and discard unused portion in obiltoxaximab vials. *Syringe:* Administer immediately. Do not store solution in syringe. Discard unused product.

COMPATIBILITY
Specific information not available. Consider specific use; consult pharmacist.

RATE OF ADMINISTRATION
Administer through a 0.22-micron in-line filter.

A single dose as an infusion over 90 minutes. See chart in Dilution for recommended total infusion volumes and infusion rates for weight-based dosing. Flush the IV line with NS after the infusion.

ACTIONS
A chimeric IgG1 kappa monoclonal antibody (mAb) that binds the protective antigen (PA) component of *Bacillus anthracis* toxin. It inhibits the binding of PA to its cellular receptors, thereby preventing the intracellular entry of the anthrax lethal factor and edema factor, the enzymatic toxin components responsible for the pathogenic effects of anthrax toxin. Steady-state volume of distribution is greater than plasma volume, suggesting some tissue distribution. Virtually no renal clearance occurs.

INDICATIONS AND USES
Treatment of inhalational anthrax due to *B. anthracis* in adult and pediatric patients. Used in combination with appropriate antibacterial drugs (e.g., ciprofloxacin [Cipro], doxycycline, levofloxacin [Levaquin]). ▪ Prophylaxis of inhalational anthrax due to *B. anthracis* when alternative therapies are not available or are not appropriate.

Limitation of use: Should only be used for prophylaxis when its benefit for prevention of inhalational anthrax outweighs the risk of hypersensitivity and anaphylaxis. ▪ Effectiveness is based solely on efficacy studies in animal models of inhalational anthrax. ▪ No studies of the safety or pharmacokinetics (PK) have been done in the pediatric population. Dosing in pediatric patients was derived using a population pharmacokinetics approach designed to match the observed adult exposure to obiltoxaximab at a 16 mg/kg dose. ▪ Does not have direct antibacterial activity. Should be used in combination with appropriate antibacterial drugs. ▪ Not expected to cross the blood-brain barrier and does not prevent or treat meningitis.

CONTRAINDICATIONS
Manufacturer states, "None."

PRECAUTIONS
For IV use only. ▪ Administered by or under the direction of a physician knowledgeable in its use and in a facility equipped to monitor the patient and respond to any medical emergency. ▪ Hypersensitivity reactions, including anaphylaxis, have been reported. ▪ A therapeutic protein, there is a potential for immunogenicity.

Monitor: Monitor for S/S of a hypersensitivity reaction (e.g., chest discomfort, cough, cyanosis, dyspnea, hypotension, postural dizziness, pruritus, rash, throat irritation, urticaria, wheezing) during the infusion and for some time following completion of the infusion. Reactions have occurred both during and after the infusion. ▪ Premedication with diphenhydramine does not prevent anaphylaxis and may mask or delay the onset of symptoms of hypersensitivity.

Patient Education: Effectiveness has been studied only in animals with inhalational anthrax. ▪ Immediately report any S/S of a hypersensitivity reaction (e.g., chest discomfort, cough, cyanosis, dyspnea, hypotension, postural dizziness, pruritus, rash, throat irritation, urticaria, wheezing) occurring during or after administration.

Maternal/Child: Pregnancy category B: use during pregnancy only if clearly needed. ▪ Use caution during breast-feeding; effects unknown. ▪ Safety and effectiveness for use in pediatric patients is based solely on efficacy studies in animal models; see Limitation of Use.

Elderly: Numbers in clinical studies are insufficient to determine whether the elderly respond differently than younger subjects.

DRUG/LAB INTERACTIONS
Coadministration of 16 mg/kg obiltoxaximab IV with IV or oral ciprofloxacin did not alter the pharmacokinetics of either ciprofloxacin or obiltoxaximab.

SIDE EFFECTS
The most frequently reported side effects in adults were cough, headache, infections of the upper respiratory tract, infusion site pain and/or swelling, nasal congestion, pain in extremity, pruritus, urticaria, and vessel puncture site bruising. Hypersensitivity reactions are the most serious side effect.

ANTIDOTE
Keep the physician informed of all side effects. Most will be treated symptomatically. If a hypersensitivity reaction occurs, discontinue the infusion immediately and treat with oxygen, epinephrine, antihistamines (e.g., IV diphenhydramine), corticosteroids, albuterol, vasopressors (e.g., dopamine), and ventilation equipment as indicated. No clinical experience with overdose. If overdose occurs, monitor patients for S/S of adverse effects. Resuscitate as necessary.

OBINUTUZUMAB BBW

(oh-bi-nue-**TOOZ**-ue-mab)

Gazyva

Monoclonal antibody
Antineoplastic

pH 6

USUAL DOSE

Hypotension may occur during obinutuzumab infusion. Consider withholding antihypertensive medications for 12 hours before and throughout each infusion and for the first hour after administration.

Premedication: Premedication required. To prevent or attenuate severe hypersensitivity reactions, premedicate according to the following chart before the indicated infusion.

Premedication for Obinutuzumab Infusion to Reduce Infusion-Related Reactions (IRR) in Patients with Chronic Lymphocytic Leukemia (CLL) and Follicular Lymphoma (FL)			
Day of Treatment Cycle	Patients Requiring Premedication	Premedication	Administration
Cycle 1: **CLL** **Day 1** **Day 2**	All patients	IV glucocorticoid: Dexamethasone 20 mg **OR** Methylprednisolone 80 mg*	Completed at least 1 hour before obinutuzumab infusion
FL **Day 1**		Acetaminophen 650 to 1,000 mg Antihistamine (e.g., diphenhydramine [Benadryl] 50 mg)	Administer at least 30 minutes before obinutuzumab infusion
All subsequent infusions	All patients	Acetaminophen 650 to 1,000 mg	Administer at least 30 minutes before obinutuzumab infusion
	Patients with an IRR (≥Grade 1 to 2) with the previous infusion	Acetaminophen 650 to 1,000 mg Antihistamine (e.g., diphenhydramine [Benadryl] 50 mg)	Administer at least 30 minutes before obinutuzumab infusion
	Patients with a Grade 3 IRR with the previous infusion **OR** With a lymphocyte count >25,000 cells/mm^3 before next treatment	IV glucocorticoid: Dexamethasone 20 mg **OR** Methylprednisolone 80 mg*	Completed at least 1 hour before obinutuzumab infusion
		Acetaminophen 650 to 1,000 mg Antihistamine (e.g., diphenhydramine [Benadryl] 50 mg)	Administer at least 30 minutes before obinutuzumab infusion

*Hydrocortisone is not recommended. It has not been effective in reducing the rate of infusion reactions.

Tumor lysis syndrome (TLS) prophylaxis: Premedicate patients who have a high tumor burden, high circulating absolute lymphocyte counts (greater than 25,000 cells/mm^3), or renal impairment with antihyperuricemics (e.g., allopurinol or rasburicase) before the start of therapy. Ensure adequate hydration. Continue prophylaxis before each subsequent obinutuzumab infusion as needed. ■ **Antimicrobial prophylaxis** is strongly recommended for patients with Grade 3 to 4 neutropenia lasting more than 1 week. Prophylaxis should continue until resolution of neutropenia to Grade 1 or 2. Consider antiviral and antifungal prophylaxis.

Obinutuzumab: Doses must be administered as an infusion through a dedicated line according to the two charts on the next page.

Continued

N-O

Dose of Obinutuzumab to Be Administered During 6 Treatment Cycles, Each of 28 Days' Duration, for Patients with CLL			
Day of Treatment Cycle		Dose of Obinutuzumab	Rate of Infusion (in Absence of Infusion Reactions/ Hypersensitivity During Previous Infusions)
Cycle 1 (loading doses)	Day 1	100 mg	Administer at 25 mg/hr over 4 hours. Do not increase the infusion rate.
	Day 2	900 mg	Administer at 50 mg/hr. The rate of the infusion can be increased in increments of 50 mg/hr every 30 minutes to a maximum rate of 400 mg/hr.
	Day 8	1,000 mg	If no infusion reaction occurred during the previous infusion and the final infusion rate was 100 mg/hr or faster, infusions can be started at a rate of 100 mg/hr and increased by 100-mg/hr increments every 30 minutes to a maximum of 400 mg/hr.
	Day 15	1,000 mg	
Cycles 2-6	Day 1	1,000 mg	

Dose of Obinutuzumab to Be Administered During 6 Treatment Cycles, Each of 28 Days' Duration, Followed by Obinutuzumab Monotherapy for Patients with FL			
Day of Treatment Cycle		Dose of Obinutuzumab	Rate of Infusion (in Absence of Infusion Reactions/Hypersensitivity During Previous Infusions)
Cycle 1 (loading doses)	Day 1	1,000 mg	Administer at 50 mg/hr. The rate of the infusion can be increased in increments of 50 mg/hr every 30 minutes to a maximum rate of 400 mg/hr.
	Day 8	1,000 mg	If no infusion reaction occurred during the previous infusion and the final infusion rate was 100 mg/hr or faster, infusions can be started at a rate of 100 mg/hr and increased by 100-mg/hr increments every 30 minutes to a maximum of 400 mg/hr.
	Day 15	1,000 mg	
Cycles 2 to 6	Day 1	1,000 mg	
Monotherapy*	Every 2 months for 2 years	1,000 mg	

*Patients with FL who achieve stable disease, complete response, or partial response to the initial 6 cycles of obinutuzumab in combination with bendamustine should continue obinutuzumab as monotherapy for 2 years.

DOSE ADJUSTMENTS

Consider treatment interruption if patients experience an infection, Grade 3 or 4 cytopenia, or a Grade 2 or greater nonhematologic toxicity. ▪ In patients with Grade 3 or 4 thrombocytopenia, consider a dose delay of obinutuzumab and chemotherapy or a dose reduction of chemotherapy. ▪ If a planned dose is missed during the first 6 cycles, administer as soon as possible and adjust dosing schedule accordingly. If appropriate, patients being treated for CLL who do not complete the Day 1 Cycle 1 dose may proceed to the Day 2 Cycle 1 dose. If a dose is missed during monotherapy in a patient being treated for FL, maintain the original dosing schedule for subsequent doses. ▪ No dose adjustment indicated based on age, weight, or moderate renal impairment. Has not been studied in patients with a CrCl less than 30 mL/min or in patients with hepatic impairment.

DILUTION

Available in a 1,000 mg/40 mL (25 mg/mL) single-use vial. Aseptic technique imperative. **CLL: *Preparation of solution for infusion on Day 1 (100 mg) and Day 2 (900 mg) of Cycle 1:*** Withdraw 4 mL (100 mg) of obinutuzumab solution from the vial. Inject into a 100-mL infusion bag of NS for immediate administration. Withdraw the remaining 36 mL (900 mg) of solution from the vial and inject into a 250-mL infusion bag of NS for use on Day 2. Mix infusion bags by gentle inversion. ***Do not shake.*** Clearly label each infusion bag; see Storage.

CLL and FL: *Preparation of 1,000-mg dose:* Withdraw 40 mL of obinutuzumab solution from the vial. Inject into a 250-mL infusion bag of NS. Mix by gentle inversion. *Do not shake or freeze.* Should be used immediately; see Storage. Final concentrations of 0.4 to 4 mg/mL are suitable for administration.

Filters: Specific information not available.

Storage: Refrigerate single-use vials at 2° to 8° C (36° to 46° F) in carton to protect from light. *Do not freeze. Do not shake.* If not used immediately, infusions diluted for use may be refrigerated for up to 24 hours, followed by 48 hours (including infusion time) at RT. Allow to come to room temperature, then use immediately.

COMPATIBILITY

Manufacturer states, "Dilute into a 0.9% sodium chloride (NS) PVC or non-PVC polyolefin infusion bag. *Do not* use other diluents such as dextrose (5%)," "Do not mix with other drugs," " Administer through a dedicated line," and "No **incompatibilities** with polyvinylchloride (PVC) or non-PVC polyolefin bags and administration sets have been observed."

RATE OF ADMINISTRATION

Do not administer as an IV push or bolus. See Usual Dose for specific rates of infusion. If an infusion reaction occurs, adjust the rate as follows.

Grade 1-2 (mild to moderate): Reduce or interrupt infusion and treat as indicated. With resolution of symptoms, continue or resume infusion. If no further reactions occur, rate may escalate as indicated for each treatment-cycle dose.

Grade 3 (severe): Interrupt infusion and manage symptoms. With resolution of symptoms, consider restarting the infusion at no more than half the rate that caused the reaction. If no further reactions occur, rate may escalate as indicated for each treatment-cycle dose. Discontinue permanently if a reaction occurs on rechallenge.

Grade 4 (life-threatening): Stop infusion immediately and discontinue therapy permanently.

ACTIONS

An antineoplastic agent. A humanized anti-CD20 monoclonal antibody of the IgG1 subclass produced by recombinant DNA technology. It targets the CD20 antigen expressed on the surface of pre B-lymphocytes and mature B-lymphocytes. Upon binding to CD20, it mediates B-cell lysis through several processes, resulting in cell death. Causes CD19 B-cell depletion. Recovery of CD19 B-cells may occur approximately 9 months after the last obinutuzumab dose, but some patients remain depleted at 18 months. Elimination occurs by a linear clearance pathway and a time-dependent nonlinear clearance pathway. Terminal half-life ranges from 26.4 to 36.8 days.

INDICATIONS AND USES

Treatment of patients with previously untreated chronic lymphocytic leukemia (CLL) in combination with chlorambucil (Leukeran). ▪ Treatment of patients with follicular lymphoma (FL) who relapsed after or are refractory to a rituximab-containing regimen. Given in combination with bendamustine followed by obinutuzumab monotherapy.

CONTRAINDICATIONS

Manufacturer states, "None."

PRECAUTIONS

For IV infusion only; do not administer as an IV push or bolus. ▪ Should be administered by or under the direction of the physician specialist in facilities equipped to monitor the patient and respond to any medical emergency. ▪ Hepatitis B virus reactivation with fulminant hepatitis, hepatic failure, and death can occur in patients treated with anti-CD20–directed cytolytic antibodies, including obinutuzumab. For patients who show evidence of hepatitis B infection, consult physician with expertise in managing hepatitis B regarding monitoring and consideration for HBV antiviral therapy; see Monitor. ▪ Progressive multifocal leukoencephalopathy (PML), including fatal PML, can occur in patients receiving obinutuzumab. JC virus infection resulting in PML was observed in patients treated with obinutuzumab. ▪ Severe and life-threatening infusion reactions have occurred within 24 hours of the first 1,000 mg infused and with subsequent infusions. ▪ Tumor lysis syndrome (TLS) has been reported within 12 to 24 hours after the first obinutuzumab infusion. S/S may include rapid reduction in tumor volume, renal insufficiency, hyperkalemia, hypocalcemia, hyperuricemia, or hyperphosphatemia. May cause acute renal failure requiring dialysis and has been fatal. ▪ TLS occurs more often in patients with a high tumor burden, a high circulating lymphocyte count (greater than 25,000/mm^3), or renal impairment. Consider prophylactic measures; see Monitor and Usual Dose. ▪ Serious bacterial, fungal, and new or reactivated viral infections can occur during and/or following therapy. Do not administer to patients with an active infection. Patients with a history of recurring or chronic infections may be at increased risk for infection. ▪ Severe and life-threatening neutropenia has been reported during treatment with obinutuzumab. May be delayed (occurring more than 28 days after completion of treatment and/or prolonged (lasting longer than 28 days). Anticipate, evaluate, and treat any S/S of developing infection. Consider administration of granulocyte colony-stimulating factors (G-CSF) in patients with Grade 3 or 4 neutropenia. ▪ Severe and life-threatening thrombocytopenia has been reported during treatment with obinutuzumab in combination with chlorambucil or bendamustine. Fatal hemorrhagic events have occurred during Cycle 1 in patients with CLL being treated with obinutuzumab. ▪ Has not been studied in patients with a CrCl less than 30 mL/min or in patients with hepatic impairment. ▪ See Drug/Lab Interactions.

Monitor: Obtain baseline CBC and platelet count and monitor at regular intervals. Repeat more frequently in patients who develop cytopenias (e.g., leukopenia, neutropenia, thrombocytopenia). ▪ Screen all patients for HBV infection before treatment initiation. Monitor HBV-positive patients during and after treatment with obinutuzumab. Monitor patients with evidence of current or prior HBV infection for clinical and laboratory signs of hepatitis or HBV reactivation during and for several months after treatment with obinutuzumab. ▪ Insufficient data exist regarding the safety of resuming obinutuzumab therapy in patients who develop HBV reactivation; see Antidote. ▪ Consider PML in patients with new-onset or changes to pre-existing neurologic manifestations; consultation with a neurologist, brain MRI, and lumbar puncture may be required for diagnosis. ▪ Monitor closely for S/S of an infusion reaction (e.g., bronchospasm, chills, diarrhea, dizziness, dyspnea, fatigue, fever, flushing, headache, hypertension, hypotension, laryngeal edema, larynx and throat irritation, nausea, tachycardia, vomiting, and wheezing). See Antidote for responses to various grades of an infusion reaction. ▪ Patients with pre-existing cardiac or pulmonary conditions may be at greater risk for severe infusion reactions; monitor closely during and after the infusion. ▪ Monitor patients for TLS, especially during the initial days of obinutuzumab treatment. Prevention and treatment of hyperuricemia due to TLS may be accomplished with adequate hydration and, if necessary, allopurinol or rasburicase and alkalinization of urine. Monitor electrolytes, renal function, and fluid status. Correct electrolyte abnormalities and provide supportive care, including dialysis, as indicated. ▪ Observe closely for signs of infection. Patients with severe and long-lasting (greater than 1 week) neutropenia are strongly recommended to receive antimicrobial prophylaxis until resolution of neutropenia to Grade 1 or 2. Antiviral and antifungal prophylaxis should also be considered. ▪ Monitor for thrombocytopenia (platelet count less than 50,000/mm^3) and hemorrhagic events, especially during the first cycle. Initiate precautions to prevent excessive bleeding (e.g., inspect IV sites, skin, and mucous membranes; use extreme care during invasive procedures; test urine, emesis, stool, and secretions for occult blood).

Patient Education: Avoid pregnancy; see Maternal/Child. ▪ Discuss health history (e.g., presence of an infection, carrier of or previous infection with hepatitis B virus, recent or scheduled vaccinations) and prescription and nonprescription medications with the health care provider administering the obinutuzumab. ▪ Avoid vaccinations with live virus vaccines. ▪ Review monitoring requirements and potential side effects before therapy. ▪ Promptly report S/S of infection (e.g., fever, cough). ▪ Promptly report S/S of infusion reactions, including breathing problems, chest pain, chills, diarrhea, dizziness, fever, nausea, and vomiting. ▪ Promptly report S/S of TLS, including diarrhea, lethargy, nausea, and vomiting, and S/S of hepatitis, including worsening fatigue or yellow discoloration of skin or eyes. ▪ Promptly report new neurologic S/S (e.g., changes in vision, loss of balance or coordination, disorientation, or confusion); could be warning signs of PML. ▪ Promptly report S/S of hepatitis (e.g., fatigue, jaundice). ▪ See Appendix D, p. 1333.

Maternal/Child: Use during pregnancy only if the potential benefit justifies the potential risk to the fetus. Obinutuzumab is likely to cause fetal B-cell depletion. Safety and timing of administration of live virus vaccines to infants born to mothers who were administered obinutuzumab during pregnancy require consultation with health care professionals. ▪ Weigh risk versus benefit when considering breast-feeding. ▪ Safety and effectiveness for use in pediatric patients not established.

Elderly: In clinical trials, the incidence of serious adverse events was higher in older patients. Effectiveness was similar to that seen in younger adults.

DRUG/LAB INTERACTIONS

Formal drug interaction studies have not been performed. ▪ Avoid vaccinations with live or attenuated virus vaccines. Immunization with live virus vaccines is not recommended during treatment and until B-cell recovery. ▪ Consider withholding concomitant medications that may increase the risk of bleeding (e.g., platelet inhibitors, anticoagulants), especially during the first cycle. ▪ Hypotension may occur during obinutuzumab infusion. Consider withholding antihypertensive medications for 12 hours before and throughout each infusion and for the first hour after administration.

SIDE EFFECTS

Anemia, cough, diarrhea, fever, infusion reactions, nausea, neutropenia, and thrombocytopenia are the most commonly reported adverse reactions in patients with CLL or FL. Arthralgia, asthenia, constipation, decreased appetite, fatigue, sinusitis, upper respiratory tract infections, urinary tract infections, and vomiting were also commonly reported in patients with FL. Infusion reactions may be life-threatening. Hepatitis B reactivation, PML, tumor lysis syndrome, and serious infections have all been reported and may be life threatening. Back pain; dyspepsia; fatal hemorrhagic events (first cycle); hyperkalemia; hypoalbuminemia; hypocalcemia; hypokalemia; hyponatremia; hypophosphatemia; increased ALT, AST, alkaline phosphatase, and creatinine; leukopenia; lymphopenia; nasal congestion; nasopharyngitis; pain in extremities; pruritus; and worsening of pre-existing cardiac conditions have also been reported.

ANTIDOTE

Keep physician informed of all side effects. May constitute a medical emergency or will be treated symptomatically as indicated. Interrupt or reduce rate of infusion for Grade 1 or 2 infusion reactions and manage symptoms. Interrupt therapy for Grade 3 infusion reactions until resolution of symptoms. Permanently discontinue therapy for any Grade 4 infusion reaction including, but not limited to, anaphylaxis. Severe infusion reactions may require epinephrine (Adrenalin), antihistamines (e.g., diphenhydramine [Benadryl]), corticosteroids (e.g., dexamethasone [Decadron]), oxygen or bronchodilators (e.g., albuterol). Maintain a patent airway. In patients who have a Grade 1, 2, or 3 infusion reaction, see Rate of Administration for rate adjustments required if treatment is to be continued. In patients who develop reactivation of HBV, immediately discontinue obinutuzumab and concomitant chemotherapy and institute appropriate treatment. Resumption of therapy should be discussed with physicians with expertise in managing hepatitis B. Discontinue obinutuzumab and consider discontinuation or reduction of concomitant chemotherapy or immunosuppressive therapy in patients who develop PML. Consider treatment interruption in the event of infection, Grade 3 or 4 cytopenia, or a hematologic toxicity equal to or greater than Grade 2. Dose delays of obinutuzumab and chemotherapy or dose reductions of chemotherapy may be indicated. Consider administration of granulocyte colony-stimulating factors (G-CSF) in patients with Grade 3 or 4 neutropenia. Tumor lysis syndrome requires correction of electrolyte abnormalities and monitoring of renal function and fluid balance. Supportive care, including dialysis, may be required. Thrombocytopenia may require transfusion of blood products (i.e., platelet transfusion). Resuscitate as indicated.

OCTREOTIDE ACETATE
(ok-**TREE**-oh-tide **AS**-ah-tayt)

Antidiarrheal
Growth hormone suppressant

Octreotide Acetate PF, Sandostatin

pH 3.9 to 4.5

USUAL DOSE

Usually given SC. Check label and confirm for IV use; Sandostatin LAR Depot is for IM use only; see Precautions. In most situations begin with a lower dose to allow gradual tolerance to GI side effects. Increase gradually based on patient response and tolerance. Begin SC or IM (LAR Depot) dosing as soon as practical.

Antidiarrheal (GI tumor): 50 mcg once or twice daily. Increase gradually if indicated.

Antidiarrheal (unlabeled for AIDS): 100 mcg as an IV bolus over 10 minutes. Follow with a continuous infusion, intermittent infusion, or bolus dose of 10 mcg/hr. Increase gradually to 100 mcg/hr. When adequate control is achieved, decrease to 75 mcg/hr. SC dose range is from 100 mcg up to 3,000 mcg/24 hr.

Carcinoid tumors: 100 to 600 mcg/24 hr in equally divided doses 2 to 4 times daily during first 2 weeks of therapy (50 to 300 mcg every 12 hours or 25 to 150 mcg every 6 hours). Average total daily dose ranges from 300 to 450 mcg, but therapeutic response is obtained with ranges from 50 to 750 mcg. Up to 1,500 mcg/day has been used in selected patients.

Carcinoid crisis (unlabeled): 100 mcg as an IV bolus. May be given to treat carcinoid crisis during anesthesia or given before induction of anesthesia as a prophylactic measure.

Vasoactive intestinal peptide tumors: Average dose range is 200 to 300 mcg/24 hr in equally divided doses 2 to 4 times daily during first 2 weeks of therapy (100 to 150 mcg every 12 hours or 50 to 75 mcg every 6 hours). Average total daily dose ranges from 150 to 750 mcg but therapeutic response usually achieved with doses under 450 mcg/24 hr.

Treatment of GI bleeding (unlabeled): Begin with a loading dose of 50 to 100 mcg. Follow with a continuous infusion of 25 to 50 mcg/hr for 1 to 5 days. Intermittent infusion or bolus doses may be substituted for the continuous infusion.

Growth hormone suppression (acromegaly): 50 mcg every 8 hours is the initial dose. Increase dose gradually as indicated by IGF-1 levels; see Monitor. Acromegaly has been suppressed at doses of 300 to 500 mcg/24 hr. May be maintained at home with infusions through an implantable IV or SC pump or SC dosing of 50 to 100 mcg every 8 hours.

Antihypoglycemic: Life-threatening hypoglycemia secondary to insulinoma (unlabeled): 100 mcg as an IV bolus.

Reduce output from GI or pancreatic fistulas (unlabeled): 50 to 200 mcg every 8 hours. In one study, 250 mcg/hr was given as a continuous infusion for 48 hours, followed with SC dosing. Fistula became dry within 72 hours and eventually closed.

PEDIATRIC DOSE

Experience is limited, and doses are **unlabeled.** See Maternal/Child.

Intractable diarrhea: 1 to 10 mcg/kg of body weight/24 hr. May be given as a single daily dose or divided and given every 12 hours. Dose may be increased within the recommended range by 0.3 mcg/kg/dose every 3 days as needed. Maximum dose is 1,500 mcg/24 hr.

Diarrhea associated with graft versus host: 1 mcg/kg/dose bolus followed by 1 mcg/kg/hr as a continuous infusion has been used.

DOSE ADJUSTMENTS

In all situations dose adjustment may be required on a daily basis to maintain symptomatic control. After initial 2 weeks of therapy, gradually decrease dose to achieve therapeutically effective maintenance dose. ■ Reduce dose in the elderly; half-life extended and clearance decreased. Start at the lower end of the dosing range. Consider the greater frequency of decreased organ function and of concomitant disease or drug therapy. ■

Half-life markedly extended in severe renal failure requiring dialysis. Reduction of maintenance dose indicated. ▪ See Drug/Lab Interactions.

DILUTION

Available in several different concentrations and formulations; read label carefully. May be given undiluted or may be diluted with 50 to 200 mL of NS or D5W and given as an intermittent infusion or further diluted and given as a continuous infusion.

Storage: Before use store in refrigerator (2° to 8° C [36° to 46° F]) or at CRT for 14 days; protect from light. May store at room temperature on day of use. Diluted solution stable for 24 hours. Multidose vial must be dated on opening and discarded after 14 days.

COMPATIBILITY   (Underline Indicates Conflicting Compatibility Information)

Consider any drug NOT listed as compatible to be INCOMPATIBLE until consulting a pharmacist; specific conditions may apply.

Manufacturer lists TPN as **incompatible** (forms a conjugate that decreases effectiveness). If used as an additive with insulin, octreotide markedly increases adsorption of insulin and reduces insulin availability.

One source suggests the following **compatibilities:**

Additive: Heparin.

Y-site: 6% Hydroxyethyl starch (Voluven), pantoprazole (Protonix IV).

RATE OF ADMINISTRATION

IV injection: A single dose over 3 minutes.

Intermittent infusion: A single dose over 15 to 30 minutes.

Continuous infusion: Give at a rate consistent with the required hourly dose in an amount of fluid appropriate for the specific patient.

ACTIONS

A long-acting octapeptide. Mimics the actions of the natural hormone somatostatin, suppressing secretion of serotonin, gastroenteropancreatic peptides (e.g., gastrin, vasoactive intestinal peptide, insulin, glucagon, secretin, motilin, pancreatic polypeptide), and growth hormone. Decreases splanchnic blood flow. Stimulates fluid and electrolyte absorption from GI tract and prolongs GI transit time. These pharmacologic actions provide a means of treating the symptoms associated with metastatic carcinoid tumors (flushing and diarrhea) and vasoactive intestinal peptide (VIP)–secreting tumors (watery diarrhea). Other actions include inhibition of gallbladder contractility and bile secretion and suppression of thyroid-stimulating hormone (TSH) secretion. Distribution from plasma is rapid. About 65% bound to plasma protein. Half-life longer than the natural hormone (1.7 to 1.9 hours compared to 1 to 3 minutes). Action may extend to 12 hours. Some excreted unchanged in urine.

INDICATIONS AND USES

To suppress or inhibit the severe diarrhea and flushing episodes associated with carcinoid tumor. ▪ Treatment of profuse watery diarrhea associated with vasoactive intestinal peptide tumors (VIPomas). ▪ Treatment of acromegaly to suppress growth hormone and achieve normalization of growth hormone and IGF-1 levels.

Unlabeled uses: Treatment of severe diarrhea in patients with AIDS; treatment of chemotherapy-induced diarrhea. Carcinoid crisis during anesthesia, adjunct to treatment of life-threatening hypoglycemia, treatment of GI bleeding. Adjunct to pancreatectomy and treatment of GI or pancreatic fistulas.

CONTRAINDICATIONS

Sensitivity to octreotide acetate or any of its components.

PRECAUTIONS

IV use is limited to emergency situations. SC injection with rotation of injection sites is preferred route of administration. ▪ Sandostatin LAR Depot must be administered intragluteally but has the advantage of extending the interval between injections to every 4 weeks. ▪ May decrease size of tumors and slow rate of growth and metastases. Data not definitive. ▪ May inhibit gallbladder contractility and decrease bile secretion. ▪ Use caution in patients with diabetes. In patients with Type 1 diabetes, octreotide is likely to affect glucose regulation, and insulin requirements may be decreased. Severe, symptomatic hypoglycemia has been reported. In nondiabetics and Type 2 diabetics with partially intact insulin reserves, octreotide may result in decreased insulin levels and hyperglycemia. Glucose tolerance and antidiabetic treatment should be closely monitored. ▪ Cardiac abnormalities (e.g., arrhythmias, bradycardia, conduction abnormalities, QT prolongation) have been reported. More common in patients with acromegaly; see Side Effects. ▪ Suppresses thyroid-stimulating hormone. May cause hypothyroidism.

Monitor: Observe for transient hyperglycemia or hypoglycemia during induction and dose changes because of changes in balance of hormones (e.g., insulin, glucagon, and growth hormone). ▪ Monitor fluids and electrolytes carefully. ▪ 5-HIAA, plasma serotonin, and plasma substance P may be useful lab studies to evaluate patient response with carcinoid tumor. Measurement of plasma vasoactive intestinal peptide will be helpful in VIPoma. ▪ In acromegaly, initial response may be monitored with growth hormone levels at 1- to 4-hour intervals for 8 to 12 hours after a dose. IGF-1 levels every 2 weeks and/or multiple growth hormone levels taken 0 to 8 hours after administration may be used to make dose adjustments. Goal is to achieve growth hormone levels less than 5 ng/mL or IGF-1 (somatomedin C) levels less than 1.9 units/mL in males and less than 2.2 units/mL in females. After stabilization, IGF-1 or growth hormone levels should be re-evaluated at 6-month intervals. ▪ In patients with acromegaly who have received irradiation, octreotide should be withdrawn yearly for 4 weeks to assess disease activity. If growth hormone or IGF-1 levels increase and S/S recur, octreotide therapy should be resumed. ▪ Can alter fat absorption and decrease gallbladder motility; observe for gallbladder disease. Baseline and periodic ultrasound of gallbladder and bile ducts indicated in long-term SC therapy. Periodic fecal fat and carotene studies also indicated. ▪ Pancreatitis has been reported. Monitor pancreatic enzymes as indicated. ▪ Depressed B_{12} levels have been observed. Monitor in prolonged therapy. ▪ Monitor baseline and periodic thyroid function tests (TSH, total, and/or free T_4), especially in long-term SC therapy. ▪ See Dose Adjustments and Drug/Lab Interactions.

Patient Education: Instruct patient and/or family in appropriate skills if self-administration indicated. To avoid or lessen incidence of GI side effects, schedule injections between meals and at bedtime. ▪ In women with acromegaly being treated with octreotide, normalization of GH and IGF-1 may restore fertility. Adequate contraception is recommended.

Maternal/Child: Category B: although studies do not indicate harm to the fetus or infants, use in pregnancy and breast-feeding only if clearly needed. ▪ Safety and effectiveness for use in pediatric patients not established; see Literature. In post-marketing reports, hypoxia, necrotizing enterocolitis, and death have been reported, most notably in pediatric patients under 2 years of age, many of which had serious underlying comorbid conditions. Relationship to octreotide not established.

Elderly: See Dose Adjustments. ▪ Response similar to that seen in younger patients; however, may be more sensitive to side effects; observe carefully.

DRUG/LAB INTERACTIONS
Use caution in patients receiving concomitant **beta-blockers** (e.g., atenolol [Tenormin], propranolol), **calcium channel blockers** (e.g., diltiazem [Cardizem], verapamil), **or any agents used for fluid and electrolyte balance.** Will require adjustment in these therapies as symptoms are controlled by octreotide. ▪ May affect absorption of **orally administered medications.** ▪ May inhibit effectiveness of **cyclosporine** and may result in transplant rejection. ▪ Markedly increases adsorption of **insulin** and reduces availability. ▪ Concurrent use with **oral antidiabetic agents, glucagon, growth hormone, or insulin** may cause hypoglycemia or hyperglycemia. Monitor patient carefully and give adjunct dose of these agents as indicated. ▪ May increase availability of **bromocriptine** (Parlodel). ▪ Suppression of growth hormones may cause a decreased clearance of drugs metabolized by selected cytochrome P_{450} enzymes. Use caution with concurrent use of **drugs metabolized by CYP3A4** (e.g., cisapride [Propulsid], erythromycin, HMG-CoA reductase inhibitors [lov-

astatin (Mevacor) and simvastatin (Zocor)], itraconazole [Sporanox], oral midazolam [Versed], quinidine, terfenadine).

SIDE EFFECTS

Most side effects are of mild to moderate severity and of short duration. Abdominal pain/discomfort, abnormal stools, anorexia, anxiety, biliary sludge, cholelithiasis, constipation, convulsions, depression, diarrhea, dizziness, drowsiness, fat malabsorption, fatigue, flatulence, fluttering sensation, GI bleeding, headache, heartburn, hepatitis, hyperesthesia, hyperglycemia, hypoglycemia, increase in liver enzymes, insomnia, irritability, jaundice, nausea, pancreatitis, pounding in the head, rectal spasm, swollen stomach, vomiting. In rare cases, GI side effects may resemble intestinal obstruction with progressive abdominal distension, severe epigastric pain, abdominal tenderness, and guarding. Many other side effects occur in fewer than 1% of patients. Side effects that occur more often in patients with acromegaly include cardiac abnormalities (e.g., sinus bradycardia, ECG changes [including QT prolongation], conduction abnormalities, and arrhythmias) and hypothyroidism.

Post-Marketing: Intestinal obstruction, thrombocytopenia.

ANTIDOTE

Keep physician informed of all side effects. A dose adjustment of either octreotide or other concomitant therapies may be required. Symptomatic and supportive treatment may be indicated. Overdose will cause hyperglycemia or hypoglycemia depending on tumor involved and endocrine status of patient. Discontinue octreotide temporarily, notify the physician, and monitor the patient carefully. Symptomatic treatment should be sufficient.

OFATUMUMAB BBW
(oh-**FAT**-oo-moo-mab)

Arzerra

Monoclonal antibody
Antineoplastic

pH 5.5

USUAL DOSE

Premedication: Patients should receive all of the following premedication agents 30 minutes to 2 hours before each infusion of ofatumumab. The premedication schedule is listed in the following chart.

Premedication Schedule for Ofatumumab					
	Previously Untreated CLL or Extended Treatment of CLL		Refractory CLL		
Infusion number	1 and 2	3 and beyond*	1, 2, and 9	3 to 8	10 to 12
IV corticosteroid (prednisolone or equivalent)	50 mg	0 to 50 mg†	100 mg	0 to 100 mg†	50 to 100 mg‡
Oral acetaminophen	1,000 mg				
Oral or IV antihistamine	Diphenhydramine 50 mg or cetirizine 10 mg (or equivalent)				

*Up to 13 infusions for previously untreated CLL; up to 14 infusions for extended treatment of CLL.
†Corticosteroid may be reduced or omitted for subsequent infusions if a Grade 3 or greater infusion-related adverse event did not occur with the preceding infusion(s).
‡Prednisolone may be given at a reduced dose of 50 to 100 mg (or equivalent) if a Grade 3 or greater infusion-related adverse event did not occur with Infusion 9.

Previously untreated chronic lymphocytic leukemia (CLL): 300 mg as the initial dose (Day 1). Follow 1 week later (on Day 8) with 1,000 mg (Cycle 1). Follow with 1,000 mg on Day 1 of subsequent 28-day cycles for a minimum of 3 cycles until best response or a maximum of 12 cycles.

Extended treatment of CLL: 300 mg on Day 1. Follow with 1,000 mg 1 week later on Day 8. Follow with 1,000 mg 7 weeks later and every 8 weeks thereafter for up to a maximum of 2 years. Given as a *single-agent* extended treatment.

Refractory CLL: 300 mg as the initial dose (Dose 1). Follow 1 week later with 2,000 mg weekly for 7 doses (Doses 2 through 8), followed 4 weeks later with 2,000 mg every 4 weeks for 4 doses (Doses 9 through 12).

DOSE ADJUSTMENTS

Ofatumumab: Interrupt infusion for an infusion reaction of any severity. Treatment may be resumed at the discretion of the treating physician using the following guidelines. ▪ If an infusion reaction resolves with interruption or remains less than or equal to Grade 2, resume infusion with the following modifications based on the initial grade of the infusion reaction: *Grade 1 or 2:* infuse at one half of the previous infusion rate. *Grade 3 or 4:* infuse at 12 mL/hr. After resuming the infusion, the rate may be increased according to the chart in Rate of Administration. ▪ Consider permanent discontinuation if the severity of the infusion reaction does not resolve to equal to or less than Grade 2 despite adequate clinical intervention. Permanently discontinue therapy in patients who develop an anaphylactic reaction. ▪ No dose adjustment is indicated for age, body weight, or gender.

Premedication: *Previously untreated CLL:* Corticosteroid dose may be reduced or omitted in subsequent infusions if a Grade 3 or greater infusion-related reaction (IRR) does not occur during the first 2 infusions. *Refractory CLL:* Do not reduce the corticosteroid dose for Doses 1, 2, and 9. ▪ Doses 3 through 8: If a Grade 3 or greater IRR did not occur with the preceding dose, the corticosteroid dose may be reduced or omitted with subsequent infusions. ▪ Doses 10 through 12: If a Grade 3 or greater infusion reaction did not occur with Dose 9, administer prednisolone 50 to 100 mg or equivalent (e.g., methylpredniso-lone [Solu-Medrol] 40 to 80 mg).

DILUTION

Do not shake ofatumumab in vial or solution. Should be a clear to opalescent colorless solution. Prepare all doses in 1,000 mL of NS.

300-mg dose: Withdraw and discard 15 mL from a 1,000-mL bag of NS. Withdraw 5 mL from each of 3 (100-mg) vials of ofatumumab and add to the bag of NS.

1,000-mg dose: Withdraw and discard 50 mL from a 1,000-mL bag of NS. Withdraw 50 mL from 1 single-use 1,000-mg vial of ofatumumab and add to the bag of NS.

2,000-mg dose: Withdraw and discard 100 mL from a 1,000-mL bag of NS. Withdraw 50 mL from each of 2 (1,000-mg) vials of ofatumumab and add to the bag of NS.

Mix all diluted solution by gentle inversion. Administer using an infusion pump and PVC administration sets.

Filters: An in-line filter is no longer provided or required; see latest prescribing information.

Storage: Refrigerate vials and prepared solutions between 2° to 8° C (36° to 46° F). Protect vials from light and do not freeze. Start infusion within 12 hours of preparation and discard the prepared solution after 24 hours.

COMPATIBILITY

Manufacturer states, "Do not mix ofatumumab with, or administer as an infusion with, other medicinal products." Flush the IV line with NS before and after each dose. "No **incompatibilities** observed with polyvinylchloride or polyolefin bags and administration sets."

RATE OF ADMINISTRATION

For IV infusion only. Use of an infusion pump and PVC administration set is required. Flush the IV line with NS before and after each dose. Interrupt infusion for infusion reactions of any severity; see Dose Adjustments.

Previously untreated CLL and extended treatment of CLL: *300-mg dose:* Initiate infusion at a rate of 3.6 mg/hr (12 mL/hr).

1,000-mg doses: Initiate infusion at a rate of 25 mg/hr (25 mL/hr). Reduce to 12 mg/hr if a Grade 3 or greater infusion-related reaction (IRR) occurred during the previous infusion. If there is no IRR, the rate may be increased every 30 minutes as described in the following chart. Do not exceed these infusion rates.

Ofatumumab Infusion Rates for Previously Untreated CLL and Extended Treatment of CLL		
Interval After Start of Infusion	Initial 300-mg Dose* (mL/hr)	Subsequent Infusions† (mL/hr)
0 to 30 minutes	12 mL/hr	25 mL/hr
31 to 60 minutes	25 mL/hr	50 mL/hr
61 to 90 minutes	50 mL/hr	100 mL/hr
91 to 120 minutes	100 mL/hr	200 mL/hr
121 to 150 minutes	200 mL/hr	400 mL/hr
151 to 180 minutes	300 mL/hr	400 mL/hr
>180 minutes	400 mL/hr	400 mL/hr

*Initial 300 mg: Median duration of infusion = 4.8 to 5.2 hours.
†Subsequent infusions of 1,000 mg: Median duration of infusion = 4.2 to 4.4 hours.

Refractory CLL: *Dose 1 (300-mg dose):* Initiate infusion at a rate of 3.6 mg/hr (12 mL/hr).
Dose 2 (2,000-mg dose): Initiate infusion at a rate of 24 mg/hr (12 mL/hr).
Doses 3 through 12 (2,000-mg doses): Initiate infusion at a rate of 50 mg/hr (25 mL/hr).

If there is no infusion reaction, the rate may be increased every 30 minutes as described in the following chart. Do not exceed these infusion rates.

Ofatumumab Infusion Rates in Refractory CLL		
Interval After Start of Infusion	Infusions 1 and 2* (mL/hr)	Subesquent Infusions† (mL/hr)
0 to 30 minutes	12 mL/hr	25 mL/hr
31 to 60 minutes	25 mL/hr	50 mL/hr
61 to 90 minutes	50 mL/hr	100 mL/hr
91 to 120 minutes	100 mL/hr	200 mL/hr
>120 minutes	200 mL/hr	400 mL/hr

*Infusions 1 and 2 (300 mg and 2,000 mg): Median duration of infusion = 6.8 hours.
†Subsequent infusions (2,000 mg): Median duration of infusion = 4.2 to 4.4 hours.

ACTIONS

A CD20-directed cytolytic monoclonal antibody (also known as an IgGlk human mono-clonal antibody). The CD20 molecule is expressed on normal B lymphocytes and on B-cell CLL. Ofatumumab binds specifically to both the small and large extracellular loops of the CD20 molecule, resulting in B-cell lysis. Possible mechanisms of cell lysis include complement-dependent cytotoxicity and antibody-dependent, cell-mediated cytotoxicity. Decreases circulating CD19-positive B-cells. Ofatumumab is eliminated through both a target-independent route and a B-cell–mediated route. With depletion of B-cells, the clearance of ofatumumab decreases substantially after subsequent infusions compared with the first infusion. The mean half-life after repeated infusions was approximately 17.1 days.

INDICATIONS AND USES

Used in combination with chlorambucil (Leukeran) for the treatment of previously un-treated patients with CLL when fludarabine-based therapy is considered inappropriate. ▪ Extended treatment of patients who are in complete or partial response after at least two lines of therapy for recurrent or progressive CLL. ▪ Treatment of patients with chronic lymphocytic leukemia (CLL) refractory to fludarabine (Fludara) and alemtuzumab (Campath).

CONTRAINDICATIONS

Manufacturer states, "None."

PRECAUTIONS

Do not administer as an IV push or bolus or SC injection. For IV infusion only. ▪ Ad-ministered under the supervision of a physician experienced in the use of antineoplastic therapy in a facility equipped to monitor the patient and respond to any medical emer-gency. ▪ Serious, including fatal, infusion reactions have occurred and seem to occur more frequently with the first 2 infusions and may occur despite premedication; see Monitor. ▪ Cardiac events (e.g., MI, acute coronary syndrome, arrhythmias) and cyto-kine release syndrome have also been reported. ▪ Severe cytopenias, including anemia, neutropenia, and thrombocytopenia, have occurred with ofatumumab. Pancytopenia, agranulocytosis, and fatal neutropenic sepsis have occurred in patients receiving ofatu-mumab in combination with chlorambucil. Grade 3 or 4 late-onset neutropenia (onset at least 42 days after the last treatment dose) and/or prolonged neutropenia (not resolved between 24 and 42 days after the last treatment dose) have been reported. ▪ Progressive multifocal leukoencephalopathy (PML) resulting in death has been reported. ▪ Hepatitis B virus (HBV) reactivation can occur in patients receiving ofatumumab and, in some cases, result in fulminant and fatal hepatitis, hepatic failure, and death. For patients who show evidence of hepatitis B infec-tion, consult physician with expertise in managing hepatitis regarding monitoring and consideration for HBV antiviral therapy. Insufficient data exist regarding the safety of ofatumumab administration in patients who develop HBV reactivation. ▪ Fatal infection due to hepatitis B in patients who have not been previously infected has also been ob-served. ▪ Tumor lysis syndrome (TLS) has been reported and has required hospitaliza-tion. Patients with a high tumor burden and/or high circulating lymphocyte counts (greater than 25,000/mm³) are at greater risk for developing TLS. ▪ A protein substance, it has the potential for producing immunogenicity. ▪ No studies of ofatumumab use in impaired hepatic or renal function have been conducted; use with caution. ▪ See Monitor.

Monitor: Obtain baseline CBC and platelet counts and monitor at regular intervals during and after conclusion of therapy. Increase the frequency of monitoring in patients who develop Grade 3 or 4 cytopenias. ▪ Monitor for S/S of infusion reactions. S/S have included abdominal pain, anaphylactoid/anaphylactic reactions, angioedema, back pain, bronchospasm, cardiac ischemia/infarction, cytokine release syndrome, dyspnea, fever, flushing, hypertension, hypotension, laryngeal edema, pulmonary edema, rash, syncope, and urticaria. ▪ Monitor for new onset of or changes in pre-existing neurologic signs or symptoms. Evaluation for PML includes consultation with a neurologist, brain MRI, and lumbar puncture. ▪ Screen patients for hepatitis B virus (HBV) before initiating therapy. Monitor patients with evidence of current or prior HBV closely for clinical and laboratory signs of hepatitis or HBV reactivation during treatment and for 6 to 12 months after the last infusion. Patients without a history of HBV should also be monitored for S/S of hepatitis. ▪ Prevention and treatment of hyperuricemia due to tumor lysis syndrome may be accomplished with adequate hydration and, if necessary, allupurinol and alkalinization of the urine. Consider initiating prophylaxis 12 to 24 hours before infusion of ofatumumab. Monitor renal function and correct any electrolyte abnormalities that may develop. ▪ Monitor for thrombocytopenia (platelet count less than 50,000/mm³). Initiate precautions to prevent excessive bleeding (e.g., inspect IV sites, skin, and mucous membranes; use extreme care during invasive procedures; test urine, emesis, stool, and secretions for occult blood). ▪ Use of prophylactic antiemetics may be indicated to reduce nausea and/or vomiting and to increase patient comfort. ▪ Observe closely for signs of infection. Prophylactic antibiotics may be indicated.

Patient Education: Potential for fetal B-cell depletion when given to a pregnant woman. ▪ Blood counts will be required at regular intervals. ▪ Avoid vaccination with live virus vaccines. ▪ Additional monitoring and possible need for treatment may be required with a history of hepatitis B infection. ▪ Promptly report symptoms of the following potential side effects: bleeding, easy bruising or petechiae, fatigue, infection (e.g., cough, fever), infusion reactions (e.g., breathing problems, chills, fever, rash that occur within 24 hours of infusion), pallor or worsening weakness, new or worsening abdominal pain or nausea, new or worsening neurologic S/S, worsening fatigue or yellow discoloration of skin or eyes. ▪ See Appendix D, p. 1333.

Maternal/Child: Use during pregnancy only if the potential benefit justifies the potential risk to the fetus. ▪ Use caution if breast-feeding. The effects of local gastrointestinal and limited systemic exposure to ofatumumab are unknown. ▪ May cause fetal B-cell depletion. Avoid administering live vaccines to neonates and infants exposed to ofatumumab in utero until B-cell recovery occurs. ▪ Safety and effectiveness for use in pediatric patients not established.

Elderly: No clinically meaningful differences in efficacy were seen between elderly and younger patients. *Previously untreated CLL:* A higher incidence of serious/severe side effects occurred in elderly patients receiving ofatumumab with chlorambucil. A higher incidence of Grade 3 or greater neutropenia and pneumonia were reported. *Refractory CLL:* Numbers of patients over 65 years of age in studies were not sufficient to determine a response that might differ from younger patients.

DRUG/LAB INTERACTIONS

Formal drug-drug interaction studies have not been conducted. ▪ Do not administer **live virus vaccines** to patients who have recently received ofatumumab. ▪ Coadministration with chlorambucil did not result in clinically relevant effects on the pharmacokinetics of chlorambucil or its active metabolite, phenylacetic acid mustard.

SIDE EFFECTS

Previously untreated CLL: Infusion reactions and neutropenia are most common. Severe cytopenias, including anemia, neutropenia, pancytopenia, thrombocytopenia, agranulocytosis, and fatal neutropenic sepsis, are the most serious side effects in combination with chlorambucil. Other side effects reported included arthralgia, asthenia, headache, herpes simplex, leukopenia, lower respiratory tract infection, and upper abdominal pain.**Extended treatment of CLL:** Infusion reactions, neutropenia, and upper respiratory infections are the most common side effects reported. **Refractory CLL:** The most common side effects are anemia, bronchitis, cough, diarrhea, dyspnea, fatigue, fever, nausea, neutropenia, pneumonia, rash, and upper respiratory infections. Fever, infections (some fatal) including pneumonia and sepsis, infusion reactions, and neutropenia were the most common serious side effects. **All diagnoses:** Other side effects reported include abdominal pain, arthralgia, asthenia, back pain, chills, edema, headache, hepatitis B infection or reactivation, herpes simplex, herpes zoster, hypertension, hypogammaglobulinemia, hypotension, influenza, insomnia, intestinal obstruction, leukopenia, lower respiratory tract infection, lymphopenia, muscle spasms, nasopharyngitis, peripheral edema, PML, sinusitis, tachycardia, thrombocytopenia, tumor lysis syndrome, and urticaria.

Post-Marketing: Cardiac arrest, porphyria cutanea tarda, Stevens-Johnson syndrome.

ANTIDOTE

Notify physician of significant side effects. Temporarily discontinue the infusion for an infusion reaction, angina, or S/S of myocardial ischemia. Delay therapy for serious infection or serious hematologic toxicity until the infection or adverse event resolves. Treatment of most reactions will be supportive. Discontinue medication permanently for severe reactions, including Grade 4 infusion reactions or S/S of PML or in patients who develop reactivation of HBV. Infusion reactions may be treated with acetaminophen, antiemetics (e.g., ondansetron [Zofran]), antihistamines (e.g., diphenhydramine [Benadryl]), or corticosteroids (e.g., hydrocortisone) as indicated. Discontinue ofatumumab and provide supportive therapy in overdose. Treat hypersensitivity reactions with epinephrine, antihistamines, and corticosteroids as needed. Resuscitate as indicated.

ONDANSETRON HYDROCHLORIDE

Antiemetic

(on-**DAN**-sih-tron hy-droh-**KLOR**-eyed)

5HT$_3$ receptor antagonist

Ondansetron HCl PF, Zofran, Zofran PF

pH 3 to 4

USUAL DOSE

Prevention of nausea and vomiting associated with emetogenic cancer chemotherapy in adult and pediatric patients 6 months to 18 years of age: Three 0.15 mg/kg of body weight doses up to a maximum of 16 mg/dose. Administer the first dose 30 minutes before giving emetogenic cancer chemotherapy (e.g., cisplatin, methotrexate). Given as an intermittent infusion over 15 minutes. Repeat 0.15 mg/kg dose up to a maximum of 16 mg/dose at 4 and 8 hours after the first dose. Concurrent use with dexamethasone may improve the effectiveness of ondansetron in controlling cisplatin-induced nausea and vomiting.

Prevention of postoperative nausea and/or vomiting in adults and pediatric patients weighing 40 kg or more: 4 mg *undiluted* before anesthesia induction or postoperatively if the patient did not receive prophylactic antiemetics and experiences nausea or vomiting within 2 hours after surgery. Although repeat doses are not recommended by the manufacturer, they have been given. Benefit of repeat dosing has not been demonstrated in studies.

PEDIATRIC DOSE

See Maternal/Child.

Nausea associated with emetogenic cancer chemotherapy agents in pediatric patients 6 months to 18 years of age: See Usual Dose.

Postoperative nausea in pediatric patients 1 month to 12 years of age: Given immediately before or following anesthesia induction or postoperatively if the patient did not receive prophylactic antiemetics and experiences nausea or vomiting shortly after surgery. See comments under Usual Dose.

Weight 40 kg or less: 0.1 mg/kg.

Weight more than 40 kg: See Usual Dose.

DOSE ADJUSTMENTS

No dose adjustment required for the elderly or in renal disease. ▪ Before emetogenic chemotherapy, a single maximum daily dose of 8 mg is suggested for patients with severe hepatic disease (Child-Pugh score of 10 or greater).

DILUTION

IV injection: 4 mg dose may be given undiluted.

Intermittent infusion: A single dose should be diluted in 50 mL of NS or D5W. See Compatibility.

Storage: Store unopened vials between 2° and 30° C (36° and 86° F). Protect from light. Stable at RT under normal lighting conditions for 48 hours after dilution. However, manufacturer recommends that the dilution not be used beyond 24 hours. Shake vigorously to resolubilize if a precipitate forms at the stopper/vial interface.

COMPATIBILITY　　　　　　　　(Underline Indicates Conflicting Compatibility Information)

Consider any drug NOT listed as compatible to be INCOMPATIBLE until consulting a pharmacist; specific conditions may apply.

Manufacturer states, "Should not be mixed with alkaline solutions as a precipitate may form" and lists as **compatible** and stable for up to 48 hours with D5W, NS, D5/¹/₂NS, D5NS, or 3% NaCl injection; see Dilution.

One source suggests the following **compatibilities:**

Additive: *Not recommended by manufacturer.* Cisplatin, cyclophosphamide (Cytoxan), cytarabine (ARA-C), dacarbazine (DTIC), dexamethasone (Decadron), doxorubicin (Adriamycin), etoposide (VePesid), hydromorphone (Dilaudid), mannitol (Osmitrol), meperidine (Demerol), meropenem (Merrem IV), methotrexate, morphine.

Y-site: Acetaminophen (Ofirmev), aldesleukin (Proleukin), amifostine (Ethyol), amikacin, azithromycin (Zithromax), aztreonam (Azactam), bleomycin (Blenoxane), carboplatin (Paraplatin), carmustine (BiCNU), caspofungin (Cancidas), cefazolin (Ancef), cefotaxime (Claforan), cefoxitin (Mefoxin), ceftaroline (Teflaro), ceftazidime (Fortaz), cefuroxime (Zinacef), chlorpromazine (Thorazine), cisatracurium (Nimbex), cisplatin, cladribine (Leustatin), clindamycin (Cleocin), cyclophosphamide (Cytoxan), cytarabine (ARA-C), dacarbazine (DTIC), dactinomycin (Cosmegen), daunorubicin (Cerubidine), dexamethasone (Decadron), dexmedetomidine (Precedex), diphenhydramine (Benadryl), docetaxel (Taxotere), dopamine, doripenem (Doribax), doxorubicin (Adriamycin), doxorubicin liposomal (Doxil), doxycycline, droperidol (Inapsine), etoposide (VePesid), etoposide phosphate (Etopophos), famotidine (Pepcid IV), fenoldopam (Corlopam), filgrastim (Neupogen), fluconazole (Diflucan), fludarabine (Fludara), fluorouracil (5-FU), gallium nitrate (Ganite), gemcitabine (Gemzar), gentamicin, heparin, hetastarch in electrolytes (Hextend), hydrocortisone sodium succinate (Solu-Cortef), hydromorphone (Dilaudid), ifosfamide (Ifex), imipenem-cilastatin (Primaxin), linezolid (Zyvox), magnesium sulfate, mannitol, mechlorethamine (nitrogen mustard), melphalan (Alkeran), meperidine (Demerol), meropenem (Merrem IV), mesna (Mesnex), methotrexate, metoclopramide (Reglan), mitomycin (Mutamycin), mitoxantrone (Novantrone), morphine, oxaliplatin (Eloxatin), paclitaxel (Taxol), pentostatin (Nipent), piperacillin/tazobactam (Zosyn), potassium chloride (KCl), prochlorperazine (Compazine), promethazine (Phenergan), ranitidine (Zantac), remifentanil (Ultiva), sodium acetate, streptozocin (Zanosar), telavancin (Vibativ), teniposide (Vumon), thiotepa, ticarcillin/clavulanate (Timentin),

O-N

topotecan (Hycamtin), vancomycin, vinblastine, vincristine, vinorelbine (Navelbine), zidovudine (AZT, Retrovir).

RATE OF ADMINISTRATION

IV injection (postoperative N/V in adults and pediatric patients): A single 4-mg dose over at least 30 seconds; 2 to 5 minutes preferred.

Intermittent infusion adults and pediatric patients: A single dose equally distributed over 15 minutes.

ACTIONS

A selective antagonist of serotonin (5-HT$_3$) receptors. 5-HT$_3$ receptors are found both peripherally on vagal nerve terminals and centrally in the chemoreceptor trigger zone. It is unclear whether antiemetic action in chemotherapy-induced nausea and vomiting is mediated centrally, peripherally, or at both sites. Chemotherapeutic agents such as cis-platin increase the release of serotonin from specific cells in the GI tract, causing emesis. By antagonizing these receptors, chemotherapy-induced nausea and vomiting are pre-vented. Lacks the activity at dopamine receptors of metoclopramide (Reglan), so it does not cause the same level of sedation. No correlation between plasma levels and anti-emetic activity. Metabolized by specific hepatic enzymes of the cytochrome P$_{450}$ isoen-zyme system; onset of action is prompt. Half-life is 3.5 to 5.5 hours. Excreted in feces and urine.

INDICATIONS AND USES

Prevention of nausea and vomiting associated with initial and repeat courses of emeto-genic cancer chemotherapy, including high-dose cisplatin in patients age 6 months and older. ▪ Prevention of postoperative nausea and/or vomiting in patients age 1 month and older. ▪ Used orally (available as liquid, tablets, and orally disintegrating tablets) for prevention of nausea and vomiting, including postoperative N/V, and N/V associated with chemotherapy and radiotherapy (including total body irradiation). Approved for IM injection as an alternative to IV in the prevention of postoperative nausea and vomiting.

CONTRAINDICATIONS

Hypersensitivity to ondansetron or any of its components. ▪ Concomitant use of apomorphine.

PRECAUTIONS

Sterile technique imperative in withdrawing a single dose from the multidose vial. Avail-able in single-dose and multidose vials and in 4- and 8-mg tablets. ▪ Hypersensitivity reactions, including anaphylaxis and bronchospasm, have been reported. Cross-sensitivity has been reported between ondansetron and other 5HT$_3$ receptor agonists (e.g., dolase-tron [Anzemet] or granisetron [Kytril]). ▪ Use with caution in patients with hepatic impairment. Clearance is decreased; see Dose Adjustments. ▪ Not indicated instead of gastric suction. Use in abdominal surgery or in patients with chemotherapy-induced nausea and vomiting may mask a progressive ileus or gastric distension. ▪ May cause ECG changes, including QT-interval prolongation (prolongs the QT interval in a dose-dependent manner). Post-marketing cases of torsades de pointes have been reported. Avoid use in patients with congenital long QT syndrome. Use with caution in patients with electrolyte abnormalities (e.g., hypokalemia, hypomagnesemia), CHF, or bradyar-rhythmias or in patients taking other medicines that may lead to QT prolongation; see Monitor and Drug/Lab Interactions. ▪ Serotonin syndrome has been reported with 5-HT$_3$ receptor antagonists. Most reports were associated with concomitant use of sero-tonergic drugs (e.g., selective serotonin reuptake inhibitors [e.g., paroxetine (Paxil), escitalopram (Lexapro)], serotonin and norepinephrine reuptake inhibitors [e.g., dulox-etine (Cymbalta), venlafaxine (Effexor XR)], monoamine oxidase inhibitors [e.g., sele-giline (Eldepryl)], mirtazapine [Remeron], fentanyl, lithium, tramadol [Ultram], and intravenous methylene blue). Some cases were fatal. ▪ Routine prophylaxis is not recommended for patients in whom there is little expectation of postoperative N/V. However, for patients in whom nausea and vomiting must be avoided during the postoperative period, prophylaxis is recommended even when the incidence of postoperative N/V is low.

Monitor: Observe closely. Ambulate slowly to avoid orthostatic hypotension. ▪ ECG monitoring is recommended in patients with electrolyte abnormalities (e.g., hypokalemia, hypomagnesemia), CHF, or bradyarrhythmias or in patients taking other medicines that may lead to QT prolongation. ▪ Monitor for S/S of a hypersensitivity reaction (e.g., chest pain, dizziness, dyspnea, fever, flushing, hypotension, nausea, pruritus, rash, rigors, urticaria). ▪ Monitor for serotonin syndrome, especially when ondansetron is used concurrently with other serotonergic drugs. Symptoms associated with serotonin syndrome may include the following combination of S/S: mental status changes (e.g., agitation, coma, delirium, hallucinations), autonomic instability (e.g., diaphoresis, dizziness, flushing, hyperthermia, labile blood pressure, tachycardia), neuromuscular symptoms (e.g., hyperreflexia, incoordination, myoclonus, rigidity, tremor), and seizures, with or without GI symptoms (e.g., diarrhea, nausea, vomiting). ▪ Stool softeners or laxatives may be required to prevent constipation.

Patient Education: May cause dizziness or fainting; request assistance to ambulate. ▪ Promptly report difficulty breathing, tightness in the chest, or wheezing. ▪ May cause cardiac arrhythmias; discuss personal and family history and all prescription and nonprescription medications with a health care professional. ▪ Promptly report S/S of serotonin syndrome (e.g., altered mental status, autonomic instability, and neuromuscular symptoms); see Precautions.

Maternal/Child: Category B: no evidence of impaired fertility or harm to fetus. Use in pregnancy only if potential benefit justifies potential risk. ▪ Use caution if required during breast-feeding. ▪ Information limited in pediatric cancer patients under 6 months of age and in pediatric surgical patients under 1 month of age. ▪ In general, surgical and cancer pediatric patients younger than 18 years tend to have a higher clearance compared with adults, leading to a shorter half-life (2.9 hours). Infants 1 to 4 months of age have a lower clearance, resulting in a longer half-life (6.7 hours). Close monitoring of patients younger than 4 months of age is recommended.

Elderly: See Dose Adjustments.

DRUG/LAB INTERACTIONS

Does not appear to induce or inhibit the **cytochrome P$_{450}$ isoenzyme system.** However, it is metabolized by this system, and medications that induce or inhibit this system may affect its clearance and half-life. Dose adjustment is not recommended. ▪ **Phenytoin** (Dilantin), **carbamazepine** (Tegretol), and **rifampin** (Rifadin) increase clearance and decrease levels of ondansetron. Dose adjustment not recommended. ▪ Concomitant use of **apomorphine** may result in profound hypotension and loss of consciousness; see Contraindications. ▪ Concomitant use with **tramadol** (Ultram) may result in reduced analgesic activity of tramadol. See Precautions and use extreme caution with **diuretics** with the potential for inducing electrolyte abnormalities (e.g., furosemide [Lasix], hydrochlorothiazide) **or antiarrhythmic drugs or other drugs that lead to prolonged QT intervals** (e.g., amiodarone [Nexterone], procainamide [Pronestyl], quinidine). ▪ Serotonin syndrome (including altered mental status, autonomic instability, and neuromuscular symptoms) has been reported following the concomitant use of 5-HT$_3$ receptor antagonists and other serotonergic drugs, including selective serotonin reuptake inhibitors (SSRIs) and serotonin and norepinephrine reuptake inhibitors (SNRIs); see Precautions. ▪ Coadministration does not affect pharmacokinetics or pharmacodynamics of **temazepam** (Restoril). ▪ Does not alter respiratory depressant effects produced by alfentanil or the degree of neuromuscular blockade produced by atracurium (Tracrium). ▪ Carmustine (BiCNU), etoposide (VePesid), etoposide phosphate (Etopophos), and cisplatin do not affect the pharmacokinetics of ondansetron. ▪ Ondansetron does not increase the concentrations of high-dose methotrexate. ▪ Has been used with cyclophosphamide (Cytoxan), doxorubicin (Adriamycin), etoposide (VePesid), fluorouracil (5-FU), ifosfamide (Ifex), methotrexate, mitoxantrone (Novantrone), and vincristine.

SIDE EFFECTS

The most common side effects reported were diarrhea, fever, and headache.

Adults: Agitation, arrhythmias (including ventricular and superventricular tachycardia, PVCs, atrial fibrillation, and bradycardia), chest pain, cold sensation, constipation, cramps, diarrhea, dizziness, drowsiness, ECG alterations (including second-degree heart block, QT-interval prolongation, and ST segment depression), faintness, fatigue, fever, flushing, headache, hypersensitivity reactions (e.g., anaphylaxis, angioedema, bronchospasm, cardiopulmonary arrest, hypotension, laryngospasm, shock, shortness of breath, stridor, urticaria), hiccups, hypokalemia, injection site reactions, oculogyric crisis, pain (abdominal, joint, musculoskeletal, rib cage, shoulder), palpitations, paresthesia, pruritus, shivering, transient blurred vision or blindness, transient elevation of AST or ALT, urinary retention. Other side effects have occurred (e.g., extrapyramidal reaction, rash) in fewer than 1% of patients. Overdose caused sudden blindness in one patient.

Infants 1 to 24 months: Bronchospasm, diarrhea, fever, postprocedural pain.

Pediatric patients 2 to 12 years of age: Anxiety/agitation, drowsiness/sedation, fever, headache, wound problems.

Post-Marketing: Arthralgia; dyspnea; ECG changes, including QT/QTc interval prolongation; erythema; hepatitis, hepatic necrosis, hepatic failure, and death (in patients receiving potentially hepatotoxic cytotoxic chemotherapy and antibiotics; etiology unclear); hyperhidrosis; increased alkaline phosphatase (ALP), gamma-glutamyl transferase (GGT), and bilirubin; jaundice; laryngeal edema; lethargy; Stevens-Johnson syndrome; torsades de pointes; toxic epidermal necrolysis; ventricular fibrillation. Serotonin syndrome has been reported as a 5-HT$_3$ class reaction.

ANTIDOTE

Most side effects will be treated symptomatically. Keep physician informed as indicated. Overdose of 10 times the usual dose has not caused significant problems. If symptoms of serotonin syndrome occur, discontinue ondansetron and initiate supportive care. Treat anaphylaxis and resuscitate as necessary.

ORITAVANCIN
(**OR**-it-**A**-van-**SIN**)

Orbactiv

Antibacterial
(lipoglycopeptide)

pH 3.1 to 4.3

USUAL DOSE
A single 1,200-mg dose administered as an infusion over 3 hours.

DOSE ADJUSTMENTS
No dose adjustment is recommended in patients with mild or moderate renal or hepatic impairment. ▪ No dose adjustment recommended based on age, gender, weight, or race.

DILUTION
Available in single-use vials containing 400 mg of oritavancin as a lyophilized powder. Three vials are required to prepare a single dose. Reconstitute each 400-mg vial with 40 mL of SWFI. Gently swirl to avoid foaming, and ensure that all oritavancin powder is completely dissolved. Concentration is 10 mg/mL in each vial. Solution should be clear and colorless to pale yellow. Withdraw and discard 120 mL from a 1,000-mL IV bag of D5W. Withdraw 40 mL from each of the three reconstituted vials and add to the D5W IV bag to bring the volume back to 1,000 mL. Final concentration is 1.2 mg/mL.
Filters: Specific information not available.
Storage: Vials may be stored at CRT. Reconstituted vials and/or fully diluted solutions may be stored at RT for up to 6 hours or refrigerated at 2° to 8° C (36° to 46° F) for up to 12 hours. Total time from reconstitution to dilution to completion of administration should not exceed 6 hours at RT or 12 hours if refrigerated.

COMPATIBILITY
Manufacturer states, "Use only D5W for dilution. Do **NOT** use NS. NS is **incompatible** with oritavancin and may cause precipitation of the drug. Other IV substances, additives, or other medications mixed in NS should not be added to oritavancin single-use vials or infused simultaneously through the same IV line or through a common IV port. In addition, drugs formulated at a basic or neutral pH may be **incompatible** with oritavancin. If the same IV line is used for sequential infusion of additional medications, the line should be flushed before and after infusion of oritavancin with D5W."

RATE OF ADMINISTRATION
A single dose as an infusion equally distributed over 3 hours. If a common IV line is used to administer other drugs in addition to oritavancin, flush the IV line before and after each oritavancin infusion with D5W. If an infusion reaction occurs, temporarily stop or slow the infusion as indicated.

ACTIONS
Oritavancin is a semi-synthetic lipoglycopeptide antibacterial drug. It exerts a concentration-dependent bactericidal activity in vitro against *Staphylococcus aureus, Streptococcus pyogenes,* and *Enterococcus faecalis.* It has three mechanisms of action (1) inhibition of the transglycosylation (polymerization) step of cell wall biosynthesis by binding to the stem peptide of peptidoglycan precursors, (2) inhibition of the transpeptidation (cross-linking) step of cell wall biosynthesis by binding to the peptide bridging segments of the cell wall, and (3) disruption of bacterial membrane integrity, leading to depolarization, permeabilization, and cell death. Approximately 85% bound to plasma proteins. Extensively distributed into tissue. Not metabolized. Terminal half-life is approximately 245 hours. Minimally excreted as unchanged drug in feces and urine.

INDICATIONS AND USES
Treatment of adult patients with acute bacterial skin and skin structure infections (ABSSSI) caused by susceptible isolates of designated Gram-positive microorganisms, including *Staphylococcus aureus* (both methicillin-susceptible [MSSA] and methicillin-resistant [MRSA] strains).

CONTRAINDICATIONS

Known hypersensitivity to oritavancin. ▪ Use of IV unfractionated heparin sodium is contraindicated for 120 hours (5 days) after oritavancin administration because aPTT test results are expected to remain falsely elevated for up to 120 hours (5 days).

PRECAUTIONS

Coadministration of oritavancin with warfarin (Coumadin) may increase exposure of warfarin, which may increase the risk of bleeding; see Drug/Lab Interactions. Use oritavancin in patients on chronic warfarin therapy only when the benefits can be expected to outweigh the risk of bleeding. ▪ The aPTT has been shown to be artificially prolonged for up to 120 hours, the PT and INR for up to 12 hours, and the activated clotting time (ACT) for up to 24 hours after administration of oritavancin. D-dimer concentrations have been shown to be elevated for up to 72 hours after administration; see Drug/Lab Interactions. ▪ Serious hypersensitivity reactions have been reported. Check history of previous hypersensitivity reactions to glycopeptides (e.g., dalbavancin [Dalvance], telavancin [Vibativ], vancomycin). Exercise caution in patients with a history of glycopeptide allergy; cross-sensitivity is possible. ▪ Infusion-related reactions have been reported; see Rate of Administration. ▪ Specific sensitivity studies are indicated to determine susceptibility of the causative organism to oritavancin. ▪ To reduce the development of drug-resistant bacteria and maintain its effectiveness, oritavancin should be used to treat only those infections proven or strongly suspected to be caused by bacteria. ▪ *Clostridium difficile*–associated diarrhea (CDAD) has been reported for nearly all systemic antibacterial agents and may range in severity from mild diarrhea to fatal colitis. Consider in patients who present with diarrhea during or after treatment with oritavancin. ▪ In clinical trials, more cases of osteomyelitis were reported in the oritavancin-treated arm than in the vancomycin-treated arm. If osteomyelitis is suspected or diagnosed, institute appropriate alternate antibacterial therapy. ▪ The pharmacokinetics of oritavancin has not been studied in patients with severe renal or hepatic impairment.

Monitor: Frequently monitor patients on chronic warfarin therapy for signs of bleeding. ▪ Monitoring of the anticoagulation effect of warfarin (e.g., PT, INR) is unreliable for up to 12 hours after oritavancin administration; see Precautions and Drug/Lab Interactions. ▪ If aPTT monitoring is required within 120 hours of oritavancin dosing, use a nonphospholipid-dependent coagulation test such as a factor Xa (chromogenic) assay, or consider an alternative anticoagulant not requiring aPTT monitoring. ▪ Monitor for S/S of hypersensitivity (e.g., hypotension, rash, urticaria, tightness of the chest, wheezing). In clinical trials, the median onset of hypersensitivity reactions was 1.2 days and the median duration of these reactions was 2.4 days. ▪ Monitor for S/S of an infusion reaction; see Rate of Administration. ▪ Monitor for S/S of osteomyelitis; see Antidote.

Patient Education: Promptly report S/S of a hypersensitivity reaction (e.g., hives, rash, shortness of breath, wheezing) or an infusion reaction (e.g., flushing of the upper body, pruritus, rash, and/or urticaria). ▪ Promptly report diarrhea or bloody stools that occur during treatment or up to several months after an antibiotic has been discontinued; may indicate CDAD and require treatment.

Maternal/Child: Category C: use during pregnancy only if the potential benefit outweighs the potential risk to the fetus. ▪ Use caution during breast-feeding. ▪ Safety and effectiveness for use in pediatric patients not established.

Elderly: Numbers in clinical studies insufficient to determine if the elderly respond differently from younger subjects. Differences have not been identified. However, greater sensitivity of some older individuals cannot be ruled out.

DRUG/LAB INTERACTIONS

Clinical drug-drug interaction studies have not been conducted. ▪ Oritavancin is a nonspecific weak inducer and weak inhibitor of selected **cytochrome P$_{450}$ enzymes**. Caution should be used when administering oritavancin with drugs that have a narrow therapeutic window and are predominantly metabolized by one of the affected CYP$_{450}$ enzymes (e.g., **warfarin** [Coumadin]). Coadministration may increase or decrease concentrations of drugs with a narrow therapeutic range. Monitor closely for signs of toxicity or lack of effectiveness (e.g., monitor patients on concomitant warfarin for bleeding). ▪ Oritavancin has been shown to artificially prolong aPTT for up to 120 hours, PT and INR for up to 12 hours, and ACT for up to 24 hours after administration of a single 1,200-mg dose by binding to and preventing the action of the phospholipid reagents that activate coagulation in commonly used laboratory coagulation tests. Oritavancin has also been shown to elevate D-dimer concentration up to 72 hours after oritavancin administration. ▪ Oritavancin does not affect chromogenic factor Xa assay, thrombin time (TT), or tests that are used for the diagnosis of heparin-induced thrombocytopenia (HIT). ▪ Oritavancin does not interfere with coagulation in vivo. ▪ Oritavancin is neither a substrate nor an inhibitor of the efflux transporter **P-glycoprotein (P-gp)**. ▪ In vitro, oritavancin demonstrated synergistic bactericidal activity in combination with gentamicin, linezolid (Zyvox), moxifloxacin (Avelox), and rifampin (Rifadin) against designated organisms.

SIDE EFFECTS
The most common side effects reported are diarrhea, headache, limb and subcutaneous abscesses, and nausea and vomiting. Hypersensitivity and/or infusion reactions and CDAD may be severe. Cellulitis, dizziness, increased ALT and AST levels, infusion site phlebitis, osteomyelitis, and tachycardia were also reported. Many other side effects occurred in fewer than 1.5% of patients.

ANTIDOTE
Notify physician of any side effects. Discontinue the drug if indicated. Treat hypersensitivity reactions as indicated (e.g., diphenhydramine [Benadryl], epinephrine [Adrenalin], albuterol) and resuscitate as necessary. Temporarily discontinue or slow infusion for infusion-related reactions. Mild cases of CDAD may respond to discontinuation of oritavancin. Treat CDAD with fluids, electrolytes, protein supplements, and oral vancomycin (Vancocin) or metronidazole (Flagyl) as indicated. In severe cases, surgical evaluation may be indicated. If osteomyelitis is suspected or diagnosed, institute appropriate alternate antibacterial therapy. Oritavancin is not removed by hemodialysis.

O-N

OXALIPLATIN BBW

(OX-al-ee-plah-tin)

Antineoplastic

Eloxatin

USUAL DOSE

Both indications: Given in combination with 5-FU and leucovorin calcium in a dose schedule that repeats every 2 weeks. When used as adjuvant therapy in patients with stage III colon cancer, a treatment period repeated every 2 weeks for 6 months is recommended (a total of 12 cycles). For advanced disease, treatment is recommended until disease progression or unacceptable toxicity. For information on 5-FU and leucovorin calcium, see respective monographs. Prehydration is not required. Premedication with antiemetics recommended; see Monitor. Some clinicians are administering magnesium and calcium before and after oxaliplatin to decrease neurotoxicity.

Day 1: Oxaliplatin 85 mg/M^2 and leucovorin calcium 200 mg/M^2, both given as an IV infusion over 120 minutes at the same time in separate bags using a Y-line. Follow with 5-FU 400 mg/M^2 IV bolus given over 2 to 4 minutes, followed by 5-FU 600 mg/M^2 in 500 mL D5W (recommended) as a 22-hour continuous infusion.

Day 2: Leucovorin calcium 200 mg/M^2 IV infusion over 120 minutes. Follow with 5-FU 400 mg/M^2 IV bolus given over 2 to 4 minutes, followed by 5-FU 600 mg/M^2 in 500 mL D5W (recommended) as a 22-hour continuous infusion.

DOSE ADJUSTMENTS

Decrease starting dose to 65 mg/M^2 in patients with severe renal impairment (CrCl less than 30 mL/min). ▪ Withhold oxaliplatin for sepsis or septic shock, and reduce dose if indicated as outlined in the following sections.

Advanced colorectal cancer: Dose adjustments are based on clinical toxicities. Reduce dose of oxaliplatin to 65 mg/M^2 in patients who experience persistent Grade 2 neurosensory events that do not resolve. (See Monitor for study-specific neurotoxicity scale.) The infusional 5-FU/leucovorin calcium regimen need not be altered. ▪ Reduce dose of oxaliplatin to 65 mg/M^2 and 5-FU to a 300 mg/M^2 bolus and 500 mg/M^2 as a 22-hour infusion in patients who develop Grade 3 or 4 gastrointestinal toxicity (despite prophylactic treatment), Grade 4 neutropenia, febrile neutropenia, or Grade 3 or 4 thrombocytopenia. Delay next dose until neutrophils are greater than or equal to 1.5 × 10^9/L [1,500 cells/mm^3] and platelets are greater than or equal to 75 × 10^9/L [75,000 cells/mm^3]).

Adjuvant therapy in stage III colon cancer (postoperative): Reduce dose of oxaliplatin to 75 mg/M^2 in patients who experience persistent Grade 2 neurosensory events that do not resolve (NCICTC scale version 1 used). The infusional 5-FU/leucovorin calcium regimen need not be altered. ▪ Reduce dose of oxaliplatin to 75 mg/M^2 and 5-FU to a 300 mg/M^2 bolus and 500 mg/M^2 as a 22-hour infusion in patients who develop Grade 3 or 4 gastrointestinal toxicity (despite prophylactic treatment), Grade 4 neutropenia, febrile neutropenia, or Grade 3 or 4 thrombocytopenia. Delay next dose until neutrophils are greater than or equal to 1.5 × 10^9/L (1,500 cells/mm^3) and platelets are greater than or equal to 75 × 10^9/L (75,000 cells/mm^3).

Both indications: Consider discontinuing therapy in patients with persistent Grade 3 neurosensory events.

DILUTION

Specific techniques required; see Precautions.

Do not reconstitute or dilute with a sodium chloride solution (e.g., NS, ½NS, ¼NS) or other chloride-containing solutions. Available as a concentrate for solution. The concentrate for solution must be further diluted with 250 to 500 mL of D5W. *Do not use NS or any chloride-containing solutions; see Compatibility.* Do not use needles or administration sets with aluminum parts; a precipitate may form, and potency may decrease.

Storage: Store vials with concentrate in the original carton at CRT. Protect vials with concentrate from light and do not freeze. After final dilution with 250 to 500 mL of D5W, the solution may be stored for up to 6 hours at RT (20° to 25° C [68° to 77° F]) or up to 24 hours under refrigeration.

COMPATIBILITY
(Underline Indicates Conflicting Compatibility Information)

Consider any drug NOT listed as compatible to be INCOMPATIBLE until consulting a pharmacist; specific conditions may apply.

Manufacturer states oxaliplatin "is **incompatible** in solution with alkaline medications or media (such as basic solutions of 5-FU) and must not be mixed with these or administered simultaneously through the same infusion line. *The infusion line should be flushed with D5W prior to administration of any concomitant medication.*" Reconstitution or final dilution must not be performed with a sodium chloride solution or other chloride-containing solutions. Do not use needles or administration sets with aluminum parts; a precipitate may form, and potency may decrease.

Sources suggest the following **compatibilities:**

Y-site: Manufacturer lists leucovorin calcium. Another source lists bumetanide, buprenorphine (Buprenex), butorphanol (Stadol), calcium gluconate, carboplatin (Paraplatin), chlorpromazine (Thorazine), cyclophosphamide (Cytoxan), dexamethasone (Decadron), diphenhydramine (Benadryl), dobutamine, docetaxel (Taxotere), dolasetron (Anzemet), dopamine, doxorubicin (Adriamycin), droperidol (Inapsine), enalaprilat (Vasotec IV), epirubicin (Ellence), etoposide phosphate (Etopophos), famotidine (Pepcid IV), fentanyl, furosemide (Lasix), gemcitabine (Gemzar), granisetron (Kytril), heparin, hydrocortisone sodium succinate (Solu-Cortef), hydromorphone (Dilaudid), ifosfamide (Ifex), irinotecan (Camptosar), leucovorin calcium, lorazepam (Ativan), magnesium sulfate, mannitol (Osmitrol), meperidine (Demerol), mesna (Mesnex), methotrexate, methylprednisolone (Solu-Medrol), metoclopramide (Reglan), mitoxantrone (Novantrone), morphine, nalbuphine, ondansetron (Zofran), paclitaxel (Taxol), palonosetron (Aloxi), potassium chloride (KCl), prochlorperazine (Compazine), promethazine (Phenergan), ranitidine (Zantac), theophylline, topotecan (Hycamtin), verapamil, vincristine, vinorelbine (Navelbine).

RATE OF ADMINISTRATION

The infusion line should be flushed with D5W prior to administration of any concomitant medication.

Day 1: Oxaliplatin and leucovorin calcium are given as infusions and equally distributed over 120 minutes. Given at the same time in separate bags using a Y-line. When complete, flush the IV line with D5W. Follow with a **5-FU bolus** administered over 2 to 4 minutes, followed by a **5-FU continuous infusion** equally distributed over 22 hours. ▪ Increasing the infusion time of oxaliplatin from 2 to 6 hours may mitigate acute toxicities. The infusion times for 5-FU and leucovorin calcium need not be altered.

Day 2: Leucovorin calcium is given as an infusion equally distributed over 120 minutes. Follow with a **5-FU bolus** administered over 2 to 4 minutes, followed by a **5-FU continuous infusion** equally distributed over 22 hours.

ACTIONS

A platinum-based antineoplastic agent. Undergoes nonenzymatic conversion to active derivatives that inhibit DNA replication and transcription. Cytotoxicity is cell-cycle nonspecific. Rapidly distributed into tissues or eliminated in the urine. Highly protein bound. Undergoes rapid and extensive nonenzymatic biotransformation. No evidence of cytochrome P_{450}-mediated metabolism. Major route of elimination is renal excretion.

INDICATIONS AND USES

Used in combination with infusional 5-FU and leucovorin calcium for the treatment of patients with advanced colorectal cancer and for adjuvant therapy of stage III colon cancer patients who have undergone complete resection of the primary tumor.

CONTRAINDICATIONS

Hypersensitivity to oxaliplatin or other platinum-containing compounds (e.g., carboplatin [Paraplatin], cisplatin).

PRECAUTIONS

Follow guidelines for handling cytotoxic agents. See Appendix A, p. 1331. ▪ Administered by or under the direction of the physician specialist. ▪ Adequate diagnostic and treatment facilities and emergency resuscitation equipment and supplies must always be available. ▪ Hypersensitivity and anaphylactic-like reactions, some fatal, have been reported and may occur within minutes of administration and during any cycle. Rechallenge is contraindicated. See Side Effects and Antidote. ▪ Use with caution in patients with renal impairment; see Dose Adjustments. ▪ Associated with two types of neuropathy. *The first type is an acute, reversible, primarily peripheral sensory neuropathy that is of early onset, occurs within hours or 1 to 2 days of dosing, resolves within 14 days, and frequently recurs with further dosing.* Symptoms may be precipitated or exacerbated by exposure to cold temperature or cold objects. Usually presents as transient paresthesia (abnormal sensation [e.g., burning, prickling]), dysesthesia (decreased sensitivity to stimulation), and hypoesthesia (impairment of any sense, especially touch) in the hands, feet, perioral area, or throat. *The second type is a persistent (lasting more than 14 days), primarily peripheral, sensory neuropathy that is usually characterized by paresthesias, dysesthesias, and hypoesthesias but may also include deficits in proprioception (stimulus of the sensory end organs [e.g., muscles, tendons]), which can interfere with daily activities (e.g., writing, buttoning, swallowing, and walking).* May occur without any prior acute neuropathy event. Symptoms may or may not improve with discontinuation of oxaliplatin. ▪ Reversible posterior leukoencephalopathy syndrome (RPLS) has been reported; see Monitor. ▪ Grade 3 or 4 neutropenia has occurred in patients treated with oxaliplatin. Sepsis, neutropenic sepsis, and septic shock have been reported. Deaths have occurred. ▪ Has been associated with pulmonary fibrosis, which may be fatal; see Monitor. ▪ Hepatotoxicity has been reported; see Monitor. ▪ QT prolongation and ventricular arrhythmias, including fatal torsades de pointes, have been reported. Avoid oxaliplatin in patients with congenital long QT syndrome; see Monitor and Drug/Lab Interactions. ▪ Rhabdomyolysis, including fatal cases, has been reported. ▪ See Drug/Lab Interactions.

Monitor: CBC with differential, platelet count, and blood chemistries (including ALT, AST, bilirubin, and creatinine) are recommended before each cycle. See Dose Adjustments and Precautions. ▪ Monitor for S/S of a hypersensitivity reaction (e.g., bronchospasm, chest pain, diaphoresis, diarrhea associated with oxaliplatin infusion, disorientation, erythema, flushing, hypotension, pruritus, rash, shortness of breath, syncope, urticaria). ▪ Monitor for S/S of RPLS; may include abnormal vision from blurriness to blindness, altered mental functioning, headache, or seizures. Diagnosis of PRES is based on confirmation by brain imaging. ▪ Monitor for unexplained respiratory symptoms such as nonproductive cough, dyspnea, crackles, or radiologic pulmonary infiltrates. Discontinue oxaliplatin until pulmonary investigation rules out interstitial lung disease or pulmonary fibrosis. ▪ Monitor for S/S of neuropathy (e.g., transient paresthesia [abnormal sensation (e.g., burning, prickling)], dysesthesia [decreased sensitivity to stimulation], and hypoesthesia [impairment of any sense, especially touch] in the hands, feet, perioral area, or throat). Neurotoxicity scale used during advanced colorectal cancer studies differed from National Cancer Institute toxicity grading. Grading scale for paresthesias/dysesthesias was as follows: Grade 1, resolved and did not interfere with functioning; Grade 2, interfered with function but not daily activities; Grade 3, pain or functional impairment that interfered with daily activities; Grade 4, persistent impairment that is disabling or life threatening. ▪ Nausea and vomiting may be significant. Prophylactic administration of antiemetics, including 5HT$_3$ blockers (e.g., ondansetron [Zofran]), with or without dexamethasone (Decadron), is recommended. ▪ Observe closely for signs of infection, sepsis, or septic shock. Prophylactic antibiotics may be indicated pending results of C/S in a febrile neutropenic patient. ▪ Monitor for S/S of hepatotoxicity. Hepatic vascular disorders should be considered in the case of abnormal liver function test results or portal hypertension that cannot be explained by liver metastases. ▪ ECG monitoring is recommended for patients with CHF, bradyarrhythmias, drugs known to prolong the QT interval, and electrolyte abnormalities. Correct hypokalemia and hypomagnesemia before initiating oxaliplatin therapy, and monitor these electrolytes periodically during therapy; see Drug/Lab Interactions. ▪ Monitor for S/S of rhabdomyolysis (muscle pain, weakness, dark urine, elevation in creatinine kinase [CK] and other serum muscle enzymes).

Patient Education: Avoid pregnancy. Nonhormonal birth control recommended. ▪ Report any neurologic symptoms (e.g., confusion or a change in the way you think; headache; numbness, pain, or tingling in extremities; seizures; vision problems; sensitivity to cold; troubled breathing or swallowing). Acute neurosensory toxicity may be precipitated or exacerbated by exposure to cold. Avoid cold drinks and use of ice. Cover exposed skin before exposure to cold temperature. ▪ Promptly report persistent vomiting, diarrhea, breathing difficulty, cough, or any sign of infection, allergic reaction, or dehydration. ▪ Use caution while driving or using machines; neurologic symptoms (e.g., dizziness), nausea and vomiting, and vision abnormalities (e.g., transient vision loss) may interfere with abilities. ▪ Manufacturer supplies a patient information leaflet; read before taking oxaliplatin. ▪ See Appendix D, p. 1333.

Maternal/Child: Category D: avoid pregnancy; may cause fetal harm. ▪ Discontinue breast-feeding. ▪ Safety and effectiveness for use in pediatric patients not established. Has been studied in a small number of solid tumors in pediatric patients. No significant response was observed. See manufacturer's literature.

Elderly: The overall rates of adverse events, including Grade 3 and 4 events, were similar for all age-groups. However, the incidence of dehydration, diarrhea, fatigue, Grade 3 to 4 granulocytopenia, hypokalemia, leukopenia, and syncope were higher in patients 65 years of age or older. Adjustment of starting dose is not required.

DRUG/LAB INTERACTIONS

Formal studies have not been performed. ▪ Do not administer **live virus vaccines** to patients receiving antineoplastic agents. ▪ Platinum-containing species are eliminated primarily through the kidney; clearance of these products may be decreased by coadministration of potentially **nephrotoxic compounds** (e.g., aminoglycosides [e.g., gentamicin], amphotericin B [all formulations], NSAIDs [e.g., ibuprofen (Advil, Motrin), naproxen (Aleve, Naprosyn)], pamidronate [Aredia], tacrolimus [Prograf]). ▪ Oxaliplatin is not metabolized by, nor does it inhibit, cytochrome P_{450} isoenzymes. P_{450}-mediated interactions are not anticipated. ▪ A prolonged PT and INR (occasionally associated with hemorrhage) has been reported when oxaliplatin is used concomitantly with **anticoagulants** (e.g., warfarin [Coumadin]); close monitoring of PT and INR recommended. ▪ Use caution when administered with **drugs known to prolong the QT interval** (e.g., Class Ia and III antiarrhythmics [e.g., disopyramide (Norpace), procainamide (Pronestyl), quinidine, amiodarone (Nexterone)], macrolide antibiotics [e.g., azithromycin (Zithromax), clarithromycin (Biaxin)], fluoroquinolones [e.g., ciprofloxacin (Cipro), levofloxacin (Levaquin)], antiemetics [e.g., dolasetron (Anzemet), ondansetron (Zofran)]). ECG monitoring recommended.

SIDE EFFECTS

Are frequent and numerous. The most common adverse reactions are anemia, diarrhea, fatigue, increased liver function tests (e.g., alkaline phosphatase, total bilirubin, and transaminases), nausea, neutropenia, peripheral sensory neuropathies, stomatitis, thrombocytopenia, and vomiting; see Precautions. Other reported reactions include abdominal pain, alopecia, angioedema, anorexia, arthralgia, back pain, chest pain, colitis (including *Clostridium difficile* diarrhea), conjunctivitis, constipation, coughing, deafness, dehydration, dizziness, dyspepsia, dyspnea, dysuria, edema, elevated serum creatinine, epistaxis, fever, flushing, gastroesophageal reflux, hand-foot syndrome, headache, hematuria, hemolytic uremic syndrome, hypersensitivity reactions (e.g., anaphylaxis, angioedema, bronchospasm, erythema, hypotension, laryngospasm, pruritus, rash, urticaria), hypertension, hypokalemia, immunoallergic hemolytic anemia, infection, injection site reaction, insomnia, intestinal obstruction, lacrimation abnormalities, metabolic acidosis, mucositis, pain, pancreatitis, persistent vomiting, pharyngitis, pulmonary fibrosis, rhinitis, rigors, secondary malignancies, taste perversion, thromboembolism, veno-occlusive disease of the liver, visual disorders (e.g., decrease of visual acuity, visual field disturbance, optic neuritis), weight gain. Many other side effects have been reported and may occur.

Overdose: Chest pain, dehydration, diarrhea, dyspnea, enlarged abdomen and Grade 4 intestinal obstruction, hypersensitivity reactions, myelosuppression, nausea and vomiting, neurotoxicity, paresthesia, respiratory failure, severe bradycardia, stomatitis, wheezing, and death.

Post-Marketing: Acute interstitial nephritis, acute tubular necrosis, acute renal failure, colitis (including *Clostridium difficile* diarrhea), convulsions, cranial nerve palsies, dysarthria, fasciculations, hemolytic uremic syndrome, ileus, immunoallergic thrombocytopenia, Lhermitte's sign, metabolic acidosis, perisinusoidal fibrosis, pulmonary fibrosis and other interstitial lung diseases (sometimes fatal), QT prolongation leading to ventricular arrhythmias (including fatal torsades de pointes), rhabdomyolysis (including fatal outcomes), reversible posterior leukoencephalopathy syndrome (RPLS), septic shock (including fatal cases), severe diarrhea/vomiting resulting in hypokalemia, transient vision loss (reversible after oxaliplatin is discontinued).

ANTIDOTE

Notify physician of all side effects. Oxaliplatin may need to be discontinued permanently or until recovery. Slowing of infusion rate may help mitigate acute toxicities. Symptomatic and supportive treatment is indicated. Administration of whole blood products (e.g., packed RBCs, platelets, leukocytes) and/or blood modifiers (e.g., darbepoetin alfa [Aranesp], epoetin alfa [Epogen], filgrastim [Neupogen, Zarxio], pegfilgrastim [Neulasta], sargramostim [Leukine]) may be indicated to treat bone marrow toxicity. Treat anaphylaxis with epinephrine, corticosteroids, oxygen, and antihistamines (diphenhydramine). There is no specific antidote. Resuscitate as indicated.

OXYMORPHONE HYDROCHLORIDE

Opioid analgesic (agonist)

(ox-ee-**MOR**-fohn hy-droh-**KLOR**-eyed)

Opana

pH 2.7 to 4.5

USUAL DOSE

Individualize dose. Consider age, general condition, and medical status of the patient as well as type and severity of pain and prior analgesic treatment experience.

0.5 mg initially. May repeat every 2 to 4 hours. Up to 1.5 mg may be required.

When seeking the required dose to achieve pain relief for an individual patient, increases in increments of at least 25% of the previous dose are suggested. Lower slightly if pain controlled but patient is too drowsy, or lower dose and increase frequency.

DOSE ADJUSTMENTS

Reduced dose or extended intervals may be required in the elderly, in hepatic or renal disease, and in emphysema. ▪ Doses appropriate for the general population may cause serious respiratory depression in vulnerable patients. ▪ Reduce dose by one third to one half in patients who are concurrently receiving other CNS depressants; see Drug/Lab Interactions. ▪ Increase doses as required if analgesia is inadequate, tolerance develops, or pain severity increases. The first sign of tolerance is usually a reduced duration of effect.

DILUTION

May be given undiluted; however, further dilution with 5 mL of SWFI or NS to facilitate titration is appropriate. May give through Y-tube or three-way stopcock of infusion set.

Storage: Store at CRT. Protect from light.

COMPATIBILITY
Specific information not available.

RATE OF ADMINISTRATION
Rapid IV administration increases the possibility of hypotension and respiratory depression.

A single dose over 2 to 5 minutes. Usually titrated according to symptom relief and respiratory rate.

ACTIONS
A semi-synthetic opioid analgesic closely related to morphine. Ten times more potent than morphine milligram for milligram. Produces a wide range of pharmacologic effects, including analgesia, anxiolysis, cough suppression, diminished GI motility, dysphoria, euphoria, physical dependence, respiratory depression, and somnolence. Onset of action is 5 to 10 minutes. Duration of action is 3 to 6 hours. Metabolized in the liver and excreted in urine and feces. Crosses placental barrier. Secreted in breast milk.

INDICATIONS AND USES
Relief of moderate to severe pain. ▪ Support of anesthesia. ▪ Obstetric analgesia. ▪ Relief of anxiety in patients with dyspnea associated with pulmonary edema secondary to acute left ventricular dysfunction.

CONTRAINDICATIONS
Acute bronchial asthma, pediatric patients under 12 years of age, diarrhea caused by poisoning until toxic material eliminated, hypercarbia, known hypersensitivity to oxymorphone or other morphine analogs (e.g., codeine), moderate to severe hepatic impairment, paralytic ileus, premature infants and labor and delivery of premature infants, pulmonary edema caused by chemical respiratory irritant, upper airway obstruction.

PRECAUTIONS
Schedule II opioid agonists, including hydromorphone, morphine, oxymorphone, oxycodone, fentanyl, and methadone, have the highest potential for abuse and risk of producing respiratory depression. Alcohol, CNS depressants, and other opioids potentiate the respiratory depressant effects of hydromorphone, increasing the risk of respiratory depression that might result in death; see Drug/Lab Interactions. ▪ Use extreme caution in patients with conditions accompanied by hypoxia, hypercapnia, or decreased respiratory reserve such as asthma, COPD, cor pulmonale, severe obesity, sleep apnea syndrome, myxedema, kyphoscoliosis, CNS depression, or coma. May decrease respiratory drive and increase airway resistance to the point of apnea. ▪ Use with caution in the elderly or debilitated and in patients known to be sensitive to CNS depressants, such as those with cardiovascular, pulmonary, renal, or hepatic disease. ▪ Use extreme caution in craniotomy, head injury, and increased intracranial pressure; respiratory depression and intracranial pressure may be further increased. ▪ Can also produce effects on pupillary response and consciousness, which may obscure neurologic signs of further increases in intracranial pressure. ▪ Use with caution in patients in circulatory shock. May further reduce cardiac output or BP. ▪ Use with caution in acute alcoholism, adrenocortical insufficiency (e.g., Addison's disease), CNS depression, delirium tremens, prostatic hypertrophy, or urethral stricture. ▪ Symptoms of acute abdominal conditions may be masked. Can cause spasm of the sphincter of Oddi. Use with caution in patients with biliary tract disease, including acute pancreatitis. ▪ May increase ventricular response rate in presence of supraventricular tachycardias. ▪ Cough reflex is suppressed. ▪ Tolerance to oxymorphone gradually increases. A marked increase in dose may precipitate seizures. ▪ Concerns about abuse, addiction, and diversion should not prevent proper management of pain.

Monitor: Oxygen, controlled respiratory equipment, and naloxone must be available. ▪ Assess baseline pain, then assess pain with vital signs and/or more frequently if needed. Reassess after administration of oxymorphone and adjust dose or interval as required. ▪ Keep patient supine; orthostatic hypotension and fainting may occur. Uncontrolled pain causes sleep deprivation, decreases pain threshold, and increases pain; when pain is

N-O

finally controlled, expect the patient to sleep more until recovery from sleep deprivation. ▪ Adhere to prescribed bowel care regimen to avoid constipation and/or impaction. Maintain adequate hydration.

Patient Education: Avoid alcohol or other CNS depressants (e.g., barbiturates, benzodiazepines [e.g., diazepam (Valium)]). ▪ May cause blurred vision, dizziness, or drowsiness; use caution in tasks that require alertness. ▪ Request assistance with ambulation. ▪ May be habit forming.

Maternal/Child: Category C: safety for use in pregnancy or breast-feeding not established; see Contraindications. ▪ Use with caution during labor. May cause respiratory depression in the newborn. ▪ Safety for use in pediatric patients under 18 years of age not established.

Elderly: See Dose Adjustments and Precautions. ▪ May be more sensitive to effects (e.g., respiratory depression, constipation, urinary retention). Adverse effects more commonly observed in the elderly include confusion, dizziness, nausea, and somnolence. ▪ Lower doses may provide effective analgesia. ▪ Consider age-related organ impairment.

DRUG/LAB INTERACTIONS

Potentiated by **phenothiazines and other CNS depressants** such as narcotic analgesics, alcohol, antihistamines, barbiturates, cimetidine (Tagamet), hypnotics, sedatives, MAO inhibitors (e.g., selegiline [Eldepryl]), neuromuscular blocking agents (e.g., atracurium [Tracrium]), and psychotropic agents. Interactive effects resulting in respiratory depression, hypotension, profound sedation, or coma may result with concomitant use. Reduced dosages of both drugs may be indicated. ▪ Administration of **agonist/antagonist analgesics** (e.g., butorphanol [Stadol], buprenorphine [Buprenex]) to an opiate-dependent patient receiving a pure opiate may reduce the analgesic effect of the pure opiate and/or precipitate withdrawal symptoms. ▪ Concomitant use with **anticholinergics or medications with anticholinergic activity** (e.g., diphenhydramine [Benadryl]) may result in an increased risk of urinary retention and/or severe constipation, which may lead to paralytic ileus. ▪ Concomitant use with **propofol** (Diprivan) for the induction of anesthesia may increase the incidence of bradycardia. ▪ Plasma **amylase and lipase determinations** may be unreliable for 24 hours following opioid administration.

SIDE EFFECTS

At equianalgesic doses, may cause more nausea, vomiting, and euphoria than morphine.

Abdominal pain, anorexia, biliary colic, blurred vision, bradycardia, bronchospasm, confusion, constipation, diplopia, dizziness, dry mouth, flushing, hallucinations, miosis, paralytic ileus, pruritus, skin rash, urinary retention, urticaria.

Major: Anaphylaxis, hypotension, respiratory depression, somnolence.

ANTIDOTE

Notify the physician of any side effect. If minor side effects progress or any major side effect occurs, discontinue the drug and notify the physician. Treat anaphylaxis as indicated or resuscitate as necessary. Naloxone hydrochloride will reverse cardiovascular, CNS, and respiratory reactions.

OXYTOCIN INJECTION BBW

(ox-eh-**TOE**-sin in-**JEK**-shun)

Pitocin

Oxytocic
Antihemorrhagic

pH 2.5 to 4.5

USUAL DOSE
Determined by uterine response and intended use, dilution, and rate of administration. Dose must be individualized and initiated at a very low level. Piggyback oxytocin into a physiologic electrolyte IV solution (e.g., NS) without oxytocin; see Precautions.

Induction of labor: 0.5 to 1 milliunit/min (mU/min) (equal to 3 to 6 mL/hr of properly diluted solution). See Dilution and Rate of Administration.

Control of postpartum bleeding: See Dilution and Rate of Administration.

Incomplete, inevitable, or elective abortion: A total of 10 units delivered at 10 to 20 mU/min. A total dose should not exceed 30 units in a 12-hour period due to the risk of water intoxication. See Dilution and Rate of Administration.

DILUTION
In all situations, rotate gently to distribute medication through solution.

Induction of labor: Dilute 1 mL (10 units) in 1 liter of NS or LR for infusion (10 mU/mL).

Control of postpartum bleeding: Dilute 1 to 4 mL (10 to 40 units) in 1 liter of above infusion fluids (10 to 40 mU/mL).

Incomplete, inevitable, or elective abortion: Dilute 1 mL (10 units) in 500 mL of NS or D5W.

Storage: Store at CRT.

COMPATIBILITY
Consider any drug NOT listed as compatible to be INCOMPATIBLE until consulting a pharmacist; specific conditions may apply.

Rapidly decomposes in the presence of sodium bisulfate.

One source suggests the following **compatibilities:**

Additive: Chloramphenicol (Chloromycetin), sodium bicarbonate, verapamil.

Y-site: Heparin, hydrocortisone sodium succinate (Solu-Cortef), insulin (regular), meperidine (Demerol), morphine, potassium chloride (KCl), warfarin (Coumadin), zidovudine (AZT, Retrovir).

RATE OF ADMINISTRATION
Given only as an IV infusion. Use of an infusion pump or other accurate control device is required. In all situations, use the minimum effective rate and monitor strength, frequency, and duration of contractions; resting uterine tone; fetal HR (in induction of labor); and maternal BP; see Monitor.

Induction of labor: Begin with 0.5 to 1 mU/min (3 to 6 mL/hr), and increase in increments of 1 to 2 mU/min at 30- to 60-minute intervals until contractions simulate normal labor. Maximum dose rarely exceeds 9 to 10 mU/min at term; average is 2 to 5 mU/min. Reduce by similar increments when desired frequency of contractions is reached and labor has progressed to 5 to 6 cm. 6 mU/min provides oxytocin levels similar to spontaneous labor. Preterm induction may require somewhat higher doses due to a lower concentration of oxytocin receptors; use caution.

Control of postpartum bleeding: Adjust rate of infusion to sustain contractions and control uterine atony.

Incomplete, inevitable, or elective abortion: 10 to 20 mU/min. Total dose should not exceed 30 units in a 12-hour period due to the risk of water intoxication.

ACTIONS
A synthetic posterior pituitary hormone that will produce rhythmic contraction of uterine smooth muscle. Has specific receptors in the myometrium, and the receptor concentration increases greatly during pregnancy. Promotes contractions by increasing the intracellular calcium. Distributed throughout the extracellular fluid. Onset of action is almost

immediate. Half-life is 1 to 6 minutes. Duration of action is approximately 1 hour. Is the drug of choice for induction of delivery. Rapidly removed from plasma via liver and kidney. Only small amounts are excreted in urine unchanged. May exhibit antidiuretic and pressor effects at higher doses. Probably crosses the placental barrier in small amounts.

INDICATIONS AND USES

Antepartum: Indicated for the initiation or improvement of uterine contractions (when these are desirable and considered suitable for reasons of fetal or maternal concern) in order to achieve vaginal delivery. Indicated for (1) induction of labor in patients with a medical indication (e.g., Rh problems, maternal diabetes, pre-eclampsia at or near term) or when membranes are prematurely ruptured and delivery is indicated; (2) stimulation or reinforcement of labor, as in selected cases of uterine inertia; and (3) as adjunctive therapy in the management of incomplete or inevitable abortion. In the first trimester, curettage is generally considered primary therapy. In second-trimester abortion, oxytocin infusion will often be successful in emptying the uterus. However, other means of therapy may be required.

Postpartum: Indicated to produce uterine contractions during the third stage of labor and to control postpartum bleeding or hemorrhage. ▪ Not indicated for elective induction of labor (i.e., the initiation of labor in a pregnant individual who has no medical indication for induction).

CONTRAINDICATIONS

Cephalopelvic disproportion, fetal malpresentation, hypersensitivity, hypertonic uterine contractions, lack of satisfactory progress with adequate uterine activity, obstetrical emergencies in which the benefit-to-risk ratio for either the fetus or the mother favors surgical intervention (e.g., abruptio placentae), or when vaginal delivery is contraindicated (e.g., active herpes genitalis, cord presentation or prolapse, invasive cervical carcinoma, total placenta previa and vasa previa). See Precautions.

PRECAUTIONS

A NS IV without oxytocin should be hung, connected by Y-tube or three-way stopcock, and ready for use in adverse reactions. ▪ Should be administered only in the hospital under continuous observation by trained personnel; the physician must be immediately available. ▪ The use of oxytocin for fetal distress, hydramnios, partial placenta previa, prematurity, borderline cephalopelvic disproportion, or any condition that may cause uterine rupture (e.g., previous major surgery on the cervix or uterus, including cesarean section, uterine overdistension, grand multiparity, or past history of uterine sepsis or traumatic delivery) is not recommended except in unusual circumstances. ▪ Maternal deaths due to hypertensive episodes, subarachnoid hemorrhage, and uterine rupture, as well as fetal deaths due to various causes, have been reported. ▪ When used for induction or reinforcement of already existing labor, patients should be carefully selected. Evaluate pelvic adequacy and maternal and fetal conditions before use.

Monitor: When properly administered, oxytocin should stimulate uterine contractions comparable to normal labor. Monitor BP, fetal heart tones, strength and timing of contractions, and resting uterine tone. Continuous observation of patient required. ▪ Electronic fetal monitoring provides the best means of early detection of overdose. A fetal scalp electrode provides a more accurate recording of fetal HR than external monitoring. ▪ Has an intrinsic antidiuretic effect, increasing water reabsorption from the glomerular filtrate. Monitor oral fluid intake and observe for signs of water intoxication. ▪ See Precautions and Drug/Lab Interactions.

Maternal/Child: There is no indication for use in the first trimester of pregnancy other than in relation to spontaneous or induced abortion. Not expected to present a risk if used as indicated; see Indications and Contraindications.

DRUG/LAB INTERACTIONS

Severe hypertension can result in the presence of a **vasoconstrictor** given in conjunction with a **local or regional anesthetic** (caudal or spinal) **and with dopamine, ephedrine, epineph-**

rine, and other vasopressors. ▪ Concurrent use with **cyclopropane anesthesia** may cause hypotension and/or sinus bradycardia with abnormal atrioventricular rhythms. ▪ **Prostaglandins** (e.g., dinoprostone [Cervidil]) may potentiate the uterine response to oxytocin, increasing the risk of uterine hyperstimulation and rupture.

SIDE EFFECTS

Maternal: Anaphylaxis; cardiac arrhythmias; fatal afibrinogenemia; fluid retention leading to water intoxication and coma, convulsion, and death; hypertension; increased blood loss; nausea; pelvic hematoma; PVCs; postpartum hemorrhage; severe uterine hypertonicity, spasm, or tetanic contraction; subarachnoid hemorrhage; uterine rupture; vomiting.

Fetal: Bradycardia, brain damage, CNS damage, death, low Apgar scores, neonatal jaundice, PVCs and other arrhythmias, retinal hemorrhage, seizures.

ANTIDOTE

Nausea and vomiting are tolerable and can be treated symptomatically. Immediately call the physician's attention to any side effect noted or suspected; many can be fatal. Discontinue the drug immediately for any signs of fetal distress, uterine hyperactivity, tetanic contractions, uterine resting tone exceeding 15 to 20 mm Hg, or water intoxication. Use of a Y-connection or three-way stopcock, allowing the oxytocin drip to be discontinued while the vein is kept open, is recommended. Turn mother on side (to prevent fetal anoxia) and administer oxygen. Restriction of fluids, diuresis, hypertonic saline solutions IV, correction of electrolyte imbalance, control of convulsions with cautious use of barbiturates, or the use of magnesium sulfate may be required. These side effects can occur during labor and delivery and into the postpartum period. Careful evaluation and selection of patients eliminate many hazards, but be prepared for an emergency.

O-N

PACLITAXEL · PACLITAXEL PROTEIN-BOUND PARTICLES FOR INJECTABLE SUSPENSION (ALBUMIN-BOUND) BBW

Antineoplastic
(taxane)

(**PACK**-lih-**tax**-el)

Onxol, Taxol ▪ Abraxane

pH 4.4 to 5.6 ▪ not available

USUAL DOSE

Assessment required before dosing: see Precautions, Monitor, and Dose Adjustments.

CONVENTIONAL PACLITAXEL

Several regimens of paclitaxel, alone or in combination with other antineoplastics, are in use. Doses vary, depending on the regimen used. Consult literature. ▪ For all uses, premedication, specific parameters, and specific equipment are required before or during administration; see Premedication, Dose Adjustments, and Precautions/Monitor.

Premedication: Must be premedicated before each dose to prevent severe hypersensitivity reactions. Usual regimen includes oral dexamethasone (Decadron) 20 mg 12 and 6 hours before; IV diphenhydramine (Benadryl) 50 mg 30 to 60 minutes before; and an H_2 antagonist (e.g., ranitidine [Zantac] 50 mg or famotidine [Pepcid IV] 20 mg) 30 to 60 minutes before dosing with paclitaxel. When premedicating patients with AIDS-related Kaposi's sarcoma, reduce the dose of dexamethasone to 10 mg at 12 and 6 hours before paclitaxel. The doses of IV diphenhydramine and IV H_2 antagonists remain as above.

Ovarian cancer in previously untreated patients: 135 mg/M^2 as an infusion over 24 hours. Follow with cisplatin 75 mg/M^2 as an infusion over 6 to 8 hours. Repeat every 3 weeks. An alternative regimen is paclitaxel 175 mg/M^2 as an infusion over 3 hours. Follow with cisplatin 75 mg/M^2 (one source suggests an infusion over 24 hours; another suggests 6 to 8 hours, which would allow for outpatient therapy). Repeat every 3 weeks. See comments under Usual Dose.

Ovarian cancer in patients previously treated with chemotherapy: 135 or 175 mg/M^2 as an infusion over 3 hours. An alternate regimen suggests the same dose given as a 24-hour infusion. Repeat every 3 weeks. Larger doses, with or without filgrastim (G-CSF, Neupogen), have produced similar responses. See comments under Usual Dose.

Adjuvant treatment of node-positive breast cancer: 175 mg/M^2 as an infusion over 3 hours. Repeat every 3 weeks for four courses. Administered sequentially to doxorubicin-containing combination therapy. Clinical trials used four courses of doxorubicin and cyclophosphamide. Administer filgrastim (G-CSF) 5 mcg/kg/dose on Days 3 through 10. See comments under Usual Dose.

Breast cancer in patients previously treated with chemotherapy: 175 mg/M^2 as an infusion over 3 hours. Repeat every 3 weeks. An alternate regimen suggests 175 to 250 mg/M^2 over 3 hours every 3 weeks. See comments under Usual Dose.

First-line treatment of non–small-cell lung cancer: 135 mg/M^2 as an infusion over 24 hours. Follow with cisplatin 75 mg/M^2 over 6 to 8 hours. Repeat every 3 weeks. See comments under Usual Dose. A Canadian source recommends 175 mg/M^2 as an infusion over 3 hours followed with cisplatin 75 mg/M^2 over 6 to 8 hours and repeated every 3 weeks.

AIDS-related Kaposi's sarcoma: 135 mg/M^2 as an infusion over 3 hours. An alternate regimen suggests the same dose given as a 24-hour infusion. Repeat every 3 weeks. Another regimen is 100 mg/M^2 as an infusion over 3 hours repeated every 2 weeks. Toxicity somewhat increased with 135 mg/M^2 dose in clinical studies. See comments under Usual Dose.

ABRAXANE

Premedication: Generally not required; see Precautions.

Metastatic breast cancer (MBC): 260 mg/M^2 as an infusion over 30 minutes every 3 weeks.

Non–small-cell lung cancer (NSCLC): 100 mg/M^2 as an infusion over 30 minutes on Days 1, 8, and 15 of each 21-day cycle. Given in combination with carboplatin on Day 1 only of each 21-day cycle, beginning immediately after the completion of Abraxane administration.

Adenocarcinoma of the pancreas: 125 mg/M^2 as an infusion over 30 to 40 minutes followed by gemcitabine 1,000 mg/M^2 as an infusion over 30 to 40 minutes on Days 1, 8, and 15 of each 28-day cycle.

DOSE ADJUSTMENTS

CONVENTIONAL PACLITAXEL

Reduce dose by 20% for subsequent courses in patients who experience severe peripheral neuropathy or severe neutropenia (neutrophils less than 500 cells/mm^3) for 1 week or longer. ▪ Withhold therapy if neutrophils below 1,500/mm^3 or platelets below 100,000/mm^3. ▪ Dose reduction not required in impaired renal function. ▪ In AIDS-related Kaposi's sarcoma the parameters are slightly different. Initiate or repeat paclitaxel only if neutrophil count is equal to or greater than 1,000/mm^3; reduce dose of dexamethasone to 10 mg/dose; reduce dose of paclitaxel by 20% in patients who experience severe neutropenia (neutrophils less than 500/mm^3 for a week or longer); use concomitant filgrastim (G-CSF) as clinically indicated. ▪ Recommendations for dose adjustment of the initial course of therapy in patients with impaired hepatic function are listed in the following chart.

Guidelines for Dose Adjustment of Paclitaxel in Impaired Hepatic Function*			
Degree of Hepatic Impairment			
Transaminase Levels		Bilirubin Levels†	Recommended TAXOL Dose‡
24-Hour Infusion			
<2 × ULN	and	≤1.5 mg/dL	135 mg/M^2
2 to <10 × ULN	and	≤1.5 mg/dL	100 mg/M^2
<10 × ULN	and	1.6-7.5 mg/dL	50 mg/M^2
≥10 × ULN	or	>7.5 mg/dL	Not recommended
3-Hour Infusion			
<10 × ULN	and	≤1.25 × ULN	175 mg/M^2
<10 × ULN	and	1.26-2 × ULN	135 mg/M^2
<10 × ULN	and	2.01-5 × ULN	90 mg/M^2
≥10 × ULN	or	>5 × ULN	Not recommended

*These recommendations are based on clinical trials of dosages for patients without hepatic impairment of 135 mg/M^2 over 24 hours or 175 mg/M^2 over 3 hours; data are not available to make dose adjustment recommendations for other regimens (e.g., for AIDS-related Kaposi's sarcoma).

†Differences in criteria for bilirubin levels between the 3- and 24-hour infusion are due to differences in clinical trial design.

‡Dosage recommendations are for the first course of therapy; further dose reduction in subsequent courses should be based on individual tolerance.

ABRAXANE

Adjustment of starting dose is not necessary in patients with mild to moderate renal impairment (CrCl equal to or greater than 30 to less than 90 mL/min). ▪ Withhold therapy in all patients if neutrophils below 1,500/mm^3. ▪ In patients with MBC, withhold therapy if platelets below 100,000/mm^3. ▪ For MBC, reduce dose to 220 mg/M^2 in patients who experience severe neutropenia (neutrophils less than 500 cells/mm^3 for 7 days or more) or severe sensory neuropathy. Further reduce dose to 180 mg/M^2 for subsequent courses if severe neutropenia (less than 500 cells/mm^3 for 7 days or more) or severe sensory neuropathy recurs. ▪ If Grade 3 sensory neuropathy occurs, withhold treatment until resolution to Grade 1 or 2 for *MBC* or until resolution to less than or equal to Grade 1 for *NSCLC,* followed by a dose reduction for all subsequent courses. ▪ No dose adjustment

Continued

is necessary for patients with mild hepatic impairment (total bilirubin greater than ULN and less than or equal to 1.5 times the ULN and AST less than or equal to 10 times the ULN), regardless of indication. ▪ Do not administer Abraxane to patients with total bilirubin greater than 5 times the ULN or AST greater than 10 times the ULN regardless of indication because these patients have not been studied. ▪ Do not administer Abraxane to patients with metastatic adenocarcinoma of the pancreas who have moderate to severe hepatic impairment. ▪ Recommendations for a starting dose in patients with hepatic impairment are shown in the following chart. Doses for subsequent cycles should be based on patient tolerance.

Abraxane Starting Dose Recommendations for Patients with Hepatic Impairment					
Degree of Hepatic Impairment	SGOT (AST) Levels	Bilirubin Levels	Abraxane Dose*		
			MBC	NSCLC‡	Pancreatic‡ Adenocarcinoma
Mild	<10 × ULN and	>ULN to ≤1.5 × ULN	260 mg/M²	100 mg/M²	125 mg/M²
Moderate	<10 × ULN and	>1.5 to ≤3 × ULN	200 mg/M²†	80 mg/M²†	N/R
Severe	<10 × ULN and	>3 to ≤5 × ULN	200 mg/M²†	80 mg/M²†	N/R
	>10 × ULN or	>5 × ULN	N/R	N/R	N/R

MBC, Metastatic breast cancer; *N/R*, Not recommended; *NSCLC*, non–small-cell lung cancer.
*Dose recommendations are for the first course of therapy. The need for further dose adjustments in subsequent courses should be based on individual tolerance.
†A dose increase to 260 mg/M² for patients with MBC or to 100 mg/M² for patients with NSCLC in subsequent courses should be considered if the patient tolerates the reduced dose for two cycles.
‡Patients with bilirubin levels above the ULN were excluded from clinical trials for pancreatic or lung cancer.

▪ In patients with NSCLC who develop severe neutropenia or thrombocytopenia, withhold therapy until counts recover to an ANC of at least 1,500 cells/mm³ and platelets of at least 100,000 cells/mm³ on Day 1 or to an ANC of at least 500 cells/mm³ and platelets of at least 50,000 cells/mm³ on Day 8 or 15 of the cycle. Upon resumption of dosing, follow dose reduction outlined in the following chart.

Permanent Abraxane Dose Reductions for Hematologic and Neurologic Adverse Drug Reactions in NSCLC			
Adverse Drug Reaction	Occurrence	Weekly Abraxane Dose (mg/M²)	Every-3-Week Carboplatin Dose (AUC mg•min/mL)
Neutropenic fever (ANC less than 500/mm³ with fever >38° C) **OR** Delay of next cycle by more than 7 days for ANC less than 1,500/mm³ **OR** ANC less than 500/mm³ for more than 7 days	First	75 mg/M²	4.5 mg•min/mL
	Second	50 mg/M²	3 mg•min/mL
	Third	Discontinue treatment	Discontinue treatment
Platelet count less than 50,000/mm³	First	75 mg/M²	4.5 mg•min/mL
	Second	Discontinue treatment	Discontinue treatment
Severe sensory neuropathy (Grade 3 or 4)	First	75 mg/M²	4.5 mg•min/mL
	Second	50 mg/M²	3 mg•min/mL
	Third	Discontinue treatment	Discontinue treatment

- Dose-level reductions for patients with adenocarcinoma of the pancreas are outlined in the following chart.

Abraxane Dose-Level Reductions for Patients with Adenocarcinoma of the Pancreas		
Dose Level	Abraxane (mg/M²)	Gemcitabine (mg/M²)
Full dose	125 mg/M²	1,000 mg/M²
1st dose reduction	100 mg/M²	800 mg/M²
2nd dose reduction	75 mg/M²	600 mg/M²
If additional dose reduction required	Discontinue	Discontinue

- Dose modifications for neutropenia and/or thrombocytopenia for patients with adenocarcinoma of the pancreas are provided in the following chart.

Dose Recommendations and Modifications for Neutropenia and/or Thrombocytopenia for Patients with Adenocarcinoma of the Pancreas				
Cycle Day	ANC* (cells/mm³)		Platelet Count (cells/mm³)	Abraxane/Gemcitabine
Day 1	<1,500	or	<100,000	Delay doses until recovery
Day 8	500 to <1,000	or	50,000 to <75,000	Reduce 1 dose level
	<500	or	<50,000	Withhold doses
Day 15: If Day 8 doses were reduced or given without modification:				
	500 to <1,000	or	50,000 to <75,000	Reduce 1 dose level from Day 8
	<500	or	<50,000	Withhold doses
Day 15: If Day 8 doses were withheld:				
	≥1,000	or	≥75,000	Reduce 1 dose level from Day 1
	500 to <1,000	or	50,000 to <75,000	Reduce 2 dose levels from Day 1
	<500	or	<50,000	Withhold doses

*ANC, Absolute neutrophil count.

- Dose modifications for other adverse reactions for patients with adenocarcinoma of the pancreas are provided in the following chart.

Dose Modifications for Other Adverse Reactions for Patients with Adenocarcinoma of the Pancreas		
Adverse Drug Reaction	Abraxane	Gemcitabine
Febrile Neutropenia: Grade 3 or 4	Withhold until fever resolves and ANC ≥1,500; resume at next lower dose level	
Peripheral Neuropathy: Grade 3 or 4	Withhold until improves to ≤Grade 1; resume at next lower dose level	No dose reduction
Cutaneous Toxicity: Grade 2 or 3	Reduce to next lower dose level; discontinue treatment if toxicity persists	
Gastrointestinal Toxicity: Grade 3 mucositis or diarrhea	Withhold until improves to ≤Grade 1; resume at next lower dose level	

DILUTION
Specific techniques required; see Precautions.
CONVENTIONAL PACLITAXEL
Must be diluted and given as an infusion. May leach the toxic plasticizer DEHP from PVC infusion bags or sets; prepare and store in bottles (glass, polypropylene) or plastic bags (polypropylene, polyolefin) and administer through polyethylene-lined administra-

tion sets. **Compatible** with NS, D5W, D5NS, or D5R. Final concentration of 0.3 to 1.2 mg/mL required. For a 135 mg/M² dose, a large adult (body surface about 2 M²) will receive 270 mg (45 mL of paclitaxel at 6 mg/mL). Will require dilution in an additional 180 mL to make a 1.2 mg/mL concentration or in an additional 855 mL to make a 0.3 mg/mL concentration. Solution may appear hazy. Do not use a chemo-dispensing pin; can cause the stopper to collapse and result in loss of sterility.

ABRAXANE
Available in single-use vials, each containing 100 mg (5 mg/mL after reconstitution with 20 mL of NS). Calculate the exact number of vials needed to achieve the total dosing volume of suspension required.

Total # of vials required = Total dose (mg) ÷ 100 mg
Dosing volume (mL) = Total dose (mg) ÷ 5 (mg/mL)

For example, a MBC patient with a body surface area (BSA) of 1.73 M² would need a dose of 449.8 mg of Abraxane. 449.8 mg divided by 100 mg equals 4.498 vials, so 5 vials of Abraxane would be needed. 449.8 mg divided by 5 (mg/mL) equals a dosing volume of 90 mL of reconstituted solution.

Reconstitute each 100-mg vial with 20 mL of NS. A specific process is required to avoid foaming or clumping. Over a minimum of 1 minute, slowly inject the NS, directing it to the inside wall of the vial. Do not allow the NS to flow directly onto the lyophilized cake (will cause foaming). Allow each vial to sit for a minimum of 5 minutes while the NS wets the cake. Gently swirl and/or invert each vial slowly for at least 2 minutes until complete dissolution. Avoid generation of foam. If foaming or clumping occurs, allow solution to stand for at least 15 minutes until foam subsides. Solution should be milky and homogenous without visible particulates. If particulates are visible, gently invert to ensure complete resuspension before use.

Withdraw the calculated volume and inject into an empty sterile polyvinyl chloride (PVC) container or a PVC or non–PVC-type infusion bag (a total dosing volume of 90 mL in the previous example). The use of medical devices containing silicone oil as a lubricant (i.e., syringes and IV bags) to reconstitute and administer Abraxane may result in the formation of proteinaceous strands. Discard suspension if proteinaceous strands, particulate matter, or discoloration are observed.

Filters: *Conventional paclitaxel:* Use of an in-line filter not greater than 0.22 microns required for administration.

Storage: *Conventional paclitaxel:* May be stored at CRT or refrigerated before dilution (may appear precipitated under refrigeration; will redissolve at room temperature). Diluted for infusion, it is stable at room temperature for up to 27 hours. ***Abraxane:*** Store vials in original package at 20° to 25° C (68° to 77° F). Protect from light. Refrigeration or freezing does not affect stability of the product. Immediate use of reconstituted solution is preferred, but reconstituted vial may be refrigerated at 2° to 8° C (36° to 46° F) for a maximum of 24 hours if necessary. If refrigeration required, return to original carton to protect from light. Ensure complete resuspension after removing from refrigerator by gently inverting. Discard unused portions of the vial. Reconstituted solution in an infusion bag should be used immediately; however, it may be refrigerated and protected from bright light for a maximum of 24 hours. The total combined refrigerated storage time of reconstituted Abraxane in the vial and in the infusion bag is 24 hours. This may be followed by storage in the infusion bag at ambient temperature and lighting conditions for a maximum of 4 hours.

COMPATIBILITY   (Underline Indicates Conflicting Compatibility Information)
Consider any drug NOT listed as compatible to be INCOMPATIBLE until consulting a pharmacist; specific conditions may apply.

CONVENTIONAL PACLITAXEL
Leaches out plasticizers; see Dilution.
One source suggests the following **compatibilities:**

CONVENTIONAL PACLITAXEL

Additive: Carboplatin (Paraplatin), <u>cisplatin</u>, doxorubicin (Adriamycin); see Drug/Lab Interactions.

Y-site: Acyclovir (Zovirax), amikacin, aminophylline, ampicillin/sulbactam (Unasyn), <u>anidulafungin (Eraxis)</u>, bleomycin (Blenoxane), butorphanol (Stadol), calcium chloride, carboplatin (Paraplatin), cefotetan, ceftazidime (Fortaz), ceftriaxone (Rocephin), cisplatin, cladribine (Leustatin), cyclophosphamide (Cytoxan), cytarabine (ARA-C), dacarbazine (DTIC), dexamethasone (Decadron), diphenhydramine (Benadryl), doripenem (Doribax), doxorubicin (Adriamycin), droperidol (Inapsine), etoposide (VePesid), etoposide phosphate (Etopophos), famotidine (Pepcid IV), fluconazole (Diflucan), fluorouracil (5-FU), furosemide (Lasix), ganciclovir (Cytovene IV), gemcitabine (Gemzar), gentamicin, granisetron (Kytril), heparin, hydrocortisone sodium succinate (Solu-Cortef), hydromorphone (Dilaudid), ifosfamide (Ifex), linezolid (Zyvox), lorazepam (Ativan), magnesium sulfate, mannitol, meperidine (Demerol), mesna (Mesnex), methotrexate, metoclopramide (Reglan), morphine, nalbuphine, ondansetron (Zofran), oxaliplatin (Eloxatin), <u>palonosetron (Aloxi)</u>, pemetrexed (Alimta), pentostatin (Nipent), potassium chloride (KCl), prochlorperazine (Compazine), propofol (Diprivan), ranitidine (Zantac), sodium bicarbonate, thiotepa, topotecan (Hycamtin), vancomycin, vinblastine, vincristine, zidovudine (AZT, Retrovir).

ABRAXANE

Manufacturer states, "Use of specialized DEHP-free solution containers or administration sets is not necessary." The use of medical devices containing silicone oil as a lubricant (i.e., syringes and IV bags) to reconstitute and administer Abraxane may result in the formation of proteinaceous strands. Additional specific information not available.

RATE OF ADMINISTRATION

CONVENTIONAL PACLITAXEL

A single dose properly diluted must be equally distributed over 3 hours or as indicated in Usual Dose. Use of an in-line filter not greater than 0.22 microns required. Use a metriset (60 gtt/mL) or an infusion pump appropriate to control flow. Rate extended to 24 hours in some regimens.

ABRAXANE

A single dose properly reconstituted and equally distributed over 30 minutes.

ACTIONS

ALL FORMULATIONS

An antineoplastic. A novel antimicrotubule inhibitor. Paclitaxel derived from the bark of Pacific yew has now been replaced by paclitaxel produced semi-synthetically from a renewable source (needles and twigs of the Himalayan yew). Both are chemically identical. Through specific processes it stabilizes microtubules by preventing depolymerization. This action inhibits the normal dynamic reorganization of the microtubule network essential for vital interphase and mitotic cellular functions. Also induces abnormal bundles of microtubules throughout the cell cycle and multiple asters of microtubules during mitosis. Distribution and/or tissue binding is extensive. Evidence suggests metabolism in the liver via the cytochrome P_{450} isoenzyme system (CYP2C8 and CYP3A4). Terminal half-life ranges from 13.1 to 27 hours. Excreted primarily as metabolites in feces and, to a lesser extent, in urine.

CONVENTIONAL PACLITAXEL

More active in patients who have not received previous chemotherapy.

ABRAXANE

Consists of albumin-bound paclitaxel nanoparticles. Highly bound to serum proteins; metabolized in the liver, primarily by CYP2C8 and, to a lesser extent, by CYP3A4. Terminal half-life ranges from 13 to 27 hours. Minimal excretion in urine and feces.

INDICATIONS AND USES

CONVENTIONAL PACLITAXEL

First-line and subsequent therapy for the treatment of advanced carcinoma of the ovary.
■ First-line treatment for ovarian cancer in combination with cisplatin. ■ Adjuvant treat-

P

ment of node-positive breast cancer administered sequentially to standard doxorubicin-containing combination chemotherapy. Most effective in estrogen- and progesterone-receptor–negative tumors. ▪ Metastatic breast cancer refractory to initial chemotherapy or for a relapse within 6 months. ▪ First-line treatment, in combination with cisplatin, for non–small-cell lung cancer in patients who are not candidates for potentially curative surgery or radiation therapy. ▪ Second-line treatment of AIDS-related Kaposi's sarcoma.

ABRAXANE

Treatment of breast cancer after failure of combination chemotherapy for metastatic disease or relapse within 6 months of adjuvant chemotherapy. Prior therapy should have included an anthracycline unless clinically contraindicated. ▪ First-line treatment of locally advanced or metastatic non–small-cell lung cancer (NSCLC) (in combination with carboplatin) in patients who are not candidates for curative surgery or radiation therapy. ▪ First-line treatment of patients with metastatic adenocarcinoma of the pancreas, in combination with gemcitabine.

Unlabeled uses: *Conventional paclitaxel:* Advanced head and neck cancer. ▪ Cancers of the bladder and cervix. ▪ Small-cell lung cancer. ▪ In combination with other agents for treatment of metastatic breast cancer. ▪ Relapsed or refractory testicular cancer and testicular germ cell tumors. ▪ Treatment of (unknown primary) adenocarcinoma. *Abraxane:* Recurrent ovarian, fallopian, and primary peritoneal cancers.

CONTRAINDICATIONS

CONVENTIONAL PACLITAXEL

Baseline neutropenia less than 1,500 cells/mm³ in patients with solid tumors or baseline neutropenia less than 1,000 cells/mm³ in patients with AIDS-related Kaposi's sarcoma. History of prior severe hypersensitivity reactions to paclitaxel or other drugs formulated in polyoxyethylated castor oil (Cremophor EL [e.g., cyclosporine, teniposide]).

ABRAXANE

Baseline neutrophil count less than 1,500 cells/mm³. ▪ Patients who experience a severe hypersensitivity reaction to Abraxane should not be rechallenged with the drug.

PRECAUTIONS

ALL FORMULATIONS

Follow guidelines for handling cytotoxic agents. See Appendix A, p. 1331. ▪ Usually administered by or under the direction of the physician specialist in a facility with adequate diagnostic and treatment facilities to monitor the patient and respond to any medical emergency.

CONVENTIONAL PACLITAXEL

Use caution in patients with cardiac conduction abnormalities, CHF, and MI within previous 6 months. ▪ Bradycardia, hypertension, and hypotension have been observed but rarely required treatment. Occasionally the infusion must be interrupted or discontinued because of initial or recurrent hypertension; see Monitor. ▪ Pre-existing neuropathies resulting from prior therapies are not a contraindication for paclitaxel therapy. ▪ Various studies show that incidence and severity of neurotoxicity and hematologic toxicity increase with dose, especially above 190 mg/M². ▪ Use with caution in patients with a total bilirubin greater than 2 times the ULN. May be at increased risk of toxicity, especially profound myelosuppression; see Dose Adjustments. ▪ See Drug/Lab Interactions.

ABRAXANE

Do not substitute for or with other paclitaxel formulations. ▪ Use of gloves recommended. Wash skin immediately if contact occurs. Flush mucous membranes thoroughly with water if contact occurs. Topical exposure may result in tingling, burning, and redness. ▪ Premedication to prevent hypersensitivity reactions is not required but may be needed in patients who have had a prior hypersensitivity reaction to Abraxane. Reports of severe and sometimes fatal hypersensitivity reactions have occurred; see Contraindications; do not rechallenge patients who have had a severe reaction. ▪ Neutropenia is dose dependent and is a dose-limiting toxicity. Do not administer Abraxane to patients with a baseline absolute neutrophil count (ANC) of less than 1,500 cells/mm³; see Dose Adjustments. ▪ Sensory neuropathy is dose dependent and schedule dependent and occurs frequently; see Dose

Adjustments. ▪ Sepsis occurred in 5% of patients, with or without neutropenia, who received Abraxane in combination with gemcitabine. Biliary obstruction or the presence of a biliary stent were risk factors for severe or fatal sepsis. ▪ Pneumonitis, including some cases that were fatal, has been reported in patients receiving Abraxane in combination with gemcitabine; see Antidote. ▪ Has not been studied in patients with severe renal dysfunction or end-stage renal disease. ▪ Use with caution in patients with hepatic impairment. May be at increased risk for toxicity, particularly myelosuppression; see Dose Adjustments. ▪ Derived from human albumin; may carry a risk of transmission of viral disease or Creutzfeldt-Jakob disease; risk considered extremely remote. ▪ Has not been studied in patients who have had a hypersensitivity reaction to conventional paclitaxel.

Monitor: ALL FORMULATIONS: Neutropenia is dose dependent and is the dose-limiting toxicity. Obtain baseline CBC with differential and platelet count. Monitor frequently during therapy and before each dose. ▪ Monitor injection site carefully; avoid extravasation. ▪ Observe closely for signs of infection. Prophylactic antibiotics may be indicated pending results of C/S in a febrile neutropenic patient. ▪ Use prophylactic antiemetics to reduce nausea and vomiting and increase patient comfort. ▪ Monitor for thrombocytopenia (platelet count less than 50,000/mm³). Initiate precautions to prevent excessive bleeding (e.g., inspect IV sites, skin, and mucous membranes; use extreme care during invasive procedures; test urine, emesis, stool, and secretions for occult blood).

CONVENTIONAL PACLITAXEL: Neutrophil nadir occurs around Day 11; see Dose Adjustments. ▪ Monitor VS frequently, particularly during the first hour of the infusion. ▪ Consider obtaining a baseline ECG; arrhythmias have occurred. Continuous cardiac monitoring required for all patients with an abnormal baseline ECG or for those who experienced conduction arrhythmias during administration of a previous dose. ▪ Monitoring of cardiac function is recommended when paclitaxel is used in combination with doxorubicin; see doxorubicin monograph. ▪ Anaphylaxis and severe hypersensitivity reactions characterized by dyspnea, hypotension requiring treatment, angioedema, and generalized urticaria have been reported. Fatal reactions have occurred despite premedication. ▪ Most severe hypersensitivity reactions occur in the first hour; chest pain, dyspnea, flushing, and tachycardia were the most frequent initial symptoms; abdominal pain, diaphoresis, extremity pain, and hypertension also occurred. Monitor all vital signs, including BP, continuously for the first 30 minutes of the infusion and at frequent intervals after that. Incidence seems to decrease with subsequent doses. ▪ Treatment can often be continued in patients with mild hypersensitivity reactions if proper premedication is given. ▪ Monitor injection site carefully; avoid extravasation. Incidence of inflammation increased with 24-hour infusions. Injection site reactions may occur during administration or be delayed by 7 to 10 days. Recurrence of skin reactions at a site of previous extravasation following administration of paclitaxel ("recall") has been reported.

ABRAXANE: Limited infusion time (30 minutes) reduces the likelihood of infusion-related reactions; however, they have been reported; monitor for S/S. ▪ Monitor for S/S of hypersensitivity reactions. ▪ Monitor for S/S of sensory neuropathy. ▪ Monitor for S/S of pneumonitis. ▪ Based on patient history, a baseline ECG may be indicated. ▪ See Precautions and Dose Adjustments.

Patient Education: ALL FORMULATIONS: Males and females should avoid conception; nonhormonal birth control recommended. ▪ Review of monitoring requirements and adverse events before therapy imperative. ▪ Report any unusual or unexpected symptoms, side effects, pain or burning at injection site, S/S of a hypersensitivity reaction (e.g., bronchospasm, difficulty breathing, rash, urticaria), signs of infection (e.g., chills, fever, night sweats), signs of sensory neuropathy (e.g., numbness, tingling, or burning in hands and/or feet), signs of pneumonitis (e.g., dry, persistent cough or shortness of breath), or signs of bleeding (e.g., bruising, tarry stools, blood in urine, pinpoint red spots on skin) as soon as possible. ▪ Avoid tasks that require mental alertness (e.g., driving, operating machinery) until the effect of the medication is known. Side effects such as fatigue, lethargy, and malaise may affect the ability to perform these tasks. ▪ See Appendix D, p. 1333. ▪ Obtain name and telephone number of a contact person for emergencies, questions, or problems. ▪ Seek resources for counseling or supportive therapy. ▪ Manufacturer provides a patient information booklet.

Maternal/Child: ALL FORMULATIONS: Category D: females should avoid pregnancy, and males should avoid fathering a child. May cause fetal harm. ▪ Discontinue breast-feeding. ▪ Safety and effectiveness for use in pediatric patients not established.

CONVENTIONAL PACLITAXEL: CNS toxicity (rarely associated with death) was reported in one pediatric trial using high-dose paclitaxel. Use of antihistamines and the ethanol contained in the paclitaxel may have contributed to toxicity noted.

Elderly: ALL FORMULATIONS: Studies suggest response is similar to that seen in younger patients.

CONVENTIONAL PACLITAXEL: Incidence of side effects, including myelosuppression, neuropathy, and cardiovascular events, may be increased in the elderly.

ABRAXANE: Increased incidence of dehydration, diarrhea, epistaxis, fatigue, and peripheral edema was seen in elderly patients receiving Abraxane as monotherapy for MBC. Incidence of myelosuppression, neuropathy, and arthralgia was more common in patients receiving Abraxane and carboplatin for treatment of NSCLC. Incidence of decreased appetite, dehydration, diarrhea, and epistaxis was more common in patients receiving Abraxane and gemcitabine for treatment of adenocarcinoma of the pancreas.

DRUG/LAB INTERACTIONS

ALL FORMULATIONS

Do not administer **chloroquine or live virus vaccines** to patients receiving antineoplastic agents.

CONVENTIONAL PACLITAXEL

Formal drug interaction studies have not been conducted. To reduce potential for profound myelosuppression when using paclitaxel and **cisplatin** concurrently, give paclitaxel first, then cisplatin. ▪ Neurotoxicity and symptomatic motor dysfunction occurring with higher doses (greater than 250 mg/M²) may be potentiated by **cisplatin and filgrastim** (G-CSF). ▪ May cause additive effects with **bone marrow–suppressing agents, radiation therapy, or agents that cause blood dyscrasias** (e.g., amphotericin B, antithyroid agents [methimazole (Tapazole)], azathioprine, chloramphenicol, ganciclovir [Cytovene], interferon, plicamycin [Mithracin], zidovudine [AZT, Retrovir]). Reduced doses may be required. ▪ May increase levels of **doxorubicin** and its active metabolite when drugs are used in combination. ▪ Metabolized by **cytochrome P₄₅₀ isoenzymes CYP3A4 and CYP2C8.** Use caution when administered concomitantly with known **substrates** (e.g., buspirone [BuSpar], eletriptan [Relpax], felodipine [Plendil], lovastatin [Mevacor], midazolam [Versed], sildenafil [Viagra, Revatio], simvastatin [Zocor], and triazolam [Halcion]), **inhibitors** (e.g., atazanavir [Reyataz], clarithromycin [Biaxin], indinavir [Crixivan], itraconazole [Sporanox], ketoconazole [Nizoral], nefazodone, nelfinavir [Viracept], ritonavir [Norvir], saquinavir [Invirase], and telithromycin [Ketek]), **and inducers** (e.g., rifampin [Rifadin] and carbamazepine [Tegretol]) **of CYP3A4.** ▪ **Other medications that are substrates and/or inducers of CYP3A4** (e.g., ritonavir [Norvir], saquinavir [Invirase], indinavir [Crixivan], and nelfinavir [Viracept]) may alter the metabolism of paclitaxel but have not been evaluated in clinical trials. ▪ Use caution when administered concomitantly with known **substrates** (e.g., repaglinide [Prandin], rosiglitazone [Avandia]), **inhibitors** (e.g., gemfibrozil [Lopid]), **and inducers** (e.g., rifampin [Rifadin]) **of CYP2C8.** ▪ Dexamethasone (Decadron), diphenhydramine (Benadryl), cimetidine (Tagamet), and ranitidine (Zantac) do not affect the protein binding of paclitaxel.

ABRAXANE

Drug interaction studies have not been conducted. See All Formulations above. ▪ Use caution when administering with medicines **known to inhibit or induce CYP2C8 or CYP3A4.** Drugs that may inhibit these enzymes include ketoconazole (Nizoral) and other imidazole antifungals, erythromycin, fluoxetine (Prozac), gemfibrozil (Lopid), cimetidine (Tagamet), ritonavir (Norvir), saquinavir (Invirase), indinavir (Crixivan), and nelfinavir (Viracept). Drugs that may induce these enzymes include rifampin (Rifadin), carbamazepine (Tegretol), phenobarbital, phenytoin (Dilantin), efavirenz (Sustiva), nevirapine (Viramune).

SIDE EFFECTS

CONVENTIONAL PACLITAXEL

Dose dependent and generally reversible, but may be fatal. All patients were premedicated to prevent hypersensitivity reactions. Abnormal ECG, alopecia, arthralgia/myalgia, asthenia, autonomic neuropathy resulting in paralytic ileus, bleeding, bone marrow suppression (anemia, leukopenia, neutropenia, thrombocytopenia), bradycardia, CHF (including cardiac dysfunction and reduction in left ventricular ejection fraction or ventricular failure [more common in patients receiving combination therapy with anthracyclines]), diarrhea, elevated alkaline phosphatase, elevated AST, elevated bilirubin, febrile neutropenia, fever, fluid retention and edema, hypersensitivity reactions (moderate [e.g., dyspnea, flushing, hypotension, rash, tachycardia]; severe [e.g., chest pain, dyspnea requiring bronchodilators, hypotension requiring treatment, generalized urticaria]), hypertension, hypotension, infections including opportunistic infections (chills, fever, night sweats), injection site reactions (cellulitis, fibrosis, induration, necrosis, phlebitis, skin exfoliation), mucositis, nausea and vomiting, numbness, optic nerve and/or visual disturbances, peripheral neuropathy, respiratory reactions (interstitial pneumonia, lung fibrosis, pleural effusions, pulmonary embolism, respiratory failure), Stevens-Johnson syndrome, toxic epidermal necrolysis, and visual disturbances. A grand mal seizure occurred in one patient. Other side effects (e.g., cardiac arrest, cardiac ischemia/infarction, CVA, hepatic necrosis, and hepatic encephalopathy leading to death; intestinal obstruction; intestinal perforation; ischemic colitis; pancreatitis; thrombosis/embolism) have been reported rarely. A higher incidence of elevated liver function tests and renal toxicity is seen in Kaposi's sarcoma patients.

Post-Marketing: Diffuse edema, thickening, and sclerosing of the skin; exacerbation of S/S of scleroderma; ototoxicity.

ABRAXANE

Single-agent use in patients with MBC: Abnormal ECG, alopecia, anemia, diarrhea, elevation of alkaline phosphate and AST, fatigue/asthenia, infections (oral candidiasis, pneumonia, and respiratory tract), myalgia/arthralgia, nausea, neutropenia, and sensory neuropathy are most common.

Combination use in patients with NSCLC: Alopecia, anemia, fatigue, nausea, neutropenia, peripheral neuropathy, and thrombocytopenia are most common. The most serious side effects reported are anemia and pneumonia. The most common side effects that result in dose reduction, the withholding of a dose, or a delay in dosing are anemia, neutropenia, and thrombocytopenia. Neutropenia, peripheral neuropathy, and thrombocytopenia sometimes resulted in permanent discontinuation of Abraxane.

Combination use in patients with adenocarcinoma of the pancreas: Alopecia, decreased appetite, dehydration, diarrhea, fatigue, fever, nausea, neutropenia, peripheral edema, peripheral neuropathy, rash, and vomiting. The most common serious side effects are dehydration, fever, pneumonia, and vomiting. The most common side effects that result in dose reduction or delay in dosing are anemia, diarrhea, fatigue, neutropenia, peripheral neuropathy, and thrombocytopenia. The most common side effects resulting in permanent discontinuation are fatigue, peripheral neuropathy, and thrombocytopenia.

All diagnoses with Abraxane: Hypersensitivity reactions have occurred but are not usually severe; premedication is not indicated. Other side effects have been reported and include bradycardia, cardiovascular events (e.g., cardiac ischemia/infarction, SVT), dehydration, extravasation, fever, hypotension, pancytopenia, pneumonitis, pneumothorax, Stevens-Johnson syndrome, toxic epidermal necrolysis, and many others. Frequency of sensory neuropathy may increase with cumulative dose.

Post-Marketing: Many of these side effects occur with paclitaxel and Abraxane and include CHF, left ventricular dysfunction, and atrioventricular block; cranial nerve palsies; hepatic necrosis and hepatic encephalopathy; injection site reactions; interstitial pneumonia; intestinal obstruction or perforation; ischemic colitis; pancreatitis; paralytic ileus;

pneumonitis; pulmonary embolism; visual disorders (reduced visual acuity); vocal cord paresis. Rare reports of severe hypersensitivity reactions have occurred with Abraxane.

ANTIDOTE

Keep physician informed of all side effects. Most will be treated symptomatically as indicated. Most hypersensitivity reactions will subside with temporary discontinuation of paclitaxel, and incidence seems to decrease with subsequent doses. Moderate reactions such as dyspnea, flushing, hypotension, skin reactions, or tachycardia do not usually require interruption of treatment. Severe reactions may require epinephrine (Adrenalin), antihistamines (e.g., diphenhydramine [Benadryl]), corticosteroids (e.g., dexamethasone [Decadron]), or bronchodilators (e.g., albuterol, theophylline [aminophylline]). Most severe reactions should not be rechallenged, but some patients tolerated subsequent doses of **conventional paclitaxel;** see Contraindications. Neutropenia can be profound, and the nadir usually occurs about Day 11 with **conventional paclitaxel.** Recovery is generally rapid and spontaneous but may be treated with filgrastim (Neupogen, Zarxio), pegfilgrastim (Neulasta). Severe thrombocytopenia (nadir Day 8 or 9 with **conventional paclitaxel**) may require platelet transfusions. Severe anemia (less than 8 Gm/dL) may require packed cell transfusions. Hypotension and bradycardia do not usually occur at the same time except in hypersensitivity. Treat only if symptomatic. Some arrhythmias (e.g., nonspecific repolarization abnormalities, sinus tachycardia, and PVCs) are common and may not require intervention. Promptly treat any serious or symptomatic arrhythmia (e.g., conduction abnormalities, ventricular tachycardia), and monitor continuously during subsequent doses. Neurologic symptoms tend to worsen with each course; see Dose Adjustments. Usually improve within several months. Severe peripheral neuropathies or seizure may necessitate discontinuation of paclitaxel. Permanently discontinue treatment with **Abraxane** and gemcitabine if pneumonitis develops. There is no specific antidote for overdose. Supportive therapy will help sustain the patient in toxicity. Resuscitate if indicated.

PALIFERMIN
(**PAL**-lih-fur-min)

Growth factor

Kepivance, KGF

pH 6.5

USUAL DOSE
Administered as an IV bolus injection for 3 consecutive days before and 3 consecutive days after myelotoxic therapy (a total of 6 doses). Do not administer within 24 hours before, during infusion of, or within 24 hours after administration of myelotoxic chemotherapy. Has resulted in increased severity and duration of oral mucositis. Myelotoxic therapy is high-dose chemotherapy, with or without radiation, that is destructive to bone marrow or any of its components. Followed by bone marrow transplant/hematopoietic stem cell support.

Pre-myelotoxic therapy (first 3 doses): Administer 60 mcg/kg/day for 3 consecutive days before beginning myelotoxic therapy, with the third dose 24 to 48 hours before myelotoxic therapy.

Post-myelotoxic therapy (last 3 doses): Administer 60 mcg/kg/day for 3 consecutive days after myelotoxic therapy is complete; the first of these doses should be administered after, but on the same day of, hematopoietic stem cell infusion and at least 4 days after the most recent administration of palifermin. See Precautions.

DOSE ADJUSTMENTS
None indicated. Gender-related differences were not observed. ▪ No dose adjustment is recommended in impaired renal function. ▪ Pharmacokinetic studies have not been performed for pediatric patients or for patients with hepatic insufficiency.

DILUTION
Available as a lyophilized powder in a 6.25-mg single vial. Reconstitute by slowly injecting 1.2 mL SWFI into vial. Final concentration is 5 mg/mL. Swirl contents gently. **Do not shake.** Dissolution should take less than 3 minutes. Solution is clear and colorless. Do not use if particulates are present or if solution is discolored.

Filters: Manufacturer states, "Do not filter the reconstituted solution during preparation or administration."

Storage: Keep vials in carton until use. Store at 2° to 8° C (36° to 46° F). Protect from light. Do not use beyond expiration date on vial. Reconstituted product should be used immediately but can be stored up to 24 hours if refrigerated and stored in its carton. Do not freeze. Solution may be warmed to RT before injection but should not be left at RT for more than 1 hour and must be protected from light.

COMPATIBILITY
Specific information not available; however, manufacturer states, "If heparin is used to maintain an IV line, saline should be used to flush the line before and after administration since palifermin has been shown to bind to heparin in vitro."

RATE OF ADMINISTRATION
A single dose administered as an IV bolus injection. If heparin is used to maintain an IV line, flush the line with NS before and after administration.

ACTIONS
Human keratinocyte growth factor (KGF) produced by recombinant DNA technology. Binding of KGF to its receptor results in proliferation, differentiation, and migration of epithelial cells. KGF receptors are present on the epithelial cells in many tissues, including the tongue, buccal mucosa, esophagus, stomach, intestine, salivary gland, lung, liver, pancreas, kidney, bladder, mammary gland, skin (hair follicles and sebaceous gland), and the lens of the eye. The KGF receptor is not present on the cells of the hematopoietic lineage. KGF stimulates the growth of cells in tissues such as the skin and the epithelial layer of the mouth, stomach, and colon. Protects the epithelial cells that line the mouth and GI tract from the damage caused by chemotherapy and radiation and stimulates the

growth and development of new epithelial cells. Average half-life is 4.5 hours (range: 3.3 to 5.7 hours).

INDICATIONS AND USES

To decrease the incidence and duration of severe oral mucositis in patients with hematologic malignancies who are receiving myelotoxic therapy (high-dose chemotherapy), with or without radiation therapy, and who require hematopoietic stem cell support. Indicated as supportive care for preparative regimens predicted to result in equal to or greater than WHO Grade 3 mucositis in the majority of patients.

Limitations of use: Safety and efficacy for use in patients with nonhematologic malignancies not established; see Precautions. ▪ Not recommended for use with melphalan 200 mg/M^2 as a conditioning regimen.

Investigational uses: Studies to determine whether palifermin can be used safely in other types of cancer are in progress.

CONTRAINDICATIONS

Manufacturer states, "None."

PRECAUTIONS

Safety and efficacy have not been established in patients with nonhematologic malignancies. Effect of palifermin on stimulation of KGF receptor–expressing, nonhematopoietic tumors in patients is not known. There is some evidence of tumor growth and stimulation in cell cultures and in animal models of nonhematopoietic human tumors.

Monitor: Monitor improvement in symptoms of oral mucositis. ▪ Monitor for the appearance of mucocutaneous adverse effects (e.g., edema, erythema, oral/perioral dysesthesia [impairment of sensitivity to touch], rash, taste alteration, tongue discoloration, tongue thickening).

Patient Education: Review possible side effects. ▪ Promptly report side effects (e.g., edema, impairment of sensitivity to touch [especially around the mouth], rash, taste alteration, tongue discoloration, tongue thickening). ▪ Inform patient of the evidence of tumor growth and stimulation in cell cultures and animal models of nonhematopoietic human tumors.

Maternal/Child: Category C: potential benefit to mother must justify potential risk to fetus. ▪ Discontinue breast-feeding. ▪ Information on dosing and safety in pediatric patients is limited. However, use in pediatric patients ages 1 to 16 years is supported by evidence from well-controlled studies in adults and from a Phase 1 study that included 27 pediatric patients with acute leukemia undergoing hematopoietic stem cell transplant. Adverse events were similar to those reported for adults, and age did not affect the pharmacokinetics of palifermin.

Elderly: Age-related differences have not been observed.

DRUG/LAB INTERACTIONS

Formal studies have not been conducted. ▪ Interacts with **unfractionated as well as low-molecular-weight heparins** (e.g., enoxaparin [Lovenox]). When coadministered, there was no significant effect of palifermin on heparin activity with respect to aPPT. However, coadministration resulted in an increased palifermin AUC and a decreased palifermin clearance, volume of distribution, and half-life. If heparin is used to maintain an IV line, NS should be used to flush the line before and after palifermin administration. ▪ Do not administer within 24 hours before, during infusion of, or within 24 hours after administration of **myelotoxic chemotherapy.** Has resulted in increased severity and duration of oral mucositis.

SIDE EFFECTS

The most common serious side effects are fever, GI events, respiratory events, and skin rash. Other commonly reported reactions include arthralgia, edema, elevated serum amylase and lipase, hypertension, oral toxicities (alteration of taste, oral/perioral dysesthesia, tongue discoloration, tongue thickening), pain, paresthesia, proteinuria, and skin toxicities (erythema, pruritus, rash). Has the potential for immunogenicity, but the clinical significance is unknown.

Post-Marketing: Anaphylaxis, cataracts, edema of the face and mouth, palmar-plantar erythrodysesthesia syndrome (dysesthesia, edema on the palms and soles, erythema), tongue disorders (e.g., bumps, edema, redness), transient hyperpigmentation of the skin, vaginal edema and erythema.

ANTIDOTE
Notify physician of all side effects. Most will be treated symptomatically.

PALONOSETRON
(**pal**-oh-**NOH**-seh-tron)

Aloxi

Antiemetic
(5-HT$_3$ receptor antagonist)

pH 4.5 to 5.5

USUAL DOSE
Chemotherapy-induced nausea and vomiting: A single dose of 0.25 mg approximately 30 minutes before the start of chemotherapy. Has been coadministered with corticosteroids (e.g., dexamethasone [Decadron]) and metoclopramide (Reglan); see Drug/Lab Interactions.
Postoperative nausea and vomiting: A single dose of 0.075 mg immediately before induction of anesthesia.

PEDIATRIC DOSE
Chemotherapy-induced nausea and vomiting: A single dose of 20 mcg/kg (maximum 1.5 mg) approximately 30 minutes before the start of chemotherapy.

DOSE ADJUSTMENTS
No dose adjustment required based on age or race or in patients with any degree of renal or hepatic impairment.

DILUTION
Available in 0.25 mg/5 mL and 0.075 mg/1.5 mL single-use vials. May be given undiluted.
Filters: No data available from manufacturer.
Storage: Before use, store at CRT. Protect from freezing and light.

COMPATIBILITY   (Underline Indicates Conflicting Compatibility Information)
Consider any drug NOT listed as compatible to be INCOMPATIBLE until consulting a pharmacist; specific conditions may apply.
Manufacturer states, "Should not be mixed with other drugs. Flush the infusion line with NS before and after administration."
    One source suggests the following **compatibilities:**
Additive: *Not recommended by manufacturer.* Dexamethasone (Decadron).
Y-site: Ampicillin/sulbactam (Unasyn), atropine, carboplatin (Paraplatin), cefazolin (Ancef), cefotetan, cisatracurium (Nimbex), cisplatin, cyclophosphamide (Cytoxan), dacarbazine (DTIC), docetaxel (Taxotere), famotidine (Pepcid IV), fentanyl, fluorouracil (5-FU), gemcitabine (Gemzar), gentamicin, glycopyrrolate (Robinul), heparin, hetastarch in electrolytes (Hextend), hydromorphone (Dilaudid), ifosfamide (Ifex), irinotecan (Camptosar), lidocaine, lorazepam (Ativan), mannitol (Osmitrol), meperidine (Demerol), metoclopramide (Reglan), metronidazole (Flagyl IV), midazolam (Versed), morphine, neostigmine, oxaliplatin (Eloxatin), paclitaxel (Taxol), potassium chloride, promethazine (Phenergan), rocuronium (Zemuron), succinylcholine (Anectine), sufentanil (Sufenta), topotecan (Hycamtin), vancomycin, vecuronium.

RATE OF ADMINISTRATION
Flush the infusion line with NS before and after administration.
Chemotherapy-induced nausea and vomiting in adults: A single dose as an IV injection equally distributed over 30 seconds.

Chemotherapy-induced nausea and vomiting in pediatric patients: A single dose as an IV infusion equally distributed over 15 minutes.

Postoperative nausea and vomiting: A single dose as an IV injection equally distributed over 10 seconds.

ACTIONS

A long-acting (up to 120 hours [5 days]) antinauseant and antiemetic agent. A selective antagonist of specific serotonin (5HT$_3$) receptors. Has a strong binding affinity for this receptor and little or no affinity for other receptors. Chemotherapeutic agents such as cisplatin increase the release of serotonin from specific cells in the GI tract, causing emesis. Postoperative nausea and vomiting is also triggered by the release of serotonin. By antagonizing serotonin receptors both on the vagus nerve in the periphery and centrally in the chemoreceptor trigger zone, the incidence and severity of chemotherapy-induced nausea and vomiting and postoperative nausea and vomiting are decreased. 62% bound to plasma protein. Partially metabolized by multiple CYP enzymes; however, palonosetron is not an inhibitor or an inducer of CYP enzyme activity. Eliminated slowly from the body through both metabolic pathways and renal excretion. Has a prolonged half-life of approximately 40 hours. 80% of a single dose was recovered in urine within 144 hours.

INDICATIONS AND USES

Prevention of acute nausea and vomiting associated with initial and repeat courses of *moderately and highly emetogenic* cancer chemotherapy in pediatric patients 1 month to less than 17 years of age and in adults. ▪ Prevention of delayed nausea and vomiting associated with initial and repeat courses of *moderately emetogenic* cancer chemotherapy in adults. Studies identified cisplatin in doses equal to or greater than 70 mg/M^2 and cyclophosphamide (Cytoxan) in doses equal to or greater than 1,100 mg/M^2 as *highly emetogenic*. Studies identified cisplatin in doses equal to or less than 50 mg/M^2, cyclophosphamide in doses less than 1,100 mg/M^2, doxorubicin (Adriamycin) in doses greater than 25 mg/M^2, methotrexate in doses greater than 250 mg/M^2, and carboplatin (Paraplatin), epirubicin (Ellence), and irinotecan (Camptosar) in standard doses as *moderately emetogenic*. ▪ Prevention of postoperative nausea and vomiting (PONV) in adults for up to 24 hours following surgery. Efficacy beyond 24 hours has not been demonstrated.

CONTRAINDICATIONS

Known hypersensitivity to palonosetron or any of its components. ▪ See Precautions.

PRECAUTIONS

Hypersensitivity reactions, including anaphylaxis, have been reported with or without known hypersensitivity to other 5-HT$_3$ receptor antagonists. Cross-sensitivity may occur with other selective 5-HT$_3$ receptor antagonists (e.g., dolasetron [Anzemet], granisetron [Kytril], ondansetron [Zofran]). ▪ Serotonin syndrome has been reported with 5-HT$_3$ receptor antagonists. Most reports were associated with concomitant use of serotonergic drugs (e.g., selective serotonin reuptake inhibitors [e.g., paroxetine (Paxil), escitalopram (Lexapro)], serotonin and norepinephrine reuptake inhibitors [e.g., duloxetine (Cymbalta), venlafaxine (Effexor XR)], monoamine oxidase inhibitors [e.g., selegiline (Eldepryl)], mirtazapine [Remeron], fentanyl, lithium, tramadol [Ultram], and intravenous methylene blue). Some cases were fatal. ▪ Routine prophylaxis is not recommended for patients in whom there is little expectation of PONV. However, for patients in whom nausea and vomiting must be avoided during the postoperative period, prophylaxis is recommended even when the incidence of PONV is low. ▪ Palonosetron does not appear to have any effect on ECG intervals, including QT$_C$ duration.

Monitor: Observe closely. Monitor VS. ▪ Monitor for serotonin syndrome, especially when palonosetron is used concurrently with other serotonergic drugs. Symptoms associated with serotonin syndrome may include the following combination of S/S: mental status changes (e.g., agitation, coma, delirium, hallucinations), autonomic instability (e.g., diaphoresis, dizziness, flushing, hyperthermia, labile blood pressure, tachycardia), neuromuscular symptoms (e.g., hyperreflexia, incoordination, myoclonus, rigidity, tremor), and seizures, with or without GI symptoms (e.g., diarrhea, nausea, vomiting). ▪

Ambulate slowly to avoid orthostatic hypotension. ▪ Stool softeners or laxatives may be required to prevent constipation.

Patient Education: Request assistance with ambulation. ▪ Used to prevent and/or treat both early and late N/V caused by chemotherapy. Report persistent N/V promptly. ▪ Maintain adequate hydration. ▪ Review prescription and nonprescription medications with health care provider. Drug interactions are possible, especially with diuretics or antiarrhythmics. ▪ Review other medical conditions with health care provider. ▪ Promptly report S/S of serotonin syndrome (e.g., altered mental status, autonomic instability, and neuromuscular symptoms); see Precautions.

Maternal/Child: Category B: use during pregnancy only if clearly needed. ▪ Safety for use during breast-feeding not established; effects unknown, but potential for tumorigenicity is a concern. Discontinue breast-feeding. ▪ Safety and effectiveness have been established for use in pediatric patients 1 month to less than 17 years of age for the prevention of acute nausea and vomiting associated with initial and repeat courses of emetogenic cancer chemotherapy, including highly emetogenic chemotherapy. Pediatric patients require a higher palonosetron dose than adults to prevent chemotherapy-induced nausea and vomiting. However, the safety profile seen in pediatric patients is consistent with the established profile in adults. ▪ Safety and effectiveness have not been established in pediatric patients for prevention of postoperative nausea and vomiting.

Elderly: Safety and effectiveness similar to younger adults; however, greater sensitivity in some elderly cannot be ruled out. No dose adjustment or special monitoring required.

DRUG/LAB INTERACTIONS

Eliminated through both renal excretion and metabolic pathways. Does not induce or inhibit the cytochrome P_{450} drug metabolizing system; potential for clinically significant drug interactions is considered to be low. ▪ Serotonin syndrome (including altered mental status, autonomic instability, and neuromuscular symptoms) has been reported following the concomitant use of 5-HT$_3$ receptor antagonists and other serotonergic drugs, including selective serotonin reuptake inhibitors (SSRIs) and serotonin and norepinephrine reuptake inhibitors (SNRIs); see Precautions. ▪ Has been safely administered with analgesics, antiemetics/antinauseants, antispasmodics, anticholinergic agents, and corticosteroids. ▪ Has been safely administered with PO metoclopramide (10 mg 4 times daily). ▪ Has been administered with oral aprepitant (Emend). ▪ Does not appear to inhibit the antitumor activity of emetogenic cancer chemotherapies (cisplatin, cyclophosphamide, cytarabine, doxorubicin, and mitomycin C have been tested in murine tumor models). ▪ See Precautions.

SIDE EFFECTS

Chemotherapy-induced nausea and vomiting in adults: The most common side effects are headache and constipation. Other reported side effects include abdominal pain, diarrhea, dizziness, fatigue, and insomnia.

Chemotherapy-induced nausea and vomiting in pediatric patients: Allergic dermatitis, dizziness, dyskinesia, headache, and infusion site pain.

Postoperative nausea and vomiting: The most common side effects, occurring in at least 2% of patients, are bradycardia, constipation, headache, and QT prolongation. Several other side effects are reported in 1% or fewer of patients.

Overdose: Doses more than 20 times the recommended dose did not cause significant problems. Collapse, convulsions, cyanosis, gasping, and pallor occurred in animal studies with rats and mice.

Post-Marketing: Rare cases of hypersensitivity reactions, including anaphylaxis, anaphylactic shock, and injection site reactions (burning, induration, pain). Serotonin syndrome has been reported as a 5-HT$_3$ class reaction.

ANTIDOTE

Most side effects will be treated symptomatically. Keep physician informed. There is no specific antidote. If symptoms of serotonin syndrome occur, discontinue palonosetron and initiate supportive care. Has a large volume of distribution; dialysis not likely to be effective in overdose. Treat hypersensitivity reactions and resuscitate as indicated.

PAMIDRONATE DISODIUM
(pah-**MIH**-droh-nayt **DYE**-so-dee-um)

APD, Aredia

Bone resorption inhibitor
Antihypercalcemic
(bisphosphonate)

pH 6 to 7.4

USUAL DOSE
Prehydration required. Do not exceed a 90-mg dose. See Precautions and Monitor.
Moderate hypercalcemia (corrected serum calcium of 12 to 13.5 mg/dL): One dose of 60 to 90 mg as an infusion.
Severe hypercalcemia (corrected serum calcium greater than 13.5 mg/dL): One dose of 90 mg as an infusion. Serum calcium levels should fall into the normal range (8.5 to 10.5 mg/100 mL [1 dL], corrected for serum albumin).

Experience is limited, but retreatment with the same dose may be considered if hypercalcemia is not fully corrected or recurs; wait at least 7 days from completion of first infusion to allow full response. Always used in conjunction with adequate hydration and appropriate testing. See Precautions/Monitor.
Paget's disease: 30 mg/day as an infusion for 3 consecutive days (total dose is 90 mg over 3 days). Selected patients have been retreated with the same dose when indicated. Experience limited. Prehydration required; see Precautions and Monitor.
Osteolytic bone lesions of multiple myeloma: 90 mg as an infusion once every 30 days. Optimal duration of therapy not known. Withhold dose if renal function has deteriorated; see Dose Adjustments, Precautions, and Monitor.
Osteolytic bone metastases of breast cancer: 90 mg as an infusion every 3 to 4 weeks. Optimum duration of therapy not known. Withhold dose if renal function has deteriorated; see Dose Adjustments, Precautions, and Monitor.

DOSE ADJUSTMENTS
Accumulation of pamidronate in renally impaired patients is not anticipated if dosed on a monthly schedule. No experience with creatinine above 5 mg/100 mL (1 dL) or in severe hepatic disease. ▪ See Precautions and Elderly.
Osteolytic bone lesions of multiple myeloma and osteolytic bone metastases of breast cancer: Withhold dose if renal function has deteriorated. Renal deterioration is defined as an increase of 0.5 mg/dL in patients with a *normal* baseline creatinine or an increase of 1 mg/dL in patients with *abnormal* baseline creatinine. One study suggests that treatment should not be resumed until SCr has returned to within 10% of baseline value.

DILUTION
Reconstitute each 30- or 90-mg vial with 10 mL SWFI. Dissolve completely (3 or 9 mg/mL).
Hypercalcemia of malignancy: Further dilute a single dose in 1,000 mL NS, ½NS, or D5W. A minimum of 500 mL diluent may be used if absolutely necessary in patients with compromised cardiovascular status.
Paget's disease: Further dilute a single daily dose in 500 mL NS, ½NS, or D5W.
Osteolytic bone lesions of multiple myeloma: Further dilute each 90-mg dose in 500 mL NS, ½NS, or D5W.
Osteolytic bone metastases of breast cancer: Further dilute each 90-mg dose in 250 mL NS, ½NS, or D5W.
Storage: Before reconstitution, store at CRT. After reconstitution, may be refrigerated for up to 24 hours. Stable after dilution for 24 hours at room temperature.

COMPATIBILITY
Manufacturer states, "Should be given in a single intravenous solution and line separate from all other drugs, and do not mix with calcium-containing solutions (e.g., Ringer's solutions)."

RATE OF ADMINISTRATION

Use of a microdrip (60 gtt/mL) or an infusion pump recommended for even distribution. Do not exceed recommended rate of infusion. Duration should be no less than 2 hours. Too-rapid infusion rate may lead to overdose, elevated BUN and creatinine levels, and renal tubular necrosis. Rate recommendations vary considerably. They are based on specific clinical trials for each diagnosis. In some trials a rate of up to 1 mg/min has been used with caution.

Hypercalcemia of malignancy: A 60-mg dose or 90-mg dose equally distributed over 2 to 24 hours. Longer infusion times (i.e., greater than 2 hours) may reduce the risk of renal toxicity, particularly in patients with pre-existing renal insufficiency.

Paget's disease: A single dose over 4 hours.

Osteolytic bone lesions of multiple myeloma: A single dose over 4 hours.

Osteolytic bone metastases of breast cancer: A single dose over 2 hours.

ACTIONS

A bisphosphonate hypocalcemic agent. Reduces serum calcium concentrations by inhibiting bone resorption. Binds to preformed bone surfaces and may block bone mineral dissolution. May also inhibit osteoclast activity. Effectively inhibits accelerated bone resorption resulting from osteoclast hyperactivity induced by various tumors. Does not inhibit bone formation and mineralization. Some reduction in calcium levels seen in 24 to 48 hours, and maximum response in 4 to 7 days. Rapidly adsorbed by bone. Is not metabolized. Half-life is approximately 21 to 35 hours. Slowly excreted in urine.

INDICATIONS AND USES

Treatment of moderate to severe hypercalcemia of malignancy in patients with or without bone metastasis, in conjunction with adequate hydration. Symptoms of hypercalcemia may include anorexia, bone pain, confusion, constipation, dehydration, depression, fatigue, lethargy, muscle weakness, nausea and vomiting, and polyuria. Severe dehydration may lead to renal insufficiency. With high levels of serum calcium, cardiac manifestations (e.g., bradycardia, cardiac arrest, ventricular arrhythmias) and neurologic symptoms (e.g., coma, seizures, and death) may occur. ■ Treatment of Paget's disease. ■ Adjunct in treatment of osteolytic lesions of multiple myeloma and osteolytic bone metastases of breast cancer.

Unlabeled uses: Prevention of bone loss associated with androgen deprivation therapy in prostate cancer.

CONTRAINDICATIONS

Hypersensitivity to pamidronate or other bisphosphonates (e.g., alendronate [Fosamax], risedronate [Actonel], zoledronic acid [Reclast, Zometa]).

PRECAUTIONS

Calcium is bound to albumin. Total serum calcium levels in patients who have hypercalcemia of malignancy may not reflect the severity of the hypocalcemia because concomitant hypoalbuminemia is commonly present. Measurement with ionized calcium levels is preferred. If unavailable, all calcium measurement should be corrected for albumin to establish a basis for treatment and evaluation of treatment. ■ Mild or asymptomatic hypercalcemia will be treated with conservative measures (e.g., saline hydration, with or without diuretics [after correcting hypovolemia]). Consider patient's cardiovascular status. Corticosteroids may be indicated if the underlying cancer is sensitive (e.g., hematologic cancers). ■ May be used adjunctively with chemotherapy, radiation, or surgery. ■ May cause renal toxicity. Deterioration in renal function progressing to renal failure has been reported and has occurred after the initial or a single dose of pamidronate. Patients with pre-existing renal impairment may be at increased risk for developing toxicity. Do not exceed dose of 90 mg. ■ Osteonecrosis of the jaw (ONJ) has been reported in patients receiving bisphosphonates. The majority of cases have been in cancer patients. Risk factors include cancer, concomitant therapy (e.g., chemotherapy, radiotherapy, corticosteroids), and comorbid conditions (e.g., anemia, coagulopathies, infection, pre-existing oral disease). Literature and case reports suggest a higher frequency of ONJ based on tumor type (breast cancer, multiple myeloma) and dental status (dental extraction, periodontal disease, local trauma, including poorly fitting dentures). Cancer patients should maintain good oral hygiene. Consider dental exam and appropriate preventive dentistry before beginning therapy with bisphosphonates. Avoid invasive dental procedures during bisphosphonate therapy. Dental surgery may exacerbate ONJ in patients who develop ONJ while on bisphosphonate therapy. ▪ Severe and occasionally incapacitating bone, joint, and/or muscle pain has been reported rarely. Onset of symptoms varied from one day to several months after beginning treatment with pamidronate. In most cases, pain resolves when pamidronate is discontinued; however, in some patients symptoms resolved slowly or persisted. ▪ Atypical subtrochanteric and diaphyseal femoral fractures have been reported. May occur after minimal or no trauma. Risk may be increased in patients receiving concurrent glucocorticoids (e.g., dexamethasone, prednisone). ▪ May be at risk for anemia, leukopenia, or thrombocytopenia; see Monitor. ▪ Patients with a history of thyroid surgery may have relative hypoparathyroidism that may predispose them to hypocalcemia with pamidronate. *Osteolytic bone lesions of multiple myeloma and osteolytic bone metastases of breast cancer:* Patients being treated for multiple myeloma and bone metastases should have the dose withheld if renal function has deteriorated; see Dose Adjustments. Use is not recommended in patients with severe renal impairment being treated for bone metastases. See Monitor and Dose Adjustments. Limited information available on use in multiple myeloma patients with a CrCl less than 30 mL/min. In clinical trials, patients with a SCr above 3 mg/dL were excluded. ▪ In the absence of hypercalcemia, patients with *multiple myeloma* or *Paget's disease of the bone* or patients with *predominantly lytic bone metastases* who are at risk for calcium and vitamin D deficiency should be given oral calcium and vitamin D to reduce the risk of hypocalcemia.

Monitor: Obtain baseline measurements of serum calcium (corrected for serum albumin), electrolytes, phosphate, magnesium, and creatinine and CBC with differential and hematocrit/hemoglobin. Monitor all closely as indicated by baseline results (may be daily). Serum phosphate levels will decrease and may require treatment. ▪ Monitor renal function before each treatment; deterioration in renal function has been reported; see Precautions. ▪ Monitor serum alkaline phosphatase during therapy for Paget's disease. ▪ Patients with cancer-related hypercalcemia are frequently dehydrated. Must be adequately hydrated orally and/or IV before treatment is initiated. Hydration with saline is preferred to facilitate renal excretion of calcium and to correct dehydration. A pretreatment urine output of 2 L/day is recommended. Maintain adequate hydration and urine output throughout treatment. ▪ Avoid overhydration in patients with compromised cardiovascular status. Observe frequently for signs of fluid overload. Correct hypovolemia before using diuretics. ▪ Monitor patients with pre-existing anemia, leukopenia, or thrombocytopenia very carefully during treatment and for the first 2 weeks following treatment. ▪ Monitor for S/S of atypical femoral fractures that may occur with minimal or no trauma. Thigh or groin pain may be experienced weeks to months before a fracture appears. Fractures are often bilateral; examine both femurs. *Osteolytic bone lesions of multiple myeloma:* Adequately hydrate patients who have marked Bence-Jones proteinuria and dehydration before pamidronate infusion.

Patient Education: Regular visits and assessment of lab tests imperative. ▪ Dietary restriction of calcium and vitamin D may be required. ▪ Take only prescribed medications. ▪ Report abdominal cramps, chills, confusion, fever, muscle spasms, sore throat, and/or any new medical problems promptly. ▪ Report development of bone, joint, or muscle pain promptly. Onset of pain is variable. ▪ Avoid pregnancy; use of nonhormonal birth control suggested.

Maternal/Child: Category D: should not be used during pregnancy. May cause fetal harm. Avoid pregnancy; use of birth control necessary during treatment and for an undetermined time after treatment; see prescribing information. ▪ Discontinue breastfeeding. ▪ Safety for use in pediatric patients not established.

Elderly: Response similar to that seen in younger patients. ▪ Use with caution based on age-related impaired organ function and concomitant disease or drug therapy; monitor renal function closely. See Dose Adjustments. ▪ Monitor fluid and electrolyte status carefully to avoid overhydration or electrolyte imbalance. Use of lower fluid volume may be required; see Dilution.

DRUG/LAB INTERACTIONS

Use caution when administered with other **potentially nephrotoxic drugs** (e.g., aminoglycosides [amikacin, tobramycin, gentamicin], cisplatin). ■ Concurrent administration with **furosemide** (Lasix) does not affect calcium-lowering action of pamidronate. ■ Does not interfere with any known primary cancer therapy. ■ Effects may be antagonized by **calcium-containing preparations or vitamin D**; avoid use. ■ Concurrent use with **thalidomide** (Thalomid) may increase risk of renal toxicity in patients with multiple myeloma.

SIDE EFFECTS

Average dose: Abdominal pain, anemia, anorexia, bone pain, confusion and visual hallucinations (sometimes in conjunction with electrolyte imbalance), constipation, fever (mild and transient), generalized pain, hypertension, hypocalcemia (abdominal cramps, confusion, muscle spasms), infusion site reaction (e.g., induration and pain on palpation, redness, swelling), musculoskeletal pain (bone, joint, and/or muscle pain), pruritus, rash, renal toxicity, seizures, urinary tract infections, vomiting. Fluid overload, hypokalemia, hypomagnesemia, and hypophosphatemia occur frequently with use of concurrent fluid and diuretics. Rare instances of hypersensitivity reactions, including anaphylaxis, angioedema, dyspnea, and hypotension, have occurred. Osteonecrosis (primarily of the jaw) has been reported (see Precautions). Anemia, leukopenia, and thrombocytopenia may occur.

Overdose: Occurs less frequently with lower dose range (30 to 60 mg). Fever (high), hypocalcemia, hypotension, leukopenia or lymphopenia (fever, chills, sore throat), transient taste perversion. Elevated BUN and CrCl levels and renal tubular necrosis may occur with excessive dose or rate of administration.

Post-Marketing: Adult respiratory distress syndrome (ARDS); atypical subtrochanteric and diaphyseal femoral fractures; bone, joint, and muscle pain (may be severe and incapacitating); conjunctivitis; focal segmental glomerulosclerosis (including the collapsing variant); glomerulonephropathies; hematuria; hypernatremia; influenza-like symptoms; interstitial lung disease; nephrotic syndrome; orbital inflammation; reactivation of herpes simplex and herpes zoster; renal tubular disorders; tubulointerstitial nephritis.

ANTIDOTE

Keep physician informed of side effects. Some may respond to symptomatic treatment. Magnesium, phosphorus, and potassium may require replacement if depletion too severe. If mild, all will probably return toward normal in 7 to 10 days. For asymptomatic or mild to moderate hypocalcemia (6.5 to 8 mg/100 mL [1 dL] corrected for serum albumin), short-term calcium therapy (e.g., calcium gluconate) may be indicated. Consider discontinuing pamidronate in patients who develop atypical fractures of the femur. Unknown if risk continues after stopping treatment. Discontinue drug for any symptoms of overdose. Monitor serum calcium and use vigorous IV hydration, with or without diuretics, for 2 to 3 days. Monitor intake and output to ensure adequacy and balance. Use short-term IV calcium therapy if indicated. High fever may respond to steroids. RBC transfusions may be required in anemia. Treat anaphylaxis and resuscitate as indicated.

PANCURONIUM BROMIDE BBW
(pan-kyou-**ROH**-nee-um **BRO**-myd)

Neuromuscular blocking agent
(nondepolarizing)
Anesthesia adjunct

pH 4

USUAL DOSE
Adjunct to general anesthesia for adults and pediatric patients: Must be individualized, depending on previous drugs administered and degree and length of muscle relaxation required. Must be used with adequate anesthesia and/or sedation and after unconsciousness induced. Succinylcholine must show signs of wearing off before pancuronium is given. 0.04 to 0.1 mg/kg of body weight initially. 0.01 mg/kg in increments as required to maintain muscle relaxation; usually 25- to 60-minute intervals.
Endotracheal intubation: 0.06 to 0.1 mg/kg.
Support of intubated mechanically ventilated or respiratory-controlled adult ICU patients (unlabeled): *IV bolus injection:* 0.1 to 0.2 mg/kg every 1 to 3 hours. *Continuous infusion:* Begin with a *loading dose* of 0.03 to 0.1 mg/kg followed by a *maintenance dose* of 0.06 to 0.1 mg/kg/hr. A lower-end or reduced dose may be indicated if administered more than 5 minutes after the start of an inhalation agent, when steady-state has been achieved, or in patients with organ dysfunction (e.g., impaired renal function). Adjust dose according to clinical assessment of the patient's response. Use of a peripheral nerve stimulator is recommended.

NEONATAL DOSE
Adjunct to general anesthesia: Extreme sensitivity to pancuronium exists during the first month of life. Begin with a test dose of 0.02 mg/kg and assess responsiveness. See Maternal/Child.

DOSE ADJUSTMENTS
See Drug/Lab Interactions; marked reduction of pancuronium dose may be required. ▪ A higher total dose may be required in biliary or hepatic disease, but onset is slower and neuromuscular block is prolonged. ▪ Clearance decreased and half-life increased in renal insufficiency. One source recommends administering 50% of a dose if CrCl is between 10 and 50 mL/min; do not use if CrCl is less than 10 mL/min.

DILUTION
May be given undiluted or diluted in D5W, D5/¹/₂NS, D5NS, NS, or LR for use as an infusion.
Storage: Best if stored in refrigerator. Will maintain potency at room temperature for up to 6 months.

COMPATIBILITY
(Underline Indicates Conflicting Compatibility Information)
Consider any drug NOT listed as compatible to be INCOMPATIBLE until consulting a pharmacist; specific conditions may apply.
One source suggests the following **compatibilities:**
Additive: Ciprofloxacin (Cipro IV), verapamil.
Y-site: Aminophylline, cefazolin (Ancef), cefuroxime (Zinacef), dexmedetomidine (Precedex), dobutamine, dopamine, epinephrine (Adrenalin), esmolol (Brevibloc), etomidate (Amidate), fenoldopam (Corlopam), fentanyl, fluconazole (Diflucan), gentamicin, heparin, hetastarch in electrolytes (Hextend), hydrocortisone sodium succinate (Solu-Cortef), isoproterenol (Isuprel), levofloxacin (Levaquin), lorazepam (Ativan), midazolam (Versed), milrinone (Primacor), morphine, nitroglycerin IV, nitroprusside sodium, propofol (Diprivan), ranitidine (Zantac), sulfamethoxazole/trimethoprim, vancomycin.

RATE OF ADMINISTRATION
Adjunct to general anesthesia: A single dose over 60 to 90 seconds.
Mechanical ventilation support in ICU: See Usual Dose for specific rates and criteria.

ACTIONS
A skeletal muscle relaxant. Causes paralysis by interfering with neural transmission at the myoneural junction. Onset of action is dose dependent. Peak effect occurs in 3 to 4 minutes and lasts 30 to 45 minutes. It may take another 30 minutes or up to several hours before complete recovery occurs. Excreted in the urine.

INDICATIONS AND USES
Adjunctive to general anesthesia to facilitate endotracheal intubation and to relax skeletal muscles during surgery or mechanical ventilation.
Unlabeled uses: Support of intubated, mechanically ventilated, or respiratory-controlled patients in ICU.

CONTRAINDICATIONS
Known hypersensitivity to pancuronium or bromides; first trimester of pregnancy.

PRECAUTIONS
Usually administered by or under the direct observation of the anesthesiologist. Appropriate emergency drugs and equipment for monitoring the patient and responding to any medical emergency must be readily available. ■ Severe anaphylactic reactions have been reported with neuromuscular blocking agents; some have been fatal. Use caution in patients who have had an anaphylactic reaction to another neuromuscular blocking agent (depolarizing or nondepolarizing); cross-reactivity has occurred. ■ Repeated doses may produce a cumulative effect. ■ Impaired pulmonary function or respiratory deficiencies can cause critical reactions. ■ Use caution in impaired liver or kidney function, in patients with tachycardia, and in any patient who might develop adverse effects from an increase in HR. ■ Myasthenia gravis increases sensitivity to drug. ■ Long-term use (i.e., intensive care) may result in prolonged paralysis or skeletal muscle weakness. ■ Acid-base and/or electrolyte imbalance, debilitation, hypoxic episodes, and/or the use of other drugs (e.g., broad-spectrum antibiotics, narcotics, steroids) may prolong the effects of pancuronium.
Monitor: All uses: This drug produces apnea. Controlled artificial ventilation with oxygen must be continuous and under direct observation at all times. Maintain a patent airway. ■ Use a peripheral nerve stimulator to monitor response to pancuronium and avoid overdose. ■ Patient may be conscious and completely unable to communicate by any means. Pancuronium has no analgesic or sedative properties. ■ Action is altered by dehydration, electrolyte imbalance, body temperatures, and acid-base imbalance. ■ Hyperkalemia may cause cardiac arrhythmias and increased paralysis. ■ See Precautions and Drug/Lab Interactions.
Mechanical ventilation support in ICU: Physical therapy is recommended to prevent muscular weakness, atrophy, and joint contracture. Muscular weakness may first be noticed during attempts to wean patients from the ventilator.
Maternal/Child: Category C: unknown potential hazards to fetus. Benefits must outweigh risks. Not recommended in first trimester. ■ Has caused rare severe skeletal muscle weakness in neonates undergoing mechanical ventilation.
Elderly: Delay in onset time may be caused by slower circulation time in cardiovascular disease, old age, or edematous states; allow more time for drug to achieve maximum effect.

DRUG/LAB INTERACTIONS
May cause severe arrhythmias with **inhalant anesthetics** (e.g., enflurane, halothane) and in patients on chronic **tricyclic antidepressant therapy** (e.g., amitriptyline [Elavil]). ■ Potentiated by **hypokalemia, some carcinomas, many antibiotics** (e.g., aminoglycosides [kanamycin, gentamicin], bacitracin, colistin [Coly-Mycin S], colistimethate [Coly-Mycin M], polymyxin-B [Aerosporin], tetracyclines, piperacillin), **calcium salts, CO_2, diuretics, diazepam** (Valium) **and other muscle relaxants, digoxin, magnesium sulfate, quinidine, morphine, lidocaine, meperidine, propranolol** (Inderal), **succinylcholine, and others.** May need to reduce dose of pancuronium; use with caution. ■ Recurrent paralysis may occur with **quinidine.** ■ Effects may be decreased by **acetylcholine, aminophylline, anticholinesterases, azathioprine, carbamazepine, and potassium.** ■ **Succinylcholine** must show signs of wearing off before pancuronium is given. Use caution.

SIDE EFFECTS

Increased HR, decrease in mean arterial pressure, prolonged action resulting in respiratory insufficiency or apnea and tachycardia. Airway closure caused by relaxation of epiglottis, pharynx, and tongue muscles. Hypersensitivity reactions are possible. Anaphylaxis, histamine release (e.g., bronchospasm, vasodilation, hypotension, cutaneous flushing), and shock may occur. Muscular weakness and atrophy may occur with long-term use (1 to 3 weeks).

ANTIDOTE

All side effects are medical emergencies. Treat symptomatically. Controlled artificial ventilation must be continuous. Pyridostigmine (Regonol) or neostigmine given with atropine will probably reverse the muscle relaxation. Not effective in all situations; may aggravate severe overdose. Resuscitate as necessary.

PANITUMUMAB BBW

(pan-i-**TUE**-moo-mab)

Antineoplastic
Immunosuppressant
Monoclonal antibody

Vectibix

pH 5.6 to 6

USUAL DOSE

Pre-testing required: Before initiating treatment, assess *RAS* mutational status in colorectal tumors and confirm the absence of a *RAS* mutation; see Precautions. See prescribing information for access to FDA-approved tests.

Panitumumab: 6 mg/kg as an infusion once every 14 days.

DOSE ADJUSTMENTS

Upon the first occurrence of a Grade 3 (NCI-CTC/CTCAE) dermatologic reaction, withhold 1 to 2 doses of panitumumab. If the reaction improves to less than Grade 3, reinitiate panitumumab at the original dose. ▪ Upon the second occurrence of a Grade 3 (NCI-CTC/CTCAE) dermatologic reaction, withhold 1 to 2 doses of panitumumab. If the reaction improves to less than Grade 3, reinitiate panitumumab at 80% of the original dose. ▪ Upon the third occurrence of a Grade 3 (NCI-CTC/CTCAE) dermatologic reaction, withhold 1 to 2 doses of panitumumab. If the reaction improves to less than Grade 3, reinitiate panitumumab at 60% of the original dose. ▪ Upon the fourth occurrence of a Grade 3 (NCI-CTC/CTCAE) dermatologic reaction, permanently discontinue panitumumab. ▪ Permanently discontinue panitumumab following the occurrence of a Grade 4 dermatologic reaction or for a Grade 3 dermatologic reaction that does not recover after withholding 1 to 2 doses.

DILUTION

Solution may contain a small amount of visible, translucent-to-white, amorphous, and proteinaceous panitumumab particulates (will be removed by in-line filter). Do not use if solution is discolored. **Do not shake.** Withdraw calculated dose from vial. Dilute to a total volume of 100 mL with NS. Doses higher than 1,000 mg should be diluted to a volume of 150 mL. (Withdraw a volume of NS equal to the volume of the calculated dose from the infusion bag.) Final concentration should not exceed 10 mg/mL. Mix diluted solution by gentle inversion. **Do not shake.**

Filters: Must be administered through a low–protein binding, 0.2- or 0.22-micron, in-line filter.

Storage: Store unopened vials in refrigerator (2° to 8° C [36° to 46° F]). Protect from direct sunlight. Do not freeze. Diluted solutions should be used within 6 hours of preparation if stored at RT and within 24 hours if stored in refrigerator. Do not freeze. Single-dose vial; discard any unused product after entry into vial.

COMPATIBILITY
Manufacturer states, "Should not be mixed with, or administered as an infusion with, other medicinal products. No other medications should be added to solutions containing panitumumab."

RATE OF ADMINISTRATION
Flush line before and after panitumumab administration with NS. **Do not administer as an IV push or bolus.** Administer with an IV infusion pump using a low–protein binding, 0.2- or 0.22-micron, in-line filter.

A single dose equally distributed over 60 minutes. If the first infusion is tolerated, administer subsequent infusions over 30 to 60 minutes. Doses over 1,000 mg should be administered over 90 minutes. Reduce rate of infusion by 50% in patients experiencing a Grade 1 or 2 infusion reaction.

ACTIONS
A genetically engineered recombinant, human IgG2 kappa monoclonal antibody that binds specifically to the human epidermal growth factor receptor (EGFR). EGFR is a transmembrane glycoprotein that is expressed in many normal epithelial tissues, including skin and hair follicles. Overexpression of EGFR is detected in many human cancers, including those of the colon and rectum. Interaction of EGFR with its normal ligands leads to a series of reactions that regulate the transcription of molecules involved with cellular growth and survival, motility, proliferation, and transformation. Panitumumab binds to EGFR on both normal and tumor cells, inhibiting the binding of normal ligands to EGFR. This competitive binding results in inhibition of cell growth, induction of apoptosis, decreased proinflammatory cytokine and vascular growth factor production, and internalization of EGFR. The end result is inhibition of growth and survival of selected human tumor cells that express EGFR. Half-life is approximately 7.5 days (range 3.6 to 10.9 days).

INDICATIONS AND USES
Treatment of patients with wild-type *KRAS* (exon 2 in codons 12 or 13) metastatic colorectal cancer (mCRC) as determined by an FDA-approved test for this use. May be used as first-line therapy in combination with FOLFOX (5-fluorouracil [5-FU], leucovorin, and oxaliplatin [Eloxatin]) or as monotherapy following disease progression after prior treatment with fluoropyrimidine (fluorouracil [5-FU])-, oxaliplatin-, and irinotecan (Camptosar)-containing chemotherapy.

Limitation of use: Not indicated for the treatment of patients with *RAS* mutant mCRC or for patients whose *RAS* mutation status is unknown.

CONTRAINDICATIONS
None known. See Precautions.

PRECAUTIONS
Panitumumab should be used only for treatment of patients with *KRAS* wild-type mCRC as determined by an FDA-approved test. In studies, patients with *KRAS*-mutant mCRC tumors receiving panitumumab in combination with FOLFOX experienced some overall survival compared with patients receiving FOLFOX alone. Perform the assessment for *KRAS* mutational status in colorectal cancer laboratories with demonstrated proficiency in the technology required for testing. ▪ Dermatologic toxicities were reported in 90% of patients and were severe (NCI-CTC/CTCAE Grade 3 or higher) in 15% of patients. Manifestations included dermatitis acneiform, dry skin, erythema, paronychia, pruritus, rash, skin exfoliation, and skin fissures. Severe dermatologic toxicities were complicated by infection. Life-threatening and fatal infectious complications, including necrotizing fasciitis, abscesses requiring incision and drainage, and sepsis, have been observed. Life-threatening and fatal bullous mucocutaneous disease with blisters, erosions, and skin sloughing has also been reported. It is unclear whether these reactions were directly related to EGFR inhibition or to idiosyncratic immune-related effects (e.g., Stevens-Johnson syndrome or toxic epidermal necrolysis). See Dose Adjustments and Antidote. ▪ Sunlight may exacerbate

dermatologic toxicity. Protection from sun is advised; see Patient Education. ▪ Infusion reactions, some severe, have been reported. Fatal reactions have been reported. Administer in a facility with adequate emergency medical equipment and medications for treating these reactions and for responding to any medical emergency; see Rate of Administration and Antidote. ▪ Increased mortality and toxicity were seen in studies in which panitumumab was administered in combination with bevacizumab (Avastin) and chemotherapy; see manufacturer's prescribing information. ▪ Electrolyte abnormalities have been reported; see Monitor. ▪ Fatal and nonfatal cases of interstitial lung disease (ILD) and pulmonary fibrosis have been reported; see Monitor. In patients with a history of interstitial pneumonitis or pulmonary fibrosis or with evidence of interstitial pneumonitis or pulmonary fibrosis, the benefit of therapy versus the risk of pulmonary complications must be considered. ▪ Severe diarrhea and dehydration leading to acute renal failure and other complications have been observed in patients treated with panitumumab in combination with chemotherapy. ▪ Keratitis and ulcerative keratitis, known risk factors for corneal perforation, have been reported. ▪ A protein substance. Potential for immunogenicity exists. Anti-panitumumab antibodies have been detected in a small number of patients. No evidence of altered safety profiles has been confirmed.

Monitor: Obtain baseline electrolytes and monitor periodically during and for 8 weeks after completion of therapy. Hypomagnesemia, hypocalcemia, and hypokalemia have been reported. Oral or IV electrolyte replacement may be required. ▪ Monitor hydration status. ▪ Monitor vital signs before, during (as needed), and at the completion of the infusion. ▪ Monitor for S/S of hypersensitivity or infusion-related reactions. Severe reactions may include anaphylaxis, bronchospasm, chills, dyspnea, fever, and hypotension; see Side Effects. Mild to moderate infusion reactions may respond to a reduction in the rate of infusion; see Rate of Administration. Utility of premedication to minimize or prevent infusion-related reactions has not been determined. ▪ Monitor skin integrity. Monitor patients who develop dermatologic or soft tissue toxicities for the development of inflammatory or infectious sequelae. ▪ Monitor lung function. Interrupt therapy in the event of acute onset or worsening of pulmonary symptoms. Discontinue therapy if ILD is confirmed. ▪ Monitor for evidence of keratitis or ulcerative keratitis.

Patient Education: Avoid pregnancy. Nonhormonal birth control recommended for both men and women during and for 6 months following completion of therapy. ▪ Review side effects, including dermatologic toxicity, infusion reactions, pulmonary fibrosis, and potential for fetal harm. ▪ Report skin or ocular changes, cough, dehydration, diarrhea, dyspnea, or infusion-related reactions promptly. ▪ Limit sun exposure during and for 2 months after the last dose of panitumumab. Use of sunscreen and hats recommended. ▪ Compliance with periodic lab work required.

Maternal/Child: Category C: safety for use in pregnancy has not been established. EGFR is thought to be involved in prenatal development and may be essential for normal organogenesis, proliferation, and differentiation in the developing embryo. Human IgG crosses the placental barrier. Therefore it is possible that panitumumab may be transmitted from the mother to the developing fetus. Appropriate contraceptive measures must be used during treatment with panitumumab; see Patient Education. ▪ Women who become pregnant during panitumumab therapy are encouraged to enroll in Amgen's Pregnancy Surveillance Program. ▪ Discontinue breast-feeding during and for 2 months after the completion of therapy. ▪ Safety and effectiveness for use in pediatric patients not established.

Elderly: When used as monotherapy, specific differences in safety and effectiveness compared with younger adults not noted. An increased incidence of serious adverse events and an increased incidence of serious diarrhea were seen in patients over the age of 65 when given panitumumab in combination with FOLFOX.

DRUG/LAB INTERACTIONS

Formal drug interaction studies have not been conducted.

SIDE EFFECTS

The most commonly reported side effects of panitumumab as **monotherapy** are diarrhea, fatigue, nausea, paronychia, and skin rash with variable presentations. The most common serious reactions, as well as the reactions that lead most often to discontinuation of therapy, were general physical health deterioration and intestinal obstruction. Side effects occurring in 5% or more of patients receiving panitumumab as monotherapy included acne, acneiform dermatitis, cough, dry skin, dyspnea, erythema, exfoliative rash, mucosal inflammation, nail disorders, rash, skin exfoliation, skin fissures, skin ulcer, stomatitis, and vomiting. The most commonly reported side effects when panitumumab was used **in combination with chemotherapy** were acneiform dermatitis, anorexia, asthenia, diarrhea, dry skin, hypokalemia, hypomagnesemia, mucosal inflammation, paronychia, pruritus, rash, and stomatitis. The most common serious reactions were diarrhea and dehydration. The most commonly reported side effects leading to discontinuation were acneiform dermatitis, diarrhea, fatigue, hypersensitivity, paresthesia, and rash. Side effects occurring in 5% or more of patients receiving panitumumab in combination with chemotherapy included acne, alopecia, conjunctivitis, dehydration, epistaxis, erythema, nail disorders, palmar-plantar erythrodysesthesia syndrome, skin fissures, and weight decrease. Other serious but less frequently reported side effects as outlined in Precautions included acute renal failure, infusion reactions, interstitial lung disease/pulmonary fibrosis, and ocular toxicity.

Post-Marketing: Angioedema, infusion reactions (fatal), keratitis/ulcerative keratitis, life-threatening and fatal bullous mucocutaneous disease, and skin necrosis.

ANTIDOTE

Notify physician of any side effects; most will be treated symptomatically. Replace electrolytes parenterally or orally as indicated. Reduce infusion rate by 50% if a mild or moderate (Grade 1 or 2) infusion reaction occurs. Discontinue panitumumab for a serious infusion reaction (Grade 3 or 4). Depending on the severity and/or persistence of the reaction, discontinue permanently. Hold or discontinue panitumumab if dermatologic or soft tissue toxicities Grade 3 or higher occur, if they are considered intolerable, or if severe or life-threatening inflammatory or infectious complications occur. See Dose Adjustments for criteria to resume or permanently discontinue treatment. Discontinue if ILD is confirmed. Interrupt or discontinue panitumumab infusion for acute or worsening keratitis. Treat hypersensitivity or infusion reaction as indicated (e.g., oxygen, antihistamines [e.g., diphenhydramine (Benadryl)], epinephrine [Adrenalin], corticosteroids, vasopressors [e.g., dopamine], ventilation equipment, and/or fluids). Resuscitate as necessary.

PANTOPRAZOLE SODIUM
(pan-**TOH**-prah-zohl **SO**-dee-um)

Protonix IV

Proton pump inhibitor
(Gastric acid inhibitor)

pH 9 to 10.5

USUAL DOSE
Given as an alternative to continued oral therapy. Resume oral therapy as soon as practical.
Treatment of gastroesophageal reflux disease (GERD): 40 mg as an infusion once daily for 7 to 10 days.
Treatment of Zollinger-Ellison syndrome (ZES): 80 mg as an infusion every 12 hours. Adjust to patient needs based on acid output measurements. If an increased dose is required, 80 mg every 8 hours is expected to maintain gastric acid output at less than 10 mEq/hr. Daily doses in excess of 240 mg or for more than 6 days have not been studied.
Recurrent gastrointestinal bleeding, prophylaxis (unlabeled): 80 mg as an IV injection followed by a continuous infusion of 8 mg/hr for 72 hours.

DOSE ADJUSTMENTS
No dose adjustments are necessary based on race or gender; in the elderly; in patients with mild, moderate, or severe renal insufficiency; in patients on hemodialysis; or in patients with mild to severe impaired hepatic function. Doses higher than 40 mg/day have not been studied in patients with hepatic impairment.

DILUTION
40-mg dose: Reconstitute each single dose with 10 mL NS. May be further diluted with 100 mL D5W, NS, or LR to achieve a final concentration of approximately 0.4 mg/mL for infusion.
80-mg dose: Combining of two 40-mg vials is required; reconstitute each 40-mg vial with 10 mL NS. This total 80-mg dose may be further diluted with 80 mL D5W, NS, or LR (a total volume of 100 mL) to achieve a final concentration of approximately 0.8 mg/mL for infusion.
Filters: No longer required.
Storage: Store unopened vials at CRT. Protect from light. Do not freeze reconstituted product. Vials reconstituted for the 2-minute infusion may be stored for up to 24 hours at RT. Vials reconstituted for the 15-minute infusion may be stored for up to 6 hours at RT prior to further dilution. Fully diluted solution may then be stored at RT but must be used within 24 hours of initial reconstitution. Protection from light is not required for reconstituted or fully diluted solutions.

COMPATIBILITY   (Underline Indicates Conflicting Compatibility Information)
Consider any drug NOT listed as compatible to be INCOMPATIBLE until consulting a pharmacist; specific conditions may apply.
Manufacturer states, "Administer through a dedicated line or through a Y-site. Should not be simultaneously administered through the same line with other intravenous solutions." See Rate of Administration. Manufacturer lists as **incompatible** at the **Y-site** with midazolam (Versed) and states, "May not be **compatible** with products containing zinc." *Discontinue if discoloration or precipitation occurs with any drug at the Y-site.*
One source suggests the following **compatibilities:**
Y-site: Ampicillin, anidulafungin (Eraxis), caspofungin (Cancidas), cefazolin (Ancef), ceftaroline (Teflaro), ceftriaxone (Rocephin), dimenhydrinate, dopamine, doripenem (Doribax), epinephrine (Adrenalin), furosemide (Lasix), insulin (regular), morphine, nitroglycerin IV, norepinephrine (Levophed), octreotide (Sandostatin), potassium chloride (KCl), telavancin (Vibativ), vasopressin.

RATE OF ADMINISTRATION
Flush IV line before and after administration of pantoprazole with **compatible** infusion solutions (D5W, NS, or LR).

Concentration determines the rate of administration.

40 mg/10 mL or 80 mg/20 mL: As an injection evenly distributed over at least 2 minutes.

40 mg/100 mL or 80 mg/100 mL: As an infusion evenly distributed over at least 15 minutes (approximately 7 mL/min).

ACTIONS

A proton pump inhibitor (PPI) that suppresses the final step in gastric acid production. Acts at the secretory surface of the gastric parietal cell. Inhibits both basal and stimulated gastric acid secretion irrespective of the stimulus. Does not accumulate and pharmacokinetics are not altered with multiple daily dosing. Onset of antisecretory activity is within 15 to 30 minutes. Half-life is approximately 1 hour. However, duration of antisecretory effect persists longer than 24 hours. Distributed mainly in extracellular fluid. Highly bound by serum protein (primarily albumin). Extensively metabolized in the liver through the cytochrome P_{450} system (primarily through CYP2C19 and, to a lesser extent, through CYP3A4). Metabolism is independent of the route of administration (intravenous or oral). Primarily excreted in urine with some excretion in feces. Secreted in breast milk.

INDICATIONS AND USES

Short-term treatment (7 to 10 days) of gastroesophageal reflux disease (GERD) with a history of erosive esophagitis, as an alternative to oral therapy. ▪ Treatment of pathologic hypersecretion associated with Zollinger-Ellison syndrome or other pathologic hypersecretory conditions.

Unlabeled uses: Prophylaxis against recurrent GI bleed (peptic ulcer bleed).

CONTRAINDICATIONS

Known hypersensitivity to pantoprazole (Protonix), other substituted benzimidazoles (e.g., esomeprazole [Nexium], omeprazole [Prilosec]), or any component of the formulation.

PRECAUTIONS

For IV use only; do not give IM or SC. ▪ Gastric malignancy may be present even though patient's symptoms improve with pantoprazole therapy. ▪ Formulation contains edetate disodium, which can chelate zinc; see Monitor. ▪ Should be discontinued as soon as the patient is able to resume treatment with pantoprazole delayed-release tablets or oral suspension. ▪ Data on safe and effective dosing for other conditions (including life-threatening upper GI bleeds) not available. 40 mg IV of pantoprazole daily does not raise gastric pH levels sufficiently to treat such life-threatening conditions. ▪ Hypersensitivity reactions, including anaphylaxis and severe skin reactions (e.g., erythema multiforme, Stevens-Johnson syndrome, and toxic epidermal necrolysis), have been reported. ▪ May be associated with an increased risk for osteoporosis-related fractures of the hip, wrist, or spine. Risk increased in patients receiving high-dose (multiple daily doses) and long-term therapy (a year or longer). Use lowest dose and shortest duration of therapy appropriate for the condition being treated. ▪ In patients treated with proton pump inhibitors (PPIs) for at least 3 months and, in most cases, after a year of treatment, hypomagnesemia (symptomatic and asymptomatic) has been reported. Serious adverse events, including arrhythmias, seizures, and tetany, have occurred. Discontinuation of the PPI and magnesium replacement have been required. ▪ May be associated with an increased risk of *Clostridium difficile*–associated diarrhea (CDAD), especially in hospitalized patients. Consider in patients who develop diarrhea that does not improve. ▪ Acute interstitial nephritis has been observed and is generally attributed to an idiopathic hypersensitivity reaction. May occur at any time during therapy. Discontinue pantoprazole if it occurs. ▪ Use caution in transplant patients receiving mycophenolate mofetil (CellCept). ▪ See Drug/Lab Interactions.

Monitor: Observe for S/S of a hypersensitivity reaction and/or severe skin reaction (e.g., acute interstitial nephritis, anaphylactic shock, anaphylaxis, angioedema, bronchospasm, urticaria). ▪ Monitor vital signs and pain levels. ▪ Concomitant use of antacids may be indicated. ▪ In hypersecretory states, acid output measurements may be indicated to guide dose adjustment. ▪ Monitor injection site. Thrombophlebitis has been reported.

- Zinc supplementation may be indicated in patients who are prone to zinc deficiency; see Precautions. ▪ Monitoring of magnesium levels may be indicated with prolonged PPI therapy; see Precautions and Drug/Lab Interactions. ▪ Change to oral dosing when appropriate. ▪ See Drug/Lab Interactions.

Patient Education: Review prescription and nonprescription drugs with your physician. ▪ Oral route preferred.

Maternal/Child: Category B: use during pregnancy only when clearly needed. ▪ Has potential for serious harm to nursing infants; discontinue breast-feeding. ▪ Safety and effectiveness for pediatric patients under 18 years of age not established.

Elderly: Safety and effectiveness similar to that of younger patients.

DRUG/LAB INTERACTIONS

Because of profound and long-lasting inhibition of gastric acid secretion, pantoprazole may interfere with the **absorption of drugs in which gastric pH is an important determinant of their bioavailability.** Absorption of **atazanavir** (Reyataz), **erlotinib** (Tarceva), **iron salts** (ferrous sulfate), **ketoconazole** (Nizoral), and **mycophenolate mofetil** (CellCept) can decrease; other drugs (e.g., **digoxin** [Lanoxin]) can increase. Coadministration of **mycophenolate mofetil** (MMF) and **omeprazole** (Prilosec) in transplant patients receiving MMF reduces the exposure to MMF's active metabolite, mycophenolic acid; see Precautions. ▪ Increases in INR and PT have been reported when administered concurrently with **warfarin** (Coumadin); monitoring of INR and PT indicated. ▪ Concurrent use with **atazanavir** (Reyataz) or **nelfinavir** (Viracept) is not recommended. Coadministration of proton pump inhibitors (e.g., esomeprazole [Nexium], pantoprazole [Protonix]) results in a significant reduction in **atazanavir** or **nelfinavir** plasma concentrations, thereby inhibiting atazanavir's therapeutic effect and increasing development of drug resistance. ▪ Long-term use may increase the risk of **digoxin** toxicity secondary to hypomagnesemia. ▪ Patients on long-term therapy receiving concomitant **diuretic therapy** may be at increased risk for hypomagnesemia. ▪ Concomitant use of proton pump inhibitors with high-dose **methotrexate** may elevate and prolong serum levels of methotrexate and/or its metabolite. May lead to methotrexate toxicity; consider withdrawal of pantoprazole. ▪ Concomitant administration of pantoprazole and clopidogrel (Plavix) had no clinically significant effect on clopidogrel-induced platelet aggregation. No dose adjustment of clopidogrel is necessary when administered with approved doses of pantoprazole. ▪ Studies suggest that with concurrent use the metabolism and serum concentrations of pantoprazole are not significantly altered by other drugs metabolized by the cytochrome P_{450} system (e.g., clarithromycin [Biaxin], diazepam [Valium], diclofenac [Apo-Diclo], metoprolol [Lopressor], midazolam [Versed], naproxen [Aleve], nifedipine [ProCardia XL], phenytoin [Dilantin], piroxicam [Feldene], theophylline). ▪ Studies also suggest that concurrent use with pantoprazole has not been found to significantly alter the metabolism and serum concentrations of the above agents as well as other drugs metabolized by a similar process (e.g., carbamazepine [Tegretol], cisapride [Propulsid], oral contraceptives). Concurrent administration should not require dose adjustment of either drug. ▪ Amoxicillin, caffeine, digoxin (Lanoxin), ethanol, glyburide (DiaBeta), and metronidazole (Flagyl IV) had no clinically relevant interactions during clinical studies. ▪ May cause false-positive **urine screening test for tetrahydrocannabinol** (THC).

SIDE EFFECTS

The most frequently occurring side effects are abdominal pain, arthralgias, diarrhea, dizziness, flatulence, headache, nausea, and vomiting. Abscess, blurred vision, chest pain, confusion, dyspnea, gastroenteritis, hemorrhage, hyperglycemia, hypokinesia, increased salivation, injection site reactions including thrombophlebitis, pruritus, rash, speech disorder, tinnitus, transient elevations of serum transaminase, urinary tract infection, and vertigo are reported. Numerous other side effects have been associated with oral pantoprazole.

Post-Marketing: Agranulocytosis, anterior ischemic optic neuropathy, asthenia, bone fracture, CDAD, elevated creatine phosphokinase (CPK), fatigue, hallucinations, hepatocellular damage leading to jaundice and hepatic failure, hypersensitivity reactions (e.g., anaphylaxis, angioedema), hypomagnesemia, hyponatremia, insomnia, interstitial nephritis, malaise, pancreatitis, pancytopenia, rhabdomyolysis, severe dermatologic reactions (e.g., erythema multiforme, Stevens-Johnson syndrome, taste disorders, toxic epidermal necrolysis [some fatal]), somnolence, weight gain.

ANTIDOTE
Keep physician informed of all side effects. May be treated symptomatically. Discontinue and initiate appropriate treatment if S/S associated with post-marketing reports occur; see Side Effects. Adverse effects from overdose (up to 240 mg/day in healthy subjects) did not occur during clinical trials. Not removed by hemodialysis.

PAPAVERINE HYDROCHLORIDE
(pah-**PAV**-er-een hy-droh-**KLOR**-eyed)

Vasodilator
(peripheral)

pH 3 to 4.5

USUAL DOSE
1 to 4 mL (30 to 120 mg) every 3 hours as indicated. Second dose may be given in 10 minutes only when treating extrasystoles.

PEDIATRIC DOSE
1.5 mg/kg of body weight every 6 hours; see Maternal/Child.

DOSE ADJUSTMENTS
See Drug/Lab Interactions.

DILUTION
May be given undiluted or may be diluted in an equal amount of SWFI. Usually not added to IV solutions. May be given through Y-tube or three-way stopcock of infusion set.

COMPATIBILITY
Consider any drug NOT listed as compatible to be INCOMPATIBLE until consulting a pharmacist; specific conditions may apply.
Will form a precipitate with LR.
   One source suggests the following **compatibilities:**
Additive: Theophylline.

RATE OF ADMINISTRATION
1 mL (30 mg) or fraction thereof over 2 minutes. Rapid IV injection may cause death.

ACTIONS
A nonnarcotic opium alkaloid, it is a direct smooth muscle relaxant and antispasmodic. Relaxation is noted in vascular system and bronchial musculature and in GI, biliary, and urinary tracts. More effective on muscle in spasm, it has an affinity for the smooth muscle of blood vessels. Affects cardiac muscle to depress conduction and increase refractory period. Improved circulation and muscle relaxation decrease pain. Metabolized in the liver and excreted in the urine.

INDICATIONS AND USES
Vascular spasm associated with an acute myocardial infarction. ▪ Peripheral or pulmonary embolism. ▪ Peripheral vascular disease and cerebral angiospastic states. ▪ Visceral spasm of ureteral, biliary, or GI colic. ▪ Angina pectoris.

CONTRAINDICATIONS
Complete AV heart block.

PRECAUTIONS
Rarely used; active therapeutic value is questioned. ▪ Rapid IV injection may cause death. ▪ IM injection is preferred. ▪ Use with caution in glaucoma and impaired liver

function. ▪ Large doses can depress AV and intraventricular conduction, resulting in arrhythmias.

Monitor: Observe patient continuously; monitor vital signs. ▪ See Drug/Lab Interactions.

Patient Education: Avoid alcohol and other CNS depressants. ▪ May cause dizziness and drowsiness; request assistance for ambulation. ▪ Use caution in any task requiring alertness.

Maternal/Child: Category C: safety for use in pregnancy and breast-feeding and in pediatric patients not established.

Elderly: Risk of hypothermia may be increased.

DRUG/LAB INTERACTIONS

May be used with **narcotics** if the relaxant effect is not adequate to relieve discomfort. Narcotic dosage should be reduced. ▪ Antagonizes effects of **levodopa.**

SIDE EFFECTS

Blurred or double vision, diaphoresis, discomfort (generalized), flushing, hypertension (slight), hypotension, respiratory depth increase, scleral jaundice, sedation, tachycardia.

Major: Respiratory depression, seizures, ventricular ectopic rhythms, sudden death.

ANTIDOTE

Notify the physician of any minor side effects. If minor symptoms progress or any major side effect appears, discontinue the drug immediately and notify the physician. Treatment of toxicity will be symptomatic and supportive. Consider diazepam (Valium) or phenytoin (Dilantin) for convulsions. Anesthesia with thiopental and paralysis with a neuromuscular blocking agent may be required. Use dopamine for hypotension. Calcium gluconate may reduce toxic cardiovascular effects. Monitor ECG. Resuscitate as necessary.

PARICALCITOL
(pair-ee-**KAL**-sih-tohl)

Zemplar

Vitamin D analog

USUAL DOSE

The currently accepted target range for intact parathyroid hormone (iPTH) in chronic kidney disease (CKD) Stage 5 patients is no more than 1.5 to 3 times the nonuremic upper limit of normal.

Recommended initial dose is 0.04 to 0.1 mcg/kg administered no more frequently than every other day at any time during dialysis. Doses as high as 0.24 mcg/kg have been safely administered.

Information supplied by the manufacturer suggests that the relative dosing of paricalcitol to calcitriol is 4:1. When converting a patient from calcitriol to paricalcitol, the initial dose of paricalcitol should be four times greater than the patient's dose of calcitriol.

PEDIATRIC DOSE

Dose recommendations are based on severity of disease in addition to body weight. A dose is administered at any time during dialysis.

Pediatric patients 5 to 19 years of age (unlabeled): Doses used in clinical trials were:

Baseline iPTH level less than 500 pg/mL: 0.04 mcg/kg 3 times a week.

Baseline iPTH level equal to or greater than 500 pg/mL: 0.08 mcg/kg 3 times a week.

See Dose Adjustments.

DOSE ADJUSTMENTS

Adults: Adjust dosing based on patient response. If a satisfactory response is not observed, dose may be increased by 2 to 4 mcg at 2- to 4-week intervals. Monitor serum calcium, phosphorus, and calcium $\times$ phosphorus product (Ca $\times$ P) frequently during any dose adjustment period. See Monitor.

Pediatric patients: Adjust dose in 0.04-mcg/kg increments based on the levels of serum iPTH, calcium, and Ca $\times$ P (from clinical trials).

Adults and pediatric patients: Reduce dose or interrupt therapy if elevated calcium level or a Ca $\times$ P product of greater than 75 is noted. Reinitiate therapy at a lower dose when parameters have normalized. ▪ Paricalcitol dose may need to be reduced as parathyroid hormone (PTH) levels decrease in response to therapy. The currently accepted target range for intact parathyroid hormone (iPTH) in patients with chronic kidney disease (CKD) is no more than 1.5 to 3 times the nonuremic upper limit of normal. Incremental dosing must be individualized and commensurate with PTH, serum calcium, and phosphorus levels. The following chart is a suggested approach to dose titration.

Paricalcitol Suggested Dosing Guidelines	
PTH Level	Paricalcitol Dose
The same or increasing	Increase
Decreasing by <30%	Increase
Decreasing by >30%, <60%	Maintain
Decreasing by >60%	Decrease
1 1/2 to 3 times the upper limit of normal	Maintain

DILUTION
May be given undiluted. Available as a 2 mg/mL and a 5 mcg/mL solution in 1- and 2-mL vials.

Filters: Not required by manufacturer; no further data available.

Storage: Store single-dose and multidose vials at CRT before use. Discard unused portions of single-dose vials. Multidose vial is stable for up to 7 days at CRT after entry into vial.

COMPATIBILITY
Specific information not available. Consider specific use; consult pharmacist.

RATE OF ADMINISTRATION
Administer as a bolus dose at any time during dialysis.

ACTIONS
A synthetic analog of calcitriol, the metabolically active form of vitamin D indicated for the prevention and treatment of secondary hyperparathyroidism associated with chronic kidney disease (CKD) Stage 5. In the diseased kidney, activation of vitamin D is diminished, resulting in a rise in parathyroid hormone (PTH), subsequently leading to secondary hyperparathyroidism and disturbances in calcium and phosphorus homeostasis. Paricalcitol binds to vitamin D receptors present in the parathyroid gland, intestine, kidney, and bone to maintain parathyroid function and calcium and phosphorus homeostasis. Studies suggest that paricalcitol may cause less hypercalcemia and hyperphosphatemia than calcitriol. Serum paricalcitol levels decrease rapidly after a bolus injection. Extensively bound to plasma proteins. Extensively metabolized by multiple hepatic and nonhepatic enzymes. Mean half-life is approximately 15 hours. Eliminated primarily by hepatobiliary excretion in feces and, to a much smaller extent, by the kidneys.

INDICATIONS AND USES
Prevention and treatment of secondary hyperparathyroidism associated with chronic kidney disease (CKD) Stage 5.

CONTRAINDICATIONS
Patients with evidence of vitamin D toxicity, hypercalcemia, or hypersensitivity to any ingredient in this product; see Precautions.

P

PRECAUTIONS

Acute overdose may cause hypercalcemia and require emergency attention. If clinically significant hypercalcemia develops, dose should be reduced or held. Chronic administration may place patient at risk of hypercalcemia, elevated Ca × P product, and metastatic calcification. Chronic hypercalcemia can lead to generalized vascular calcification and other soft tissue calcification. See Side Effects and Antidote. ▪ Phosphate or vitamin D–related compounds should not be taken concomitantly with paricalcitol. High intake of calcium and phosphate concomitant with vitamin D compounds (paricalcitol) may lead to serum abnormalities and require more frequent monitoring and individualized dose titration. ▪ Adynamic bone lesions may develop if PTH levels are suppressed to abnormal levels. ▪ Avoid chronic administration of aluminum-containing preparations (e.g., antacids, phosphate binders); may increase blood levels of aluminum and cause aluminum bone toxicity.

Monitor: During initiation of therapy, obtain baseline serum calcium and phosphorus levels and determine levels at least twice a week. Once dosage has been established, serum calcium and phosphorus should be monitored at least monthly. See Dose Adjustments. ▪ Calculate Ca × P (should be less than 75). ▪ Measurements of serum or plasma PTH are recommended every 3 months. ▪ Monitor for signs and symptoms of hypercalcemia. See Side Effects.

Patient Education: Report symptoms of hypercalcemia promptly (e.g., constipation, difficulty thinking clearly, fatigue, increased thirst, increased urination, loss of appetite, nausea or vomiting, weight loss). Dose adjustment or treatment may be required. Strict adherence to dietary supplementation of calcium and restriction of phosphorus is required to ensure optimal effectiveness of therapy. Phosphate-binding compounds (e.g., calcium acetate [Phos-lo], sevelamer [Renagel]) may be needed to control serum phosphorus levels in patients with CKD, but excessive use of aluminum-containing products (e.g., aluminum hydroxide gel [Alternagel]) should be avoided.

Maternal/Child: Category C: safety for use in pregnancy not established. Benefits must outweigh risks. ▪ Discontinue breast-feeding. ▪ Has not been studied in pediatric patients under 5 years of age.

Elderly: No overall differences in effectiveness or safety have been observed in the elderly.

DRUG/LAB INTERACTIONS

Specific interaction studies have not been performed. ▪ Paricalcitol is partially metabolized by the **cytochrome P₄₅₀ enzyme CYP3A.** Use with caution when administered concomitantly **with known inhibitors of this enzyme** (e.g., atazanavir [Reyataz], clarithromycin [Biaxin], indinavir [Crixivan], itraconazole [Sporanox], ketoconazole [Nizoral], nefazodone, nelfinavir [Viracept], ritonavir [Norvir], saquinavir [Invirase], telithromycin [Ketek], voriconazole [VFEND]). ▪ Digitalis toxicity is potentiated by hypercalcemia. Use caution when paricalcitol is prescribed concomitantly with **digoxin** compounds. ▪ **Phosphate or vitamin D–related compounds** should not be taken concomitantly with paricalcitol; see Precautions. ▪ May reduce **serum total alkaline phosphatase** levels.

SIDE EFFECTS

The most commonly reported side effects include arthralgia, chills, dry mouth, edema, fever, gastrointestinal hemorrhage, influenza, malaise, nausea, palpitations, pneumonia, sepsis, and vomiting. Many other side effects occurred in fewer than 2% of patients. Overdose or chronic administration may lead to hypercalcemia. Signs and symptoms of vitamin D intoxication associated with hypercalcemia include: **Early:** bone pain, constipation, dry mouth, headache, metallic taste, muscle pain, nausea, somnolence, vomiting, and weakness. **Late:** Anorexia, cardiac arrhythmias, conjunctivitis (calcific), death, decreased libido, ectopic calcification, elevated AST and ALT, elevated BUN, hypercholesterolemia, hypertension, hyperthermia, overt psychosis (rare), pancreatitis, photophobia, pruritus, rhinorrhea, somnolence, and weight loss.

Post-Marketing: Hypersensitivity reactions (e.g., angioedema [including laryngeal edema]), rash, urticaria.

ANTIDOTE

Notify physician of any side effects. Treatment should consist of general supportive measures and serial serum electrolyte determinations (especially calcium). Monitor rate of urinary calcium excretion. Treatment of patients with clinically significant hypercalcemia consists of immediate dose reduction or interruption of the therapy and includes a low-calcium diet, withdrawal of calcium supplements, patient mobilization, attention to fluid and electrolyte imbalances, assessment of electrocardiographic abnormalities (critical in patients receiving digoxin), and hemodialysis or peritoneal dialysis against a calcium-free dialysate, as warranted. Monitor serum calcium levels frequently until calcium levels return to within normal limits. Paricalcitol may be restarted at a lower dose when serum calcium levels return to within normal limits. Not significantly removed by dialysis.

PEGASPARGASE ▪ ASPARAGINASE
Erwinia chrysanthemi
(peg-**AS**-par-gays) ▪ (as-**PAR**-a-jin-ase)

Antineoplastic
(miscellaneous)
Enzyme

Oncaspar, PEG-L-Asparaginase ▪ Erwinaze

pH 7.3 (Oncaspar)

USUAL DOSE (International units [IU])

Adult and pediatric patients: Oncaspar: 2,500 international units (IU)/M^2 as an infusion. Do not administer more frequently than every 14 days. Most frequently used as a component of a multiple-agent protocol.

Erwinaze: *To substitute for a dose of pegaspargase:* 25,000 international units (IU)/M^2 3 times a week (Monday/Wednesday/Friday) for 6 doses.

To substitute for a dose of native E. coli asparaginase: 25,000 international units (IU)/M^2 for each scheduled dose of native *E. coli* asparaginase within a treatment.

Both products: May be administered IV or IM; see prescribing information for IM specifics.

DOSE ADJUSTMENTS

Dose adjustment recommendations are not provided by the manufacturer. Other sources recommend possible dose adjustment based on patient response and toxicity; see literature.

DILUTION (International units [IU])

Oncaspar: Available preservative free in 5-mL vials containing 750 IU/mL. Must be further diluted with 100 mL of NS or D5W and administered through the Y-tube or three-way stopcock of a free-flowing infusion of similar solutions (NS or D5W). Do not shake; mix gently. Use only clear solutions.

Erwinaze: Available as a lyophilized powder in 3-mL vials containing 10,000 IU. Reconstitute each vial by slowly injecting 1 or 2 mL of preservative-free NS against the inner vial wall. Do not inject directly onto or into the powder. 1 mL of diluent yields a concentration of 10,000 IU/mL; 2 mL of diluent yields a concentration of 5,000 IU/mL. Gently mix or swirl; *do not shake or invert vial*. A clear, colorless solution. Calculate the required dose and volume required and withdraw into a polypropylene syringe within 15 minutes of reconstitution. Slowly inject the calculated dose into a 100-mL IV infusion bag of NS. *Do not shake or squeeze the infusion bag.*

Storage: *Both products:* Refrigerate unopened vials, protect from light, and do not use after expiration date on vial. For single-dose use only. Do not re-enter vial; discard unused portions. *Oncaspar: Do not administer* if drug has been frozen, stored at RT for more than 48 hours, or shaken or vigorously agitated. Immediate use preferred, but the diluted solution may be refrigerated. Storage after dilution should not exceed 48 hours from the time of preparation to completion of administration. Protect infusion bag from direct sunlight. Discard if cloudy or discolored.

Erwinaze: Do not freeze or refrigerate after reconstitution and dilution, and administer within 4 hours or discard.

COMPATIBILITY

Oncaspar: Specific information not available. Consider specific use and toxicity; consult pharmacist.

Erwinaze: Manufacturer states, "Do not infuse other IV drugs through the same IV line."

RATE OF ADMINISTRATION

Both products: A single dose evenly distributed over 1 to 2 hours.

ACTIONS

Oncaspar is L-asparaginase (L-asparagine amidohydrolase) that is covalently conjugated to monomethoxpolyethylene glycol (MPEG). It is a modified form of *E. coli*–derived asparaginase that has a longer half-life than the native enzyme and is less immunogenic. *Erwinaze* contains an asparagine-specific enzyme derived from *Erwinia chrysanthemi*. Asparaginase is cycle specific for the G1 phase of the cell cycle. It breaks down asparagine, rapidly depleting it from cells. Some malignant cells have a metabolic defect that makes them unable to synthesize asparagine as normal cells do. They are dependent on exogenous asparagine for survival. Depletion of asparagine kills the leukemic cells without affecting normal cells that synthesize their own asparagine. Plasma half-life of *Oncaspar* after IM administration is approximately 5.8 days. Mean half-life of *Erwinaze* after IV administration is approximately 7.51 hours. Half-lives are longer when administered IM.

INDICATIONS AND USES

Oncaspar: First-line treatment of patients with acute lymphoblastic leukemia (ALL). ■ Treatment of patients with ALL and hypersensitivity to native forms of L-asparaginase. Used as a component of a multiagent regimen for both indications.

Erwinaze: A component of a multiagent chemotherapeutic regimen for the treatment of patients with ALL who have developed hypersensitivity to *E. coli*-derived asparaginase. **Unlabeled uses:** *Oncaspar:* Treatment of acute lymphocytic leukemia.

CONTRAINDICATIONS

Both products: History of serious thrombosis or serious hemorrhagic events associated with prior L-asparaginase therapy. History of serious hypersensitivity reactions to either product.

Oncaspar: History of pancreatitis with prior L-asparaginase therapy.

Erwinaze: History of *serious* pancreatitis with prior L-asparaginase therapy.

PRECAUTIONS

Both products: Administered by or under the direction of a physician specialist in a facility with adequate diagnostic and treatment facilities to monitor the patient and respond to any medical emergency. ■ Serious hypersensitivity reactions can occur. Risk increased in patients with known hypersensitivity to other forms of L-asparaginase. ■ Serious thrombotic events, including sagittal sinus thrombosis and pulmonary embolism (PE), have occurred. ■ Pancreatitis has been reported. ■ Glucose intolerance has occurred; may be irreversible. ■ As with all therapeutic proteins, there is a potential for immunogenicity. ■ See Monitor, Drug/Lab Interactions, and Antidote.

Oncaspar: Increased PT, PTT, or hypofibrinogenemia is possible. ■ Hepatotoxicity and abnormal liver function (including elevations of AST, ALT, alkaline phosphatase, and bilirubin [direct and indirect]) and depression of serum albumin and plasma fibrinogen can occur.

Erwinaze: Fibrinogen, protein C activity, protein S activity, and anti-thrombin III decreased in a majority of patients after a 2-week course of Erwinaze by IM administration.

Monitor: *Both products:* Obtain baseline CBC with differential, coagulation parameters (e.g., fibrinogen, PT, PTT), liver function tests, amylase, lipase, triglycerides, and serum glucose and monitor periodically during treatment. ■ Monitor for S/S of hemorrhage or thrombosis. ■ Evaluate patients with abdominal pain for evidence of pancreatitis. ■ Monitor for S/S of hypersensitivity reactions (e.g., bronchospasm, hypotension, laryngeal edema, local erythema or swelling, systemic rash, urticaria). *Oncaspar* manufacturer recommends observing patient carefully during and for at least 1 hour after infusion. *Erwinaze:* With IV use, consider monitoring nadir (pre-dose) serum asparaginase activity (NSAA) levels and switching to IM administration if desired NSAA levels are not achieved.

Patient Education: Report all side effects promptly, especially abdominal pain, hypersensitivity reactions (e.g., dizziness, feeling faint, flushing, hives, itching, nausea, pruritus, rash, shortness of breath), bleeding, increased thirst or urination, or S/S of thrombosis (arm or leg swelling, chest pain, headache, shortness of breath); incidence of hypersensitivity reactions is significant and risk of bleeding is increased. ■ See Appendix D, p. 1333.

Maternal/Child: Category C: effect on fetus unknown. Use during pregnancy only if clearly needed. ■ Discontinue breast-feeding. ■ Safety and effectiveness for use in pediatric patients were established with clinical studies.

Elderly: *Oncaspar:* Numbers in clinical studies insufficient to determine if the elderly respond differently from younger subjects. *Erwinaze:* Safety and effectiveness not studied in geriatric patients.

DRUG/LAB INTERACTIONS

Both products: Manufacturers state that specific drug interaction studies have not been performed. Other sources suggest the following interactions: Asparaginase may increase the serum concentration of **dexamethasone** (Decadron). ■ Coadministration with **bexarotene** (Targretin) may increase the risk of pancreatitis. ■ Coadministration with **thalidomide** (Thalomid) may increase the risk of thromboembolism.

SIDE EFFECTS

Both products: The most common adverse reactions reported include elevated transaminases, hyperbilirubinemia, hypersensitivity reactions (including anaphylaxis), hyperglycemia, pancreatitis, and thrombosis.

Oncaspar: Additional most common adverse reactions reported include central nervous system (CNS) thrombosis, coagulopathy.

Erwinaze: Additional most common adverse reactions reported include abdominal pain/discomfort, diarrhea, fever, local reactions, nausea, thrombosis (including pulmonary embolism [PE] and cerebrovascular accident [CVA]), and vomiting.

ANTIDOTE

Both products: Notify physician of all side effects. Discontinue if coagulopathies or a thrombotic or hemorrhagic event occurs. Symptomatic and supportive treatment is indicated. If the event is mild and symptoms resolve, it may be possible to resume therapy. Administer insulin therapy as necessary in patients with hyperglycemia. Discontinue in patients who experience severe hypersensitivity reactions. Treat hypersensitivity reactions as indicated; may require epinephrine, airway management, oxygen, IV fluids, antihistamines (e.g., diphenhydramine [Benadryl]), corticosteroids (e.g., hydrocortisone sodium succinate [Solu-Cortef]), and pressor amines (e.g., dopamine). Consider administration of fresh frozen plasma (FFP) to patients with severe or symptomatic coagulopathy. There is no specific antidote. *Oncaspar:* Discontinue in patients with pancreatitis. *Erwinaze:* Discontinue in patients with severe or hemorrhagic pancreatitis manifested by abdominal pain greater than 72 hours and amylase elevation of equal to or greater than 2 times the ULN. In cases of mild pancreatitis, hold therapy until the S/S subside and amylase levels return to normal. After resolution, treatment with Erwinaze may be resumed. Discontinue for a thrombotic or hemorrhagic event until symptoms resolve; after resolution, treatment with Erwinaze may be resumed.

PEGLOTICASE BBW

(peg-**LOE**-ti-kase)

Antigout agent

Krystexxa

USUAL DOSE

Discontinue oral urate-lowering medications before beginning therapy; see Precautions and Drug/Lab Interactions.

Gout flare prophylaxis: Use of an NSAID or oral colchicine is recommended beginning at least 1 week before the start of pegloticase therapy and lasting at least 6 months unless medically contraindicated or not tolerated.

Premedication: Patients should be premedicated before each dose with antihistamines and corticosteroids to reduce the risk of infusion reactions, including anaphylaxis or other hypersensitivity reactions. An oral antihistamine, an IV corticosteroid, and/or acetaminophen have been used.

Pegloticase: 8 mg as an IV infusion every 2 weeks. Optimum treatment duration not established.

DOSE ADJUSTMENTS

No dose adjustment is required based on age, gender, race, or renal impairment.

DILUTION

Withdraw 1 mL (8 mg) from the 2-mL vial. A clear, colorless solution that must be further diluted by injecting it into a 250-mL bag of NS or ½NS for infusion. Ensure thorough mixing by inverting the infusion bag a number of times. Do not shake. If diluted solution has been refrigerated, bring to RT before administration (do not subject to artificial heating [e.g., hot water, microwave]).

Filters: No study data available; if filtering is necessary, contact manufacturer.

Storage: Before use, refrigerate in carton at 2° to 8° C (36° to 46° F). Protect from light. Do not shake or freeze. Do not use beyond the expiration date stamped. Diluted infusion bags are stable for 4 hours refrigerated or at RT (20° to 25° C [68° to 77° F]). Manufacturer recommends storing under refrigeration (not frozen), protected from light, and used within 4 hours of dilution. Discard unused product remaining in the 2-mL vial.

COMPATIBILITY

Manufacturer states, "Do not mix or dilute with other drugs."

RATE OF ADMINISTRATION

A single dose properly diluted as an infusion over no less than 2 hours; see Antidote.

Do not administer by IV push or as a bolus. Administer by gravity feed, with a syringe-type pump or infusion pump.

ACTIONS

A uric acid–specific enzyme; a PEGylated product that consists of recombinant modified mammalian urate oxidase (uricase) produced by a genetically modified strain of *Escherichia coli*. Achieves its therapeutic effect by catalyzing the oxidation of uric acid to allantoin, thereby lowering serum uric acid. Duration of suppression of plasma uric acid appears to be dose related. Allantoin is an inert and water-soluble purine metabolite that is readily eliminated, primarily by renal excretion.

INDICATIONS AND USES

Treatment of chronic gout in adult patients refractory to conventional therapy. Gout refractory to conventional therapy occurs in patients who have failed to normalize serum uric acid and in patients whose S/S are inadequately controlled with xanthine oxidase inhibitors (e.g., allopurinol [Aloprim]) at the maximum medically appropriate dose or for whom these drugs are contraindicated.

Limitation of use: Not recommended for the treatment of asymptomatic hyperuricemia.

CONTRAINDICATIONS
Patients with glucose-6-phosphate dehydrogenase (G6PD) deficiency due to risk of hemolysis and methemoglobinemia.

PRECAUTIONS
Administer under the direction of a physician knowledgeable in its use in a facility with adequate diagnostic and treatment facilities to monitor the patient and respond to any medical emergency. ▪ Anaphylaxis and infusion reactions have been reported to occur during and after administration of pegloticase. ▪ Anaphylaxis may occur with any infusion, including a first infusion, and generally manifests within 2 hours of the infusion. However, delayed-type hypersensitivity reactions have also been reported. ▪ Infusion reactions, including anaphylaxis, occurred in patients premedicated with one or more doses of an oral antihistamine and an IV corticosteroid and/or acetaminophen. ▪ Risk of infusion reaction, including anaphylaxis, is higher in patients who have lost therapeutic response (e.g., uric acid levels increase to above 6 mg/dL). ▪ Concomitant use of oral urate-lowering agents (e.g., allopurinol [Aloprim], febuxostat [Uloric]) and pegloticase may blunt the rise of serum uric acid levels. Discontinue oral urate-lowering medications and do not institute oral urate-lowering agents while taking pegloticase. ▪ An increase in gout flares is often observed with the initiation of antihyperuricemic therapy because changing serum uric acid levels result in the mobilization of urate from tissue deposits. Gout flare prophylaxis with an NSAID (e.g., indomethacin [Indocin], ketoprofen, naproxen [Aleve, Naprosyn]) or colchicine is recommended. Pegloticase does not need to be discontinued because of a gout flare. ▪ Exacerbation of CHF has occurred; use with caution in patients with CHF. ▪ Data not available for safety and efficacy of retreatment with pegloticase after stopping treatment for longer than 4 weeks. May increase risk of infusion reactions, including anaphylaxis. ▪ Antipegloticase antibodies developed in most patients treated. High titers were associated with a failure to maintain pegloticase-induced normalization of uric acid. These patients also had a higher incidence of infusion reactions. Anti-PEG antibodies were also detected; the impact on patients' responses to other PEG-containing therapeutics is unknown. ▪ Effects of either renal or hepatic impairment on pegloticase pharmacokinetics were not studied.

Monitor: Before initiating treatment, screening for G6PD deficiency is recommended in patients at higher risk (e.g., African or Mediterranean ancestry); see Contraindications. ▪ Monitor serum uric acid levels before each infusion. Consider discontinuing treatment if levels increase to above 6 mg/dL, particularly when two consecutive levels above 6 mg/dL are observed. ▪ Closely monitor for S/S of potential anaphylaxis for an appropriate period (e.g., during and for at least 1 hour after administration). Manifestations of anaphylaxis have included hemodynamic instability, perioral or lingual edema, and wheezing with or without rash or urticaria. S/S of infusion reactions have included chest discomfort or pain, dyspnea, erythema, flushing, and urticaria. S/S of infusion reactions may overlap with those of anaphylaxis. Infusion reactions can occur at any time during therapy, with approximately 3% occurring with the first infusion and approximately 91% occurring during the time of infusion. Slow or stop the infusion (depending on the severity) if an infusion reaction occurs. ▪ Closely monitor patients with a history of CHF during and after infusion. ▪ Patients being restarted on therapy after a drug-free interval longer than 4 weeks should be monitored carefully.

Patient Education: Immediately report S/S of an infusion or hypersensitivity reaction (e.g., chest pain, dizziness, dyspnea, fever, flushing, hypotension, nausea, pruritus, rash, rigors, urticaria). ▪ Review prescription and nonprescription drugs with physician. Report use of oral urate-lowering agents. ▪ Report side effects of pegloticase that are bothersome or do not go away (e.g., nausea, vomiting). ▪ Patients of African or Mediterranean descent may require testing for G6PD deficiency. ▪ Gout flares may increase with initiation of pegloticase; prophylactic medications recommended.

Maternal/Child: Category C: use during pregnancy only if clearly needed. ▪ Not recommended for use during breast-feeding. ▪ Safety and effectiveness for use in pediatric patients under 18 years of age not established.

Elderly: Response similar to other age-groups; however, greater sensitivity in the elderly cannot be ruled out.

DRUG/LAB INTERACTIONS

Formal drug interaction studies have not been conducted. ▪ Concomitant use of oral **urate-lowering agents** (allopurinol [Aloprim], febuxostat [Uloric]) and pegloticase may blunt the rise of serum uric acid levels; discontinue oral urate-lowering medications and do not institute oral urate-lowering agents while taking pegloticase. ▪ Anti-pegloticase antibodies appear to bind to the PEG portion of the drug; there may be the potential for binding with other PEGylated products (e.g., interferon alpha [Pegasys, Peg-Intron], L-asparaginase [Oncaspar], recombinant methionyl human granulocyte colony-stimulating factor [Neulasta], liposome-containing doxorubicin [Doxil, Caelyx]). Impact of anti-PEG antibodies on patients' responses to other PEG-containing therapeutics is unknown.

SIDE EFFECTS

The most common side effects include anaphylaxis, chest pain, constipation, contusion or ecchymosis, gout flares, infusion reactions, nasopharyngitis, nausea, pain, and vomiting. Most serious reactions are infusion reactions, including anaphylaxis or other hypersensitivity reactions.

ANTIDOTE

Keep physician informed of all side effects. Some will be tolerated or treated symptomatically. Discontinue immediately for any acute serious infusion or hypersensitivity reaction and treat as appropriate; may require epinephrine (Adrenalin), airway management, oxygen, antihistamines (e.g., diphenhydramine [Benadryl]), vasopressors (e.g., dopamine), corticosteroids, albuterol, IV fluids, and ventilation equipment as indicated. Resuscitate as necessary. Slow or stop the infusion (depending on the severity) if an infusion reaction occurs. May be restarted at a slower rate if symptoms subside. Pegloticase does not need to be discontinued because of a gout flare. No specific antidote; monitor and support as indicated in overdose. Resuscitate as necessary.

PEMBROLIZUMAB

(**PEM**-broe-**LIZ**-ue-mab)

Keytruda

Antineoplastic
Monoclonal antibody

pH 5.5

USUAL DOSE

Patient selection for non–small-cell lung cancer (NSCLC): Select patients for second line or greater treatment of metastatic NSCLC based on the presence of positive PD-L1 expression. Information about FDA-approved tests for the detection of PD-L1 expression in NSCLC is available at http://www.fda.gov/CompanionDiagnostics.

Pembrolizumab dose (both indications): 2 mg/kg administered as an IV infusion over 30 minutes every 3 weeks until disease progression or unacceptable toxicity.

DOSE ADJUSTMENTS

Withhold pembrolizumab for any of the following: (1) Grade 2 pneumonitis, (2) Grade 2 or 3 colitis, (3) Grade 3 or 4 endocrinopathies, (4) Grade 2 nephritis, (5) Grade 3 hyperthyroidism, (6) aspartate aminotransferase (AST) or alanine aminotransferase (ALT) greater than 3 and up to 5 times the upper limit of normal (ULN) or total bilirubin greater than 1.5 and up to 3 times the ULN, and (7) any other severe or Grade 3 treatment-related adverse reaction. ▪ Resume pembrolizumab in patients whose adverse reactions recover to Grade 0 to 1. ▪ No dose adjustment is recommended for patients with renal impairment or mild hepatic impairment. In addition, gender, race, and tumor burden do not affect the clearance of pembrolizumab. ▪ See Precautions, Monitor, and Antidote.

DILUTION

Available in single-use vials containing 100 mg/4 mL of pembrolizumab in solution or in single-use vials containing 50 mg of pembrolizumab as a lyophilized powder. Calculate the number of vials required for the recommended dose. Reconstitute each 50-mg vial with 2.3 mL of SWFI. Inject the SWFI along the walls of the vial and not directly on the lyophilized powder (resulting concentration is 25 mg/mL). Slowly swirl the vial. Allow up to 5 minutes for the bubbles to clear. *Do not shake.* A clear to slightly opalescent, colorless to slight yellow solution. Discard reconstituted vial if extraneous particulate matter other than translucent to white proteinaceous particles is observed. Withdraw the required volume from the vial(s) of pembrolizumab and transfer into an IV bag or container of NS or D5W. Mix diluted solution by gentle inversion. The final concentration of the diluted solution should be between 1 and 10 mg/mL. A 2-mg/kg dose for a 70-kg patient would require 140 mg of 25 mg/mL or 5.6 mL of pembrolizumab. Dilution of this 140-mg dose in 50 or 100 mL of NS would still be within the required concentration limits.

Filters: Must be administered using IV tubing that contains a sterile, nonpyrogenic, low–protein-binding, 0.2- to 5-micron in-line or add-on filter.

Storage: Before use, refrigerate both formulations at 2° to 8° C (36° to 46° F). Store 100 mg/4 mL single-use vials in the carton to protect from light. Do not freeze or shake. Does not contain a preservative. Store the reconstituted and/or diluted solutions at RT for no more than 6 hours or refrigerate for no more than 24 hours. Storage times reflect time from initial manipulation of product (reconstitution of lyophilized powder or dilution of solution) through administration of dose. If diluted solution is refrigerated, allow it to come to RT before administration. Discard any unused portion left in a vial.

COMPATIBILITY

Manufacturer states, "Do not coadminister other drugs through the same infusion line."

RATE OF ADMINISTRATION

A single dose as an infusion equally distributed over 30 minutes. If diluted solution for administration has been refrigerated, allow it to come to RT before administration. If a common IV line is used to administer other drugs in addition to pembrolizumab, flush the IV line before and after each infusion of pembrolizumab with NS. Administer through an IV tubing that contains a sterile, nonpyrogenic, low–protein-binding, 0.2- to 5-micron in-line or add-on filter.

ACTIONS

An antineoplastic agent. Pembrolizumab is a humanized monoclonal antibody and an IgG4 kappa immunoglobulin that binds to the programmed death receptor-1 (PD-1 receptor) found on the T-cells, thereby inhibiting T-cell proliferation and cytokine production. Up-regulation of PD-1 ligands occurs in some tumors, and signaling through this pathway can contribute to the inhibition of active T-cell immune surveillance of tumors. Pembrolizumab binds to the PD-1 receptor and blocks its interaction with PD-L1 and PD-L2, releasing PD-1 pathway–mediated inhibition of the immune response, including the antitumor immune response. In syngeneic mouse tumor models, blocking PD-1 activity resulted in decreased tumor growth. Mean elimination half-life is 27 days. Steady-state concentrations were reached by 19 weeks of repeated dosing. Clearance increased with increasing body weight. Age, gender, renal impairment, mild hepatic impairment, and tumor burden had no clinically important effect on the clearance of pembrolizumab.

INDICATIONS AND USES

Treatment of patients with unresectable or metastatic melanoma. ▪ Treatment of patients with metastatic non–small-cell lung cancer (NSCLC) whose tumors express PD-L1 as determined by an FDA-approved test with disease progression on or after platinum-containing chemotherapy. Patients with EGFR or ALK genomic tumor aberrations should have disease progression on FDA-approved therapy for these aberrations before receiving pembrolizumab. (This indication is approved under accelerated approval based on tumor response rate and durability of response. An improvement in survival or disease-related symptoms has not yet been established. Continued approval may be contingent upon verification and description of clinical benefit in confirmatory trials.)

CONTRAINDICATIONS

Manufacturer states, "None."

PRECAUTIONS

Immune-mediated pneumonitis, including fatal cases, has occurred with pembrolizumab. In the NSCLC trial, pneumonitis occurred more frequently in patients with a history of asthma or chronic obstructive pulmonary disease and in patients with a prior history of thoracic irradiation than in patients without a history of these conditions/treatments. ▪ Immune-mediated colitis has occurred with pembrolizumab. ▪ Immune-mediated hepatitis has occurred with pembrolizumab. ▪ Immune-mediated endocrinopathies, including hypophysitis (inflammation of the pituitary gland), thyroid disorders, and type 1 diabetes mellitus have occurred with pembrolizumab. ▪ Immune-mediated nephritis has occurred with pembrolizumab. ▪ Numerous other immune-mediated adverse reactions were reported in fewer than 1% of patients. ▪ Severe and life-threatening infusion-related reactions have been reported. ▪ See Dose Adjustments, Monitor, and Antidote for required dose adjustments, indicated criteria and medications for treatment of adverse reactions, and criteria for discontinuation of pembrolizumab. ▪ Pembrolizumab has not been studied in patients with moderate or severe hepatic impairment. ▪ A protein substance; has a potential for immunogenicity.

Monitor: Obtain serum electrolytes and glucose, baseline liver function tests (e.g., ALT, AST, alkaline phosphatase, total bilirubin), serum creatinine, and thyroid function tests before initiating treatment, and monitor periodically during treatment and as indicated based on clinical evaluation. ▪ Monitor for S/S of infusion-related reactions (e.g., chills, fever, flushing, hypotension, hypoxemia, pruritus, rash, rigors, and wheezing); see Antidote. ▪ Monitor patients for S/S of pneumonitis (e.g., chest pain, new or worsening cough, or shortness of breath). Evaluate patients with suspected pneumonitis with radiographic imaging, and administer corticosteroids (initial dose of 1 to 2 mg/kg/day prednisone or equivalent, followed by a taper) for Grade 2 or greater pneumonitis. Withhold pembrolizumab for moderate (Grade 2) pneumonitis; see Dose Adjustments and Antidote. ▪ Monitor patients for S/S of colitis. Administer corticosteroids (initial dose of 1 to 2 mg/kg/day prednisone or equivalent, followed by a taper) for Grade 2 or greater colitis. Withhold pembrolizumab for moderate (Grade 2) or severe (Grade 3) colitis; see Dose Adjustments and Antidote. ▪ Monitor patients for changes in liver function and S/S of hepatitis (e.g., easy bruising or bleeding, jaundice, lethargy, pain on right side of the abdomen, severe nausea or vomiting). Administer corticosteroids (initial dose of 0.5 to 1 mg/kg/day [for Grade 2 hepatitis] or 1 to 2 mg/kg/day [for Grade 3 or greater hepatitis] prednisone or equivalent, followed by a taper) and, based on severity of liver enzyme elevations, withhold or discontinue pembrolizumab; see Dose Adjustments and Antidote. ▪ Monitor for S/S of hypophysitis (e.g., fatigue, headache, dizziness or fainting, changes in vision, low levels of the hormones produced by the pituitary [adrenocorticotropic hormone (ACTH), thyroid-stimulating hormone (TSH), follicle-stimulating hormone (FSH), luteinizing hormone (LH), growth hormone (GH), prolactin]). Administer corticosteroids and hormone replacement as clinically indicated. Withhold pembrolizumab for moderate (Grade 2) hypophysitis, and withhold or discontinue pembrolizumab for severe (Grade 3) hypophysitis; see Dose Adjustments and Antidote. ▪ Thyroid disorders can occur at any time during treatment. Monitor patients for changes in thyroid function. Administer replacement hormones for hypothyroidism, and manage hyperthyroidism with thionamides and beta-blockers as appropriate. Withhold or discontinue pembrolizumab for severe (Grade 3) or life-threatening (Grade 4) hyperthyroidism; see Dose Adjustments and Antidote. ▪ Monitor for hyperglycemia or other S/S of diabetes (e.g., increased thirst, urination). Administer insulin for type 1 diabetes, and withhold pembrolizumab and administer antihyperglycemics in patients with severe hyperglycemia; see Dose Adjustments and Antidote. ▪ Monitor patients for changes in renal function. Administer corticosteroids (initial dose of 1 to 2 mg/kg/day prednisone or equivalent, followed by a taper) for Grade 2 or greater nephritis. Withhold pembrolizumab for moderate (Grade 2) nephritis; see Dose Adjustments and Antidote. ▪ Monitor patient for other clinically significant immune-mediated adverse reactions. Examples of immune-mediated adverse reactions that have occurred include arthritis, bullous pemphigoid, exfoliative dermatitis, Guillain-Barré syndrome, hemolytic anemia, myasthenic syndrome, myositis, pancreatitis, partial seizures arising in a patient with inflammatory foci in brain parenchyma, rash, serum sickness, uveitis, and vasculitis. ▪ For any suspected immune-mediated adverse reactions, ensure adequate evaluation to confirm etiology or to exclude other causes. Based on the severity of the adverse reaction, withhold pembrolizumab and administer corticosteroids. With improvement to Grade 1 or less, begin corticosteroid taper and continue to taper over at least 1 month. Based on limited data from clinical trials in patients whose immune-related adverse reactions could not be controlled with corticosteroids, administration of other systemic immunosuppressants can be considered. Restart pembrolizumab if the adverse reaction remains at Grade 1 or less following taper; see Dose Adjustments and Antidote.

Patient Education: Review manufacturer's medication guide. ▪ Highly effective contraception required during treatment with pembrolizumab and for at least 4 months following the last dose of pembrolizumab. ▪ Promptly report a known or suspected pregnancy. ▪ Immediately report any S/S of infusion-related reactions (e.g., chills, fever, flushing, hypotension, hypoxemia, pruritus, rigors, and wheezing). ▪ Some side effects may require corticosteroid treatment and interruption or discontinuation of pembrolizumab. ▪ Promptly report S/S of pneumonitis (e.g., chest pain, new or worsening cough, or shortness of breath). ▪ Promptly report S/S of colitis (e.g., diarrhea or severe abdominal pain). ▪ Promptly report S/S of hepatitis (e.g., easy bruising or bleeding, jaundice, lethargy, pain on right side of the abdomen, severe nausea or vomiting). ▪ Promptly report S/S of hypophysitis (e.g., dizziness or fainting, extreme weakness, persistent or unusual headache, vision changes) or of hypothyroidism, hyperthyroidism, or type 1 diabetes mellitus (e.g., constipation, dizziness or fainting, extreme tiredness, feeling cold, hair loss, headaches that will not go away, increased thirst or urination, weight gain or loss). ▪ Promptly report S/S of kidney dysfunction (e.g., blood in urine, decreased urine output, loss of appetite, swelling in ankles). ▪ Keeping scheduled appointments for blood work or other laboratory tests is imperative.

Maternal/Child: Has the potential to be transmitted from the mother to the developing fetus. Based on its mechanism of action and data from animal studies, pembrolizumab can cause fetal harm when administered to a pregnant woman; see Patient Education. ■ Discontinue breast-feeding. ■ Safety and effectiveness for use in pediatric patients have not been established.

Elderly: No overall differences in safety or efficacy were reported between elderly patients and younger adults.

DRUG/LAB INTERACTIONS

No formal pharmacokinetic drug interaction studies have been conducted with pembrolizumab.

SIDE EFFECTS

The most common adverse reactions (reported in at least 20% of patients) were constipation, cough, decreased appetite, diarrhea, dyspnea, fatigue, nausea, pruritus, and rash. Other reported side effects included abdominal pain; anemia; arthralgia; asthenia; back pain; chills; decreased bicarbonate; dizziness; dyspnea; fever; headache; hypercholesterolemia; hyperglycemia; hypertriglyceridemia; hypoalbuminemia; hypocalcemia; hyponatremia; increased alkaline phosphatase, ALT, AST; insomnia; lymphopenia; myalgia; pain in extremity; peripheral edema; sepsis; upper respiratory tract infection; vitiligo; and vomiting.

ANTIDOTE

Keep physician informed of all side effects. May constitute a medical emergency or will be treated symptomatically as indicated. Permanently discontinue pembrolizumab in patients with any of the following: (1) any life-threatening adverse reaction (excluding endocrinopathies controlled with hormone replacement therapy), (2) severe (Grade 3) or life-threatening (Grade 4) pneumonitis or recurrent pneumonitis of Grade 2 severity, (3) severe (Grade 3) or life-threatening (Grade 4) nephritis, (4) AST or ALT greater than 5 times the ULN or total bilirubin greater than 3 times the ULN (for patients with liver metastasis who begin treatment with Grade 2 AST or ALT, if AST or ALT increases by 50% or more relative to baseline and lasts for at least 1 week), (5) Grade 3 or 4 infusion-related reactions, (6) any severe or Grade 3 treatment-related adverse reaction that recurs, (7) inability to reduce corticosteroid dose to 10 mg or less of prednisone or equivalent per day within 12 weeks, and (8) persistent Grade 2 or 3 treatment-related adverse reactions (excluding endocrinopathies controlled with hormone replacement therapy) that do not recover to Grade 0 to 1 within 12 weeks after last dose of pembrolizumab. Treat these side effects aggressively; see Precautions and Monitor. Treat severe infusion reactions as indicated (e.g., epinephrine [Adrenalin], diphenhydramine [Benadryl], IV fluids, oxygen).

PEMETREXED
(peh-meh-**TREX**-ed)

Alimta

Antineoplastic
(Antifolate)

pH 6.6 to 7.8

USUAL DOSE

PREMEDICATION REQUIRED

Regimen begins 1 week before the first infusion of pemetrexed.

Folic acid supplementation: Prophylaxis to reduce treatment-related hematologic and GI toxicity (pemetrexed is an antifolate; severe myelosuppression can occur); 400 to 1,000 mcg of folic acid *must* be taken daily for 7 days *before* the first dose of pemetrexed. Must be continued daily throughout the treatment regimen and for 21 days after treatment is complete. May be taken as a folic acid preparation or as a multivitamin with folic acid. The most commonly used dose of oral folic acid in clinical trials was 400 mcg.

Vitamin B$_{12}$ supplementation: Prophylaxis to reduce treatment-related hematologic and GI toxicity; 1,000 mcg of vitamin B$_{12}$ *must* be given as an injection 1 week *before* the first dose of pemetrexed. Repeat this dose every 3 cycles (about every 9 weeks) during treatment; subsequent doses may be given on the same day as the pemetrexed infusion. *Do not substitute oral vitamin B$_{12}$ for intramuscular vitamin B$_{12}$.*

Corticosteroid: To reduce the incidence and severity of dermatologic toxicity, administer dexamethasone (Decadron) 4 mg PO (or equivalent) twice daily the day before, the day of, and the day after the pemetrexed infusion. Repeat with each planned dose of pemetrexed.

Prehydration: Required with cisplatin; see cisplatin monograph.

PRETESTING REQUIRED

See Monitor. Do not begin a new cycle of treatment unless the ANC (absolute neutrophil count) is equal to or greater than 1,500 cells/mm^3, the platelet count is equal to or greater than 100,000 cells/mm^3, and the CrCl is equal to or greater than 45 mL/min.

PEMETREXED

Nonsquamous non–small-cell lung cancer (NSCLC) and malignant pleural mesothelioma: *Pemetrexed:* 500 mg/M^2 as an infusion over 10 minutes on Day 1 of each 21-day cycle.

Cisplatin: Begin 30 minutes after the end of the pemetrexed infusion. 75 mg/M^2 as an infusion over 2 hours.

As a single agent in nonsquamous NSCLC: *Pemetrexed:* 500 mg/M^2 as an infusion over 10 minutes on Day 1 of each 21-day cycle.

DOSE ADJUSTMENTS

Other than those recommended for all patients, no dose adjustments are required based on age, gender, or race or in patients with a CrCl equal to or greater than 45 mL/min. ■ Dose Adjustments are based on the nadir hematologic counts of the previous dose cycle for hematologic toxicities and the common toxicity criteria (CTC) for nonhematologic toxicities and neurotoxicity. Therapy may be delayed to allow sufficient time for recovery; when recovery occurs, reinitiate therapy according to the following charts:

Pemetrexed/Cisplatin Dose Reduction (Single Agent or in Combination): Hematologic Toxicities	
ANC and Platelet Count	Dose of Pemetrexed (mg/M^2) and Cisplatin (mg/M^2)
Nadir ANC <500/mm^3 and nadir platelets ≥50,000/mm^3	75% of previous dose (both drugs)
Nadir platelets <50,000/mm^3 without bleeding, regardless of nadir ANC	75% of previous dose (both drugs)
Nadir platelets <50,000/mm^3 with bleeding, regardless of nadir ANC	50% of previous dose (both drugs)

Continued

Pemetrexed and Cisplatin Dose Reduction (Single Agent or in Combination) in Neurotoxicity		
CTC Grade*	Dose of Pemetrexed (mg/M²)	Dose of Cisplatin (mg/M²)
0 or 1	100% of previous dose	100% of previous dose
2	100% of previous dose	50% of previous dose
3 or 4	Discontinue therapy	Discontinue therapy

*Common Terminology Criteria for Adverse Events (CTCAE).

Excluding neurotoxicity, if patients develop nonhematologic toxicities equal to or greater than Grade 3, pemetrexed should be withheld until pretherapy values are achieved. Resume treatment according to the following chart.

Pemetrexed and Cisplatin Dose Reduction (Single Agent or in Combination): Nonhematologic Toxicities*		
CTC Grade†	Dose of Pemetrexed (mg/M²)	Dose of Cisplatin (mg/M²)
Any Grade 3 or 4 toxicities except mucositis	75% of previous dose	75% of previous dose
Any diarrhea requiring hospitalization or Grade 3 or 4 diarrhea	75% of previous dose	75% of previous dose
Grade 3 or 4 mucositis	50% of previous dose	100% of previous dose

*Excluding neurotoxicity.
†Common Terminology Criteria for Adverse Events (CTCAE).

Discontinue therapy if hematologic or nonhematologic Grade 3 or 4 toxicity occurs after two dose reductions or immediately if Grade 3 or 4 neurotoxicity is observed.

DILUTION

Specific techniques required; see Precautions. Calculate the dose and number of vials needed. Reconstitute each 100-mg vial with 4.2 mL of preservative-free NS and each 500-mg vial with 20 mL of preservative-free NS. Concentration equals 25 mg/mL. Gently swirl to completely dissolve the powder. Solution ranges in color from colorless to yellow or green-yellow. Withdraw the required volume to provide the calculated dose of pemetrexed. *Must* be further diluted to a total volume of 100 mL with preservative-free NS.
Filters: No data available from manufacturer.
Storage: Store unopened vials at CRT. Reconstituted and diluted solutions are chemically and physically stable for 24 hours refrigerated. Contains no preservatives; discard unused portions.

COMPATIBILITY

Consider any drug NOT listed as compatible to be INCOMPATIBLE until consulting a pharmacist; specific conditions may apply.
Manufacturer states, "Is physically **incompatible** with diluents containing calcium, including lactated Ringer's and Ringer's injection. Coadministration with other diluents has not been studied." **Compatible** with standard PVC administration sets and bags.
   One source suggests the following **compatibilities:**
Y-site: Acyclovir (Zovirax), amifostine (Ethyol), amikacin, aminophylline, ampicillin, ampicillin/sulbactam (Unasyn), aztreonam (Azactam), bumetanide, buprenorphine (Buprenex), butorphanol (Stadol), carboplatin (Paraplatin), ceftriaxone (Rocephin), cefuroxime (Zinacef), cisplatin, clindamycin (Cleocin), cyclophosphamide (Cytoxan), cytarabine (ARA-C), dexamethasone (Decadron), dexrazoxane (Zinecard), diphenhydramine (Benadryl), docetaxel (Taxotere), dopamine, enalaprilat (Vasotec IV), famotidine (Pepcid IV), fluconazole (Diflucan), fluorouracil (5-FU), ganciclovir (Cytovene IV), granisetron (Kytril), heparin, hydromorphone (Dilaudid), ifosfamide (Ifex), leucovorin calcium, lorazepam (Ativan), mannitol (Osmitrol), meperidine (Demerol), mesna (Mesnex), methylprednisolone (Solu-Medrol), metoclopramide (Reglan), morphine, paclitaxel (Taxol),

potassium chloride (KCl), promethazine (Phenergan), ranitidine (Zantac), sodium bicarbonate, sulfamethoxazole/trimethoprim, ticarcillin/clavulanate (Timentin), vancomycin,
vinblastine, vincristine, zidovudine (AZT, Retrovir).

RATE OF ADMINISTRATION
A single dose as an infusion equally distributed over 10 minutes.

ACTIONS
An antifolate antineoplastic agent. It disrupts folate-dependent metabolic processes essential for cell replication. Transported into cells by both the reduced folate carrier and the
membrane folate-binding protein transport systems. Converts to polyglutamate forms,
which are inhibitors of folate-dependent enzymes involved in the de novo biosynthesis of
thymidine and purine nucleotides. Polyglutamation is a time- and concentration-dependent
process that occurs in tumor cells and, to a lesser extent, in normal tissues. Polyglutamated
metabolites have an increased intracellular half-life, resulting in prolonged drug action in
malignant cells. Inhibited the in vitro growth of mesothelioma cell lines and showed synergistic effects when used concurrently with cisplatin. Folic acid and vitamin B_{12} supplementation is required during treatment. 81% bound to plasma protein. Not appreciably
metabolized. Half-life is 3.5 hours. Primarily eliminated in urine as an unchanged drug.
Clearance decreases and exposure (AUC) increases as renal function decreases.

INDICATIONS AND USES
Used in combination with cisplatin for the treatment of malignant pleural mesothelioma in
patients whose disease is unresectable or who are not candidates for curative surgery. ▪ As
a single agent for treatment of patients with locally advanced or metastatic nonsquamous
NSCLC after prior chemotherapy. ▪ Used in combination with cisplatin for the initial
treatment of patients with locally advanced or metastatic nonsquamous NSCLC. ▪ Maintenance treatment of patients with locally advanced or metastatic nonsquamous NSCLC
whose disease has not progressed after 4 cycles of platinum-based first-line chemotherapy.
Limitation of use: Not indicated for treatment of squamous cell NSCLC.

CONTRAINDICATIONS
History of severe hypersensitivity reaction to pemetrexed or any of its components. ▪ Should not be administered to patients with a CrCl less than 45 mL/min.

PRECAUTIONS
Follow guidelines for handling cytotoxic agents. See Appendix A, p. 1331. ▪ Use of
gloves recommended. If a solution of pemetrexed contacts the skin, wash the skin immediately and thoroughly with soap and water. If there is contact with mucous membrane, flush
thoroughly with water. ▪ Should be administered by or under the direction of a physician
specialist in a facility equipped to monitor the patient and respond to any medical emergency. ▪ Use caution in patients with a CrCl less than 80 mL/min if NSAIDs (e.g., ibuprofen [Advil, Motrin], naproxen [Aleve, Naprosyn]) are administered concurrently. ▪ Bone
marrow suppression (e.g., anemia, neutropenia, thrombocytopenia) is a dose-limiting toxicity; see Dose Adjustments. ▪ Folic acid and vitamin B_{12} supplementation is required; a
prophylactic measure to reduce treatment-related hematologic and GI toxicity. ▪ In patients with pleural effusion and/or ascites, consider drainage of third-space fluid before
administration; the effects of this fluid accumulation on pemetrexed are not known. ▪ Coadministration with cisplatin has not been studied in patients with moderate renal impairment. ▪ Cutaneous reactions (skin rash) occur more frequently in patients not pretreated
with a corticosteroid. ▪ See Contraindications and Drug/Lab Interactions.
Monitor: Pretreatment with folic acid, vitamin B_{12}, dexamethasone, and adequate hydration required; see Usual Dose. ▪ Obtain baseline CBC, including platelet count, CrCl,
and liver function tests. Repeat CBC and platelet count before each dose and on Days 8
and 15 of each cycle. Do not begin a new cycle of treatment unless the ANC is equal to
or greater than 1,500 cells/mm^3, the platelet count is equal to or greater than
100,000 cells/mm^3, and the CrCl is equal to or greater than 45 mL/min. ▪ Monitor CBC
and platelets for nadir and recovery. Time to ANC nadir ranged between 8 and 9.6 days.
Return to baseline ANC occurred 4.2 to 7.5 days after the nadir. Has no cumulative effect

on ANC nadir over multiple treatment cycles. ▪ Repeat CrCl before each dose to evaluate renal function. Plasma clearance of pemetrexed given concurrently with cisplatin decreases as renal function decreases; see Dose Adjustments and Contraindications. ▪ No effect of elevated AST, ALT, or total bilirubin on the pharmacokinetics of pemetrexed was seen. However, formal studies to examine the effects of hepatic impairment on the pharmacokinetics of pemetrexed have not been conducted. ▪ Monitor patients who have been or are taking NSAIDs carefully for signs of toxicity, especially myelosuppression and renal or GI toxicity; see Drug/Lab Interactions. ▪ Monitor for thrombocytopenia (platelet count less than 50,000/mm³). Initiate precautions to prevent excessive bleeding (e.g., inspect IV sites, skin, and mucous membranes; use extreme care during invasive procedures; test urine, emesis, stool, and secretions for occult blood). ▪ See Precautions, Drug/Lab Interactions, and Antidote.

Patient Education: Avoid pregnancy; use of nonhormonal birth control recommended. See Maternal/Child. Women should report a suspected pregnancy immediately. ▪ Adherence to regimen (medication [folic acid, vitamin B_{12}, dexamethasone, avoidance or limiting of aspirin or NSAIDs], required lab work, follow-up visits with health care professional) is imperative. ▪ Promptly report S/S of anemia, bleeding, dehydration from diarrhea or vomiting, fatigue, infection (e.g., fever), rash, redness or sores in the mouth, trouble swallowing, or other symptoms. ▪ Review manufacturer's supplied patient information guide. ▪ See Appendix D, p. 1333.

Maternal/Child: Category D: avoid pregnancy; may cause fetal harm. Fetotoxic and teratogenic in mice. ▪ Reduced fertility, hypospermia, and testicular atrophy occurred in mice. ▪ Discontinue breast-feeding. ▪ Safety and effectiveness for use in pediatric patients not established.

Elderly: See Dose Adjustments; required only based on general patient criteria. ▪ Incidence of CTCAE Grade 3 and 4 for anemia, fatigue, hypertension, neutropenia, and thrombocytopenia was greater in patients 65 years of age or older even though they were fully supplemented with vitamins.

DRUG/LAB INTERACTIONS

Concomitant use with **nephrotoxic agents** (e.g., aminoglycosides [e.g., gentamicin], amphotericin B, cisplatin, NSAIDs, vancomycin) and **agents that are tubularly secreted** (e.g., probenecid) may delay clearance of pemetrexed. ▪ **NSAIDs** (e.g., ibuprofen [Advil, Motrin], naproxen [Aleve, Naprosyn]) decrease clearance and increase AUC in patients with normal renal function. Ibuprofen 400 mg four times daily was administered to patients with normal renal function (CrCl equal to or greater than 80 mL/min) who were receiving pemetrexed. Effects of larger doses unknown; see Precautions. All patients taking NSAIDs should avoid taking them for from 2 days (short-acting NSAIDs) to 5 days (long-acting NSAIDs) before, the day of, and at least 2 days after a dose of pemetrexed. Monitoring for hematologic, renal, and GI toxicity required. ▪ Pharmacokinetics of both drugs (pemetrexed and cisplatin) are not affected by each other. ▪ Coadministration of oral folic acid or IM vitamin B_{12} does not adversely affect pemetrexed. ▪ Is not a clinically significant inhibitor of drugs metabolized by cytochrome P_{450} enzymes. Used as recommended (every 21 days), it would not be expected to cause any significant enzyme induction. ▪ May be used concurrently with aspirin in low to moderate doses (325 mg every 6 hours). Effect of higher doses not known.

SIDE EFFECTS

The most common side effects with single-agent use are anorexia, fatigue, and nausea. When used in combination with cisplatin, additional common side effects include constipation, hematologic toxicity (anemia, leukopenia, neutropenia, thrombocytopenia), pharyngitis, stomatitis, and vomiting. Bone marrow suppression (anemia, leukopenia, neutropenia, thrombocytopenia), selected nonhematologic toxicities (e.g., Grade 3 or 4 toxicities, diarrhea requiring hospitalization, mucositis), and neurotoxicity are dose-limiting toxicities. Other frequently occurring side effects include fever, infection (including sepsis), and rash with desquamation. Infections and rash leading to bullous conditions (e.g., Stevens-Johnson syndrome and toxic epidermal necrolysis) have been fatal. Other side effects may include hypersensitivity reactions, alopecia, anorexia, arthralgia, chest pain, decreased CrCl, dehydration, depression, diarrhea, dysphagia, dyspnea, edema, elevated ALT, elevated AST, embolism or thrombosis, esophagitis, fatigue, febrile neutropenia, mood alteration, myalgia, neuropathy (sensory), odynophagia (pain produced by swallowing), renal failure.

Overdose: Bone marrow suppression (e.g., anemia, neutropenia, thrombocytopenia), diarrhea, infection with or without fever, mucositis, rash.

Post-Marketing: Colitis, edema, esophagitis, immune-mediated hemolytic anemia, interstitial pneumonitis, pancreatitis, radiation recall.

ANTIDOTE

Keep physician informed of dose parameters and other side effects. Pemetrexed may be delayed or discontinued based on the degree of side effects. Symptomatic and supportive therapy is indicated. Death may occur from the progression of some side effects. Begin leucovorin treatment immediately for Grade 4 thrombocytopenia, bleeding associated with Grade 3 thrombocytopenia, or Grade 3 or 4 mucositis. Leucovorin treatment is also indicated if Grade 4 neutropenia or Grade 4 leukopenia lasting 3 or more days occurs. Regimen recommended is leucovorin 100 mg/M^2 IV as an initial dose followed by 50 mg/M^2 IV every 6 hours for 8 days. Administration of whole blood products (e.g., packed RBCs, platelets, leukocytes) and/or blood modifiers (e.g., darbepoetin alfa [Aranesp], epoetin alfa [Epogen], filgrastim [Neupogen, Zarxio], pegfilgrastim [Neulasta], sargramostim [Leukine]) may be indicated to treat bone marrow toxicity. Effect of hemodialysis on pemetrexed is unknown.

PENICILLIN G AQUEOUS

(pen-ih-**SILL**-in **A**-kwe-us)

Penicillin G Potassium, Penicillin G Sodium, Pfizerpen

Antibacterial
(penicillin)

pH 5.5 to 8

USUAL DOSE

Adults and pediatric patients 12 years of age and older: 1 million to 20 million units/24 hr equally distributed over 24 hours as a continuous infusion or equally divided in 4 to 6 intermittent infusions (250,000 to 5 million units every 6 hours or 166,000 to 3,333,333 units every 4 hours). Doses up to 80 million units/24 hr have been given in life-threatening infections. (400,000 units equals approximately 250 mg.) See package insert for specific indications.

PEDIATRIC DOSE

Administration by intermittent infusion over 15 to 30 minutes is preferred. Dose is based on age or weight and the severity of the infection.

Serious infections (e.g., pneumonia, endocarditis): 25,000 units/kg every 4 hours or 37,500 units/kg every 6 hours (150,000 units/kg/24 hr).

Meningitis: 41,666 units/kg every 4 hours (250,000 units/kg/24 hr). Continue treatment for 7 to 14 days. Maximum dose is 12 to 20 million units/24 hr.

Disseminated gonococcal infections (arthritis), weight less than 45 kg: 25,000 units/kg every 6 hours (100,000 units/kg/24 hr) for 7 to 10 days.

Disseminated gonococcal infections (meningitis), weight less than 45 kg: 41,666 units/kg every 4 hours (250,000 units/kg/24 hr) for 10 to 14 days.

Disseminated gonococcal infections (endocarditis), weight less than 45 kg: 41,666 units/kg every 4 hours (250,000 units/kg/24 hr) for 4 weeks.

Disseminated gonococcal infections (arthritis, meningitis, endocarditis), weight 45 kg or greater: 2,500,000 units every 6 hours (10,000,000 units/24 hr). Duration of therapy is dependent on diagnosis.

Continued

Syphilis (congenital or neurosyphilis) after the newborn period: 50,000 units/kg every 4 to 6 hours (200,000 to 300,000 units/kg/24 hr). Continue treatment for 10 to 14 days.

Diphtheria (adjunctive to antitoxin and prevention of carrier state): 37,500 to 62,500 units/kg every 6 hours (150,000 to 250,000 units/kg/24 hr) for 7 to 10 days.

Rat-bite fever, Haverhill fever (caused by a specific organism): 25,000 to 41,666 units/kg every 4 hours (150,000 to 250,000 units/kg/24 hr) for 4 weeks.

The American Association of Pediatrics (AAP) recommends:

Pediatric patients from 1 month to under 12 years of age: *Mild to moderate bacterial infections:* 6,250 to 12,500 units/kg every 6 hours (25,000 to 50,000 units/kg/24 hr).

Severe bacterial infections and Group B streptococcal meningitis: 62,500 to 100,000 units/kg every 6 hours or 41,666 to 66,666 units/kg every 4 hours (250,000 to 400,000 units/kg/24 hr).

Another source recommends:

Pediatric patients under 12 years of age: 100,000 to 400,000 units/kg/24 hr in equally divided doses every 4 to 6 hours as an intermittent infusion (25,000 to 100,000 units/kg every 6 hours or 16,666 to 66,666 units/kg every 4 hours). Dosage can vary greatly and must be adjusted according to the severity of the infection. Maximum dose is 24,000,000 units/24 hr.

Treatment of congenital syphilis over 4 weeks of age: 50,000 to 75,000 units/kg every 6 hours (200,000 to 300,000 units/kg/24 hr). Total course of treatment is 10 to 14 days.

NEONATAL DOSE

Administration by intermittent infusion over 15 to 30 minutes is preferred. Dose is based on weight and age and the severity of the infection.

The American Academy of Pediatrics (AAP) has recommended 25,000 to 50,000 units/dose. Adjust the dosing intervals based on the neonate's weight and age as follows:

Moderate to severe bacterial infections:

Weight less than 1,200 Gm; 4 weeks of age or younger: Every 12 hours.

Weight 1,200 to 2,000 Gm; under 7 days of age: Every 12 hours.

Weight 1,200 to 2,000 Gm; 1 to 4 weeks of age: Every 8 hours.

Weight over 2,000 Gm; under 7 days of age: Every 8 hours.

Weight over 2,000 Gm; 1 to 4 weeks of age: Every 6 hours.

Meningitis caused by beta streptococci:

7 days of age or younger: 83,333 to 133,333 units/kg every 8 hours (250,000 to 400,000 units/kg/24 hr).

Older than 7 days of age: 112,500 units/kg every 6 hours (450,000 units/kg/24 hr).

Treatment of congenital syphilis; under 4 weeks of age: 50,000 units/kg every 12 hours (100,000 units/kg/24 hr) for the first week, then 50,000 units/kg every 8 hours (150,000 units/kg/24 hr) for an additional 3 to 7 days. Total course of treatment is 10 to 14 days.

DOSE ADJUSTMENTS

Reduce dose in severe impaired renal function; additional reductions may be indicated if liver function is also impaired. ▪ If CrCl is greater than 10 mL/min in uremic patients, give a full loading dose followed by one-half loading dose every 4 to 5 hours. ▪ If CrCl is less than 10 mL/min/1.73 M^2, administer a full loading dose followed by one half of the loading dose every 8 to 10 hours. Another source recommends giving 75% of a normal dose every 4 to 6 hours to patients with a CrCl of 10 to 50 mL/min and 20% to 50% of a normal dose every 4 to 6 hours to patients with a CrCl less than 10 mL/min. ▪ See Drug/Lab Interactions.

DILUTION

Available as a premixed frozen solution, or reconstitute each vial with SWFI or NS. Direct flow of diluent against sides of the vial while gently rotating vial. Shake vigorously. Directions on vial should be followed to provide desired number of units per milliliter. Available with 1, 5, 10, and 20 million units per vial. May be added to NS or dextrose solutions for infusion. See chart on inside back cover.

Storage: Dry powder stored at CRT. Reconstituted solutions of penicillin G potassium are stable for 1 week if refrigerated. Reconstituted solutions of penicillin G sodium are stable for 3 days if refrigerated. Infusion solutions are stable at CRT for 24 hours. Store pre-mixed frozen solution at or below $-20°$ C ($-4°$ F). The thawed solution is stable for 14 days refrigerated or for 24 hours at RT. Do not refreeze.

COMPATIBILITY
(Underline Indicates Conflicting Compatibility Information)

Consider any drug NOT listed as compatible to be INCOMPATIBLE until consulting a pharmacist; specific conditions may apply.

Penicillins are rapidly inactivated in alkaline carbohydrate solutions, reducing agents, alcohols, and glycols; optimum pH range is 6 to 7. To preserve bactericidal action, consult pharmacist before mixing other agents with penicillin in the infusion solution. May form a precipitate with vancomycin. Inactivated in solution with aminoglycosides (e.g., amikacin, gentamicin). Do not mix in the same solution. Appropriate spacing and/or separate sites required. See Drug/Lab Interactions.

One source suggests the following **compatibilities:**

PENICILLIN G POTASSIUM

Additive: *See general comments under Compatibility.* Amikacin, ascorbic acid, calcium chloride, calcium gluconate, chloramphenicol (Chloromycetin), colistimethate (Coly-Mycin M), dimenhydrinate, diphenhydramine (Benadryl), ephedrine, erythromycin (Erythrocin), heparin, hydrocortisone sodium succinate (Solu-Cortef), lidocaine, lincomycin (Lincocin), magnesium sulfate, methylprednisolone (Solu-Medrol), metronidazole (Flagyl IV), potassium chloride (KCl), prochlorperazine (Compazine), promethazine (Phenergan), ranitidine (Zantac), sodium bicarbonate, verapamil.

Y-site: Acyclovir (Zovirax), amiodarone (Nexterone), cyclophosphamide (Cytoxan), diltiazem (Cardizem), enalaprilat (Vasotec IV), esmolol (Brevibloc), fluconazole (Diflucan), foscarnet (Foscavir), heparin, hydrocortisone sodium succinate (Solu-Cortef), hydromorphone (Dilaudid), labetalol, magnesium sulfate, meperidine (Demerol), morphine, nicardipine (Cardene IV), potassium chloride (KCl), tacrolimus (Prograf), theophylline, verapamil.

PENICILLIN G SODIUM

Additive: *See general comments under Compatibility.* Calcium chloride, calcium gluconate, chloramphenicol (Chloromycetin), colistimethate (Coly-Mycin M), dextran 40, diphenhydramine (Benadryl), erythromycin (Erythrocin), gentamicin, heparin, hydrocortisone sodium succinate (Solu-Cortef), lincomycin (Lincocin), potassium chloride (KCl), ranitidine (Zantac), verapamil.

Y-site: Levofloxacin (Levaquin).

RATE OF ADMINISTRATION

Penicillin is not given by IV injection. Administer as ordered as continuous IV drip; for example, 5 million units in 1,000 mL of D5W over 12 hours. Is sometimes given by intermittent infusion ($^{1}/_{6}$ or $^{1}/_{4}$ of a daily dose in 100 mL over 1 to 2 hours every 4 to 6 hours). Because of its short half-life, frequent dosing is required to maintain serum concentration above the MIC (minimum inhibitory concentration) for most of the dosing interval. Too-rapid administration or excessive doses may cause electrolyte imbalance and/or seizures. Stable at room temperature for at least 24 hours.

Pediatric rate: Administration by intermittent infusion over 15 to 30 minutes is preferred for infants and children.

ACTIONS

Bactericidal against penicillin-sensitive microorganisms during the stage of active multiplication. Inhibits bacterial cell wall synthesis. Distributed into most body fluids. Distribution into spinal fluid is minimal unless inflammation is present. Half-life is approximately 40 minutes. Crosses the placental barrier. Excreted in the urine via glomerular filtration and tubular secretion. Secreted in breast milk. Available in a potassium salt containing 1.02 mEq of potassium and 0.3 mEq sodium in 1 million units or a sodium salt containing 2 mEq sodium in 1 million units.

INDICATIONS AND USES

Severe infections caused by penicillin G–sensitive gram-positive, gram-negative, and anaerobic microorganisms (e.g., streptococcal, pneumococcal, Vincent's gingivitis, spirochetal infections, meningitis, endocarditis).

Unlabeled uses: Arthritis, carditis.

CONTRAINDICATIONS

Known sensitivity to any penicillin or cephalosporin (not absolute; see Precautions).

PRECAUTIONS

Hypersensitivity reactions, including fatalities, have been reported in patients undergoing penicillin therapy; most likely to occur in patients with a history of penicillin allergy or sensitivity to multiple allergens. There have been reports of individuals with a history of penicillin hypersensitivity experiencing severe reactions when treated with cephalosporins. Check history of previous hypersensitivity reactions to penicillins, cephalosporins, or other allergens. Actual incidence of cross-allergenicity not established but may be more common with first-generation cephalosporins. ▪ Sensitivity studies necessary to determine susceptibility of the causative organism to penicillin. ▪ To reduce the development of drug-resistant bacteria and maintain its effectiveness, penicillin should be used to treat or prevent only those infections proven or strongly suspected to be caused by bacteria. ▪ Continue treatment for 48 to 72 hours after symptoms subside. To reduce the risk of rheumatic fever, patients being treated for Group A beta-hemolytic streptococcal infections should be treated for at least 10 days. ▪ Avoid prolonged use of drug; superinfection caused by overgrowth of nonsusceptible organisms may result. ▪ *Clostridium difficile*–associated diarrhea (CDAD) has been reported. May range from mild diarrhea to fatal colitis. Consider in patients who present with diarrhea during or after treatment with penicillin. ▪ Potassium penicillin most frequently used. Doses over 10,000,000 units may cause fatal hyperkalemia, especially in patients with renal insufficiency.

Monitor: Periodic evaluation of renal, hepatic, and hematopoietic systems is recommended in prolonged therapy. ▪ Test patients with gonococcal infections and syphilis for HIV. Test patients with gonococcal infections for syphilis. ▪ Electrolyte imbalance from potassium or sodium content is very possible. Monitor closely. Penicillin G potassium contains 1.02 mEq sodium/million units. May aggravate CHF. ▪ May cause thrombophlebitis; observe carefully and rotate infusion sites. ▪ See Drug/Lab Interactions.

Patient Education: May require alternate birth control. ▪ Promptly report diarrhea or bloody stools that occur during treatment or up to several months after an antibiotic has been discontinued; may indicate CDAD and require treatment.

Maternal/Child: Category B: use only if clearly needed. ▪ May cause diarrhea, candidiasis, or allergic response in nursing infants. ▪ Elimination rate markedly reduced in neonates.

Elderly: Response similar to that seen in younger adults. ▪ Consider age-related organ impairment and concomitant disease or drug therapy. Monitor renal function. ▪ See Dose Adjustments.

DRUG/LAB INTERACTIONS

Synergistic when used in combination with **aminoglycosides** (e.g., amikacin, gentamicin). Synergism may be inconsistent; see Compatibility. ▪ May be antagonized by **bacteriostatic antibiotics** (e.g., chloramphenicol, erythromycin, tetracyclines); may interfere with bactericidal action. ▪ **ASA, ethacrynic acid** (Edecrin), **furosemide** (Lasix), **indomethacin** (Indocin), **sulfonamides** (Bactrim), **and thiazide diuretics** (e.g., chlorothiazide [Diuril]) may interfere with tubular secretion of penicillin, increasing serum concentration and risk of toxicity. ▪ Risk of bleeding with **anticoagulants** (e.g., heparin) is increased. ▪ **Probenecid** decreases elimination of penicillin, resulting in prolonged half-life and increased serum levels. May be desirable or may cause toxicity. ▪ May decrease effectiveness of **oral contraceptives**; breakthrough bleeding or pregnancy could result. ▪ Concomitant use with **potassium supplements, potassium-sparing diuretics** (e.g., spironolactone [Aldactone]), **or ACE inhibitors** (e.g., enalapril [Vasotec]) may increase risk of hyperkalemia. ■ May decrease clearance and increase toxicity of **methotrexate.** ■ May cause false values in common **lab tests;** see literature.

SIDE EFFECTS
Arthralgia, chills, edema, fever, pain at the injection site, prostration, skin rash, thrombophlebitis, urticaria.
Major: Acute interstitial nephritis, anaphylaxis, convulsions, hemolytic anemia, hyperreflexia, neurotoxicity, potassium poisoning with coma, sodium-induced congestive heart failure. Hypersensitivity myocarditis (fever, eosinophilia, rash, sinus tachycardia, ST-T changes, and cardiomegaly) and CDAD can occur. Higher-than-normal doses may cause neurologic adverse effects including convulsions, especially with impaired renal function.

ANTIDOTE
For all side effects, discontinue the drug, treat hypersensitivity reactions or resuscitate as necessary, and notify the physician. Treat minor side effects symptomatically according to physician's order. Mild cases of CDAD may respond to discontinuation of the drug. Treat CDAD with fluids, electrolytes, protein supplements, and oral vancomycin (Vancocin) or metronidazole (Flagyl) as indicated. In severe cases, surgical evaluation may be indicated. Removed by hemodialysis.

PENTAMIDINE ISETHIONATE
(pen-**TAM**-ih-deen is-ah-**THIGH**-oh-nayt)

Antiprotozoal

pH 4.09 to 5.4

USUAL DOSE
Treatment of *Pneumocystis jiroveci:* 4 mg/kg of body weight once daily for 14 days. See Precautions/Monitor. Has been used up to 21 days; benefits not defined.
Pneumocystis prophylaxis: 4 mg/kg once each month. May be given every 2 weeks if indicated.
Leishmania, visceral (unlabeled): 2 to 4 mg/kg once daily for up to 15 days.
Leishmania, cutaneous (unlabeled): 2 to 4 mg/kg once or twice a week until lesions heal.
Trypanosoma gambiense (unlabeled): 4 mg/kg once daily for 10 days.

PEDIATRIC DOSE
Pneumocystis jiroveci: 4 mg/kg once daily for 12 to 14 days.
Pneumocystis prophylaxis: See Usual Dose.
Leishmania donovani: 2 to 4 mg/kg once daily for 15 days. Up to 21 days have been suggested, but risks with therapy over 14 days may be increased.
Trypanosoma gambiense: See Usual Dose.

DOSE ADJUSTMENTS
Reduced dose in renal failure may be indicated. One source recommends 4 mg/kg every 24 hours with a CrCl of 10 to 50 mL/min or 4 mg/kg every 24 to 36 hours with a CrCl less than 10 mL/min.

DILUTION
Initially dilute each 300 mg or fraction thereof in 3 to 5 mL SWFI or D5W. A single dose must be further diluted in 50 to 250 mL of D5W and given as an infusion.
Storage: Stable at room temperature for 24 hours. Discard unused portion. Protect dry product and reconstituted solution from light.

P

COMPATIBILITY

Consider any drug NOT listed as compatible to be INCOMPATIBLE until consulting a pharmacist; specific conditions may apply.

Will form a precipitate with NS; do not use for dilution or infusion. Manufacturer states, "Do not mix pentamidine solutions with any other drugs."

One source suggests the following **compatibilities:**

Y-site: Diltiazem (Cardizem), zidovudine (AZT, Retrovir).

RATE OF ADMINISTRATION

A single dose should be evenly distributed over 60 minutes.

Leishmania, visceral and cutaneous: A single dose evenly distributed over 1 to 2 hours.

ACTIONS

An antiprotozoal agent. Specifically active against *Pneumocystis jiroveci*. It is thought to interfere with nuclear metabolism and inhibit the synthesis of DNA, RNA, phospholipids, and proteins. Route of metabolism is unknown. Excreted partially in urine. May accumulate in renal failure.

INDICATIONS AND USES

Treatment and prophylaxis of *Pneumocystis jiroveci* pneumonia (PCP).

Unlabeled uses: Treatment of trypanosomiasis and visceral and cutaneous leishmaniasis. Aerosol used prophylactically to prevent PCP in high-risk patients.

CONTRAINDICATIONS

None if the diagnosis of *Pneumocystis jiroveci* pneumonia is confirmed.

PRECAUTIONS

Specific use only; establish correct diagnosis. ■ Sulfamethoxazole/trimethoprim is the drug of choice for treatment of *Pneumocystis* pneumonia. Pentamidine causes numerous and serious side effects and is indicated only if the patient does not respond to or tolerate SMZ-TMP. ■ Use extreme caution in patients with hypertension, hypotension, hypoglycemia, hyperglycemia, hypocalcemia, leukopenia, thrombocytopenia, anemia, hepatic or renal dysfunction, ventricular tachycardia, pancreatitis, and Stevens-Johnson syndrome. **Monitor:** Before, during, and after therapy obtain a BUN and SCr (daily), CBC, platelet count, alkaline phosphatase, bilirubin, AST, ALT, serum calcium, and ECG. ■ Has caused fatalities resulting from severe hypotension, hypoglycemia, and cardiac arrhythmias even with the administration of the first dose. Keep patient supine, observe continuously for any sign of adverse reaction, and monitor BP continuously during infusion and afterward until stable. ■ Emergency equipment for resuscitation must be immediately available. ■ Monitor blood glucose levels daily during therapy and several times after therapy is complete. Pancreatic necrosis and very high plasma insulin levels have occurred. May also cause hyperglycemia and diabetes mellitus.

Patient Education: May cause severe hypotension; remain lying down until BP is stable. ■ Report any unusual bleeding or bruising.

Maternal/Child: Category C: use only when clearly needed during pregnancy and breast-feeding. Hazards to fetus or infant are unknown. ■ Discontinue breast-feeding.

DRUG/LAB INTERACTIONS

Nephrotoxic effects may be additive with concomitant use with **other nephrotoxic drugs** (e.g., aminoglycosides [e.g., gentamicin], amphotericin B, cisplatin, foscarnet [Foscavir], vancomycin). Monitoring of renal function, dose reductions, and/or dose interval adjustments may be required.

SIDE EFFECTS

Occur in over 50% of patients and may be life threatening. Some occur after course of treatment is completed. Acute renal failure, anemia, anorexia, bad taste in mouth, cardiac arrhythmias including ventricular tachycardia, confusion, dizziness, elevated SCr and liver function tests, fever, hallucinations, hyperglycemia, hyperkalemia, hypocalcemia, hypoglycemia, hypotension, leukopenia, nausea, neuralgia, phlebitis, rash, thrombocytopenia.

ANTIDOTE

Discontinue drug for any life-threatening side effects. Notify physician of all side effects. Symptomatic treatment indicated. Resuscitate as necessary.

PENTOBARBITAL SODIUM
(**PEN**-toh-**bar**-bih-tal **SO**-dee-um)

Barbiturate
Sedative-hypnotic
Anticonvulsant

Nembutal Sodium

pH 9 to 10.5

USUAL DOSE
100 mg initially. Wait 1 full minute between each dose to determine drug effect. Additional doses in increments of 25 to 50 mg may be given as indicated. Maximum dosage ranges from 200 to 500 mg.

Barbiturate coma: *Loading dose:* 3 to 10 mg/kg over 30 minutes to 3 hours.
Maintenance dose: 1.5 to 2 mg/kg every 1 to 2 hours or an infusion of 0.5 to 3 mg/kg/hr. Adjust to maintain pentobarbital blood level between 110 and 177 mm/L (25 to 40 mg/dL) or ICP below 25 Torr.

PEDIATRIC DOSE
See Maternal/Child.

1 to 3 mg/kg slowly until asleep. Maximum dose 100 mg/24 hr.

Barbiturate coma: See Usual Dose. An alternate source suggests *Loading dose:* 10 to 15 mg/kg over 1 to 2 hours. *Maintenance dose:* Begin with 1 mg/kg/hr; increase to 2 to 3 mg/kg/hr to maintain EEG burst suppression.

DOSE ADJUSTMENTS
Reduce dose in impaired renal or hepatic function; usually required in the debilitated or elderly. ▪ See Drug/Lab Interactions.

DILUTION
May be given undiluted or, preferably, may be further diluted in SWFI, NS, or Ringer's injection. Any desired amount of diluent may be used. 9 mL of diluent with 1 mL of pentobarbital (50 mg) equals 5 mg/mL. Use only absolutely clear solutions.

COMPATIBILITY
Consider any drug NOT listed as compatible to be INCOMPATIBLE until consulting a pharmacist; specific conditions may apply.

Manufacturer states, "Should not be admixed with any other medication or solution." Do not mix in a syringe with pentazocine (Talwin); precipitation will occur. May precipitate in acidic solutions.

One source suggests the following **compatibilities:**

Additive: *Not recommended by manufacturer.* Amikacin, aminophylline, calcium chloride, chloramphenicol (Chloromycetin), dimenhydrinate, erythromycin (Erythrocin), lidocaine, verapamil.

Y-site: Acyclovir (Zovirax), insulin (regular), linezolid (Zyvox), propofol (Diprivan).

RATE OF ADMINISTRATION
50 mg or fraction thereof over 1 minute. Titrate slowly to desired effect. Rapid injection rate may cause symptoms of overdose (e.g., serious respiratory depression).

Barbiturate coma: See specific dose recommendations.

ACTIONS
A sedative, hypnotic barbiturate of short duration with anticonvulsant effects. Pentobarbital is a CNS depressant. Onset of action is prompt by the IV route and lasts about 3 to 4 hours. Will effectively depress the motor cortex if adequate doses are administered. Pain perception is unimpaired. Reportedly reduces cerebral blood flow and thus reduces cerebral edema and intracranial pressure. Detoxified in the liver and excreted fairly quickly in the urine in changed form. Crosses the placental barrier. Secreted in breast milk.

INDICATIONS AND USES
Preanesthetic sedation. ▪ Dental and minor surgical sedation. ▪ Control of convulsions caused by disease and drug poisoning. ▪ Short-term hypnotic. ▪ Sedation in psychotic states.

Unlabeled uses: High doses have been used to induce coma in the management of cerebral ischemia and increased intracranial pressure. Has been most effective in patients under 35 years of age or in closed head injuries.

CONTRAINDICATIONS

Acute or chronic pain, delivery (when maximum drug effect would be at the time of delivery), history of porphyria, known hypersensitivity to barbiturates, severely impaired liver function especially with any signs of hepatic coma, severe respiratory disease or respiratory depression.

PRECAUTIONS

IV route usually reserved for critical situations. ■ Use caution in status asthmaticus, shock, severe renal or liver disease, depressive states after convulsions, shock, and in the elderly. ■ Use caution in acute or chronic pain. ■ Status epilepticus can occur from too-rapid withdrawal. ■ May be habit forming. Use caution in the presence of fever, diabetes, hyperthyroidism, or severe anemia; may increase side effects. ■ Benzodiazepines (diazepam [Valium], midazolam [Versed]) generally preferred for sedation.

Monitor: Record BP, pulse, and respirations every 3 to 5 minutes. Keep patient under constant observation. ■ Maintain a patent airway. ■ Treat the cause of a convulsion. ■ Highly alkaline; determine absolute patency of vein; use of large veins preferred to prevent thrombosis. Avoid extravasation. Intra-arterial injection will cause gangrene. ■ Monitor phenytoin and barbiturate levels when both drugs are used concurrently. ■ Monitor hematopoietic, renal, and hepatic systems in extended therapy. ■ See Drug/Lab Interactions.

Patient Education: Avoid alcohol and other CNS depressants (e.g., antihistamines, diazepam [Valium]). ■ May be habit forming. ■ May require alternate birth control.

Maternal/Child: Category D: avoid pregnancy; will cause birth defects. ■ May cause drowsiness in the nursing infant. ■ See Contraindications. ■ May cause paradoxical excitement in pediatric patients.

Elderly: Often have increased sensitivity to barbiturates; may cause marked excitement, depression, confusion, and increased risk of barbiturate-induced hypothermia. ■ See Dose Adjustments and Precautions. ■ Consider age-related hepatic or renal impairment and concomitant disease or drug therapy.

DRUG/LAB INTERACTIONS

Use extreme caution if any **other CNS depressants** have been given, such as alcohol, narcotic analgesics, anesthetics, antidepressants, antihistamines, hypnotics, MAO inhibitors, phenothiazines, sedatives, aminoglycoside antibiotics, or tranquilizers; potentiation with respiratory depression may occur. ■ Inhibits effectiveness of **propranolol, corticosteroids, doxycycline, oral anticoagulants, oral contraceptives, quinidine, and theophylline.** Capable of innumerable interactions with many drugs. ■ May increase orthostatic hypotension with **furosemide** (Lasix). ■ Monitor **phenytoin** and barbiturate levels when both drugs are used concurrently. ■ May inhibit **vitamin D** metabolism with extended use.

SIDE EFFECTS

Average dose: Depression, dermatitis, facial edema, fever, hypotension, neonatal apnea, pain at or below injection site, respiratory depression (hypoventilation), thrombocytopenic purpura.

Overdose: Apnea, coma, cough reflex depression, flat EEG (reversible unless hypoxic damage has occurred), hypotension, laryngospasm, lowered body temperature, pulmonary edema, renal shutdown, respiratory depression, sluggish or absent reflexes.

ANTIDOTE

Discontinue drug immediately for pain at or below injection site. Notify the physician of any side effects. Symptomatic and supportive treatment is most important in overdose. Maintain an adequate airway with artificial ventilation if indicated. Keep the patient warm. IV volume expanders (dextran) and IV fluids will help maintain adequate circulation. Diuretics or hemodialysis will promote the elimination of the drug. Vasopressors (dopamine) will maintain BP.

PENTOSTATIN BBW
(**PEN**-toh-**stah**-tin)

2-Deoxycoformycin, Nipent

Antineoplastic
(antibiotic)

pH 7 to 8.5

USUAL DOSE
Evaluation and prehydration are required before administration; see Monitor.

4 mg/M² every other week. Do not exceed recommended dose; see Precautions. If there is no major toxicity and improvement is continuous, treat until a complete response is achieved, then administer two additional doses. Do not treat beyond 12 months.

DOSE ADJUSTMENTS
Reduced dose and benefit-versus-risk assessment may be required with impaired renal function (CrCl below 60 mL/min); insufficient data available. Two patients with impaired renal function (CrCl 50 to 60 mL/min) achieved complete response without unusual adverse events when treated with 2 mg/M². ▪ Withhold dose if SCr elevated; obtain CrCl. ▪ Withhold dose if the absolute neutrophil count falls from a baseline of greater than 500 cells/mm³ before therapy to less than 200 cells/mm³ during treatment. Resume treatment when count returns to predose levels.

DILUTION
Specific techniques required; see Precautions. Diluent (5 mL SWFI) provided; dissolve completely; will yield 2 mg/mL. May be given by IV injection or further diluted in 25 to 50 mL NS or D5W; 25 mL yields 0.33 mg/mL, 50 mL yields 0.18 mg/mL. Treat spills or waste with a 5% sodium hypochlorite solution before disposal.

Storage: Refrigerate before initial reconstitution. Store at room temperature and use within 8 hours after initial reconstitution or dilution for infusion.

COMPATIBILITY
Consider any drug NOT listed as compatible to be INCOMPATIBLE until consulting a pharmacist; specific conditions may apply.

Does not interact with PVC infusion containers or administration sets at concentrations specified for dilution.

One source suggests the following **compatibilities:**

Y-site: Melphalan (Alkeran), ondansetron (Zofran), paclitaxel (Taxol), sargramostim (Leukine). Physically **compatible** at the **Y-site** with fludarabine (Fludara); however, the two drugs are not recommended for concurrent use; see Drug/Lab Interactions.

RATE OF ADMINISTRATION
Follow each dose with an additional 500 mL of prehydration infusion fluids.

IV injection: A single dose over 1 minute.

Infusion: A single dose over 20 to 30 minutes.

ACTIONS
Mechanism of action is not known, but it is cytotoxic as a result of its potent inhibition of the enzyme adenosine deaminase (ADA). Blocks DNA and RNA synthesis and causes DNA damage. Average terminal half-life of 6 hours is extended to 18 hours in patients with impaired renal function (CrCl less than 50 mL/min). Inhibits ADA for up to 1 week; actual response may not occur for months. Primarily excreted in urine.

INDICATIONS AND USES
Single-agent treatment of both untreated patients and alpha-interferon–refractory hairy cell leukemia (HCL) patients with active disease as defined by clinically significant anemia, neutropenia, thrombocytopenia, or disease-related symptoms.

Unlabeled uses: Treatment of chronic lymphocytic leukemia, prolymphocytic leukemia, non-Hodgkin's lymphoma, cutaneous T-cell lymphoma, and peripheral T-cell lymphomas.

CONTRAINDICATIONS
Hypersensitivity to pentostatin; see Drug/Lab Interactions.

PRECAUTIONS

Follow guidelines for handling cytotoxic agents. See Appendix A, p. 1331. ▪ Assess drug profile before administration. ▪ Severe renal, liver, pulmonary, and CNS toxicities have occurred at higher doses; do not exceed recommended dose. ▪ Usually administered by or under the supervision of a physician specialist. ▪ Myelosuppression, especially neutropenia, is most severe during the first few courses of treatment. ▪ Must consider risk/benefit in patients with some bone marrow suppression, the possibility of chickenpox or herpes zoster, a history of gout or urate renal stones, renal function impairment, or previous cytotoxic drug or radiation therapy. Use extreme caution. ▪ After 6 months of treatment, assess for response; if partial or complete response is not evident, discontinue treatment. If partial response is evident, re-evaluate as indicated but do not treat beyond 12 months.

Monitor: Monitor CBC (including differential and platelet count) and SCr before each dose and as indicated. Blood chemistries, including serum uric acid, and a CrCl assay are required before and during treatment. ▪ Prehydration with 500 to 1,000 mL D5/^{1}/$_2$NS or an equivalent is required. An additional 500 mL is required postadministration. ▪ Treatment of patients with infection may exacerbate symptoms and cause death. Control infection before treatment is initiated. Withhold treatment if an active infection occurs; resume when infection is controlled. ▪ Prophylactic antiemetics recommended (e.g., prochlorperazine [Compazine], ondansetron [Zofran]); continue for 48 to 72 hours. ▪ Observe closely for severe rashes, nervous system toxicity, and myelosuppression (especially after initial cycles); pentostatin may have to be withheld or discontinued. ▪ For severe neutropenia beyond the initial cycles, evaluate for disease status, including a bone marrow examination. ▪ Assess response to treatment with periodic monitoring of peripheral blood for hairy cells. Bone marrow aspirates and biopsies may be required at 2- to 3-month intervals. ▪ Monitor for thrombocytopenia (platelet count less than 50,000/mm^3). Initiate precautions to prevent excessive bleeding (e.g., inspect IV sites, skin, and mucous membranes; use extreme care during invasive procedures; test urine, emesis, stool, and secretions for occult blood).

Patient Education: Consider birth control options; nonhormonal birth control recommended. ▪ Report rashes, symptoms of infection, or bruising and bleeding immediately. ▪ See Appendix D, p. 1333.

Maternal/Child: Category D: avoid pregnancy; can cause fetal harm. ▪ Discontinue breastfeeding. ▪ Safety for use in pediatric patients under 18 years of age not established.

Elderly: Consider decreased renal function.

DRUG/LAB INTERACTIONS

Assess drug profile before administration. ▪ Do not use with **fludarabine** (Fludara); may increase risk of fatal pulmonary toxicity. ▪ Combination therapy with **carmustine** (BiCNU), **etoposide** (VePesid), **and high-dose cyclophosphamide** as part of the ablative regimen for bone marrow transplant has caused acute pulmonary edema and hypotension. Deaths have occurred. ▪ Pentostatin enhances the effects of **vidarabine** (Ara-A). Combined use of these agents may result in an increase in adverse reactions associated with each drug. The therapeutic benefit of this drug combination has not been established. ▪ May cause skin rash with **allopurinol.** ▪ Elevates **liver function tests;** usually reversible. ▪ Do not administer **live virus vaccines** to patients receiving antineoplastic drugs. ▪ Uric acid levels may increase; increased dose of **gout agents** (e.g., colchicine, probenecid, sulfinpyrazone [Anturane]) may be indicated. ▪ Leukopenia and thrombocytopenia increased by **agents causing blood dyscrasias** (e.g., anticonvulsants [phenytoin (Dilantin)], penicillins, phenothiazines, and many others).

SIDE EFFECTS

Anemia, anorexia, chills, cough, diarrhea, fatigue, fever, GU disorders, headache, hepatic disorders/elevated liver function tests, hypersensitivity reactions, infection, leukopenia, lung disorders, myalgia, nausea, neurologic disorders/CNS, pain, rashes, skin disorders, thrombocytopenia, upper respiratory infections, and vomiting occur in 10% of patients and may require discontinuation of treatment. Abdominal pain; abnormal ECG; abnormal thinking; abnormal vision; anxiety; arthralgia; asthenia; back pain; bronchitis; cardiac arrhythmias; chest pain; confusion; conjunctivitis; constipation; depression; dizziness; dry skin; dyspnea; dysuria; ear pain; ecchymosis; eczema; elevated BUN, creatinine, and LDH; epistaxis; eye pain; flatulence; flu syndrome; hematuria; hemorrhage; herpes simplex; herpes zoster; insomnia; lung edema; lymphadenopathy; maculopapular rash; malaise; neoplasm; nervousness; paresthesia; peripheral edema; petechia; pharyngitis; pneumonia; pruritus; rhinitis; seborrhea; sinusitis; skin discoloration; somnolence; stomatitis; sweating; thrombophlebitis; vesiculobullous rash; weight loss; and death have occurred in 3% to 10% or more of patients.

ANTIDOTE

Keep physician informed of all side effects; most will be treated symptomatically if indicated. Withhold dose and notify physician for elevated SCr, absolute neutrophil count below 200 cells/mm^3, myelosuppression, infection, CNS toxicity, or severe rash. Administration of whole blood products (e.g., packed RBCs, platelets, leukocytes) and/or blood modifiers (e.g., darbepoetin alfa [Aranesp], epoetin alfa [Epogen], filgrastim [Neupogen, Zarxio], pegfilgrastim [Neulasta], sargramostim [Leukine]) may be indicated to treat bone marrow toxicity. Overdose may cause death due to severe renal, hepatic, pulmonary, or CNS toxicity. There is no specific antidote. Supportive therapy as indicated will help sustain the patient.

PERAMIVIR

(per-**AM**-i-vir)

Rapivab

Antiviral

(Influenza virus neuraminidase inhibitor)

pH 5.5 to 8.5

USUAL DOSE

Administer peramivir within 2 days of onset of symptoms of influenza.

A single dose of 600 mg administered as an IV infusion over 15 to 30 minutes.

DOSE ADJUSTMENTS

No dose adjustment is required in patients with a creatinine clearance of 50 mL/min or higher. ▪ Reduce dose in patients with a baseline creatinine clearance below 50 mL/min using the recommendations in the following chart.

| Dose Adjustment of Peramivir in Impaired Renal Function ||
Creatinine Clearance (mL/min)	Recommended Dose (mg)
≥50 mL/min	600 mg
30 to 49 mL/min	200 mg
10 to 29 mL/min	100 mg
Patients with chronic renal impairment maintained on hemodialysis	Administer after dialysis at a dose adjusted based on renal function.

▪ No dose adjustment is required based on gender, impaired hepatic function, weight, or race (was evaluated primarily in Asians and Caucasians).

DILUTION

Available in single-use vials containing 200 mg/ 20 mL (10 mg/mL) as a clear, colorless solution. Contains no preservatives. Do not use if seal over bottle opening is broken or missing. Calculate the number of vial(s) required for the recommended dose, and withdraw the required volume of peramivir and dilute by transferring into an IV bag or container of NS, $^1/_2$NS, D5W, or LR to a maximum volume of 100 mL.

Filters: No data available from manufacturer.

Storage: Before use, store in original cartons at CRT. Administer fully diluted solutions immediately or refrigerate at 2° to 8° C (36° to 46° F) for up to 24 hours. If refrigerated, allow the diluted solution to reach room temperature, then administer immediately. Discard any unused diluted solution of peramivir after 24 hours.

COMPATIBILITY

Compatible with NS, $^1/_2$NS, D5W, or LR. Also **compatible** with materials commonly used for administration such as polyvinylchloride (PVC) bags and PVC-free bags, polypropylene syringes, and polyethylene tubing. Manufacturer states, "Do not mix or co-infuse with other intravenous medications."

RATE OF ADMINISTRATION

A single dose as an infusion equally distributed over 15 to 30 minutes.

ACTIONS

Peramivir is an antiviral drug with activity against the influenza virus. It is an inhibitor of the influenza virus neuraminidase, an enzyme that releases viral particles from the plasma membrane of infected cells. The relationship between the antiviral activity in cell culture, the inhibitory activity in the neuraminidase assay, and the inhibition of influenza virus replication in humans has not been established. Maximum serum concentration is reached by the end of the infusion. In vitro binding to human plasma proteins is less than 30%. Not significantly metabolized in humans. Elimination half-life is approximately 20 hours. Primarily excreted as unchanged drug in urine.

INDICATIONS AND USES

Treatment of acute uncomplicated influenza in patients 18 years or age and older who have been symptomatic for no more than 2 days.

Limitations of use: Efficacy of peramivir is based on clinical trials of naturally occurring influenza in which the predominant influenza infections were influenza A virus; a limited number of subjects infected with influenza B virus were enrolled. ▪ Influenza viruses change over time. Emergence of resistance substitutions could decrease drug effectiveness. Other factors (e.g., changes in viral virulence) might also diminish the clinical benefit of antiviral drugs. Prescribers should consider available information on influenza drug susceptibility patterns and treatment effects when deciding whether to use peramivir. ▪ The use of peramivir was not shown to provide benefit to patients with serious influenza requiring hospitalization.

CONTRAINDICATIONS

Manufacturer states, "None."

PRECAUTIONS

Rare cases of serious skin and hypersensitivity reactions, including erythema multiforme, have been reported. ▪ Influenza can be associated with a variety of neurologic and behavioral symptoms that can include events such as abnormal behavior, delirium, and hallucinations, which in some cases result in fatal outcomes. These events may occur in the setting of encephalitis or encephalopathy but also can occur in uncomplicated influenza. Neuropsychiatric events (e.g., delirium and abnormal behavior) have been reported in patients with influenza who are receiving neuraminidase inhibitors, including peramivir. The contribution of peramivir to these events has not been established. ▪ There is no evidence for the efficacy of peramivir in any illness caused by agents other than influenza viruses. Serious bacterial infections may begin with influenza-like symptoms or may coexist with or occur as complications during the course of influenza. Peramivir has not been shown to prevent such complications. ▪ Circulating seasonal influenza strains expressing neuraminidase resistance–associated substitutions have been observed in individuals who have not received peramivir. Prescribers should consider available information from the CDC on influenza virus drug susceptibility patterns and treatment effects when deciding whether to use peramivir. ▪ Has not been studied in patients with impaired hepatic function; however, because peramivir is cleared in urine by glomerular filtration, no clinically relevant problems are expected. ▪ Cross-resistance between peramivir (Rapivab), oseltamivir (Tamiflu), and zanamivir (Relenza) was observed in neuraminidase biochemical assays and cell culture assays. The clinical impact of this reduced susceptibility is unknown.

Monitor: Monitor for serious skin reactions. Appropriate treatment should be instituted if a serious skin reaction occurs or is suspected. ▪ Monitor for potential secondary bacterial infections and treat with antibiotics as appropriate. ▪ Monitor for S/S of a hypersensitivity reaction (e.g., hypotension, rash, urticaria, tightness of the chest, wheezing). ▪ Patients with influenza should be closely monitored for signs of abnormal behavior.

Patient Education: There is a risk of serious skin reactions. Seek immediate medical attention if a skin reaction occurs. ▪ There is a risk of neuropsychiatric events in patients with influenza. Patients should contact their physician if they experience signs of abnormal behavior after receiving peramivir. ▪ Promptly report S/S of a hypersensitivity reaction (e.g., hives, rash, shortness of breath, wheezing).

Maternal/Child: Category C: use during pregnancy only if clearly needed. ▪ It is not known whether peramivir is excreted in human milk; use caution during breast-feeding. ▪ Safety and effectiveness in pediatric patients under 18 years of age have not been established. ▪ In a single-arm trial conducted in Japan, pediatric patients with uncomplicated influenza (28 days to 16 years of age) were treated with a single dose of peramivir 10 mg/kg. The most common clinical and laboratory adverse events included decreased neutrophil count, diarrhea, and vomiting.

Elderly: Numbers in clinical studies were insufficient to determine if elderly patients respond differently than do younger subjects.

DRUG/LAB INTERACTIONS

The concurrent use of peramivir with **live attenuated influenza vaccine** (LAIV) intranasal has not been evaluated. Because of the potential for interference between these two products, avoid the use of LAIV within 2 weeks before or 48 hours after administration of peramivir unless medically indicated. For LAIV, antiviral drugs may inhibit viral replication and may reduce vaccine efficacy. ▪ Inactivated influenza vaccine can be administered at any time. ▪ Not a substrate for CYP enzymes, does not affect glucuronidation, and is not a substrate or inhibitor of P-glycoprotein–mediated transport. ▪ No evidence of drug-drug interactions when peramivir was administered with oral rimantadine (Flumadine), oral oseltamivir (Tamiflu), or oral contraceptives containing ethinyl estradiol and levonorgestrel or when peramivir IM was administered with oral probenecid.

SIDE EFFECTS

The most common adverse reaction is diarrhea. Serious skin and hypersensitivity reactions and neuropsychiatric events have occurred. Constipation; decreased neutrophils; hypertension; increased ALT, AST, creatine phosphokinase, and serum glucose; and insomnia were also reported.

Post-Marketing: Abnormal behavior, exfoliative dermatitis, hallucination, rash, and Stevens-Johnson syndrome.

ANTIDOTE

Notify physician of any side effects. Discontinue the drug if indicated. Treat overdose with general supportive measures, including monitoring of vital signs and observation of the clinical status of the patient. There is no specific antidote. Treat hypersensitivity reactions as indicated (e.g., diphenhydramine [Benadryl], epinephrine [Adrenalin], albuterol) and resuscitate as necessary. Removed by hemodialysis.

PERTUZUMAB BBW
(per-**TOOZ**-ue-mab)

Perjeta

Recombinant monoclonal antibody
Antineoplastic

pH 6

USUAL DOSE
Preassessment is required; see Monitor. Pertuzumab is given in combination with trastuzumab (Herceptin) and docetaxel (Taxotere). See docetaxel and trastuzumab monographs; preassessment and premedication indicated. Pertuzumab, trastuzumab, and docetaxel should be administered sequentially. Pertuzumab and trastuzumab can be given in any order. Docetaxel should be administered after pertuzumab and trastuzumab infusions are complete. An observation period of 30 to 60 minutes is recommended after each pertuzumab infusion and before beginning any subsequent infusion of trastuzumab or docetaxel.

METASTATIC BREAST CANCER (MBC)
Initial doses: *Pertuzumab:* 840 mg as an infusion over 60 minutes; see Monitor; preassessment required.
Trastuzumub: 8 mg/kg as an infusion over 90 minutes.
Docetaxel: 75 mg/M^2 as an infusion over 60 minutes.
Subsequent doses: Begin 3 weeks after initial doses.
Pertuzumab: 420 mg administered as an infusion over 30 to 60 minutes and repeated every 3 weeks.
Trastuzumub: 6 mg/kg as an infusion over 30 to 90 minutes and repeated every 3 weeks.
Docetaxel: If the initial dose is well tolerated, the dose may be escalated to 100 mg/M^2 and repeated every 3 weeks.

NEOADJUVANT TREATMENT OF BREAST CANCER
Administer pertuzumab every 3 weeks for 3 to 6 cycles as part of one of the following treatment regimens for early breast cancer. *Actual initial and subsequent doses of pertuzumab, trastuzumab, and docetaxel are the same as above in MBC.* Note all comments under Usual Dose.
* Four preoperative cycles of pertuzumab in combination with trastuzumab and docetaxel followed by 3 postoperative cycles of fluorouracil, epirubicin, and cyclophosphamide (FEC).
* Three preoperative cycles of FEC alone followed by 3 preoperative cycles of pertuzumab in combination with docetaxel and trastuzumab.
* Six preoperative cycles of pertuzumab in combination with docetaxel, carboplatin, and trastuzumab (TCH) (escalation of docetaxel above 75 mg/M^2 is not recommended).
Following surgery, patients should continue to receive trastuzumab to complete 1 year of treatment.

DOSE ADJUSTMENTS
If a dose is delayed or missed and the time between two infusions is less than 6 weeks, administer the 420-mg dose. Do not wait until the next planned dose. ■ If the time between two infusions is 6 weeks or more, readminister the initial dose of 840 mg and follow with the subsequent dose regimen of 420 mg beginning in 3 weeks. ■ Discontinue immediately for a serious hypersensitivity reaction. ■ Withhold pertuzumab and trastuzumab for at least 3 weeks if there is a drop in left ventricular ejection fraction (LVEF) to less than 45% or a LVEF of 45% to 49% with a 10% or greater absolute decrease below pretreatment values, and reassess LVEF in 3 weeks. Pertuzumab may be resumed if the LVEF recovers to greater than 49%, or if it recovers to between 45% and 49% if associated with less than a 10% absolute decrease below pretreatment values. If after a repeat assessment within approximately 3 weeks the LVEF has not improved or has declined further, pertuzumab and trastuzumab should be discontinued unless benefits

outweigh risks for the individual patient. ▪ Pertuzumab should be discontinued if trastuzumab treatment is discontinued. ▪ Dose reductions are not recommended for pertuzumab. ▪ See docetaxel monograph for docetaxel dose adjustments. ▪ No dose adjustment is indicated in patients with mild or moderate renal impairment. In patients with severe renal impairment (CrCl less than 30 mL/min), no dose adjustments can be recommended because of the limited pharmacokinetic data available. ▪ See Rate of Administration, Precautions, Monitor, and Antidote.

DILUTION

Withdraw the calculated dose of pertuzumab from the vial(s) and inject into a 250-mL PVC or non-PVC polyolefin infusion bag of NS. Invert diluted solution gently to mix. **Do not shake.** Dilute only with NS. Do not use D5W. Immediate use is preferred.

Filters: Not required by manufacturer; additional data not available.

Storage: Store vials in carton in refrigerator at 2° to 8° C (36° to 46° F). Do not freeze. Do not shake. Protect from light. Immediate use preferred; if the diluted solution is not used immediately, however, it can be refrigerated for 24 hours.

COMPATIBILITY

Manufacturer states, "Do not mix pertuzumab with other drugs" and lists as **incompatible** with D5W.

RATE OF ADMINISTRATION

For IV infusion only; do not administer as an IV push or IV bolus. The rate of infusion may be slowed or interrupted if the patient develops an infusion-associated reaction. Discontinue immediately for a serious hypersensitivity reaction.

Pertuzumab: Administer the *initial dose* over 60 minutes. Administer *subsequent doses* over 30 to 60 minutes. An observation period of 30 to 60 minutes is recommended after each pertuzumab infusion and before beginning any subsequent infusion of trastuzumab or docetaxel.

Trastuzumab: Administer the *initial dose* over 90 minutes. Administer *subsequent doses* over 30 to 90 minutes. May be administered before or after pertuzumab.

Docetaxel: Each dose equally distributed over 60 minutes. Administer after pertuzumab and trastuzumab infusions have been completed.

ACTIONS

A recombinant humanized monoclonal antibody. It targets the human epidermal growth factor receptor 2 protein (HER2) and blocks ligand-dependent heterodimerization of HER2 with other HER family members, including EGFR, HER3, and HER4. By inhibiting specific pathways, cell growth arrest and apoptosis can occur. Pertuzumab also mediates antibody-dependent, cell-mediated cytotoxicity. Using pertuzumab alone inhibits the proliferation of human tumor cells, whereas the combination of pertuzumab and trastuzumab greatly augments antitumor activity in HER2-overexpressing xenograft models. Steady-state concentration can be reached after the first maintenance dose.

INDICATIONS AND USES

Pertuzumab in combination with trastuzumab and docetaxel is indicated for the treatment of patients with HER2-positive metastatic breast cancer who have not received prior anti-HER2 therapy or chemotherapy for metastatic disease. ▪ Pertuzumab in combination with trastuzumab and docetaxel is indicated for the neoadjuvant treatment of patients with HER2-positive, locally advanced, inflammatory, or early-stage breast cancer (either greater than 2 cm in diameter or node positive) as part of a complete treatment regimen for early breast cancer. This indication is based on demonstration of an improvement in pathologic complete response rate. Data demonstrating improvement in event-free survival or overall survival is not available.

Limitations of use: The safety of pertuzumab as part of a doxorubicin-containing regimen has not been established. ▪ The safety of pertuzumab administered for more than 6 cycles for early breast cancer has not been established.

CONTRAINDICATIONS

Known hypersensitivity to pertuzumab or to any of its excipients.

P

PRECAUTIONS

For IV infusion only; do not administer as an IV push or IV bolus. ▪ Assess HER2 status before beginning pertuzumab therapy. Testing should be done by a laboratory with demonstrated proficiency in the testing process using FDA-approved tests. In clinical studies, the only patients who have received benefit from pertuzumab therapy are those with HER2 protein overexpression. ▪ Can cause fetal harm when administered to pregnant women; see Patient Education and Maternal/Child. ▪ Administered by or under the direction of a physician specialist. ▪ Adequate laboratory and supportive medical resources must be available. ▪ Emergency equipment and drugs for treatment of left ventricular dysfunction and/or hypersensitivity or infusion reactions must be immediately available; see Antidote. ▪ Can result in subclinical and clinical cardiac failure. Evaluate left ventricular function in all patients before and during treatment with pertuzumab. Decreases in LVEF with drugs that block HER2 activity, including pertuzumab, have been reported. Patients who have received prior anthracyclines or radiotherapy to the chest wall may be at higher risk for decreased LVEF. ▪ Hypersensitivity reactions, including anaphylaxis, and infusion reactions have occurred. ▪ Trastuzumab and docetaxel also have extensive precautions and monitoring requirements; a review of their monographs is imperative. ▪ Effects on patients with severe renal impairment and/or hepatic impairment have not been studied. ▪ A protein substance; has the potential for immunogenicity.

Monitor: Verify pregnancy status before beginning pertuzumab therapy ▪ Assess LVEF before beginning therapy and at regular intervals during treatment (e.g., every 3 months in the metastatic setting and every 6 weeks in the neoadjuvant setting) to verify that it remains within expected parameters; see Dose Adjustments. ▪ Monitor for S/S of a hypersensitivity reaction (e.g., chest pain, chills, dizziness, dyspnea, fever, flushing, hypotension, nausea, pruritus, rash, urticaria) or infusion reaction (e.g., asthenia, chills, dysgeusia, fatigue, fever, headache, myalgia, vomiting). Observe closely for 60 minutes after the first infusion and for at least 30 minutes after subsequent infusions. ▪ Trastuzumab and docetaxel have additional monitoring requirements.

Patient Education: Avoid pregnancy; effective contraception required while receiving therapy and for 7 months following the last dose. ▪ During infusion, promptly report chills and/or fever and other S/S of an infusion or hypersensitivity reaction (e.g., chest pain, dizziness, feeling faint, flushing, hives, itching, nausea, pruritus, rash, shortness of breath). ▪ Promptly report new onset or worsening of shortness of breath, cough, swelling of ankles/legs, swelling of the face, palpitations, weight gain of more than 5 pounds in 24 hours, dizziness, or loss of consciousness. ▪ Report a suspected pregnancy immediately. If a pregnancy occurs during therapy, if pertuzumab is administered during a pregnancy, or if pregnancy occurs within 7 months of the last dose of pertuzumab, report exposure immediately to the Genentech Adverse Event Line. ▪ See Appendix D, p. 1333.

Maternal/Child: Category D: avoid pregnancy; may cause fetal harm. Exposure can result in embryo-fetal death and birth defects. Studies in animals have resulted in oligohydramnios, delayed renal development, and embryo-fetal deaths; see Patient Education. ▪ Encourage patients who are exposed during pregnancy or who become pregnant within 7 months after the last dose of pertuzumab to enroll in the MotHER Pregnancy Registry. ▪ Discontinue breastfeeding. ▪ Safety and effectiveness for use in pediatric patients not established.

Elderly: No differences in safety and effectiveness noted compared with younger adults.

DRUG/LAB INTERACTIONS

No formal drug interaction studies have been done. ▪ No drug-to-drug interactions observed between pertuzumab and trastuzumab or between pertuzumab and docetaxel.

SIDE EFFECTS

The most common side effects when pertuzumab was administered in combination with trastuzumab and docetaxel were alopecia, diarrhea, fatigue, nausea, neutropenia, peripheral neuropathy, and rash. Anemia, thrombocytopenia, and vomiting were reported when carboplatin was added to the regimen. The most common Grade 3 and 4 adverse reactions were anemia, asthenia, diarrhea, fatigue, febrile neutropenia, leukopenia, neutropenia, and peripheral neuropathy. Adverse events occurring in 10% or more of patients treated with pertuzumab include arthralgia, constipation, decreased appetite, dizziness, dry skin, dysgeusia, dyspnea, headache, increased lacrimation, insomnia, itching, mucosal inflammation, myalgia, nail disorders, nasopharyngitis, stomatitis, upper respiratory tract infections, and vomiting. Clinically relevant adverse events reported in fewer than 10% of patients include left ventricular dysfunction (including symptomatic left ventricular systolic dysfunction), hypersensitivity and/or infusion reactions, paronychia, and pleural effusion. Adverse reactions were reported less frequently after discontinuation of docetaxel treatment.

ANTIDOTE

Notify physician of all side effects. Most will be treated symptomatically. If signs of an infusion reaction occur, slow or interrupt the infusion and treat appropriately. Monitor patients carefully until symptoms resolve. Discontinue immediately for a serious hypersensitivity reaction. Discontinue pertuzumab for a confirmed clinically significant decrease in left ventricular function. If treatment with pertuzumab and trastuzumab has been withheld because of a drop in LVEF and if LVEF has not improved or has declined further after a repeat assessment within approximately 3 weeks, pertuzumab and trastuzumab should be discontinued unless benefits outweigh risks for the individual patient. Administration of whole blood products (e.g., packed RBCs, platelets, leukocytes) and/or blood modifiers (e.g., darbepoetin alfa [Aranesp], epoetin alfa [Epogen], filgrastim [Neupogen, Zarxio], pegfilgrastim [Neulasta], sargramostim [Leukine]) may be indicated to treat bone marrow toxicity from concurrent antineoplastics. Treat hypersensitivity reactions with epinephrine, antihistamines, corticosteroids, bronchodilators, and oxygen. Resuscitate as indicated.

PHENOBARBITAL SODIUM
(fee-no-**BAR**-bih-tal **SO**-dee-um)

Barbiturate
Sedative-hypnotic
Anticonvulsant

Luminal Sodium

pH 8.5 to 10.5

USUAL DOSE

Use only enough medication to achieve the desired effect. May take up to 15 minutes to reach peak levels in the brain; guard against overdose and excessive respiratory depression.

Hypnotic: 100 to 325 mg.

Sedative: 30 to 120 mg/day in 2 or 3 divided doses (15 to 60 mg every 12 hours or 10 to 40 mg every 8 hours).

Anticonvulsant: 200 to 320 mg. May be repeated if necessary. Maximum dose usually does not exceed 600 mg.

Status epilepticus: *Loading dose:* 10 to 20 mg/kg in single or divided doses. May give an additional 5 mg/kg every 15 to 30 minutes up to a maximum dose of 30 mg/kg.

Maintenance dose: 1 to 3 mg/kg/24 hr or 0.5 to 1.5 mg/kg every 12 hours.

PEDIATRIC DOSE

See comments under Usual Dose.

Preoperative sedation: 1 to 3 mg/kg of body weight 60 to 90 minutes before procedure.

Status epilepticus: *Loading dose:* 15 to 18 mg/kg as a single dose or in divided doses. May give an additional 5 mg/kg every 15 to 30 minutes up to a maximum total dose of 30 mg/kg.

Maintenance dose: Infants: 2.5 to 3 mg/kg every 12 hours.

Ages 1 to 5: 3 to 4 mg/kg every 12 hours.

Ages 6 to 12: 2 to 3 mg/kg every 12 hours.

Over 12 years of age: 0.5 to 1.5 mg/kg every 12 hours. Up to 12 mg/kg/24 hours has been used in maintenance doses. *Continued*

NEONATAL DOSE
See comments under Usual Dose.

Status epilepticus: *Loading dose:* 15 to 20 mg/kg as a single dose or in divided doses. ***Maintenance dose:*** 1.5 to 2 mg/kg every 12 hours; may be increased to 2.5 mg/kg every 12 hours if needed. Therapeutic range is 15 to 40 mg/L. Because of its long half-life, it may take 2 to 3 weeks to reach steady-state levels.

DOSE ADJUSTMENTS
Reduce dose in impaired renal or hepatic function; usually required in the debilitated or elderly. ▪ See Drug/Lab Interactions.

DILUTION
Sterile powder must be slowly diluted with SWFI. Use a minimum of 3 mL of diluent. Also available in sterile vials and tubexes. Best if further diluted up to 10 mL with SWFI. Solutions from powder form must be freshly prepared. Use only absolutely clear solutions. Discard powder or solution exposed to air for 30 minutes.

COMPATIBILITY
(Underline Indicates Conflicting Compatibility Information)

Consider any drug NOT listed as compatible to be INCOMPATIBLE until consulting a pharmacist; specific conditions may apply.

One source suggests the following **compatibilities:**

Additive: Amikacin, aminophylline, calcium chloride, calcium gluconate, colistimethate (Coly-Mycin M), dimenhydrinate, meropenem (Merrem IV), verapamil.

Y-site: Doripenem (Doribax), doxapram (Dopram), enalaprilat (Vasotec IV), fentanyl, fosphenytoin (Cerebyx), hydromorphone (Dilaudid), levofloxacin (Levaquin), linezolid (Zyvox), meropenem (Merrem IV), methadone (Dolophine), morphine, propofol (Diprivan).

RATE OF ADMINISTRATION
60 mg (gr 1) or fraction thereof over 1 minute. Titrate slowly to desired effect. Rapid injection rate may cause symptoms of overdose (e.g., serious respiratory depression).

Status epilepticus: A single loading dose over 10 to 15 minutes.

ACTIONS
A sedative, hypnotic barbiturate of long duration with potent anticonvulsant effects. Phenobarbital is a CNS depressant. Onset of action is prompt by the IV route and becomes rapidly more intense. Effects last from 6 to 10 hours. Will effectively depress the motor cortex with small doses. Pain perception is unimpaired. Rapidly absorbed by all body tissues and excreted in changed form in the urine. Excreted more readily in alkaline urine. Crosses the placental barrier. Secreted in breast milk.

INDICATIONS AND USES
Prolonged sedation (medical and psychiatric). ▪ Anticonvulsant.

CONTRAINDICATIONS
History of porphyria, impaired renal function, impaired hepatic function especially with any signs of hepatic coma, known hypersensitivity to barbiturates, previous addiction, severe respiratory depression including dyspnea, obstruction, or cor pulmonale.

PRECAUTIONS
IV route usually reserved for critical situations. ▪ Use caution in elderly and debilitated patients and those with asthma, pulmonary disease, shock, and impaired renal or hepatic function. ▪ Status epilepticus can occur from too-rapid withdrawal. ▪ May be habit forming. Use caution in acute or chronic pain. ▪ Benzodiazepines (diazepam [Valium], midazolam [Versed]) generally preferred for sedation.

Monitor: Keep patient under constant observation. Record vital signs every hour, or more often if indicated. ▪ Maintain a patent airway. ▪ Monitor hematopoietic, renal and hepatic systems in any extended therapy. ▪ Treat the cause of a convulsion. ▪ Keep equipment for artificial ventilation available. ▪ Highly alkaline. Determine absolute patency of vein; use of large veins preferred to prevent thrombosis. Avoid extravasation. Intra-arterial injection will cause gangrene. ▪ Monitor serum levels as indicated; the therapeutic range in adults is 20 to 40 mcg/mL (15 to 40 mcg/mL in pediatric patients). Because of its long half-life, it may take 2 to 3 weeks to reach steady-state levels. ▪ See Drug/Lab Interactions.

Patient Education: Avoid alcohol or other CNS depressants (e.g., antihistamines, diazepam [Valium]). May be habit forming. ▪ May require alternate birth control.

Maternal/Child: Category D: avoid pregnancy; will cause birth defects. ▪ May cause drowsiness in the nursing infant. ▪ See Precautions.

Elderly: See Dose Adjustments and Precautions. ▪ Often have increased sensitivity to barbiturates; may cause marked excitement, depression, confusion, and increased risk of barbiturate-induced hypothermia. ▪ Consider age-related hepatic or renal impairment and concomitant disease or drug therapy.

DRUG/LAB INTERACTIONS
Use extreme caution if any other **CNS depressants** have been given, such as alcohol, aminoglycoside antibiotics, narcotic analgesics, anesthetics, antidepressants, antihistamines, hypnotics, MAO inhibitors, phenothiazines, sedatives, tranquilizers. Potentiation with respiratory depression may occur. ▪ Inhibits effectiveness of **corticosteroids, doxycycline, oral anticoagulants, oral contraceptives, propranolol, quinidine, and theophylline.** Capable of innumerable interactions with many drugs. ▪ May increase orthostatic hypotension with **furosemide** (Lasix). ▪ Monitor **phenytoin** (Dilantin), **felbamate** (Felbatol), **carbamazepine** (Tegretol), **valproic acid and phenobarbital** levels when any combination of these drugs is used concurrently. ▪ May decrease the pharmacologic effect of **vitamin D.** ▪ May decrease plasma concentrations and effectiveness of **triazole antifungals** (e.g., itraconazole [Sporanox]).

SIDE EFFECTS
Rarely occur with slow injection of average doses.

Average dose: Depression, dermatitis, facial edema, fever, headache, hypotension, nausea, neonatal apnea, respiratory depression (hypoventilation), thrombocytopenic purpura, vertigo.

Overdose: Apnea, coma, cough reflex depression, delirium, flat EEG (reversible unless hypoxic damage has occurred), hypotension, laryngospasm, lowered body temperature, pulmonary edema, renal shutdown, respiratory depression, sluggish or absent reflexes, stupor.

ANTIDOTE
Notify the physician of any side effects. Symptomatic and supportive treatment is most important in overdose. Maintain an adequate airway with artificial ventilation if indicated. Keep the patient warm. IV volume expanders (dextran) and other IV fluids will help maintain adequate circulation. Diuretics may promote the elimination of the drug. Vasopressors (e.g., dopamine) will maintain BP.

P

PHENYLEPHRINE HYDROCHLORIDE BBW

(fen-ill-**EF**-rin hy-droh-**KLOR**-eyed)

Vasopressor

Neo-Synephrine, Vazculep

pH 3 to 6.5

USUAL DOSE

Perioperative setting: *Bolus:* 40 to 100 mcg by IV bolus administration. May repeat every 1 to 2 minutes as needed, not to exceed a total dose of 200 mcg.

A second manufacturer lists an initial bolus of 50 to 100 mcg with a range of 50 to 250 mcg.

Continuous infusion: If BP is below target goal, begin a continuous infusion of 10 to 35 mcg/min, not to exceed 200 mcg/min.

A second manufacturer lists a rate of 0.5 to 1.4 mcg/kg/min. Titrate to blood pressure goal.

Septic or other vasodilatory shock *(no longer recommended for routine use for this indication):* Do not administer a bolus. Begin with a continuous infusion of 0.5 to 6 mcg/kg/min. Titrate to blood pressure goal. Doses above 6 mcg/kg/min do not show a significant incremental increase in blood pressure.

Another source recommends:

Begin infusion at 100 to 180 mcg/min (0.1 to 0.18 mg/min) until BP is stabilized at a low normal for specific individual. Maintain with 40 to 60 mcg/min (0.04 to 0.06 mg/min). Titrate to desired effect.

DOSE ADJUSTMENTS

Patients with liver cirrhosis (Child-Pugh Class B and Class C) may have decreased responsiveness to phenylephrine. Higher-end doses may be required to achieve BP goal. ■ Patients with end-stage renal disease may have increased responsiveness to phenylephrine. Initiate dosing at lower end of dosing range.

DILUTION

IV bolus: Dilute 10 mg (1 mL of a 10 mg/mL solution) with 99 mL of NS or D5W to provide a final concentration of 100 mcg/mL. Withdraw an appropriate dose from this solution prior to bolus administration.

Infusion: Dilute 10 mg in 500 mL of NS or D5W to provide a final concentration of 20 mcg/mL.

Storage: Store unopened vials at CRT in carton. Protect from light. Diluted solution should not be held for more than 4 hours at RT or for more than 24 hours under refrigeration. Discard any unused portion.

COMPATIBILITY

(Underline Indicates Conflicting Compatibility Information)

Consider any drug NOT listed as compatible to be INCOMPATIBLE until consulting a pharmacist; specific conditions may apply.

One source suggests the following **compatibilities:**

Additive: Chloramphenicol (Chloromycetin), dobutamine, lidocaine, potassium chloride (KCl), sodium bicarbonate.

Y-site: Amiodarone (Nexterone), anidulafungin (Eraxis), argatroban, bivalirudin (Angiomax), caspofungin (Cancidas), cisatracurium (Nimbex), dexmedetomidine (Precedex), doripenem (Doribax), etomidate (Amidate), famotidine (Pepcid IV), fenoldopam (Corlopam), hetastarch in electrolytes (Hextend), levofloxacin (Levaquin), micafungin (Mycamine), propofol (Diprivan), remifentanil (Ultiva), telavancin (Vibativ), vasopressin, zidovudine (AZT, Retrovir).

RATE OF ADMINISTRATION

IV injection: Administer by slow injection.

Infusion: See Usual Dose. Titrate to maintain individual's low-normal BP. Use an infusion pump or microdrip (60 gtt/mL) to administer. Central line preferred.

ACTIONS

An alpha-1 adrenergic receptor agonist. Interacts with the receptors on the vascular smooth muscle cells, resulting in vasoconstriction. Increases in systolic blood pressure, diastolic blood pressure, mean arterial blood pressure, and total peripheral vascular resistance are observed within minutes of administration. As blood pressure increases, vagal activity also increases, resulting in a reflex bradycardia. Active on most vascular beds, including renal, pulmonary, and splanchnic arteries. Duration of effect is 15 to 20 minutes. Terminal half-life is 2.5 hours. Metabolized primarily by monoamine oxidase and sulfotransferase. Excreted in urine, primarily as inactive metabolites.

INDICATIONS AND USES

Treatment of clinically important hypotension resulting primarily from vasodilation in settings such as septic shock or anesthesia. *(No longer recommended for routine use in treatment of hypotension related to septic shock.)*

CONTRAINDICATIONS

Hypersensitivity to phenylephrine or any of its components.

PRECAUTIONS

Usually administered by or under the supervision of a physician knowledgeable in its use. ■ Intravascular volume depletion should be corrected. ■ Correct acidosis. Acidosis may reduce effectiveness of phenylephrine. ■ Because of its pressor effects, phenylephrine can precipitate angina in patients with severe arteriosclerosis or history of angina, exacerbate underlying heart failure, and increase pulmonary arterial pressure. ■ Avoid extravasation. Can cause necrosis or sloughing of tissue. ■ Can cause peripheral and visceral vasoconstriction and ischemia to vital organs, particularly in patients with extensive peripheral vascular disease. ■ Can cause severe bradycardia and decreased cardiac output. ■ Can increase the need for renal replacement therapy in patients with septic shock. ■ The pressor response to adrenergic drugs, including phenylephrine, can be increased in patients with autonomic dysfunction, such as may occur with spinal cord injuries. ■ Contains bisulfites; use caution in allergic individuals. ■ See Drug/Lab Interactions.

Monitor: Monitor vital signs. ■ Check infusion site for free flow. Discontinue IV administration if vein infiltrates or is thrombosed. ■ Monitor renal function. ■ See Precautions, Drug/Lab Interactions.

Maternal/Child: Category C: safety for use in pregnancy or breast-feeding not established. ■ Safety and effectiveness for use in pediatric patients not established.

Elderly: See Precautions; may have increased sensitivity to effects.

DRUG/LAB INTERACTIONS

Oxytocic drugs (e.g., oxytocin) potentiate the increasing blood pressure effects of sympathomimetic pressor amines, including phenylephrine, with the potential for hemorrhagic stroke. ■ The pressor effect of phenylephrine is also increased in patients receiving **MAO inhibitors** (e.g., selegiline [Eldepryl]), **tricyclic antidepressants** (e.g., desipramine [Norpramin]), **angiotensin, aldosterone, atropine, steroids** (e.g., hydrocortisone), **norepinephrine transporter inhibitors** (e.g., atomoxetine), **ergot alkaloids** (e.g., methylergonovine maleate [Methergine]). ■ The pressor effect of phenylephrine is decreased in patients receiving **alpha-adrenergic antagonists** (e.g., doxazosin [Cardura], prazosin [Minipress]), **phosphodiesterase type 5 inhibitors** (e.g., sildenafil [Viagra]), **mixed alpha- and beta-receptor antagonists** (e.g., labetalol [Trandate], carvedilol [Coreg]), **calcium channel blockers** (e.g., diltiazem [Cardizem], nifedipine [Procardia]), **benzodiazepines** (e.g., diazepam [Valium], midazolam [Versed]), **ACE inhibitors** (e.g., enalapril [Vasotec], lisinopril [Zestril, Prinivil]), **centrally acting sympatholytic agents** (e.g., reserpine, guanfacine [Intuniv]).

SIDE EFFECTS

The most common side effects are headache, nausea, and vomiting. Other reported side effects include arrhythmias, blurred vision, chest pain, diaphoresis, dyspnea, epigastric pain, extravasation, fullness of head, hypersensitivity (sulfite sensitivity), hypertension, hypertensive crisis, ischemia, lower cardiac output, neck pain, nervousness, paresthesia, pruritus, pulmonary edema, rales, reflexive bradycardia, skin blanching, skin necrosis with extravasation, and tremor.

ANTIDOTE

To prevent sloughing and necrosis in areas of extravasation, with a fine hypodermic needle inject 5 to 10 mg of phentolamine (Regitine) diluted in 10 to 15 mL of NS liberally throughout the tissue in the extravasated area. Treatment should be started as soon as extravasation is recognized. Notify the physician of all side effects. IM injection may be preferable. Treat hypertension with phentolamine (Regitine). Treat cardiac arrhythmias as indicated. Treat bradycardia with atropine. Resuscitate as necessary.

PHENYTOIN SODIUM BBW

(**FEN**-ih-toyn **SO**-dee-um)

Dilantin

Hydantoin

Anticonvulsant

pH 12

USUAL DOSE

In all situations, transfer to oral therapy 12 to 24 hours after a loading dose or as soon as practical. See Precautions and Monitor.

Status epilepticus, anticonvulsant: A *loading dose* of 10 to 15 mg/kg. Do not exceed a total dose of 1.5 Gm. Lethal dose estimated at 2 to 5 Gm. Another source suggests that 15 to 20 mg/kg is generally recommended. Follow with **maintenance doses** of 100 mg every 6 to 8 hours. Adjust dose based on phenytoin levels; see Monitor. Other measures, including concomitant administration of an IV benzodiazepine (such as diazepam) or an IV short-acting barbiturate, will usually be necessary for rapid control of seizures because of the required slow rate of administration of phenytoin. If seizure is not terminated, consider other anticonvulsants, barbiturates, or anesthesia.

PEDIATRIC DOSE

Status epilepticus, anticonvulsant: 15 to 20 mg/kg as a *loading dose.* Follow with a *maintenance dose for age* (listed below):

Neonates: Begin with 5 mg/kg/24 hr in equally divided doses every 12 hours. Range is 5 to 8 mg/kg/24 hr (2.5 to 4 mg/kg every 12 hours).

Infants and other pediatric patients: Begin with 5 mg/kg/24 hr in equally divided doses every 8 to 12 hours (2.5 mg/kg every 12 hours or 1.67 mg/kg every 8 hours). Range varies according to age:

6 months to 3 years: 8 to 10 mg/kg/24 hr (4 to 5 mg/kg every 12 hours or 2.67 to 3.33 mg/kg every 8 hours).

4 to 6 years: 7.5 to 9 mg/kg/24 hr (3.75 to 4.5 mg/kg every 12 hours or 2.5 to 3 mg/kg every 8 hours).

7 to 9 years: 7 to 8 mg/kg/24 hr (3.5 to 4 mg/kg every 12 hours or 2.3 to 2.6 mg/kg every 8 hours).

10 to 16 years: 6 to 7 mg/kg/24 hr (3 to 3.5 mg/kg every 12 hours or 2 to 2.3 mg/kg every 8 hours).

DOSE ADJUSTMENTS

Use caution, lower dose, and slower rate of administration in the seriously ill, elderly, and cachectic patients. ▪ Lower doses may also be required in patients with renal or hepatic disease or in those with hypoalbuminemia. Monitoring of unbound (free) phenytoin concentrations may be a better dosing guide. ▪ See Drug/Lab Interactions.

DILUTION

Available in 100- or 250-mg ampules or vials and in 100-mg syringes. After verifying patency, may be administered directly into a large peripheral or central vein through a large-gauge catheter. Alternately, may be further diluted in NS to a concentration of no less than 5 mg/mL and administered as an infusion. Use solution only when completely dissolved and clear.

Filters: Manufacturer recommends use of an in-line filter (0.22 to 0.55 microns) when administered as an infusion.

Storage: Store between 15° and 30° C. Infusion solutions should be administered immediately after preparation and must be completed within 1 to 4 hours. Do not refrigerate infusion solutions.

COMPATIBILITY

Consider any drug NOT listed as compatible to be INCOMPATIBLE until consulting a pharmacist; specific conditions may apply.

Manufacturer recommends not adding to IV solutions other than NS or mixing with other medications and states that "the addition of phenytoin to dextrose or dextrose-containing solutions will result in precipitation." Always flush line with NS before and after administration of any other drug through the same IV line. See Dilution.

One source suggests the following **compatibilities:**

Additive: *Not recommended by manufacturer.* Verapamil.

Y-site: Esmolol (Brevibloc), famotidine (Pepcid IV), fluconazole (Diflucan), tacrolimus (Prograf).

RATE OF ADMINISTRATION

Because of the risk of local toxicity, IV phenytoin should be administered directly into a large peripheral or central vein through a large-gauge catheter. Before administration, the patency of the IV should be tested with a sterile saline flush. Follow the administration of phenytoin with a saline flush to avoid local venous irritation due to the alkalinity of the solution.

Adults: Administer slowly at a rate of 25 to 50 mg or fraction thereof over 1 minute. Do not exceed 50 mg/min.

Pediatric patients: Do not exceed 1 to 3 mg/kg/min. Another source suggests 0.5 mg/kg/min in neonates or 1 mg/kg/min in infants and other pediatric patients not to exceed 50 mg/min.

Elderly: Limit rate to 25 mg/min.

Infusion: Should be completed within 1 to 4 hours. Do not exceed 25 to 50 mg/min rate. Best if piggybacked to a **compatible** primary IV so phenytoin can be discontinued if side effects occur, but IV can be kept open.

ACTIONS

A synthetic anticonvulsant, chemically related to barbiturates. Selectively stabilizes seizure threshold and depresses seizure activity in the motor cortex. Mechanism of action may be due to increasing efflux or decreasing influx of sodium ions across the cell membrane during generation of the action potential. Phenytoin reduces the maximum activity of the brain stem centers responsible for the tonic phase of generalized tonic-clonic seizures. Effective control in emergency treatment of seizures may take 15 to 20 minutes because of rate of injection required. Highly protein bound. Metabolized by cytochrome P_{450} enzymes CYP2C9 and CYP2C19 and is excreted in changed form in the urine. Half-life ranges from 10 to 15 hours. Crosses the placental barrier. Secreted in breast milk.

INDICATIONS AND USES

Control of generalized tonic-clonic status epilepticus and prevention and treatment of seizures during neurosurgery. Parenteral phenytoin should be used only when oral phenytoin administration is not possible.

CONTRAINDICATIONS

Known hypersensitivity to phenytoin or other hydantoin products. ■ Bradycardia; sinoatrial, second-, or third-degree heart block; Stokes-Adams syndrome. ■ Coadministration with delavirdine (Rescriptor).

PRECAUTIONS

Discontinue immediately for hypersensitivity reactions; with caution, substitute a nonhydantoin anticonvulsant. When substituting a new anticonvulsant, consideration should be given to avoiding structurally related drugs such as carboxamides (e.g., carbamazepine), barbiturates, succinimides, and oxazolidinediones (e.g., trimethadione). ▪ Abrupt withdrawal may cause increased seizure activity. Gradually reduce dose, discontinue, or substitute alternative antiepileptic agents. ▪ Not effective for absence seizures; combined therapy is required if both conditions are present. ▪ Not indicated for seizures due to hypoglycemia or other metabolic causes. ▪ Severe hypotension and cardiac arrhythmias have occurred with rapid infusion. Risk increases with increased rates, but adverse cardiac events have been reported at or below the recommended infusion rates. Careful cardiac monitoring is required during and after IV administration. Because of the risks of cardiac and local toxicity associated with IV phenytoin, oral phenytoin should be used whenever possible. ▪ Use caution in hypotension and severe myocardial insufficiency. ▪ Use caution with low serum albumin level, and adjust dose as indicated. Phenytoin is highly bound to serum protein (approximately 80% to 90% or more) and a reduced albumin causes an increase in free drug availability. ▪ Drug reaction with eosinophilia and systemic symptoms (DRESS), also known as multiorgan hypersensitivity, has been reported. Usually presents with fever, rash, and/or lymphadenopathy in association with other organ system involvement such as hepatitis, nephritis, hematologic abnormalities, myocarditis, or myositis. Eosinophilia is often present. Deaths have been reported. ▪ Serious and sometimes fatal dermatologic reactions, including toxic epidermal necrolysis (TEN) and Stevens-Johnson syndrome (SJS), have been reported. Onset of symptoms is usually within 28 days but can occur later. ▪ Discontinue phenytoin if skin rash appears unless the rash is clearly not drug related. ▪ Selected patients of Asian ancestry (e.g., Han Chinese, Filipino, Malaysian, South Asian Indian, and Thai descent) with a specific human leukocyte antigen allele may have an increased risk of serious skin reactions (e.g., Stevens-Johnson syndrome, toxic epidermal necrolysis) from phenytoin therapy. ▪ Cases of acute hepatotoxicity, including hepatic failure, have been reported. These events may be part of the spectrum of DRESS or may occur in isolation. Reactions have included elevated liver function tests, eosinophilia, fever, hepatomegaly, jaundice, leukocytosis, and lymphadenopathy. Discontinue immediately and substitute alternative anticonvulsant therapy. ▪ Hematopoietic complications, some fatal, have been reported (e.g., agranulocytosis, granulocytopenia, leukopenia, thrombocytopenia, or pancytopenia with or without bone marrow suppression). ▪ Some reports suggest a relationship between phenytoin and the development of lymphadenopathy (local or generalized). Lymph node involvement may occur with or without S/S resembling DRESS. In all cases of lymphadenopathy, follow-up observation for an extended period is indicated, and alternative anticonvulsant therapy should be strongly considered. ▪ Local toxicity, including purple glove syndrome (edema, discoloration, and pain distal to the injection site), has occurred and may or may not be associated with extravasation. Irritation may range from slight tenderness to extensive necrosis and sloughing. ▪ Inhibits insulin release and may increase serum glucose; monitoring indicated in patients with diabetes. ▪ Use with caution in patients with porphyria. Phenytoin may exacerbate this disease. ▪ Antiepileptic drugs (AEDs) increase the risk of suicidal thoughts or behavior in patients taking these drugs for any indication. Patients treated with any AED for any indication should be monitored for the emergence or worsening of depression, suicidal thoughts or behavior, and/or any unusual changes in mood or behavior. Some psychotic symptoms and/or behavioral changes resolved without intervention. Others required dose reduction or discontinuation of the antiepileptic agent.

Monitor: Narrow margin of error between therapeutic and toxic dose. Plasma levels above 10 mcg/mL usually control seizure activity. The acceptable range is 5 to 20 mcg/mL. Consider monitoring free phenytoin levels in patients with hypoalbuminemia or renal or hepatic insufficiency (therapeutic range is 1 to 2 mcg/mL). Toxicity begins with nystagmus and may be seen at levels less than 20 mcg/mL. Serum levels sustained above the optimum range may produce confusional states referred to as delirium, psychosis, encephalopathy, or rarely irreversible cerebellar dysfunction. ▪ Observe patient closely for signs of CNS side effects. ▪ Periodic monitoring of CBC, platelets, albumin, urinalysis, and hepatic and renal function is recommended. ▪ Monitor ECG and BP continuously. ▪ Closely monitor patients who are gravely ill, have impaired liver function, or are elderly. May show early signs of toxicity. ▪ Observation of patient symptoms and effectiveness of all medications is imperative. ▪ Observe for rash and discontinue if one appears; see Precautions. ▪ Determine absolute patency of vein. Avoid extravasation. Very alkaline; follow each injection with sterile NS to reduce local venous irritation. ▪ Patients maintained with phenytoin should be given a dose the morning of surgery to maintain adequate serum levels. ▪ See Precautions and Drug/Lab Interactions.

Patient Education: May increase the risk of suicidal thoughts and behavior. Promptly report emergence or worsening of S/S of depression, any unusual changes in mood or behavior, or thoughts about self-harm. ▪ Women who are pregnant or who become pregnant should be encouraged to enroll in the North American Antiepileptic Drug (NAAED) Pregnancy Registry.

Maternal/Child: Category D: avoid pregnancy. Prenatal exposure to phenytoin may increase the risk for congenital malformations and other adverse development outcomes. Consider risks versus benefit. ▪ Alterations in phenytoin kinetics in pregnant women may necessitate periodic monitoring of serum levels. ▪ Newborns whose mothers received phenytoin during pregnancy may develop a life-threatening bleeding disorder that can be prevented by giving vitamin K to the mother before delivery and to the neonate after birth. ▪ Discontinue breast-feeding.

Elderly: See Dose Adjustments and Rate of Administration. ▪ Clearance tends to decrease with increasing age. ▪ Low serum albumin causing a decrease in protein binding may result in increased sensitivity to phenytoin.

DRUG/LAB INTERACTIONS

Interactions are numerous and potentially life threatening. Review of drug profile by pharmacist imperative. ▪ Coadministration with **delavirdine** (Rescriptor) is contraindicated. Has potential for loss of virologic response and possible resistance to delavirdine or to the class of nonnucleoside reverse transcriptase inhibitors. ▪ Serum levels may be increased by **alcohol** (acute ingestion), **amiodarone** (Nexterone), **antiepileptic agents** (e.g., ethosuximide [Zarontin], felbamate [Felbatol], methsuximide [Celontin], oxcarbazepine [Trileptal], topiramate [Topamax]), **azoles** (e.g., fluconazole [Diflucan], itraconazole [Sporanox], ketoconazole [Nizoral], miconazole [Oravig], voriconazole [VFEND]), **capecitabine** (Xeloda), **chloramphenicol** (Chloromycetin), **chlordiazepoxide** (Librium), **disulfiram** (Antabuse), **estrogens, fluorouracil** (5-FU), **fluoxetine** (Prozac), **fluvastatin** (Lescol), **fluvoxamine** (Luvox), **H₂ antagonists** (e.g., cimetidine [Tagamet]), **halothane, isoniazid** (INH), **methylphenidate** (Ritalin), **omeprazole** (Prilosec), **phenothiazines** (e.g., prochlorperazine [Compazine]), **salicylates** (aspirin), **sertraline** (Zoloft), **succinimides, sulfonamides** (e.g., sulfadiazine, sulfamethoxazole/trimethoprim [Bactrim], sulfaphenazole), **ticlopidine** (Ticlid), **tolbutamide** (Orinase), **trazodone** (Desyrel), **and warfarin** (Coumadin). ▪ Serum levels and effectiveness may be decreased by **antineoplastics** usually in combination (e.g., bleomycin [Blenoxane], carboplatin [Paraplatin], cisplatin, doxorubicin [Adriamycin], methotrexate), **carbamazepine** (Tegretol), **chronic alcohol abuse, diazepam** (Valium), **diazoxide** (Proglycem), **folic acid, fosamprenavir** (Lexiva), **nelfinavir** (Viracept), **reserpine, rifampin** (Rifadin), **ritonavir** (Norvir), **St. John's wort, theophylline, and vigabatrin** (Sabril). ▪ Phenytoin serum levels may be increased or decreased by **phenobarbital** (Luminal), **valproate sodium** (Depacon), **and valproic acid** (Depakene). Similarly, phenytoin may unpredictably affect the levels and efficacy of these drugs. ▪ The addition of withdrawal of drugs while patients are undergoing phenytoin therapy may require an adjustment of the phenytoin dose. ▪ Phenytoin will inhibit the effects of **azoles** (e.g., fluconazole, itraconazole, ketoconazole, posaconazole [Noxafil], voriconazole), **corticosteroids, doxycycline, estrogens, furosemide** (Lasix), **irinotecan** (Camptosar), **oral contraceptives, paclitaxel** (Taxol), **paroxetine** (Paxil), **quinidine, rifampin** (Rifadin), **sertraline** (Zoloft), **teniposide** (Vumon), **theoph-**

ylline, and vitamin D. Dose adjustment of these agents may be indicated. ▪ Phenytoin decreases plasma concentrations of **active metabolites of albendazole** (Albenza), **HIV antivirals** (e.g., efavirenz [Sustiva], lopinavir/ritonavir [Kaletra], indinavir [Crixivan], nelfinavir [Viracept], ritonavir [Norvir], saquinavir [Invirase]), **antiepileptic agents** (e.g., carbamazepine [Tegretol], felbamate [Felbatol], lamotrigine [Lamictal], oxcarbazepine [Trileptal], quetiapine [Seroquel], topiramate [Topomax]), **atorvastatin** (Lipitor), **chlorpropamide** (Diabinese), **clozapine** (Clozaril), **cyclosporine** (Sandimmune), **digoxin** (Lanoxin), **fluvastatin** (Lescol), **folic acid, methadone** (Dolophine), **mexiletine, nifedipine** (Procardia), **nimodipine, nisoldipine** (Sular), **praziquantel** (Biltricide), **simvastatin** (Zocor), **and verapamil**. Adjust doses of these agents as indicated. ▪ Phenytoin when given with **fosamprenavir** alone may decrease the concentration of **amprenavir** (Agenerase), the active metabolite. Phenytoin when given with the combination of **fosamprenavir and ritonavir** may increase the concentration of **amprenavir** (Agenerase). ▪ May increase or decrease PT/INR responses when coadministered with **warfarin** (Coumadin). ▪ Chronically administered phenytoin may cause resistance to the neuromuscular blocking action of **nondepolarizing neuromuscular blocking agents** (e.g., cisatracurium [Nimbex], pancuronium, rocuronium [Zemuron], and vecuronium). Monitor patients closely; recovery from neuromuscular blockade may be more rapid than expected, and infusion rate requirements may be higher. ▪ Alters **some clinical laboratory tests** (e.g., may decrease T_4; may increase glucose, alkaline phosphatase, and GGT; and may produce low results in dexamethasone or metyrapone tests).

SIDE EFFECTS

Altered tatste sensation, ataxia, confusion, constipation, decreased coordination, dizziness, drowsiness, dyskinesias, fever, headache, hyperplasia of gums, insomnia, nausea, nervousness, nystagmus, paresthesia, skin eruptions, slurred speech, somnolence, tremors, vertigo, visual disturbances, vomiting.

Major: Acute hepatic failure, bradycardia, cardiac arrest, cardiovascular collapse, CNS depression, dermatologic reactions (including local toxicity, Stevens-Johnson syndrome, and toxic epidermal necrolysis), DRESS, heart block, hematopoietic complications, hypotension, lymphadenopathy, Peyronie's disease, respiratory arrest, tonic seizures, toxic hepatitis, ventricular fibrillation. Hypersensitivity reactions, including anaphylaxis, have been reported (rare). Psychotic symptoms, including aggression, agitation, anger, anxiety, apathy, depersonalization, depression, emotional lability, hallucinations, hostility, irritability, and suicidal tendencies, have occurred with antiepileptic agents.

Overdose: Ataxia, blurred vision, dysarthria, hyperreflexia, lethargy, nausea, nystagmus, slurred speech, tremor, and vomiting.

ANTIDOTE

Notify the physician of any side effects. If minor symptoms progress or any major side effect occurs, discontinue the drug and notify the physician; see Precautions. Maintain a patent airway and resuscitate as necessary. Symptoms of heart block or bradycardia may be reversed with IV atropine. Epinephrine may also be useful. Decrease rate or discontinue infusion for severe hypotension or cardiac arrhythmias. Hemodialysis may be useful in overdose.

PHOSPHATE

(**FOS**-fayt)

Potassium Phosphate, Sodium Phosphate

pH 5 to 7.8

USUAL DOSE

Dependent on individual needs of the patient.

TPN, adults and pediatric patients: 10 to 15 mM (310 to 465 mg) of phosphorus/liter of TPN solution should maintain normal serum phosphate. Larger amounts may be required. 1 mM equals 31 mg.

Acute hypophosphatemia: Adults and pediatric patients: 0.08 to 0.32 mM/kg of body weight as a *loading dose* equally distributed over 6 hours. *Maintain pediatric patients* with 0.5 to 1.5 mM/kg/24 hr. *Maintain adults* with 48.4 to 64.5 mM/24 hr.

INFANT DOSE

Infants receiving TPN: 1.5 to 2 mM/kg of body weight/day.

DOSE ADJUSTMENTS

Lower-end initial doses may be indicated in the elderly based on the potential for decreased organ function and concomitant disease or drug therapy.

DILUTION

Must be diluted in a larger volume of suitable IV solution and given as an infusion. Soluble in most commonly used IV solutions (see chart on inside back cover) except protein hydrolysate. Mix thoroughly. See Compatibility.

COMPATIBILITY (Underline Indicates Conflicting Compatibility Information)

Consider any drug NOT listed as compatible to be INCOMPATIBLE until consulting a pharmacist; specific conditions may apply.

ALL FORMULATIONS

Mix thoroughly after each addition of supposedly **compatible** drugs or solutions. TPN solutions requiring the addition of phosphates and calcium salts must be mixed by the pharmacist to avoid a precipitate of calcium phosphate. Specific amounts, calculations, order, and temperature (precipitate forms more readily at room temperature) are required. Deaths have been reported.

One source suggests the following **compatibilities:**

POTASSIUM PHOSPHATE

Additive: *See comments under All Formulations.* Mix thoroughly. Metoclopramide (Reglan), verapamil.

Y-site: Diltiazem (Cardizem), enalaprilat (Vasotec IV), esmolol (Brevibloc), famotidine (Pepcid IV), 6% hydroxyethyl starch (Voluven), labetalol, micafungin (Mycamine), nicardipine (Cardene IV), nitroprusside sodium, telavancin (Vibativ).

SODIUM PHOSPHATE

Y-site: Doripenem (Doribax), micafungin (Mycamine), telavancin (Vibativ).

RATE OF ADMINISTRATION

A usual dose is usually equally distributed over 6 hours. Other sources suggest administering up to 15 mM over 2 hours, up to 30 mM over 4 hours, and up to 45 mM over 6 hours. Potassium phosphate will be further limited by the maximum rate for potassium. Consider sodium/potassium content. Infuse slowly. Rapid infusion may cause phosphate or potassium intoxication. Serum calcium may be reduced rapidly, causing hypocalcemic tetany.

ACTIONS

Involved in bone deposition. Helps to maintain calcium levels, has a buffering effect on acid-base equilibrium, and influences renal excretion of the hydrogen ion. Normal levels in adults, 3 to 4.5 mg/dL of serum; in pediatric patients, 4 to 7 mg/dL. Excreted in urine.

P

INDICATIONS AND USES
To prevent or correct hypophosphatemia in patients with restricted or no oral intake.

CONTRAINDICATIONS
Any disease with high phosphate or low calcium levels, hyperkalemia (potassium phosphate), hypernatremia (sodium phosphate).

PRECAUTIONS
Rapid infusion may cause phosphate, sodium, or potassium intoxication. Serum calcium may be reduced, rapidly causing hypocalcemic tetany. ▪ Use sodium phosphate with caution in renal impairment, cirrhosis, cardiac failure, or any edematous, sodium-retaining state. ▪ Use potassium phosphate with caution in cardiac disease, renal disease, and digitalized patients. ▪ See Compatibility.

Monitor: Monitor serum calcium, potassium, phosphate, chlorides, and sodium. Discontinue when serum phosphate exceeds 2 mg/dL. ▪ See Drug/Lab Interactions.

Maternal/Child: Category C: safety for use in pregnancy not established.

Elderly: Differences in response between elderly and younger patients have not been identified. Lower-end initial doses may be appropriate in the elderly; see Dose Adjustments.

DRUG/LAB INTERACTIONS
May cause hyperkalemia with **potassium-sparing diuretics** (e.g., amiloride) **or angiotensin-converting enzyme inhibitors** (e.g., enalapril [Vasotec]).

SIDE EFFECTS
Elevated phosphates, reduced calcium levels and hypocalcemic tetany, elevated potassium levels causing cardiac arrhythmias, flaccid paralysis, heaviness of the legs, hypotension, listlessness, mental confusion, paresthesia of the extremities.

ANTIDOTE
For any side effect, discontinue the drug and notify the physician. Restore serum calcium with calcium gluconate or chloride. Shift potassium from serum to cells with 150 mL of $^1/6$ M sodium lactate or 10% to 20% dextrose with 10 units regular insulin for each 20 Gm dextrose at 300 to 500 mL/hr. Correct acidosis with sodium bicarbonate. Reduce sodium by restriction, diuretics, or hemodialysis. Resuscitate as necessary.

PHYSOSTIGMINE SALICYLATE
(fye-zoh-**STIG**-meen sah-**LIS**-ah-layt)

Cholinergic
Cholinesterase inhibitor
Antidote

pH 5.8

USUAL DOSE
Postanesthesia: 0.5 to 1 mg initially. Repeat at 10- to 30-minute intervals until desired results obtained.

Anticholinergic toxicity: 0.5 to 2 mg initially. 1 to 4 mg may be repeated as necessary as life-threatening signs recur (arrhythmias, convulsions, deep coma). Maximum dose is 4 mg in 30 minutes.

PEDIATRIC DOSE
To be used in life-threatening situations only. 0.02 mg/kg/dose. May be repeated at 5- to 10-minute intervals only if toxic effects persist and there is no sign of cholinergic effects. Maximum total dose is 2 mg. See Maternal/Child.

DILUTION
May be given undiluted. Do not add to IV solutions. May be given through Y-tube or three-way stopcock of infusion set.

COMPATIBILITY
Specific information not available. Consider specific use; consult pharmacist.

RATE OF ADMINISTRATION
Rapid IV administration may cause bradycardia, hypersalivation, respiratory distress, and convulsions.

1 mg or fraction thereof over 1 to 3 minutes.

Pediatric rate: 0.5 mg or fraction thereof over at least 1 minute.

ACTIONS
An extract of *Physostigma venenosum* seeds. It inhibits the destructive action of acetylcholinesterase and prolongs and exaggerates the effects of acetylcholine. Stimulates parasympathetic nerve stimulation (pupil contraction, increased intestinal musculature tonus, bronchial constriction, salivary and sweat gland stimulation). Does enter the CNS. Onset of action occurs in 5 minutes and lasts about 1 hour. Rapidly hydrolyzed by cholinesterases.

INDICATIONS AND USES
To reverse CNS toxic effects caused by drugs capable of producing anticholinergic poisoning (e.g., atropine), other anticholinergic/antispasmodic agents (e.g., phenothiazines, antihistamines), anticholinergic antiparkinson agents (e.g., benztropine [Cogentin], trihexyphenidyl [Artane]), and tricyclic antidepressants (e.g., imipramine [Tofranil]).
Unlabeled uses: Treatment of delirium tremens.

CONTRAINDICATIONS
Asthma, cardiovascular disease, diabetes, gangrene, mechanical obstruction of the intestines or urogenital tract, vagotonic states, patients receiving choline esters, depolarizing neuromuscular blocking agents (succinylcholine), or tricyclic antidepressants (e.g., amitriptyline [Elavil]).

PRECAUTIONS
Rapid IV administration may cause bradycardia, hypersalivation, respiratory distress, and convulsions. ▪ Contains bisulfites; use caution in allergic individuals.

Monitor: Atropine must always be available. ▪ Monitor vital signs. ▪ See Drug/Lab Interactions.

Maternal/Child: Safety for use in pregnancy and breast-feeding not established. ▪ Has caused muscular weakness in neonates of mothers treated with other cholinesterase inhibitors for myasthenia gravis. ▪ May contain benzyl alcohol; do not use in neonates.

DRUG/LAB INTERACTIONS

Potentiates **succinylcholine** and **other choline esters** (e.g., bethanecol). ▪ May antagonize CNS depressant effects of **diazepam** (Valium). ▪ May cause serious complications, including death, with **tricyclic antidepressants** (e.g., amitriptyline [Elavil]).

SIDE EFFECTS

Anxiety, bradycardia, cholinergic crisis (overdose), coma, convulsions, defecation, delirium, disorientation, emesis, hallucinations, hyperactivity, hypersalivation, hypersensitivity, nausea, respiratory distress, salivation, seizures, sweating, urination.

ANTIDOTE

Keep physician informed of side effects. For excessive nausea or sweating, reduce dose. Discontinue drug for bradycardia; convulsions; excessive defecation, emesis, salivation, or urination; or respiratory distress. Treat cholinergic side effects (e.g., arrhythmias, bronchoconstriction) or hypersensitivity with the specific antagonist atropine sulfate in doses of 0.6 mg IV. May be repeated every 3 to 10 minutes. Endotracheal intubation or tracheostomy are considered prophylactic in anesthesia or crisis. Artificial ventilation, oxygen therapy, cardiac monitoring, adequate suctioning, and treatment of shock or convulsions must be instituted and maintained as necessary.

PHYTONADIONE BBW
(fye-toe-nah-**DYE**-ohn)

Vitamin (prothrombinogenic)
Antidote
Antihemorrhagic

Vitamin K₁

pH 5 to 7

USUAL DOSE

Should be given by the SC or oral route whenever possible; parenteral route administration has caused death; see Precautions. A single dose is preferred, but it may be repeated if clinically indicated.

Vitamin K deficiency: Up to 10 mg may be added to TPN solutions as indicated.

Anticoagulant-induced (warfarin or dicumarol) hypoprothrombinemia: 2.5 to 10 mg. Doses up to 25 mg and, rarely, 50 mg may be needed. May repeat in 6 to 8 hours if initial response is not adequate. Doses as low as 1 to 2 mg may be effective. Use the smallest dose that achieves effective results to prevent clotting hazards.

Hypoprothrombinemia from other causes: 2 to 25 mg (rarely 50 mg), depending on the severity of the deficiency and the response obtained.

PEDIATRIC DOSE

See Usual Dose, Precautions, and Maternal/Child.

Vitamin K deficiency: 1 to 2 mg may be added to TPN solutions as indicated.

Anticoagulant-induced (warfarin or dicumarol) hypoprothrombinemia in infants and children: 1 to 2 mg/dose.

Hypoprothrombinemia from other causes in infants and children: A single dose of 1 to 2 mg.

NEWBORN DOSE

See Usual Dose, Precautions, and Maternal/Child. Rarely given IV in the newborn. SC injection preferred.

Prophylaxis of hemorrhagic disease of the newborn: 0.5 to 1 mg IM within 1 hour of birth.

Treatment of hemorrhagic disease of the newborn: 1 to 2 mg/24 hr SC or IM. Higher doses may be necessary if the mother has been receiving oral anticoagulants (e.g., warfarin [Coumadin]) or anticonvulsants (e.g., phenytoin [Dilantin]). Whole blood or blood components may be indicated for excessive bleeding. Give phytonadione concurrently to correct the underlying disorder.

DOSE ADJUSTMENTS

See Drug/Lab Interactions.

DILUTION

Use only preservative-free solutions. May be diluted only with NS, D5NS, or D5W. Dilution with at least 10 mL of diluent is recommended to facilitate prescribed rate of administration. Photosensitive; protect from light in all dilutions. Use immediately after preparation.

Filters: Not required by manufacturer; however, there should be no significant loss of potency with the use of a 0.22-micron filter.

Storage: Photosensitive; protect from light before use and in all dilutions. Store unopened ampules below 40° C (104° F), preferably between 15° C and 30° C (59° F and 86° F). Protect from light and freezing. Discard diluted solution and drug remaining in ampule after single use.

COMPATIBILITY

Consider any drug NOT listed as compatible to be INCOMPATIBLE until consulting a pharmacist; specific conditions may apply.

One source suggests the following **compatibilities:**

Additive: Amikacin, chloramphenicol (Chloromycetin), sodium bicarbonate.

Y-site: Ampicillin, epinephrine (Adrenalin), famotidine (Pepcid IV), heparin, hydrocortisone sodium succinate (Solu-Cortef), potassium chloride (KCl).

RATE OF ADMINISTRATION

Each 1 mg or fraction thereof over 1 minute or longer. Too-rapid injection has caused severe reactions, including fatalities.

ACTIONS

Vitamin K, a fat-soluble vitamin, is essential for hepatic production of four blood coagulation factors including prothrombin. These are required for normal blood clotting. Onset of action is within 1 to 2 hours. Usually controls hemorrhage in 3 to 6 hours; normal prothrombin levels should be obtained in 12 to 14 hours. Metabolized by the liver and eliminated in urine and bile.

INDICATIONS AND USES

Coagulation disorders due to faulty formation of factors II, VII, IX, and X when caused by vitamin K deficiency or interference with vitamin K activity. Indicated in anticoagulant-induced prothrombin deficiency (warfarin or dicumarol). ■ Prophylaxis and treatment of hemorrhagic disease of the newborn. ■ Hypoprothrombinemia resulting from antibacterial therapy. ■ Hypoprothrombinemia secondary to factors limiting the absorption or synthesis of vitamin K (e.g., obstructive jaundice, biliary fistula, sprue, ulcerative colitis, celiac disease, intestinal resection, cystic fibrosis of the pancreas, and regional enteritis). ■ Other drug-induced hypoprothrombinemia where it is definitely shown that the result is due to interference with vitamin K metabolism (e.g., salicylates).

CONTRAINDICATIONS

Hypersensitivity to components.

PRECAUTIONS

IV and/or IM is not the route of choice; used only when SC or oral route cannot be used. Use extreme caution; has caused severe reactions, including death, with the first injection, even when the product has been diluted and infused slowly. ■ As an alternative to administering phytonadione, discontinuation or reduction of the doses of drugs interfering with coagulation mechanisms (e.g., antibiotics, salicylates) should be considered. The severity of the coagulation disorder should determine if phytonadione is required in addition to discontinuing or reducing the doses of interfering drugs. To correct excess anticoagulation after the use of warfarin (Coumadin) (e.g., returning an increased INR to the desired range), consider the degree of elevation and the presence of clinically significant bleeding. ■ Supplement with whole blood transfusion or blood components if indicated. ■ Now the only vitamin K product for IV use. ■ Do not use to counteract anticoagulant effects of heparin; not effective. Protamine sulfate is indicated. ■ Does not restore abnormal platelet function to normal. ■ Does not correct hypoprothrombinemia due to hepatocellular damage. ■ When phytonadione is used in a patient for whom anticoagulant therapy is indicated, the same clotting hazards that existed before beginning anticoagulant therapy will recur. Use the smallest dose of phytonadione possible and monitor PT.

Monitor: See Neonatal Dose, Precautions, and Drug/Lab Interactions. ▪ Dose and effect determined by PT/INR. Repeat PT/INR 6 to 8 hours after a dose. Keep the physician informed. ▪ Pain and swelling at injection site can occur.

Maternal/Child: Category C: safety for use not established. ▪ Use caution during breast-feeding. ▪ Use extreme caution in premature infants and neonates. Hemolysis, jaundice, and hyperbilirubinemia in newborns may be related to the dose of phytonadione. The recommended dose should not be exceeded. Severe hemolytic anemia, hemoglobinuria, kernicterus, brain damage, and death may occur. ▪ Neonates with hemorrhagic disease of the newborn should respond to administration of phytonadione with a shortening of the PT within 2 to 4 hours. If shortening of the PT is not seen, consider other coagulation disorders. ▪ May contain benzyl alcohol. When used as recommended, there is no evidence to suggest that this small amount is associated with toxicity.

DRUG/LAB INTERACTIONS

Discontinue drugs **adversely affecting the coagulation mechanism** if possible (e.g., salicylates, antibiotics). ▪ May cause temporary resistance to **prothrombin-depressing oral anticoagulants** by increasing amount of phytonadione in the liver and blood. Anticoagulation will require larger doses of same or use of heparin sodium.

SIDE EFFECTS

Cyanosis, diaphoresis, dizziness, dyspnea, hyperbilirubinemia, hypotension, injection site reactions, peculiar taste sensations, rapid and weak pulse, tachycardia, transient flushing sensation. Anaphylaxis, cardiac and/or respiratory arrest, shock, and death have occurred with parenteral route.

ANTIDOTE

Should not be necessary if dosage is accurately calculated before administration. Action can be reversed by warfarin or heparin if indicated. Discontinue the drug and notify the physician of any side effects. For most side effects the physician will probably choose to continue the drug at a decreased rate of administration. Treat hypersensitivity reactions as necessary.

PIPERACILLIN SODIUM AND TAZOBACTAM SODIUM	Antibacterial (extended-spectrum penicillin and beta-lactamase inhibitor)

PIPERACILLIN SODIUM AND TAZOBACTAM SODIUM

(pie-**PER**-ah-sill-in **SO**-dee-um and tay-zoh-**BAC**-tam **SO**-dee-um)

Antibacterial
(extended-spectrum penicillin
and beta-lactamase inhibitor)

Zosyn

USUAL DOSE

Measurement of both drugs is included in the total dose; for every 1 Gm of piperacillin there is 0.125 Gm of tazobactam (8:1 ratio).

12 Gm piperacillin/1.5 Gm tazobactam/24 hours given as 3.375 (3 Gm piperacillin/0.375 Gm tazobactam) every 6 hours. Usual duration of therapy is 7 to 10 days, based on severity of infection and patient progress.

Nosocomial pneumonia: 4.5 Gm every 6 hours. Also use an aminoglycoside. Continue aminoglycoside if *P. aeruginosa* is isolated; may be discontinued if it is not isolated. Usual duration of therapy is 7 to 14 days.

PEDIATRIC DOSE

2 months to 9 months of age: 80 mg piperacillin/10 mg tazobactam per kg of body weight every 8 hours.

Over 9 months of age weighing up to 40 kg: 100 mg piperacillin/12.5 mg tazobactam per kg of body weight every 8 hours.

Pediatric patients over 40 kg: See Usual Dose.

DOSE ADJUSTMENTS

No dose adjustment needed in impaired liver function. ■ Dose reduction may be required in the elderly. ■ Adjust dose in adult patients with impaired renal function based on the following chart. ■ Dose recommendations for pediatric patients with impaired renal function are not available.

Piperacillin/Tazobactam Dose Guidelines in Adults with Impaired Renal Function		
Renal Function (Creatinine Clearance, mL/min)	All Indications (Except Nosocomial Pneumonia)	Nosocomial Pneumonia
>40 mL/min	3.375 Gm q 6 hr	4.5 Gm q 6 hr
20-40 mL/min*	2.25 Gm q 6 hr	3.375 Gm q 6 hr
<20 mL/min*	2.25 Gm q 8 hr	2.25 Gm q 6 hr
Hemodialysis†	2.25 Gm q 12 hr	2.25 Gm q 8 hr
CAPD	2.25 Gm q 12 hr	2.25 Gm q 8 hr

*Creatinine clearance for patients not receiving hemodialysis.
†Hemodialysis removes 30% to 40% of piperacillin/tazobactam. Give an additional dose of 0.75 Gm following each dialysis session. No additional dose is necessary for CAPD patients.

DILUTION

Available in two different formulations: one with EDTA (edetate disodium dihydrate) and one without. **Compatibility** information differs; consult pharmacist. See Compatibility.

Each 1 Gm of piperacillin content should be reconstituted with at least 5 mL of suitable diluent (e.g., SWFI or NS with or without preservatives, or D5W). Swirl until dissolved. Should be further diluted to desired volume (50 to 150 mL) with **compatible** infusion solutions (NS, SWFI, Dextran 6% in Saline, or D5W).

EDTA-containing formulation of Zosyn is compatible with all of the previously listed solutions plus LR. If further diluted with SWFI, maximum recommended volume of SWFI per dose is 50 mL. Also available premixed and in ADD-Vantage vials for use with ADD-Vantage infusion containers. May be used in ambulatory IV infusion pumps. Considered stable at

RT for 12 hours when reconstituted and diluted to a final volume of 25 or 37.5 mL. See manufacturer's literature for additional information.

Storage: Store unopened vials at RT. Use single-dose vials immediately after reconstitution; discard any unused portion after 24 hours at room temperature or 48 hours if refrigerated. Do not freeze vials after reconstitution. Stable for 24 hours at RT or for up to 7 days after dilution if refrigerated. Also available as a frozen premixed solution. Store frozen solution at $-20°$ C $(-4°$ F). Frozen solutions should be thawed at RT or under refrigeration. Do not force thaw. Thawed solutions are stable for 24 hours at RT or for 14 days if refrigerated. Do not refreeze.

COMPATIBILITY
(Underline Indicates Conflicting Compatibility Information)

Consider any drug NOT listed as compatible to be INCOMPATIBLE until consulting a pharmacist; specific conditions may apply.

Manufacturer states, "Should not be mixed with other drugs in a syringe or infusion bottle. Not chemically stable in solutions containing only sodium bicarbonate and/or solutions that significantly alter the pH. **Incompatible** with LR *(the EDTA-free formulation of Zosyn only)* and should not be added to blood products or albumin hydrolysates." One source recommends temporarily discontinuing other solutions infusing at the same site to avoid compatibility problems. May be inactivated in solution with aminoglycosides (e.g., amikacin, gentamicin). Do not mix in the same solution. Separate administration required. Formulation containing EDTA **may be compatible** at the **Y-site** with amikacin or gentamicin. Selected doses, specific diluents, and amounts of diluent are required. Consult pharmacist or manufacturer's literature. See Drug/Lab Interactions.

One source suggests the following **compatibilities:**

Y-site: *See general comments under Compatibility.* Acetaminophen (Ofirmev), aminophylline, anidulafungin (Eraxis), aztreonam (Azactam), bivalirudin (Angiomax), bleomycin (Blenoxane), bumetanide, buprenorphine (Buprenex), butorphanol (Stadol), calcium gluconate, carboplatin (Paraplatin), carmustine (BiCNU), cisatracurium (Nimbex), clindamycin (Cleocin), cyclophosphamide (Cytoxan), cytarabine (ARA-C), dexamethasone (Decadron), dexmedetomidine (Precedex), diphenhydramine (Benadryl), docetaxel (Taxotere), dopamine, enalaprilat (Vasotec IV), etoposide (VePesid), etoposide phosphate (Etopophos), fenoldopam (Corlopam), fluconazole (Diflucan), fludarabine (Fludara), fluorouracil (5-FU), furosemide (Lasix), gallium nitrate (Ganite), granisetron (Kytril), heparin, hetastarch in electrolytes (Hextend), hydrocortisone sodium succinate (Solu-Cortef), hydromorphone (Dilaudid), ifosfamide (Ifex), leucovorin calcium, linezolid (Zyvox), lorazepam (Ativan), magnesium sulfate, mannitol, meperidine (Demerol), mesna (Mesnex), methotrexate, methylprednisolone (Solu-Medrol), metoclopramide (Reglan), metronidazole (Flagyl IV), milrinone (Primacor), morphine, ondansetron (Zofran), potassium chloride (KCl), ranitidine (Zantac), remifentanil (Ultiva), sargramostim (Leukine), sodium bicarbonate, sulfamethoxazole/trimethoprim, telavancin (Vibativ), thiotepa, tigecycline (Tygacil), vancomycin (Vancocin), vasopressin, vinblastine, vincristine, zidovudine (AZT, Retrovir).

RATE OF ADMINISTRATION
A single dose over 30 minutes as an intermittent infusion. Discontinue primary IV infusion during administration.

Extended infusion method (unlabeled dosing): 3.375 to 4.5 Gm IV over 4 hours every 8 hours.

ACTIONS
An antimicrobial agent that combines the extended-spectrum penicillin piperacillin with the potent beta-lactamase inhibitor tazobactam. May be used in suspected polymicrobial infections due to its broad spectrum of activity. Acts by inhibiting septum formation and cell wall synthesis of susceptible bacteria. Bactericidal against gram-positive aerobes, gram-negative aerobes, and anaerobes that may be resistant to other antibiotics. Widely distributed into most body fluids and tissues. Mean tissue concentrations are 50% to 100% of plasma concentrations. Peak levels are achieved immediately at the completion of an infusion. Plasma half-life ranges from 0.7 to 1.2 hours. Metabolized and ex-

creted in urine and, to a small extent, in bile. Crosses the placental barrier. Secreted in breast milk.

INDICATIONS AND USES

Treatment of infections caused by piperacillin/tazobactam–susceptible, beta-lactamase–producing strains of specific microorganisms in the following conditions: intra-abdominal (e.g., appendicitis complicated by rupture or abscess and peritonitis), gynecologic (e.g., postpartum endometritis and pelvic inflammatory disease), skin and skin structure (complicated and uncomplicated [e.g., cellulitis, cutaneous abscesses, and ischemic/diabetic foot infection]), community-acquired pneumonia (moderate severity only), and nosocomial pneumonia (moderate to severe severity). ▪ Used in combination with aminoglycosides for nosocomial pneumonia caused by susceptible organisms, including *Pseudomonas aeruginosa.*

Unlabeled uses: Treatment of septicemia.

CONTRAINDICATIONS

History of hypersensitivity reaction to any penicillin, cephalosporin, or beta-lactamase inhibitors (not absolute; see Precautions).

PRECAUTIONS

Hypersensitivity reactions, including fatalities, have been reported in patients on penicillin therapy; most likely to occur in patients with a history of penicillin, cephalosporin, or carbapenem allergy or sensitivity to multiple allergens. There have been reports of individuals with a history of penicillin hypersensitivity experiencing severe reactions when treated with cephalosporins. Check history of previous hypersensitivity reactions to penicillins, cephalosporins, or other allergens. Actual incidence of cross-allergenicity not established but may be more common with first-generation cephalosporins. ▪ Serious skin reactions such as Stevens-Johnson syndrome, toxic epidermal necrolysis, drug reaction with eosinophilia and systemic symptoms (DRESS), and generalized exanthematous pustulosis have been reported. ▪ Sensitivity studies indicated to determine susceptibility of the causative organism to piperacillin. ▪ To reduce the development of drug-resistant bacteria and maintain its effectiveness, piperacillin/tazobactam should be used to treat or prevent only those infections proven or strongly suspected to be caused by bacteria. ▪ Avoid prolonged use of drug; superinfection caused by overgrowth of nonsusceptible organisms may result. ▪ Bleeding manifestations have been reported and may be associated with abnormal coagulation tests (e.g., clotting time, platelet aggregation, and PT). Patients with impaired renal function may be at increased risk for bleeding tendencies. ▪ Leukopenia/neutropenia has been reported, most commonly with prolonged therapy. ▪ Use caution in patients with CHF or those with a history of bleeding disorders or GI disease (e.g., colitis). ▪ *Clostridium difficile*–associated diarrhea (CDAD) has been reported. May range from mild diarrhea to fatal colitis. Consider in patients who present with diarrhea during or after treatment with piperacillin/tazobactam. ▪ Incidence of side effects (e.g., fever and rash) may be increased in patients with cystic fibrosis. ▪ Administration of higher than recommended doses has resulted in neuromuscular excitability and convulsions. Patients with renal impairment are at increased risk. ▪ Continue at least 2 days after symptoms of infection disappear.

Monitor: Watch for early symptoms of a hypersensitivity reaction. ▪ Closely monitor patients who develop a skin rash. Discontinue therapy if lesions progress. ▪ Periodic evaluation of renal, hepatic, and hematopoietic systems and electrolytes recommended, especially with prolonged therapy. May cause hypokalemia; monitor closely. ▪ Contains 2.79 mEq (64 mg) of sodium/Gm. At the usual recommended doses, patients would receive 33.5 to 44.6 mEq (768 to 1,024 mg) per day. Observe for electrolyte imbalance and cardiac irregularities. May aggravate CHF. ▪ May cause thrombophlebitis; observe carefully and rotate infusion sites. ▪ Observe for increased bleeding tendencies in all patients, especially those with impaired renal function. ▪ See Drug/Lab Interactions.

Patient Education: Report promptly: fever, rash, sore throat, unusual bleeding or bruising, severe stomach cramps and/or diarrhea, seizures. ▪ May require alternate birth control. ▪ Promptly report diarrhea or bloody stools that occur during treatment or up to several months after an antibiotic has been discontinued; may indicate CDAD and require treatment.

Maternal/Child: Category B: use during pregnancy only if clearly needed. ▪ Use caution in breast-feeding. May cause diarrhea or candidiasis in nursing infants. ▪ Safety and effectiveness for use in pediatric patients under 2 months of age not established.

Elderly: No problems documented. Consider age-related organ function and concomitant disease or drug therapy.

DRUG/LAB INTERACTIONS

Synergistic when used in combination with **aminoglycosides** (e.g., amikacin, gentamicin). Synergism may be inconsistent; see Compatibility. ▪ Coadministration with aminoglycosides in patients with end-stage renal disease requiring hemodialysis may result in significant reduction of aminoglycoside concentrations. Monitor closely. ▪ Does not affect pharmacokinetics of vancomycin; may be given without dose adjustment. ▪ Concomitant administration with **probenecid** decreases rate of elimination of piperacillin/tazobactam, resulting in higher and more prolonged blood levels. Avoid coadministration unless benefit outweighs risk. ▪ Use caution with **anticoagulants** (e.g., heparin, warfarin [Coumadin]), **medications that affect platelet aggregation** (e.g., aspirin, clopidogrel [Plavix], dextran, dipyridamole, glycoprotein GPIIb/IIIa receptor antagonists [e.g., abciximab (ReoPro), eptifibatide (Integrilin), tirofiban (Aggrastat)], NSAIDs [e.g., ibuprofen (Advil, Motrin), naproxen (Aleve, Naprosyn)]). Risk of bleeding may be increased. Monitoring of coagulation tests may be indicated. ▪ May be antagonized by **bacteriostatic antibiotics** (e.g., chloramphenicol, erythromycin, and tetracyclines); may interfere with bactericidal action. ▪ May decrease clearance and increase toxicity of **methotrexate;** monitor methotrexate levels. ▪ May inhibit effectiveness of **oral contraceptives;** could result in breakthrough bleeding or pregnancy. ▪ May prolong neuromuscular blockade with **vecuronium** or other nondepolarizing muscle relaxants. ▪ May cause **false-positive glucose** with Clinitest. ▪ **False-positive test results** using the Bio-Rad Laboratories Platelia Aspergillus EIA test in patients receiving piperacillin/tazobactam (Zosyn) have been reported. ▪ See Side Effects.

SIDE EFFECTS

The most common side effects include constipation, diarrhea, headache, insomnia, and nausea. Abdominal pain; abnormal coagulation tests (e.g., increased bleeding time, prolonged PT and PTT); abscess; agitation; anxiety; CDAD; chest pain; cholestatic jaundice; constipation; diarrhea; dizziness; dyspnea; dyspepsia; edema; electrolyte abnormalities, including hypokalemia; fever; headache; hematuria; hematologic abnormalities (agranulocytosis, anemia, hemolytic anemia, pancytopenia, thrombocytopenia, thrombocytosis); hypertension; increased AST, BUN, and serum creatinine; insomnia; local reactions; moniliasis; nausea; pain; pharyngitis; positive Coombs test; pruritus; pseudomembranous colitis; rash (e.g., bullous, eczematoid, maculopapular, urticarial); rhinitis; seizures; and vomiting have been reported. Anaphylaxis can occur. Transient leukopenia and eosinophilia can occur with prolonged therapy.

Post-Marketing: Agranulocytosis, dermatologic reactions (including acute generalized exanthematous pustulosis, erythema multiforme, DRESS, Stevens-Johnson syndrome, and toxic epidermal necrolysis), hemolytic anemia, hepatitis, hypersensitivity reactions (including anaphylactic/anaphylactoid reactions), interstitial nephritis, jaundice, and pancytopenia.

ANTIDOTE

Notify the physician immediately of any adverse symptoms. For severe symptoms, discontinue the drug, treat hypersensitivity reactions (antihistamines, epinephrine, corticosteroids, airway management, oxygen), and resuscitate as necessary. Use anticonvulsants (e.g., diazepam [Valium]) or barbiturates (e.g., phenobarbital) for seizures. Treat CDAD with fluids, electrolytes, protein supplements, and oral vancomycin (Vancocin) or metronidazole (Flagyl) as indicated. In severe cases, surgical evaluation may be indicated. Mild cases may respond to drug discontinuation alone. Hemodialysis is effective in overdose.

PLASMA PROTEIN FRACTION
(**PLAZ**-ma **PRO**-teen **FRAK**-shun)

Plasma volume expander

Plasmanate, Plasmatein, Protenate

pH 6.7 to 7.3

USUAL DOSE
Variable, depending on indication for use, condition of patient, and response to therapy. Range is from 250 to 1,500 mL/24 hr. Each 500-mL bottle yields 25 Gm of plasma protein. Suggested initial doses are as follows:

Shock: 250 to 500 mL.

Burns: 500 to 1,000 mL.

Hypoproteinemia: 1,000 to 1,500 mL/24 hr.

PEDIATRIC DOSE
Treatment of acute shock (unlabeled): See Maternal/Child. One source recommends 10 to 30 mL/kg of body weight.

DILUTION
Available as a 5% solution buffered with saline in 250- and 500-mL bottles with injection sets. Plasmanate also available in a 50-mL size. No further dilution is required. Do not use if solution is turbid or a sediment is visible. Use immediately after opening and discard any unused portion. Contains no preservatives.

Storage: Store at CRT.

COMPATIBILITY
Consider any drug NOT listed as compatible to be INCOMPATIBLE until consulting a pharmacist; specific conditions may apply.

Manufacturer lists as **incompatible** with solutions containing alcohol, protein hydrolysates, or amino acid products. Manufacturer states, "**Compatible** with the usual carbohydrate and electrolyte solutions."

RATE OF ADMINISTRATION
Variable, depending on indication, present blood volume, and patient response. Adjust or slow rate according to clinical response and rising BP. Averages are:

Normal blood volume: 1 mL/min.

Treatment of shock and burns in adult: 5 to 8 mL/min. Higher rates may be tolerated if necessary. Rapid infusion (over 10 mL/min) may cause hypotension. Decrease flow rate as patient improves.

Treatment of shock in infants and other pediatric patients: 5 to 10 mL/min. Do not exceed 10 mL/min in pediatric patients.

Treatment of hypoproteinemia: Single 500-mL dose over 1 hour. For larger amounts the maximum rate is 100 mL/hr.

ACTIONS
A sterile, natural, plasma protein substance containing at least 83% albumin, no more than 17% alpha and beta globulins, and no more than 1% gamma globulin. Contains 130 to 160 mEq sodium/liter. It expands intravascular volume, prevents marked hemoconcentration, and maintains appropriate electrolyte balance in burns.

INDICATIONS AND USES
Emergency treatment of hypovolemic shock caused by burns, infections, surgery, or trauma (may also be due to dehydration in infants and other pediatric patients). ▪ Temporary treatment of hemorrhage when whole blood unavailable. ▪ Hypoproteinemia until cause determined and corrected. ▪ Prevention of hemoconcentration and maintenance of electrolyte balance in burn patients.

CONTRAINDICATIONS
Cardiac failure, cardiopulmonary bypass, history of hypersensitivity reactions to albumin, normal or increased intravascular volume, severe anemia.

PRECAUTIONS

May be given without regard to blood group or type. ▪ Not effective for coagulation mechanism defects. ▪ Added protein, fluid, and sodium load requires caution in hepatic or renal impairment. ▪ If continuous protein loss occurs or edema is present, normal serum albumin (25%) may be the preferred product.

Monitor: Monitor vital signs (including central venous pressure if possible) and urine output every 5 to 15 minutes for 1 hour and hourly thereafter depending on condition. ▪ For treatment of shock, observe carefully for bleeding points that may not have been evident at lower pressures. ▪ Whole blood may be indicated for considerable RBC loss or anemia caused by administration of large amounts of plasma protein fraction. ▪ Additional fluids are required for dehydrated patients. Tissue dehydration caused by osmotic action of plasma proteins can be acute. ▪ May cause vascular overload; monitor for signs of pulmonary edema or heart failure (e.g., dyspnea, fluid in the lungs, abnormal increases in BP or CVP). ▪ Hemoglobin, hematocrit, electrolyte, and serum protein evaluations are necessary during therapy.

Maternal/Child: Category C: safety for use in pregnancy not established. ▪ Safety and effectiveness for use in pediatric patients not established.

DRUG/LAB INTERACTIONS

May cause an **elevated alkaline phosphatase** level.

SIDE EFFECTS

Hypersensitivity and/or pyrogenic reactions can occur. Incidence of toxicity is low when administered with appropriate caution. Slight nausea can occur. Hypotension can be sudden if administered too rapidly.

ANTIDOTE

Notify the physician of all symptoms and side effects. Discontinue infusion for sudden hypotension. Decrease flow rate if indicated and treat symptomatically. Resuscitate as necessary.

POOLED PLASMA (HUMAN)
(**POOLD PLAZ**-ma **HUE**-man)

Plasma replacement and exchange

Octaplas

USUAL DOSE

Administer pooled plasma (Octaplas) based on ABO blood group compatibility.

Pooled Plasma (Octaplas) Dose Guidelines	
Indication	Dose
Replacement of multiple coagulation factors in patients with acquired deficiencies	10 to 15 mL/kg* Adjust dose based on the desired clinical response
Plasma exchange in patients with thrombotic thrombocytopenic purpura (TTP)	1 to 1.5 plasma volumes (40 to 60 mL/kg)†

*Patient's plasma coagulation factor levels should increase by approximately 15% to 25%. If hemostasis is not achieved, use higher doses.

†Completely replace plasma volume removed during plasmapheresis with Octaplas. In general, 1 to 1.5 plasma volumes corresponds to 40 to 60 mL/kg.

DOSE ADJUSTMENTS

Replacement of multiple coagulation factors in patients with acquired deficiencies: Adjust dose based on desired clinical response.

DILUTION

Available as a frozen solution for infusion (specific to blood group A, B, AB, or O) containing 45 to 70 mg human plasma proteins per mL in a 200-mL volume. Administer after thawing using an infusion set with a filter. Avoid shaking.

To thaw in a water bath: Thaw in outer wrapper for up to 30 minutes in a circulating water bath at 30° to 37° C (86° to 98.6° F). An overwrap bag may be used to provide further protection of contents if appropriate. Prevent water from contaminating the entry port. Thawing should not take more than 30 minutes.

To thaw by a dry tempering system: See specific instructions in prescribing information.

Filters: Administration through an in-line filter required.

Storage: Store at −18° C (−0.4° F) or lower, protected from light. Thaw according to manufacturer's instructions. Use thawed product within 12 hours if stored at 2° to 4° C (35.6° to 39.2° F) or within 3 hours if stored at 20° to 25° C (68° to 77° F). Do not refreeze Octaplas. Discard unused product. Discard after expiration date on container label.

COMPATIBILITY

Manufacturer states, "Do not inject drugs containing calcium in the same IV line with Octaplas because precipitates may block the line."

RATE OF ADMINISTRATION

Infusion rate should not exceed 0.020 to 0.025 mmol citrate/kg/min (i.e., less than 1 mL pooled plasma [Octaplas]/kg/min); see Precautions.

ACTIONS

Octaplas replaces human plasma proteins. It is a sterile, pyrogen-free, frozen solution of solvent/detergent (S/D) treated, pooled human plasma. It is manufactured from pooled plasma of a single ABO blood group (A, B, AB, or O). The finished product is tested for coagulation factors II, V, VII, VIII, X, and XI; protein C; protein S; alpha 2-antiplasmin (plasmin inhibitor); fibrinogen; and ADAMTS13. The content and distribution of plasma proteins in Octaplas are comparable to reference ranges for healthy blood donors, except for Protein S and alpha 2-antiplasmin, which are labile to S/D treatment and are controlled to ensure levels in the final product of equal to or greater than 0.4 IU/mL. Coagulation factor activities are controlled to obtain levels within the range of normal human plasma.

INDICATIONS AND USES

Replacement of multiple coagulation factors in patients who have acquired deficiencies due to liver disease or are undergoing cardiac surgery or liver transplant. ▪ Plasma exchange in patients with thrombotic thrombocytopenic purpura (TTP).

CONTRAINDICATIONS

History of hypersensitivity to fresh frozen plasma (FFP) or plasma-derived products, including any plasma protein. ▪ History of hypersensitivity reaction to Octaplas. ▪ IgA deficiency. ▪ Severe deficiency of Protein S.

PRECAUTIONS

Administration of Octaplas must be based on ABO blood group compatibility. Transfusion reactions can occur with ABO blood group mismatches. ▪ Administer in a facility with equipment for monitoring the patient and responding to any medical emergency. ▪ High infusion rates can induce hypervolemia with consequent pulmonary edema or cardiac failure. ▪ Excessive bleeding due to hyperfibrinolysis can occur due to low levels of alpha 2-antiplasmin (plasmin inhibitor). ▪ Thrombosis can occur due to low levels of Protein S. ▪ Citrate toxicity can occur with volumes exceeding 1 mL/kg/min. ▪ Made from human plasma and may contain infectious agents (e.g., HIV, Creutzfeldt-Jakob disease, hepatitis B, hepatitis C). Numerous steps in the manufacturing process are used to make the potential for infection extremely remote. Report suspected infections to manufacturer or FDA.

Monitor: *Replacement of multiple coagulation factors in patients with acquired deficiencies:* Obtain baseline aPTT, PT, and/or specific coagulation factors and monitor response with additional measurements.

All indications: Monitor for S/S of a hypersensitivity reaction (e.g., chest pain, chills, dizziness, dyspnea, fever, flushing, hypotension, nausea, pruritus, rash, urticaria). ▪ Monitor for S/S of pulmonary edema or cardiac failure. ▪ Monitor for S/S of thrombosis in patients at risk. ▪ Monitor for S/S of citrate toxicity (hypocalcemia [e.g., fatigue, muscle spasms, paresthesia]). Potential for citrate toxicity may be increased in patients with impaired hepatic function.

Liver transplant patients: Monitor for S/S of excessive bleeding; may be due to hyperfibrinolysis.

Patient Education: Promptly report S/S of a hypersensitivity reaction (e.g., chest pain, chills, dizziness, dyspnea, fever, flushing, hypotension, nausea, pruritus, rash, urticaria). ▪ Report development of edema or volume overload, including shortness of breath and/or difficulty breathing.

Maternal/Child: Category C: use during pregnancy only if clearly needed. ▪ Use caution in labor and delivery and during breast-feeding; safety and effectiveness unknown. ▪ Safety and effectiveness for use in pediatric patients not evaluated.

Elderly: Safety and effectiveness for use in geriatric patients not evaluated.

DRUG/LAB INTERACTIONS
May form a precipitate with **drugs containing calcium** (e.g., calcium gluconate).

SIDE EFFECTS
Headache, nausea, paresthesia, pruritus, and urticaria are most common. Anaphylactic shock, citrate toxicity, and severe hypotension are the most serious side effects reported.

Post-Marketing: Abdominal pain, alkalosis, bronchospasm, cardiac arrest or failure, chest discomfort or pain, chills, circulatory overload, dyspnea, erythema, fever, hyperfibrinolysis, hypersensitivity reactions (including anaphylaxis), pulmonary edema, rash, respiratory arrest or failure, seroconversions (passive transfer of antibodies), tachycardia, tachypnea, thromboembolism, and vomiting have been reported.

ANTIDOTE
Notify the physician of all side effects. Minor side effects may be tolerated and treated symptomatically. For major side effects (e.g., hypervolemia, hyperfibrinolysis, thrombosis), discontinue Octaplas and treat symptomatically. Treat anaphylaxis immediately with oxygen, epinephrine (Adrenalin), antihistamines (e.g., diphenhydramine [Benadryl]), vasopressors (e.g., dopamine), corticosteroids, albuterol, IV fluids, and ventilation equipment as indicated. Treat citrate toxicity with calcium gluconate IV into another vein. Resuscitate as necessary.

PORFIMER SODIUM
(**POOR**-fih-mer **SO**-dee-um)

Photofrin

Photosensitizing agent
Antineoplastic

pH 7 to 8

USUAL DOSE
A course is a two-stage process requiring administration of both drug and light.

Stage one: Administration of porfimer: A single IV injection of 2 mg/kg. No further injection of porfimer sodium should be given in any one course of therapy.

Stage two: Illumination: Illumination with nonthermal laser light at 40 to 50 hours postinjection.

Esophageal and Endobronchial Cancer
2 mg/kg of porfimer sodium as an IV injection. Approximately 40 to 50 hours after the injection, standard endoscopic techniques are used for light administration and débridement. The laser system must be approved for delivery of a stable power output at a wavelength of 630 ± 3 nm. Light is delivered to the tumor by cylindrical OPTIGUIDE

fiber-optic diffusers passed through the operating channel of an endoscope/bronchoscope. The choice of diffuser tip length depends on the length of the tumor. Diffuser length should be sized to avoid exposure of nonmalignant tissue to light and to prevent overlapping of previously treated malignant tissue. A second laser light application may be given 96 to 120 hours after injection. Before providing a second laser light treatment, the residual tumor should be gently débrided. Vigorous débridement may cause esophageal tumor bleeding; see Precautions.

Up to three courses may be given, but each must be separated by at least 30 days. Evaluate patients with esophageal cancer for the presence of a tracheoesophageal or bronchoesophageal fistula before each course. Evaluate all patients for possible erosion of the tumor into a major blood vessel.

Esophageal cancer: 2 mg/kg of porfimer sodium as an IV injection. A light dose of 300 joules/cm of diffuser length should be delivered by the specific process outlined previously. Light exposure time is set to 12 minutes and 30 seconds. Débridement of tumor may be performed 2 to 3 days later; see Precautions.

Endobronchial non–small-cell lung cancer: 2 mg/kg of porfimer sodium as an IV injection. A light dose of 200 joules/cm of diffuser length should be delivered by the specific process outlined previously. Light exposure time is set to 8 minutes and 20 seconds. Débridement of tumor should be performed 2 to 3 days later; see Precautions.

High-Grade Dysplasia (HGD in Barrett's Esophagus [BE])

2 mg/kg of porfimer sodium as an IV injection. Approximately 40 to 50 hours after the injection, administration of light should be delivered by an X-cell Photodynamic Therapy (PDT) balloon with a fiber-optic diffuser. The choice of fiber-optic/balloon diffuser combination will depend on the length of Barrett's mucosa to be treated (see manufacturer's information). The objective of therapy is to expose and treat all areas of HGD and the entire length of Barrett's esophagus. The light dose administered is 130 joules/cm of diffuser length. Acceptable light intensity for the balloon/diffuser combinations ranges from 200 to 270 mW/cm of diffuser. Treatment time is dependent on the fiber-optic/balloon diffuser combination used (see manufacturer's information). A maximum of 7 cm of esophageal mucosa may be treated at the first light session. If possible, the area treated should include normal tissue margins of a few millimeters at both the proximal and distal ends. Nodules are pretreated at a light dose of 50 joules/cm of diffuser length with a short (2.5 cm) fiber-optic diffuser placed directly against the nodule. A second laser light application may be given to a previously treated segment that shows a "skip" area using a 2.5-cm fiber-optic diffuser at a light dose of 50 joules/cm of the diffuser length. Patients with Barrett's esophagus greater than 7 cm should have the remaining untreated length of Barrett's epithelium treated with a second PDT course at least 90 days later. See Precautions.

Up to 3 courses (each separated by 90 days) may be given to a previously treated segment that still shows high-grade dysplasia, low-grade dysplasia, or Barrett's metaplasia, or to a new segment if the initial Barrett's segment was greater than 7 cm in length.

DOSE ADJUSTMENTS
No adjustments required.

DILUTION
Specific techniques required; see Precautions. Prepare immediately before use. Each vial of porfimer sodium must be reconstituted with 31.8 mL of D5W or NS. Concentration will be 2.5 mg/mL. Shake well until dissolved. An opaque solution; detection of particulate matter by visual inspection is difficult. Withdraw desired dose. Must be protected from bright light and used immediately.

Storage: Store unopened vials at CRT in carton to protect from light.

COMPATIBILITY
Manufacturer states, "Do not mix porfimer sodium with other drugs in the same solution."

RATE OF ADMINISTRATION
A single dose equally distributed over 3 to 5 minutes.

ACTIONS

The first light-activated drug (photosensitizing agent) for use in photodynamic therapy (PDT) to be approved in the United States. Treatment consists of a two-step process involving administration of drug and light. Cytotoxic and antitumor actions are light dependent and oxygen dependent and are the result of the propagation of radical reactions. PDT with porfimer causes direct intracellular damage by initiating radical chain reactions that damage intracellular membranes and mitochondria. After IV infusion of drug, it is allowed to circulate. It accumulates and is retained in tumors, skin, and organs of the reticuloendothelial system (e.g., liver, spleen) while largely clearing from other tissues. Has no apparent effect on tumors until it is activated by selective delivery of light (usually 40 to 50 hours postinfusion). Light activation induces a photochemical, not a thermal, effect that produces an active form of oxygen and releases thromboxane A_2. This process causes vasoconstriction, activation and aggregation of platelets, and increased clotting that contribute to ischemic necrosis leading to tissue and tumor death. The necrotic reaction and associated inflammatory response may evolve over several days. In patients with esophageal cancer, ability to swallow is improved, as is quality of life. Elimination half-life is very prolonged, up to several weeks. Highly protein bound.

INDICATIONS AND USES

Palliative treatment of patients with completely obstructing esophageal cancer or partially obstructing esophageal cancers that are unsuitable for treatment with thermal laser therapy. ▪ Treatment of microinvasive endobronchial non–small-cell lung cancer (NSCLC) in patients for whom surgery and radiotherapy are not indicated. ▪ Reduction of obstruction and palliation of symptoms in patients with completely or partially obstructing endobronchial non–small-cell lung cancer. ▪ Ablation of high-grade dysplasia (HGD) of Barrett's esophagus patients who do not undergo esophagectomy.

Unlabeled uses: Treatment of AIDS-related cutaneous Kaposi's sarcoma, primary or recurrent basal cell carcinoma, and squamous cell carcinoma.

CONTRAINDICATIONS

Known allergies to porphyrins, an existing tracheoesophageal or bronchoesophageal fistula, porphyria, or tumors eroding into a major blood vessel. ▪ Photodynamic therapy (PDT) is not suitable for emergency treatment of patients with severe acute respiratory distress caused by an obstructing endobronchial lesion because 40 to 50 hours are required between injection with porfimer sodium and laser light treatment. ▪ PDT is not suitable for patients with esophageal or gastric varices or for patients with esophageal ulcers greater than 1 cm in diameter.

PRECAUTIONS

Use rubber gloves and eye protection during preparation and administration. Avoid any skin or eye contact since that area will become photosensitive. Wipe up spills with a damp cloth. Dispose of all contaminated materials in a polyethylene bag to avoid accidental contact by others. Protection from light will be necessary if accidental exposure or overexposure occurs. See process in Patient Education. ▪ Administered by or under the direction of the physician specialist with appropriate knowledge of the selected laser system. Facilities for monitoring the patient and responding to any medical emergency must be available. ▪ Requires laser systems and a fiber-optic diffuser to activate. The FDA has approved several photodynamic lasers and the OPTIGUIDE fiber-optic diffuser for use with porfimer sodium. ▪ Avoid exposure of skin and eyes to direct sunlight or bright indoor light; see Patient Education. ▪ Porfimer elimination may be prolonged in patients with hepatic or renal impairment, and they may require longer precautionary measures for photosensitivity. ▪ In the original studies for esophageal tumors, some experienced investigators indicated that natural sloughing action in the esophagus might be sufficient and débridement could needlessly traumatize the area. However, débridement may be performed after each light activation to minimize the potential for obstruction caused by necrotic debris. ▪ A minimum of 4 weeks after completion of radiation therapy is recommended before treatment with PDT. This allows the acute inflammation produced by radiotherapy to subside. ▪ 2 to 4 weeks should be allowed after PDT is complete before beginning any radiotherapy. ▪ Thromboembolic events can occur following PDT with porfimer. More common in patients with other risk factors for thromboembolism (e.g., advanced cancer, cardiovascular disease, after a major surgery, or prolonged immobilization).

Esophageal tumors: Not recommended if the esophageal tumor is eroding into the trachea or bronchial tree; tracheoesophageal or bronchoesophageal fistula may result from treatment. Serious and sometimes fatal gastrointestinal and esophageal necrosis and perforation can occur after treatment. ▪ Use extreme caution in patients with esophageal varices. Light should not be given directly to the variceal area because of the high risk of bleeding.

Endobronchial cancer: Interstitial fiber placement is preferred to intraluminal activation in noncircumferential endobronchial tumors that are soft enough to penetrate. Results in less exposure of the normal bronchial mucosa to light. ▪ Patients with obstructing lung cancer who have received prior radiation therapy or who have tumors that are large, centrally located, cavitating, or extensive and extrinsic to the bronchus have a higher incidence of fatal hemoptysis. ▪ An endobronchial tumor that invades deeply into the bronchial wall may create a fistula as the tumor resolves. ▪ Use with extreme caution in endobronchial tumors located where treatment-induced inflammation could obstruct the airway (e.g., long or circumferential tumors of the trachea, tumors of the carina that involve both mainstem bronchi circumferentially, or circumferential tumors in the mainstem bronchus in patients with prior pneumonectomy).

HGD in Barrett's esophagus: Before initiating treatment with porfimer PDT, a diagnosis of HGD in Barrett's esophagus should be confirmed by a GI pathologist. ▪ Long-term effect of PDT on HGD in Barrett's esophagus is unknown. There may be a risk of leaving cancerous cells behind or of leaving residual abnormal epithelium beneath the new squamous cell epithelium. ▪ Esophageal strictures are a common adverse effect seen in patients treated with PDT for HGD in Barrett's esophagus. Nodule pretreatment and retreatment of the same mucosal segment more than once may influence the risk of developing an esophageal stricture. Usually occur within 6 months following PDT. May be managed with esophageal dilation; several dilations may be required.

Monitor: Obtain baseline CBC and monitor for anemia due to tumor bleeding. ▪ Prevent extravasation at the injection site. Should extravasation occur, area must be protected from light. ▪ Opiates may be required to control pain. ▪ Observe patients carefully; most are critically ill, and many complications could occur. Monitor patients with ***endobronchial tumors*** closely between the laser light therapy and the mandatory débridement bronchoscopy for any evidence of respiratory distress, inflammation, mucositis, or necrotic debris that may cause obstruction of the airway. Immediate bronchoscopy may be required to remove secretions and debris to open the airway. ▪ Monitor for hemoptysis; may be a sign of progressive disease, or may result from resolution of a tumor that has eroded into a pulmonary artery. ▪ In patients who have received PDT for ***HGD in Barrett's esophagus,*** endoscopic biopsy surveillance should be conducted every 3 months until 4 consecutive negative evaluations for HGD have been recorded. Further follow-up should be performed every 6 to 12 months. ▪ Photosensitivity not transferable through skin to caregivers. ▪ See Precautions, Patient Education, and Drug/Lab Interactions.

Patient Education: Must observe precautions to avoid exposure of skin and eyes to direct sunlight or bright indoor light for at least 30 days. Some patients may remain photosensitive for up to 90 or more days. Photosensitivity is due to residual drug, which is present in all parts of the skin. Ambient indoor light is beneficial as it gradually inactivates the remaining drug through a photobleaching reaction. Do not remain in a darkened room. Do expose skin to ambient indoor light. Avoid bright indoor light from examination lamps, dental lamps, operating room lamps, and unshaded light bulbs. Limit time outdoors to necessary excursions, and completely cover body with clothing and shade face before going out. Conventional ultraviolet sunscreens are of no value because photoactivation is caused by visible light, not UV rays. Eyes will be sensitive to sun, bright lights, and car headlights; wear dark sunglasses with an average white light transmittance of less than 4%. After several weeks and before exposing any area of skin to direct sunlight or bright indoor light, test a small area of skin (not the face) for residual photosensitivity. Expose the small area of skin for 10 minutes. If no photosensitivity reaction (redness, swelling, or blistering) occurs within 24 hours, gradually resume normal outdoor activities. Exercise caution and increase skin exposure gradually. If some photosensitivity reaction occurs, continue precautions for 2 more weeks and then retest. Retest level of photosensitivity if traveling to a different geographic area with greater sunshine. ▪ Report chest pain (caused by inflammatory response within the area of treatment); may require prescription pain medication. ▪ Effective contraception necessary for women of childbearing age.

Maternal/Child: Category C: use during pregnancy only if benefits justify potential risk to fetus. Effective contraception necessary for women of childbearing age. Has caused maternal and fetal toxicity in rats and rabbits (increased resorptions, decreased litter size, and reduced fetal body weight). ▪ Discontinue breast-feeding; not known if it is secreted in breast milk, but serious reactions could occur in the infant. ▪ Safety and effectiveness for use in pediatric patients not established.

Elderly: Dose modification based on age is not required.

DRUG/LAB INTERACTIONS

No specific studies have been completed, but the following interactions are likely to occur. ▪ Use with **other photosensitizing agents** (e.g., griseofulvin, fluoroquinolones [e.g., ciprofloxacin (Cipro IV)], phenothiazines [e.g., prochlorperazine (Compazine)], sulfonamides [sulfisoxazole (Gantrisin), ophthalmic solutions (AK-Sulf)], sulfonylurea hypoglycemic agents [tolbutamide], tetracyclines [doxycycline], thiazide diuretics [chlorothiazide (Diuril)]) could increase the photosensitivity reaction. ▪ Antitumor activity may be decreased by **dimethyl sulfoxide, beta-carotene, ethanol, formate, mannitol.** ▪ Antitumor activity may also be decreased by **allopurinol** (Aloprim), **calcium channel blockers** (e.g., diltiazem [Cardizem]), **prostaglandin synthesis inhibitors** (NSAIDs [e.g., ibuprofen (Advil, Motrin), naproxen (Aleve, Naprosyn)]), **and tissue ischemia.** ▪ Effectiveness may be reduced by **drugs that decrease clotting, vasoconstriction** (e.g., nicardipine [Cardene]), **or platelet aggregation** (e.g., dipyridamole [Persantine], ticlopidine [Ticlid]). ▪ **Glucocorticoid hormones** (e.g., dexamethasone [Decadron]) given before or with PDT may reduce the effectiveness of porfimer by inhibiting the production of thromboxane A_2.

SIDE EFFECTS

All diagnoses: May cause constipation. Most toxicities are local effects in the region of illumination and occasionally in surrounding tissues. Usually an inflammatory response induced by the photodynamic effects. Photosensitivity reactions occurred in 20% of patients in clinical studies. Reactions were usually mild to moderate erythema, but also included blisters, burning sensation, itching, and swelling. Less common skin manifestations included increased hair growth, skin discoloration, skin nodules, increased wrinkles, and skin fragility. Cases of fluid imbalance and thromboembolic events have been reported. Cataracts have been reported in one man with a family history of cataracts. Relationship to porfimer sodium unknown.

Post-Marketing: Infusion reactions (bradycardia, dizziness, hypertension, hypotension, urticaria).

Esophageal tumors: Bronchoesophageal or tracheoesophageal fistula can occur as a result of the disease or treatment, including débridement. Abdominal pain, anemia (more prevalent if tumor is located in the lower third of the esophagus), anorexia, arrhythmias (atrial fibrillation [more prevalent if tumor is located in the middle third of the esophagus], tachycardia), candidiasis, chest pain, coughing, dyspepsia, dysphagia, dyspnea, edema, eructation, esophageal edema (more prevalent if tumor is located in the upper third of the esophagus), esophageal tumor bleeding, esophageal stricture, esophagitis, fever, hematemesis, hypertension, hypotension, insomnia, nausea, pleural effusion, and vomiting may occur, as well as numerous others.

Endobronchial tumors: Coughing, dysphagia, dyspnea (may be life threatening), mucositis reaction (e.g., edema, exudate, and mucous plug obstruction), stricture, ulceration. Fatal hemoptysis has occurred (higher incidence in patients who have received radiation therapy).

High-grade dysplasia (HGD in Barrett's esophagus [BE]): Esophageal narrowing and esophageal stricture are common side effects and may require multiple dilations. Other side effects may include abdominal pain, anorexia, anxiety, arthralgia, back pain, chest discomfort or pain, dehydration, depression, diarrhea, dyspepsia, dysphagia, dyspnea, eructation, esophageal pain, fatigue, fever, headache, hiccups, hypertension, infections (bronchitis, sinusitis), insomnia, nausea and vomiting, odynophagia (pain on swallowing), pleural effusion.

ANTIDOTE

If an overdose of porfimer sodium is given, do not give the laser light treatment. Porfimer sodium is not dialyzable. Increased side effects and damage to normal tissue can be expected if an overdose of light is given. Keep physician informed of all side effects; most will be treated symptomatically. Some may be life threatening. Respiratory obstruction may require immediate bronchoscopy and removal of the obstruction with suction or forceps. Stent placement may be required in endobronchial stricture. Chest pain may require the use of opiates.

POSACONAZOLE
(**POE**-sa-**KON**-a-zole)

Noxafil

Antifungal
(azole derivative)

USUAL DOSE

Should be administered via a central venous line (e.g., central venous catheter or peripherally inserted central catheter [PICC]); see Precautions. Duration of treatment is based on recovery from immunosuppression or neutropenia and on clinical response. Obtain baseline electrolytes and correct calcium, magnesium, and potassium deficiencies before initiating posaconazole.

Posaconazole dose: 300 mg as an IV infusion twice a day on the first day. Beginning on the second day, administer 300 mg once each day.

Oral formulations may be substituted when appropriate.

DOSE ADJUSTMENTS

No dose adjustment is required in patients with an estimated glomerular filtration rate (eGFR) of 50 mL/min or greater; however, the intravenous vehicle Betadex Sulfobutyl Ether Sodium (SBECD) accumulates in patients with an eGFR of less than 50 mL/min. Use of oral posaconazole is recommended in these patients; see Precautions and Monitor. ■ No dose adjustment recommended in patients with mild to severe hepatic impairment (Child-Pugh Class A, B, or C); however, specific studies have not been conducted. ■ No dose adjustment indicated based on age or gender. ■ Patients weighing more than 120 kg may have lower posaconazole levels. Monitor for breakthrough fungal infections.

DILUTION

Bring the 300-mg vial of posaconazole solution to RT. Aseptically transfer the contents of the vial (16.7 mL [18 mg/mL]) to a bag or bottle of ½NS, NS, D5W, D5½NS, D5NS, or D5W with 20 mEq KCl. Final concentration should be 1 to 2 mg/mL. Solution will be colorless to yellow.

Filters: Must be administered through a 0.22-micron polyethersulfone (PES) or polyvinylidene difluoride (PVDF) filter.

Storage: Refrigerate unopened vials at 2° to 8° C (36° to 46° F). Contains no preservatives; immediate use of the admixed product is preferred, but it may be refrigerated for up to 24 hours. Discard any unused solution.

COMPATIBILITY

Posaconazole and coadministered drug products should be prepared only in the solutions listed under Dilution. Use of other infusion solutions may result in particulate formation. Do not coadminister any products or diluents that are not listed by the manufacturer.

Manufacturer states that posaconazole is **compatible** with and can be infused at the same time through the same IV line **(Y-site)** as the following products prepared in D5W or NS: amikacin, caspofungin (Cancidas), ciprofloxacin (Cipro IV), daptomycin (Cubicin), dobutamine, famotidine (Pepcid), filgrastim (Neupogen), gentamicin, hydromorphone (Dilaudid), levofloxacin (Levaquin), lorazepam (Ativan), meropenem (Merrem IV), micafungin (Mycamine), morphine, norepinephrine (Levophed), potassium chloride, and vancomycin (Vancocin).

Manufacturer states that posaconazole is **incompatible** with and must not be diluted with LR, D5LR, and 4.2% sodium bicarbonate.

RATE OF ADMINISTRATION

Do not administer as an IV bolus. Administer through a 0.22-micron polyethersulfone (PES) or polyvinylidene difluoride (PVDF) filter.

Central venous catheter: Each dose as an IV infusion equally distributed over 90 minutes. **Single or initial dose (if a central venous catheter is not available):** A single dose as an IV infusion equally distributed over 30 minutes.

ACTIONS

An azole antifungal agent. It blocks the synthesis of ergosterol, a key component of the fungal cell membrane, by inhibiting the cytochrome P_{450}–dependent enzyme lanosterol 14α-demethylase, which is responsible for the conversion of lanosterol to ergosterol. The depletion of ergosterol results in weakening of the structure and function of the fungal cell membrane (antifungal activity). Primarily circulates as the parent compound in plasma. Highly bound to human plasma proteins, predominantly albumin. Primarily metabolized via UDP glucuronidation and is a substrate for p-glycoprotein (P-gp) efflux. Mean terminal half-life is 27 hours. Primarily eliminated in feces as parent compound. Some minor excretion of metabolites occurs in urine and feces.

INDICATIONS AND USES

Prophylaxis of invasive *Aspergillus* and *Candida* infections in patients 18 years of age and older who are at high risk for developing these infections due to being severely immunocompromised, such as hematopoietic stem cell transplant (HSCT) recipients with graft-versus-host disease (GVHD) or patients with hematologic malignancies with prolonged neutropenia from chemotherapy.

CONTRAINDICATIONS

Known hypersensitivity to posaconazole or other azole antifungal agents. ▪ Concomitant administration with sirolimus. ▪ Concomitant administration with CYP3A4 substrates that prolong the QT interval (e.g., pimozide [Orap], quinidine). ▪ Coadministration with HMG-CoA reductase inhibitors primarily metabolized through CYP3A4 (e.g., atorvastatin [Lipitor], lovastatin [Mevacor], simvastatin [Zocor]). ▪ Coadministration with ergot alkaloids (e.g., ergotamine [Ergomar], dihydroergotamine [D.H.E.]). ▪ See Drug/Lab Interactions.

PRECAUTIONS

Should be administered via a central venous line (e.g., central venous catheter or peripherally inserted central catheter [PICC]). If necessary, the initial dose may be administered through a peripheral IV line in advance of central venous line placement or to bridge the period during which a central venous line is replaced or is in use for other treatment. In clinical trials, multiple peripheral infusions resulted in infusion site reactions. *Do not administer as an IV bolus.* ▪ Avoid use in patients with moderate or severe renal impairment (eGFR less than 50 mL/min) unless an assessment of the benefit versus risk to the patient justifies use; see Dose Adjustments. ▪ Concomitant administration with cyclosporine (Sandimmune) or tacrolimus (Prograf) increases the whole blood trough concentrations of these calcineurin inhibitors; see Drug/Lab Interactions. Nephrotoxicity and leukoencephalopathy (including deaths) have been reported in patients with elevated cyclosporine or tacrolimus concentrations. ▪ Has been associated with prolongation of the QT interval. Torsades de pointes has been reported. Use with caution in patients with potentially proarrhythmic conditions. Do not administer with drugs that are known to prolong the QTc interval and are metabolized through CYP3A4. Correct electrolyte abnormalities before administration. ▪ Hepatic toxicity (e.g., mild to moderate elevations in ALT, AST, alkaline phosphatase, total bilirubin, and/or clinical hepatitis) has been reported. Cases of more severe hepatic reactions, including cholestasis or hepatic failure (including deaths), have been reported in patients with serious underlying medical conditions (e.g., hematologic malignancy). Consider discontinuing posaconazole in patients who develop S/S of hepatic toxicity. ▪ Use with midazolam (Versed) may prolong hypnotic and sedative effects of midazolam; see Drug/Lab Interactions. Benzodiazepine receptor antagonists should be available (e.g., flumazenil [Romazicon]). ▪ Hypersensitivity reactions have been reported. ▪ Cross-resistance between azoles may occur; clinical significance unknown.

Monitor: Rigorous attempts to correct calcium, magnesium, and potassium should be made before starting posaconazole. ▪ Obtain baseline CBC, platelets, serum creatinine, and electrolytes. Monitor as indicated during therapy; however, monitor electrolytes frequently. ▪ Obtain baseline liver function tests and monitor throughout treatment. If elevations in ALT, AST, alkaline phosphatase, or total bilirubin occur, monitor for S/S of more severe hepatic injury. ▪ Monitor serum creatinine levels closely in patients with moderate or severe renal impairment who receive posaconazole. ▪ Monitor for S/S of hypersensitivity reactions (e.g., chest pain, dizziness, dyspnea, fever, flushing, hypotension, nausea, pruritus, rash, rigors, urticaria). ▪ Closely monitor patients weighing more than 120 kg for breakthrough fungal infections, they may have lower posaconazole plasma drug exposure. ▪ See Drug/Lab Interactions.

Patient Education: Review of health history and complete medication profile, including over-the-counter medicines, vitamins, and herbal supplements, is imperative. ▪ Do not start a new medicine without consulting your health care provider. ▪ Review FDA-approved Patient Information. ▪ Use of nonhormonal birth control may be indicated. ▪ Promptly report S/S of a hypersensitivity reaction (e.g., itching, hives, shortness of breath). ▪ Promptly report S/S of liver toxicity (e.g., feeling very tired, flu-like symptoms, itchy skin, nausea or vomiting, yellowing of the eyes). ▪ Additional precautions may be required with transfer to oral posaconazole.

Maternal/Child: Use during pregnancy only if benefits justify potential risk to fetus. ▪ Discontinue breast-feeding. ▪ Safety and effectiveness for use in pediatric patients under 18 years of age not established.

Elderly: Safety profile similar to younger adults; dose adjustment not indicated.

DRUG/LAB INTERACTIONS

Interactions are numerous. Review of drug profile by pharmacist imperative.

Primarily metabolized via **UDP glucuronosyltransferase** and is a **substrate of p-glycoprotein** (P-gp) efflux. Inhibitors or inducers of these clearance pathways may affect posaconazole plasma concentrations. ▪ A strong **inhibitor of CYP3A4**. May increase plasma concentrations of drugs predominantly metabolized by CYP3A4. ▪ Concomitant administration with **sirolimus** is **contraindicated.** Blood concentrations of sirolimus may be increased approximately ninefold and result in sirolimus toxicity. ▪ Concomitant administration with **CYP3A4 substrates that prolong the QT interval** (e.g., pimozide [Orap], quinidine) is **contraindicated.** May result in increased plasma concentrations of the CYP3A4 substrates, leading to QTc prolongation and torsades de pointes. ▪ Coadministration with **HMG-CoA reductase inhibitors primarily metabolized through CYP3A4** (e.g., atorvastatin [Lipitor], lovastatin [Mevacor], simvastatin [Zocor]) is **contraindicated.** Increased plasma concentrations of these drugs can lead to rhabdomyolysis. ▪ Coadministration with **ergot alkaloids** (e.g., ergotamine [Ergomar], dihydroergotamine [D.H.E.]) is **contraindicated.** Increased plasma concentration of ergot alkaloids may lead to ergotism. ▪ Concomitant administration with **cyclosporine** (Sandimmune) or **tacrolimus** (Prograf) increases the whole blood trough concentrations of these calcineurin-inhibitors. Reduce dose of cyclosporine to approximately three fourths of the original dose and reduce the dose of tacrolimus to approximately one third of the original dose. Monitor concentrations frequently. ▪ Concomitant use with **midazolam** (Versed) increases midazolam plasma concentrations by approximately five-fold and prolongs the hypnotic and sedative effects of midazolam. **Other benzodiazepines** metabolized by CYP3A4 (e.g., alprazolam [Xanax], triazolam [Halcion]) could also result in increased plasma concentrations. If concomitant administration of these drugs with posaconazole is indicated, monitor patients closely, and a benzodiazepine receptor antagonist (e.g., flumazenil [Romazicon]) should be available. ▪ **Efavirenz** (Sustiva), **rifabutin** (Mycobutin), and **phenytoin** (Dilantin) induce UDP-glucuronidase and significantly decrease posaconazole plasma concentrations. Avoid concomitant use unless benefit outweighs risks. Monitor patients for breakthrough fungal infections. ▪ **Rifabutin** (Mycobutin) is metabolized by CYP3A4; coadministration with posaconazole increases rifabutin plasma concentrations. If concomitant administration is indicated, monitor closely for breakthrough fungal infections and monitor full blood counts to avoid side effects (e.g., uveitis, leukopenia) from increased rifabutin plasma concentrations. ▪ **Phenytoin** (Dilantin) is metabolized by CYP3A4; coadministration with posaconazole increases phenytoin plasma concentrations. If concomitant administration is indicated, monitor closely for breakthrough fungal infections and monitor phenytoin concentrations frequently. Consider dose reduction of phenytoin. ▪ **Atazanavir** (Reyataz) and **ritonavir** (Norvir) are metabolized by CYP3A4, and posaconazole increases their plasma concentrations. Monitor frequently for adverse effects and toxicity of atazanavir and ritonavir if coadministration is indicated. ▪ Concomitant administration with **fosamprenavir** (Lexiva) may decrease posaconazole plasma concentrations; monitoring for breakthrough fungal infections is recommended. ▪ **Vinca alkaloids** (e.g., vincristine, vinblastine) are substrates of CYP3A4; posaconazole may increase their plasma concentrations, leading to neurotoxicity. Consider dose adjustment of the vinca alkaloid. ▪ Posaconazole may increase the plasma concentrations of **calcium channel blockers** metabolized by CYP3A4 (e.g., diltiazem [Cardizem], felodipine [Plendil], nicardipine [Cardene], nifedipine [Procardia], verapamil [Calan]). If coadministration is indicated, monitor frequently for side effects associated with calcium channel blockers. Dose reduction of the calcium channel blocker may be indicated. ▪ May increase plasma concentrations of **digoxin** (Lanoxin). Monitor digoxin plasma concentrations during coadministration. ▪ Dose adjustment is not required with coadministration of **glipizide** (Glucotrol); however, monitoring of serum glucose is recommended.

SIDE EFFECTS

Diarrhea, fever, hypokalemia, and nausea and vomiting are most common. Most serious side effects include arrhythmias and QT prolongation, hepatic toxicity, and hypersensitivity (including anaphylaxis). Abdominal pain, anemia, chills, constipation, cough, decreased appetite, dyspnea, epistaxis, fatigue, headache, hypertension, hypomagnesemia, peripheral edema, petechiae, rash, and thrombocytopenia have also been reported.

ANTIDOTE

Notify physician of all side effects; most will be treated symptomatically. If a hypersensitivity reaction occurs, discontinue the infusion and treat with oxygen, epinephrine, antihistamines (e.g., diphenhydramine [Benadryl]), corticosteroids (e.g., dexamethasone [Decadron]), or bronchodilators (e.g., albuterol) as indicated. Consider discontinuation of posaconazole if liver function tests are elevated and/or clinical S/S of liver disease attributable to posaconazole develop. No known specific antidote. Not removed by hemodialysis. Resuscitate as indicated.

POTASSIUM ACETATE AND POTASSIUM CHLORIDE

(po-**TASS**-ee-um **AS**-ah-tayt,
po-**TASS**-ee-um **KLOR**-eyed)

Electrolyte replenisher
Antihypokalemic

pH 4 to 8

USUAL DOSE

Concentrated potassium solutions must be diluted before administration; direct injection of any concentrated solution can be instantly fatal.
Dose and rate of administration are dependent on specific patient condition.

Normal daily requirements: *Adults:* 40 to 80 mEq/24 hr.

Starting dose based on losses, desired replacement, or maintenance. 20 to 60 mEq/24 hr. 200 mEq/24 hr is usually not exceeded. Up to 400 mEq/24 hr has been given in selected situations (e.g., serum potassium less than 2 mEq/L) with extreme caution. Potassium acetate may contain up to 200 mcg/L of aluminum; see Precautions.

PEDIATRIC DOSE

Normal daily requirements: *Newborn:* 2 to 6 mEq/kg/24 hr. *Other pediatric patients:* 2 to 3 mEq/kg/24 hr.

1 to 4 mEq/kg of body weight/24 hr. Do not exceed 40 mEq/day. Potassium acetate may contain up to 200 mcg/L of aluminum; see Precautions and Maternal/Child.

DOSE ADJUSTMENTS

Reduce dose in impaired renal function. ▪ Lower-end initial doses may be appropriate in the elderly based on potential for decreased organ function and concomitant disease or drug therapy.

DILUTION

Each individual dose must be diluted in a larger volume of suitable IV solution and given as an infusion. Check labels for aluminum content; see Precautions. Soluble in commonly used IV solutions; see chart on inside back cover. 40 mEq/L is the preferred dilution. 80 mEq/L is the usual maximum concentration and must be administered with caution. In replacement therapy more concentrated doses may be used and must be administered with extreme caution. 40 mEq/100 mL is commonly used and must be controlled by an infusion pump. *Up to 100 mEq/100 mL has been administered through a central line (to avoid phlebitis); must be controlled by an infusion pump.* **Direct injection of any concentrated solution can be instantly fatal.** Avoid layering of potassium by thoroughly agitating the prepared IV solution. Do not add potassium to an IV bottle in the hanging position; remove from hanger to guarantee dispersion throughout solution. In severe hypokalemia, solutions without dextrose are preferred (dextrose might decrease serum potassium level). Use only clear solutions.

COMPATIBILITY
(Underline Indicates Conflicting Compatibility Information)

Consider any drug NOT listed as compatible to be INCOMPATIBLE until consulting a pharmacist; specific conditions may apply.

One source suggests the following **compatibilities:**

POTASSIUM ACETATE

Additive: Metoclopramide (Reglan).

Y-site: Ciprofloxacin (Cipro IV).

POTASSIUM CHLORIDE

Additive: <u>Amikacin,</u> aminophylline, amiodarone (Nexterone), atracurium (Tracrium), calcium gluconate, cefepime (Maxipime), ceftazidime (Fortaz), chloramphenicol (Chloromycetin), ciprofloxacin (Cipro IV), clindamycin (Cleocin), cytarabine (ARA-C), dimenhydrinate, <u>dobutamine,</u> dopamine, enalaprilat (Vasotec IV), erythromycin (Erythrocin), fluconazole (Diflucan), foscarnet (Foscavir), fosphenytoin (Cerebyx), furosemide (Lasix), heparin, hydrocortisone sodium succinate (Solu-Cortef), hydromorphone (Dilaudid), isoproterenol (Isuprel), lidocaine, magnesium sulfate, methyldopa, metoclopramide (Reglan), mitoxantrone (Novantrone), nafcillin (Nallpen), nicardipine (Cardene

IV), norepinephrine (Levophed), oxacillin (Bactocill), penicillin G potassium, penicillin G sodium, phenylephrine (Neo-Synephrine), ranitidine (Zantac), sodium bicarbonate, vancomycin, verapamil.

Y-site: Acetaminophen (Ofirmev), acyclovir (Zovirax), aldesleukin (Proleukin), allopurinol (Aloprim), amifostine (Ethyol), aminophylline, amiodarone (Nexterone), ampicillin, anidulafungin (Eraxis), atropine, aztreonam (Azactam), bivalirudin (Angiomax), calcium gluconate, caspofungin (Cancidas), ceftaroline (Teflaro), chlorpromazine (Thorazine), ciprofloxacin (Cipro IV), cisatracurium (Nimbex), cladribine (Leustatin), dexamethasone (Decadron), dexmedetomidine (Precedex), digoxin (Lanoxin), diltiazem (Cardizem), diphenhydramine (Benadryl), dobutamine, docetaxel (Taxotere), dopamine, doripenem (Doribax), doxorubicin liposomal (Doxil), droperidol (Inapsine), edrophonium (Enlon), enalaprilat (Vasotec IV), epinephrine (Adrenalin), ertapenem (Invanz), esmolol (Brevibloc), estrogens, conjugated (Premarin), ethacrynic acid (Edecrin), etoposide phosphate (Etopophos), famotidine (Pepcid IV), fenoldopam (Corlopam), fentanyl, filgrastim (Neupogen), fludarabine (Fludara), fluorouracil (5-FU), furosemide (Lasix), gallium nitrate (Ganite), gemcitabine (Gemzar), gentamicin, granisetron (Kytril), heparin, hetastarch in electrolytes (Hextend), hydralazine, 6% hydroxyethyl starch (Voluven), idarubicin (Idamycin), indomethacin (Indocin IV), isoproterenol (Isuprel), labetalol, levofloxacin (Levaquin), lidocaine, linezolid (Zyvox), lorazepam (Ativan), magnesium sulfate, melphalan (Alkeran), meperidine (Demerol), meropenem (Merrem IV), methylprednisolone (Solu-Medrol), micafungin (Mycamine), midazolam (Versed), milrinone (Primacor), morphine, neostigmine, nicardipine (Cardene IV), nitroprusside sodium, norepinephrine (Levophed), ondansetron (Zofran), oxacillin (Bactocill), oxaliplatin (Eloxatin), oxytocin (Pitocin), paclitaxel (Taxol), palonosetron (Aloxi), pantoprazole (Protonix IV), pemetrexed (Alimta), penicillin G potassium, pentazocine (Talwin), phytonadione (vitamin K$_1$), piperacillin/tazobactam (Zosyn), procainamide (Pronestyl), prochlorperazine (Compazine), promethazine (Phenergan), propofol (Diprivan), propranolol, quinupristin/dalfopristin (Synercid in KCl 40 mEq/L), remifentanil (Ultiva), sargramostim (Leukine), sodium bicarbonate, succinylcholine, tacrolimus (Prograf), telavancin (Vibativ), teniposide (Vumon), theophylline, thiotepa, tigecycline (Tygacil), tirofiban (Aggrastat), vinorelbine (Navelbine), warfarin (Coumadin), zidovudine (AZT, Retrovir).

RATE OF ADMINISTRATION

A maximum of 10 mEq/hr of potassium chloride in any given amount of infusion fluid should not be exceeded. With serious potassium depletion (under 2 mEq/L serum), 20 to 40 mEq/hr has been given with extreme caution. Use of an infusion pump is recommended in all situations and required with any dose exceeding 60 mEq/24 hr. Too-rapid infusion of hypertonic solutions may cause local pain and, rarely, vein irritation. Adjust rate of administration according to patient tolerance.

Pediatric rate: 0.5 to 1 mEq/kg/hr. Do not exceed 10 mEq/hr.

ACTIONS

Potassium: Principal cation of intracellular fluid. Important for maintenance of body fluid composition and electrolyte balance. Participates in carbohydrate utilization and protein synthesis. Critical in the regulation of nerve conduction and muscle contraction, particularly in the heart. The normal serum potassium range is 3.5 to 5 mEq/L. The kidney normally regulates potassium balance but does not conserve potassium balance as well as or as promptly as it conserves sodium. Excreted in urine.

Chloride: The major extracellular anion. Closely follows the metabolism of sodium. Changes in the acid-base balance of the body are reflected by the changes in chloride concentration.

Acetate: An alternate source of bicarbonate by metabolic conversion in the liver.

INDICATIONS AND USES

Prophylaxis or treatment of potassium deficiency (e.g., hypokalemia due to diuretic therapy, adjunct to treatment of digoxin toxicity, low dietary potassium intake, vomiting and diarrhea, diabetic acidosis, metabolic alkalosis, corticosteroid therapy, increased renal excretion resulting from acidosis, hemodialysis). ▪ Utilized when oral replacement therapy is not feasible.

CONTRAINDICATIONS
Any disease or condition in which high potassium levels may occur through potassium retention or other processes (e.g., acute dehydration, adrenocortical insufficiency [untreated Addison's disease]), adynamica episodica hereditaria [periodic loss of strength or weakness], anuria, azotemia, crush syndrome, heat cramps, hyperkalemia from any cause, oliguria, patients taking digoxin with severe or complete heart block, postoperative oliguria (early [except during GI drainage]), renal failure, severe hemolytic reactions.

PRECAUTIONS
Impaired renal function or adrenal insufficiency can cause potassium intoxication, which can develop rapidly and without symptoms. ▪ Loss of chloride usually accompanies potassium depletion and may cause hypochloremic alkalosis. Treat cause of potassium depletion in addition to giving potassium. ▪ Potassium phosphate is preferred for specific intracellular deficiency not caused by alkalosis, since phosphate is the usual ion attached to potassium in the body. Not used in the presence of kidney failure. ▪ Alkalyzing potassiums (e.g., acetate, citrate) are preferred for potassium-deficient patients with renal tubular acidosis. Metabolic acidosis and hyperchloremia are most likely present. ▪ Use potassium acetate with caution in patients with metabolic or respiratory alkalosis and in patients with severe hepatic insufficiency. ▪ Administration of IV solutions can cause fluid and/or solute overload, resulting in dilution of serum electrolyte concentrations, overhydration, congested states, or pulmonary edema. The risk of dilutional states is inversely proportional to the electrolyte concentration (increased fluids may dilute electrolyte concentration). The risk of solute overload causing congested states with peripheral and pulmonary edema is directly proportional to the electrolyte concentration (higher electrolytes pull in fluid, leading to fluid overload). ▪ Use solutions containing potassium with caution in patients with cardiac disease, particularly in the presence of renal disease. Cardiac monitoring is recommended. ▪ Some solutions of potassium may contain aluminum. In impaired kidney function, aluminum may reach toxic levels. Premature neonates are particularly at risk because of their immature kidneys and requirement for calcium and phosphate, which also contain aluminum. Research indicates that patients with impaired renal function who receive more than 4 to 5 mcg/kg/day of parenteral aluminum are at risk for developing CNS or bone toxicity associated with aluminum accumulation.

Monitor: Monitor changes in fluid balance, electrolyte concentration, and acid-base balance (e.g., serum potassium, sodium, chloride, bicarbonate, urinary output, pH). Only extracellular potassium can be measured; intracellular potassium equals 98% of total body potassium. Entire clinical picture must be considered. ▪ Potassium replacement should be monitored whenever possible by continuous or serial ECG, especially in patients taking digoxin. Serum potassium levels are not necessarily dependable indicators of tissue potassium levels. ▪ Continuous cardiac monitoring is preferable for infusion of over 10 mEq of potassium in 1 hour. ▪ Confirm absolute patency of vein. Extravasation will cause necrosis. Local pain and phlebitis may occur with concentrations greater than 40 mEq/L. ▪ See Drug/Lab Interactions.

Patient Education: Report burning or stinging at IV site promptly.

Maternal/Child: Category C: effect unknown; use caution and only if clearly needed in pregnancy and breast-feeding. ▪ Safety and effectiveness for use of KCl in pediatric patients not established. However, use for treatment of potassium deficiency when oral therapy is not feasible is referenced in medical literature. Safety and effectiveness of potassium acetate for use in pediatric patients have been established.

Elderly: See Dose Adjustments. Monitoring of renal function suggested. ▪ Increased risk of hyperkalemia.

DRUG/LAB INTERACTIONS

Potentiated by **angiotensin-converting enzyme inhibitors** (e.g., captopril, enalapril [Vasotec], lisinopril [Zestril]) and **angiotensin receptor blockers** (e.g., losartan [Cozaar], valsartan [Diovan]); risk of hyperkalemia increased. ▪ Digitalis intoxication may occur with hypokalemia. Use caution if discontinuing potassium after stabilization in patients taking **digoxin.** ▪ **Potassium-sparing diuretics** (e.g., spironolactone [Aldactone], triamterene [Dyrenium], amiloride [Midamor], and a component of Dyazide and Maxzide) may cause hyperkalemia.

SIDE EFFECTS

Abdominal pain, diarrhea, nausea, and vomiting are common side effects of potassium administration and may progress to potassium intoxication. Extravasation, fever, hyperkalemia, hypervolemia, infection or pain at the site of injection, phlebitis, or venous thrombosis may occur.

Potassium intoxication: Areflexia (absence of reflexes), cardiac arrest, cardiac arrhythmias (e.g., bradycardia, ventricular fibrillation), ECG abnormalities (including increased amplitude of T wave, decreased amplitude of R wave, below-baseline depression of S wave, disappearing P wave, PR prolongation), heart block, hypotension, mental confusion, muscular or respiratory paralysis, paresthesias of the extremities, weakness. Progression of side effects may cause death.

Potassium deficit: Disruption of neuromuscular function, intestinal ileus, and dilatation.

ANTIDOTE

For any side effect, discontinue the drug and notify the physician. Death may result from potassium levels of 8 mEq/L. For severe hyperkalemia (over 6.5 mEq/L plasma), use IV sodium bicarbonate 40 to 160 mEq over 5 minutes to correct acidosis. Repeat in 10 to 15 minutes if ECG still abnormal. Initially, one ampule of 50% dextrose may be given into a large vein. Follow with IV dextrose, 10% to 25%, containing 10 units of regular insulin per 20 Gm of dextrose and infuse at 300 to 500 mL over 1 hour. 150 mL of $1/6$ M sodium lactate is rarely used as a substitute. Eliminate potassium-containing foods and medicines. Monitor ECG continuously. If P waves are absent, give calcium gluconate or chloride 0.5 to 1 Gm over 2 minutes (exceeds usual rate of administration). Do not use if patient is receiving digoxin. All of these measures cause a shift of potassium into the cells and may be used simultaneously. Sodium polystyrene sulfonate (Kayexalate) orally or as retention enemas is used to actually remove potassium from the body. Hemodialysis or peritoneal dialysis may be useful. Use caution in the digitalized patient; too-rapid removal of potassium may cause digoxin toxicity. Resuscitate as necessary. For extravasation, apply warm, moist compresses.

PRALATREXATE

(pral-a-**TREX**-ate)

Folotyn

Antineoplastic
(Antifolate)

pH 7.5 to 8.5

USUAL DOSE

Premedication: 10 days before starting pralatrexate, begin folic acid 1 to 1.25 mg PO daily. Continue daily throughout the full course of therapy and for 30 days after the last dose of pralatrexate. Administer vitamin B_{12} (1 mg) IM within the 10 weeks before starting pralatrexate and every 8 to 10 weeks thereafter. Subsequent vitamin B_{12} injections may be given the same day as pralatrexate.

Pralatrexate: 30 mg/M^2 by IV push over 3 to 5 minutes via the side port of a free-flowing infusion of NS. Administer once weekly for 6 weeks in 7-week cycles until progressive disease or unacceptable toxicity occurs. Management of severe or intolerable side effects may require dose omission or reduction or interruption of therapy; see Dose Adjustments.

DOSE ADJUSTMENTS

Before administering any dose of pralatrexate, mucositis should be equal to or less than Grade 1, platelet count should be equal to or more than 100,000 cells/mm³ for the first dose and equal to or greater than 50,000 cells/mm³ for all subsequent doses, and the absolute neutrophil count (ANC) should be equal to or greater than 1,000 cells/mm³. Doses may be omitted or reduced based on patient tolerance. Do not make up omitted doses at the end of the cycle, and do not re-escalate once a dose reduction occurs for toxicity. See the following charts for dose modifications based on patient symptoms.

Guidelines for Pralatrexate Dose Modifications for Mucositis		
Mucositis Grade* on Day of Treatment	Action	Dose on Recovery to ≤ Grade 1
Grade 2	Omit dose	Continue prior dose
Grade 2 recurrence	Omit dose	20 mg/M^2
Grade 3	Omit dose	20 mg/M^2
Grade 4	Stop therapy	

*Per National Cancer Institute Common Terminology Criteria for Adverse Events (NCI CTCAE), Version 4.0.

Guidelines for Pralatrexate Dose Modifications for Hematologic Toxicities			
Blood Count on Day of Treatment	Duration of Toxicity	Action	Dose on Restart
Platelets <50,000/mm³	1 week	Omit dose	Continue prior dose
	2 weeks	Omit dose	20 mg/M^2
	3 weeks	Stop therapy	
ANC 500 to 1,000/mm³ and no fever	1 week	Omit dose	Continue prior dose
ANC 500 to 1,000/mm³ with fever or ANC <500/mm³	1 week	Omit dose, give G-CSF or GM-CSF support	Continue prior dose with G-CSF or GM-CSF support
	2 weeks or recurrence	Omit dose, give G-CSF or GM-CSF support	20 mg/M^2 with G-CSF or GM-CSF support
	3 weeks or 2nd recurrence	Stop therapy	

Continued

Guidelines for Pralatrexate Dose Modifications for All Other Treatment-Related Toxicities		
Toxicity Grade* on Day of Treatment	Action	Dose Upon Recovery to ≤ Grade 2
Grade 3	Omit dose	20 mg/M²
Grade 4	Stop therapy	

*Per National Cancer Institute Common Terminology Criteria for Adverse Events (NCI CTCAE), Version 4.0.

DILUTION

Specific techniques for handling required; see Precautions. A clear yellow solution. *Do Not Dilute.* Aseptically withdraw the calculated dose directly into a syringe for immediate use. Available in vials containing 20 mg or 40 mg. Concentration of both is 20 mg/mL.

Filters: Specific information not available.

Storage: Refrigerate vials at 2° to 8° C (36° to 46° F) in original carton to protect from light until use. Unopened vial(s) are stable in original carton at RT for up to 72 hours. Discard if left at RT for more than 72 hours.

COMPATIBILITY

Manufacturer recommends administration via the side port of a free-flowing infusion of NS.

RATE OF ADMINISTRATION

A single dose by IV push over 3 to 5 minutes via the side port of a free-flowing infusion of NS.

ACTIONS

A folate analog metabolic inhibitor. It interferes with the growth of and leads to the destruction of cancer cells. It competitively inhibits dihydrofolate reductase and folylpolyglutamyl synthetase. This inhibition results in the depletion of thymidine and other biologic molecules. May also affect healthy cells. Approximately 67% bound to plasma proteins. Half-life is 12 to 18 hours. Some drug excreted unchanged in urine (approximately 31%).

INDICATIONS AND USES

Treatment of patients with relapsed or refractory peripheral T-cell lymphoma (PTCL).

CONTRAINDICATIONS

Manufacturer states, "None."

PRECAUTIONS

Follow guidelines for handling cytotoxic agents; see Appendix A, p. 1331. ■ Administered under the direction of a physician knowledgeable in its use and in a facility with adequate diagnostic and treatment facilities to monitor the patients and respond to any medical emergency. ■ Bone marrow suppression can occur (e.g., anemia, neutropenia, and thrombocytopenia). Dose modification based on ANC and platelet count is required before each dose; see Dose Adjustments. ■ May cause mucositis; see Dose Adjustments. ■ To potentially reduce treatment-related hematologic toxicity and mucositis, folic acid and vitamin B₁₂ supplementation is required. ■ Severe dermatologic reactions, including skin exfoliation, toxic epidermal necrolysis, and ulceration, have been reported. May increase in severity with continued treatment, may involve skin and subcutaneous sites of known lymphoma, and may result in death. ■ Tumor lysis syndrome has been reported. ■ Has not been studied in patients with moderate to severe renal impairment. May be at greater risk for increased exposure and toxicity; administer with caution. ■ Serious drug reactions, including toxic epidermal necrolysis and mucositis, were reported in patients with ESRD undergoing dialysis. ■ Avoid pralatrexate use in patients with ESRD, including those undergoing dialysis, unless the potential benefit justifies the potential risk. ■ Can cause hepatic toxicity and liver function abnormalities. Persistent liver function test abnormalities may be indicators of liver toxicity. Has not been studied in patients with hepatic impairment, and patients with selected liver test elevations were excluded from clinical trials.

Monitor: Obtain baseline CBC and platelets and serum chemistry tests, including renal and hepatic function. Monitor CBC and platelets and severity of mucositis weekly before each dose. Repeat serum chemistry tests, including renal and hepatic function, before the start of the first and fourth dose of a given cycle. ▪ Monitor patients with moderate to severe renal function closely. Adjust dose accordingly; see Dose Adjustments. ▪ Monitor patients with elevated liver enzymes closely (e.g., AST, ALT, transaminases). If liver function test abnormalities are greater than or equal to Grade 3, omit or modify dose; see Dose Adjustments. ▪ Observe for S/S of skin reactions (e.g., blisters, peeling and loss of skin, rash, sores); see Antidote. ▪ Monitor closely for S/S of tumor lysis syndrome (e.g., flank pain, hematuria, hyperkalemia, hyperphosphatemia, hyperuricemia, hypocalcemia, metabolic acidosis, urate crystalluria, and renal failure) and treat as appropriate. Allopurinol and alkalinization of urine may be indicated for prevention and/or treatment of hyperuricemia. ▪ Monitor for thrombocytopenia (platelet count less than $50,000/mm^3$). Initiate precautions to prevent excessive bleeding (e.g., inspect IV sites, skin, and mucous membranes; use extreme care during invasive procedures; test urine, emesis, stool, and secretions for occult blood). ▪ Use prophylactic antiemetics to reduce nausea and/or vomiting and increase patient comfort. ▪ Observe closely for signs of infection. Prophylactic antibiotics may be indicated pending results of C/S in a febrile neutropenic patient.

Patient Education: A patient information guide is available from the manufacturer. ▪ Avoid pregnancy; nonhormonal birth control is recommended. ▪ Blood counts will be required at regular intervals. ▪ Take folic acid and vitamin B_{12} as prescribed to help reduce side effects. ▪ Report soreness in the mouth, redness of mucous membranes, difficulty swallowing, or ulcerations in the mouth. Discuss ways to avoid and/or manage mucositis with a health care professional. ▪ Promptly report S/S of infection (e.g., fever), S/S of bleeding (e.g., anemia, bruising), and S/S of tumor lysis syndrome (e.g., flank pain, hematuria). ▪ Promptly report S/S of skin reactions (e.g., blisters, peeling and loss of skin, rash, sores). ▪ Discuss medications (prescription and nonprescription) with a health care professional; see Drug/Lab Interactions. ▪ Avoid vaccination with live virus vaccines. ▪ See Appendix D, p. 1333.

Maternal/Child: Category D: avoid pregnancy. Can cause fetal harm. ▪ Discontinue breast-feeding. ▪ Safety and effectiveness for use in pediatric patients not established.

Elderly: No overall differences in effectiveness or safety based on age. ▪ No dose adjustment required in elderly patients with normal renal function; however, dose selection should be cautious. Consider age-related organ impairment (e.g., bone marrow reserve, renal, hepatic) and monitor closely.

DRUG/LAB INTERACTIONS

Coadministration with **probenecid** (an inhibitor of multiple transporter systems, including the multidrug resistance–associated protein 2 [MRP2] efflux transporter) resulted in delayed renal clearance and an increase in pralatrexate exposure. ▪ Concomitant administration of drugs that are substantially cleared by the renal system (e.g., **NSAIDs** [e.g., ibuprofen (Advil, Motrin), naproxen (Aleve, Naprosyn)] **and sulfamethoxazole/ trimethoprim**) may result in delayed clearance of pralatrexate. ▪ Do not administer **live virus vaccines** to patients receiving antineoplastic drugs. ▪ Not a substrate, inhibitor, or inducer of CYP_{450} isoenzymes and has a low potential for drug-drug interactions with drugs metabolized by these isoenzymes.

SIDE EFFECTS

The most common side effects are fatigue, mucositis, nausea, and thrombocytopenia. The most common serious side effects are dehydration, dyspnea, febrile neutropenia, fever, mucositis (stomatitis or mucosal inflammation of the GI and GU tracts), sepsis, and thrombocytopenia. Mucositis and thrombocytopenia were the most common reasons for discontinuing treatment. Other reported side effects include abdominal pain, abnormal liver function tests (e.g., AST, ALT, transaminases), anemia, anorexia, asthenia, back pain, constipation, cough, diarrhea, edema, epistaxis, hypokalemia, leukopenia, neutropenia, night sweats, pain in extremities, pharyngolaryngeal pain, pruritus, rash, tachycardia, tumor lysis syndrome, upper respiratory infection, vomiting.

Post-Marketing: Dermatologic reactions (e.g., skin exfoliation, toxic epidermal necrolysis, and ulceration).

ANTIDOTE

Treatment of most side effects will be supportive and may require dose adjustment or discontinuation. Discontinue pralatrexate if toxicity from side effects occurs (e.g., dermatologic reactions, Grade 4 treatment-related toxicities [e.g., mucositis], hematologic toxicities [persisting for 3 weeks], uncontrolled tumor lysis syndrome) and notify the physician; see Dose Adjustments. Administration of blood products and/or blood modifiers (e.g., darbepoetin [Aranesp], epoetin alfa [Epogen], filgrastim [Neupogen, Zarxio], pegfilgrastim [Neulasta], sargramostim [Leukine]) may be indicated to treat bone marrow toxicity. Treat hypersensitivity reactions with epinephrine, antihistamines, and corticosteroids as needed. In addition to initiating supportive measures, leucovorin calcium (citrovorum factor, folinic acid) may be given PO, IM, or IV promptly to counteract inadvertent overdose. Resuscitate as indicated.

PRALIDOXIME CHLORIDE

(prah-lih-**DOX**-eem **KLOR**-eyed)

Protopam Chloride

Antidote
(anticholinesterase antagonist)

pH 3.5 to 4.5

USUAL DOSE

In poisonings, correct any existing hypoxemia, then administer atropine as directed in the following paragraphs. After the effects of atropine have become apparent, pralidoxime may be administered. See Contraindications. If IV administration is not possible, may be given IM or SC.

ORGANOPHOSPHATE PESTICIDE POISONING

Atropine: Must be given before pralidoxime and as soon as possible after adequate ventilation has been established (hypoxemia corrected). Ventricular fibrillation can occur if oxygenation is inadequate. Give atropine, 2 to 4 mg IV, after cyanosis disappears, then give initial dose of pralidoxime. Repeat atropine every 10 minutes until atropine toxicity (delirium, dilated pupils, dry mouth, muscle twitching, pulse 140 beats/min). Maintain atropinization for at least 48 hours.

Pralidoxime: 1 to 2 Gm initially after hypoxemia has been corrected, initial dose of atropine has been given, and effects of atropine are apparent (secretions are inhibited). Repeat in 1 hour if indicated. If muscle weakness continues, additional doses can be given with extreme caution, usually every 10 to 12 hours (has been given more frequently). Evidence suggests that a loading dose followed by a continuous infusion may maintain therapeutic levels longer than the traditional short intermittent infusion therapy; see prescribing information for studied regimens.

ORGANOPHOSPHATE CHEMICAL POISONING

Usually administered IM by an autoinjector system (survival technology). Atropine must be given first. After the effects of atropine are apparent (e.g., dry mouth), give pralidoxime 600 mg. Repeat both drugs at 15-minute intervals times 2 if indicated. If muscle weakness persists, seek medical help; IV doses may be required.

ANTICHOLINESTERASE OVERDOSE (E.G., NEOSTIGMINE, PYRIDOSTIGMINE)

1 to 2 Gm followed by 250 mg every 5 minutes.

PEDIATRIC DOSE

See Maternal/Child.

Organophosphate pesticide/chemical poisoning: Give **atropine** 0.05 to 0.1 mg/kg. See Usual Dose for order of administration and specific criteria.

Pralidoxime—Loading dose followed by a continuous infusion: Administer a loading dose of 20 to 50 mg/kg (not to exceed 2,000 mg) over 15 to 30 minutes. Follow with a continuous infusion of 10 to 20 mg/kg/hr.

Pralidoxime—Intermittent Infusion: Administer 20 to 50 mg/kg (not to exceed 2,000 mg) over 15 to 30 minutes. May repeat dose in 1 hour if muscle weakness has not been relieved. Repeat every 10 to 12 hours as needed.

DOSE ADJUSTMENTS

Reduce dose in renal impairment. ▪ Lower-end initial doses may be indicated in the elderly. Dose selection should be cautious in the elderly. Consider age-related organ impairment and concomitant disease or drug therapy.

DILUTION

Each 1 Gm of sterile powder is diluted with 20 mL of SWFI. Should be further diluted in 100 mL of NS and given as an IV infusion. If reduced fluids are indicated (e.g., pulmonary edema is present) or rapid administration is required, a 5% solution (1 Gm in 20 mL SWFI) given over no less than 5 minutes may be used.

Storage: Store at CRT. Use promptly after reconstitution; discard remaining solution.

COMPATIBILITY

Specific information not available. Consider specific use; consult pharmacist.

RATE OF ADMINISTRATION

Too-rapid injection may cause laryngospasm, muscle rigidity, or tachycardia. Do not exceed a rate of 200 mg/min.

IV injection diluted in 20 mL SWFI: Each 1 Gm or fraction thereof over no less than 5 minutes. Used only if pulmonary edema present or infusion not practical.

Infusion (diluted in 100 mL NS, preferred): A single dose over 15 to 30 minutes.

ACTIONS

An anticholinesterase antagonist that reactivates cholinesterase inhibited by phosphate esters. Slows the conversion of phosphorylated cholinesterase to a nonreactivatable form and detoxifies certain organophosphates by direct chemical reaction. Its most critical effect is in relieving paralysis of the respiratory muscles. Because pralidoxime is less effective in relieving depression of the respiratory center, atropine is always required concomitantly to block the effect of accumulated acetylcholine at this site. Rapidly dispersed throughout body fluids. Onset of action is within 10 to 40 minutes; half-life is short (about 1.2 hours), requiring repeated doses as more poison is absorbed. Partially metabolized by the liver. Most of a single dose is excreted within 6 hours in the urine.

INDICATIONS AND USES

Principal indications for the use of pralidoxime are muscle weakness and respiratory depression. In severe poisoning, respiratory depression may be due to muscle weakness. ▪ An antidote (treatment adjunct) in organophosphate pesticide or chemical poisoning. Primarily useful for many phosphate ester insecticide poisons with anticholinesterase activity (e.g., diazinon, malathion) or chemicals with anticholinesterase activity (e.g., nerve gas). ▪ Control of overdose of anticholinesterase drugs used to treat myasthenia gravis. Confirm diagnosis with edrophonium (Tensilon).

CONTRAINDICATIONS

No known absolute contraindications to use of pralidoxime. Relative contraindications include known hypersensitivity to pralidoxime or any component of the product. ▪ See Precautions.

PRECAUTIONS

In poisoning: Most effective if administered immediately after poisoning. May be ineffective if more than 36 hours have passed since exposure; some response may be obtained in severe poisoning; see Contraindications. ▪ Not recommended in carbamate poisoning (increases toxicity of Sevin [carbamate insecticide]). ▪ Not effective for treatment of poisoning with phosphorus, inorganic phosphates, or organophosphates not having anticholinesterase activity. ▪ Rapid IV administration may lead to temporary worsening of cholinergic manifestations. Continuous or intermittent infusion is preferred; see Rate of Administration. ▪ Caregivers must protect themselves from contamination. Wear gowns and gloves. ▪ Remove contaminated clothing and cleanse contaminated skin surfaces, hair, and fingernails with water, sodium bicarbonate solution, or alcohol. ▪ Gently flush eyes with water for at least 15 minutes. ▪ Diazepam (Valium) may be required to stop convulsions. ▪ Use caution in myasthenia gravis; may cause a myasthenic crisis.

Monitor: Before any medication is given, establish and maintain an adequate airway and controlled respiration as indicated. Suctioning of secretions and oxygen usually required. Cardiovascular support, correction of metabolic abnormalities, and seizure control may be necessary. ▪ Draw blood samples for baseline RBC acetylcholinesterase and pseudo-cholinesterase concentrations. ▪ In suspected poisoning, initiate treatment without waiting for lab confirmation of diagnosis. Combined with a history of possible poisoning, a RBC cholinesterase concentration less than 50% of normal is indicative of organophosphate ester poisoning. ▪ Gastric lavage and activated charcoal are indicated if organophosphates are ingested; most effective if started within 30 minutes of ingestion. Avoid emesis as patient may lose consciousness and aspirate. ▪ Monitor vital signs and ECG continuously. ▪ Maintain adequate urine output. ▪ In cases of ingested poison, toxicity may recur as poison is absorbed from bowel; monitor for 48 to 72 hours. ▪ In all cases of organophosphate poisoning, patient should be observed for at least 48 to 72 hours. ▪ See Drug/Lab Interactions.

Maternal/Child: Category C: effects not known; use only if clearly needed. ▪ Safety for breast-feeding not established. ▪ Efficacy in pediatric patients is extrapolated from the adult population and is supported by nonclinical studies, pharmacokinetic studies in adults, and experience in pediatric patients. Muscle fasciculations, apnea, and convulsions have been reported; see Rate of Administration.

Elderly: Response similar to younger adults. ▪ Dose selection should be cautious; see Dose Adjustments.

DRUG/LAB INTERACTIONS

Used in combination with **atropine.** Signs of atropinization (e.g., dryness of mouth and nose, flushing, mydriasis, tachycardia) may occur earlier than when atropine is used alone. ▪ **CNS depressants** (e.g., anticonvulsants, antihistamines, muscle relaxants, narcotics, reserpine compounds, phenothiazines) and xanthines (e.g., aminophylline, caffeine) will intensify the effects of organophosphate poisoning and defeat effectiveness of treatment. ▪ **Barbiturates** are potentiated by anticholinesterases; use with caution in treatment of seizures. ▪ **Succinylcholine** may cause prolonged respiratory paralysis. ▪ **Thiamine** delays excretion of pralidoxime.

SIDE EFFECTS

Blurred vision, diplopia, dizziness, drowsiness, headache, hyperventilation, impaired accommodation, increased diastolic and systolic BP, laryngospasm, muscle rigidity, muscular weakness, nausea, pharyngeal pain, tachycardia, transient elevated AST, ALT, and CPK. Excitement and manic behavior may occur (atropinization) if pralidoxime is delayed after atropine has been given.

ANTIDOTE

Has not been needed. Patient should be observed for atropine intoxication. Artificial ventilation and other supportive therapy should be administered as needed.

PROCAINAMIDE HYDROCHLORIDE

Antiarrhythmic

(proh-**KAYN**-ah-myd hy-droh-**KLOR**-eyed)

Pronestyl

pH 4 to 6

USUAL DOSE

Loading dose: 0.2 to 1 Gm (100 mg/mL). 100 mg every 5 minutes or 20 mg every 1 minute may be given as an infusion until arrhythmia is suppressed or 500 mg is administered. Wait 10 minutes to allow adequate distribution, then resume dosing until arrhythmia is suppressed, maximum initial dose of 1 Gm is reached, or side effects appear (e.g., hypotension, QRS complex widening by 50%). Dose cautiously to avoid a hypotensive response. AHA recommends 20 mg/min as an infusion to a maximum total dose of 17 mg/kg. *Maintenance dose:* After arrhythmia is suppressed or maximum dose is reached, follow initial dose with an infusion of 1 to 4 mg/min (may require up to 6 mg/min). Titrate to control arrhythmias. Maintain with oral procainamide as soon as possible but at least 4 hours after last IV dose.

Recurrent VT/VF: AHA recommends 20 mg/min as an infusion. Up to 50 mg/min may be used in urgent situations. Maximum total dose is 17 mg/kg.

PEDIATRIC DOSE

See Maternal/Child; pediatric doses are unlabeled.

2 to 5 mg/kg of body weight. Do not exceed 100 mg/dose. Repeat as indicated every 10 to 30 minutes. Maximum dose in 24 hours is 30 mg/kg or 2 Gm. An alternate dose regimen is 2 to 6 mg/kg as a *loading dose* given over 5 minutes; follow with a *maintenance infusion* of 20 to 80 mcg/kg/min to control arrhythmias.

Supraventricular tachycardia (SVT), atrial flutter, VT with pulse: AHA recommends 15 mg/kg over 30 to 60 minutes.

DOSE ADJUSTMENTS

Maintenance dose may be reduced in impaired or reduced renal function and in individuals over 50 years of age. ▪ See Drug/Lab Interactions.

DILUTION

IV injection: Dilute each 100 mg with 5 to 10 mL of D5W.

Infusion: Add 1 Gm of procainamide to 50, 250, or 500 mL of D5W. Yields 20 mg/mL, 4 mg/mL, or 2 mg/mL respectively. 20 mg/mL should be used only as a loading dose. 2 and 4 mg/mL dilutions may be used for loading or maintenance based on fluid restrictions. Solution should be clear; may be light yellow. Discard if darker than light amber.

Pediatric infusion: *Loading dose:* Add a calculated loading dose (2 to 5 mg/kg) to a minimum of 10 mL D5W for each 100 mg or fraction thereof. More diluent may be used based on size of child and fluid restriction.

Maintenance infusion: See chart under Rate of Administration (Pediatric).

Storage: Photosensitive; protect from light. Store at CRT.

COMPATIBILITY

(Underline Indicates Conflicting Compatibility Information)

Consider any drug NOT listed as compatible to be INCOMPATIBLE until consulting a pharmacist; specific conditions may apply.

One source suggests the following **compatibilities:**

Additive: *Consider individualized rate adjustments necessary to achieve desired effects.* Amiodarone (Nexterone), atracurium (Tracrium), dobutamine, flumazenil (Romazicon), lidocaine, verapamil.

Y-site: Amiodarone (Nexterone), bivalirudin (Angiomax), cisatracurium (Nimbex), dexmedetomidine (Precedex), diltiazem (Cardizem), famotidine (Pepcid IV), fenoldopam (Corlopam), heparin, hetastarch in electrolytes (Hextend), hydrocortisone sodium succinate (Solu-Cortef), metoprolol (Lopressor), nitroprusside sodium, potassium chloride (KCl), ranitidine (Zantac), remifentanil (Ultiva), vasopressin.

P

RATE OF ADMINISTRATION

20 mg or fraction thereof over 1 minute. Use an infusion pump or a microdrip (60 gtt/mL) for infusion to deliver a constant rate. Up to 50 mg may be given by IV injection over 1 minute with extreme caution. After stabilized with loading dose, follow with a maintenance infusion at 1 to 6 mg/min.

Procainamide Infusion Rate (Adult)						
Desired Dose	1 Gm in 500 mL D5W 2 mg/mL			1 Gm in 250 mL D5W 4 mg/mL		
mg/min	mg/hr	mL/min	mL/hr	mg/hr	mL/min	mL/hr
1 mg/min	60	0.5	30	60	0.25	15
2 mg/min	120	1	60	120	0.5	30
3 mg/min	180	1.5	90	180	0.75	45
4 mg/min	240	2	120	240	1	60
5 mg/min	300	2.5	150	300	1.25	75
6 mg/min	360	3	180	360	1.5	90

Procainamide Infusion Rate (Pediatric)		
Desired Dose	200 mg in 500 mL D5W 400 mcg/mL	200 mg in 125 mL D5W 1,600 mcg/mL
mcg/kg/min	mL/kg/min × kg = mL/min	mL/kg/min × kg = mL/min
20 mcg/kg/min	0.05 × wt in kg	0.0125 × wt in kg
30 mcg/kg/min	0.075 × wt in kg	0.01875 × wt in kg
40 mcg/kg/min	0.1 × wt in kg	0.025 × wt in kg
50 mcg/kg/min	0.125 × wt in kg	0.03125 × wt in kg
60 mcg/kg/min	0.15 × wt in kg	0.0375 × wt in kg
70 mcg/kg/min	0.175 × wt in kg	0.04375 × wt in kg
80 mcg/kg/min	0.2 × wt in kg	0.05 × wt in kg

Example: To deliver 30 mcg/kg/min of a 400 mg/mL solution to a child weighing 20 kg, multiply 0.075 (mL/kg/min) × 20 (wt in kg) = an infusion rate of 1.5 mL/min.

ACTIONS

A procaine derivative. Exerts a depressing antiarrhythmic action on the heart, slowing the rate, slowing conduction, reducing myocardial irritability, and prolonging the refractory period. Decreases membrane permeability of the cell and prevents loss of sodium and potassium ions. Onset of action should occur in 2 to 3 minutes. Half-life is 3 to 4 hours. Crosses the placental barrier. Plasma levels decrease slowly; partially metabolized to the active metabolite NAPA; remaining drug excreted in the urine.

INDICATIONS AND USES

Suppress PVCs and recurrent ventricular tachycardia when lidocaine is contraindicated or has not suppressed ventricular arrhythmias. ■ Treat wide-complex tachycardias difficult to distinguish from VT (lidocaine preferred). ■ Rarely used in atrial fibrillation, paroxysmal atrial tachycardia, or arrhythmias caused by anesthesia. Safer drugs (e.g., verapamil, diltiazem) are readily available.

CONTRAINDICATIONS

Complete atrioventricular heart block, second- and third-degree AV block unless an electrical pacemaker is operative, pre-existing QT prolongation, torsades de pointes, known sensitivity to procainamide or any other local anesthetic of the ester type, myasthenia gravis, systemic lupus erythematosus.

PRECAUTIONS

Oral or IM administration is the route of choice; IV route for emergencies only. ▪ Use extreme caution in first- or second-degree blocks, ventricular tachycardia after a myocardial infarction, digoxin intoxication, CHF, any structural heart disease, and impaired liver or reduced kidney function. ▪ Predigitalize or cardiovert patients with atrial flutter or fibrillation to reduce incidence of sudden increase in ventricular rate as atrial rate is slowed. Use caution if used concurrently with other drugs that prolong QT interval (e.g., amiodarone [Nexterone]). ▪ Some clinicians recommend giving a dose the night before surgery and then discontinuing until after surgery. If an arrhythmia occurs, use lidocaine for ventricular arrhythmias and calcium channel blockers (e.g., diltiazem, verapamil) or beta-blockers (e.g., atenolol, propranolol) for supraventricular arrhythmias. Resume dosing after surgery and utilize oral dosing as soon as possible.

Monitor: Monitor the patient's ECG and BP continuously. Keep patient in a supine position. Avoid a hypotensive response. ▪ Discontinue IV use when the cardiac arrhythmia is interrupted or when the ventricular rate slows without regular atrioventricular conduction. ▪ Small emboli may be dislodged when atrial fibrillation is corrected. ▪ Monitor blood levels of procainamide and NAPA (active metabolite) in patients with renal impairment and in any patient receiving a constant infusion over 3 mg/min for more than 24 hours. ▪ Monitor CBC, including WBC, differential, and platelets with continued use; fatal blood dyscrasias have occurred with usual doses. ▪ See Drug/Lab Interactions.

Maternal/Child: Category C: safety for use in pregnancy and breast-feeding and in pediatric patients not established. Consider quinidine as an alternate for use during pregnancy.

Elderly: Half-life of parent drug and active metabolite is prolonged; renal excretion reduced about 25% at age 50 and 50% at age 75. ▪ Increased risk of hypotension.

DRUG/LAB INTERACTIONS

Potentiates or is potentiated by **neuromuscular blocking antibiotics** (e.g., kanamycin), **anticholinergics** (e.g., atropine), **thiazide diuretics, antihypertensive agents, muscle relaxants, succinylcholine, cimetidine** (Tagamet), **and others.** ▪ May cause serious arrhythmias (e.g., prolongation of QT interval or other additive effects) with **other antiarrhythmic agents** (e.g., amiodarone (Nexterone), digoxin, disopyramide [Norpace], lidocaine, quinidine). Lower doses of both drugs may be required. ▪ Antagonizes **anticholinesterases** (e.g., neostigmine). ▪ **Alcohol** may increase hepatic metabolism. ▪ May **elevate AST levels.**

SIDE EFFECTS

Anorexia, bleeding, bruising, chills, dizziness, fever, flushing, giddiness, hallucinations, joint swelling or pain, mental confusion, nausea, skin rash, tremor, vomiting, weakness. May indicate onset of more serious side effects.

Major: Blood dyscrasias (e.g., agranulocytosis, bone marrow suppression, hypoplastic anemia, neutropenia, thrombocytopenia); hypotension with a BP drop over 15 mm Hg, lupus erythematosus-like symptoms, PR interval prolongation, QRS complex widening, QT interval prolongation, ventricular asystole, ventricular fibrillation, ventricular tachycardia.

ANTIDOTE

Notify the physician of any side effect. If minor symptoms progress or any major side effect appears, discontinue the drug immediately and notify the physician. Use dopamine or phenylephrine hydrochloride (Neo-Synephrine) to correct hypotension. Treatment of toxicity is symptomatic and supportive. Infusion of $^1/_6$ M sodium lactate injection may reduce cardiotoxic effects. Hemodialysis may be indicated or urinary acidifiers may increase renal clearance. Resuscitate as necessary. Depending on arrhythmia, quinidine or lidocaine is an effective alternate. Consider insertion of a ventricular pacing electrode as a precautionary measure in case serious AV block develops.

PROCHLORPERAZINE EDISYLATE
(proh-klor-**PAIR**-ah-zeen eh-**DIS**-ah-layt)

Phenothiazine
Antiemetic
Antipsychotic

Compazine

pH 4.2 to 6.2

USUAL DOSE

A single IV dose should not exceed 10 mg. The maximum daily IV dose should not exceed 40 mg.

Control of severe nausea and vomiting: 2.5 to 10 mg; may be repeated one time in 1 to 2 hours if indicated.

Control of severe nausea and vomiting in adult surgical patients: 5 to 10 mg 15 to 30 minutes before induction of anesthesia or to control symptoms during or after surgery. Repeat once if necessary. Another source suggests 20 mg diluted in 1 L solution (see Dilution) during and/or after surgery.

Management of nausea and vomiting in emetic-inducing chemotherapy (unlabeled): One source suggests 10 to 20 mg 30 minutes before and 3 hours after treatment. Another source suggests 30 to 40 mg 30 minutes before and 3 hours after treatment. A third source suggests 0.8 mg/kg 30 minutes before and 3 hours after treatment and cites precipitous hypotension with larger doses; but another source suggests 2 mg/kg for highly emetogenic agents (e.g., cisplatin, dacarbazine) and 1 mg/kg for less emetogenic agents. Begin 30 minutes before chemotherapy, repeat every 2 hours for 2 doses, then every 3 hours for 3 doses. Treat extrapyramidal symptoms with diphenhydramine (Benadryl) IM. These doses have not been recommended by the manufacturer and exceed the recommended maximum daily IV dose of 40 mg/24 hr. In addition, recommended doses of newer agents (e.g., ondansetron [Zofran]) may be more effective.

Control of severe vascular and tension headaches (unlabeled): 10 mg given as an injection over 2 minutes. Sometimes given concurrently with dihydroergotamine 1 mg as an infusion over 30 minutes. Another regimen administers 3.5 mg of prochlorperazine over 5 minutes followed by dexamethasone 20 mg over 10 minutes.

PEDIATRIC DOSE

IV route not recommended for pediatric patients; safety has not been established; see Contraindications, Precautions, and Maternal/Child.

DOSE ADJUSTMENTS

Lower-end initial doses and more gradual adjustments may be indicated in the elderly and in debilitated or emaciated patients. ▪ See Drug/Lab Interactions.

DILUTION

May be given undiluted or each 5 mg (1 mL) may be diluted with 9 mL of NS to facilitate titration. 1 mL will equal 0.5 mg. Larger amounts of NS may be used. May add doses over 10 mg to 50 mL to 1 liter of commonly used IV solution (e.g., D5W, NS, D5/$\frac{1}{2}$NS, Ringer's or LR), and give as an intermittent or prolonged infusion. Handle carefully; may cause contact dermatitis. Slightly yellow color does not affect potency. Discard if markedly discolored.

Storage: Store below 40° C and protect from light and freezing.

COMPATIBILITY

Consider any drug NOT listed as compatible to be INCOMPATIBLE until consulting a pharmacist; specific conditions may apply.

Manufacturer recommends not mixing with other agents in a syringe.

One source suggests the following **compatibilities:**

Additive: Amikacin, ascorbic acid, calcium gluconate, dexamethasone (Decadron), dimenhydrinate, erthyromycin (Erythrocin), ethacrynic acid (Edecrin), lidocaine, nafcillin (Nallpen), penicillin G potassium, sodium bicarbonate.

Y-site: Acetaminophen (Ofirmev), calcium gluconate, cisatracurium (Nimbex), cladribine (Leustatin), dexmedetomidine (Precedex), docetaxel (Taxotere), doxorubicin liposomal (Doxil), fluconazole (Diflucan), granisetron (Kytril), heparin, hetastarch in electrolytes (Hextend), hydrocortisone sodium succinate (Solu-Cortef), linezolid (Zyvox), melphalan (Alkeran), ondansetron (Zofran), oxaliplatin (Eloxatin), paclitaxel (Taxol), potassium chloride (KCl), propofol (Diprivan), remifentanil (Ultiva), sargramostim (Leukine), teniposide (Vumon), thiotepa, topotecan (Hycamtin), vinorelbine (Navelbine).

RATE OF ADMINISTRATION
IV injection: Each 5 mg or fraction thereof over 1 minute.

Infusion: May be given at ordered rate, or rate may be increased or decreased as symptoms indicate. Use an infusion pump for infusion.

Management of nausea and vomiting associated with emetic-inducing chemotherapy: A single dose over 15 to 20 minutes as an *intermittent IV.*

ACTIONS
A phenothiazine derivative approximately six times more potent than chlorpromazine (Thorazine), with effects on the central, autonomic, and peripheral nervous systems. Has weak anticholinergic effects, moderate sedative effects, and strong extrapyramidal effects. A potent antiemetic, acting both centrally at the chemoreceptor trigger zone and peripherally by blocking the vagus nerve in the GI tract. Onset of action is prompt and lasting. Metabolized in the liver and excreted in urine and feces. Crosses placental barrier. Secreted in breast milk.

INDICATIONS AND USES
Control of severe nausea and vomiting. ▪ Used IM or PO in the treatment of schizophrenia and nonpsychotic anxiety.

Unlabeled uses: Use of higher doses to control nausea and vomiting associated with emetic-inducing chemotherapy. ▪ Treatment of severe vascular and tension headaches.

CONTRAINDICATIONS
Pediatric patients under 2 years or 10 kg (22 lb); pediatric patients with conditions that do not have an established dose; comatose or severely depressed states or in the presence of large amounts of CNS depressants (e.g., alcohol, barbiturates, narcotics); hypersensitivity to phenothiazines; breast-feeding and pregnancy, except labor and delivery; do not use in pediatric surgery.

PRECAUTIONS
Use IV only when absolutely necessary. IV not recommended for pediatric patients. ▪ Extrapyramidal symptoms caused by prochlorperazine may be confused with undiagnosed disease (e.g., Reye's syndrome, encephalopathy). ▪ May mask diagnosis of other conditions, including Reye's syndrome, brain tumor, drug intoxication, and intestinal obstruction. ▪ May produce ECG changes (e.g., prolonged QT interval, changes in T waves). ▪ Use caution in coronary disease, glaucoma, severe hypertension or hypotension, and in patients with bone marrow suppression. ▪ Use caution in patients with epilepsy. May lower the seizure threshold. ▪ Neuroleptic malignant syndrome (NMS), characterized by hyperpyrexia, muscle rigidity, autonomic instability, and altered mental status, has been reported with phenothiazine use. ▪ Tardive dyskinesia (potentially irreversible involuntary dyskinetic movements) may develop. Use the smallest doses and shortest duration of therapy to minimize risk. ▪ Anticholinergic and cardiac effects may be troublesome during anesthesia. For patients receiving phenothiazines, taper and discontinue preoperatively if they will not be continued after surgery. ▪ May discolor urine pink to reddish brown. ▪ Photosensitivity of skin is possible. ▪ May cause paradoxical excitation in pediatric patients and the elderly. ▪ Do not re-expose patients who have experienced jaundice, skin reactions, or blood dyscrasias in reaction to a phenothiazine. Cross-sensitivity may occur. ▪ May contain sulfites; use caution in patients with allergies.

Monitor: Keep patient in supine position and monitor BP and pulse before administration and between doses. ■ Cough reflex may be suppressed. Monitor closely if nauseated or vomiting to prevent aspiration. ■ See Drug/Lab Interactions.

Patient Education: Avoid use of alcohol or other CNS depressants (e.g., antihistamines, barbiturates). ■ Request assistance for ambulation; may cause dizziness or fainting. ■ Use caution performing tasks that require alertness. ■ May cause skin and eye photosensitivity. Avoid unprotected exposure to sun.

Maternal/Child: Safety for use in pregnancy, breast-feeding, and pediatric patients not established; see Contraindications. ■ Has been used during pregnancy for intractable nausea and vomiting; physician must decide if benefit outweighs risk. ■ Use near term may cause maternal hypotension and adverse neonatal effects (e.g., extrapyramidal syndrome, hyperreflexia, hyporeflexia, jaundice). ■ Fetuses and infants have a reduced capacity to metabolize and eliminate. ■ Pediatric patients may metabolize antipsychotic agents more rapidly than adults. ■ Incidence of extrapyramidal reactions is relatively high in pediatric patients, especially in the presence of acute illness (e.g., measles, chickenpox, gastroenteritis).

Elderly: See Dose Adjustments and Precautions. ■ Have a reduced capacity to metabolize and eliminate and may have increased sensitivity to postural hypotension, anticholinergic and sedative effects. ■ Increased risk of extrapyramidal side effects (e.g., tardive dyskinesia, parkinsonism).

DRUG/LAB INTERACTIONS

Use with **epinephrine** not recommended; may cause precipitous hypotension. ■ Increased CNS respiratory depression and hypotensive effects with **narcotics, alcohol, anesthetics, barbiturates;** reduced doses of these agents usually indicated. ■ Additive effects with **MAO inhibitors** (e.g., selegiline [Eldepryl]), **anticholinergics, antihistamines, antihypertensives, hypnotics, muscle relaxants, phenytoin** (Dilantin), **propranolol, rauwolfia alkaloids, and thiazide diuretics;** dose adjustment may be necessary. ■ Risk of cardiotoxicity increased with **pimozide** (Orap) and **sparfloxacin** (Zagam); concurrent use not recommended. ■ Risk of additive QT interval prolongation, cardiac depressant effects, and cardiac arrhythmias increased with **amiodarone** (Nexterone), **disopyramide** (Norpace), **erythromycin, probucol** (Lorelco), **procainamide** (Pronestyl), **and quinidine.** ■ Concurrent use with **antidepressants** (e.g., fluoxetine [Prozac], paroxetine [Paxil]), **tricyclic antidepressants** (e.g., amitriptyline [Elavil], imipramine [Tofranil]), or **MAO inhibitors** may increase effects of both drugs; risk of neuroleptic malignant syndrome may be increased. ■ Encephalopathic syndrome has been reported with concurrent use of **lithium;** monitor for S/S of neurologic toxicity. ■ May diminish effects of **oral anticoagulants.** ■ May lower seizure threshold. Dose adjustment of **anticonvulsants** may be necessary. ■ Use with **metrizamide** (Amipaque) may lower seizure threshold; discontinue prochlorperazine 48 hours before **myelography,** and do not resume for 24 hours after test is completed. ■ Use caution during anesthesia with **barbiturates** (e.g., methohexital, thiopental); may increase frequency and severity of hypotension and neuromuscular excitation. ■ Capable of innumerable other interactions.

SIDE EFFECTS

Usually transient if drug discontinued but may require treatment if severe: anaphylaxis, blurring of vision, cardiac arrest, dermatitis, dizziness, drowsiness, dryness of mouth, dysphagia, elevated BP, extrapyramidal symptoms (e.g., abnormal positioning, extreme restlessness, pseudoparkinsonism, weakness of extremities), excitement, fever without etiology, hematologic toxicities (e.g., agranulocytosis, aplastic anemia, leukopenia, thrombocytopenia), hypersensitivity reactions, hypotension, photosensitivity, slurred speech, spastic movements (especially about the face), tachycardia, tardive dyskinesia, tightness of the throat, tongue discoloration, tongue protrusion, and many others. Overdose can cause convulsions, hallucinations, and death.

ANTIDOTE

Discontinue the drug at onset of any side effect and notify the physician. Discontinue prochlorperazine and all drugs not essential to concurrent therapy immediately if NMS occurs. Will require intensive symptomatic treatment, medical monitoring, and management of concomitant medical problems. Counteract hypotension with IV fluids and norepinephrine (Levophed) or phenylephrine (Neo-Synephrine); counteract extrapyramidal symptoms with benztropine mesylate (Cogentin) or diphenhydramine (Benadryl). Maintain a clear airway and adequate hydration. *Epinephrine is contraindicated for hypotension.* Further hypotension will occur. Use diazepam (Valium) for convulsions or hyperactivity. Follow with phenytoin. Phenytoin may be helpful in ventricular arrhythmias. In treating respiratory depression and unconsciousness, avoid analeptics such as doxapram (Dopram); they may cause convulsions. Not removed by dialysis. Resuscitate as necessary.

PROMETHAZINE HYDROCHLORIDE BBW

(proh-**METH**-ah-zeen hy-droh-**KLOR**-eyed)

Phenothiazine
Antiemetic
Sedative-hypnotic

Phenergan

pH 4 to 5.5

USUAL DOSE

A vesicant; see Dilution, Rate of Administration, Contraindications, Precautions, Monitor, and Antidote. Deep IM injection is the preferred route of administration.

All uses: The Institute for Safe Medication Practices (ISMP) recommends 6.25 to 12.5 mg as a starting IV dose and suggests considering the use of alternate drugs (e.g., 5-HT$_3$ receptor antagonists [e.g., dolasetron (Anzemet), granisetron (Kytril), ondansetron (Zofran)]).

Nausea and vomiting: 12.5 to 25 mg every 4 to 6 hours as needed.

Allergic conditions: 25 mg. May repeat in 2 hours if necessary. Change to oral therapy as soon as possible.

Sedation, nighttime: 25 to 50 mg.

Sedation, perioperative: 25 to 50 mg. May combine with a reduced dose of narcotic analgesic and an anticholinergic drug (e.g., atropine).

Sedation, labor and delivery: 50 mg during early stage of labor. When labor fully established, may administer 25 to 75 mg with a reduced dose of a narcotic analgesic. May repeat every 4 hours to a maximum dose of 100 mg in a 24-hour period.

PEDIATRIC DOSE

IV use is rare and is limited to pediatric patients 2 years of age or older; see Contraindications and Maternal/Child. Adjust dose to the age, weight, and severity of condition. Use the minimum effective dose and avoid concomitant administration with other drugs with respiratory depressant effects. Do not exceed one half of adult dose. One source suggests a maximum dose of 25 mg. If given IV, administer separately from other medications (e.g., appropriately reduced doses of barbiturates or narcotics, and an appropriate dose of an anticholinergic agent).

Adjunct to premedication: 1.1 mg/kg/dose.

Nausea and vomiting (unlabeled): 0.25 to 1 mg/kg/dose every 6 hours as needed.

DOSE ADJUSTMENTS

Reduced dose may be indicated in the elderly. See Drug/Lab Interactions.

DILUTION

May be given undiluted or may dilute with NS. Concentration should never exceed 25 mg/mL. 1 mL (25 to 50 mg) diluted with 9 mL of NS equals 2.5 to 5 mg/mL. The ISMP recommends further dilution with an additional 10 to 20 mL of NS or in a 50-mL minibag of NS. Slightly yellow color does not alter potency. Discard if greatly discolored. Administer through Y-tube or three-way stopcock of a free-flowing IV.

Storage: Store at CRT. Protect from light.

COMPATIBILITY   (Underline Indicates Conflicting Compatibility Information)
Consider any drug NOT listed as compatible to be INCOMPATIBLE until consulting a pharmacist; specific conditions may apply.

May form a precipitate with heparin; flush heparinized infusion sets with SWFI or NS before and after administration.

One source suggests the following **compatibilities:**

Additive: Amikacin, ascorbic acid, hydromorphone (Dilaudid), penicillin G potassium.

Y-site: Amifostine (Ethyol), aztreonam, bivalirudin (Angiomax), ceftaroline (Teflaro), ciprofloxacin (Cipro IV), cisatracurium (Nimbex), cladribine (Leustatin), dexmedetomidine (Precedex), docetaxel (Taxotere), etoposide phosphate (Etopophos), fenoldopam (Corlopam), filgrastim (Neupogen), fluconazole (Diflucan), fludarabine (Fludara), gemcitabine (Gemzar), granisetron (Kytril), heparin, hetastarch in electrolytes (Hextend), hydrocortisone sodium succinate (Solu-Cortef), linezolid (Zyvox), melphalan (Alkeran), ondansetron (Zofran), oxaliplatin (Eloxatin), palonosetron (Aloxi), pemetrexed (Alimta), potassium chloride (KCl), remifentanil (Ultiva), sargramostim (Leukine), teniposide (Vumon), thiotepa, vinorelbine (Navelbine).

RATE OF ADMINISTRATION

The ISMP recommends administration of a single dose over 10 to 15 minutes administered at a port farthest from the patient vein; observe continuously if given in a peripheral vein.

A maximum rate of 25 mg or fraction thereof over 1 minute is suggested by the manufacturer.

ACTIONS

A phenothiazine derivative with effects on the central, autonomic, and peripheral nervous systems. It has antihistaminic, antiemetic, anticholinergic, and sedative effects. As an antihistamine, it competitively blocks the H_1 histamine receptor, antagonizing most of the effects of histamine to at least some degree. Potentiates respiratory depression, sedative, and hypotensive effects of narcotics and other CNS depressants. Has no analgesic effects and does not potentiate analgesic effects of narcotics. Onset of action is prompt. Duration of action is 4 to 6 hours. Half-life ranges from 9 to 16 hours. Primarily metabolized in the liver and excreted in the urine.

INDICATIONS AND USES

Prophylaxis or treatment of minor transfusion reactions. ▪ Treatment of or an adjunct to the treatment of hypersensitivity reactions (including anaphylaxis and other immediate-type reactions) after acute symptoms have been controlled with epinephrine and other standard measures. Consider for use if oral administration is impossible or contraindicated. ▪ Treatment of acute nausea, vomiting, and motion sickness. ▪ Sedation to meet surgical and obstetric needs. ▪ Adjunct to analgesics for control of postoperative pain. ▪ Sedation and relief of apprehension; production of a light sleep from which a patient can be easily aroused. ▪ An adjunct to anesthesia and analgesia in selected surgical situations (e.g., repeated bronchoscopy, ophthalmologic surgery, and poor-risk patients). Given in conjunction with reduced amounts of narcotic analgesics.

CONTRAINDICATIONS

Comatose or severely depressed states, hypersensitivity or an idiosyncratic reaction to phenothiazines, and pediatric patients under 2 years of age. Never inject into an artery; may cause arteriospasm resulting in gangrene. *Do not* administer SC; chemical irritation may result in necrotic lesions.

PRECAUTIONS

Ampule must state "for IV use." Deep IM injection preferred. ▪ Use with extreme caution in pediatric patients and the elderly; see Maternal/Child and Elderly. ▪ Can cause severe chemical irritation and tissue damage regardless of route of administration. Irritation and damage can result from perivascular extravasation, unintentional intra-arterial injection, and intraneuronal or perineuronal infiltration. Adverse event reports include abscesses, burning, erythema, gangrene, pain, palsies, paralysis, sensory loss, severe spasm of the distal vessels, swelling, thrombophlebitis, tissue necrosis, and venous thrombosis. ▪ Use should be avoided in patients with compromised respiratory function or in patients at risk for respiratory failure (e.g., COPD, sleep apnea); risk of potentially fatal respiratory depression is increased. ▪ May cause paradoxical excitation in pediatric patients and the elderly. ▪ Use phenothiazines with extreme caution in pediatric patients with a history of sleep apnea, a family history of sudden infant death syndrome, or in the presence of Reye's syndrome. ▪ Use with caution in patients with asthma, bladder neck obstruction, bone marrow suppression, cardiovascular disease, glaucoma, liver dysfunction, prostatic hypertrophy, pyloroduodenal obstruction, or stenosing peptic ulcer disease. ▪ May produce ECG changes (e.g., prolonged QT interval, changes in T waves). ▪ May mask diagnosis of other conditions, including Reye's syndrome, brain tumor, drug intoxication, and intestinal obstruction. ▪ May lower seizure threshold; use extreme caution in patients with known seizure disorders and with narcotics or local anesthetics that also lower seizure threshold. ▪ May contain sulfites; use caution in patients with allergies. ▪ Neuroleptic malignant syndrome (NMS), a rare syndrome manifested by hyperpyrexia, muscle rigidity, irregular BP and HR, and altered mental status, has been reported in association with promethazine alone or in combination with antipsychotic drugs.

Monitor: A vesicant; determine absolute patency of vein; extravasation will cause necrosis; see Contraindications and Precautions. ISMP suggests administering through large-bore veins but prefers use of a central venous catheter. Administration through hand or wrist veins is strongly discouraged. ▪ Monitor frequently for S/S of extravasation (e.g., burning, erythema, pain, palsies, sensory loss, and swelling along IV site), especially along peripheral sites. ▪ Keep patient in supine position. Monitor BP and pulse before administration and between doses. ▪ Sedative effect may require ambulation to be monitored. ▪ See Drug/Lab Interactions.

Patient Education: Avoid use of alcohol or other CNS depressants (e.g., antihistamines, barbiturates). ▪ Request assistance for ambulation; may cause dizziness or fainting. ▪ Use caution performing tasks that require alertness. ▪ May cause skin and eye photosensitivity. Avoid unprotected exposure to sun. ▪ Report stinging or burning at IV site promptly. ▪ Report any involuntary muscle movements.

Maternal/Child: Category C: safety for use in pregnancy and pediatric patients not established. Use only when clearly needed. ▪ Discontinue breast-feeding. ▪ Contraindicated in pediatric patients under 2 years of age. Post-marketing cases of respiratory depression and death (not directly related to individualized weight-based dosing) have been reported. Concomitant administration with other respiratory depressants increases this risk. ▪ Use caution in pediatric patients 2 years of age or older. Use the minimum effective dose. ▪ Do not use for vomiting of unknown etiology in pediatric patients. Antiemetics are not recommended for treatment of uncomplicated vomiting in pediatric patients. Use should be limited to prolonged vomiting of known etiology. Extrapyramidal symptoms that can occur secondary to promethazine administration may be confused with CNS signs of an undiagnosed primary disease (e.g., encephalopathy or Reye's syndrome). ▪ Avoid use in pediatric patients with S/S suggestive of Reye's syndrome or other hepatic diseases. ▪ Excessively large doses of antihistamines in pediatric patients have caused hallucinations, convulsions, and death. ▪ Pediatric patients metabolize antipsychotic agents more rapidly than adults. ▪ Incidence of extrapyramidal reactions is relatively high in pediatric patients, especially in the presence of acute illness (e.g., measles, chickenpox, gastroenteritis). ▪ See Precautions and Contraindications.

Elderly: See Dose Adjustments and Precautions. ▪ Have a reduced capacity to metabolize and eliminate. ▪ May cause confusion, dizziness, hyperexcitability, hypotension, and/or sedation. ▪ Increased sensitivity to anticholinergic effects (e.g., dry mouth, urinary retention). ▪ Increased risk of extrapyramidal side effects (e.g., tardive dyskinesia, parkinsonism).

DRUG/LAB INTERACTIONS

Increased CNS depression and hypotensive effects with **narcotics, alcohol, anesthetics, and barbiturates;** reduced doses of these agents usually indicated. ▪ Additive effects with **MAO inhibitors** (e.g., selegiline [Eldepryl]), **anticholinergics, antihistamines, antihypertensives, hypnotics, muscle relaxants, and propranolol;** dose adjustments may be necessary. ▪ Use with **epinephrine** not recommended; may cause precipitous hypotension. ▪ Risk of cardiotoxicity increased with **pimozide** (Orap), **quinidine, and sparfloxacin** (Zagam); concurrent use not recommended. ▪ Risk of additive QT interval prolongation, cardiac depressant effects, and cardiac arrhythmias increased with **amiodarone** (Nexterone), **disopyramide** (Norpace), **erythromycin, procainamide** (Pronestyl), **and quinidine.** ▪ Concurrent use with **antidepressants** (e.g., fluoxetine [Prozac], paroxetine [Paxil]), **tricyclic antidepressants** (e.g., amitriptyline [Elavil]), **or MAO inhibitors** may increase effects of both drugs. ▪ Concurrent use with **other neuroleptic agents** (e.g., haloperidol [Haldol]) may increase the risk of NMS. ▪ May lower seizure threshold. Dose adjustment of **anticonvulsants** may be necessary. ▪ Capable of innumerable other interactions. ▪ Selected **pregnancy tests** may show a false-negative or false-positive result. ▪ May cause an increase in blood glucose; consider when a **glucose tolerance test** is indicated.

SIDE EFFECTS

Average dose: Blurring of vision, bradycardia, confusion, dizziness, drowsiness, dryness of mouth, extrapyramidal symptoms, faintness, hallucinations, hematologic side effects (e.g., agranulocytosis, leukopenia, thrombocytopenia, thrombocytopenic purpura), hyperexcitability, hypersensitivity reactions, hypertension (rare), hypotension (mild), lassitude, nightmares, photosensitivity, sedation, somnolence, tachycardia, tinnitus, tremors.
Overdose: Anaphylaxis, cardiac arrest, coma, convulsions, deep sedation, respiratory depression. All side effects of phenothiazines are possible, but rarely occur. See prochlorperazine (Compazine).

ANTIDOTE

Discontinue the drug immediately at onset of any side effect and notify the physician. Sympathetic block and heparinization have been used during acute management of promethazine extravasation (unintentional intra-arterial injection or perivascular extravasation). In some cases surgical intervention, including fasciotomy, skin graft, and/or amputation, has been required. Counteract hypotension with IV fluids, Trendelenburg position, norepinephrine (Levophed), or phenylephrine (Neo-Synephrine); counteract extrapyramidal symptoms with benztropine mesylate (Cogentin) or diphenhydramine (Benadryl). Epinephrine is contraindicated for hypotension; further hypotension will occur. Use diazepam (Valium) or phenobarbital for convulsions or hyperactivity. In treating respiratory depression and unconsciousness, avoid analeptics such as doxapram (Dopram); they may cause convulsions. Treatment of NMS includes discontinuation of all unnecessary drugs and intensive symptomatic treatment and monitoring. Dialysis does not appear to be helpful in overdose situations. Resuscitate as necessary.

PROPOFOL INJECTION

(**PROH**-poh-fohl in-**JEK**-shun)

General anesthetic
Anesthesia adjunct
Sedative-hypnotic

Diprivan

pH 7 to 8.5

USUAL DOSE

Lidocaine may be administered to minimize pain on injection of propofol. Administer before propofol injection or add to propofol immediately before administration. Do not exceed more than 20 mg lidocaine to 200 mg propofol.

INDUCTION OF ANESTHESIA

Must be individualized and titrated to desired response. Allow 3 to 5 minutes between dose adjustments to allow for and assess clinical effects.

Healthy adults under 55 years of age: 40 mg every 10 seconds until induction onset (approximately 2 to 2.5 mg/kg).

Adults over 55 years of age, debilitated, or ASA III or IV risk patients: 20 mg every 10 seconds until induction onset (approximately 1 to 1.5 mg/kg).

Cardiac anesthesia: 20 mg every 10 seconds until induction onset (0.5 to 1.5 mg/kg).

Neurosurgical patients: 20 mg every 10 seconds until induction onset (approximately 1 to 2 mg/kg). Infusion or slow injection (20 mg over 10 seconds) is used to avoid significant hypotension and decrease in cerebral perfusion pressure. If increased intracranial pressure is suspected, hyperventilation and hypocarbia should accompany administration.

MAINTENANCE OF ANESTHESIA

Must be individualized and titrated to desired response. Allow 3 to 5 minutes between dose adjustments to allow for and assess clinical effects.

Adults under 55 years of age: Immediately follow induction with an infusion of 100 to 200 mcg/kg/min (6 to 12 mg/kg/hr) or an intermittent bolus in increments of 25 to 50 mg as needed.

Adults over 55 years of age, debilitated, or ASA III or IV risk patients: Immediately follow induction with an infusion of 50 to 100 mcg/kg/min (3 to 6 mg/kg/hr). Do NOT use a rapid intermittent bolus in these patients.

Cardiac anesthesia: Most patients require 100 to 150 mcg/kg/min in combination with an opioid (primary propofol with an opioid secondary). An alternate regimen is an opioid primary with low-dose propofol 50 to 100 mcg/kg/min (3 to 6 mg/kg/hr).

Neurosurgical patients: Immediately follow induction with an infusion of 100 to 200 mcg/kg/min (6 to 12 mg/kg/hr). Do NOT use a rapid intermittent bolus in these patients.

INITIATION OF MONITORED ANESTHESIA CARE (MAC) SEDATION

Must be individualized and titrated to desired response. Allow 3 to 5 minutes between dose adjustments to allow for and assess clinical effects. MAC sedation rates are approximately 25% of those used for anesthesia.

Healthy adults under 55 years of age: An infusion of 100 to 150 mcg/kg/min (6 to 9 mg/kg/hr) over 3 to 5 minutes or a slow injection of 0.5 mg/kg over 3 to 5 minutes. Slow infusion or slow injection techniques are preferable to rapid bolus administration.

Adults over 55 years of age, debilitated, or ASA III or IV risk patients: Most patients require doses similar to healthy adults. Must be given over 3 to 5 minutes as a slow infusion (preferred) or as a slow injection over 3 to 5 minutes. Do NOT give as a rapid bolus.

MAINTENANCE OF MAC SEDATION

Healthy adults under 55 years of age: Maintain with an infusion (preferred) of 25 to 75 mcg/kg/min (1.5 to 4.5 mg/kg/hr) or incremental bolus doses of 10 to 20 mg.

Continued

Adults over 55 years of age, debilitated, or ASA III or IV risk patients: Reduce dose to 80% of usual dose; an infusion of 20 to 60 mcg/kg/min (1.2 to 3.6 mg/kg/hr). Do NOT use bolus doses.

SEDATION OF INTUBATED, MECHANICALLY VENTILATED ICU PATIENTS

Must be individualized and titrated to desired response. Given as a continuous infusion. Begin with an initial dose of 5 mcg/kg/min (0.3 mg/kg/hr) for 5 minutes. Allow at least 5 minutes between adjustments to reach peak drug effect and to avoid hypotension. Increase slowly over 5 to 10 minutes by 5 to 10 mcg/kg/min (0.3 to 0.6 mg/kg/hr) to desired level of sedation. Individualize to patient condition, response, blood lipid profile, and vital signs. Some clinicians recommend reducing dose by approximately one half for elderly (over 55 years) and debilitated. Check urinalysis and urine sediment before administration of propofol in patients at risk for renal failure; see Precautions and Monitor.

MAINTENANCE OF SEDATION IN MECHANICALLY VENTILATED OR RESPIRATORY-CONTROLLED ICU PATIENTS

5 to 50 mcg/kg/min (0.3 to 3 mg/kg/hr) or higher as a continuous infusion slowly titrated to desired level of sedation. Use caution with doses higher than 50 mcg/kg/min; may increase risk of hypotension. Bolus doses of 10 to 20 mg may be used to rapidly increase the depth of sedation in patients in whom hypotension is not likely to occur. Temporarily reduce dose once each day to assess neurologic and respiratory function and to determine minimum dose required for desired level of sedation. Average maintenance dose *under 55 years* is 38 mcg/kg/min; *over 55 years*, 20 mcg/kg/min. Average maintenance dose for *post–coronary artery bypass graft (CABG) patients* is usually low (median of 11 mcg/kg/min) because of high intraoperative opiates.

RELIEF OF PRURITUS ASSOCIATED WITH USE OF SPINAL OPIATES OR CHOLESTASIS (UNLABELED)

Subhypnotic doses of 10 to 15 mg as an IV injection or 0.5 to 1.5 mg/kg/hr as an infusion.

MANAGEMENT OF REFRACTORY STATUS EPILEPTICUS (UNLABELED)

Administer doses of 1 to 2 mg/kg as an IV injection over 5 minutes; may be repeated if seizure activity recurs. If indicated, follow with a maintenance infusion of 2 to 10 mg/hr. Adjust to achieve the lowest rate needed to suppress seizure activity. Decrease gradually to prevent withdrawal seizures.

PEDIATRIC DOSE

To minimize pain on injection of propofol in pediatric patients, administer through larger veins or pretreat smaller veins with lidocaine. See Maternal/Child.

INDUCTION OF ANESTHESIA IN HEALTHY PEDIATRIC PATIENTS 3 TO 16 YEARS OF AGE

Must be individualized and titrated to desired response. 2.5 to 3.5 mg/kg administered over 20 to 30 seconds. *Induction with propofol is indicated only in pediatric patients 3 years of age or older. In pediatric patients from 2 months to 3 years of age, induction must be achieved by supplementing with another agent (literature suggests nitrous oxide 60% to 70%).* See Dose Adjustments.

MAINTENANCE OF ANESTHESIA IN HEALTHY PEDIATRIC PATIENTS FROM 2 MONTHS TO 16 YEARS OF AGE

Must be titrated to desired clinical effect. (See statement under induction in healthy pediatric patients in the previous paragraph, and see Indications and Uses.) Administered as a variable-rate infusion supplemented with nitrous oxide 60% to 70% for most pediatric patients.

Pediatric patients 2 months of age and older: Immediately follow induction dose with an infusion of 125 to 300 mcg/kg/min (7.5 to 18 mg/kg/hr). Initially, a rate of 200 to 300 mcg/kg/min may be indicated and can usually be reduced to 125 to 150 mcg/kg/min after the first half-hour. Decrease infusion rate if clinical signs of light anesthesia are not present after 30 minutes of maintenance; see Rate of Administration. Younger pediatric patients may require higher maintenance infusion rates than older pediatric patients. See Dose Adjustments.

DOSE ADJUSTMENTS

All situations: Reduce induction and maintenance doses for pediatric patients classified as ASA III or IV. ■ See Usual Dose for specific reduced doses required for adults over 55 years of age; debilitated, ASA III, or ASA IV risk patients; or patients with circulatory disorders. ▪ Reduced dose required in presence of other CNS depressants. See Drug/Lab Interactions. ▪ No dose adjustment required for gender, chronic hepatic cirrhosis, or chronic renal failure.

ICU sedation: Adjust infusion to maintain a light level of sedation through the wake-up assessment or weaning process.

DILUTION

Supplied in ready-to-use vials containing 10 mg/mL. Shake well before use. May be further diluted only with D5W. Do not dilute to a concentration less than 2 mg/mL (4 mL diluent to 1 mL propofol yields 2 mg/mL). More stable in glass than in plastic. Strict aseptic technique imperative; emulsion supports rapid growth of microorganisms. Failure to use strict aseptic technique has been associated with microbial contamination of the product with resultant fever, infection, sepsis, other life-threatening illnesses, and/or death. Do not use with evidence of emulsion separation. Prepare immediately before each use. Flush IV line at end of every 6 hours in extended procedures to remove residual propofol.

Filters: Use filters with caution. The pore size should be equal to or greater than 5 microns. Filters with a pore size less than 5 microns may impede the flow of propofol and/or cause a breakdown of the emulsion.

Storage: Protect from light and store below 22° C (72° F) but do not refrigerate. Discard infusion and tubing every 12 hours or every 6 hours if propofol has been transferred from the original container.

COMPATIBILITY   (Underline Indicates Conflicting Compatibility Information)

Consider any drug NOT listed as compatible to be INCOMPATIBLE until consulting a pharmacist; specific conditions may apply.

Manufacturer states, "Should not be mixed with other therapeutic agents prior to administration. **Compatibility** with blood/serum/plasma has not been established."

Y-site: Manufacturer lists as **compatible** at the **Y-site** with the following solutions: D5W, LR, D5LR, D5½NS, D5¼NS. Other sources list acyclovir (Zovirax), alfentanil, aminophylline, ampicillin, atracurium (Tracrium), atropine, aztreonam (Azactam), bumetanide, buprenorphine (Buprenex), butorphanol (Stadol), calcium gluconate, carboplatin (Paraplatin), cefazolin (Ancef), cefotaxime (Claforan), cefotetan, cefoxitin (Mefoxin), ceftaroline (Teflaro), ceftazidime (Fortaz), ceftriaxone (Rocephin), cefuroxime (Zinacef), chlorpromazine (Thorazine), cisatracurium (Nimbex), cisplatin, clindamycin (Cleocin), cyclophosphamide (Cytoxan), cyclosporine (Sandimmune), cytarabine (ARA-C), dexamethasone (Decadron), dexmedetomidine (Precedex), diphenhydramine (Benadryl), dobutamine, dopamine, doxycycline, droperidol (Inapsine), enalaprilat (Vasotec IV), ephedrine, epinephrine (Adrenalin), esmolol (Brevibloc), famotidine (Pepcid IV), fenoldopam (Corlopam), fentanyl, fluconazole (Diflucan), fluorouracil (5-FU), furosemide (Lasix), ganciclovir (Cytovene IV), glycopyrrolate (Robinul), granisetron (Kytril), heparin, hydrocortisone sodium succinate (Solu-Cortef), hydromorphone (Dilaudid), 6% hydroxyethyl starch (Voluven), ifosfamide (Ifex), imipenem-cilastatin (Primaxin), insulin (regular), isoproterenol (Isuprel), ketamine (Ketalar), labetalol, lidocaine, lorazepam (Ativan), magnesium sulfate, mannitol, meperidine (Demerol), midazolam (Versed), milrinone (Primacor), morphine, nafcillin (Nallpen), nalbuphine, naloxone, nitroglycerin IV, nitroprusside sodium, norepinephrine (Levophed), paclitaxel (Taxol), pancuronium, pentobarbital (Nembutal), phenobarbital (Luminal), phenylephrine (Neo-Synephrine), potassium chloride (KCl), prochlorperazine (Compazine), propranolol, ranitidine (Zantac), sodium bicarbonate, succinylcholine, sufentanil (Sufenta), telavancin (Vibativ), ticarcillin/clavulanate (Timentin), vancomycin, vecuronium.

RATE OF ADMINISTRATION

Use of a syringe pump or volumetric pump recommended to provide controlled infusion rates. See Usual Dose for specific rates for specific age and/or indication. Decrease rate based on age, debilitation, or calculated risk. Must be individualized and titrated to desired level of sedation and changes in vital signs. Monitor respiratory function continuously. Continuous administration preferable to intermittent to avoid periods of undersedation or oversedation. Too-rapid administration (bolus dosing, too-rapid increase in infusion rate, overdose) can cause severe cardiorespiratory complications, especially in pediatric patients, adults over 55 years, debilitated or ASA III or IV risk patients. In all anesthesia, higher rates are generally required for the first 15 minutes, then appropriate responses can usually be maintained with a decrease of 30% to 50%. Always titrate rates downward until there is a mild response to surgical stimulation. This avoids administration at rates higher than clinically necessary. Control increased response to surgical stimulation or lightening of anesthesia (increased pulse rate, BP, sweating and/or tearing) with bolus injections of 25 to 50 mg *(adults under 55 years of age only),* slow injection of reduced doses, or by increasing the infusion rate *(adults under or over 55 years of age)* or by increasing the infusion rate *(pediatric patients).* If control not effective within 5 minutes, consider use of an opioid, barbiturate, or inhalation agent.

ACTIONS

A potent emulsified IV sedative hypnotic agent. Action is dose dependent and rate dependent. Can provide conscious (verbal contact maintained) or unconscious sedation, depending on dose. Produces hypnosis rapidly and smoothly with minimal excitation, usually within 40 seconds. Depth of sedation easily and rapidly controlled by adjusting rate of infusion. Rapid onset of action facilitates accurate titration and minimizes oversedation. Due to extensive redistribution from the central nervous system to other tissues and high metabolic clearance, recovery from anesthesia or sedation is rapid. Time to awakening is dependent on duration of infusion. Discontinuation of an infusion after maintenance of anesthesia for 1 hour or sedation in the ICU for 1 day will result in rapid awakening. Prolonged infusions (e.g., 10 days in ICU) will result in drug accumulation and an increased time to awakening. Terminal half-life after a 10-day infusion is 1 to 3 days. Other effects include decreased systemic vascular resistance, myocardial blood flow, and oxygen consumption; a decrease in cerebral blood flow and intracranial pressure; and a decrease in intraocular pressure. Also has antiemetic properties. Has minimal impact on cardiac output, but changes may occur because of assisted or controlled ventilation. Hypotension, oxyhemoglobin desaturation, apnea, and airway obstruction can occur. Addition of an opioid may further decrease cardiac output or respiratory drive. Metabolized in the liver and excreted as metabolites in urine. Crosses placental barrier. Secreted in breast milk.

INDICATIONS AND USES

Adults: Induce and/or maintain anesthesia as part of a balanced anesthetic technique for inpatient and outpatient surgery. ▪ Initiate and maintain monitored anesthesia care (MAC) during diagnostic procedures (e.g., colonoscopy, dental procedures) and in conjunction with local/regional anesthesia during surgical procedures. ▪ Continuous sedation and control of stress responses in intubated, mechanically ventilated ICU patients (e.g., post-CABG, postsurgical, neuro/head trauma, ARDS, COPD, asthma, status epilepticus, tetanus). Continuous infusion of low doses allows controlled recovery of consciousness when required and for assessment.

Pediatric patients: Induction of anesthesia as a part of a balanced anesthetic technique for inpatient and outpatient surgery in pediatric patients over 3 years of age. ▪ Maintenance of anesthesia as part of a balanced anesthetic technique for inpatient and outpatient surgery in pediatric patients over 2 months of age. ▪ Not recommended for induction of anesthesia for pediatric patients under 3 years of age or for maintenance of anesthesia under 2 months of age. ▪ Not indicated for use in pediatric patients for ICU sedation or for MAC sedation for surgical, nonsurgical, or diagnostic procedures.

Unlabeled uses: Subhypnotic doses used for relief of pruritus associated with use of spinal opiates or cholestasis; treatment of status epilepticus refractory to standard anticonvulsant therapy.

CONTRAINDICATIONS

Known hypersensitivity to propofol or its components (e.g., soybean oil, glycerol, egg lecithin, sodium hydroxide) or any time general anesthesia or sedation is contraindicated.

PRECAUTIONS

All situations: For IV use only. ▪ Administered by or under the direct observation of the anesthesiologist. Must have responsibility only for anesthesia during surgery and/or procedures. In the ICU setting, may be administered to intubated, mechanically ventilated patients by persons skilled in medical management of critically ill patients and trained in cardiovascular resuscitation and airway management. Both life-threatening and fatal anaphylactoid and anaphylactic reactions have been reported. ▪ Strict aseptic technique required; see Dilution. ▪ Use caution in patients with compromised myocardial function, intravascular volume depletion, or abnormally low vascular tone (e.g., sepsis); may be more susceptible to hypotension. ▪ Avoid rapid bolus administration in the elderly, debilitated, or ASA-PS III or IV patients. May cause undesirable cardiopulmonary depression, including apnea, airway obstruction, hypotension, and oxygen desaturation. ▪ An emulsion; use caution in patients with lipid metabolism disorders (e.g., diabetic hyperlipidemia, pancreatitis, and primary hyperlipoproteinemia). ▪ May cause convulsions during recovery phase in patients with epilepsy. ▪ Use caution in patients with increased intracranial pressure or impaired cerebral circulation. Decrease in mean arterial pressure may cause decreases in cerebral perfusion. ▪ Propofol infusion syndrome has been reported and is characterized by severe metabolic acidosis, hyperkalemia, lipemia, rhabdomyolysis, hepatomegaly, and cardiac and renal failure. Deaths have occurred. Most often associated with prolonged, high-dose infusions in ICU but has been observed following large-dose, short-term infusions during surgical anesthesia. Consider alternative means of sedation when there is a prolonged need for sedation, when large doses of propofol are required to maintain a desired level of sedation, or if a patient develops metabolic acidosis. ▪ Has no analgesic properties; provide pain relief or local anesthetic as indicated. Has been used successfully with midazolam (Versed), 1 to 3 mg, for initial induction. Midazolam provides better amnesia and causes less pain on injection, whereas propofol sustains sedation and allows more rapid recovery. ▪ May contain sulfites; use caution in patients with allergies.

Monitor: *All situations:* Correct fluid volume deficiencies before administration. ▪ Will cause transient local pain during IV injection; minimize by using larger veins and lidocaine previous to injection. Use with midazolam reduces awareness of this pain. ▪ Apnea may occur during induction and last for more than 60 seconds. Intubation equipment, controlled ventilation equipment, oxygen, and facilities for resuscitation and life support must be available. Maintain a patent airway and ascertain adequate ventilation at all times. ▪ All vital signs must be monitored continuously. Use of a respiratory monitor required. ▪ Hypotension common during first 60 minutes; monitor closely. Significant hypotension or cardiovascular depression can be profound. ▪ To prevent profound bradycardia, anticholinergic agents (e.g., atropine, glycopyrrolate) may be required to modify increases in vagal tone due to concomitant agents (e.g., succinylcholine) or surgical stimulation. ▪ Bed rest required for a minimum of 3 hours after IV injection, or satisfy specific hospital rules for discharge. ▪ See Precautions and Drug/Lab Interactions.

ICU sedation: Observe for signs and symptoms of pain; may indicate need for opioids or analgesia, not an increase in propofol dose. ▪ Benzodiazepines (e.g., diazepam [Valium]) and/or neuromuscular blocking agents (e.g., atracurium [Tracrium], succinylcholine) may also be used. ▪ Monitor triglycerides with long-term use (ICU sedation). Adjust if fat is inadequately cleared from body, and reduce other lipid administration. 1 mL of propofol contains approximately 0.1 Gm of fat (1.1 kcal). ▪ Dose may be reduced carefully to allow patient to awaken to a lighter level of sedation, allowing neurologic and respiratory assessment daily. Avoid rapid awakening; will cause anxiety, agitation, and resistance to mechanical ventilation. ▪ Monitor urinalysis and urine sediment on alternate days in patients at risk for renal impairment. ▪ Some formulations contain EDTA, a trace metal chelator. Formulations containing EDTA should not be infused for longer than 5 days without providing a drug holiday to safely replace estimated or measured zinc losses. Consider zinc supplementation in patients who may be predisposed (e.g., patients with burns, diarrhea, or major sepsis). ▪ Discontinue opioids and paralytic agents and optimize respiratory function before weaning from mechanical ventilation. ▪ Maintain light sedation until 15 minutes before extubation.

Patient Education: Avoid alcohol or other CNS depressants (e.g., antihistamines, benzodiazepines) for 24 hours following anesthesia. ▪ Do not perform tasks requiring mental alertness (e.g., driving, operating hazardous machinery, or signing legal documents) until the day after surgery or longer. All effects must have subsided.

Maternal/Child: Category B: use during pregnancy only if clearly needed. ▪ Not recommended for use in obstetric procedures, including cesarean section; no assurance of safety for fetus. ▪ Not recommended for use during breast-feeding. ▪ Has been approved for induction of anesthesia in pediatric patients 3 years to 16 years of age. Has been approved for maintenance of anesthesia in pediatric patients 2 months to 16 years of age. ▪ Distribution and clearance in pediatric patients 3 years to 12 years of age is similar to that seen in adults. ▪ Serious bradycardia may result with concomitant administration of fentanyl. ▪ Serious adverse effects (e.g., metabolic acidosis) occurred during ICU sedation in pediatric patients with respiratory infections and/or with doses in excess of recommendations for adults. Fatalities have occurred. ▪ A recent study identified an increase in deaths with propofol versus standard sedative agents. Manufacturer has issued a warning letter stating that propofol should not be used for sedation of pediatric patients in ICU. ▪ See Side Effects.

Elderly: Dose requirements decrease after age 55 due to reduced clearance and volume distribution and higher blood levels. Minimize undesirable cardiorespiratory depression (hypotension, apnea, airway obstruction, and/or oxygen desaturation) by using reduced doses and rates of administration. Avoid rapid single or repeated bolus doses; see Precautions. See Usual Dose and Dose Adjustments.

DRUG/LAB INTERACTIONS

Potentiated by **inhalational anesthetics** (e.g., enflurane, halothane, isoflurane, nitrous oxide), **narcotics** (e.g., morphine, meperidine [Demerol], fentanyl), **sedatives** (e.g., barbiturates, benzodiazepines [e.g., diazepam (Valium), midazolam (Versed)], chloral hydrate, droperidol [Inapsine]). Anesthetic and sedative effects increased; systolic, diastolic, mean arterial pressure, and cardiac output are decreased. Dose adjustment may be indicated with concomitant use. ▪ No significant adverse interactions noted to date with neuromuscular blocking agents (e.g., atracurium [Tracrium], succinylcholine). ▪ Competition for chemoreceptor binding sites may occur if used in combination with **droperidol;** use of propofol as a single agent is suggested to control nausea and vomiting. ▪ In pediatric patients, serious bradycardia may result with concomitant administration of **fentanyl.**

SIDE EFFECTS

Adults and pediatric patients: More likely to occur during loading boluses, with supplemental boluses, or during higher rate of administration. Apnea; bradycardia (profound); cough; dyspnea; headache; hypotension; hypoventilation; injection site burning, pain, stinging; nausea, and upper airway obstruction are most common. Urine may be green. Abdominal cramping, anaphylaxis (including bronchospasm, erythema, and hypotension), bucking/jerking/thrashing, clonic/myclonic movement (rarely including convulsions and opisthotonus), dizziness, fever, flushing, hiccups, hypertension, tingling/numbness/coldness at injection site, twitching, and vomiting may occur.

Pediatric patients: Increased incidences of agitation, bradycardia, and jitteriness have occurred; apnea has been observed frequently. Abrupt discontinuation following prolonged infusion may result in agitation, flushing of the hands and feet, hyperirritability, and tremulousness.

Overdose: Cardiorespiratory depression (hypotension, apnea, airway obstruction, and/or oxygen desaturation).

ANTIDOTE

Keep physician informed of all side effects. Reduction of dose may be required or will be treated symptomatically. Discontinue the drug for major side effects, paradoxical reactions, or accidental overdose. A short-acting drug, a patent airway, and continuous controlled ventilation with oxygen until normal function assured should be adequate. Treat bradycardia and/or hypotension with increased rate of IV fluids, Trendelenburg position, vasopressors (e.g., dopamine). Anticholinergic agents (e.g., atropine or glycopyrrolate) may be required. Treat hypersensitivity reactions and resuscitate as necessary.

PROPRANOLOL HYDROCHLORIDE

(proh-**PRAN**-oh-lohl hy-droh-**KLOR**-eyed)

Beta-adrenergic blocking agent
Antiarrhythmic

pH 2.8 to 3.5

USUAL DOSE

1 to 3 mg given 1 mg at a time under careful monitoring (e.g., CVP, ECG); see Monitor and Rate of Administration. Do not give additional propranolol if the desired change in rate or rhythm is achieved. If there is no change in rhythm for at least 2 minutes after the initial dose, cycle may be repeated one time. (AHA recommends 0.5 to 1 mg over 1 minute, repeated as needed up to a total dose of 0.1 mg/kg.) *No further propranolol may be given by any route for at least 4 hours.* Best results achieved if administered within 2 to 4 hours of symptom onset or thrombolytic therapy. Transfer to oral therapy as soon as possible.

PEDIATRIC DOSE (UNLABELED)

0.01 to 0.1 mg/kg/dose over 10 minutes. Maximum dose is 1 mg for infants and 3 mg for other pediatric patients. Repeat at 6- to 8-hour intervals if needed.

Tetralogy spells (hypercyanotic spells): 0.15 to 0.25 mg/kg/dose may be given slowly. May repeat once in 15 minutes. Another source recommends 0.01 to 0.2 mg/kg/dose. Should not exceed 5-mg dose.

DOSE ADJUSTMENTS

Lower-end initial doses may be indicated in the elderly based on potential for decreased organ function and concomitant disease or drug therapy. ▪ Consider dose reduction in patients with impaired hepatic function. ▪ See Drug/Lab Interactions. ▪ Reduce dose gradually to avoid rebound angina, myocardial infarction, or ventricular arrhythmias.

DILUTION

May be given undiluted; however, further dilution of each 1 mg in 10 mL D5W or NS is preferred to facilitate titration of an exact dose while monitoring effect. May be diluted in 50 mL of D5W, D5/½NS, D5NS, or NS for infusion.

Storage: Store at CRT. Protect from freezing or excessive heat.

COMPATIBILITY

Consider any drug NOT listed as compatible to be INCOMPATIBLE until consulting a pharmacist; specific conditions may apply.

One source suggests the following **compatibilities:**

Additive: Dobutamine, verapamil.

Y-site: Alteplase (tPA, Activase), fenoldopam (Corlopam), heparin, hydrocortisone sodium succinate (Solu-Cortef), linezolid (Zyvox), meperidine (Demerol), milrinone (Primacor), morphine, nesiritide (Natrecor), potassium chloride (KCl), propofol (Diprivan), tacrolimus (Prograf), tirofiban (Aggrastat).

RATE OF ADMINISTRATION

Each 1 mg or fraction thereof must be given over 1 minute to avoid excessive hypotension and/or cardiac standstill. A single dose may be given as an infusion over 10 to 15 minutes. Allow adequate time for distribution; consider slow circulation time. Observe monitor and discontinue propranolol as soon as rhythm change occurs.

Pediatric rate: Extend rate of administration of a single dose by injection to a minimum of 5 minutes in pediatric patients.

ACTIONS

Propranolol is a nonselective beta-adrenergic blocker with antiarrhythmic effects. Cardiac response to sympathetic nerve stimulation is inhibited, slowing the HR (especially ventricular rate) by inhibiting atrioventricular conduction. Decreases the force of cardiac contractility, and decreases arterial pressure and cardiac output. Blockade of beta$_2$-adrenergic receptors found predominantly in smooth muscle (e.g., vascular, bronchial, gastrointestinal, and genitourinary); leads to constriction in these tissues. Well distributed throughout the body, the onset of action occurs within 1 to 2 minutes and lasts about 4 hours. Half-life is 2 to 5.5 hours. Metabolized in the liver. Excreted primarily in the urine. Secreted in breast milk.

INDICATIONS AND USES

Reserve IV use for life-threatening situations or for those occurring under anesthesia. ■ Short-term treatment to decrease the ventricular rate in supraventricular tachycardia, including Wolff-Parkinson-White syndrome and thyrotoxicosis. ■ Treatment of persistent and symptomatic PVCs that do not respond to conventional measures. ■ Use in patients with atrial flutter or atrial fibrillation should be reserved for arrhythmias unresponsive to standard therapy or when more prolonged control is required. ■ Control of ventricular rate in life-threatening, digoxin-induced arrhythmias (severe bradycardia may occur). ■ Treatment of tachyarrhythmias due to excessive catecholamine action during anesthesia when other measures fail. ■ Not the drug of first choice for treatment of ventricular arrhythmias unless the arrhythmia is induced by catecholamines or digoxin. In critical situations, when cardioversion or other drugs are not indicated or effective, propranolol may be used with caution. (Use a low dose and administer very slowly so the failing heart maintains some sympathetic drive to maintain myocardial tone. May respond with NSR, but a reduction in ventricular rate is more likely.) ■ Numerous other uses PO.

Unlabeled uses: Other beta-blockers (e.g., atenolol, esmolol) have been used in the perioperative period to reduce cardiac morbidity and mortality in patients at risk; propranolol was not used in these studies. ■ Has been used for adjunctive treatment of pheochromocytoma following primary treatment with an alpha-adrenergic blocking agent (e.g., phenoxybenzamine [Dibenzyline], phentolamine [Regitine]) and for treatment of other refractory arrhythmias when benefit outweighs risk.

CONTRAINDICATIONS

Cardiogenic shock, sinus bradycardia, greater than first-degree heart block, bronchial asthma, known hypersensitivity to propranolol.

PRECAUTIONS

Oral administration is preferred. Use IV administration only when necessary. ■ Not considered the drug of choice for arrhythmias in myocardial infarction. ■ Used concurrently with digoxin or alpha-adrenergic blockers as indicated. ■ Use with caution in overt CHF. May precipitate more severe failure. ■ Use with extreme caution in asthmatics or in patients with lung disease or bronchospasm; can block bronchodilation produced by endogenous and exogenous catecholamine stimulation of beta receptors. ■ Use with caution in patients with diabetes or in patients with a history of hypoglycemia. May cause hypoglycemia and mask the symptoms. ■ Beta blockade can mask symptoms of hyperthyroidism. Abrupt withdrawal of propranolol may be followed by exacerbation of symptoms, including thyroid storm. ■ Use caution in patients with hepatic or renal impairment. ■ May cause arrhythmia, angina, MI, or death if stopped abruptly. ■ Beta-adrenergic receptor blockade can cause a reduction in intraocular pressure. Withdrawal of propranolol may lead to a return of elevated intraocular pressure. May also interfere with the screening test for glaucoma. ▪ IV dose used during surgery to replace an oral dose should be one-tenth of the oral dose. ▪ May cause severe bradycardia in patients with Wolff-Parkinson-White syndrome. See Drug/Lab Interactions.

Monitor: Continuous ECG and BP monitoring is mandatory during administration of IV propranolol. Monitoring of pulmonary wedge pressure or central venous pressure is recommended. Discontinue the drug when a rhythm change is noted and wait to note full effect before giving additional medication if indicated. ▪ See Precautions and Drug/Lab Interactions.

Patient Education: Report any breathing difficulty promptly.

Maternal/Child: Category C: safety for use in pregnancy and breast-feeding and in pediatric patients not established. Use only when clearly indicated. ▪ Bradycardia, hypoglycemia, and respiratory depression have been seen in neonates whose mothers received propranolol during labor or delivery.

Elderly: Lower-end initial doses may be indicated; see Dose Adjustments. ▪ Response of elderly versus younger patients not documented. ▪ Use with caution in age-related peripheral vascular disease; risk of hypothermia increased. ▪ May exacerbate mental impairment.

DRUG/LAB INTERACTIONS

Metabolism involves multiple pathways in the **cytochrome P$_{450}$ system.** Interactions with inhibitors, inducers, or substrates of this system are documented. ▪ Blood levels of propranolol **increased** when administered concurrently **with substrates or inhibitors** such as amiodarone (Nexterone), cimetidine (Tagamet), ciprofloxacin (Cipro IV), delavirdine (Rescriptor), fluconazole (Diflucan), fluoxetine (Prozac), fluvoxamine (Luvox), imipramine (Tofranil), isoniazid (INH), paroxetine (Paxil), quinidine, ritonavir (Norvir), rizatriptan (Maxalt), teniposide (Vumon), theophylline, tolbutamide, zileuton (Zyflo), zolmitriptan (Zomig). ▪ Blood levels of propranolol **decreased** when administered concurrently with **inducers** such as cigarette smoke, ethanol, and rifampin (Rifadin). ▪ Concurrent use with **propafenone** may produce additive negative inotropic and beta-blocking effects. ▪ Concurrent administration with **quinidine** results in additive negative inotropic effects and beta-blockade and postural hypotension. ▪ Concurrent use with **disopyramide** (Norpace) has been associated with additive hypotension, severe bradycardia, asystole, and heart failure. ▪ Concurrent use with **amiodarone** (Nexterone) results in additive negative chronotropic properties. ▪ Decreases **lidocaine** clearance; lidocaine toxicity has been reported with concurrent use. ▪ Effects additive when given with **other agents that slow A-V nodal conduction** (e.g., digoxin [Lanoxin], lidocaine). ▪ Concurrent use with **calcium channel blockers** that have negative inotropic and/or chronotropic activity (e.g., diltiazem [Cardizem], verapamil) may further depress myocardial contractility and A-V nodal conduction. Bradycardia, heart failure, and cardiovascular collapse have been reported with verapamil and beta-blockers. Bradycardia, hypotension, heart block, and heart failure have been reported with coadministration of diltiazem and beta-blockers. ▪ Antihypertensive effects of **clonidine** may be antagonized by propranolol. Use with clonidine may precipitate acute hypertension or aggravate rebound hypertension if clonidine is stopped abruptly; discontinue propranolol several days before gradual withdrawal of clonidine. Monitor BP with concurrent use. ▪ First-dose hypotension may be prolonged with **prazosin** (Minipress). Postural hypotension has been reported when used concurrently with **doxazosin** (Cardura) **and terazosin** (Hytrin). ▪ Coadministration with **reserpine** (a catecholamine-depleting drug) may result in hypotension, bradycardia, vertigo, syncope, or orthostatic hypotension. ▪ Avoid concurrent use with **epinephrine.** Beta-blockade may lead to unopposed alpha-receptor stimulation, resulting in uncontrolled hypertension. ▪ **Dobutamine or isoproterenol** (Isuprel) may be administered to reverse the effects of propranolol. However, patients may experience protracted, severe hypotension. ▪ **Anesthetic agents** (e.g., methoxyflurane and trichloroethylene) may depress myocardial contractility when administered with propranolol. ▪ **ACE inhibitors** (enalapril [Vasotec], lisinopril [Zestril]) may increase bronchial hyperactivity when given concurrently with propranolol. ▪ Hypotension and cardiac arrest have been reported with concurrent use of **haloperidol** and propranolol. ▪ Propranolol may increase serum levels of **theophylline and diazepam** (Valium). ▪ Potentiates **ergot alkaloids** (e.g., dihydroergotamine [D.H.E. 45]); monitor for peripheral ischemia; reduce ergot dose or discontinue beta-blocker. ▪ Added hypotensive effect with **diuretics** (e.g., furosemide), **other antihypertensive agents** (e.g., enalapril, nitroglycerin), some **phenothiazines** (e.g., chlorpromazine [Thorazine]), **and reserpine.** Reduced dose of one or both drugs may be indicated. ▪ May prolong effects of **nondepolarizing muscle relaxants** (e.g., pancuronium). ▪ May increase anticoagulant effects of **warfarin.** ▪ May mask symptoms of hypoglycemia with **insulin and sulfonylureas** and result in prolonged hypoglycemia. ▪ Can interfere with **numerous diagnostic and physiologic tests.** Consult literature. ▪ May alter **thyroid function tests** and cause **elevations in BUN, serum potassium, triglycerides, serum transaminases, and alkaline phosphatase.** ▪ Metabolism and release of catecholamines increased in **smokers;** increased doses may be required. May also interfere with therapeutic effects in **treatment of angina.** ▪ Patients taking beta-blockers who are exposed to a potential allergen may be unresponsive to the usual dose of **epinephrine** used to treat a hypersensitivity reaction.

SIDE EFFECTS

AV conduction delays, bradyarrhythmias, bronchospasm, cardiac failure, cardiac standstill, erythematous rash, hallucination, hypotension, laryngospasm, nausea, paresthesia of the hands, respiratory distress, syncopal attacks, vertigo, visual disturbances. Many other side effects have been reported with oral propranolol and could be seen with the IV route; see manufacturer's literature.

ANTIDOTE

For any side effect or excessive dosage, discontinue the drug and notify the physician immediately. Treat bradycardia with atropine 0.25 to 1 mg. Isoproterenol (Isuprel) may be used with caution if no response to vagal blockade. Serious bradycardia may require pacing. Treat cardiac failure with digitalization and diuretics. Treat hypotension or depressed myocardial function with glucagon. Administer 50 to 150 mcg/kg IV followed by an infusion of 1 to 5 mg/hr (see glucagon monograph for correct dilution). Isoproterenol (Isuprel) and dopamine may also be useful; see Drug/Lab Interactions. Treat bronchospasm with isoproterenol and aminophylline. Treat other side effects symptomatically. Monitor ECG, HR, neurobehavioral status, and intake and output until stable. Not significantly removed by hemodialysis or peritoneal dialysis. Resuscitate as necessary.

PROTAMINE SULFATE BBW

(**PROH**-tah-meen **SUL**-fayt)

Antidote
(heparin antagonist)

pH 6 to 7

USUAL DOSE

Following a serious heparin overdose, discontinue heparin and administer protamine immediately.

Pretreatment: Corticosteroids and antihistamines can be used for patients at risk for protamine hypersensitivity.

IV heparin overdose: 1 mg of IV protamine neutralizes approximately 100 USP units of heparin. May be repeated if needed in 10 to 15 minutes. Never exceed 50 mg in any 10-minute period. Dose adjusted as indicated by coagulation studies. Any dose over 100 mg in 2 hours should be justified by coagulation studies (has its own anticoagulant effect). Because heparin disappears rapidly from the circulation, the dose of protamine required decreases rapidly with the time elapsed after heparin injection (e.g., 30 minutes after IV heparin, 0.5 mg [or one half of the dose] of protamine may be sufficient to neutralize 100 USP units of heparin).

Subcutaneous heparin overdose: 1 to 1.5 mg IV protamine per 100 units of heparin. Some clinicians recommend a loading dose of 25 to 50 mg given slowly over 10 minutes followed by administration of the remainder of the calculated dose as a continuous infusion over 8 to 16 hours (the continuous infusion covers the absorption time seen with administration of SC heparin). See comments under IV heparin overdose.

Low-molecular-weight heparin overdose (unlabeled): 1 mg IV protamine for every 100 antifactor Xa units of LMWH. If PTT remains prolonged 2 to 4 hours after the first dose, or if bleeding continues, consider administration of a second dose of 0.5 mg protamine for every 100 antifactor Xa units. Only 60% to 75% of antifactor Xa activity is neutralized. Excessive protamine doses can worsen bleeding potential. See comments under IV heparin overdose.

DOSE ADJUSTMENTS

Because heparin disappears rapidly from the system, reduce dose of protamine based on length of time elapsed since heparin dose (up to one half if 30 minutes has elapsed). ▪ Prompt administration of protamine sulfate may also decrease dose requirements.

DILUTION

May be given undiluted or may be further diluted with NS or D5W.

Storage: Store at CRT. Do not freeze. Discard remaining medication or diluted solution.

COMPATIBILITY

Consider any drug NOT listed as compatible to be INCOMPATIBLE until consulting a pharmacist; specific conditions may apply.

Manufacturer recommends not mixing with other drugs unless **compatibility** is known, and lists as **incompatible** with some antibiotics, including several cephalosporins and penicillins. Consider individualized rate adjustment necessary to produce desired effects.

One source suggests the following **compatibilities:**

Additive: Ranitidine (Zantac), verapamil.

RATE OF ADMINISTRATION

50 mg (5 mL) or fraction thereof over 10 minutes. Do not exceed 50 mg in 10 minutes. As an infusion, may be given over 2 to 3 hours with dosage titrated according to coagulation studies. Increase duration of infusion to 8 to 16 hours for treatment of SC heparin overdose. Use infusion pump or microdrip (60 gtt/mL) to administer. Too-rapid administration, high doses, or repeated doses can cause anaphylaxis, bradycardia, cardiovascular collapse, catastrophic pulmonary vasoconstriction, pulmonary hypertension, dyspnea, flushing, noncardiogenic pulmonary edema, sensation of warmth, or severe hypotension. Hypertension has also occurred.

ACTIONS

An anticoagulant if administered alone. In the presence of heparin, protamine forms a stable salt, neutralizing the anticoagulant effect of both drugs. Does not bind to low-molecular-weight fragments of LMWH preparations, leading to incomplete neutralization of antifactor Xa. Each 1 mg of protamine can neutralize approximately 100 USP units of heparin. Onset of action is within 0.5 to 1 minute. Neutralization of heparin occurs within 5 minutes. Duration of action is about 2 hours.

INDICATIONS AND USES

To neutralize the anticoagulant activity of heparin in severe heparin overdosage.

Unlabeled uses: Neutralization of heparin administered during extracorporeal circulation in arterial and cardiac surgery or dialysis procedures. ▪ Heparin neutralization in pregnant women near delivery. ▪ Treatment of overdose of low-molecular-weight heparin (e.g., dalteparin, enoxaparin, tinzaparin). Neutralization of LMWH is not complete.

CONTRAINDICATIONS

Known hypersensitivity to protamine. ▪ Do not use for bleeding that occurs without prior exposure to heparin.

PRECAUTIONS

For IV use only. Can cause severe hypotension, cardiovascular collapse, noncardiogenic pulmonary edema, catastrophic pulmonary vasoconstriction, and pulmonary hypertension. Risk factors include high dose or overdose, rapid administration, repeated doses, previous administration of protamine, and current or previous use of protamine-containing drugs (e.g., NPH insulin, protamine zinc insulin, and certain beta-blockers). Allergy to fish, previous vasectomy (may have antiprotamine antibodies), severe left ventricular dysfunction, and abnormal preoperative pulmonary hemodynamics also may be risk factors. In patients with any of these risk factors, the risk versus benefit of protamine sulfate administration should be carefully considered. See Rate of Administration and Usual Dose. ▪ Must be administered in a facility equipped to monitor the patient and respond to any medical emergency. ▪ Pulmonary edema and/or circulatory collapse may occur in patients undergoing cardiac bypass surgery; etiology unknown. ▪ Protamine sulfate should not be given when bleeding occurs without prior heparin use.

Monitor: Coagulation studies (e.g., aPTT, ACT, heparin titration test with protamine, plasma thrombin time) may be indicated to monitor therapeutic response. ▪ Facilities to treat shock must be available; see Precautions. ▪ After cardiac surgery or dialysis procedures, even with adequate neutralization, further bleeding may occur any time within 24 hours (heparin "rebound"). Observe the patient continuously. Additional protamine sulfate may be indicated.

Maternal/Child: Category C: safety for use in pregnancy, breast-feeding, or pediatric patients not established.

DRUG/LAB INTERACTIONS

Specific information not available.

SIDE EFFECTS

Occur more frequently with too-rapid injection; anaphylaxis, back pain, bradycardia, dyspnea, feeling of warmth, flushing, lethargy, nausea, vomiting, severe hypertension or hypotension. Acute pulmonary hypertension, noncardiogenic pulmonary edema, catastrophic pulmonary vasoconstriction, circulatory collapse, capillary leak, or pulmonary edema may occur.

ANTIDOTE

Discontinue the drug and notify the physician, who may recommend a decrease in rate of administration or, if side effects are severe, symptomatic treatment such as administration of whole blood, vasopressors (e.g., dopamine) for hypotension, atropine for bradycardia, and oxygen for dyspnea. Resuscitate as necessary.

PROTEIN AMINO ACIDS, DEXTROSE, FAT EMULSION, AND ELECTROLYTES BBW

Nutritional therapy

(**PROH**-teen ah-**MEE**-noh **AS**-ids)

Kabiven ▪ Perikabiven

USUAL DOSE

Obtain baseline labs; see Monitor. Correct severe fluid, electrolyte, and acid-base disorders before initiating therapy.

Kabiven: 19 to 38 mL/kg/day. Do not exceed 40 mL/kg/day.

Perikabiven: 27 to 40 mL/kg/day. Do not exceed 40 mL/kg/day.

Maximum infusion rate is based on the dextrose component. Individualize dose based on patient's clinical condition (ability to adequately metabolize amino acids, dextrose, and lipids), on patient's body weight and nutritional/fluid requirements, as well as on additional energy given orally/enterally to the patient. Dosage selection is based on fluid requirements, which can be used in conjunction with the nutritional requirements to determine final dosage. Products meet total nutritional requirements for protein, dextrose, and lipids in stable patients and can be individualized to meet specific needs with the addition of nutrients. Treatment may be continued for as long as is required by the patient's condition.

The recommended daily nutritional requirements for protein, dextrose, and lipids compared to the amount of nutrition provided by each product are shown in the following chart. See Rate of Administration for additional dosing instructions.

Nutritional Comparison				
	Nutrition Provided by Kabiven Recommended Dosage	Nutrition Provided by Perikabiven Recommended Dosage	Recommended Nutritional Requirements	
			Stable Patients	Critically Ill Patients*
Fluid (mL/kg/day)	19 to 38	27 to 40	30 to 40	Minimum needed to deliver adequate macronutrients
Protein† (Gm/kg/day)	0.6 to 1.3	0.64 to 0.94	0.8 to 1	1.5 to 2
Nitrogen (Gm/kg/day)	0.1 to 0.2	0.1 to 0.15	0.13 to 0.16	0.24 to 0.3
Dextrose (Gm/kg/day)	1.9 to 3.7	1.8 to 2.7	≤10	≤5.8
Lipids (Gm/kg/day)	0.7 to 1.5	0.95 to 1.4	1	≤1
Total energy requirement (kcal/kg/day)	16 to 32	18 to 27	20 to 30	25 to 30

*Do not use in patients with conditions that are contraindicated; see Contraindications.

†Protein provided as amino acids. When infused IV, amino acids are metabolized and utilized as the building blocks of protein.

DOSE ADJUSTMENTS

Stop infusion in patients with a serum triglyceride concentration above 400 mg/dL. Monitor levels. Once serum triglycerides are less than 400 mg/dL, restart infusion at a reduced rate. Advance rate in smaller increments toward target dosage, checking the triglyceride levels before each adjustment. ▪ Administer the recommended dosage in
Continued

patients with renal impairment. Renal patients not needing dialysis require 0.6 to 0.8 Gm of protein/kg/day. Patients undergoing hemodialysis or continuous renal replacement therapy should receive 1.2 to 1.8 Gm of protein/kg/day up to a maximum of 2.5 Gm of protein/kg/day based on nutritional status and estimated protein losses. Dosage may require adjustment based on fluid, protein, and electrolyte requirements in these patients. Adjust dosage based on treatment for renal impairment, supplementing protein as indicated. If required, additional amino acids may be added to the Kabiven or Perikabiven bag or infused separately; see Compatibility. ▪ Lower-end initial dosing may be appropriate in the elderly based on the potential for decreased hepatic, renal, or cardiac function and on concomitant disease or drug therapy.

DILUTION

Kabiven and Perikabiven are sterile, hypertonic emulsions in a three-chamber container. The individual chambers contain one of the following, respectively: amino acids and electrolytes, dextrose, or lipid injectable emulsion. Available in multiple volumes. Process of activation is extensive. See manufacturer's prescribing information for **contents** of Kabiven and Perikabiven when mixed and for *Preparation Instructions* and *Instructions for Use.* An instructional video is available at www.KabivenUSA.com.

Inspect the bag before activation and discard if any of the following conditions exists: there is evidence of damage to the bag, more than one chamber is white, the solution is yellow, or any seal is already broken. *After activating the bag*, add any **compatible** additives (e.g., MVI and trace elements) via the additive port (white port) using an 18- to 23-gauge needle with a maximum length of 1.5 inches (40 mm). Mix thoroughly after each addition by inverting the bag to ensure a homogenous admixture. Visually inspect for particulate matter and discoloration before administration. Ensure that precipitates have not formed and that the emulsion has not separated. (Separation of the emulsion can be visibly identified by a yellowish streaking or the accumulation of yellowish droplets in the mixed emulsion.)

Filters: Use of a 1.2-micron in-line filter required.

Storage: *Kabiven and Perikabiven:* Before use, store at CRT. Avoid excessive heat and protect from freezing. If accidentally frozen, discard. Do not remove container from the overpouch until intended for use. Product should be used immediately after mixing and the introduction of additives. If not used immediately, the storage time and conditions before use should not be longer than 24 hours refrigerated at 2° to 8° C (36° to 46° F). After removal from refrigeration, the admixture should be infused within 24 hours. Any mixture remaining must be discarded.

Kabiven: In the absence of additives, once activated, the product remains stable for 48 hours at 25° C (77° F). If not used immediately, the activated bag can be stored for up to 7 days under refrigeration. After removal from refrigeration, the activated bag should be used within 48 hours.

COMPATIBILITY

Consider any drug NOT listed as compatible to be INCOMPATIBLE until consulting a pharmacist; specific conditions may apply.

Manufacturer states, "Ceftriaxone (Rocephin) *must not be administered* simultaneously with calcium-containing intravenous solutions such as Kabiven or Perikabiven via a Y-site due to precipitation. However, may be administered sequentially if the infusion lines are thoroughly flushed between infusions with a **compatible** fluid. *Do not use administration sets and lines that contain DEHP.* Administration sets that contain polyvinyl chloride (PCV) components have DEHP as a plasticizer." ▪ **Compatibility** of additions should be evaluated by a pharmacist, and questions may be directed to Fresenius Kabi USA, LLC, Vigilance and Medical Affairs.

RATE OF ADMINISTRATION

For IV infusion only. Use a dedicated line without any connections. Multiple connections could result in air embolism. Use a 1.2-micron in-line filter. Use a nonvented infusion set or close the air inlet on a vented set. (Use of a vented intravenous administration set with a vent in the open position could result in air embolism.)

Kabiven: Maximum infusion rate is 2.6 mL/kg/hr via a **central vein.**

Perikabiven: Maximum infusion rate is 3.7 mL/kg/hr via a **central or peripheral vein.**

The maximum infusion rates listed correspond to 0.09 Gm/kg/hr of amino acids, 0.25 Gm/kg/hr of dextrose (the rate-limiting factor), and 0.1 Gm/kg/hr of lipids. The recommended duration of infusion is between 12 and 24 hours, depending on the clinical situation.

Dosing Instructions: 1. After determining the fluid requirements to be delivered (see preceding chart in Usual Dose), select the corresponding bag that will supply the correct volume of solution. 2. Determine the preferred duration of infusion (12 to 24 hours). 3. Ensure that the rate of infusion in mL/kg/day divided by the preferred duration of infusion in hours does not exceed the maximum infusion rate for the patient (i.e., 2.6 mL/kg/hr for **Kabiven** and 3.7 mL/kg/hr for **Perikabiven**). The infusion rate may need to be reduced and the duration of infusion increased in order not to exceed the maximum infusion rate. 4. Once the infusion rate in mL/kg/hr has been selected, calculate the infusion rate (mL/hr) using the patient's weight. 5. Compare the patient's nutrient requirements with the amount supplied by Kabiven or Perikabiven. Discuss any additions that may be required with a pharmacist or dietitian.

Example:

1. A stable, ambulatory 50-kg patient is to receive Kabiven at a rate of 30 mL/kg/day.

   30 mL/kg/day × 50 kg = 1,500 mL/day. A 1,540 mL bag is chosen.

2. To accommodate different therapies, an infusion duration of 12 hours is chosen.
3. Verify that the maximum rate has not been exceeded: 30 mL/kg/day ÷ 12 = 2.5 mL/kg/hr.
4. 2.5 mL/kg/hr × 50 kg = 125 mL/hr.

ACTIONS

Kabiven and Perikabiven are used as a supplement or as the sole source of nutrition in patients, providing macronutrients (amino acids, dextrose, and lipids) and micronutrients (electrolytes) parenterally. The amino acids provide the structural units that make up proteins and are used to synthesize proteins and other biomolecules or are oxidized to urea and carbon dioxide as a source of energy. Dextrose is oxidized to carbon dioxide and water, yielding energy. Lipids provide biologically utilizable sources of calories and essential fatty acids. Fatty acids serve as an important substrate for energy production. Fatty acids are important for membrane structure and function, as precursors for bioactive molecules (such as prostaglandins), and as regulators of gene expression. The disposition of amino acids, dextrose, and electrolytes is essentially the same as those supplied by ordinary food. The elimination and oxidation rates of infused lipids depend on the patient's clinical condition. Elimination is faster and utilization is increased in postoperative patients and with sepsis, burns, and trauma, whereas patients with renal impairment and hypertriglyceridemia may show lower utilization of exogenous lipid emulsions.

INDICATIONS AND USES

Indicated as a source of calories, protein, electrolytes, and essential fatty acids for adult patients requiring parenteral nutrition when oral or enteral nutrition is not possible, is insufficient, or is contraindicated. May be used to prevent essential fatty acid deficiency or to treat negative nitrogen balance.

Limitation of use: Not recommended for use in pediatric patients under 2 years of age, including preterm infants, because the fixed content of the formulation does not meet the nutritional requirements of this age-group; see Maternal/Child.

CONTRAINDICATIONS

Known hypersensitivity to egg, soybean proteins, peanut proteins, corn or corn products, or any of the active substances or excipients. ▪ Severe hyperlipidemia or severe disorders of lipid metabolism characterized by hypertriglyceridemia (serum triglyceride concentration greater than 1,000 Gm/dL). ▪ Inborn error of amino acid metabolism. ▪ Cardiopulmonary instability (including pulmonary edema, cardiac insufficiency, myocardial infarction, acidosis, and hemodynamic instability requiring significant vasopressor support). ▪ Hemophagocytic syndrome.

PRECAUTIONS

For intravenous infusion only. **Kabiven** is indicated for administration into a *central vein* only (e.g., superior vena cava). Infusion of hypertonic nutrient injections into a peripheral vein may result in vein irritation, vein damage, and/or thrombosis. **Perikabiven** may be administered into a *peripheral or central vein*. Peripheral catheters should not be used for solutions with osmolarity of 900 mOsm/L or greater. The primary complication of peripheral access is venous thrombophlebitis. ▪ Not recommended for pediatric patients under 2 years of age, including preterm infants; see Maternal/Child. ▪ Stop infusion immediately for S/S of hypersensitivity reaction. ▪ Patients who require parenteral nutrition are at high risk for infections due to malnutrition and their underlying disease state. Decrease risk of septic complications with a heightened emphasis on aseptic technique in catheter placement and maintenance, as well as with aseptic technique in the preparation of the nutritional formula. ▪ A reduced or limited ability to metabolize the lipid contained in Kabiven and Perikabiven accompanied by prolonged plasma clearance may result in fat overload syndrome. Syndrome is characterized by a sudden deterioration in the patient's condition accompanied by fever, anemia, leukopenia, thrombocytopenia, coagulation disorders, hyperlipidemia, liver fatty infiltrations (hepatomegaly), deteriorating liver function, and central nervous system manifestations (e.g., coma). Cause of fat overload syndrome is unclear but is usually reversible with discontinuation of the lipid emulsion. ▪ Refeeding syndrome, characterized by the intracellular shift of potassium, phosphorus, and magnesium, may occur when refeeding severely undernourished patients with parenteral nutrition. Thiamine deficiency and fluid retention may also develop. Increase intake gradually to avoid overfeeding and to prevent these complications. ▪ Use with caution in patients with diabetes mellitus or hyperglycemia. Hyperglycemia or hyperosmolar syndrome may develop. Administration of dextrose at a rate exceeding the patient's utilization rate may lead to hyperglycemia, coma, and death; see Rate of Administration. ▪ Hepatobiliary disorders, including cholecystitis, cholelithiasis, cholestasis, hepatic steatosis, fibrosis, and cirrhosis, possibly leading to hepatic failure, have developed in patients without pre-existing liver disease who receive parenteral nutrition. Increase of blood ammonia levels and hyperammonemia may occur in patients receiving amino acid solutions. May indicate hepatic insufficiency or the presence of an inborn error of amino acid metabolism. A clinician knowledgeable in liver diseases should assess patients developing signs of hepatobiliary disorders. ▪ Parenteral nutrition–associated liver disease (PNALD) has been reported in patients receiving parenteral nutrition for extended periods. Exact etiology is unknown; see Antidote. ▪ Use with caution in patients with impaired liver function. ▪ Use with caution in patients with renal impairment, such as prerenal azotemia, renal obstruction, and protein-losing nephropathy. May be at increased risk for electrolyte and fluid volume imbalance. Patients developing signs of renal impairment should be assessed by a clinician knowledgeable in renal disease. ▪ Close monitoring of triglyceride levels is required to avoid consequences associated with hypertriglyceridemia. Serum triglyceride levels above 1,000 mg/dL have been associated with an increased risk of pancreatitis. ▪ Impaired lipid metabolism with hypertriglyceridemia may occur with conditions such as inherited lipid disorders, obesity, diabetes mellitus, and metabolic syndrome. In these cases, increased triglycerides can also be increased by dextrose and/or overfeeding; see Monitor and Dose Adjustments. ▪ Kabiven and Perikabiven contain no more than 25 mcg/L of aluminum. In impaired kidney function, aluminum may reach toxic levels. Research indicates that patients with impaired renal function who receive greater than 4 to 5 mcg/kg/day of parenteral aluminum are at risk for developing CNS or bone toxicity associated with aluminum accumulation. Tissue loading may occur at even lower rates of administration of total parenteral nutrition products.

Monitor: Frequent clinical evaluation and laboratory determinations are necessary for proper monitoring during administration. ▪ Obtain baseline labs, including electrolytes, serum triglycerides, blood glucose, liver/kidney function (BUN, SCr, liver function tests, ammonia), serum osmolarity, and CBC, including platelet and coagulation parameters. Repeat frequently as indicated by clinical condition. ▪ Monitor fluid status closely in patients with heart failure, pulmonary edema, or renal impairment. ▪ Evaluate patient's ability to eliminate and metabolize infused lipid emulsion by measuring serum triglyceride levels at baseline, with each increase in dosage, and regularly throughout treatment. ▪ Monitor patients for S/S of essential fatty acid deficiency. Laboratory tests are available to determine serum fatty acid levels. ▪ Monitor for S/S of a hypersensitivity reaction (e.g., altered mentation, bronchospasm, chills, cyanosis, dizziness, dyspnea, erythema, fever, flushing, headache, hypotension, hypoxia, nausea, rash, sweating, tachycardia, tachypnea, urticaria, vomiting). ▪ Monitor for S/S of early infection (e.g., fever, chills, hyperglycemia, leukocytosis). Check parenteral access device frequently. ▪ Monitor for S/S of fat overload syndrome. ▪ Monitor severely undernourished patients for S/S of refeeding syndrome. ▪ Monitor blood glucose levels and treat hyperglycemia to maintain optimum levels while infusing parenteral nutrition. Insulin may be administered or adjusted to maintain optimum blood glucose levels during parenteral nutrition administration. ▪ Monitor for thrombophlebitis, which may manifest as erythema, pain, tenderness, or a palpable cord. ▪ Monitor for S/S of hepatobiliary disorders (e.g., elevated LFTs/ammonia, jaundice). ▪ Monitor overall energy intake and other sources of lipid and dextrose, as well as drugs that may interfere with lipid and dextrose metabolism.

Patient Education: Report S/S of hyperglycemia, hypersensitivity reaction (e.g., bronchospasm, itching, rash, wheezing), hypoglycemia, infection (e.g., fever), nausea, vomiting, or fluid retention. ▪ Periodic laboratory tests and routine follow-up with health care provider required. ▪ Report any changes in prescription or nonprescription medications and supplements.

Maternal/Child: Category C: use during pregnancy only if clearly needed. Parenteral nutrition should be considered in cases of severe maternal malnutrition in which nutritional requirements cannot be fulfilled by enteral route because of the risks to the fetus associated with severe malnutrition, such as preterm delivery, low birth weight, intrauterine growth restriction, congenital malformations, and perinatal mortality. ▪ Use caution during breast-feeding. ▪ Safety and effectiveness in pediatric patients have not been established. Deaths in preterm infants after infusion of IV lipid emulsions have been reported. Autopsy findings included intravascular fat accumulation in the lungs. Preterm infants and low-birth-weight infants have poor clearance of IV lipid emulsion and increased free fatty acid plasma levels following lipid emulsion infusion. ▪ Not recommended for use in pediatric patients under 2 years of age, including preterm infants, because the fixed content of the formulation does not meet the nutritional requirements of this age-group.

Elderly: Differences in response between the elderly and younger patients have not been identified. Dose selection should be cautious; see Dose Adjustment.

DRUG/LAB INTERACTIONS

High levels of lipid in plasma may interfere with **some laboratory blood tests,** such as hemoglobin, triglycerides, bilirubin, LDH, and oxygen saturation, if blood is sampled before lipid has been cleared from the bloodstream. Lipids are normally cleared after a lipid-free interval of 5 to 6 hours in most patients. ▪ Kabiven and Perikabiven contain vitamin K, which can reverse coumarin and coumarin derivatives, including **warfarin.** Monitor laboratory parameters for anticoagulant activity in patients who are taking both Kabiven or Perikabiven and warfarin.

SIDE EFFECTS

Kabiven: The most common adverse reactions are decreased hemoglobin, decreased total protein, fever, hypertension, hypokalemia, increased gamma glutamyltransferase (GGT), nausea, vomiting. Less frequently reported reactions include decreased blood calcium, hyperglycemia, increased blood alkaline phosphatase, prolonged PT, pruritus, tachycardia.

Perikabiven: The most common adverse reactions are fever, hyperglycemia, hypokalemia, and increased blood triglycerides. Less frequently reported reactions include hypoalbuminemia, increased alanine aminotransferase (ALT), increased blood alkaline phosphatase, increased BUN, increased C-reactive protein, increased GGT, nausea, phlebitis, and pruritus. A number of other reactions occurred in 1% or fewer of patients. See Precautions for serious adverse reactions that have been reported with Kabiven or Perikabiven. **Post-Marketing:** *Kabiven:* Cholestasis, hypersensitivity reaction (including anaphylaxis), infection, subependymal hemorrhage.

Perikabiven: Abdominal distension, abdominal pain, chest tightness, cholestasis, flushed face, infection.

ANTIDOTE

Notify the physician immediately of any adverse symptoms. Stop infusion for severely elevated electrolyte levels or triglyceride levels above 400 mg/dL. Monitor electrolytes and triglycerides. Reinitiate infusion at a reduced rate when laboratory values are within normal limits. Consider discontinuation or dosage reduction in patients who develop liver test abnormalities. Stop infusion immediately at the first sign of a hypersensitivity reaction and treat as indicated (antihistamines, epinephrine, corticosteroids, airway management, oxygen). Resuscitate as necessary. In the event of an overdose, fat overload syndrome may result. Stop infusion and allow lipids to clear from serum. Effects are usually reversible after the lipid infusion is stopped. The lipid administered and the fatty acids produced are not dialyzable.

PROTEIN C CONCENTRATE (HUMAN)
(**PROH**-teen C **KON**-sen-trayt)

Anticoagulant
Antithrombotic

Ceprotin

pH 6.7 to 7.3

USUAL DOSE

(International units [IU])

Dose, administration frequency, and duration of treatment depend on the severity of the protein C deficiency, the patient's age, the clinical condition of the patient, and the patient's plasma level of protein C. Initiate therapy as directed in the chart below and adjust the dosage regimen according to the pharmacokinetic profile for each patient. See Dose Adjustments and Monitor.

Protein C Concentrate Dosing Schedule for Acute Episodes, Short-Term Prophylaxis, and Long-Term Prophylaxis			
	Initial Dose*	Subsequent 3 Doses*	Maintenance Dose*
Acute episodes/ short-term prophylaxis†	100 to 120 IU/kg	60 to 80 IU/kg every 6 hours	45 to 60 IU/kg every 6 or 12 hours
Long-term prophylaxis	N/A	N/A	45 to 60 IU/kg every 12 hours

*Dose regimen should be adjusted according to the pharmacokinetic profile for each individual patient.
†Continue therapy until the desired anticoagulation is achieved.

PEDIATRIC AND NEONATAL DOSE

See Usual Dose and Maternal/Child.

DOSE ADJUSTMENTS

For treatment of acute episodes or with short-term prophylaxis, adjust dose according to the pharmacokinetic profile of the patient. Adjust to maintain a target peak protein C activity of 100%. After resolution of the acute episode, continue patient on the same dose to maintain a trough protein C activity above 25% for the duration of treatment. ▪ Higher peak protein C activity levels may be required for situations in which there is an increased risk of thrombosis (e.g., infection, surgical intervention, trauma). Maintaining trough protein C activity levels above 25% is recommended. ▪ Use in renal and hepatic impairment has not been studied. See Precautions.

DILUTION (International units [IU])

Available in single-dose vials that contain 500 or 1,000 international units (IU) of protein C. Reconstitute the 500-IU vial with 5 mL of SWFI and the 1,000-IU vial with 10 mL of SWFI to provide a single dose of human protein C at a concentration of 100 IU/mL. Vials also contain human albumin, trisodium citrate dihydrate, and sodium chloride as excipients. Bring the vials of protein C and SWFI (supplied diluent) to room temperature. Remove tops of vials and cleanse stoppers. Insert one end of the manufacturer-supplied double-ended transfer needle through the center of the diluent vial stopper. Invert the diluent vial and insert the free end of the double-ended transfer needle into the protein C vial. The vacuum in the vial should pull in the diluent. If a vacuum is not present, do not use the vial. Remove the double-ended transfer needle from the diluent vial, then from the protein C vial. Gently swirl the protein C vial until the powder is completely dissolved. The powder must be completely dissolved to prevent active materials from being removed by the filter needle during infusion. Solution should be colorless to slightly yellowish and clear to slightly opalescent. Attach manufacturer-supplied filter needle to a disposable syringe. Withdraw plunger to admit air into the syringe and inject air into the protein C vial. Withdraw reconstituted solution from the vial into the syringe. Remove the filter needle and attach a suitable needle or infusion set for administration. The filter needle is intended to filter the contents of a single vial of protein C.

Filters: Filtering required; see Dilution.

Storage: Refrigerate unopened vials in original carton at 2° to 8° C (36° to 46° F); protect from light. Shelf life is 3 years. Do not use beyond expiration date. Do not freeze. Administer reconstituted product within 3 hours of reconstitution. Single-dose vial; discard any unused product after entry into vial.

COMPATIBILITY

Specific information not available. Consider specialized use.

RATE OF ADMINISTRATION

Administer as an infusion.

Adults and pediatric patients over 10 kg: Maximum rate 2 mL/min.

Pediatric patients less than 10 kg: Maximum rate 0.2 mL/kg/min.

ACTIONS

A precursor of the vitamin K–dependent anticoagulant glycoprotein (serine protease) that is synthesized in the liver. Manufactured from human plasma. Numerous processes are used during manufacturing to minimize the risk for viral transmission; see Precautions. Protein C is converted to activated protein C (APC), a serine protease with potent anticoagulant effects. APC exerts its effect by inactivation of the activated forms of factors V and VIII, which leads to a decrease in thrombin formation. APC also has been shown to have profibrinolytic effects. A complete absence of protein C is not compatible with life. A severe deficiency of this protein leads to unchecked coagulation activation, resulting in thrombin generation and intravascular clot formation and thrombosis. An increase in plasma levels of protein C can be seen within $1/2$ hour after administration of protein C concentrate. Replacement of protein C in protein C–deficient patients is expected to control or, if given prophylactically, prevent thrombotic complications. In clinical studies, patients with severe congenital protein C deficiency were treated more effectively with protein C concentrate than those treated with modalities such as fresh-frozen plasma or conventional anticoagulants. Half-life ranges from 4.9 to 14.7 hours, with a median of 9.8 hours. In patients with acute thrombosis, purpura fulminans, and skin necrosis, both the half-life and the increase in protein C plasma level may be reduced.

INDICATIONS AND USES

Prevention and treatment of venous thrombosis and purpura fulminans in patients with severe congenital protein C deficiency. A replacement therapy for pediatric and adult patients.

CONTRAINDICATIONS

None known.

PRECAUTIONS

Initiate treatment under the supervision of a physician experienced in replacement therapy with coagulation factors/inhibitors and in a facility where monitoring of protein C activity is available. ▪ Half-life of protein C concentrate may be shortened in certain clinical conditions such as acute thrombosis, purpura fulminans, and skin necrosis. Patients treated during the acute phase of their disease may display much lower increases in protein C activity. ▪ May contain trace amounts of mouse protein and heparin due to the manufacturing process. Hypersensitivity reactions are possible; see Monitor and Antidote. ▪ Manufactured from pooled human plasma. Special screening and purification techniques are used to minimize the risk of transmitting infectious agents (e.g., hepatitis A, human parvovirus B19, Creutzfeldt-Jakob disease [CJD]), but transmission cannot be completely ruled out. Appropriate vaccination (hepatitis A and B) should be considered for patients receiving human-derived protein C. ▪ Contains heparin. Discontinue if heparin-induced thrombocytopenia (HIT) is suspected; see Monitor. ▪ Use with caution in patients who may be sensitive to a sodium load (e.g., patients with hypertension or CHF); see Monitor. ▪ Patients being started on anticoagulant therapy with a vitamin K–antagonist anticoagulant (e.g., warfarin) may experience a transient hypercoagulable state before desired anticoagulation is reached. Patients may be at increased risk for warfarin-induced skin necrosis. Initiate warfarin therapy at a low dose and adjust incrementally as indicated by INR monitoring. Continue protein C replacement until stable anticoagulation with warfarin is reached. ▪ Bleeding episodes have been reported. Simultaneous administration with alteplase (Activase, tPA) and/or anticoagulants (e.g., warfarin, heparin) may increase the risk of bleeding; see Drug Interactions. ▪ Use with caution in patients with renal and/or hepatic impairment. Has not been studied.

Monitor: Measure protein C activity using a chromogenic assay before and during treatment. ▪ In the case of an acute thrombotic event, it is recommended that protein C activity measurements be obtained immediately before the next injection until the patient is stabilized. Once stabilized, continue monitoring to maintain the trough protein C level above 25%. ▪ Coagulation parameters (e.g., INR/PT) should be monitored. However, a correlation between coagulation parameters and protein C activity levels has not been determined. ▪ Discontinue therapy and check platelet count if heparin-induced thrombocytopenia is suspected. ▪ Contains more than 200 mg of sodium. Monitor fluid and electrolyte status, especially in patients on a low-sodium diet and/or in patients with renal impairment. ▪ Monitor for S/S of hypersensitivity reactions (e.g., anaphylaxis, hives, hypotension, generalized itching, tightness of the chest, and/or wheezing).

Patient Education: Manufactured from pooled human plasma. Risk of transmission of infectious agents cannot be ruled out. Discuss risk versus benefit of therapy with physician. ▪ Review vaccination status with physician. Vaccination against hepatitis A and B should be considered. ▪ Contains sodium. ▪ Report S/S of hypersensitivity reaction immediately (e.g., hives, generalized itching, tightness of the chest, wheezing). ▪ Consultation with a physician is required if abdominal pain, chills, drowsiness, fever, jaundice, nausea and vomiting, prolonged poor appetite, runny nose, tiredness, or dark urine occurs.

Maternal/Child: Category C: safety for use in pregnancy and lactation has not been established. ▪ Has been used in patients as young as 2 days of age. ▪ Pharmacokinetics in the very young may differ from that of older pediatric patients and adults. Systemic exposure (Cmax and AUC) may be reduced due to a faster clearance, larger volume of distribution, and/or shorter half-life. Doses must be individualized based on protein C activity levels; see Dose Adjustments.

Elderly: Specific differences in safety and efficacy have not been identified.

DRUG/LAB INTERACTIONS

Formal drug interaction studies have not been conducted. ▪ Simultaneous use with **alteplase** (Activase, tPA) and **anticoagulants** (e.g., warfarin, heparin) may increase the risk of bleeding. ▪ Patients being started on anticoagulant therapy with a **vitamin K–antagonist anticoagulant** (e.g., warfarin) may experience a transient hypercoagulable state before desired anticoagulation is reached; see Precautions.

SIDE EFFECTS

The most commonly reported side effects are itching, light-headedness, and rash.

Post-Marketing: Fever, hemothorax, hyperhidrosis, hypotension, and restlessness.

ANTIDOTE

Notify physician of any side effects; most will be treated symptomatically. Discontinue protein C concentrate for any serious reaction (e.g., HIT, hypersensitivity). Treat hypersensitivity reactions as indicated (e.g., oxygen, diphenhydramine, epinephrine, corticosteroids, vasopressors, and/or fluids). Resuscitate as necessary.

P

PROTHROMBIN COMPLEX CONCENTRATE (HUMAN) BBW

Antihemorrhagic

(**PRO**-throm-bin **KOM**-plex **KAN**-sen-trayt [**HUE**-man])

Kcentra

USUAL DOSE

(International Units [IU])

Dosing should be individualized based on the patient's baseline International Normalized Ratio (INR) value and body weight.

Vitamin K: Administer vitamin K (phytonadione) concurrently to maintain vitamin K–dependent factor levels once the effects of the prothrombin complex concentrate (human) have diminished.

Prothrombin complex concentrate (human): Coagulation factor levels may be unstable in patients with acute major bleeding who are receiving vitamin K. Obtain baseline INR (close to time of dosing). Using this INR and the patient's weight, individualize dose as shown in the following chart.

Prothrombin Complex Concentrate (Human) Dosing Guidelines			
	Pretreatment INR		
	2 to Less Than 4	4 to 6	Greater Than 6
Dose of prothrombin complex concentrate [human]* (units† of factor IX/kg body weight)	25 IU/kg	35 IU/kg	50 IU/kg
Maximum dose (units of factor IX)‡	Not to exceed 2,500 IU	Not to exceed 3,500 IU	Not to exceed 5,000 IU

*Dose is based on body weight. Dose is also based on actual potency as stated on the carton, which will vary from 20 to 31 factor IX units/mL.

†Units refer to international units.

‡Dose is based on body weight up to but not exceeding 100 kg. For patients weighing more than 100 kg, maximum dose should not be exceeded.

Example dosing calculation for an 80-kg patient with a baseline INR of 5:

35 units of Factor IX/kg × 80 kg = 2,800 units of Factor IX required

For a vial with an actual potency of 30 units/mL factor IX, 93 mL would be given:

2,800 units ÷ 30 units/mL = 93 mL

Repeat dosing with prothrombin complex concentrate is not supported by clinical data and is not recommended.

DILUTION

Available in a kit that contains 500 units of prothrombin complex concentrate in a single-use vial, a 20-mL vial of SWFI, a Mix2Vial filter transfer set, and an alcohol swab. The actual potency per vial of factors II, VII, IX, and X and of proteins C and S is stated on the carton (potency in IU is defined by factor IX content). When reconstituted, the final concentration of drug product in factor IX units will range from 20 to 31 units/mL (400 to 620 units/vial) depending on actual potency, which is listed on the carton. Nominal potency is 500 units per vial, which is approximately 25 units/mL after reconstitution. Record the lot number of the product in the patient's medical record when prothrombin complex concentrate is administered.

Begin the reconstitution process by bringing prothrombin complex concentrate and diluent vial to room temperature. Use of aseptic technique required. Remove vial tops and wipe stoppers with the alcohol swab. Open the Mix2Vial transfer set package, leaving transfer set in the clear package. Place *diluent vial* on a flat surface and hold vial tightly. Grip the Mix2Vial transfer set together with the clear package and push the plastic spike at the *blue end of the transfer set* firmly through the center of the diluent vial stopper. Carefully remove the clear package from the Mix2Vial transfer set. With the *prothrombin complex concentrate vial* firmly on a flat surface, invert the diluent vial with the transfer set attached and push the plastic spike of the *transparent adapter* firmly through the center of the stopper of the prothrombin complex concentrate vial. The diluent will automatically transfer into the prothrombin complex concentrate vial. With both vials still attached to the transfer set, gently swirl the prothrombin complex concentrate vial to ensure complete dissolution. *Do not shake.* Solution should be colorless, clear to slightly opalescent, and free from visible particles. With one hand, grasp the prothrombin complex concentrate side of the Mix2Vial transfer set, and with the other hand grasp the blue diluent side of the Mix2Vial transfer set, and unscrew the set into two pieces. Draw air into an empty, sterile syringe. While the prothrombin complex concentrate vial is upright, screw the syringe to the Mix2Vial transfer set. Inject air into the vial. While keeping the syringe plunger pressed, invert the system upside down and draw the concentrate into the syringe by pulling the plunger back slowly. Unscrew the syringe from the transfer set and attach to a suitable intravenous administration set. If the same patient is to receive more than one vial, contents of multiple vials may be pooled. Use a separate, unused Mix2Vial transfer set for each product vial.

Storage: Store lyophilized powder in carton at 2° to 25° C (36° to 77° F); protect from light and freezing. Stable for 36 months from date of manufacture. Do not use beyond the expiration date on the carton and vial labels. Product must be used within 4 hours following reconstitution. Reconstituted product can be stored at 2° to 25° C. If cooled, the solution should be warmed to 20° to 25° C (68° to 77° F, approximate room temperature) before administration. Do not freeze reconstituted product. Discard partially used vials.

COMPATIBILITY
Manufacturer states, "Do not mix with other medicinal products; administer through a separate infusion line. No blood should enter the syringe, as there is a possibility of fibrin clot formation."

RATE OF ADMINISTRATION
Administer at room temperature at a rate of 0.12 mL/kg/min (approximately 3 units/kg/min), up to a maximum of 8.4 mL/min (approximately 210 units/min).

ACTIONS
A purified, heat-treated, nanofiltered, and lyophilized nonactivated four-factor prothrombin complex concentrate prepared from human U.S. Source Plasma. Contains the vitamin K–dependent coagulation factors II, VII, IX, and X (together known as the prothrombin complex) and the antithrombotic proteins C and S. Factor IX is the lead factor for the potency of the preparation. (Human antithrombin III, heparin and human albumin, sodium chloride, and sodium citrate are listed as excipients.) A dose-dependent acquired deficiency of the vitamin K–dependent coagulation factors occurs during vitamin K antagonist (VKA) treatment. Vitamin K antagonists exert anticoagulant effects by lowering both factor synthesis and function. Administration of prothrombin complex concentrate rapidly increases plasma levels of the vitamin K–dependent coagulation factors II, VII, IX, and X as well as the antithrombotic proteins C and S. In clinical trials, prothrombin complex concentrate restored the decreased vitamin K–dependent clotting factors significantly faster than plasma in patients on warfarin. A single dose of prothrombin complex concentrate produced a rapid and sustained increase in plasma levels of factors II, VII, IX, and X within 30 minutes posttreatment with 87% less volume than with plasma. In addition, infusion time with prothrombin complex concentrate was seven times faster than with plasma. In most subjects, prothrombin complex concentrate decreased INR to less than or equal to 1.3 within 30 minutes. The relationship between this or other INR values and clinical hemostasis in patients has not been established.

INDICATIONS AND USES

Indicated for the urgent reversal of acquired coagulation factor deficiency induced by vitamin K antagonists (e.g., warfarin) therapy in adult patients with acute major bleeding. Not indicated for urgent reversal of vitamin K antagonist anticoagulation in patients without acute major bleeding.

CONTRAINDICATIONS

Patients with known anaphylactic or severe systemic reactions to prothrombin complex concentrate or any of its components, including heparin; factors II, VII, IX, and X; proteins C and S; antithrombin III; and human albumin. ▪ Patients with disseminated intravascular coagulation (DIC). ▪ Patients with known heparin-induced thrombocytopenia (HIT). Prothrombin complex concentrate contains heparin.

PRECAUTIONS

For IV use only. ▪ Hypersensitivity reactions have been reported. ▪ Both fatal and nonfatal arterial and venous thromboembolic complications have been reported. Patients being treated with VKA therapy have underlying disease states that predispose them to thromboembolic events. The potential benefits of reversing VKA should be weighed against the potential risks of thromboembolic events, especially in patients with a history of a thromboembolic event. Resumption of anticoagulation should be carefully considered as soon as the risk of thromboembolic events outweighs the risk of acute bleeding. ▪ Prothrombin complex concentrate has not been studied in subjects who have had a thromboembolic event, myocardial infarction, disseminated intravascular coagulation, cerebrovascular accident, transient ischemic attack, unstable angina pectoris, or severe peripheral vascular disease within the previous 3 months. Prothrombin complex concentrate may not be suitable in patients who have had a thromboembolic event in the previous 3 months. ▪ Made from human blood and may contain infectious agents (e.g., HIV, Creutzfeldt-Jakob disease, hepatitis B, hepatitis C). Numerous steps in the manufacturing process are used to make the potential for transmission of infectious agents extremely remote. ▪ Prothrombin complex concentrate has not been studied in patients with congenital factor deficiencies.

Monitor: Monitor INR and clinical response during and after treatment. ▪ Standard clinical assessments (e.g., VS, hemoglobin measurements, CT assessments relevant to the type of bleeding [e.g., GI, cerebral]) may be used to evaluate effective hemostasis. ▪ Monitor for S/S of hypersensitivity reactions (e.g., angioedema, anxiety, bronchospasm, dyspnea, flushing, hypotension, nausea, pulmonary edema, tachycardia, urticaria, wheezing, vomiting). ▪ Monitor for signs and symptoms of thromboembolic events (e.g., deep venous thrombosis, pulmonary embolism, stroke) during and after administration of prothrombin complex concentrate.

Patient Education: Report any S/S of hypersensitivity promptly (e.g., hives, rash, tightness of chest, wheezing). ▪ Report S/S of thrombosis (e.g., limb or abdominal swelling and/or pain, chest pain or pressure, shortness of breath, loss of sensation or motor power, altered consciousness, vision, or speech). ▪ Prothrombin complex concentrate is made from human blood and may carry a remote risk of transmitting infectious agents. See Precautions.

Maternal/Child: Category C: safety for use during pregnancy, labor and delivery, and during breast-feeding not established; use only if clearly indicated. ▪ Safety and effectiveness for use in pediatric patients not established.

Elderly: Response similar to other age-groups.

DRUG/LAB INTERACTIONS

Specific information not available.

SIDE EFFECTS

The most common side effects observed were arthralgia, headache, hypotension, nausea, and vomiting. The most serious side effects were thromboembolic events, including deep vein thrombosis, pulmonary embolism, and stroke. Other side effects included abnormal breath sounds, chest pain, constipation, dyspnea, fluid overload, hypertension, hypokalemia, hypoxia, insomnia, intracranial hemorrhage, mental status changes, myocardial infarction, myocardial ischemia, pulmonary edema, respiratory distress, and tachycardia.

Post-Marketing: Hypersensitivity or allergic reactions (e.g., angioedema, anxiety, broncho-spasm, dyspnea, flushing, hypotension, nausea, pulmonary edema, tachycardia, urticaria, vomiting, wheezing) and thromboembolic complications (arterial thromboembolic events [arterial thrombosis, acute MI], venous thromboembolic events [pulmonary embolism and venous thrombosis], and DIC).

ANTIDOTE

Notify physician of any side effect. If a severe hypersensitivity or anaphylactic-type reaction occurs, immediately discontinue administration and institute appropriate treatment (e.g., oxygen, hydrocortisone, epinephrine (Adrenalin), diphenhydramine (Benadryl), an H_2 antagonist [e.g., famotidine (Pepcid), ranitidine (Zantac)]).

QUINUPRISTIN/DALFOPRISTIN
(kwin-oo-**PRIS**-tin/**DAL**-foh-**pris**-tin)

Synercid

Antibacterial
(Streptogramin)

pH 4.5 to 4.75

USUAL DOSE

Complicated skin and skin structure infection: 7.5 mg/kg every 12 hours. Minimum recommended duration of therapy is 7 days.

PEDIATRIC DOSE

Safety and effectiveness for use in pediatric patients under 16 years of age not established; however, the manufacturer recommends a dose of 7.5 mg/kg every 12 hours for pediatric patients (12 to less than 18 years of age). Dose recommendations for patients less than 12 years of age are not available. Doses of 7.5 mg/kg every 8 or 12 hours have been used under emergency-use conditions in a limited number of pediatric patients.

DOSE ADJUSTMENTS

No dose adjustments required in the elderly, pediatric patients, patients with renal insufficiency, or patients undergoing hemodialysis or peritoneal dialysis. See Maternal/Child. ▪ Dose reduction may be required in patients with hepatic cirrhosis (Child-Pugh Class A or B). Exact recommendations are not currently available, but one source recommends decreasing dose to 5 mg/kg in patients who cannot tolerate the usual dose. ▪ Patients experiencing arthralgias and myalgias may respond to a reduction in dose frequency to every 12 hours; see Precautions. ▪ See Drug/Lab Interactions.

DILUTION

Reconstitute the 500-mg single-dose vial by slowly adding 5 mL of D5W or SWFI. Swirl gently to limit foam formation. Do not shake. Allow solution to sit until foam has disappeared. Final concentration of reconstituted solution is 100 mg/mL. Must be further diluted; withdraw calculated dose and add to 250 mL of D5W. Desired concentration is approximately 2 mg/mL. If moderate to severe venous irritation occurs following peripheral administration, consideration should be given to increasing infusion volume to 500 to 750 mL of D5W; see Precautions. An infusion volume of 100 mL may be used for central line infusions.

Storage: Store unopened vials in refrigerator at 2° to 8° C (36° to 46° F). Reconstituted solution should be used within 30 minutes. Diluted solution is stable for 5 hours at RT and for 54 hours if refrigerated.

COMPATIBILITY   (Underline Indicates Conflicting Compatibility Information)

Consider any drug NOT listed as compatible to be INCOMPATIBLE until consulting a pharmacist; specific conditions may apply.

Manufacturer lists saline solutions and heparin as **incompatible** and recommends administering quinupristin/dalfopristin separately. Always flush line with D5W before and after administration of any other drug through the same IV line.

Manufacturer lists **Y-site compatibility** with specific concentrations of aztreonam (Azactam [20 mg/mL]), ciprofloxacin (Cipro IV [1 mg/mL]), fluconazole (Diflucan [2 mg/mL]), metoclopramide (Reglan [5 mg/mL]), and potassium chloride (KCl [40 mEq/L]). Another source adds <u>anidulafungin (Eraxis)</u>, <u>caspofungin (Cancidas)</u>, and fenoldopam (Corlopam).

RATE OF ADMINISTRATION

Flush IV line with D5W before and after administration. A single dose properly diluted over 60 minutes. Use of an infusion pump or device to control rate of infusion is recommended. In animal studies toxicity was higher when administered as a bolus. Studies in humans have not been performed.

ACTIONS

A streptogramin antimicrobial agent composed of two semi-synthetic pristinamycin derivatives, quinupristin and dalfopristin, in a ratio of 30:70 (w:w). Quinupristin and dalfopristin bind to the bacterial ribosome, thereby inhibiting protein synthesis. When combined, the two components act synergistically. The compound is bactericidal against strains of methicillin-susceptible and methicillin-resistant staphylococci. Cross-resistance between quinupristin/dalfopristin and other antibacterial agents such as beta-lactams, aminoglycosides, glycopeptides, quinolones, macrolides, lincosamides, and tetracyclines has not been reported. Metabolized in the liver via nonenzymatic processes to several active metabolites. Elimination half-life of quinupristin and dalfopristin is approximately 0.85 and 0.7 hours, respectively. Although the elimination half-life for each component is short, the combination exhibits a prolonged postantibiotic effect of 10 hours with *Staphylococcus aureus* and 9.1 hours with *Streptococcus pneumoniae.* Fecal excretion is the primary elimination route for both components and their metabolites. Urinary excretion accounts for about 15% of the quinupristin and 19% of the dalfopristin dose.

INDICATIONS AND USES

Treatment of complicated skin and skin structure infections caused by *Staphylococcus aureus* (methicillin susceptible) or *Streptococcus pyogenes.*

CONTRAINDICATIONS

Known hypersensitivity to quinupristin/dalfopristin or to other streptogramins (e.g., pristinamycin or virginiamycin).

PRECAUTIONS

C/S indicated to determine susceptibility of causative organism to quinupristin/dalfopristin. ▪ Flush line with D5W after completion of peripheral infusion to minimize vein irritation. If moderate to severe venous irritation occurs with 250-mL infusion, consider increasing volume to 500 or 750 mL of D5W, changing the infusion site, or infusing by a peripherally inserted central catheter (PICC) or a central venous catheter; see Dilution. Concomitant administration of hydrocortisone or diphenhydramine does ***not*** appear to alleviate venous irritation. ▪ Episodes of arthralgia and myalgia have been reported. In some patients, improvement was noted with a reduction in dose frequency to every 12 hours; see Dose Adjustments. ▪ Superinfection caused by the overgrowth of nonsusceptible organisms may occur with antibiotic use. Treat as indicated. ▪ *Clostridium difficile*–associated diarrhea (CDAD) has been reported. May range from mild diarrhea to fatal colitis. Consider in patients who present with diarrhea during or after treatment with quinupristin/dalfopristin.

Monitor: Monitor total bilirubin. Levels greater than 5 times the upper limit of normal were reported in approximately 25% of patients. ▪ Monitor infusion site for any sign of irritation or inflammation; see Precautions.

Patient Education: Report pain at injection site or any other side effect promptly. ▪ Promptly report diarrhea or bloody stools that occur during treatment or up to several months after an antibiotic has been discontinued; may indicate CDAD and require treatment.

Maternal/Child: Category B: safety for use in pregnancy and breast-feeding not established. Use caution. ▪ Safety and effectiveness in pediatric patients under 16 years of age not established. Has been used in a limited number of pediatric patients under emergency-use conditions. Dose adjustment does not appear to be required; see Pediatric Dose.

Elderly: No apparent differences in frequency, type, or severity of side effects. Dose adjustment not required.

DRUG/LAB INTERACTIONS

Quinupristin/dalfopristin significantly inhibits cytochrome P_{450} 3A4 metabolism of **cyclosporin A** (Sandimmune), **midazolam** (Versed), **nifedipine** (Procardia), **and tacrolimus** (Prograf) and increases their plasma concentrations; dose adjustments may be indicated. Monitoring of cyclosporine and/or tacrolimus serum levels to determine therapeutic dose should be performed when cyclosporine or tacrolimus must be used concomitantly with quinupristin/dalfopristin. ▪ It is reasonable to expect that quinupristin/dalfopristin would **inhibit other drugs that are metabolized by the P_{450} 3A4 enzyme system.** Use caution if being coadministered with **drugs that have a narrow therapeutic index** (e.g., cyclosporine) and are metabolized via this pathway. Effects may be prolonged, side effects may be increased, and dose adjustments may be indicated. Some drugs that are predicted to have elevated plasma concentrations when coadministered with quinupristin/dalfopristin are **carbamazepine** (Tegretol), **cisapride** (Propulsid), **delavirdine** (Rescriptor), **diazepam** (Valium), **dihydropyridines** (e.g., nifedipine [Procardia]), **diltiazem** (Cardizem), **disopyramide** (Norpace), **docetaxel** (Taxotere), **HMA-CoA reductase inhibitors** (e.g., lovastatin [Mevacor], simvastatin [Zocor]), **lidocaine, quinidine, indinavir** (Crixivan), **methylprednisolone** (Solu-Medrol), **nevirapine** (Viramune), **paclitaxel** (Taxol), **ritonavir** (Norvir), **verapamil, vinca alkaloids** (e.g., vinblastine). ▪ Concomitant medications metabolized by the P_{450} 3A4 enzyme system that **may prolong the QTc interval** should be avoided. ▪ May increase **digoxin** levels. If S/S of digoxin toxicity occur, monitor digoxin levels. ▪ In vitro combination testing of quinupristin/dalfopristin with aztreonam, cefotaxime (Claforan), ciprofloxacin, and gentamicin against *Enterobacteriaceae* and *Pseudomonas aeruginosa* did not show antagonism. ▪ In vitro combination testing of quinupristin/dalfopristin prototype drugs with aminoglycosides (gentamicin), beta-lactams (cefepime, ampicillin, and amoxicillin), glycopeptides (vancomycin), quinolones (ciprofloxacin), tetracyclines (doxycycline), and also chloramphenicol against enterococci and staphylococci did not show antagonism. See Actions.

SIDE EFFECTS

Allergic reaction; arthralgia; diarrhea; edema, inflammation, and/or pain at infusion site; elevated total and conjugated bilirubin; headache; myalgia; nausea; pain; pruritus; rash; thrombophlebitis; thrombus; and vomiting are reported most frequently. Numerous other side effects have been reported in fewer than 1% of patients. CDAD has been reported. ▪ Numerous laboratory abnormalities were noted during studies but were not significantly different from those seen in the comparator group. See literature.

ANTIDOTE

Notify physician of any side effects. Discontinue drug if indicated. Treat hypersensitivity reactions as indicated. Observation and supportive therapy are indicated in an overdose situation. Is not removed by hemodialysis or peritoneal dialysis. Treat CDAD with fluids, electrolytes, protein supplements, and oral vancomycin (Vancocin) or metronidazole (Flagyl) as indicated. In severe cases, surgical evaluation may be indicated. Resuscitate as necessary.

RAMUCIRUMAB BBW

Recombinant monoclonal antibody
Angiogenesis inhibitor
Antineoplastic

Cyramza   pH 6

USUAL DOSE

Premedication: Before each infusion, premedicate all patients with an intravenous histamine H_1 antagonist (e.g., diphenhydramine [Benadryl]). For patients who have experienced a Grade 1 or 2 infusion reaction, also premedicate with dexamethasone (or equivalent) and acetaminophen before each infusion.

Ramucirumab dose: *Gastric cancer:* 8 mg/kg every 2 weeks administered as an infusion over 60 minutes. Continue until disease progression or unacceptable toxicity. May be given as a single agent or in combination with paclitaxel. Administer prior to paclitaxel infusion. (In studies, paclitaxel 80 mg/M² was administered on Days 1, 8, and 15 of each 28-day cycle.)

NSCLC: 10 mg/kg administered as an infusion over 60 minutes on Day 1 of a 21-day cycle. Administer prior to docetaxel infusion. (Docetaxel dose was 60 to 75 mg/M² in studies.) Continue until disease progression or unacceptable toxicity.

Colorectal cancer: 8 mg/kg administered every 2 weeks as an infusion over 60 minutes before FOLFIRI (irinotecan, folinic acid, and 5-fluorouracil) administration. Continue until disease progression or unacceptable toxicity.

DOSE ADJUSTMENTS

No dose adjustments are recommended for patients with impaired renal function or mild to moderate impaired hepatic function; see Precautions. ▪ Permanently discontinue for Grade 3 or 4 infusion-related reactions (IRR), urine protein levels greater than 3 Gm/24 hr, or in the setting of nephrotic syndrome, severe hypertension that cannot be controlled with antihypertensive therapy, GI perforation, Grade 3 or 4 bleeding, or an arterial thromboembolic event. ▪ Interrupt therapy for severe hypertension until controlled with medical management. ▪ Interrupt ramucirumab therapy before scheduled surgery until the wound is fully healed. ▪ Interrupt therapy for urine protein levels 2 Gm/24 hr or higher. Once urine protein level returns to less than 2 Gm/24 hr, reinitiate treatment at a reduced dose as outlined in the following chart. If a urine protein level of 2 Gm/24 hr or higher recurs, interrupt therapy and further reduce the dose as outlined in the following chart once the urine protein level returns to less than 2 Gm/24 hr.

Ramucirumab Dose Reductions for Proteinuria		
Initial Ramucirumab Dose	First Dose Reduction to:	Second Dose Reduction to:
8 mg/kg	6 mg/kg	5 mg/kg
10 mg/kg	8 mg/kg	6 mg/kg

▪ For toxicities related to paclitaxel, docetaxel, or the components of FOLFIRI, refer to current prescribing information. ▪ See Rate of Administration, Precautions, Monitor, and Antidote.

DILUTION

Available as a 10 mg/mL solution in 10- or 50-mL single-use vials. Calculate desired dose and choose the appropriate vial or combination of vials. Withdraw the required volume of ramucirumab and further dilute only with NS to a final volume of 250 mL. Gently invert container to ensure adequate mixing. *Do not shake infusion solution.*

Filters: Administration through a protein-sparing, 0.22-micron filter is recommended.

Storage: Store in original carton in refrigerator at 2° to 8° C (36° to 46° F). Protect from light. Do not shake or freeze. Diluted solutions may be stored for up to 24 hours refrigerated or for up to 4 hours at RT. Contains no preservatives; unused portions must be discarded.

COMPATIBILITY

Manufacturer states, "Do not use dextrose-containing solutions. Do not dilute with other solutions or co-infuse with other electrolytes or medications." Administer through a separate infusion line and flush the line with NS at the end of the infusion.

RATE OF ADMINISTRATION

Do not administer as an IV push or bolus. Use of a separate line and administration through a protein-sparing, 0.22-micron filter recommended. Administer as an infusion via an infusion pump evenly distributed over 60 minutes. Reduce rate of infusion by 50% for Grade 1 or 2 infusion-related reactions. Flush line with NS at end of infusion.

ACTIONS

A recombinant human IgG$_1$ monoclonal antibody that specifically binds to vascular endothelial growth factor receptor 2 (VEGFR2). Acts as an antagonist, blocking the binding of VEGFR ligands, VEGF-A, VEGF-C, and VEGF-D. As a result, it inhibits ligand-stimulated activation of VEGF Receptor 2, thereby inhibiting ligand-induced proliferation and migration of human endothelial cells. Ramucirumab inhibits angiogenesis in an in vivo animal model. Mean elimination half-life was 15 to 23 days.

INDICATIONS AND USES

As a single agent or in combination with paclitaxel for the treatment of patients with advanced or metastatic, gastric or gastroesophageal junction adenocarcinoma with disease progression during or after prior fluoropyrimidine- or platinum-containing chemotherapy. ▪ In combination with docetaxel for the treatment of patients with metastatic non–small-cell lung cancer (NSCLC) with progression during or after platinum-based chemotherapy. Patients with *EGFR* or *ALK* genomic tumor aberrations should have disease progression during FDA-approved therapy for these aberrations before receiving ramucirumab. ▪ In combination with FOLFIRI (irinotecan, folinic acid, and 5-fluorouracil) for treatment of patients with metastatic colorectal cancer (mCRC) with progression on or after therapy with bevacizumab, oxaliplatin, and a fluoropyrimidine.

CONTRAINDICATIONS

Manufacturer states, "No known contraindications." However, ramucirumab must be discontinued if an arterial thrombotic event, Grade 3 or 4 bleeding, a Grade 3 or 4 infusion-related reaction, GI perforation, greater than 3 Gm urinary protein/24 hr, nephrotic syndrome, hypertensive crisis, or reversible posterior leukoencephalopathy syndrome (RPLS) develops.

PRECAUTIONS

Do not administer as an IV push or bolus. ▪ Should be administered by or under the direction of a physician specialist in a facility equipped to monitor the patient and respond to any medical emergency. ▪ Ramucirumab increases the risk of hemorrhage and gastrointestinal hemorrhage, including severe and sometimes fatal hemorrhagic events. Patients with gastric cancer receiving NSAIDs were excluded from clinical trials; therefore the risk of gastric hemorrhage in these patients is unknown. Patients with NSCLC receiving therapeutic anticoagulation, chronic therapy with NSAIDs, or other antiplatelet therapy (other than a once-daily aspirin) and patients with radiographic evidence of major airway or blood vessel invasion or intra-tumor cavitation were excluded from studies; therefore the risk of pulmonary hemorrhage in these patients is unknown. ▪ Serious and sometimes fatal arterial thromboembolic events, including MI, cardiac arrest, cerebrovascular accident, and cerebral ischemia, have been reported. ▪ An increased incidence of severe hypertension occurred in patients receiving ramucirumab. Control hypertension before initiating therapy; see Monitor and Dose Adjustment. ▪ Infusion reactions have occurred and can be severe. The majority of reactions occurred during or after the first or second infusion. Premedication is recommended; see Usual Dose, Monitor, and Antidote. ▪ Ramucirumab is an antiangiogenic therapy that can increase the risk of GI perforation, a potentially fatal event. GI perforation was reported during clinical trials. Consider GI perforation in any patient with complaints of abdominal pain associated with constipation, fever, nausea, and vomiting. ▪ Ramucirumab has not been studied in patients with serious or nonhealing wounds. However, as an antiangiogenic therapy it has the potential to adversely affect wound healing. Impaired wound healing can occur with antibodies inhibiting the VEGF pathway. Withhold ramucirumab therapy before surgery. Resume following the surgical intervention based on clinical judgment of adequate wound healing. If a patient develops wound-healing complications during therapy, discontinue ramucirumab until the wound is fully healed. ▪ Use with caution and only if potential benefit outweighs risk in patients with Child-Pugh Class B or C cirrhosis. Clinical deterioration manifested by new-onset or worsening encephalopathy, ascites, or hepatorenal syndrome has been reported in these patients. ▪ Reversible posterior leukoencephalopathy syndrome (RPLS) has been reported. May present with blindness and other visual and neurologic disturbances, confusion, headache, lethargy, and seizures. Mild to severe hypertension may be present. MRI is required to confirm diagnosis. Symptoms usually resolve gradually with discontinuation of ramucirumab and treatment of hypertension; however, some patients with RPLS experienced ongoing neurologic sequelae or death. ▪ Proteinuria occurred during studies; however, it occurred more frequently in patients treated with ramucirumab in combination with FOLFIRI; see Dose Adjustments. ▪ A protein substance, it has the potential to produce an immune response. Anti-ramucirumab antibodies have been detected in a small number of patients; clinical significance is not known. ▪ See Antidote.

Monitor: Obtain baseline BP, CBC with differential and platelets, electrolytes, liver function tests, thyroid function tests, and urinalysis. ▪ Monitor for S/S of an infusion reaction (e.g., back pain/spasms, chest pain or tightness, chills, dyspnea, flushing, hypoxia, paresthesia, rigors/tremors, wheezing). In severe cases, S/S have included bronchospasm, hypotension, and supraventricular tachycardia. ▪ Monitor VS and BP at least every 2 weeks; monitor more frequently in patients with hypertension. ▪ Repeat CBC with differential and platelets and electrolytes as indicated. ▪ Monitor proteinuria by urine dipstick and/or urinary protein creatinine ratio for the development of worsening proteinuria; see Dose Adjustments. ▪ Check surgical wounds for wound dehiscence and monitor for S/S of bleeding or GI perforation (e.g., abdominal pain, constipation, fever, hypotension, nausea and vomiting). ▪ Monitor thyroid function during treatment; hypothyroidism has been reported. ▪ Monitor for thrombocytopenia (platelet count less than 50,000 mm^3). Initiate precautions to prevent excessive bleeding (e.g., inspect IV sites, skin, and mucous membranes; use extreme care during invasive procedures; test urine, emesis, stool, and secretions for occult blood). ▪ See Dose Adjustments, Rate of Administration, Precautions, and Antidote.

Patient Education: Avoid pregnancy during treatment and for at least 3 months after the last dose of ramucirumab. Nonhormonal birth control recommended; see Maternal/Child. Women should report a suspected pregnancy immediately. ▪ Increases risk of ovarian failure and may impair fertility. ▪ Full disclosure of health history is imperative. ▪ Do not undergo any type of surgery without first discussing the risk of impaired wound healing with the health care provider. ▪ Report any unusual or unexpected symptoms or side effects promptly (e.g., abdominal pain, bleeding from any source, constipation, dyspnea, persistent cough, sudden onset of worsening neurologic function, vomiting, wound separation). ▪ Routine monitoring of BP required. ▪ See Appendix D, p. 1333.

Maternal/Child: Can cause fetal harm; avoid pregnancy. Animal models link angiogenesis, VEGF, and VEGF receptor 2 (VEGFR2) to critical aspects of female reproduction, embryo-fetal development, and postnatal development. Use effective contraception during treatment with ramucirumab and for at least 3 months after the last dose. ▪ May impair fertility. ▪ Discontinue breast-feeding during treatment with ramucirumab. ▪ Safety and effectiveness for use in pediatric patients not established.

Elderly: No overall differences in safety or efficacy were observed between elderly patients and younger patients being treated for gastric cancer or mCRC. Hazard ratio for overall survival was slightly increased in elderly treated for NSCLC.

DRUG/LAB INTERACTIONS

Drug interaction studies have not been completed. No pharmacokinetic interactions were observed between ramucirumab and paclitaxel or between ramucirumab and docetaxel.

SIDE EFFECTS

Single agent: The most common side effects observed were diarrhea and hypertension. The most common serious side effects observed were anemia and intestinal obstruction. Less frequently reported side effects included arterial thromboembolic events, clinical deterioration in patients with Child-Pugh Class B or C cirrhosis (ascites, encephalopathy, hepatorenal syndrome), epistaxis, GI perforation, headache, hemorrhage, hyponatremia, impaired wound healing, infusion-related reactions, neutropenia, proteinuria, rash, reversible posterior leukoencephalopathy syndrome (RPLS).

In combination with paclitaxel: The most common side effects observed were diarrhea, epistaxis, fatigue, and neutropenia. The most common serious side effects were neutropenia and febrile neutropenia. Neutropenia and thrombocytopenia were the most common reasons for discontinuation of therapy. Less frequently reported side effects included GI hemorrhagic events, hypertension, hypoalbuminemia, peripheral edema, proteinuria, sepsis, stomatitis, and thrombocytopenia.

In combination with docetaxel: The most common side effects observed were asthenia/fatigue, neutropenia, and stomatitis/mucosal inflammation. The most common serious side effects were neutropenia, febrile neutropenia, and pneumonia. Infusion-related reactions and epistaxis were the most common reasons for discontinuation of therapy. Less frequently reported side effects included hypertension, hyponatremia, increased lacrimation, peripheral edema, and thrombocytopenia.

In combination with FOLFIRI: The most common side effects observed were decreased appetite, diarrhea, epistaxis, neutropenia, and stomatitis. The most common serious side effects were diarrhea, febrile neutropenia, and intestinal obstruction. Neutropenia and thrombocytopenia were the most common reasons for discontinuation of any component of treatment, and gastrointestinal perforation and proteinuria were the most common reasons for permanent discontinuation. Other reported side effects included GI hemorrhage events, hypertension, hypoalbuminemia, hypothyroidism, palmar-plantar erythrodysesthesia syndrome, and peripheral edema.

ANTIDOTE

Keep physician informed of all side effects. May constitute a medical emergency or will be treated symptomatically as indicated. Permanently discontinue ramucirumab in patients who experience severe bleeding, in patients with impaired wound healing, and in any of the following: Grade 3 or 4 infusion-related reactions, severe hypertension that cannot be controlled with antihypertensive therapy, or in patients with hypertensive crisis or hypertensive encephalopathy, GI perforation, urine protein level greater than 3 Gm/24 hr or in the setting of nephrotic syndrome, a severe arterial thromboembolic event, or reversible posterior leukoencephalopathy syndrome. Treat these side effects aggressively; see Precautions and Monitor. Treat severe infusion reactions as indicated (e.g., epinephrine [Adrenalin], diphenhydramine [Benadryl], IV fluids, oxygen). Temporarily discontinue if moderate to severe proteinuria (equal to or greater than 2 Gm/24 hr) occurs. Resume therapy when proteinuria is less than 2 Gm/24 hr; see Dose Adjustment. Temporarily discontinue for severe hypertension until controlled with medical management; see Monitor and Precautions.

Q-R

RANITIDINE
(rah-**NIH**-tih-deen)

H₂ antagonist
Antiulcer agent
Gastric acid inhibitor

Zantac

pH 6.7 to 7.3

USUAL DOSE
IV injection or intermittent infusion: 50 mg (2 mL) every 6 to 8 hours. Increase frequency of dose, not amount, if necessary for pain relief. 50 mg every 8 to 12 hours may be used short term to replace an oral dose of 150 mg every 12 hours in patients unable to take oral meds. Do not exceed 400 mg/day.

Continuous infusion: 150 mg may be given as a continuous infusion equally distributed over 24 hours. To maintain intergastric acid secretion rates at 10 mEq/hr or less, dose range may be higher in patients with pathologic hypersecretory syndrome (Zollinger-Ellison). Literature suggests an initial dose of 1 mg/kg/hr. Measure gastric acid output in 4 hours. If above 10 mEq/hr or symptoms recur, adjust dose upward in 0.5 mg/kg/hr increments. Up to 2.5 mg/kg/hr has been used.

Additive for total parenteral nutrition (TPN [unlabeled]): 70% to 100% of an average 24-hour dose has been used equally distributed over 24 hours as a continuous infusion. May be supplemented with intermittent doses as needed.

Perioperatively to prevent pulmonary aspiration during anesthesia (unlabeled): 45 to 50 mg 60 minutes before anesthesia.

Prophylaxis and/or control of GI hemorrhage associated with stress ulcers (unlabeled): 150 mg over 24 hours.

PEDIATRIC DOSE
Safety for selective use in pediatric patients from 1 month to 16 years of age established; see Indications.

One source suggests:

Infants and other pediatric patients: 2 to 4 mg/kg/24 hr in equally divided doses every 6 to 8 hours (0.5 to 1 mg/kg every 6 hours or 0.67 to 1.3 mg/kg every 8 hours). Do not exceed 50 mg/dose.

NEONATAL DOSE
Safety for use of IV ranitidine in neonates under 1 month of age not established; see Maternal/Child.

2 mg/kg every 12 to 24 hours or as a continuous infusion.

Another source suggests 2 mg/kg/24 hr in equally divided doses every 6 to 8 hours (0.5 mg/kg every 6 hours or 0.67 mg/kg every 8 hours).

DOSE ADJUSTMENTS
Dose selection should be cautious in the elderly. ▪ If the CrCl is less than 50 mL/min, reduce dose to 50 mg every 18 to 24 hours. Gradually increase to 50 mg every 12 hours, or 6 hours with caution if indicated. Adjust schedule to be given after dialysis.

DILUTION
IV injection: Each vial containing 50 mg (2 mL) must be diluted with 18 mL of NS or other **compatible** infusion solution for injection (D5W, D10W, LR, 5% sodium bicarbonate). Concentration of solution must be no greater than 2.5 mg/mL. Additional diluent may be used.

Intermittent infusion: Available premixed as a 1 mg/mL solution in 50 mL. May be given without further dilution. Or each 50 mg may be diluted in 100 mL (0.5 mg/mL) of D5W or other **compatible** infusion solution and given piggyback. Concentration of solution should be no greater than 0.5 mg/mL. Manufacturer recommends discontinuing primary IV during intermittent infusion to avoid **incompatibilities**. Do not use premixed plastic containers in series connections; may cause air embolism.

Continuous infusion: Total daily dose may be diluted in 250 mL of D5W or other **compatible** infusion solution. For Zollinger-Ellison patients, concentration of solution must be no greater than 2.5 mg/mL. In all situations, avoid any contact with aluminum (e.g., needles) during administration. Inspect for color and clarity. Slight darkening of solution does not affect potency. **Compatible** in selected TPN solutions for 24 hours (consult pharmacist).

Storage: Store at CRT protected from light. Stable at room temperature for 48 hours after dilution.

COMPATIBILITY   (Underline Indicates Conflicting Compatibility Information)

Consider any drug NOT listed as compatible to be INCOMPATIBLE until consulting a pharmacist; specific conditions may apply.

Manufacturer states, "Additives should not be introduced into the premixed solution, and the primary IV should be discontinued during ranitidine infusion."

Solution: D5¹/₂NS, IV fat emulsion 10%, selected TNA and TPN solutions; see Dilution.
     One source suggests the following **compatibilities:**

Additive: *See previous comments under Compatibility.* Acetazolamide (Diamox), amikacin, aminophylline, ampicillin, chloramphenicol (Chloromycetin), chlorothiazide (Diuril), ciprofloxacin (Cipro IV), clindamycin (Cleocin), colistimethate (Coly-Mycin M), dexamethasone (Decadron), digoxin (Lanoxin), dobutamine, dopamine, doxycycline, epinephrine (Adrenalin), erythromycin (Erythrocin), flumazenil (Romazicon), furosemide (Lasix), gentamicin, heparin, isoproterenol (Isuprel), lidocaine, lincomycin (Lincocin), meropenem (Merrem IV), methylprednisolone (Solu-Medrol), midazolam (Versed), nitroprusside sodium, norepinephrine (Levophed), penicillin G potassium and sodium, potassium chloride (KCl), protamine sulfate, quinidine gluconate, tobramycin, vancomycin, zidovudine (AZT, Retrovir).

Y-site: Acetaminophen (Ofirmev), acyclovir (Zovirax), aldesleukin (Proleukin), allopurinol (Aloprim), amifostine (Ethyol), aminophylline, anidulafungin (Eraxis), atracurium (Tracrium), aztreonam (Azactam), bivalirudin (Angiomax), cefazolin (Ancef), cefoxitin (Mefoxin), ceftaroline (Teflaro), ceftazidime (Fortaz), ciprofloxacin (Cipro IV), cisatracurium (Nimbex), cladribine (Leustatin), dexmedetomidine (Precedex), diltiazem (Cardizem), dobutamine, docetaxel (Taxotere), dopamine, doripenem (Doribax), doxapram (Dopram), doxorubicin liposomal (Doxil), enalaprilat (Vasotec IV), epinephrine (Adrenalin), esmolol (Brevibloc), etoposide phosphate (Etopophos), fenoldopam (Corlopam), fentanyl, filgrastim (Neupogen), fluconazole (Diflucan), fludarabine (Fludara), foscarnet (Foscavir), furosemide (Lasix), gallium nitrate (Ganite), gemcitabine (Gemzar), granisetron (Kytril), heparin, hetastarch in electrolytes (Hextend), hydromorphone (Dilaudid), idarubicin (Idamycin), labetalol, linezolid (Zyvox), lorazepam (Ativan), melphalan (Alkeran), meperidine (Demerol), midazolam (Versed), milrinone (Primacor), morphine, nicardipine (Cardene IV), nitroglycerin IV, norepinephrine (Levophed), ondansetron (Zofran), oxaliplatin (Eloxatin), paclitaxel (Taxol), pancuronium, pemetrexed (Alimta), piperacillin/tazobactam (Zosyn), procainamide (Pronestyl), propofol (Diprivan), remifentanil (Ultiva), sargramostim (Leukine), tacrolimus (Prograf), telavancin (Vibativ), teniposide (Vumon), theophylline, thiotepa, tigecycline (Tygacil), vecuronium, vinorelbine (Navelbine), warfarin (Coumadin), zidovudine (AZT, Retrovir).

RATE OF ADMINISTRATION

Too-rapid administration has precipitated rare instances of bradycardia, tachycardia, and PVCs.

IV injection: Each 50 mg or fraction thereof at a rate not to exceed 4 mL/min diluted solution (20 mL over 5 min).

Intermittent infusion: Each 50-mg dose over 15 to 20 minutes.

Continuous infusion: Total daily dose equally distributed over 24 hours. Should not exceed a rate of 6.25 mg/hr (10.7 mL/hr if 150 mg [6 mL ranitidine] is diluted in 250 mL). Use of infusion pump preferred to avoid complications of overdose or too-rapid administration.

ACTIONS

A histamine H_2 antagonist, it inhibits both daytime and nocturnal basal gastric acid secretion. It also inhibits gastric acid secretion stimulated by food, histamine, bentazole, and pentagastrin. Not an anticholinergic agent. Does not lower calcium levels in hypercalcemia. Onset of action is prompt and effective for 6 to 8 hours. 5 to 12 times more potent than cimetidine. Half-life is 2 to 2.5 hours. Metabolized in the liver. Excreted in the urine. 70% of a dose is recovered in urine as unchanged drug. Crosses placental barrier. Secreted in breast milk.

INDICATIONS AND USES

Short-term treatment of intractable duodenal ulcers and pathologic hypersecretory conditions in the hospitalized patient. ▪ Treatment of active benign gastric ulcers in those patients unable to take oral medication. ▪ Treatment of duodenal ulcers in pediatric patients from 1 month to 16 years of age. Safety for use in pathologic hypersecretory conditions not established. ▪ Oral dosing for treatment of duodenal and gastric ulcers, maintenance of healing of duodenal and gastric ulcers, and treatment of GERD and erosive esophagitis has been approved for pediatric patients from 1 month to 16 years of age; see package insert.

Unlabeled uses: Perioperatively to suppress gastric acid secretion, prevent stress ulcers, and prevent aspiration pneumonitis. ▪ Reduce the incidence of GI hemorrhage associated with stress ulcers. ▪ Additive to TPN to simplify fluid and electrolyte management (decreases the volume and chloride content of gastric secretions).

CONTRAINDICATIONS

Known hypersensitivity to ranitidine or its components.

PRECAUTIONS

Use antacids concomitantly to relieve pain. ▪ Gastric malignancy may be present even though patient's symptoms improve on ranitidine therapy. ▪ Use caution in patients with impaired hepatic or renal function. ▪ Avoid use in patients with acute porphyria; may precipitate acute porphyric attacks. ▪ Gastric pain and ulceration may recur after medication is stopped. ▪ Effects maintained with oral dosage. Total treatment usually discontinued after 6 weeks.

Monitor: Observe frequently; monitor vital signs and pain levels. ▪ Obtain baseline SCr. Monitor periodically during extended course of treatment. ▪ Monitor ALT if therapy exceeds 400 mg for over 5 days. ▪ Change to oral dose when appropriate. ▪ See Drug/Lab Interactions.

Patient Education: Stop smoking or at least avoid smoking after the last dose of the day. ▪ May increase blood alcohol levels.

Maternal/Child: Category B: use during pregnancy or breast-feeding only when clearly needed. ▪ No significant difference in pharmacokinetic parameter values between pediatric patients over 1 month of age and healthy adults when correction is made for body weight. ▪ Safety for use of IV ranitidine in neonates under 1 month of age not established; however, limited data suggest that ranitidine may be useful and safe in increasing gastric pH for infants at risk of GI hemorrhage. ▪ Half-life in neonates averages 6.6 hours.

Elderly: Use caution in dose selection; monitoring of renal function suggested; see Dose Adjustments. ▪ Half-life is prolonged (3.1 hours) and total clearance is decreased due to reduced renal function. ▪ Differences in response between elderly and younger patients not identified; greater sensitivity of some elderly cannot be ruled out. ▪ Agitation, confusion (reversible), depression, and hallucination have been reported.

DRUG/LAB INTERACTIONS

Concurrent use with **warfarin** may result in increased or decreased PT and/or INR. Close monitoring is recommended. ▪ High doses of ranitidine may reduce the renal excretion of **procainamide;** monitoring for procainamide toxicity is suggested if ranitidine doses exceed 300 mg/day. ▪ May increase serum concentrations of **sulfonylureas** (e.g., glipizide); monitor blood glucose and adjust dose as indicated. ▪ Increased pH may reduce the antibiotic effectiveness of selected **cephalosporins** (e.g., cefpodoxime [Vantin], cefuroxime [Zinacef]). ▪ Increased pH may impair the absorption of **atazanavir** (Reyataz) **and delavirdine** (Rescriptor). ▪ Effectiveness of **gefitinib** (Iressa) may be reduced if coadministered with ranitidine and sodium bicarbonate. ▪ Reduces the plasma concentrations and antibiotic effectiveness of **enoxacin** (Penetrex). ▪ Monitor for excessive sedation with concurrent administration of selected **benzodiazepines** (e.g., midazolam [Versed], triazolam [Halcion]). ▪ May potentiate the effects of **alcohol.** ▪ May inhibit gastric absorption of **itraconazole** (Sporanox) and **ketoconazole** (Nizoral) and reduce antifungal effects. ▪ Clinical effect (inhibition of nocturnal gastric secretions) may be reversed by **cigarette smoking.** ▪ Elevated **ALT, slight elevation in SCr,** and a **false-positive for urine protein** with Multistix may occur.

SIDE EFFECTS
Abdominal discomfort, burning and itching at IV site, constipation, diarrhea, headache (severe), and nausea and vomiting are the most common side effects. Hypersensitivity reactions (bronchospasm, fever, rash, eosinophilia) can occur. Acute interstitial nephritis, agitation, alopecia, arthralgias, bradycardia, confusion, depression, dizziness, elevated ALT, erythema multiforme, galactorrhea (rare), gynecomastia (rare), hallucinations, hepatitis (reversible), impotence, insomnia, malaise, muscular pain, pneumonia, PVCs, somnolence, tachycardia, vasculitis, and vertigo occur rarely. See Drug/Lab Interactions.

ANTIDOTE
Notify physician of all side effects. May be treated symptomatically or may respond to decrease in frequency of dosage. Discontinue ranitidine if S/S of hepatitis with or without jaundice occur. Resuscitate as necessary for overdose. Hemodialysis or peritoneal dialysis may be indicated in overdose.

RASBURICASE BBW
(ras-**BYOUR**-ih-kase)

Elitek

Antihyperuricemic
Enzyme, urate-oxidase
(recombinant)

USUAL DOSE
Prehydration required; see Monitor.
0.2 mg/kg as a single daily dose each day for up to 5 days. Safety and effectiveness of other schedules have not been evaluated. Dosing beyond 5 days and/or administration of more than one course of rasburicase is not recommended. Alternate unlabeled single- and multiple-dose regimens have been used; see literature.

PEDIATRIC DOSE
Same as adult dose; see Maternal/Child.

DOSE ADJUSTMENTS
No dose adjustments recommended.

DILUTION
Available in 1.5- and 7.5-mg vials with manufacturer-supplied diluent (SWFI and Poloxamer 188). Determine the vial size and/or number of vials needed to provide the calculated dose. Reconstitute each 1.5-mg vial with 1 mL of diluent and each 7.5-mg vial with 5 mL of diluent. Final concentration is 1.5 mg/mL. Mix by swirling gently. *Do not shake.* Withdraw the calculated dose of reconstituted solution and inject into an infusion bag containing the appropriate volume of NS to achieve a final total volume of 50 mL. (For example a 20-kg child would receive a dose of 4 mg [20 kg × 0.2 mg/kg = 4 mg]. Reconstitute 3 vials, each with 1 mL of the diluent provided. Withdraw 2.7 mL of reconstituted solution and add to an infusion bag containing 47.3 mL of NS.)
Filters: *No filters should be used for the infusion.*

Q-R

Storage: Refrigerate unopened lyophilized drug product and diluent. Do not freeze; protect from light. Both the reconstituted and diluted product may be stored for 24 hours if refrigerated. Discard any unused product.

COMPATIBILITY

Manufacturer states, "Should be infused through a different line than that used for the infusion of other concomitant medications. If use of a separate line is not possible, the line should be flushed with at least 15 mL of NS prior to and after infusion with rasburicase."

RATE OF ADMINISTRATION

A single dose as an infusion equally distributed over 30 minutes.
Do not administer as a bolus infusion. Do not filter infusion.

ACTIONS

A recombinant urate-oxidase enzyme produced by genetic engineering. Catalyzes enzymatic oxidation of uric acid into an inactive and soluble metabolite (allantoin). Onset of action is 4 hours. Mean terminal half-life is similar between pediatric and adult patients and ranges from 15.7 to 22.5 hours.

INDICATIONS AND USES

Initial management of plasma uric acid levels in pediatric and adult patients with leukemia, lymphoma, and solid tumor malignancies who are receiving anticancer therapy that is expected to result in tumor lysis and subsequent elevation of plasma uric acid.
Limitation of use: Indicated only for a single course of treatment.

CONTRAINDICATIONS

Glucose-6-phosphatase dehydrogenase (G6PD) deficiency or a history of anaphylaxis or severe hypersensitivity, hemolytic reactions, or methemoglobinemia reactions to rasburicase.

PRECAUTIONS

May cause severe hypersensitivity reactions, including anaphylaxis. Reactions may occur at any time during treatment, including with the first dose; see Monitor and Antidote. ▪ Has caused severe hemolytic reactions in patients with G6PD deficiency. It is recommended that patients at higher risk for G6PD deficiency (e.g., patients of African or Mediterranean descent) be screened before starting rasburicase therapy. See Contraindications and Antidote. ▪ Methemoglobinemia has been reported. Patients developed serious hypoxemia, requiring intervention and medical support. See Antidote. ▪ As with all therapeutic proteins, there is the potential for immunogenicity. May elicit antibodies that inhibit the activity of rasburicase.
Monitor: Monitor serum uric acid levels, electrolytes, and renal function before and during therapy. ▪ Patients should be hydrated intravenously according to standard medical practice for the management of plasma uric acid in patients at risk for tumor lysis syndrome (TLS). ▪ Maintain urine at neutral or slightly alkaline pH. ▪ Observe for symptoms of TLS (e.g., hyperuricemia, hyperkalemia, hyperphosphatemia, and hypocalcemia). If untreated, may develop acute uric acid nephropathy, leading to renal failure. ▪ Monitor for S/S of a hypersensitivity reaction (e.g., anaphylaxis, bronchospasm, chest pain, dyspnea, hypotension, hypoxia, shock, urticaria). ▪ Screen patients at risk for hemolysis; see Contraindications and Precautions. Monitor for S/S of hemolysis (e.g., anemia, jaundice with increased indirect bilirubin and LDH, pallor, reduced haptoglobin). In studies, severe hemolytic reactions occurred within 2 to 4 days of the start of therapy. ▪ Monitor for S/S of methemoglobinemia (e.g., cyanosis, dyspnea, headache, hypoxemia, lethargy, methemoglobin). ▪ Will cause enzymatic degradation of uric acid within blood samples left at room temperature, resulting in falsely low uric acid levels. To ensure accurate measurement, blood must be collected into prechilled tubes containing heparin anticoagulant and immediately *immersed and maintained* in an ice water bath. Plasma samples must be prepared by centrifugation in a precooled centrifuge (4° C [39° F]). Plasma samples must be analyzed within 4 hours of sample collection.
Patient Education: Report blood in urine, painful urination, or signs of a hypersensitivity reaction promptly.

Maternal/Child: Category C: studies have not been performed. Potential benefits must justify potential risks to fetus. ▪ Discontinue breast-feeding. ▪ Studied in pediatric patients from 1 month to 17 years of age. Pediatric patients under 2 years of age had a higher mean uric acid AUC and a lower rate of success at achieving normal uric acid concentrations by 48 hours than did older pediatric patients.

Elderly: No overall differences in pharmacokinetics, safety, and effectiveness were observed between elderly and younger patients.

DRUG/LAB INTERACTIONS

Studies have not been conducted. ▪ Does not metabolize allopurinol (Aloprim), cytarabine (ARA-C), methylprednisolone (Solu-Medrol), methotrexate, 6-mercaptopurine (Purinethol), thioguanine, etoposide (VePesid), etoposide phosphate (Etopophos), daunorubicin (Cerubidine), cyclophosphamide, or vincristine in vitro. Metabolic-based drug interactions are not anticipated with these agents. ▪ Did not affect the activity of P_{450} isoenzymes in preclinical in vivo studies. Clinically relevant P_{450}-mediated drug-drug interactions are not anticipated. ▪ Will cause enzymatic degradation of uric acid within blood samples left at room temperature, resulting in **falsely low uric acid levels;** see Monitor.

SIDE EFFECTS

The most common adverse reactions are abdominal pain, anxiety, constipation, diarrhea, fever, headache, nausea, peripheral edema, and vomiting. Serious adverse reactions observed are hemolysis, hypersensitivity reactions (e.g., anaphylaxis, chest pain, dyspnea, hypotension, urticaria), methemoglobinemia, and severe rash. Other observed reactions include abdominal and GI infections, acute renal failure, fluid overload, hyperbilirubinemia, hyperphosphatemia, hypophosphatemia, increased ALT, ischemic coronary artery disorders, mucositis, neutropenia with or without fever, pharyngolaryngeal pain, pulmonary hemorrhage, rash, respiratory distress/failure, sepsis, and supraventricular arrhythmias.

Post-Marketing: Convulsions, muscle contractions (involuntary).

ANTIDOTE

Notify physician of all side effects. Should be immediately and permanently discontinued in patients who experience severe hypersensitivity reactions, hemolysis, or methemoglobinemia. Do not rechallenge. Treat anaphylaxis with epinephrine, corticosteroids (e.g., dexamethasone [Decadron]), oxygen, and antihistamines (diphenhydramine [Benadryl]). Hemolysis or methemoglobinemia may require transfusion support. Methylene blue may be required for treatment of methemoglobinemia. There is no specific antidote. Resuscitate as indicated.

RAXIBACUMAB
(rack-see-**BACK**-u-mab)

Monoclonal antibody
Antidote

ABthrax

USUAL DOSE

Premedication in adults: Premedicate with diphenhydramine 25 to 50 mg within 1 hour before raxibacumab infusion to prevent or attenuate infusion reactions. May be given IV or PO depending on proximity to the start of the raxibacumab infusion.

Adults: A single dose of 40 mg/kg as an infusion over 2 hours and 15 minutes.

PEDIATRIC DOSE

Premedication in pediatric patients: Premedicate with an appropriate dose of diphenhydramine within 1 hour before raxibacumab infusion to prevent or attenuate infusion reactions. May be given IV or PO depending on proximity to the start of the raxibacumab infusion.

Dosage for pediatric patients: *Weight more than 50 kg:* A single dose of 40 mg/kg.

Weight more than 15 kg and up to 50 kg: A single dose of 60 mg/kg.

Weight 15 kg or less: A single dose of 80 mg/kg.

DOSE ADJUSTMENTS

No dose adjustments indicated based on age, gender, or race.

DILUTION

Available as a single-use vial that contains 1700 mg/34 mL (50 mg/mL). The recommended dose is weight-based and is given as an intravenous infusion after appropriate dilution in a **compatible** solution. The following chart outlines dose, diluent, total infusion volume, and infusion rate based on patient body weight.

Raxibacumab Dose, Diluent, Infusion Volume, and Rate by Body Weight					
	Preparation			Administration	
Body Weight (kg)	Dose (mg/kg)	Total Infusion Volume (mL)	Type of Diluent	Infusion Rate (mL/hr) First 20 Minutes	Infusion Rate (mL/hr) Remaining Infusion
1 kg or less	80 mg/kg	7 mL	1/2 NS or NS	0.5 mL/hr	3.5 mL/hr
1.1 to 2 kg	80 mg/kg	15 mL	1/2 NS or NS	1 mL/hr	7 mL/hr
2.1 to 3 kg	80 mg/kg	20 mL	1/2 NS or NS	1.2 mL/hr	10 mL/hr
3.1 to 4.9 kg	80 mg/kg	25 mL	1/2 NS or NS	1.5 mL/hr	12 mL/hr
5 to 10 kg	80 mg/kg	50 mL	1/2 NS or NS	3 mL/hr	25 mL/hr
11 to 15 kg	80 mg/kg	100 mL	NS	6 mL/hr	50 mL/hr
16 to 30 kg	60 mg/kg	100 mL	NS	6 mL/hr	50 mL/hr
31 to 40 kg	60 mg/kg	250 mL	NS	15 mL/hr	125 mL/hr
41 to 50 kg	60 mg/kg	250 mL	NS	15 mL/hr	125 mL/hr
Greater than 50 kg or adult	40 mg/kg	250 mL	NS	15 mL/hr	125 mL/hr

Weight in kg × Dose in mg/kg = Calculated dose of raxibacumab in mg

Calculated dose in mg ÷ Raxibacumab concentration (50 mg/mL) =
Required volume of raxibacumab in mL

Based on total infusion volume from the previous chart, prepare either a syringe or infusion bag as appropriate.

Bag preparation: Select the appropriate size bag of **compatible** solution. Withdraw a volume of solution from the bag equal to the calculated volume in milliliters of raxibacumab and discard. Withdraw the calculated dose of raxibacumab from the vial and transfer into the prepared infusion bag. Gently invert bag to mix. *Do not shake.*

Syringe preparation: Select an appropriate size syringe for the total volume of infusion to be administered. Using this syringe, withdraw the calculated raxibacumab dose. Then withdraw an appropriate amount of **compatible** solution to prepare a total volume infusion syringe as specified in the chart. Gently mix. *Do not shake.*

Filters: Not required by manufacturer; additional data not available.

Storage: Store in original carton until time of use to protect from light. Refrigerate at 2° to 8° C (36° to 46° F). Do not freeze. Discard unused raxibacumab. Prepared solution stable for 8 hours at RT.

COMPATIBILITY
Specific information not available; consider specific use; consult pharmacist.

RATE OF ADMINISTRATION
Administer as outlined in the chart under Dilution. Total infusion time is 2 hours and 15 minutes. Slow or interrupt the infusion for infusion-related symptoms or other side effects.

ACTIONS
A human IgG1λ monoclonal antibody. Produced by recombinant DNA technology in a murine cell expression system. It does not have direct antibacterial activity but binds to the protective antigen (PA) of *B. anthracis* toxin. Raxibacumab inhibits the binding of the PA to its cellular receptor. This prevents the intracellular entry of the anthrax lethal factor and edema factor, the enzymatic toxin components responsible for the pathogenic effects of the anthrax toxin. Mean steady-state volume of distribution was greater than plasma volume, suggesting some tissue distribution. Virtually no renal clearance occurs.

INDICATIONS AND USES
Treatment of adult and pediatric patients with inhalation anthrax due to *Bacillus anthracis* in combination with the appropriate antibacterial drugs. ▪ Prophylaxis of inhalation anthrax when alternative therapies are not appropriate or available for use.

Limitations of use: Effectiveness based solely on efficacy studies in animal models of inhalational anthrax. ▪ Does not cross the blood-brain barrier and does not prevent or treat meningitis. ▪ Does not have direct antibacterial activity. Should be used in combination with appropriate antibacterial drugs. ▪ See Maternal/Child.

CONTRAINDICATIONS
Manufacturer states, "None."

PRECAUTIONS
Infusion-related reactions have been reported; see Monitor and Antidote. ▪ A protein product; has the potential for immunogenicity. ▪ Adequate laboratory and supportive medical resources must be available.

Monitor: Premedication required; see Usual Dose. ▪ Monitor for infusion-related reactions during administration (e.g., dyspnea, pruritus, rash, urticaria) and slow or interrupt infusion as indicated.

Patient Education: Promptly report S/S of an infusion reaction (e.g., hives, itching, rash, shortness of breath). ▪ The effectiveness of raxibacumab is based on studies done in animals and has not been tested in humans with anthrax.

Maternal/Child: Category B: safety for use in pregnancy, breast-feeding, and pediatric patients not established. Use raxibacumab only if clearly needed. ▪ As in adults, effectiveness in pediatric patients is based solely on efficacy studies in animal models. There are no studies of safety or pharmacokinetics in pediatric patients.

Elderly: Numbers in clinical studies insufficient to determine if the elderly respond differently compared with younger subjects.

DRUG/LAB INTERACTIONS
The pharmacokinetics of ciprofloxacin and raxibacumab was not altered with coadministration of 40 mg/kg raxibacumab IV and either IV or oral ciprofloxacin.

In a study determining the efficacy of the drugs in the treatment of animals with systemic anthrax disease, the pharmacokinetics of levofloxacin and raxibacumab was unaffected by product coadministration.

SIDE EFFECTS

The most frequently reported side effects were pain in extremities, pruritus, rash, and somnolence. Anemia, back pain, dizziness, fatigue, flushing, hypertension, increased blood amylase and blood creatine phosphokinase, infusion site pain, insomnia, leukopenia, lymphadenopathy, muscle spasms, palpitations, peripheral edema, prolonged PT, and vasovagal syncope have been reported.

ANTIDOTE

Notify physician of all side effects. Most will be treated symptomatically. If signs of an infusion reaction occur, slow or interrupt the infusion and treat appropriately. No cases of overdose have been observed. If overdose occurs, monitor for any signs or symptoms of adverse effects and apply appropriate medical therapies.

RESLIZUMAB `BBW`

Interleukin-5 antagonist
Monoclonal antibody (IgG4$_\kappa$)

Cinqair

pH 5.5

USUAL DOSE

3 mg/kg once every 4 weeks as an infusion over 20 to 50 minutes.

DOSE ADJUSTMENTS

No dose adjustments required based on age, gender, or race. Clinical studies have not been conducted to assess the effect of hepatic or renal impairment on the pharmacokinetics of reslizumab.

DILUTION

Supplied as a clear to slightly hazy/opalescent, colorless to slightly yellow solution in single-use vials containing 100 mg/10 mL (10 mg/mL). May contain a few translucent-to-white amorphous particulates. *Do not shake.* Aseptic technique required. Allow solution to reach room temperature. Withdraw the proper volume of reslizumab from the vial(s) based on the recommended weight-based dose and slowly add to a 50-mL infusion bag of NS. Gently invert to mix the solution. *Do not shake.*

Filters: Use of an infusion set with an in-line, low–protein-binding, 0.2-micron filter is required. **Compatible** with polyethersulfone (PES), polyvinylidene fluoride (PVDF), nylon, and cellulose acetate in-line infusion filters.

Storage: Before use, refrigerate at 2° to 8° C (36° to 46° F) in original carton to protect from light. Do not freeze. *Do not shake.* Administer diluted solution immediately after preparation or may be refrigerated or kept at RT (up to 25° C [77° F]), protected from light, for up to 16 hours. Time between preparation and administration should not exceed 16 hours. If refrigerated before administration, allow the diluted solution to reach RT. Discard unused portion.

COMPATIBILITY

Manufacturer states, "Do not mix or dilute with other drugs. Do not infuse concomitantly in the same IV line with other agents." **Compatible** with polyvinylchloride (PVC) or poly-olefin infusion bags and with polyethersulfone (PES), polyvinylidene fluoride (PVDF), nylon, and cellulose acetate in-line infusion filters.

RATE OF ADMINISTRATION

For IV infusion only. Do not administer as an IV push or bolus. Use of an infusion set with an in-line, low–protein-binding, 0.2-micron filter is required.

Administer a single dose as an infusion over 20 to 50 minutes. Infusion time varies based on weight-based dosing. After administration, flush the IV line with NS to ensure that all of the reslizumab has been administered.

ACTIONS
Inflammation is an important component in the pathogenesis of asthma. Multiple cell types and mediators are involved in inflammation. Reslizumab is a humanized interleukin-5 antagonist monoclonal antibody (IgG4, kappa). IL-5 is the major cytokine responsible for the growth and differentiation, recruitment, activation, and survival of eosinophils. Reslizumab binds to IL-5, inhibiting the bioactivity of IL-5. By inhibiting IL-5 signaling, reslizumab reduces the production and survival of eosinophils, one of the cell types implicated in the inflammation seen with asthma. Specific mechanism of action not definitively established. Following administration of reslizumab, reductions in blood eosinophil counts were observed and maintained through 52 weeks of treatment. There is minimal distribution into the extravascular tissues. Reslizumab is degraded by enzymatic proteolysis into small peptides and amino acids. Half-life is approximately 24 days.

INDICATIONS AND USES
Add-on maintenance treatment of patients with severe asthma who have an eosinophilic phenotype and are 18 years of age or older.

Limitation of use: Not indicated for the treatment of other eosinophilic conditions. ▪ Not indicated for the relief of acute bronchospasm or status asthmaticus.

CONTRAINDICATIONS
Known hypersensitivity to reslizumab or any of its excipients.

PRECAUTIONS
For IV use only. ▪ Administered by or under the direction of a physician knowledgeable in its use and in a facility equipped to monitor the patient and respond to any medical emergency. ▪ Hypersensitivity reactions, including anaphylaxis, have been reported. ▪ Should not be used to treat acute asthma symptoms or acute exacerbations. Do not use to treat acute bronchospasm or status asthmaticus. ▪ Malignant neoplasms have been reported. The majority were diagnosed within less than 6 months of exposure to reslizumab. ▪ No clinical studies have been conducted to assess the reduction of maintenance corticosteroid doses following administration of reslizumab. Do not discontinue systemic or inhaled corticosteroids abruptly upon initiation of reslizumab therapy. ▪ Eosinophils may be involved in the immunologic response to some helminth infections. The effects of reslizumab on the immune response against parasitic infections are unknown. Patients with known parasitic infections were excluded from clinical studies. ▪ A therapeutic protein, there is a potential for immunogenicity. ▪ See Monitor.

Monitor: Monitor for S/S of a hypersensitivity reaction during and following completion of the infusion. In clinical trials, anaphylaxis was observed during or within 20 minutes after completion of the infusion and was reported as early as the second dose of reslizumab. Manifestations included decreased oxygen saturation, dyspnea, skin and mucosal involvement (including urticaria), vomiting, and wheezing. ▪ Reductions in corticosteroid dose, if appropriate, should be gradual and under physician supervision. Monitor for systemic withdrawal symptoms and/or conditions previously suppressed by systemic corticosteroid therapy. ▪ Treat pre-existing helminth infections before initiating reslizumab. Discontinue treatment until infection resolves in patients who become infected during therapy and do not respond to anti-helminth treatment.

Patient Education: Immediately report any S/S of a hypersensitivity reaction (e.g., chest discomfort, cough, dyspnea, postural dizziness, pruritus, rash, throat irritation, urticaria, wheezing) occurring during or after administration. ▪ Does not treat acute asthma symptoms or acute exacerbations. Seek medical advice if asthma remains uncontrolled or worsens after initiation of treatment with reslizumab. ▪ Malignancies have been reported. ▪ Do not discontinue or reduce the dose of maintenance systemic or inhaled corticosteroids except under the direct supervision of a physician.

Maternal/Child: Use during pregnancy only if clearly needed. In women with poorly or moderately controlled asthma, evidence demonstrates an increased risk of pre-eclampsia in the mother and an increased risk of prematurity, low birth weight, and smaller for gestational age in the neonate. The level of asthma control should be closely monitored in pregnant women and treatment adjusted as necessary to maintain optimal control. Monoclonal antibodies such as reslizumab cross the placental barrier. The potential effects on a fetus are likely to be greater during the second and third trimester of pregnancy. Consider the long half-life of reslizumab. ▪ Use caution during breast-feeding; effects unknown. ▪ Safety and effectiveness for use in pediatric patients 17 years of age or younger not established.

Elderly: No overall differences in safety or effectiveness observed between younger patients and patients 65 years of age and older. No dose adjustment is necessary.

DRUG/LAB INTERACTIONS

No formal drug interaction studies have been performed. Population pharmacokinetics analyses indicate that concomitant use of either leukotriene antagonists (e.g., montelukast [Singulair]) or corticosteroids does not affect the pharmacokinetics of reslizumab.

SIDE EFFECTS

Oropharyngeal pain is the most common side effect. Less commonly reported adverse reactions include myalgia and transient creatine phosphokinase (CPK) elevations. Hypersensitivity reactions (including anaphylaxis) and malignancy are the most serious side effects.

ANTIDOTE

Keep the physician informed of all side effects. Most will be treated symptomatically. If a hypersensitivity reaction occurs, discontinue the infusion immediately and treat with oxygen, epinephrine, antihistamines (e.g., IV diphenhydramine [Benadryl]), corticosteroids, albuterol, vasopressors (e.g., dopamine), and ventilation equipment as indicated. Symptoms of overdose were not noted in clinical trials. If overdose occurs, monitor patients for S/S of adverse effects. Resuscitate as necessary.

RETEPLASE RECOMBINANT
(**REE**-teh-place re-**KOM**-buh-nant)

Retavase, r-PA

Thrombolytic agent
(recombinant)

pH 7 to 7.4

USUAL DOSE
Administered concomitantly with heparin. Give a 5,000-unit IV bolus of heparin before the initial injection of reteplase, then give 10 units (10 mL) of reteplase as an IV injection. Follow with a 1,000 unit/hr continuous IV infusion of heparin for at least 24 hours. Give a second 10-unit bolus of reteplase 30 minutes after the first. See Dilution, Compatibility, and Rate of Administration. Aspirin is also used either during or following heparin treatment; an initial dose of 160 to 350 mg is followed by doses of 75 to 350 mg.

DOSE ADJUSTMENTS
The second bolus should not be given if serious bleeding in a critical location (e.g., intracranial, gastrointestinal, retroperitoneal, pericardial) occurs before it is due to be given.

DILUTION
Supplied in a kit with all components for reconstitution. Each kit contains a package insert and two of each of the following: single-use reteplase vials (10.8 units each), single-use diluent vials of SWFI (10 mL each), sterile 10-mL syringes with 20-gauge needles attached, sterile dispensing pins, sterile 20-gauge needles for administration, and alcohol swabs. Withdraw diluent with 20-gauge needle. Discard needle and put dispensing pin on syringe of diluent. Transfer diluent to vial of reteplase. Pin and syringe should remain in place while vial is swirled to dissolve reteplase. **Do not shake.** When completely dissolved, withdraw 10 mL reconstituted solution into the syringe (vials are 0.7 mL overfilled). Remove dispensing pin and replace with a 20-gauge needle for administration.

Storage: Kit should remain sealed to protect contents from light. Store at 2° to 25° C (36° to 77° F). Do not use beyond expiration date. Contains no preservatives; should be reconstituted immediately before use, but may be stored at room temperature if used within 4 hours. Discard all unused solution and supplies.

COMPATIBILITY
Manufacturer states, "Should be given via an IV line in which no other medication is being simultaneously injected or infused. No other medication should be added to the injection solution containing reteplase. **Incompatible** with heparin; do not administer heparin in the same IV line unless the line is flushed through with NS or D5W before and after reteplase."

RATE OF ADMINISTRATION
Heparin: First 1,000 units over 1 minute. After this test dose, the balance of 4,000 units may be given over 1 minute. Follow with an infusion of 1,000 units/hr.

Reteplase: A single dose evenly distributed over 2 minutes. To avoid **incompatibilities** and ensure delivery of both doses, be sure to flush line with a minimum of 30 to 50 mL NS or D5W before and after each injection.

ACTIONS
A recombinant plasminogen activator. Exerts its thrombolytic action by generating plasmin from plasminogen through a specific process. Plasmin then degrades the fibrin matrix of the thrombus. Potency is expressed in units that are specific to reteplase. With therapeutic doses, a decrease in circulating fibrinogen makes the patient susceptible to bleeding. Onset of action is prompt, effecting patency of the vessel within 90 minutes in most patients. The FDA has allowed the manufacturer to claim superiority over alteplase at achieving patency within 90 minutes. Prompt opening of arteries increases probability of improved cardiac function. Half-life is 13 to 16 minutes. Cleared from the plasma

by the liver and kidneys. Mean fibrinogen level should return to baseline value within 48 hours.

INDICATIONS AND USES

Management of acute myocardial infarction (AMI) in adults for the improvement of ventricular function following AMI, the reduction of the incidence of congestive failure, and the reduction of mortality associated with AMI. Treatment should begin as soon as possible after the onset of symptoms of AMI. ▪ Current AHA and JAMA recommendations identify thrombolytic agents as Class I therapy in patients younger than 70 years with recent onset of chest pain (within 6 hours) consistent with AMI and at least 0.1 mV of ST segment elevation in at least two ECG leads. Use in all other patients based on age, accurate diagnosis, and time from onset of chest pain.

CONTRAINDICATIONS

Active internal bleeding, arteriovenous malformation or aneurysm, bleeding diathesis, history of cerebral vascular accident, intracranial or intraspinal surgery or trauma within 2 months, intracranial neoplasm, severe uncontrolled hypertension.

PRECAUTIONS

Administered under the direction of a physician knowledgeable in its use and with appropriate emergency drugs and diagnostic and laboratory facilities available. ▪ Reperfusion arrhythmias occur frequently (e.g., sinus bradycardia, accelerated idioventricular rhythm, PVCs, ventricular tachycardia); have antiarrhythmic medications available at bedside. ▪ A greater alteration of hemostatic status than with heparin. Strict bed rest indicated to reduce risk of bleeding. Use extreme care with the patient; avoid any excessive or rough handling or pressure (including too-frequent BPs); avoid invasive procedures (e.g., arterial puncture, venipuncture, IM injection). If these procedures are absolutely necessary, use extreme precautionary methods (use radial artery instead of femoral; small-gauge catheters and needles, and sites that are easily observed and compressible where bleeding can be controlled; avoid handling of catheter sites, and use extended pressure application of up to 30 minutes). Minor bleeding occurs often at catheter insertion sites. Avoid use of razors and toothbrushes. ▪ Use extreme caution and weigh risks against anticipated benefits in the following situations: recent major surgery (e.g., coronary artery bypass graft, obstetric delivery, organ biopsy), previous puncture of noncompressible vessels (e.g., jugular, subclavian), cerebrovascular disease, recent GI or GU bleeding, recent trauma, hypertension (e.g., systolic BP equal to or greater than 180 mm Hg and/or diastolic BP equal to or greater than 110 mm Hg), high likelihood of left heart thrombus (e.g., mitral stenosis with atrial fibrillation), acute pericarditis, subacute bacterial endocarditis, hemostatic defects including those secondary to severe hepatic or renal disease, severe hepatic or renal dysfunction, pregnancy, diabetic hemorrhagic retinopathy or other hemorrhagic ophthalmic conditions, septic thrombophlebitis or occluded AV cannula at a seriously infected site, advanced age, patients currently receiving oral anticoagulants (e.g., warfarin [Coumadin]), any other condition in which bleeding constitutes a significant hazard or would be particularly difficult to manage because of its location. ▪ Simultaneous therapy with continuous infusion of heparin is used to reduce the risk of rethrombosis. Markedly increases risk of bleeding. ▪ Standard treatment for myocardial infarction continues simultaneously with reteplase therapy except if temporarily contraindicated (e.g., arterial blood gases unless absolutely necessary). ▪ No experience with patients receiving repeat courses of reteplase. ▪ Cholesterol embolization has been reported and may be fatal.

Monitor: Best to establish separate IV lines for reteplase and heparin. If not appropriate, be sure to flush the IV line before and after each injection of reteplase. ▪ Baseline ECG, CPK, and clotting studies (TT, PTT, CBC, fibrinogen level, platelets) and baseline assessment (patient condition, pain, hematomas, petechiae, or recent wounds) should be completed before administration. Type and cross-match may also be ordered. ▪ Monitor ECG continuously, and record strips with greatest ST segment elevation initially and every 15 minutes for at least 4 hours. A 12-lead ECG is indicated when therapy is complete. ▪ Maintain strict bed rest; monitor the patient carefully and frequently for anginal pain and signs of bleeding; observe catheter sites at least every 15 minutes and apply pressure dressings to any recently invaded site; watch for hematuria, hematemesis, bloody stool, petechiae, hematoma, flank pain, muscle weakness; do neuro checks every hour. Continue until normal clotting function returns. ▪ Watch for extravasation. ▪ See Precautions and Drug/Lab Interactions.

Patient Education: Compliance with all measures to minimize bleeding (e.g., strict bed rest) is very important. ▪ Avoid use of razors, toothbrushes, and other sharp items. ▪ Use caution while moving to avoid excessive bumping. ▪ Report all episodes of bleeding and apply local pressure if indicated. Expect oozing from IV sites.

Maternal/Child: Category C: has resulted in hemorrhage leading to spontaneous abortions in rabbits. Safety for use in pregnancy, breast-feeding, and pediatric patients not established.

Elderly: See Indications and Precautions. ▪ May have poorer prognosis following AMI and pre-existing conditions that may increase risk of intracranial bleeding. Select patients carefully to maximize benefits.

DRUG/LAB INTERACTIONS
Interaction of reteplase with other cardioactive drugs has not been studied. Risk of bleeding may be increased by **any medicine that affects blood clotting,** including anticoagulants (e.g., heparin, warfarin [Coumadin]); **any medication that may cause hypoprothrombinemia, thrombocytopenia, or GI ulceration or bleeding** (e.g., selected antibiotics [e.g., cefotetan], aspirin, NSAIDs [e.g., ibuprofen (Advil, Motrin), naproxen (Aleve, Naprosyn)]); **and/or any other medication that inhibits platelet aggregation** (e.g., clopidogrel [Plavix], dipyridamole [Persantine], glycoprotein GPIIb/IIIa receptor antagonists [e.g., abciximab (ReoPro), eptifibatide (Integrilin), tirofiban (Aggrastat)], plicamycin [Mithracin], sulfinpyrazone [Anturane], ticlopidine [Ticlid], valproic acid [Depacon]). Concurrent use not recommended with the exception of heparin and aspirin (in AMI) to reduce the risk of rethrombosis. If concurrent or subsequent use is indicated (e.g., management of acute coronary syndrome, percutaneous coronary intervention), monitor PT and aPTT closely. ▪ **Coagulation tests will be unreliable;** specific procedures can be used; notify the lab of reteplase use.

SIDE EFFECTS
Bleeding is most common: internal (GI tract, GU tract, intracranial, respiratory, or retroperitoneal sites), epistaxis, gingival, and superficial or surface bleeding (venous cutdowns, arterial punctures, sites of recent surgical intervention). Reperfusion arrhythmias are common; other serious arrhythmias may occur. A few hypersensitivity reactions, as well as fever, hypotension, nausea, and vomiting, have occurred. Cholesterol embolism has been reported and may be fatal. Clinical S/S may include acute renal failure, gangrenous digits, hypertension, infarctions (e.g., bowel, cerebral, myocardial, or spinal cord), pancreatitis, "purple toe" syndrome, renal artery occlusion.

ANTIDOTE
Notify physician of all side effects. Note even the most minute bleeding tendency. Oozing at IV sites is expected. Control minor bleeding by local pressure. For severe bleeding in a critical location, discontinue second dose of reteplase if it has not been given and any heparin therapy immediately. Whole blood, packed RBCs, cryoprecipitate, fresh frozen plasma, platelets, desmopressin, tranexamic acid, and aminocaproic acid may all be indicated. Topical preparations of aminocaproic acid may stop minor bleeding. Consider protamine if heparin has been used. Treat bradycardia with atropine, reperfusion arrhythmias with lidocaine or procainamide; VT or VF may require cardioversion. Treat minor hypersensitivity reactions symptomatically. Discontinue drug and treat anaphylaxis as indicated; resuscitate as necessary. Discontinue therapy if any symptoms of cholesterol embolism occur.

Q-R

Rh$_0$(D) IMMUNE GLOBULIN INTRAVENOUS (HUMAN) BBW
(ih-**MUNE GLAW**-byoo-lin **IN**-trah-ve-nes)

Immunizing agent
(passive)
Platelet count stimulator

Rh$_0$(D)-IGIV, Rhophylac, WinRho SDF

pH 6.5 to 7.6

USUAL DOSE

(International units [IU])

Pregnancy, predelivery: *Rhophylac and WinRho SDF:* Confirm Rh$_0$(D) negative status of patient. May be given IV or IM. 1,500 IU (300 mcg) at 28 weeks' gestation. If *WinRho SDF* is administered early in the pregnancy, it should be repeated at 12-week intervals to maintain an adequate level of passively acquired anti-Rh.

Pregnancy, postdelivery: Confirm Rh$_0$(D) negative status of patient. May be given IV or IM. Administer as soon as possible after delivery of a confirmed Rh$_0$(D)-positive baby. Usually given no later than 72 hours postdelivery. If the Rh status of the infant is unknown at 72 hours, administer to the mother at that time. Should be given as soon as possible up to 28 days after delivery. This second dose postdelivery (first dose given predelivery; see above) can reduce treatment failure.

Rhophylac: 1,500 IU (300 mcg).

WinRho SDF: 600 IU (120 mcg).

Postabortion, amniocentesis (after 34 weeks' gestation), or any other manipulation late in pregnancy (after 34 weeks' gestation): Confirm Rh$_0$(D) negative status of patient. May be given IV or IM. Administer immediately after abortion or procedure associated with increased risk of Rh isoimmunization. Must be given within 72 hours. One half of a dose (a mini-dose [IM product]) may be given if a pregnancy terminates before 13 weeks' gestation, administration within 3 hours is preferred. According to the literature, this mini-dose can provide 100% effectiveness in preventing Rh immunization.

Rhophylac: 1,500 IU (300 mcg).

WinRho SDF: 600 IU (120 mcg).

Postamniocentesis before 34 weeks' gestation or after chorionic villus sampling: Confirm Rh$_0$(D) negative status of patient. May be given IV or IM. *Rhophylac or WinRho SDF:* 1,500 IU (300 mcg) immediately after the procedure. Repeat *WinRho SDF* every 12 weeks during the pregnancy.

Threatened abortion: Confirm Rh$_0$(D) negative status of patient. May be given IV or IM. ***Rhophylac or WinRho SDF:*** 1,500 IU (300 mcg) as soon as possible.

Transfusion or fetal hemorrhage: Confirm Rh$_0$(D) negative status of patient. May be given IV or IM. Administer within 72 hours of an incompatible event involving Rh$_0$(D) positive blood such as exposure to incompatible blood transfusions (Rh+ whole blood or Rh+ red blood cells) or massive fetal hemorrhage.

Rhophylac: Give 100 IU (20 mcg) per each 2 mL transfused blood or per 1 mL erythrocyte concentrate. In cases of known or suspected excessive feto-maternal hemorrhage, the number of fetal red blood cells in the maternal circulation should be determined. If testing is not feasible and excessive feto-maternal hemorrhage cannot be excluded, administer a dose of 1,500 IU (300 mcg).

WinRho SDF: Give up to 3,000 IU (600 mcg) every 8 hours IV or 6,000 IU (1,200 mcg) every 12 hours IM until the total dose is administered. Total IV dose is 45 IU (9 mcg) for every milliliter of Rh+ whole blood exposure or 90 IU (18 mcg) for every milliliter of Rh+ red blood cell exposure. Total IM dose is 60 IU (12 mcg) for every milliliter of Rh+ whole blood exposure or 120 IU (24 mcg) for every milliliter of Rh+ red blood cell exposure.

Treatment of immune thrombocytopenic purpura (ITP); Adults and pediatric patients: *WinRho SDF:* Confirm Rh$_0$(D)-positive status of patient. Must be given IV. Hemoglobin should be greater than 10 Gm/dL. Give 250 IU/kg (50 mcg/kg) of body weight as the initial dose. May be given as a single dose or divided in half and given on two consecutive days.

If response to the initial dose is adequate, maintenance doses of 125 to 300 IU/kg (25 to 60 mcg/kg) may be given. If response to the initial dose is inadequate, see Dose Adjustments. Dose and frequency based on patient's clinical response (e.g., RBC, hemoglobin, reticulocyte levels, and platelet counts); see Dose Adjustments.

PEDIATRIC DOSE
Treatment of ITP: *WinRho SDF:* See Usual Dose and Dose Adjustments.

DOSE ADJUSTMENTS   (International units [IU])
Pregnancy and obstetrical conditions: *WinRho SDF* suggests protection must be maintained throughout pregnancy once Rh$_0$(D) immune globulin is administered. Level of passively acquired anti-Rh$_0$(D) should not fall below levels required to prevent an immune response to Rh$_0$(D)+ blood. Additional doses should be given every 12 weeks during pregnancy and at delivery unless the previous dose was administered within 3 weeks and there is less than 15 mL of fetomaternal red blood cell hemorrhage during delivery.

Suppression of Rh isoimmunization: *Rhophylac and WinRho SDF:* A large fetomaternal hemorrhage may cause an incorrect evaluation by standard tests of the amount of Rh$_0$(D) IGIV required. Assess the amount of hemorrhage and adjust dose accordingly.

Treatment of ITP: Adults and pediatric patients: *WinRho SDF:* If the hemoglobin level is less than 10 Gm/dL before or after the initial dose, reduce the initial dose and/or maintenance doses to 125 to 200 IU (25 to 40 mcg)/kg to minimize the risk of increasing the severity of anemia in the patient. ▪ In patients with adequate platelet response to the initial dose, adjust maintenance doses based on platelet and hemoglobin levels. ▪ If response to the initial dose is inadequate, adjust subsequent doses as follows:

Hemoglobin above 10 Gm/dL: redose with 250 to 300 IU (50 to 60 mcg)/kg.
Hemoglobin is 8 to 10 Gm/dL: redose with 125 to 200 IU (25 to 40 mcg)/kg.
Hemoglobin below 8 Gm/dL: use with caution; may increase severity of anemia.

DILUTION   (International units [IU])
Rhophylac: Available in a prefilled 2-mL syringe containing 1,500 IU (300 mcg) for single-dose use. Bring to room or body temperature before use.
WinRho SDF: Available as a ready-to-use liquid. 5 IU equals 1 mcg. Withdraw the entire contents of the vial to obtain the labeled dose. If indicated, calculate a partial dose, then discard the excess from the syringe. The target fill volume of each vial is included in the following chart.

WinRho SDF Target Fill Volumes/Vial	
Vial Size	Target Fill Volume
600 IU (120 mcg)	0.5 mL
1,500 IU (300 mcg)	1.3 mL
2,500 IU (500 mcg)	2.2 mL
5,000 IU (1,000 mcg)	4.4 mL
15,000 IU (3,000 mcg)	13 mL

Storage: *Rhophylac:* Refrigerate syringes before use. Protect from light. Should not be used after expiration date. Discard unused product in syringe. *WinRho SDF:* Store unopened vials in refrigerator. Note expiration date. Do not freeze. Discard unused portion.

COMPATIBILITY
Rhophylac: Specific information not available.
WinRho SDF: Manufacturer states, "Should be administered separately from other drugs." Dilute only with NS.

RATE OF ADMINISTRATION
Rhophylac: A single dose as a slow IV injection.
WinRho SDF: A single dose as an IV injection over 3 to 5 minutes.

ACTIONS
(International units [IU])

Rhophylac and WinRho SDF: Specialty immunoglobulins. A gamma globulin (IgG) fraction containing antibodies to the Rh$_O$(D) antigen (D Antigen). Reduces the incidence of Rh immunization of an Rh$_O$(D)-negative mother by an Rh$_O$(D)-positive infant before, during, and after delivery; reduces the likelihood of hemolytic disease in an Rh$_O$(D)-positive infant in present and future pregnancies. Has also been shown to increase platelet counts in nonsplenectomized Rh$_O$(D)-positive patients with immune thrombocytopenic purpura (ITP). A 1,500-IU vial or syringe contains 300 mcg of anti-Rh$_O$(D), which can effectively suppress the immunizing potential of approximately 15 to 17 mL of Rh$_O$(D)-positive blood cells, and, in addition, contains 25 to 40 mg of nonspecific gammaglobulin. Pooled from source plasma selected for high titers of Rh$_O$(D) antibody. Purified and standardized by several methods (e.g., solvent-detergent viral inactivation process to decrease the possibility of transmission of blood-borne pathogens [e.g., HIV, hepatitis]). Similar to native IgG that normally circulates in human plasma.

Rhophylac: Is thimerosol free, mercury free, and latex free. Contains albumin as a stabilizer. Half-life is 12 to 20 days. Anti-D IgG titers were measurable up to 9 weeks after injection.

WinRho SDF: Has also been shown to increase platelet counts in nonsplenectomized Rh$_O$(D)-positive patients with immune thrombocytopenic purpura (ITP). Platelet counts usually begin to rise in 1 to 2 days with peak effect in 7 to 14 days. Some effects last about 30 days. Contains 25 to 40 mg of nonspecific gammaglobulin. The liquid form contains maltose as a stabilizer; the lyophilized powder is stabilized with glycine, NaCl, and polysorbate 80. Half-life is 24 days. Crosses the blood-brain barrier.

INDICATIONS AND USES

Rhophylac and WinRho SDF: Suppression of Rh isoimmunization in nonsensitized Rh$_O$(D)-negative women during the normal course of pregnancy, within 72 hours after spontaneous or induced abortions, amniocentesis, chorionic villus sampling, ruptured tubal pregnancy, abdominal trauma or transplacental hemorrhage, unless the blood type of the fetus or father is known to be Rh$_O$(D)-negative. ■ Suppression of Rh isoimmunization in Rh$_O$(D)-negative female pediatric patients and female adults in their childbearing years transfused with Rh$_O$(D)-positive red blood cells or blood components containing Rh$_O$(D)-positive RBCs.

WinRho SDF: Treatment of nonsplenectomized Rh$_O$(D)-positive pediatric patients with acute or chronic immune thrombocytopenic purpura (ITP), adults with chronic ITP, pediatric patients and adults with ITP secondary to HIV infection in clinical situations requiring an increase in platelet counts to prevent excessive hemorrhage.

CONTRAINDICATIONS

Rhophylac and WinRho SDF: *All uses:* History of a prior severe hypersensitivity reaction to human immune globulin preparations or their components (*Rhophylac* contains albumin, *WinRho SDF* may contain thimerosol); patients with isolated IgA deficiency or preexisting IgA antibodies (benefits must outweigh risks; risk of anaphylaxis is greater).

Suppression of Rh isoimmunization in pregnancy: For suppression of Rh isoimmunization in the mother. *Do not administer to the infant.* Not recommended for use in Rh$_O$(D)-negative individuals shown to be Rh immunized by standard screening tests.

WinRho SDF: *Treatment of ITP:* Not recommended for use in Rh$_O$(D)-negative or splenectomized individuals.

PRECAUTIONS

All uses: Confirm vial or syringe label—must state for IV or IV/IM use; several similar products are for IM use only (e.g., RhoGam). ■ May risk transmission of infectious agents (e.g., hepatitis, HIV, possibly the Creutzfeldt-Jakob disease [CJD] agent); see Actions. ■ May contain trace amounts of anti-A, anti-B, anti-C, and anti-E blood group antibodies. ■ Use caution and weigh benefit versus risk in patients with known hypogammaglobulinemia or selective IgA deficiency; risk of severe allergic reactions or anaphylaxis is increased. ■ Not intended for use in Rh+ individuals (with the exception of *WinRho SDF* in the treatment of ITP). ■ Use with caution and monitor renal function in patients at risk for renal insufficiency. IGIV products have been reported to produce renal dysfunction in patients who are predisposed to acute renal failure or in those who have renal insufficiency. Most reports involve products that contain sucrose as a stabilizer. WinRho SDF does not contain sucrose.

Suppression of Rh isoimmunization in pregnancy: More than 1 dose of Rh$_O$(D) immune globulin may be required. A fetal RBC count can be done on maternal blood to determine the required dose. ▪ If a large fetomaternal hemorrhage occurs late in pregnancy or after delivery Rh$_O$(D) IGIV should be administered in sufficient doses if there is any doubt about the mother's blood type (e.g., presence of passively administered anti-Rh$_O$(D) in maternal or fetal blood [positive Coombs test]). ▪ See Monitor. ▪ Manufacturer recommends IM or IV use. Another source recommends IM injection when Rh$_O$(D) is used as an immunizing agent. ▪ Not effective in Rh$_O$(D)-negative females who have already been sensitized to the Rh$_O$(D) erythrocyte factor; however, if administered, the risk of side effects is not increased.

Treatment of ITP: IV route required for ITP. ▪ Rare cases of intravascular hemolysis have been reported. Usually occurs within 4 hours of administration. Complications may include clinically compromising anemia and multisystem organ failure, including ARDS. Fatalities have occurred. Serious complications, including severe anemia, acute renal insufficiency, renal failure, and DIC, have also been reported. Even if previous infusions have been uneventful, intravascular hemolysis and its complications may occur with subsequent infusions. ▪ If the hemoglobin level is less than 8 Gm/dL, use with extreme caution; may increase severity of anemia.

Monitor: All uses: See Precautions. ▪ Observe patient for at least 20 to 30 minutes after injection.

Suppression of Rh isoimmunization in pregnancy: Maintain accurate records of Rh factor and Rh$_O$(D)-IGIV. ▪ Obtain CBC and other appropriate lab work based on procedure or situation. ▪ Monitor vital signs if indicated.

Treatment of ITP: Obtain baseline RBC, hemoglobin, reticulocyte levels, and platelet counts. Monitor during therapy to determine clinical response. ▪ Given to Rh$_O$(D)-positive patients in this situation, interaction with RBC usually causes some degree of RBC hemolysis; observe carefully. Monitor for S/S of intravascular hemolysis (back pain, chills, fever, hemoglobinuria) for at least 8 hours after infusion. Perform a dipstick urinalysis at baseline, at 2 and 4 hours, and before the end of the monitoring period. ▪ Monitor for complications of intravascular hemolysis (IVH), including clinically compromising anemia (decreased hemoglobin, hypotension, pallor, and tachycardia), acute renal insufficiency (anuria, dyspnea, edema, or oliguria), or DIC (increased bruising and prolongation of bleeding or clotting time). ▪ If S/S of IVH or its complications occur, lab tests should be performed to confirm the diagnosis. Tests include but are not limited to CBC with platelets, haptoglobin, plasma hemoglobin, urine dipstick, BUN, SCr, LDH, direct and indirect bilirubin, and DIC-specific tests (e.g., D-dimer, fibrin degradation products [FDP], fibrin split products [FSP]). ▪ If transfusion is required, use Rh$_O$(D)-negative RBCs to avoid exacerbating ongoing IVH. Platelet products may contain RBCs; use caution if platelets from an Rh$_O$(D)+ donor are used.

Patient Education: Report S/S of a hypersensitivity reaction (e.g., feeling of fainting, hives, itching, tightness in the chest, wheezing). ▪ Report feelings of dizziness, tiredness, weakness. **ITP:** May cause a considerable drop in hemoglobin; follow-up testing important. ▪ Immediately report symptoms of back pain, chills, decreased urine output, discolored urine or hematuria, fever, sudden weight gain, fluid retention/edema, and/or shortness of breath. May indicate onset of intravascular hemolysis (IVH).

Maternal/Child: Category C: use only if clearly needed. ▪ Rhophylac is not secreted in breast milk. Specific information is not available for WinRho SDF on safety during breast-feeding. ▪ For the suppression of Rh isoimmunization in the mother; do not administer to the infant.

Elderly: When used for treatment of ITP, fatal outcomes associated with IVH and its complications occurred most frequently in patients over 65 years of age with comorbid conditions.

Q-R

DRUG/LAB INTERACTIONS

Interaction with other drugs has not been evaluated. ▪ Antibodies contained in Rh$_0$(D) immune globulin may interfere with the body's immune response to certain **live virus vaccines.** Do not administer live virus vaccines (e.g., measles, mumps, polio, or rubella) for at least 3 months after Rh$_0$(D) administration. ▪ Trace amounts of anti-A, anti-B, anti-C, and anti-E blood group antibodies may be detectable in **direct and indirect antiglobulin (Coombs) tests** following treatment with Rh$_0$(D). ▪ May affect outcomes of **blood typing and antibody testing** in neonates. ▪ The liquid formulation of WinRho SDF contains maltose, which may give **falsely high blood glucose levels** with certain types of blood glucose testing systems. Only testing systems that are glucose specific should be used to monitor blood glucose levels in patients receiving maltose-containing parenteral products such as WinRho SDF.

SIDE EFFECTS

All uses: Abdominal or back pain, arthralgias, asthenia, chills, diarrhea, dizziness, fever, headache, hyperkinesia, hypertension, hypotension, increased LDH, pruritus, rash, somnolence, and sweating. Hypersensitivity reactions, including anaphylaxis, have been reported rarely. Made from human plasma donors, transmission of selected diseases possible but not probable; see Precautions.

Suppression of Rh isoimmunization in pregnancy: Side effects are infrequent in Rh$_0$(D)-negative individuals. Only a few women have had treatment failures resulting in development of Rh$_0$(D) antibodies.

ITP: Destruction of Rh$_0$(D) red cells resulting in decreased hemoglobin (range was 0.4 to 6.1 Gm/dL). IVH (back pain, shaking chills, hemoglobinuria), acute onset and exacerbation of anemia, and renal insufficiency have been reported in Rh$_0$(D)-positive patients. Has rarely resulted in death.

ANTIDOTE

Keep physician informed of side effects; may require symptomatic treatment. Discontinue immediately if an allergic reaction occurs; treat as indicated (e.g., maintain airway, administer fluids, oxygen, epinephrine [Adrenalin], diphenhydramine [Benadryl], corticosteroids [e.g., dexamethasone (Decadron)]). *ITP:* Treatment may have to be discontinued if drop in hemoglobin too severe. Transfusion may be required.

RIFAMPIN
(rih-**FAM**-pin)

Rifadin

Antibacterial
(antituberculosis)

pH 7.8 to 8.8

USUAL DOSE

Dose and schedule may vary depending on treatment regimen selected. IV doses are the same as oral. Use oral dose form as soon as practical.

Tuberculosis (adults and pediatric patients 15 years of age or older): 10 mg/kg once a day when used in conjunction with other antituberculosis agents in a daily regimen, or 10 mg/kg not to exceed 600 mg/dose two or three times a week when used in an intermittent multiple-drug regimen. Do not exceed 600 mg/day. Prescribed concurrently with other antituberculin drugs (e.g., ethambutol [Myambutol], isoniazid [INH], pyrazinamide, or streptomycin). Consult current CDC guidelines for suggested treatment regimens.

Meningococcal carriers: 600 mg every 12 hours for 2 days.

PEDIATRIC DOSE

Tuberculosis: 10 to 20 mg/kg of body weight once a day when used in conjunction with other antituberculosis agents in a daily regimen, or two or three times a week when used in an intermittent multiple-drug regimen. Do not exceed 600 mg/day. Prescribed concurrently with other antituberculin drugs (e.g., ethambutol [Myambutol], isoniazid [INH], pyrazinamide, or streptomycin).

Meningococcal carriers: *Under 1 month of age:* 5 mg/kg every 12 hours for 2 days. *Over 1 month of age:* 10 mg/kg every 12 hours for 2 days.

DOSE ADJUSTMENTS

To reduce hepatotoxicity, a reduced dose may be required in impaired hepatic function. ▪ No dose adjustment is necessary in impaired renal function; serum concentrations do not change. ▪ See Drug/Lab Interactions.

DILUTION

Each 600-mg vial must be initially diluted in 10 mL of SWFI (60 mg/mL). Swirl gently to dissolve. Withdraw desired dose and further dilute in 500 mL or 100 mL of D5W or NS; see Storage.

Storage: Store vials at CRT. Avoid excessive heat (temperatures above 40° C [104° F]). Protect from light. Reconstituted solution stable at RT for 24 hours. Use solution diluted in D5W within 4 hours; solution diluted in NS stable for 24 hours.

COMPATIBILITY

Manufacturer states, "May form a precipitate with diltiazem (Cardizem) at the **Y-site.**" Infusion solutions other than D5W or NS are not recommended.

RATE OF ADMINISTRATION

A single dose equally distributed as an infusion over 3 hours. In selected situations a single dose diluted in 100 mL may be administered over 30 minutes.

ACTIONS

A semi-synthetic antibiotic derivative of rifamycin. Has bactericidal action against slow and intermittently growing *Mycobacterium tuberculosis* organisms. Inhibits bacterial DNA-dependent RNA polymerase activity in susceptible *M. tuberculosis* organisms but does not inhibit the mammalian enzyme. Rapidly distributed throughout the body and present in many organs and body fluids, including CSF. 80% protein bound. Metabolized in the liver. Undergoes enterohepatic circulation. Excreted in bile and urine. Half-life following repeated dosing is 3 to 4 hours. Crosses the placental barrier. Secreted in breast milk.

INDICATIONS AND USES

Treatment or retreatment of tuberculosis when the drug cannot be taken by mouth. ▪ Treatment of asymptomatic carriers of *Neisseria* meningitis. Not indicated for treatment of meningococcal infection because of rapid emergence of resistant meningococci.

Unlabeled uses: Used in combination with other agents in the treatment of certain atypical mycobacterial infections (e.g., *Mycobacterium avium*). ▪ Used in combination with other antistaphylococcal agents to treat serious staphylococcal infections.

CONTRAINDICATIONS
Hypersensitivity to rifampin or any of its components or to any rifamycins. Individuals with liver disease are at higher risk for complications. ▪ Contraindicated in patients receiving ritonavir-boosted saquinavir; risk for severe hepatocellular toxicity is increased. ▪ Concomitant use with atazanavir (Reyataz), darunavir (Prezista), fosamprenavir (Lexiva), saquinavir (Invirase), and tipranavir (Aptivus); see Drug/Lab Interactions.

PRECAUTIONS
For IV use only. Do not administer IM or SC. ▪ Obtain cultures before starting therapy to confirm susceptibility of the organism to rifampin. Repeat cultures periodically during therapy to monitor for the emergence of resistance. ▪ Resistance can emerge rapidly; appropriate susceptibility tests should be performed in the event of persistent positive cultures. ▪ Susceptibility tests also required before use as treatment for asymptomatic carriers of *Neisseria* meningitis. ▪ To reduce the development of drug-resistant bacteria and maintain its effectiveness, rifampin should be used to treat or prevent only those infections proven or strongly suspected to be caused by bacteria. ▪ Organisms resistant to rifampin are likely to be resistant to other rifamycins. ▪ Has been shown to produce liver dysfunction. Risk of liver damage is markedly increased if impaired liver function is present. Hepatotoxicity, hepatic encephalopathy, and death associated with jaundice have occurred in patients with liver disease and when rifampin is given with other hepatotoxic agents (e.g., isoniazid [INH], halothane). Discontinue one or both drugs if signs of hepatocellular damage occur. ▪ May exacerbate porphyria. ▪ Use with caution in patients with diabetes; diabetes management may be more difficult. ▪ Not recommended for intermittent therapy; interruption of daily dosage regimen has resulted in rare renal hypersensitivity reactions when therapy was resumed. ▪ Urine, feces, sputum, sweat, and tears may be colored red-orange. Soft contact lenses may be permanently stained. CSF may be light yellow. ▪ Pseudomembranous colitis has been reported. May range from mild to life threatening. Consider in patients who present with diarrhea during or after treatment with rifampin.

Monitor: Obtain baseline measurements of hepatic enzymes (e.g., ALT and AST), bilirubin, SCr, CBC, and platelet count. Routine lab monitoring in patients with normal baseline labs is generally not necessary. However, patients should be seen monthly and questioned about symptoms that may indicate adverse reactions. ▪ Monitor liver function every 2 to 4 weeks in patients with pre-existing liver impairment. ▪ Monitor blood glucose closely in patients with diabetes. ▪ Notify physician immediately if flu-like symptoms develop; may be due to hepatotoxicity. ▪ Thrombocytopenia has occurred. Reversible if rifampin is discontinued as soon as purpura occurs. Cerebral hemorrhage has occurred when rifampin has been continued or resumed after the appearance of purpura. Contact physician immediately if purpura occurs. ▪ Confirm patency of IV; avoid extravasation. Restart IV at a new site for any signs of inflammation or irritation. ▪ Do all lab tests and affected radiology studies before daily dose of medication. ▪ See Drug/Lab Interactions.

Patient Education: Reliability of hormonal contraceptives may be affected; use of nonhormonal contraceptives recommended. ▪ Avoid use of alcohol or other hepatotoxic agents (e.g., acetaminophen [Anacin-3, Tylenol], NSAIDs [ibuprofen (Advil, Motrin), naproxen (Aleve, Naprosyn)], phenothiazines [e.g., promethazine (Phenergan)], some antineoplastic agents, sulfonamides). ▪ Review side effects with health care professional and promptly report darkened urine, fever, loss of appetite, malaise, nausea and vomiting, pain or swelling of the joints, or yellowish discoloration of the skin and eyes. ▪ May cause reddish-orange discoloration of feces, sputum, sweat, urine, and tears. ▪ May discolor soft contact lenses. ▪ Do not interrupt daily dosage regimen.

Maternal/Child: Category C: has teratogenic potential. Safety for use during pregnancy not established. Benefit must outweigh risk. See literature for best combinations with least known risk. ▪ Administration during the last few weeks of pregnancy may cause post-natal hemorrhages in mother and infant; treatment with vitamin K may be required. ▪ Closely monitor neonates of rifampin-treated mothers for adverse effects. ▪ Discontinue breast-feeding if mother requires treatment.

Elderly: Differences in response between elderly and younger patients have not been identified. ▪ See Dose Adjustments.

DRUG/LAB INTERACTIONS

Interactions are numerous and potentially life threatening. Review of drug profile by pharmacist imperative. ▪ Hepatotoxicity, hepatic encephalopathy, and death associated with jaundice have occurred when rifampin is given with **other hepatotoxic agents** (e.g., alcohol, isoniazid [INH], halothane). Discontinue one or both drugs for signs of hepatocellular damage. ▪ Concurrent use of rifampin with **saquinavir/ritonavir** (ritonavir-boosted saquinavir) is **contraindicated;** significant hepatocellular toxicity with markedly increased transaminase elevations has been reported. ▪ Concurrent administration with **atazanavir** (Reyataz), **darunavir** (Prezista), **fosamprenavir** (Lexiva), **saquinavir** (Invirase), and **tipranavir** (Aptivus) is **contraindicated;** rifampin may substantially decrease plasma concentrations of these antiviral agents. Loss of antiviral effectiveness and/or development of viral resistance may result. ▪ Rifampin increases metabolism and clearance and decreases serum levels and effectiveness of numerous drugs. Manufacturer lists **antiarrhythmics** (e.g., disopyramide [Norpace], mexiletine, quinidine, tocainide [Tonocard]), **anticonvulsants** (e.g., phenytoin [Dilantin]), **antifungals** (e.g., fluconazole [Diflucan], itraconazole [Sporanox], ketoconazole [Nizoral]), **barbiturates** (e.g., phenobarbital), **beta-blockers** (e.g., propranolol), **calcium channel blockers** (e.g., diltiazem [Cardizem], nifedipine [Procardia], verapamil), **cardiac glycoside preparations** (e.g., digoxin [Lanoxin], digitoxin), **chloramphenicol** (Chloromycetin), **clarithromycin** (Biaxin), **clofibrate** (Atromid-S), **corticosteroids** (e.g., prednisone), **cyclosporine** (Sandimmune), **dapsone, diazepam** (Valium), **doxycycline, fluoroquinolones** (e.g., ciprofloxacin [Cipro IV]), **haloperidol** (Haldol), **levothyroxine** (Synthroid), **methadone, narcotic analgesics, oral anticoagulants** (e.g., warfarin [Coumadin]), **oral hypoglycemic agents** (e.g., sulfonylureas [e.g., glyburide (DiaBeta), tolbutamide]), **oral or other systemic hormonal contraceptives, progestins** (e.g., progesterone), **quinine, tacrolimus** (Prograf), **theophylline** (aminophylline), **tricyclic antidepressants** (e.g., amitriptyline [Elavil], nortriptyline [Aventyl]), **zidovudine.** Other sources add **amiodarone** (Nexterone), **amprenavir** (Agenerase), **benzodiazepines** (e.g., midazolam [Versed], in addition to diazepam), **buspirone** (BuSpar), **estrogens, lamotrigine** (Lamictal), **losartan** (Cozaar), **ondansetron** (Zofran), **and zolipidem** (Ambien). Increased doses of these drugs may be required. Monitor carefully; obtain prothrombin daily when used with **anticoagulants** (e.g., warfarin); use of **nonhormonal contraceptives** recommended during rifampin therapy; and **diabetes** may be more difficult to control. ▪ May reduce analgesic effects of **morphine and methadone.** Monitor carefully; an alternate analgesic may be required (see earlier statement). ▪ Treatment failure of **ketoconazole** (Nizoral) **or rifampin** may occur when given concomitantly. ▪ Concomitant use of rifampin and **macrolide antibiotics** (e.g., clarithromycin) may decrease the metabolism of rifampin and increase the metabolism of the macrolide antibiotic. ▪ Potentiated by **probenecid and co-trimoxazole.** ▪ May decrease concentrations of enalaprilat, the active metabolite of **enalapril** (Vasotec), resulting in hypertension. Adjust dose as required. ▪ When taken concomitantly, decreased concentrations of **atovaquone** (Mepron) and increased concentration of rifampin have been observed. ▪ May induce metabolism of endogenous substrates including **adrenal hormones, thyroid hormones, and vitamin D.** Reduced levels of vitamin D may be accompanied by decreased serum calcium and phosphate and increased parathyroid hormone. ▪ Concomitant administration with **sulfasalazine** may cause a decrease in sulfapyridine levels. ▪ Cross-reactivity and false-positive urine screening **tests for opiates** have been reported when using certain assays. Gas chromatography or mass spectrometry will distinguish rifampin from opiates. ▪ May cause an early rise in bilirubin during initial days of treatment; should subside. Throughout treatment transient abnormalities in **liver function tests** will occur. Monitor laboratory trends and patient's clinical condition. ▪ Therapeutic levels inhibit microbiologic assays of **serum folate and vitamin B₁₂.** ▪ Reduced biliary excretion of contrast media for **gallbladder studies** may occur. Perform test prior to dose of rifampin.

SIDE EFFECTS

Average dose: Anaphylaxis may occur even with repeat doses. Abnormal liver function tests, anorexia, ataxia, behavioral changes, conjunctivitis (exudative), cramps, diarrhea, DIC, dizziness, edema of face and extremities, epigastric distress, eosinophilia, fatigue, flu-like symptoms (e.g., chills, fever, headache, malaise, muscle and bone pain), flushing, gas, heartburn, hematuria, hemolytic anemia, hepatic reactions, hepatitis or a shocklike syndrome and abnormal liver function tests (rare), hypersensitivity reactions (e.g., pruritus, rash, Stevens-Johnson syndrome, toxic epidermal necrolysis, urticaria), hypotension, jaundice, leukopenia, menstrual disturbances, mental confusion, myopathy (rare), muscle weakness, nausea, numbness (generalized), pain in extremities, pseudomembranous colitis, psychosis, purpura, renal failure (acute), shortness of breath, sore mouth and tongue, thrombocytopenia, visual disturbances, vomiting, wheezing.

Overdose: Abdominal pain; bilirubin levels and/or liver enzymes may increase rapidly; brown-red discoloration of feces, skin, sweat, tears, and urine is proportional to amount of overdose; headache, lethargy, nausea, and vomiting are immediate; pruritus; unconsciousness. Liver enlargement, possibly with tenderness, can develop within a few hours after severe overdose; bilirubin levels may increase and jaundice may develop rapidly. Arrhythmias, cardiac arrest, hypotension, and seizures have been reported in fatal overdoses.

ANTIDOTE

With increasing severity of any side effect, alterations in liver function tests, flu-like symptoms, purpura, thrombocytopenia, or symptoms of overdose, discontinue the drug and notify the physician immediately. Antiemetics (e.g., ondansetron [Zofran], prochlorperazine [Compazine]) may be required to control nausea and vomiting. Forced diuresis will promote excretion. Hemodialysis may be indicated. If hemodialysis is not available, peritoneal dialysis can be used along with forced diuresis. In severe overdose or acute toxicity, maintain an adequate airway and confirm adequate respiratory exchange. Treat anaphylaxis and resuscitate as necessary.

RITUXIMAB BBW
(rih-**TUK**-sih-mab)

Rituxan

Recombinant monoclonal antibody
Antineoplastic

pH 6.5

USUAL DOSE

Premedication: *Use recommended for all indications.* Acetaminophen (Tylenol) and diphenhydramine (Benadryl) are recommended before each dose to prevent or attenuate severe hypersensitivity and/or infusion reactions. Additional premedication (e.g., methylprednisolone 100 mg IV or equivalent) is required for patients with rheumatoid arthritis (RA). Patients with granulomatosis with polyangiitis (GPA [Wegener's granulomatosis (WG)]) and microscopic polyangiitis (MPA) require additional premedication with methylprednisolone IV 1,000 mg. See Precautions for PCP prophylaxis and/or antiherpetic viral prophylaxis required in specific indications.

Relapsed or refractory, low-grade or follicular, CD20-positive, B-cell non-Hodgkin's lymphoma (NHL): Single agent: *Initial therapy:* 375 mg/M² as an infusion once a week for 4 or 8 doses. See Drug/Lab Interactions. Risk of Grade 3 or 4 adverse events increased with treatment with 8 doses as compared to treatment with 4 doses. *Retreatment therapy:* Patients who subsequently develop progressive disease may be retreated with 375 mg/M² as an IV infusion once each week for 4 doses. Incidence of adverse events similar to initial therapy. Data on more than 2 courses are limited.

Previously untreated follicular, CD20-positive, B-cell NHL: 375 mg/M² as an infusion, given on Day 1 of each cycle of CVP chemotherapy for up to 8 doses. In patients with complete or partial response, initiate rituximab maintenance 8 weeks after completion of rituximab in combination with chemotherapy. Administer rituximab as a single agent every 8 weeks for 12 doses.

Nonprogressing, low-grade, CD20-positive, B-cell NHL (after first-line CVP chemotherapy): In patients who have not progressed following 6 to 8 cycles of CVP chemotherapy (stable disease), 375 mg/M² may be administered as an infusion once a week for 4 doses every 6 months for up to 16 doses.

Diffuse large B-cell, CD20-positive NHL: 375 mg/M² as an infusion on Day 1 of each cycle of chemotherapy for up to 8 doses.

Chronic lymphocytic leukemia (CLL): 375 mg/M² the day before the initiation of FC chemotherapy (fludarabine [Fludara] and cyclophosphamide [Cytoxan]) in the first cycle, then 500 mg/M² on Day 1 of Cycles 2 through 6 (every 28 days); see Precautions.

Rheumatoid arthritis: Administer *glucocorticoids* (e.g., methylprednisolone [Solu-Medrol] 100 mg IV) 30 minutes before each infusion of rituximab to reduce the incidence and severity of infusion reactions. Follow with a *rituximab* infusion of 1,000 mg. Repeat entire sequence one time in 2 weeks. Given in combination with methotrexate. Subsequent courses should be administered every 24 weeks or based on clinical evaluation, but not sooner than every 16 weeks.

Granulomatosis with polyangiitis (GPA [Wegener's granulomatosis (WG)]) and microscopic polyangiitis (MPA):

Methylprednisolone: 1,000 mg/day IV for 1 to 3 days followed by oral prednisone 1 mg/kg/day (not to exceed 80 mg/day and tapered per clinical need) is recommended to treat severe vasculitis symptoms. This regimen should begin within 14 days before or with the initiation of rituximab and may continue during and after the 4-week course of treatment.

Rituximab: 375 mg/M² as an infusion once weekly for 4 weeks. Safety and effectiveness of subsequent courses not established. See Precautions.

Therapeutic regimen with ibritumomab tiuxetan: 250 mg/M² as an IV infusion. Given in a specific protocol in combination with Y-90 ibritumomab tiuxetan (Zevalin); see ibritumomab monograph on the Evolve website.

DOSE ADJUSTMENTS

No dose adjustments recommended. Has not been formally studied in patients with renal or hepatic impairment. See Rate of Administration. ■ Interrupt or slow infusion rate for infusion reactions. Continue the infusion at one-half the previous rate when symptoms subside.

DILUTION

Each single dose must be further diluted to a final concentration of 1 to 4 mg/mL with NS or D5W. 500 mg (50 mL) in 450 mL will yield 1 mg/mL; 500 mg (50 mL) in 75 mL will yield 4 mg/mL. Gently invert to mix solution. Contains no preservatives; discard any unused portion left in vial.

Storage: Refrigerate vials at 2° to 8° C (36° to 46° F); protect from light and freezing. Do not shake. Do not use beyond expiration date. Diluted solutions may be refrigerated for 24 hours and are stable at room temperature for an additional 24 hours.

COMPATIBILITY

Manufacturer states, "Rituximab should not be mixed or diluted with other drugs." No **incompatibilities** with polyvinylchloride or polyethylene bags have been observed.

RATE OF ADMINISTRATION

Must be given as an infusion. *Do not administer as an IV push or bolus.* Hypersensitivity (non–IgE-mediated) and/or infusion reactions are a common occurrence and may be prevented or lessened with premedication and a reduced rate of infusion.

Q-R

First infusion: Begin with an initial rate of 50 mg/hr (at this rate a 500-mg dose would be infused over 10 hours). If no discomfort or adverse effects occur, may be gradually increased by 50-mg/hr increments at 30-minute intervals to a maximum rate of 400 mg/hr. At any time that discomfort or adverse effects occur, interrupt or reduce the rate of infusion. When symptoms have completely resolved, the infusion can be restarted at half the previous rate. Discontinue the infusion for severe reactions and treat as indicated; see Antidote.

Subsequent infusions: If the patient did not tolerate the first infusion well, follow instructions under first infusion. If no discomfort or adverse effects occurred with the first infusion, use the following guidelines:

Standard infusion: Subsequent infusions may begin with an initial rate of 100 mg/hr and increased by 100-mg/hr increments at 30-minute intervals to a maximum rate of 400 mg/hr. See all precautionary measures under First Infusion (see above).

Previously untreated follicular NHL and diffuse large B-cell lymphoma (DLBCL) patients: If a Grade 3 or 4 infusion-related reaction did not occur during the first infusion, a subsequent 90-minute infusion can be administered with a glucocorticoid-containing chemotherapy regimen. Administer the corticosteroid, acetaminophen, and diphenhydramine; follow with rituximab. Administer 20% of rituximab dose equally distributed over the first 30 minutes and the remaining 80% of the dose equally distributed over 60 minutes. If this initial subsequent 90-minute infusion is tolerated, it can be repeated in the remaining infusions of the protocol. ▪ Patients who have clinically significant cardiovascular disease or who have a circulating lymphocyte count equal to or greater than 5,000/mm^3 before Cycle 2 should not be administered the 90-minute infusion.

ACTIONS

An antineoplastic agent. A humanized (Ig)G$_1$ monoclonal antibody produced by recombinant DNA technology. Designed to bind to the CD20 antigen found on the surface of normal (pre-B-lymphocytes and mature B-lymphocytes) and malignant B-lymphocytes. Upon binding to CD20, rituximab mediates B-cell lysis. Results in a rapid and sustained depletion (cytotoxity) of circulating and tissue-based B-cells. Cell lysis may be the result of complement-dependent cytotoxicity and antibody-dependent cellular cytotoxicity. May sensitize drug-resistant human B-cell lymphoma cell lines to cytotoxic chemotherapy. Detected in serum for 3 to 6 months after completion of therapy. B-cell depletion was sustained for 6 to 9 months posttreatment in 83% of patients. B-cell recovery begins at approximately 6 months, and most levels return to normal by 12 months following completion of treatment. B-cells are believed to play a role in the pathogenesis of rheumatoid arthritis (RA) and associated chronic synovitis. In this setting, B-cells may act at multiple sites in the autoimmune/inflammatory process, including through production of rheumatoid factor and other auto-antibodies, antigen presentation, T-cell activation, and/or pro-inflammatory cytokine production. In RA it induces depletion of peripheral B-lymphocytes, with near-complete depletion occurring in most patients within 2 weeks of the first dose. This B-lymphocyte depletion lasted for at least 6 months, followed by a gradual recovery. Treatment with rituximab in patients with RA was associated with a reduction of certain biologic markers for inflammation. A few patients had prolonged peripheral B-cell depletion lasting more than 3 years after a single course of treatment. Median half-life ranged from 18 to 32 days depending on diagnosis. Crosses the placental barrier. May be secreted in breast milk.

INDICATIONS AND USES

As a single agent in the treatment of patients with relapsed or refractory low-grade or follicular CD20-positive, B-cell NHL. ▪ In combination with CHOP (cyclophosphamide, doxorubicin [hydroxydaunorubicin], vincristine, and prednisone) or other anthracycline-based chemotherapy regimens for treatment in previously untreated diffuse large B-cell, CD20-positive NHL. ▪ Treatment of previously untreated follicular, CD20-positive, B-cell NHL in combination with first-line chemotherapy and as a single-agent maintenance therapy in patients achieving a complete or partial response to rituximab in combination with chemotherapy. ▪ Treatment of nonprogressing (including stable disease), low-grade, CD20-positive, B-cell NHL as a single agent after first-line CVP chemotherapy. ▪ Treatment of patients with previously untreated and previously treated CD20-positive CLL. Used in combination with FC chemotherapy (fludarabine and cyclophosphamide). ▪ In combination with glucocorticoids for the treatment of adult patients with granulomatosis with polyangiitis (GPA [Wegener's granulomatosis (WG)]) and microscopic polyangiitis (MPA). ▪ In combination with ibritumomab tiuxetan as part of a therapeutic regimen for the treatment of patients with relapsed or refractory low-grade or follicular B-cell NHL. ▪ In combination with methotrexate to reduce S/S and to slow the progression of structural damage in adult patients with moderate to severe RA who have had an inadequate response to one or more TNF (tumor necrosis factor) antagonist therapies.

Limitation of use: Not recommended for patients with severe active infections.

Unlabeled uses: To postpone relapses in patients with NHL.

CONTRAINDICATIONS

Manufacturer states, "None." Known IgE-mediated hypersensitivity or anaphylactic reactions to murine proteins, rituximab, or any of its components.

PRECAUTIONS

Has been given on an outpatient basis; however, rituximab should be administered by or under the direction of the physician specialist in facilities equipped to monitor the patient and respond to any medical emergency. ▪ Severe infusion reactions and hypersensitivity reactions have occurred for up to 24 hours after initiating rituximab infusions, and some have been fatal. Most severe reactions occur within 30 minutes to 2 hours of beginning the first infusion. S/S of severe reactions may include hypotension, angioedema, hypoxia, urticaria, or bronchospasm. More severe manifestations may include anaphylactic and anaphylactoid events, pulmonary infiltrates, acute respiratory distress syndrome, myocardial infarction, ventricular fibrillation, and cardiogenic shock. ▪ Use caution in patients who either have or develop HAMA/HACA titers. Clinical relevance of HACA formation in rituximab-treated patients is unclear. ▪ Tumor lysis syndrome (TLS) has been reported within 12 to 24 hours after the first rituximab infusion in patients with NHL. S/S are rapid reduction in tumor volume, renal insufficiency, hyperkalemia, hypocalcemia, hyperuricemia, or hyperphosphatemia. May cause acute renal failure requiring dialysis and has been fatal. ▪ TLS occurs more often in patients with high numbers of circulating malignant cells or high tumor burden. Consider prophylactic measures; see Monitor. ▪ Renal toxicity occurs more frequently in patients with high numbers of circulating malignant cells, high tumor burden, and/or TLS. Severe, including fatal, renal toxicity has occurred in patients with NHL. ▪ Safety of immunization with vaccines, particularly live virus vaccines, following rituximab therapy has not been studied. Review vaccination status. Administration of live virus vaccines is not recommended. Weigh benefit versus risk in NHL patients if a delay in treatment may occur for vaccination. ▪ Administer any CDC-recommended, non–live virus vaccinations to RA patients at least 4 weeks before initiating treatment with rituximab. ▪ In CLL patients, *Pneumocystis jiroveci* pneumonia (PCP) and antiherpetic viral prophylaxis is recommended during treatment and for up to 12 months following treatment. ▪ In GPA (WG) and MPA patients, *Pneumocystis jiroveci* pneumonia (PCP) prophylaxis is recommended during treatment and for at least 6 months following the last rituximab infusion. ▪ Mucocutaneous reactions (including lichenoid dermatitis, paraneoplastic pemphigus, Stevens-Johnson syndrome, toxic epidermal necrolysis, and vesiculobullous dermatitis), some with fatal outcomes, have been reported. Onset of reaction has been variable and includes reports of onset on the first day of rituximab exposure. ▪ Hepatitis B virus reactivation with fulminant hepatitis, hepatic failure, and death has been reported. For patients who show evidence of hepatitis B infection, consult physician with expertise in managing hepatitis regarding monitoring and consideration for HBV antiviral therapy; see Monitor. ▪ Not recommended for use in patients with severe active infections. ▪ Serious (including fatal) bacterial, fungal, and new or reactivated viral infections can occur during and following rituximab therapy. Infections have been reported in some patients with prolonged hypogammaglobulinemia (defined as hypogammaglobulinemia more than 11 months after rituximab exposure). New or reactivated viral infections have included JC virus (progressive multifocal leukoencephalopathy [PML], cytomegalovirus, herpes simplex virus, parvovirus B19, varicella zoster virus, West Nile virus, and hepatitis B and C). Deaths have occurred. ▪ JC virus infection resulting in PML and death can occur in rituximab-treated patients who have hematologic malignancies or autoimmune diseases. PML is a rare, progressive, demyelinating disease of the CNS. Usually leads to death or severe disability, and there is no effective treatment. Has been reported in patients receiving rituximab for both approved and unlabeled indications. Most of these patients received rituximab in combination with chemotherapy, prior to or concurrent with immunosuppressive therapy, or as part of a hematopoietic stem cell transplant. However, PML has also been reported in patients with autoimmune diseases (e.g., rheumatoid arthritis) who have been treated previously or concurrently with immunosuppressive therapy. ▪ RA patients may have an increased risk of cardiovascular events. ▪ Not indicated for use in patients with RA who have responded to treatment with TNF antagonists (e.g., adalimumab [Humira], etanercept [Enbrel]). ▪ Abdominal pain, bowel obstruction, and perforation have been reported in patients receiving rituximab in combination with chemotherapy. Death has occurred. Mean time to GI perforation was 6 days (range 1 to 77 days) in patients with NHL. ▪ Use of concomitant immunosuppressants other than corticosteroids has not been studied in GPA (WG) or MPA patients exhibiting peripheral B-cell depletion following treatment with rituximab. ▪ See Rate of Administration, Drug/Lab Interactions, and Antidote.

Monitor: In patients with lymphoid malignancies who are receiving rituximab monotherapy, obtain a baseline CBC and platelet count and repeat before each course of therapy. In patients treated with rituximab and chemotherapy, obtain baseline CBC and platelet count at weekly to monthly intervals. Repeat more frequently in patients who develop cytopenias (e.g., leukopenia, neutropenia, thrombocytopenia). In RA, GPA (WG), or MPA patients, obtain a baseline CBC and platelet count and repeat at 2- to 4-month intervals during therapy. Duration of cytopenias may extend months beyond the treatment period. ▪ Observe patient continuously for symptoms of hypersensitivity and/or infusion reactions, which are more common during the first infusion but can occur at any time; see Antidote. ▪ Monitor HR and BP frequently. ▪ ECG and pulmonary monitoring required during and in the immediate posttreatment period in patients with pre-existing cardiac or pulmonary conditions, in any patient who develops or has previously developed a clinically significant cardiopulmonary adverse event during treatment, and in patients with RA. ▪ Monitor patients with high numbers of circulating malignant cells (greater than or equal to 25,000/mm³) with or without other evidence of high tumor burden for infusion reaction and tumor lysis syndrome. Monitoring of serum electrolytes and renal function indicated. ▪ Prevention and treatment of hyperuricemia due to TLS may be accomplished with adequate hydration and, if necessary, allopurinol (Aloprim) and alkalinization of urine; see Drug/Lab Interactions. ▪ Prevention and/or treatment of hyperphosphatemia, hyperkalemia, and hypocalcemia due to TLS is also indicated. ▪ Monitor closely for signs of renal failure, and discontinue rituximab in patients with a rising SCr or oliguria. ▪ Assess neurologic status frequently. Consider PML in patients with new-onset neurologic manifestations; consultation with a neurologist, brain MRI, and lumbar puncture may be required for diagnosis. ▪ Screen all patients for HBV infection before treatment initiation. Monitor patients with evidence of current or prior HBV for clinical and laboratory signs of hepatitis or HBV reactivation during and for several months after treatment with rituximab. ▪ Observe closely for signs of infection. Prophylactic antibiotics may be indicated pending results of C/S in a febrile neutropenic patient. ▪ Monitor for signs of mucocutaneous reactions. ▪ Use prophylactic antiemetics to reduce nausea and vomiting and increase patient comfort. ▪ Monitor for thrombocytopenia (platelet count less than 50,000/mm³). Initiate precautions to prevent excessive bleeding (e.g., inspect IV sites, skin, and mucous membranes; use extreme care during invasive procedures; test urine, emesis, stool, and secretions for occult blood). ▪ Monitor patients with diffuse large B-cell, CD20-positive NHL treated with R-CHOP closely for abdominal pain and repeated vomiting, especially early in the course of treatment. A thorough diagnostic evaluation is indicated; treat appropriately to prevent bowel obstruction and perforation. ▪ See Premedication in Usual Dose, Rate of Administration, Precautions, Drug/Lab Interactions, and Antidote.

Patient Education: Avoid pregnancy; nonhormonal birth control recommended; report a suspected pregnancy immediately. See Maternal/Child. ▪ Read manufacturer's patient information sheet before each infusion. ▪ Discuss health history (e.g., presence of an infection, carrier of or had a previous hepatitis B virus infection, heart or lung problems, recent or scheduled vaccinations, scheduled surgeries) and prescription and nonprescription medications with the health care provider administering the rituximab. ▪ Review monitoring requirements and potential side effects before therapy. ▪ Promptly report S/S of infection (e.g., fever), blisters, cough, difficulty breathing, dizziness, drowsiness, headache, hives, peeling skin, painful sores, ulcers, swelling, or wheezing; immediate medical treatment may be indicated. ▪ New neurologic S/S (e.g., changes in vision, loss of balance or coordination, disorientation, or confusion) could be warning signs of PML. Report them promptly. ▪ See Appendix D, p. 1333.

Maternal/Child: Category C: avoid pregnancy; women of childbearing age should use birth control during treatment and for up to 12 months after completion of treatment. B-cell lymphocytopenia generally lasting less than 6 months has occurred in infants exposed to rituximab in utero. Use only if clearly needed. ▪ Use caution if breast-feeding; weigh risk versus benefit. ▪ Safety and effectiveness for use in pediatric patients not established. Hypogammaglobulinemia has been observed in pediatric patients treated with rituximab.

Elderly: No overall differences in effectiveness were observed between different age-groups of patients treated for diffuse large B-cell NHL. Cardiac and pulmonary adverse reactions (e.g., supraventricular arrhythmia, pneumonia, pneumonitis) occurred more frequently in the elderly. ▪ The numbers of elderly treated for low-grade or follicular NHL were insufficient to determine differences. ▪ The incidence of Grade 3 and 4 adverse reactions was higher in patients over 70 years of age treated for CLL with R-FC. No observed benefit was seen with the addition of rituximab to FC in patients over 70 years of age. ▪ In older patients being treated for RA, GPA, or MPA, the incidence of side effects was similar to younger adults; however, the rate of serious side effects, including serious infection, malignancies, and cardiovascular events, was higher.

DRUG/LAB INTERACTIONS
Formal drug interaction studies have not been performed. ▪ May inhibit the generation of an anamnestic (immunologic memory) or humoral (development of antibodies in the blood) response to any **vaccine.** ▪ Pharmacokinetics of rituximab remained similar to rituximab alone when given in combination with CHOP chemotherapy (cyclophosphamide, doxorubicin, vincristine, prednisone). ▪ Risk of renal toxicity increased in patients receiving concomitant therapy with **cisplatin** (the combination of cisplatin and rituximab is not an approved treatment regimen). ▪ Concurrent use with **CHOP chemotherapy** has resulted in an increase in fatal infections in HIV-related lymphoma patients. ▪ Data on the safety of the use of biologic agents or **disease-modifying antirheumatic drugs** (DMARDs) other than methotrexate in RA patients are limited. Monitor patients closely for signs of infection with concurrent use of biologic agents or DMARDs other than methotrexate.

SIDE EFFECTS
CD20-positive, B-cell NHL: The most common side effects are asthenia, chills, fever, infection, infusion reactions, and lymphopenia.

Diffuse large B-cell, CD20-positive NHL: In addition to the previously listed side effects, anemia, neutropenia, viral infection, and Grade 3 or 4 respiratory symptoms and thrombocytopenia occurred more frequently among patients on the R-CHOP regimen. Patients on this regimen 60 years of age and over reported increased incidences of cardiac events (e.g., supraventricular arrhythmias, tachycardia), chills, fever, and respiratory symptoms.

CLL: The most common side effects during clinical trials were infusion reactions and neutropenia.

Major side effects for the previously listed indications include angina, bowel obstruction and perforation, cardiac arrhythmias (e.g., supraventricular and ventricular tachycardia, ventricular fibrillation), hepatitis B reactivation with fulminant hepatitis and other viral infections (including JC virus infection resulting in PML), hypersensitivity reactions (e.g., hypotension, bronchospasm, and angioedema), infusion reactions, mucocutaneous reactions (e.g., lichenoid dermatitis, paraneoplastic pemphigus, Stevens-Johnson syndrome, toxic epidermal necrolysis, and vesiculobullous dermatitis), renal failure, and tumor lysis syndrome (may occur within 12 to 24 hours). Hypersensitivity or infusion-related side effects generally occur within 30 minutes to 2 hours of beginning of first infusion. Other side effects include abdominal pain, angioedema, anorexia, anxiety, arthralgia, back pain, bone marrow suppression (e.g., anemia, leukopenia, neutropenia, thrombocytopenia, prolonged pancytopenia, and marrow hypoplasia), cough, diarrhea, dizziness, dyspnea, elevated LDH, flushing, headache, hyperglycemia, hypertension, hypotension, infections (with or without neutropenia), myalgia, nausea, night sweats, pain at disease sites, peripheral edema, pruritus, rash, respiratory symptoms (e.g., acute infusion-related bronchospasm, acute pneumonitis 1 to 4 weeks post-rituximab infusion, bronchiolitis obliterans [one case ended in death]), rhinitis, sinusitis, tachycardia, throat irritation, urticaria, and vomiting. Incidence of abdominal pain, anemia, dyspnea, hypotension, and neutropenia is higher in patients with bulky disease lesions equal to or greater than 10 cm.

Rheumatoid arthritis: Similar to those seen in patients with NHL. Major side effects include infusion reactions, cardiac events, immunogenicity, and infections (e.g., bronchitis, nasopharyngitis, sinusitis, URI, UTI). Other more frequently reported side effects include abdominal pain (upper), anxiety, arthralgia, asthenia, chills, dyspepsia, fever, hypercholesterolemia, hypertension, migraine headache, nausea, paresthesia, pruritus, rhinitis, throat irritation, urticaria.

GPA (WG) and MPA: Most common side effects reported include anemia, diarrhea, headache, infections, muscle spasm, and peripheral edema. Other commonly reported side effects include arthralgia, cough, dyspnea, epistaxis, fatigue, hypertension, hypogammaglobulinemia, increased ALT, insomnia, leukopenia, nausea, and rash. All major side effects associated with rituximab (e.g., infusion reactions, infections) may occur.

Post-Marketing: Bowel obstruction and perforation, bronchiolitis obliterans (fatal), cardiac failure (fatal), disease progression of Kaposi's sarcoma, Grade 3 to 4 prolonged or late-onset neutropenia, hyperviscosity syndrome in Waldenström's macroglobulinemia, hypogammaglobulinemia (prolonged), increase in fatal infections in HIV-associated lymphoma and a reported increased incidence of Grade 3 and 4 infections in patients with previously treated lymphoma without known HIV infection, lupus-like syndrome, marrow hyperplasia, mucocutaneous reactions (severe), neutropenia (late onset), optic neuritis, pancytopenia (prolonged), pleuritis, pneumonitis (including interstitial pneumonitis), polyarticular arthritis, serum sickness, systemic vasculitis, uveitis, vasculitis with rash, and viral infections, including PML.

ANTIDOTE

Keep physician informed of all side effects. May constitute a medical emergency or will be treated symptomatically as indicated. Hypersensitivity or infusion-related side effects generally resolve with slowing or interruption of the rituximab infusion and with supportive care (IV saline; diphenhydramine; bronchodilators such as albuterol or aminophylline; and acetaminophen). Most patients who have had non–life-threatening reactions have been able to complete the full course of therapy. Restart the infusion at half the previous rate after symptoms have resolved completely. Discontinue the infusion immediately for any life-threatening side effect (e.g., clinically significant bronchospasm, cardiac arrhythmias, Grade 3 or 4 infusion reactions, hypersensitivity reactions, hypotension, tumor lysis syndrome, or severe mucocutaneous reaction). Discontinue rituximab in any patient who develops a serious infection or experiences HBV reactivation. Initiate appropriate antiviral/anti-infective therapy as indicated. Discontinue treatment in patients who develop severe mucocutaneous reactions. Skin biopsy may be required to diagnose mucocutaneous reaction and guide treatment. Safety of readministration of rituximab to patients with severe mucocutaneous reactions has not been determined. Discontinue treatment in patients who develop PML; consider reduction or discontinuation of concomitant chemotherapy or immunosuppressive therapy. Discontinue treatment in patients with a rising SCr or oliguria. Treat anaphylaxis with oxygen, antihistamines (diphenhydramine), epinephrine, and corticosteroids. Maintain a patent airway. Treat arrhythmias if indicated and monitor ECG until recovery and with subsequent doses. Treat hypotension with IV fluids, Trendelenburg position, and, if necessary, vasopressors (e.g., norepinephrine [Levophed], dopamine). Blood modifiers (e.g., darbepoetin alfa [Aranesp], epoetin alfa [Epogen], filgrastim [Neupogen, Zarxio], pegfilgrastim [Neulasta], sargramostim [Leukine]) may be indicated to treat bone marrow toxicity. Tumor lysis syndrome requires correction of electrolyte abnormalities and monitoring of renal function and fluid balance. Supportive care, including dialysis, may be required. Resuscitate if indicated.

ROMIDEPSIN
(**ROE**-mi-**DEP**-sin)

Istodax

Antineoplastic
(HDAC inhibitor)

USUAL DOSE
14 mg/M^2 as an infusion over 4 hours. Administer on Days 1, 8, and 15 of a 28-day cycle; see Monitor. Cycles may be repeated every 28 days provided the patient continues to benefit from and tolerates the drug. Discontinuation or interruption with or without dose reduction to 10 mg/M^2 may be needed to manage adverse drug reactions; see Dose Adjustments.

DOSE ADJUSTMENTS

Romidepsin Dose Modification for Nonhematologic Toxicities Except Alopecia		
CTCAE* Grade on Day of Treatment	Action	Dose on Recovery
Grade 2 or 3 toxicity	Delay dose until toxicity returns to ≤ Grade 1 or baseline	14 mg/M^2
Grade 3 toxicity recurrence	Delay dose until toxicity returns to ≤ Grade 1 or baseline	Permanently reduce dose to 10 mg/M^2
Grade 4 toxicity	Delay dose until toxicity returns to ≤ Grade 1 or baseline	Permanently reduce dose to 10 mg/M^2
Grade 3 or 4 toxicities recur after dose reduction	Discontinue therapy	

*Per Common Terminology Criteria for Adverse Events (CTCAE), Version 4.0.

Romidepsin Dose Modification for Hematologic Toxicities		
CTCAE* Grade on Day of Treatment	Action	Dose on Recovery
Grade 3 or 4 neutropenia or thrombocytopenia	Delay dose until ANC ≥1,500/mm^3 and/or platelet count ≥75,000/mm^3	14 mg/M^2
Grade 4 febrile (≥38.5° C) neutropenia or thrombocytopenia that requires platelet transfusion	Delay dose until the specific cytopenia returns to ≤ Grade 1 or baseline	Permanently reduce dose to 10 mg/M^2

*Per Common Terminology Criteria for Adverse Events (CTCAE), Version 4.0.

No dose adjustments required based on age; gender; race; mild, moderate, or severe renal impairment; or mild hepatic impairment.

Q-R

DILUTION
Special techniques required; see Precautions: Reconstitute each 10-mg vial with 2 mL of the supplied diluent. Inject diluent slowly into the vial of romidepsin and swirl contents until there are no visible particles. Concentration equals 5 mg/mL. Withdraw the calculated dose and further dilute in 500 mL NS.

Filters: Specific information not available.

Storage: Store vials in carton at CRT. Reconstituted solution is stable for up to 8 hours at RT. Diluted solutions are stable at RT for 24 hours, but use soon after dilution is recommended.

COMPATIBILITY
Manufacturer states, "The diluted solution is **compatible** with polyvinyl chloride (PVC), ethylene vinyl acetate (EVA), polyethylene (PE) infusion bags as well as glass bottles." No additional information available; consider specific use and consult pharmacist.

RATE OF ADMINISTRATION
A single dose as an infusion equally distributed over 4 hours.

ACTIONS
A histone deacetylase (HDAC) inhibitor. HDACs catalyze the removal of acetyl groups from acetylated lysine residues in histones, resulting in the modulation of gene expression. Induces cell cycle arrest and apoptosis of some cancer cell lines. Mechanism of antineoplastic effect not fully characterized. Highly protein bound. It undergoes extensive metabolism in vitro by CYP3A4 with minor contributions from other cytochrome P_{450} isoenzymes. Half-life is approximately 3 hours. No accumulation of plasma concentrations observed after repeated dosing.

INDICATIONS AND USES
Treatment of cutaneous T-cell lymphoma (CTCL) and peripheral T-cell lymphoma (PTCL) in patients who have received at least one prior systemic therapy. These indications are based on response rates. Improvement in overall survival has not been demonstrated.

CONTRAINDICATIONS
Manufacturer states, "None."

PRECAUTIONS
Follow guidelines for handling cytotoxic agents. See Appendix A, p. 1331. ▪ Administered under the direction of a physician knowledgeable in its use in a facility with adequate diagnostic and treatment facilities to monitor the patients and respond to any medical emergency. ▪ Bone marrow suppression can occur (e.g., anemia, lymphopenia, neutropenia, and thrombocytopenia). Dose modification based on ANC, and platelet count is required; see Dose Adjustments. ▪ Serious and sometimes fatal infections, including pneumonia, sepsis, and viral reactivation (including Epstein-Barr and hepatitis B viruses), have been reported during or within 30 days of therapy. Patients with a history of prior treatment with monoclonal antibodies directed against lymphocyte antigens and patients with disease involvement of the bone marrow may be at increased risk for developing a life-threatening infection. ▪ Reactivation of Epstein-Barr viral infection leading to liver failure has occurred. In one case, ganciclovir prophylaxis failed to prevent Epstein-Barr viral reactivation. ▪ Several treatment-emergent ECG changes have been reported (e.g., T-wave and ST-segment changes, QT prolongation). Use caution in patients with congenital long QT syndrome or a history of significant CV disease or in patients taking antiarrhythmic or other medicines that can lead to significant QT prolongation; see Drug/Lab Interactions. ▪ Tumor lysis syndrome has been reported. ▪ Use with caution in patients with moderate or severe hepatic impairment. ▪ Renal impairment is not expected to influence romidepsin exposure. Effect on end-stage renal disease (ESRD) has not been studied; use with caution in patients with ESRD.

Monitor: Due to the risk of QT prolongation, potassium and magnesium should be within the normal range before administration of romidepsin. ▪ Obtain baseline CBC, platelets, and electrolytes. Baseline CrCl or SCr and liver function tests may be indicated. ▪ Monitor CBC, platelets, and electrolytes during treatment and modify dose as indicated; see

Dose Adjustments. ▪ Consider ECG monitoring and more frequent monitoring of electrolytes in at-risk cardiac patients; see Precautions. ▪ Monitor for signs of tumor lysis syndrome. Prevention and treatment of hyperuricemia may be accomplished with adequate hydration and, if necessary, allopurinol and alkalinization of urine. ▪ Monitor for thrombocytopenia (platelet count less than 50,000/mm³). Initiate precautions to prevent excessive bleeding (e.g., inspect IV sites, skin, and mucous membranes; use extreme care during invasive procedures; test urine, emesis, stool, and secretions for occult blood). ▪ Use prophylactic antiemetics to reduce nausea and/or vomiting and increase patient comfort. ▪ Observe closely for signs of infection. Prophylactic antibiotics may be indicated pending results of C/S in a febrile neutropenic patient. ▪ Monitoring for hepatitis B reactivation and administration of antiviral prophylaxis should be considered in patients with evidence of prior hepatitis B infection.

Patient Education: Read patient insert carefully. ▪ Avoid pregnancy; nonhormonal birth control recommended; see Drug/Lab Interactions. ▪ Blood counts will be required at regular intervals. ▪ Report any history of hepatitis B before starting therapy. ▪ Maintain high fluid intake for at least 72 hours after each dose to decrease the risks associated with tumor lysis syndrome. ▪ Promptly report unusual bleeding, abnormal heartbeat, chest pain, or shortness of breath. ▪ Report burning on urination, cough, fever, flu-like symptoms, muscle aches, or worsening of skin problems. ▪ Nausea and vomiting are common. Prophylactic antiemetics are recommended. ▪ Discuss medications (prescription, nonprescription, and herbal) with a health care professional; see Drug/Lab Interactions. ▪ See Appendix D, p. 1333.

Maternal/Child: Category D: avoid pregnancy; may cause fetal harm. If the drug is used during pregnancy or the patient becomes pregnant during therapy, inform the patient of the potential hazard to the fetus. ▪ Discontinue breast-feeding. ▪ Safety and effectiveness for use in pediatric patients not established.

Elderly: No differences in safety and effectiveness compared with younger patients were noted; however, greater sensitivity of some older patients cannot be ruled out.

DRUG/LAB INTERACTIONS
Concurrent use with **warfarin** (Coumadin) may prolong PT and elevate INR. Monitoring of PT and INR recommended. ▪ **Strong CYP3A4 inhibitors** (e.g., atazanavir [Reyataz], clarithromycin [Biaxin], indinavir [Crixivan], itraconazole [Sporanox], ketoconazole [Nizoral], nefazodone, nelfinavir [Viracept], ritonavir [Norvir], saquinavir [Invirase], telithromycin [Ketek], and voriconazole [VFEND]) may increase concentrations of romidepsin; monitor for toxicity and follow dose modifications for toxicity; see Dose Adjustments. Use caution with concomitant use of **moderate CYP3A4** inhibitors (aprepitant [Emend], verapamil). ▪ Avoid coadministration with **rifampin (a strong CYP3A4 inducer).** In a pharmacokinetic drug interaction trial, romidepsin exposure was *increased* when coadministered with rifampin. Typically, coadministration of CYP3A4 inducers decreases concentrations of drugs metabolized by CYP3A4. The increase in exposure seen after coadministration with rifampin is likely due to rifampin's inhibition of an undetermined hepatic uptake process that is predominantly responsible for the disposition of romidepsin. It is unknown if other **potent CYP3A4 inducers** (e.g., carbamazepine [Tegretol], dexamethasone [Decadron], phenobarbital [Luminal], phenytoin [Dilantin], rifabutin [Mycobutin], rifapentine [Priftin], and St. John's wort) would alter the exposure of romidepsin. Avoid coadministration with other potent CYP3A4 inducers if possible. ▪ Use caution with **drugs that inhibit the efflux transporter P-glycoprotein (P-gp, ABCB1)** (e.g., protease inhibitors [e.g., nelfinavir (Viracept)]); may increase concentrations of romidepsin. ▪ Do not administer **live virus vaccines** to patients receiving antineoplastic drugs. ▪ Concurrent use with other **drugs that prolong the QT interval** (e.g., antiarrhythmics [e.g., amiodarone (Nexterone), disopyramide (Norpace), ibutilide (Corvert), mexiletine, procainamide (Pronestyl), quinidine], antihistamines, azole antifungals [e.g., itraconazole (Sporanox)], fluoroquinolones [e.g., levofloxacin (Levaquin)], phenothiazines [e.g., thioridazine (Mellaril)], and tricyclic antidepressants [e.g., amitriptyline (Elavil), imipramine (Tofranil)]) may cause torsades de pointes and could be fatal.

SIDE EFFECTS

Most common side effects are anorexia, bone marrow suppression (e.g., anemia, lymphopenia, neutropenia, thrombocytopenia), ECG T-wave changes, fatigue, infections, nausea, and vomiting. Anemia, dyspnea, elevated AST, fatigue, hypomagnesemia, infection, QT prolongation, and thrombocytopenia were the most common reasons for discontinuing therapy. Adverse reactions categorized as severe included abdominal pain, acute renal failure, cardiopulmonary failure, cellulitis, central line infection, chest pain, deep venous thrombosis, dehydration, dyspnea, edema, elevated ALT and AST, fatigue, febrile neutropenia, fever, hyperbilirubinemia, hypersensitivity, hyperuricemia, hypoalbuminemia, hypocalcemia, hypophosphatemia, hypotension, hypoxia, infection, leukopenia, lymphopenia, nausea, neutropenia, pneumonitis, pulmonary embolism, reactivation of hepatitis B infection, sepsis, supraventricular arrhythmia, syncope, thrombocytopenia, ventricular arrhythmia, and vomiting. Other side effects reported include asthenia, constipation, dermatitis, diarrhea, dysgeusia, exfoliative dermatitis, hyperglycemia, hypermagnesemia, hypokalemia, hyponatremia, and pruritus.

ANTIDOTE

Treatment of most side effects will be supportive and may require dose adjustment or discontinuation. Discontinue if Grade 3 or 4 toxicities recur after dose reduction. Keep physician informed. Administration of blood products and/or blood modifiers (e.g., darbepoetin [Aranesp], epoetin alfa [Epogen], filgrastim [Neupogen, Zarxio], pegfilgrastim [Neulasta], sargramostim [Leukine]) may be indicated to treat bone marrow toxicity. Treat hypersensitivity reactions with epinephrine, antihistamines, and corticosteroids as needed. No known antidote. Discontinue romidepsin and provide supportive therapy in overdose. Not known if romidepsin is dialyzable. Resuscitate if indicated.

SARGRAMOSTIM
(sar-**GRAM**-oh-stim)

Colony-stimulating factor
Antineutropenic

GM-CSF, Human Granulocyte-Macrophage Colony-Stimulating Factor, Leukine

pH 7.1 to 7.7

USUAL DOSE

Myeloid reconstitution after allogeneic or autologous bone marrow transplantation: 250 mcg/M^2/day as a 2-hour infusion daily for 21 days. Initial infusion must begin 2 to 4 hours after bone marrow infusion and not less than 24 hours after the last dose of chemotherapy and 12 hours after the last dose of radiation. Post–marrow infusion absolute neutrophil count (ANC) should be less than 500 cells/mm^3.

Engraftment delay or failure of bone marrow transplantation: 250 mcg/M^2/day as a 2-hour infusion daily for 14 days. Wait for 7 days; if engraftment has not occurred, repeat 14-day course of 250 mcg/M^2/day. Wait an additional 7 days; if engraftment has still not occurred, give a 14-day course of 500 mcg/M^2/day. If engraftment does not occur, further courses or dose increases are not indicated. Note time restrictions on chemotherapy and radiation above and in Drug/Lab Interactions.

Neutrophil recovery following chemotherapy in acute myelogenous leukemia (AML) in adults 55 years of age or older: 250 mcg/M^2/day as an infusion over 4 hours. Begin on Day 11 or 4 days after induction chemotherapy is complete. Day 10 bone marrow should be hypoplastic with fewer than 5% blasts. Repeat sargramostim daily until absolute neutrophil count (ANC) is greater than 1,500/mm^3 for three consecutive days or a maximum of 42 days. Use same criteria if a second cycle of induction chemotherapy is indicated.

Mobilization of peripheral blood progenitor cells: 250 mcg/M^2/day as a 24-hour continuous infusion (or give SC once daily). Continue at the same dose until adequate numbers of progenitor stem cells are collected. Collection of progenitor cells (apheresis) usually begins about Day 5 and is repeated daily. All cells are stored until predetermined targets are achieved. After immunosuppression with selected antineoplastic bone marrow suppressant agents to neutralize remaining tumor cells or ineffective leukocytes, the collected progenitor stem cells are reinfused into the patient by IV infusion. This process has been used primarily in patients who were not candidates for bone marrow transplant; however, it is increasingly being used instead of bone marrow transplant.

Post–peripheral blood progenitor cell transplantation: 250 mcg/M^2/day as a 24-hour continuous infusion (or give SC once daily). Begin immediately following infusion of harvested progenitor cells and continue until an ANC is greater than 1,500/mm^3 for three consecutive days. Neutrophil recovery occurs somewhat sooner in patients receiving sargramostim stimulation. Results in a shorter time to platelet and RBC transfusion independence.

DOSE ADJUSTMENTS
May require reduced dose in impaired renal or hepatic function. Based on individual patient response. ▪ For an ANC above 20,000 cells/mm^3, WBC above 50,000 cells/mm^3, or a platelet count above 500,000/mm^3, reduce dose by one half or temporarily discontinue. ▪ See Antidote.

DILUTION
Now available in liquid form (reconstituted) or each 250- or 500-mcg vial of the dry product must be reconstituted with 1 mL SWFI with or without preservative. Confirm expiration date to ensure valid product. Direct diluent to the side of the vial and swirl gently. Avoid foaming or vigorous agitation. Do not shake. Either product must be further diluted in NS for infusion. If the final concentration of sargramostim will be below 10 mcg/mL, albumin (human) must be added to the NS before addition of the sargramostim (1 mL of 5% albumin to each 50 mL NS). This will prevent adsorption of the drug into the components of the IV delivery system. Liquefied product contains benzyl alcohol. Use sterile technique; enter vial only to dilute and/or to withdraw a single dose. Discard any unused portion. Should be clear and colorless.

Filters: Manufacturer states, *"An in-line membrane filter should not be used for IV infusion of sargramostim."*

Storage: Must be refrigerated in all forms; do not freeze or shake. Reconstituted with SWFI without preservatives or any diluted solution should be used within 6 hours. Reconstituted with bacteriostatic SWFI (benzyl alcohol preservative) or the new liquid preparation can be refrigerated for up to 20 days.

COMPATIBILITY   (Underline Indicates Conflicting Compatibility Information)
Consider any drug NOT listed as compatible to be INCOMPATIBLE until consulting a pharmacist; specific conditions may apply.

Manufacturer recommends that no medication other than albumin be added to the infusion solution and that only NS be used to prepare IV solutions until specific **compatibility** data are available.

One source suggests the following **compatibilities:**

Y-site: Amikacin, aminophylline, amphotericin B (conventional), aztreonam (Azactam), bleomycin (Blenoxane), butorphanol (Stadol), calcium gluconate, carboplatin (Paraplatin), carmustine (BiCNU), cefazolin (Ancef), cefotaxime (Claforan), cefotetan, ceftazidime (Fortaz), ceftriaxone (Rocephin), cefuroxime (Zinacef), cisplatin, clindamycin (Cleocin), cyclophosphamide (Cytoxan), cyclosporine (Sandimmune), cytarabine (ARA-C), dacarbazine (DTIC), dactinomycin (Cosmegen), dexamethasone (Decadron), diphenhydramine (Benadryl), dopamine, doxorubicin (Adriamycin), doxycycline, droperidol (Inapsine), etoposide (VePesid), famotidine (Pepcid IV), fentanyl, fluconazole (Diflucan), fluorouracil (5-FU), furosemide (Lasix), gentamicin, granisetron (Kytril), heparin, idarubicin (Idamycin), ifosfamide (Ifex), immune globulin IV (e.g., Gamunex-C), magnesium sulfate, mannitol, mechlorethamine (nitrogen mustard), meperidine (Demerol), mesna (Mesnex), methotrexate, metoclopramide (Reglan), metronidazole (Flagyl IV), mitoxantrone (Novantrone), pentostatin (Nipent), piperacillin/tazobactam

(Zosyn), potassium chloride (KCl), prochlorperazine (Compazine), promethazine (Phenergan), ranitidine (Zantac), sulfamethoxazole/trimethoprim, teniposide (Vumon), ticarcillin/clavulanate (Timentin), <u>vancomycin</u>, vinblastine, vincristine, zidovudine (AZT, Retrovir).

RATE OF ADMINISTRATION

See Usual Dose. Each single dose must be evenly distributed over 2, 4, or 24 hours. Do not use an in-line membrane filter. Reduce rate or temporarily discontinue for onset of any side effects that cause concern (e.g., hypersensitivity reactions).

ACTIONS

Colony-stimulating factors are glycoproteins that bind to specific hematopoietic cell surface receptors and stimulate proliferation, differentiation commitment, and some end-cell functional activation. Utilizing recombinant DNA technology, sargramostim is produced in a yeast *(Saccharomyces cerevisiae)*. It differs slightly from endogenous G-CSF. It induces partially committed progenitor cells to divide and differentiate in the granulocyte-macrophage pathways. Can also activate mature granulocytes and macrophages. It is a multilineage factor and has dose-dependent effects. It increases the cytotoxicity of monocytes toward certain neoplastic cell lines and activates polymorphonuclear neutrophils to inhibit the growth of tumor cells. It significantly improves the time to neutrophil recovery (engraftment), decreases length of hospitalization, shortens the duration of infectious episodes, and decreases antibiotic usage. Patients with fewer impaired organs have the best opportunity for improvement in survival. Detected in the serum in 5 minutes; peak levels are reached 2 hours after injection and last at least 6 hours.

INDICATIONS AND USES

Acceleration of hematopoietic recovery (myeloid engraftment) in patients undergoing allogeneic or autologous bone marrow transplantation. ▪ Bone marrow transplantation failure or engraftment delay. ▪ Neutrophil recovery following chemotherapy in acute myelogenous leukemia (AML); safety for use in adults under 55 years not established. ▪ Mobilization of peripheral blood progenitor cells. ▪ Stimulate neutrophil recovery post–peripheral blood progenitor cell transplantation.

Unlabeled uses: Increase WBC in myelodysplastic syndromes and in AIDS patients receiving zidovudine. ▪ Correct neutropenia in aplastic anemia. ▪ Decrease transplantation-associated organ system damage, especially in kidney and liver transplants.

CONTRAINDICATIONS

Hypersensitivity to any components of sargramostim or yeast products; patients with leukemic myeloid blasts in the bone marrow or peripheral blood equal to 10% or more.

PRECAUTIONS

Should be administered under the direction of a physician knowledgeable about appropriate use. ▪ Use caution if considered for use in any malignancy with myeloid characteristics. Can act as a growth factor for any tumor type, particularly myeloid malignancies. ▪ Can be effective in patients receiving purged bone marrow if the purging process preserves a sufficient number of progenitors. ▪ Effects may be limited in patients previously exposed to intensive chemotherapy or radiation therapy. ▪ Neutralizing antibodies may form after receiving sargramostim and may inhibit therapeutic effect.

Monitor: Obtain a CBC with differential before administration and twice weekly thereafter to monitor for excessive leukocytosis (WBC above 50,000 cells/mm³; or an absolute neutrophil count [ANC] above 20,000 cells/mm³). ▪ If blast cells appear or disease progression occurs, treatment should be discontinued. ▪ Anemia, leukocytopenia, and thrombocytopenia occur as side effects of various procedures; monitor carefully. ▪ Observe for fluid retention; may cause peripheral edema, pleural effusion, and/or pericardial effusion. May occur more frequently in individuals with pre-existing lung disease or cardiac disease, including a history of arrhythmias. Use with caution. ▪ Use with caution in patients with pre-existing renal or hepatic dysfunction; an increased SCr or increased bilirubin and hepatic enzymes may occur. Reversible if drug discontinued.

Monitor renal and hepatic function biweekly. ▪ Flushing, hypotension, and syncope may occur, especially with the initial dose. Reduce rate or stop temporarily.

Patient Education: Promptly report any symptoms of infection (e.g., fever) or hypersensitivity reactions (e.g., itching, swelling, redness at the injection site).

Maternal/Child: Category C: safety for use in pregnancy and breast-feeding not established; use only if clearly needed. ▪ Has been used in more than 100 pediatric patients from 4 months to 18 years of age with similar experience to the adult population, even though literature says safety not established. ▪ Liquefied product contains benzyl alcohol; do not use in neonates.

DRUG/LAB INTERACTIONS

Do not administer within 24 hours preceding or following **chemotherapy** or within 12 hours preceding or following **radiotherapy.** Rapidly dividing cells and the success of the treatment would be adversely affected by chemotherapy and radiation. ▪ Myeloproliferative effects may be potentiated by **lithium or corticosteroids;** use with caution.

SIDE EFFECTS

Asthenia, diarrhea, malaise, peripheral edema, rash, and urinary tract disorders are most common. Hypersensitivity reactions, including anaphylaxis, are possible; arthralgia, capillary leak syndrome, dyspnea, fever, headache, hypoxia, local injection site reactions, myalgia, pericardial effusion, peripheral edema, pleural effusion, and supraventricular arrhythmias have been reported.

ANTIDOTE

Discontinue sargramostim for anaphylaxis, if blast cells appear, or there is progression of underlying disease. A maximum dose limit has not been determined; for accidental overdose, discontinue and monitor for WBC increase and respiratory symptoms. For an ANC above 20,000 cells/mm^3, WBC above 50,000 cells/mm^3, or a platelet count above 500,000/mm^3, reduce dose by one half or temporarily discontinue. Blood cell count should return to baseline level in 3 to 7 days. For any side effect that causes concern, reduce dose or temporarily discontinue. Keep physician informed. Treat anaphylaxis and resuscitate as necessary.

SILDENAFIL BBW*

(sil-DEN-a-fil)

Revatio

Vasodilating agent
Antihypertensive (pulmonary)

*This drug is on the Black Box Warning list; however, a BBW is not provided in the parenteral prescribing information.

USUAL DOSE

2.5 mg (3.125 mL) or 10 mg (12.5 mL) as an IV bolus 3 times daily. Administer doses 4 to 6 hours apart. A 10-mg IV dose of sildenafil is equivalent to a 20-mg oral dose. Resume oral therapy as soon as tolerated. In a study evaluating lower doses, there were no significant differences in the effects on hemodynamic variables compared with higher doses. Treatment with doses higher than 10 mg IV (20 mg PO) three times a day is not recommended.

DOSE ADJUSTMENTS

No dose adjustments required for age, gender, race, weight, renal impairment (mild, moderate, or severe), or hepatic impairment (mild or moderate). Has not been studied in patients with severe hepatic impairment.

DILUTION

May be given undiluted. Aseptically withdraw the dose directly into a syringe for immediate use.

Filters: Specific information not available.

Storage: Store vials at CRT.

COMPATIBILITY

Specific information not available. Manufacturer made no recommendations.

RATE OF ADMINISTRATION

A single dose as an IV bolus.

ACTIONS

An inhibitor of cGMP-specific phosphodiesterase type 5 (PDE-5) in the smooth muscle of the pulmonary vasculature where PDE5 is responsible for degradation of cGMP. Sildenafil increases cGMP within pulmonary vascular smooth muscle cells, resulting in relaxation. In patients with pulmonary hypertension, this can lead to vasodilation of the pulmonary vascular bed and, to a lesser degree, vasodilation in the systemic circulation. PDE5 is also found in other tissues, including vascular and visceral smooth muscle, and in platelets. Sildenafil and its major metabolite are approximately 96% protein bound. Metabolized in the liver predominantly by CYP3A4 and other hepatic microsomal isoenzymes. Terminal half-life is about 4 hours. Findings suggest a lower clearance and/or a higher bioavailability of sildenafil in patients with pulmonary hypertension compared with healthy volunteers. Primarily excreted in feces and approximately 13% in urine.

INDICATIONS AND USES

Treatment of pulmonary arterial hypertension (PAH) (WHO Group 1) in patients who are currently prescribed oral sildenafil and are temporarily unable to take oral medications. Intended to improve exercise ability and delay clinical worsening. Delay in clinical worsening demonstrated with concurrent use of epoprostenol (Flolan). Studies establishing effectiveness included predominantly patients with NYHA Functional Class II-III symptoms and idiopathic etiology or associated with connective tissue disease.

Limitation of use: Adding sildenafil to bosentan (Tracleer) therapy in the treatment of PAH does not result in any beneficial effect on exercise capacity.

CONTRAINDICATIONS

Known hypersensitivity to sildenafil or any component of the product. ▪ Concomitant use of organic nitrates in any form, either regularly or intermittently, because of the greater risk of hypotension. ▪ Concomitant use of riociguat (Adempas), a guanylate cyclase stimulator. PDE5 inhibitors, including sildenafil, may potentiate the hypotensive effects of riociguat.

PRECAUTIONS

Has vasodilatory properties, resulting in mild and transient decreases in BP. Use with caution in patients with resting hypotension (BP less than 90/50 mm Hg), fluid depletion, severe left ventricular outflow obstruction, autonomic dysfunction, and in patients undergoing antihypertensive therapy. ▪ Increase in mortality with increasing dose noted in pediatric patients; see Maternal/Child. ▪ Not recommended for use in patients with pulmonary veno-occlusive disease (PVOD); it may significantly worsen their cardiac status. Consider the possibility of associated PVOD if signs of pulmonary edema occur. ▪ Epistaxis has been reported in patients with PAH secondary to connective tissue disease (CTD) and in patients treated with a concomitant oral vitamin K antagonist (warfarin [Coumadin]). ▪ Safety for use in patients with bleeding disorders or active peptic ulceration is unknown. ▪ Sudden loss of vision in one or both eyes has been reported. Nonarteritic anterior ischemic optic neuropathy (NAION), a cause of decreased vision (including permanent loss of vision), has been reported in temporal association with PDE-5 inhibitors (sildenafil [Revatio, Viagra], vardenafil [Levitra], tadalafil [Cialis]). Use with caution in patients with retinitis pigmentosa. ▪ Sudden decrease or loss of hearing has been reported; may be accompanied by dizziness and tinnitus. ▪ Use with caution in patients with an anatomic deformation of the penis (e.g., angulation, cavernosal fibrosis, or Peyronie's disease) or in patients with conditions that may predispose them to priapism (e.g., sickle cell anemia, multiple myeloma, or leukemia). Penile tissue damage and permanent loss of potency can result from priapism lasting more than 6 hours. ▪ Effectiveness and safety of sildenafil in pulmonary hypertension secondary to sickle cell anemia has not been established. Increased incidence of vaso-occlusive crisis requiring hospitalization has been reported in this patient population. ▪ See Drug/Lab Interactions.

Monitor: Obtain baseline studies as indicated by specific patient history. ▪ Monitor VS closely to note unsafe drops in BP. Monitoring of BP is especially important when sildenafil is coadministered with other BP-lowering drugs. ▪ Monitor for cardiovascular and cerebrovascular events, especially in patients with risk factors. ▪ Monitor for vision and/or hearing loss. ▪ See Precautions, Patient Education, and Drug/Lab Interactions.

Patient Education: Read manufacturer's patient education booklet carefully. ▪ Never take sildenafil with nitrate medicines or guanylate cyclase stimulators (e.g., riociguat [Adempas]); may cause a sudden and unsafe drop in BP. ▪ Do not take Viagra or other similar medications for erectile dysfunction with sildenafil. ▪ Seek immediate medical attention with a sudden loss of vision in one or both eyes. ▪ Seek prompt medical attention in the event of a sudden decrease or loss of hearing. ▪ Seek emergency help if an erection lasts for more than 4 hours. ▪ Discuss medications (prescription, nonprescription, and herbal) with a health care professional; see Drug/Lab Interactions.

Maternal/Child: Category B: use during pregnancy only if clearly needed. ▪ Use during labor and delivery has not been studied. ▪ Not known if sildenafil is secreted in human milk; use caution if required during breast-feeding. ▪ Use in pediatric patients, particularly chronic use, is not recommended. In a long-term study, mortality increased; deaths were first observed after about 1 year.

Elderly: Major differences in response compared with younger adults have not been identified; however, healthy elderly volunteers had a reduced clearance resulting in higher plasma concentrations. Dosing should be cautious. Consider age-related organ impairment and concomitant disease or drug therapy.

DRUG/LAB INTERACTIONS

Sildenafil is also marketed as Viagra. Do not take **Viagra or other PDE5 inhibitors** (e.g., tadalafil [Cialis], vardenafil [Levitra]) concurrently with sildenafil (Revatio). ▪ Potentiates the hypotensive effects of nitrates. Concurrent use with **nitrates** in any form is *contraindicated.* Nitrates are medicines that treat chest pain (angina) (e.g., nitroglycerin in any form, isosorbide mononitrate [Monoket, Imdur], isosorbide dinitrate [Isordil, Dilatrate-SR], street drugs called "poppers" [amyl nitrate or nitrite]). May result in an unsafe drop in BP. ▪ Potentiates the hypotensive effects of **riociguat** (Adempas), a guanylate cyclase stimulator used to treat pulmonary hypertension. ▪ Concurrent use with **alpha-adrenergic blocking agents** (e.g., alfuzosin [Uroxatral], doxazosin [Cardura], phentolamine, prazosin [Minipress], tamsulosin [Flomax], terazosin [Hytrin]) can lower BP significantly and lead to symptomatic hypotension. BP may be lowered further with this combined use of vasodilators by other variables, including intravascular volume depletion and concomitant use of other **antihypertensive drugs** (e.g., calcium channel blockers [amlodipine (Norvasc), diltiazem (Cardizem)]). ▪ Concomitant use of sildenafil with **ritonavir** (Norvir) **and other potent CYP3A4 inhibitors** (e.g., atazanavir [Reyataz], clarithromycin [Biaxin], indinavir [Crixivan], itraconazole [Sporanox], ketoconazole [Nizoral], nefazodone, nelfinavir [Viracept], saquinavir [Invirase], telithromycin [Ketek], and voriconazole [VFEND]) *is not recommended.* ▪ **Cimetidine** (Tagamet) and **erythromycin** may cause an increase in sildenafil plasma concentrations. ▪ **Potent CYP3A4 inducers** (e.g., carbamazepine [Tegretol], dexamethasone [Decadron], phenytoin [Dilantin], phenobarbital [Luminal], rifabutin [Mycobutin], rifapentine [Priftin], rifampin [Rifadin], and St. John's wort) may increase sildenafil clearance and reduce its effectiveness. ▪ **Bosentan** (Tracleer) may also increase sildenafil clearance; see Limitations of Use. ▪ Concurrent use with epoprostenol (Flolan) did not have a significant effect on sildenafil pharmacokinetics; effect on epoprostenol not known. ▪ Does not potentiate the increase in bleeding time caused by aspirin. ▪ Did not potentiate hypotensive effects with alcohol in healthy volunteers. ▪ Has been given with atorvastatin [Lipitor], oral contraceptives, and tolbutamide without effect.

SIDE EFFECTS

Manufacturer does not distinguish between side effects caused by oral dosing versus injectable dosing. Most common side effects are dyspepsia, dyspnea, epistaxis, erythema, flushing, headache, insomnia, and rhinitis. Serious side effects include hearing loss, hypotension, indigestion, priapism, vaso-occlusive crisis, and vision loss. Other side effects reported include diarrhea, fever, gastritis, myalgia, paresthesia, and sinusitis. Sildenafil combined with epoprostenol (Flolan) added edema (including peripheral edema), nasal congestion, nausea, and pain in extremities. Retinal hemorrhage occurred in patients with risk factors for hemorrhage, including concurrent anticoagulant therapy. Most hypersensitivity reactions have been nonserious. Serious hypersensitivity reactions (e.g., anaphylaxis, shock) have been rare.

Post-Marketing: Serious cardiovascular, cerebrovascular, and vascular events, including MI, cerebrovascular hemorrhage, hypertension, pulmonary hemorrhage, subarachnoid and intracerebral hemorrhages, TIA, ventricular arrhythmia, and sudden cardiac death; NAION (with decreased vision, including permanent vision loss); sudden decrease or loss of hearing; seizure; and seizure recurrence.

ANTIDOTE

Treatment of most side effects will be supportive. Notify physician immediately if a serious side effect occurs (e.g., hearing loss, hypersensitivity, hypotension, priapism, vision loss). Treat hypersensitivity reactions with epinephrine, antihistamines, and corticosteroids as needed. Hemodialysis is not expected to be effective in overdose.

SILTUXIMAB

Monoclonal antibody
Interleukin-6 (IL-6)
antagonist

Sylvant

pH 5.2

USUAL DOSE

Pre-testing required: Absolute neutrophil count (ANC), platelet count, and hemoglobin testing required before each dose for the first 12 months and every 3 dosing cycles thereafter. Treatment criteria are outlined in the following chart. If criteria are not met, consider delaying treatment. ***Do not reduce dose.***

	Siltuximab Treatment Criteria	
Laboratory Parameter	Requirements Before the First Siltuximab Infusion	Retreatment Criteria for Every-3-Week Infusions
Absolute neutrophil count	$\geq 1 \times 10^9$/L	$\geq 1 \times 10^9$/L
Platelet count	$\geq 75 \times 10^9$/L	$\geq 50 \times 10^9$/L
Hemoglobin	<17 Gm/dL	<17 Gm/dL

Siltuximab: 11 mg/kg as an IV infusion equally distributed over 1 hour. Administer every 3 weeks until treatment failure.

DOSE ADJUSTMENTS

No initial dosage adjustment is necessary for patients with CrCl greater than or equal to 15 mL/min. ▪ No initial dosage adjustment is necessary for patients with mild to moderate hepatic impairment.

DILUTION

Siltuximab is available as a lyophilized powder in 100-mg and 400-mg single-use vials for intravenous infusion. Determine the number of vials required using the following calculations:

Weight in kg × Dose/kg ÷ 100 or 400 mg/vial = # of vials required

A 60-kg man requiring 11 mg/kg would require 660 mg. 660 mg ÷ 100 mg/vial = 6.6 (÷ 400 mg/vial = 1.65) vials required. After patient is weighed and appropriate dose is calculated, remove vials from the refrigerator and allow to come to RT for 30 minutes. Use of a 21-gauge $1^1/_2$-inch needle is recommended for preparation. Aseptically reconstitute each siltuximab vial as instructed in the following chart.

Instructions for Reconstituting Vials of Siltuximab		
Strength	Amount of SWFI Required	Concentration in mg/mL
100-mg vial	5.2 mL	20 mg/mL
400-mg vial	20 mL	20 mg/mL

Gently swirl reconstituted vials. ***Do Not Shake or Swirl Vigorously.*** Powder may take up to 60 minutes to dissolve. Must be further diluted for infusion within 2 hours of the initial reconstitution. Maintain at RT. Do not use if particles or solution discoloration is present or if solution is visibly opaque. To further dilute, withdraw a volume of D5W equal to the calculated volume of the siltuximab dose from a 250-mL infusion bag of D5W and slowly add the siltuximab solution. Gently invert to mix the solution. Infusion bags must be made of either polyvinyl chloride (PVC) with di(2-ethylhexyl) phthalate (DEHP) or polyolefin (PO).

Filters: Use of a 0.2-micron inline polyethersulfone (PES) filter required.

Storage: Store unopened vials at 2° to 8° C (36° to 46° F) in original cartons to protect from light. Do not use beyond expiration date located on the carton and vial. Complete infusion within 4 hours of dilution. Discard any unused portion of the reconstituted product or the infusion solution. Waste material should be disposed of in accordance with local requirements.

COMPATIBILITY

Manufacturer states, "Do not infuse siltuximab concomitantly in the same intravenous line with other agents." **Compatible** only with infusion bags of polyvinyl chloride (PVC) with di(2-ethylhexyl) phthalate (DEHP) or polyolefin (PO) and administration sets lined with PVC, DEHP, or polyurethane (PU).

RATE OF ADMINISTRATION

A single dose equally distributed over 1 hour as an IV infusion. Stop the infusion if the patient develops a mild to moderate infusion reaction. If the reaction resolves, siltuximab may be restarted at a lower infusion rate. Consider premedication with antihistamines, acetaminophen, and corticosteroids as indicated. Discontinue siltuximab if patient does not tolerate the infusion following these interventions. Complete infusion within 4 hours of dilution.

ACTIONS

Siltuximab is a human-mouse chimeric monoclonal antibody produced by Chinese hamster ovary cells. It binds human interleukin-6 (IL-6) and prevents the binding of IL-6 to both soluble and membrane-bound IL-6 receptors. Overproduction of IL-6 has been linked to systemic manifestations in patients with multicentric Castleman's disease (MCD). With the first infusion, peak serum concentration occurs close to the end of the infusion. With the once-every-3-week dosing regimen, siltuximab steady-state is achieved by the sixth infusion. The mean terminal half-life for siltuximab in patients after the first infusion is 20.6 days (range 14.2 to 29.7 days).

INDICATIONS AND USES

Treatment of patients with multicentric Castleman's disease (MCD) who are human immunodeficiency virus (HIV) negative and human herpesvirus-8 (HHV-8) negative.

Limitation of use: Siltuximab was not studied in patients with MCD who are HIV-positive or HHV-8 positive because siltuximab did not bind to virally produced IL-6 in a nonclinical study.

CONTRAINDICATIONS

Severe hypersensitivity reaction to siltuximab or any of its excipients.

PRECAUTIONS

Administered under the direction of a physician knowledgeable in its use in a facility with adequate diagnostic and treatment facilities to monitor the patient and respond to any medical emergency. ■ Do not administer siltuximab to patients with severe infections until the infection resolves. May mask signs and symptoms of acute inflammation, including suppression of fever and of acute-phase reactants such as C-reactive protein (CRP). ■ Hypersensitivity and/or infusion reactions, including anaphylaxis, may occur. ■ Do not administer live virus vaccines to patients receiving siltuximab. IL-6 inhibition may interfere with the normal immune response to new antigens. ■ Use with caution in patients who may be at increased risk for GI perforation. ■ May increase hemoglobin. ■ Effects of severe renal impairment (CrCl less than 15 mL/min) on siltuximab pharmacokinetics have not been determined. ■ Patients with severe hepatic impairment (Child-Pugh Class C) were not included in clinical trials. ■ A protein substance, it has the potential for producing an immune response. Anti-siltuximab antibodies have been detected in a small number of patients; clinical significance unknown.

Monitor: Obtain ANC, platelets, and hemoglobin before each dose for the first 12 months and every 3 dosing cycles thereafter. Consider delay of treatment if established parameters are not met. Do not reduce dose; see Usual Dose. ■ Monitor closely for S/S of infections.

Prompt anti-infective therapy is recommended. Do not administer further siltuximab until the infection resolves. ▪ Monitor for S/S of a hypersensitivity reaction (e.g., chest pain, chills, dizziness, dyspnea, fever, flushing, hypotension, nausea, pruritus, rash, urticaria) or infusion reaction (e.g., back pain, chest pain or discomfort, erythema, flushing, palpitations, nausea and vomiting). ▪ Promptly evaluate patients presenting with symptoms that may be associated or suggestive of GI perforation. ▪ Monitor uric acid levels as indicated. May be treated with adequate hydration and, if necessary, with allopurinol and alkalinization of urine. ▪ Assess patient's overall health at each treatment visit.

Patient Education: Review manufacturer's medication guide before each dose. ▪ Discuss recommended vaccinations before treatment with siltuximab. ▪ Promptly report S/S of serious hypersensitivity or infusion reaction during the infusion. S/S include chest tightness, difficulty breathing, severe dizziness or light-headedness, swelling of the lips, skin rash, and wheezing. ▪ May lower resistance to infections; promptly report S/S of infection (e.g., fever, sore throat, unusual redness around a sore). ▪ Report any S/S of new or worsening medical conditions. ▪ Avoid pregnancy. Women of childbearing potential should use contraception during treatment and for 3 months after treatment.

Maternal/Child: Category C: avoid pregnancy; use during pregnancy only if potential benefit justifies the risk to the fetus. ▪ Use of contraception indicated during and for 3 months after treatment is complete. ▪ Infants born to pregnant women taking siltuximab may be at an increased risk for infection. Caution is advised in the administration of live virus vaccines to these infants. ▪ Discontinue breast-feeding. ▪ Safety and effectiveness for use in pediatric patients not established.

Elderly: Differences in response compared with younger adults have not been identified, but greater sensitivity of older individuals cannot be ruled out.

DRUG/LAB INTERACTIONS

No in vitro or in vivo drug-drug interaction studies have been conducted with siltuximab. ▪ Inhibition of IL-6 signaling in patients treated with siltuximab may increase metabolism of CYP_{450} substrates. When initiating or discontinuing siltuximab in patients being treated with CYP_{450} substrates with a narrow therapeutic index, monitoring of effect (e.g., INR with warfarin [Coumadin]) or drug concentrations (e.g., cyclosporine [Sandimmune], theophylline) may be required. Adjust dose as needed. The effect of siltuximab on CYP_{450} enzyme activity can persist for several weeks after stopping therapy. Use caution when siltuximab is coadministered with CYP3A4 substrates when a decrease in effectiveness would be undesirable (e.g., atorvastatin [Lipitor], lovastatin [Mevacor], oral contraceptives). ▪ Do not administer live virus vaccines to patients receiving siltuximab.

SIDE EFFECTS

The most commonly reported side effects were hyperuricemia, increased weight, pruritus, rash (rash generalized, rash maculopapular, rash popular, and rash pruritic), and upper respiratory tract infection. Concurrent active serious infections as well as hypersensitivity and/or infusion-related reactions may occur. Other side effects reported include arthralgia, constipation, diarrhea, dry skin, eczema, edema (generalized, localized), fatigue, headache, hypercholesterolemia, hypertriglyceridemia, hypotension, lower respiratory tract infection, oropharyngeal pain, pain in extremities, psoriasis, renal impairment, and thrombocytopenia.

ANTIDOTE

Keep physician informed of side effects; may be treated symptomatically if indicated. Based on the severity of the reaction, slow the infusion rate, temporarily interrupt, or discontinue the infusion. Manage acute reactions that require intervention by either temporarily interrupting or discontinuing the infusion and administering antihistamines, antipyretics, or corticosteroids as necessary. Discontinue siltuximab in patients with severe hypersensitivity and/or infusion-related reactions, anaphylaxis, or cytokine release syndromes. Do not reinstitute treatment. Treat with oxygen, epinephrine (Adrenalin), antihistamines (e.g., diphenhydramine [Benadryl]), vasopressors (e.g., dopamine), corticosteroids, albuterol, IV fluids, and ventilation equipment as indicated. Resuscitate as necessary.

SIPULEUCEL-T
Provenge

Autologous cellular immunotherapy
Antineoplastic

USUAL DOSE

An autologous (derived from the same individual) cellular immunotherapy. Each infusion of sipuleucel-T is preceded by a leukapheresis procedure and a specific preparation procedure by the manufacturer; see Dilution and Actions. Three complete doses are administered at approximately 2-week intervals (range of 1 to 15 weeks in clinical trials).

Approximately 3 days before the desired infusion date: *Leukapheresis:* Peripheral blood mononuclear cells are obtained via a standard leukapheresis procedure. These cells are then sent to the manufacturer (Dendreon) to be prepared for reinfusion into the patient.

Day of infusion: *Premedication:* Administer oral acetaminophen and an antihistamine (e.g., diphenhydramine [Benadryl]) 30 minutes before administration to minimize potential acute infusion reactions (e.g., chills, fever).

Sipuleucel-T: For autologous IV use only. Do **not** use a cell filter. Confirm that the patient's identity matches the patient identifiers on the infusion bag and the Cell Product Disposition Form (CPDF). Each dose contains a minimum of 50,000,000 autologous CD54+ cells activated with PAP-GM-CSF and suspended in 250 mL of LR in a sealed, patient-specific infusion bag. Do **not** infuse until confirmation of product release has been received from Dendreon; see Dilution. Infusion must begin before the expiration date and time on the Cell Product Disposition Form (CPDF).

DILUTION

Will be shipped directly to the infusing provider in packaging intended to protect the infusion bag and maintain storage temperatures until infusion. Verify the product and patient-specific labels located on top of the insulated container. Do **not** remove from the shipping box or open the lid of the insulated container until the patient is ready for infusion. The manufacturer will send to the infusion site a CPDF that contains the patient identifiers, expiration date and time, and disposition status (approved for infusion or rejected). When all preparations have been made for infusion and the CPDF has been received and verified, remove the sipuleucel-T infusion bag from the insulated container and inspect for signs of leakage. Contents will be slightly cloudy and a cream-to-pink color. Gently mix and resuspend contents, inspecting for clumps and clots. Small clumps of cellular material should disperse with gentle manual mixing. Do **not** administer if the bag leaks during handling or if clumps remain in the bag.

Filters: Do not use a cell filter.

Storage: After removal from the insulated container, the infusion must be complete within 3 hours at RT. Do not return to the shipping container. Do not initiate infusion of expired sipuleucel-T.

COMPATIBILITY

Specific information not available; however, specific use indicates it should be administered separately; consult pharmacist.

RATE OF ADMINISTRATION

A single dose of 250 mL as an infusion equally distributed over 1 hour. Do **not** use a cell filter. If an infusion reaction occurs, decrease rate or interrupt infusion depending on the severity of the reaction; see Antidote.

ACTIONS

An autologous cellular immunotherapy. The patient's own immune cells are obtained through leukapheresis. Active components of sipuleucel-T are autologous peripheral blood mononuclear cells, including antigen-presenting cells (APCs) and PAP-GM-CSF (prostatic acid phosphatase [PAP], an antigen expressed in prostate cancer tissue, linked to granulocyte-macrophage colony-stimulating factor [GM-CSF], an immune cell activator). The recombinant antigen can bind to and be processed by APCs into smaller protein fragments. The recombinant antigen is designed to target APCs and may help direct the immune response to PAP. The final product contains T-cells, B cells, natural killer (NK) cells and other cells.

INDICATIONS AND USES

Treatment of asymptomatic or minimally symptomatic metastatic hormone refractory prostate cancer.

CONTRAINDICATIONS

Manufacturer states, "None."

PRECAUTIONS

Intended solely for autologous use. For IV use only. ▪ Administered under the direction of a physician knowledgeable in its use in a facility with adequate diagnostic and treatment facilities to monitor the patient and respond to any medical emergency. ▪ Concurrent use of immunosuppressive agents may alter the effectiveness and/or safety of sipuleucel-T; see Drug/Lab Interactions. ▪ Health care professionals must use universal precautions when handling leukapheresis material and sipuleucel-T. Neither is routinely tested for transmissible infectious diseases and thus may carry the risk of infectious disease transmission to health professionals during handling of the products. ▪ Acute infusion reactions (reported within 1 day of infusion) occur frequently and range from mild to serious; see Monitor. Incidence increased with the second infusion and decreased after the third infusion.

Monitor: Obtain baseline vital signs and repeat as indicated. ▪ Observe the patient for S/S of an acute infusion reaction (e.g., bronchospasm, chills, fatigue, fever, hypertension, joint aches, nausea, tachycardia) during the infusion and for at least 30 minutes after the infusion. If an acute infusion reaction occurs, the infusion may be interrupted or slowed depending on the severity of the reaction. Do not resume the infusion if the bag will be held at RT for more than 3 hours. ▪ Closely monitor patients with cardiac or pulmonary conditions. ▪ If the patient is unable to receive a scheduled infusion, the patient will need to undergo an additional leukapheresis procedure. ▪ Monitor for extravasation.

Patient Education: Maintain all scheduled appointments. ▪ An additional leukapheresis procedure will be required if a scheduled infusion cannot be completed. ▪ A central venous line may be required if peripheral venous access is not adequate to accommodate the leukapheresis procedure and/or the infusion. ▪ Promptly report S/S of an infusion reaction (e.g., breathing problems, chills, dizziness, fatigue, fever, headache, hypertension, muscle aches, nausea, or vomiting). ▪ Report S/S that may indicate a cardiac arrhythmia (e.g., very slow or rapid pulse). ▪ Review prescription and nonprescription drug profile with a physician; see Drug/Lab Interactions.

Maternal/Child: Not indicated for use in these populations.

Elderly: Safety similar to that seen in younger adults.

DRUG/LAB INTERACTIONS

Drug interaction studies have not been performed. ▪ Use of either **chemotherapy or immunosuppressive agents** (such as systemic corticosteroids) given concurrently with the leukapheresis procedure or sipuleucel-T has not been studied. ▪ Sipuleucel-T is designed to stimulate the immune system, and concurrent use of **immunosuppressive agents** may alter the effectiveness and/or safety of sipuleucel-T. Evaluate patients carefully for the medical appropriateness of reducing or discontinuing immunosuppressive agents before treatment.

SIDE EFFECTS

The most common events of backache, chills, fatigue, fever, headache, joint aches, and nausea are usually mild or moderate and generally resolve within 2 days. Other side effects included anemia, anorexia, citrate toxicity, constipation, cough, diarrhea, hematuria, hot flush, influenza-like illness, insomnia, muscle aches and spasms, pain (back, bone, chest [musculoskeletal], extremity, and neck), paresthesia (oral, extremity), peripheral edema, rash, sweating, tremor, URIs, UTIs, weight loss. Acute infusion reactions (mild to moderate) occur frequently. Severe acute infusion reactions (Grade 3) add asthenia, bronchospasm, dizziness, dyspnea, hypertension, hypoxia, and vomiting. Cerebro-vascular events (e.g., hemorrhagic and ischemic strokes) and single reports of eosino-philia, myasthenia gravis, myositis, rhabdomyolysis, and tumor flare have been reported.

ANTIDOTE

Keep the physician informed of significant side effects and treat as appropriate. For acute infusion reactions, the infusion may be interrupted or slowed depending on the severity of the reaction. Do not resume the infusion if the bag will be held at RT for more than 3 hours. In controlled clinical trials, acute infusion reactions were treated with acetamino-phen, IV antihistamines (e.g., diphenhydramine [Benadryl]) and/or H$_2$ blockers (e.g., ranitidine [Zantac]) and low-dose IV meperidine. Resuscitate as indicated.

SODIUM ACETATE
(**SO**-dee-um **AS**-ah-tayt)

Electrolyte replenisher
Antihyponatremic
Alkalizing agent

pH 6 to 7

USUAL DOSE

Determined by nutritional needs, evaluation of electrolytes, and degree of hyponatremia. Some solutions may contain aluminum; see Precautions. Available in 2 mEq and 4 mEq/mL concentrations. Each mL provides 2 or 4 mEq each of sodium and acetate.

DOSE ADJUSTMENTS

Lower-end initial doses may be appropriate in the elderly based on the potential for de-creased organ function and concomitant disease or drug therapy.

DILUTION

Must be added to larger volumes of IV infusion solutions including total parenteral nutri-tion. Use only clear solutions. Check labels for aluminum content; see Precautions.

Storage: Store at room temperature. Discard unused portion.

COMPATIBILITY

Consider any drug NOT listed as compatible to be INCOMPATIBLE until consulting a pharmacist; specific conditions may apply.

One source suggests the following **compatibilities:**

Y-site: Enalaprilat (Vasotec IV), esmolol (Brevibloc), labetalol, nicardipine (Cardene IV), ondansetron (Zofran).

RATE OF ADMINISTRATION

Administer at prescribed rate for infusion solutions. Rapid or excessive administration may produce sodium overload, water retention, alkalosis, or hypokalemia.

ACTIONS

An alkalizing agent and sodium salt. Sodium is the predominant cation of extracellular fluid. It controls water distribution throughout the body. Hypothalamus osmoreceptors, sensitive to osmolarity changes in the blood, control serum sodium concentration (142 mEq/L). Body fluid is lost when sodium content decreases and retained when so-dium content increases. Sodium is excreted by the kidney. The acetate ion is metabolized to bicarbonate, thus providing a source of bicarbonate. It also acts as a hydrogen ion receptor.

INDICATIONS AND USES

To prevent or correct hyponatremia in patients with restricted intake, especially in indi-vidualized IV formulations when basic needs are not met by standard solutions. ▪ Treat-ment of mild to moderate acidotic states. ▪ Source of sodium ions in hemodialysis and peritoneal dialysis.

CONTRAINDICATIONS
Patients with hypernatremia or water retention.

PRECAUTIONS
Use with caution in impaired renal function, congestive heart failure, hypertension, peripheral or pulmonary edema, any condition resulting in salt retention, and in patients receiving corticosteroids. ▪ Use acetate-containing solutions with extreme caution in patients with metabolic or respiratory alkalosis and/or impaired hepatic function. ▪ Temporary therapy in acidosis. Treatment of primary condition must be instituted. ▪ Sodium bicarbonate is the drug of choice for use in severe acidosis that requires immediate correction. ▪ Some solutions of sodium acetate contain aluminum. In impaired kidney function, aluminum may reach toxic levels. Premature neonates are particularly at risk because of their immature kidneys and requirement for calcium and phosphate, which also contain aluminum. Research indicates that patients with impaired renal function who receive more than 4 to 5 mcg/kg/day of parenteral aluminum are at risk for developing CNS or bone toxicity associated with aluminum accumulation.

Monitor: Evaluate electrolytes frequently during treatment. ▪ Evaluate fluid balance. ▪ Rapid or excessive administration may produce alkalosis or hypokalemia. Cardiac arrhythmias may result from an intracellular shift of potassium. Many other complications may arise from electrolyte imbalance.

Maternal/Child: Category C: safety not established; use only if clearly needed.

Elderly: Differences in response between elderly and younger patients have not been identified. Lower-end initial doses may be appropriate in the elderly; see Dose Adjustments.

DRUG/LAB INTERACTIONS
Alkalinization of urine may increase the renal elimination and decrease the effects of many drugs, including **tetracyclines, chlorpropamide, lithium carbonate, methotrexate, salicylates,** and may decrease the renal elimination and prolong the effects of others, including **anorexiants** (e.g., amphetamines), **flecainide, mecamylamine, quinidine, sympathomimetics** (e.g., dopamine, ephedrine).

SIDE EFFECTS
Hypernatremia, sodium level over 147 mEq/L, is most common (congestive heart failure, delirium, dizziness, edema, fever, flushing, headache, hypotension, oliguria, pulmonary edema, reduced salivation and lacrimation, respiratory arrest, restlessness, swollen tongue, tachycardia, thirst, weakness). Alkalosis and fluid or solute overload can occur.

ANTIDOTE
Notify the physician of any side effect. Reduce rate and notify physician at first sign of congestion or fluid overload. May be treated by sodium restriction and/or use of diuretics (e.g., furosemide [Lasix]) or dialysis. Resuscitate as necessary.

SODIUM BICARBONATE

(**SO**-dee-um bye-**KAR**-bon-ayt)

Electrolyte replenisher
Alkalizing agent

pH 7 to 8.5

USUAL DOSE

Adjusted according to pH, $Paco_2$, calculated base deficit, clinical response, and fluid limitations of the patient. In the presence of a low CO_2 content, adjust gradually to avoid unrecognized alkalosis. Correction to a CO_2 of 20 mEq/L within 24 hours will most likely result in a normal pH if the cause of acidosis is controlled and normal kidney function is present. Average dose for most indications is 2 to 5 mEq/kg/24 hr in adults and pediatric patients.

Cardiac arrest: 1 mEq/kg of body weight, only when appropriate (see Precautions; evidence supports little benefit and use may be detrimental). Repeat half dose in 10 minutes if indicated by blood pH and $Paco_2$.

PEDIATRIC DOSE

0.5 to 1 mEq/kg. For neonates and children up to 2 years of age, dose must never exceed 8 mEq/kg/24 hr of a 4.2% or more dilute solution; see Usual Dose, Monitor, and Maternal/Child.

DILUTION

4.2% sodium bicarbonate solution: 5 mEq/10 mL (0.5 mEq/mL).
5% sodium bicarbonate solution: 297.5 mEq/500 mL (0.595 mEq/mL).
7.5% sodium bicarbonate solution: 44.6 mEq/50 mL (0.892 mEq/mL).
8.4% sodium bicarbonate solution: 50 mEq/50 mL (1 mEq/mL).
neut (4% sodium bicarbonate solution): 2.4 mEq/5 mL (0.48 mEq/mL). Use limited to a buffering solution. Will raise pH of IV fluids and medications. Never used as a systemic alkalinizer.

May be given in prepared solutions. 7.5% and 8.4% solutions should be diluted with equal amount of water for injection, or diluted with **compatible** IV solutions, depending on desired dosage and desired rate of administration. 4.2% or a more dilute solution is preferred for infants and children. Use only clear solutions.

COMPATIBILITY

(Underline Indicates Conflicting Compatibility Information)

Consider any drug NOT listed as compatible to be INCOMPATIBLE until consulting a pharmacist; specific conditions may apply.

Will form a precipitate with many drugs, including epinephrine. *If coadministration with epinephrine is indicated, give at separate sites.*

One source suggests the following **compatibilities:**

Additive: Amikacin, aminophylline, amphotericin B (conventional), atropine, calcium chloride, cefoxitin (Mefoxin), ceftazidime (Fortaz), ceftriaxone (Rocephin), chloramphenicol (Chloromycetin), clindamycin (Cleocin), cytarabine (ARA-C), erythromycin (Erythrocin), esmolol (Brevibloc), furosemide (Lasix), heparin, levofloxacin (Levaquin), lidocaine, magnesium sulfate, mannitol, meperidine (Demerol), methotrexate, methyldopate, multivitamins (M.V.I.), nafcillin (Nallpen), oxytocin (Pitocin), penicillin G potassium, phenylephrine (Neo-Synephrine), phytonadione (vitamin K_1), potassium chloride (KCl), prochlorperazine (Compazine), verapamil.

Y-site: Acyclovir (Zovirax), amifostine (Ethyol), aztreonam (Azactam), bivalirudin (Angiomax), ceftaroline (Teflaro), ceftriaxone (Rocephin), ciprofloxacin (Cipro IV), cisatracurium (Nimbex), cladribine (Leustatin), cyclophosphamide (Cytoxan), cytarabine (ARA-C), daunorubicin (Cerubidine), dexamethasone (Decadron), dexmedetomidine (Precedex), diltiazem (Cardizem), docetaxel (Taxotere), doripenem (Doribax), doxorubicin (Adriamycin), etoposide (VePesid), etoposide phosphate (Etopophos), famotidine (Pepcid IV), filgrastim (Neupogen), fludarabine (Fludara), gallium nitrate (Ganite), gemcitabine (Gemzar), granisetron (Kytril), heparin, hydrocortisone sodium succinate (Solu-Cortef), 6% hydroxyethyl starch (Voluven), ifosfamide (Ifex), indomethacin (Indocin IV), insulin (regular), levofloxacin (Levaquin), linezolid (Zyvox), melphalan (Alkeran), mesna (Mesnex), methylprednisolone (Solu-Medrol), milrinone (Primacor), morphine, paclitaxel (Taxol), pemetrexed (Alimta), piperacillin/tazobactam (Zosyn), potassium chloride (KCl), propofol (Diprivan), remifentanil (Ultiva), tacrolimus (Prograf), telavancin (Vibativ), teniposide (Vumon), thiotepa, vancomycin, vasopressin.

RATE OF ADMINISTRATION
Flush IV line thoroughly before and after administration. Usual rate of administration of any solution is 2 to 5 mEq/kg over 4 to 8 hours. Do not exceed 50 mEq/hr. Decrease rate for pediatric patients. See Pediatric Dose. Rapid or excessive administration may produce alkalosis, hypernatremia, hypocalcemia, and hypokalemia. Cardiac arrhythmias may result from an intracellular shift of potassium. Will also produce pain and irritation along injection site.

Cardiac arrest: Up to 1 mEq/kg properly diluted over 1 to 3 minutes.

ACTIONS
An alkalizing agent and sodium salt. Helps to maintain osmotic pressure and ion balance. It is the buffering agent in blood. Bicarbonate ion elevates blood pH promptly. 99% reabsorbed with normal kidney function. Only 1% is excreted in the urine.

INDICATIONS AND USES
Metabolic acidosis (blood pH below 7.2 or plasma bicarbonate of 8 mEq/L or less) caused by circulatory insufficiency resulting from shock or severe dehydration, extracorporeal circulation of blood, severe renal disease, cardiac arrest (see Precautions), uncontrolled diabetes with ketoacidosis (low-dose insulin preferred), and primary lactic acidosis. ■ Hyperkalemia. ■ Hemolytic reactions requiring alkalinization of urine to reduce nephrotoxicity. ■ Severe diarrhea. ■ Barbiturate, methyl alcohol, or salicylate intoxication. ■ Buffering solution to raise pH of IV fluids and medications.

CONTRAINDICATIONS
Diuretics known to produce hypochloremic alkalosis (e.g., thiazides), edema, hypertension, hypocalcemia (alkalosis may produce CHF, convulsions, hypertension, and tetany), hypochloremia (from vomiting, GI suction, or diuretics), hypernatremia, impaired renal function, metabolic alkalosis, respiratory alkalosis or acidosis, and any situation in which the administration of sodium could be clinically detrimental.

PRECAUTIONS
Temporary therapy in metabolic acidosis. Treatment of primary condition must be instituted. Best to partially correct acidosis and allow compensatory mechanisms to complete the correction. ■ Use with caution in cardiac, liver, or renal disease; CHF; fluid/solute overload; elderly and postoperative patients with renal or cardiovascular insufficiency; and in patients receiving corticosteroids. ■ Use in cardiac arrest indicated only in cases of prolonged resuscitation with effective ventilation or after return of spontaneous circulation after a long arrest interval. ■ Adequate alveolar ventilation should control acid-base balance in most arrest situations except prolonged cardiac arrest, arrested patients with pre-existing metabolic acidosis, hyperkalemia, or tricyclic or barbiturate overdose.

Monitor: Confirm absolute patency of vein. Extravasation may cause chemical cellulitis, necrosis, ulceration, or sloughing. ■ Flush IV line thoroughly before and after administration; many **incompatibilities.** ■ Determine blood pH, Po_2, Pco_2, and electrolytes several times daily during intensive treatment and daily in most other situations. Determine base excess or deficit in infants and children (dose = 0.3 × kg × base deficit). Notify physician of all results. ■ Rapid or excessive administration may produce alkalosis, hypokalemia, and hypocalcemia. Cardiac arrhythmias may result from an intracellular shift of potassium. Many other complications may arise from electrolyte imbalance. ■ Use only 50-mL ampules in cardiac arrest to prevent accidental overdose. Recent practice indicates smaller doses may be appropriate when indicated in cardiac arrest and may prevent secondary alkalosis. Adequate alveolar ventilation is imperative. Evaluate patient response and blood gases.

S

Maternal/Child: Category C: safety for use in pregnancy not established; use only if clearly needed. ▪ Use caution in breast-feeding. ▪ Doses in excess of 8 mEq/kg/24 hr and/or given too rapidly (10 mL/min) may cause intracranial hemorrhage, hypernatremia, and decrease in cerebrospinal fluid pressure in neonates and children under 2 years.

Elderly: Contains sodium; use caution in the elderly with renal or cardiovascular insufficiency with or without CHF; see Precautions.

DRUG/LAB INTERACTIONS

Alkalinization of urine may increase the renal elimination and decrease the effects of many drugs, including **tetracyclines, chlorpropamide, lithium carbonate, methotrexate, salicylates,** and may decrease the renal elimination and prolong the effects of others, including **anorexiants** (e.g., amphetamines), **flecainide, mecamylamine, quinidine, sympathomimetics** (e.g., dopamine, ephedrine).

SIDE EFFECTS

Rare when used with caution: alkalosis (hyperirritability and tetany), hypernatremia (edema, CHF), hypokalemia, local site venous irritation.

ANTIDOTE

Discontinue the drug and notify the physician of any side effect. Hypokalemia usually occurs with alkalosis. Sodium and potassium chloride must be supplemented as indicated for correction. Treatment of alkalosis often results in more alkalosis. Rebreathing expired air from a paper bag may help to control beginning symptoms of alkalosis. Calcium gluconate may help in severe alkalosis. Administration of a balanced hypotonic electrolyte solution (Isolyte H, Normosol-M, Plasma-lyte 56) with sodium and potassium chloride added may help to excrete the bicarbonate ion in the urine. Ammonium chloride may be indicated. Treat tetany as indicated (calcium gluconate). For extravasation, discontinue infusion; aspirate fluid, drug, and/or 3 to 5 mL of blood through the in-place needle, then remove the needle. Elevate the extremity and apply warm, moist compresses. Resuscitate as necessary.

SODIUM CHLORIDE
(**SO**-dee-um **KLOR**-eyed)

Electrolyte replenisher
Antihyponatremic

pH 4.5 to 7

USUAL DOSE

Highly individualized and dependent on age, weight, clinical condition of patient, concentration of salts in the plasma, and/or loss of body fluids.

Hypotonic: (0.45% [½NS], 4.5 Gm of sodium chloride/L or 77 mEq of sodium and 77 mEq of chloride [approximately 155 mOsm/L]) 2 to 4 L/24 hr.

Isotonic: (0.9% [NS], 9 Gm of sodium chloride/L or 154 mEq of sodium and 154 mEq of chloride [approximately 310 mOsm/L]) 1.5 to 3 L/24 hr.

Bacteriostatic isotonic NS contains benzyl alcohol as a preservative. It is used in small amounts (usually 1 to 2 mL) as a diluent for injectable drugs (IV, IM, SC) or to flush IV lines. One study suggests that up to 30 mL/dose may be used in adults. However, the amount of benzyl alcohol that is tolerated within 24 hours in adults without toxic effects has not been determined. *Use only preservative-free sodium chloride in newborns for all indications.*

Hypertonic: Calculate sodium deficit. Total body water (TBW) is 45% to 50% in females and 50% to 60% in males.

Na deficit in mEq = TBW [desired − observed plasma Na]

Hypertonic (3%, 30 Gm of sodium chloride/L or 513 mEq of sodium and 513 mEq of chloride [approximately 1,030 mOsm/L] or 5%, 50 Gm of sodium chloride/L or 855 mEq of sodium and 855 mEq of chloride [approximately 1,710 mOsm/L]), 200 to 400 mL/24 hr. To correct *acute serious hyponatremia,* hypertonic sodium chloride is used to correct the serum sodium in 5 mEq/L/dose increments at a rate of no more than 0.5 mEq/hr until serum sodium is 125 mEq/L or neurologic symptoms improve. In the first 3 to 4 hours, an increase of plasma sodium at rates up to 1 mEq/L/hr may be tolerated in patients with distressing symptoms. To prevent an overly rapid correction, an increase in plasma sodium of less than 10 mEq/L in the first 24 hours and an increase of less than 18 mEq/L in the first 48 hours is desired. See Precautions.

Concentrated: To be used only as an additive in parenteral fluid therapy (14.6% contains 2.5 mEq of sodium and chloride/mL; 23.4% contains 4 mEq of sodium and chloride/mL).

DOSE ADJUSTMENTS

Dose selection should be cautious in the elderly, especially with hypertonic or concentrated solutions. Start at the lower end of the desired dosing range; consider the greater frequency of decreased organ function and of concomitant disease or drug therapy.

DILUTION

Available as *hypotonic* 25 mL, 50 mL, 150 mL, 250 mL, 500 mL, 1 L; *isotonic* (2 mL, 3 mL, 5 mL, 10 mL, 20 mL, 25 mL, 30 mL, 50 mL, 100 mL, 150 mL, 250 mL, 500 mL, 1 L); or *hypertonic* (500 mL) solution in vials and/or bottles for injection or infusion and ready for use. Isotonic and hypotonic sodium chloride are frequently combined with 5% or 10% dextrose. *Concentrated* must be diluted before use. Used only as an additive in parenteral fluids. Permits specific mEq for mEq replacement of sodium and chloride without contributing to fluid overload. Available in 14.6% strength in 20 mL, 40 mL, and 200 mL; 23.4% strength in 30 mL, 50 mL, 100 mL, and 200 mL.

Bacteriostatic isotonic available in 2-mL, 10-mL, and 30-mL vials ready for use as a diluent. Never use in neonates.

Storage: Store at CRT. Do not freeze.

COMPATIBILITY

Consider any drug NOT listed as compatible to be INCOMPATIBLE until consulting a pharmacist; specific conditions may apply.

One source suggests the following **compatibility** for concentrations of 14.6% and 23.4%:

Y-site: Ciprofloxacin (Cipro IV).

RATE OF ADMINISTRATION

IV infusions in flexible plastic containers: Do not hang in series connection, do not pressurize to increase flow rates without first fully evacuating residual air from the container, and do not use vented IV administration sets. All may result in air embolism.

Isotonic and hypotonic: A single daily dose equally distributed over 24 hours. Rate is dependent on age, weight, and clinical condition of the patient.

Hypertonic: One-half the calculated dose over at least 8 hours. Do not exceed 100 mL over 1 hour. Too-rapid infusion may cause local pain and venous irritation; reduce rate for tolerance; see Usual Dose.

Concentrated: Properly diluted in parenteral fluids and equally distributed over 24 hours. Never exceed hypertonic rate (see above) based on actual mEq of sodium chloride.

ACTIONS

Sodium: The predominant cation of extracellular fluid. It controls water distribution throughout the body. Hypothalamus osmoreceptors, sensitive to osmolarity changes in the blood, control serum sodium concentration (142 mEq/L). Body fluid is lost when sodium content decreases and retained when sodium content increases.

Chloride: The major extracellular anion. Closely follows the metabolism of sodium. Changes in the acid-base balance of the body are reflected by the changes in chloride concentration.

Distribution and excretion of sodium and chloride are largely under control of the kidney, which maintains a balance between intake and output.

INDICATIONS AND USES

Replace lost fluid or sodium and chloride ions in the body (e.g., hyponatremia, low salt syndrome, dehydration). ▪ Maintain fluid and electrolyte balance.

Hypotonic: Water replacement without increase of osmotic pressure or serum sodium levels; treatment of hyperosmolar diabetes requiring considerable fluid without excess sodium.

Isotonic: To replace sodium and chloride lost from vomiting because of obstructions and/or aspiration of GI fluids; treatment of metabolic alkalosis with fluid loss and sodium depletion. ▪ Diluent in parenteral preparations. ▪ To initiate and terminate blood transfusions without hemolyzing RBCs. ▪ Maintain patency and perform routine irrigations of many types of intravascular devices (e.g., catheters, implanted ports). ▪ Antidote for drug-induced hypercalcemia. Given concurrently with furosemide (Lasix). ▪ Priming solution in hemodialysis procedures.

Hypertonic: Used only when high sodium and/or chloride content without large amounts of fluid is required (e.g., electrolyte and fluid loss replaced with sodium-free fluids, excessive water intake resulting in drastic dilution of body water, emergency treatment of severe salt depletion, addisonian crisis, diabetic coma).

Concentrated: Used to meet the specific requirements of patients with unusual fluid and electrolyte needs (e.g., special problems of sodium electrolyte intake or excretion).

CONTRAINDICATIONS

Hypernatremia; fluid retention; situations where sodium or chloride could be detrimental. 3% and 5% sodium chloride solutions are contraindicated with elevated, normal, or slightly decreased serum sodium and chloride levels. Bacteriostatic sodium chloride is contraindicated in newborns.

PRECAUTIONS

Use caution in circulatory insufficiency, congestive heart failure, edema with sodium retention, kidney dysfunction, hepatic disease, hypoproteinemia, in the elderly or debilitated individuals, and in patients receiving corticosteroids. ▪ Use with caution in surgical patients; see Monitor. ▪ More than 1 liter of NS may cause hypernatremia, which can result in loss of bicarbonate ions and acidosis. ▪ All uses require preservative-free solutions except the limited use of bacteriostatic NS as a diluent or flushing agent. ▪ Inadvertent direct injection or absorption of concentrated sodium chloride may cause sudden hypernatremia, cardiovascular shock, CNS disorders, extensive hemolysis, cortical necrosis of the kidneys, and severe local tissue necrosis with extravasation. Use extreme caution; see Dilution. ▪ Administration of IV solutions can cause fluid and/or solute overload, resulting in dilution of serum electrolyte concentrations, overhydration, congested states, or pulmonary edema. The risk of dilutional states is inversely proportional to the electrolyte concentration (increased fluids may dilute electrolyte concentration). The risk of solute overload causing congested states with peripheral and pulmonary edema is directly proportional to the electrolyte concentration (higher electrolytes pull in fluid, leading to fluid overload). ▪ Overly rapid correction of severe hyponatremia (plasma sodium less than 110 to 115 mEq/L) may lead to a neurologic disorder (osmotic demyelination syndrome [central pontine myelinolysis]), which may be irreversible; see Usual Dose.

Monitor: Maintain accurate intake and output; monitor electrolytes and acid-base balance, especially in prolonged therapy. ▪ Monitor vital signs as indicated. ▪ Monitor for signs of hyponatremia (sodium less than 135 mEq/L [e.g., disorientation, headache, lethargy, nausea, weakness]). May progress to coma and seizures. ▪ Excessive administration of potassium-free solutions may cause hypokalemia. ▪ Before and during use of hypertonic or concentrated sodium chloride, determine osmolar concentrations and chloride and bicarbonate content of the serum. Observe patient continuously to prevent pulmonary edema. ▪ Hypertonic solutions can cause vein damage; use a small needle and a large vein to reduce venous irritation and avoid extravasation; see Precautions.

Maternal/Child: Category C: safety for use during pregnancy not established; use only if clearly needed. ▪ Use caution in breast-feeding. ▪ Benzyl alcohol preservative in bacteriostatic sodium chloride has caused toxicity in newborns. Do not use. ▪ Is used in pediatric patients. Safety and effectiveness based on similarity of clinical conditions of pediatric and adult populations. Use caution in neonates or very small infants; the volume of fluid may affect fluid and electrolyte balance.

Elderly: Lower-end initial doses may be indicated in the elderly; see Dose Adjustments. ▪ Incidence of adverse reactions may be increased; monitor carefully, especially with renal or cardiac insufficiency with or without CHF. ▪ See Precautions.

DRUG/LAB INTERACTIONS
High sodium intake may reduce serum **lithium** concentrations.

SIDE EFFECTS
Fever, hypovolemia, and injection site reactions may occur.

Osmotic demyelination syndrome (central pontine myelinolysis) secondary to too-rapid correction with hypertonic solutions.

Due to sodium excess: Aggravation of existing acidosis, anorexia, cellular dehydration, deep respiration, disorientation, distension, edema, hydrogen loss, hyperchloremic acidosis, hypertension, increased BUN, nausea, oliguria, potassium loss, pulmonary edema, water retention, weakness. Excessive excretion of crystalloids to maintain normal osmotic pressure will increase excretion of potassium and bicarbonate and further increase acidosis. Other salts (e.g., iodide and bromide) used for therapy will also be excreted rapidly.

ANTIDOTE
Discontinue or decrease rate of infusion; notify the physician of side effects. Sodium excess can be treated by sodium restriction and/or use of diuretics or hemodialysis to remove excessive amounts. Observe patient carefully and treat symptomatically. Save balance of fluid for examination.

SODIUM FERRIC GLUCONATE COMPLEX	Antianemic Iron supplement
(**SO**-dee-um **FAIR**-ick **GLUE**-koh-nayt **KOM**-pleks)	
Ferrlecit	pH 7.7 to 9.7

USUAL DOSE
Dose is represented in terms of mg of elemental iron. Given as an infusion and may be administered during the dialysis session.

Treatment of iron deficiency in hemodialysis patients: 125 mg (10 mL)/dose. Doses above 125 mg may be associated with a higher incidence and/or severity of adverse events; see Side Effects. A minimum cumulative dose of 1 Gm of elemental iron is required by most patients. May be administered over eight sessions at sequential dialysis treatments to achieve a favorable hemoglobin or hematocrit response. Additional doses as necessary are indicated to maintain target levels of hemoglobin, hematocrit, and laboratory parameters of iron storage within acceptable limits. Use the lowest dose that achieves this goal.

PEDIATRIC DOSE
1.5 mg/kg (0.12 mL/kg) of elemental iron as a 1-hour infusion. Do not exceed 125-mg dose. Administer at 8 sequential dialysis sessions. See Maternal/Child.

DOSE ADJUSTMENTS
Begin at the low end of the dosing range in elderly patients. Consider decreased cardiac, hepatic, or renal function, and concomitant disease or other drug therapy.

DILUTION
Available in ampules or vials containing 62.5 mg/5 mL (12.5 mg/mL) of elemental iron.

S

Therapeutic dose: 125-mg (10-mL) dose may be diluted in 100 mL NS or may be given undiluted; see Rate of Administration.

Pediatric therapeutic dose: Dilute calculated dose in 25 mL of NS.

Filters: Specific studies not available from manufacturer. Filter needle not required by FDA for drug approval; however, use of a filter needle to withdraw it from an ampule should not have an adverse effect.

Storage: Store ampules at CRT. Do not freeze. Use immediately after dilution in NS.

COMPATIBILITY

Manufacturer states, "Do not mix with other medications or add to parenteral nutrition solutions." Known to be **compatible** only with NS.

RATE OF ADMINISTRATION

Too-rapid administration may cause hypotension associated with fatigue; light-headedness; malaise; severe pain in the chest, back, flanks, or groin; and weakness.

Therapeutic dose: *Injection (adults only):* A single dose (undiluted) as a slow IV injection. May be given at a rate up to 12.5 mg/min (1 mL/min).

Infusion (adults and pediatric patients): A single dose as an infusion properly diluted and equally distributed over 60 minutes.

ACTIONS

A stable macromolecular complex in sucrose injection. Contains elemental iron as the sodium salt of a ferric ion carbohydrate complex. Used to replete the total body content of iron. Iron is critical for normal hemoglobin synthesis to maintain oxygen transport and necessary for metabolism and synthesis of DNA and various other processes. Half-life is approximately 1 hour. Doses of 1 mg/day are adequate to replenish losses in healthy non-menstruating adults. Iron complex is not dialyzable.

INDICATIONS AND USES

Treatment of iron-deficiency anemia in adult patients and pediatric patients 6 years of age or older with chronic kidney disease who are receiving hemodialysis and supplemental erythropoietin therapy (e.g., EPO, Epogen, Procrit); see Maternal/Child.

CONTRAINDICATIONS

All anemias not associated with iron deficiency. Hypersensitivity to sodium ferric gluconate complex or any of its components.

PRECAUTIONS

Use only when truly indicated to avoid excess storage of iron. Not recommended for use in patients with iron overload. ■ Too-rapid administration may cause clinically significant hypotension; see Rate of Administration and Side Effects. ■ Studies have included patients who have had prior iron dextran exposure with hypersensitivity reactions to at least one form of iron dextran (InFeD or DexFerrum). The majority of these patients tolerated Ferrlecit therapy without a subsequent hypersensitivity reaction. ■ There have been rare occurrences of severe hypersensitivity reactions, including anaphylactic-type reactions, some of which have been life threatening and fatal. Administer in a facility equipped to monitor the patient and respond to any medical emergency. ■ Serum iron levels greater than 300 mcg/dL combined with transferrin oversaturation may indicate iron poisoning; see Side Effects.

Monitor: Recumbent position during and after injection may help to prevent postural hypotension. Hypotensive effects may be additive to transient hypotension during dialysis and/or from too-rapid rate of infusion; monitor closely. Hypotensive reactions associated with fatigue; light-headedness; malaise; severe pain in the back, chest, flanks, or groin; and weakness may occur with IV iron. These symptoms may or may not be indicative of a hypersensitivity reaction and usually resolve within 1 or 2 hours. ■ Observe continuously for a hypersensitivity reaction during an infusion and after administration for at least 30 minutes and until clinically stable. Monitor vital signs. ■ Periodic monitoring of hemoglobin and hematocrit and iron storage levels recommended. Doses in excess of iron needs may lead to accumulation of iron in iron storage sites and iatrogenic hemosiderosis.

Patient Education: Report S/S of a hypersensitivity reaction (e.g., difficulty breathing, rash, shortness of breath) promptly. Report pain at injection site.

Maternal/Child: Category B: use during pregnancy only if potential benefit justifies potential risk to fetus. ▪ Safety for use during breast-feeding and in pediatric patients under 6 years of age not established. ▪ Contains benzyl alcohol; should not be used in neonates. Benzyl alcohol present in maternal serum may cross into human milk and may be orally absorbed by a breast-feeding infant.

Elderly: No age differences identified. Caution in the elderly suggested; see Dose Adjustments.

DRUG/LAB INTERACTIONS

May reduce absorption of concomitantly administered **oral iron preparations.** ▪ Concurrent administration of iron therapy with **dimercaprol** (BAL in Oil) will result in the formation of a toxic complex. Either postpone iron therapy to at least 24 hours after dimercaprol or consider transfusions.

SIDE EFFECTS

Hypotension associated with fatigue; light-headedness; malaise; severe pain in the chest, back, flanks, or groin; and weakness may be caused by too-rapid infusion. Severe hypersensitivity reactions (e.g., angioedema, bronchospasm, cardiac arrest, cardiovascular collapse, dyspnea, edema [oral or pharyngeal], muscle spasm, pain [back or chest], pruritus, urticaria) have been reported rarely. Most commonly reported side effects include abdominal pain, back pain, chest pain, cramps, diarrhea, dizziness, dyspnea, fever, headache, hypersensitivity reactions, hypertension, hypotension, infection, injection site reactions, nausea and vomiting, pain, pharyngitis, pruritus, rhinitis, tachycardia, and thrombosis. Many other side effects occurred in less than 1% of patients and may or may not be attributable to sodium ferric gluconate complex.

Post-Marketing: Anaphylaxis, convulsions, dysgeusia, hypoesthesia, loss of consciousness, pallor, phlebitis, shock, and skin discoloration have been identified. In addition, post-marketing reports have identified that individual doses exceeding 125 mg may result in a higher incidence and/or severity of side effects, including abdominal pain, chest pain, diarrhea, dizziness, dyspnea, hypotension, nausea, paresthesia, peripheral swelling, and urticaria.

Overdose: Serum iron levels greater than 300 mcg/dL may indicate iron poisoning. May result in hemosiderosis, and excess iron may increase susceptibility to infection. If acute toxicity is seen, it may present as abdominal pain, diarrhea, or vomiting progressing to pallor or cyanosis, lassitude, drowsiness, hyperventilation due to acidosis, iatrogenic hemosiderosis, and cardiovascular collapse.

ANTIDOTE

Reduce rate or temporarily discontinue infusion for hypotension; volume expanders (e.g., albumin, hetastarch [Hespan]) may be indicated. Restart when resolved. Discontinue drug and treat hypersensitivity reactions or resuscitate as necessary; notify physician. Epinephrine (Adrenalin) and diphenhydramine (Benadryl) should always be available. In overdose, monitor CBC, iron studies, vital signs, blood gases, and glucose and electrolytes. Maintain fluid and electrolyte balance. Correct acidosis with sodium bicarbonate. Iron complex is not dialyzable.

SODIUM PHENYLACETATE AND SODIUM BENZOATE

Ammonia detoxicant

(**SO**-dee-um fen-ill-**AH**-seh-tate and **SO**-dee-um **BEN**-zoh-ate)

Ammonul

pH 6 to 8

USUAL DOSE

Must be diluted and administered through a central line. Administration through a peripheral line may cause burns. Given in combination with arginine (dose is dependent on the specific urea cycle disorder [UCD] and is contraindicated in patients with arginase deficiency); see Dilution, Rate of Administration, Precautions, and Monitor. Urea cycle disorders can result from decreased activity of any of the following enzymes: *N*-acetylglutamate synthetase (NAGS), carbamyl phosphate synthetase (CPS), argininosuccinate synthetase (ASS), ornithine transcarbamylase (OTC), argininosuccinate lyase (ASL), or arginase (ARG); dose and treatment may vary for each. Sodium phenylacetate and sodium benzoate (AMMONUL) infusion should be started as soon as the diagnosis of hyperammonemia is made.

Discontinue analogous oral drugs (e.g., sodium phenylbutyrate [Buphenyl]) before sodium phenylacetate and sodium benzoate (AMMONUL) infusion.

A **loading dose** as an infusion is administered over 90 to 120 minutes, followed by an **equivalent maintenance dose** as an infusion administered over 24 hours. Treatment also requires caloric supplementation and restriction of dietary protein. Nonprotein calories should be supplied principally as glucose (8 to 10 mg/kg/min), with intravenous fat (e.g., Intralipid) added to maintain a caloric intake of greater than 80 cal/kg/day.

The dose of sodium phenylacetate and sodium benzoate (AMMONUL) is based on mg/kg in neonates, infants, and younger pediatric patients weighing up to 20 kg and on body surface area for older pediatric patients, adolescents, and adults weighing more than 20 kg as described in the following chart.

Dose and Administration Guidelines for Sodium Phenylacetate and Sodium Benzoate (AMMONUL)					
Patient Population	Components of Infusion Solution AMMONUL must be diluted with D10W at equal to or greater than 25 mL/kg before administration		Dosage Provided		
	Ammonul	Arginine HCl Injection, 10%	Sodium Phenylacetate	Sodium Benzoate	Arginine HCl
WEIGHT EQUAL TO OR LESS THAN 20 KG:					
CPS and OTC Deficiency					
Loading dose: Over 90 to 120 minutes **Maintenance:** Over 24 hours	2.5 mL/kg	2 mL/kg	250 mg/kg	250 mg/kg	200 mg/kg
ASS and ASL Deficiency					
Loading dose: Over 90 to 120 minutes **Maintenance:** Over 24 hours	2.5 mL/kg	6 mL/kg	250 mg/kg	250 mg/kg	600 mg/kg

Dose and Administration Guidelines for Sodium Phenylacetate and Sodium Benzoate (AMMONUL)—cont'd					
Patient Population	Components of Infusion Solution AMMONUL must be diluted with D10W at equal to or greater than 25 mL/kg before administration	Dosage Provided			
	Ammonul	Arginine HCl Injection, 10%	Sodium Phenylacetate	Sodium Benzoate	Arginine HCl
WEIGHT MORE THAN 20 KG:					
CPS and OTC Deficiency					
Loading dose: Over 90 to 120 minutes **Maintenance:** Over 24 hours	55 mL/M^2	2 mL/kg	5.5 Gm/M^2	5.5 Gm/M^2	200 mg/kg
ASS and ASL Deficiency					
Loading dose: Over 90 to 120 minutes **Maintenance:** Over 24 hours	55 mL/M^2	6 mL/kg	5.5 Gm/M^2	5.5 Gm/M^2	600 mg/kg

Repeat loading doses should not be administered because plasma levels achieved by phenylacetate are prolonged. Continue maintenance infusions until elevated plasma ammonia levels have been normalized or oral nutrition and medications can be tolerated. Mean duration of treatment was 4.6 days per episode and ranged from 1 to 72 days.

DOSE ADJUSTMENTS
No specific recommendations; see Precautions.

DILUTION
Must be diluted with D10W. Do not administer undiluted product.
Loading dose: Dilute with an amount of D10W equal to or more than 25 mL/kg of body weight per dose.
Equivalent maintenance dose: Also requires dilution with an amount of D10W equal to or more than 25 mL/kg of body weight per dose.
  A 4-kg neonate would require a minimum of 100 mL of D10W for dilution of the loading dose given over 90 to 120 minutes and a minimum of 100 mL of D10W for dilution of the maintenance dose given over 24 hours. An 80-kg adult would require a minimum of 2,000 mL of D10W for dilution of the loading dose over 90 to 120 minutes and a minimum of 2,000 mL D10W for dilution of the maintenance dose given over 24 hours.
Filters: Use of a 0.22-micron filter has been used to inject Ammonul into D10W.
Storage: Store unopened vials at CRT. Diluted solutions are stable at CRT and room lighting conditions for up to 24 hours.

COMPATIBILITY
May be mixed in the same container with 10% arginine HCl injection. Manufacturer states, "Other infusion solutions and drug products should not be administered together with sodium phenylacetate and sodium benzoate." May be prepared in glass or PVC containers.

RATE OF ADMINISTRATION
Loading dose infusion rates are relatively high, especially for infants; monitor closely.
Loading dose: A single dose properly diluted as an infusion and equally distributed over 90 to 120 minutes.
Maintenance dose: Each single dose properly diluted as an infusion and equally distributed over 24 hours.

ACTIONS

Sodium phenylacetate and sodium benzoate are metabolically active compounds that can provide an alternative pathway for nitrogen disposal in patients without a fully functioning urea cycle. Two moles of nitrogen are removed per mole of phenylacetate when it is conjugated with glutamine, and one mole of nitrogen is removed per mole of benzoate when it is conjugated with glycine. Has been shown to decrease elevated plasma ammonia levels. Considered to be the result of the reduction in nitrogen overload through glutamine and glycine scavenging by sodium phenylacetate and sodium benzoate (AMMONUL) in combination with appropriate dietary and other supportive measures.
Phenylacetate: Conjugates with glutamine in the liver and kidneys to form phenylacetylglutamine. It is then excreted by the kidneys via glomerular filtration and tubular secretion. Each mole of phenylacetylglutamine contains two moles of waste nitrogen. The nitrogen content of phenylacetylglutamine per mole is identical to that of urea (2 moles of nitrogen). Plasma levels remain higher and are present for a longer period of time than plasma levels of benzoate.
Benzoate: Conjugates with glycine to form hippuric acid, which is rapidly excreted by the kidneys by glomerular filtration and tubular secretion. One mole of hippuric acid contains one mole of waste nitrogen. The formation of hippurate from benzoate occurs more rapidly than that of phenylacetylglutamine from phenylacetate, and the rate of elimination of hippurate appears to be more rapid than that of phenylacetylglutamine.

INDICATIONS AND USES

Adjunctive therapy for the treatment of acute hyperammonemia and associated encephalopathy in adult and pediatric patients with deficiencies in enzymes of the urea cycle. UCDs can result from decreased activity of any of the following enzymes: N-acetylglutamate synthetase (NAGS), carbamyl phosphate synthetase (CPS), argininosuccinate synthetase (ASS), ornithine transcarbamylase (OTC), argininosuccinate lyase (ASL), or arginase (ARG). In acute hyperammonemic episodes, arginine supplementation, caloric supplementation, dietary protein restriction, hemodialysis, and other ammonia-lowering therapies should be considered.

CONTRAINDICATIONS

Manufacturer states, "None."

PRECAUTIONS

For IV infusion only. Must be infused through a central line. Administration through a peripheral line may cause burns. ▪ Acute symptomatic hyperammonemia should be treated as a life-threatening emergency. Treatment may require hemodialysis to remove a large burden of ammonia. Uncontrolled hyperammonemia can rapidly result in brain damage or death, and prompt use of all therapies necessary to reduce ammonia levels is essential. ▪ Administered under the direction of a physician knowledgeable in its use and in the treatment of diseases resulting from inborn errors in metabolism. Should be administered in a facility with adequate diagnostic and treatment facilities to monitor the patient and respond to any medical emergency. In addition, facilities for hemodialysis, nutritional support, and medical support are required. ▪ Patients with a large ammonia burden or patients who are not responsive to sodium phenylacetate and sodium benzoate (AMMONUL) require aggressive therapy, including hemodialysis. ▪ Metabolized in the liver and kidneys and excreted by the kidneys. Use caution in patients with impaired renal or hepatic function. ▪ Use with extreme caution, if at all, in patients with CHF or severe renal insufficiency and in clinical states where there is sodium retention with edema; contains 30.5 mg of sodium/mL of undiluted product; see Antidote. ▪ Bioavailability of both benzoate and phenylacetate may be slightly higher in females than in males. ▪ See Monitor, Maternal/Child, and Drug/Lab Interactions.

Monitor: Plasma and urine amino acid analyses are used to diagnose ASS and ASL and to provide a preliminary diagnosis of CPS, OTC, or ARG. Blood citrulline levels are very low or absent in OTC and CPS, very high in ASS, and normal to moderately high in ASL and ARG. High urine levels of an unusual amino acid (argininosuccinic acid [ASA]) may distinguish ASL; however, ASA may be difficult to detect on initial examination. Specific studies are required to separate it from other amino acids. ARG is characterized by high urine levels of arginine. A liver biopsy is indicated for definitive diagnosis of CPS and OTC. RBC enzyme analysis is needed to confirm a diagnosis of ARG. ■ Monitor catheter infusion site closely. Extravasation may lead to skin necrosis. If extravasation is suspected, discontinue the infusion and, if necessary, resume at a different site. ■ Monitor plasma ammonia, glutamine, quantitative plasma amino acids, blood glucose, ABGs, AST, and ALT during and after infusion. ■ Ongoing assessment of clinical response includes monitoring of neurologic status, Glasgow Coma Scale, tachypnea, CT or MRI scan or fundoscopic evidence of cerebral edema, and/or gray matter and white matter damage. In patients responding to therapy, mean ammonia levels decreased significantly within 4 hours of initiation of therapy. ■ May be used in combination with dialysis. Hemodialysis is the most commonly used and can either be instituted immediately while waiting for a more definitive diagnosis or used as a recommended addition to treatment for those patients who fail to have a significant reduction in plasma ammonia levels within 4 to 8 hours after receiving sodium phenylacetate and sodium benzoate (AMMONUL). High levels of ammonia can be reduced quickly when sodium phenylacetate and sodium benzoate (AMMONUL) is used with dialysis. The ammonia scavenging of sodium phenylacetate and sodium benzoate (AMMONUL) suppresses the production of ammonia from catabolism of endogenous protein, and dialysis eliminates the ammonia and ammonia conjugates. ■ Monitor serum electrolytes and maintain within normal range. Monitor plasma potassium levels carefully and treat as indicated; urine potassium loss is enhanced by excretion of the nonresorbable anions phenylacetylglutamine and hippurate. ■ May cause side effects associated with salicylate overdose (e.g., hyperventilation, metabolic acidosis). Obtain baseline and monitor blood chemistry profiles, blood pH, and Pco$_2$. ■ Use with high-dose arginine may cause hyperchloremic acidosis. Obtain baseline and monitor chloride and bicarbonate levels; administer bicarbonate as indicated. ■ Use prophylactic antiemetics to reduce nausea and vomiting. ■ Neurotoxicity has been reported (e.g., disorientation, exacerbation of a preexisting neuropathy, fatigue, headaches, hypoacusis [partial loss of hearing], impaired memory, light-headedness, somnolence). Onset may be acute, and symptoms should improve when therapy is discontinued. ■ Closely monitor patients with impaired renal function; drug therapy may be less effective due to poor clearance of drug metabolites and, subsequently, ammonia. ■ See Precautions, Maternal/Child, and Drug/Lab Interactions.

Patient Education: Compliance with dietary restrictions and supplemental medications is imperative. ■ Obtain identification (e.g., a bracelet) with UCD diagnosis.

Maternal/Child: Category C: use during pregnancy and/or labor and delivery only if clearly needed. Effects on fetus unknown. ■ Not known if it is secreted in human milk; use caution if required during breast-feeding. Has the potential for serious harm to infant. ■ Is used as a treatment for acute hyperammonemia in pediatric patients, including patients in the early neonatal period. ■ The most commonly presented symptoms of UCD in neonates include edema, lethargy, neurologic changes, poor feeding, respiratory distress, and seizures. Milder forms of UCDs may not present until late childhood, adolescence, or adulthood. Symptoms, including hyperammonemic crisis with coma, delirium, and/or lethargy, are often precipitated by viral illness, high-protein diet, stress, or trauma.

Elderly: Relevant information not available. Oldest patient in studies was 53 years of age. Average age in studies was 8.54 years. ■ Monitoring of renal and hepatic function is suggested.

DRUG/LAB INTERACTIONS

Formal drug interaction studies have not been performed. ■ Concurrent use with **corticosteroids** (e.g., dexamethasone [Decadron]) may cause the breakdown of body protein and increase plasma ammonia levels in patients with an impaired ability to form urea. ■ Some **antibiotics** (e.g., penicillin) may compete with phenylacetylglutamine and hippurate for active secretion by renal tubules. This competition may affect the overall disposition of either of the infused drugs. ▪ **Probenecid** is known to inhibit the renal transport of many drugs and may inhibit the renal excretion of phenylacetylglutamine and hippurate, reducing its effectiveness. ▪ **Valproic acid** has been reported to induce hyperammonemia. Administration to patients with UCD may exacerbate their condition and antagonize the effectiveness of sodium phenylacetate and sodium benzoate (AMMONUL).

SIDE EFFECTS

The most commonly reported side effects include convulsions, hyperglycemia, hypokalemia, mental impairment, and vomiting. Acidosis, agitation, anemia, coma, diarrhea, DIC, edema of the brain, fever, hyperammonemia, hypocalcemia, hypotension, injection site reactions, metabolic acidosis, nausea, respiratory distress, and urinary tract infections were also reported frequently. Injection site reactions and metabolic acidosis were dose-limiting reactions in several patients. Incidence and severity of side effects tend to be increased in patients with enzyme deficiencies occurring earlier in the urea cycle (i.e., OTC and CPS). Incidence of side effects was also specific to age and diagnosis as follows.

Pediatric patients 30 days of age or less: Blood and lymphatic system disorders (e.g., anemia, DIC) and hypotension.

Patients more than 30 days of age: GI disorders (e.g., diarrhea, nausea, and vomiting).

Patients with OTC, ASS, CPS, and diagnoses characterized as other: Side effects were primarily the ones most frequently reported.

Patients with OTC and CPS: Nervous system disorders (e.g., coma, convulsions, edema of the brain, mental impairment) were most common.

Overdose: Cardiovascular collapse, encephalopathy (progressive), hypernatremia, hyperosmolarity, hyperventilation, large anion gap, metabolic acidosis (severe and compensated) with a respiratory component, obtundation (in the absence of hyperammonemia), and death. Causes of death from overdose were cardiorespiratory failure/arrest, error in dialysis procedure, hyperammonemia, hypotension (intractable) with probable sepsis, increased intracranial pressure, pneumonitis with septic shock and coagulopathy.

ANTIDOTE

Keep physician informed of all side effects. Many may be life threatening and immediate, and appropriate treatment is required. If an adverse reaction occurs due to sodium content, discontinue infusion, evaluate the patient, and treat as indicated. If extravasation is suspected, discontinue the infusion and, if necessary, resume at a different site. Treat extravasation by aspirating the residual drug from the catheter, elevating the limb (if a limb is involved), and applying intermittent cold packs. If overdose occurs, discontinue the drug, and monitor and treat as indicated by symptoms. In severe cases, hemodialysis (procedure of choice) and/or peritoneal dialysis (when hemodialysis is not available) may be indicated. Resuscitate as indicated.

SOTALOL HYDROCHLORIDE BBW
(**SO**-tuh-lol hy-droh-**KLOR**-eyed)

Beta-adrenergic blocking agent
Antiarrhythmic

pH 6 to 7

USUAL DOSE
To minimize the risk of induced arrhythmia, patients initiated or reinitiated on sotalol and patients who are converted from IV to oral administration should be hospitalized in a facility that can provide cardiac resuscitation and continuous ECG monitoring. CrCl must be greater than 60 mL/min. Baseline studies and correction of electrolyte abnormalities required before initiating therapy; see Precautions, Monitor, and Dose Adjustments.

Initial dose: 75 mg twice daily. If symptomatic arrhythmia is not controlled and dose is tolerated without excessive QTc prolongation (i.e., greater than 500 msec), may increase dose to 112.5 mg twice daily after 3 days. Continuous ECG monitoring required during dose escalation.

Dose for ventricular arrhythmias: 75 mg twice daily. Dose may be increased in increments of 75 mg/day every 3 days. Usual therapeutic effect is seen with doses of 75 to 150 mg twice daily. However, doses as high as 225 to 300 mg have been required in patients with refractory life-threatening arrhythmias.

Dose for symptomatic atrial fibrillation/atrial flutter (AFIB/AFL): 112.5 mg twice daily was found to be the most effective dose in studies. If symptomatic arrhythmia is not controlled and this dose is tolerated without excessive QTc prolongation (i.e., greater than 520 msec), increase dose to 150 mg twice daily.

Conversion from oral to intravenous sotalol: Patients who have been stabilized on oral sotalol and are unable to take oral medications may be converted to IV sotalol using the following conversion chart.

Conversion from Oral Sotalol to IV Sotalol	
Oral Dose	Intravenous Dose
80 mg	75 mg (5 mL sotalol injection)
120 mg	112.5 mg (7.5 mL sotalol injection)
160 mg	150 mg (10 mL sotalol injection)

DOSE ADJUSTMENTS
Increase dosing interval to every 24 hours in patients with a CrCl between 40 and 60 mL/min. Sotalol is not recommended in patients with a CrCl less than 40 mL/min. ■ Titrate dose upward or downward as needed based on clinical effect, QT interval, or adverse reactions as described in Usual Dose.

DILUTION
Available in vials containing 150 mg/10 mL. Dilute required dose with NS, D5W, or LR as described in the following chart.

S

Sotalol Infusion Preparation to Compensate for Dead Space in the Infusion Set				
Target Dose	Sotalol Injection	Diluent	Volume Prepared	Volume to Infuse
75 mg	6 mL	114 mL	120 mL	100 mL
112.5 mg	9 mL	111 mL		
150 mg	12 mL	108 mL		
75 mg	6 mL	294 mL	300 mL	250 mL
112.5 mg	9 mL	291 mL		
150 mg	12 mL	288 mL		

Storage: Store at CRT. Protect from light and freezing.

COMPATIBILITY

Specific information not available. Consult pharmacist; specific conditions may apply.

RATE OF ADMINISTRATION

A single dose equally distributed over 5 hours. Use of an infusion pump recommended.

ACTIONS

An antiarrhythmic with Class II (beta-adrenoreceptor blocking) and Class III (cardiac action potential duration prolongation) properties. The beta-blocking effect is noncardio-selective. Slows heart rate, decreases AV nodal conduction, and increases AV nodal refractoriness. ECG shows dose-related increase in QT and QTc. Produces a reduction in systolic and diastolic blood pressures and cardiac index and an increase in pulmonary capillary wedge pressure. Does not bind to plasma proteins and is not metabolized. Half-life is 12 hours. Excreted predominantly via the kidney in unchanged form. Crosses the placenta. Secreted in breast milk.

INDICATIONS AND USES

A substitute for oral sotalol in patients who are unable to take oral medications. ▪ Maintenance of normal sinus rhythm in patients with a history of highly symptomatic AFIB/AFL. ▪ Treatment of documented life-threatening ventricular arrhythmias.

CONTRAINDICATIONS

Bradycardia (HR below 50 beats/min), sick sinus syndrome, or second- or third-degree AV block unless a functioning pacemaker is present. ▪ Congenital or acquired long QT syndromes, QT interval greater than 450 msec. ▪ Cardiogenic shock, uncontrolled heart failure. ▪ CrCl less than 40 mL/min. ▪ Serum potassium less than 4 mEq/L. ▪ Bronchial asthma or related bronchospastic conditions. ▪ Known hypersensitivity to sotalol.

PRECAUTIONS

To minimize the risk of induced arrhythmia, patients initiated or reinitiated on sotalol and patients who are converted from IV to oral administration should be hospitalized for at least 3 days (or until steady-state drug levels are reached) in a facility that can provide cardiac resuscitation and continuous ECG monitoring. Personnel trained in the management of serious ventricular arrhythmias must be present. ▪ Can cause serious ventricular arrhythmias, primarily torsades de pointes (TdP), a polymorphic ventricular tachycardia associated with QTc prolongation. QTc prolongation is directly related to the concentration of sotalol. Factors that may increase the risk of TdP include a reduced CrCl, larger doses, female gender, sustained VT, and a history of cardiomegaly or CHF. ▪ The use of sotalol in conjunction with other drugs that prolong the QT interval has not been studied and is not recommended; see Drug/Lab Interactions. ▪ May cause bradycardia, which increases risk of TdP. ▪ Increased risk of TdP in patients with AFIB and sinus node dysfunction, especially after cardioversion. Sotalol increases bradycardia and QTc following cardioversion. ▪ Produces significant reductions in both systolic and diastolic BP. May cause deterioration in cardiac performance in patients with marginal cardiac compensation. ▪ Use caution in CHF. Beta blockade may depress myocardial contractility and precipitate or exacerbate heart failure. ▪ Use caution in the presence of heart failure controlled by digoxin. Both drugs slow AV conduction. ▪ Experience with use following acute MI is limited. Use caution, titrate dose carefully, and monitor patient closely. ▪ May cause angina, arrhythmia, or MI if discontinued abruptly; gradually reduce over 1 to 2 weeks if possible. ▪ May mask tachycardia occurring with hypoglycemia in diabetes and tachycardia of hyperthyroidism. ▪ In general, patients with bronchospastic disease should not receive beta-blockers. If sotalol is to be administered, use the smallest effective dose; see Contraindications. ▪ Use caution in patients with renal impairment; see Dose Adjustments. ▪ Patients with atrial fibrillation should be anticoagulated according to usual medical practice.

Monitor: Obtain baseline ECG to determine the QT interval. If baseline QT interval is greater than 450 msec, sotalol is not recommended. Monitor QT interval after the completion of each infusion. If the QT interval increases to 500 msec or greater, reduce the dose, decrease the infusion rate, or discontinue therapy. ▪ Measure and normalize serum potassium and magnesium levels before initiating therapy and as required during therapy. Pay special attention to electrolytes and acid-base status in patients with prolonged diarrhea or in patients receiving concomitant diuretics. ▪ Obtain baseline SCr and calculate CrCl to establish dosing interval. ▪ Monitor HR and BP. Monitor hemodynamics in patients with marginal cardiac compensation. ▪ In patients with life-threatening ventricular arrhythmias, the response to treatment should be evaluated by a suitable method (e.g., programmed electrical stimulation [PES] or Holter monitoring) at steady-state blood levels of the drug before continuing the patient on chronic therapy.

Patient Education: Do not discontinue therapy abruptly. ▪ Promptly report any breathing difficulty, syncope, or pain at injection site.

Maternal/Child: Category B: use during pregnancy only if clearly needed. ▪ Discontinue breast-feeding. ▪ Safety for use in pediatric patients not established. See prescribing information for unlabeled suggested oral doses for use in pediatric patients.

Elderly: Age-related differences in safety and effectiveness not identified; however, greater sensitivity of some elderly cannot be ruled out. Dose with caution, taking into account decreased renal function; see Dose Adjustments.

DRUG/LAB INTERACTIONS

Proarrhythmic events were more common in sotalol-treated patients also receiving **digoxin.** Unclear as to whether this is a drug interaction or is related to the presence of heart failure, which is a known risk factor for arrhythmias. ▪ Concurrent use with **calcium channel blockers** (e.g., diltiazem [Cardizem], verapamil) is expected to have additive effects on AV conduction, ventricular function, and BP. ▪ Beta-adrenergic blocking agents may be continued during the perioperative period in most patients; however, use caution with **selected anesthetic agents** that may depress the myocardium. Protracted severe hypotension and difficulty in restoring and maintaining normal cardiac rhythm after anesthesia have been reported. ▪ Concurrent use with **clonidine** may precipitate acute hypertension if one or both agents are stopped abruptly. ▪ Coadministration with **catecholamine-depleting drugs** (e.g., reserpine and guanethidine) may result in hypotension, bradycardia, vertigo, syncope, or orthostatic hypotension. ▪ Hyperglycemia may occur. Dosage of **insulin and other antidiabetic drugs** may require adjustment. ▪ Symptoms of **hypoglycemia may be masked.** ▪ Increased doses of **beta-agonists** such as albuterol, terbutaline, and isoproterenol may be required when administered concomitantly with sotalol. ▪ Patients taking **beta-blockers** who are exposed to a potential allergen may be unresponsive to the usual dose of epinephrine used to treat a hypersensitivity reaction. ▪ The use of sotalol in conjunction with other **drugs that prolong the QT interval** has not been studied and is not recommended. Such drugs include some phenothiazines (e.g., prochlorperazine [Compazine], promethazine [Phenergan]), tricyclic antidepressants (e.g., amitriptyline [Elavil], imipramine [Tofranil]), certain oral macrolides (e.g., erythromycin [E-Mycin], clarithromycin [Biaxin]), Class I antiarrhythmic (e.g., disopyramide [Norpace], procainamide [Pronestyl], quinidine), and Class III antiarrhythmics (e.g., amiodarone [Nexterone]). **Class I and III antiarrhythmic agents** should be withheld for at least three half-lives before dosing with sotalol. In studies, sotalol was not administered to patients who had been previously treated with **oral amiodarone** (Nexterone) for more than 1 month in the previous 3 months. ▪ Interactions with hydrochlorothiazide and warfarin were not observed. ▪ The presence of sotalol in the urine may result in **falsely elevated levels of urinary metanephrine** by certain methods.

SIDE EFFECTS

There is no clinical experience with IV sotalol. Side effects should be similar to those seen with oral sotalol therapy. The most common side effects (dose related) are asthenia, bradycardia, chest pain, dizziness, dyspnea, fatigue, headache, light-headedness, nausea, QT prolongation, and palpitations. Ventricular arrhythmia, primarily TdP, is the most common serious side effect. Other reported side effects include abdominal distension and pain, abnormal ECG, angina, bradycardia, cough, decreased appetite, diarrhea, dyspepsia, edema, fever, heart failure, hyperhidrosis, hypotension, infection, insomnia, musculoskeletal pain, tracheobronchitis, upper respiratory infection, visual disturbance, vomiting, and weakness. Other reactions have been reported.

Overdose: Bradycardia, bronchospasm, cardiac asystole, CHF, hypoglycemia, hypotension, premature ventricular complexes, prolongation of the QT interval, TdP, and ventricular arrhythmia.

ANTIDOTE

Notify physician of any side effects. If the QT interval increases to 500 msec or greater, reduce the dose, decrease the infusion rate, or discontinue therapy. Atropine, another anticholinergic drug, a beta-adrenergic agonist, or transvenous cardiac pacing may be used to treat bradycardia or cardiac asystole. A transvenous cardiac pacemaker may be required for second- or third-degree heart block. Epinephrine may be useful for treatment of hypotension. Aminophylline or aerosol beta-2–receptor stimulants (e.g., albuterol) may be useful for treatment of bronchospasm. DC cardioversion, magnesium sulfate, and potassium replacement may be required for treatment of TdP. Once TdP is terminated, transvenous cardiac pacing or an isoproterenol infusion may be used to increase heart rate.

STREPTOZOCIN BBW
(strep-toe-**ZOH**-sin)

Zanosar

Antineoplastic
(alkylating agent/nitrosurea)

pH 3.5 to 4.5

USUAL DOSE
500 mg/M^2 for 5 consecutive days; see Monitor. Repeat every 6 weeks until maximum benefit or treatment-limiting toxicity observed. May also give 1,000 mg/M^2 weekly for 2 doses. May then increase up to 1,500 mg/M^2 to achieve therapeutic response if significant toxicity not observed. Overall cumulative dose to onset of response is 2,000 mg/M^2. Maximum response is usually achieved with 4,000 mg/M^2 total cumulative dose.

DOSE ADJUSTMENTS
Reduce dose in impaired renal function; see Precautions/Monitor. ▪ Reduce dose or discontinue drug if mild proteinuria occurs. Lower-end initial doses may be appropriate in the elderly; consider the potential for decreased organ function and concomitant disease or drug therapy. ▪ Can be used with other antineoplastic drugs in reduced doses to achieve tumor remission.

DILUTION
Specific techniques required; see Precautions. Each 1-Gm vial must be diluted with 9.5 mL NS or D5W (100 mg/mL). Usually further diluted in larger amounts (50 to 250 mL) of the same solutions.

Storage: Store in refrigerator before and after dilution. Discard within 12 hours of dilution. Contains no preservatives. Protect from light.

COMPATIBILITY
Consider any drug NOT listed as compatible to be INCOMPATIBLE until consulting a pharmacist; specific conditions may apply.

One source suggests the following **compatibilities:**

Y-site: Amifostine (Ethyol), etoposide phosphate (Etopophos), filgrastim (Neupogen), gemcitabine (Gemzar), granisetron (Kytril), melphalan (Alkeran), ondansetron (Zofran), teniposide (Vumon), thiotepa, vinorelbine (Navelbine).

RATE OF ADMINISTRATION
A single dose in minimum diluent given over 5 to 15 minutes is recommended. Increase injection time somewhat if additional diluent used or if indicated for patient comfort. Has been given as a continuous infusion over 5 days. Some side effects may be reduced, but CNS side effects (e.g., confusion, depression, lethargy) may be increased.

ACTIONS
An alkylating agent of the nitrosurea group with antitumor activity, cell cycle phase nonspecific. Has a diabetogenic (hyperglycemic) effect resulting from selective uptake into and toxicity to pancreatic islet beta cells. Disappears from the blood rapidly. Concentrates in the liver and kidneys. Excreted primarily in urine.

INDICATIONS AND USES
Suppress or retard neoplastic growth in metastatic pancreatic islet cell carcinoma. Use limited by renal toxicity to those with symptomatic or progressive metastatic disease.

Unlabeled uses: Treatment of adrenocortical and colon cancers and Hodgkin's lymphoma.

CONTRAINDICATIONS
Hypersensitivity to streptozocin. Severely impaired liver or renal function may be a contraindication.

PRECAUTIONS
Follow guidelines for handling cytotoxic agents. See Appendix A, p. 1331. ▪ Administered by or under the direction of the physician specialist. ▪ Adequate diagnostic and treatment facilities must be readily available. ▪ Consider risk of known toxic effects versus benefit before initiating therapy. ▪ Marked decrease in leukocyte and platelet counts has occurred and may be fatal. ▪ Risk of nephrotoxicity may be reduced by decreasing renal and urinary concentration of strep-

S

tozocin and its metabolites with adequate hydration. ▪ Avoid concomitant use with other potential nephrotoxins (e.g., aminoglycosides [e.g., gentamicin], amphotericin B). ▪ Liver dysfunction and diarrhea have been observed in some patients.

Monitor: Renal toxicity is dose related, cumulative, and can be fatal. Monitor renal function before, weekly, and for 4 weeks after each course of therapy (serial urinalysis, BUN, plasma creatinine, serum electrolytes, CrCl). Reduce dose or discontinue drug if mild proteinuria occurs. Further deterioration of renal function may occur; see Precautions. ▪ Determine absolute patency and quality of vein and adequate circulation of extremity. Local inflammation (e.g., burning, edema, erythema, tenderness), severe cellulitis, and/or necrosis may result from extravasation. If extravasation occurs, discontinue injection; use another vein. ▪ Have IV dextrose available especially with the first dose. Sudden release of insulin may precipitate hypoglycemia. Monitor serum glucose at periodic intervals. ▪ Monitor CBC and liver function tests weekly. ▪ Nausea and vomiting have occurred in all patients and can be severe. Prophylactic administration of antiemetics recommended. ▪ Observe for any signs of infection. Use of prophylactic antibiotics may be indicated pending results of C/S in a febrile neutropenic patient. ▪ Maintain hydration; see Precautions. ▪ Monitor for thrombocytopenia (platelet count less than 50,000/mm³). Initiate precautions to prevent excessive bleeding (e.g., inspect IV sites, skin, and mucous membranes; use extreme care during invasive procedures; test urine, emesis, stool, and secretions for occult blood). ▪ See Drug/Lab Interactions.

Patient Education: Avoid pregnancy; nonhormonal birth control recommended. ▪ Report IV site burning or stinging promptly. ▪ Use caution in tasks that require alertness, such as driving or using complex machinery. ▪ See Appendix D, p. 1333.

Maternal/Child: Category D: avoid pregnancy. Produces teratogenic effects in rats. Has mutagenic potential. ▪ Discontinue breast-feeding.

Elderly: Differences in response compared to younger adults not observed. Lower-end initial doses may be appropriate; see Dose Adjustments.

DRUG/LAB INTERACTIONS

Do not administer **live virus vaccines** to patients receiving antineoplastic drugs. ▪ Concurrent use with **hepatotoxic or nephrotoxic medications and radiation therapy** may increase toxicity and could be fatal. ▪ Toxicity may be additive when used in combination with **other cytotoxic drugs** (e.g., cyclophosphamide [Cytoxan], doxorubicin [Adriamycin, Doxil]). ▪ May prolong the elimination half-life of **doxorubicin** and lead to severe bone marrow suppression. A reduced dose of doxorubicin may be indicated. ▪ Concurrent use with **phenytoin** (Dilantin) may decrease therapeutic effects of streptozocin.

SIDE EFFECTS

Anemia, decreased platelet count (precipitous), diarrhea, elevated AST and LDH, hepatic toxicity (usually reversible), hypoalbuminemia, hypoglycemia, insulin shock, leukopenia (precipitous), nausea and vomiting (severe), proteinuria, thrombocytopenia. Two cases of diabetes insipidus have been reported.

ANTIDOTE

Notify physician of all side effects. Nausea and vomiting, hematologic changes, and renal toxicity (proteinuria) may require dose reduction or discontinuation of the drug. There is no specific antidote. Supportive therapy as indicated will help sustain the patient in toxicity. Administration of whole blood products (e.g., packed RBCs, platelets, leukocytes) and/or blood modifiers (e.g., darbepoetin alfa [Aranesp], epoetin alfa [Epogen], filgrastim [Neupogen, Zarxio], pegfilgrastim [Neulasta], sargramostim [Leukine]) may be indicated to treat bone marrow toxicity. For extravasation, elevate extremity, consider injection of long-acting dexamethasone (Decadron LA) throughout extravasated tissue. Use a 27- or 25-gauge needle. Apply warm, moist compresses.

SUGAMMADEX
(soo-**GAM**-ma-dex)

Antidote
Selective relaxant binding agent

Bridion

pH 7 to 8

USUAL DOSE
A peripheral nerve stimulator should be used to determine when sugammadex should be initiated. Doses and timing of sugammadex administration should be based on monitoring for twitch responses and the extent of spontaneous recovery that has occurred. Before sugammadex administration and up until complete recovery of neuromuscular function, the patient should be well ventilated and a patent airway maintained. The recommended dose of sugammadex does not depend on the anesthetic regimen. Sugammadex can be used to reverse different levels of rocuronium-induced or vecuronium-induced neuromuscular blockade. Base dose on actual body weight.

For rocuronium and vecuronium: *Deep blockade:* 4 mg/kg as a single IV bolus injection is recommended if spontaneous recovery of the twitch response has reached 1 to 2 posttetanic counts (PTCs) and there are no twitch responses to train-of-four (TOF) stimulation following neuromuscular blockade.

Moderate blockade: 2 mg/kg as a single IV bolus injection is recommended if spontaneous recovery has reached the reappearance of the second twitch (T_2) in response to TOF stimulation following neuromuscular blockade.

Immediate reversal of rocuronium only: 16 mg/kg as a single IV bolus injection is recommended if there is a clinical need to reverse neuromuscular blockade soon (approximately 3 minutes) after administration of a single dose of 1.2 mg/kg rocuronium. The efficacy of the 16 mg/kg dose following administration of vecuronium has not been studied.

DOSE ADJUSTMENTS
Individualize dose based on extent of spontaneous recovery at time of administration (rocuronium and vecuronium) and whether there is a need to rapidly reverse the neuromuscular blocking agent (rocuronium only). ▪ Use of lower than recommended doses of sugammadex may lead to an increased risk of recurrence of neuromuscular blockade after initial reversal and is not recommended. ▪ No dose adjustment is recommended in patients with mild to moderate renal impairment. Sugammadex is not recommended for use in patients with severe renal impairment. ▪ No dose adjustment is recommended in patients with hepatic impairment, pulmonary complications, or cardiac disease (e.g., patients with ischemic heart disease, chronic heart failure, cardiac arrhythmias); see Precautions.

DILUTION
Available as a 100 mg/mL solution in a 2- or 5-mL single-dose vial. Solution is clear and colorless to slightly yellow-brown. Withdraw the calculated dose and inject into the IV line of a running infusion.

Filters: No data available from the manufacturer.

Storage: Store at CRT. Protect from light. If not protected from light, the vial must be used within 5 days.

COMPATIBILITY
May inject into the IV line of a running infusion with the following IV solutions: NS, D5W, D2.5/¹/₂NS, D5NS, Isolyte P in D5W, RL, and Ringer's solution. Flush line with a **compatible** solution (e.g., NS) before and after administration of sugammadex. Manufacturer states that sugammadex should not be administered with other products and that it is physically **incompatible** with ondansetron (Zofran), ranitidine (Zantac), and verapamil.

RATE OF ADMINISTRATION
Administer intravenously as a single bolus injection over 10 seconds. May administer into an existing IV line. Flush line with a **compatible** solution (e.g., NS) before and after administration of sugammadex.

ACTIONS

A modified gamma-cyclodextrin. Sugammadex forms a complex with rocuronium and vecuronium, thereby reducing the amount of neuromuscular blocking agent (NMBA) available to bind to nicotinic cholinergic receptors in the neuromuscular junction. This results in the reversal of neuromuscular blockade induced by rocuronium and vecuronium. Neither sugammadex nor the complex of sugammadex and the NMBA binds to plasma proteins or erythrocytes. Sugammadex is not metabolized by the liver. No metabolites of sugammadex have been observed, and the only route of elimination observed is renal excretion of the unchanged product. Elimination half-life is about 2 hours.

INDICATIONS AND USES

Reversal of the neuromuscular blockade induced by rocuronium bromide and vecuronium bromide in adults undergoing surgery.

Limitation of use: Sugammadex has not been studied for reversal following rocuronium or vecuronium administration in the ICU. ▪ Sugammadex should not be used to reverse neuromuscular blockade induced by nonsteroidal NMBAs such as succinylcholine or benzylisoquinolinium compounds (e.g., atracurium, cisatracurium, mivacurium) or to reverse neuromuscular blockade induced by steroidal NMBAs other than rocuronium or vecuronium.

CONTRAINDICATIONS

Known hypersensitivity to sugammadex or any of its components.

PRECAUTIONS

For IV administration only. ▪ Should be administered by a trained health care provider familiar with the use, actions, characteristics, and complications of NMBAs and neuromuscular block reversal agents. ▪ Ventilatory support is mandatory for patients until adequate spontaneous respiration is restored and the ability to maintain a patent airway is ensured. Should neuromuscular blockade persist after sugammadex administration or recur following extubation, appropriate steps should be taken to provide adequate ventilation. ▪ Because of the possibility of hypersensitivity reactions or cardiovascular events, medications and equipment to monitor the patient and respond to any medical emergency should be readily available. ▪ Hypersensitivity reactions have occurred in patients treated with sugammadex and can range from isolated skin reactions to serious systemic reactions (i.e., anaphylaxis, anaphylactic shock). Anaphylaxis has resulted in prolonged hospitalization, the use of vasopressors for circulatory support, and/or the use of additional respiratory support until full recovery (reintubation, prolonged intubation, manual or mechanical ventilation). Hypersensitivity reactions can be fatal. ▪ Cases of marked bradycardia, some of which have resulted in cardiac arrest, have been observed within minutes after the administration of sugammadex. ▪ Delayed or minimal response to sugammadex has been reported in a small number of patients. ▪ A minimum waiting time is necessary before administration of a steroidal neuromuscular blocking agent after the administration of sugammadex. After reversal with up to 4 mg/kg of sugammadex, a minimum waiting time of 5 minutes is required before a dose of 1.2 mg/kg of rocuronium can be readministered. When this dose of rocuronium is administered within 30 minutes of sugammadex administration, the onset of the neuromuscular blockade may be delayed up to approximately 4 minutes, and the duration of neuromuscular blockade may be shortened by up to approximately 15 minutes. ▪ After reversal with up to 4 mg/kg of sugammadex, a minimum waiting time of 4 hours is required before a dose of 0.6 mg/kg of rocuronium or 0.1 mg/kg of vecuronium can be readministered. This wait time should be extended to 24 hours in patients with mild or moderate renal impairment. If a shorter wait time is required, the rocuronium dose for a new neuromuscular blockade should be increased to 1.2 mg/kg. ▪ After administration of a 16 mg/kg dose of sugammadex, a waiting time of 24 hours is suggested before readministration of rocuronium or administration of vecuronium. ▪ If neuromuscular blockade is required before the recommended waiting time has elapsed, a nonsteroidal NMBA (e.g., cisatricurium or mivacurium) should be used. ▪ The onset of a depolarizing NMBA (e.g., succinylcholine) may be slower than expected because a substantial fraction of postjunctional nicotinic receptors can still be occupied by the NMBA. ▪ Has been associated with increases in aPTT and PT/INR of up to 25% for up to 1 hour. Patients receiving thromboprophylaxis with heparin or low-molecular-weight heparin (LMWH) who received 4 mg/kg of sugammadex did not experience an increased incidence of blood loss or anemia. Higher doses of sugammadex, thromboprophylaxis with agents other than heparin or LMWH, and patients receiving therapeutic anticoagulation were not studied. ▪ Use with caution in patients with hepatic impairment accompanied by coagulopathy. ▪ Sugammadex is not recommended for use in patients with severe renal impairment, including those requiring dialysis. ▪ See Drug/Lab Interactions.

Monitor: Obtain baseline SCr. ▪ Monitor the patient to ensure adequate ventilation and maintenance of a patent airway. Even if recovery from neuromuscular blockade is complete, other drugs used in the perioperative and postoperative period could depress respiratory function and necessitate the need for continued ventilator support. ▪ A peripheral nerve stimulation device capable of delivering a train-of-four (TOF) stimulus is required. ▪ TOF monitoring alone should not be relied on to determine the adequacy of neuromuscular blockade reversal as related to a patient's ability to adequately ventilate and maintain a patent airway following tracheal extubation. Satisfactory recovery should be determined through the assessment of skeletal muscle tone and respiratory measurements in addition to the response to the peripheral nerve stimulator. ▪ Monitor for S/S of a hypersensitivity reaction. The most commonly reported hypersensitivity reactions were nausea, pruritus, and urticaria. Other reported hypersensitivity reactions have included bronchospasm, conjunctival edema, dermatologic reactions (erythema, flushing, rash, skin eruption), reduction in peak expiratory flow, and swelling of the pharynx, tongue, and/or uvula. ▪ Monitor for hemodynamic changes during and after reversal of neuromuscular blockade; see Antidote. ▪ Monitor coagulation parameters (e.g., aPTT, PT/INR) in patients with known coagulopathies, patients being treated with therapeutic anticoagulation, patients receiving thromboprophylaxis drugs other than heparin or LMWH, or patients receiving any thromboprophylaxis drugs and sugammadex at a dose of 16 mg/kg.

Patient Education: May reduce the efficacy of hormonal contraceptives. Women of reproductive potential who are using hormonal contraceptives should use an additional, nonhormonal contraceptive (e.g., condom, spermicide) for 7 days following sugammadex administration.

Maternal/Child: Use during pregnancy only if clearly needed. ▪ Use caution during breast-feeding. ▪ Safety and efficacy in pediatric patients have not been established.

Elderly: Dose adjustment is not generally needed in elderly patients with normal organ function, but an extended monitoring period to ensure complete reversal may be warranted. Risk of adverse events may be greater in patients with renal impairment. May be useful to monitor renal function.

DRUG/LAB INTERACTIONS

Toremifene (Fareston) has a high binding affinity for sugammadex. May cause displacement of vecuronium and rocuronium from the complex with sugammadex, thereby decreasing the effectiveness of sugammadex. Monitor for recurrence of neuromuscular blockade. ▪ Sugammadex may bind to **progestogen**, thereby decreasing progestogen exposure and effectiveness. Patients using **hormonal forms of contraception** (oral and nonoral) who receive sugammadex must use an additional, nonhormonal contraceptive method or backup method of contraception for the next 7 days. ▪ Sugammadex may interfere with the **serum progesterone assay**.

SIDE EFFECTS

The most common side effects are headache, hypotension, nausea, pain, and vomiting. Other side effects include abnormal QT interval, airway complication of anesthesia, anesthetic complication, anxiety, bradycardia, chills, cough, decreased red blood cell count, depression, dizziness, dry mouth, erythema, fever, flatulence, hypersensitivity reactions (including anaphylaxis), hypertension, hypocalcemia, hypoesthesia, increased blood creatine phosphokinase, insomnia, myalgia, procedural complications, pruritus, recurrence of prolonged neuromuscular blockade, restlessness, tachycardia, and wound hemorrhage.

Post-Marketing: Bradycardia, cardiac arrest, cardiac arrhythmias, dyspnea, hypersensitivity reactions (including anaphylaxis), laryngospasm, pulmonary edema, respiratory arrest, and wheezing.

ANTIDOTE

Treat anaphylaxis immediately with oxygen, epinephrine (Adrenalin), antihistamines (e.g., diphenhydramine [Benadryl]), vasopressors (e.g., dopamine), corticosteroids, albuterol, IV fluids, and ventilation equipment as indicated. Treatment with an anticholinergic such as atropine should be administered if clinically significant bradycardia is observed. Sugammadex can be removed using hemodialysis with a high-flux filter but not a low-flux filter. Resuscitate as necessary.

SULFAMETHOXAZOLE AND TRIMETHOPRIM

Antibacterial
Antiprotozoal

(sul-fah-meh-**THOX**-ah-zohl and try-**METH**-oh-prim)

SMZ-TMP, TMP-SMZ   pH 10

USUAL DOSE

Doses listed are based on the trimethoprim component of the drug.

Severe urinary tract infections and shigellosis in adults and pediatric patients over 2 months of age: 8 to 10 mg/kg/24 hr in equally divided doses every 6, 8, or 12 hours (2 to 2.5 mg/kg every 6 hours, 2.67 to 3.33 mg/kg every 8 hours, or 4 to 5 mg/kg every 12 hours). Administer for 14 days (urinary tract infections) or 5 days (shigellosis). Maximum recommended dose is 960 mg trimethoprim and 4,800 mg sulfamethoxazole/24 hr (60 mL/24 hr).

***Pneumocystis jiroveci* pneumonitis in adults and pediatric patients over 2 months of age:** 15 to 20 mg/kg/24 hr in equally divided doses every 6 or 8 hours (3.75 to 5 mg/kg every 6 hours or 5 to 6.67 mg/kg every 8 hours) for up to 14 days.

DOSE ADJUSTMENTS

Reduce dose by one half for CrCl between 15 and 30 mL/min; see Contraindications. ▪ Reduced dose may be indicated in the elderly. ▪ See Monitor and Drug/Lab Interactions.

DILUTION

Each 5-mL ampule (16 mg trimethoprim/mL [80 mg/5 mL], 80 mg sulfamethoxazole/mL [400 mg/5 mL]) must be diluted in 125 mL D5W and given as an infusion. Reduce diluent to 75 mL for each ampule only if fluid restriction required. Standard dilution must be used within 6 hours; fluid restriction dilution must be used within 2 hours. Available in 5-, 10-, 20-, and 30-mL vials. Concentration per mL same as 5-mL ampule. Discard if cloudiness or crystallization is present.

Storage: Store at room temperature; do not refrigerate.

COMPATIBILITY   (Underline Indicates Conflicting Compatibility Information)

Consider any drug NOT listed as compatible to be INCOMPATIBLE until consulting a pharmacist; specific conditions may apply.

Manufacturer states, "Do not mix with other drugs or solutions."

One source suggests the following **compatibilities:**

Y-site: Acyclovir (Zovirax), aldesleukin (Proleukin), allopurinol (Aloprim), amifostine (Ethyol), amphotericin B cholesteryl (Amphotec), anidulafungin (Eraxis), atracurium (Tracrium), aztreonam (Azactam), bivalirudin (Angiomax), ceftaroline (Teflaro), cisatracurium (Nimbex), cyclophosphamide (Cytoxan), dexmedetomidine (Precedex), diltiazem (Cardizem), docetaxel (Taxotere), doxorubicin liposomal (Doxil), enalaprilat (Vasotec IV), esmolol (Brevibloc), etoposide phosphate (Etopophos), fenoldopam (Corlopam), filgrastim (Neupogen), fludarabine (Fludara), foscarnet (Foscavir), gallium nitrate (Ganite), gemcitabine (Gemzar), granisetron (Kytril), hetastarch in electrolytes (Hextend), hydromorphone (Dilaudid), labetalol, lorazepam (Ativan), magnesium sulfate, melphalan (Alkeran), meperidine (Demerol), morphine, nicardipine (Cardene IV), pancuronium, pemetrexed (Alimta), piperacillin/tazobactam (Zosyn), remifentanil (Ultiva), sargramostim (Leukine), tacrolimus (Prograf), teniposide (Vumon), thiotepa, vecuronium, zidovudine (AZT, Retrovir).

RATE OF ADMINISTRATION
A single dose must be infused over 60 to 90 minutes. When administered by an infusion device, thoroughly flush all lines used to remove any residual sulfamethoxazole/trimethoprim. Avoid rapid infusion or bolus injection.

ACTIONS
A broad-spectrum antibacterial and antiprotozoal combination agent with bactericidal action effective against gram-positive and gram-negative organisms. Blocks sequential steps in the folic acid pathway, preventing the synthesis of nucleic acids and proteins essential to many bacteria. Combination contains 400 mg sulfamethoxazole and 80 mg trimethoprim per each 5 mL. Widely distributed in all body fluids and tissues, including cerebrospinal fluid, sputum, and bile. Onset of action is prompt and serum levels are maintained up to 10 hours. Metabolized in the liver and up to 60% is excreted in urine in 24 hours. Crosses placental barrier. Secreted in breast milk. Partially removed by hemodialysis.

INDICATIONS AND USES
Severe urinary tract infections. ▪ *Pneumocystis jiroveci* pneumonia. ▪ Shigellosis. ▪ Prophylaxis in neutropenic patients. ▪ Used orally in HIV and other immunocompromised patients to prevent pneumonia.
Unlabeled uses: Treatment of cholera and salmonella-type infections. ▪ An alternative agent in the treatment of meningitis caused by susceptible organisms.

CONTRAINDICATIONS
CrCl less than 15 mL/min, hypersensitivity to trimethoprim or sulfonamides, megaloblastic anemia resulting from folate deficiency, nursing mothers, pregnancy at term and infants under 2 months of age (may cause hemolytic anemia, jaundice, and kernicterus), streptococcal pharyngitis.

PRECAUTIONS
Sensitivity studies indicated to determine susceptibility of the causative organism to sulfamethoxazole/trimethoprim. ▪ Not for IM use. ▪ Use caution in impaired liver or renal function, possible folate deficiency, allergic individuals, bronchial asthma, porphyria, glucose 6-phosphate dehydrogenase (G-6PD) deficiency, and in the elderly. ▪ A sulfonamide drug; hypersensitivity reactions can occur. Use caution in patients with a history of hypersensitivity to furosemide (Lasix), thiazide diuretics (e.g., chlorothiazide), sulfonylureas (e.g., tolbutamide), or carbonic anhydrase inhibitors (e.g., acetazolamide). ▪ Some products contain bisulfites; use caution in patients with allergies. ▪ Incidence of side effects markedly increased in AIDS patients. May not tolerate or respond to this drug. ▪ *Clostridium difficile*–associated diarrhea (CDAD) has been reported. May range from mild diarrhea to fatal colitis. Consider in patients who present with diarrhea during or after treatment with sulfamethoxazole/trimethoprim.
Monitor: Maintain adequate hydration to prevent crystalluria and stone formation. ▪ CBC required before and during therapy. Discontinue for any significant reduction in a blood-forming element. Urinalysis and renal function tests also indicated. ▪ If extravasation occurs, discontinue and restart at a new site. May cause phlebitis. ▪ Monitor closely if any signs of rash appear or have appeared in previous infusions. Several cases of life-threatening reactions have occurred. ▪ See Precautions and Drug/Lab Interactions.
Patient Education: Maintain adequate hydration. ▪ Report bruising or bleeding, fever, rash, or sore throat promptly. ▪ Possible skin photosensitivity. Avoid unprotected expo-

sure to sunlight. ▪ Promptly report diarrhea or bloody stools that occur during treatment or up to several months after an antibiotic has been discontinued; may indicate CDAD and require treatment.

Maternal/Child: Category C: no adequate studies. May interfere with folic acid metabolism in mother and fetus. Benefits must outweigh risks. ▪ May contain benzyl alcohol. ▪ See Contraindications. ▪ Discontinue breast-feeding. ▪ Two infants who developed a rash had life-threatening reactions when sulfamethoxazole/trimethoprim was restarted.

Elderly: See Dose Adjustments. ▪ Increased risk of severe side effects (e.g., bone marrow suppression, decrease in platelets with or without purpura, skin reactions), especially in impaired renal or liver function or with other drugs (e.g., diuretics).

DRUG/LAB INTERACTIONS

May be potentiated by **probenecid.** ▪ May inhibit **cyclosporine** (Sandimmune) and increase nephrotoxicity. ▪ May potentiate **warfarin** (Coumadin), **phenytoin** (Dilantin), **oral hypoglycemics, dapsone, and zidovudine** (AZT, Retrovir). ▪ The sulfa component may displace **methotrexate** from its binding sites, increasing free fraction of methotrexate and its potential for toxicity. The trimethoprim component inhibits methotrexate metabolism and increases toxicity. ▪ May decrease effectiveness of **tricyclic antidepressants** (e.g., amitriptyline [Elavil]). ▪ Concurrent use with **folate antagonists** (e.g., hydantoins [e.g., phenytoin], methotrexate) is not recommended. May increase possibility of megaloblastic anemia. ▪ Concurrent use with **leucovorin calcium** may cause treatment failure and increased morbidity in HIV-infected patients being treated for *Pneumocystis jiroveci* pneumonia. ▪ Concurrent use with **bone marrow suppressants** (e.g., antineoplastics [e.g., busulfan, cisplatin], amphotericin B [all formulations], ganciclovir [Cytovene]) may increase leukopenic or thrombocytopenic effects. Monitor differential blood count. ▪ Serum levels of **digoxin** may be increased with concurrent use; monitor digoxin levels. ▪ Concurrent use with **hemolytics** (e.g., doxapram [Dopram], methyldopa, procainamide [Pronestyl], quinidine) may increase potential for toxic side effects. ▪ Concurrent use with **hepatotoxic agents** (e.g., amiodarone [Nexterone], erythromycins, fluconazole [Diflucan]) may increase incidence of hepatotoxicity. Risk increased with prolonged use or in patients with a history of liver disease. ▪ May form an insoluble precipitate in acid urine or cause crystalluria with **methenamine** (Mandelamine); concurrent use not recommended. ▪ May decrease clearance and increase serum concentrations of **N-acetylprocainamide** (NAPA) **and procainamide** (Pronestyl). ▪ Concurrent use with **rifampin** (Rifadin) will increase elimination, reduce serum concentrations, and shorten half-life of trimethoprim. ▪ Concurrent use with **thiazide diuretics** (e.g., chlorothiazide) in the elderly may result in an increased incidence of thrombocytopenia with purpura. ▪ May interfere with **serum methotrexate assay and Jaffe assay for creatinine.** ▪ See Precautions.

SIDE EFFECTS

All side effects of sulfonamides, including hypersensitivity reactions, are possible. Nausea, vomiting, and rash occur most frequently. Ataxia, convulsions, tremors, and respiratory depression are symptoms of major toxicity. With high doses or administration over an extended period of time, bone marrow suppression (leukopenia, megaloblastic anemia, thrombocytopenia) may occur. CDAD has been reported.

ANTIDOTE

Notify the physician of any side effect. Discontinue the drug at any sign of major toxicity or bone marrow suppression. Some sources recommend leucovorin calcium 5 to 15 mg daily for treatment of bone marrow suppression. Peritoneal dialysis is not effective in toxicity; hemodialysis may be moderately effective in reducing serum levels. Acidification of urine may increase excretion. Treat anaphylaxis with epinephrine, corticosteroids, antihistamines, and vasopressors. Treat CDAD with fluids, electrolytes, protein supplements, and oral vancomycin (Vancocin) or metronidazole (Flagyl) as indicated. In severe cases, surgical evaluation may be indicated.

TACROLIMUS BBW

Immunosuppressant

(tah-**KROH**-lih-mus)

Prograf

USUAL DOSE

See Precautions. IV route used for patients unable to take oral medications; risk of anaphylaxis increased with IV administration. Transfer to oral therapy as soon as tolerated, usually within 2 to 3 days.

For all indications: Dose regimens vary among transplant centers and approved or investigational use (range 0.01 to 0.05 mg/kg/day). Begin no sooner than 6 hours after transplantation in liver and heart transplant patients. In kidney transplant patients, initial dose may be administered within 24 hours of transplantation but should be delayed until renal function has recovered. Adults usually receive doses at the lower end of the range. Pediatric patients may require doses at the upper end of the range. Individualized adjustment based on clinical assessment of rejection or patients' tolerance is imperative and may be required on a daily basis. Adjunctive adrenal corticosteroid therapy early posttransplant is recommended. Initiate oral tacrolimus therapy as soon as feasible. Oral doses vary with specific organ transplant and in adults and pediatric patients (see literature). Total dose in mg/kg/day is given in equally divided doses every 12 hours. Begin 8 to 12 hours after IV tacrolimus is discontinued. Lower doses may be sufficient for maintenance therapy.

Prophylaxis of organ rejection in heart transplant: The recommended starting dose is 0.01 mg/kg/day as a continuous infusion. Used in combination with azathioprine or mycophenolate (CellCept) in addition to adrenal corticosteroids. See all comments and protocol under For All Indications above.

Prophylaxis of organ rejection in kidney transplant: The recommended starting dose is 0.03 to 0.05 mg/kg/day as a continuous infusion. Used in combination with azathioprine or mycophenolate (CellCept) in addition to adrenal corticosteroids. See all comments and protocol under For All Indications above.

Prophylaxis of organ rejection in liver transplant: The recommended starting dose is 0.03 to 0.05 mg/kg/day as a continuous infusion. Used in combination with adrenal corticosteroids. See all comments and protocol under For All Indications above.

PEDIATRIC DOSE

Has been used successfully in pediatric patients up to 16 years of age in liver transplants. See Usual Dose for mg/kg/day dose recommendations. Studies indicate that higher doses may be required to maintain blood trough concentrations similar to adults. Experience in pediatric heart and kidney transplant patients is limited. See Dilution and Maternal/Child.

DOSE ADJUSTMENTS

Dosing should be titrated based on clinical assessments of rejection and tolerability. ▪ Use lowest dosing range initially for patients with impaired renal or hepatic function (pretransplant or posttransplant). Nephrotoxicity may be increased and further reductions may be required. Half-life prolonged and clearance decreased in patients with severe hepatic impairment (Child-Pugh greater than or equal to 10). Dose reduction may be required. ▪ In kidney transplant patients with postoperative oliguria, the initial dose of tacrolimus should be administered no sooner than 6 hours and within 24 hours of transplantation, but it may be delayed until renal function shows evidence of recovery. ▪ Lower doses may be appropriate for maintenance. ▪ Black patients who have undergone a kidney transplant may require a higher dose to obtain trough concentrations comparable to those seen in white patients. ▪ See Monitor and Drug/Lab Interactions.

DILUTION

Specific techniques required; see Precautions. Available as a 5-mg/mL solution in a 1-mL ampule. A 24-hour dose must be diluted with an appropriate amount of NS or D5W.

Desired concentration is between 4 and 20 mcg/mL. May leach phthalate from polyvinylchloride containers; mix in glass or polyethylene infusion bottles. Use PVC-free IV tubing in pediatric patients. The following chart provides some dose and dilution examples.

Tacrolimus Dose and Dilution Examples				
Desired Dose	Weight	Total Dose	Amount of Diluent	mcg/mL
0.01 mg/kg	70 kg	0.7 mg/24 hr	100 mL	7 mcg/mL
0.03 mg/kg	100 kg	3 mg/24 hr	250 mL	12 mcg/mL
0.05 mg/kg	60 kg	3 mg/24 hr	500 mL	6 mcg/mL
			250 mL	12 mcg/mL

Storage: Store between 5° and 25° C (41° and 77° F) before dilution. Discard diluted solution in 24 hours.

COMPATIBILITY   (Underline Indicates Conflicting Compatibility Information)
Consider any drug NOT listed as compatible to be INCOMPATIBLE until consulting a pharmacist; specific conditions may apply.
Manufacturer states, "Should not be mixed with solutions of pH 9 or greater (e.g., acyclovir [Zovirax], ganciclovir [Cytovene IV])." See Dilution.

One source suggests the following **compatibilities:**

Y-site: Aminophylline, amphotericin B (conventional), ampicillin, ampicillin/sulbactam (Unasyn), anidulafungin (Eraxis), benztropine (Cogentin), calcium gluconate, caspofungin (Cancidas), cefazolin (Ancef), cefotetan, ceftazidime (Fortaz), ceftriaxone (Rocephin), cefuroxime (Zinacef), chloramphenicol (Chloromycetin), ciprofloxacin (Cipro IV), clindamycin (Cleocin), dexamethasone (Decadron), digoxin (Lanoxin), diphenhydramine (Benadryl), dobutamine, dopamine, doripenem (Doribax), doxycycline, erythromycin (Erythrocin), esmolol (Brevibloc), fluconazole (Diflucan), furosemide (Lasix), gentamicin, heparin, hydrocortisone sodium succinate (Solu-Cortef), hydromorphone (Dilaudid), imipenem-cilastatin (Primaxin), insulin (regular), isoproterenol (Isuprel), leucovorin calcium, lorazepam (Ativan), methylprednisolone (Solu-Medrol), metoclopramide (Reglan), metronidazole (Flagyl IV), micafungin (Mycamine), morphine, multivitamins (M.V.I.), mycophenolate (CellCept IV), nitroglycerin IV, nitroprusside sodium, oxacillin (Bactocill), penicillin G potassium, phenytoin (Dilantin), potassium chloride (KCl), propranolol, ranitidine (Zantac), sodium bicarbonate, sulfamethoxazole/trimethoprim, tobramycin, vancomycin.

RATE OF ADMINISTRATION
A single dose properly diluted and equally distributed over 24 hours as a continuous infusion. Use of a metriset (60 gtt/min) or infusion pump suggested.

ACTIONS
A potent immunosuppressive agent. Prolongs survival of allogeneic heart, kidney, and liver transplants. Inhibition of T-lymphocyte activation results in immunosuppression. Highly protein bound. Metabolized primarily by the P_{450} enzyme system (CYP3A). Half-life ranges from 32 to 55 hours. Primarily excreted in feces. Minimal excretion in urine. Crosses the placental barrier. Secreted in breast milk.

INDICATIONS AND USES
Prophylaxis of organ rejection in allogeneic heart, kidney, and liver transplants in conjunction with adrenal corticosteroids. In heart and kidney transplant patients, concomitant use with azathioprine or mycophenolate is recommended in addition to the adrenal corticosteroids.

Limitations of use: Should not be used simultaneously with cyclosporine. ▪ Should be reserved for patients unable to take oral tacrolimus. ▪ Use with sirolimus (Rapamune) is not recommended in liver and heart transplant patients. Safety and effectiveness of tacrolimus with sirolimus in kidney transplant patients have not been established.

Unlabeled uses: Treatment of autoimmune diseases (i.e., rheumatoid arthritis). ▪ Prevention and treatment of acute graft-versus-host disease.

CONTRAINDICATIONS

Hypersensitivity to tacrolimus or polyoxyl 60 hydrogenated castor oil.

PRECAUTIONS

Follow guidelines for handling hazardous agents. See Appendix A, p. 1331. ▪ For IV use only. ▪ Oral dosing preferred; begin as soon as feasible. Risk of anaphylaxis is increased by IV route versus oral route; use caution. *Reserve for patients unable to take oral medication.* ▪ Usually administered in the hospital by or under the direction of a physician experienced in immunosuppressive therapy and management of organ transplant patients. ▪ Adequate laboratory and supportive medical resources must be available. ▪ Use caution in impaired renal function; increases in SCr may require dose reduction or use of an alternate immunosuppressant. ▪ Use caution in severe hepatic dysfunction (mean Pugh score: greater than 10); clearance decreased. ▪ Can cause nephrotoxicity and neurotoxicity, particularly at higher doses; see Monitor. ▪ Posterior reversible encephalopathy syndrome (PRES), delirium, and coma have been reported; see Monitor. ▪ Hypertension is a common adverse effect and may require hypertensive therapy; see Drug/Lab Interactions. ▪ Use combination immunosuppressant therapy with caution; may oversuppress the immune system and increase susceptibility to infection. ▪ Immunosuppressed patients are at increased risk for bacterial, viral, fungal, and protozoal infections, including opportunistic infections. ▪ Opportunistic infections may include latent viral infections such as polyoma virus infections. Polyoma virus infections may result in polyoma virus–associated nephropathy (PVAN) and JC virus–associated progressive multifocal leukoencephalopathy (PML). PVAN is associated with serious outcomes, including deteriorating renal function and kidney graft loss. PML is a serious progressive neurologic disorder caused by infection of the CNS by JC virus, a member of the papovavirus family. It typically occurs in immunocompromised patients. PML is rare but may result in irreversible neurologic deterioration and death, and there is no known effective treatment. Hemiparesis, apathy, confusion, cognitive deficiencies, and ataxia are the most commonly observed clinical signs. ▪ Patients receiving immunosuppression are at increased risk for developing cytomegalovirus (CMV) viremia and CMV disease. ▪ Antiviral prophylaxis (e.g., ganciclovir, valganciclovir) may be advisable in some patients. ▪ Concurrent use with sirolimus (Rapamune) is not recommended in liver or heart transplant patients. Regimen is associated with an increased risk of wound healing complications, renal function impairment, and insulin-dependent, posttransplant diabetes mellitus in heart transplant patients; regimen is associated with excess mortality, graft loss, and hepatic artery thrombosis in liver transplant patients. The safety and efficacy of tacrolimus and sirolimus have not been established in kidney transplant patients. ▪ Post–liver transplant patients experiencing hepatic impairment may be at increased risk of developing renal insufficiency related to elevated tacrolimus concentrations. ▪ May cause lymphomas and other malignancies (especially of skin). Risk appears to be related to intensity and duration of immunosuppression. Has also been associated with a posttransplant lymphoproliferative disorder (PTLD), usually related to Epstein-Barr virus infection. ▪ New-onset diabetes mellitus has been reported in tacrolimus-treated heart, kidney, and liver transplant patients. May be reversible over 1 to 2 years in some patients. Black and Hispanic kidney transplant patients may be at an increased risk; see Monitor. ▪ Myocardial hypertrophy has been reported in pediatric patients and adults. Reversible in most cases with dose reduction or discontinuation of tacrolimus. ▪ May prolong the QT/QTc interval and cause torsades de pointes. Avoid use in patients with congenital long QT syndrome. Patients with CHF, bradyarrhythmias, or electrolyte abnormalities (e.g., hypokalemia, hypocalcemia, hypomagnesemia) and patients taking medicinal products that may lead to QT prolongation may be at increased risk; see Monitor and Drug/Lab Interactions. ▪ Pure red cell aplasia (PRCA) has been reported. ▪ GI perforation has been reported. All reported cases were considered to be a complication of transplant surgery or accompanied by infection, diverticulum, or malignant neoplasm. ▪ See Drug/Lab Interactions.

Monitor: Obtain baseline CBC, differential, platelets, electrolytes, fasting glucose, BUN, SCr, and liver function tests. Monitor regularly during therapy. ▪ Contains a castor oil derivative and alcohol; observe continuously for signs of a hypersensitivity reaction (e.g., acute respiratory distress syndrome [ARDS], dyspnea, pruritus, rash) for the first 30 minutes of the infusion and frequently thereafter. A source of oxygen and epinephrine must always be available. ▪ Monitor urine output and SCr carefully. Overt nephrotoxicity occurs more frequently early after transplant. Nephrotoxicity may be acute or chronic. Acute nephrotoxicity is characterized by increasing SCr, hyperkalemia, and/or a decrease in urine output and is usually reversible. Chronic nephrotoxicity is usually progressive and is associated with increased SCr, decreased kidney graft life, and characteristic histologic changes on renal biopsy. Consider changing to another immunosuppressive therapy in patients with persistent elevations of SCr who are unresponsive to dose adjustments. ▪ Monitor for S/S of neurotoxicity (e.g., changes in motor or sensory function, changes in mental status, coma, delirium, headache, paresthesias, tremors, seizures). ▪ Monitor for S/S of PRES (e.g., altered mental status, headache, hypertension, seizures, and visual disturbances). Diagnosis may be confirmed by MRI. Maintain BP control, and an immediate decrease of immunosuppression is advised. Symptoms have reversed when immunosuppression is reduced or discontinued. ▪ Monitor for S/S of PML; apathy, ataxia, cognitive deficiencies, confusion, and hemiparesis are the most commonly observed clinical signs. Consultation with a neurologist may be indicated. ▪ Tacrolimus whole blood trough concentrations in conjunction with other laboratory parameters and clinical parameters are used to evaluate rejection, toxicity, need for dose reduction, and patient compliance. Risk of toxicity (e.g., nephrotoxicity, neurotoxicity, posttransplant diabetes mellitus) is increased with higher trough concentrations. Whole blood median trough concentrations may vary considerably during the first week but then stabilize. Most patients are stable when trough whole blood concentrations are between 5 and 20 ng/mL depending on indication and length of time since the transplant. The trough concentrations described above and in the manufacturer's prescribing information pertain only to oral administration of tacrolimus. Monitoring tacrolimus concentrations during a continuous IV infusion of tacrolimus may have some utility; however, the observed concentrations will not represent exposures comparable to those estimated by the trough concentrations observed in patients on oral therapy. ▪ Monitor all parameters to evaluate possibility of organ rejection. ▪ Monitor BP; antihypertensives may be indicated; see Drug/Lab Interactions. ▪ Monitor electrolyte concentrations. May cause hyperkalemia or hypomagnesemia. ▪ In patients with CHF, bradyarrhythmias, or electrolyte abnormalities (e.g., hypokalemia, hypocalcemia, hypomagnesemia) and in patients taking certain antiarrhythmics or other medicinal products that may lead to QT prolongation, consider obtaining an electrocardiogram and monitoring electrolytes periodically during treatment. ▪ May cause hyperglycemia. Monitor carefully; treatment may be required. ▪ Observe for signs of infection (e.g., fever, sore throat, tiredness) or unusual bleeding or bruising. ▪ Consider echocardiographic evaluation in patients who develop renal failure or clinical manifestations of ventricular dysfunction. Consider dose reduction or discontinuation of tacrolimus if myocardial hypertrophy is diagnosed. ▪ See Precautions and Drug/Lab Interactions.

Patient Education: Review manufacturer's medication guide. ▪ Nonhormonal birth control preferred to oral contraceptives to reduce complications of drug interactions. ▪ Emphasize need for frequent routine lab work; compliance imperative. ▪ Interacts with many medications. Discuss any changes in drug regimen (prescription or nonprescription) with doctor or pharmacist. ▪ Promptly report any side effects (e.g., hypertension, nephrotoxicity, neurotoxicity, S/S of infection). ▪ Review S/S of diabetes mellitus. ▪ Inform patient of increased risk of neoplasia, including malignant skin changes. Limit exposure to sunlight and ultraviolet light. ▪ See Appendix D, p. 1333.

Maternal/Child: Category C: use only if necessary; benefits must outweigh risk to fetus. Has been associated with hyperkalemia and renal dysfunction in the fetus. ▪ Discontinue breast-feeding. ▪ Safety and effectiveness for use in pediatric kidney and heart transplant patients not established. ▪ Appears to be an increased risk for lymphoprolif-erative disorder (LPD) and primary Epstein-Barr virus infection in immunosuppressed pediatric patients.

Elderly: Consider age-related organ impairment.

DRUG/LAB INTERACTIONS

Used concurrently with **adrenocorticosteroids and azathioprine or mycophenolate (CellCept).** *Do not use simultaneously with cyclosporine (Sandimmune).* If a change of immunosuppres-sants is indicated (tacrolimus to cyclosporine or cyclosporine to tacrolimus), avoid addi-tive nephrotoxicity by waiting for at least 24 hours before starting the alternate drug. If elevated blood concentrations are present, further extend the interval between the two drugs. ▪ Concurrent use with **sirolimus** (Rapamune) is not recommended; see Precau-tions. ▪ Coadministration with **strong CYP3A4 inhibitors** (e.g., azole antifungal agents [e.g., itraconazole (Sporanox), ketoconazole (Nizoral), voriconazole (VFEND)], boceprevir [Victrelis], clarithromycin [Biaxin], ritonavir [Norvir], telaprevir [Incivek]) **and strong inducers** (e.g., rifampin [Rifadin], rifabutin [Mycobutin]), **including those that prolong the QT interval** (e.g., azole antifungals, clarithromycin), is not recommended with-out adjustments in tacrolimus dosing and close monitoring of tacrolimus whole blood trough concentration and associated side effects. ▪ Concurrent use with **other drugs that prolong the QT interval** may require dose adjustment and monitoring of the QT interval and trough concentrations. **Amiodarone** (Nexterone) has been reported to increase tacrolimus whole blood concentration with or without concurrent QT prolongation. ▪ Use extreme caution with **other nephrotoxic agents** (e.g., aminoglycosides [gentamicin, tobramycin], amphotericin B [conventional], cisplatin, ganciclovir [Cytovene], nucleotide reverse transcriptase inhibitors [e.g., tenofovir (Viread)], and protease inhibitors [e.g., ritonavir (Norvir), indinavir (Crixivan)]). ▪ Do not use **potassium-sparing diuretics** (e.g., spirono-lactone [Aldactone]); increases risk of hyperkalemia. Other agents associated with hyperkalemia (e.g., **ACE inhibitors** [enalapril (Vasotec)] and **angiotensin receptor blockers** [e.g., losartan (Cozaar)]) should be used with caution. ▪ **Calcium channel blockers** (e.g., diltiazem [Cardizem], nicardipine [Cardene], nifedipine [Procardia], verapamil), **bro-mocriptine** (Parlodel), **chloramphenicol** (Chloromycetin), **cimetidine** (Tagamet), **danazol** (Cyclomen), **erythromycin, estradiol** (Estrace), **herbal products containing schisandra sphen-anthera extracts, lansoprazole** (Prevacid), **methylprednisone** (Solu-Medrol), **metoclopramide** (Reglan), **metronidazole** (Flagyl), **omeprazole** (Prilosec), **protease inhibitors** (e.g., ritonavir [Norvir], saquinavir [Invirase]), **theophylline, and troleandomycin** (TAO) may inhibit the P_{450} enzyme system and increase tacrolimus blood levels, increasing toxicity potential. Tacrolimus toxicity may also be increased if given concurrently with **nefazodone.** ▪ Avoid concomitant use with **nelfinavir** unless benefits outweigh risks. ▪ When initiating therapy with **posaconazole or voriconazole** in patients already receiving tacrolimus, decrease tacro-limus dose to one third of the original dose. Adjust subsequent tacrolimus doses based on tacrolimus whole blood concentrations. ▪ **Anticonvulsants** (e.g., carbamazepine [Tegretol], phenobarbital, phenytoin [Dilantin]), **caspofungin** (Cancidas), **rifamycins** (e.g., rifabutin [Mycobutin], rifampin [Rifadin]), **and St. John's wort** may induce the P_{450} enzyme system, decreasing effectiveness and leading to decreased tacrolimus blood lev-els and organ rejection. ▪ Tacrolimus may increase serum concentrations of **phenytoin** (Dilantin). ▪ **Grapefruit juice** may affect certain enzymes of the P_{450} system and should be avoided. ▪ **Do not use live virus vaccines** in patients receiving tacrolimus.

SIDE EFFECTS

Heart transplant: Abnormal renal function, anemia, bronchitis, CMV infection, diabetes mellitus, hyperglycemia, hyperlipidemia, hypertension, infection, leukopenia, pericardial effusion, tremor, and urinary tract infection are most common.

Kidney transplant: Abdominal pain, abnormal renal function, constipation, diarrhea, head-ache, hypertension, infection, insomnia, nausea, and tremor are most common.

Liver transplant: Abdominal pain, abnormal renal function, anemia, asthenia, diarrhea, fever, headache, hyperglycemia, hyperkalemia, hypertension, hypomagnesemia, insom-nia, nausea, pain, paresthesia, and tremor are most common. The above side effects are most common by diagnosis, but any of them may occur with any patient receiving a heart, liver, or kidney transplant. Side effects occur in a majority of patients and are more pronounced at higher doses. May improve somewhat over time. Nephrotoxicity (abnormal renal function with increased SCr and BUN, oliguria) and neurotoxicity (delirium, headache, insomnia, paresthesia, tremor, seizures) may be dose limiting. Abnormal ECG, abnormal liver function tests, acute kidney failure, albuminuria, anorexia, arrhythmias, ascites, atelectasis, back pain, blood dyscrasias, CHF, coma, cushingoid features, dyspnea, gastroenteritis, glycosuria, hearing loss (including deafness), hemolytic-uremic syndrome, hypokalemia, hypophosphatemia, impaired wound healing, leukocytosis, leukoencephalopathy, myocardial hypertrophy, neuralgia, pancreatitis, peripheral edema, peritonitis, photosensitivity, pleural effusion, pruritus, pulmonary edema, QT prolongation, rash, seizures, Stevens-Johnson syndrome, thrombocytopenia, thrombophlebitis, torsades de pointes, vertigo, and vomiting have also been reported. Many other side effects have occurred in fewer than 3% of patients.

Post-Marketing: Acute respiratory distress syndrome, agranulocytosis, cardiac arrhythmia, cerebral infarction, DIC, enterocolitis, gastroesophageal reflux disease, GI perforation, hemolytic anemia, hepatotoxicity, interstitial lung disease, posterior reversible encephalopathy syndrome (PRES), PRCA, primary graft dysfunction, progressive multifocal leukoencephalopathy (PML), and PVAN nephropathy are some of the many additional side effects reported.

ANTIDOTE
Notify the physician of all side effects. Most will be treated symptomatically. Tacrolimus may be decreased or discontinued or alternate immunosuppressive agents substituted. Nephrotoxicity, neurotoxicity, or hematopoietic depression may require temporary reduction of dose or discontinuation of therapy. Reduction in immunosuppression should be considered for patients who develop evidence of PVAN, PML, or CMV viremia and/or CMV disease. However, the risk that reduced immunosuppression represents to the functioning allograft must also be considered. If S/S of PRES occur, maintain BP control, and an immediate decrease of immunosuppression is advised. Consider discontinuing tacrolimus if PRCA is diagnosed. Dialysis is not effective in overdose. Discontinue immediately if anaphylaxis occurs and treat with oxygen, epinephrine, corticosteroids, and/or antihistamines (e.g., diphenhydramine [Benadryl]). Resuscitate as necessary.

TALIGLUCERASE ALFA
(tal-e-**GLUE**-sir-ace **AL**-fa)

Elelyso

Enzyme replenisher
(glucocerebrosidase)

pH 6

USUAL DOSE
Treatment-naïve adults and pediatric patients 4 years of age and older: 60 units/kg of body weight administered once every 2 weeks as a 60- to 120-minute IV infusion.

Patients switching from imiglucerase: Patients currently being treated with imiglucerase for Type 1 Gaucher disease can be switched to taliglucerase alfa. Patients on a stable dose of imiglucerase may transfer to the same unit/kg dose of taliglucerase alfa. Administer dose every other week as a 60- to 120-minute IV infusion.

DOSE ADJUSTMENTS
Patients switching from imiglucerase: Dose may increase or decrease based on achievement of each patient's therapeutic goals. Optimal goal is to establish the lowest dose that is effective in maintaining control of the disease and preventing a recurrence of symptoms for each patient.

DILUTION
Available as a lyophilized powder in 200-unit vials. Determine the number of vials required using the following calculations:

Weight in kg × Dose/kg desired ÷ 200 (units/vial) = # of vials required

A 60-kg man requiring 60 units/kg would require 3,600 units. The number of vials required would be 18. If necessary, round up to the next whole vial. After patient is weighed and appropriate dose is calculated, remove sufficient vials from refrigerator. Do not leave vials at RT for longer than 24 hours before reconstitution.

Each 200-unit vial must be reconstituted with 5.1 mL of SWFI to yield a reconstituted product with a concentration of 40 units/mL and an extractable volume of 5 mL. Gently swirl to mix the solution. **Do not shake.** Withdraw exactly 5 mL (40 units/mL) from each 200-unit vial. A total dose must be further diluted with NS to a total volume of 100 to 200 mL. For **pediatric patients**, a final volume of 100 to 120 mL should be used. For **adult patients**, a final volume of 130 to 150 mL may be used. However, if the volume of the reconstituted product alone is equal to or greater than 130 to 150 mL, then the final volume should not exceed 200 mL. Mix gently; **do not shake.** Do not use if discolored or opaque or if particulate matter is present. After dilution, slight flocculation (thin translucent fibers) may occur.

Filters: Should be administered through an in-line, low–protein-binding, 0.2-micron filter.

Storage: Before use, refrigerate at 2° to 8° C (36° to 46° F). Protect from light. Do not freeze. Do not use after expiration date on bottle. Contains no preservative. Following reconstitution, immediate use is preferred; however, reconstituted and/or diluted vials may be refrigerated for up to 24 hours at 2° to 8° C (36° to 46° F) protected from light. Reconstituted vials are stable for up to 4 hours at 20° to 25° C (68° to 77° F) without protection from light. Store reconstituted and/or diluted product for no more than 24 hours protected from light. Do not freeze, and discard any unused product.

COMPATIBILITY
Specific information not available. Consider specific use; consult pharmacist.

RATE OF ADMINISTRATION
Use of an infusion set with an in-line, low–protein-binding, 0.2-micron filter is required. Use of an infusion pump is helpful. Flush the IV line with NS at the end of the infusion to ensure the total dose is received. Administer as an infusion over 60 to 120 minutes as outlined in the following paragraphs.

Pediatric patients: Begin with a rate of 1 mL/min. If the patient tolerates the initial infusion rate, it may be increased to 2 mL/min. Total time of the infusion should be no less than 1 hour.

Adult patients: Begin with a rate of 1.2 mL/min. If the patient tolerates the initial infusion rate, it may be increased to 2.2 mL/min. Total time of the infusion should be no less than 1 hour. Reduction in the rate of infusion may be helpful in the event of side effects or infusion reactions.

ACTIONS

A hydrolytic lysosomal glucocerebroside-specific enzyme. It is produced by recombinant DNA technology using plant cell culture (carrot). An active form of the lysosomal enzyme β-glucocerebrosidase. It catalyzes the hydrolysis of glucocerebroside to glucose and ceramide, reducing the amount of accumulated glucocerebroside normally seen in patients with Gaucher disease. In clinical trials, spleen and liver size were reduced, and anemia and thrombocytopenia were improved. Median terminal half-life was 32.5 minutes in pediatric patients and 28.7 minutes in adult patients. No significant accumulation was noted with repeated dosing.

INDICATIONS AND USES

Treatment of patients with a confirmed diagnosis of Type 1 Gaucher disease.

CONTRAINDICATIONS

Manufacturer states, "None."

PRECAUTIONS

Should be used under the direction of a physician knowledgeable in the management of Gaucher disease and administered in a facility with adequate diagnostic and treatment facilities to monitor the patient and respond to any medical emergency. ▪ Hypersensitivity reactions, including anaphylaxis, have occurred; see Monitor and Antidote. ▪ A therapeutic protein product, patients have developed IgG antidrug antibodies (ADA) to taliglucerase alfa. The relationship between ADA and hypersensitivity reactions is not fully understood. Monitoring for ADA to taliglucerase alfa may be useful in ADA-positive patients or in patients who have experienced hypersensitivity reactions to taliglucerase alfa. Neutralizing antibodies have also been detected in some patients receiving taliglucerase alfa. Clinical relevance as it relates to therapeutic effect is unclear.

Monitor: Obtain weight before each dose (used to calculate dose). Monitor vital signs. ▪ Observe patient during and after the infusion for S/S of a hypersensitivity reaction. In clinical trials, serious hypersensitivity reactions, including anaphylaxis, occurred during the infusion. S/S included chest tightness, dizziness, flushing, hypotension, nausea, urticaria, vomiting, and wheezing. Other hypersensitivity reactions occurred up to 3 hours after the start of the infusion and included angioedema, chest tightness, cough, erythema, flushing, nausea, pruritus, rash, throat irritation, and vomiting. Discontinue the infusion immediately if anaphylaxis occurs; consider the risk versus benefit of readministering taliglucerase in patients who have experienced a severe reaction. Caution should be exercised upon rechallenge. ▪ Decreasing the infusion rate, temporarily stopping the infusion, and/or administering antihistamines, antipyretics, and/or corticosteroids is recommended. Pretreatment with antihistamines and/or corticosteroids may prevent subsequent reactions in these patients. ▪ Observe patient closely for signs of improvement (e.g., improvement in hemoglobin and platelet counts, reduction in size of liver and/or spleen).

Patient Education: Enzyme replacement therapy is required for life. ▪ Promptly report S/S of a hypersensitivity or infusion reaction (e.g., chills, dizziness, fatigue, fever, headache, itching, nausea, rash, shortness of breath, wheezing). Reactions may occur during or after infusion. ▪ Pretreatment with antihistamines or corticosteroids may be used to prevent reactions.

Maternal/Child: Consider risk versus benefit. Women with Type 1 Gaucher disease have an increased risk of spontaneous abortion if disease symptoms are not treated and controlled before conception and during pregnancy. Pregnancy can exacerbate existing Type 1

Gaucher disease symptoms, and Type 1 Gaucher disease manifestations may lead to adverse pregnancy outcomes ▪ Safety for use during breast-feeding not established. Not known if taliglucerase alfa is secreted in breast milk. The effects on the breast-fed infant or on milk production are also unknown. ▪ Safety and effectiveness for use in pediatric patients under 4 years of age not established. Pediatric patients experienced a higher frequency of vomiting than adult patients. Frequencies of other adverse reactions were similar between adult and pediatric patients.

Elderly: Numbers in clinical studies insufficient to determine if the elderly respond differently than do younger adults.

DRUG/LAB INTERACTIONS
Specific information not available.

SIDE EFFECTS
The most commonly reported adverse reactions in clinical trials were abdominal pain, arthralgia, dizziness, extremity pain, fatigue, flushing, headache, nausea, pruritus, rash, urticaria, and vomiting. Back pain, diarrhea, and hypersensitivity reactions have also been reported.

Post-Marketing: Anaphylaxis.

ANTIDOTE
Keep physician informed of side effects; may be treated symptomatically if indicated. Based on the severity of the reaction, temporarily interrupt or discontinue infusion for clinical evidence of a hypersensitivity reaction. Patients have successfully continued therapy after mild hypersensitivity reactions with a reduction in rate of administration and/or treatment or pretreatment with antipyretics, antihistamines (e.g., diphenhydramine [Benadryl]), and/or corticosteroids (e.g., dexamethasone [Decadron]). Discontinue infusion immediately for anaphylaxis and treat with oxygen, epinephrine (Adrenalin), antihistamines (e.g., diphenhydramine [Benadryl]), vasopressors (e.g., dopamine), corticosteroids, albuterol, IV fluids, and ventilation equipment as indicated. Resuscitate as necessary.

TEDIZOLID PHOSPHATE
(te-**DIZ**-oh-lid **FOS**-fayt)

Sivextro

Antibacterial
(oxazolidinone)

USUAL DOSE
200 mg once daily for 6 days as an infusion over 1 hour. Alternately, may be given orally (with or without food).

DOSE ADJUSTMENTS
No dose adjustment necessary when changing from IV to oral doses. ▪ If a dose is missed or delayed, it should be administered as soon as possible any time up to 8 hours before the next scheduled dose. If less than 8 hours remain before the next dose, wait until the next scheduled dose. ▪ No dose adjustments indicated based on age, gender, weight, race, or any degree of hepatic or renal impairment.

DILUTION
Available in single-use vials containing 200 mg of tedizolid as a lyophilized powder. Reconstitute the 200-mg vial with 4 mL of SWFI. Gently swirl the contents and let the vial stand until completely dissolved and any foam disperses. Solution should be clear and colorless to pale yellow. Tilt the upright vial and insert a needle attached to a syringe to the bottom corner of the vial. Withdraw 4 mL of the reconstituted solution. *Do not invert the vial during extraction* of its contents. Further dilute by slowly injecting the 4 mL into a 250-mL bag of NS. Invert the bag gently to mix. *Do NOT shake*; may cause foaming.

Filters: Specific information not available.

Storage: Before use, vials may be stored at CRT. Total time from reconstitution to dilution to completion of administration of both reconstituted vials and/or fully diluted solutions should not exceed 24 hours at RT or under refrigeration at 2° to 8° C (36° to 46° F).

COMPATIBILITY
Tedizolid is **compatible** only with NS. Manufacturer states, "Other IV substances, additives, or other medications should not be added to tedizolid single-use vials or infused simultaneously through the same IV line or through a common IV port. If the same IV line is used for sequential infusion of additional medications, the line should be flushed before and after infusion of tedizolid with NS." It is **incompatible** with any solution containing divalent cations (e.g., calcium, magnesium), including LR injection and Hartmann's solution.

RATE OF ADMINISTRATION
A single dose as an infusion equally distributed over 1 hour. **Do not administer as an IV push or bolus.** If a common IV line is used to administer other drugs in addition to tedizolid, flush the IV line before and after each tedizolid infusion with NS.

ACTIONS
Tedizolid phosphate belongs to the oxazolidinone class of antibacterial drugs. It is a phosphate prodrug and is converted to tedizolid by phosphatases. Its antibacterial activity is mediated by binding to the 50S subunit of the bacterial ribosome, resulting in inhibition of protein synthesis. This mechanism of action is different from that of other non-oxazodidinone class antibacterial drugs; therefore cross-resistance between tedizolid and other classes of antibacterial drugs is unlikely. Bacteriostatic against designated strains of *Staphylococcus, Streptococcus,* and *Enterococcus*; see Indications. Peak plasma concentrations are achieved at the end of the 1-hour infusion. Penetrates into the interstitial space fluid of adipose and skeletal muscle tissue with exposure similar to free-drug exposure in plasma. Approximately 70% to 90% bound to human plasma proteins. Half-life is approximately 12 hours. The majority of elimination occurs via the liver. Primarily excreted as a microbiologically inactive sulfate conjugate in feces with some excretion in urine.

INDICATIONS AND USES

Treatment of adult patients with acute bacterial skin and skin structure infections (ABSSSI) caused by susceptible isolates of designated gram-positive microorganisms, including *Staphylococcus aureus* (both methicillin-susceptible [MSSA] and methicillin-resistant [MRSA] strains).

CONTRAINDICATIONS

Manufacturer states, "None."

PRECAUTIONS

For IV use only. ▪ Safety and efficacy for use in patients with neutropenia (neutrophil counts less than 1,000 cells/mm³) have not been adequately evaluated. In an animal model of infection, the antibacterial activity of tedizolid was reduced in the absence of granulocytes. Consider alternative therapy when treating patients with neutropenia and ABSSSI. ▪ Specific sensitivity studies are indicated to determine susceptibility of the causative organism to tedizolid. ▪ To reduce the development of drug-resistant bacteria and maintain its effectiveness, tedizolid should be used to treat only those infections proven or strongly suspected to be caused by bacteria. ▪ *Clostridium difficile*–associated diarrhea (CDAD) has been reported for nearly all systemic antibacterial agents and may range in severity from mild diarrhea to fatal colitis. Consider in patients who present with diarrhea during or after treatment with tedizolid.

Monitor: Obtain baseline CBC with differential and platelets. ▪ Monitor for S/S of hypersensitivity (e.g., hypotension, rash, urticaria, tightness of the chest, wheezing).

Patient Education: Promptly report S/S of a hypersensitivity reaction (e.g., hives, rash, shortness of breath, wheezing). ▪ Promptly report diarrhea or bloody stools that occur during treatment or up to several months after an antibiotic has been discontinued; may indicate CDAD and require treatment.

Maternal/Child: Category C: use during pregnancy only if the potential benefit outweighs the possible risk to the fetus. ▪ Use caution during breast-feeding. ▪ Safety and effectiveness for use in pediatric patients not established.

Elderly: Numbers in clinical studies insufficient to determine if the elderly respond differently than do younger subjects. No overall differences in pharmacokinetics were observed between elderly subjects and younger subjects.

DRUG/LAB INTERACTIONS

Tedizolid did not detectably inhibit or induce the metabolism of **cytochrome P₄₅₀ enzyme substrates.** There was no degradation of tedizolid in human liver microsomes, indicating that tedizolid is unlikely to be a substrate for hepatic CYP₄₅₀ enzymes. ▪ During in vitro studies, no clinically significant inhibition of any transporter (e.g., the efflux transporter **P-glycoprotein ([P-gp], selected OAT, OCT, or ABCG2)** was observed. ▪ A reversible inhibitor of monoamine oxidase. Not evaluated because subjects taking MAO inhibitors were excluded from trials. ▪ In in vitro studies, tedizolid did not demonstrate synergy or antagonism with amphotericin B (conventional), aztreonam (Azactam), ceftazidime (Fortaz), ceftriaxone (Rocephin), ciprofloxacin (Cipro), clindamycin (Cleocin), daptomycin (Cubicin), gentamicin, imipenem-cilastin (Primaxin), ketoconazole (Nizoral), minocycline (Minocin), rifampin (Rifadin), terbinafine (Lamsil), sulfamethoxazole/trimethoprim (Bactrim), or vancomycin.

SIDE EFFECTS

The most common adverse reactions are diarrhea, dizziness, headache, nausea, and vomiting. CDAD, decreased WBC, dermatitis, eye disorders (e.g., asthenopia, blurred vision, visual impairment, vitreous floaters), flushing, hypersensitivity reactions, hypertension, hypoesthesia, increased hepatic transaminases, infusion-related reactions, insomnia, myelosuppression (anemia, neutropenia, thrombocytopenia), oral candidiasis, palpitations, paresthesia, pruritus, seventh nerve paralysis, tachycardia, urticaria, and vulvovaginal mycotic infection have been reported. Peripheral and optic neuropathy have been described in patients treated with another member of the oxazolidinone class (e.g., linezolid [Zyvox]) for longer than 28 days.

ANTIDOTE

Notify physician of any side effects. Discontinue the drug if indicated. Treat hypersensitivity reactions as indicated (e.g., diphenhydramine [Benadryl], epinephrine [Adrenalin], albuterol) and resuscitate as necessary. Mild cases of CDAD may respond to discontinuation of tedizolid. Treat CDAD with fluids, electrolytes, protein supplements, and oral vancomycin (Vancocin) or metronidazole (Flagyl) as indicated. In severe cases, surgical evaluation may be indicated. In the event of an overdose, discontinue tedizolid and provide supportive treatment as needed. Is not effectively removed from the circulation by hemodialysis.

TELAVANCIN BBW

(tel-a-**VAN**-sin)

Vibativ

Antibacterial
(lipoglycopeptide)

pH 4 to 5

USUAL DOSE

Complicated skin and skin structure infections (cSSSI): 10 mg/kg as an infusion once every 24 hours for 7 to 14 days. Duration of therapy is dependent on severity and site of infection and on the patient's clinical progress.

Hospital-acquired and ventilator-associated bacterial pneumonia (HABP/VABP): 10 mg/kg as an infusion once every 24 hours for 7 to 21 days. Duration of therapy is dependent on severity and site of infection and on the patient's clinical progress.

DOSE ADJUSTMENTS

Dose adjustment required in renal impairment as outlined in the following chart.

Telavancin Dosage Adjustment in Adult Patients with Renal Impairment	
Creatinine Clearance* (mL/min)	Telavancin Dosage Regimen
>50 mL/min	10 mg/kg every 24 hours
30 to 50 mL/min	7.5 mg/kg every 24 hours
10 to <30 mL/min	10 mg/kg every 48 hours

*Calculate using Cockcroft-Gault formula and ideal body weight. Use actual body weight if it is less than ideal body weight.

There is insufficient information to make specific dose recommendations for patients with end-stage renal disease (CrCl less than 10 mL/min), including patients undergoing hemodialysis. ▪ Reduced doses may be indicated in the elderly based on age-related renal impairment. ▪ No dose adjustment is recommended based on gender or in patients with mild or moderate hepatic impairment. Has not been studied in patients with severe hepatic impairment.

DILUTION

Reconstitute each 250-mg vial with 15 mL of D5W, SWFI, or NS (45 mL for a 750-mg vial). Resultant solution has a final concentration of 15 mg/mL. To minimize foaming during reconstitution, allow the vacuum of the vial to pull the diluent from the syringe into the vial. Do not forcefully inject the diluent into the vial. Do not forcefully shake the vial. Reconstitution time is generally under 2 minutes but can occasionally take as long as 20 minutes. Mix thoroughly to dissolve contents completely. Discard vial if vacuum does not pull diluent into vial. Doses of 150 to 800 mg must be further diluted in 100 to 250 mL of D5W, NS, or LR. Doses less than 150 mg or greater than 800 mg must be diluted in a sufficient volume to provide a final concentration of 0.6 to 8 mg/mL. Do not shake the final infusion solution.

Storage: Store unopened vials in refrigerator at 2° to 8° C (36° to 46° F). Excursions up to 25° C (77° F) are acceptable. Reconstituted and diluted solutions are stable for 12 hours at RT and for 7 days refrigerated. Total time in the vial plus the time in the infusion bag should not exceed 12 hours at RT and 7 days under refrigeration. The diluted solution can also be stored at −30° to −10° C (−22° to −14° F) for up to 32 days.

COMPATIBILITY   (Underline Indicates Conflicting Compatibility Information)

Consider any drug NOT listed as compatible to be INCOMPATIBLE until consulting a pharmacist; specific conditions may apply.

Manufacturer states, "Additives or other medications should not be added to telavancin single-use vials or infused simultaneously through the same IV line. If the same IV line is used for sequential infusion of additional medications, the line should be flushed before and after infusions of telavancin with D5W, NS, or LR."

One source suggests the following **compatibilities:**

Y-site: *Not recommended by manufacturer.* Amphotericin B lipid complex (Abelcet), ampicillin/sulbactam (Unasyn), azithromycin (Zithromax), calcium gluconate, caspofungin (Cancidas), cefepime (Maxipime), ceftazidime (Fortaz), ceftriaxone (Rocephin), ciprofloxacin (Cipro IV), colistimethate (Coly-Mycin M), cyclosporine (Sandimmune), dexamethasone (Decadron), diltiazem (Cardizem), dobutamine, dopamine, doripenem (Doribax), doxycycline, ertapenem (Invanz), famotidine (Pepcid IV), fluconazole (Diflucan), gentamicin, heparin, hydrocortisone sodium succinate (Solu-Cortef), imipenem-cilastatin (Primaxin), labetalol, magnesium sulfate, mannitol (Osmitrol), meropenem (Merrem IV), methylprednisolone (Solu-Medrol), metoclopramide (Reglan), milrinone (Primacor), norepinephrine (Levophed), ondansetron (Zofran), pantoprazole (Protonix IV), phenylephrine (Neo-Synephrine), piperacillin/tazobactam (Zosyn), potassium chloride (KCl), potassium phosphates, propofol (Diprivan), ranitidine (Zantac), sodium bicarbonate, sodium phosphates, tigecycline (Tygacil), tobramycin, vasopressin.

RATE OF ADMINISTRATION

A single dose equally distributed as an infusion over 60 minutes. Rapid IV infusions can cause "red man syndrome"–like infusion-related reactions, including flushing of the upper body, urticaria, pruritus, or rash. Stopping or slowing the infusion may result in cessation of these reactions.

ACTIONS

A lipoglycopeptide antibacterial that is a synthetic derivative of vancomycin. Bactericidal against gram-positive organisms, including susceptible strains of staphylococci, streptococci, and vancomycin-susceptible enterococci. Exerts bactericidal action through inhibition of cell wall synthesis. Highly protein bound, primarily to albumin. The metabolic pathway for telavancin has not been identified. Half-life is 6.6 to 9.6 hours. Primarily excreted by the kidney.

INDICATIONS AND USES

Treatment of adult patients with complicated skin and skin structure infections (cSSSI) caused by susceptible isolates of gram-positive microorganisms, including *Staphylococcus aureus* (including methicillin-susceptible and methicillin-resistant isolates), *Streptococcus pyogenes, Streptococcus agalactiae, Streptococcus anginosus* group, or *Enterococcus faecalis* (vancomycin-susceptible isolates only). ▪ Treatment of adult patients with hospital-acquired and ventilator-associated bacterial pneumonia (HABP/VABP) caused by susceptible isolates of *Staphylococcus aureus* (including methicillin-susceptible and methicillin-resistant isolates). Reserve use for when alternative treatments are not suitable.

CONTRAINDICATIONS

Known hypersensitivity to telavancin. ▪ Use of IV unfractionated heparin sodium is contraindicated; see Drug/Lab Interactions.

PRECAUTIONS

To reduce the development of drug-resistant bacteria and maintain its effectiveness, telavancin should be used to treat or prevent only those infections proven or strongly suspected to be caused by bacteria. ▪ Sensitivity studies are necessary to determine susceptibility of the causative organism to telavancin. ▪ Combination therapy may be clinically indicated if the documented or presumed pathogens include gram-negative organisms. ▪ Prolonged use of drug may result in superinfection caused by overgrowth of nonsusceptible organisms. ▪ New-onset or worsening renal impairment has been reported. Patients with underlying renal dysfunction or risk factors for renal dysfunction (diabetes mellitus, CHF, or hypertension) may be at increased risk. Patients who received concomitant medications known to affect kidney function (e.g., NSAIDs, ACE inhibitors, and loop diuretics) may also be at higher risk; see Drug Interactions. ▪ Patients with pre-existing moderate to severe renal impairment (CrCl less than or equal to 50 mL/min) who were treated with telavancin for HABP/VABP had increased mortality observed versus vancomycin. Use of telavancin in patients with pre-existing moderate to severe renal impairment should be considered only when the anticipated benefit to the patient outweighs the potential risk. ▪ Data from cSSSI trials suggest that clinical cure rates were lower in patients with baseline CrCl less than or equal to 50 mL/min. The same decrease in clinical cure rates was not seen in vancomycin-treated patients. These data should be considered when selecting antibacterial therapy for use in patients with baseline moderate/severe renal impairment. ▪ Serious and sometimes fatal hypersensitivity reactions, including anaphylactic reactions, may occur after the first dose or subsequent doses. Telavancin is a semi-synthetic derivative of vancomycin; it is unknown if patients with hypersensitivity reactions to vancomycin will experience cross-reactivity to telavancin. Use with caution in patients with known hypersensitivity to vancomycin. ▪ *Clostridium difficile*–associated diarrhea (CDAD) has been reported. May range from mild diarrhea to fatal colitis. Consider in patients who present with diarrhea during or after treatment with telavancin. ▪ Infusion-related reactions have been reported; see Rate of Administration and Monitor. ▪ Has caused prolongation of the QTc interval. Use with caution in patients who are taking drugs known to prolong the QTc interval. Avoid use in patients with congenital long QT syndrome, known prolongation of the QTc interval, uncompensated heart failure, or severe left ventricular hypertrophy. ▪ Does not interfere with coagulation. Increased risk of bleeding and effects on platelet aggregation have not been observed. However, has been shown to affect certain anticoagulation tests; see Drug/Lab Interactions. ▪ There is no known cross-resistance between telavancin and other classes of antibiotics. Some vancomycin-resistant enterococci have a reduced susceptibility to telavancin. ▪ See Maternal/Child.

Monitor: Obtain baseline CBC with differential and SCr. Monitor SCr every 48 to 72 hours, or more frequently if indicated, and at the end of therapy. If renal function deteriorates, the risk versus benefit of continuing therapy should be assessed. ▪ Monitor for possible infusion-related reactions. ▪ Monitor for S/S of hypersensitivity reactions.

Patient Education: Review manufacturer-supplied medication guide. ▪ Women of childbearing potential should have a pregnancy test before initiating therapy. Effective birth control should be used throughout therapy. A pregnancy registry has been established to monitor the outcomes of women who become pregnant while receiving telavancin. ▪ Report all side effects promptly. ▪ Promptly report diarrhea or bloody stools that occur during treatment or up to several months after telavancin has been discontinued; may indicate CDAD and require treatment.

Maternal/Child: Category C: adverse developmental outcomes in three animal species at clinically relevant doses raise concerns about potential adverse developmental outcomes in humans. Avoid use during pregnancy unless potential benefit justifies potential risk. ▪ Women with childbearing potential should have a serum pregnancy test before receiving telavancin. A pregnancy registry has been established to monitor pregnancy outcomes in women exposed to telavancin during pregnancy. ▪ Safety for use in breast-feeding not established and effects unknown; use caution. ▪ Safety and effectiveness for use in pediatric patients have not been studied.

Elderly: In cSSSI trials, lower clinical cure rates were seen in patients over 65 years of age. Overall, treatment-emergent adverse events occurred with similar frequencies in patients of all age-groups studied. However, adverse events indicative of renal impairment occurred more frequently in the elderly. In HABP/VABP trials, treatment-emergent adverse events, deaths, and other serious adverse events occurred more often in patients 65 years of age or older. Consider age-related renal impairment; see Dose Adjustments.

DRUG/LAB INTERACTIONS
Use with caution in patients taking **medications known to prolong the QTc interval** (e.g., amiodarone [Nexterone] and other antiarrhythmics, diphenhydramine [Benadryl], fosphenytoin [Cerebyx], furosemide [Lasix], itraconazole [Sporanox]). Effects may be additive. ▪ Concomitant use with **other agents that can affect renal function** (e.g., NSAIDs [e.g., ibuprofen (Advil, Motrin), naproxen (Naprosyn, Aleve)], diuretics [e.g., furosemide (Lasix)], and ACE inhibitors [e.g., lisinopril (Zestril), enalapril (Vasotec)]) may increase the risk of renal toxicity. ▪ Has been administered with aztreonam (Azactam) and piperacillin/tazobactam (Zosyn). There was no effect on the pharmacokinetics of either drug. ▪ In vitro studies demonstrate no antagonism between telavancin and amikacin, aztreonam (Azactam), cefepime (Maxipime), ceftriaxone (Rocephin), ciprofloxacin (Cipro), gentamicin, imipenem-cilastatin (Primaxin), meropenem (Merrem), oxacillin (Bactocil), rifampin (Rifadin), and sulfamethoxazole/trimethoprim when tested against telavancin-susceptible staphylococci, streptococci, and enterococci. ▪ May affect **certain anticoagulation tests.** Increases in PT, INR, aPTT, ACT, and coagulation-based factor X activity assays have been observed. Effects dissipate over time. Interference seen when using samples drawn between 0 and 18 hours after telavancin administration. Collect blood samples for these coagulation tests immediately before a patient's next telavancin dose to minimize interaction. Because aPPT test results are expected to be artificially prolonged after televancin administration, concurrent use of intravenous unfractionated **heparin** is contraindicated. ▪ Interferes with **urine qualitative dipstick protein assays** and **quantitative dye methods** (e.g., pyrogallol red-molybdate). However, microalbumin assays are not affected and can be used to monitor urinary protein excretion.

SIDE EFFECTS
The most common side effects include diarrhea, foamy urine, nausea, taste disturbances, and vomiting. Most serious side effects include cardiac events, CDAD, infusion-related reactions, nephrotoxicity (increased SCr, renal insufficiency, renal failure), and respiratory events. The most common events leading to discontinuation of therapy were acute renal failure, nausea, QTc prolongation, and rash. Other reported side effects include abdominal pain, decreased appetite, dizziness, infusion site pain and erythema, pruritus, and rigors.

Post-Marketing: Hypersensitivity reactions, including anaphylaxis.

ANTIDOTE
Notify the physician of all side effects. Initiate supportive care as indicated. Infusion-related reactions may respond to temporarily discontinuing or slowing the rate of infusion. Consider alternative antimicrobial therapy in patients who develop renal toxicity. Discontinue telavancin at the first sign of skin rash or other sign of hypersensitivity. Treat CDAD with fluids, electrolytes, protein supplements, and oral vancomycin (Vancocin) or metronidazole (Flagyl) as indicated. In severe cases, surgical evaluation may be indicated. There is no information on the use of hemodialysis or continuous venovenous hemofiltration in toxicity.

TEMOZOLOMIDE
(te-moe-**ZOE**-loe-mide)

Antineoplastic
(alkylating agent)

Temodar

USUAL DOSE

IV and oral doses are therapeutically equivalent if the IV dose is administered equally distributed over 90 minutes. The oral form should be used as soon as tolerated by the patient.

Newly diagnosed glioblastoma multiforme (GBM): *Concomitant phase:* 75 mg/M^2 daily for 42 days. Given concomitantly with focal radiotherapy. No dose reductions are recommended during the concomitant phase; however, dose interruptions or discontinuation may occur based on toxicity. The temozolomide dose should be continued throughout the 42-day concomitant period up to 49 days if all of the following conditions are met:

- Absolute neutrophil count must be equal to or greater than 1.5 × 10^9/L (1,500/mm^3).
- Platelet count must be equal to or greater than 100 × 10^9/L (100,000/mm^3).
- Nonhematologic toxicity must be equal to or less than Grade 1 (except for alopecia, nausea, and vomiting).
- CBC and platelet count should be obtained weekly.
- Interrupt or discontinue temozolomide dosing based on the hematologic and nonhematologic criteria in the following chart.

Temozolomide (TMZ) Dosing Interruption or Discontinuation During Concomitant Radiotherapy		
Toxicity	TMZ Interruption*	TMZ Discontinuation
Absolute neutrophil count	≥0.5 and <1.5 × 10^9/L	<0.5 × 10^9/L
Platelet count	≥10 and <100 × 10^9/L	<10 × 10^9/L
CTCAE nonhematologic toxicity (except for alopecia, nausea, vomiting)	CTCAE Grade 2	CTCAE Grade 3 or 4

TMZ, Temozolomide; *CTCAE*, Common Terminology Criteria for Adverse Events.
*Treatment with concomitant TMZ could be continued when all of the following conditions are met: ANC ≥1.5 × 10^9/L, platelet count ≥100 × 10^9/L, CTCAE nonhematologic toxicity Grade ≤1 (except for alopecia, nausea, vomiting).

Prophylaxis against *Pneumocystis jiroveci* pneumonia (PCP): Required for all patients during this concomitant therapy. PCP prophylaxis should be continued in patients who develop lymphocytopenia until they recover from lymphocytopenia (CTCAE Grade ≤1).

Newly diagnosed glioblastoma multiforme (GBM): *Maintenance phase:* 4 weeks after completing the temozolomide plus focal radiotherapy phase, temozolomide is administered for an additional 6 cycles of maintenance.

Cycle 1: The initial dose is 150 mg/M^2 once daily for 5 days followed by 23 days without treatment (a 28-day cycle).

Cycles 2 through 6: The dose can be increased to 200 mg/M^2 if the following conditions are met:

- Absolute neutrophil count is equal to or greater than 1.5 × 10^9/L (1,500/mm^3)
- Platelet count is equal to or greater than 100 × 10^9/L (100,000/mm^3)
- Nonhematologic toxicity is equal to or less than Grade 2 (except for alopecia, nausea, and vomiting).

The dose remains at 200 mg/M^2 per day for the first 5 days of each subsequent cycle except if toxicity occurs. If the dose was not increased at Cycle 2, it should not be increased for subsequent cycles. See Dose Adjustments for dose reduction or discontinuation during maintenance.

Refractory anaplastic astrocytoma: 150 mg/M^2 once daily for 5 consecutive days for each 28-day treatment cycle. This dose may be increased to 200 mg/M^2/day if both the nadir and day of dosing (Day 29, Day 1 of next cycle) ANC are equal to or greater than 1.5 × 10^9/L (1,500/mm^3) and the nadir and day of dosing (Day 29, Day 1 of next cycle) platelet count are equal to or greater than 100 × 10^9/L (100,000/mm^3). During treatment, a CBC should be obtained on Day 22 (21 days after the Day 1 dose of temozolomide) or within 48 hours of that day for each cycle. Repeat weekly until the ANC is above 1.5 × 10^9/L (1,500/mm^3) and the platelet count exceeds 100 × 10^9/L (100,000/mm^3). The next cycle of temozolomide should not be started until the ANC and platelet count exceed these levels. If the ANC falls to <1 × 10^9/L (1,000/mm^3) or the platelet count is <50 × 10^9/L (50,000/mm^3) during any cycle, reduce the next cycle by 50 mg/M^2 but not below 100 mg/M^2 (the lowest recommended dose). Therapy can be continued until disease progression. See the flow chart in Dose Adjustments.

DOSE ADJUSTMENTS

Newly diagnosed glioblastoma multiforme (GBM): Temozolomide dose must be adjusted according to the nadir ANC and platelet counts in the previous cycle and the ANC and platelet counts at the time of initiating the next cycle. Obtain a CBC and platelet count weekly during the concomitant phase and as indicated during the 4-week interim before beginning the maintenance phase. Obtain a baseline CBC and platelet count before beginning a cycle and repeat on Day 22 (21 days after the first dose of temozolomide in the cycle or within 48 hours of that day). Repeat weekly until the ANC is above 1.5 × 10^9/L (1,500/mm^3) and the platelet count exceeds 100 × 10^9/L (100,000/mm^3). The next cycle of temozolomide should not be started until the ANC and platelet count exceed these levels. This sequence is repeated for Cycles 1 through 6 of maintenance dosing. Base dose reductions during the next cycle on the lowest blood counts and worst nonhematologic toxicity during the previous cycle. Dose reductions or discontinuations during maintenance should be applied according to the following two charts.

Temozolomide Dose Levels for Maintenance Treatment		
Dose Level	Dose (mg/M^2/day)	Remarks
−1	100 mg/M^2/day	Reduction for prior toxicity
0	150 mg/M^2/day	Dose during Cycle 1
1	200 mg/M^2/day	Dose during Cycles 2 through 6 in absence of toxicity

Temozolomide Dose Reduction or Discontinuation During Maintenance Treatment		
Toxicity	Reduce TMZ by 1 Dose Level*	Discontinue TMZ
ANC	<1 × 10^9/L	See † in footnote
Platelet count	<50 × 10^9/L	See † in footnote
CTCAE nonhematologic toxicity (except for alopecia, nausea, vomiting)	CTCAE Grade 3	CTCAE Grade 4

TMZ, Temozolomide; *CTCAE*, Common Terminology Criteria for Adverse Events.
*See preceding chart for temozolomide dose levels for maintenance treatment.
†TMZ is to be discontinued if a dose reduction to <100 mg/M^2 is required or if the same Grade 3 nonhematologic toxicity (except for alopecia, nausea, vomiting) recurs after dose reduction.

See the next page for temozolomide dose modifications for refractory anaplastic astrocytoma. *Continued*

Temozolomide Dose Modification Table for Refractory Anaplastic Astrocytoma:

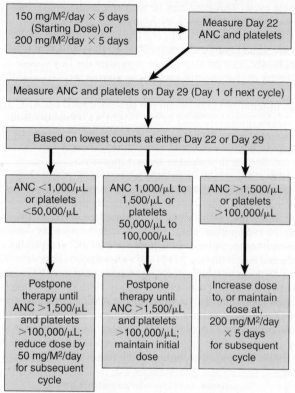

DILUTION

Specific techniques required; see Precautions. Bring vial(s) to room temperature before reconstitution. Reconstitute each 100-mg vial with 41 mL of SWFI. Swirl gently to dissolve; *do not shake;* will yield a concentration of 2.5 mg/mL of temozolomide. **Do not further dilute** the reconstituted solution. Withdraw up to 40 mL from each vial and transfer into an empty 250-mL PVC infusion bag for delivery with an infusion pump.

Filters: Specific information not available.

Storage: Refrigerate single-use vials at 2° to 8° C (36° to 46° F). Store reconstituted product at RT. Reconstituted solution must be used within 14 hours, including infusion time.

COMPATIBILITY

No **compatibility** data available. Manufacturer states, "Other medications should not be infused simultaneously through the same IV line." May be administered only in the same infusion line as NS.

RATE OF ADMINISTRATION

A single dose equally distributed over 90 minutes. Use of an infusion pump is recommended. Bioequivalence was established only with the 90-minute infusion. Infusion over a longer or shorter period may result in suboptimal dosing. In addition, the possibility of an increase in infusion-related adverse reactions cannot be ruled out. Flush IV lines before and after temozolomide infusion. Infusion must be complete within 14 hours of reconstitution.

ACTIONS

An imidazotetrazine derivative and alkylating agent. It is not directly active but undergoes rapid nonenzymatic conversion, as dacarbazine does, to the reactive compound 5-(3-methyl triazen-1-yl)-imidazole-4-carboxamide (MTIC) and to temozolomide acid metabolite. Cytotoxicity is thought to be due primarily to alkylation of DNA. Weakly bound to plasma proteins. Rapidly eliminated with a mean elimination half-life of 1.8 hours. Some excretion in urine and a very small amount in feces.

INDICATIONS AND USES

Treatment of adults with newly diagnosed glioblastoma multiforme. Initially given concomitantly with radiotherapy and then continued as maintenance treatment. ▪ Treatment of adults with refractory anaplastic astrocytoma (i.e., adults who have experienced disease progression on a drug regimen containing nitrosourea and procarbazine).

CONTRAINDICATIONS

Known history of hypersensitivity reaction to temozolomide or any of its components (e.g., urticaria, allergic reaction including anaphylaxis, toxic epidermal necrolysis, and Stevens-Johnson syndrome). ▪ Known history of hypersensitivity to dacarbazine.

PRECAUTIONS

Follow guidelines for handling cytotoxic agents. See Appendix A, p. 1331. ▪ Usually administered by or under the direction of the physician specialist in a facility with adequate diagnostic and treatment facilities to monitor the patient and respond to any medical emergency. ▪ Myelosuppression may be severe and dose limiting. May include prolonged pancytopenia, which may result in aplastic anemia. Deaths have been reported. Risk may be increased with concomitant use of other medications associated with aplastic anemia (e.g., carbamazepine [Tegretol], phenytoin [Dilantin], sulfamethoxazole/trimethoprim [Bactrim]). ▪ Risk of myelosuppression increased in women and the elderly. ▪ Cases of myelodysplastic syndrome and secondary malignancies, including myeloid leukemia, have been observed. ▪ Prophylaxis against *Pneumocystis jiroveci* pneumonia (PCP) is required for all patients being treated for newly diagnosed glioblastoma multiforme (a 42-day regimen). The longer dosing regimen may increase the risk of PCP; however, all patients, particularly those receiving steroids, should be monitored for symptoms of PCP regardless of the regimen. ▪ Severe, sometimes fatal hepatotoxicity have been reported. ▪ Use caution in patients with severe renal or hepatic impairment.

Monitor: Obtain a baseline CBC and platelet count. See Usual Dose for minimum levels required before administration of temozolomide. ▪ Obtain baseline liver function tests. Repeat midway through the first cycle, before each subsequent cycle, and approximately 2 to 4 weeks after the last dose of temozolomide.

Patients with newly diagnosed GBM: Obtain a CBC and platelet count weekly during the concomitant phase and as indicated during the 4-week interim before beginning the maintenance phase. Obtain a baseline CBC and platelet count before beginning a maintenance dose (28-day cycles) and repeat on Day 22 (21 days after the first maintenance dose of temozolomide or within 48 hours of that day). Repeat weekly until the ANC is above 1.5 × 10⁹/L (1,500/mm³) and the platelet count exceeds 100 × 10⁹/L (100,000/mm³). This sequence is repeated for Cycles 1 through 6 of maintenance dosing.

Patients with refractory anaplastic astrocytoma: Obtain a CBC and platelet count on Day 1 of each cycle. During treatment (28-day cycles), a CBC should be obtained on Day 22 (21 days after the Day 1 dose of temozolomide or within 48 hours of that day for each cycle). Repeat weekly until the ANC is above 1.5 × 10⁹/L (1,500/mm³) and the platelet count exceeds 100 × 10⁹/L (100,000/mm³). Myelosuppression usually occurred within the first few cycles of therapy and was not cumulative. It occurred late in the treatment cycle and returned to normal, on average, within 14 days of nadir counts. (The median nadirs occurred at 26 days for platelets and 28 days for neutrophils.)

All indications: Nausea and vomiting may be significant. Prophylactic antiemetics may reduce nausea and vomiting and increase patient comfort. ▪ Observe closely for signs of infection. Prophylactic antibiotics may be indicated pending results of C/S in a febrile neutropenic patient. ▪ Monitor for thrombocytopenia (platelet count less than 50,000/mm³). Initiate precautions to prevent excessive bleeding (e.g., inspect IV sites, skin, and mucous membranes; use extreme care during invasive procedures; test urine, emesis, stool, and secretions for occult blood). ▪ Regardless of the regimen, monitor all patients, particularly those receiving steroids, for symptoms of PCP (dyspnea; fever; dry, nonproductive cough; characteristic x-ray).

Patient Education: Avoid pregnancy; use of nonhormonal birth control is recommended. ▪ Promptly report a rash; swelling of the face, throat, or tongue; severe skin reaction; or troubled breathing. ▪ Report IV site burning or stinging promptly. ▪ Secondary malignancies have been reported. ▪ See Appendix D, p. 1333. ▪ Additional precautions are required with the capsule form.

Maternal/Child: Category D: avoid pregnancy; can cause fetal harm. ▪ Discontinue breast-feeding. ▪ Safety and effectiveness for use in pediatric patients not established. A 5-day regimen every 28 days using the oral formulation has been studied in selected pediatric patients from 3 to 18 years of age. Toxicity profile was similar to that seen in adults.

Elderly: Numbers in clinical studies are insufficient to determine if the elderly respond differently than younger subjects. Dose selection should be cautious based on the potential for decreased organ function and concomitant disease or drug therapy. *In newly diagnosed patients with glioblastoma multiforme,* side effects were similar to those seen in younger patients. In the *anaplastic astrocytoma study,* patients 70 years or older had a higher incidence of Grade 4 neutropenia and Grade 4 thrombocytopenia in the first cycle of therapy.

DRUG/LAB INTERACTIONS

Valproic acid decreases the oral clearance of temozolomide by about 5%; clinical significance is not known. ▪ Administration of **live attenuated viral or bacterial vaccines** should be avoided.

SIDE EFFECTS

Newly diagnosed glioblastoma multiforme: Myelosuppression may be severe and dose limiting. May include prolonged pancytopenia, which may result in aplastic anemia; deaths have been reported. Alopecia, anorexia, constipation, headache, nausea and vomiting, and thrombocytopenia were the most frequently reported side effects. The most commonly reported severe or life-threatening reactions were convulsions, fatigue, headache, and thrombocytopenia. Abdominal pain, arthralgia, blurred vision, confusion, coughing, diarrhea, dizziness, dry skin, dyspnea, erythema, hypersensitivity reactions (including anaphylaxis), insomnia, memory impairment, pruritus, radiation injury, rash, stomatitis, taste perversion, and weakness have also been reported.

Refractory anaplastic astrocytoma: Fatigue, headache, and nausea and vomiting were the most frequently reported side effects. Myelosuppression (neutropenia and thrombocytopenia) was the dose-limiting adverse reaction. Abdominal pain, abnormal coordination, abnormal gait, abnormal vision (blurred vision, vision changes, visual deficit), adrenal hypercorticism, amnesia, anemia, anorexia, anxiety, asthenia, ataxia, back pain, breast pain (female), confusion, constipation, convulsions (local and general), coughing, depression, diarrhea, diplopia, dizziness, dysphasia, fever, hemiparesis, insomnia, lymphopenia, myalgia, paresis, paresthesia, peripheral edema, pharyngitis, pruritus, rash, sinusitis, somnolence, URI, urinary incontinence, UTI, viral infection, and weight increase have been reported.

Injection site reactions: Erythema, irritation, pain, pruritus, swelling, and warmth at the infusion site; hematoma; and petechiae.

Post-Marketing: Alveolitis, cholestasis, diabetes insipidus, elevation of liver enzymes, erythema multiforme, hepatitis, hepatotoxicity (severe and sometimes fatal), hyperbilirubinemia, hypersensitivity reactions (including anaphylaxis), opportunistic infections (including pneumocystis pneumonia [PCP], primary and reactivated cytomegalovirus [CMV], and reactivation of hepatitis B), interstitial pneumonitis, pneumonitis, prolonged pancytopenia that may result in aplastic anemia with fatal outcomes, pulmonary fibrosis, Stevens-Johnson syndrome, and toxic epidermal necrolysis.

ANTIDOTE

Keep physician informed of all side effects and CBC results. Temozolomide may need to be reduced or discontinued. Symptomatic and supportive treatment is indicated. Administration of whole blood products (e.g., packed RBCs, platelets, leukocytes) and/or blood modifiers (e.g., darbepoetin alfa [Aranesp], epoetin alfa [Epogen], filgrastim [Neupogen, Zarxio], pegfilgrastim [Neulasta], sargramostim [Leukine]) may be indicated to treat bone marrow toxicity. Precautions are indicated for cancer patients with erythropoietin-stimulating agents (ESAs); see darbepoetin alfa and epoetin alfa monographs. Treat hypersensitivity reactions and/or anaphylaxis as indicated (e.g., epinephrine, corticosteroids, oxygen, and antihistamines [diphenhydramine]). There is no specific antidote. Resuscitate as indicated.

TEMSIROLIMUS
(**TEM**-sir-**OH**-li-mus)

Torisel

Antineoplastic
(kinase inhibitor)

USUAL DOSE

Premedication: To minimize the incidence of hypersensitivity reactions, administer diphenhydramine (Benadryl) 25 to 50 mg IV (or similar antihistamine) 30 minutes before the start of each dose of temsirolimus; see Precautions and Monitor.

Temsirolimus: 25 mg as an infusion once a week until disease progression or unacceptable toxicity.

DOSE ADJUSTMENTS

Hold for absolute neutrophil count (ANC) less than 1,000/mm³, platelet count less than 75,000/mm³, or CTCAE Grade 3 or greater adverse reactions. Once toxicities have resolved to Grade 2 or less, restart therapy with the dose reduced by 5 mg/week to a dose no lower than 15 mg/week. ▪ Consider dose reduction to 12.5 mg/week when coadministered with a strong CYP3A4 inhibitor; see Drug Interactions. If the strong inhibitor is discontinued, wait approximately 1 week before adjusting the temsirolimus dose upward to the indicated dose. ▪ Consider a dose increase to 50 mg/week when coadministered with a strong CYP3A4 inducer; see Drug Interactions. If the strong inducer is discontinued, the temsirolimus dose should be returned to the dose used prior to initiation of the strong CYP3A4 inducer. ▪ Decrease dose to 15 mg/week in patients with mild hepatic impairment (bilirubin greater than 1 to 1.5 ULN or AST greater than ULN but bilirubin equal to or less than ULN); see Contraindications. ▪ No dose adjustment indicated based on age, race, gender, or renal status. Not studied in hemodialysis patients.

DILUTION

Specific techniques required; see Precautions and Compatibility. Available as a kit containing a vial of temsirolimus and a vial of a manufacturer-supplied diluent. Temsirolimus and diluent vials contain overfill. A two-step dilution process is required. Reconstitute the temsirolimus vial with 1.8 mL of the provided diluent. Invert the vial several times to mix thoroughly. Allow time for foam to subside. Final concentration in temsirolimus vial is 10 mg/mL. Solution will be clear to slightly turbid and colorless to yellow. Withdraw the required amount of reconstituted temsirolimus and inject into a 250-mL container *(glass, polyolefin, or polypropylene)* of NS. Invert bag to mix; **see Compatibility.** Avoid excessive shaking. Use of non-DEHP, non-polyvinylchloride (PVC) tubing (polyethylene-lined administration set is recommended) with appropriate filter is recommended. If a PVC administration set must be used, it should not contain DEHP. Temsirolimus contains polysorbate 80 when diluted, which increases the rate of DEHP extraction from PVC.

Filter: Use of an in-line polyethersulfone filter with a pore size not greater than 5 microns is recommended. If an administration set with an in-line filter is not available, a poly-ethersulfone end-filter should be used. The use of both an in-line and end-filter is not recommended.

Storage: Store unopened vials at 2° to 8° C (36° to 46° F). Protect from light. During handling and preparation, protect from excessive room light or sunlight. The temsirolimus/diluent mixture (10 mg/mL) is stable for up to 24 hours below 25° C (77° F) in the temsirolimus vial. Administration of the final product diluted in NS should be completed within 6 hours of adding the temsirolimus/diluent mixture to the NS.

COMPATIBILITY

Manufacturer states, "Final dilution for infusion should be stored in bottles (glass, polypropylene) or plastic bags (polypropylene, polyolefin) and administered through polyethylene-lined administration sets." Non–DEHP-containing materials must be used for administration. Manufacturer also states that undiluted temsirolimus should not be added directly to aqueous infusion solutions. A precipitate will form. In addition, "The stability of temsirolimus in other infusion solutions has not been evaluated. Addition of other drugs or nutritional agents to admixtures of temsirolimus in NS has not been evaluated and should be avoided. Temsirolimus is degraded by both acids and bases, and thus combinations of temsirolimus with agents capable of modifying solution pH should be avoided."

RATE OF ADMINISTRATION

A single dose as an infusion equally distributed over 30 to 60 minutes. Use of an infusion pump is recommended. Increase duration of infusion to 60 minutes in patients who experience a hypersensitivity reaction.

ACTIONS

An inhibitor of mTOR (mammalian target of rapamycin). Binds to an intracellular protein (FKBP-12); this protein-drug complex inhibits the activity of mTOR that controls cell division. Results in a cell cycle–specific (G1) growth arrest in treated tumor cells. In in vitro studies, temsirolimus inhibited the activity of mTOR and resulted in reduced levels of hypoxia-inducible factors HIF-1α and HIF-2α and the vascular endothelial growth factor. Both temsirolimus and sirolimus are extensively partitioned into formed blood elements. Extensively metabolized, primarily by cytochrome P_{450} 3A4. Sirolimus is the principal metabolite and is active. Elimination is primarily via the feces and to a small extent via urine. Mean half-lives of temsirolimus and sirolimus were 17.3 and 54.6 hours, respectively.

INDICATIONS AND USES

Treatment of advanced renal cell carcinoma.

CONTRAINDICATIONS

Bilirubin greater than 1.5 ULN; see Dose Adjustments and Precautions.

PRECAUTIONS

Follow guidelines for handling cytotoxic agents. See Appendix A, p. 1331. ■ Should be administered by or under the direction of the physician specialist in facilities equipped to monitor the patient and respond to any medical emergency. ■ Hypersensitivity/infusion reactions have been reported. May occur early in the first infusion but may also occur with subsequent infusions. Premedication required to minimize the chance of a reaction; see Usual Dose. Use with caution in patients with known hypersensitivity to temsirolimus or its metabolites (including sirolimus) or to any components of the product. Use caution in patients who cannot receive prophylactic treatment with an antihistamine for medical reasons; see Monitor. ■ Patients with moderate and severe hepatic impairment had increased rates of adverse reactions and deaths. Use caution when treating patients with mild hepatic impairment; see Dose Adjustments and Contraindications. ■ Hyperglycemia/glucose intolerance is common. Initiation of or an increase in the dose of insulin and/or oral hypoglycemic agent therapy may be required. ■ Elevated cholesterol and triglycerides are common. Initiation or adjustment of existing therapy may be required.

▪ May cause immunosuppression, thus increasing the risk of infections, including opportunistic infections. *Pneumocystis jiroveci* pneumonia (PJP), including fatalities, has been reported. May be associated with concomitant use of corticosteroids or other immunosuppressants. ▪ Cases of interstitial lung disease, some resulting in death, have been reported. ▪ Cases of fatal bowel perforation have been reported. ▪ Rapidly progressive and sometimes fatal acute renal failure has occurred. ▪ Has been associated with abnormal wound healing. Exercise caution when temsirolimus is used in the perioperative period. ▪ Patients who have CNS tumors and/or are receiving anticoagulation therapy may be at increased risk of intracerebral bleeding. ▪ The use of live virus vaccines and close contact with those who have received live virus vaccines should be avoided. See Drug Interactions.

Monitor: Obtain baseline and weekly CBC with differential and platelet count. Obtain a baseline chemistry panel, including bilirubin and liver function tests (ALT, AST), and repeat every 2 weeks. Obtain baseline radiographic assessment by lung CT or chest x-ray. Repeat assessments periodically. ▪ Monitor for S/S of a hypersensitivity/infusion reaction (e.g., anaphylaxis, apnea, bronchospasm, chest pain, dyspnea, flushing, hypotension, loss of consciousness, rash). If a reaction occurs, the infusion should be stopped and the patient should be observed for at least 30 to 60 minutes (depending on the severity of the reaction). At the discretion of the physician, and after a benefit-risk assessment, treatment may be resumed with the administration of an H_1-receptor antagonist (such as diphenhydramine [Benadryl]) if not previously administered and/or an H_2-receptor antagonist (e.g., ranitidine [Zantac] 50 mg IV or famotidine [Pepcid] 20 mg IV) approximately 30 minutes before restarting the temsirolimus infusion. The infusion may be resumed at a slower rate; see Rate of Administration. ▪ Monitor serum glucose, cholesterol, and triglycerides before and during therapy. ▪ Monitor for S/S of infection. ▪ Consider prophylaxis of PJP when concomitant use of corticosteroids or other immunosuppressive agents are required. ▪ Monitor respiratory status. Patients may present with symptoms such as dyspnea, cough, hypoxia, and fever or may be asymptomatic. If clinically significant respiratory symptoms develop, consider withholding temsirolimus until after recovery of symptoms and improvement of radiographic findings related to pneumonitis. Opportunistic infections such as PJP should be considered in the differential diagnosis. Empiric treatment with corticosteroids and/or antibiotics may be considered. ▪ Monitor for S/S of bowel perforation (abdominal pain, acute abdomen, bloody stools, diarrhea, fever, metabolic acidosis). ▪ Monitor for thrombocytopenia (platelet count less than $50,000/mm^3$); see Dose Adjustments and Contraindications. Initiate precautions to prevent excessive bleeding (e.g., inspect IV sites, skin, and mucous membranes; use extreme care during invasive procedures; test urine, emesis, stool, and secretions for occult blood).

Patient Education: Review medical history with health care provider. Temsirolimus may affect existing medical conditions (e.g., diabetes, high cholesterol, hyperlipidemia). Therapy may need to be adjusted. ▪ Review medication list (prescription, over-the-counter, and herbal [including past or present use of corticosteroids or immunosuppressants]) with health care provider. Interactions are possible. ▪ Promptly report any S/S of a hypersensitivity reaction (chest tightness, dyspnea, flushing, pruritus, rash, urticaria). ▪ Avoid pregnancy during and for 3 months after completion of therapy. Men with partners of childbearing potential should use reliable contraception during treatment and for 3 months after completion of therapy. ▪ Report excessive thirst or any increase in volume or frequency of urination. ▪ Promptly report S/S of infection, new or worsening respiratory symptoms, new or worsening abdominal pain, or blood in stools. ▪ Wound healing complications may occur while on therapy. ▪ The use of live virus vaccines and close contact with those who have received live virus vaccines should be avoided. ▪ Increased risk of intracerebral bleed in patients who have CNS tumors and/or are receiving anticoagulants.

Maternal/Child: Category D: avoid pregnancy; may cause fetal harm. ▪ Potential for tumorigenicity. Discontinue breast-feeding. ▪ Safety and effectiveness for use in pediatric patients not established.

Elderly: Elderly patients may be more likely to experience certain side effects, including diarrhea, edema, and pneumonia.

DRUG/LAB INTERACTIONS

Concomitant use of **strong CYP3A4 inhibitors** (e.g., amprenavir [Agenerase], atazanavir [Reyataz], clarithromycin [Biaxin], delavirdine [Rescriptor], indinavir [Crixivan], itraconazole [Sporanox], ketoconazole [Nizoral], nefazodone, nelfinavir [Viracept], ritonavir [Norvir], saquinavir [Invirase], telithromycin [Ketek], or voriconazole [VFEND]) may increase plasma concentrations of the active metabolite sirolimus. Avoid concomitant use if possible. If required, consider a dose reduction of temsirolimus to 12.5 mg/week and monitor closely for acute toxicity. If the strong inhibitor is discontinued, a washout period of approximately 1 week should be allowed before adjusting the temsirolimus dose upward to the indicated dose; see Dose Adjustments. ▪ **Grapefruit juice** may increase plasma concentrations of sirolimus (a major metabolite of temsirolimus) and should be avoided. ▪ **CYP3A4/5 inducers** (e.g., carbamazepine [Tegretol], dexamethasone [Decadron], phenobarbital [Luminal], phenytoin [Dilantin], rifabutin [Mycobutin], rifampin [Rifadin]) may decrease plasma concentrations of the active metabolite sirolimus, thus decreasing effectiveness. Avoid concomitant use if possible. If required, consider a dose increase to 50 mg/week. If the strong inducer is discontinued, the temsirolimus dose should be returned to the dose used before initiating the strong CYP3A4 inducer; see Dose Adjustments. ▪ Angioneurotic edema-type reactions (including delayed reactions occurring 2 months after initiation of therapy) have been observed in some patients with concurrent administration of ACE inhibitors (e.g., enalapril [Vasotec]). ▪ **St. John's wort** may decrease temsirolimus plasma concentrations, decreasing effectiveness. Avoid use. ▪ Use caution with other **drugs that inhibit the efflux transporter P-glycoprotein (P-gp, ABCB1)** (e.g., protease inhibitors [e.g., nelfinavir (Viracept)]); may increase concentrations of temsirolimus. ▪ Temsirolimus inhibits P-gp in vitro. Coadministration with drugs that are substrates of P-gp may result in increased concentration of substrates. ▪ The combination of sunitinib (Sutent) and temsirolimus resulted in dose-limiting toxicity. ▪ Do not administer **live virus vaccines** to patients receiving temsirolimus, and avoid close contact with those who have received live virus vaccines. ▪ No clinically significant effect is anticipated when temsirolimus is coadministered with agents that are metabolized by CYP2D6 or CYP3A4.

SIDE EFFECTS

The most common side effects include anemia, anorexia, asthenia, edema, elevated alkaline phosphatase and AST, elevated SCr, hyperglycemia, hyperlipemia, hypertriglyceridemia, hypophosphatemia, leukopenia, lymphopenia, mucositis, nausea, rash, and thrombocytopenia. Other commonly reported side effects include abdominal pain, acne, arthralgia, chest pain, chills, constipation, convulsions, cough, depression, diarrhea, dry skin, dysgeusia, dyspnea, edema, epistaxis, fever, headache, hemorrhage (GI, rectal), hypokalemia, increased bilirubin, increased total cholesterol, increased triglycerides, infection (pneumonia, URI, wound [including postoperative] sepsis), insomnia, nail disorder, neutropenia, pain, pericardial effusion, pleural effusion, pneumonitis, pruritus, rash, vomiting, and weight loss. The most serious side effects include bowel perforation, hyperglycemia/glucose intolerance, hyperlipemia, hypersensitivity reactions, hypertension, interstitial lung disease, intracerebral hemorrhage, renal failure, venous thromboembolism (including DVT and pulmonary embolus [including fatal outcomes]), and wound healing complications.

Post-Marketing: Complex regional pain syndrome (reflex sympathetic dystrophy); extravasation with erythema, pain, swelling, and warmth; injection site reactions; rhabdomyolysis; Stevens-Johnson syndrome.

ANTIDOTE

Keep physician informed of all side effects. Most minor side effects will be treated symptomatically. Monitor patient closely. Discontinue temsirolimus at the first sign of a hypersensitivity reaction. Monitor patient for 30 to 60 minutes. Treatment may be resumed at the discretion of the physician; see Monitor. Treat severe hypersensitivity reactions as indicated; may require epinephrine, airway management, oxygen, IV fluids, antihistamines (e.g., diphenhydramine [Benadryl]), corticosteroids (e.g., hydrocortisone sodium succinate [Solu-Cortef]), and pressor amines (e.g., dopamine). Treat the development of interstitial lung disease as indicated. May require discontinuation of temsirolimus and/or treatment with corticosteroids and/or antibiotics. Some patients have been able to continue therapy without additional intervention.

TENECTEPLASE

(teh-**NECK**-teh-plays)

TNKase

Thrombolytic agent
(recombinant)

pH 7.3

USUAL DOSE

Initiate therapy as soon as possible after the onset of acute myocardial infarction (AMI) symptoms. Total dose is based on patient weight and should not exceed 50 mg. See the following chart.

Tenecteplase Dosing Guidelines		
Patient Weight (kg)	Tenecteplase (mg)	Volume of Tenecteplase* to Be Administered (mL)
<60 kg	30 mg	6 mL
≥60 to <70 kg	35 mg	7 mL
≥70 to <80 kg	40 mg	8 mL
≥80 to <90 kg	45 mg	9 mL
≥90 kg	50 mg	10 mL

*From one vial of tenecteplase reconstituted with 10 mL of SWFI.

Concurrent administration of heparin and aspirin has been used in MI patients receiving tenecteplase therapy. In the ASSENT-2 trial, the following doses were used.

Aspirin: 150 to 325 mg as soon as possible was followed by 150 to 325 mg daily.

Heparin IV: Was administered based on weight. *Patients weighing 67 kg or less* received a heparin loading dose of 4,000 units followed by an infusion at 800 units/hr. *Patients weighing more than 67 kg* received a heparin loading dose of 5,000 units followed by an infusion at 1,000 units/hr. Heparin was continued for 48 to 72 hours with the infusion rate adjusted to maintain the aPPT at 50 to 75 seconds.

DOSE ADJUSTMENTS

None noted.

DILUTION

Remove the shield assembly from the manufacturer-supplied B-D® 10-mL syringe with TwinPak™ dual Cannula Device. Aseptically withdraw 10 mL of SWFI from the supplied diluent vial using the red hub cannula syringe filling device. Do not use bacteriostatic water for injection. Do not discard the shield assembly. Inject the 10 mL of SWFI into the tenecteplase vial, directing the diluent stream into the powder. Slight foaming may occur. Allow product to stand for several minutes. Gently swirl until contents are completely dissolved. Do not shake. The reconstituted preparation is colorless to pale yellow and contains tenecteplase 50 mg/10 mL. Withdraw the desired dose from the vial using the syringe. Once the appropriate dose is drawn into the syringe, stand the shield vertically on a flat surface with the green side down and passively recap the red hub cannula. Remove the entire shield assembly, including the red hub cannula, by twisting counterclockwise. **Note:** The shield assembly also contains the clear-ended blunt plastic cannula; retain for split septum IV access. The supplied syringe is **compatible** with a conventional needle and with needleless IV systems. See package insert for complete instructions for administration.

Storage: Store unopened vial at CRT or under refrigeration (at 2° to 8° C [(36° to 46° F]). Reconstitution immediately before use preferred, or may be refrigerated for up to 8 hours.

COMPATIBILITY

Manufacturer states, "Precipitation may occur when tenecteplase is administered in an IV line containing dextrose. Dextrose-containing lines should be flushed with a saline-containing solution prior to and following single bolus administration of tenecteplase."

RATE OF ADMINISTRATION

A single bolus dose over 5 seconds. Flush line with saline-containing solution to ensure delivery of entire dose.

ACTIONS

A tissue plasminogen activator and enzyme produced by recombinant DNA technology. Binds to fibrin in a thrombus and converts plasminogen to plasmin. Plasmin digests fibrin and dissolves the clot. Onset of action is prompt. Cleared via hepatic metabolism. Terminal half-life is 90 to 130 minutes.

INDICATIONS AND USES

For use in the reduction of mortality associated with acute myocardial infarction (AMI). Treatment should be initiated as soon as possible after the onset of AMI symptoms.

CONTRAINDICATIONS

Active internal bleeding, history of cerebrovascular accident, intracranial or intraspinal surgery or trauma within the past 2 months, intracranial neoplasm, arteriovenous malformation or aneurysm, known bleeding diathesis, and severe uncontrolled hypertension.

PRECAUTIONS

Administered under the direction of a physician knowledgeable in its use and with appropriate emergency drugs and diagnostic and laboratory facilities available. ▪ Most common complication is bleeding. May be internal bleeding or superficial or surface bleeding. Strict bed rest indicated to reduce risk of bleeding. Use extreme care with the patient; avoid any excessive or rough handling or pressure; avoid invasive procedures (e.g., arterial puncture, venipuncture, IM injection). If these procedures are absolutely necessary, use extreme precautionary methods (use radial artery instead of femoral; use small-gauge catheters and needles, and sites that are easily observed and compressible where bleeding can be controlled; avoid handling catheter sites; and use extended pressure application of up to 30 minutes). Minor bleeding occurs often at catheter insertion sites. Avoid use of razors and toothbrushes. If serious bleeding (not controlled by local pressure) occurs, discontinue any concomitant heparin or antiplatelet agents immediately. ▪ Use extreme caution in the following situations: recent major surgery (e.g., CABG), previous puncture of noncompressible vessels, organ biopsy or trauma, cerebrovascular disease, recent GI or GU bleeding, hypertension (systolic BP above 180 and/or diastolic BP above 110), high likelihood of left heart thrombus (e.g., mitral stenosis with atrial fibrillation), acute pericarditis, subacute bacterial endocarditis, hemostatic defects (including those secondary to severe hepatic or renal disease), severe hepatic dysfunction, pregnancy or recent childbirth, diabetic hemorrhagic retinopathy, septic thrombophlebitis or occluded AV cannula at a seriously infected site, advanced age, patients currently receiving oral anticoagulants (e.g., warfarin), recent administration of GPIIb/

IIIa inhibitors (e.g., abciximab [ReoPro], eptifibatide [Integrilin]), or any other condition in which bleeding constitutes a significant hazard or would be particularly difficult to manage because of its location. In the presence of any of these situations, the risk versus benefit of tenecteplase therapy must be evaluated. ▪ Cholesterol embolism has been reported rarely in patients treated with all types of thrombolytic agents. See Side Effects. ▪ Reperfusion arrhythmias (e.g., sinus bradycardia, accelerated idioventricular rhythm, ventricular premature depolarization, ventricular tachycardia) may occur following coronary thrombolysis. Manage with standard antiarrhythmic measures. Have antiarrhythmic medications readily available. ▪ Standard management of MI should be implemented concomitantly with tenecteplase therapy. Simultaneous therapy with heparin and aspirin is used to reduce the risk of rethrombosis. Increases risk of bleeding; see Usual Dose. ▪ Readministration of tenecteplase to patients who have received prior plasminogen activator therapy has not been studied. Use caution if deemed necessary, and monitor for signs of hypersensitivity or anaphylactic reactions.

Monitor: Obtain appropriate clotting studies (e.g., PT, PTT, aPTT, fibrinogen levels), CBC, and platelet count. ▪ Diagnosis-specific baseline studies (e.g., ECG, CPK with isoenzymes, troponin) are indicated. Baseline assessment (patient condition, pain, hematomas, petechiae, or recent wounds) should be completed before administration. ▪ Type and cross-match may also be ordered. ▪ Maintain strict bed rest; monitor the patient carefully and frequently for pain and signs of bleeding; observe catheter sites at least every 15 minutes and apply pressure dressings to any recently invaded site; watch for hematuria, hematemesis, bloody stool, petechiae, hematoma, flank pain, muscle weakness; and do neuro checks every hour (or more frequently if indicated). Continue until normal clotting function returns. ▪ Monitor ECG continuously. ▪ See Precautions and Drug/Lab Interactions.

Patient Education: Compliance with all measures to minimize bleeding (e.g., strict bed rest) is very important. ▪ Avoid use of razors, toothbrushes, and other sharp items. Use caution while moving to avoid excessive bumping. ▪ Report all episodes of bleeding and apply local pressure if indicated. Expect oozing from IV sites.

Maternal/Child: Category C: safety for use in pregnancy, breast-feeding and pediatric patients not established.

Elderly: See Indications and Precautions. May have poorer prognosis following AMI and with pre-existing conditions that may increase the risk of adverse events, including bleeding. Select patients carefully to maximize benefits.

DRUG/LAB INTERACTIONS

Formal studies have not been performed. ▪ Risk of bleeding may be increased by **any medicine that affects blood clotting,** including anticoagulants (e.g., heparin, warfarin [Coumadin]); **any medication that may cause hypoprothrombinemia, thrombocytopenia, or GI ulceration or bleeding** (e.g., selected antibiotics [e.g., cefotetan], aspirin, NSAIDs [e.g., ibuprofen (Advil, Motrin), naproxen (Aleve, Naprosyn)]); **and/or any other medication that inhibits platelet aggregation** (e.g., clopidogrel [Plavix], dipyridamole [Persantine], glycoprotein GPIIb/IIIa receptor antagonists [e.g., abciximab (ReoPro), eptifibatide (Integrilin), tirofiban (Aggrastat)], plicamycin [Mithracin], sulfinpyrazone [Anturane], ticlopidine [Ticlid], valproic acid [Depacon, Depakene]). Concurrent use not recommended with the exception of heparin and aspirin to reduce the risk of rethrombosis. If concurrent or subsequent use indicated (e.g., management of acute coronary syndrome, percutaneous coronary intervention), monitor PT and aPTT closely. ▪ **Coagulation test will be unreliable;** specific procedures can be used; notify the lab of tenecteplase use.

SIDE EFFECTS

Bleeding is most common: internal (GI tract, GU tract, retroperitoneal, or intracranial), epistaxis, gingival, and superficial or surface bleeding (venous cutdowns, arterial punctures, sites of recent surgical intervention). Hypersensitivity reactions (e.g., anaphylaxis, angioedema, laryngeal edema, rash, and urticaria) have been reported rarely. Fever, hypotension, nausea and vomiting, and reperfusion arrhythmias have occurred. Cholesterol embolization can occur with thrombolytic therapy, but has been reported rarely. Clinical features may include livedo reticularis; "purple toe" syndrome; acute renal failure; gangrenous digits; hypertension; pancreatitis; MI; cerebral, spinal cord, or bowel infarction; retinal artery occlusion; and rhabdomyolysis. Several other adverse events have been reported. These reactions are frequently sequelae of the underlying disease, and the effect of tenecteplase on the incidence of these events is unknown.

ANTIDOTE

Notify physician of all side effects. Note even the most minute bleeding tendency. Oozing at IV sites is expected. Control minor bleeding by local pressure. For severe bleeding in a critical location or suspected intracranial bleeding, discontinue any heparin therapy immediately. Obtain PT, aPTT, platelet count, and fibrinogen. Draw blood for type and cross-match. Platelets and cryoprecipitate are most commonly used but whole blood, packed red blood cells, fresh frozen plasma, desmopressin, tranexamic acid, or aminocaproic acid may be indicated. Topical preparations of aminocaproic acid may stop minor bleeding. Consider protamine if heparin has been used. Treat bradycardia with atropine, and treat reperfusion arrhythmias with lidocaine, procainamide, or other standard antiarrhythmic therapy; VT or VF may require cardioversion. If hypotension occurs, vasopressors (e.g., dopamine), Trendelenburg position, and suitable plasma expanders (e.g., albumin, plasma protein fraction [Plasmanate], or hetastarch) may be indicated. Treat minor hypersensitivity reactions symptomatically. Discontinue drug and treat anaphylaxis as indicated; resuscitate as necessary.

TENIPOSIDE BBW

(teh-**NIP**-ah-side)

VM-26, Vumon

Antineoplastic
(mitotic inhibitor)

pH 5

USUAL DOSE

Adults: *All indications and doses are unlabeled.*

Acute lymphoblastic leukemia: 165 mg/M^2 by IV infusion on Days 1, 4, 8, and 11 during consolidation on the "Linker" regimen.

Refractory non-Hodgkin's lymphoma: Given as an IV infusion. Dosage schedules include 30 mg/M^2 for 10 days or 50 to 100 mg/M^2 weekly as a single agent; or 60 to 70 mg/M^2 weekly in combination with other chemotherapy agents.

PEDIATRIC DOSE

See Precautions and Maternal/Child. Optimum dose not established.

Acute lymphocytic leukemia (ALL): 165 mg/M^2 in combination with cytarabine 300 mg/M^2. Both drugs are given twice weekly for 8 to 9 doses. An alternate regimen includes teniposide 250 mg/M^2 and vincristine 1.5 mg/M^2 once each week for 4 to 8 weeks plus prednisone 40 mg/M^2 PO daily for 28 days.

DOSE ADJUSTMENTS

Reduce dose by one half in patients with Down's syndrome and leukemia (increased sensitivity to myelosuppressive chemotherapy). Higher doses may be used in subsequent courses based on degree of myelosuppression and mucositis. Must be individualized. ■ Reduced dose may be necessary in severe renal or hepatic impairment.

DILUTION

Specific techniques required; see Precautions. Must be diluted and given as an infusion. May leach the toxic plasticizer DEHP from PVC infusion bags or sets; prepare and store in bottles (glass, polypropylene) or plastic bags (polypropylene, polyolefin) and administer through polyethylene-lined administration sets (e.g., lipid administration sets or low DEHP–containing nitroglycerin IV sets). Undiluted tenoposide has caused acrylic or ABS plastic devices to crack and leak; handle carefully during dilution process.

Compatible with NS or D5W. Final concentration of 0.1, 0.2, 0.4, or 1 mg/mL desired. Contains 10 mg/mL. 100 mg (10 mL) in 990 mL yields 0.1 mg/mL, in 490 mL yields 0.2 mg/mL, in 240 mL yields 0.4 mg/mL, in 90 mL yields 1 mg/mL. Precipitation may occur at recommended concentrations, especially with excessive agitation. Avoid contact of diluted solution with any other drugs or fluids; flush IV line with D5W or NS before and after administration.

Storage: Refrigerate unopened ampules in original packaging. Do not refrigerate diluted solutions; 1 mg/mL should be administered within 4 hours; all other dilutions are stable at RT for up to 24 hours.

COMPATIBILITY

Consider any drug NOT listed as compatible to be INCOMPATIBLE until consulting a pharmacist; specific conditions may apply.

Manufacturer states, "Heparin solution can cause precipitation of teniposide; flush IV line thoroughly with D5W or NS before and after administration of teniposide. Because of potential for precipitation, **compatibility** with other drugs, infusion materials, or IV pumps cannot be ensured." See Dilution, Rate of Administration, and Precautions/Monitor.

One source suggests the following **compatibilities:**
Y-site: *Not recommended by manufacturer.* Acyclovir (Zovirax), allopurinol (Aloprim), amifostine (Ethyol), amikacin, aminophylline, amphotericin B (conventional), ampicillin, ampicillin/sulbactam (Unasyn), aztreonam (Azactam), bleomycin (Blenoxane), bumetanide, buprenorphine (Buprenex), butorphanol (Stadol), calcium gluconate, carboplatin (Paraplatin), carmustine (BiCNU), cefazolin (Ancef), cefotaxime (Claforan), cefotetan, cefoxitin (Mefoxin), ceftazidime (Fortaz), ceftriaxone (Rocephin), cefuroxime (Zinacef), chlorpromazine (Thorazine), ciprofloxacin (Cipro IV), cisplatin, cladribine (Leustatin), clindamycin (Cleocin), cyclophosphamide (Cytoxan), cytarabine (ARA-C), dacarbazine (DTIC), dactinomycin (Cosmegen), daunorubicin (Cerubidine), dexamethasone (Decadron), diphenhydramine (Benadryl), doxorubicin (Adriamycin), doxycycline, droperidol (Inapsine), enalaprilat (Vasotec IV), etoposide (VePesid), etoposide phosphate (Etopophos), famotidine (Pepcid IV), fluconazole (Diflucan), fludarabine (Fludara), fluorouracil (5-FU), furosemide (Lasix), gallium nitrate (Ganite), ganciclovir (Cytovene IV), gemcitabine (Gemzar), gentamicin, granisetron (Kytril), hydrocortisone sodium succinate (Solu-Cortef), hydromorphone (Dilaudid), ifosfamide (Ifex), imipenem-cilastatin (Primaxin), leucovorin calcium, lorazepam (Ativan), mannitol, mechlorethamine (nitrogen mustard), melphalan (Alkeran), meperidine (Demerol), mesna (Mesnex), methotrexate, methylprednisolone (Solu-Medrol), metoclopramide (Reglan), metronidazole (Flagyl IV), mitomycin (Mutamycin), mitoxantrone (Novantrone), morphine, nalbuphine, ondansetron (Zofran), potassium chloride (KCl), prochlorperazine (Compazine), promethazine (Phenergan), ranitidine (Zantac), sargramostim (Leukine), sodium bicarbonate, streptozocin (Zanosar), sulfamethoxazole/trimethoprim, thiotepa, ticarcillin/clavulanate (Timentin), tobramycin, vancomycin, vinblastine, vincristine, vinorelbine (Navelbine), zidovudine (AZT, Retrovir).

RATE OF ADMINISTRATION

Total desired dose, properly diluted and evenly distributed over at least 30 to 60 minutes. Infusion time may be extended. Flush IV line with D5W or NS before and after administration to avoid precipitation of teniposide in IV catheter. Rapid infusion may cause marked hypotension or increased nausea and vomiting.

ACTIONS

An antineoplastic agent. A semi-synthetic derivative of podophyllotoxin related to etoposide. Cell cycle–specific for the late S or early G_2 phase, thus preventing cells from entering mitosis. Cytotoxic effects are related to the relative number of single- and double-strand DNA breaks produced in cells. Has a broad spectrum of in vivo antitumor activity against murine tumors, including hematologic malignancies and various solid tumors. Active against certain murine leukemias with acquired resistance to cisplatin, doxorubicin, amsacrine, daunorubicin, mitoxantrone, or vincristine. Highly protein bound; limits distribution within the body (a beneficial effect). Plasma levels increase with dose. Terminal half-life is 5 hours. Metabolized primarily in the liver. Only about 10% excreted as unchanged drug in urine.

INDICATIONS AND USES

Induction therapy in refractory childhood acute lymphoblastic leukemia. Used in combination with other antineoplastic agents.

Unlabeled uses: Has been used as an unlabeled agent in several adult protocols (e.g., refractory non-Hodgkin's lymphoma and neuroblastoma).

CONTRAINDICATIONS

Hypersensitivity to teniposide, etoposide (no cross-sensitivity to date), or a history of prior severe hypersensitivity reactions to other drugs formulated in Cremophor EL (e.g., cyclosporine, paclitaxel).

PRECAUTIONS

Follow guidelines for handling cytotoxic agents. See Appendix A, p. 1331. Always wear impervious gloves when handling ampules containing tenoposide. After contact with skin, wash immediately and thoroughly with soap and water; after contact with mucous membranes, flush immediately and thoroughly with water. ▪ Usually administered by or under the direction of the physician specialist. ▪ Adequate diagnostic and treatment facilities must be readily available. ▪ May cause severe myelosuppression with resulting infection or bleeding. ▪ Causes severe myelosuppression when used in combination with other chemotherapeutic agents. Sepsis, sometimes fatal, may result. ▪ Use caution in patients with impaired hepatic or renal function; may reduce plasma clearance and increase toxicity. ▪ Hypersensitivity reactions, including anaphylaxis, may occur with initial dosing or with repeated exposure. ▪ Incidence of hypersensitivity may be increased in patients with brain tumors or neuroblastoma. ▪ Acute CNS depression, hypotension, and metabolic acidosis occurred in patients receiving high-dose teniposide pretreated with antiemetic drugs; use caution. ▪ Pediatric patients with ALL in remission on teniposide maintenance therapy have shown an increased risk of developing secondary acute nonlymphocytic leukemia (ANLL). ▪ Reduce dose in patients with Down's syndrome. ▪ See Drug/Lab Interactions.

Monitor: Bone marrow suppression; occurs early with indicated doses and can be profound. Obtain baseline hemoglobin, WBC count with differential, and platelet count. Monitor frequently during therapy, before each dose, and after therapy. See Dose Adjustments. ▪ Severe hypersensitivity reactions can occur with teniposide and may be life threatening. Epinephrine, oxygen, and other emergency supplies must be at the bedside. Monitor patient continuously and take vital signs very frequently during the first hour and at intervals thereafter. ▪ Monitor renal and hepatic function tests before and during therapy. ▪ Determine absolute patency and quality of vein and adequate circulation of extremity. Avoid extravasation; can cause local tissue necrosis and thrombophlebitis. ▪ Precipitation sufficient to occlude central venous access catheters has occurred; monitor infusion closely, and flush thoroughly before and after administration. ▪ Use prophylactic antiemetics to increase patient comfort. ▪ Steady-state volume of distribution increases with a decrease in plasma albumin levels; monitor pediatric patients with hypoalbuminemia carefully. ▪ If severe myelosuppression occurs, bone marrow examination should be repeated before a decision to continue therapy is made. ▪ Monitor for thrombocytopenia (platelet count less than 50,000/mm^3). Initiate precautions to prevent excessive bleeding (e.g., inspect IV sites, skin, and mucous membranes; use extreme care during invasive procedures; test urine, emesis, stool, and secretions for occult blood). ▪ Observe closely for signs of infection. Prophylactic antibiotics may be indicated pending results of C/S in a febrile neutropenic patient.

Patient Education: Report IV site burning or stinging promptly. ▪ Avoid pregnancy; non-hormonal birth control recommended for males and females. ▪ Males should consider the possibility of storing sperm for future artificial insemination. ▪ Report any signs of hypersensitivity promptly (e.g., chills, difficult breathing, fever, flushing, rapid heartbeat, rash). ▪ Secondary acute nonlymphocytic leukemia (ANLL) has been reported (see

Precautions). ▪ Interacts with many medications. Discuss all drugs (prescription or non-prescription) with doctor or pharmacist. ▪ See Appendix D, p. 1333.

Maternal/Child: Category D: avoid pregnancy. May cause fetal harm; see Patient Education. ▪ Potential for serious adverse reactions in nursing infants; discontinue breast-feeding. ▪ Contains benzyl alcohol; not recommended for use in premature infants. ▪ Intended for use in pediatric patients, but see Precautions/Monitor. ▪ When used as a single agent, side effects in pediatric patients from 2 weeks to 20 years of age are similar to other age-groups.

Elderly: Monitor renal, hepatic, and hematologic function closely.

DRUG/LAB INTERACTIONS

Concomitant use with **vincristine sulfate** has resulted in neurotoxicity, including severe cases of neuropathy. ▪ **Sodium salicylate, sulfamethizole, and tolbutamide** displace teniposide from protein-binding sites. Can cause substantial increases in free drug levels and increase toxicity of teniposide. ▪ May result in clinically significant drug interactions with **other drugs highly bound to protein** (e.g., buprenorphine, calcium channel blocking agents [e.g., diltiazem, verapamil], phenothiazines [e.g., prochlorperazine (Compazine)]). ▪ May increase plasma clearance and increase intracellular levels of **methotrexate**. ▪ **Phenobarbital, fosphenytoin** (Cerebyx), **and phenytoin** (Dilantin) increase clearance of teniposide; may reduce effectiveness. ▪ Depressant and hypotensive effects of **antiemetics** may be additive with alcohol in teniposide. ▪ May cause additive effects with **bone marrow–suppressing agents or agents that cause blood dyscrasias** (e.g., amphotericin B, antithyroid agents [methimazole (Tapazole)], azathioprine, chloramphenicol, ganciclovir [Cytovene], interferon, plicamycin [Mithracin], zidovudine [AZT, Retrovir]) **and radiation therapy.** ▪ Do not administer **live virus vaccines.**

SIDE EFFECTS

Most are reversible if detected early. Hypersensitivity reactions (e.g., bronchospasm, chills, confusion, dyspnea, facial flushing, fever, headache, hypertension, hypotension, tachycardia, urticaria) have occurred and can be fatal if not treated promptly. Myelosuppression (anemia, leukopenia, neutropenia, thrombocytopenia) occurs early, can be profound, and recovery can be delayed. Alopecia, asthenia, bleeding, diarrhea, fever, hypotension/cardiovascular, infection, mucositis, nausea and vomiting, rash, thrombophlebitis. Hepatic dysfunctions, metabolic abnormalities, neurotoxicity, and renal dysfunction have occurred in fewer than 1% of patients.

Overdose: Acute CNS depression, hypotension, and metabolic acidosis.

ANTIDOTE

Keep physician informed of all side effects. Symptomatic treatment is often indicated. Discontinue teniposide and treat hypersensitivity reactions immediately (epinephrine [Adrenalin], antihistamines [e.g., diphenhydramine (Benadryl)], cimetidine [Tagamet], corticosteroids [e.g., dexamethasone (Decadron)], bronchodilators [e.g., theophylline (Aminophylline)], IV fluids). Consider risk/benefit before rechallenging any patient who has had a severe hypersensitivity reaction. Pretreatment with corticosteroids and antihistamines and constant observation are imperative. Administration of whole blood products (e.g., packed RBCs, platelets, leukocytes) and/or blood modifiers (e.g., darbepoetin alfa [Aranesp], epoetin alfa [Epogen], filgrastim [Neupogen, Zarxio], pegfilgrastim [Neulasta], sargramostim [Leukine]) may be indicated to treat bone marrow toxicity. Consider diazepam (Valium) or phenytoin (Dilantin) for seizures. Hypotension is usually due to a rapid infusion rate; discontinue temporarily. Trendelenburg position and IV fluids should reverse the hypotension; vasopressors (e.g., dopamine) may be required. In addition to antiemetics (e.g., ondansetron [Zofran]), rate reduction may reduce nausea and vomiting. For extravasation, discontinue the drug immediately and administer into another site. Resuscitate as necessary.

THIAMINE HYDROCHLORIDE
(**THIGH**-ah-min hy-droh-**KLOR**-eyed)

Vitamin B$_1$

Nutritional supplement
(vitamin)

pH 2.5 to 4.5

USUAL DOSE
Transfer to PO doses when practical; see Precautions. Administer before dextrose solutions in the poorly nourished to avoid the development of acute symptoms of thiamine deficiency.

Thiamine deficiency (prophylaxis): Administered as part of a TPN program and based on individual patient needs (average daily requirement in a normal healthy adult is 1 mg). Average supplementation in TPN is 6 mg/day; may be increased to 25 to 50 mg/day in patients with a history of alcohol abuse. In critically ill adults, an initial dose of up to 100 mg has been used. May be followed with 50 to 100 mg daily until a regular balanced diet can be eaten. IV dextrose solutions or high carbohydrate diets increase thiamine requirements and may worsen symptoms in patients who are thiamine deficient.

Beriberi: 5 to 30 mg IV or IM 3 times daily for up to 2 weeks. Continue PO for 1 month.

Alcohol withdrawal syndrome: 100 mg IV or IM daily for several days. Administer concurrently with IV glucose. Follow with 50 to 100 mg/day PO.

Wernicke's encephalopathy: An initial dose of 100 mg IV. Larger doses may be required in the first 24 hours with extreme caution. Follow with 50 to 100 mg daily until a normal diet is resumed.

PEDIATRIC DOSE
Thiamine deficiency (prophylaxis and/or treatment): Administered as part of a TPN program and based on individual patient needs (average daily requirement in a normal healthy infant or child ranges from 0.2 mg in infants to 0.9 mg in 9- to 13-year-olds). Up to 10 to 25 mg/24 hr may be used in critically ill pediatric patients. See comments under Usual Dose.

Beriberi: 10 to 25 mg/24 hr. Follow with 10 to 50 mg PO daily for 2 weeks, then 5 to 10 mg PO daily for 1 month.

DILUTION
May be given by IV injection or added to most IV solutions and given as an infusion. See chart on inside back cover.

Storage: Can be refrigerated; protect from freezing and from light.

COMPATIBILITY
Consider any drug NOT listed as compatible to be INCOMPATIBLE until consulting a pharmacist; specific conditions may apply.

Manufacturer states, "Unstable in neutral or alkaline solutions. Do not use in combination with alkaline solutions (e.g., acetates, barbiturates [e.g., phenobarbital (Luminal)], carbonates, citrates, copper ions). **Incompatible** with solutions containing sulfites and other oxidizing and reducing agents."

One source suggests the following **compatibilities:**

Y-site: Famotidine (Pepcid IV).

RATE OF ADMINISTRATION
100 mg or fraction thereof over 5 minutes. For 100 mg or larger doses, equal distribution over an extended time as an infusion is preferred.

ACTIONS
A water-soluble vitamin, thiamine is necessary to most metabolic processes in humans, especially carbohydrate metabolism. Widely distributed in all body tissues, metabolized in the liver, and excreted in urine.

INDICATIONS AND USES
Prophylaxis or treatment of thiamine deficiency syndromes including beriberi (wet or dry), Wernicke's encephalopathy, or peripheral neuritis.

CONTRAINDICATIONS

Known hypersensitivity to thiamine hydrochloride.

PRECAUTIONS

Not commonly administered IV; PO or IM is preferred. ▪ Rarely used alone, it is more often administered as a multiple B vitamin. ▪ In thiamine deficiency, administer thiamine before giving any glucose load to prevent the sudden onset of Wernicke's encephalopathy or add 100 mg to each of the first few liters of IV fluid to avoid precipitating heart failure. ▪ Requirements may be increased in certain conditions (e.g., alcoholism, burns, GI disease, or malabsorption). ▪ Supplementation is necessary in patients receiving total parenteral nutrition (usually administered as a multivitamin). ▪ S/S of thiamine deficiency (e.g., ataxia, edema, heart failure, neuritis, ocular signs) may respond within hours of thiamine administration and disappear within days. Confusion and psychosis may be slower to respond and may not improve if nerve damage has occurred.

Patient Education: Dietary consultation indicated to prevent relapse.

Maternal/Child: Category A: use only if clearly needed. ▪ Use caution in breast-feeding.

SIDE EFFECTS

Anaphylaxis and death caused by hypersensitivity reaction can occur with IV administration. Recent studies have shown that hypersensitivity reactions can occur with equal frequency by any route. Incidence after IV administration is less than 0.1%. May increase in frequency with repeat injections. Other reactions include feeling of warmth, nausea, pain, pruritus, sweating, urticaria, and weakness.

ANTIDOTE

Discontinue the drug, treat hypersensitivity reactions or resuscitate as necessary, and notify the physician.

THIOTEPA
(thigh-oh-**TEP**-ah)

Antineoplastic
(alkylating agent/nitrosurea)

pH 5.5 to 7.5

USUAL DOSE

Dose must be carefully individualized. A slow response does not necessarily indicate a lack of response. After maximum benefit is obtained by initial therapy, it is necessary to continue the patient on maintenance therapy (1- to 4-week intervals). Initially the higher dose in the given range is commonly administered. The maintenance dose should be adjusted weekly on the basis of pretreatment control blood counts and subsequent blood counts.

Dose: 0.3 to 0.4 mg/kg every 1 to 4 weeks. Dose based on average weight in presence of ascites or edema.

DOSE ADJUSTMENTS

Reduce dose or discontinue if WBC or platelet count falls rapidly. ▪ Usually contraindicated but can be used with extreme caution and in low doses in patients with existing hepatic, renal, or bone marrow damage if benefits outweigh risks.

DILUTION

Specific techniques required; see Precautions. Each 15 mg of drug is reconstituted with 1.5 mL of SWFI (10 mg/mL). Shake solution gently and allow to stand until clear. A hypotonic solution; further dilute with NS before administration. Must be filtered through a 0.22-micron filter before administration. May then be given through Y-tube or three-way stopcock of a free-flowing IV infusion. Final solution should be clear; do not use if hazy, opaque, or a precipitate is present.

Filters: Filter through a 0.22-micron filter before administration. See Dilution.

Storage: Must be refrigerated before and after reconstitution. Protect from light at all times. Use reconstituted solution within 8 hours. Use diluted solution immediately.

COMPATIBILITY

Consider any drug NOT listed as compatible to be INCOMPATIBLE until consulting a pharmacist; specific conditions may apply.

One source suggests the following **compatibilities:**

Y-site: Acyclovir (Zovirax), allopurinol (Aloprim), amifostine (Ethyol), amikacin, aminophylline, amphotericin B (conventional), ampicillin, ampicillin/sulbactam (Unasyn), aztreonam (Azactam), bleomycin (Blenoxane), bumetanide, buprenorphine (Buprenex), butorphanol (Stadol), calcium gluconate, carboplatin (Paraplatin), carmustine (BiCNU), cefazolin (Ancef), cefotaxime (Claforan), cefotetan, cefoxitin (Mefoxin), ceftazidime (Fortaz), ceftriaxone (Rocephin), cefuroxime (Zinacef), chlorpromazine (Thorazine), ciprofloxacin (Cipro IV), clindamycin (Cleocin), cyclophosphamide (Cytoxan), cytarabine (ARA-C), dacarbazine (DTIC), dactinomycin (Cosmegen), daunorubicin (Cerubidine), dexamethasone (Decadron), diphenhydramine (Benadryl), dobutamine, dopamine, doxorubicin (Adriamycin), doxycycline, droperidol (Inapsine), enalaprilat (Vasotec IV), etoposide (VePesid), etoposide phosphate (Etopophos), famotidine (Pepcid IV), fluconazole (Diflucan), fludarabine (Fludara), fluorouracil (5-FU), furosemide (Lasix), gallium nitrate (Ganite), ganciclovir (Cytovene IV), gemcitabine (Gemzar), gentamicin, granisetron (Kytril), heparin, hydrocortisone sodium succinate (Solu-Cortef), hydromorphone (Dilaudid), idarubicin (Idamycin), ifosfamide (Ifex), imipenem-cilastatin (Primaxin), leucovorin calcium, lorazepam (Ativan), magnesium sulfate, mannitol, melphalan (Alkeran), meperidine (Demerol), mesna (Mesnex), methotrexate, methylprednisolone (Solu-Medrol), metoclopramide (Reglan), metronidazole (Flagyl IV), mitomycin (Mutamycin), mitoxantrone (Novantrone), morphine, nalbuphine, ondansetron (Zofran), paclitaxel (Taxol), piperacillin/tazobactam (Zosyn), potassium chloride (KCl), prochlorperazine (Compazine), promethazine (Phenergan), ranitidine (Zantac), sodium bicarbonate, streptozocin (Zanosar), sulfamethoxazole/trimethoprim, teniposide (Vumon), ticarcillin/clavulanate (Timentin), tobramycin, vancomycin, vinblastine, vincristine, zidovudine (AZT, Retrovir).

RATE OF ADMINISTRATION

Use of a 0.22-micron filter required. A single dose by rapid IV administration.

ACTIONS

An alkylating agent chemically and pharmacologically related to nitrogen mustard. Has antitumor activity and is cell-cycle phase–nonspecific. The radiomimetic action is thought to occur through the release of ethylenimine radicals which, like irradiation, disrupt DNA bonds. Results in inhibition of protein, RNA, and DNA synthesis. It is metabolized extensively in the liver and has one major active metabolite (TEPA). Half-life is approximately 2 hours. Is excreted as metabolites in the urine.

INDICATIONS AND USES

To suppress or retard neoplastic growth in adenocarcinomas of the breast and ovary. ▪ For controlling intracavitary effusions secondary to diffuse or localized neoplastic diseases of various serosal cavities. ▪ Treatment of superficial papillary carcinoma of the urinary bladder. ▪ Although now largely superseded by other treatments, thiotepa has been effective against other lymphomas, such as lymphosarcoma and Hodgkin's disease.

CONTRAINDICATIONS

Hepatic, renal, or bone marrow damage unless need is greater than the risk; known hypersensitivity to thiotepa.

PRECAUTIONS

Follow guidelines for handling cytotoxic agents. See Appendix A, p. 1331. ▪ Administered by or under the direction of the physician specialist. ▪ Highly toxic to the hematopoietic system. Death from septicemia and hemorrhage has occurred as a direct result of hematopoietic depression. ▪ Death has occurred after intravesical administration, caused by bone marrow depression from the systematically absorbed drug. ▪ See Dose Adjustments and Side Effects.

Monitor: Obtain baseline and weekly CBC and platelet counts during therapy and for at least 3 weeks after therapy has been discontinued. ▪ Obtain baseline SCr, BUN, and/or liver function tests in patients with renal or hepatic impairment and monitor during treatment. ▪ Be alert for signs of bone marrow suppression or infection. Use of prophylactic antibiotics may be indicated pending results of C/S in a febrile neutropenic patient. ▪ Prophylactic antiemetics may increase patient comfort. ▪ Monitor for thrombocytopenia (platelet count less than 50,000/mm^3). Initiate precautions to prevent excessive bleeding (e.g., inspect IV sites, skin, and mucous membranes; use extreme care during invasive procedures; test urine, emesis, stool, and secretions for occult blood). ▪ See Drug/Lab Interactions.

Patient Education: Effective contraception should be used during therapy if either the patient or the partner is of childbearing potential. ▪ Promptly report S/S of bleeding (e.g., black stools, bruising, change in urine color, epistaxis), infection (e.g., fever, chills), or suspected pregnancy. ▪ See Appendix D, p. 1333.

Maternal/Child: Category D: avoid pregnancy. Can cause fetal harm; see Patient Education. Has a mutagenic potential. ▪ Discontinue breast-feeding. ▪ Safety and effectiveness for use in pediatric patients not established.

Elderly: Studies did not include sufficient numbers of subjects over age 65 years to determine whether elderly subjects respond differently than younger subjects. Differences have not been seen. Dose selection should be cautious, taking into account age-related organ impairment and concomitant disease states or drug therapy.

DRUG/LAB INTERACTIONS

Possible pharmacokinetic interactions with any concomitantly administered medications have not been formally investigated. ▪ Avoid combination, either simultaneously or sequentially, with **cancer chemotherapeutic agents or therapeutic modalities** (e.g., nitrogen mustard, cyclophosphamide, radiation therapy) that have the same mechanism of action. Will increase toxicity without increasing therapeutic benefit. Allow complete recovery verified by WBC count before using a second agent. ▪ **Other drugs that cause bone marrow suppression** (e.g., amphotericin B [all formulations], ganciclovir [Cytovene]) should be avoided. ▪ May potentiate **succinylcholine.** May cause prolonged apnea. ▪ Do not administer **live virus vaccines** to patients receiving antineoplastic drugs.

SIDE EFFECTS

Frequency of adverse events was not defined. Side effects have included abdominal pain, alopecia, amenorrhea, anorexia, blurred vision, conjunctivitis, contact dermatitis, dizziness, dysuria, fatigue, fever, headache, hives, hyperuricemia, interference with spermatogenesis, nausea, pain at injection site, skin rash, throat tightness, urinary retention, vomiting.

Major: Hemorrhage, hypersensitivity reactions (e.g., anaphylaxis, asthma, laryngeal edema, rash, urticaria, wheezing), intestinal perforation, septicemia. Bone marrow suppression (anemia, leukopenia, thrombocytopenia) may be life threatening, is dose related, and can occur with usual doses.

ANTIDOTE

Minor side effects will be treated symptomatically if necessary. Discontinue the drug and notify the physician of major side effects. If platelet count falls below 150,000/mm^3 or WBCs fall below 3,000/mm^3, discontinue use and notify physician. Administration of whole blood products (e.g., packed RBCs, platelets, or leukocytes) and/or blood modifiers (e.g., darbepoetin alfa [Aranesp], epoetin alfa [Epogen], filgrastim [Neupogen, Zarxio], pegfilgrastim [Neulasta], sargramostim [Leukine]) may be indicated to treat bone marrow toxicity. Treat hypersensitivity reactions as indicated. Thiotepa is dialyzable.

TIGECYCLINE FOR INJECTION BBW
(tye-ge-**SYE**-kleen)

Tygacil

Antibacterial
(glycylcycline)

pH 7.8

USUAL DOSE
100 mg as an initial dose. Follow with 50 mg every 12 hours. Recommended duration of treatment is 5 to 14 days for complicated skin and skin structure infections and complicated intra-abdominal infections and 7 to 14 days for community-acquired bacterial pneumonia. Duration of treatment is based on the severity and site of the infection and the patient's clinical and bacteriologic progress.

DOSE ADJUSTMENTS
In patients with severe impaired liver function (Child-Pugh Class C [score 10 to 15]), the initial dose remains the same, but subsequent doses should be reduced to 25 mg every 12 hours. ■ No dose adjustment is indicated for impaired renal function, for mild to moderate impaired liver function (Child-Pugh Class A and Child-Pugh Class B [score 5 to 9]), or in patients undergoing hemodialysis. ■ No dose adjustment is indicated based on age, gender, or race.

DILUTION
Reconstitute each 50-mg vial with 5.3 mL of NS, D5W, or LR (yields 10 mg/mL). Use 2 vials for the 100-mg dose. Swirl gently until lyophilized powder is dissolved. Reconstituted solution should be yellow to orange in color. Immediately withdraw 5 mL from each of two vials for the 100-mg dose (vials have overfill) or from one vial for the 50-mg dose and add to a 100-mL IV bag of D5W, NS, or LR for infusion. Maximum concentration should be 1 mg/mL.

Filters: No data available from manufacturer.

Storage: Store unopened vials at CRT. Reconstituted solution may be stored at RT for up to 6 hours. Fully diluted solution in the IV bag may be stored at RT for up to 24 hours or for 6 hours in the vial and the remaining time in the IV bag, or the fully diluted solution in either D5W or NS may be refrigerated at 2° to 8° C (36° to 46° F) for up to 48 hours following immediate transfer of the reconstituted solution into the IV bag.

COMPATIBILITY
(Underline Indicates Conflicting Compatibility Information)

Consider any drug NOT listed as compatible to be INCOMPATIBLE until consulting a pharmacist; specific conditions may apply.

Manufacturer states, "The following drugs *should not* be administered simultaneously through the same **Y-site** as tigecycline: amphotericin B (conventional), amphotericin B lipid complex (Abelcet), diazepam (Valium), esomeprazole (Nexium IV), and omeprazole (Prilosec)."

Y-site: Manufacturer lists as **compatible** at the **Y-site** with amikacin, dobutamine, dopamine, gentamicin, LR solution, lidocaine, metoclopramide (Reglan), morphine, norepinephrine (Levophed), piperacillin/tazobactam (Zosyn), potassium chloride, propofol (Diprivan), ranitidine (Zantac), theophylline (Aminophylline), and tobramycin.

Another source adds **compatibility** at the **Y-site** with azithromycin (Zithromax), aztreonam (Azactam), cefepime (Maxipime), cefotaxime (Claforan), ceftazidime (Fortaz), ceftriaxone (Rocephin), ciprofloxacin (Cipro IV), doripenem (Doribax), epinephrine (Adrenalin), ertapenem (Invanz), fluconazole (Diflucan), heparin, imipenem-cilastatin (Primaxin), linezolid (Zyvox), metoclopramide (Reglan), telavancin (Vibativ), vancomycin.

RATE OF ADMINISTRATION
Flush IV line with D5W, NS, or LR before and after infusion of tigecycline if other drugs are administered through the same line; see Compatibility. Consider **compatibility** of other drugs when flushing the line.

A single dose as an infusion over 30 to 60 minutes.

ACTIONS

A broad-spectrum tetracycline class antibacterial agent that is bacteriostatic against specific aerobic gram-positive and gram-negative microorganisms and specific anaerobic microorganisms; see prescribing information. Inhibits protein translation in bacteria by binding to a specific ribosomal subunit and blocking entry of specific molecules into the A site of the ribosome. Plasma protein binding is approximately 71% to 89%. Extensively distributed beyond the plasma volume and into tissues. For example, concentrations have been identified in the bone, colon, gallbladder, synovial fluid, and lung. Mean half-life is 42.4 hours. Not extensively metabolized. 59% of a dose is excreted in bile and feces, and 33% is excreted in urine.

INDICATIONS AND USES

Treatment of patients 18 years of age and older with infections caused by susceptible strains of designated microorganisms in complicated skin and skin structure infections, complicated intra-abdominal infections, and community-acquired bacterial pneumonia. **Limitations of use:** Tigecycline is not indicated for treatment of diabetic foot infections. ▪ Tigecycline is not indicated for treatment of hospital-acquired or ventilator-associated pneumonia. In a comparator clinical trial, greater mortality and decreased efficacy were reported in the patients treated with tigecycline.

CONTRAINDICATIONS

Known hypersensitivity to tigecycline. Contains no excipients or preservatives.

PRECAUTIONS

An increase in all-cause mortality has been observed in a meta-analysis of Phase 3 and 4 clinical trials in tigecycline-treated patients versus comparator-treated patients. The cause of this increase has not been established. Tigecycline should be reserved for use in situations in which alternative treatments are not suitable. ▪ A trial of patients with hospital-acquired (including ventilator-associated) pneumonia failed to demonstrate the efficacy of tigecycline; see Limitations of Use. ▪ Sensitivity studies are indicated to determine susceptibility of the causative organism to tigecycline. Treatment may begin after culture and sensitivity studies are drawn. Re-evaluate after results are known. ▪ To reduce the development of drug-resistant bacteria and maintain its effectiveness, tigecycline should be used to treat only those infections proven or strongly suspected to be caused by bacteria. ▪ Cross-resistance and/or antagonism between tigecycline and other antibiotics has not been observed. ▪ Not affected by resistance mechanisms seen with other antibiotics (e.g., β-lactamases or ribosomal protection and efflux seen with other tetracyclines). However, some ESBL-producing isolates may confer resistance to tigecycline via other resistance mechanisms. ▪ Structurally similar to the tetracycline class of antibiotics; may have similar side effects (e.g., antianabolic action [which has led to acidosis, azotemia, hyperphosphatemia, and increased BUN], photosensitivity, and pseudotumor cerebri). ▪ Anaphylactic reactions have been reported. Should be avoided in patients with a history of hypersensitivity to tetracyclines; may have cross-sensitivity. ▪ Acute pancreatitis, including fatalities, has been reported. ▪ Monotherapy with tigecycline should be avoided in patients with complicated intra-abdominal infections secondary to clinically apparent intestinal perforation; sepsis/septic shock has occurred. ▪ Abnormalities in total bilirubin, PT, and transaminases have been seen in patients treated with tigecycline. Isolated cases of significant hepatic dysfunction and hepatic failure have also been reported; see Monitor. ▪ May cause permanent discoloration of the teeth during tooth development; see Maternal/Child. ▪ Avoid prolonged use of drug; superinfection caused by overgrowth of nonsusceptible organisms may result. ▪ Use caution in patients with severe liver impairment. Reduced dose and monitoring for treatment response is indicated; see Dose Adjustments. ▪ *Clostridium difficile*–associated diarrhea (CDAD) has been reported. May range from mild diarrhea to fatal colitis. Consider in patients who present with diarrhea during or after treatment with tigecycline.

Monitor: Monitor vital signs carefully. ▪ Obtain baseline CBC with differential, and monitor as indicated. ▪ Monitor liver function. If abnormal liver function tests develop, monitor closely for worsening hepatic function and evaluate for risk/benefit of continuing therapy. Hepatic dysfunction may occur after tigecycline is discontinued. ▪ Monitor for S/S or laboratory abnormalities suggestive of acute pancreatitis. ▪ Observe for signs of hypersensitivity reactions (e.g., chills, fever, hives, rash, shortness of breath). ▪ See Precautions and Drug/Lab Interactions.

Patient Education: Avoid pregnancy; use effective contraceptive measures; see Drug/Lab Interactions. Should pregnancy occur, notify physician immediately and discuss potential hazards. ▪ Promptly report diarrhea or bloody stools that occur during treatment or up to several months after an antibiotic has been discontinued; may indicate CDAD and require treatment. ▪ Promptly report S/S of hypersensitivity (e.g., chills, fever, hives, rash, shortness of breath) and/or S/S of liver dysfunction (e.g., jaundice or yellow sclera).

Maternal/Child: Category D: avoid pregnancy. May cause fetal harm; use of effective contraception required; see Drug/Lab Interactions. Use during pregnancy only if benefits justify potential risk to the fetus. ▪ Use during tooth development (the last half of pregnancy, infancy, and childhood to the age of 8 years) may cause permanent discoloration of the teeth and is not recommended. ▪ Not known if tigecycline is secreted in breast milk; use caution. ▪ Safety and effectiveness for use in pediatric patients under 18 years of age have not been evaluated due to the observed increase in mortality associated with tigecycline in adult patients. Tigecycline should not be used in pediatric patients unless no alternative antibacterial drugs are available. Under these circumstances, the following doses are suggested: *Pediatric patients 8 to 11 years of age* should receive 1.2 mg/kg every 12 hours (not to exceed 50 mg every 12 hours). *Pediatric patients over 11 years of age* should receive 50 mg every 12 hours.

Elderly: Response similar to that seen in younger adults; however, the potential for greater sensitivity to side effects cannot be disregarded.

DRUG/LAB INTERACTIONS

Digoxin (Lanoxin) and tigecycline do not affect each other's pharmacokinetics; no dose adjustment of either drug is indicated. ▪ May decrease clearance of warfarin. Prothrombin time or other suitable anticoagulation tests should be monitored if tigecycline is administered with warfarin. ▪ May render **oral contraceptives** less effective, resulting in pregnancy or breakthrough bleeding. ▪ Tigecycline does not inhibit the metabolism mediated by any of the following six cytochrome P_{450} (CYP) isoforms: 1A2, 2C8, 2C9, 2C19, 2D6, and 3A4; it is not expected to alter the metabolism of drugs metabolized by these enzymes. In addition, because tigecycline is not extensively metabolized, its clearance is not expected to be affected by drugs that induce or inhibit the activity of these P_{450} isoforms. ▪ No reported interactions with lab tests.

SIDE EFFECTS

Nausea and vomiting are the most common side effects and are the primary reason for discontinuing therapy. Other commonly reported side effects include abdominal pain, diarrhea, headache, and increased ALT. Less commonly reported side effects include abnormal healing; abscess; acute pancreatitis; anemia; asthenia; bilirubinemia; CDAD; dizziness; dyspepsia; hyponatremia; hypoproteinemia; increased alkaline phosphatase, amylase, AST, and BUN; infection; phlebitis; pneumonia; rash. Sepsis/septic shock and death occurred in a few patients with complicated infections.

Post-Marketing: Acute pancreatitis, anaphylactic reactions, hepatic cholestasis, jaundice, severe skin reactions (including Stevens-Johnson syndrome), and symptomatic hypoglycemia in patients with and without diabetes.

Overdose: Increased incidence of nausea and vomiting.

ANTIDOTE

Keep physician informed of all side effects. Most minor side effects will be treated symptomatically; monitor closely. If minor side effects are progressive or if any major side effect occurs, discontinue the drug, treat hypersensitivity reactions, or resuscitate as necessary. Mild cases of CDAD may respond to discontinuation of tigecycline. Treat CDAD with fluids, electrolytes, protein supplements, and oral vancomycin (Vancocin) or metronidazole (Flagyl) as indicated. In severe cases, surgical evaluation may be indicated. Not removed by hemodialysis.

TIROFIBAN HYDROCHLORIDE
(ty-roh-**FYE**-ban hy-droh-**KLOR**-eyed)

Aggrastat

Antiplatelet agent

pH 5.5 to 6.5

USUAL DOSE
Tirofiban: A *loading infusion* of 25 mcg/kg administered within 5 minutes followed by a *maintenance infusion (CrCl over 60 mL/min)* of 0.15 mcg/kg/min for up to 18 hours; see Dose Adjustments for dosing in patients with a CrCl equal to or less than 60 mL/min. Has been used in combination with aspirin, clopidogrel (Plavix), and heparin or bivalirudin (Angiomax).

DOSE ADJUSTMENTS
Reduce maintenance dose to 0.075 mcg/kg/min for up to 18 hours in patients with a CrCl equal to or less than 60 mL/min. ▪ No dose adjustment indicated based on age, race, gender, or hepatic impairment.

DILUTION
Available premixed in a plastic container in a 50 mcg/mL concentration (5 mg/100 mL and 12.5 mg/250 mL). Remove overwrap. Plastic may be somewhat opaque due to sterilization process. Opacity should diminish. Squeeze inner container to check for leak. Discard if leakage noted; sterility is impaired. Do not use plastic containers in a series connection.
Storage: Store unopened or premixed containers at 25° C (77° F). Variations from 15° to 30° C (59° to 86° F) are acceptable (CRT). Protect from light during storage. Do not freeze. Discard unused solution.

COMPATIBILITY
Consider any drug NOT listed as compatible to be INCOMPATIBLE until consulting a pharmacist; specific conditions may apply.
Manufacturer states, "Do not add other drugs or remove solution directly from the bag with a syringe. Should not be administered in the same IV line as diazepam (Valium)."

Manufacturer indicates **compatibility** at the **Y-site** with atropine, dobutamine, dopamine, epinephrine (Adrenalin), famotidine (Pepcid IV), furosemide (Lasix), lidocaine, midazolam (Versed), morphine, nitroglycerin IV, potassium chloride, propranolol. Another source adds amiodarone (Nexterone), argatroban (Acova), bivalirudin (Angiomax), and heparin.

RATE OF ADMINISTRATION
Loading infusion: 25 mcg/kg administered within 5 minutes.
Maintenance infusion: *CrCl greater than 60 mL/min:* 0.15 mcg/kg/min for up to 18 hours.
CrCl equal to or less than 60 mL/min: 0.075 mcg/kg/min for up to 18 hours.

Tirofiban Infusion Rates Based on Weight (in kg) and CrCl			
	Within 5 Minutes (All Patients) (mL)	Maintenance Infusion Rate (mL/hr)	
Patient Weight (kg)		CrCl >60 mL/min	CrCl ≤60 mL/min
30 to 37 kg	17 mL	6 mL/hr	3 mL/hr
38 to 45 kg	21 mL	7.5 mL/hr	3.75 mL/hr
46 to 54 kg	25 mL	9 mL/hr	4.5 mL/hr
55 to 62 kg	29 mL	10.5 mL/hr	5.25 mL/hr
63 to 70 kg	33 mL	12 mL/hr	6 mL/hr
71 to 79 kg	37.5 mL	13.5 mL/hr	6.75 mL/hr
80 to 87 kg	42 mL	15 mL/hr	7.5 mL/hr

Continued

	Tirofiban Infusion Rates Based on Weight (in kg) and CrCl—cont'd		
Patient Weight (kg)	Within 5 Minutes (All Patients) (mL)	Maintenance Infusion Rate (mL/hr)	
		CrCl >60 mL/min	CrCl ≤60 mL/min
88 to 95 kg	46 mL	16.5 mL/hr	8.25 mL/hr
96 to 104 kg	50 mL	18 mL/hr	9 mL/hr
105 to 112 kg	54 mL	19.5 mL/hr	9.75 mL/hr
113 to 120 kg	58 mL	21 mL/hr	10.5 mL/hr
121 to 128 kg	62 mL	22.5 mL/hr	11.25 mL/hr
129 to 137 kg	66.5 mL	24 mL/hr	12 mL/hr
138 to 145 kg	71 mL	25.5 mL/hr	12.75 mL/hr
146 to 153 kg	75 mL	27 mL/hr	13.5 mL/hr

ACTIONS

A nonpeptide antagonist of the platelet glycoprotein GPIIb/IIIa receptor. It inhibits platelet aggregation by preventing the binding of fibrinogen to the receptor site on activated platelets. Inhibits platelet aggregation in a dose- and concentration-dependent manner. When given according to the recommended regimen, greater than 90% inhibition is attained within 10 minutes. Bleeding time is prolonged. Inhibition is reversible, with aggregation returning to baseline in more than 90% of patients within 4 to 8 hours following cessation of the infusion. Half-life is approximately 2 hours. Cleared from the plasma primarily by renal excretion, with about 65% of the unchanged drug appearing in the urine and about 25% appearing in feces. Metabolism is limited.

INDICATIONS AND USES

Indicated to reduce the rate of thrombotic cardiovascular events (combined end point of death, myocardial infarction, or refractory ischemia/repeat cardiac procedure) in patients with non–ST elevation acute coronary syndrome (NSTE-ACS).

CONTRAINDICATIONS

Severe hypersensitivity (e.g., anaphylaxis) to tirofiban. ▪ A history of thrombocytopenia following prior exposure to tirofiban. ▪ Active internal bleeding or a history of bleeding diathesis, major surgical procedure, or severe physical trauma within the previous month.

PRECAUTIONS

Bleeding is the most common complication encountered during therapy. Most bleeding associated with tirofiban occurs at the arterial access site for cardiac catheterization; see Monitor. Fatal bleeding events have been reported. ▪ Concomitant use of fibrinolytics, oral anticoagulants, and antiplatelet drugs increases the risk of bleeding; see Drug/Lab Interactions. ▪ Profound thrombocytopenia has been reported. Previous exposure to GPIIb/IIIa receptor antagonists (e.g., abciximab [ReoPro], eptifibatide [Integrilin], tirofiban [Aggrastat]) may increase the risk of developing thrombocytopenia. ▪ Patients treated with tirofiban plus heparin were more likely to experience decreases in platelet counts than were patients on heparin alone. ▪ Plasma clearance is decreased in patients with moderate to severe renal insufficiency; see Dose Adjustments. Safety and effectiveness not established for use in patients on hemodialysis. ▪ Hypersensitivity reactions, including anaphylaxis, have been reported in post-marketing. They have occurred during initial infusion and during readministration.

Monitor: Obtain platelet count, hemoglobin, and hematocrit before therapy, within 6 hours following the loading infusion, and at least daily thereafter. More frequent monitoring may be indicated. ▪ If platelet count drops to below 90,000/mm^3, additional platelet counts should be performed to exclude pseudothrombocytopenia. If thrombocytopenia is confirmed, heparin and tirofiban should be discontinued and appropriate therapy initiated. ▪ Obtain an aPTT before treatment and carefully monitor the anticoagulant effects of heparin by repeated determinations of aPTT; adjust heparin dose accordingly. ▪ Monitor for S/S of hypersensitivity or infusion-related reactions (e.g., anaphylaxis, hypotension, pruritus, rash, urticaria, or wheezing). ▪ Monitor the patient for signs of bleeding; take vital signs (avoiding automatic BP cuffs); observe any invaded sites at least every 15 minutes (e.g., sheaths, IV sites, cutdowns, punctures, epidural sites, Foleys, NGs); watch for hematuria, hematemesis, bloody stool, petechiae, hematoma, flank pain, muscle weakness. Perform neuro checks frequently. If during therapy bleeding cannot be controlled with pressure, tirofiban and heparin infusions should be discontinued. ▪ Use care in handling patient; minimize use of urinary catheters, nasotracheal intubation, and nasogastric tubes. Avoid arterial puncture, venipuncture, epidural procedures, and IM injection. Use extreme precautionary methods and only compressible sites if these procedures are absolutely necessary (i.e., avoid subclavian or jugular veins). Apply pressure for 30 minutes to any invaded site and then apply pressure dressings. Saline or heparin locks suggested to facilitate blood draws.

Patient Education: Compliance with all measures to minimize bleeding (e.g., strict bed rest, positioning) is imperative. ▪ Avoid use of razors, toothbrushes, and other sharp items. ▪ Use caution while moving to avoid excessive bumping. ▪ Promptly report S/S of a hypersensitivity reaction (e.g., hives, rash, shortness of breath or troubled breathing, swelling of eyelids, lips, or face) and all episodes of bleeding, and apply local pressure if indicated. ▪ Expect oozing from IV sites.

Maternal/Child: Category B: safety for use in pregnancy not established. Benefits must outweigh risks. ▪ Discontinue breast-feeding until 24 hours after completion of tirofiban therapy. ▪ Safety and efficacy for use in pediatric patients not established.

Elderly: Effectiveness similar to that seen in younger patients. ▪ Dose adjustment based solely on age is not necessary. Consider age-related renal impairment; see Dose Adjustments.

DRUG/LAB INTERACTIONS

Studies with tirofiban included the use of **aspirin, clopidogrel** (Plavix), and **heparin** or **bivalirudin** (Angiomax). Concomitant use, although indicated, increases the risk of bleeding. ▪ Use caution when given with drugs that affect hemostasis (e.g., **anticoagulants** [e.g., heparin, warfarin (Coumadin)], **NSAIDs** [e.g., ibuprofen (Advil, Motrin), naproxen (Aleve, Naprosyn)], **platelet aggregation inhibitors** [e.g., clopidogrel (Plavix), dipyridamole (Persantine), ticlopidine (Ticlid)], or **thrombolytic agents** [e.g., alteplase (tPA, Activase), reteplase (Retavase), streptokinase (Streptase)]). Risk of bleeding is increased.

SIDE EFFECTS

Bleeding is the most frequent adverse event. Laboratory findings related to bleeding include decrease in hemoglobin, hematocrit, and platelet count and occult blood in urine and feces. Other side effects that occur at an incidence of greater than 1%, regardless of drug relationship, are bradycardia, dissection of the coronary artery, dizziness, edema, hypersensitivity reactions (e.g., hives, rash), leg pain, nausea, pelvic pain, sweating, thrombocytopenia, and vasovagal reflex.

Post-Marketing: Hypersensitivity reactions (including anaphylaxis), severe thrombocytopenia. Fatal bleeding events have been reported.

ANTIDOTE

Keep physician informed of laboratory values and side effects. Discontinue the infusion of tirofiban and heparin if any serious bleeding not controllable with pressure occurs. If platelet count drops to below 90,000 mm^3, obtain additional platelet counts to exclude pseudothrombocytopenia. If thrombocytopenia is confirmed, discontinue tirofiban and heparin. Platelet transfusion may be required. If a hypersensitivity reaction should occur, discontinue the infusion and treat as indicated by severity (e.g., epinephrine, dopamine, theophylline, antihistamines [e.g., diphenhydramine (Benadryl)], and/or corticosteroids as necessary).

No specific antidote is available. Overdosage should be treated by assessment of the patient's clinical condition and cessation or adjustment of the drug infusion as appropriate. Hemodialysis may be useful in an overdose situation.

TOBRAMYCIN SULFATE `BBW`
(toe-brah-**MY**-sin **SUL**-fayt)

Antibacterial
(aminoglycoside)

pH 3 to 6.5

USUAL DOSE
3 mg/kg of body weight/24 hr equally divided into 3 doses and given every 8 hours (1 mg/kg every 8 hours). Up to 5 mg/kg equally divided into 3 or 4 doses may be given in life-threatening infections (1.25 mg/kg every 6 hours or 1.67 mg/kg every 8 hours). Reduce to usual dose as soon as feasible. For obese patients, the dosing weight used to calculate the mg/kg dose is achieved by adding the ideal or lean body weight (IBW) to 40% of the excess over IBW.

$$\text{Dosing weight} = \text{IBW} + 0.4 \,(\text{Total body weight} - \text{IBW})$$

Do not exceed 5 mg/kg/day unless serum levels are monitored.

Studies suggest that in certain populations a single daily dose of 5 to 7 mg/kg (instead of divided into 2 to 3 doses) may provide higher peak levels and enhance drug effectiveness while actually reducing or having no adverse effects on risk of toxicity. Various procedures for monitoring blood levels are in use. Some health facilities are monitoring with trough levels; others may draw levels at predetermined times and plot the concentration on nomograms. Depending on the protocol in place, doses or intervals may be adjusted. See Dose Adjustments and Precautions.

Patients with cystic fibrosis: One source suggests 7.5 to 10.5 mg/kg/24 hr equally divided into 3 doses and given every 8 hours for 7 to 21 days (2.5 to 3.5 mg/kg every 8 hours).

PEDIATRIC DOSE
In pediatric and neonatal patients, monitor serum levels. Wide interpatient variability; see Monitor and Maternal/Child.

Over 1 week of age: 6 to 7.5 mg/kg of body weight/24 hr in 3 or 4 equally divided doses (1.5 to 1.89 mg/kg every 6 hours or 2 to 2.5 mg/kg every 8 hours). Another source suggests the same as adult dose.

A single daily dose is also being used in pediatric patients. See comments under Usual Dose.

Severe cystic fibrosis: 10 mg/kg/day in equally divided doses every 6 hours (2.5 mg/kg every 6 hours).

NEONATAL DOSE
1 week of age or less: Up to 4 mg/kg of body weight/24 hr in two equal doses every 12 hours (up to 2 mg/kg every 12 hours). Lower doses may be safer because of immature kidney function. 2.5 mg/kg every 18 hours or 3 mg/kg every 24 hours may provide acceptable peak and trough levels in neonates weighing less than 2,000 Gm. See Maternal/Child.

DOSE ADJUSTMENTS
Reduce daily dose commensurate with amount of renal impairment and/or increase intervals between injections. Measurement of serum concentrations following a loading dose of 1 mg/kg is suggested. Adjust subsequent doses accordingly. ▪ Once-daily dosing is not usually used in patients with ascites, burns covering more than 20% of the total body surface area, CrCl less than 40 mL/min (including patients requiring dialysis), CrCl greater than 120 mL/min, cystic fibrosis, endocarditis, mycobacterium infections, or in infants or during pregnancy. ▪ Reduced doses or extended intervals may be required in the elderly. ▪ See Drug/Lab Interactions.

DILUTION
Prepared solutions equal 10 or 40 mg/mL. Further dilute each single dose in 50 to 100 mL of NS or D5W and administer through an additive tubing. Also available in ADD-Vantage vials for use with ADD-Vantage infusion containers. Reduce volume of diluent proportionately for pediatric patients.
Storage: Store at CRT.

COMPATIBILITY   (Underline Indicates Conflicting Compatibility Information)
Consider any drug NOT listed as compatible to be INCOMPATIBLE until consulting a pharmacist; specific conditions may apply.
Manufacturer states, "Do not physically premix with other drugs; administer separately." Inactivated in solution with beta-lactam antibiotics (e.g., cephalosporins, penicillins) and vancomycin; do not mix in the same solution. Appropriate spacing required because of physical **incompatibilities.** See Drug/Lab Interactions.
   One source suggests the following **compatibilities:**
Additive: *Not recommended by manufacturer.* Aztreonam (Azactam), bleomycin (Blenoxane), calcium gluconate, cefoxitin (Mefoxin), ciprofloxacin (Cipro IV), clindamycin (Cleocin), dextran 40, furosemide (Lasix), imipenem-cilastatin (Primaxin), linezolid (Zyvox), mannitol (Osmitrol), metronidazole (Flagyl IV), ranitidine (Zantac), verapamil.
Y-site: Acyclovir (Zovirax), alprostadil, amifostine (Ethyol), amiodarone (Nexterone), anidulafungin (Eraxis), aztreonam (Azactam), bivalirudin (Angiomax), caspofungin (Cancidas), cefepime (Maxipime), ceftaroline (Teflaro), ceftazidime (Fortaz), ciprofloxacin (Cipro IV), cisatracurium (Nimbex), cyclophosphamide (Cytoxan), dexmedetomidine (Precedex), diltiazem (Cardizem), docetaxel (Taxotere), doripenem (Doribax), doxorubicin liposomal (Doxil), enalaprilat (Vasotec IV), esmolol (Brevibloc), etoposide phosphate (Etopophos), fenoldopam (Corlopam), filgrastim (Neupogen), fluconazole (Diflucan), fludarabine (Fludara), foscarnet (Foscavir), furosemide (Lasix), gemcitabine (Gemzar), granisetron (Kytril), hetastarch in electrolytes (Hextend), hydromorphone (Dilaudid), insulin (regular), labetalol, linezolid (Zyvox), magnesium sulfate, melphalan (Alkeran), meperidine (Demerol), midazolam (Versed), milrinone (Primacor), morphine, nicardipine (Cardene IV), remifentanil (Ultiva), tacrolimus (Prograf), telavancin (Vibativ), teniposide (Vumon), theophylline, thiotepa, tigecycline (Tygacil), vinorelbine (Navelbine), zidovudine (AZT, Retrovir).

RATE OF ADMINISTRATION
Each single dose, properly diluted, over a minimum of 20 and a maximum of 60 minutes.

ACTIONS
An aminoglycoside antibiotic with potential neuromuscular blocking action. Inhibits protein synthesis in bacterial cells. Bactericidal against specific gram-negative bacilli, including *Escherichia coli, Klebsiella, Proteus,* and *Pseudomonas.* Well distributed through all body fluids. Usual half-life is 2 to 2.5 hours. Half-life is prolonged in infants, postpartum females, fever, liver disease and ascites, spinal cord injury, cystic fibrosis, and the elderly; shorter in severe burns. Crosses the placental barrier. Excreted in the kidneys.

INDICATIONS AND USES
Short-term treatment of serious infections caused by susceptible organisms. Indicated infections include septicemia; lower respiratory tract infections; CNS infections (meningitis); intra-abdominal infections (including peritonitis); skin, bone, and skin structure infections; and complicated and recurrent urinary tract infections. ■ Primarily used when penicillin and other less toxic antibiotics are ineffective or contraindicated. ■ Concurrent therapy with a penicillin or cephalosporin sometimes indicated.

CONTRAINDICATIONS
Known tobramycin or aminoglycoside sensitivity. Sulfite sensitivity may be a contraindication.

PRECAUTIONS

Use extreme caution if therapy is required over 7 to 10 days. ▪ Sensitivity studies necessary to determine susceptibility of causative organism to tobramycin. ▪ To reduce the development of drug-resistant bacteria and maintain its effectiveness, tobramycin should be used to treat or prevent only those infections proven or strongly suspected to be caused by bacteria. ▪ Superinfection may occur from overgrowth of nonsusceptible organisms. ▪ Use caution in infants, children, the elderly, and patients with congestive heart failure, extensive burns, or muscular disorders. ▪ May contain sulfites; use caution in patients with asthma. ▪ Potentially nephrotoxic, ototoxic, and neurotoxic. Risk for neurotoxicity (e.g., auditory and vestibular ototoxicity) increased in patients with pre-existing renal damage or in normal renal function with prolonged use. Partial or total irreversible deafness may continue to develop after tobramycin is discontinued. ▪ Aminoglycosides are nephrotoxic; risk for nephrotoxicity increased in patients with impaired renal function and in patients who receive high doses or prolonged therapy. ▪ Single daily dosing has been used effectively in abdominal, pelvic inflammatory, and GU infections in patients with normal renal function. Not recommended in bacteremia caused by *Pseudomonas aeruginosa,* endocarditis, meningitis, during pregnancy, or in patients less than 6 weeks postpartum. Limited data available for use in all other situations (e.g., burns, pediatric patients or the elderly, cystic fibrosis, renal impairment). ▪ *Clostridium difficile*–associated diarrhea (CDAD) has been reported. May range from mild diarrhea to fatal colitis. Consider in patients who present with diarrhea during or after treatment with tobramycin.

Monitor: Watch for decrease in urine output, rising BUN and SCr, and declining CrCl levels. Dose may need to be reduced. ▪ Closely monitor renal and eighth cranial nerve function, especially in patients with known or suspected reduced renal function at onset of therapy and in patients who develop signs of renal dysfunction during therapy. Monitor urine for decreased specific gravity, increased protein, and the presence of cells or casts. Serial audiograms are recommended, particularly in high-risk patients. ▪ Closely monitor patients with impaired renal function for nephrotoxicity and neurotoxicity (e.g., auditory and vestibular ototoxicity, convulsions, muscle twitching, numbness, tingling); nephrotoxicity may be reversible. ▪ Routine evaluation of hearing is recommended. ▪ Narrow range between toxic and therapeutic levels. Periodically monitor peak and trough concentrations to avoid peak serum concentrations above 12 mcg/mL and trough concentrations above 2 mcg/mL (indicates accumulation). With traditional dosing, therapeutic levels are between 4 and 8 mcg/mL depending on site and severity of infection. Accumulation, excessive peak concentrations, advanced age, cumulative doses, and dehydration may contribute to ototoxicity and nephrotoxicity. ▪ Maintain good hydration. ▪ Monitor serum calcium, magnesium, potassium, and sodium; levels may decline. ▪ Closely monitor patients with impaired renal function for nephrotoxicity and neurotoxicity (e.g., auditory and vestibular ototoxicity); nephrotoxicity may be reversible. ▪ In extended treatment, monitoring of serum levels, electrolytes, renal, auditory, and vestibular functions daily is recommended. ▪ See Drug/Lab Interactions.

Patient Education: Report promptly dizziness, hearing loss, weakness, or any changes in balance. ▪ Consider birth control options. ▪ Promptly report diarrhea or bloody stools that occur during treatment or up to several months after an antibiotic has been discontinued; may indicate CDAD and require treatment.

Maternal/Child: Category D: avoid pregnancy; use during pregnancy and breast-feeding only when absolutely necessary. Potential hazard to fetus. ▪ Peak concentrations are generally lower in infants and young children. ▪ Use extreme caution in premature infants and neonates; immature kidney function will result in prolonged half-life. ▪ See Precautions.

Elderly: Consider less toxic alternatives. ▪ Monitor renal function and drug levels carefully. Measurement of CrCl more useful than BUN or SCr to assess renal function. ▪ Half-life prolonged; longer intervals between doses may be more important than reduced doses. ▪ See Precautions, Dose Adjustments, and Side Effects.

DRUG/LAB INTERACTIONS

Synergistic when used in combination with **beta-lactam antibiotics** (e.g., cephalosporins, penicillins) **and vancomycin.** Synergism may be inconsistent; see Compatibility. ▪

Concurrent and/or sequential use topically or systemically with any other neurotoxic, ototoxic, or nephrotoxic agents should be avoided. May have dangerous additive effects with **anesthetics** (e.g., enflurane), **other neuromuscular blocking antibiotics** (e.g., other aminoglycosides [e.g., kanamycin]), **diuretics** (e.g., furosemide [Lasix]), **beta-lactam antibiotics** (e.g., cephalosporins), **vancomycin, and many others.** ▪ Neuromuscular blocking muscle relaxants (e.g., atracurium [Tracrium], succinylcholine) are potentiated by aminoglycosides. *Apnea can occur.* ▪ May be antagonized by **bacteriostatic antibiotics** (e.g., chloramphenicol, erythromycin, and tetracycline); bactericidal action may be affected. ▪ **Magnesium sulfate** may reduce the antibiotic activity of tobramycin. ▪ Aminoglycosides are potentiated by **anticholinesterases** (e.g., edrophonium), **antineoplastics** (e.g., nitrogen mustard, cisplatin). ▪ See Side Effects.

SIDE EFFECTS

Occur more frequently with impaired renal function, higher doses, prolonged administration, dehydration, in the elderly, and in patients receiving other ototoxic or nephrotoxic drugs.

Dizziness; fever; headache; increased AST, ALT, and serum bilirubin; itching; lethargy; rash; roaring in the ears; seizures; urticaria; vomiting.

Major: Apnea; blood dyscrasias; CDAD; cylindruria; elevated BUN, nonprotein nitrogen (NPN), and creatinine; hearing loss; leukocytosis; neuromuscular blockade; oliguria; proteinuria; seizures (large doses); tinnitus; vertigo.

ANTIDOTE

Notify the physician of all side effects. If minor side effects persist or any major symptom appears, discontinue the drug and notify the physician. Evidence of impaired renal, vestibular, or auditory function requires discontinuation of tobramycin or a dose adjustment. Treatment is symptomatic or a reduction in dose may be required. Mild cases of CDAD may respond to discontinuation of drug. Treat CDAD with fluids, electrolytes, protein supplements, and oral vancomycin (Vancocin) or metronidazole (Flagyl) as indicated. In severe cases, surgical evaluation may be indicated. In overdose hemodialysis may be indicated. Monitor fluid balance, CrCl, and plasma levels carefully. Complexation with ticarcillin may be as effective as hemodialysis. Consider exchange transfusion in the newborn. Calcium salts or neostigmine may reverse neuromuscular blockade. Resuscitate as necessary.

TOCILIZUMAB BBW
(**TOE**-si-**LIZ**-oo-mab)

Antirheumatic
Monoclonal antibody

Actemra

pH 6.5

USUAL DOSE

Before initial use, the absolute neutrophil count (ANC) should be equal to or greater than 2,000/mm³, platelet count should be equal to or greater than 100,000/mm³, and ALT and AST should be no more than 1.5 times the ULN.

Rheumatoid arthritis (RA): Initial adult dose in rheumatoid arthritis: 4 mg/kg as an IV infusion once every 4 weeks. Increase dose to 8 mg/kg every 4 weeks based on clinical response. May be used as monotherapy or in combination with methotrexate or other nonbiologic, disease-modifying, antirheumatic drugs (DMARDs) as an IV infusion or SC injection. Doses above 800 mg per infusion are not recommended.

Polyarticular juvenile idiopathic arthritis (PJIA): *Weight less than 30 kg:* 10 mg/kg.

Weight at or above 30 kg: 8 mg/kg. Administer as an IV infusion once every 4 weeks. May be used alone or in combination with methotrexate. Do not adjust dose based on a single-visit body weight; weight may fluctuate. SC administration is not approved for PJIA.

Systemic juvenile idiopathic arthritis (SJIA): *Weight less than 30 kg:* 12 mg/kg.

Weight equal to or more than 30 kg: 8 mg/kg. Administer as an IV infusion once every 2 weeks. May be used alone or in combination with methotrexate. Do not adjust dose based on a single-visit body weight; weight may fluctuate. SC administration is not approved for SJIA.

DOSE ADJUSTMENTS

There is a trend toward a higher clearance with increasing body weight; see Usual Dose. No specific dose adjustments required based on age, gender, race, or mild renal impairment. ▪ Hold therapy in patients with severe infections, an opportunistic infection, or sepsis until infection is controlled. ▪ Dose reduction has not been studied in PJIA or SJIA. Dose interruptions are recommended for liver enzyme abnormalities, low neutrophil counts, and low platelet counts in patients with PJIA or SJIA at levels similar to those outlined in the following charts for patients with rheumatoid arthritis (RA). May require interruption or discontinuation of tocilizumab and/or other concomitant medications (e.g., methotrexate) until evaluation of the clinical situation. The decision to discontinue tocilizumab for a lab abnormality should be based on medical assessment of the individual. ▪ The effects of moderate to severe renal impairment or hepatic impairment have not been studied. ▪ The following charts outline dose adjustments for adults with RA based on ANC, platelets, and liver function tests.

Tocilizumab Dose Recommendations for Adults with RA with a Low Absolute Neutrophil Count (ANC)	
Lab Value (cells/mm³)	Recommendation
ANC >1,000/mm³	Maintain dose.
ANC 500 to 1,000/mm³	Hold tocilizumab dosing. When ANC >1,000/mm³, resume tocilizumab at 4 mg/kg and increase to 8 mg/kg as clinically appropriate.
ANC <500/mm³	Discontinue tocilizumab.

Tocilizumab Dose Recommendations for Adults with RA with a Low Platelet Count	
Lab Value (cells/mm³)	Recommendation
Platelet count 50,000 to 100,000/mm³	Hold tocilizumab dosing. When platelet count is >100,000/mm³, resume tocilizumab at 4 mg/kg and increase to 8 mg/kg as clinically appropriate.
Platelet count <50,000/mm³	Discontinue tocilizumab.

Tocilizumab Dose Recommendations for Adults with RA with Liver Enzyme Abnormalities	
Lab Value	Recommendation
>1 to 3 × ULN	Dose modify concomitant DMARDs if appropriate. For persistent increases in this range, reduce tocilizumab dose to 4 mg/kg or hold dosing until ALT and/or AST have normalized.
>3 to 5 × ULN (confirmed by repeat testing)	Hold tocilizumab dosing until <3 × ULN, and follow recommendations above for >1 to 3 × ULN. For persistent increases >3 × ULN, discontinue tocilizumab.
>5 × ULN	Discontinue tocilizumab.

DILUTION

Available as a solution for single use (20 mg/mL). For adults and PJIA and SJIA patients weighing 30 kg or more, the solution must be further diluted to 100 mL in NS. For PJIA and SJIA patients weighing less than 30 kg, dilute to 50 mL in NS. From a 100-mL (or 50-mL) infusion bag or bottle, withdraw a volume of NS equal to the volume of solution required for the calculated dose. Slowly add tocilizumab and avoid foaming by gently inverting the bag or bottle. Bring fully diluted solution to RT before administration.

For Intravenous Use: Volume of Tocilizumab Injection per kg of Body Weight		
Dose	Indication	Volume of Tocilizumab Injection per kg of Body Weight
4 mg/kg	Adult RA	0.2 mL/kg
8 mg/kg	Adult RA PJIA and SJIA (>30 kg of body weight)	0.4 mL/kg
10 mg/kg	PJIA (<30 kg of body weight)	0.5 mL/kg
12 mg/kg	SJIA (<30 kg of body weight)	0.6 mL/kg

Filters: Specific information not available.

Storage: Refrigerate unopened vials in original carton at 2° to 8° C (36° to 46° F). Do not use beyond expiration date. Protect from light. Do not freeze. Fully diluted solution may be refrigerated or stored at RT for up to 24 hours. Protect from light. Discard unused solution.

COMPATIBILITY

Manufacturer states, "Fully diluted solutions are **compatible** with polypropylene, polyethylene, and polyvinyl chloride infusion bags and glass infusion bottles. Tocilizumab should not be infused concomitantly in the same intravenous line with other drugs."

RATE OF ADMINISTRATION

A single dose as an infusion equally distributed over 60 minutes.

ACTIONS

A recombinant humanized antihuman interleukin 6 (IL-6) receptor monoclonal antibody. Binds specifically to both soluble and membrane-bound IL-6 receptors. Inhibits IL-6–mediated signaling through these receptors. IL-6 is a pro-inflammatory cytokine produced by a variety of cell types. IL-6 is also produced by synovial and endothelial cells leading to local production of IL-6 in joints affected by inflammatory processes such as rheumatoid arthritis. IL-6 has been shown to be involved in diverse physiologic processes such as T-cell activation, induction of immunoglobulin secretion, initiation of hepatic acute-phase protein synthesis, and stimulation of hematopoietic precursor cell proliferation and differentiation. Following administration, increases in hemoglobin and decreases in C-reactive protein, rheumatoid factor, erythrocyte sedimentation rate, and serum amyloid A were observed. ANC counts decreased to the nadir 3 to 5 days after administration, and neutrophils recovered toward baseline in a dose-dependent manner. Steady state is reached with the first administration. It undergoes biphasic elimination from the circulation. Half-life is concentration dependent and ranges from 11 to 13 days in adults depending on the dose administered. Half-life in pediatric patients ranges from 16 to 23 days.

INDICATIONS AND USES

Treatment of adults with moderately to severely active rheumatoid arthritis who have had an inadequate response to one or more disease-modifying antirheumatic drugs (DMARDs), such as cyclophosphamide (Cytoxan), cyclosporine (Sandimmune), methotrexate, and biologics (e.g., adalimumab [Humira], etanercept [Enbrel], infliximab [Remicade], rituximab [Rituxan]). ■ Treatment of patients 2 years of age and older with active polyarticular juvenile idiopathic arthritis (PJIA). ■ Treatment of patients 2 years of age and older with active systemic juvenile idiopathic arthritis (SJIA).

CONTRAINDICATIONS

Known hypersensitivity to tocilizumab.

PRECAUTIONS

Administered under the direction of a physician knowledgeable in its use in a facility with adequate diagnostic and treatment facilities to monitor the patients and respond to any medical emergency. ■ Serious and sometimes fatal infections due to bacterial, mycobacterial, invasive fungal, viral, protozoal, or other opportunistic pathogens have been reported. Deaths have occurred. The most common serious infections included bacterial arthritis, cellulitis, diverticulitis, gastroenteritis, herpes zoster, pneumonia, sepsis, and UTIs. Opportunistic infections reported with tocilizumab include aspergillosis, candidiasis, cryptococcus, pneumocystosis, and tuberculosis (TB). Patients were often taking concomitant immunosuppressants such as methotrexate or corticosteroids, which may have predisposed them to infection. ■ Do not administer tocilizumab to patients with an active infection, including localized infections. Assess the risks and benefits of tocilizumab before initiating in patients with chronic or recurrent infection, patients who have been exposed to tuberculosis, patients with a history of a serious or an opportunistic infection, patients who have resided or traveled in areas of endemic tuberculosis or endemic mycoses, or patients with underlying conditions that may predispose them to infection. ■ Evaluate patients for TB risk factors and latent TB before initiating therapy; see Monitor. ■ Viral reactivation has been reported with immunosuppressive biologic therapies. Cases of herpes zoster exacerbation have been reported with tocilizumab. Cases of hepatitis B reactivation have not been reported, but patients who screened positive for hepatitis were excluded from studies. ■ Has not been studied in patients with active hepatic disease or hepatic impairment, including patients with positive HBV (hepatitis B virus) or HCV (hepatitis C virus) serology. Use is not recommended. ■ Has not been studied in patients with moderate to severe renal impairment. ■ Use caution in patients who may be at risk for GI perforation (e.g., diverticulitis [primarily in RA patients]) and in patients with pre-existing or recent-onset demyelinating disorders (e.g., multiple sclerosis, chronic inflammatory demyelinating polyneuropathy). ■ Hypersensitivity reactions, including anaphylaxis and death, have been reported. Emergency medical equipment and medications for treating these reactions must be readily available. ■ Tocilizumab is associated with a higher incidence of neutropenia and elevated transaminases, a reduction in platelet counts, and increases in lipids; see Monitor and Dose Adjustments. ■ Infusion-related reactions have occurred; see Side Effects. ■ A small number of patients have developed binding antibodies to tocilizumab. Hypersensitivity reactions leading to withdrawal have been reported. ■ Treatment may result in an increased risk of malignancy.

Monitor: Evaluate patients for TB risk factors and latent TB with a TB skin test before tocilizumab use and during therapy. Patients testing positive in TB screening should be treated with a standard TB regimen before initiating therapy with tocilizumab. Consider treatment in patients with a history of latent or active TB when an adequate course of treatment cannot be confirmed and in patients who have a negative test for latent TB but have risk factors for TB. Consultation with a specialist in TB diagnosis and treatment is encouraged. Closely monitor all patients for S/S of tuberculosis. May present with pulmonary or extrapulmonary disease. ▪ Screening for viral hepatitis may be indicated. ▪ In RA patients, obtain baseline CBC, platelets, and liver function tests (e.g., ALT, AST, bilirubin). Consider obtaining a baseline bilirubin. Monitor neutrophils, platelets, ALT, and AST 4 to 8 weeks after start of therapy and every 3 months thereafter. In PJIA and SJIA patients, obtain baseline CBC, platelets, and liver function tests. Monitor neutrophils, platelets, ALT, and AST before the second infusion and every 4 to 8 weeks for PJIA and every 2 to 4 weeks for SJIA. ▪ In RA, PJIA, and SJIA patients, obtain baseline lipid studies (e.g., cholesterol [HDL, LDL, and total], triglycerides). Repeat in 4 to 8 weeks and then at 24-week intervals. Elevated lipids respond to lipid-lowering agents (e.g., simvastatin [Zocor]). ▪ Closely monitor for S/S of infection during and after treatment with tocilizumab; patients with invasive fungal infections may present with disseminated, rather than localized, disease; S/S may be lessened due to suppression of the acute-phase reactants. Hold tocilizumab if a serious infection, an opportunistic infection, or sepsis develops, and appropriate evaluation and treatment should be initiated promptly. ▪ Monitor for S/S of hypersensitivity or infusion-related reactions (e.g., anaphylaxis, hypotension, pruritus, rash, urticaria, or wheezing); most hypersensitivity reactions have occurred between the second and fourth infusion but can occur at any time, even if they have not occurred with earlier infusions. Have occurred in patients who received premedication; see Side Effects. ▪ Monitor for S/S of GI perforation (e.g., new-onset abdominal pain). ▪ Monitor for S/S potentially indicative of demyelinating disorders. ▪ Do not administer live virus vaccines. All patients, especially PJIA and SJIA patients, should be brought up-to-date with all immunizations before beginning therapy. ▪ See Precautions and Drug/Lab Interactions.

Patient Education: Read FDA-approved medication guide before starting therapy. ▪ Promptly report S/S of an allergic reaction (e.g., rash, itching, wheezing), infusion reaction (e.g., dizziness, headache), or infection (e.g., chill, cough, with or without a fever). Report severe, persistent abdominal pain promptly. ▪ Discuss previous infections, current infections, or exposure to TB. ▪ Routine laboratory monitoring required. ▪ All vaccinations should be brought up-to-date before starting tocilizumab.

Maternal/Child: Category C: use during pregnancy only if the potential benefit justifies the potential risk to the fetus. ▪ A pregnancy registry has been established; contact manufacturer. ▪ Discontinue breast-feeding. ▪ Safety and effectiveness have been established for use only in pediatric patients 2 years of age or older with SJIA and PJIA.

Elderly: Incidence of infection is higher in the elderly. Use caution; see Precautions.

DRUG/LAB INTERACTIONS

Formal drug interaction studies have not been conducted. ▪ Avoid concurrent use with **biological DMARDS** such as TNF antagonists (e.g., adalimumab [Humira], etanercept [Enbrel], infliximab [Remicade]), IL-1R antagonists, anti-CD20 monoclonal antibodies, and selective costimulation modulators; may increase immunosuppression and risk of infection. ▪ Methotrexate, NSAIDs (e.g., naproxen [Naprosyn, Aleve], ibuprofen [Advil, Motrin]), and corticosteroids (e.g., prednisone) do not appear to influence tocilizumab clearance. ▪ Has no clinically significant effect on methotrexate exposure. ▪ Increased frequency and magnitude of LFT elevations may be seen when tocilizumab is coadministered with other potentially **hepatotoxic medications** (e.g., methotrexate). ▪ Inhibition of IL-6 signaling in patients treated with tocilizumab may restore CYP450 activities to higher levels, resulting in an increased metabolism of drugs that are CYP450 substrates. Concurrent use showed an increase in metabolism and lower serum concentrations of **omeprazole** (Prilosec) and **simvastatin** (Zocor). This effect may be clinically relevant with CYP450 substrates with a narrow therapeutic index, in which the dose is individually adjusted (e.g., **warfarin** [Coumadin], **cyclosporine** [Sandimmune], **theophylline**). Therapeutic monitoring of effect (INR) and/or serum concentrations is indicated to adjust the dose of these drugs with initiation or termination of tocilizumab. Use caution with CYP3A4 substrate drugs in which a decrease in effectiveness is undesirable (e.g., **atorvastatin** [Lipitor], **lovastatin** [Mevacor], **oral contraceptives**). The effect of tocilizumab on CYP450 enzyme activity may persist for several weeks after therapy is discontinued. ▪ Do not administer **live virus vaccines.**

SIDE EFFECTS

RA: The most common adverse reactions include headache, hypertension, increased transaminases (ALT, AST), nasopharyngitis, and upper respiratory tract infections. The most common serious infections include bacterial arthritis, cellulitis, diverticulitis, gastroenteritis, herpes zoster, pneumonia, sepsis, and UTIs. The most common side effects that required discontinuation of therapy were increased hepatic transaminase values and serious infections. Infusion-related reactions have been reported. Hypertension frequently occurred during infusion, and headache and skin reactions (e.g., pruritus, rash, urticaria) were reported within the next 24 hours. Hypersensitivity reactions (e.g., anaphylactoid and anaphylactic) did occur in a few patients. Other side effects reported include bronchitis, conjunctivitis, cough, dizziness, dyspnea, elevated lipids, gastric ulcer, gastritis, GI perforation, hypothyroidism, increased total bilirubin, increased weight, leukopenia, mouth ulceration, nephrolithiasis, neutropenia, oral herpes simplex, peripheral edema, stomatitis, thrombocytopenia, and upper abdominal pain.

PJIA: Side effects consistent with those seen in RA and SJIA patients.

SJIA: The most common adverse reactions included diarrhea, headache, nasopharyngitis, and upper respiratory tract infections. Anaphylaxis, decreased platelet count, development of anti-tocilizumab antibodies, increased liver function tests and lipids, infections, infusion reactions, macrophage activation syndrome (MAS), and neutropenia have been reported.

Post-Marketing: Fatal anaphylaxis, Stevens-Johnson syndrome.

ANTIDOTE

Notify physician of any side effects; most will be treated symptomatically. During clinical studies, most infusion-related reactions were mild to moderate. Interrupt therapy for decreases in ANC and platelets and increases in liver function studies as outlined in Dose Adjustments. Therapy may need to be interrupted in patients who develop infections. Discontinue tocilizumab for any serious reaction or infection. Treat infusion and hypersensitivity reactions as indicated (e.g., oxygen, diphenhydramine, epinephrine, corticosteroids, vasopressors, and/or fluids). Resuscitate as necessary.

TOPOTECAN HYDROCHLORIDE BBW

(toh-poh-**TEE**-kan hy-droh-**KLOR**-eyed)

Hycamtin

Antineoplastic
(topoisomerase I inhibitor)

pH 2.5 to 3.5

USUAL DOSE

Verify dose using body surface area before dispensing. Recommended dose should generally not exceed 4 mg IV. Before giving the initial dose, the baseline neutrophil count must be at least 1,500/mm³ and baseline platelet count must be at least 100,000/mm³.

Ovarian cancer and small-cell lung cancer: 1.5 mg/M² as an infusion each day for 5 consecutive days (Days 1 through 5 of a 21-day course). Begin the second course on Day 22. See Dose Adjustments.

Cervical cancer: 0.75 mg/M² as an infusion on Days 1, 2, and 3. On Day 1 follow with cisplatin 50 mg/M². Repeat every 21 days. See cisplatin monograph for prehydration requirements.

Non–small-cell lung cancer (unlabeled): 1.5 mg/M² as an infusion each day for 5 consecutive days. Repeat every 21 days.

DOSE ADJUSTMENTS

Do not begin subsequent courses of topotecan until neutrophils recover to more than 1,000/mm³, platelets recover to 100,000/mm³, and hemoglobin recovers to 9 mg/dL (with transfusion if necessary). ■ **For single-agent use,** reduce dose to 1.25 mg/M² for (1) neutrophil counts less than 500 cells/mm³, or administer granulocyte-colony stimulating factor (G-CSF) starting no sooner than 24 hours after the last dose of topotecan; or (2) platelet counts less than 25,000 cells/mm³ during the previous cycle. ■ **For combination use with cisplatin,** reduce dose to 0.6 mg/M² (and further to 0.45 mg/M² if necessary) for (1) febrile neutropenia (defined as neutrophil counts less than 1,000 cells/mm³ with temperature greater than or equal to 38° C [100.4° F]), or administer G-CSF starting no sooner than 24 hours after the last dose of topotecan; or (2) platelet counts less than 25,000 cells/mm³ during the previous cycle. See cisplatin monograph for specific dose adjustments. ■ **For single-agent use,** reduce dose to 0.75 mg/M² in patients with moderate impaired renal function (CrCl 20 to 39 mL/min). There are inadequate data at this time to recommend a dose in severe renal impairment. ■ Dose adjustment may be required in the elderly because of age-related renal impairment.

DILUTION

Specific techniques required; see Precautions. Available as a 4-mg lyophilized powder in a single-dose vial. Reconstitute each 4-mg vial with 4 mL of SWFI (1 mg/mL). Also available as a generic in a 4 mg/4 mL solution in a single-use vial. Withdraw the calculated dose and further dilute in NS or D5W.

Filters: No data available from manufacturer.

Storage: *Hycamtin:* Store unopened vials in cartons protected from light between 20° and 25° C (68° and 77° F). Reconstituted solutions contain no preservative; use immediately. Solutions diluted for infusion are stable at room temperature in soft light for 24 hours. *Generic:* Store unopened vials in cartons protected from light and refrigerated between 2° and 8° C (36° and 46° F). Solutions diluted for infusion are stable for no more than 4 hours at RT or for 12 hours if refrigerated.

COMPATIBILITY

(Underline Indicates Conflicting Compatibility Information)

Consider any drug NOT listed as compatible to be INCOMPATIBLE until consulting a pharmacist; specific conditions may apply.

One source suggests the following **compatibilities:**

Y-site: Carboplatin (Paraplatin), cisplatin, cyclophosphamide (Cytoxan), doxorubicin (Adriamycin), etoposide (VePesid), gemcitabine (Gemzar), granisetron (Kytril), ifosfamide (Ifex), methylprednisolone (Solu-Medrol), metoclopramide (Reglan), ondansetron (Zofran), oxaliplatin (Eloxatin), paclitaxel (Taxol), palonosetron (Aloxi), prochlor-perazine (Compazine), ticarcillin/clavulanate (Timentin), vincristine.

RATE OF ADMINISTRATION
A single dose as an infusion evenly distributed over 30 minutes.

ACTIONS
A class of antineoplastic agent that inhibits the enzyme topoisomerase I required for DNA replication. It is a semi-synthetic derivative of camptothecin. Causes cell death by damaging DNA produced during the S-phase of the cell cycle. Undergoes pH-dependent hydrolysis in plasma, and minor additional metabolism occurs in the liver. Terminal half-life is 2 to 3 hours. Moderately bound to plasma protein (35%). Excreted in urine and, to a lesser extent, in feces.

INDICATIONS AND USES
As a single agent for treatment of patients with metastatic carcinoma of the ovary after disease progression on or after initial or subsequent chemotherapy. ■ As a single agent for treatment of patients with small-cell lung cancer with platinum-sensitive disease who progressed at least 60 days after initiation of first-line chemotherapy. ■ In combination with cisplatin for treatment of patients with stage IV-B, recurrent, or persistent carcinoma of the cervix not amenable to curative treatment.

Unlabeled uses: Treatment of non–small-cell lung cancer.

CONTRAINDICATIONS
History of severe hypersensitivity reactions to topotecan.

PRECAUTIONS
Follow guidelines for handling cytotoxic agents. See Appendix A, p. 1331. ■ Administered by or under the direction of the physician specialist. ■ Adequate diagnostic and treatment facilities must be available to meet any medical emergency. ■ May cause severe myelosuppression. Bone marrow suppression (primarily neutropenia) is the dose-limiting toxicity. Severe myelotoxicity has been reported when topotecan is administered in combination with cisplatin. Anemia, neutropenia, febrile neutropenia, pancytopenia, and thrombocytopenia have been reported; see Monitor. ■ Use with caution in impaired renal function; clearance decreased. ■ Neutropenic enterocolitis (typhlitis) has been reported. Fatalities have occurred; see Monitor. ■ Interstitial lung disease (ILD), including fatalities, has occurred; risk increased in patients with a history of ILD, lung cancer, pulmonary fibrosis, thoracic irradiation, and the use of pneumotoxic drugs and/or colony-stimulating factors; see Monitor.

Monitor: Baseline neutrophil count must be at least 1,500/mm^3 and platelets at least 100,000/mm^3 before the initial dose. ■ Obtain a baseline CBC with differential and platelets. ■ Monitor before each course and frequently during treatment. Platelet count must be 100,000/mm^3, neutrophils 1,000/mm^3, and hemoglobin 9 mg/dL before a course of therapy can be repeated. Anemia is frequent and transfusion is often indicated. ■ Baseline CrCl and BUN suggested. ■ Monitor vital signs. ■ Maintain adequate hydration. ■ Nausea and vomiting can be frequent and may be severe; use prophylactic administration of antiemetics to increase patient comfort. ■ Observe closely for S/S of infection. Prophylactic antibiotics may be indicated pending results of C/S in a febrile neutropenic patient. ■ Not a vesicant, but monitor injection site for inflammation and/or extravasation. Severe cases have been reported. If S/S of extravasation occur, discontinue infusion and manage as indicated. ■ Monitor for S/S of ILD (e.g., cough, dyspnea, fever, and/or hypoxia). ■ Monitor for signs of neutropenic colitis (e.g., fever, neutropenia, and abdominal pain). ■ Monitor for thrombocytopenia (platelet count less than 50,000/mm^3). Platelet transfusions may be required. Initiate precautions to prevent excessive bleeding (e.g., inspect IV sites, skin, and mucous membranes; use extreme care during invasive procedures; test urine, emesis, stool, and secretions for occult blood).

Patient Education: Females should use effective contraception during treatment and for at least 1 month after the last dose of topotecan. ■ May damage spermatozoa. Males with a female sexual partner of reproductive potential should use effective contraception during and for 3 months after treatment with topotecan. ■ Potential risk for impaired fertility in both male and female patients. Discuss family planning options if appropriate. ▪ Report any unusual or unexpected symptoms or side effects as soon as possible (e.g., signs of infection [e.g., chills, fever, night sweats] or signs of bleeding [e.g., bruising, black tarry stools]). ▪ May cause loss of strength or fatigue. Use caution when driving or operating machinery. ▪ See Appendix D, p. 1333.

Maternal/Child: Avoid pregnancy; can cause fetal harm; see Patient Education. ▪ Discontinue breast-feeding. ▪ Safety and effectiveness for use in pediatric patients not established.

Elderly: Safety and effectiveness similar to younger adults. ▪ Consider age-related renal impairment; see Dose Adjustments. Monitoring of renal function may be useful.

DRUG/LAB INTERACTIONS

May cause severe prolonged myelosuppression and Grade 3 or 4 nonhematologic effects (e.g., diarrhea, lethargy, nausea, vomiting) with **cisplatin.** ▪ Concurrent administration of **G-CSF (filgrastim)** can prolong the duration of neutropenia. If used, do not administer until at least 24 hours after the final dose of topotecan. ▪ Concurrent or consecutive administration of **other bone marrow suppressants** (e.g., cyclophosphamide [Cytoxan], paclitaxel [Taxol]) **or radiation therapy** may produce additive bone marrow suppression. Dose reduction may be required based on blood cell counts. ▪ Concurrent use with **hydantoins** (e.g., phenytoin [Dilantin]) may decrease plasma concentrations of topotecan. Specific guidelines for topotecan dose adjustment are not available. Consider alternatives to phenytoin when possible. ▪ Do not administer **palifermin** (Kepivance) within 24 hours before or after topotecan; coadministration may increase the severity and duration of oral mucositis. ▪ Do not administer **live virus vaccines.**

SIDE EFFECTS

Bone marrow suppression, primarily neutropenia, is the dose-limiting toxicity of topotecan.

Ovarian cancer: The most common hematologic adverse reactions were anemia (Grade 3 and 4), febrile neutropenia, neutropenia (Grade 4), and thrombocytopenia (Grade 4). The most common nonhematologic adverse reactions were diarrhea, dyspnea, fatigue, nausea, and vomiting. Other reported reactions included abdominal pain, asthenia, constipation, elevated bilirubin and hepatic enzymes, intestinal obstruction, pain, and sepsis.

Small-cell lung cancer: The most common hematologic adverse reactions were anemia (Grade 3 and 4), febrile neutropenia, neutropenia (Grade 4), and thrombocytopenia (Grade 4). The most common nonhematologic adverse reactions were abdominal pain, asthenia, dyspnea, fatigue, nausea, and pneumonia. Other reported reactions included elevated bilirubin and hepatic enzymes, pain, and sepsis.

Cervical cancer: The most common hematologic adverse reactions were anemia (Grade 3 and 4), neutropenia (Grade 3 and 4), and thrombocytopenia (Grade 3 and 4). The most common nonhematologic adverse reactions were infection/febrile neutropenia, pain, and vomiting. Other reported reactions included asthenia, chills, fatigue, fever, lethargy, malaise, rigors, stomatitis-pharyngitis, sweating, and weight gain or loss.

Post-Marketing: Abdominal pain associated with neutropenic enterocolitis, extravasation, hypersensitivity reactions (including anaphylaxis), interstitial lung disease, severe bleeding, skin and subcutaneous tissue disorders (e.g., angioedema, severe dermatitis, severe pruritus).

ANTIDOTE

Keep physician informed of all side effects. Withhold topotecan until myelosuppression has improved to minimum requirements. Neutropenia recovery may be aided by G-CSF (filgrastim, pegfilgrastim [Neulasta]) under specific conditions; see Dose Adjustments or Drug/Lab Interactions. Anemia often required RBC or whole blood tranfusions. Thrombocytopenia may require platelet transfusion. Death can result from the progression of many side effects. Discontinue topotecan if a new diagnosis of ILD is confirmed. No known antidote for overdose. If an overdose is suspected, monitor for bone marrow suppression and institute supportive care measures (e.g., prophylactic G-CSF and antibiotic therapy) as appropriate. Treat hypersensitivity reactions with oxygen, epinephrine, corticosteroids, and antihistamines.

TORSEMIDE INJECTION
(**TOR**-seh-myd in-**JEK**-shun)

Diuretic (loop)
Antihypertensive

Demadex

pH over 8.3

USUAL DOSE
IV and oral doses are therapeutically equivalent. Oral dose can replace an IV dose at any time. If diuretic response is not adequate, titrate the recommended dose upward by doubling the dose until desired response achieved or maximum suggested dose reached.

Edema of congestive heart failure: 10 to 20 mg once daily. See general instructions above; single doses over 200 mg have not been adequately studied.

Edema of chronic renal failure: 20 mg once daily. See general instructions above; single doses over 200 mg have not been adequately studied.

Hepatic cirrhosis with ascites: 5 to 10 mg once daily. To prevent hypokalemia and metabolic alkalosis give in combination with an aldosterone antagonist (e.g., spironolactone [Aldactone]) or a potassium-sparing diuretic (e.g., dyazide). See general instructions above; single doses over 40 mg have not been adequately studied.

Hypertension: 5 mg once daily. May be increased to 10 mg in 4 to 6 weeks if BP reduction is inadequate. If response is still inadequate, the addition of other antihypertensive agents is recommended instead of larger doses of torsemide. Usually given PO.

Continuous infusion: Studies used a 100-mg dose divided as follows. A *loading dose* of 25 mg (2.5 mL) as an IV injection over 2 minutes (25% of total daily dose). Follow with an infusion at 3.1 mg/hr (10 mL/hr) or 75% of total daily dose equally distributed over 24 hours.

DOSE ADJUSTMENTS
Higher doses may be required in renal failure. See Drug/Lab Interactions.

DILUTION
Available as 10 mg/mL. May be given undiluted. May be given through Y-tube or three-way stopcock of infusion set. May be further diluted in NS, $1/2$NS, or D5W. For a 75-mg dose (75% of the 100-mg total daily dose), dilute 7.5 mL to a total volume of 240 mL. 200 mg in 250 mL diluent yields 0.8 mg/mL. 50 mg in 500 mL diluent yields 0.1 mg/mL.

Storage: Store at CRT. Do not freeze.

COMPATIBILITY
Consider any drug NOT listed as compatible to be INCOMPATIBLE until consulting a pharmacist; specific conditions may apply.

Manufacturer recommends flushing the IV line before and after torsemide injection to avoid **incompatibilities** caused by alkaline pH.

One source suggests the following **compatibilities:**

Y-site: Milrinone (Primacor), nesiritide (Natrecor).

RATE OF ADMINISTRATION
Ototoxicity (usually reversible) has occurred with too-rapid injection and doses over 200 mg. Flush IV line with NS before and after administration.

IV injection: Each 200 mg or fraction thereof over 2 minutes.

Continuous infusion: Balance of daily dose after loading dose equally distributed over 24 hours. For a 75-mg dose, the rate would be 3.1 mg (10 mL/hr) for 24 hours.

ACTIONS
A sulfonamide type loop diuretic. Acts from within the ascending portion of the loop of Henle to excrete water, sodium, chlorides, and some potassium. Diuretic action correlates better with the rate of drug excretion in urine than with plasma concentration. Will produce diuresis in alkalosis or acidosis. Effects begin within 10 minutes and peak within 1 hour. Diuresis lasts 6 to 8 hours. Highly protein bound. Metabolized by the liver (80%).

20% eliminated via urinary excretion. Other loop diuretics cross the placental barrier and are secreted in breast milk; specific information not available for torsemide.

INDICATIONS AND USES
Treatment of edema associated with congestive heart failure, cirrhosis of the liver with ascites, and chronic renal failure. Used when a rapid onset of diuresis is desired or when oral administration is impractical. ▪ Treatment of hypertension.

CONTRAINDICATIONS
Known hypersensitivity to torsemide or to sulfonylureas and in anuric patients.

PRECAUTIONS
Tests to determine serum levels of torsemide not widely available. ▪ In patients with congestive heart failure and/or renal failure, a smaller dose is actually delivered to the ascending loop of Henle, resulting in less response at any given dose. ▪ Use caution and improve basic condition first in hepatic coma, electrolyte depletion, and advanced cirrhosis of the liver. Initiation of therapy in the hospital is preferred. ▪ Use extreme caution in patients sensitive to bumetanide, furosemide (Lasix), or sulfonamides (including thiazide diuretics); may also be sensitive to torsemide. ▪ In patients with hepatic disease with cirrhosis and ascites use a potassium-sparing diuretic (e.g., dyazide) or an aldosterone antagonist (e.g., spironolactone) concurrently to prevent hypokalemia and metabolic alkalosis. ▪ Use caution in acute MI; excessive diuresis may precipitate shock. ▪ In nonanuric renal failure, may cause marked increases in water and sodium excretion without impacting steady-state fluid retention. High doses (500 to 1,200 mg) have caused seizures. ▪ May activate or exacerbate systemic lupus erythematosus. Chronic use in renal or hepatic disease has not been adequately studied. ▪ Antihypertensive effects greater in black patients.

Monitor: Monitor BP frequently, especially during initial therapy. May precipitate excessive diuresis with water and electrolyte depletion. Dehydration, electrolyte imbalance, hypovolemia, prerenal axotemia, embolism, or thrombosis can occur. Routine checks on electrolyte panel, CO_2, and BUN are necessary during therapy. Potassium chloride and/or magnesium replacement may be required. ▪ Risk of hypokalemia greatest in patients with cirrhosis of the liver, during brisk diuresis, with inadequate oral electrolyte intake, or with concurrent administration of corticosteroids (e.g., prednisone). ▪ May increase blood glucose, serum cholesterol, and triglycerides. ▪ Slight increases in BUN, SCr, and uric acid may occur but usually reverse when therapy is discontinued. Sudden changes in fluid and electrolyte balance may precipitate hepatic coma in patients with hepatic disease and ascites. ▪ Rarely precipitates an attack of gout. ▪ See Drug/Lab Interactions.

Patient Education: Hypotension may cause dizziness; request assistance with ambulation. ▪ May cause a decrease in potassium levels and require a supplement. ▪ Possible skin photosensitivity. Avoid unprotected exposure to sunlight. ▪ Report cramps, dizziness, muscle weakness, or nausea promptly.

Maternal/Child: Category B: use only if clearly needed during pregnancy; safety for use not established. ▪ Safety for use during breast-feeding not established; other loop diuretics suggest discontinuing breast-feeding. ▪ Safety and effectiveness for use in pediatric patients under 18 years of age not established. Administration of other loop diuretics to premature infants with edema due to patent ductus arteriosus and hyaline membrane disease may have caused renal calcifications; also other loop diuretics may have increased the risk of persistent patent ductus arteriosus in premature infants with hyaline membrane disease. Torsemide has not been studied in these situations.

Elderly: No specific age-related differences; dose adjustment not indicated. May be more susceptible to dehydration; observe carefully. ▪ Avoid rapid contraction of plasma volume and hemoconcentration. May cause thromboembolic episodes (e.g., CVA, pulmonary emboli).

DRUG/LAB INTERACTIONS
Concurrent administration with **high-dose salicylates** may cause salicylate toxicity. ▪ Probenecid decreases the diuretic activity of torsemide. ▪ May reduce renal clearance of

spironolactone, but dose adjustment not required. ▪ Has been administered with beta-blockers (e.g., atenolol), ACE inhibitors (e.g., captopril), calcium-channel blockers (e.g., diltiazem), cimetidine (Tagamet), digoxin, and nitrates (e.g., nitroglycerin) without new or unexpected adverse events; however, torsemide has caused severe hypotension with **ACE inhibitors** in sodium- or volume-depleted patients. ▪ Does not affect protein binding of glyburide (DiaBeta) or coumarin derivatives (e.g., warfarin). ▪ May cause excessive potassium depletion with **amphotericin B** (Abelcet, conventional), **corticosteroids, thiazide diuretics** (e.g., hydrochlorothiazide). Monitor electrolytes closely. ▪ May cause cardiac arrhythmias with **digoxin and other antiarrhythmic agents** secondary to potassium and magnesium depletion. ▪ **NSAIDs** (e.g., indomethacin [Indocin], ibuprofen [Advil, Motrin], naproxen [Aleve, Naprosyn]) **or salicylates** (e.g., aspirin) may cause retention of sodium and water and may decrease diuretic and antihypertensive effects. ▪ Antihypertensive effects may be increased by any **hypotension-producing agent** (e.g., lidocaine, nitroglycerin, nitroprusside sodium, paclitaxel); reduced dose of the antihypertensive agent or both drugs may be indicated. ▪ May potentiate **propranolol, salicylates, muscle relaxants** (e.g., atracurium [Tracrium]), and hypotensive effect of **other diuretics.** ▪ May increase ototoxicity in doses exceeding the usual or in conjunction with **ototoxic drugs** (e.g., cisplatin, aminoglycosides [e.g., amikacin, streptomycin, gentamicin], ethacrynic acid [Edecrin]). ▪ May increase nephrotoxicity if given concurrently with **any other nephrotoxic agent** (e.g., amphotericin B, aminoglycosides [e.g., gentamicin], foscarnet [Foscavir], rifampin [Rifadin]). Concurrent use with **amphotericin B** is not recommended, especially in patients with some impaired renal function. ▪ Effects of **warfarin** (Coumadin) are increased; may require dose adjustment. ▪ May be inhibited by **phenytoin** (Dilantin). ▪ May reduce excretion of **lithium** and cause lithium toxicity. ▪ May increase or decrease effectiveness of **theophyllines.**

SIDE EFFECTS
Arthralgia, constipation, cough, diarrhea, dizziness, dyspepsia, ECG abnormalities, edema, electrolyte imbalance, esophageal hemorrhage, excessive thirst, excessive urination, headache, hyperglycemia, hyperuricemia, hypokalemia, impotence, insomnia, myalgia, nervousness, ototoxicity (usually reversible), rhinitis, sore throat, and tinnitus have all been reported. Hypersensitivity reactions can occur. Hypocalcemia and hypomagnesemia have been minimal with usual doses.

Major: Anorexia; dizziness; drowsiness; dryness of the mouth; hypotension; increased BUN; lethargy; mental confusion; muscle cramps, fatigue, or pain; nausea and vomiting; oliguria; restlessness; tachycardia; thirst; or weakness may indicate severe electrolyte imbalance, hypovolemia, or prerenal azotemia.

Overdose: Circulatory collapse, dehydration, excessive diuresis, hemoconcentration, hypochloremic alkalosis, hyperchloremia or hypochloremia, hyperkalemia or hypokalemia, hypomagnesemia, hypernatremia or hyponatremia, hypotension, hypovolemia, vascular thrombosis, and embolism.

ANTIDOTE
Notify the physician of any side effect. Depending on severity the physician may treat the side effects symptomatically and either continue or discontinue torsemide. Fluid and electrolyte replacement may be indicated. If side effects are progressive or any major side effects or signs of overdose appear, discontinue the drug immediately and notify the physician. Treatment of overdose is symptomatic and aggressive. Hemodialysis is not effective in overdose. Resuscitate as necessary. Torsemide may be restarted at a lower dose after the patient is stable.

TRABECTEDIN
(tra-**BEK**-te-din)

Yondelis

Antineoplastic
(alkylating agent)

pH 3.6 to 4.2

USUAL DOSE
Premedication: Dexamethasone 20 mg IV 30 minutes before each dose of trabectedin.
Trabectedin: 1.5 mg/M^2 administered as an infusion over 24 hours through a central venous line every 21 days (3 weeks), until disease progression or unacceptable toxicity, to patients with normal bilirubin and AST or ALT less than or equal to 2.5 times the ULN.
There is no recommended dose of trabectedin in patients with serum bilirubin levels above the institutional ULN.

DOSE ADJUSTMENTS
No dose adjustment is recommended in patients with mild (CrCl 60 to 89 mL/min) or moderate (CrCl 30 to 59 mL/min) renal impairment. ▪ ***First-dose reduction:*** Reduce trabectedin dose to 1.2 mg/M^2 every 3 weeks. ▪ ***Second-dose reduction:*** Reduce trabectedin dose to 1 mg/M^2 every 3 weeks. ▪ Once reduced, the dose of trabectedin should not be increased in subsequent treatment cycles. ▪ Recommended dose modifications for laboratory results and adverse reactions are listed in the following chart.

Recommended Dose Modifications for Laboratory Results or Adverse Reactions to Trabectedin		
Laboratory Result or Adverse Reaction	DELAY Next Dose of Trabectedin for Up to 3 Weeks	REDUCE Next Dose of Trabectedin by One Dose Level for Adverse Reaction(s) During Prior Cycle
Platelets	Less than 100,000 platelets/mm^3	Less than 25,000 platelets/mm^3
Absolute neutrophil count	Less than 1,500 neutrophils/mm^3	Less than 1,000 neutrophils/mm^3 with fever/infection Less than 500 neutrophils/mm^3 lasting more than 5 days
Total bilirubin	Greater than the ULN	Greater than the ULN
AST or ALT	More than 2.5 times the ULN	More than 5 times the ULN
Alkaline phosphatase (ALP)	More than 2.5 times the ULN	More than 2.5 times the ULN
Creatine phosphokinase	More than 2.5 times the ULN	More than 5 times the ULN
Decreased left ventricular ejection fraction	• Less than the lower limit of normal OR • Clinical evidence of cardiomyopathy	• Absolute decrease of 10% or more from baseline and less than the lower limit of normal OR • Clinical evidence of cardiomyopathy
Other nonhematologic adverse reactions	Grade 3 or 4	Grade 3 or 4

Permanently discontinue trabectedin for (1) persistent adverse reactions requiring a delay in dosing of more than 3 weeks, (2) adverse reactions requiring a dose reduction after trabectedin administration at 1 mg/M^2, (3) severe liver dysfunction (all of the following: bilirubin 2 times the ULN, AST or ALT 3 times the ULN, and alkaline phosphatase less than 2 times the ULN in the previous treatment cycle), (4) rhabdomyolysis, or (5) symptomatic cardiomyopathy or persistent left ventricular dysfunction that does not recover to the lower limit of normal within 3 weeks.

DILUTION

Specific techniques required; see Precautions. Available as a lyophilized powder in a single-dose vial containing 1 mg of trabectedin. Using aseptic technique, inject 20 mL of SWFI into the vial. Shake the vial until complete dissolution. The reconstituted solution is clear, colorless to pale brownish-yellow, and contains 0.05 mg/mL of trabectedin. Inspect for particulate matter and discoloration before further dilution. Discard vial if particles or discoloration are observed. Immediately following reconstitution, withdraw the calculated volume of trabectedin and further dilute in 500 mL of NS or D5W.

Filters: Use of a 0.2-micron polyethersulfone (PES) in-line filter is recommended to reduce the risk of exposure to adventitious pathogens that may be introduced during solution preparation.

Storage: Before use, store vials in a refrigerator at 2° to 8° C (36° to 46° F). Discard any unused portion of the reconstituted solution, and discard any remaining diluted solution within 30 hours of reconstituting the lyophilized powder.

COMPATIBILITY

Manufacturer states, "Do not mix trabectedin with other drugs." Trabectedin diluted solution is **compatible** with Type I colorless glass vials; polyvinylchloride (PVC) and polyethylene (PE) bags and tubing; PE and polypropylene (PP) mixture bags; polyethersulfone (PES) in-line filters; titanium, platinum, or plastic ports; silicone and polyurethane catheters; and pumps having contact surfaces made of PVC, PE, or PE/PP.

RATE OF ADMINISTRATION

Infuse the reconstituted, diluted solution over 24 hours through a central venous line using an infusion set with a 0.2-micron PES in-line filter. Complete infusion within 30 hours of initial reconstitution.

ACTIONS

Trabectedin is an alkylating drug that binds guanine residues in the minor groove of DNA, forming adducts and resulting in a bending of the DNA helix toward the major groove. Adduct formation triggers a cascade of events that can affect the subsequent activity of DNA binding proteins, resulting in perturbation of the cell cycle and eventual cell death. Highly protein bound (97%). Terminal elimination half-life is approximately 175 hours. No accumulation in plasma is observed with repeated administrations every 3 weeks. Extensively metabolized with negligible unchanged drug in urine and feces following administration.

INDICATIONS AND USES

Treatment of patients with unresectable or metastatic liposarcoma or leiomyosarcoma who received a prior anthracycline-containing regimen.

CONTRAINDICATIONS

Known severe hypersensitivity, including anaphylaxis, to trabectedin.

PRECAUTIONS

Follow guidelines for handling cytotoxic agents. See Appendix A, p. 1331. ▪ Administered under the direction of a physician knowledgeable in its use in a facility with adequate diagnostic and treatment facilities to monitor the patient and respond to any medical emergency. ▪ Neutropenic sepsis, including fatal cases, can occur. Grade 3 or 4 neutropenia, febrile neutropenia, and sepsis have been reported. ▪ Rhabdomyolysis and musculoskeletal toxicity have occurred. Has led to renal failure and death in some cases. ▪ Hepatotoxicity, including hepatic failure, has occurred. Patients with serum bilirubin levels above the ULN or AST or ALT levels greater than 2.5 times the ULN were excluded from clinical trials. ▪ Cardiomyopathy, including cardiac failure, congestive heart failure, decreased ejection fraction, diastolic dysfunction, or right ventricular dysfunction, has been reported. Patients with a history of New York Heart Association Class II to IV heart failure or abnormal left ventricular ejection fraction (LVEF) at baseline were excluded from clinical trials. ▪ Extravasation resulting in tissue necrosis and requiring debridement can occur. Evidence of tissue necrosis can occur more than 1 week after the extravasation. Use of a central venous line required. ▪ Based on its mechanism of action, trabectedin can cause fetal harm; see Patient Education and Maternal/Child.

Monitor: Premedication required; see Usual Dose. ▪ Obtain baseline CBC with differential and platelets, SCr, and liver function tests (LFTs). ▪ Obtain CBC, including differential and platelet count, before each dose of trabectedin and periodically throughout the treatment cycle. Withhold trabectedin for neutrophil counts of less than 1,500 cells/mm³ on the day of dosing. Permanently reduce the dose of trabectedin for life-threatening or prolonged, severe neutropenia in the preceding cycle; see Dose Adjustments. ▪ Obtain creatine phosphokinase (CPK) levels before each dose of trabectedin. Withhold trabectedin for serum CPK levels more than 2.5 times the ULN. Permanently discontinue trabectedin if rhabdomyolysis occurs; see Dose Adjustments. ▪ Assess LFTs before each dose of trabectedin. Monitor for S/S of hepatotoxicity (e.g., abdominal pain [upper right], jaundice, lethargy, nausea, vomiting). Manage elevated LFTs with treatment interruption, dose reduction, or permanent discontinuation based on severity and duration of LFT abnormality; see Dose Adjustments. ▪ Assess left ventricular ejection fraction (LVEF) by echocardiogram or multigated acquisition (MUGA) scan before initiation of trabectedin and at 2- to 3-month intervals thereafter until trabectedin is discontinued. Monitor for S/S of cardiomyopathy (e.g., chest pain; dyspnea; edema of the legs, ankles, or feet; heart palpitations). Withhold trabectedin for LVEF below the lower limit of normal; see Dose Adjustments. Permanently discontinue trabectedin for symptomatic cardiomyopathy or persistent left ventricular dysfunction that does not recover to the lower limit of normal within 3 weeks. ▪ Monitor for S/S of hypersensitivity reactions (e.g., anaphylaxis, hypotension, pruritus, rash, urticaria, or wheezing). ▪ Monitor IV site for any sign of extravasation. ▪ Effects of any degree of hepatic impairment, severe renal impairment, or ESRD on trabectedin exposure is unknown.

Patient Education: Review manufacturer's medication guide. ▪ Females of reproductive potential must use effective contraception during therapy and for at least 2 months after the last dose of trabectedin. Notify your health care provider if you become pregnant or suspect a pregnancy. ▪ Males with female partners of reproductive potential must use effective contraception during therapy and for at least 5 months after the last dose of trabectedin. ▪ Immediately report S/S of a hypersensitivity reaction (e.g., difficulty breathing, chest tightness, wheezing, severe dizziness or light-headedness, swelling of the lips, or skin rash). ▪ Promptly report discomfort, itchiness, leaking, redness, or swelling at the injection site. ▪ Promptly report fever, unusual bruising, bleeding, severe muscle pain or weakness, tiredness, or paleness. ▪ Promptly report S/S of hepatotoxicity (e.g., yellowing of the skin and eyes [jaundice], pain in the upper right quadrant, severe nausea or vomiting, difficulty concentrating, disorientation, or confusion). ▪ Promptly report new-onset chest pain, shortness of breath, fatigue, lower extremity edema, or heart palpitations. ▪ See Appendix D, p. 1333.

Maternal/Child: Based on its mechanism of action, trabectedin can cause fetal harm; effective contraception is required for females and males; see Patient Education. May damage spermatozoa, resulting in possible genetic and fetal abnormalities, and may result in decreased fertility in males and females. ▪ Discontinue breast-feeding. ▪ Safety and effectiveness in pediatric patients not established.

Elderly: Numbers insufficient to determine differences in response in elderly patients compared with younger adults.

DRUG/LAB INTERACTIONS

Coadministration of trabectedin with **strong CYP3A inhibitors** increases the systemic exposure of trabectedin. Avoid the use of strong CYP3A inhibitors (e.g., atazanavir [Reyataz], boceprevir [Victrelis], clarithromycin [Biaxin], conivaptan [Vaprisol], indinavir (Crixivan), itraconazole [Sporanox], ketoconazole [Nizoral], lopinavir/ritonavir [Kaletra], nefazodone, nelfinavir (Viracept), posaconazole [Noxafil], ritonavir [Norvir], saquinavir [Invirase], telaprevir [Incivek], telithromycin [Ketek], and voriconazole [VFEND]). If a **strong CYP3A inhibitor** must be used for a short time (fewer than 14 days), wait to administer until 1 week after the trabectedin infusion, and discontinue the day before the next scheduled infusion. ▪ Avoid **grapefruit and/or grapefruit juice** during therapy. ▪ Coadministration with **strong CYP3A inducers** decreases the systemic exposure of trabectedin. Avoid the use of strong CYP3A inducers (e.g., phenobarbital [Luminal], rifampin [Rifadin], St. John's wort).

SIDE EFFECTS

The most common adverse reactions are constipation, decreased appetite, diarrhea, dyspnea, fatigue, headache, nausea, peripheral edema, and vomiting. Other clinically important adverse reactions include hypoesthesia, paresthesia, peripheral neuropathy, and pulmonary embolism. The most common Grades 3 to 4 laboratory abnormalities are anemia; hypoalbuminemia; increased AST, ALT, alkaline phosphatase, CPK, and creatinine; neutropenia; and thrombocytopenia.

ANTIDOTE

Keep physician informed of all side effects. May constitute a medical emergency or will be treated symptomatically as indicated. Withhold trabectedin as indicated in Dose Adjustments (e.g., neutrophil counts less than 1,500 cells/mm^3; total bilirubin greater than the ULN; AST, ALT, ALP, and CPK more than 2.5 times the ULN; LVEF less than the lower limit of normal; cardiomyopathy; or other Grade 3 or 4 adverse reactions) on the day of dosing. Permanently reduce the dose of trabectedin for life-threatening or prolonged severe neutropenia in the preceding cycle. Discontinue administration at the first sign of a serious hypersensitivity reaction and treat as indicated (e.g., oxygen, diphenhydramine, epinephrine, corticosteroids, vasopressors, and/or fluids). Discontinue permanently for (1) persistent adverse reactions requiring a delay in dosing of more than 3 weeks, (2) adverse reactions requiring a dose reduction after trabectedin administration at 1 mg/M^2, (3) severe liver dysfunction (all of the following: bilirubin 2 times the ULN, AST or ALT 3 times the ULN, and alkaline phosphatase less than 2 times the ULN in the previous treatment cycle), (4) rhabdomyolysis, or (5) symptomatic cardiomyopathy or persistent left ventricular dysfunction that does not recover to the lower limit of normal within 3 weeks. See Precautions and Monitor. Administration of whole blood products (e.g., packed RBCs, platelets, leukocytes) and/or blood modifiers (e.g., darbepoetin alfa [Aranesp], epoetin alfa [Epogen], filgrastim [Neupogen, Zarxio], pegfilgrastim [Neulasta], sargramostim [Leukine]) may be indicated to treat bone marrow toxicity. There is no specific antidote for trabectedin. Hemodialysis is not expected to enhance the elimination of trabectedin because trabectedin is highly bound to plasma proteins and not significantly renally excreted. Resuscitate as indicated.

TRANEXAMIC ACID
(**TRAN**-eks-am-ik **AS**-id)

Cyklokapron

Antifibrinolytic
Antihemorrhagic

pH 6.5 to 8

USUAL DOSE

Dental extraction in adults and pediatric patients with hemophilia: *Preoperative:* Normal renal function required. 10 mg/kg IV immediately before surgery. *Postoperative:* 10 mg/kg IV every 6 to 8 hours for 2 to 8 days.

Trauma-associated hemorrhage (unlabeled): A loading dose of 1,000 mg IV over 10 minutes followed by an infusion of 1,000 mg over 8 hours. Treatment should begin within 8 hours of injury.

Total knee replacement surgery, blood loss reduction (unlabeled): Several regimens have been studied and include:

10 mg/kg IV over 30 minutes before inflation of the tourniquet followed by 10 mg/kg IV 3 hours after the first dose

OR

10 mg/kg IV administered 30 minutes before deflation of the tourniquet followed by an infusion of 1 mg/kg/hr. Infusion begins at the end of surgery and continues for 6 hours postoperatively.

DOSE ADJUSTMENTS

Lower-end initial and/or reduced doses may be indicated in the elderly based on the potential for decreased organ function and concomitant disease or drug therapy. ■ Reduce dose in impaired renal function according to the following chart.

Tranexamic Dose Guidelines in Impaired Renal Function	
Serum Creatinine (mg/dL)	Dose
1.36-2.83 mg/dL	10 mg/kg two times per day
2.83-5.66 mg/dL	10 mg/kg once per day
>5.66 mg/dL	10 mg/kg every 48 hours or 5 mg/kg every 24 hours

DILUTION

100 mg equals 1 mL of prepared solution. Further dilute a single dose with at least 50 mL **compatible** infusion solutions (e.g., NS, dextrose solutions in water or various concentrations of NS; see Compatibility. Prepare solution immediately before use; discard any unused solution.

Storage: Store ampules at CRT. Prepare the same day it is to be administered.

COMPATIBILITY

Consider any drug NOT listed as compatible to be INCOMPATIBLE until consulting a pharmacist; specific conditions may apply.

Manufacturer states, "Do not mix with blood and do not mix with solutions containing penicillins." See Drug/Lab Interactions.

Solutions: Manufacturer states, "May be mixed with IV solutions, including solutions containing electrolytes, carbohydrates, amino acids, or dextran."

Additive: Manufacturer lists as **compatible** with heparin.

RATE OF ADMINISTRATION

100 mg or fraction thereof over at least 1 minute. Too-rapid infusion may cause hypotension.

ACTIONS

An inhibitor of fibrinolysis. Inhibits plasminogen activation and, at higher concentrations, inhibits plasmin. About 10 times more potent than aminocaproic acid. Onset of action is prompt. Half-life approximately 2 hours. Excreted in urine primarily as unchanged drug. Crosses the placental barrier. Secreted in breast milk.

INDICATIONS AND USES

Reduce or prevent hemorrhage and reduce the need for replacement therapy in hemophilia patients during and following tooth extraction.

Unlabeled uses: Trauma-associated hemorrhage, prevention of perioperative bleeding associated with cardiac surgery and spinal surgery, reduction of blood loss associated with orthopedic surgery or cesarean section.

CONTRAINDICATIONS

Acquired defective color vision, active intravascular clotting, subarachnoid hemorrhage, and hypersensitivity to tranexamic acid or its ingredients.

PRECAUTIONS

For short-term use only (2 to 8 days). ■ Focal areas of retinal degeneration have been seen in animals, and visual abnormalities have been noted in post-marketing reports; see Monitor. ■ Rapid administration in any form may cause hypotension. ■ Whole blood transfusions may be given if necessary but must be given through a second infusion site. ■ In patients with upper urinary tract bleeding, ureteral obstruction due to clot formation has been reported. ■ Risk of venous or arterial thrombosis increased in patients with a previous history of thromboembolic disease. ▪ Thromboembolic events (e.g., central retinal artery and vein obstruction, cerebral thrombosis, deep vein thrombosis, pulmonary embolism) have been reported rarely in patients receiving tranexamic acid for indications other than hemorrhage prevention in patients with hemophilia. ▪ Patients with DIC being treated with tranexamic acid require the strict supervision of a physician specialist. ▪ Convulsions have been reported with tranexamic acid treatment. ▪ See Compatibility and Drug/Lab Interactions.

Monitor: Use only in conjunction with general and specific tests to determine the amount of fibrinolysis present. ▪ In repeated treatment or if treatment will last more than several (2 to 3) days, a complete ophthalmologic examination (visual acuity, color vision, eyeground, visual fields) should be done before and at regular intervals during treatment. Discontinue use if changes are found.

Patient Education: May produce dizziness; request assistance with ambulation and use caution performing tasks that require alertness (e.g., driving or operating machinery).

Maternal/Child: Category B: use caution and only if clearly needed in pregnancy and breast-feeding. ▪ Use in pediatric patients has been limited. Available data suggest that the mg/kg dose for adults can be used.

Elderly: Lower-end initial or reduced doses may be indicated; see Dose Adjustments. ▪ Monitoring of renal function suggested.

DRUG/LAB INTERACTIONS
No formal Drug Interaction studies between tranexamic acid and other drugs have been conducted. ▪ Concomitant use with **factor IX complex** (e.g., AlphaNine SD, Mononine, Konyne) or **anti-inhibitor coagulant concentrates** (e.g., Feiba) is not recommended; may increase the risk for venous or arterial thrombosis.

SIDE EFFECTS
Allergic dermatitis, diarrhea, giddiness, hypotension, nausea and vomiting. Thromboembolic events (e.g., central retinal artery and vein obstruction, cerebral thrombosis, deep vein thrombosis, pulmonary embolism) have been reported rarely.

Post-Marketing: Chromatopsia and visual impairment, convulsions, and thromboembolic events as above have been reported.

ANTIDOTE
All side effects may subside with reduced dosage or rate of administration. Discontinue use of drug if any changes are found during follow-up ophthalmologic examinations. Resuscitate as necessary.

TRASTUZUMAB BBW
(traz-**TOO**-zah-mab)

Herceptin

Monoclonal antibody
Antineoplastic

pH 6

USUAL DOSE
DO NOT administer as an IV push or bolus. DO NOT mix trastuzumab with other drugs. DO NOT substitute trastuzumab for or with ado-trastuzumab emtansine.

Premedication: Pretreatment with antihistamines (e.g., diphenhydramine [Benadryl]) and/or corticosteroids (e.g., dexamethasone [Decadron]) may be indicated and is suggested for patients being retreated after a hypersensitivity reaction or a severe infusion reaction; see Precautions. Pretreatment may not be successful; hypersensitivity reaction and/or infusion reaction may recur. Preassessment required; see Monitor. Combination therapies may require additional premedication; refer to product monographs.

Adjuvant treatment of breast cancer: Administer according to one of the following dose regimens and schedules for a total of 52 weeks of trastuzumab therapy (extending adjuvant treatment beyond 1 year is not recommended):

1. *During and following paclitaxel, docetaxel, or docetaxel/carboplatin:* Administer an initial dose of *trastuzumab* 4 mg/kg as an infusion over 90 minutes. Follow with a dose of 2 mg/kg as an infusion over 30 minutes at weekly intervals for the first 12 weeks when given in combination with *paclitaxel or docetaxel* or for 18 weeks when given in combination with *docetaxel/carboplatin.* Beginning 1 week after the last 2-mg/kg weekly dose of *trastuzumab,* administer *trastuzumab* 6 mg/kg as an infusion over 30 to 90 minutes every 3 weeks.

2. *As a single agent within 3 weeks of completion of multimodality, anthracycline-based chemotherapy regimens,* administer an initial dose of *trastuzumab* 8 mg/kg as an infusion over 90 minutes. Follow with a dose of 6 mg/kg as an infusion over 30 to 90 minutes every 3 weeks.

3. See clinical studies in prescribing information for different treatment regimens used. In all studies, *trastuzumab* was initiated *after completion of the doxorubicin and cyclophosphamide treatment cycles.*

Metastatic breast cancer: *Initial dose:* 4 mg/kg as an infusion over 90 minutes. Follow with a *maintenance dose* of 2 mg/kg as an infusion over 30 minutes at weekly intervals. Trastuzumab is administered until tumor progression.

Metastatic breast cancer in combination therapy with paclitaxel: *Trastuzumab* dose as above. *Paclitaxel dose:* 175 mg/M^2 over 3 hours every 21 days for at least 6 cycles. See paclitaxel monograph.

Metastatic gastric cancer in combination with cisplatin and capecitabine or 5-fluorouracil: *Initial dose:* 8 mg/kg as an infusion over 90 minutes. Follow with a dose of 6 mg/kg as an infusion over 30 to 90 minutes every 3 weeks until disease progression. See individual monographs and specific protocol for doses of cisplatin and capecitabine (Xeloda) or 5-fluorouracil (5-FU).

DOSE ADJUSTMENTS

Withhold trastuzumab dose for at least 4 weeks for either (1) equal to or greater than a 16% absolute decrease in left ventricular ejection fraction (LVEF) from baseline assessment, or (2) LVEF below institutional limits of normal and equal to or greater than 10% absolute decrease in LVEF from baseline assessment.

May resume trastuzumab if within 4 to 8 weeks the LVEF returns to normal limits and the absolute decrease from baseline is equal to or less than 15%. Discontinue permanently for a persistent (more than 8 weeks) LVEF decline or for suspension of trastuzumab dosing on more than three occasions for cardiomyopathy. ▪ See prescribing information for recommended actions if a dose is missed.

DILUTION

Check vial labels to ensure use of trastuzumab and **not** ado-trastuzumab emtansine.

Manufacturer supplies a vial of bacteriostatic water for injection (BWFI). Confirm content of vial; 20 mL is required to obtain the correct concentration. Inject diluent slowly directed at the lyophilized cake. Swirl gently; *do not shake* (is sensitive to agitation or rapid expulsion from a syringe). Allow vial to stand for 5 minutes; slight foaming is permissible. Will yield a multidose solution containing 21 mg/mL. Label vial immediately with a "do not use after" date 28 days from date of reconstitution. SWFI may be used to reconstitute trastuzumab for patients with a known hypersensitivity to benzyl alcohol, but the calculated dose must be withdrawn, used immediately, and the balance of the reconstituted solution discarded. Reconstituted solution must be further diluted and given as an infusion. Withdraw the calculated dose from the reconstituted vial (21 mg/mL) and add it to an infusion bag containing 250 mL of NS. Gently invert to mix the solution.

Filters: In-line filters are not necessary but may be used (0.2-micron filters were evaluated).

Storage: Refrigerate unopened and reconstituted vials at 2° to 8° C (36° to 46° F). Vials reconstituted in supplied diluent are stable for 28 days after reconstitution. Discard remaining diluent. Discard reconstituted trastuzumab after expiration date written or stamped on vial. Solutions diluted in NS may be refrigerated for 24 hours before use. Do not freeze reconstituted trastuzumab.

COMPATIBILITY

Manufacturer states, "Do not reconstitute with drugs other than BWFI or SWFI. Further dilute infusion with NS. Infusions should not be administered or mixed with dextrose solutions. Do not mix with other drugs." Is **compatible** with polyethylene and polyvinyl-chloride infusion bags and tubing.

RATE OF ADMINISTRATION

Use of a microdrip (60 gtt/min) or other IV controller suggested. For infusion only; *do not administer* as an IV push or bolus. Decrease rate of infusion for mild or moderate infusion reactions.

Initial dose: A single dose as an infusion over a minimum of 90 minutes. Observe for chills, fever, or other infusion-associated symptoms; see Precautions/Monitor.

Maintenance dose: If the initial dose was well tolerated, administer a single dose as an infusion over 30 to 90 minutes (based on regimen; see Usual Dose).

ACTIONS

A recombinant DNA–derived humanized monoclonal antibody that selectively binds with high affinity to the extracellular domain of the human epidermal growth factor receptor 2 (HER2) protein. Inhibits proliferation and mediates an antibody-dependent cellular toxicity in cancer cells that overexpress the HER2 protein. Half-life increases and clearance decreases with increasing doses. May cross the placental barrier. May be secreted in breast milk.

INDICATIONS AND USES

Indicated for adjuvant treatment of breast cancer that is HER2-overexpressing, node-positive or node-negative (ER/PR-negative or with one high-risk feature). May be used as part of a treatment regimen that may consist of (1) doxorubicin (Adriamycin), cyclophosphamide (Cytoxan), and either paclitaxel (Taxol) or docetaxel (Taxotere); (2) a regimen with docetaxel and carboplatin (Paraplatin); or (3) a single agent following multimodal anthracycline-based therapy. ▪ As a single agent for treatment of patients with metastatic breast cancer whose tumors overexpress the HER2 protein and who have received one or more chemotherapy regimens for their metastatic disease. ▪ In combination with paclitaxel (Taxol) for the first-line treatment of patients with metastatic breast cancer whose tumors overexpress the HER2 protein and who have not received chemotherapy for their metastatic disease. ▪ In combination with cisplatin and capecitabine (Xeloda) or 5-fluorouracil (5-FU) for treatment of patients with HER2-overexpressing metastatic gastric or gastroesophageal junction adenocarcinoma who have not received prior treatment for metastatic disease.

CONTRAINDICATIONS

None known when used as indicated; see Precautions.

PRECAUTIONS

Do not administer as an IV push or bolus. ▪ Trastuzumab should be used only in patients whose tumors have HER2 overexpression. Tumor histology differs; use FDA-approved tests for specific tumor type (breast or gastric/gastroesophageal adenocarcinoma) to assess HER2 overexpression and HER2 gene amplification. Must be performed in laboratories with demonstrated proficiency in the specific technology. ▪ Administered by or under the direction of the physician specialist. May be given on an outpatient basis. ▪ Adequate laboratory and supportive medical resources must be available. ▪ Emergency equipment and drugs for treatment of left ventricular dysfunction and/or infusion reactions must be immediately available; see Antidote. ▪ Use with caution in patients with known hypersensitivity to trastuzumab, Chinese hamster ovary cell proteins, benzyl alcohol, or any component of this product. ■ Serious and fatal infusion reactions and pulmonary toxicity have been reported. Retreatment after full recovery from an infusion reaction has been tried following pretreatment with antihistamines and/or corticosteroids. Some tolerated treatment; others had another severe reaction. ■ Can cause subclinical and clinical cardiac failure. Incidence of cardiac dysfunction was highest in patients who received trastuzumab with an anthracycline-containing chemotherapy regimen (e.g., doxorubicin [Adriamycin]) and in the elderly. ■ Can cause left ventricular cardiac dysfunction, arrhythmias, hypertension, disabling cardiac failure, cardiomyopathy, and cardiac death. May also cause asymptomatic decline in left ventricular ejection fraction (LVEF). ■ Use extreme caution in treating patients with pre-existing cardiac dysfunction or pulmonary compromise. Pre-existing cardiac disease or prior cardiotoxic therapy (e.g., anthracyclines), radiation therapy to the chest, or pre-existing pulmonary compromise secondary to intrinsic lung disease and/or malignant pulmonary involvement may decrease ability to tolerate trastuzumab. ■ May exacerbate chemotherapy-induced neutropenia.

Monitor: Obtain baseline CBC with differential and platelet count and repeat as needed. ■ Monitor all vital signs before and during therapy. ■ Treatment with trastuzumab can result in the development of ventricular dysfunction and CHF. Evaluate left ventricular function before and during treatment. For all treatment regimens (monotherapy and/or combination therapies), patients should have a thorough baseline cardiac assessment, including a history and physical exam and determination of LVEF by an echocardiogram or a MUGA scan. Monitoring and assessment may not identify all patients at risk for developing cardiotoxicity. ■ Monitor closely throughout treatment for S/S of deteriorating cardiac function (e.g., cough, dyspnea, paroxysmal nocturnal dyspnea, peripheral edema, S_3 gallop, or reduced ejection fraction [symptomatic or asymptomatic]). Suggested monitoring schedule includes a repeat evaluation of left ventricular function (echocardiogram or MUGA scan) every 3 months during treatment with trastuzumab and at least every 6 months for 2 years after completion of treatment if trastuzumab was used as a component of adjuvant therapy. More frequent monitoring should be used for patients with pre-existing cardiac dysfunction and/or if S/S of deteriorating cardiac function develop; see Dose Adjustments. ■ Onset and clinical course of infusion reactions are variable. Most occur during or immediately following the infusion or within 24 hours. Monitor patient until symptoms completely resolve. Chills and/or fever occur in 40% of patients during the first infusion. May be treated with acetaminophen (Tylenol), diphenhydramine (Benadryl), and meperidine (Demerol) with or without reduction in the rate of infusion. During infusion, monitor closely; asthenia, bronchospasm, dizziness, dyspnea, headache, hypotension (may be severe), hypoxia, nausea, pain (may be at tumor site), rash, rigors, and vomiting have also occurred. ■ Monitor closely; in addition to the symptoms of infusion reaction previously noted, severe and sometimes fatal hypersensitivity reactions (e.g., anaphylaxis, angioedema, bronchospasm, hypotension, urticaria) and pulmonary reactions (e.g., dyspnea, interstitial pneumonitis, pulmonary infiltrates, pleural effusions, noncardiogenic pulmonary edema, pulmonary fibrosis, pulmonary insufficiency, hypoxia, and ARDS) have occurred during and after the infusion. ■ Monitor for thrombocytopenia (platelet count less than 50,000/mm³). Initiate precautions to prevent excessive bleeding (e.g., inspect IV sites, skin, and mucous membranes; use extreme care during invasive procedures; test urine, emesis, stool, and secretions for occult blood). ■ Not a vesicant; if extravasation occurs, discontinue infusion and restart using another vein.

Patient Education: During infusion, promptly report chills and/or fever and other S/S of infusion reaction. ■ Promptly report cough, difficulty breathing, weight gain, and swelling of extremities. ■ Avoid pregnancy; use effective contraception during treatment and for at least 7 months after the last dose of trastuzumab. ■ See Appendix D, p. 1333.

Maternal/Child: Avoid pregnancy. Verify pregnancy status of females of reproductive potential before initiating trastuzumab. Can cause fetal harm. Increases the risk for oligohydramnios and oligohydramnios sequence manifesting as pulmonary hypoplasia, skeletal abnormalities, and neonatal death. Pregnant women who receive trastuzumab are encouraged to enroll in the

MotHER Pregnancy Registry and to report the trastuzumab exposure to the manufacturer (Genentech).There is no information on the presence of trastuzumab in human milk, the effects on the breast-fed infant, or the effects on milk production. Consider the developmental and health benefits of breast-feeding along with the mother's clinical need for trastuzumab treatment and any potential adverse effects on the breast-fed child from trastuzumab or from the underlying maternal condition. This consideration should also take into account the trastuzumab washout period of 7 months. ▪ Discontinue breast-feeding during trastuzumab therapy. ▪ Safety and effectiveness in pediatric patients not established.

Elderly: Advanced age may increase the risk of cardiac dysfunction.

DRUG/LAB INTERACTIONS
No formal drug interaction studies have been done. Use with **paclitaxel** may decrease trastuzumab clearance and increase serum levels. Paclitaxel concentration is not affected. ▪ The plasma concentration of capecitabine, carboplatin, cisplatin, docetaxel, doxorubicin, and paclitaxel was not altered when used in combination with trastuzumab. ▪ Risk of cardiotoxicity increased with concurrent use or previous use of **anthracyclines** (e.g., doxorubicin). Patients who receive anthracycline after stopping trastuzumab may also be at increased risk for cardiac dysfunction. ▪ Bone marrow toxicity may be additive with **other antineoplastic agents** (e.g., anthracyclines, cyclophosphamide).

SIDE EFFECTS
Cardiomyopathy, pulmonary toxicity, infusion reactions, and exacerbation of chemotherapy-induced neutropenia are the most serious side effects. Anemia, chills, cough, diarrhea, dysgeusia, dyspnea, fatigue, fever, headache, infections, infusion reactions, insomnia, mucosal inflammation, myalgia, nasopharyngitis, nausea, neutropenia, rash, stomatitis, thrombocytopenia, upper respiratory tract infections, vomiting, and weight loss are most common. Side effects that cause interruption or discontinuation of therapy include severe infusion reactions, pulmonary toxicity, congestive heart failure, and a decline in left ventricular cardiac function. Abdominal pain, accidental injury, acne, anorexia, arthralgia, asthenia, back pain, bone pain, depression, dizziness, edema, flu syndrome, headache, herpes simplex, hypersensitivity reactions, hypotension, neuropathy, pain (may be at tumor site), paresthesia, peripheral edema, peripheral neuritis, pharyngitis, rash, rhinitis, sinusitis, and tachycardia have been reported in more than 5% of patients. Many other serious side effects have been reported in some patients (e.g., cardiac arrest, coagulation disorder, death, hypersensitivity reactions [e.g., angioedema, bronchospasm, dyspnea, urticaria, wheezing], hypertension, hypotension, noncardiogenic pulmonary edema, pancytopenia, pericardial or pleural effusion, pulmonary infiltrates, pulmonary insufficiency and hypoxemia requiring O_2 and/or ventilatory support, shock arrhythmia, syncope, vascular thrombosis).

Post-Marketing: Serious adverse events including hypersensitivity reactions and infusion reactions, including some with a fatal outcome; and pulmonary events including ARDS and death. Symptoms occurred most commonly during the infusion, but some occurred 24 hours or more after the infusion. Renal toxicity (glomerulopathy) and immune thrombocytopenia have also been reported. Cases of oligohydramnios, and oligohydramnios sequence manifesting as pulmonary hypoplasia, skeletal abnormalities, and neonatal death, have been reported when trastuzumab has been administered to pregnant women.

ANTIDOTE
Notify physician of all side effects. Most will be treated symptomatically. Decrease rate of infusion for mild or moderate infusion reactions. Interrupt infusion if dyspnea or clinically significant hypotension occurs. Discontinue trastuzumab for severe or life-threatening infusion reactions. Discontinue infusion in patients who develop anaphylaxis, angioedema, ARDS, and interstitial pneumonitis. Discontinue trastuzumab in patients receiving adjuvant therapy, and withhold therapy in patients with metastatic disease for clinically significant decrease in left ventricular function. Safety of continuation or resumption of therapy has not been studied. Treatment may include diuretics, ACE inhibitors (e.g., lisinopril [Zestril], enalapril [Vasotec]), inotropic

agents (e.g., digoxin, inamrinone, isoproterenol [Isuprel]), beta-blockers (e.g., atenolol [Tenormin], propranolol), and/or supplemental oxygen. Infusion reaction is treated with acetaminophen, diphenhydramine, and meperidine. Administration of whole blood products (e.g., packed RBCs, platelets, leukocytes) and/or blood modifiers (e.g., darbepoetin alfa [Aranesp], epoetin alfa [Epogen], filgrastim [Neupogen, Zarxio], pegfilgrastim [Neulasta], sargramostim [Leukine]) may be indicated to treat bone marrow toxicity from concurrent antineoplastics. Treat hypersensitivity reactions (may be more frequent with coadministration of paclitaxel) with epinephrine, antihistamines, corticosteroids, bronchodilators, and oxygen. To treat extravasation, apply cold compresses and elevate extremity. Resuscitate as indicated.

TROMETHAMINE   Alkalizing agent
(troh-**METH**-ah-meen)

Tham-E   pH 8.6

USUAL DOSE
Limit dose to amount needed to increase blood pH to normal limits (7.35 to 7.45) and to correct acid-base derangements. Evaluate the need for repeat doses by serial determinations of existing base deficit, pH, and clinical observations. Tham-E contains electrolytes.
Acidosis: Required dose (mL of 0.3 molar solution) equal to body weight in kilograms $\times$ base deficit in mEq/L $\times$ 1.1.
Acidosis in cardiac bypass surgery: 9 mL/kg (324 mg/kg) of body weight. 500 mL (18 Gm) is an average adult dose. Up to 1,000 mL has been used. Never exceed 500 mg/kg in any individual dose over less than 1 hour.
Correct acidity of ACD (acid-citrate-dextrose) priming blood: Stored blood has a pH of 6.22 to 6.8. An average of 60 mL (15 to 77 mL) tromethamine to each 500 mL of stored blood is required to correct pH to 7.4.
Acidosis in cardic arrest: Use only if indicated. Never inject into cardiac muscle. Initial dose in an open chest is 62 to 185 mL (2 to 6 Gm). Additional doses should be based on evaluation of base deficit. If the chest is not open, give 111 to 333 mL (3.6 to 10.8 Gm); use a large peripheral vein. After arrest is reversed, additional amounts may be needed to control persistent acidosis.

PEDIATRIC DOSE
Correction of metabolic acidosis associated with respiratory distress syndrome (RDS) in neonates and infants: 1 mL/kg of body weight for each pH unit below 7.4. Repeat doses may be given according to changes in Pao_2, pH, and Pco_2.

DOSE ADJUSTMENTS
Lower-end initial doses may be appropriate in the elderly based on the potential for decreased organ function and concomitant disease or drug therapy.

DILUTION
Supplied as a 0.3 molar solution. Each 100 mL contains tromethamine 3.6 Gm in water for injection. May be given undiluted as an infusion or added to pump oxygenator blood, other priming fluid, or ACD blood.
Storage: Store at CRT. Single-use container; discard unused solution.

COMPATIBILITY
Specific information not available. Consider specific use; consult pharmacist.

RATE OF ADMINISTRATION
Slow IV infusion recommended. 5 mL or less/min would deliver up to 300 mL in 1 hour. Rate dictated by patient's condition and intended use; see Usual Dose and Precautions. Reduced rate may control venospasm.

ACTIONS

Acts as a proton acceptor. Prevents or corrects acidosis by actively binding hydrogen ions in metabolic acids and carbonic acid. Releases bicarbonate anions. Rapidly excreted in the urine, it has an osmotic diuretic effect, increases urine output, urine pH, and excretion of fixed acids, CO_2, and electrolytes. Also capable of neutralizing acidic ions of the intracellular fluid.

INDICATIONS AND USES

Prevention and correction of metabolic acidosis, particularly metabolic acidosis associated with cardiac bypass surgery, correction of acidity of ACD blood in cardiac bypass surgery, and cardiac arrest.

CONTRAINDICATIONS

Hypersensitivity to tromethamine, anuria, and uremia. In neonates it is also contraindicated in chronic respiratory acidosis and salicylate intoxication.

PRECAUTIONS

Intended for short-term use only (1 day). ▪ Sodium bicarbonate or sodium lactate is effective in most acidotic situations and has fewer side effects. ▪ Use extreme caution in impaired renal function or decreased urine output.

Monitor: Determine blood pH, P_{CO_2}, bicarbonate, glucose, and electrolytes before, during, and after administration. ▪ Avoid overdose (total drug or too-rapid rate). Severe alkalosis and/or prolonged hypoglycemia may result. ▪ May cause fluid and/or solute overload, resulting in dilution of serum electrolyte concentrations, overhydration, congested states, or pulmonary edema. ▪ Use a large peripheral vein. Determine absolute patency of vein; necrosis may result from extravasation. ▪ May severely depress respiration. Incidence may be increased in patients who have chronic hypoventilation or those who have been treated with drugs that depress respiration. Oxygen and controlled ventilation equipment must always be available. ▪ ECG monitoring and frequent serum potassium measurements are required to rule out hyperkalemia in impaired renal function or decreased urine output. Decreased excretion of tromethamine may also occur, resulting in toxicity.

Maternal/Child: Category C: safety for use not established. Benefits must outweigh risks. ▪ Use caution or discontinue breast-feeding. ▪ Has been used to treat severe cases of metabolic acidosis with concurrent respiratory acidosis because it does not raise P_{CO_2} as bicarbonate does in neonates and infants with respiratory failure. It has also been used in neonates and infants with hypernatremia and metabolic acidosis to avoid the additional sodium given with the bicarbonate. However, because the osmotic effects of tromethamine are greater and large continuous doses are required, bicarbonate is preferred to tromethamine in the treatment of acidotic neonates and infants with RDS. ▪ Severe hypoglycemia may occur in premature or full-term infants. ▪ Infusion via low-lying umbilical venous catheters has been associated with hepatocellular necrosis.

Elderly: Lower-end initial doses may be appropriate in the elderly; see Dose Adjustments. Differences in response between elderly and younger patients have not been identified.

DRUG/LAB INTERACTIONS

Potentiates **amphetamines, ephedrine, and quinidine.** ▪ Inhibits **lithium, methotrexate, and salicylates.** ▪ Incidence of respiratory depression may be increased in patients receiving **drugs that depress respiration** (e.g., narcotic analgesics [morphine]). ▪ May **increase coagulation time.**

SIDE EFFECTS

Hyperkalemia, hypoglycemia, phlebitis, respiratory depression, and thrombosis.

Overdose: Alkalosis, overhydration, severe prolonged hypoglycemia, solute overload. May be due to total drug or too-rapid rate of administration.

ANTIDOTE

Notify physician of all side effects. Reduced rate of infusion may prevent hypoglycemia. Use glucose if indicated. Discontinue drug immediately for hyperkalemia or extravasation. Local infiltration with 1% procaine with phentolamine may reduce tissue necrosis. Use a number 25 needle. Symptomatic treatment is indicated. Alternate drugs are indicated (sodium bicarbonate, sodium lactate).

VACCINIA IMMUNE GLOBULIN INTRAVENOUS (HUMAN) BBW

Immunizing agent
(passive)

(vack-**SIN**-ee-ah ih-**MUNE GLAW**-byoo-lin IV)

VIGIV

USUAL DOSE
100 mg/kg (2 mL/kg) as a single-dose IV infusion; see Monitor. May be repeated based on the severity of symptoms and on individual patient response. Higher doses (200 mg/kg or 500 mg/kg) may be considered in patients who do not respond to the initial 100 mg/kg dose; see Precautions.

DOSE ADJUSTMENTS
Because of sucrose content, doses higher than 400 mg/kg are not recommended in patients with potential renal problems.

DILUTION
Contains sucrose; see Precautions. A ready-to-use liquid preparation supplied in a 50-mL vial containing 50 mg VIGIV/mL or 2,500 mg VIGIV/vial. Solution should be colorless, free of particulate matter, and not turbid. *Do not shake vial; avoid foaming.* Further dilution before or during administration is not recommended. Infusion should begin within 6 hours of entering the vial and be complete within 12 hours of entering the vial. Use of a dedicated IV line, a 0.22-micron in-line filter, and a constant infusion pump is recommended. If necessary, it may be piggybacked into a pre-existing IV line containing NS or D2½W, D5W, D10W, or D20W with or without NaCl added; see Compatibility. VIGIV should not be diluted more than 1:2 (v/v) with any of these solutions.

Filters: Use of a 0.22-micron in-line filter is recommended; see Dilution.

Storage: Store between 2° and 8° C (35.6° and 46.4° F). Do not use after expiration date. Infusion must begin within 6 hours and be complete within 12 hours of entering the vial. Discard partially used vials. Do not use if turbid or has been frozen.

COMPATIBILITY
Manufacturer states, "Administer separately from other drugs or medications." If necessary, it may be piggybacked into a pre-existing IV line containing NS or D2½W, D5W, D10W, or D20W with or without NaCl added. Flush line before and after administration. VIGIV should not be diluted more than 1:2 (v/v) with any of these solutions.

RATE OF ADMINISTRATION
Flush line before and after administration.

Administer 1 mL/kg/hr for the first 30 minutes. If no discomfort or adverse effects, it may be increased to 2 mL/kg/hr for the next 30 minutes and then to 3 mL/kg/hr for the remainder of the infusion, as tolerated. Infusion of 100 mg/kg (2 mL/kg) should take approximately 70 minutes in a 70-kg patient. Do not exceed these rates. Too-rapid infusion may cause infusion rate–related reactions (e.g., arthralgia, back pain, chills, fever, flushing, muscle cramps, nausea, vomiting, wheezing). *In patients at risk for developing renal dysfunction, administer at the minimum concentration available and the minimum rate of infusion practicable.* Use of a dedicated IV line, a 0.22-micron in-line filter, and a constant infusion pump (i.e., an IVAC pump or equivalent) is recommended.

ACTIONS
An immunoglobulin (Ig). Obtained from human plasma, purified, and standardized. Donors had received booster immunizations with the Dryvax smallpox vaccine. Specific methods (e.g., cold ethanol fractionation, detergents, nanofiltration, solvents) inactivate bloodborne viruses (e.g., hepatitis, HIV). Tested and found negative for antibodies against HIV, hepatitis, Creutzfeldt-Jakob disease, and others. Contains increased levels of protective antibodies against the vaccinia virus—the live virus used in the currently available smallpox vaccine. When use is necessary, can help to minimize possible risks

associated with this highly effective smallpox vaccine. Half-life is approximately 22 days but may be decreased by fever or infection (increased catabolism or consumption).

INDICATIONS AND USES

Treatment and/or modification of the following conditions: aberrant infections induced by the vaccinia virus that include accidental implantation in the eyes (excluding isolated keratitis; see Contraindications), mouth, or other areas where vaccinia infection would be hazardous; eczema vaccinatum; progressive vaccinia; severe generalized vaccinia; and vaccinia infections in individuals who have skin conditions such as burns, impetigo, varicella-zoster, or poison ivy or in individuals who have eczematous skin lesions because of the activity or extensiveness of such lesions.

CONTRAINDICATIONS

Presence of isolated vaccinia keratitis. ▪ Individuals known to have an allergic response to this or other human immunoglobulin preparations. ▪ Contains trace amounts of IgA. Patients with isolated or selective IgA deficiency can develop antibodies to IgA and have an increased risk of anaphylactic reactions with subsequent exposure to blood products that contain IgA. ▪ Not considered effective for the treatment of postvaccinal encephalitis.

PRECAUTIONS

For IV infusion only. ▪ Hypersensitivity reactions are possible and have occurred with other IGIV preparations; administer in a facility with adequate equipment and supplies to monitor the patient and respond to any medical emergency. ▪ Use extreme caution in individuals with a history of prior systemic hypersensitivity reactions. Incidence of anaphylaxis may be increased, especially with repeated injections. ▪ Use caution when treating complications that include vaccinia keratitis; may cause increased corneal scarring. ▪ IGIV products have been associated with renal dysfunction, acute renal failure, osmotic nephrosis, and death. Use extreme caution in patients with any degree of renal insufficiency; in patients 65 years of age and older; in patients with diabetes mellitus, paraproteinemia, sepsis, or volume depletion; and/or in patients receiving known nephrotoxic drugs. If used, should be administered at the minimum concentration available and at the minimum rate of infusion practicable. *Products containing sucrose as a stabilizer have demonstrated an increased risk of renal dysfunction.* Consider benefit versus risk before use. ▪ May cause aseptic meningitis syndrome (AMS), which may begin from 2 hours to 2 days after treatment. Symptoms are drowsiness, fever, headache (severe), nausea and vomiting, nuchal rigidity, painful eye movements, and photophobia. Symptoms resolve if VIGIV is discontinued. A neurologic exam to rule out other causes of meningitis is indicated. ▪ IGIV products have been associated with thrombotic events; use caution in patients with a history of cardiovascular disease or thrombotic episodes and in patients with thrombotic risk factors (e.g., cerebrovascular disease, coronary artery disease, diabetes, hypertension). Baseline assessment of blood viscosity should be made in patients at risk for hyperviscosity, including chylomicronemia, markedly high triglycerides, or monoclonal gammopathies. ▪ Hemolysis and hemolytic anemia may develop. ▪ Noncarcinogenic pulmonary edema (transfusion-related acute lung injury ([TRALI]) has been reported with other IGIV preparations; see Monitor. ▪ Interacts with some glucose-monitoring systems; see Monitor and Drug/Lab Interactions.

Monitor: Use of larger veins may reduce infusion site discomfort. ▪ Correct volume depletion before administration. ▪ Recording the lot number on vials is helpful. ▪ Monitor vital signs and observe patient continuously during infusion. A precipitous drop in BP or anaphylaxis can occur at any time. Emergency equipment and supplies must be at bedside. ▪ Monitor renal function (e.g., BUN, SCr) and urine output in patients at increased risk for renal failure. Obtain baseline studies, monitor at intervals, and discontinue future VIGIV therapy if renal function deteriorates. See Precautions. ▪ Monitor for S/S of hemolysis (e.g., anemia, lysis of red blood cells, liberation of hemoglobin). ▪ Monitor for S/S of TRALI (e.g., fever, hypoxemia, normal left ventricular function, pulmonary edema, severe respiratory distress). Usually occurs within 1 to 6 hours after completion of the transfusion. Manage with oxygen and adequate ventilatory support. If TRALI is suspected, test for the presence of antineutrophil antibodies in product and patient serum. ▪ Some types of blood glucose testing systems (e.g., those based on the glucose dehydrogenase pyrroloquinoline quinone [GDH-PQQ] or glucose-dye-oxidoreductase methods) could falsely interpret the maltose contained in VIGIV as glucose. To avoid this interference by maltose contained in VIGIV, blood glucose measurements in patients receiving VIGIV must be done with a glucose-specific method (monitor and test strips); see Drug/Lab Interactions.

Patient Education: Report a burning sensation in the head, chills, cyanosis, diaphoresis, dyspnea, faintness or light-headedness, fatigue, fever, hives, itching or rash, neck pain or difficulty moving neck, tachycardia, wheezing. ▪ Report chest pain or tightness, difficulty passing urine, decreased urine output, edema, fluid retention, shortness of breath, or sudden weight gain.

Maternal/Child: Category C: use during pregnancy only if clearly needed. ▪ Safety for use in breast-feeding not established. ▪ Safety and effectiveness for use in pediatric patients not established.

Elderly: Not tested for safety and effectiveness in the elderly. Use with caution. Incidence of renal insufficiency and other side effects may be increased due to age, potential for decreased organ function, and pre-existing medical conditions; see Precautions.

DRUG/LAB INTERACTIONS

Defer administration of **live virus vaccines** for approximately 6 months after administration of VIGIV. ▪ Concurrent use with **nephrotoxic drugs** (e.g., aminoglycosides [e.g., gentamicin], amphotericin B [Amphotec, conventional], cidofovir [Vistide], rifampin [Rifadin]) may increase the risk of renal insufficiency. ▪ Maltose in IVIG products has been shown to give falsely high blood glucose levels. Use could result in inappropriate doses of insulin, resulting in life-threatening hypoglycemia or untreated hypoglycemia masked by falsely elevated glucose readings. Review product information of the blood glucose testing system, including test strips, to determine if the system is appropriate for use with maltose-containing parenteral products. ▪ Additional drug/lab interaction studies have not been completed.

SIDE EFFECTS

Headache and mild to moderate urticaria are most frequently observed. A full range of hypersensitivity symptoms, including anaphylaxis, is possible. Backache, dizziness, injection site reaction, nausea, and upper respiratory infections also occur. A precipitous hypotensive reaction can occur and is most commonly associated with a too-rapid rate of injection. Serious side effects reported with other IGIV products should be considered and include acute renal failure, acute tubular necrosis, osmotic nephrosis, and proximal tubular nephropathy (may result in death); aseptic meningitis syndrome; hemolytic anemia (reversible); increased BUN and SCr (may occur as soon as 1 to 2 days following infusion); noncarcinogenic pulmonary edema (transfusion-related acute lung injury [TRALI]); severe reactions (e.g., circulatory collapse, fever, loss of consciousness, nausea and vomiting, sudden onset of dyspnea), which are more common in patients with antibody deficiencies; thromboembolism. Made from human plasma; the manufacturing process attempts to eliminate the risk of bloodborne viruses (e.g., hepatitis, HIV infection, Creutzfeldt-Jakob disease), but the potential for infection cannot be ruled out.

ANTIDOTE

Reduce rate or temporarily interrupt infusion for patient discomfort or any sign of adverse reaction. Reduce rate in patients at risk for renal insufficiency. Loop diuretics (e.g., furosemide [Lasix]) may be helpful in the management of fluid overload. If patient continues to experience adverse reactions after rate has been reduced, other IGIV preparations suggest premedicating with hydrocortisone 1 to 2 mg/kg 30 minutes before the immune globulin infusion. Pretreatment with acetaminophen (Tylenol) and diphenhydramine (Benadryl) may also be useful. Discontinue the drug immediately for any signs of a hypersensitivity reaction. Notify the physician. May be treated symptomatically and infusion resumed at slower rate if symptoms subside. Treat anaphylaxis immediately. Epinephrine (Adrenalin), diphenhydramine (Benadryl), oxygen, vasopressors (e.g., dopamine), corticosteroids, and ventilation equipment must always be available. Manage TRALI with oxygen and ventilatory support. Resuscitate as necessary.

VALPROATE SODIUM BBW

(val-**PROH**-ayt **SO**-dee-um)

Anticonvulsant

Depacon

pH 7.6

USUAL DOSE

Adults and pediatric patients 10 years of age or older: For all indications optimal clinical response is usually achieved with doses less than 60 mg/kg/24 hr. Usual therapeutic range of plasma levels is 50 to 100 mcg/mL. A total daily dose exceeding 250 mg should be given in divided doses every 6 hours (studies used an every-6-hour regimen). See Precautions, Monitor, and Drug/Lab Interactions. Use of IV formulation for more than 14 days has not been studied. Transfer to oral dosing as soon as practical. Oral and IV doses are considered to be equivalent and should be given at previously established intervals (e.g., every 6 or 8 hours). See Precautions.

Complex partial seizures (monotherapy [initial]): Begin with an initial dose of 10 to 15 mg/kg/24 hr. May be increased by 5 to 10 mg/kg/week until desired clinical response achieved or until side effects are dose limiting.

Complex partial seizures (conversion to monotherapy): Begin with an initial dose of 10 to 15 mg/kg/24 hr. May be increased by 5 to 10 mg/kg/week until desired clinical response achieved or until side effects are dose limiting. Concomitant antiepilepsy drug (AED) dosage can usually be reduced by 25% every 2 weeks. Dose of AEDs may be decreased at the beginning of valproate therapy or decrease may be delayed for 1 to 2 weeks to avoid unwanted seizures.

Complex partial seizures (adjunctive therapy): Begin with an initial dose of 10 to 15 mg/kg/24 hr. May be increased by 5 to 10 mg/kg/week until desired clinical response achieved. Has been used in combination with either carbamazepine (Tegretol) or phenytoin (Dilantin). Dose adjustment of these drugs is not usually needed; however, drug interactions may occur; monitor plasma concentrations, especially during early therapy.

Simple and complex absence seizures: Begin with an initial dose of 15 mg/kg/24 hr. May be increased by 5 to 10 mg/kg/week until seizures are controlled or side effects are dose limiting.

PEDIATRIC DOSE

No IV dose recommendations available for pediatric patients under 10 years of age. See Maternal/Child.

DOSE ADJUSTMENTS

Monitor plasma concentrations when transferring from oral to IV or IV to oral; dose increases or decreases may be indicated. ▪ Reduce initial dose in the elderly; base subsequent doses on clinical response and/or development of side effects. ▪ Reduced dose or discontinuation of therapy may be indicated if there is evidence of decreased food or fluid intake or excessive somnolence in the elderly. ▪ Reduced dose or discontinuation of therapy may be indicated if there is evidence of bruising, hemorrhage, or a disorder of hemostasis/coagulation. ▪ No dose adjustments required for impaired renal function, gender, or race. ▪ See Maternal/Child.

DILUTION

Each single dose should be diluted with at least 50 mL of D5W, NS, or LR.

Storage: Store vials at CRT. Diluted solutions stable at CRT for 24 hours. No preservative added; discard unused contents of vial.

COMPATIBILITY

Consider any drug NOT listed as compatible to be INCOMPATIBLE until consulting a pharmacist; specific conditions may apply.

One source suggests the following **compatibilities:**

Additive: Levetiracetam (Keppra).

Y-site: Cefepime (Maxipime), ceftazidime (Fortaz).

RATE OF ADMINISTRATION

A single dose as an infusion over 60 minutes. Manufacturer has recommended that a rate of 20 mg/min not be exceeded; however, results of a single study suggest that selected patients tolerated rates from 1.5 to 3 mg/kg/min, allowing administration of up to 15 mg/kg/dose over 5 to 10 minutes. Incidence of side effects may be increased with too-rapid infusion.

ACTIONS

An anticonvulsant. A sodium salt of valproic acid. Therapeutic effect in epilepsy may result from increased brain concentrations of gamma-aminobutyric acid (GABA). Peak effect occurs at the end of a 60-minute infusion or 4 hours after an oral dose. Plasma protein binding is high and is concentration dependent. Concentration in CSF is similar to unbound concentrations in plasma (10%). Half-life range is 13 to 19 hours. The half-life will be in the lower part of the range in patients receiving other enzyme-inducing antiepileptic agents (e.g., carbamazepine [Tegretol], phenobarbital [Luminal], phenytoin [Dilantin]). Metabolized in the liver. 30% to 50% excreted in changed form in urine. Crosses placental barrier. Secreted in breast milk.

INDICATIONS AND USES

Use of IV product indicated in the following specific conditions when oral administration of valproate products (e.g., divalproex sodium [Depakote]) is temporarily not feasible. ■ Treatment of complex partial seizures occurring in isolation or with other seizures (monotherapy or adjunctive therapy). ■ Treatment of simple and complex absence seizures (monotherapy or adjunctive therapy). ■ Adjunctive treatment of multiple seizure types that include absence seizures.

Unlabeled uses: Used alone or in combination with other antiepileptic drugs for treatment of patients with status epilepticus (refractory) who have not responded to other therapies.

Limitations of use: Because of the risk to the fetus of decreased IQ, neural tube defects, and other major congenital malformations, valproate products should not be administered to a woman of childbearing potential unless it is essential to the management of her medical condition.

CONTRAINDICATIONS

Known hypersensitivity to valproate products. ■ Patients with hepatic disease or significant hepatic dysfunction. ■ Patients known to have mitochrondrial disorders caused by mutations in mitochondrial DNA polymerase γ (POLG) gene (e.g., Alpers-Huttenlocher syndrome), and children under 2 years of age who are suspected of having a POLG-related disorder. ■ Patients with known urea cycle disorders.

PRECAUTIONS

Use of IV valproate for more than 14 days has not been studied. Safety of doses above 60 mg/kg/day is not known. ■ Has caused fatal hepatic failure. Incidents usually occur during the first 6 months of treatment. Patients with a history of hepatic disease, patients taking multiple anticonvulsants, pediatric patients, patients with congenital metabolic disorders, patients with severe seizure disorders accompanied by cognitive impairment, and patients with organic brain disease may be at particular risk. Pediatric patients under 2 years of age are at the greatest risk. If valproate is used in pediatric patients under 2 years of age with or without these increased risk factors, benefits must outweigh risks; use only as a sole agent and with extreme caution. Incidence of fatal hepatotoxicity decreases in progressively older patient groups. ■ Cases of life-threatening pancreatitis have been reported in both pediatric patients and adults receiving valproate. Some of the cases have been described as hemorrhagic with rapid progression from initial symptoms to death. May occur at any time from shortly after initiation of therapy to years later. If pancreatitis is diagnosed, valproate should be discontinued. ■ Patients with hereditary neurometabolic syndromes caused by DNA mutations of the mitochondrial DNA polymerase γ (POLG) gene (e.g., Alpers-Huttenlocher syndrome) have an increased risk of valproate-induced liver failure and death; see Contraindications and Monitor. ■ Hyperammonemic encephalopathy, sometimes fatal, has been reported in patients with urea cycle disorders (UCD). Before starting valproate, consider a possible diagnosis of UCD in patients with a history of unexplained encephalopathy or coma, encephalopathy associated with a protein load, pregnancy-related or postpartum encephalopathy, unexplained cognitive impairment, a history of elevated plasma ammonia or glutamine, cyclical vomiting or lethargy, episodic extreme irritability, ataxia, low BUN, protein avoidance, a family history of UCD or unexplained infant deaths, or any other S/S of UCD. ▪ Hyperammonemia may be present even with normal liver function tests. Hyperammonemic encephalopathy should be considered in patients who present with lethargy and vomiting or altered mental status. Hyperammonemia should also be considered in patients who present with hypothermia (unintentional drop in body temperature to less than 35° C [95° F]). Elevation of ammonia may also be asymptomatic. ▪ Hyperammonemia with or without encephalopathy has been reported with concomitant administration of valproic acid and topiramate (Topamax). Has occurred in patients who have tolerated either drug alone. S/S in most cases are abated with discontinuation of either drug. ▪ Hypothermia has occurred with valproate therapy both in conjunction with and in the absence of hyperammonemia. Can also occur in patients using concomitant topiramate with valproate after starting topiramate therapy or after increasing the dose of topiramate. ▪ Antiepileptic drugs (AEDs) increase the risk of suicidal thoughts or behavior in patients taking these drugs for any indication. Patients treated with any AED for any indication should be monitored for the emergence or worsening of depression, suicidal thoughts or behavior, and/or any unusual changes in mood or behavior. Some behavioral changes resolved without intervention. Others required dose reduction or discontinuation of valproate. ▪ The frequency of adverse events (particularly elevated liver enzymes and thrombocytopenia) may be dose-related. The benefit of improved therapeutic effect with higher doses should be weighed against the possibility of a greater incidence of adverse reactions. ▪ Incidence of thrombocytopenia increases at total trough concentrations greater than 110 mcg/mL in females and greater than 135 mcg/mL in males. ▪ Drug reaction with eosinophilia and systemic symptoms (DRESS), also known as multiorgan hypersensitivity, has been reported in patients receiving valproate therapy. May be fatal or life threatening. Initial S/S include fever, rash, and/or lympadenopathy associated with other organ system involvement (e.g., arthralgia, hematologic abnormalities, hepatitis, myocarditis, myositis, nephritis). Eosinophilia is often present. Discontinue valproate and use alternative therapy. ▪ Plasma protein binding is decreased and free fraction is increased in the elderly, in hyperlipidemic patients, in chronic hepatic disease, in impaired renal function, and in the presence of other drugs; see Drug/Lab Interactions. Total plasma concentrations may be normal, but free concentrations may be substantially elevated in these patients. ▪ Antiepilepsy drugs should not be abruptly discontinued in patients being treated for major seizure activity. Reduce AED doses gradually to prevent status epilepticus. ▪ Can cause major congenital malformations, particularly neural tube defects (e.g., spina bifida). Do not administer to a woman of childbearing potential unless essential to the management of her medical condition. Consider benefit versus risk to the fetus in women of childbearing age. Do not use to treat non–life-threatening conditions (e.g., migraine). See Maternal/Child. ▪ In vitro studies suggest that valproate may stimulate the replication of the HIV and CMV viruses under certain experimental conditions. The clinical significance of this is unknown but should be kept in mind when evaluating patients with HIV or CMV. ▪ Not recommended for use in patients with acute head trauma for the prophylaxis of posttraumatic seizures.

Monitor: Thrombocytopenia, inhibition of the secondary phase of platelet aggregation, and abnormal coagulation parameters (e.g., low fibrinogen, coagulation factor deficiencies, acquired von Willebrand disease) have been reported. Obtain baseline platelet counts and coagulation tests and monitor during therapy. Repeat before planned surgery and during pregnancy. ▪ Obtain baseline serum liver testing and monitor frequently during therapy, especially during the first 6 months. ▪ Observe closely for S/S of hepatotoxicity (e.g., anorexia, facial edema, lethargy, loss of seizure control, malaise, weakness, vomiting). ▪ Abdominal pain, anorexia, nausea, and vomiting may be symptoms of pancreatitis and should be evaluated promptly. ▪ Valproate products should be used only after other anticonvulsants have failed in patients over 2 years of age who are clinically suspected of having a hereditary mitochondrial disease. Closely monitor during treatment for the development of acute liver injury with regular clinical assessments and serum liver testing. Perform POLG mutation screening as indicated (e.g., family history, unexplained encephalopathy, refractory epilepsy [focal, myoclonic], status epilepticus at presentation, developmental delays, psychomotor regression, axonal sensorimotor neuropathy, myopathy cerebellar ataxia, ophthalmoplegia, or complicated migraine with occipital aura). ▪ Therapeutic serum levels for most patients will range from 50 to 100 mcg/mL; however, a good correlation has not been established between daily dose, serum levels, and therapeutic effect. Some patients may be controlled with lower or higher serum concentrations. One contributing factor is the nonlinear, concentration-dependent protein binding of valproate, which affects the clearance of the drug. ▪ Monitor antiepileptic concentrations more frequently whenever concomitant AEDs are being introduced or withdrawn, and observe closely for seizure activity. ▪ When used as replacement therapy, the equivalence shown between the IV and oral formulations was evaluated only in an every-6-hour regimen. If valproate sodium is given twice or three times daily, close monitoring of trough plasma levels may be needed to ensure therapeutic levels are being maintained. ▪ Monitor serum concentrations more frequently if any of the risk factors listed in Dose Adjustments or Precautions are present, and when any drugs that affect hepatic enzymes are introduced or discontinued; see Drug/Lab Interactions. ▪ Evaluate for S/S of UCD; see Precautions and Antidote. ▪ Consider hyperammonemia encephalopathy in patients who develop unexplained lethargy and vomiting or changes in mental status. Consider hyperammonemia in patients who present with hypothermia. Elevations of ammonia may be asymptomatic; monitor plasma ammonia levels closely; see Antidote. Treat hyperammonemia and assess for underlying UCD. ▪ Observe patient closely for signs of CNS side effects; see Precautions. ▪ Monitor for S/S of DRESS. ▪ Total serum valproic acid concentration is affected by variable free-fractions of drug; consider hepatic metabolism and protein binding when interpreting valproic acid concentrations. ▪ See Dose Adjustments, Precautions, and Drug/Lab Interactions for additional monitoring requirements.

Patient Education: May cause drowsiness; determine effects before driving or operating any machinery. ▪ Avoid pregnancy; use effective contraception; see Maternal/Child. ▪ Read the patient information leaflet provided by manufacturer, and discuss your medical history and concurrent prescription and nonprescription medications with your health care provider. ▪ Promptly report symptoms such as abdominal pain, anorexia, changes in mental state, fever, jaundice, lethargy, lymphadenopathy, nausea, rash, unexplained lethargy, unintentional drop in body temperature to less than 35° C (95° F), or vomiting; may be symptoms of serious side effects (e.g., hepatotoxicity, hyperammonemia, hypersensitivity, pancreatitis) and require prompt evaluation and treatment. ▪ May increase the risk of suicidal thoughts and behavior. Promptly report emergence or worsening of the S/S of depression, any unusual changes in mood or behavior, or thoughts about self-harm. ▪ Women who are pregnant or who become pregnant should be encouraged to enroll in the North American Antiepileptic Drug (NAAED) Pregnancy Registry. ▪ See Maternal/Child.

Maternal/Child: Category D: avoid pregnancy. Valproate products should be used during pregnancy only if other anticonvulsants have failed to control symptoms or are otherwise unacceptable. There is an increased risk for major congenital malformations, particularly neural tube defects (e.g., spina bifida) and other birth defects such as craniofacial defects, cardiovascular malformation, hypospadias, and limb malformations; in addition, there is a risk for decreased IQ in infants exposed to valproate sodium and related products in utero. The incidence of congenital malformations associated with the use of valproate by women with seizure disorders during pregnancy is higher than in women with seizure disorders who use other AEDs. The increased teratogenic risk from valproate in women with epilepsy is expected to be reflected in an increased risk in other indications (e.g., bipolar disorder, migraine). Use during pregnancy only if essential for management of a serious medical condition (e.g., seizures). ▪ Evidence suggests that folic acid supplementation before conception and during the first trimester decreases the risk for congenital neural tube defects in the general population. Tests to detect neural tube and other defects should be considered as part of routine prenatal care in pregnant women receiving valproate. Dietary folic acid supplementation before conception and during pregnancy is recommended. ▪ To prevent major seizures, do not discontinue valproate abruptly in these patients; can precipitate status epilepticus, resulting in maternal and fetal hypoxia and a threat to life. ▪ When used during pregnancy, valproate has caused clotting abnormalities in the mother that may result in hemorrhagic complications in the neonate. Deaths have been reported. If clotting parameters are abnormal in the mother, then these parameters should also be monitored in the neonate; see Monitor. ▪ Has caused hepatic failure in infants exposed to valproate in utero. ▪ Has caused hypoglycemia in infants exposed to valproate in utero. ▪ Use with caution during breast-feeding. ▪ Neonates under 2 months have a markedly decreased ability to eliminate valproate compared to older pediatric patients and adults. ▪ Pediatric patients 3 months to 10 years of age have 50% higher clearance rates based on weight. ▪ Younger pediatric patients, especially those receiving enzyme-inducing drugs (e.g., carbamazepine, phenobarbital, phenytoin) will require larger maintenance doses to achieve therapeutic valproic acid concentrations. ▪ IV product has not been studied in pediatric patients under 2 years of age. If used, use as a sole agent with extreme caution. ▪ Children under 2 years of age are at an increased risk for developing fatal hepatotoxicity. ▪ See Precautions and Monitor.

Elderly: May be more prone to adverse events. Initial dose should be lower, and dosage should be increased slowly. Rate of clearance decreased, free fraction increased; see Dose Adjustments. ▪ Monitor for fluid and nutritional intake, dehydration, somnolence, and other adverse events. Dose reduction or discontinuation of valproate should be considered in patients with decreased food or fluid intake and in patients with excessive somnolence. ▪ A higher percentage of patients over 65 years of age reported accidental injury, infection, pain, somnolence, and tremor.

DRUG/LAB INTERACTIONS

Clearance increased and effectiveness reduced by **drugs that induce hepatic enzymes** (e.g., phenytoin [Dilantin], carbamazepine [Tegretol], phenobarbital [Luminal], primidone [Mysoline], ritonavir [Norvir]); increased monitoring of valproate and concomitant drug concentrations indicated. ▪ **Aspirin** decreases protein binding, inhibits metabolism, and increases free concentration of valproate; use caution and monitor valproate concentrations if administered concomitantly. ▪ Peak concentrations increased if coadministered with **felbamate** (Felbatol); reduced dose of valproate indicated. ▪ Metabolism may be decreased and serum levels increased when given concurrently with **erythromycin.** ▪ **Carbapenem antibiotics** (e.g., doripenem [Doribax], ertapenem [Invanz], meropenem [Merrem]) may reduce serum valproic acid concentrations to subtherapeutic levels, resulting in loss of seizure control. Monitor valproic acid levels. Consider alternative antibacterial or anticonvulsant therapy if serum valproate concentrations drop significantly or seizure control deteriorates. ▪ **Rifampin** (Rifadin) may increase clearance of valproate and require dose adjustment. ▪ Inhibits metabolism of **barbiturates** (e.g., phenobarbital) **and primidone,** increasing their effects. Monitor for neurologic toxicity; obtain barbiturate serum levels and reduce barbiturate dose as indicated. ▪ May decrease serum levels of carbamazepine. **Carbamazepine** decreases plasma concentrations of valproate, and a loss of seizure control may occur; monitor carefully and increase valproate dose if indicated. ▪ Concomitant use with **clonazepam** (Klonopin) may induce absence status in patients with a history of absence-type seizures. ▪ **Displaces some protein-bound drugs** (e.g., carbamazepine, diazepam [Valium], phenytoin, tolbutamide, warfarin [Coumadin]). In addition to decreasing protein binding, may also decrease the metabolism of diazepam and phenytoin. Dose adjustments and serum concentrations may be indicated. ▪ **Phenytoin** with valproate has caused breakthrough seizures in patients with epilepsy; adjust dose of phenytoin as indicated by serum concentrations. ▪ Hyperammonemia with or without encephalopathy, as well as hypothermia, has been reported with concomitant administration of valproic acid and **topiramate** (Topamax); see Precautions. ▪ Monitor coagulation tests if administered with **anticoagulants** (e.g., warfarin). ▪ CNS effects may be increased when given concurrently with **CNS depressants** (e.g., benzodiazepines [e.g., diazepam (Valium)] **and tricyclic antidepressants** [e.g., amitriptyline (Elavil)]). ▪ May decrease clearance and increase effects of **amitriptyline** (Elavil) **and nortriptyline** (Aventyl). Dose reduction of these drugs may be required. ▪ Inhibits metabolism of **ethosuximide** (Zarontin); monitor serum concentrations of both drugs with concomitant administration. ▪ Concurrent administration of **lamotrigine** (Lamictal) and valproate may increase lamotrigine levels. Serious skin reactions have been reported. Dose adjustments of lamotrigine may be required. ▪ Decreases clearance and may increase toxicity of **zidovudine** (AZT, Retrovir). ▪ Rufinamide (Banzel) clearance is decreased by valproate. Concentrations were increased by less than 16% to 70% depending on the concentration of valproate. Patients stabilized on rufinamide before initiating valproate therapy should begin valproate at a low dose and titrate to a clinically effective dose. Similarly, patients on valproate should begin rufinamide at a dose lower than 10 mg/kg/day (pediatric patients) or 400 mg/day (adults). ▪ See package insert for additional information about many drugs that do not present significant clinical interactions. ▪ May alter **thyroid function tests.** ▪ May cause **false-positive urine ketone test.**

SIDE EFFECTS

Abdominal pain; alopecia; amblyopia/blurred vision; amnesia; anorexia with weight loss; asthenia; ataxia; bronchitis; constipation; depression; diarrhea; diplopia; dizziness; dyspepsia; dyspnea; ecchymosis; emotional lability; fever; flu syndrome; headache; increased appetite with weight gain; infection; insomnia; nausea; nervousness; nystagmus; peripheral edema; pharyngitis; rhinitis; somnolence; thinking abnormally; thrombocytopenia; tinnitus; tremor; and vomiting are most common. Accidental injury, back pain, chest pain, euphoria, hypesthesia, injection site inflammation, injection site pain, rash, sweating, taste perversion, and vasodilation were the next most commonly reported side effects. Psychiatric symptoms, including aggression, agitation, anger, anxiety, apathy, depersonalization, depression, emotional lability, hallucinations, hostility, irritability, and suicidal tendencies, have also been reported. Frequency of elevated liver enzymes and thrombocytopenia may be dose related. Fatal hepatotoxicity (anorexia, facial edema, lethargy, loss of seizure control, malaise, sweating, vasodilation, vomiting, weakness) has occurred. Encephalopathy with or without fever has caused fatalities in patients with hyperammonemic encephalopathy and/or underlying UCD disorder. See Precautions for other reported serious adverse events.

Overdose: Somnolence, deep coma, heart block, and hypernatremia. Some fatalities have been reported.

Post-Marketing: Many adverse reactions have been reported during postapproval use of valproate sodium. The frequency of reactions and/or causal relationship to valproate may be difficult to determine. Some of the reported reactions have included dermatologic reactions (e.g., erythema multiforme, nail and nail bed disorders, photosensitivity, Stevens-Johnson syndrome, toxic epidermal necrolysis), endocrine abnormalities (e.g., elevated testosterone, hirsutism, hyperandrogenism, secondary amenorrhea), enuresis, Fanconi's syndrome, hair color and texture changes, hematologic reactions (e.g., anemia including macrocytic with or without folate deficiency, aplastic anemia, bone marrow suppression), hypersensitivity reactions (including anaphylaxis), osteopenia, osteoporosis, reproductive reactions (e.g., aspermia, azoospermia, male infertility), and weight gain.

ANTIDOTE

Keep physician informed of all side effects. Some may respond to a decrease in the rate of administration. Discontinue immediately if signs of suspected or apparent significant hepatic dysfunction appear (e.g., hyperammonemia, elevated liver function tests) or S/S of underlying UCD. Hepatic dysfunction may progress after valproate is discontinued. Discontinue if S/S of DRESS occur. Initiate alternate therapy. Reduce dose or discontinue if bruising, hemorrhage, or abnormal coagulation parameters occur (e.g., thrombocytopenia). Discontinue if S/S of pancreatitis occur. All of the above situations may be life threatening and will require immediate symptomatic treatment. Maintain a patent airway and resuscitate as indicated. Support patient as required in treatment of overdose; monitor and maintain adequate urine output. Hemodialysis is effective in overdose. Naloxone may reverse CNS depressant effects in overdose but may also reverse antiepilepsy effects of valproate. Psychotic symptoms may require dose reduction or discontinuation of valproate.

VANCOMYCIN HYDROCHLORIDE
(van-koh-**MY**-sin hy-droh-**KLOR**-eyed)

Antibacterial
(tricylic-glycopeptide)

pH 2.4 to 5

USUAL DOSE

7.5 mg/kg or 500 mg every 6 hours or 15 mg/kg or 1 Gm every 12 hours for 7 to 10 days. Maximum dosage of 3 to 4 Gm/24 hr used only in extreme situations. Normal renal function required.

Prevention of bacterial endocarditis in selected penicillin-allergic patients having GI, biliary, or GU surgery or instrumentation:

Adults and adolescents: 1 Gm IV before the procedure. Give gentamicin 1.5 mg/kg IV concurrently in high-risk patients (not to exceed 120 mg). Infusion must be administered over at least 60 minutes and should be completed within 30 minutes of starting the procedure. Gentamicin may not be necessary in moderate-risk patients. Both doses may be repeated in 8 to 12 hours for high-risk patients. Vancomycin alone may be indicated in selected patients having dental procedures or upper respiratory tract surgery or instrumentation. Consult recent recommendations of the American Heart Association or the American Dental Association.

Treatment of patients with methicillin-resistant or methicillin-susceptible staphylococcal endocarditis who have a native cardiac valve: 30 mg/kg/24 hr equally divided into 2 doses (15 mg/kg every 12 hours) for 6 weeks or longer. If more than 2 Gm/day are required, monitoring of serum concentrations of vancomycin is recommended.

Treatment of patients with methicillin-resistant or methicillin-susceptible staphylococcal endocarditis who have a prosthetic valve or other prosthetic material: 30 mg/kg/24 hr equally divided into 2 doses (15 mg/kg every 12 hours) or 4 doses (7.5 mg/kg every 6 hours) for 6 weeks or longer. If more than 2 Gm/day are required, monitoring of serum concentrations of vancomycin is recommended. Given in conjunction with oral rifampin 300 mg every 8 hours for 6 weeks or longer and IM or IV gentamicin 1 mg/kg every 8 hours during the first 2 weeks of vancomycin therapy.

Treatment of endocarditis caused by viridans streptococci or *Streptococcus bovis*: 30 mg/kg/24 hr equally divided into 2 doses (15 mg/kg every 12 hours) for 4 weeks. If more than 2 Gm/day are required, monitoring of serum concentrations of vancomycin is recommended.

Treatment of enterococcal endocarditis: 30 mg/kg/24 hr equally divided into 2 doses (15 mg/kg every 12 hours) for 4 to 6 weeks. If more than 2 Gm/day are required, monitoring of serum concentrations of vancomycin is recommended. Given in conjunction with IM or IV gentamicin 1 mg/kg every 8 hours for 4 to 6 weeks.

Perioperative prophylaxis in selected surgeries (e.g., cardiac, prosthetic valve, coronary artery bypass, joint replacement, craniotomy) when a cephalosporin cannot be used or there is a high incidence of methicillin-resistant staphylococci at the institution (unlabeled use): 1 Gm IV over 1 to 2 hours; should be completed within 30 minutes before the start of surgery. May be repeated one or more times if surgery is prolonged or major blood loss occurs. Postoperative doses are considered generally unnecessary and are not recommended.

Prevention of neonatal Group B streptococcal disease: Used for women with penicillin hypersensitivity who should not receive β-lactam anti-infectives or if resistance to clindamycin or erythromycin is known or suspected. 1 Gm every 12 hours until delivery. Initiate at the beginning of labor or rupture of membranes.

PEDIATRIC DOSE

Pediatric patients 1 month of age or older: *Mild to moderate infections:* 40 mg/kg of body weight/24 hr equally divided and given every 6, 8, or 12 hours (10 mg/kg every 6 hours, 13.33 mg/kg every 8 hours, or 20 mg/kg every 12 hours) for 7 to 10 days.

Severe infections: Up to 60 mg/kg/24 hr (15 mg/kg every 6 hours, 20 mg/kg every 8 hours, or 30 mg/kg every 12 hours) has been used if there is CNS involvement. Do not exceed 2 Gm in 24 hours.

Prevention of bacterial endocarditis in selected penicillin-allergic patients having GI, biliary, or GU surgery or instrumentation: 20 mg/kg before the procedure. Give gentamicin 1.5 mg/kg concurrently in high-risk patients (not to exceed 120 mg). Gentamicin may not be necessary in moderate-risk patients. Infusion must be administered over at least 60 minutes and should be complete within 30 minutes of starting the procedure. Both doses may be repeated in 8 to 12 hours for high-risk patients. Note comments about dental and upper respiratory surgery or instrumentation under Usual Dose.

NEONATAL DOSE

15 mg/kg as an initial dose. See Maternal/Child. Follow with 10 mg/kg. Adjust interval based on age and/or weight as follows:

Infants up to 1 week of age: Give every 12 hours.

Infants 1 week to 1 month of age: Give every 8 hours.

The American Academy of Pediatrics recommends 10 to 15 mg/kg. Adjust dose and interval based on weight and/or age as follows:

Postnatal Weight and Age	Dose and Interval
Less than 1.2 kg and less than 7 days of age	15 mg/kg/dose every 24 hours
Less than 1.2 kg and 7 days of age or older	15 mg/kg/dose every 24 hours
1.2 to 2 kg and less than 7 days of age	10 to 15 mg/kg/dose every 12 to 18 hours
1.2 to 2 kg and 7 days of age or older	10 to 15 mg/kg/dose every 8 to 12 hours
Over 2 kg and less than 7 days of age	10 to 15 mg/kg/dose every 8 to 12 hours
Over 2 kg and 7 days of age or older	15 to 20 mg/kg/dose every 6 to 8 hours

DOSE ADJUSTMENTS

Reduce total daily dose in premature infants and the elderly. Greater dose reductions than expected may be necessary in these patients because of impaired renal function. ▪ Dose reduction required in impaired renal function. In all renal impaired patients (including functionally anephric and anuric patients), the initial dose should be no less than 15 mg/kg. *See prescribing information;* dose is reduced for every decrease of 10 mL/min in the CrCl. Subsequent doses of 250 to 1,000 mg every several days are suggested for functionally anephric patients. Subsequent doses of 1,000 mg every 7 to 10 days are suggested for anuric patients. Monitoring of serum levels is recommended.

DILUTION

Available premixed, premixed and frozen, or reconstitute each 500-mg vial with 10 mL of SWFI. Each 500 mg must be further diluted with 100 mL of NS or D5W and given as an intermittent infusion. Also **compatible** in D5NS, LR, D5LR, D5 Normosol-M, Isolyte E, and acetated Ringer's injection. Concentrations greater than 5 mg/mL are not recommended. If absolutely necessary, 1 to 2 Gm may be further diluted in sufficient amounts of the same infusion fluids and given over 24 hours. Not recommended. Also available in ADD-Vantage vials for use with ADD-Vantage infusion containers.

Storage: Store in refrigerator after initial dilution. Maintains potency for 2 weeks in D5W or NS, 96 hours for other infusion solutions. Solutions prepared from ADD-Vantage vials stable at room temperature for 24 hours.

COMPATIBILITY   (Underline Indicates Conflicting Compatibility Information)

Consider any drug NOT listed as compatible to be INCOMPATIBLE until consulting a pharmacist; specific conditions may apply.

Several sources recommend not admixing with other drugs. They suggest it is **incompatible** with alkaline solutions (e.g., aminophylline, aztreonam [Azactam], barbiturates [e.g., pentobarbital (Nembutal)], chloramphenicol [Chloromycetin], dexamethasone [Decadron], sodium bicarbonate) and may form a precipitate with heavy metals. May inactivate aminoglycosides; should also not be combined in the same solution with albumin, selected cephalosporins, foscarnet (Foscavir), or selected penicillins; if administered concurrently, administer at separate sites or separate intervals (flush IV line with a **compatible** solution before and after administration).

One source suggests the following **compatibilities:**

Additive: *See general comments under Compatibility.* Acetaminophen (Ofirmev), amikacin, aminophylline, atracurium (Tracrium), aztreonam (Azactam), calcium gluconate, cefepime (Maxipime), dimenhydrinate, famotidine (Pepcid IV), heparin, hydrocortisone sodium succinate (Solu-Cortef), meropenem (Merrem IV), potassium chloride (KCl), ranitidine (Zantac), verapamil.

Y-site: *See general comments under Compatibility.* Acyclovir (Zovirax), aldesleukin (Proleukin), allopurinol (Aloprim), alprostadil, amifostine (Ethyol), amiodarone (Nexterone), ampicillin, ampicillin/sulbactam (Unasyn), anidulafungin (Eraxis), atracurium (Tracrium), aztreonam (Azactam), caspofungin (Cancidas), cefazolin (Ancef), cefepime (Maxipime), cefotaxime (Claforan), cefotetan, cefoxitin (Mefoxin), ceftazidime (Fortaz), ceftriaxone (Rocephin), cefuroxime (Zinacef), cisatracurium (Nimbex), cyclophosphamide (Cytoxan), dexmedetomidine (Precedex), diltiazem (Cardizem), docetaxel (Taxotere), doripenem (Doribax), doxapram (Dopram), doxorubicin liposomal (Doxil), enalaprilat (Vasotec IV), esmolol (Brevibloc), etoposide phosphate (Etopophos), fenoldopam (Corlopam), filgrastim (Neupogen), fluconazole (Diflucan), fludarabine (Fludara), foscarnet (Foscavir), gallium nitrate (Ganite), gemcitabine (Gemzar), granisetron (Kytril), heparin, hetastarch in electrolytes (Hextend), hydromorphone (Dilaudid), insulin (regular), labetalol, levofloxacin (Levaquin), linezolid (Zyvox), lorazepam (Ativan), magnesium sulfate, melphalan (Alkeran), meperidine (Demerol), meropenem (Merrem IV), methotrexate, midazolam (Versed), milrinone (Primacor), morphine, mycophenolate (CellCept IV), nafcillin (Nallpen), nicardipine (Cardene IV), ondansetron (Zofran), paclitaxel (Taxol), palonosetron (Aloxi), pancuronium, pemetrexed (Alimta), piperacillin/tazobactam (Zosyn), propofol (Diprivan), remifentanil (Ultiva), sargramostim (Leukine), sodium bicarbonate, tacrolimus (Prograf), teniposide (Vumon), theophylline, thiotepa, ticarcillin/clavulanate (Timentin), tigecycline (Tygacil), vecuronium, vinorelbine (Navelbine), warfarin (Coumadin), zidovudine (AZT, Retrovir).

RATE OF ADMINISTRATION

Severe hypotension, with or without red blotching of the face, neck, chest, and extremities, and cardiac arrest can occur with too-rapid injection.

A single dose properly diluted (concentration of no more than 5 mg/mL) at a rate not to exceed 10 mg/min or 60 minutes, whichever is longer. Another reference suggests infusion over 1 to 2 hours. This intermittent infusion is the preferred route of administration because of high incidence of thrombophlebitis.

Pediatric rate: A single dose over a minimum of 60 minutes.

ACTIONS

A very potent tricyclic glycopeptide antibiotic, it is bactericidal against gram-positive organisms. Bactericidal action results from the inhibition of cell wall synthesis. Also alters bacterial cell-membrane permeability and RNA synthesis. Well distributed in most body tissues and fluids, including pleural, pericardial, ascitic, and synovial fluids; in urine; in peritoneal dialysis fluid; and in atrial appendage tissue. Penetration into the CSF occurs when the meninges are inflamed. Half-life is 4 to 6 hours in patients with normal renal function. Vancomycin is excreted in biologically active form in the urine. Crosses the placental barrier. Secreted in breast milk.

INDICATIONS AND USES

Serious gram-positive infections (e.g., staphylococcal infections), including endocarditis, septicemia, bone, lower respiratory tract, and skin and skin structure infections that do not respond or are resistant to other less toxic antibiotics, such as penicillins or cephalosporins (e.g., methicillin-resistant staphylococci). ■ Penicillin-allergic patients. ■ Treatment of endocarditis caused by *Streptococcus viridans* or *S. bovis* concurrently with an aminoglycoside antibiotic; endocarditis caused by diphtheroids or *S. epidermidis* concurrently with rifampin and/or an aminoglycoside. ▪ Parenteral form used orally for pseudomembranous colitis/staphylococcal enterocolitis caused by *C. difficile.*

Unlabeled uses: Prophylaxis against bacterial endocarditis in moderate or high-risk (prosthetic heart valves, congenital or rheumatic heart disease) penicillin-allergic patients undergoing GI, biliary, or GU surgery or instrumentation. Given in combination with gentamicin in GI or GU procedures.

CONTRAINDICATIONS
Known hypersensitivity to vancomycin. Solutions containing dextrose may be contraindicated in patients with allergies to corn or corn products.

PRECAUTIONS
To reduce the development of drug-resistant bacteria and maintain its effectiveness, vancomycin should be used only to treat or prevent infections proven or strongly suspected to be caused by bacteria. ▪ Sensitivity studies necessary to determine susceptibility of the causative organism to vancomycin. ▪ Prolonged use of drug may result in superinfection caused by overgrowth of nonsusceptible organisms. ▪ May be ototoxic and nephrotoxic. Some clinicians feel the risk of ototoxicity and nephrotoxicity is minimal in patients with normal renal function who receive vancomycin as a single agent. ▪ Use caution in impaired hearing, impaired renal function, pregnancy, breast-feeding, neonates, and the elderly. ▪ *Clostridium difficile*–associated diarrhea (CDAD) has been reported. May range from mild diarrhea to fatal colitis. Consider in patients who present with diarrhea during or after treatment with vancomycin. ▪ Oral vancomycin has a local effect only (e.g., in the bowel); not for systemic use. ▪ A syndrome of chemical peritonitis has been reported in patients receiving intraperitoneal vancomycin during CAPD.

Monitor: Monitoring of serum levels and SCr may be indicated in patients at increased risk for developing nephrotoxicity and/or ototoxicity (e.g., underlying renal dysfunction, or receiving concomitant aminoglycosides [e.g., gentamicin]). ▪ Determine absolute patency of vein. Necrosis and sloughing will result from extravasation. Rotate injection sites every 2 to 3 days. ▪ Observe for furry tongue, diarrhea, and foul-smelling stools. ▪ Severe hypotension, with or without red blotching of the face, neck, chest, and extremities, and cardiac arrest can occur with too-rapid injection (red man or red neck syndrome). ▪ Monitor BP continuously during infusion to prevent a precipitous drop. ▪ Auditory testing indicated with prolonged use. ▪ Periodic monitoring of leukocyte count recommended in prolonged therapy. ▪ See Drug/Lab Interactions.

Patient Education: Report all side effects promptly. ▪ Promptly report diarrhea or bloody stools that occur during treatment or up to several months after an antibiotic has been discontinued; may indicate CDAD and require treatment.

Maternal/Child: Category C: studies not conclusive. Use only if clearly needed. ▪ Safety for use in breast-feeding not established; discontinue breast-feeding. ▪ Neonates have immature renal function; blood levels may be excessive. Confirmation of desired serum concentrations suggested in premature and full-term neonates.

Elderly: Systemic and renal clearance may be reduced; dosage reduction required.

DRUG/LAB INTERACTIONS
Synergistic with **aminoglycosides** (e.g., amikacin, gentamicin, tobramycin) against many strains of *Staphylococcus aureus* and streptococci; see package insert. Combined use may increase risk of ototoxicity and nephrotoxicity. ▪ Use caution with **dimenhydrinate,** which can mask ototoxicity. ▪ Additive toxicities may occur with *systemic or topical* use of **other nephrotoxic, neurotoxic, or ototoxic drugs** (e.g., aminoglycosides, amphotericin B, bacitracin, cisplatin, colistin, ethacrynic acid [Edecrin], furosemide [Lasix], polymyxin B). Use with caution in combination with vancomycin; serial monitoring of renal and auditory systems indicated. ▪ May enhance neuromuscular blockade with **nondepolarizing muscle relaxants** (e.g., pancuronium). ▪ May cause erythema and histamine-like flushing in pediatric patients with **anesthetics.** Use with anesthetics may also increase the risk of hypersensitivity reactions, including anaphylaxis and infusion reactions. Administration of vancomycin as a 1-hour infusion before anesthetic induction may reduce this

interaction. ▪ May inhibit **methotrexate** excretion and increase methotrexate toxicity. May occur even if 10 days have elapsed since vancomycin was administered. Adjust methotrexate dose as indicated.

SIDE EFFECTS

Chills, dizziness, fever, macular rashes, pain at injection site, pruritus, tinnitus, urticaria. **Major:** Anaphylaxis, cardiac arrest, CDAD, dyspnea, eosinophilia, hearing loss, hypotension, infusion-related events (anaphylactoid reactions, dyspnea, flushing of the upper body, pruritus, urticaria, wheezing), interstitial nephritis, neutropenia, red neck or red man syndrome, renal failure, Stevens-Johnson syndrome (erythema multiforme [flu-like symptoms that can be fatal]), thrombophlebitis, wheezing.

Post-Marketing: Drug rash with eosinophilia and systemic symptoms (DRESS).

ANTIDOTE

Notify the physician of all side effects. Hearing loss may progress even if drug is discontinued. If minor side effects are progressive or any major side effect occurs, discontinue the drug, treat hypersensitivity reaction, or resuscitate as necessary. Prevent severe hypotension by slowing infusion rate to 2 hours. Fluids, antihistamines, corticosteroids, and vasopressors (e.g., dopamine) may be required. Mild cases of CDAD may respond to discontinuation of drug. Treat CDAD with fluids, electrolytes, protein supplements, and oral vancomycin (Vancocin) or metronidazole (Flagyl) as indicated. In severe cases, surgical evaluation may be indicated. Hemodialysis or CAPD will not decrease blood levels in toxicity.

VASOPRESSIN INJECTION
(vay-so-**PRESS**-in in-**JEK**-shun)

Hormone
Antidiuretic
Vasopressor
(unlabeled)

Pitressin, Pressyn ✦

pH 2.5 to 4.5

USUAL DOSE

ALL IV DOSES AND USES ARE UNLABELED.

Treatment of shock-resistant VF or pulseless VT during cardiac arrest in adult patients: AHA Emergency Cardiovascular Care recommends 40 units by IV push or through the endotracheal tube for one dose only (may replace the first or second dose of epinephrine).

Hemodynamic support during vasodilatory shock (e.g., septic shock): AHA guidelines recommend a continuous infusion of 0.02 to 0.04 units/min. Other sources in the literature recommend low-dose vasopressin infusions in vasodilatory shock refractory to catecholamines. 0.04 units/min as an infusion (range was 0.01 to 0.1 units/min). Doses greater than 0.08 units/min showed no added benefit. Continue infusion until the patient is stabilized. Mean duration in a study was 18 to 168 hours.

GI hemorrhage: 0.2 units/min as an infusion. Increase each hour by 0.2 units/min until hemorrhage is controlled. Doses up to 1 unit/min are suggested. Another source suggests 0.2 to 0.4 units/min as an infusion. Gradually increase dose as needed to a maximum dose of 0.9 units/min.

PEDIATRIC DOSE

All IV doses and uses are unlabeled; however, studies in pediatric patients have been conducted.

Hemodynamic support during vasodilatory shock: 0.0003 to 0.002 units/kg/min as an infusion (range is 0.018 to 0.12 units/kg/hr). Continue infusion until the patient and concurrently administered catecholamine infusions are stabilized. Mean duration in a study was 6 to 144 hours. AHA guidelines recommend a continuous infusion of 0.0002 to 0.002 units/kg/min (0.2 to 2 milliunits/kg/min).

Treatment of shock-resistant VF or pulseless VT during cardiac arrest: Recommended for use in adult patients only. AHA guidelines recommend 0.4 to 1 unit/kg IV push (maximum dose 40 units).

GI hemorrhage: 0.002 to 0.005 units/kg/min as an infusion. Gradually increase dose as needed to a maximum dose of 0.01 units/kg/min.

DILUTION

AHA guidelines do not mention the use of a diluent, which suggests that vasopressin may be given undiluted. Another source recommends dilution for IV use to a 0.1 to 1 unit/mL dilution with NS or D5W. 38 mL diluent with 2 mL vasopressin (40 units) yields 1 unit/mL. 398 mL diluent with 2 mL vasopressin (40 units) yields 0.1 unit/mL.

Storage: Store unopened vials at CRT.

COMPATIBILITY   (Underline Indicates Conflicting Compatibility Information)

Consider any drug NOT listed as compatible to be INCOMPATIBLE until consulting a pharmacist; specific conditions may apply.

Consider specific use and unlabeled IV use.

One source suggests the following **compatibilities:**

Additive: Verapamil.

Y-site: Amiodarone (Nexterone), argatroban, caspofungin (Cancidas), ceftaroline (Teflaro), ciprofloxacin (Cipro IV), diltiazem (Cardizem), dobutamine, dopamine, epinephrine (Adrenalin), fluconazole (Diflucan), gentamicin, heparin, 6% hydroxyethyl starch (Voluven), imipenem-cilastatin (Primaxin), insulin (regular), lidocaine, linezolid (Zyvox), meropenem (Merrem IV), metronidazole (Flagyl IV), micafungin (Mycamine), milrinone (Primacor), moxifloxacin (Avelox), nitroglycerin IV, norepinephrine (Levophed), pantoprazole (Protonix IV), phenylephrine (Neo-Synephrine), piperacillin/tazobactam (Zosyn), procainamide (Pronestyl), sodium bicarbonate, telavancin (Vibativ), voriconazole (VFEND IV).

RATE OF ADMINISTRATION

Injection: A single dose IV push; see Precautions.

Infusion: See Usual Dose for recommended rates for each diagnosis. Use of a central venous catheter is recommended. Titrate rate so that perfusion remains adequate while BP is optimized. Do not discontinue abruptly; one source recommends tapering over 2 to 3 hours while monitoring effects.

ACTIONS

Synthetic vasopressin of the posterior pituitary gland standardized to 20 units/mL. An antidiuretic. Also a potent vasoconstrictor. Causes smooth muscle contraction of all parts of the vascular bed (e.g., capillaries, small arterioles, and venules). Has a lesser effect on the smooth muscles of larger arteries and veins. This direct contractile effect on the smooth muscle of the vascular system is not antagonized by adrenergic blocking agents (e.g., atenolol [Tenormin], metoprolol [Lopressor]) and is not prevented by vascular denervation (loss of nerve impulse to the vascular system). Its IV use is as an alternative pressor agent to epinephrine. Not effective in normotensive patients; however, promotes an effective increase in BP in hypotensive patients, even when other agents have failed. Rapidly degraded by enzymes in the liver and kidneys. Plasma half-life is 10 to 35 minutes. A small amount is excreted unchanged in the urine.

INDICATIONS AND USES

Used IM or SC as an antidiuretic in central diabetes insipidus or as a diagnostic aid in diabetes insipidus.

Unlabeled uses: The AHA Handbook of Emergency Cardiovascular Care recommends use in the treatment of adult shock-refractory ventricular fibrillation (Class IIb) (an alternative pressor agent to epinephrine) and for hemodynamic support in vasodilatory shock (e.g., septic shock). Has also been used for treatment of GI hemorrhage.

CONTRAINDICATIONS

Hypersensitivity to vasopressin or any of its components; see Precautions. AHA guidelines state "not recommended for responsive patients with coronary heart disease."

PRECAUTIONS

IV uses are unlabeled. ▪ May cause ischemia of other organs (e.g., GI tract, kidneys) if fluid intake is not adequate. ▪ Use with extreme caution in patients with vascular disease, especially coronary artery disease; may cause cardiac ischemia. Small doses may precipitate anginal pain, and larger doses may cause myocardial infarction. ▪ May produce water intoxication; use with caution in patients with asthma, chronic nephritis and nitrogen retention, epilepsy, heart failure, migraine, or any conditions in which a rapid addition to extracellular water could be hazardous.

Monitor: In addition to management of airway, oxygenation, and blood gas determinations, the continuous monitoring of ECG, vital signs, and fluid and electrolyte status is mandatory. ▪ Monitor IV site very closely, especially if it is a peripheral site; a central venous catheter is preferred. Produces intense vasoconstriction. Avoid extravasation; vasoconstriction that may result in severe tissue necrosis and gangrene can occur. ▪ Maintain adequate fluid intake to avoid ischemia of other organs. ▪ Use of vasopressin in vasodilatory shock may permit reduction or discontinuation of other vasopressors. ▪ Use an indwelling urinary catheter to confirm urine output and monitor closely. ▪ Fluid restriction may be indicated; initial signs of water intoxication include drowsiness, listlessness, and headache, which can rapidly progress to terminal coma and convulsions. ▪ See Rate of Administration, Precautions, and Drug/Lab Interactions.

Maternal/Child: Category C: safety for use during pregnancy not established; use only if clearly needed. ▪ Safety for use during breast-feeding not established. ▪ Safety and effectiveness for use in pediatric patients not established; however, it has been used successfully in selected critically ill pediatric patients with catecholamine-resistant hypotension.

Elderly: See Precautions; elderly may be more sensitive to adverse effects.

DRUG/LAB INTERACTIONS

Vasodilators (e.g., nitroglycerin, nitroprusside sodium) counteract the vasoconstrictive effects of vasopressin. ▪ Additive pressor response with **ganglionic blocking agents** (e.g., trimethaphan [Arfonad (rarely used antihypertensive)]). ▪ Antidiuretic effect may be increased with concurrent use of **carbamazepine** (Tegretol), **chlorpropamide** (Diabinese), **clofibrate** (Atromid-S), **fludrocortisone** (Florinef), **tricyclic antidepressants** (e.g., amitriptyline [Elavil]), **urea.** ▪ Antidiuretic effect may be decreased with concurrent use of **alcohol, demeclocycline** (Declomycin), **heparin, lithium** (Carbolith), **norepinephrine** (Levophed).

SIDE EFFECTS

Arrhythmias, bradycardia, hypertension, and MI have resulted from high doses. Abdominal cramps, angina, arrhythmias, bronchial constriction, cardiac arrest, circumoral pallor, cutaneous gangrene, decreased cardiac output, diaphoresis, flatus, gangrene, headache (pounding), hypersensitivity reactions (including anaphylaxis), hyponatremia, injection site ischemia resulting in severe tissue necrosis and gangrene, ischemic skin and mucous membrane lesions, myocardial ischemia, nausea, organ ischemia (e.g., GI, kidney), peripheral vasoconstriction, shock, sweating, tremor, urticaria, venous thrombosis, vertigo, and vomiting.

Overdose: Water intoxication.

ANTIDOTE

In an emergency cardiac care situation, all side effects can present life-threatening additional problems. Monitor the patient closely and observe all S/S that may indicate further deterioration. Treat symptomatically according to AHA guidelines. Monitor fluid intake and urine output to ensure adequate hydration. Extravasation and/or ischemia at the injection site should be reported immediately to prevent tissue necrosis and gangrene. If water intoxication should occur, treat with water restriction and discontinue vasopressin. If possible, discontinue gradually as described in Rate of Administration to prevent a rapid fall in BP. If severe, may require osmotic diuresis with mannitol, hypertonic dextrose, or urea alone or with furosemide (Lasix).

VECURONIUM BROMIDE BBW

(veh-kyour-**OH**-nee-um **BRO**-myd)

Neuromuscular blocking agent
(nondepolarizing)
Anesthesia adjunct

Norcuron ♣   pH 4

USUAL DOSE

Adjunct to general anesthesia: Must be individualized, depending on previous drugs administered and degree and length of muscle relaxation required. 0.08 to 0.1 mg/kg (80 to 100 mcg/kg) of body weight initially as an IV bolus. Must be used with adequate anesthesia and/or sedation and after unconsciousness induced. One source suggests using IBW for obese patients (equal to or greater than 30% of IBW). Determine need for *maintenance dose* based on beginning symptoms of neuromuscular blockade reversal determined by a peripheral nerve stimulator. *IV bolus injection:* 0.01 to 0.015 mg/kg (10 to 15 mcg/kg) will be required in approximately 25 to 40 minutes and every 12 to 20 minutes thereafter to maintain muscle relaxation. Higher doses (0.15 to 0.28 mg/kg) at longer intervals have been given with proper ventilation without causing adverse cardiac effects. *Continuous infusion:* 1 mcg/kg/min. Begin in 20 to 40 minutes after initial bolus dose.

Support of intubated, mechanically ventilated, or respiratory-controlled adult ICU patients (unlabeled): *IV bolus injection:* 0.1 to 0.2 mg/kg (100 to 200 mcg/kg) every 1 hour. *Continuous infusion:* Begin with a loading dose of 0.1 mg/kg (100 mcg/kg) followed by a *maintenance dose* of 0.05 to 0.1 mg/kg/hr (50 to 100 mcg/kg/hr). A lower-end or reduced dose may be indicated if administered more than 5 minutes after the start of an inhalation agent, when steady-state has been achieved, or in patients with organ dysfunction (e.g., impaired liver function). Adjust dose according to clinical assessment of the patient's response. Use of a peripheral nerve stimulator is recommended. Vecuronium may be the preferred agent for patients with renal failure.

PEDIATRIC DOSE

Adjunct to general anesthesia: 1 to 10 years of age: May require high end of initial adult dose, and maintenance dose may be required on a more frequent basis.

DOSE ADJUSTMENTS

Reduce dose by 15% if administered more than 5 minutes after inhalation general anesthetics. ▪ Reduce dose to 0.04 to 0.06 mg/kg if following succinylcholine administration. Succinylcholine must show signs of wearing off before vecuronium is given. Use caution. ▪ Reduced dose required with numerous drugs; see Drug/Lab Interactions. ▪ Reduced dose may be required in renal or hepatic impairment. Preparation by dialysis before surgery is recommended for patients with renal failure. In an emergency surgery when dialysis cannot be accomplished, consider a lower initial dose. ▪ Infants between 7 weeks and 1 year may require a slightly lower dose, and recovery time will be extended.

DILUTION

Each 10 mg must be diluted with 5 mL SWFI (supplied). May be given by IV injection or 10 (20) mg may be further diluted in up to 100 mL NS, D5W, D5NS, or LR and given as an infusion of 0.1 (0.2) mg/mL concentration. Titrated to symptoms of neuromuscular blockade reversal.

Storage: Stable at room temperature before reconstitution. Store under refrigeration. Discard after 24 hours except if reconstituted with bacteriostatic water; stable refrigerated up to 5 days.

COMPATIBILITY   (Underline Indicates Conflicting Compatibility Information)

Consider any drug NOT listed as compatible to be INCOMPATIBLE until consulting a pharmacist; specific conditions may apply.

Manufacturer states, "Has an acid pH. Reconstituted vecuronium should not be mixed with alkaline solutions (e.g., barbiturates) in the same syringe or administered simultaneously during IV infusion through the same needle or the same IV line."

One source suggests the following **compatibilities:**

Additive: Ciprofloxacin (Cipro IV).

Y-site: Alprostadil, aminophylline, amiodarone (Nexterone), cefazolin (Ancef), cefuroxime (Zinacef), dexmedetomidine (Precedex), diltiazem (Cardizem), dobutamine, dopamine, epinephrine (Adrenalin), esmolol (Brevibloc), fenoldopam (Corlopam), fentanyl, fluconazole (Diflucan), gentamicin, heparin, hetastarch in electrolytes (Hextend), hydrocortisone sodium succinate (Solu-Cortef), hydromorphone (Dilaudid), isoproterenol (Isuprel), labetalol, linezolid (Zyvox), lorazepam (Ativan), midazolam (Versed), milrinone (Primacor), morphine, nicardipine (Cardene IV), nitroglycerin IV, nitroprusside sodium, norepinephrine (Levophed), palonosetron (Aloxi), propofol (Diprivan), ranitidine (Zantac), sulfamethoxazole/trimethoprim, vancomycin.

RATE OF ADMINISTRATION

Adjunct to general anesthesia: A single dose as an IV bolus over 30 to 60 seconds. If maintenance dose is given as an infusion, adjust rate to specific dose desired, usually 1 mcg/kg/min. See the following chart.

Vecuronium Guidelines for Infusion During General Anesthesia		
Desired Vecuronium Delivery Rate (mcg/kg/min)	Vecuronium Infusion Delivery Rate (mL/kg/min)	
	0.1 mg/mL*	0.2 mg/mL†
0.7 mcg/kg/min	0.007 mL/kg/min	0.0035 mL/kg/min
0.8 mcg/kg/min	0.008 mL/kg/min	0.0040 mL/kg/min
0.9 mcg/kg/min	0.009 mL/kg/min	0.0045 mL/kg/min
1.0 mcg/kg/min	0.010 mL/kg/min	0.0050 mL/kg/min
1.1 mcg/kg/min	0.011 mL/kg/min	0.0055 mL/kg/min
1.2 mcg/kg/min	0.012 mL/kg/min	0.0060 mL/kg/min
1.3 mcg/kg/min	0.013 mL/kg/min	0.0065 mL/kg/min

*10 mg of vecuronium in 100 mL solution.
†20 mg of vecuronium in 100 mL solution.

Mechanical ventilation support in ICU: Dose must be calculated; the preceding chart is for use during general anesthesia only. See Usual Dose for specific rates and criteria.

ACTIONS

A nondepolarizing skeletal muscle relaxant about one-third more potent than pancuronium with a shorter duration of neuromuscular blockade. Acts by competing for cholinergic receptors at the motor end plate. Onset of action is within 30 seconds, is dose dependent, produces maximum neuromuscular blockade (paralysis) within 3 to 5 minutes, and lasts about 25 minutes. It may take up to 60 minutes or more before complete recovery occurs. Up to three times the therapeutic dose has been given without significant changes of hemodynamic parameters in good-risk surgical patients. Excreted as metabolites in bile and urine. Crosses the placental barrier.

INDICATIONS AND USES

Adjunctive to general anesthesia, to facilitate endotracheal intubation and to relax skeletal muscles during surgery or mechanical ventilation.

Unlabeled uses: Support of intubated, mechanically ventilated, or respiratory-controlled patients in ICU.

CONTRAINDICATIONS

Known hypersensitivity to vecuronium.

PRECAUTIONS

For IV use only. ■ Administered by or under the direct observation of the anesthesiologist. ■ Appropriate emergency drugs and equipment for monitoring the patient and responding to any medical emergency must be readily available. ■ Repeated doses have no cumulative effect if recovery is allowed to begin before administration. ■ Use extreme caution in patients with cirrhosis, cholestasis, obesity, or circulatory insufficiency. ■ Myasthenia gravis and other neuromuscular diseases increase sensitivity to drug. Can cause critical reactions. ■ Severe anaphylactic reactions have been reported with neuromuscular blocking agents; some have been fatal. Use caution in patients who have had an anaphylactic reaction to another neuromuscular blocking agent (depolarizing or nondepolarizing); cross-reactivity has occurred. ■ Acid-base and/or electrolyte imbalance, debilitation, hypoxic episodes, and/or the use of other drugs (e.g., broad-spectrum antibiotics, narcotics, steroids) may prolong the effects of vecuronium.
Monitor: *All uses:* This drug produces apnea. Controlled artificial ventilation with oxygen must be continuous and under direct observation at all times. Maintain a patent airway. ■ Use a peripheral nerve stimulator to monitor response to vecuronium and avoid overdose. Have reversal agents available (e.g., edrophonium, neostigmine, pyridostigmine with atropine or glycopyrrolate); see Antidote. ■ Patient may be conscious and completely unable to communicate by any means. Has no analgesic or sedative properties. Respiratory depression with morphine may be preferred in some patients requiring mechanical ventilation. ■ Action is altered by dehydration, electrolyte imbalance, body temperatures, and acid-base imbalance. ■ Recovery time extended in infants 7 weeks to 1 year. ■ See Drug/Lab Interactions. *Mechanical ventilation support in ICU:* Physical therapy is recommended to prevent muscular weakness, atrophy, and joint contracture. Muscular weakness may be first noticed during attempts to wean patients from the ventilator.
Maternal/Child: Category C: use in pregnancy only if use justifies potential risk to fetus. Has been used during cesarean section; monitor infant carefully. Action may be enhanced by magnesium administered for the management of toxemia of pregnancy. ■ Use caution during breast-feeding. ■ Safety for use in infants under 7 weeks of age not established. ■ Some preparations contain benzyl alcohol; do not use in premature infants. ■ See Dose Adjustments.
Elderly: Differences in response compared to younger adults not observed. Lower-end initial doses may be appropriate based on the potential for decreased organ function and concomitant disease or drug therapy. ■ Duration of neuromuscular block may be prolonged.

DRUG/LAB INTERACTIONS

Potentiated by **acidosis, hypokalemia, some carcinomas, general anesthetics** (e.g., enflurane, isoflurane, halothane), **many antibiotics** (e.g., clindamycin [Cleocin]), **aminoglycosides** (e.g., kanamycin, gentamicin), **polypeptide antibiotics** (e.g., bacitracin, colistimethate), **tetracyclines, diuretics, diazepam** (Valium) **and other muscle relaxants, magnesium sulfate, quinidine, morphine, meperidine, succinylcholine, verapamil, and others.** May need to reduce dose of vecuronium. Use with caution. ■ Effects may be decreased by **acetylcholine, alkalosis, anticholinesterases, azathioprine, carbamazepine, phenytoin, and theophylline.** ■ **Succinylcholine** must show signs of wearing off before vecuronium is given. Use caution.

SIDE EFFECTS

No side effects have occurred except with overdose: prolonged action resulting in respiratory insufficiency or apnea, airway closure caused by relaxation of epiglottis, pharynx, and tongue muscles. Hypersensitivity reactions including anaphylaxis are possible. Muscular weakness and atrophy may occur with long-term use (1 to 3 weeks).

ANTIDOTE

All side effects are medical emergencies. Treat symptomatically. Controlled artificial ventilation must be continuous until full muscle control returns. Edrophonium (Enlon), pyridostigmine (Regonol), or neostigmine given with atropine or glycopyrrolate will probably reverse the muscle relaxation but should not be required because of short time of effectiveness. Not effective in all situations; may aggravate severe overdose. Resuscitate as necessary.

VEDOLIZUMAB

Integrin receptor antagonist
Monoclonal antibody

Entyvio

pH 6.3

USUAL DOSE

Before initiating treatment with vedolizumab, patients should be brought up-to-date with all immunizations.

300 mg as an IV infusion over 30 minutes at 0, 2, and 6 weeks and then every 8 weeks thereafter. Discontinue in patients who show no evidence of therapeutic benefit by Week 14. Consider pretreatment with standard medical therapy in patients who experience mild to moderate infusion-related reactions or hypersensitivity reactions; see Antidote.

DOSE ADJUSTMENTS

No dose adjustments indicated. ▪ Pharmacokinetics in patients with renal or hepatic insufficiency has not been studied.

DILUTION

Available as a lyophilized powder in a 20-mL, single-use vial containing 300 mg. Bring vial to room temperature before reconstitution. Reconstitute with 4.8 mL SWFI using a syringe with a 21- to 25-gauge needle. Direct the SWFI to the glass wall of the vial to avoid excessive foaming. Gently swirl the vial for at least 15 seconds to dissolve the powder. *Do not vigorously shake or invert.* Allow solution to sit for up to 20 minutes. May be gently swirled. If not fully dissolved, allow another 10 minutes. Do not use if not fully dissolved within 30 minutes. Solution should be clear or opalescent, colorless to light brownish yellow. Before withdrawing the reconstituted solution, gently invert the vial 3 times. Using a syringe with a 21- to 25-gauge needle, withdraw 5 mL (300 mg) from the vial and add to an infusion bag or bottle containing 250 mL of NS.

Filters: Specific information not available.

Storage: Refrigerate unopened vials at 2° to 8° C (36° to 46° F). Retain in original package to protect from light. Immediate use after reconstitution and dilution is preferred; however, the infusion solution may be refrigerated for up to 4 hours. Do not freeze. Discard any unused portion.

COMPATIBILITY

Manufacturer states, "Do not add other medicinal products to the prepared infusion solution or intravenous infusion set."

RATE OF ADMINISTRATION

Do not administer as an IV push or bolus; for IV infusion only.

Administer a single dose (300 mg) as an IV infusion equally distributed over 30 minutes.

Flush line before the infusion and after infusion is complete with 30 mL of NS.

ACTIONS

A recombinant humanized monoclonal antibody, vedolizumab is an integrin receptor antagonist. It specifically binds to the $\alpha 4\beta 7$ integrin and blocks the interaction of $\alpha 4\beta 7$ integrin with mucosal addressin cell adhesion molecule-1 (MAdCAM-1) and inhibits the migration of memory T-lymphocytes across the endothelium into inflamed gastrointestinal parenchymal tissue. Does not bind to or inhibit function of the $\alpha 4\beta 1$ and $\alpha E\beta 7$ integrins and does not antagonize the interaction of $\alpha 4$ integrins with vascular cell adhesion molecule-1 (VCAM-1). The interaction of the $\alpha 4\beta 7$ integrin with MAdCAM-1 has been implicated as an important contributor to the chronic inflammation that is a hallmark of ulcerative colitis and Crohn's disease. A reduction in GI inflammation has been observed in rectal biopsy specimens. Clearance depends on both linear and nonlinear pathways. Serum half-life is approximately 25 days.

INDICATIONS AND USES

Treatment of adults with moderate to severe ulcerative colitis (UC) to induce and maintain clinical response and clinical remission, improve the endoscopic appearance of the mucosa, and achieve corticosteroid-free remission. ▪ Treatment of adults with moderate to severe Crohn's disease (CD) to achieve clinical response and clinical remission and corticosteroid-free remission. ▪ Indicated in adults with UC and CD who have had an inadequate response to, lost response to, or were intolerant of a tumor necrosis factor (TNF) blocker or immunomodulator or who had an inadequate response to, were intolerant of, or demonstrated dependence on corticosteroids.

CONTRAINDICATIONS

Known serious or severe hypersensitivity reaction to vedolizumab or any of its excipients.

PRECAUTIONS

Do not administer as an IV push or bolus; for IV infusion only ▪ Administered under the direction of a physician knowledgeable in its use in a facility with adequate diagnostic and treatment facilities to monitor the patient and respond to any medical emergency. ▪ Has been associated with infusion-related reactions and hypersensitivity reactions, including anaphylaxis. Reactions may occur during or several hours after the infusion. ▪ Effects on the immune system may increase the risk of infection, including opportunistic infection. ▪ Not recommended for patients with active, severe infections until the infections are controlled. ▪ Use caution in patients with a history of recurring severe infections. Consider screening for tuberculosis (TB). ▪ Progressive multifocal leukoencephalopathy (PML) has been reported with another integrin receptor antagonist; see Monitor. ▪ Elevations of transaminase and/or bilirubin have occurred. May be a predictor of severe liver injury that may lead to death or the need for a liver transplant; see Monitor. ▪ Update all vaccinations before initiating treatment with vedolizumab. Non–live virus vaccines (e.g., influenza) may be administered if indicated. No data on the secondary transmission of infection by live virus vaccines. ▪ Anti-vedolizumab antibodies may develop and should be considered if there is an inadequate response or a reduced therapeutic effect to treatment.

Monitor: Monitor for S/S of a hypersensitivity reaction (e.g., bronchospasm, dyspnea, hypertension, rash, tightness of the chest, urticaria, wheezing) during the infusion and for several hours after completion. ▪ Assess neurologic status frequently. S/S associated with PML are diverse and occur over days to weeks. May include progressive weakness on one side of the body, clumsiness of the limbs, disturbances of vision, or changes in thinking, memory, and orientation leading to confusion and personality changes. Progression of deficits usually leads to severe disability or death over weeks to months. Withhold vedolizumab if PML is suspected; consultation with a neurologist is indicated. If PML is confirmed, discontinue vedolizumab permanently. ▪ Monitor for S/S of liver injury (e.g., elevated bilirubin, elevated liver function tests, jaundice). Discontinue vedolizumab in patients with jaundice or other evidence of significant liver injury. ▪ Monitor for S/S of infection.

Patient Education: Read medication guide carefully. ▪ Review medical conditions and medications with health care provider before beginning treatment. ▪ Promptly report any new medical problems (e.g., new or sudden change in thinking, eyesight, balance, or strength). ▪ Report infections. ▪ Report jaundice and any symptoms of infusion or hypersensitivity reactions immediately (e.g., difficulty breathing, dizziness, feeling faint, itching, nausea). ▪ Discuss potential risks and benefits of treatment (e.g., risk of PML).

Maternal/Child: Category B: use during pregnancy only if the benefits to the mother outweigh the risk to the fetus. A pregnancy exposure registry has been created. Contact manufacturer for information. ▪ Not known if vedolizumab is secreted in human milk; use caution if required during breast-feeding. ▪ Safety and effectiveness for use in pediatric patients not established.

Elderly: Safety and effectiveness similar to that seen in younger adults.

DRUG/LAB INTERACTIONS

Because of the potential for increased risk of PML and other infections, avoid the concomitant use of vedolizumab with **natalizumab** (Tysabri). ▪ Because of the increased risk of infections, avoid the concomitant use of vedolizumab with **TNF blockers** (e.g., infliximab [Remicade]). ▪ Benefits must outweigh risks if **live virus vaccines** are to be administered concurrently with vedolizumab; see Precautions. ▪ Prior treatment with **TNF blockers** (e.g., infliximab [Remicade]), coadministered **immunomodulators** (including azathioprine, 6-mercaptopurine, methotrexate), and coadministered **aminosalicylates** did not have a clinically meaningful effect on the pharmacokinetics of vedolizumab.

SIDE EFFECTS

Arthralgia, back pain, bronchitis, cough, fatigue, fever, headache, influenza, nasopharyngitis, nausea, oropharyngeal pain, pain in extremities, pruritus, rash, sinusitis, and upper respiratory tract infection are most common. Infusion-related reactions and hypersensitivity reactions, including anaphylaxis, have occurred. Other serious side effects include liver injury (e.g., hepatitis), PML, and serious infections such as anal abscess, cytomegaloviral colitis, giardiasis, Listeria meningitis, salmonella sepsis, sepsis (some fatal), and tuberculosis.

ANTIDOTE

Keep physician informed of all side effects. Most will be treated symptomatically. Discontinue vedolizumab at the first sign of liver injury. Discontinue infusion if any S/S of a serious hypersensitivity or infusion reaction occur. Treat with epinephrine, corticosteroids, diphenhydramine, bronchodilators, and oxygen as indicated. In clinical trials, patients with mild to moderate infusion-related reactions or hypersensitivity reactions were pretreated with standard medical therapy (e.g., acetaminophen, antihistamines, and/or hydrocortisone) before the next infusion. Withhold vedolizumab if S/S suggestive of PML occur; if diagnosis is confirmed, discontinue permanently. Consider withholding vedolizumab if a severe infection occurs.

VERAPAMIL HYDROCHLORIDE

(ver-**AP**-ah-mil hy-droh-**KLOR**-eyed)

Calcium channel blocker
Antiarrhythmic

pH 4.1 to 6

USUAL DOSE

5 to 10 mg initially (0.075 to 0.15 mg/kg of body weight). May cause transient bradycardia or hypotension. 10 mg (0.15 mg/kg) may be repeated in 30 minutes if needed to achieve appropriate response. Maximum total dose is 20 mg. AHA recommendation is 2.5 to 5 mg as an initial dose. Repeat 5 to 10 mg if needed every 15 to 30 min. Maximum dose 20 mg. Alternately, give 5 mg every 15 min to a total dose of 30 mg.

PEDIATRIC DOSE

ECG and BP monitoring mandatory. See Maternal/Child.

Infants up to 1 year of age: 0.1 to 0.2 mg/kg of body weight (usually 0.75 to 2 mg). Repeat in 30 minutes if indicated.

1 to 15 years of age: 0.1 to 0.3 mg/kg (usually 2 to 5 mg). Do not exceed 5 mg. Repeat in 30 minutes if response not adequate. Repeat dose should not exceed 10 mg as a single dose.

DOSE ADJUSTMENTS

Reduced dose may be required in hepatic or renal disease, especially with repeat dosing. ▪ Dose selection should be cautious in the elderly. Reduced doses may be indicated based on the potential for decreased organ function and concomitant disease or drug therapy. ▪ See Drug/Lab Interactions.

DILUTION

IV injection: May be given undiluted through Y-tube or three-way stopcock of tubing containing D5W, NS, or Ringer's solution for infusion.

Filters: No data available from manufacturer.

Storage: Store between 15° and 30° C (59° and 86° F). Protect from light and freezing. Do not use if discolored or particulate matter present. Discard unused solution.

COMPATIBILITY   (Underline Indicates Conflicting Compatibility Information)

Consider any drug NOT listed as compatible to be INCOMPATIBLE until consulting a pharmacist; specific conditions may apply.

Manufacturer states, "Not recommended for dilution with sodium lactate in polyvinyl chloride bags. Will precipitate in any solution with a pH greater than 6." Lists as **incompatible** with albumin, amphotericin B (conventional), hydralazine, sulfamethoxazole/trimethoprim.

One source suggests the following **compatibilities:**

Additive: Amikacin, amiodarone (Nexterone), ampicillin, ascorbic acid, atropine, calcium chloride, calcium gluconate, cefazolin (Ancef), cefotaxime (Claforan), cefoxitin (Mefoxin), chloramphenicol (Chloromycetin), clindamycin (Cleocin), dexamethasone (Decadron), dextran 40, diazepam (Valium), digoxin (Lanoxin), dobutamine, dopamine, epinephrine (Adrenalin), erythromycin (Erythrocin), furosemide (Lasix), gentamicin, heparin, hydrocortisone sodium succinate (Solu-Cortef), hydromorphone (Dilaudid), isoproterenol (Isuprel), lidocaine, magnesium sulfate, mannitol, meperidine (Demerol), methyldopate, methylprednisolone (Solu-Medrol), metoclopramide (Reglan), morphine, multivitamins (M.V.I.), nafcillin (Nallpen), naloxone, nitroglycerin IV, nitroprusside sodium, norepinephrine (Levophed), oxacillin (Bactocill), oxytocin (Pitocin), pancuronium, penicillin G potassium and sodium, pentobarbital (Nembutal), phenobarbital (Luminal), phentolamine (Regitine), phenytoin (Dilantin), potassium chloride (KCl), potassium phosphates, procainamide (Pronestyl), propranolol, protamine sulfate, quinidine gluconate, sodium bicarbonate, theophylline, tobramycin, vancomycin, vasopressin.

Y-site: Argatroban, bivalirudin (Angiomax), ciprofloxacin (Cipro IV), dexmedetomidine (Precedex), dobutamine, dopamine, famotidine (Pepcid IV), fenoldopam (Corlopam), hetastarch in electrolytes (Hextend), hydralazine, linezolid (Zyvox), meperidine (Demerol), milrinone (Primacor), nesiritide (Natrecor), oxaliplatin (Eloxatin), penicillin G potassium.

RATE OF ADMINISTRATION

IV injection: A single dose over a minimum of 2 minutes for adults and pediatric patients. Extend to 3 minutes in the elderly.

ACTIONS

A calcium (and possibly sodium) ion inhibitor through slow channels into conductile and contractile myocardial cells and vascular smooth muscle cells. Slows conduction through SA and AV nodes, prolongs effective refractory period in the AV node, and reduces ventricular rates. Prevents re-entry phenomena through the AV node. Reduces myocardial contractility, afterload, arterial pressure, vascular tone, and oxygen demand. Effective within 1 to 5 minutes. Hemodynamic effects last about 20 minutes, but antiarrhythmic effects may last up to 6 hours. Does not alter total serum calcium levels. Metabolized in the liver. Half-life range is 2 to 5 hours. Crosses the placental barrier. Excreted in urine and feces. Secreted in breast milk.

INDICATIONS AND USES

Treatment of supraventricular tachyarrhythmias including conversion to normal sinus rhythm of paroxysmal supraventricular tachycardia (includes Wolff-Parkinson-White and Lown-Ganong-Levine syndromes). ▪ Temporary control of rapid ventricular rate in atrial flutter or atrial fibrillation.

Unlabeled uses: Alternative drug after adenosine to terminate re-entry SVT with narrow QRS complex and adequate BP and preserved LV function (AHA guidelines).

CONTRAINDICATIONS

SA nodal function impairment or atrial fibrillation or flutter when associated with an accessory bypass tract (e.g., Wolff-Parkinson-White or Lown-Ganong-Levine syndromes), cardiogenic shock, congestive heart failure (severe) unless secondary to supraventricular tachyarrhythmia treatable with verapamil, known hypersensitivity to verapamil, second- or third-degree AV block (unless functioning artificial pacemaker is in place), severe hypotension, sick sinus syndrome (unless functioning artificial pacemaker in place), patients receiving IV beta-adrenergic blocking drugs (e.g., propranolol) within a few hours, and ventricular tachycardia.

PRECAUTIONS

Administer in a facility with adequate personnel, equipment, and supplies to monitor the patient and respond to any medical emergency. ▪ Valsalva maneuver recommended before use of verapamil in all paroxysmal supraventricular tachycardias if clinically appropriate. ▪ May produce hypotension. Usually transient and asymptomatic, but can cause dizziness. ▪ Has rarely caused second- and third-degree AV block and, in extreme cases, asystole. ▪ Caution required in hepatic and renal disease, especially if repeated dosing is required. ▪ Use extreme caution in patients with hypertrophic cardiomyopathy. ▪ May cause ventricular fibrillation in patients with wide-complex ventricular tachycardia. ▪ May precipitate respiratory muscle failure in patients with muscular dystrophy or increase intracranial pressure during anesthesia induction in patients with supratentorial tumors. Use caution and monitor closely. ▪ Use with caution in patients with severe aortic stenosis and acute MI with pulmonary congestion documented by x-ray. ▪ Reduction of myocardial contractility may worsen CHF in patients with severe left ventricular dysfunction. ▪ Continue regular dosing on day of surgery and thereafter unless otherwise specified by physician. May cause severe angina or MI if discontinued. ▪ Recent studies indicate that verapamil inhibits thrombus formation and platelet aggregation.

Monitor: Continuous ECG and BP monitoring recommended. ▪ Document cardiac rhythm before therapy, with any significant change in type or rate, and at least every 4 hours. See PR interval. ▪ Monitor BP and HR very closely, every 5 minutes times 3 or until reasonably stabilized, every 15 minutes times 4, and hourly thereafter. May need more frequent checks with increased drip rate. ▪ Emergency resuscitation drugs and equipment must always be available. ▪ When heart failure is not severe or rate related, it should be controlled with digoxin and diuretics before using verapamil. ▪ Patients with pulmonary wedge pressure above 20 mm Hg and/or ejection fraction below 30% may experience acute worsening of heart failure. ▪ Maintain bed rest until effects on HR, BP, and potential dizziness are evaluated. ▪ Monitor for side effects (AV block) and digoxin levels when used concurrently with digoxin. ▪ Monitor for any unusual bleeding or bruising. ▪ See Drug/Lab Interactions.

Maternal/Child: Category C: safety for use in pregnancy not yet established; use only when clearly indicated. ▪ Discontinue breast-feeding. ▪ Controlled studies have not been conducted in pediatric patients. Severe hemodynamic side effects (e.g., bradycardia, hypotension, or a rapid ventricular rate in atrial flutter/fibrillation) can occur in infants and neonates. Use caution and monitor closely.

Elderly: May have an increased hypotensive effect; see Rate of Administration. ▪ Half-life may be prolonged; see Dose Adjustments. ▪ May cause drug-induced tinnitus.

DRUG/LAB INTERACTIONS

Potentiates **digoxin;** lower dose may be appropriate. Both drugs slow AV conduction. Monitor for AV block and bradycardia. ▪ Do not give comcomitantly (within a few hours) with **IV beta-adrenergic blocking drugs** (e.g., propranolol); see Contraindications. Use with extreme caution with **oral or ophthalmic beta blockers.** Both drugs depress myocardial contractility and AV node conduction; monitor patient closely. ▪ Do not administer **disopyramide** (Norpace) within 48 hours before or 24 hours after verapamil. ▪ Use caution with **inhalation anesthetics.** Both depress cardiovascular activity. Titrate each carefully to avoid excessive cardiovascular depression. ▪ Coadministration with **amiodarone**

(Nexterone) may result in bradycardia and decreased cardiac output. Monitor closely. ▪ Potentiates **cyclosporine, carbamazepine, and theophyllines.** Monitor serum levels of these drugs and adjust dose as needed. ▪ Potentiates **nondepolarizing muscle relaxants** (e.g., vecuronium); dose reduction of either drug may be required. ▪ Metabolism may be decreased and serum concentrations may be increased by **itraconazole** (Sporanox). ▪ Verapamil may increase serum concentrations of **dofetilide** (Tikosyn). One source says avoid use; another says concurrent use contraindicated. ▪ Verapamil may increase serum concentrations of **HMG-CoA reductase inhibitors** (e.g., atorvastatin [Lipitor], simvastatin [Zocor]), **imipramine** (Tofranil), **prazosin** (Minipress), **sirolimus** (Rapamune), **tacrolimus** (Prograf). Monitor serum levels and/or monitor for S/S of toxicity; adjust dose as needed. ▪ Concomitant use of **HMG-CoA reductase inhibitors** (e.g., atorvastatin [Lipitor], lovastatin [Mevacor], simvastatin [Zocor]) has been associated with reports of myopathy and rhabdomyolysis. In patients receiving verapamil, limit dose of simvastatin to 10 mg daily and limit lovastatin dose to 40 mg daily. Dose reductions for other HMG-CoA reductase inhibitors may also be required. ▪ May increase effects of certain **benzodiazepines** (e.g., midazolam [Versed], triazolam [Halcion]) and **buspirone** (BuSpar); monitor and adjust doses as indicated. ▪ May cause excessive hypotension with **other antihypertensive drugs** (vasodilators and diuretics). ▪ Serum concentrations and effectiveness of verapamil may be decreased by **barbiturates** (e.g., phenobarbital), **calcium salts, phenytoin** (Dilantin), **sulfinpyrazone** (Anturane). ▪ Concomitant use with **IV dantrolene** (Dantrium) may result in cardiovascular collapse. ▪ Use caution with **quinidine**; may cause hypotension. ▪ Hypotension and bradycardia have been observed with concurrent **telithromycin** (Ketek). ▪ Highly protein bound; use with caution with **other highly protein-bound drugs** (e.g., oral hypoglycemics, warfarin). ▪ Variable effects when administered with **lithium.** Has caused decreased effectiveness of lithium and may cause neurotoxicity. ▪ Monitor heart rate with concurrent use of verapamil with **clonidine;** has resulted in sinus bradycardia requiring pacemaker insertion. ▪ **Grapefruit juice** may affect certain enzymes of the P_{450} enzyme system and increase the serum concentrations of verapamil and should be avoided.

SIDE EFFECTS
Abdominal discomfort, asystole, bradycardia, dizziness, headache, second- and third-degree heart block, heart failure, hypersensitivity reactions (including anaphylaxis), rapid ventricular rate (Wolff-Parkinson-White and Lown-Ganong-Levine syndromes), hypotension (symptomatic), increased ventricular response in atrial flutter, nausea, PVCs, skin eruptions (including rare reports of erythema multiforme), tachycardia.

ANTIDOTE
Discontinue verapamil and notify physician promptly if hypotension, bradycardia, or second- or third-degree heart block occurs. Keep physician informed of all side effects. Treatment will depend on clinical situation. Calcium chloride may reverse effects of verapamil and can be used in toxicity. Glucagon may also be used in toxicity; see glucagon monograph. Rapid ventricular response in atrial flutter/fibrillation should respond to cardioversion, procainamide, and/or lidocaine. Treat bradycardia, AV block, and asystole with standard AHA protocol (atropine, pacing). Norepinephrine (Levarterenol) or dopamine will reverse hypotension. Treat hypersensitivity reactions or resuscitate as necessary. Not removed by hemodialysis.

VERTEPORFIN
(ver-teh-**POR**-fin)

Visudyne

Photosensitizing agent
Macular degeneration
therapy adjunct

USUAL DOSE

A course is a *two-stage process* requiring administration of both drug and light. Each course may be repeated every 3 months as indicated. Body surface area, lesion size determination, and spot size determination of the choroidal neovascularization (CNV) are used by the retina specialist to calculate dosing of verteporfin. The greatest linear dimension of the lesion is estimated by fluorescein angiography and color fundus photography. The treatment spot size should be 1,000 microns larger than the greatest linear dimension of the lesion on the retina to allow a 500-micron border. The nasal edge of the treatment spot must be positioned at least 200 microns from the temporal edge of the optic disc.

First stage: 6 mg/M^2 of verteporfin as a single IV infusion.

Second stage: Activation of verteporfin using a recommended light dose of 50 J/cm^2 of neovascular lesion administered at an intensity of 600 mW/cm^2 over 83 seconds. Initiate 689 ± 3 nm wavelength laser light delivery 15 minutes after the start of the verteporfin infusion. Light is delivered to the retina as a single circular spot via a fiber optic and a slit lamp, using a suitable ophthalmic magnification lens. Light dose, light intensity, ophthalmic lens magnification factor, and zoom lens setting are important parameters for the appropriate delivery of light to the predetermined treatment spot. Follow the laser system manuals for procedure setup and operation.

Concurrent bilateral treatment: In patients who present with eligible lesions in both eyes without prior verteporfin therapy, treat only one eye (the most aggressive lesion) during the first course. One week after the first course, if no significant safety issues are identified, the second eye can be treated, using the same treatment regimen including a verteporfin infusion and light activation. Approximately 3 months later, both eyes can be evaluated, and concurrent treatment following a new verteporfin infusion can be started if both lesions still show evidence of leakage. When treating both eyes concurrently, the more aggressive lesion should be treated first, at 15 minutes after the start of infusion. Immediately at the end of light application to the first eye, the laser settings should be adjusted to introduce the treatment parameters for the second eye, with the same light dose and intensity as for the first eye, starting no later than 20 minutes from the start of the infusion.

DOSE ADJUSTMENTS

No adjustments required. See Precautions.

DILUTION

Specific techniques required; see Precautions. Reconstitute each vial of verteporfin with 7 mL of SWFI to provide 7.5 mL of opaque, dark-green solution containing 2 mg/mL. Withdraw the desired dose from the vial and further dilute with D5W to a total infusion volume of 30 mL.

Filters: Use of a 1.2-micron in-line filter is required for administration.

Storage: Store between 20° and 25° C (68° and 77° F). Reconstituted and diluted solution must be protected from light and used within 4 hours.

COMPATIBILITY

Manufacturer states, "May precipitate in saline solutions. Do not use NS or other parenteral solutions. Do not mix in same solution with other drugs." Use only SWFI and D5W as listed under Dilution.

RATE OF ADMINISTRATION

A 30-mL infusion equally distributed over 10 minutes (3 mL/min) using an appropriate syringe pump and a 1.2-micron in-line filter.

ACTIONS

A light-activated drug (photosensitizing agent) for use in photodynamic therapy (PDT). Transported in the plasma by lipoproteins. Endothelial cells of the abnormal choroidal blood vessels, which have high concentrations of lipoprotein receptors, take up the lipoprotein-verteporfin complex. Light activation in the presence of O_2 induces a photochemical reaction, generating highly reactive singlet oxygen and reactive oxygen radicals that cause local damage to the neovascular endothelium. The damaged endothelium releases procoagulant and vasoactive factors through the lipo-oxygenase (leukotriene) and cyclo-oxygenase (eicosanoids such as thromboxane) pathways, resulting in platelet aggregation, fibrin clot formation, vasoconstriction, and ultimately, vessel occlusion. Verteporfin appears to preferentially accumulate in neovasculature, including chorioidal neovasculature. However, animal models indicate that the drug is also present in the retina. Therefore, there may be collateral damage to retinal structures following photoactivation. Terminal elimination half-life of verteporfin is 5 to 6 hours. It is metabolized to a small extent by liver and plasma esterases and is eliminated primarily by the fecal route as unchanged drug. May be secreted in breast milk.

INDICATIONS AND USES

Treatment of patients with predominantly classic subfoveal choroidal neovascularization due to age-related macular degeneration (AMD), pathologic myopia, or presumed ocular histoplasmosis. Slows retinal damage; does not reverse loss of vision in eyes damaged by AMD. ▪ Not recommended for use in treatment of predominantly occult subfoveal choroidal neovascularization; evidence insufficient.

CONTRAINDICATIONS

Patients with porphyria or a known hypersensitivity to any component of this preparation.

PRECAUTIONS

Use rubber gloves and eye protection during preparation and administration. Avoid any skin or eye contact since that area will become photosensitive. Wipe up spills with a damp cloth. Dispose of all contaminated materials in a polyethylene bag to avoid accidental contact by others. Protection from light will be necessary if accidental exposure or overexposure occurs. Note process in Patient Education. ▪ Administered by or under the direction of the physician specialist with appropriate knowledge of the selected laser system. Facilities for monitoring the patient and responding to any medical emergency must be available. ▪ Requires laser systems and a fiber-optic diffuser to activate. *Coherent Opal Photoactivator Laser Console and LaserLink Adapter, Zeiss VISULAS 690s laser and VISILINK PDT adapter, Ceralas I laser system and Ceralink Slit Lamp Adapter, and Quantel Activis laser console and the ZSL30 ACTTM, ZSL120 ACTTM, and HSBMBQ ACTTM slit lamp adapters* are the laser systems that have been tested for **compatibility** with verteporfin and are approved for delivery of a stable power output at a wavelength of 689 ± 3 nm. Use of **incompatible** lasers that do not provide the required characteristics of light could result in incomplete treatment due to partial photoactivation, overtreatment due to overactivation, or damage to surrounding normal tissue. ▪ Following verteporfin administration, care should be taken to avoid exposure of skin or eyes to direct sunlight or bright indoor light for 5 days. If emergency surgery is necessary within 48 hours after treatment, as much of the internal tissue as possible should be protected from intense light. ▪ Patients who experience severe decrease of vision of 4 lines or more within 1 week after treatment should not be retreated, at least until their vision completely recovers to pretreatment levels. Potential risk versus benefit of any subsequent treatment should be considered. ▪ Use with caution in patients with moderate to severe hepatic impairment or biliary obstruction, and in anesthetized patients. There is no clinical experience with these patient populations. ▪ Older patients, patients with dark irides, patients with occult lesions or patients with less than 50% classic CNV may be less likely to benefit from verteporfin therapy. ▪ Safety and efficacy of verteporfin beyond 2 years has not been demonstrated; however, it has been used up to 5 years in extension studies.

Monitor: Standard precautions should be taken to avoid extravasation (e.g., establish a free-flowing IV line in a large arm vein, preferably the antecubital vein). If extravasation occurs, the infusion should be stopped immediately and cold compresses applied. The extravasation area must be thoroughly protected from direct light until the swelling and discoloration have faded in order to prevent the occurrence of a local burn, which could be severe. Oral analgesics may be indicated. ▪ Monitor patient during infusion. Verteporfin has caused a concentration-dependent increase in complement activation in human blood in vitro. S/S consistent with complement activation (chest pain, dyspnea, flushing, syncope) have been reported. ▪ Patient should be re-evaluated every 3 months; if choroidal neovascular leakage is detected on fluorescein angiography, therapy should be repeated. ▪ See Usual Dose, Precautions, Patient Education, and Drug/Lab Interactions.

Patient Education: ▪ Must observe precautions to avoid exposure of skin and eyes to direct sunlight or bright indoor light for 5 days. Photosensitivity is due to residual drug, which is present in all parts of the skin. Ambient indoor light is beneficial as it gradually inactivates the remaining drug through a photobleaching reaction. Do not remain in a darkened room. Do expose skin to ambient indoor light. Avoid bright indoor light from examination lamps, dental lamps, operating room lamps, bright halogen lighting, and unshaded light bulbs. Limit time outdoors to necessary excursions and completely cover body with clothing and shade face before going out. Ultraviolet sunscreens are of no value because photoactivation is caused by visible light, not UV rays. Eyes will be sensitive to sun, bright lights, and car headlights; wear dark sunglasses with an average white light transmittance of less than 4%. ▪ Visual disturbances may develop and interfere with the ability to drive or operate machinery. Avoid these activities as long as visual symptoms persist.

Maternal/Child: Category C: use during pregnancy only if benefits justify potential risk to fetus. Effective contraception necessary for women of childbearing age. Has caused maternal and fetal toxicity in rats and rabbits. ▪ Discontinue breast-feeding. ▪ Safety and effectiveness for use in pediatric patients not established.

Elderly: Reduced treatment effect was seen with increasing age (75 years of age or older).

DRUG/LAB INTERACTIONS

Formal drug interaction studies have not been performed. Based on the mechanism of action of verteporfin, many drugs used concomitantly could influence the effect of verteporfin therapy. ▪ **Calcium channel blockers** (e.g., diltiazem [Cardizem], verapamil, nicardipine [Cardene]), **polymyxin B, or radiation therapy** could enhance the rate of verteporfin uptake by the vascular endothelium. ▪ Use with **other photosensitizing agents** (e.g., griseofulvin, phenothiazines [e.g., prochlorperazine (Compazine)], sulfonamides [sulfisoxazole (Gantrisin)], ophthalmic solutions (AK-Sulf)], sulfonylurea hypoglycemic agents [tolbutamide], tetracyclines [doxycycline], thiazide diuretics [chlorothiazide (Diuril)]) could increase the potential for a photosensitivity reaction. ▪ Compounds that quench active oxygen species or scavenge radicals (e.g., **dimethyl sulfoxide** [DMSO], **beta-carotene, ethanol, formate, mannitol**) would be expected to decrease verteporfin activity. ▪ Effectiveness may be reduced by **drugs that decrease clotting** (e.g., heparin, alteplase [tPA]), **vasoconstriction** (e.g., nicardipine [Cardene]) **or platelet aggregation** (e.g., clopidogrel [Plavix], dipyridamole [Persantine], ticlopidine [Ticlid]).

SIDE EFFECTS

The most frequently reported side effects are headache, injection site reactions (e.g., edema, extravasation, hemorrhage with discoloration, pain, and rashes), self-resolving photosensitivity, and visual disturbances (e.g., blurred vision, decreased visual acuity, and visual field defects). Less frequently reported side effects include abnormal white blood cell count (decreased or increased), albuminuria, anemia, arthralgia, arthrosis, asthenia, atrial fibrillation, back pain (primarily during infusion), blepharitis, cataracts, chest pain, conjunctivitis, constipation, decreased hearing, diplopia, dizziness, dry eyes, dyspnea, eczema, elevated liver function tests, eye hemorrhage (subconjunctival, subretinal, or vitreous), fever, flu-like syndrome, flushing, hyperesthesia, hypersensitivity reactions, hypertension, increased creatinine, lacrimation disorder, malaise, myasthenia, nausea, ocular itching, peripheral vascular disorder, pharyngitis, photosensitivity, pneumonia, prostatic disorder, pruritus, retinal detachment (nonrhegmatogenous), retinal or choroidal vessel nonperfusion, retinal pigment epithelial tear, severe vision loss (may be equivalent of 4 lines or more within 7 days of treatment and occur with or without subretinal/retinal or vitreous hemorrhage), sleep disturbance, sweating, syncope, urticaria, varicose veins, vasovagal reactions, and vertigo.

Overdose: Overdose of drug and/or light may result in nonperfusion of normal retinal vessels with the possibility of severe decrease in vision that could be permanent. May also result in prolongation of the time during which the patient will be photosensitive.

ANTIDOTE
Keep the physician informed of all side effects; most will be treated symptomatically. In the event of an overdose of drug and/or light, extend the photosensitivity precautions for a time proportional to the overdose.

VINBLASTINE SULFATE BBW
(vin-**BLAS**-teen **SUL**-fayt)

VLB

Antineoplastic
(mitotic inhibitor-vinca alkaloid)

pH 3.5 to 5

USUAL DOSE
Auxiliary labeling required; see Precautions.

3.7 mg/M^2 initially. Administered once every 7 days, increasing the dose to specific amounts (5.5, 7.4, 9.25, 11.1 mg/M^2) by a single step each week until the WBC count is decreased to 3,000 cells/mm^3, remission is achieved, or a maximum dose of 18.5 mg/M^2 is reached. Maintenance dose is one step below any dose that causes leukopenia (3,000 cells/mm^3 or less), once every 7 to 14 days. Usually 5.5 to 7.4 mg/M^2. Continue treatment for 4 to 6 weeks. Up to 12 weeks often necessary.

PEDIATRIC DOSE
See Maternal/Child.

One source suggests 2.5 mg/M^2 initially. Use same procedure as for adult dose using steps to 3.75, 5, 6.25, and 7.5 mg/M^2. Maximum dose is 12.5 mg/M^2. Maintenance dose is calculated by same parameters as Usual Dose (above). Usually differs with each individual. Other sources suggest that initial doses vary depending on the schedule used, use of vinblastine as a single agent, or its use in a combination regimen. Some suggested doses are:

Letterer-Siwe disease (unlabeled): As a single agent, an initial dose of 6.5 mg/M^2.

Hodgkin's disease: An initial dose of 6 mg/M^2 in combination with other chemotherapeutic agents.

Testicular cancer: An initial dose of 3 mg/M^2 in combination with other chemotherapeutic agents.

DOSE ADJUSTMENTS
Reduce dose by 50% if serum bilirubin above 3 mg/dL. ▪ Often used with other antineoplastic drugs and corticosteroids in reduced doses and/or extended intervals to achieve tumor remission.

DILUTION
Specific techniques required; see Precautions. Each 10 mg is diluted with 10 mL of NS for injection. 1 mg equals 1 mL. Also available in liquid form (1 mg/mL). May be given by IV injection or through Y-tube or three-way stopcock of a free-flowing IV infusion.

Storage: Store in refrigerator before and after dilution. Potency maintained for 28 days after dilution if reconstituted with bacteriostatic NS.

U-Z

COMPATIBILITY

Consider any drug NOT listed as compatible to be INCOMPATIBLE until consulting a pharmacist; specific conditions may apply.
Manufacturer suggests that the pH not be altered from between 3.5 to 5 by an additive or a diluent, and it recommends NS as a diluent and not admixing with other drugs in the same container.

One source suggests the following **compatibilities:**
Additive: *Not recommended by manufacturer.* Bleomycin (Blenoxane).
Y-site: Allopurinol (Aloprim), amifostine (Ethyol), amphotericin B cholesteryl (Amphotec), aztreonam (Azactam), bleomycin (Blenoxane), cisplatin, cyclophosphamide (Cytoxan), doxorubicin (Adriamycin), doxorubicin liposomal (Doxil), droperidol (Inapsine), etoposide phosphate (Etopophos), filgrastim (Neupogen), fludarabine (Fludara), fluorouracil (5-FU), gemcitabine (Gemzar), granisetron (Kytril), heparin, leucovorin calcium, melphalan (Alkeran), methotrexate, metoclopramide (Reglan), mitomycin (Mutamycin), ondansetron (Zofran), paclitaxel (Taxol), pemetrexed (Alimta), piperacillin/tazobactam (Zosyn), sargramostim (Leukine), teniposide (Vumon), thiotepa, vincristine, vinorelbine (Navelbine).

RATE OF ADMINISTRATION

IV injection: Total desired dose, properly diluted, over 1 minute.

ACTIONS

An alkaloid of the periwinkle plant with antitumor activity. Cell cycle–specific for M phase. Thought to interfere with the metabolic pathways of amino acids. Sometimes pharmacologically effective without any noticeable improvement in symptoms of malignancy. Cell energy production and synthesis of nucleic acid may also be inhibited. Half-life is 24.8 hours. Metabolism mediated by the hepatic cytochrome P_{450} isoenzymes in the CYP 3A subfamily. Some excretion through bile and urine.

INDICATIONS AND USES

To suppress or retard neoplastic growth. Remission and probable cure have been achieved with bleomycin and cisplatin in testicular malignancies. Response has been noted in Hodgkin's disease, non-Hodgkin's lymphomas, choriocarcinoma, Kaposi's sarcoma, mycosis fungoids, breast and renal cell malignancies. ▪ Used to treat many other malignancies.

CONTRAINDICATIONS

Bacterial infection or leukopenia below 3,000 cells/mm³.

PRECAUTIONS

Follow guidelines for handling cytotoxic agents. See Appendix A, p. 1331. ▪ Usually administered by or under the direction of the physician specialist. ▪ Manufacturer provides an auxiliary sticker labeled "Fatal if given intrathecally, for IV use only" and an overwrap labeled "Do not remove covering until moment of injection. Fatal if given intrathecally. For intravenous use only." Each and every syringe containing a specific dose and prepared in advance of actual administration must be labeled with the provided auxiliary sticker and packaged in this overwrap. If intrathecal injection should occur, immediate neurosurgical intervention is required; consult package insert for immediate steps to be taken. ▪ May cause corneal ulceration with accidental contact to the eye. ▪ Use caution in presence of ulcerated skin areas, cachexia, or impaired liver function. ▪ Leukocyte and platelet counts have fallen precipitously in patients with malignant-cell infiltration of the bone marrow following moderate doses of vinblastine. Further administration is not recommended. ▪ Acute pulmonary reactions including acute shortness of breath and severe bronchospasm have been reported in patients receiving vinca alkaloids. Occurs most frequently when given in combination with mitomycin C. Onset of reaction may occur minutes to hours after vinca administration and up to 2 weeks following the mitomycin dose.

Monitor: Determine absolute patency, quality of vein, and adequate circulation of extremity. Severe cellulitis may result from extravasation. Rinse syringe and needle with venous blood before withdrawal from the vein; see Antidote. ▪ Leukopenia is dose-limiting toxicity. Nadir occurs 5 to 10 days after therapy. Recovery occurs within another 7 to 14 days. ▪ WBC count must be checked before each dose. Must be above 4,000 cells/mm³. ▪ Be alert for signs of bone marrow suppression or infection. ▪ Prophylactic antibiotics may be indicated pending results of C/S in a febrile neutropenic patient. ▪ Thrombocytopenia is rare, but may occur in patients whose bone marrow has been impaired by prior radiation therapy or other bone marrow suppressants. If platelet count is less than 50,000/mm³, initiate precautions to prevent excessive bleeding (e.g., inspect IV sites, skin, and mucous membranes; use extreme care during invasive procedures; test urine, emesis, stool, and secretions for occult blood). ▪ Observe for increased uric acid levels; may require increased doses of antigout agents; allopurinol (Aloprim) preferred. ▪ Maintain adequate hydration. ▪ Prophylactic antiemetics may increase patient comfort. ▪ See Drug/Lab Interactions.

Patient Education: Avoid pregnancy; nonhormonal birth control recommended. ▪ Report IV site burning or stinging promptly. ▪ Report chills, fever, sore mouth, or throat promptly. ▪ Maintain adequate hydration; avoid constipation. ▪ See Appendix D, p. 1333.

Maternal/Child: Category D: avoid pregnancy. May produce teratogenic effects on the fetus. Has a mutagenic potential. ▪ Discontinue breast-feeding. ▪ Do not use diluents containing benzyl alcohol in premature infants.

Elderly: Leukopenic response may be increased in malnutrition or with skin ulcers.

DRUG/LAB INTERACTIONS

Inhibited by **some amino acids, glutamic acid, and tryptophan.** ▪ Potentiated by **other bone marrow suppressants** (e.g., antineoplastics, radiation therapy). ▪ Do not administer **live virus vaccines** to patients receiving antineoplastic drugs. ▪ Acute pulmonary reactions can occur with **Mitomycin-C;** see Precautions. ▪ May inhibit effects of **phenytoin** (Dilantin); increased doses of phenytoin may be needed. ▪ **Erythromycin** decreases metabolism and increases toxicity of vinblastine. ▪ Use caution with **any drug that inhibits P₄₅₀ enzymes** (e.g., calcium channel blockers [e.g., diltiazem (Cardizem), nicardipine (Cardene), verapamil], antifungal agents [e.g., fluconazole (Diflucan), itraconazole (Sporanox), ketoconazole (Nizoral)], bromocriptine [Parlodel], cimetidine [Tagamet], clarithromycin [Biaxin], cyclosporine [Sandimmune], danazol [Medrol], metoclopramide [Reglan]); may increase vinblastine blood levels and increase toxicity. ▪ Effect of **bleomycin** is significantly enhanced if vinblastine is administered 6 to 8 hours before bleomycin administration.

SIDE EFFECTS

Usually dose related and not always reversible: abdominal pain, alopecia, anorexia, cellulitis, constipation, convulsions, diarrhea, dizziness, extravasation, gonadal suppression, headache, hemorrhage, ileus, leukopenia (severe), malaise, mental depression, myelosuppression, nausea, numbness, oral lesions, paresthesias, peripheral neuritis, pharyngitis, Raynaud's syndrome, reflex depression (deep tendon), skin lesions, thrombophlebitis, tumor site pain, vomiting, weakness.

ANTIDOTE

For extravasation, discontinue the drug immediately and administer into another vein. Hyaluronidase should be injected locally into extravasated area. Use a fine hypodermic needle. Elevate extremity. Moist heat may be helpful. Notify the physician of all side effects; symptomatic treatment is often indicated. Administration of whole blood products (e.g., packed RBCs, platelets, leukocytes) and/or blood modifiers (e.g., darbepoetin alfa [Aranesp], epoetin alfa [Epogen], filgrastim [Neupogen, Zarxio], pegfilgrastim [Neulasta], sargramostim [Leukine]) may be indicated to treat bone marrow toxicity. Glutamic acid blocks toxicity of vinblastine but also blocks its antineoplastic activity.

VINCRISTINE SULFATE BBW
VINCRISTINE SULFATE LIPOSOME INJECTION BBW

Antineoplastic
(mitotic inhibitor-vinca alkaloid)

(vin-**KRIS**-teen **SUL**-fayt)
(vin-**KRIS**-teen **SUL**-fayt **LIP**-oh-sohm in-**JEK**-shun)

VCR, Vincasar PFS ▪ Marqibo

pH 3.5 to 5.5 • pH not available

USUAL DOSE
CONVENTIONAL VINCRISTINE
Auxiliary labeling required; see Precautions.

Neurotoxicity appears to be dose related. Use extreme care in calculating and administering vincristine. Overdose may be fatal.

1.4 mg/M^2 administered once every 7 days. Various dosage schedules have been used with caution.

MARQIBO (LIPOSOMAL VINCRISTINE)
2.25 mg/M^2 as an IV infusion over 1 hour once every 7 days. Liposomal vincristine has different dosage recommendations than conventional vincristine. Verify drug name and dose before preparation and administration.

PEDIATRIC DOSE
CONVENTIONAL VINCRISTINE
Weight over 10 kg: 1.5 to 2 mg/M^2 once each week.

Weight 10 kg (22 lb) or less: 0.05 mg/kg of body weight once a week. See comments under Usual Dose.

MARQIBO (LIPOSOMAL VINCRISTINE)
Safety and effectiveness for use in pediatric patients not established.

DOSE ADJUSTMENTS
CONVENTIONAL VINCRISTINE: In impaired hepatic function, reduce initial doses by 50% if direct bilirubin above 3 mg/dL. May be increased gradually based on individual response. ▪ Usually given with other antineoplastic drugs and corticosteroids in reduced doses to achieve tumor remission. ▪ See Drug/Lab Interactions.

MARQIBO (LIPOSOMAL VINCRISTINE)

Recommended Dose Modifications for Marqibo-Related Peripheral Neuropathy	
Severity of Peripheral Neuropathy Signs/Symptoms*	Modification of Marqibo Dose and Regimen
Patient develops Grade 3 (severe symptoms, limiting self-care activities of daily living [ADL]†) or persistent Grade 2 (moderate symptoms, limiting instrumental ADL‡) peripheral neuropathy.	Interrupt Marqibo. If the peripheral neuropathy remains at Grade 3 or 4, discontinue Marqibo. If the peripheral neuropathy recovers to Grade 1 or 2, reduce the Marqibo dose to 2 mg/M^2.
Patient has persistent Grade 2 peripheral neuropathy after the first dose reduction to 2 mg/M^2.	Interrupt Marqibo for up to 7 days. If the peripheral neuropathy increases to Grade 3 or 4, discontinue Marqibo. If peripheral neuropathy recovers to Grade 1, reduce the Marqibo dose to 1.825 mg/M^2.
Patient has persistent Grade 2 peripheral neuropathy after the second dose reduction to 1.825 mg/M^2.	Interrupt Marqibo for up to 7 days. If the peripheral neuropathy increases to Grade 3 or 4, discontinue Marqibo. If the toxicity recovers to Grade 1, reduce the Marqibo dose to 1.5 mg/M^2.

*Grading based on the National Cancer Institute Common Terminology Criteria for Adverse Events (NCI CTCAE), v4.0.
†Self-care ADL: Refers to bathing, dressing/undressing, feeding self, using the toilet, taking medications, not bedridden.
‡Instrumental ADL: Refers to preparing meals, shopping for groceries and clothes, using telephone, managing money, etc.

DILUTION

CONVENTIONAL VINCRISTINE: *Specific techniques required; see Precautions.* Apply auxiliary label and package in manufacturer-supplied overwrap; see Precautions. Available in preservative-free solutions (1 mg/mL). May be given by IV injection or through Y-tube or three-way stopcock of a free-flowing IV infusion. Occasionally further diluted in 50 mL or more NS or D5W and given as an infusion. To reduce the potential for fatal medication errors due to incorrect route of administration, vincristine should be diluted in a flexible plastic container and prominently labeled as indicated for intravenous use only.

MARQIBO (LIPOSOMAL VINCRISTINE): *Specific techniques required; see Precautions.* Marqibo will be prepared in the pharmacy by a very specific process that takes approximately 60 to 90 minutes. Dedicated, uninterrupted time is required due to extensive monitoring of temperature and time required for preparation. When prepared according to directions, each single-dose vial contains 5 mg/31 mL (0.16 mg/mL). Refer to manufacturer's literature for a detailed outline of the preparation procedure. Contact manufacturer if questions arise about preparation.

Items required by the pharmacy to prepare Marqibo include:
- Marqibo kit
- Water bath*
- Calibrated thermometer (0° to 100° C)*
- Calibrated electronic timer*
- Sterile venting needle or other suitable device equipped with a sterile 0.2-micron filter
- 1-mL or 3-mL sterile syringe with needle, and a 5-mL sterile syringe with needle

*Manufacturer will send the water bath, calibrated thermometer, and calibrated electronic timer to the medical facility at the initial order of Marqibo and will replace them every 2 years.

Filters: *Marqibo (liposomal vincristine):* 0.2-micron filter required during preparation; however, *do not use with in-line filters.*

Storage: *Conventional vincristine:* Store in refrigerator. Retain in carton to protect from light. Store upright. Solutions diluted with NS to a concentration of 0.0015 to 0.08 mg/mL are stable for 24 hours when protected from light or for 8 hours under normal light at 25° C (77° F).

Marqibo (liposomal vincristine): Store Marqibo kit in refrigerator at 2° to 8° C (36° to 46° F). *Do not freeze.* Once prepared, may be stored at CRT for no more than 12 hours.

COMPATIBILITY   (Underline Indicates Conflicting Compatibility Information)

Consider any drug NOT listed as compatible to be INCOMPATIBLE until consulting a pharmacist; specific conditions may apply.

CONVENTIONAL VINCRISTINE

Manufacturer suggests that the pH not be altered from between 3.5 to 5.5 by an additive or a diluent, and it recommends NS or D5W as a diluent and not admixing with other drugs in the same container.

One source suggests the following **compatibilities:**

Additive: *Not recommended by manufacturer.* Bleomycin (Blenoxane), cytarabine (ARA-C), doxorubicin (Adriamycin), fluorouracil (5-FU), methotrexate.

Y-site: Allopurinol (Aloprim), amifostine (Ethyol), amphotericin B cholesteryl (Amphotec), anidulafungin (Eraxis), aztreonam (Azactam), bleomycin (Blenoxane), caspofungin (Cancidas), cisplatin, cladribine (Leustatin), cyclophosphamide (Cytoxan), doxorubicin (Adriamycin), doxorubicin liposomal (Doxil), droperidol (Inapsine), etoposide phosphate (Etopophos), filgrastim (Neupogen), fludarabine (Fludara), fluorouracil (5-FU), gemcitabine (Gemzar), granisetron (Kytril), heparin, leucovorin calcium, linezolid (Zyvox), melphalan (Alkeran), methotrexate, metoclopramide (Reglan), mitomycin (Mutamycin), ondansetron (Zofran), oxaliplatin (Eloxatin), paclitaxel (Taxol), pemetrexed (Alimta), piperacillin/tazobactam (Zosyn), sargramostim (Leukine), teniposide (Vumon), thiotepa, topotecan (Hycamtin), vinblastine, vinorelbine (Navelbine).

MARQIBO (LIPOSOMAL VINCRISTINE)

Manufacturer states, "Do not mix with other drugs."

RATE OF ADMINISTRATION

CONVENTIONAL VINCRISTINE

"Fatal if given intrathecally; for IV use only."

IV injection: Total desired dose, properly diluted, over 1 minute.

Infusion: A single dose over 5 to 10 minutes or as a continuous infusion (based on specific protocols).

MARQIBO (LIPOSOMAL VINCRISTINE)

For IV use only; fatal if given by other routes. A single dose as an IV infusion equally distributed over 1 hour. Administer through a secure and free-flowing venous access line.

ACTIONS

CONVENTIONAL VINCRISTINE: An alkaloid of the periwinkle plant with antitumor activity. Cell cycle–specific for the M phase. It binds to tubulin, altering the tubulin polymerization equilibrium and resulting in altered microtubule structure and function. It stabilizes the spindle apparatus, preventing chromosome segregation and triggering metaphase arrest and inhibition of mitosis. Well distributed except in spinal fluid. Extensively metabolized with a half-life of 85 hours. Primarily excreted through feces.

MARQIBO (LIPOSOMAL VINCRISTINE): Vincristine encapsulated in sphingomyelin/cholesterol liposomes. Its mechanism of action, distribution, and elimination is similar to conventional vincristine.

INDICATIONS AND USES

CONVENTIONAL VINCRISTINE: Treatment of acute leukemia. ▪ Useful in combination with other oncolytic agents for Hodgkin's disease, non-Hodgkin's malignant lymphomas, rhabdomyosarcoma, neuroblastoma, and Wilms' tumor.

MARQIBO (LIPOSOMAL VINCRISTINE): Treatment of adults with Philadelphia chromosome-negative (Ph-) acute lymphoblastic leukemia (ALL) in second or greater relapse or adults whose disease has progressed following two or more antileukemia therapies. Indication based on overall response rate; clinical benefit such as improvement in overall survival not verified.

Unlabeled uses: Conventional vincristine: Treatment of idiopathic thrombocytopenic purpura; treatment of Kaposi's sarcoma, breast and bladder cancer.

CONTRAINDICATIONS

Both formulations: Demyelinating form of Charcot-Marie-Tooth syndrome.

Marqibo (liposomal vincristine): Hypersensitivity to vincristine sulfate or any of the components of Marqibo.

PRECAUTIONS

BOTH FORMULATIONS: Follow guidelines for handling cytotoxic agents. See Appendix A, p. 1331. ▪ Administered by or under the direction of the physician specialist. ▪ Sensory and motor neuropathies are common and cumulative. Risk of neurologic toxicity is greater in patients with pre-existing neuromuscular disorders or when other potentially neurotoxic drugs are coadministered; see Monitor. ▪ Myelosuppression may require dose adjustment. ▪ Tumor lysis syndrome leading to acute uric acid nephropathy has occurred; see Monitor.

CONVENTIONAL VINCRISTINE: Manufacturer provides an auxiliary sticker labeled "Fatal if given intrathecally, for IV use only" and an overwrap labeled "Do not remove covering until moment of injection. For intravenous use only. Fatal if given by other routes." Each and every infusion bag or syringe containing a specific dose and prepared in advance of actual administration must be labeled with the provided auxiliary sticker and packaged in this overwrap. If intrathecal injection should occur, immediate neurosurgical intervention is required; consult package insert for immediate steps to be taken. ▪ If central nervous system leukemia is diagnosed, additional agents may be required because vincristine does not appear to cross the blood-brain barrier in adequate amounts. ▪ Acute shortness of breath and severe bronchospasm have been reported following administration of vinca alkaloids. These reactions occur most frequently when the vinca alkaloid is administered in combination with mitomycin-C. Onset of these reactions may occur minutes to several hours after the vinca alkaloid is injected and may occur up to 2 weeks after the dose of mitomycin. Progressive dyspnea requiring chronic therapy may occur. Reaction may require aggressive treatment, especially if pre-existing pulmonary dysfunction is present. Vincristine should not be readministered. ▪ Use extreme caution in combination with radiation therapy. Should not be given to patients while they are receiving radiation therapy through radiation ports that include the liver. ▪ May cause corneal ulceration with accidental contact to the eye; flush eyes with water immediately. ▪ Use caution in pre-existing neuromuscular disease or impaired liver function. ▪ Not recommended for use in patients receiving radiation therapy that involves the liver.

MARQIBO (LIPOSOMAL VINCRISTINE): For IV use only; fatal if given by other routes. ▪ Death has occurred with intrathecal administration. ▪ Has different dose recommendations than conventional vincristine. Verify drug name and dose before preparation and administration to avoid overdose. ▪ Constipation and bowel obstruction have occurred. ▪ Can cause severe fatigue requiring dose delay, reduction, or discontinuation of therapy. ▪ Fatal liver toxicity and elevated AST have occurred. ▪ The influence of renal impairment and severe hepatic impairment has not been evaluated.

Monitor: *Both Formulations:* Determine absolute patency and quality of vein and adequate circulation of extremity. Severe cellulitis may result from extravasation; see Antidote. ▪ Monitor CBC and platelets, bilirubin, and liver function tests before therapy and at frequent intervals. ▪ Be alert for signs of bone marrow suppression or infection. Prophylactic antibiotics may be indicated pending results of C/S in a febrile neutropenic patient. ▪ Monitor neurologic status before therapy and at frequent intervals. Symptoms of neuropathy may include areflexia, arthralgia, burning sensation, cranial neuropathy, decreased vibratory sense, hyperesthesia, hypoesthesia, hyporeflexia, ileus, jaw pain, muscle spasm, myalgia, neuralgia, paresthesia, or weakness. ▪ Observe for increased uric acid levels; may require increased doses of antigout agents (allopurinol [Aloprim] preferred) and may require alkalinization of urine. Monitor for early signs of tumor lysis syndrome (e.g., flank pain and hematuria). ▪ Maintain adequate hydration. ▪ Prophylactic antiemetics may increase patient comfort. ▪ Monitor for hyponatremia and inappropriate secretion of antidiuretic hormone (ADH); may require fluid limitation. ▪ Institute a prophylactic bowel regimen to prevent potential constipation, bowel obstruction, and/or paralytic ileus. ▪ Monitor for thrombocytopenia (platelet count less than 50,000/mm³). Initiate precautions to prevent excessive bleeding (e.g., inspect IV sites, skin, and mucous membranes; use extreme care during invasive procedures; test urine, emesis, stool, and secretions for occult blood). ▪ See Drug/Lab Interactions.

Patient Education: *Both formulations:* Avoid pregnancy; nonhormonal birth control recommended. ▪ Report IV site burning or stinging promptly. ▪ See Appendix D, p. 1333. ▪ Use adequate dietary fiber, hydration, stool softeners and, if necessary, laxatives to avoid constipation.

Maternal/Child: *Both formulations:* Category D: avoid pregnancy. Can cause fetal harm. ▪ Discontinue breast-feeding.

Marqibo (liposomal vincristine): Safety and effectiveness for use in pediatric patients not established.

Elderly: *Both formulations:* Neurotoxicity may be more severe (observe closely for constipation, ileus, and urinary retention). Dose selection should be cautious.

DRUG/LAB INTERACTIONS

Studies have not been conducted for Marqibo, but it is expected to have interactions similar to conventional vincristine. ▪ Acute pulmonary reactions can occur with **mitomycin-C.** ▪ Do not administer **live virus vaccines** to patients receiving antineoplastic drugs. ▪ May decrease levels and effectiveness of **digoxin and phenytoin.** Monitor serum levels of digoxin and phenytoin; increased doses of these drugs may be required. ▪ A substrate for cytochrome P_{450} isoenzymes (CYP3A). Avoid concurrent use of **drugs known to inhibit cytochrome P_{450} isoenzymes** (e.g., atazanavir [Reyataz], clarithromycin [Biaxin], indinavir [Crixivan], itraconazole [Sporanox], ketoconazole [Nizoral], nefazodone, nelfinavir [Viracept], ritonavir [Norvir], saquinavir [Invirase], telithromycin [Ketek]) and **inducers of cytochrome P_{450} enzymes** (e.g., carbamazepine [Tegretol], dexamethasone (Decadron), phenobarbital (Luminal), phenytoin [Dilantin], rifabutin [Mycobutin], rifampin [Rifadin], St. John's wort). ▪ Although not yet studied, it is likely that there will be interactions, and concomitant use should be avoided with **inhibitors of P-gp** (e.g., amiodarone [Nexterone], clarithromycin, diltiazem [Cardizem], erythromycin [Erythrocin], itraconazole, ketoconazole, protease inhibitors [e.g., nelfinavir, ritonavir], quinidine, sirolimus [Rapamune], tacrolimus [Prograf]) and **inducers of P-gp** (e.g., rifampin, St. John's wort).

SIDE EFFECTS

CONVENTIONAL VINCRISTINE: Frequently dose related and not always reversible: abdominal pain, alopecia, anemia (rare), ataxia, bronchospasm, cellulitis, constipation, convulsions, cranial nerve damage, diarrhea, dysuria, extravasation, fever, foot-drop, gonadal suppression, headache, hepatic veno-occlusive disease, hypersensitivity reactions (e.g., anaphylaxis, edema, rash), hypertension, hypotension, leukopenia (rare), muscle wasting, nausea, neuritic pain, oral lacerations, paralytic ileus, paresthesias, polyuria, reflex changes, sensory impairment, shortness of breath, SIADH, thrombocytopenia (rare), thrombophlebitis, tingling and numbness of extremities, upper colon impaction, uric acid nephropathy, vomiting, weakness, weight loss.

MARQIBO (LIPOSOMAL VINCRISTINE): Anemia, constipation, decreased appetite, diarrhea, fatigue, febrile neutropenia, fever, insomnia, nausea, and peripheral sensory and motor neuropathy are most common. Asthenia, bowel obstruction, cardiac arrest, hypotension, ileus, increased AST, mental status changes, muscle weakness, neutropenia, pain, pneumonia, renal disorders, respiratory distress and/or failure, septic shock, staphylococcal bacteremia, and thrombocytopenia have also been reported. Extravasation, hepatic toxicity, and tumor lysis syndrome have occurred.

ANTIDOTE

For extravasation, discontinue the drug immediately and administer into another vein. Hyaluronidase may be injected locally into extravasated area. Use a fine hypodermic needle. Elevate extremity; moist heat may be helpful. Notify the physician of all side effects; symptomatic treatment is often indicated. Will probably reduce dose at earliest signs of neurologic toxicity (tingling and numbness of extremities). Discontinue for inappropriate ADH secretion or hyponatremia. Treat with fluid restriction and diuretics. Phenobarbital may be needed for convulsions. Use enemas or cathartics to treat constipation or prevent ileus. Folinic acid, 100 mg IV every 3 hours for 24 hours and then every 6 hours for at least 48 hours, may be helpful in overdose. Supportive measures still required. Administration of whole blood products (e.g., packed RBCs, platelets, leukocytes) and/or blood modifiers (e.g., darbepoetin alfa [Aranesp], epoetin alfa [Epogen], filgrastim [Neupogen, Zarxio], pegfilgrastim [Neulasta], sargramostim [Leukine]) may be indicated to treat bone marrow toxicity. Hemodialysis is not likely to be helpful in an overdose situation.

VINORELBINE TARTRATE BBW

(vin-**OR**-el-been **TAHR**-trayt)

Navelbine, NVB

Antineoplastic
(mitotic inhibitor-vinca alkaloid)

pH 3.5

USUAL DOSE

Auxiliary labeling required; see Precautions.

30 mg/M^2 administered once each week until disease progression or dose-limiting toxicity. Calculate carefully in presence of edema or ascites. Vinorelbine 25 mg/M^2 weekly has been used in combination with cisplatin 100 mg/M^2 every 4 weeks. Vinorelbine 30 mg/M^2 weekly has also been used in combination with cisplatin 120 mg/M^2 on Days 1 and 29 and then once every 6 weeks. Premedication with dexamethasone (Decadron) may be beneficial in patients who experience acute or subacute pulmonary reactions. See cisplatin monograph.

DOSE ADJUSTMENTS

Reduce or withhold dose based on hematologic toxicity or hepatic insufficiency (e.g., hyperbilirubinemia) on the day of treatment. For patients with both hematologic toxicity and hepatic insufficiency, administer the lower of the doses determined appropriate from the following charts.

Vinorelbine Dose Adjustments for Hematologic Toxicity	
Granulocytes (cells/mm^3) on Day of Treatment	Dose of Vinorelbine
≥1,500 cells/mm^3	100%
1,000 to 1,499 cells/mm^3	50%
<1,000 cells/mm^3	Do not administer. Repeat count in 1 week. If 3 consecutive weekly doses are held because granulocyte count is <1,000 cells/mm^3, discontinue vinorelbine.
For patients who during treatment with vinorelbine have experienced fever and/or sepsis while granulocytopenic or had 2 consecutive weekly doses held due to granulocytopenia, subsequent doses of vinorelbine should be:	
≥1,500 cells/mm^3	75%
1,000 to 1,499 cells/mm^3	37.5%
<1,000 cells/mm^3	Same as <1,000 above

Vinorelbine Dose Adjustments for Impaired Hepatic Function	
Total Bilirubin (mg/dL)	Dose of Vinorelbine
≤2 mg/dL	100%
2.1 to 3 mg/dL	50%
>3 mg/dL	25%

Appropriate dose reductions for cisplatin should be made when vinorelbine is used in combination. During studies, most patients required a 50% dose reduction of vinorelbine by Day 15 and a 50% dose reduction of cisplatin by Cycle 3. ■ No dose adjustment is required for impaired renal function. ■ If Grade 2 or greater neurotoxicity develops, discontinue vinorelbine.

DILUTION

Specific techniques required; see Precautions.

IV injection: Each 10 mg (1 mL) must be further diluted with a minimum of 2 to 5 mL NS or D5W. Desired concentration is 1.5 to 3 mg/mL (2 mL diluent yields 3 mg/mL concentration, 5 mL yields 1.5 mg/mL concentration). Must be given into the side-arm port of a free-flowing IV infusion.

Intermittent infusion: Each 10 mg (1 mL) must be further diluted with 4 to 19 mL NS or D5W, ½NS, D5/½NS, R, or LR. Desired concentration is 0.5 to 2 mg/mL (4 mL diluent yields 2 mg/mL concentration, 19 mL yields 0.5 mg/mL concentration). Other references recommend diluting a single dose to a minimum total volume of 100 mL. Must be given into the side-arm port of a free-flowing IV infusion or may be given directly into a large central vein.

Storage: Refrigerate vials and protect from light; are stable at room temperature for up to 72 hours. Diluted solution stable for 24 hours at 5° to 30° C (41° to 86° F).

COMPATIBILITY   (Underline Indicates Conflicting Compatibility Information)

Consider any drug NOT listed as compatible to be INCOMPATIBLE until consulting a pharmacist; specific conditions may apply.

Manufacturer recommends mixing only with solutions listed under Dilution.

One source suggests the following **compatibilities:**

Y-site: Amikacin, aztreonam (Azactam), bleomycin (Blenoxane), bumetanide, buprenorphine (Buprenex), butorphanol (Stadol), calcium gluconate, carboplatin (Paraplatin), carmustine (BiCNU), cefotaxime (Claforan), ceftazidime (Fortaz), chlorpromazine (Thorazine), cisplatin, clindamycin (Cleocin), cyclophosphamide (Cytoxan), cytarabine (ARA-C), dacarbazine (DTIC), dactinomycin (Cosmegen), daunorubicin (Cerubidine), dexamethasone (Decadron), diphenhydramine (Benadryl), doxorubicin (Adriamycin), doxorubicin liposomal (Doxil), doxycycline, droperidol (Inapsine), enalaprilat (Vasotec IV), etoposide (VePesid), famotidine (Pepcid IV), filgrastim (Neupogen), fluconazole (Diflucan), fludarabine (Fludara), gallium nitrate (Ganite), gemcitabine (Gemzar), gentamicin, granisetron (Kytril), heparin, hydrocortisone sodium succinate (Solu-Cortef), hydromorphone (Dilaudid), idarubicin (Idamycin), ifosfamide (Ifex), imipenem-cilastatin (Primaxin), lorazepam (Ativan), mannitol, mechlorethamine (nitrogen mustard), melphalan (Alkeran), meperidine (Demerol), mesna (Mesnex), methotrexate, metoclopramide (Reglan), metronidazole (Flagyl IV), mitoxantrone (Novantrone), morphine, nalbuphine, ondansetron (Zofran), oxaliplatin (Eloxatin), potassium chloride (KCl), prochlorperazine (Compazine), promethazine (Phenergan), ranitidine (Zantac), streptozocin (Zanosar), teniposide (Vumon), ticarcillin/clavulanate (Timentin), tobramycin, vancomycin, vinblastine, vincristine, zidovudine (AZT, Retrovir).

RATE OF ADMINISTRATION

Inadequate flushing of the vein after administration may increase the risk of phlebitis.

IV injection: Total desired dose, properly diluted over 6 to 10 minutes through the side-arm port of a free-flowing IV. After administration, flush with at least 75 to 125 mL of diluent solution over 10 minutes or more. Up to 300 mL has been used as a flush.

Intermittent infusion: Total desired dose, properly diluted over 6 to 10 minutes. Other references recommend over 20 minutes. Must be given into the side-arm port of a free-flowing IV infusion or may be given directly into a large central vein. Flush according to directions for IV injection.

ACTIONS

An antineoplastic agent. A semi-synthetic vinca alkaloid with chemical differences from other vinca alkaloids that may provide unique clinical benefits with a lower incidence of clinical neurotoxicity. Causes depolymerization of microtubules and inhibits microtubule assembly. May be more specific to mitotic microtubules. Cell cycle–specific and produces a blockade in the cell-cycle progression in G_2 and M phase. Widely distributed in the body. Elimination half-life is 27 to 43 hours. Metabolized in the liver by hepatic cytochrome P_{450} isoenzymes in the CYP3A subfamily. Excreted in bile, feces, and urine.

INDICATIONS AND USES

Treatment of unresectable advanced non–small-cell lung cancer (ANSCLC), in ambulatory patients. Used as a single agent or in combination with cisplatin. ▪ Indicated as a single agent or in combination with cisplatin in patients with Stage IV NSCLC and in combination with cisplatin in patients with Stage III NSCLC.

Unlabeled uses: Treatment of breast, cervical, and epithelial ovarian cancers; treatment of desmoid tumors and fibromatosis, and advanced Kaposi's sarcoma.

CONTRAINDICATIONS

Patients with pretreatment granulocyte counts less than 1,000 cells/mm^3.

PRECAUTIONS

Follow guidelines for handling cytotoxic agents. See Appendix A, p. 1331. ▪ Severe irritation of the eye has been reported with accidental exposure to another vinca alkaloid. If exposure occurs, thoroughly flush eye with water immediately. ▪ Administered by or under the direction of the physician specialist. ▪ Manufacturer provides an auxiliary sticker labeled "Fatal if given intrathecally, for IV use only" and an overwrap labeled "Do not remove covering until moment of injection. Fatal if given intrathecally. For Intravenous use only." Each and every syringe containing a specific dose and prepared in advance of actual administration must be labeled with the provided auxiliary sticker and packaged in this overwrap. If intrathecal injection should occur, immediate neurosurgical intervention is required; consult package insert for immediate steps to be taken. ▪ Adequate diagnostic and treatment facilities must be readily available. ▪ May cause severe granulocytopenia resulting in increased susceptibility to infection. ▪ Use extreme caution in patients with hepatic impairment, pre-existing neuromuscular disease, pre-existing peripheral neuropathies, or those taking other neurotoxic drugs (e.g., antineoplastics [cisplatin], phenothiazines [prochlorperazine]). ▪ Acute SOB and severe bronchospasm have been reported, most commonly when vinorelbine was used with mitomycin. May require treatment with oxygen, bronchodilators (e.g., albuterol), and/or corticosteroids (e.g., hydrocortisone). Incidence may be increased when there is pre-existing pulmonary dysfunction. ▪ Prior radiation therapy or treatment with other antineoplastic agents may cause an increase in myelotoxicity; use with extreme caution. ▪ Administration to patients with prior radiation therapy may result in radiation recall reactions. ▪ See Monitor and Drug/Lab Interactions.

Monitor: Monitor CBC, differential, platelets, and bilirubin on each day of treatment to determine correct dose and 1 or 2 times weekly; granulocytopenia is dose-limiting. Temporary leukopenia is an expected effect. Maximum depression usually occurs in 7 to 10 days after the dose, and recovery should occur within the following 7 to 14 days. ▪ Cases of interstitial pulmonary changes and adult respiratory distress syndrome (ARDS), most of which were fatal, have been reported. Onset of symptoms has occurred in 3 to 8 days. Promptly evaluate patients with alterations in their baseline pulmonary symptoms or with new onset of cough, dyspnea, hypoxia, or other symptoms. ▪ Monitor AST frequently. ▪ Evaluate neurologic status frequently (e.g., constipation, decreased deep tendon reflexes, paresthesia). ▪ Closely monitor patients who have had symptoms of neuropathy with previous drug regimens (e.g., paclitaxel [Taxol]) for new or worsening neuropathy. ▪ Determine absolute patency and quality of vein and adequate circulation of extremity. Local tissue necrosis and/or thrombophlebitis can result from extravasation; see Antidote. ▪ Be alert for any sign of infection. Infections must be brought under control before beginning therapy with vinorelbine. ▪ Use of prophylactic antibiotics may be indicated pending results of C/S in a febrile neutropenic patient. ▪ Maintain adequate hydration. ▪ Prophylactic antiemetics may increase patient comfort; haloperidol and oral dexamethasone have benefited some patients. ▪ May cause severe (Grade 3-4) constipation, paralytic ileus, intestinal obstruction, necrosis, and/or perforation. Use a laxative to prevent constipation. Monitor bowel sounds. ▪ Monitor for hyponatremia and syndrome of inappropriate secretion of antidiuretic hormone (SIADH). ▪ Monitor for thrombocytopenia (platelet count less than 50,000/mm³). Initiate precautions to prevent excessive bleeding (e.g., inspect IV sites, skin, and mucous membranes; use extreme care during invasive procedures; test urine, emesis, stool, and secretions for occult blood). ▪ See Precautions and Drug/Lab Interactions.

Patient Education: Report burning or stinging at IV site promptly. ▪ Report chills, fever, difficulty breathing, or shortness of breath promptly. ▪ Avoid pregnancy; nonhormonal birth control recommended. ▪ Take laxatives consistently to avoid constipation. ▪ See Appendix D, p. 1333.

Maternal/Child: Category D: avoid pregnancy; may cause fetal harm. ▪ Discontinue breast-feeding. ▪ Safety and effectiveness for use in pediatric patients have not been established but have been investigated. In one study, vinorelbine was considered to be ineffective when used in doses similar to those used in adults in a limited number of pediatric patients with recurrent solid malignant tumors (e.g., rhabdomyosarcoma/undifferentiated sarcoma, neuroblastoma, and CNS tumors). Toxicities were similar to those reported in adults.

Elderly: The pharmacokinetics of vinorelbine in elderly and younger adult patients is similar. No relationship among age, systemic exposure, and hematologic toxicity has been observed.

DRUG/LAB INTERACTIONS

Neurotoxicity may be increased by **other neurotoxic drugs** (e.g., antineoplastics [such as cisplatin, paclitaxel (Taxol)] and phenothiazines [prochlorperazine]); may require dose reduction or discontinuation of vinorelbine. Vestibular and auditory deficits have been observed, usually when vinorelbine is used in combination with cisplatin. ▪ Do not administer **live virus vaccines** to patients receiving antineoplastic drugs. ▪ **Mitomycin-C** may cause or aggravate acute pulmonary reactions (e.g., acute shortness of breath, bronchospasm). May require oxygen, bronchodilators, and/or corticosteroids. ▪ Granulocytopenia significantly higher when used in combination with **cisplatin.** ▪ Additive bone marrow suppression may occur with **radiation therapy and/or other bone marrow–suppressing agents** (e.g., azathioprine, chloramphenicol, melphalan [Alkeran]); dose reductions may be required. ▪ Leukopenic effects may be increased by **agents that cause similar blood dyscrasias** (e.g., anticonvulsants, antidepressants, phenothiazines). ▪ **Drugs that inhibit the cytochrome P₄₅₀ isoenzymes in the CYP3A subfamily** (e.g., azole antifungals [e.g., itraconazole (Sporanox)], macrolides [e.g., erythromycin (Erythrocin), troleandomycin (TAO)]) may inhibit the metabolism of vinorelbine and increase its toxicity. *Other vinca alkaloids cause interactions with the following drugs; vinorelbine has not been studied.* ▪ Use with **asparaginase or doxorubicin** may not be recommended or may require specific scheduling. ▪ May be potentiated by **calcium channel blockers** (e.g., verapamil). ▪ May inhibit **digoxin and phenytoin;** increased doses of these drugs may be required. ▪ See Precautions.

SIDE EFFECTS

Granulocytopenia is the major dose-limiting toxicity and may be significantly greater in combination regimens. Alopecia (12%, mild); anemia (87%, mild to moderate); ARDS, auditory deficits, bronchospasm, chest pain (7%); constipation (35%); diarrhea; dyspnea (2%) (acute and reversible shortness of breath may occur within a few hours); elevated total bilirubin and AST; fatigue; hematologic toxicity (99%) (leukopenia and neutropenia are the most frequent and are dose-limiting); hemorrhagic cystitis (rare); hypertension; hypotension; intestinal obstruction, necrosis, and/or perforation; jaw pain; loss of deep tendon reflexes (5%); nausea and vomiting (50% [23%]); pain and redness at injection site (38%); pancreatitis, paralytic ileus (less than 2%); peripheral neuropathy (31%), mild to moderate paresthesia and hypesthesia, phlebitis (10%); pulmonary edema; radiosensitizing effects in patients with prior or concomitant radiation therapy; SIADH (few);

subacute pulmonary reactions (4%, e.g., cough, dyspnea, hypoxemia, and interstitial infiltrates on chest x-ray); thrombocytopenia (rare), thrombocytosis (asymptomatic), tumor pain, vestibular deficits. Pattern of side effects similar when vinorelbine is used as a single agent or in combination.

ANTIDOTE

For severe reactions, discontinue vinorelbine or reduce subsequent doses. If Grade 2 or greater neurotoxicity develops, discontinue vinorelbine. For extravasation, discontinue the drug immediately and administer into another vein. Elevate the extremity. Moist heat may be helpful. Notify the physician of all side effects; symptomatic treatment is often indicated. Discontinue for hyponatremia or SIADH; may require fluid limitation and diuretics (e.g., furosemide [Lasix]). Bone marrow toxicity is reversible after discontinuing vinorelbine. Administration of whole blood products (e.g., packed RBCs, platelets, leukocytes) may be indicated. Darbepoetin alfa (Aranesp), epoetin alfa (Epogen), filgrastim (Neupogen, Zarxio), pegfilgrastim (Neulasta), or sargramostim (Leukine) may be used to promote bone marrow recovery but may not be given within 24 hours of a dose of cytotoxic therapy or until 24 hours after a dose of cytotoxic therapy. Acute or chronic pulmonary reactions may be allergic phenomena; corticosteroids (e.g., hydrocortisone sodium succinate [Solu-Cortef]), oxygen, and bronchodilators (e.g., albuterol) may be helpful. Neurologic toxicity may be reversible.

VON WILLEBRAND FACTOR/COAGULATION FACTOR VIII COMPLEX (HUMAN)

Antihemorrhagic

(von **WILL**-a-brand **FAK**-tor/koh-**AG**-yoo-**LAY**-shun **FAK**-tor VIII **KOM**-plex) (**HYOO**-man)

Wilate

USUAL DOSE
(International Units [IU])

One IU of von Willebrand factor:Ristocetin Cofactor (VWF:RCo) is approximately equal to the level of VWF:RCo activity found in 1 mL of fresh human plasma. The ratio between VWF:RCo and FVIII activities in Wilate is approximately 1:1. When using a FVIII-containing VWF product, continued treatment may cause an excessive rise in FVIII activity; see Monitor.

Calculate the required dose using the following formula:

$$\text{Required IU} = \text{Body weight (kg)} \times \text{Desired VWF:RCo rise (\%) (IU/dL)} \times 0.5 \text{ (IU/kg per IU/dL)}$$

Adjust dose and frequency of administration according to the clinical effectiveness in each patient. The following chart provides estimated doses for minor and major hemorrhages.

Guide to Wilate Dosing for Treatment of Minor and Major Hemorrhages			
Type of Hemorrhage	Loading Dose (IU VWF:RCo/kg)	Maintenance Dose (IU VWF:RCo/kg)	Therapeutic Goal
Minor Hemorrhages	20 to 40 IU/kg	20 to 30 IU/kg every 12 to 24 hours*	VWF:RCo and FVIII activity trough levels of >30%
Major Hemorrhages	40 to 60 IU/kg	20 to 40 IU/kg every 12 to 24 hours*	VWF:RCo and FVIII activity trough levels of >50%

*Maintenance doses may need to be continued for up to 3 days for minor hemorrhages and 5 to 7 days for major hemorrhages. Repeat doses may be administered for as long as needed based on repeated monitoring of appropriate clinical and laboratory measures.

Recommendations for dosing in minor and major surgeries is provided in the following chart.

Guide to Wilate Dosing for Treatment in Minor and Major Surgeries in All vWD* Types						
Type of Surgery	Loading Dose (IU VWF: RCo/kg) (Within 3 Hours Before Surgery)	VWF:RCo Peak Levels (% of Normal)	Maintenance Dose (IU VWF: RCo/kg)	VWF:RCo Trough Levels (% of Normal)	Frequency of Doses (hours)	Duration of Therapy (days)
Minor (including tooth extraction)	30 to 60 IU/kg	50%	15 to 30 IU/kg or half the loading dose	Greater than 30%	12 to 24 hours	Until wound healing achieved, up to 3 days
Major	40 to 60 IU/kg	100%	20 to 40 IU/kg or half the loading dose	Greater than 50%	12 to 24 hours (at least 2 doses within the first 24 hours after the start of surgery)	Until wound healing achieved, up to 6 days or more

*vWD, von Willebrand disease.

See prescribing information for an alternate formula to determine loading dose based on patient's individual in vivo recovery (IVR) determined before surgery.

Performing appropriate lab tests once a day after surgery is recommended to ensure adequate VWF:RCo and FVIII activity levels are reached and maintained. To decrease the risk of perioperative thrombosis, FVIII activity levels should not exceed 250%.

PEDIATRIC DOSE

Follow the general recommendations for dosing and administration for adults. See Usual Dose and Maternal/Child.

DOSE ADJUSTMENTS

Adjust dose according to the extent and location of bleeding and the patient's clinical condition. ▪ vWD Type 3 patients with GI bleeding may require higher doses.

DILUTION

Available in 5-mL and 10-mL vials containing either 500 or 1,000 IU VWF:RCo and 500 or 1,000 IU FVIII activities. Provided as a kit containing a single-dose vial of powder, a vial of diluent, a Mix2Vial transfer device, a 10-mL syringe, an infusion set, and 2 alcohol swabs. Consult instructions for reconstitution and injection in the package insert. Warm to room temperature (25° C) before dilution and maintain throughout reconstitution. If a water bath is used for warming (temperature should not exceed 37° C [98° F]), do not allow water to come into contact with the latex-free rubber stopper or vial caps. The total number of IUs available is clearly marked on each vial. Record the batch number of each vial. Should be used immediately after reconstitution. Solution should be clear or slightly opalescent.

Filters: Incorporated into the Mix2Vial.

Storage: Store in original carton to protect from light. Stable for 36 months from date of manufacture when refrigerated at 2° to 8° C (36° to 46° F). Do not freeze. May be stored at RT (maximum of 25° C [77° F]) for up to 6 months. Label vial with date removed from refrigeration. Once stored at RT, do not return to refrigeration. Shelf life expires 6 months from date of removal from refrigeration or on the expiration date on the product vial, whichever is earlier. Administer immediately after reconstitution. Discard any unused solution.

COMPATIBILITY

Manufacturer states, "Must not be mixed with other medicinal products or administered simultaneously with other IV preparations in the same infusion set."

RATE OF ADMINISTRATION

A single dose as an infusion at 2 to 4 mL/min. Reduce rate of administration or interrupt the infusion if a marked increase in pulse occurs.

ACTIONS

A purified, lyophilized von Willebrand factor (VWF) and coagulation factor VIII complex that is obtained from pooled human plasma. VWF and FVIII are normal constituents of human plasma. Patients with vWD have a deficiency or abnormality of VWF; this results in low FVIII activity and an abnormal platelet function, which causes excessive bleeding. VWF promotes platelet aggregation and platelet adhesion on damaged vascular endothelium; it also serves as a stabilizing carrier protein for the procoagulant protein FVIII, an essential cofactor in the activation of factor X, leading to the formation of thrombin and fibrin. VWF activity is measured with an assay that uses an agglutinating cofactor called Ristocetin (RCo). The VWF:RCo assay provides a quantitative measurement of VWF function by determining how well VWF helps platelets adhere to one another. Reduced VWF:RCo activity indicates a deficiency of VWF. Half-life varies based on type of vWD (1, 2, or 3).

INDICATIONS AND USES

On-demand treatment and control of bleeding episodes and perioperative management of bleeding in pediatric patients and adults with von Willebrand disease.

Limitation of use: Not indicated for the treatment of hemophilia A.

CONTRAINDICATIONS

History of anaphylactic or severe systemic reactions to plasma-derived products, any ingredient in the formulation, or components of the container.

PRECAUTIONS

For IV use only. ▪ Administered under the direction of a physician knowledgeable in the treatment of coagulation disorders in a facility with adequate diagnostic and treatment facilities to monitor the patient and respond to any medical emergency. ▪ Hypersensitivity reactions, including anaphylaxis, have occurred; see Monitor. ▪ Manufactured from human plasma. Risk of transmitting infectious agents (e.g., HIV, hepatitis and, theoretically, Creutzfeldt-Jakob disease) has been greatly reduced by screening, testing, and manufacturing techniques. However, risk of transmission cannot be totally eliminated. ▪ Hepatitis A and B vaccines are recommended for patients receiving plasma derivatives. ▪ Thrombotic events have been reported. Use caution in patients with known risk factors for thrombosis. ▪ Inhibitors may develop with large or frequent doses; see Monitor.

Monitor: Monitor BP and pulse during infusion. If a marked increase in pulse occurs, either reduce rate of infusion or interrupt the infusion. ▪ Throughout the infusion, monitor for S/S of a hypersensitivity reaction (e.g., angioedema, burning and stinging at injection site, chills, fever, flushing, headache, hives, hypotension, nausea, tachycardia, tightness of the chest, urticaria, vomiting, wheezing). Evaluate for the presence of inhibitors if an anaphylactic reaction occurs. ▪ Appropriate laboratory tests should be performed on the patient's plasma at suitable intervals to ensure that adequate VWF:RCo and FVIII activity levels have been reached and are maintained. Monitoring is also required to avoid sustained excessive VWF and FVIII activity. When using a VWF product that contains FVIII, continued treatment may cause an excessive rise in FVIII activity. Excessive activity levels may increase the risk of thrombotic events. In the postsurgery period, monitoring should be done daily if possible, and FVIII levels should not exceed 250%. ▪ Monitor for development of VWF and FVIII inhibitors (neutralizing antibodies). Consider formation of inhibitors and perform assays if bleeding is not controlled with usual doses.

Patient Education: Review manufacturer's medication guide. ▪ Prophylactic hepatitis A and hepatitis B vaccines recommended. ▪ Promptly report S/S of a hypersensitivity reaction (e.g., dizziness, hives, itching, rash, tightness of the chest). ▪ Frequent blood tests (e.g., monitoring of VWF:RCo and FVIII activity) are required to ensure effectiveness and reduce the risk of thrombotic events. ▪ Inhibitors may develop if expected VWF activity plasma levels are not attained or if bleeding is not controlled with adequate or repeat dosing; notify treating physician. ▪ Report symptoms of possibly transmitted viral infections immediately. Symptoms may include anorexia, arthralgias, fatigue, jaundice, low-grade fever, nausea, or vomiting.

Maternal/Child: Use during pregnancy or labor and delivery only if clearly needed. ▪ Safety for use during breast-feeding is unknown; consider benefit versus risk. ▪ Approved for use in pediatric patients. No dose adjustment is required.

Elderly: Numbers insufficient to determine differences in response compared with younger adults.

DRUG/LAB INTERACTIONS
Specific information not available.

SIDE EFFECTS
The most common side effects reported are dizziness, hypersensitivity reactions, and urticaria. The most serious adverse reactions were hypersensitivity reactions.

Post-Marketing: Abdominal pain, anaphylactic reaction, chest discomfort, chills, cough, dyspnea, factor VIII inhibition, fever, flushing, headache, hypotension, nausea, paresthesia, rash, tachycardia, and vomiting.

ANTIDOTE
Keep the physician informed of side effects. Slow or interrupt infusion for a marked increase in pulse rate or mild hypersensitivity reaction. Discontinue the infusion immediately if a severe hypersensitivity reaction or thrombotic event (e.g., chest pain, dyspnea, leg pain, MI) occurs, and evaluate for the presence of inhibitors. Treat hypersensitivity as necessary (e.g., antihistamines, epinephrine, corticosteroids), and treat thrombotic events with appropriate measures. Resuscitate as necessary.

VON WILLEBRAND FACTOR (RECOMBINANT)

Antihemorrhagic

(von **WILL**-a-brand **FAK**-tor)

Vonvendi

USUAL DOSE
(International Units [IU])

Each vial is labeled with the actual amount of recombinant von Willebrand factor (rVWF) activity in international units (IU) as measured with the Ristocetin cofactor assay (VWF:RCo). Hemostasis cannot be ensured until factor VIII coagulation activity (FVIII:C) level reaches 0.4 IU/mL (40% of normal activity).

If the patient's baseline plasma FVIII:C level is below 40% or unknown, it is necessary to administer an approved recombinant, non–VWF-containing factor VIII (e.g., Advate) with the first infusion of recombinant von Willebrand factor (rVWF) in order to achieve a hemostatic plasma level of FVIII:C.

If an immediate rise in FVIII:C is not necessary or if the baseline FVIII:C level is sufficient to ensure hemostasis, recombinant von Willebrand factor (rVWF) may be administered without recombinant factor VIII.

Initial dose: 40 to 80 IU/kg. For each bleeding episode, administer an approved recombinant, non–VWF-containing factor VIII (e.g., Advate) within 10 minutes of the initial dose of rVWF if factor VIII baseline levels are below 40% or unknown. A ratio of 1.3:1 (30% more) VWF to factor VIII is recommended. The following chart provides estimated doses for minor and major hemorrhages.

Vonvendi Dosing Guidelines for Treatment of Minor and Major Hemorrhages		
Hemorrhagic Event	Initial Dose*	Subsequent Dose
Minor (e.g., readily managed epistaxis, oral bleeding, menorrhagia)	40 to 50 IU/kg	40 to 50 IU/kg every 8 to 24 hours (as clinically required)
Major† (e.g., severe or refractory epistaxis, menorrhagia, GI bleeding, CNS trauma, hemarthrosis, or traumatic hemorrhage)	50 to 80 IU/kg	40 to 60 IU/kg every 8 to 24 hours for approximately 2 to 3 days (as clinically required). Maintain trough levels of VWF:RCo greater than 50% for as long as necessary.

*If recombinant factor VIII is administered, see its package insert for reconstitution and administration instructions.
†A bleed can be considered major if RBC transfusion is either required or potentially indicated or if bleeding occurs in a critical anatomic site (e.g., intracranial or GI hemorrhage).

The initial dose of rVWF should achieve greater than 60% VWF levels (based on VWF:RCo greater than 0.6 IU/mL), and an infusion of recombinant factor VIII should achieve factor VIII levels greater than 40% (FVIII:C greater than 0.4 IU/mL). To calculate specific doses using the correct ratio of 1.3:1, the following formula is recommended:

$$\text{Vonvendi dose (IU)} = \text{Dose in (IU/kg)} \times \text{Weight (kg)}$$
$$\text{Recombinant factor VIII dose (IU)} = \text{Vonvendi dose} \div 1.3$$

DOSE ADJUSTMENTS
Adjust dose according to the extent and location of bleeding. ■ Administer subsequent doses as long as clinically required.

DILUTION
Provided as a kit containing a single-dose vial of powder, a vial of diluent, and a Mix2Vial reconstitution device. Consult instructions for reconstitution and administration in the package insert. Use of plastic syringes is recommended. Warm to room temperature (25° C) before dilution and maintain throughout reconstitution. The total num-

ber of IUs available is clearly marked on each vial (approximately 650 or 1,300 IU of VWF:RCo). Record the batch number of each vial. Should be used immediately after reconstitution. Solution should be clear or slightly opalescent. Use a new Mix2Vial transfer set and syringe for each vial of drug.

If more than one vial is required, the contents of each vial must be drawn into individual syringes that should be left attached to the vial until ready to infuse to reduce the risk of contamination.

Filters: Incorporated into the Mix2Vial.

Storage: Store refrigerated at 2° to 8° C (36° to 46° F) in original carton to protect from light. Do not freeze. May be stored at RT (maximum of 30° C [86° F]) for up to 12 months. Label vial with date removed from refrigeration. Once stored at RT, do not return to refrigeration. Do not use beyond the expiration date on the product vial. Administer immediately after reconstitution, or store at RT not to exceed 27° C (81° F) for up to 3 hours. Do not refrigerate after reconstitution. Discard after 3 hours.

COMPATIBILITY
Manufacturer states, "Do not mix with other medicinal products. Use plastic syringes; proteins in the product tend to stick to the surface of glass syringes."

RATE OF ADMINISTRATION
A single dose may be administered as an infusion up to a maximum rate of 4 mL/min; consider patient comfort. Reduce rate of administration or interrupt the infusion if an increase in heart rate occurs.

ACTIONS
A purified, recombinant von Willebrand factor (rVWF) expressed in Chinese hamster ovary (CHO) cells. Patients with von Willebrand disease (vWD) have a deficiency or abnormality of VWF; this results in low factor VIII activity and an abnormal platelet function, which causes excessive bleeding. VWF re-establishes platelet adhesion at the site of vascular damage, providing primary hemostasis (shortening of bleeding time occurs immediately), and it stabilizes factor VIII by binding to it and preventing its rapid degradation. This latter action is slightly delayed. VWF activity is measured with an assay that uses an agglutinating cofactor called Ristocetin (RCo). The VWF:RCo assay provides a quantitative measurement of VWF function by determining how well VWF helps platelets adhere to one another. Reduced VWF:RCo activity indicates a deficiency of VWF. A sustained increase of factor VIII coagulation activity (FVIII:C) was observed 6 hours after a single infusion of rVWF. Half-life ranged from 19.1 to 21.9 hours depending on the dose administered.

INDICATIONS AND USES
On-demand treatment and control of bleeding episodes in adults (age 18 and older) diagnosed with von Willebrand disease.

CONTRAINDICATIONS
Life-threatening hypersensitivity reactions to von Willebrand factor (recombinant) or constituents of the product or to hamster or mouse proteins.

PRECAUTIONS
For IV use only. ▪ Administered under the direction of a physician knowledgeable in the treatment of coagulation disorders in a facility with adequate diagnostic and treatment facilities to monitor the patient and respond to any medical emergency. ▪ Hypersensitivity reactions, including anaphylaxis, have occurred; see Monitor. ▪ Thrombotic events, including disseminated intravascular coagulation (DIC), venous thrombosis, pulmonary embolism, MI, and stroke, can occur, particularly in patients with known risk factors for thrombosis. ▪ Neutralizing antibodies (inhibitors) to VWF and/or factor VIII can occur; see Monitor.

Monitor: Monitor BP and heart rate during infusion. If an increase in heart rate occurs, either reduce rate of infusion or interrupt the infusion. ▪ Throughout the infusion, monitor for S/S of a hypersensitivity reaction (e.g., acute respiratory distress, angioedema, chest tightness, hypotension, lethargy, nausea, paresthesia, pruritus, restlessness, urticaria, vomiting, wheezing). ▪ Appropriate laboratory tests should be performed on the patient's plasma at suitable intervals. If expected VWF activity plasma levels are not attained or if bleeding episode is not controlled with an appropriate dose, perform an assay that measures the presence of VWF or factor VIII inhibitors. ■ Monitor plasma levels of VWF:RCo and factor VIII activities to avoid sustained excessive VWF and/or factor VIII activity levels, which may increase the risk of thrombotic events. ■ Monitor for early S/S of thrombotic events such as cough, discoloration, dyspnea, hemoptysis, pain, swelling, and syncope.

Patient Education: Review manufacturer's medication guide. ■ Promptly report S/S of a hypersensitivity reaction (e.g., dizziness, hives, itching, rash, tightness of the chest). ■ Frequent blood tests (e.g., monitoring of VWF:RCo and FVIII activity) are required to reduce the risk of thrombotic events. ■ Report a lack of clinical response to therapy; may be a manifestation of an inhibitor. ■ If traveling, bring an adequate supply of medication based on current treatment regimen.

Maternal/Child: Use during pregnancy or labor and delivery only if clearly needed. ■ Safety for use during breast-feeding not known; consider benefit versus risk. ■ Safety and effectiveness for use in pediatric patients less than 18 years of age not established.

Elderly: Numbers insufficient to determine differences in response compared with younger adults.

DRUG/LAB INTERACTIONS
Specific information not available.

SIDE EFFECTS
The most common side effect is generalized pruritus. Chest discomfort, dizziness, dysgeusia, hot flush, hypertension, infusion site paresthesia, nausea, tachycardia, and tremor have occurred.

ANTIDOTE
Keep the physician informed of side effects. Slow or interrupt infusion for an increase in heart rate or mild hypersensitivity reaction. Discontinue the infusion immediately if a severe hypersensitivity reaction or thrombotic event (e.g., chest pain, dyspnea, leg pain, MI) occurs. Treat hypersensitivity as necessary (e.g., antihistamines, epinephrine, corticosteroids), and treat thrombotic events with appropriate measures. Resuscitate as necessary.

VORICONAZOLE

(**vor**-ih-**KOH**-nah-zohl)

VFEND IV

Antifungal
(azole derivative)

USUAL DOSE

Duration of treatment is based on severity of the underlying disease, recovery from immunosuppression, and clinical response. Pretesting required; see Precautions and Monitor. Obtain baseline electrolytes and correct calcium, magnesium, and potassium deficiencies before initiating voriconazole.

		Voriconazole Dose Guidelines	
Infection	Loading Dose	IV Maintenance Dose[f]	Oral Maintenance Dose[f]
Invasive aspergillosis[e, g]	6 mg/kg q 12 hr for the first 24 hours	4 mg/kg q 12 hr	200 mg q 12 hr[c]
Candidemia in nonneutropenic patients and in other deep tissue *Candida* infections	6 mg/kg q 12 hr for the first 24 hours	3 to 4 mg/kg q 12 hr[a, b]	200 mg q 12 hr[a, b, c]
Esophageal candidiasis			200 mg q 12 hr[c, d]
Scedosporiosis and fusariosis[g]	6 mg/kg q 12 hr for the first 24 hours	4 mg/kg q 12 hr	200 mg q 12 hr[c]

[a]In clinical trials, patients with candidemia received 3 mg/kg q 12 hr as primary therapy, and patients with other deep tissue *Candida* infections received 4 mg/kg as salvage therapy. Appropriate dose should be based on the severity and nature of the infection.
[b]Treat for at least 14 days following resolution of symptoms or following last positive culture, whichever is longer.
[c]Patients who weigh 40 kg or more should receive an oral maintenance dose of 200 mg q 12 hr. Adult patients who weigh less than 40 kg should receive an oral maintenance dose of 100 mg q 12 hr.
[d]Treat for a minimum of 14 days and for at least 7 days following the resolution of symptoms.
[e]In a clinical study of invasive aspergillosis, the median duration of IV voriconazole was 10 days (range 2 to 85 days). Median duration of oral therapy was 76 days (range 2 to 232 days).
[f]In healthy volunteer studies, a 200-mg oral dose every 12 hours provided an exposure (AUC) similar to a 3-mg/kg IV dose every 12 hours; a 300-mg oral dose every 12 hours provided an exposure (AUC) similar to a 4-mg/kg IV dose every 12 hours.
[g]IV therapy should be continued for at least 7 days.

For all indications: A switch between IV and oral formulations is appropriate because of high bioavailability of oral formulations. Depending on diagnosis, may switch to oral formulation when a patient has shown clinical improvement and can tolerate oral therapy; see Patient Education.

DOSE ADJUSTMENTS

In patients with an inadequate response weighing 40 kg or more, increase the oral maintenance dose from 200 mg every 12 hours (similar to 3 mg/kg IV every 12 hours) to 300 mg every 12 hours (similar to 4 mg/kg every 12 hours). If unable to tolerate the 300-mg oral dose, decrease it by 50-mg increments to a minimum of 200 mg orally every 12 hours. For adult patients with an inadequate response weighing less than 40 kg, increase the oral maintenance dose from 100 mg every 12 hours to 150 mg every 12 hours. If unable to tolerate the 150-mg dose, decrease it to 100 mg orally every 12 hours. ▪ Reduce the IV maintenance dose to 3 mg/kg every 12 hours in patients unable to tolerate treatment. ▪ If phenytoin (Dilantin) is being administered concurrently, increase the IV maintenance dose of voriconazole to 5 mg/kg every 12 hours or from 200 to 400 mg orally every 12 hours (or 100 mg to 200 mg orally every 12 hours in patients weighing less than 40 kg); see Drug/Lab Interactions. ▪ When voriconazole is coadministered
Continued

with efavirenz (Sustiva), increase voriconazole oral maintenance dose to 400 mg every 12 hours and decrease efavirenz dose to 300 mg every 24 hours. ▪ No dose adjustment is indicated based on age or gender or in patients with baseline liver function tests (ALT, AST) up to 5 times the ULN (see Precautions and Monitor). ▪ In patients with mild to moderate hepatic cirrhosis (Child-Pugh Class A and B), use the standard loading dose but reduce the maintenance dose by one half and administer every 12 hours based on tolerance of treatment and/or concurrent medication. ▪ No dose adjustment is required in patients with a CrCl of 50 mL/min or greater; however, the intravenous vehicle, sulfobutyl ether beta-cyclodextrin sodium (SBECD), accumulates in patients with a CrCl of less than 50 mL/min. Use of oral voriconazole is recommended in these patients; see Precautions and Monitor. ▪ A 4-hour hemodialysis session does not remove a sufficient amount of voriconazole to warrant dose adjustment.

DILUTION

Reconstitute each vial with exactly 19 mL SWFI. Use of a standard 20-mL (nonautomated) syringe is recommended to facilitate exact measurement. Volume will be 20 mL (10 mg/mL). Discard the vial if a vacuum is not present to pull the diluent into the vial. Shake until all powder is dissolved. Calculate the required dose based on patient weight (see the following chart). Must be further diluted for infusion in D5W, D5LR, LR, NS, D5/½NS, D5NS, ½NS, or D5W with 20 mEq KCl. Withdraw a volume equal to the calculated dose of voriconazole from an infusion bag or bottle (30 mL in the following example). The volume of diluent left in the infusion bag or bottle should be enough to allow a final concentration of not less than 0.5 mg/mL or greater than 5 mg/mL after voriconazole is added. Withdraw the required volume of reconstituted drug and add to the infusion bag or bottle. For example, a patient weighing 50 kg will require a loading dose of 300 mg (6 mg/kg × 50 kg), which equals 30 mL of reconstituted drug (1½ vials). Withdraw and discard 30 mL of solution from a 100-mL infusion bag and add the 30 mL of reconstituted drug. Final concentration equals 3 mg/mL.

Required Volumes of 10 mg/mL Voriconazole Concentrate			
Volume of Voriconazole Concentrate (10 mg/mL) required for:			
Body Weight (kg)	3 mg/kg Dose (number of vials)	4 mg/kg Dose (number of vials)	6 mg/kg Dose (number of vials)
30 kg	9 mL (1 vial)	12 mL (1 vial)	18 mL (1 vial)
35 kg	10.5 mL (1 vial)	14 mL (1 vial)	21 mL (2 vials)
40 kg	12 mL (1 vial)	16 mL (1 vial)	24 mL (2 vials)
45 kg	13.5 mL (1 vial)	18 mL (1 vial)	27 mL (2 vials)
50 kg	15 mL (1 vial)	20 mL (1 vial)	30 mL (2 vials)
55 kg	16.5 mL (1 vial)	22 mL (2 vials)	33 mL (2 vials)
60 kg	18 mL (1 vial)	24 mL (2 vials)	36 mL (2 vials)
65 kg	19.5 mL (1 vial)	26 mL (2 vials)	39 mL (2 vials)
70 kg	21 mL (2 vials)	28 mL (2 vials)	42 mL (3 vials)
75 kg	22.5 mL (2 vials)	30 mL (2 vials)	45 mL (3 vials)
80 kg	24 mL (2 vials)	32 mL (2 vials)	48 mL (3 vials)
85 kg	25.5 mL (2 vials)	34 mL (2 vials)	51 mL (3 vials)
90 kg	27 mL (2 vials)	36 mL (2 vials)	54 mL (3 vials)
95 kg	28.5 mL (2 vials)	38 mL (2 vials)	57 mL (3 vials)
100 kg	30 mL (2 vials)	40 mL (2 vials)	60 mL (3 vials)

Filters: No data available from manufacturer.

Storage: Store unopened vials at CRT. Immediate use of reconstituted vials is preferred; however, they may be refrigerated up to 24 hours at 2° to 8° C (37° to 46° F). Discard partially used vials.

COMPATIBILITY (Underline Indicates Conflicting Compatibility Information)
Consider any drug NOT listed as compatible to be INCOMPATIBLE until consulting a pharmacist; specific conditions may apply.

Manufacturer states, "Must not be infused concomitantly with any blood product or short-term infusion of concentrated electrolytes, even if the two infusions are running in separate IV lines or cannulas. Electrolyte disturbances such as hypokalemia, hypomagnesemia, and hypocalcemia should be corrected before initiation of voriconazole; see Precautions." Voriconazole can be infused at the same time as other IV solutions containing (nonconcentrated) electrolytes but must be infused through a separate line. Voriconazole can be infused at the same time as total parenteral nutrition (TPN) but must be infused in a separate line. If infused through a multiple-lumen catheter, TPN needs to be administered using a different port from the one used for voriconazole. Manufacturer states that voriconazole should not be diluted with 4.2% sodium bicarbonate solution. **Compatibility** with other concentrations of sodium bicarbonate is unknown; do not use.

One source suggests the following **compatibilities:**

Y-site: Anidulafungin (Eraxis), caspofungin (Cancidas), ceftaroline (Teflaro), doripenem (Doribax), vasopressin.

RATE OF ADMINISTRATION
A single dose as an infusion over 1 to 2 hours. Do not exceed a rate of 3 mg/kg/hr.

ACTIONS
A triazole antifungal agent. Inhibits a fungal cytochrome P_{450}-mediated essential step in fungal ergosterol biosynthesis. With a loading dose regimen, peak and trough plasma concentrations close to steady-state concentrations are achieved within the first 24 hours. Extensively distributed into tissues. Plasma protein binding (estimated at 58%) is not affected by varying degrees of hepatic and renal insufficiency. Metabolized by cytochrome P_{450} enzymes (CYP2C19 is significantly involved). Terminal half-life is dose dependent and is not useful in predicting accumulation or elimination. Eliminated via hepatic metabolism; less than 2% is excreted unchanged in urine.

INDICATIONS AND USES
For use in patients 12 years of age and older in treatment of the following infections: Treatment of invasive aspergillosis caused by *Aspergillus fumigatus* and other species of *Aspergillus*. ▪ Treatment of candidemia in nonneutropenic patients and the following *Candida* infections: disseminated infections in the skin and infections in the abdomen, kidney, bladder wall, and wounds. ▪ Treatment of serious fungal infections caused by *Scedosporium apiospermum* and *Fusarium* species, including *Fusarium solani*, in patients intolerant of or refractory to other therapy. ▪ Treatment of esophageal candidiasis.

CONTRAINDICATIONS
Hypersensitivity to voriconazole or any of its components. Use caution in patients exhibiting hypersensitivity to other azoles (e.g., fluconazole [Diflucan], itraconazole [Sporanox], ketoconazole [Nizoral]); see Precautions. ▪ Coadministration is specifically **contraindicated** with CYP3A4 substrates (e.g., cisapride [Propulsid], pimozide [Orap], and quinidine [astemizole and terfenadine would be included but are no longer commercially available]); increased plasma concentrations of these drugs may result in QT prolongation and torsades de pointes. ▪ Coadministration is **contraindicated** with the following drugs: barbiturates (long-acting [e.g., phenobarbital (Luminal)]), carbamazepine (Tegretol), efavirenz (Sustiva) 400 mg every 24 hours or higher with a *standard dose* of voriconazole, ergot alkaloids (ergotamine and dihydroergotamine [D.H.E. 45]), rifabutin (Mycobutin), rifampin (Rifadin), high-dose (400 mg every 12 hours) ritonavir (Norvir), sirolimus (Rapamune), and St. John's wort; see Drug Interactions.

PRECAUTIONS

Do not give as an IV bolus; for infusion only. ▪ Specimens for fungal culture, serologic testing, and histopathologic testing should be obtained before therapy to isolate and identify causative organisms. Therapy may begin as soon as all specimens are obtained and before results are known. Reassess after test results are known. ▪ Correct electrolyte disturbances such as hypokalemia, hypomagnesemia, and hypocalcemia before initiation of voriconazole. ▪ Infusion-related hypersensitivity reactions, including anaphylaxis, chest tightness, dyspnea, faintness, fever, flushing, nausea, pruritus, rash, sweating, and tachycardia have occurred. Usually appear at the beginning of the infusion. If a hypersensitivity reaction occurs, discontinue the infusion. ▪ Consider use in patients with severe hepatic insufficiency only if the benefit outweighs potential risk; monitor carefully for drug toxicity. ▪ Serious hepatic reactions (including clinical hepatitis, cholestasis, and fulminant hepatic failure, including fatalities) have occurred. Usually occur in patients with serious underlying medical conditions (e.g., hematologic malignancy); however, hepatic reactions, including hepatitis and jaundice, have occurred in patients with no other identifiable risk factors. Liver function usually improves with discontinuation of voriconazole. ▪ Pancreatitis has been reported; see Monitor. ▪ Consider use of IV formulation in patients with a CrCl less than 50 mL/min only if the benefit outweighs potential risk. Accumulation of SBECD may occur with the IV formulation; use of the oral formulation is recommended. ▪ Acute renal failure has been reported, usually in patients receiving concomitant nephrotoxic drugs or in patients who have concurrent medical conditions that may result in decreased renal function; see Drug/Lab Interactions. ▪ May cause prolongation of the QT interval on ECG and, rarely, torsades de pointes. Use with caution in patients with proarrhythmic conditions (e.g., congenital or acquired QT prolongation, cardiotoxic chemotherapy, cardiomyopathy [in particular when heart failure is present], sinus bradycardia, existing symptomatic arrhythmias, hypokalemia, and concomitant medications that may also prolong the QT interval). ▪ Because of the enzymes involved in metabolism, Asian populations may be poor metabolizers, and serum concentrations may be elevated from 2 to 4 times higher than normal metabolizers. Some whites and blacks are also poor metabolizers. ▪ Blurred vision, color vision changes, and/or photophobia are common but may be associated with higher serum concentrations and/or doses. Usually resolves within 2 weeks of the end of voriconazole therapy. If therapy continues beyond 28 days, the effects of voriconazole therapy on visual function are not known. Prolonged visual adverse effects, including optic neuritis and papilledema, have been reported. ▪ Serious exfoliative cutaneous reactions, such as Stevens-Johnson syndrome, have been reported. ▪ Photosensitivity skin reactions have been reported. If a phototoxic reaction occurs, the patient should be referred to a dermatologist. If therapy is continued despite the occurrence of phototoxicity-related skin lesions, dermatologic evaluation should be performed on a systematic and regular basis to allow for early detection and management of premalignant lesions. Squamous cell carcinoma and melanoma have been reported during long-term therapy; see Patient Education and Maternal/Child. ▪ Fluorosis (mottled enamel of human teeth caused by flouride) and periostitis (inflammation of the periosteum) have been reported during long-term therapy. Discontinue treatment in patients who develop skeletal pain or radiographic findings consistent with either of these diagnoses. ▪ Fungi with reduced susceptibility to one azole antifungal agent may also be less susceptible to other azole derivatives. Cross-resistance may occur and may require alternative antifungal therapy. ▪ Oral maintenance doses adjusted based on weight (above or below 40 kg); see product literature.

Monitor: Obtain baseline electrolytes and make rigorous attempts to correct calcium, magnesium, and potassium before initiating voriconazole. Monitor electrolytes during therapy; may cause hypocalcemia, hypokalemia, and hypomagnesemia. ▪ Obtain baseline liver function tests (e.g., alkaline phosphatase, ALT, AST, bilirubin), serum creatinine, and electrolytes in all patients. Monitor liver function tests at least weekly for the first month of treatment. May decrease monitoring to monthly during continued use if no clinically significant changes are noted. ▪ Monitor pancreatic function (e.g., serum amylase) in adults and children with risk factors for acute pancreatitis (e.g., recent chemotherapy, hematopoietic stem cell transplantation [HSCT]). ▪ Monitor serum creatinine during therapy, more frequently in patients with a CrCl less than 50 mL/min. If an increase in serum creatinine occurs, consider changing to the oral formulation. ▪ Monitor for S/S of hypersensitivity reactions; see Precautions and Antidote. ▪ Monitor visual acuity, visual field, and color perception if treatment continues beyond 28 days. ▪ If a rash develops, serious cutaneous reactions (e.g., Stevens-Johnson syndrome) may develop; see Side Effects and monitor closely. Consider discontinuing voriconazole. ▪ See Precautions, Drug/Lab Interactions, and Antidote.

Patient Education: Review of health history and medication profile is imperative. ▪ Avoid pregnancy; nonhormonal birth control recommended; see Drug/Lab Interactions. Should pregnancy occur, notify physician immediately and discuss potential hazards. ▪ Do not drive at night; changes to vision, including blurring and/or photophobia, may occur. Ophthalmologic monitoring is required with prolonged use. ▪ If a change in vision occurs, avoid hazardous tasks, such as driving or operating machinery. ▪ Avoid strong, direct sunlight; protective clothing and sunscreen with a high SPF are recommended. ▪ Promptly report S/S of a hypersensitivity reaction (e.g., itching, hives, shortness of breath) or a serious skin reaction (e.g., severe sunburn, blistering or peeling of skin). ▪ Additional precautions required with transfer to oral voriconazole.

Maternal/Child: Category D: avoid pregnancy; may cause fetal harm. Teratogenic in rats and embryotoxic in rabbits. Use of effective contraception is required in women of childbearing age. ▪ Discontinue breast-feeding. ▪ Safety and effectiveness for use in pediatric patients under 12 years of age not established. ▪ Frequency of phototoxicity reactions is higher in pediatric patients. Stringent measures for photoprotection are warranted; see Patient Education. In children experiencing photoaging injuries, sun avoidance and dermatologic follow-up are recommended, even after discontinuation of therapy.

Elderly: Safety profile similar to younger adults. ▪ Use caution; consider decreased cardiac, hepatic, or renal function and effects of concomitant disease or other drug therapy. ▪ Monitor liver and renal function closely.

DRUG/LAB INTERACTIONS

Interactions are numerous and potentially life threatening. Review of drug profile by pharmacist is imperative.

Contraindicated with CYP3A4 substrates (e.g., **cisapride** [Propulsid], **pimozide** [Orap], and **quinidine** [astemizole and terfenadine would be included but are no longer commercially available]); increased plasma concentrations of these drugs may result in QT prolongation and torsades de pointes. ▪ **Contraindicated** with **long-acting barbiturates** (e.g., phenobarbital [Luminal]), **carbamazepine** (Tegretol), **rifampin** (Rifadin), **and St. John's wort**; these drugs may significantly increase metabolism and decrease serum concentrations of voriconazole. ▪ **Contraindicated** with **high-dose (400 mg every 12 hours) ritonavir** (Norvir); decreases serum concentrations of voriconazole. **Low-dose ritonavir (100 mg every 12 hours)** reduces voriconazole concentration to a lesser extent. Coadministration should be avoided unless assessment of the benefit versus risk to the patient justifies voriconazole use. ▪ **Contraindicated** with **sirolimus** (Rapamune); metabolism of sirolimus is decreased, and serum concentrations are significantly increased by voriconazole. ▪ **Contraindicated** with **rifabutin** (Mycobutin); voriconazole significantly increases the serum concentrations of rifabutin, and rifabutin significantly decreases voriconazole serum concentrations. ▪ Coadministration of standard doses of voriconazole with **efavirenz** (Sustiva) doses of 400 mg every 24 hours or higher is **contraindicated**. Voriconazole increases serum concentrations of efavirenz, and efavirenz decreases serum concentrations of voriconazole. If coadministration is required, dose adjustment of both drugs is indicated. Increase voriconazole oral maintenance dose to 400 mg every 12 hours and decrease efavirenz to 300 mg every 24 hours. Restore the initial dose of efavirenz when treatment with voriconazole is discontinued. ▪ **Contraindicated** with **ergot alkaloids** (e.g., ergotamine and dihydroergotamine [D.H.E. 45]); serum concentrations of ergot alkaloids may be increased and may lead to ergotism. ▪ Avoid concomitant use with **fluconazole** (Diflucan). Potential for voriconazole toxicity remains if voriconazole is initiated within 24 hours of the last dose of fluconazole. ▪ May decrease the metabolism and increase serum levels of **cyclosporine** (Sandimmune). If concurrent administration with voriconazole is indicated, reduce the dose of cyclosporine by one half and monitor cyclosporine serum levels frequently. When voriconazole is discontinued, monitor cyclosporine levels frequently and increase the dose as necessary. ▪ May decrease the metabolism and increase serum levels of **methadone** (Dolophine) and increase risk of QT prolongation. If concurrent administration with voriconazole is indicated, monitor closely and decrease dose of methadone as necessary. ▪ Increases concentration and half-life of **alfentanil** (Alfenta), **fentanyl**, **oxycodone** (ETH-Oxydose), **and sufentanil** (Sufenta). Dose reduction and extended monitoring recommended. ▪ May decrease the metabolism and increase serum levels of **tacrolimus** (Prograf). If concurrent administration with voriconazole is indicated, reduce the dose of tacrolimus by one third and monitor tacrolimus serum levels frequently. When voriconazole is discontinued, monitor tacrolimus levels frequently and increase the dose as necessary. ▪ Concurrent use with **warfarin** (Coumadin) or oral coumarin preparations may cause a significant increase in PT or INR. Monitor PT or INR closely and adjust warfarin dose as necessary. ▪ May decrease the metabolism and increase serum concentrations of CYP3A4 substrates, such as selected **HMG-CoA reductase inhibitors** (statins such as lovastatin [Mevacor]), **selected benzodiazepines** (e.g., alprazolam [Xanax], midazolam [Versed], triazolam [Halcion]), **selected calcium channel blockers** (e.g., felodipine [Plendil]), **vinca alkaloids** (e.g., vinblastine, vincristine), and CYP2C9 substrates such as **sulfonylureas** (e.g., glipizide [Glucotrol XL], glyburide [DiaBeta], tolbutamide) and **NSAIDs** (e.g., ibuprofen [Motrin], diclofenac [Voltaren]). To reduce the potential for toxic effects that may be caused by these drugs (e.g., rhabdomyolysis, prolonged sedative effect, cardiac toxicity, GI toxicity, neurotoxicity, hypoglycemia), close monitoring for toxic effects of all of these drugs is indicated, and in most cases dose reduction is indicated during concomitant administration of voriconazole. ▪ Concomitant administration with **everolimus** (Afinitor), a CYP3A4 inhibitor and substrate and a P-pg substrate, is not recommended; plasma exposure of everolimus is likely to be increased. ▪ Concurrent use with **phenytoin** (Dilantin) may require dose adjustments of both drugs. Phenytoin increases metabolism and decreases serum concentrations of voriconazole. An increased dose of voriconazole is indicated; see Dose Adjustments. Voriconazole decreases the metabolism of phenytoin and increases serum concentrations. Monitor phenytoin serum concentrations and reduce dose as necessary to avoid toxicity. ▪ May decrease the metabolism and increase serum levels of **selected HIV protease inhibitors** (e.g., amprenavir [Agenerase], nelfinavir [Viracept], saquinavir [Invirase]). Selected HIV protease inhibitors (e.g., amprenavir, saquinavir) may decrease the metabolism of voriconazole and increase its serum levels. Monitor frequently for drug toxicity with coadministration of voriconazole and HIV protease inhibitors. No dose adjustment is required with indinavir (Crixivan). ▪ May decrease the metabolism and increase serum levels of **omeprazole** (Prilosec). If concurrent administration with voriconazole is indicated, reduce a dose of omeprazole of 40 mg or more by one half. The metabolism of other selected proton pump inhibitors may react similarly. ▪ **Nonnucleoside reverse transcriptase inhibitors** (NNRTIs) such as delavirdine (Rescriptor) may decrease the metabolism of voriconazole and increase its serum concentrations. Voriconazole may inhibit the metabolism of the same NNRTIs and increase their serum levels. Monitor frequently for drug toxicity with coadministration of voriconazole and NNRTIs. ▪ Concurrent use with **other nephrotoxic drugs** (e.g., aminoglycosides, cyclosporine) may result in decreased renal function or acute renal failure. ▪ Concurrent use with **oral contraceptives** may increase concentrations of both drugs. Monitor for adverse events related to each drug. Should not reduce the effectiveness of oral contraception. ▪ May have minor interactions with **cimetidine** (Tagamet), **macrolide antibiotics** (e.g., azithromycin, erythromycin), **and ranitidine** (Zantac); however, no dose adjustments are required. ▪ No significant interactions have been observed with prednisolone, digoxin (Lanoxin), and mycophenolate (CellCept).

SIDE EFFECTS
Abdominal pain, chills, diarrhea, dyspnea, fever, hallucinations, headache, hypokalemia, increases in liver function tests, nausea, peripheral edema, rash, respiratory disorders, sepsis, tachycardia, visual disturbances, and vomiting occur most frequently. Side effects that most often led to discontinuation of therapy include elevated liver function tests, rash, and visual disturbances. Blurred vision, color vision change, and/or photophobia are common but may be associated with higher serum concentrations and/or doses. Hypersensitivity reactions, including anaphylaxis, have been reported. Rarely, Stevens-Johnson syndrome and photosensitivity skin reactions have been reported. In patients with photosensitivity reactions, squamous cell cancer and melanoma have been reported. Numerous other side effects may occur, including QT prolongation and, rarely, torsades de pointes.

Post-Marketing: Pancreatitis in pediatric patients, prolonged visual adverse events, including optic neuritis and papilledema.

ANTIDOTE
Notify physician of all side effects; most will be treated symptomatically. If a hypersensitivity reaction (e.g., an infusion reaction) occurs, discontinue the infusion and treat with oxygen, epinephrine, antihistamines (e.g., diphenhydramine [Benadryl]), corticosteroids (e.g., dexamethasone [Decadron]), or bronchodilators (e.g., albuterol) as indicated. Consider discontinuation of voriconazole if liver function tests are elevated and/or clinical S/S of liver disease attributable to voriconazole develop, if visual disturbances occur, if an increase in serum creatinine occurs, if a rash develops (may be the first sign of an exfoliative skin disorder), or if a phototoxic reaction occurs. No known specific antidote. Hemodialysis may assist in the removal of some voriconazole in accidental overdose and in the removal of SBECD. Resuscitate as indicated.

WARFARIN SODIUM BBW
(WAR-far-in SO-dee-um)

Coumadin

Anticoagulant
(vitamin K antagonist)

pH 8.1 to 8.3

USUAL DOSE

Used primarily for patients on Coumadin when oral dosing is not feasible. IV and oral doses are the same, and administration of the IV formulation should not provide any increased effect or an earlier onset of action. ▪ Dose must be individualized and adjusted based on PT/international normalized ratio (INR) and the condition being treated. Consult the latest evidence-based clinical practice guidelines regarding the duration and intensity of anticoagulation for the indicated condition. For most conditions, the warfarin dose should be adjusted to achieve a target INR of 2.5 (INR range of 2 to 3). A higher INR (target INR of 3, with a range of 2.5 to 3.5) may be indicated in select patients with specific types of heart valves. An INR of greater than 4 appears to provide no additional benefit in most patients and is associated with a higher risk of bleeding. Routine use of loading doses is not recommended because this practice may increase the incidence of complications and does not offer more rapid protection against clot formation. ▪ Heparin is preferred in situations requiring prompt anticoagulation because the onset of anticoagulant action for warfarin is 24 to 72 hours, and full therapeutic effect is not reached for 5 to 7 days. Conversion to warfarin therapy may begin concomitantly with heparin therapy or may be delayed 3 to 6 days. To ensure continuous anticoagulation, overlap therapy until warfarin has produced a therapeutic response as determined by PT/INR. Discontinue heparin when therapeutic response is achieved. ▪ Duration of treatment is individualized. In general, it should continue until the danger of thrombosis and embolism has passed. See prescribing information and the latest evidence-based clinical practice guidelines for suggested durations of therapy for different indications and/or risk factors. Aspirin may or may not be a component of therapy depending on indication and risk factors. ▪ Not all factors causing warfarin dose variability are known. The maintenance dose needed to achieve a target PT/INR is influenced by clinical factors that include age, race, body weight, gender, concomitant medications, comorbidities, and genetic factors (CYP2C9 and VKORC1 genotypes). See prescribing information and Dose Adjustments for dosing related to specific genotypes.

Initial dose: Select the starting dose based on the expected maintenance dose, taking into account the above factors. If the patient's CYP2C9 and VKORC1 genotypes are not known, the initial dose is usually 2 to 5 mg/day. Adjust dose based on patient-specific clinical factors and PT/INR determination.

Maintenance dose: 2 to 10 mg/day. Adjust dose to maintain desired INR.

PEDIATRIC DOSE

Safety for use in pediatric patients under 18 years of age not established, but is used. Usually given PO. See Maternal/Child.

DOSE ADJUSTMENTS

Use low initial doses in elderly, debilitated, or Asian patients and in patients with expected increased PT/INR responses. ▪ Patients with genetic factors (CYP2C9 and VKORC1 genotypes) may require a reduced dose because these alleles may be associated with reduced clearance of warfarin. ▪ Use lower end of dose range in patients at increased risk of bleeding or those on aspirin therapy. ▪ Reduced dose may be required in impaired hepatic function due to the impaired synthesis of clotting factors and the decreased metabolism of warfarin. ▪ No dose adjustment is required in impaired renal function. ▪ Higher doses may be required in selected situations (e.g., patients with recurrent systemic embolism or mechanical prosthetic valves).

DILUTION

Available as a 5-mg lyophilized powder in a single-use vial. Reconstitute the 5-mg vial with 2.7 mL of SWFI to obtain a solution with a final concentration of 2 mg/mL.

Storage: Protect from light by storing in carton at CRT. Store reconstituted solution at room temperature and use within 4 hours. Do not refrigerate; discard any unused solution.

COMPATIBILITY   (Underline Indicates Conflicting Compatibility Information)

Consider any drug NOT listed as compatible to be INCOMPATIBLE until consulting a pharmacist; specific conditions may apply.

Some adsorption may occur in PVC containers and tubing when diluted in D5W or NS.

One source suggests the following **compatibilities:**

Y-site: Amikacin, ammonium chloride, ascorbic acid, bivalirudin (Angiomax), cefazolin (Ancef), ceftriaxone (Rocephin), dopamine, epinephrine (Adrenalin), heparin, lidocaine, morphine, nitroglycerin IV, oxytocin (Pitocin), potassium chloride (KCl), ranitidine (Zantac), vancomycin.

RATE OF ADMINISTRATION

A single dose as an injection into a peripheral vein over 1 to 2 minutes.

ACTIONS

An anticoagulant that acts by inhibiting the synthesis of vitamin K–dependent coagulation factors (e.g., factor II, VII, IX, and X) and the anticoagulant proteins C and S in the liver, resulting in a depression of their activities. An anticoagulant effect occurs within 24 hours; however, peak anticoagulant effect may be delayed for 72 to 96 hours. Approximately 99% bound to plasma proteins. Effective half-life ranges from 20 to 60 hours, with a mean of 40 hours. Effects may be more pronounced as daily maintenance doses overlap. Well-established clots are not dissolved, but growth is prevented. Metabolized by hepatic microsomal enzymes (cytochrome P_{450} system) to inactive metabolites and reduced metabolites. Excreted primarily in urine. Crosses the placental barrier.

INDICATIONS AND USES

Prophylaxis and/or treatment of venous thrombosis and its extension, pulmonary embolism (PE). ■ Prophylaxis and treatment of the thromboembolic complications associated with atrial fibrillation (AF) and/or cardiac valve replacement. ■ Reduction in the risk of death, recurrent myocardial infarction (MI), and thromboembolic events such as stroke or systemic embolization after myocardial infarction. ■ Treatment of patients receiving oral warfarin who are unable to take oral medication.

Limitation of use: Warfarin has no direct effect on an established thrombus, nor does it reverse ischemic tissue damage. Once a thrombus has occurred, however, the goals of anticoagulant treatment are to prevent further extension of the formed clot and to prevent secondary thromboembolic complications that may result in serious and possibly fatal sequelae.

CONTRAINDICATIONS

Pregnancy, except in women with mechanical heart valves, who are at high risk of thromboembolism; see Maternal/Child. ■ Patients with (1) hemorrhagic tendencies or blood dyscrasias; (2) recent or contemplated surgery of the CNS or eye or traumatic surgery resulting in large open surfaces; (3) bleeding tendencies associated with active ulceration or overt bleeding of GI, GU, or respiratory tracts; central nervous system hemorrhage; cerebral aneurysm; dissecting aorta; pericarditis; pericardial effusions; and bacterial endocarditis; (4) threatened abortion, eclampsia, or pre-eclampsia; (5) conditions associated with a potentially high level of noncompliance (unsupervised patients); (6) spinal puncture and other diagnostic or therapeutic procedures with the potential for uncontrollable bleeding; (7) hypersensitivity to warfarin; (8) major regional or lumbar block anesthesia; (9) malignant hypertension.

PRECAUTIONS

For IV use only; do not administer IM. ■ Warfarin can cause major or fatal bleeding. Hemorrhage in any tissue or organ is one of the most serious risks associated with warfarin therapy. Bleeding is more likely to occur within the first month of therapy and with higher doses (resulting in a higher INR). Risk factors for hemorrhage include an INR greater than 4 or a history of highly variable INRs, elderly patients age 65 or older, history of GI bleed, hypertension, cerebrovascular disease, anemia, malignancy, trauma, renal impairment, certain genetic factors, concomitant drugs that affect hemostasis, and a long duration of therapy. ▪ Necrosis and/or gangrene is an uncommon but serious risk associated with warfarin therapy. Necrosis appears to be associated with local thrombosis and usually appears within a few days of initiation of therapy. In severe cases, débridement or amputation may be required. ▪ Anticoagulation with warfarin may enhance the release of atheromatous plaque emboli. Systemic atheroemboli and cholesterol microemboli can present with a variety of S/S depending on the site of embolization. S/S may include abdominal, back, or flank pain; abrupt and intense pain in the leg, foot, or toes; cerebral ischemia; foot ulcers; gangrene; hematuria; hypertension; livedo reticularis (reddish blue mottling of skin on exposure to cold); myalgias; pancreatitis; "purple toes syndrome"; rash; and renal insufficiency. The kidney is the most commonly involved visceral organ, followed by the pancreas, spleen, and liver. Some cases have progressed to necrosis and death. ▪ Do not use warfarin as initial therapy in patients with heparin-induced thrombocytopenia (HIT) or in patients with heparin-induced thrombocytopenia with thrombosis syndrome (HITTS). Cases of venous limb ischemia, necrosis, and gangrene have occurred in patients with HIT or HITTS when heparin was discontinued and warfarin was started or continued. Treatment with warfarin can be considered after the platelet count has normalized. ▪ Warfarin may increase the aPTT, even in the absence of heparin. A severe aPTT elevation (greater than 50 seconds) with a PT/INR in the normal range is an indicator of increased risk of postoperative hemorrhage. ▪ Use caution in elderly or debilitated patients or in patients with moderate to severe hepatic impairment, moderate to severe hypertension, diabetes mellitus, indwelling catheters, infectious diseases or disturbances of the intestinal flora (e.g., sprue, antibiotic therapy), polycythemia vera, vasculitis, or known or suspected deficiency in protein C anticoagulant response. ▪ Increased PT/INR response may occur in patients with diarrhea, hepatic disorders, poor nutritional state, steatorrhea, or vitamin K deficiency. ▪ Decreased PT/INR response may occur with increased vitamin K intake or in patients with hereditary warfarin resistance. ▪ If dental procedures or other minor surgical procedures are necessary, the PT/INR should be adjusted to the lower end of the therapeutic range. Monitor PT/INR just before treatment. Operative site should be limited so local procedures for hemostasis can be used. Warfarin therapy may have to be interrupted; consider risks versus benefits. ▪ Limit IM injections of concomitant medications to the upper extremities to permit easy access for manual compression, inspection for bleeding, and the use of pressure bandages.

Monitor: Obtain baseline PT/INR. Frequent monitoring of PT/INR is required. Usually repeated daily during initiation of therapy and then every 1 to 4 weeks after PT/INR has stabilized in the therapeutic range. Monitor with any change in patient regimen that may affect treatment (e.g., diet, illness, change in drug regimen). Draw blood for prothrombin just before a heparin dose being given concomitantly. If heparin is given as a continuous infusion, PT/INR may be drawn at any time; see Precautions. ▪ Because heparin may affect the PT/INR in patients receiving both heparin and warfarin, PT/INR determinations should be drawn 5 hours after the last IV bolus dose of heparin, 4 hours after a heparin infusion has been discontinued, or 24 hours after the last SC injection of heparin. ▪ Patients at high risk for bleeding may benefit from more frequent monitoring of INR, careful dose adjustments to desired INR, and a shorter duration of therapy. However, maintenance of INR in the therapeutic range does not eliminate the risk of bleeding. ▪ Monitor for S/S of hemorrhage, necrosis, cholesterol microembolization, and the possible sequelae; see Precautions. ▪ Has a narrow therapeutic range that can be affected by other drugs and dietary vitamin K. See Drug/Lab Interactions. ▪ Determinations of whole blood clotting and bleeding times are not effective measures for monitoring warfarin therapy. ▪ See Maternal/Child.

Patient Education: Read manufacturer's medication guide. ▪ Effective contraception is required during treatment and for at least 1 month after the final dose of warfarin. ▪ Adhere to dose schedule; do not take or discontinue any prescription or over-the-counter medication, including herbal products, without physician's approval. ▪ Confirm procedure for missed dose. ▪ Avoid alcohol. Eat a normal balanced diet, maintaining a consistent vitamin K intake. Avoid cranberry products. ▪ Avoid any activity or sport that may result in traumatic injury. ▪ Regular PT/INR testing and physician visits are imperative. ▪ Notify physician of unusual bleeding (e.g., increased menstrual flow, nosebleeds, tarry stools), any illness (e.g., diarrhea, infection, fever), headache, dizziness, or weakness. ▪ Carry an ID stating that warfarin is being taken.

Maternal/Child: Warfarin is contraindicated in women who are pregnant, except in pregnant women with mechanical heart valves, who are at high risk of thromboembolism and for whom the benefits of warfarin may outweigh the risks to the fetus. Warfarin can cause fetal harm. Exposure during pregnancy caused a recognized pattern of major congenital malformations (warfarin embryopathy and fetotoxicity), fatal fetal hemorrhage, and an increased risk of spontaneous abortion and fetal mortality. ▪ Verify the pregnancy status of females of reproductive potential before initiating warfarin therapy. ▪ Limited data suggest that warfarin is not present in breast milk. However, because of the potential adverse effects on the breast-fed infant, caution is advised. Monitor breast-feeding infants for bruising or bleeding. ▪ Safety and effectiveness for use in pediatric patients not established; however, use is well documented for prevention and treatment of thromboembolic events. Dosing of warfarin in pediatric patients varies with age, with infants generally having the highest and adolescents having the lowest mg/kg dose requirements to maintain target INRs. Difficulty in achieving and maintaining a therapeutic PT/INR in pediatric patients has been reported. More frequent PT/INR determinations are recommended. ▪ Infants and children receiving vitamin K–supplemented nutrition, including infant formulas, may be resistant to warfarin therapy, whereas infants fed human milk may be sensitive to warfarin therapy.

Elderly: No overall differences in effectiveness or safety were observed between elderly patients and younger patients, but greater sensitivity of some older individuals cannot be ruled out. Less warfarin is required to produce a therapeutic level of anticoagulation in patients over 60 years of age; may have a greater-than-expected PT/INR response; see Dose Adjustments and Precautions. ▪ Not recommended for use in an unsupervised patient with senility.

DRUG/LAB INTERACTIONS

Drugs, dietary changes, and other factors affect INR levels achieved with warfarin. Monitor PT/INR carefully when drugs are added or discontinued or diet is modified. *Interactions are numerous and potentially life threatening. Review of drug profile by pharmacist is imperative.* ▪ Drugs may interact with warfarin through pharmacodynamic or pharmacokinetic mechanisms. Pharmacodynamic mechanisms include synergism (impaired hemostasis, reduced clotting factor synthesis), competitive antagonism (vitamin K), and alteration of the physiologic control loop for vitamin K metabolism (hereditary resistance). Pharmacokinetic mechanisms for drug interactions are mainly enzyme induction or inhibition and reduced plasma protein binding. Some drugs may interact by more than one mechanism. ▪ Some of the most significant drug interactions are listed in the following chart. *This list is not all-inclusive.* See manufacturer's prescribing information for additional medications that may interact with warfarin, and consult the labeling of all concurrently used drugs to obtain further information. ▪ The three more important CYP450 isozymes involved in the metabolism of warfarin are CYP2C9, CYP1A2 and CYP3A4. **Inhibitors of these enzymes** have the potential to increase the effect (increase the INR) of warfarin. **Inducers of these enzymes** have the potential to decrease the effect (decrease the INR) of warfarin. The following chart lists examples of inhibitors and inducers of these enzymes.

Examples of CYP450 Interactions with Warfarin		
Enzyme	Inhibitors	Inducers
CYP2C9	Amiodarone, capecitabine, cotrimoxazole, etravirine, fluconazole, fluvastatin, fluvoxamine, metronidazole, miconazole, oxandrolone, sulfinpyrazone, tigecycline, voriconazole, zafirlukast	Aprepitant, bosentan, carbamazepine, phenobarbital, rifampin
CYP1A2	Acyclovir, allopurinol, caffeine, cimetidine, ciprofloxacin, disulfiram, enoxacin, famotidine, fluvoxamine, methoxsalen, mexiletine, norfloxacin, oral contraceptives, phenylpropanolamine, propafenone, propranolol, terbinafine, thiabendazole, ticlopidine, verapamil, zileuton	Montelukast, moricizine, omeprazole, phenobarbital, phenytoin, cigarette smoking
CYP3A4	Alprazolam, amiodarone, amlodipine, amprenavir, aprepitant, atorvastatin, atazanavir, bicalutamide, cilostazol, cimetidine, ciprofloxacin, clarithromycin, conivaptan, cyclosporine, darunavir/ritonavir, diltiazem, erythromycin, fluconazole, fluoxetine, fluvoxamine, fosamprenavir, imatinib, indinavir, isoniazid, itraconazole, ketoconazole, lopinavir/ritonavir, nefazodone, nelfinavir, nilotinib, oral contraceptives, posaconazole, ranitidine, ranolazine, ritonavir, saquinavir, telithromycin, tipranavir, voriconazole, zileuton	Armodafinil, amprenavir, aprepitant, bosentan, carbamazepine, efavirenz, etravirine, modafinil, nafcillin, phenytoin, pioglitazone, prednisone, rifampin, rufinamide

- Examples of drugs that can increase the risk of bleeding when given concomitantly with warfarin are listed in the following chart.

Examples of Drugs That Can Increase the Risk of Bleeding	
Drug Class	Specific Drugs
Anticoagulants	Argatroban, dabigatran, bivalirudin, desirudin, heparin, lepirudin
Antiplatelet agents	Aspirin, cilostazol, clopidogrel, dipyridamole, prasugrel, ticlopidine
NSAIDs	Celecoxib, diclofenac, diflunisal, fenoprofen, ibuprofen, indomethacin, ketoprofen, ketorolac, mefenamic acid, naproxen, oxaprozin, piroxicam, sulindac
Serotonin reuptake inhibitors	Citalopram, desvenlafaxine, duloxetine, escitalopram, fluoxetine, fluvoxamine, milnacipran, paroxetine, sertraline, venlafaxine, vilazodone

- There have been reports of changes in INR in patients taking warfarin and **antibiotics or antifungals**, but clinical pharmacokinetic studies have not shown consistent effects of these agents on plasma concentrations of warfarin. Closely monitor INR when starting or stopping any antibiotic or antifungal. ▪ Some herbal products (e.g., **garlic** and **Ginkgo biloba**) may have anticoagulant, antiplatelet, and/or fibrinolytic properties. Consider the possibility of additive effects if administered concomitantly with warfarin. ▪ Some herbal products may decrease the effects of warfarin (e.g., **co-enzyme Q10, St. John's wort, ginseng**). ▪ Some botanicals and foods can interact with warfarin through CYP450 interactions (e.g., **Echinacea, grapefruit juice, ginkgo, goldenseal, St. John's wort**). ▪ **Foods rich in vitamin K** (e.g., green, leafy vegetables) inhibit the anticoagulant effect of warfarin. Maintain a balanced diet with a consistent intake of vitamin K.

SIDE EFFECTS

Fatal and nonfatal hemorrhage from any tissue or organ is the most common adverse reaction seen with warfarin. Other serious reactions may include necrosis and/or gangrene of skin and other tissues and complications from systemic atheroemboli and cholesterol microemboli (e.g., "purple toes syndrome"). Other reported side effects include abdominal pain, alopecia, bloating, chills, dermatitis (including bullous eruptions), diarrhea, flatulence, hepatobiliary disorders (e.g., elevated liver enzymes, hepatitis, and cholestatic hepatitis [when warfarin has been administered concomitantly with ticlopidine]), nausea, pruritus, rash, syncope, taste perversion, tracheal or tracheobronchial calcification, vasculitis, and vomiting. Hypersensitivity reactions, including anaphylaxis and urticaria, have been reported.

ANTIDOTE

Keep physician informed of all side effects; some may be life threatening. Discontinue if warfarin is suspected to be the cause of developing necrosis or if S/S of systemic atheroemboli and/or cholesterol microemboli (e.g., "purple toes syndrome") develop; consider alternative drugs if continued anticoagulation therapy is required. The treatment of excessive anticoagulation is based on the level of the INR, the presence or absence of bleeding, and clinical circumstances. Withhold warfarin or administer an antidote as clinically indicated. Phytonadione (vitamin K_1) is a specific antagonist and may be indicated in overdose or desired warfarin reversal (e.g., severe bleeding, need for emergent surgery). May be given via the parenteral or oral route. Dose will depend on clinical situation and may range from 0.5 to 10 mg. (Refer to evidence-based guidelines for recommended dosing based on INR and the clinical situation.) The use of phytonadione will impede subsequent anticoagulant therapy, and patients are at risk for returning to a pretreatment thrombotic status following rapid reversal of a prolonged PT/INR. Fresh frozen plasma or four-factor prothrombin complex concentrate (Kcentra) may be indicated for urgent reversal in patients with acute major bleeding or a need for an urgent surgery/invasive procedure.

ZIDOVUDINE BBW

(zye-**DOH**-vyou-deen)

Azidothymidine, AZT, Retrovir

USUAL DOSE

Treatment of HIV infection (symptomatic or asymptomatic): 1 mg/kg every 4 hours. Initiate oral therapy as soon as possible (100 mg PO approximately equal to 1 mg/kg IV). Impaired renal or hepatic function may increase toxicity. Usually part of a multidrug regimen; see Drug/Lab Interactions.

Prevention of maternal-fetal HIV transmission: 2 mg/kg of total body weight over 1 hour when labor begins. Follow with an infusion of 1 mg/kg/hr (of total body weight) until umbilical cord is clamped.

PEDIATRIC DOSE

See Maternal/Child.

To avoid medication errors when preparing pediatric doses, use extra care to calculate the appropriate dose based on body weight (kg). Follow with oral therapy; see comments in Usual Dose.

Treatment of HIV infections in pediatric patients 4 weeks to less than 18 years of age, weight greater than 4 kg: Recommendations for pediatric oral dosing (capsules, tablets, or syrup) can be found in the prescribing information. Should not exceed the recommended adult dose. See Dose Adjustments.

NEONATAL DOSE

See Maternal/Child.

Treatment of HIV infections (unlabeled): Oral dosing preferred but may be given IV.

Premature neonates (gestational age less than 30 weeks) younger than 6 weeks of age: 1.5 mg/kg IV every 12 hours. Increase to 2.3 mg/kg every 12 hours at 4 weeks of age.

Premature neonates (gestational age 30 to 35 weeks) younger than 6 weeks of age: 1.5 mg/kg IV every 12 hours. Increase to 2.3 mg/kg IV every 12 hours at 15 days of age.

Full-term infants (gestational age 35 weeks or more) younger than 6 weeks of age: 3 mg/kg IV every 12 hours.

Prevention of maternal-fetal HIV transmission: Start neonatal dosing within 12 hours after birth and continue through 6 weeks of age. Oral dosing preferred but may be given IV. Consider impaired hepatic or renal function; see Precautions.

Recommended Neonatal Doses of Zidovudine		
Route	Total Daily Dose	Dose and Frequency
Oral	8 mg/kg/day	2 mg/kg every 6 hours
IV	6 mg/kg/day	1.5 mg/kg infused over 30 minutes every 6 hours

DOSE ADJUSTMENTS

Dose selection should be cautious in the elderly based on the potential for decreased organ function and concomitant disease or drug therapy. ▪ Reduce dose to 1 mg/kg every 6 to 8 hours in patients with a CrCl less than 15 mL/min or in patients with ESRD who are being maintained on hemodialysis or peritoneal dialysis. ▪ Dose reduction may be required in patients with hepatic impairment. Monitor for hematologic toxicity. ▪ Dose interruption may be required in the presence of significant anemia or neutropenia. ▪ Dose adjustment may be required in anemia and/or with other drugs. See Monitor, Drug/Lab Interactions, and Antidote.

DILUTION

Each vial of zidovudine contains 200 mg in 20 mL (10 mg/mL). Withdraw the calculated dose and add to a sufficient volume of D5W to achieve a final concentration no greater than 4 mg/mL. To avoid medication errors when preparing a pediatric dose, use extra care to calculate the appropriate dose in mL based on body weight (kg).

Filters: Not required by manufacturer; no further data available from manufacturer.

Storage: Store undiluted vials at 15° to 25° C (59° to 77° F). Protect from light. Chemically and physically stable after dilution for 24 hours at RT or 48 hours refrigerated at 2° to 8° C (36° to 46° F). However, as an added precaution against microbial contamination, manufacturer recommends use within 8 hours if stored at 25° C (77° F) and 24 hours if refrigerated.

COMPATIBILITY   (Underline Indicates Conflicting Compatibility Information)
Consider any drug NOT listed as compatible to be INCOMPATIBLE until consulting a pharmacist; specific conditions may apply.

Manufacturer states, "Admixture in biologic or colloidal fluids (e.g., blood products, protein solutions) is not recommended."

One source suggests the following **compatibilities:**

Additive: Dobutamine, meropenem (Merrem IV), ranitidine (Zantac).

Y-site: Acyclovir (Zovirax), allopurinol (Aloprim), amifostine (Ethyol), amikacin, amphotericin B (conventional), amphotericin B cholesteryl (Amphotec), anidulafungin (Eraxis), aztreonam (Azactam), ceftazidime (Fortaz), ceftriaxone (Rocephin), cisatracurium (Nimbex), clindamycin (Cleocin), dexamethasone (Decadron), dobutamine, docetaxel (Taxotere), dopamine, doripenem (Doribax), doxorubicin liposomal (Doxil), erythromycin (Erythrocin), etoposide phosphate (Etopophos), filgrastim (Neupogen), fluconazole (Diflucan), fludarabine (Fludara), gemcitabine (Gemzar), gentamicin, granisetron (Kytril), heparin, imipenem-cilastatin (Primaxin), linezolid (Zyvox), lorazepam (Ativan), melphalan (Alkeran), meropenem (Merrem IV), metoclopramide (Reglan), morphine, nafcillin (Nallpen), ondansetron (Zofran), oxacillin (Bactocill), oxytocin (Pitocin), paclitaxel (Taxol), pemetrexed (Alimta), pentamidine, phenylephrine (Neo-Synephrine), piperacillin/tazobactam (Zosyn), potassium chloride (KCl), ranitidine (Zantac), remifentanil (Ultiva), sargramostim (Leukine), sulfamethoxazole/trimethoprim, teniposide (Vumon), thiotepa, tobramycin, vancomycin, vinorelbine (Navelbine).

RATE OF ADMINISTRATION
Intermittent infusion: Each single dose properly diluted must be delivered at a constant rate over 1 hour. Avoid rapid infusion or IV bolus.

Continuous infusion: Prevention of maternal-fetal HIV transmission: 2 mg/kg equally distributed over 1 hour, followed by 1 mg/kg/hr until umbilical cord clamped.

Neonates: A single dose infused over 30 minutes.

ACTIONS
A pyrimidine nucleoside analog active against HIV. Through a specific process this thymidine analog interferes with reverse transcriptase, thus inhibiting viral replication. Metabolized by glucuronidation in the liver and excreted through the kidneys. Oral dosing half-life is approximately 0.5 to 3 hours in adults. Crosses the placental barrier. Secreted in breast milk.

INDICATIONS AND USES
Treatment of HIV-1 infection in combination with other antiretroviral agents. ▪ Prevention of maternal-fetal HIV-1 transmission. In most cases, should be given in combination with other antiretroviral drugs. Protocol includes oral zidovudine beginning between week 14 and week 34 of gestation, continuing until labor begins, IV dosing during labor, and zidovudine syrup or IV dosing to the newborn; see Maternal/Child.

CONTRAINDICATIONS
Life-threatening hypersensitivity reactions to any of the components.

PRECAUTIONS
For IV use only. Do not give IM or SC. ▪ Incidence of adverse reactions appears to increase with disease progression. ▪ Has been associated with hematologic toxicity, including neutropenia and severe anemia, particularly in patients with advanced HIV. ▪ Use with caution in patients with bone marrow compromise as indicated by a granulocyte count of less than 1,000/mm³ or hemoglobin below 9.5/dL. Hematologic toxicities appear to be related to

Z-U

pretreatment bone marrow reserve and to dose and duration of therapy. ■ Prolonged use of zidovudine has been associated with symptomatic myopathy and myositis with pathologic changes similar to those produced by HIV disease. ■ Lactic acidosis and severe hepatomegaly with steatosis have been reported with the use of some nucleoside analogs, including zidovudine when used alone or in combination. Deaths have occurred. Female gender, obesity, and prolonged exposure to antiretroviral nucleoside analogs may increase risk. Has also been reported in patients with no known risk factors. Exercise particular caution in any patient with hepatomegaly, hepatitis, or other risk factors for liver disease. Suspend therapy in any patient who develops clinical or laboratory findings suggestive of lactic acidosis or pronounced hepatotoxicity (which may include hepatomegaly and steatosis, even in the absence of marked transaminase elevations). ■ Use with caution in patients with severe hepatic impairment; may be at increased risk for hematologic toxicity. ■ Hepatic decompensation has occurred in HIV/HCV co-infected patients receiving combination antiretroviral therapy for HIV and interferon alfa with or without ribavirin (Rebetol) for HCV. ■ Use with caution in patients with severely impaired renal function (CrCl less than 15 mL/min); see Dose Adjustments. ■ Immune reconstitution syndrome has been reported in patients treated with combination antiretroviral therapy, including zidovudine. Patients may develop an inflammatory response to indolent opportunistic infections (e.g., *Mycobacterium avium*, CMV, PCP, or tuberculosis). May require further evaluation and treatment. ■ Autoimmune disorders (e.g., Graves' disease, polymyositis, and Guillain-Barré syndrome) have been reported in the setting of immune reconstitution; may occur months after initiation of therapy. ■ Vial stoppers contain natural rubber latex; may cause hypersensitivity reactions in latex-sensitive individuals. ■ See Drug/Lab Interactions.

Monitor: Observe closely; not a cure for HIV infections. Patients may acquire illnesses associated with AIDS or AIDS-related complex (ARC), including opportunistic infections. ■ Frequent blood cell counts are required. Hematologic toxicity, including neutropenia, severe anemia, and occasionally reversible pancytopenia are common. Anemia may occur as early as 2 to 4 weeks. Neutropenia usually occurs after 6 to 8 weeks of therapy; dosage adjustments and/or transfusions may be required. ■ Monitor liver function. ■ Obtain baseline CD4 lymphocyte count and monitor as indicated. ■ Closely monitor patients receiving zidovudine and interferon alfa, with or without ribavirin (Rebetol), for treatment-associated toxicities, especially hepatic decompensation, neutropenia, and anemia. Discontinuation of zidovudine and dose reduction or discontinuation of interferon, ribavirin, or both may be required if worsening clinical toxicities are seen (e.g., hepatic decompensation [e.g., Child-Pugh score greater than 6]). ■ See Drug/Lab Interactions.

Patient Education: Zidovudine is not a cure. Remain under the care of a physician when using zidovudine, and avoid actions that can spread HIV-1 infection to others. ■ Report abdominal pain, jaundice, muscle weakness, shortness of breath, or rapid breathing promptly. ■ Major side effects are neutropenia and/or anemia. ■ Requires frequent lab work and close follow-up with physician; keep all appointments. ■ Check with physician before taking any other medications.

Maternal/Child: Category C: safety for use during pregnancy has been evaluated. Risk versus benefit appears justified only in HIV-infected mothers. Congenital deformities not increased in studies; however, long-term consequences of in utero and neonatal exposure to zidovudine are unknown. Because the fetus is most susceptible to the potential teratogenic effects of drugs during the first 10 weeks of gestation and because the risks of therapy with zidovudine during this period are not fully known, women in the first trimester of pregnancy who do not require immediate initiation of antiretroviral therapy for their own health may consider delaying use. (Indication for prevention of maternal-fetal HIV-1 transmission is based on use after 14 weeks of gestation.) ■ Prevention of HIV-1 transmission in women who have received zidovudine for a prolonged period before pregnancy has not been evaluated. ■ Discontinue breast-feeding to reduce incidence of HIV transmission and potential for serious adverse reactions in nursing infants. ■ Has been studied in HIV-infected pediatric patients over 6 weeks of age who have HIV-related symptoms or are asymptomatic with abnormal lab values, indicating significant HIV-related immunosuppression. Has also been studied in neonates perinatally exposed to HIV. ▪ To monitor maternal-fetal outcomes, an Antiretroviral Pregnancy Registry has been established. See prescribing information.

Elderly: Dose selection should be cautious; see Dose Adjustments. Consider impaired hepatic and renal function.

DRUG/LAB INTERACTIONS

Do not use in combination with other products that contain zidovudine (e.g., lamivudine/zidovudine [Combivir], abacavir/lamivudine/zidovudine [Trizivir]). ▪ **Probenecid** may inhibit glucuronidation or reduce renal excretion of zidovudine, increasing zidovudine toxicity. ▪ Use with **protease inhibitors** (e.g., nelfinavir [Viracept], ritonavir [Norvir]) may decrease serum concentrations of zidovudine; monitoring indicated; dose adjustment of zidovudine is not indicated. ▪ Use with **atovaquone** (Mepron), **fluconazole** (Diflucan), **methadone** (Dolophine), or **valproic acid** (Depacon, Depakene) may increase zidovudine serum concentrations; monitoring indicated; dose adjustment of zidovudine is not indicated. ▪ **Rifamycins** (e.g., rifampin [Rifadin], rifabutin [Mycobutin]) may increase clearance, reduce zidovudine serum levels, and reduce effectiveness. ▪ Antagonized by **doxorubicin** (Adriamycin), **stavudine** (Zerit), **and ribavirin** (Rebetol). Avoid concurrent use. ▪ Exacerbation of anemia due to ribavirin has been seen in patients co-infected with HIV/HCV when zidovudine is part of the HIV regimen; coadministration is not advised. ▪ Hematologic toxicity increased with **ganciclovir** (Cytovene), **interferons, or other bone marrow suppressants or cytotoxic agents** (e.g., amphotericin B [conventional], dapsone, doxorubicin [Adriamycin], flucytosine, interferon, pentamidine, ribavirin [Rebetol], vinblastine, vincristine). Close clinical and laboratory monitoring indicated if coadministration is necessary. ▪ **Phenytoin** levels may increase or decrease; monitor carefully to ensure proper dosing. ▪ **Phenytoin** may also increase zidovudine levels by decreasing clearance. ▪ Use with **acyclovir** may cause neurotoxicity (drowsiness, lethargy). ▪ Combination therapy with zidovudine and **interferon alfa,** with or without **ribavirin** (Rebetol), may increase risk of hepatic decompensation, neutropenia, and anemia. ▪ Prescribing information states that dose modification is also not warranted with coadministration of **clarithromycin** (Biaxin), **lamivudine** (Epivir), **probenecid, or rifampin** (Rifadin). Other sources suggest drug adjustments with some adverse reactions.

SIDE EFFECTS

Frequency and severity of adverse events are greater in patients with more advanced infection at the time of initiation of treatment. Anorexia, headache, malaise, nausea, and vomiting are most common with oral and IV administration. Anemia and neutropenia were reported frequently with IV administration. Abdominal cramps, abdominal pain, anaphylaxis, anorexia, arthralgia, asthenia, chills, constipation, dyspepsia, fatigue, granulocytopenia, hepatomegaly (severe), hyperbilirubinemia, increased liver function tests (e.g., ALT, AST, alkaline phosphatase), injection site reaction (e.g., pain, redness), insomnia, musculoskeletal pain, myalgia, neuropathy, pancytopenia (reversible), and thrombocytopenia have also been reported. Side effects most commonly reported in *pediatric patients* were anemia, cough, fever, and neutropenia.

ANTIDOTE

Notify physician of all side effects; most will be treated symptomatically. Moderate anemia or granulocytopenia may respond to a reduction in dose. Interrupt zidovudine therapy for severe anemia (less than 7.5 Gm/dL or a 25% reduction from baseline) or severe granulocytopenia (less than 750/mm^3 or 50% reduction from baseline). Transfusions may be required. If marrow recovery occurs following dose interruption, resumption of therapy may be appropriate using adjunctive measures such as epoetin alfa (Epogen). Suspend treatment if clinical or laboratory findings suggestive of lactic acidosis or pronounced hepatotoxicity occur. Rash may be the first sign of a more serious reaction (e.g., anaphylaxis, Stevens-Johnson syndrome); notify physician and treat with diphenhydramine (Benadryl), epinephrine (Adrenalin), and corticosteroids as indicated. Antimicrobial therapy may be indicated to treat opportunistic infections. Not removed by hemodialysis or peritoneal dialysis.

ZIV-AFLIBERCEPT BBW
(**ZIV**-a-**FLIB**-er-sept)

Angiogenesis inhibitor
Vascular endothelial growth factor (VEGF) inhibitor
Antineoplastic

Zaltrap

pH 6.2

USUAL DOSE
4 mg/kg as an infusion over 1 hour every 2 weeks. Administer before any component of the FOLFIRI regimen (5-fluorouracil, leucovorin, and irinotecan) on the day of treatment. Continue until disease progression or unacceptable toxicity. See Monographs for 5-fluorouracil, leucovorin, and irinotecan to incorporate all requirements into this regimen.

DOSE ADJUSTMENTS

Ziv-Aflibercept Dose Adjustments*	
Indication	Recommended Dose or Action
Neutrophil count less than 1,500/mm^3 (1.5 × 10^9/L)	Withhold or delay dosing until neutrophil count is at or above 1.5 × 10^9/L (1,500/mm^3).
Elective surgery	Withhold for at least 4 weeks before elective surgery.
Recurrent or severe hypertension	Withhold until hypertension is controlled, then resume at a permanently reduced dose of 2 mg/kg.
Proteinuria at or above 2 Gm/24 hr	Withhold ziv-aflibercept. Resume when proteinuria decreases to less than 2 Gm/24 hr.
Recurrent proteinuria	Withhold ziv-aflibercept until proteinuria is less than 2 Gm/24 hr, then resume at a permanently reduced dose of 2 mg/kg.
Severe hemorrhage, GI perforation, compromised wound healing, fistula formation, hypertensive crisis or hypertensive encephalopathy, arterial thromboembolic events, nephrotic syndrome or thrombotic microangiopathy, and/or reversible posterior leukoencephalopathy syndrome (RPLS)	Discontinue ziv-aflibercept.
Age, gender, or race; mild, moderate, or severe renal impairment or mild or moderate hepatic impairment; see Precautions.	No dose adjustment required.

*For toxicities related to irinotecan, 5-FU, or leucovorin, refer to individual monographs.

DILUTION
Available in single-use vials containing 100 mg/4 mL or 200 mg/8 mL (25 mg/mL). A clear, colorless to pale yellow solution. Do not use if the solution is discolored or cloudy or contains particles. Do not re-enter the vial after the initial puncture. Withdraw the prescribed dose from the vial and dilute in NS or D5W to achieve a final concentration of 0.6 to 8 mg/mL. For example, in a 70-kg patient:

Weight in kg × Dose in mg/kg = Calculated dose of drug

(70 kg × 4 mg/kg = 280 mg)

Calculated dose in mg ÷ Drug concentration (25 mg/mL) = Volume of drug required

(280 mg ÷ 25 mg/mL = 11.2 mL of drug)

Dilution in a 50-mL infusion bag plus the 11.2 mL of drug would yield 4.6 mg/mL. Dilution in a 250-mL infusion bag plus the 11.2 mL of drug would yield 1.1 mg/mL. Use PVC infusion bags containing DEHP or polyolefin infusion bags.

Filters: Administer through a 0.2-micron polyethersulfone filter. Do not use filters made of polyvinylidene fluoride (PVDF) or nylon.

Storage: Store vials in refrigerator at 2° to 8° C (36° to 46° F). Keep in original carton to protect from light. Diluted solution may be stored refrigerated for up to 24 hours or stored at RT (20° to 25° C [68° to 77° F]) for up to 8 hours. Discard any unused portion left in vial or infusion bag.

COMPATIBILITY

Manufacturer states, "Do not combine ziv-aflibercept with other drugs in the same infusion bag or intravenous line."

RATE OF ADMINISTRATION

Administer using an infusion set made of PVC containing DEHP, DEHP-free PVC containing trioctyl-trimellitate (TOTM), polypropylene, polyethylene-lined PVC, or polyurethane through a 0.2-micron polyethersulfone filter. Do not use filters made of polyvinylidene fluoride (PVDF) or nylon.

A single dose as an infusion over 1 hour.

ACTIONS

A recombinant fusion protein consisting of vascular endothelial growth factor (VEGF)–binding portions from the extracellular domains of human VEGF receptors 1 and 2 fused to the Fc portion of the human IgG1. It is a soluble receptor that binds to specific components of human VEGF. Inhibits the binding and activation of the specific receptors, resulting in decreased neovascularization and decreased vascular permeability. In animals ziv-aflibercept was shown to inhibit the proliferation of endothelial cells, thereby inhibiting the growth of new blood vessels. Elimination half-life is approximately 6 days (range 4 to 7 days). Steady-state concentrations reached by the second dose.

INDICATIONS AND USES

Treatment of metastatic colorectal cancer (mCRC) that is resistant to or has progressed following an oxaliplatin-containing regimen. Used in combination with 5-fluorouracil, leucovorin, and irinotecan (FOLFIRI).

CONTRAINDICATIONS

Manufacturer states, "None."

PRECAUTIONS

Do not administer as an IV push or bolus. ▪ Severe and sometimes fatal hemorrhagic events have been reported in patients who have received ziv-aflibercept in combination with FOLFIRI. Do not administer to patients with severe hemorrhage. ▪ GI perforation, including fatal GI perforation, can occur. ▪ Can impair wound healing in patients receiving ziv-aflibercept/FOLFIRI. Withhold ziv-aflibercept for at least 4 weeks before elective surgery and do not resume for at least 4 weeks after major surgery and until the surgical wound is fully healed. For minor surgery (e.g., CV access port placement, biopsy, tooth extraction), ziv-aflibercept may be resumed once the surgical wound is fully healed. ▪ Incidence of fistula formation is increased. Anal, enterovesical, enterocutaneous, colovaginal, and intestinal site fistulas have been reported. ▪ Risk of Grade 3 or 4 hypertension is increased. Grade 3 is defined as requiring an adjustment in existing antihypertensive therapy or treatment with more than one drug. Grade 4 is defined as a hypertensive crisis. ▪ Risk of arterial thromboembolic events is increased. ▪ Severe proteinuria, nephrotic syndrome, and thrombotic microangiopathy (TMA) have been reported. ▪ Risk of neutropenic complications (e.g., febrile neutropenia and neutropenic infection) is increased. ▪ Incidence of severe diarrhea and dehydration is increased. ▪ Reversible posterior leukoencephalopathy syndrome (RPLS) has been reported. ▪ A protein product; has potential for immunogenicity. ▪ No data available for patients with severe hepatic impairment. ▪ See Monitor and Antidote.

Monitor: Obtain baseline CBC with differential and repeat every 2 weeks before each dose of ziv-aflibercept. Withhold or delay dosing until neutrophil count is at or above 1.5×10^9/L (1,500/mm³). ▪ Obtain baseline BP history and monitor BP a minimum of every

2 weeks or more frequently as clinically indicated. ▪ Management with antihypertensive medications is indicated. Closely monitor patients already taking hypertensive medications. ▪ Monitor for S/S of bleeding (e.g., GI hemorrhage, hematuria, hemoptysis, intracranial hemorrhage, postprocedural hemorrhage, pulmonary hemorrhage). ▪ Monitor for S/S of GI perforation. ▪ Monitor for S/S of fistula formation. ▪ Monitor for S/S of arterial thromboembolic events (e.g., transient ischemic attack [TIA], cerebrovascular accident [CVA], and angina pectoris). ▪ Monitor proteinuria by urine dipstick analysis and/or urinary protein creatinine ratio (UPCR) for development or worsening of proteinuria. Obtain a 24-hour urine collection in patients with a UPCR greater than 1 or a dipstick for protein of 2+ or more. ▪ Diarrhea may be severe; monitor bowel history and encourage adequate hydration to prevent dehydration. ▪ Monitor for neurologic S/S that may be consistent with RPLS (e.g., confusion, headache, seizures, visual changes). Diagnosis confirmed by MRI. ▪ See Dose Adjustments, Precautions, and Antidote.

Patient Education: May cause hypertension; monitor BP. ▪ Promptly report abdominal pain, bleeding, elevated BP, fever or other signs of infection, light-headedness, neurologic symptoms, severe diarrhea, severe headache, or vomiting. ▪ Wound healing is compromised; do not undergo surgery or procedures (including tooth extractions) without the knowledge of a health care provider. ▪ Risk of chest pain, TIAs, and CVAs increased. ▪ Risk of fetal harm; highly effective contraception required in males and females during and for at least 3 months following the last dose of therapy. If a pregnancy occurs in patient or partner, notify health care provider immediately.

Maternal/Child: Category C. However, ziv-aflibercept was embryotoxic and teratogenic in rabbits at doses lower than required for humans. Use only if potential benefit justifies potential risk to fetus. Highly effective contraception required in both males and females; see Patient Education. ▪ Discontinue breast-feeding. ▪ Safety and effectiveness for use in pediatric patients not established.

Elderly: Incidence of asthenia, dehydration, diarrhea, dizziness, and weight loss increased. Monitor closely for dehydration and diarrhea.

DRUG/LAB INTERACTIONS

No drug-drug interaction studies have been conducted. ▪ No clinically important pharmacokinetic drug-drug interactions have been found between ziv-aflibercept and **irinotecan/SN-38 or 5-FU.**

SIDE EFFECTS

Abdominal pain, decreased appetite, diarrhea, dysphonia, epistaxis, fatigue, headache, hypertension, increased AST and ALT, increased SCr, leukopenia, neutropenia, proteinuria, stomatitis, thrombocytopenia, and weight loss are most common. The most serious side effects include arterial thrombotic events, compromised wound healing, diarrhea and dehydration, fistula formation, GI perforation, hemorrhage, hypertension, neutropenia and neutropenic complications, proteinuria, and RPLS. Asthenia, dyspnea, hemorrhoids, oropharyngeal pain, palmar-plantar erythrodysesthesia syndrome, proctalgia, rectal hemorrhage, rhinorrhea, skin hyperpigmentation, upper abdominal pain, and urinary tract infections have been reported.

Post-Marketing: Osteonecrosis of the jaw.

ANTIDOTE

Keep physician informed of all side effects. May constitute a medical emergency or will be treated symptomatically as indicated. Discontinue for severe hemorrhage, GI perforation, compromised wound healing, fistula formation, hypertensive crisis or hypertensive encephalopathy, arterial thromboembolic events, nephrotic syndrome or thrombotic microangiopathy, and/or reversible posterior leukoencephalopathy syndrome (RPLS). See Dose Adjustments for instructions on resuming treatment. Treat anaphylaxis with oxygen, antihistamines (diphenhydramine [Benadryl]), epinephrine (Adrenalin), and corticosteroids. Maintain a patent airway. Resuscitate if indicated.

ZOLEDRONIC ACID

Bisphosphonate

(**ZOH**-leh-dron-ick **AS**-id)

Reclast ▪ **Zometa**

pH 6 to 7 ▪ pH 2

USUAL DOSE

(International Units [IU])

RECLAST AND ZOMETA

Prehydration required. Always used with adequate hydration and appropriate monitoring. See Dose Adjustments, Precautions, and Monitor.

RECLAST

Administration of acetaminophen after Reclast administration may reduce the incidence of acute-phase reaction symptoms; see Side Effects. In clinical studies, a standard dose of acetaminophen was given with the infusion and for the next 72 hours as needed.

Treatment of Paget's disease: One dose of 5 mg as an infusion over no less than 15 minutes. Supplemental calcium and vitamin D are required, particularly during the 2 weeks following administration.

Calcium: 1,500 mg daily in divided doses (750 mg two times a day or 500 mg three times a day).

Vitamin D: 800 IU/day.

An extended remission period has been observed after a single treatment. Specific retreatment data not available; however, retreatment may be considered for patients who have relapsed based on increases in serum alkaline phosphatase, for patients who did not achieve normalization of their serum alkaline phosphatase, and for patients with symptoms.

Treatment of osteoporosis in men and postmenopausal women and treatment and prevention of glucocorticoid-induced osteoporosis: A single dose of 5 mg given once a year as an infusion over at least 15 minutes. 1,200 mg of calcium and 800 to 1,000 IU of vitamin D daily are recommended. If the calcium and vitamin D are not obtained by dietary means, oral supplementation is indicated.

Prevention of osteoporosis in postmenopausal women: A single dose of 5 mg given every 2 years as an infusion over at least 15 minutes. Postmenopausal women require an average of 1,200 mg of calcium and 800 to 1,000 IU of vitamin D daily.

ZOMETA

Hypercalcemia of malignancy (corrected serum calcium equal to or greater than 12 mg/dL [3 mmol/L]): One dose of 4 mg as an infusion over no less than 15 minutes.

Experience is limited, but retreatment with the same dose may be considered if serum calcium does not return to normal or remain normal after initial treatment. Wait at least 7 days from completion of the first infusion to allow full response.

Multiple myeloma and metastatic bone lesions from solid tumors: 4 mg as an infusion over no less than 15 minutes every 3 to 4 weeks. A CrCl greater than 60 mL is required; see Dose Adjustments. Optimal duration of therapy is unknown. Concurrent daily administration of PO calcium 500 mg and a multivitamin with 400 units vitamin D is recommended.

DOSE ADJUSTMENTS

RECLAST AND ZOMETA

Dose adjustment is not indicated based on age or race. Studies have not been conducted in patients with hepatic or severe renal impairment; see Dilution, Precautions, and Elderly.

RECLAST

No dose adjustment required in patients with a CrCl of 35 mL/min or greater.

Continued

Z-N

ZOMETA

Hypercalcemia of malignancy: Dose adjustments are not necessary in patients with mild to moderate renal impairment before beginning treatment (SCr less than 4.5 mg/dL). If renal function deteriorates, consider if the potential benefit of continued treatment outweighs the possible risk.

Multiple myeloma and metastatic bone lesions from solid tumors: Reduce the initial and following doses in patients with mild to moderate renal impairment based on the following chart:

Zometa Dose Adjustments in Multiple Myeloma and Metastatic Bone Lesions	
Baseline Creatinine Clearance	Zoledronic Acid Recommended Dose
Greater than 60 mL/min	4 mg
50 to 60 mL/min	3.5 mg
40 to 49 mL/min	3.3 mg
30 to 39 mL/min	3 mg

Measure SCr before each Zometa dose and withhold if renal condition deteriorates; see Monitor. When the CrCl has returned to within 10% of the baseline value, resume dosing at the same dose administered before treatment interruption.

In patients who experience a decrease in renal function after receiving the initial dose of Zometa, delayed dosing is required before retreatment as follows:

Normal serum creatinine (SCr) before treatment: If SCr has increased 0.5 mg/dL within 2 weeks of planned retreatment, withhold retreatment dose until recovery to within 10% of baseline SCr value.

Abnormal SCr before treatment: If SCr has increased 1 mg/dL within 2 weeks of planned retreatment, withhold retreatment dose until the SCr is within 10% of baseline value.

DILUTION

RECLAST

A 5-mg dose is available prediluted in 100 mL of water for injection for administration as an infusion. If previously refrigerated, allow solution to reach room temperature before administration.

ZOMETA

Available in two formulations: (1) a single-use prediluted solution containing 4 mg in 100-mL solution, and (2) a concentrate containing 4 mg in 5 mL.

Single-use, ready-to-use-bottle: 100 mL of solution equals a 4-mg dose of zoledronic acid and may be administered without further dilution.

Single-Use, Ready-to-Use Bottle Zometa Dilution Recommendations for Reduced Doses in Patients with a CrCl Less Than or Equal to 60 mL/min		
Remove and discard the following Zometa ready-to-use solution (mL)	Replace with the following volume of NS or D5W (mL)	Dose (mg)
12 mL	12 mL	3.5
18 mL	18 mL	3.3
25 mL	25 mL	3

Concentrate with 4 mg in 5 mL for single use: Vials contain overfill; measure accurately. Withdraw desired volume from vial as outlined in the following chart. Must be further diluted immediately in 100 mL of NS or D5W and given as an infusion.

4-mg Concentrate in 5 mL for Single Use Zometa Dilution Recommendations for Reduced Doses in Patients with a CrCl Less Than or Equal to 60 mL/min	
Recommended Dose (mg)	Volume of Zometa (mL)
4 mg	5 mL
3.5 mg	4.4 mL
3.3 mg	4.1 mL
3 mg	3.8 mL

Filters: Not required by manufacturer; however, use of a filter should not have an adverse effect.

Storage: *Reclast:* Store at CRT. Stable for 24 hours refrigerated at 2° to 8° C (36° to 46° F) after opening. *Zometa:* Store vials and ready-to-use container in carton at CRT. Use immediately after dilution or manipulation of ready-to-use container is preferred. Diluted solution may be refrigerated but must be used and the infusion completed within 24 hours of mixing. If refrigerated, bring to RT before administration. Do not store undiluted solution in a syringe (to avoid inadvertent injection).

COMPATIBILITY
RECLAST AND ZOMETA
Novartis manufactures both Reclast and Zometa and states, "Must not be mixed with calcium or other divalent cation–containing infusion solutions (e.g., LR). Should be administered as a single IV solution in a line separate from all other drugs."
RECLAST
A vented IV set is required.

RATE OF ADMINISTRATION
A single dose equally distributed over no less than 15 minutes. After infusion is finished, flush IV line with 10 mL NS. An increase in renal toxicity that can progress to renal failure can result from shorter infusion times.

ACTIONS
ZOLEDRONIC ACID
A bisphosphonate that inhibits osteoclast-mediated bone resorption. Used as a bone resorption inhibitor in Paget's disease (Reclast) and as a hypocalcemic agent to reduce hypercalcemia in oncology patients (Zometa). After administration, it rapidly partitions to the bone and localizes preferentially at sites of high bone turnover. Inhibits osteoclastic (destructive to bone) activity and induces osteoclast apoptosis (fragmentation of a cell into particles for elimination). Blocks the osteoclastic resorption of mineralized bone and cartilage through its binding to bone and inhibits the increased osteoclastic activity and skeletal calcium release induced by various tumors. Decreases serum calcium and phosphorus and increases urinary calcium and phosphorus excretion. Plasma protein binding of zoledronic acid is low. Not metabolized. Most bound to bone and slowly released back into the systemic circulation. Primarily excreted intact via the kidney. Half-life is triphasic with a terminal half-life of 146 hours.
RECLAST
In Paget's disease, it localizes preferentially at sites of high bone turnover and promotes bone of normal quality with no evidence of impaired bone remodeling or mineralization effect. Returns patients to normal levels of bone turnover; see Indications.

ZOMETA

In oncology patients with hypercalcemia, it reduces serum calcium concentrations by inhibiting bone resorption. Reduction in calcium levels is seen in 24 to 48 hours, but maximum response may take up to 7 days.

INDICATIONS AND USES

RECLAST

Treatment of Paget's disease of the bone in men and women. Treatment indicated to induce remission (normalization of serum alkaline phosphatase) in patients with elevations in serum alkaline phosphatase of two times or higher than the upper limit of the age-specific reference range and in patients who are symptomatic or are at risk for complications from their disease. Paget's disease of the bone is a chronic focal skeletal disorder characterized by greatly increased and disorderly bone remodeling. Excessive osteoclastic bone resorption is followed by irregular osteoblastic new bone formation, which leads to replacement of the normal bone architecture by disorganized, enlarged, and weakened bone structure. ▪ Prevention and treatment of osteoporosis in postmenopausal women. In osteoporosis diagnosed by a bone mineral density test or prevalent vertebral fractures, Reclast reduces the incidence of hip, vertebral, and nonvertebral osteoporosis-related fractures. In patients at high risk for fracture (defined as a recent low-trauma hip fracture), Reclast reduces the incidence of new clinical fractures. ▪ Treatment to increase bone mass in men with osteoporosis. ▪ Treatment and prevention of glucocorticoid-induced osteoporosis in men and women who are initiating or continuing systemic glucocorticoids in a daily dose that is equivalent to 7.5 mg or more of prednisone and who are expected to remain on glucocorticoids for at least 12 months.

Limitation of use: Safety and effectiveness for treatment of osteoporosis is based on 3 years of clinical data. Optimal duration of therapy is unknown. Re-evaluate the need for continued therapy on a periodic basis. Consider discontinuation of therapy after 3 to 5 years in patients at low risk for fracture. Patients who discontinue therapy should have their risk for fracture re-evaluated periodically.

ZOMETA

Treatment of hypercalcemia of malignancy (HCM), which is defined as an albumin-corrected calcium [cCa] greater than or equal to 12 mg/dL [3 mmol/L] using the following formula:

$$cCa \text{ in mg/dL} = Ca \text{ in mg/dL} + 0.8 [4 \text{ Gm/dL} - \text{Patient albumin (Gm/dL)}]$$

▪ Treatment of patients with multiple myeloma and patients with documented bone metastases from solid tumors in conjunction with chemotherapy. Prostate cancer should have progressed after treatment with at least one hormonal therapy.

Limitation of use: Safety for use in the treatment of hypercalcemia associated with hyperparathyroidism or with other non–tumor-related conditions has not been established.

CONTRAINDICATIONS

RECLAST AND ZOMETA

Hypersensitivity to zoledronic acid or any of its components.

RECLAST

Hypocalcemia, pregnancy, lactation, in patients with a CrCl less than 35 mL/min, and in patients with evidence of acute renal impairment.

PRECAUTIONS

RECLAST AND ZOMETA

A patient being treated with Zometa should not be treated with Reclast or another bisphosphonate (e.g., ibandronate [Boniva], pamidronate [Aredia]). A patient being treated with Reclast should not be treated with Zometa or another bisphosphonate (e.g., ibandronate [Boniva], pamidronate [Aredia]). ▪ Bisphosphonates have been associated with deterioration of renal function and potential renal failure. Multiple cycles of zoledronic acid, doses over 4 or 5 mg, and/or a rate of administration less than 15 minutes increase this risk. Patients who are elderly, are dehydrated, are receiving diuretics or other nephrotoxic drugs, or have pre-existing renal impairment may also be at increased risk. ▪ Use with caution in patients with aspirin-sensitive asthma; although not seen in zoledronic acid trials, bronchoconstriction has been reported when other bisphosphonates have been given to these patients. ▪ Osteonecrosis of the jaw (ONJ) has been reported in patients receiving bisphosphonates. The majority of cases have been in cancer patients undergoing dental procedures. Risk factors include cancer, concomitant therapy (e.g., chemotherapy, radiotherapy, corticosteroids, angiogenesis inhibitors), and comorbid conditions (e.g., anemia, coagulopathies, infection, pre-existing oral disease). Risk may also increase with duration of exposure to bisphosphonates. Post-marketing experience suggests a greater frequency of reports based on tumor type (advanced breast cancer or multiple myeloma); see Drug/Lab Interactions. ▪ A routine oral exam is recommended before beginning therapy with bisphosphonates. Patients, especially cancer patients, should consider appropriate preventive dentistry and avoid invasive dental procedures during bisphosphonate therapy. Dental surgery may exacerbate ONJ in patients who develop ONJ while undergoing bisphosphonate therapy. ▪ Severe and occasionally incapacitating bone, joint, and/or muscle pain has been reported. Onset of symptoms may be days to months after initiation of therapy. Symptoms usually resolve when zoledronic acid is discontinued; however, in some patients symptoms resolved slowly or persisted. ▪ Atypical subtrochanteric and diaphyseal femoral fractures have been reported in bisphosphonate-treated patients. May be bilateral. Many patients report prodromal pain in the affected area (usually presenting as dull, aching thigh pain) weeks to months before a complete fracture occurs. Patients presenting with thigh or groin pain in the absence of trauma should be evaluated to rule out an incomplete femur fracture. Patients presenting with an atypical fracture should also be assessed for S/S of fracture in the contralateral limb. ▪ See Monitor.

RECLAST

Hypocalcemia may occur. Pre-existing hypocalcemia must be treated by adequate intake of calcium and vitamin D before initiating therapy. Concurrent dosing with calcium and vitamin D during therapy is required and is especially important in the 2 weeks following Reclast administration. ▪ Effectively treat disturbances of calcium and mineral metabolism (e.g., hypoparathyroidism, thyroid surgery, parathyroid surgery, malabsorption syndromes, excision of the small intestine) before initiating therapy with Reclast.

ZOMETA

Calcium is bound to serum protein; concentration fluctuates with changes in blood volume. Changes in serum calcium (especially during rehydration) may not reflect true plasma levels. Measurement with ionized calcium levels is preferred. If unavailable, all calcium measurement should be corrected for albumin to establish a basis for treatment and evaluation of treatment. ▪ Hypocalcemia has been reported. Cardiac arrhythmias and adverse neurologic events (numbness, seizures, tetany) have been reported secondary to severe hypocalcemia. Correct hypocalcemia before beginning Zometa therapy. Adequately supplement with calcium and vitamin D. ▪ Mild or asymptomatic hypercalcemia will be treated with conservative measures (e.g., saline hydration, with or without diuretics [after correcting hypovolemia]). Consider patient's cardiovascular status. Corticosteroids may be indicated if the underlying cancer is sensitive (e.g., hematologic cancers). ▪ Not recommended for patients with bone metastases with a SCr greater than 3 mg/dL (265 micromol/L) or for patients with hypercalcemia of malignancy with a SCr greater than 4.5 mg/dL (400 micromol/L). These patients were excluded from the studies. After considering other treatment options, use only if benefit outweighs risk of renal failure. ▪ Retreatment may increase potential for renal failure; before retreatment, consider other available treatment options and risk versus benefit; evaluate serum creatinine before each dose. ▪ May be used adjunctively with chemotherapy, radiation, or surgery.

Monitor: RECLAST AND ZOMETA: Serum phosphate levels may decrease (hypophosphatemia) and may require treatment. Short-term supplemental therapy may also be required for hypocalcemia or hypomagnesemia. ▪ See Precautions and Drug/Lab Interactions.

RECLAST: S/S of Paget's disease range from no symptoms to severe morbidity due to bone pain, bone deformity, pathologic fractures, and neurologic and other complications. Serum alkaline phosphatase provides an objective measure of disease severity and response to therapy. Diagnosis can be confirmed by radiographic evidence. ▪ Obtain baseline measurement of serum alkaline phosphatase, serum calcium, electrolytes, phosphate, magnesium, and SCr. Monitor as indicated. Obtain serum creatinine and calculate CrCl before each dose. ▪ Supplemental calcium and vitamin D required; see Usual Dose. Very important in the 2 weeks following Reclast administration. ▪ Adequate hydration required; a minimum of two glasses of liquid is recommended before dosing on day of administration. Additional hydration is required in patients undergoing diuretic therapy. ▪ Monitor calcium and mineral levels closely in patients with disturbances of calcium and mineral metabolism (e.g., hypoparathyroidism, thyroid surgery, parathyroid surgery, malabsorption syndromes, excision of the small intestine). Bone mineral density should be evaluated 1 to 2 years after initiation of therapy in patients being treated for osteoporosis.

ZOMETA: Obtain baseline measurements of serum calcium (corrected for serum albumin), electrolytes, phosphate, magnesium, SCr, and CBC with differential. Monitor all closely as indicated by baseline results (may be daily). ▪ Monitor SCr before each dose to identify renal deterioration. During clinical studies, deterioration was considered as an increase of 0.5 mg/dL if the patient had a normal baseline; if the patient had an abnormal baseline, deterioration was considered as an increase of 1 mg/dL. ▪ Patients with cancer-related hypercalcemia are often dehydrated. Must be adequately hydrated orally and/or IV before treatment is initiated. Hydration with saline is preferred to facilitate the renal excretion of calcium and to correct dehydration. A pretreatment urine output of 2 L/day is recommended. Maintain adequate hydration and urine output throughout treatment. ▪ Correct hypovolemia before using diuretics. ▪ Avoid overhydration in patients with compromised cardiovascular status. Observe frequently for signs of fluid overload.

Patient Education: RECLAST AND ZOMETA: Review manufacturer's medication guide. Avoid pregnancy; use of nonhormonal birth control recommended. Report a suspected pregnancy; may cause fetal harm. ▪ Regular visits and assessment of lab tests imperative. ▪ Take only prescribed medications. Discuss all medications, allergies, and medical history with physician. ▪ Adequate hydration required. Drink at least two glasses of fluid before infusion. ▪ Report abdominal cramps, chills, confusion, fever, muscle spasms, sore throat, and/or any new medical problems promptly. ▪ Flu-like symptoms may occur within the first 3 days of therapy. Usually resolve within 3 days of onset but may last for up to 7 to 14 days. Administration of acetaminophen may reduce incidence of symptoms. ▪ Good dental hygiene and routine dental care required. Obtain a dental exam before initiating therapy, and avoid invasive dental procedures during therapy. ▪ Report development of bone, joint, or muscle pain promptly. Onset of pain is variable. ▪ Report thigh or groin pain promptly.

RECLAST: Calcium and vitamin D supplementation required to maintain calcium levels. ▪ Tell your physician if you have had surgery to remove some or all of the parathyroid glands in your neck, have had sections of your intestine removed, or are unable to take calcium supplements. ▪ Promptly report muscle spasms and/or numbness or tingling sensations (especially around the mouth); may indicate hypocalcemia.

ZOMETA: Dietary restriction of calcium and vitamin D may be required in hypercalcemia of malignancy. ▪ An oral calcium supplement of 500 mg and a multivitamin with 400 IU of vitamin D are recommended for patients with multiple myeloma and bone metastasis of solid tumors.

Maternal/Child: Category D: avoid pregnancy; may cause fetal harm. ▪ Discontinue breast-feeding. ▪ Not indicated for use in pediatric patients. Because of long-term retention in bone, zoledronic acid should be used in pediatric patients only when potential benefit outweighs potential risk. Has been used in pediatric patients with severe osteogenesis imperfecta; see manufacturer's prescribing information.

Elderly: Response similar to that seen in younger patients. ▪ Use with caution based on age-related impaired organ function and concomitant disease or other drug therapy. Monitor renal function closely. Elderly patients are at increased risk for acute renal failure. ▪ Monitor fluid and electrolyte status. ▪ Acute-phase reactions occur less frequently in the elderly; see Side Effects.

DRUG/LAB INTERACTIONS
RECLAST AND ZOMETA
Concurrent use with **loop diuretics** (e.g., furosemide [Lasix]) may increase risk of hypocalcemia or nephrotoxicity. ▪ Concurrent use with **aminoglycosides** (e.g., gentamicin) or **calcitonin** may have an additive hypocalcemic effect that may persist for a prolonged period. ▪ Use caution when administered with other potentially **nephrotoxic drugs** (e.g., aminoglycosides [gentamicin, tobramycin], cisplatin, NSAIDs [ibuprofen (Advil), naproxen (Aleve)]); the risk of renal deterioration is increased. Consider monitoring of SCr. ▪ Use with caution when administered with **renally eliminated drugs** (e.g., digoxin). Possible development of renal impairment may lead to increased exposure of these drugs. Use caution and consider monitoring of SCr. ▪ In vitro studies indicate that it does not inhibit microsomal CYP_{450} enzymes. ▪ Concomitant administration of **drugs associated with ONJ** (e.g., angiogenesis inhibitors [bevacizumab (Avastin), everolimus (Afinitor), pazopanib (Votrient), sorafenib (Nexavar), sunitinib (Sutent)], denosumab [Prolia, Xgeva]) may increase the risk of ONJ.

ZOMETA
Does not interfere with any known primary cancer therapy. ▪ Concurrent use with **thalidomide** does not result in a significant change in the pharmacokinetics or creatinine clearance of zoledronic acid; no dose adjustment indicated. ▪ Effects may be antagonized by **calcium-containing preparations or vitamin D;** avoid use.

SIDE EFFECTS
RECLAST AND ZOMETA
Abdominal pain, anorexia, atypical femur fracture, conjunctivitis, constipation, dehydration, diarrhea, dyspnea, episcleritis, flu-like syndrome (e.g., arthralgias and/or bone pain, chills, fever, flushing, and myalgias), headache, hypersensitivity reactions (including rare case of anaphylaxis, angioedema, and urticaria), hypocalcemia (abdominal cramps, confusion, muscle spasms), hypomagnesemia, hypophosphatemia, hypotension, injection site reactions, nausea, ocular inflammation (e.g., iritis, uveitis, scleritis, orbital inflammation and edema), osteonecrosis (primarily of the jaw), rash, renal impairment, and vomiting. In addition to the previously noted side effects, an acute-phase reaction (e.g., chills, fever, headache, or muscle, bone, or joint pain) and nausea and vomiting were reported. Symptoms may be significant and lead to dehydration. May occur within the first 3 days, is usually mild to moderate, and lasts only a few days. However, in some patients the resolution of symptoms may take 7 to 14 days or longer.

RECLAST
Hypocalcemia is the most serious side effect. Dizziness, fatigue, and nausea were commonly reported. Abdominal distension, anemia, asthenia, atrial fibrillation, back pain, dyspepsia, hypertension, lethargy, musculoskeletal stiffness, pain, paresthesia, peripheral edema, and vertigo have also been reported.

ZOMETA
The most commonly reported side effects are anemia, bone pain, constipation, dyspnea, fatigue, fever, nausea, and vomiting. In addition to the previously noted side effects, agitation, anxiety, bronchoconstriction, chest pain, confusion, cough, dehydration, dysphagia, edema, granulocytopenia, hypokalemia, increased serum creatinine, musculoskeletal pain (e.g., bone pain and/or arthralgia and myalgias, which may be severe), pancytopenia, pleural effusion, pruritus, somnolence, thrombocytopenia, urinary tract infection, and weakness have occurred in 10% or more of patients. Fluid overload, hypokalemia, hypomagnesemia, and hypophosphatemia may occur more often with the use of concurrent fluid and diuretics.

Post-Marketing: Acute renal failure; angioneurotic edema; asthma exacerbation; atypical subtrochanteric and diaphyseal femoral fractures; blurred vision; bradycardia; bronchospasm; dehydration secondary to diuretic therapy, fever, or GI losses; dry mouth; hematuria; hyperesthesia; hyperkalemia; hypernatremia; hypersensitivity reactions (including anaphylactic reaction/shock, angioedema, bronchoconstriction, Stevens-Johnson syndrome, toxic epidermal necrolysis, and urticaria); hypertension; hypocalcemia (cardiac arrhythmias, numbness, seizures, and tetany have occurred with severe hypocalcemia); increased SCr; increased sweating; influenza-like illness (asthenia, fatigue or malaise, fever persisting for more than 30 days); interstitial lung disease (ILD) with positive rechallenge; proteinuria; and weight increase.

Overdose: Clinically significant hypocalcemia (e.g., abdominal cramps; confusion; irregular heartbeats; muscle cramps in the hands, arms, feet, legs, or face; numbness and tingling around the mouth, fingertips, or feet), hypophosphatemia (e.g., unusual tiredness or weakness), and hypomagnesemia (e.g., muscle trembling or twitching) may occur. Elevated SCr levels and renal tubular necrosis may occur with excessive dose or rate of administration.

ANTIDOTE

RECLAST AND ZOMETA

Keep physician informed of side effects. According to the manufacturer, no specific treatment was required in most cases of flu-like syndrome, GI symptoms, and infusion site reactions, and the symptoms subsided in 24 to 48 hours. Some side effects may respond to symptomatic treatment. IV fluids may be required for dehydration. Magnesium and phosphorus may require replacement if depletion is too severe. If mild, all will probably return toward normal in 7 to 10 days. For asymptomatic or mild to moderate hypocalcemia (6.5 to 8 mg/100 mL [1 dL] corrected for serum albumin), short-term calcium therapy (e.g., calcium gluconate) may be indicated. Discontinue drug for any symptoms of hypersensitivity or overdose. Discontinue for severe bone, joint, or muscle pain. Treat anaphylaxis and resuscitate as indicated.

ZOMETA

Monitor serum calcium and use vigorous IV hydration, with or without diuretics, for 2 to 3 days. Monitor intake and output to ensure adequacy and balance. Use short-term IV calcium therapy if indicated. Potassium phosphate and/or magnesium sulfate may be required to treat hypophosphatemia and hypomagnesemia. High fever may respond to steroids. RBC transfusions may be required in anemia.

APPENDIX A
Recommendations for the Safe Use and Handling of Cytotoxic Drugs

Numerous references are available on the topic of guidelines, recommendations, and regulations for handling antineoplastic and other hazardous agents.

The Department of Health and Human Services in the Centers for Disease Control and Prevention has publications and other references that cover all aspects of the topic at www.cdc.gov/niosh. Click on Hazards & Exposures, then click on Antineoplastic Agents. In 2004, the National Institute for Occupational Safety and Health (NIOSH) published *Preventing Occupational Exposure to Antineoplastic and Other Hazardous Drugs in Health Care Settings*, which can be found at www.cdc.gov/niosh/docs/2004-165. In 2014, NIOSH updated and published the *NIOSH List of Antineoplastic and Other Hazardous Drugs in Healthcare Settings, 2014*, which can be found at http://www.cdc.gov/niosh/docs/2014-138/pdfs/2014-138_v3.pdf. This document discusses the criteria used to define hazardous drugs and places drugs into three different groups: (1) antineoplastic drugs, (2) nonantineoplastic drugs that meet one or more of the NIOSH criteria for a hazardous drug, and (3) drugs that primarily pose a reproductive risk to men and women who are actively trying to conceive and women who are pregnant or breast-feeding. This publication also provides some general guidance on personal protective equipment and engineering controls when working with hazardous drugs in health care settings.

The United States Pharmacopeia published General Chapter <800> on February 1, 2016, in the First Supplement to USP 39–NF 34. The purpose of this chapter is to describe practice and quality standards for handling hazardous drugs in health care settings and to help promote patient safety, worker safety, and environmental protection. The new general chapter defines processes intended to minimize the exposure to hazardous drugs in health care settings. The official implementation date of this new chapter is July 1, 2018. This delay allows facilities additional time needed to implement the standard.

Other frequently cited guidelines on handling hazardous drugs are available from the American Society of Hospital-System Pharmacists, the Oncology Nursing Society, and the International Society of Oncology Pharmacy Practitioners.

Together these guidelines and regulations represent the recommendations of many diverse groups and have been established to promote not only patient safety but also worker safety and environmental protection.

APPENDIX B
FDA Pregnancy Categories

No drug should be used during pregnancy unless clearly needed and the risks to the fetus are outweighed by the benefits to the mother.

Category A   Adequate studies have not demonstrated a risk to the fetus in any trimester.
Category B   May have caused adverse effects in animals, but no adverse effects have been demonstrated in humans in any trimester or no demonstrated risk in animals but there are no adequate studies in pregnant women.
Category C   Animal studies have shown an adverse effect but there are no adequate studies in pregnant women or no animal studies and no studies in pregnant women.
Category D   Definite fetal risks. May be given in spite of risks if needed in life-threatening conditions.
Category X   Will cause fetal abnormalities. Risk of use outweighs benefits. Not recommended for use at any time during pregnancy. Consider alternatives before treating a pregnant woman.

Consider all men and women capable of conception when any drug in Category D or Category X is to be administered. Discuss birth control options to avoid pregnancy if a specific drug in these categories must be administered. Some drugs require birth control for months after all dosing is complete. Research complete information and keep patient informed.

APPENDIX C
U.S. Department of Health and Human Services, National Institutes of Health, National Cancer Institute Common Terminology Criteria for Adverse Events (CTCAE)

In Appendix C we have in the past incorporated the Common Toxicity Criteria (CTC) provided by the U.S. Department of Health and Human Services, the National Institutes of Health, and the National Cancer Institute. It was referred to throughout the text as the National Cancer Institute Common Toxicity Grading Criteria (NCI CTGC). This listing has been expanded and updated by these organizations and is too expansive to be included in an appendix. Web access to this material is available at www.cancer.gov. Search for CTCAE (Common Terminology Criteria for Adverse Events Version 4.0). Printed copies are available free of charge; call 1-800-4-CANCER (1-800-422-6237).

APPENDIX D
Information for Patients Receiving Immunosuppressive Agents

- Report allergic or sensitivity reactions you may have had to drugs or food.
- Report other medical problems you may have (e.g., exposure to chickenpox, herpes zoster, infections, bone marrow, heart, kidney, or liver problems).
- Provide a complete list of all medications you take, prescription and nonprescription.
- In most situations birth control is essential and may be required for both patient and partner. Nonhormonal birth control reduces the possibility of drug interactions, but compliance is imperative. If there is any possibility you or your partner may be pregnant, inform your physician promptly.
- Discontinue breast-feeding.
- Take only prescribed medication(s) in the exact amounts prescribed and at the times prescribed. This will help to maintain correct blood levels and avoid drug interactions.
- Confirm procedure if you should miss a dose. If any questions, notify physician.
- Confirm procedure for correct storage of your medication(s).
- Close monitoring by your physician is very important; keep all appointments and have all required lab work done on schedule. Your medications may interfere with some test results. Discuss with your physician.
- Do not take any immunizations without your physician's approval. Polio vaccine is especially virulent in your condition; request family members to defer immunization, and either avoid friends who have been immunized or wear a protective mask covering your nose and mouth while visiting.
- Dental procedures may need to be completed before starting therapy or deferred until therapy is completed. Use caution with your toothbrush, toothpicks, or dental floss. Alternate methods of dental hygiene may be necessary should your gums become tender, inflamed, or bleed.
- Review all side effects with your physician. Confirm those that may be a special problem for you and discuss solutions and expectations.
- Avoid anyone with an infection or fever. Report symptoms such as chills, fever, cough, hoarseness, lower back or side pain, painful or difficult urination.
- Wash hands before touching your eyes or the inside of your nose.
- Report unusual bleeding, bruising, black tarry stools, blood in urine, or pinpoint red spots on your skin (petechiae).
- Report redness, swelling, or soreness in the mouth (symptoms of stomatitis).
- Report mild hair loss, nausea and vomiting, rash, tiredness, weakness.
- Avoid accidental cuts whenever possible (e.g., razors, fingernail and toenail clippers).
- Avoid contact sports in which you might be bruised or injured.
- Drink adequate amounts of fluids to prevent increases in serum uric acid concentrations. Allopurinol (Zyloprim) and/or alkalinization of urine may be required.
- Anesthesia during dental, surgical, or emergency treatment may be a problem. It is best to consult with your physician, but inform all health care professionals about the medications you are taking before they treat you in any way.

APPENDIX E
Recently Approved Drugs

BRIVARACETAM
Anticonvulsant

Briviact
pH 5.5

USUAL DOSE
When initiating treatment, gradual dose escalation is not required. IV injection may be used when oral administration is temporarily not feasible and should be administered at the same dose and frequency as oral brivaracetam. Use of the IV formulation beyond 4 consecutive days of treatment has not been studied.

Patients 16 years of age and older: 50 mg twice daily (100 mg/day) is the recommended starting dose. Based on individual patient tolerability and therapeutic response, the dose may be adjusted down to 25 mg twice daily (50 mg/day) or up to 100 mg twice daily (200 mg/day).

DOSE ADJUSTMENTS
See Usual Dose. ▪ Recommended starting dose for all stages of hepatic impairment is 25 mg twice daily (50 mg/day), with a recommended maximum dose of 75 mg twice daily (150 mg/day). ▪ For patients receiving concomitant rifampin (Rifadin), increase the dose by up to 100% (i.e., double the dose); see Drug/Lab Interactions. ▪ No dose adjustment required for patients with impaired renal function; see Precautions.

DILUTION
A clear, colorless solution available as 50 mg/5 mL (10 mg/mL) in a single-use vial. Withdraw the desired dose. May be administered without further dilution or may be further diluted with NS, D5W, or LR and given as an infusion.

Filters: Specific information not available.

Storage: Store at CRT before use. Do not freeze. Diluted solution should not be stored for more than 4 hours at RT; may be stored in polyvinyl chloride (PVC) bags. Discard any unused portion of vial.

COMPATIBILITY
Specific information not available. Consider specific use; consult pharmacist.

RATE OF ADMINISTRATION
A single dose as an IV injection or infusion over 2 to 15 minutes. Flush IV line before and after injection.

ACTIONS
An antiepileptic (anticonvulsant) drug. The precise mechanism of action is unknown. Displays a high and selective affinity for synaptic vesicle protein 2A (SV2A) in the brain, which may contribute to the anticonvulsant effect. Weakly bound to plasma proteins. Primarily metabolized by hydrolysis and secondarily by hydroxylation. The hydrolysis reaction is mediated by hepatic and extrahepatic amidase. The hydroxylation pathway is mediated primarily by CYP2C19. Terminal plasma half-life is approximately 9 hours. Eliminated primarily by metabolism and by excretion in urine.

INDICATIONS AND USES
Adjunctive therapy in the treatment of partial-onset seizures in patients 16 years of age and older with epilepsy. IV injection may be used when oral administration is temporarily not feasible.

CONTRAINDICATIONS
Known hypersensitivity to brivaracetam or any of its inactive ingredients.

PRECAUTIONS
For IV use only. ▪ Antiepileptic drugs (AEDs) increase the risk of suicidal thoughts or behavior in patients taking these drugs for any indication. Patients treated with any AED for any indication should be monitored for the emergence or worsening of depression, suicidal thoughts or behavior, and/or any unusual changes in mood or behavior. Some behavioral changes may resolve without intervention. Others may require dose reduction or discontinuation of brivaracetam. ▪ Associated with CNS side effects (somnolence, fatigue, dizziness, coordination difficulties [abnormal gait, ataxia, balance disorder, incoordination]). The risk is greatest early in treatment but can occur at any time; see Monitor and Patient Education. ▪ Has been associated with behavioral and psychiatric abnormalities (e.g., aggression, agitation, anxiety, apathy, depression, emotional lability, irritability, nervousness, and psychotic symptoms, including paranoia, acute psychosis, and suicidal ideation). ▪ Hypersensitivity reactions have been reported. ▪ Avoid abrupt withdrawal to minimize the risk of increased seizure frequency and status epilepticus. ▪ Not recommended for use in patients with end-stage renal disease who are undergoing dialysis; data not available.

Monitor: Monitor for the emergence or worsening of depression, suicidal thoughts or behavior, and/or any unusual changes in mood or behavior. ▪ Observe for seizure activity. ▪ Observe closely for signs of CNS side effects; see Precautions. ▪ Monitor for S/S of a hypersensitivity reaction; angioedema and bronchospasm have been reported. If a reaction occurs, discontinue brivaracetam.

Patient Education: Review manufacturer's medication guide. ▪ May cause dizziness, coordination difficulties, and somnolence; use caution when performing tasks that require alertness or coordination (e.g., operating machinery, driving). ▪ May increase the risk of suicidal thoughts and behavior. Promptly report the emergence or worsening of S/S of depression, any unusual changes in mood or behavior, or thoughts of self-harm. ▪ Promptly report S/S of a hypersensitivity reaction (e.g., hypotension, rash, tightness of the chest, urticaria, wheezing). ▪ Women who are pregnant or who become pregnant should be encouraged to enroll in the North American Antiepileptic Drug (NAAED) Pregnancy Registry. ▪ Do not discontinue without consulting a health care provider. Must be gradually withdrawn to reduce the potential for increased seizure frequency and status epilepticus.

Maternal/Child: Category C: use during pregnancy only if the potential benefit justifies the potential risk to the fetus. ▪ Effect of use during labor and delivery unknown. ▪ Discontinue breast-feeding. ▪ Safety and effectiveness for use in patients 16 years of age and older have been established. ▪ Safety and effectiveness for use in pediatric patients younger than 16 years of age have not been established.

Elderly: Numbers in clinical studies insufficient to determine if elderly patients respond differently than younger patients. Dose selection should usually start at the low end. Consider decreased hepatic, renal, or cardiac function and concomitant disease or other drug therapy.

DRUG/LAB INTERACTIONS
Coadministration with rifampin decreases brivaracetam plasma concentrations. Brivaracetam dose should be increased by up to 100% while patients are receiving concomitant treatment with rifampin. ▪ Coadministration with carbamazepine (Tegretol) may increase exposure to the active metabolite of carbamazepine. Consider carbamazepine dose reduction if tolerability issues arise. ▪ Increases plasma concentrations of phenytoin. Monitor phenytoin levels when concomitant brivaracetam is added to or discontinued from ongoing phenytoin therapy. ▪ Coadministration of brivaracetam with levetiracetam (Keppra) provided no added therapeutic benefit.

SIDE EFFECTS
Dizziness, fatigue, nausea, sedation, somnolence, and vomiting are most common. Constipation, decreased neutrophil count, decreased white blood cell count, dysgeusia, euphoric mood, feeling drunk, and infusion site pain and irritability have also been reported. See Precautions.

ANTIDOTE
Keep physician informed of all side effects. Some may not require intervention, and others may improve with a reduced dose or discontinuation of brivaracetam. Treat hypersensitivity reactions immediately with oxygen, epinephrine (Adrenalin), antihistamines (e.g., diphenhydramine [Benadryl]), vasopressors (e.g., dopamine), corticosteroids, albuterol, IV fluids, and ventilation equipment as indicated. Support patient as required in overdose. There is no specific antidote. Ensure adequate airway, oxygenation, and ventilation and monitor vital signs, cardiac rate, and rhythm. Hemodialysis is not expected to enhance clearance. Resuscitate as necessary.

CROTALIDAE IMMUNE F(ab^9)$_2$ (EQUINE)   Antivenin
(kro-**TAL**-ih-day im **MYOUN** fab)

Anavip   pH not available

USUAL DOSE
Contact a regional poison control center for individual treatment advice.
Adult and pediatric patients: Administer as soon as possible after a rattlesnake bite in patients who develop any signs of envenomation (e.g., local injury, coagulation abnormality, or systemic signs of envenomation). The amount of antivenin required to treat a snakebite is highly variable and depends on venom burden, potency of the venom, and the time to health care presentation. Blood work required before administration; see Monitor.
Initial dose: 10 vials is the initial recommended dose. Monitor the patient for at least 60 minutes after completion of the infusion for any hypersensitivity reaction and to determine that local signs of envenomation are not progressing, systemic symptoms have resolved, and coagulation parameters have normalized or are trending toward normal; see Monitor.
Repeat doses: Administer an additional 10 vials if needed to arrest the progressive symptoms. Observe patient following each infusion as previously outlined and in Monitor. May repeat every hour if needed. There is no known maximum dose.
Observation and late dosing: Monitor patients in a health care setting for at least 18 hours following the initial control of signs and symptoms. Re-emerging symptoms, including coagulopathies, may be suppressed with an additional 4 vials as needed.

DOSE ADJUSTMENTS
Antivenin dose following a snakebite is expected to be the same in pediatric patients and adults; no dose adjustment for age is required.

DILUTION
Initial dose (10 vials), repeat doses (10 vials), observation and late dosing (4 vials): Available as a sterile lyophilized preparation in a single-use vial. Reconstitute each vial with 10 mL of NS. Gently swirl to dissolve; should take less than 1 minute. Solution should be clear to yellow/green and opalescent. Do not use if discolored or turbid. Promptly combine the contents of the reconstituted vials (all 10 vials or all 4 vials) and further dilute with NS to a total volume of 250 mL. Fluid volumes may need to be adjusted for very small children or infants; consult a regional poison control center.
Filters: Specific information not available.

Storage: Store unopened vials at RT (up to 25° C [77° F]). Brief excursions are permitted up to 40° C (104° F). Do not freeze. Discard unused reconstituted and/or diluted product.

COMPATIBILITY
Specific information not available. Administration through a dedicated line is appropriate because of specific use and the potential for anaphylaxis.

RATE OF ADMINISTRATION
Administer as an infusion over 60 minutes. Infuse at 25 to 50 mL/hr for the first 10 minutes, carefully monitoring for any hypersensitivity reaction, including anaphylaxis. If no reactions occur, the infusion rate may be increased to deliver the full 250 mL/hr rate until completion. If there is any hypersensitivity reaction at any time, stop the infusion, treat accordingly, and reassess risk to benefit before continuing the infusion; see Antidote.

ACTIONS
A sterile, lyophilized, polyvalent preparation of equine immunoglobulin F(ab')₂ fragments manufactured from the plasma of horses immunized with the venom of *Bothrops asper* and *Crotalus durissus*. Manufacturing procedures contribute to the reduced risk of viral transmission. Contains venom-specific F(ab⁹)₂ fragments of immunoglobulin G (IgG) that bind and neutralize venom toxins, facilitating redistribution away from target tissues and elimination from the body. Mean elimination half-life is approximately 133 hours.

INDICATIONS AND USES
An equine-derived antivenin for the management of adult and pediatric patients with North American rattlesnake envenomation.

CONTRAINDICATIONS
Manufacturer states, "None."

PRECAUTIONS
For IV use only. ▪ Usually administered in the hospital by or under the direction of a physician knowledgeable in its use and in a facility equipped to monitor the patient and respond to any medical emergency. ▪ May cause hypersensitivity reactions, including anaphylaxis. Patients with known allergies to horse protein are at particular risk for an anaphylactic reaction. ▪ May cause delayed hypersensitivity reactions or serum sickness; see Monitor. ▪ Made from equine (horse) plasma and may carry a risk of transmitting infectious agents (e.g., viruses). ▪ Contains trace amounts of cresol. Localized reactions and generalized myalgias have been reported with the use of cresol as an injectable excipient.
Monitor: Before initiating treatment, obtain a CBC, platelet count, PT, PTT, serum fibrinogen level, and routine serum chemistries. Repeat as indicated to gauge response to therapy and anticipate additional dosing. ▪ Use supportive measures to treat other manifestations of rattlesnake envenomation, such as pain, swelling, hypotension, and wound infection. ▪ Monitor for S/S of a hypersensitivity reaction (e.g., dyspnea, hypotension, rash, tightness of the chest, urticaria, wheezing) during the infusion and for at least 1 hour after completion of the infusion. ▪ After completion of the infusion, monitor for at least 1 hour to determine that local signs of envenomation are not progressing (leading edge of local injury not progressing), systemic symptoms have resolved, and coagulation parameters have normalized or are trending toward normal. ▪ Monitor for S/S of a delayed hypersensitivity reaction or serum sickness (e.g., arthralgia, fever, myalgia, pruritus, rash, urticarial rash) and treat appropriately if indicated.
Patient Education: Immediately report any S/S of delayed hypersensitivity reactions or serum sickness (e.g., arthralgia, fever, myalgia, pruritus, rash, shortness of breath, or urticaria occurring after discharge). ▪ Promptly report unusual bruising or bleeding (e.g., nosebleeds, excessive bleeding after toothbrushing or superficial injuries, blood in stools or urine, excessive menstrual bleeding, petechiae).
Maternal/Child: Category C: use during pregnancy only if clearly needed. ▪ Use caution during breast-feeding. ▪ Safety and effectiveness for use in pediatric patients similar to adults.
Elderly: Effectiveness in elderly adult similar to that in younger patients.

DRUG/LAB INTERACTIONS
Specific information not available.

SIDE EFFECTS
The most common adverse reactions include arthralgia, erythema, headache, myalgia, nausea, pain in extremity, peripheral edema, pruritus, rash, and vomiting. In pediatric patients, fever, itching, nausea, and vomiting were most common. Hypersensitivity reactions, including anaphylaxis, have been reported. Anxiety, blisters, chills, dehydration, dyspnea, fever, insomnia, and thrombocytopenia have also occurred.

ANTIDOTE
Keep the physician informed of all side effects and the extent or progression of envenomation. Reduce the rate of administration if infusion-related reactions occur (e.g., low back pain, fever, nausea, wheezing). Monitor closely and discontinue the infusion if symptoms worsen or a hypersensitivity reaction occurs. Treat hypersensitivity reactions and/or anaphylaxis immediately with oxygen, epinephrine, antihistamines (e.g., IV diphenhydramine [Benadryl]), corticosteroids, albuterol, vasopressors (e.g., dopamine), and ventilation equipment as indicated. Reassess risk to benefit before continuing the infusion. Recurrent coagulopathy may require rehospitalization and additional antivenin administration. Resuscitate as necessary.

DEFIBROTIDE

Antiplatelet agent
Thrombolytic agent

Defitelio

pH 6.8 to 7.8

USUAL DOSE
Adult and pediatric patients: Before administration, confirm that the patient is not experiencing clinically significant bleeding and is hemodynamically stable on no more than one vasopressor.
Defibrotide: 6.25 mg/kg every 6 hours given as a 2-hour infusion. Base dose on patient's baseline body weight, which is defined as the patient's weight before the preparative regimen for hematopoietic stem cell transplantation (HSCT). Administer for a minimum of 21 days. If after 21 days S/S of veno-occlusive disease (VOD) have not resolved, continue defibrotide until resolution of VOD or up to a maximum of 60 days.

DOSE ADJUSTMENTS
Treatment modification, including temporary or permanent discontinuation, is outlined in the following chart.

Defibrotide Treatment Modifications for Toxicity or Invasive Procedures	
Event	**Recommended Action**
Hypersensitivity Reaction	
Severe or life-threatening (anaphylaxis)	Discontinue defibrotide permanently; do not resume treatment.
Bleeding	
Persistent, severe, or potentially life threatening	Withhold defibrotide. Treat the cause of bleeding and give supportive care as clinically indicated. Consider resuming treatment (at the same dose and infusion volume) when bleeding has stopped and the patient is hemodynamically stable.
Recurrent significant bleeding	Discontinue defibrotide permanently; do not resume treatment.
Invasive Procedures	
	There is no known reversal agent for the profibrinolytic effects of defibrotide. Discontinue defibrotide infusion at least 2 hours before an invasive procedure. Resume defibrotide treatment after the procedure, as soon as any procedure-related risk of bleeding is resolved.

DILUTION

Available in a 200 mg/2.5 mL (80 mg/mL) single-patient-use vial; a clear and light yellow to brown solution. Determine the dose based on patient's baseline weight, which is defined as the patient's weight before the preparative regimen for hematopoietic stem cell transplantation (HSCT). Calculate the volume of defibrotide needed and withdraw this amount from the vial(s). Add this volume to an infusion bag containing NS or D5W. Final concentration of the prepared solution should be 4 to 20 mg/mL. Mix gently.

Filter: 0.2-micron in-line filter required.

Storage: Store unopened vials at CRT. Diluted solution should be used within 4 hours if stored at room temperature or within 24 hours if stored under refrigeration. Up to 4 doses of defibrotide may be prepared at one time if refrigerated. Discard any partially used vials.

COMPATIBILITY

Manufacturer states, "Do not coadminister Defitelio and other intravenous drugs concurrently within the same intravenous line."

RATE OF ADMINISTRATION

Administer using an infusion set equipped with a 0.2-micron in-line filter. Flush the IV administration line with NS or D5W immediately before and after administration.

Administer each single dose as a constant infusion equally distributed over 2 hours.

ACTIONS

An oligonucleotide mixture with profibrinolytic properties. The mechanism of action of defibrotide has not been fully elucidated. In vitro, it enhances the enzymatic activity of plasmin to hydrolyze fibrin clots. It also increases tissue plasminogen activator (t-PA) and thrombomodulin expression and decreases von Willebrand factor (vWF) and plasminogen activator inhibitor-1 (PAI-1) expression, thereby reducing endothelial cell (EC) activation and increasing endothelial cell–mediated fibrinolysis. Highly bound to plasma proteins. Metabolism followed by urinary excretion is likely the main route of elimination. The exact pathway of metabolism is unknown, but in vitro studies show that defibrotide does not undergo appreciable metabolism by hepatocyte cells. Half-life is less than 2 hours.

INDICATIONS AND USES

Treatment of adult and pediatric patients with hepatic VOD, also known as sinusoidal obstruction syndrome (SOS), with renal or pulmonary dysfunction after HSCT.

CONTRAINDICATIONS

Concomitant administration with systemic anticoagulant or fibrinolytic therapy. ▪ Known hypersensitivity to defibrotide or to any of its excipients.

PRECAUTIONS

May increase the risk of bleeding in patients with VOD after HSCT. Do not initiate defibrotide in patients with active bleeding. Withhold or discontinue defibrotide in patients who develop bleeding. Treat the underlying cause and provide supportive care until the bleeding has stopped; see Dose Adjustments. ▪ Hypersensitivity reactions have been reported. Anaphylaxis was reported in a patient who had previously received defibrotide. ▪ See Drug/Lab Interactions.

Monitor: Monitor patient for signs of bleeding. ▪ Monitor for S/S of a hypersensitivity reaction, especially if there is a history of previous exposure to defibrotide. Reported hypersensitivity reactions have included anaphylaxis, angioedema, rash, and urticaria.

Patient Education: May increase the risk of hemorrhage. Promptly report any S/S of bleeding (e.g., altered vision, blood in urine or stool, confusion, easy bruising, headache, slurred speech, or unusual bleeding). ▪ Inform health care provider of any previous defibrotide use. ▪ Promptly report S/S of a hypersensitivity reaction (e.g., itching, hives, rash, shortness of breath, wheezing).

Maternal/Child: Information on use during pregnancy and breast-feeding is not available. Animal studies suggest a potential risk of miscarriage if administered during pregnancy. ▪ Because of the risk of serious adverse reactions, including bleeding in a breast-fed infant, breast-feeding is not recommended during treatment with defibrotide. ▪ Safety and effectiveness have been established in pediatric patients.

Elderly: Studies did not include sufficient numbers of subjects 65 years of age and older to determine whether they respond differently than younger subjects. Differences in response have not been identified.

DRUG/LAB INTERACTIONS

Concomitant use with a **systemic anticoagulant** (e.g., apixaban [Eliquis], heparin, rivaroxaban [Xarelto], warfarin [Coumadin]) or **fibrinolytic therapy** (e.g., alteplase [Activase], tenecteplase [TNKase]), not including use for routine maintenance or reopening of central venous lines, may increase the risk of bleeding. Discontinue anticoagulants and fibrinolytic agents before defibrotide treatment, and consider delaying the start of defibrotide administration until the effects of the anticoagulant have abated; see Contraindications. ▪ May enhance the pharmacodynamic activity of **antithrombotic/fibrinolytic drugs** such as heparin or alteplase. Concomitant use is contraindicated because of an increased risk of hemorrhage. ▪ In vitro studies demonstrate that defibrotide does not induce (CYP1A2, CYP2B6, CYP3A4, UGT1A1) or inhibit (CYP1A2, CYP2B6, CYP3A4, CYP2C8, CYP2C9, CYP2C19, CYP2D6, UGT1A1, UGT2B7) the major drug-metabolizing enzymes and is not a substrate or inhibitor of the major drug uptake transporters (OAT1, OAT3, OCT1, OCT2, OATP1B1, OATP1B3) or efflux transporters (P-gp and BCRP).

SIDE EFFECTS

The most common adverse reactions were diarrhea, epistaxis, hypotension, nausea, and vomiting. The most common serious adverse reactions were hypotension and pulmonary alveolar hemorrhage. Other reported adverse reactions included cerebral hemorrhage, gastrointestinal hemorrhage, graft-versus-host disease, hyperuricemia, infection, intracranial hemorrhage, lung infiltration, pneumonia, pulmonary hemorrhage, and sepsis.

ANTIDOTE

Notify physician of any side effects; most will be treated symptomatically. Discontinue defibrotide if bleeding develops. Treat underlying cause and provide supportive care as indicated. Discontinue defibrotide if a severe hypersensitivity reaction occurs. Treat hypersensitivity reactions as indicated (e.g., oxygen, diphenhydramine, epinephrine, corticosteroids, vasopressors, and/or fluids). Resuscitate as necessary. Defibrotide is not removed by hemodialysis.

INDEX

Color type indicates generic drug name.
Italic type indicates drug categories and listings.
*See http://evolve.elsevier.com/IVMeds for detailed information.

Color type indicates generic drug name.
Italic type indicates drug categories and listings.
*See http://evolve.elsevier.com/IVMeds for detailed information.

Color type indicates generic drug name.
Italic type indicates drug categories and listings.
*See http://evolve.elsevier.com/IVMeds for detailed information.

Color type indicates generic drug name.
Italic type indicates drug categories and listings.
*See http://evolve.elsevier.com/IVMeds for detailed information.

Color type indicates generic drug name.
Italic type indicates drug categories and listings.
*See http://evolve.elsevier.com/IVMeds for detailed information.

Color type indicates generic drug name.
Italic type indicates drug categories and listings.
*See http://evolve.elsevier.com/IVMeds for detailed information.

Color type indicates generic drug name.
Italic type indicates drug categories and listings.
*See http://evolve.elsevier.com/IVMeds for detailed information.

Color type indicates generic drug name.
Italic type indicates drug categories and listings.
*See http://evolve.elsevier.com/IVMeds for detailed information.

Color type indicates generic drug name.
Italic type indicates drug categories and listings.
*See http://evolve.elsevier.com/IVMeds for detailed information.

Color type indicates generic drug name.
Italic type indicates drug categories and listings.
*See http://evolve.elsevier.com/IVMeds for detailed information.

Color type indicates generic drug name.
Italic type indicates drug categories and listings.
*See http://evolve.elsevier.com/IVMeds for detailed information.

Color type indicates generic drug name.
Italic type indicates drug categories and listings.
*See http://evolve.elsevier.com/IVMeds for detailed information.

Color type indicates generic drug name.
Italic type indicates drug categories and listings.
*See http://evolve.elsevier.com/IVMeds for detailed information.

Color type indicates generic drug name.
Italic type indicates drug categories and listings.
*See http://evolve.elsevier.com/IVMeds for detailed information.

Color type indicates generic drug name.
Italic type indicates drug categories and listings.
*See http://evolve.elsevier.com/IVMeds for detailed information.

Color type indicates generic drug name.
Italic type indicates drug categories and listings.
*See http://evolve.elsevier.com/IVMeds for detailed information.

Color type indicates generic drug name.
Italic type indicates drug categories and listings.
*See http://evolve.elsevier.com/IVMeds for detailed information.

Color type indicates generic drug name.
Italic type indicates drug categories and listings.
*See http://evolve.elsevier.com/IVMeds for detailed information.

Color type indicates generic drug name.
Italic type indicates drug categories and listings.
*See http://evolve.elsevier.com/IVMeds for detailed information.

Color type indicates generic drug name.
Italic type indicates drug categories and listings.
*See http://evolve.elsevier.com/IVMeds for detailed information.

Color type indicates generic drug name.
talic type indicates drug categories and listings.
*See http://evolve.elsevier.com/IVMeds for detailed information.

Color type indicates generic drug name.
Italic type indicates drug categories and listings.
*See http://evolve.elsevier.com/IVMeds for detailed information.

Solution Compatibility Chart

Intravenous Medication	D2½W	D5W	D10W	D5/¼NS	D5/½NS	D5NS	NS	½NS	R	LR	D5R	D5LR	Dextran 6%/D5W/NS	Fruc 10%/W/NS	Invert sug 10%/W/NS	
Acetazolamide	C	C	C	C	C	C	C	C	C	C	C	C	C	C	C	C
Acyclovir		C		C	C	C			C							
Aminophylline	C	C	C	C	C	C	C	C	C	C	C	C	C			C
Antithymocyte Globulin	C	C	C	C	C	C	C	C								
Ascorbic Acid	C	C	C	C	C	C	C	C	C	C	C	C	C	C	C	C
Aztreonam		C	C	C	C	C			C	C	C					C
Calcium Chloride		C	C	C	C	C			C	C	C	C				
Calcium Gluconate		C	C			C	C			C		C		W		C
Cefazolin Na		C	C	C	C	C	C		C	C		C			W	
Cefoperazone Na		C	C	C			C			C		C				
Cefotaxime Na		C	C	C	C	C	C			C					W	C
Cefotetan		C					C									
Cefoxitin Na		C	C	C	C	C	C		C	C		C			C	C
Ceftazidime		C	C	C	C	C	C		C	C					W	C
Ceftriaxone Na		C	C			C			C						W	C
Cefuroxime Na		C	C	C	C	C	C		C	C					W	C
Clindamycin		C	C		C	C	C		C	C						
Dexamethasone		C					C									
Dobutamine HCl		C	C		C	C	C	C		C		C				C
Dopamine HCl		C	C		C	C	C			C		C				C
Doxycycline		C					C	C		C					W	
Epinephrine	C	C	C	C	C	C	C		C	C	C	C	C	C	C	C
Famotidine		C	C				C			C						
Fentanyl		C					C									
Folic Acid		C					C									
Furosemide		C	C			C	C			C		C				C
Gentamicin		C	C				C		C	C						
Heparin Na	C	C*		C	C	C	C*	C	C		C	C	C	C	C	
Hydrocortisone Phosphate		C	C				C	C								
Hydrocortisone Na Succinate	C	C	C	C	C	C	C	C	C	C	C	C	C	C	C	C
Hydromorphone HCl		C	C		C	C	C	C	C	C	C	C			W	C
Imipenem-Cilastatin		C[4]	C[4]	C[4]	C[4]	C[4]	C[10]									
Insulin (Regular)		C[p]	C		C		C[p]			C	C					
Isoproterenol	C	C[p]	C	C	C	C	C[p]	C	C	C	C	C	C	C	C	C
Kanamycin		C	C			C	C			C						
Labetalol		C		C		C	C		C	C	C	C				
Lidocaine		C[p]			C	C	C	C		C		C				
Magnesium Sulfate		C					C			C						
Meperidine HCl	C	C	C	C	C	C	C	C	C	C	C	C	C	C	C	C
Meropenem		C[1]	C[1]	C[1]		C[1]	C[4]		C[4]	C[4]		C[1]				C[2]

beef, water chestnut & rice soup

VARIATION

Omit the rice for a lighter soup
that is an ideal starter for an
Oriental meal of many courses.
For a more substantial soup that
would be a meal in its own right,
add diced vegetables such as
carrot, pepper or courgette.

1 Carefully trim away any fat from the beef. Cut the beef into thin strips and then place in a large saucepan.

2 Pour over the stock and add the cinnamon, star anise, soy sauce, sherry, tomato purée and water chestnuts. Bring to the boil, skimming away any surface scum with a slotted spoon. Cover the saucepan and simmer gently for 20 minutes, or until the beef is tender.

3 Skim the soup with a slotted spoon again to remove any scum. Remove and discard the cinnamon and star anise and blot the surface with kitchen paper to remove any fat.

4 Stir in the rice, orange rind and juice. Adjust the seasoning if necessary. Heat through for 2–3 minutes before ladling into warmed bowls. Serve garnished with strips of orange rind and snipped chives.

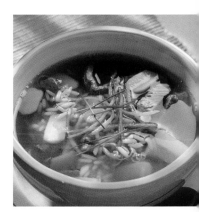

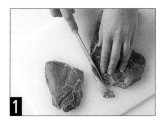

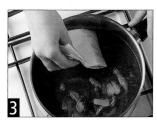

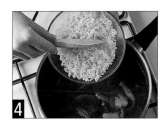

chunky potato & beef soup

serves four

2 tbsp vegetable oil

225 g/8 oz lean braising or
    frying steak, cut into strips

225 g/8 oz new potatoes, halved

1 carrot, diced

2 celery sticks, sliced

2 leeks, sliced

850 ml/1½ pints beef stock

8 baby corn cobs, sliced

1 bouquet garni

2 tbsp dry sherry

salt and pepper

chopped fresh parsley, to garnish

crusty bread, to serve

COOK'S TIP

Make double the quantity of
soup and freeze the remainder in
a rigid container for later use.
When ready to use, leave in the
refrigerator to thaw thoroughly,
then heat until piping hot.

---

1 Heat the vegetable oil in a
large saucepan. Add the strips
of steak and cook for 3 minutes,
turning constantly.

2 Add the potatoes, carrot, celery
and leeks. Cook, stirring
constantly, for a further 5 minutes.

3 Pour in the stock and bring to the
boil over a medium heat. Reduce
the heat until the liquid is simmering
gently, then add the baby corn cobs
and the bouquet garni.

4 Cook the soup for a further
20 minutes, or until the meat and
all the vegetables are tender.

5 Remove the bouquet garni from
the saucepan and discard. Stir the
sherry into the soup and season to
taste with salt and pepper. Pour the
soup into warmed soup bowls and
garnish with parsley. Serve
immediately with crusty bread.

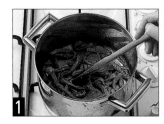

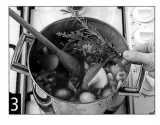

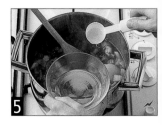

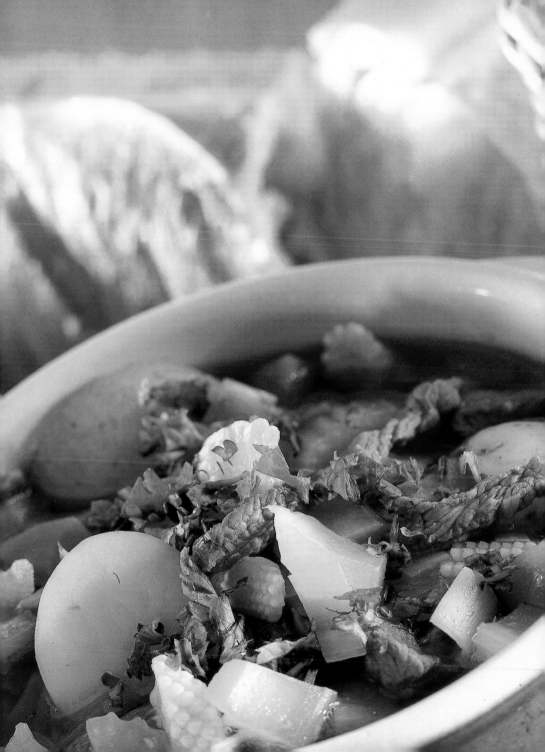

veal & ham soup

serves four

55 g/2 oz butter

1 onion, diced

1 carrot, diced

1 celery stick, diced

450 g/1 lb veal, very thinly sliced

450 g/1 lb ham, thinly sliced

55 g/2 oz plain flour

1 litre/1¾ pints beef stock

1 bay leaf

8 black peppercorns

pinch of salt

3 tbsp redcurrant jelly

150 ml/5 fl oz cream sherry

100 g/3½ oz dried vermicelli

garlic croûtons (see Cook's Tip),
   to garnish

COOK'S TIP

To make garlic croûtons, cut
3 slices of day-old crustless white
bread into small cubes. Stir-fry
1–2 chopped garlic cloves
in 3 tablespoons of oil for
1–2 minutes. Remove the garlic
and cook the bread, stirring,
until golden. Remove and drain.

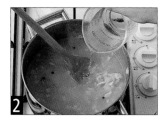

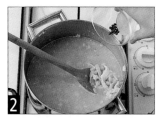

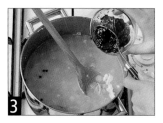

1 Melt the butter in a large
saucepan. Add the onion, carrot,
celery, veal and ham and cook over a
low heat for 6 minutes.

2 Sprinkle over the flour and cook,
stirring constantly, for a further
2 minutes. Gradually stir in the stock,
then add the bay leaf, peppercorns and
salt. Bring to the boil and simmer for
1 hour.

3 Remove the saucepan from the
heat and add the redcurrant
jelly and sherry, stirring to combine.
Set aside for about 4 hours.

4 Discard the bay leaf. Reheat
the soup over a very low heat
until warmed through. Meanwhile,
cook the vermicelli in a saucepan
of lightly salted boiling water for
10–12 minutes, or until just tender.
Stir into the soup and transfer to
bowls. Garnish with garlic croûtons.

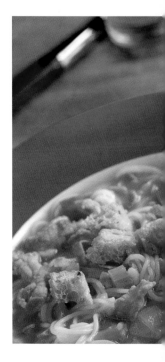

tuscan veal broth

serves four

55 g/2 oz dried peas, soaked for
2 hours and drained

900 g/2 lb boned neck of veal,
diced

1.2 litres/2 pints beef stock

600 ml/1 pint water

55 g/2 oz pearl barley, washed

salt and pepper

1 large carrot, diced

1 small turnip (about 175 g/6 oz),
diced

1 large leek, thinly sliced

1 red onion, finely chopped

100 g/3½ oz tomatoes, chopped

1 fresh basil sprig

100 g/3½ oz dried vermicelli

1 Put the peas, veal, stock and
water into a large saucepan and
bring to the boil over a low heat. Using
a slotted spoon, skim off any scum that
rises to the surface of the liquid.

2 When all of the scum has been
removed, add the pearl barley
and a pinch of salt to the mixture.
Simmer gently over a low heat for
25 minutes.

3 Add the carrot, turnip, leek,
onion, tomatoes and basil to the
saucepan and season to taste with salt
and pepper. Leave to simmer for about
2 hours, skimming the surface, using a
slotted spoon, from time to time.
Remove the saucepan from the heat
and set aside for 2 hours.

4 Set the saucepan over a medium
heat and bring to the boil. Add
the vermicelli and cook for 12 minutes,
or until just tender. Taste and adjust the
seasoning, and remove and discard the
basil. Ladle into warmed soup bowls
and serve immediately.

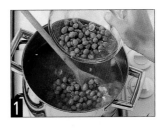

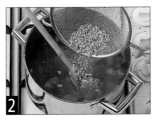

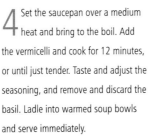

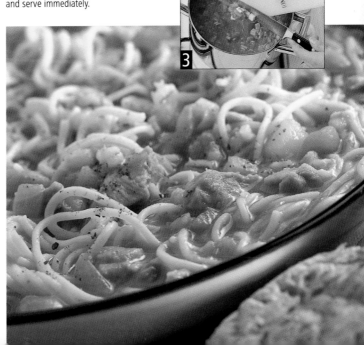

chinese potato & pork broth

serves four

1 litre/1¾ pints chicken stock

2 large potatoes, diced

2 tbsp rice wine vinegar

2 tbsp cornflour

4 tbsp water

125 g/4½ oz pork fillet, sliced

1 tbsp light soy sauce

1 tsp sesame oil

1 carrot, cut into very thin strips

1 tsp chopped fresh root ginger

3 spring onions, thinly sliced

1 red pepper, deseeded and sliced

225 g/8 oz canned bamboo
   shoots, drained

COOK'S TIP

For extra heat, add 1 chopped
fresh red chilli or 1 teaspoon
of chilli powder to the
soup in Step 5.

1 Place the stock, potatoes and 1 tablespoon of the vinegar in a saucepan and bring to the boil. Reduce the heat until the stock is just simmering.

2 Mix the cornflour with the water, then stir into the hot stock.

3 Return the stock to the boil, stirring until thickened, then reduce the heat until it is just simmering again.

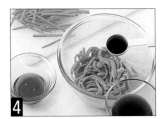

4 Place the pork slices in a dish and season with the remaining vinegar, the soy sauce and the oil.

5 Add the pork slices, carrot strips and ginger to the stock and cook for 10 minutes. Stir in the spring onions, pepper and bamboo shoots. Cook for a further 5 minutes. Pour the soup into warmed bowls and serve immediately.

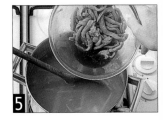

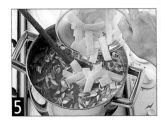

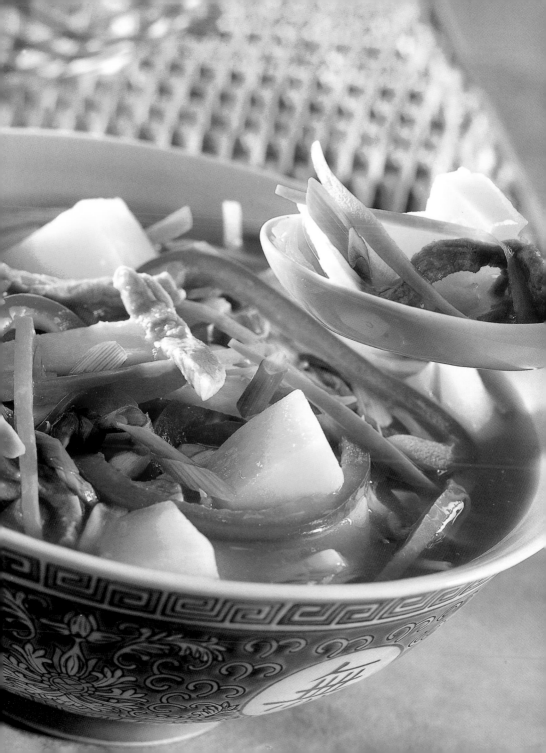

pork chilli soup

serves three

2 tsp olive oil

500 g/1 lb 2 oz fresh lean
 pork mince

salt and pepper

1 onion, finely chopped

1 celery stick, finely chopped

1 pepper, deseeded and
 finely chopped

2–3 garlic cloves, finely chopped

400 g/14 oz canned chopped
 tomatoes in juice

3 tbsp tomato purée

450 ml/16 fl oz chicken or
 meat stock

⅛ tsp ground coriander

⅛ tsp ground cumin

¼ tsp dried oregano

1 tsp mild chilli powder, or to taste

chopped fresh coriander leaves or
 parsley, to garnish

soured cream, to serve

COOK'S TIP

For a festive presentation, offer
additional accompaniments, such
as grated cheese, chopped spring
onion and guacamole.

1 Heat the oil in a large saucepan over a medium–high heat. Add the pork and season to taste with salt and pepper then cook until no longer pink, stirring frequently. Reduce the heat to medium and add the onion, celery, pepper and garlic. Cover and cook for 5 minutes, stirring occasionally, until the onion is softened.

2 Add the tomatoes, tomato purée and the stock, then add the coriander, cumin, oregano and chilli powder. Stir the ingredients in to combine well.

3 Bring just to the boil, then reduce the heat to low, cover and simmer for 30–40 minutes, or until all the vegetables are very tender. Taste and adjust the seasoning, adding more chilli powder if you like it hotter.

4 Ladle the chilli into warmed bowls and sprinkle with coriander or parsley. Hand the soured cream round separately, or top each serving with a spoonful.

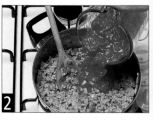

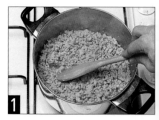

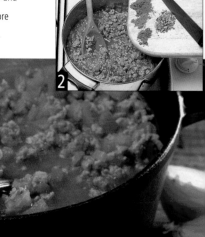

spicy lamb soup with chickpeas

serves four–five

1–2 tbsp olive oil

450 g/1 lb lean boneless lamb, such as shoulder or neck fillet, trimmed of fat and cut into 1-cm/½-inch cubes

1 onion, finely chopped

2–3 garlic cloves, crushed

1.2 litres/2 pints water

400 g/14 oz canned chopped tomatoes in juice

1 bay leaf

½ tsp dried thyme

½ tsp dried oregano

⅛ tsp ground cinnamon

¼ tsp ground cumin

¼ tsp ground turmeric

1 tsp harissa, or to taste

400 g/14 oz canned chickpeas, rinsed and drained

1 carrot, diced

1 potato, diced

1 courgette, quartered lengthways and sliced

100 g/3½ oz fresh shelled or thawed frozen peas

chopped fresh mint or coriander leaves, to garnish

1 Heat the oil in a large saucepan or cast-iron casserole over a medium–high heat. Add the lamb, in batches if necessary to avoid crowding the saucepan, and cook until evenly browned on all sides, adding a little more oil if needed. Remove the meat with a slotted spoon when browned.

2 Reduce the heat and add the onion and garlic. Cook, stirring frequently, for 1–2 minutes.

3 Add the water and return all the meat to the pan. Bring just to the boil and skim off any scum that rises to the surface. Reduce the heat and stir in the tomatoes, bay leaf, thyme, oregano, cinnamon, cumin, turmeric and harissa. Simmer for 1 hour, or until the meat is very tender. Remove and discard the bay leaf.

4 Stir in the chickpeas, carrot and potato and simmer for 15 minutes. Add the courgette and peas and continue simmering for 15–20 minutes, or until all the vegetables are tender.

5 Adjust the seasoning, adding more harissa, if wished. Ladle the soup into warmed bowls and garnish with mint or coriander.

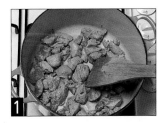

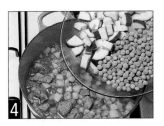

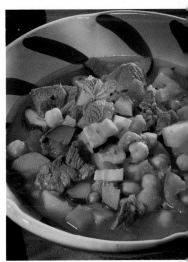

rich beef stew

serves four

1 tbsp oil

1 tbsp butter

225 g/8 oz baby onions, peeled
and halved

600 g/1 lb 5 oz stewing steak, diced
into 4-cm/1½-inch chunks

300 ml/10 fl oz beef stock

150 ml/5 fl oz red wine

4 tbsp chopped fresh oregano

1 tbsp sugar

1 orange

25 g/1 oz dried porcini or other
dried mushrooms

4 tbsp warm water

225 g/8 oz fresh plum tomatoes

cooked rice or potatoes, to serve

VARIATION

Instead of fresh tomatoes, try
using sun-dried tomatoes, cut
into wide strips, if you prefer.

1 Preheat the oven to 180°C/350°F/
Gas Mark 4. Heat the oil and
butter in a large frying pan. Add the
onions and cook for 5 minutes, or until
golden. Remove with a slotted spoon,
set aside and keep warm.

2 Add the beef to the frying pan
and cook, stirring, for 5 minutes,
or until browned all over.

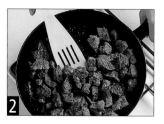

3 Return the onions to the frying
pan and add the stock, wine,
oregano and sugar, stirring to mix
well. Transfer the mixture to an
ovenproof casserole.

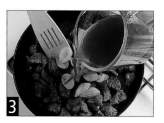

4 Pare the rind from the orange and
cut it into strips. Slice the orange
flesh into rings. Add the orange rings
and the rind to the casserole. Cook in
the oven for 1¼ hours.

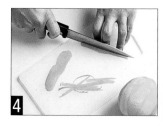

5 Soak the mushrooms for
30 minutes in a small bowl
containing the warm water.

6 Peel and halve the tomatoes. Add
the tomatoes, mushrooms and
their soaking liquid to the casserole.
Cook for a further 20 minutes, or until
the beef is tender and the juices have
thickened. Serve with rice or potatoes.

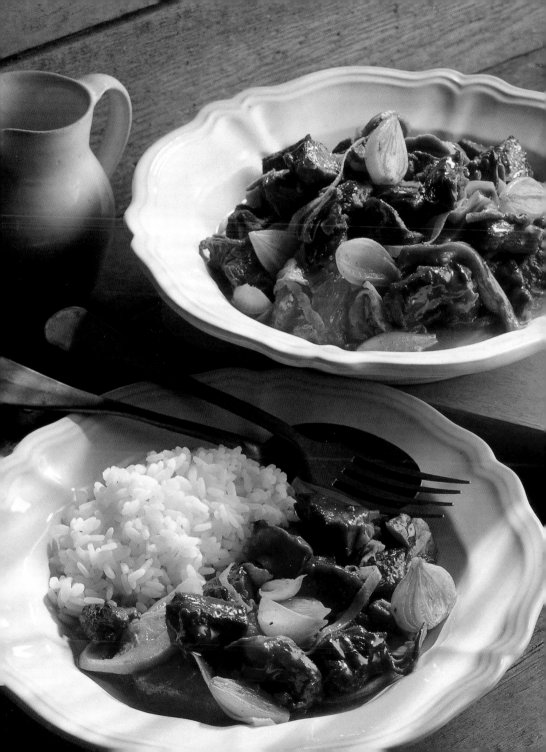

beef & orange curry

serves four

1 tbsp vegetable oil

225 g/8 oz shallots, halved

2 garlic cloves, crushed

450 g/1 lb lean rump or sirloin beef, trimmed and cut into 2-cm/ ¾-inch cubes

3 tbsp curry paste

450 ml/16 fl oz beef stock

4 oranges

2 tsp cornflour

salt and pepper

2 tbsp chopped fresh coriander, to garnish

boiled basmati rice, to serve

RAITA

½ cucumber, finely diced

3 tbsp chopped fresh mint

150 ml/5 fl oz low-fat natural yogurt

1 Heat the oil in a large saucepan. Add the shallots, garlic and beef cubes and cook over a low heat, stirring occasionally, for 5 minutes, or until the beef is evenly browned all over.

2 Blend together the curry paste and stock. Add the mixture to the beef and stir to mix thoroughly. Bring to the boil, cover and simmer for about 1 hour.

3 Grate the rind of 1 orange. Extract the juice from the orange and from 1 other. Peel the other 2 oranges, removing the pith. Slice between each segment and remove the flesh.

4 Blend the cornflour with the orange juice. At the end of the cooking time, stir the orange rind into the beef with the orange and cornflour mixture. Bring to the boil and simmer, stirring constantly, for 3–4 minutes, or until the sauce thickens. Season to taste with salt and pepper and stir in the orange segments.

5 To make the raita, mix the cucumber with the mint and stir in the yogurt. Season to taste with salt and pepper.

6 Serve the curry with rice and the cucumber raita, garnished with the chopped coriander.

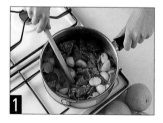
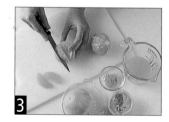
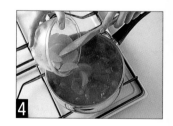

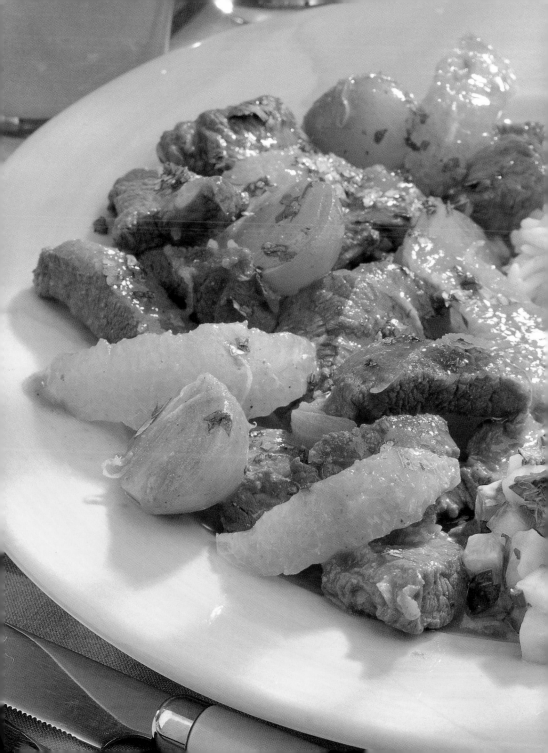

beef & tomato gratin

serves four

350 g/12 oz fresh lean beef mince

1 large onion, finely chopped

1 tsp dried mixed herbs

1 tbsp plain flour

300 ml/10 fl oz beef stock

1 tbsp tomato purée

salt and pepper

2 large tomatoes, thinly sliced

4 courgettes, thinly sliced

2 tbsp cornflour

300 ml/10 fl oz skimmed milk

150 ml/5 fl oz low-fat natural

    fromage frais

1 egg yolk

4 tbsp freshly grated

    Parmesan cheese

TO SERVE

crusty bread

steamed vegetables

1 Preheat the oven to 190°C/375°F/ Gas Mark 5. In a large frying pan, dry-fry the beef and onion for 4–5 minutes, or until browned.

2 Stir in the herbs, flour, stock and tomato purée, and season to taste with salt and pepper. Bring to the boil, then reduce the heat and simmer for 30 minutes, or until thickened.

3 Transfer the beef mixture to an ovenproof gratin dish. Cover with a layer of the sliced tomatoes and then add a layer of sliced courgettes. Set aside until required.

4 Blend the cornflour with a little of the milk in a small bowl. Pour the remaining milk into a saucepan and bring to the boil. Add the cornflour mixture and cook, stirring, for 1–2 minutes, or until thickened. Remove from the heat and beat in the fromage frais and egg yolk. Season well.

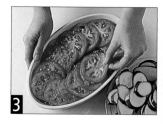

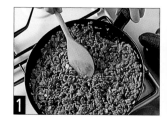

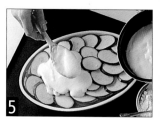

5 Spread the white sauce over the layer of courgettes. Place the dish on a baking sheet and sprinkle with Parmesan cheese. Bake in the oven for 25–30 minutes, or until golden brown. Serve with crusty bread and steamed vegetables.

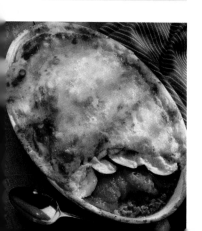

michoacan beef

serves four–six

about 3 tbsp plain flour

salt and pepper

1 kg/2 lb 4 oz stewing beef, cut into
   large bite-sized pieces

2 tbsp vegetable oil

2 onions, chopped

5 garlic cloves, chopped

400 g/14 oz tomatoes, diced

1½ dried chipotle chillies,
   reconstituted (see Cook's Tip,
   page 78), deseeded and cut into
   thin strips, or a few shakes of
   bottled chipotle salsa

1.5 litres/2¾ pints beef stock

350 g/12 oz green beans

pinch of sugar

TO SERVE

cooked kidney beans

freshly cooked rice

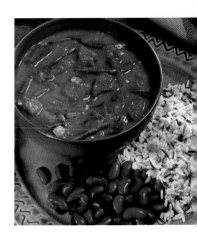

COOK'S TIP

This is traditionally made with nopales – edible cactus – which gives the dish a distinctive flavour. Look out for them in specialist shops. For this recipe you need 350–400 g/12–14 oz canned nopales, or fresh nopales, peeled, sliced and blanched. Add them to the stew with the tomatoes.

1 Place the flour in a large bowl and season to taste with salt and pepper. Add the beef and toss to coat well. Remove the beef from the bowl, shaking off the excess flour.

2 Heat the oil in a frying pan. Add the beef and brown briefly over a high heat. Reduce the heat to medium, add the onions and garlic and cook for 2 minutes.

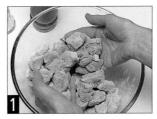

3 Add the tomatoes, chillies and stock, then cover and simmer over a low heat for 1½ hours, or until the meat is very tender, adding the green beans and sugar 15 minutes before the end of the cooking time. Skim off any fat that rises to the surface from time to time.

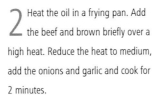

4 Transfer to individual warmed bowls and serve with kidney beans and rice.

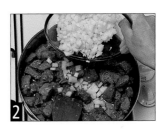

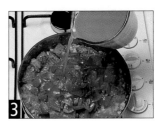

beef cooked in whole spices

serves four

300 ml/10 fl oz oil

3 onions, finely chopped

2.5-cm/1-inch piece fresh root
   ginger, grated

4 garlic cloves, sliced

2 cinnamon sticks

3 green cardamoms

3 cloves

4 black peppercorns

6 dried red chillies

150 ml/5 fl oz natural yogurt

450 g/1 lb lean beef, cubed

3 fresh green chillies, chopped

600 ml/1 pint water

VARIATION

Substitute lamb for the beef in
this recipe, if you prefer.

---

1 Heat the oil in a frying pan, add the onions and fry, stirring, until golden brown.

2 Reduce the heat, add the ginger, garlic, cinnamon sticks, cardamoms, cloves, peppercorns and dried chillies to the frying pan and stir-fry for 5 minutes. In a bowl, whisk the yogurt with a fork. Add the yogurt to the onion mixture in the pan and stir to combine.

3 Add the beef and 2 of the fresh chillies to the frying pan and stir-fry the mixture for 5–7 minutes.

4 Gradually add the water to the frying pan, stirring well. Cover and cook the beef and spice mixture for 1 hour, stirring and adding more water if necessary.

5 When thoroughly cooked through, remove the frying pan from the heat and transfer the beef and spice mixture to a warmed serving dish. Garnish with the remaining chopped fresh chilli.

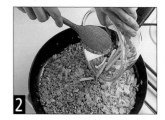

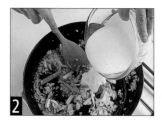

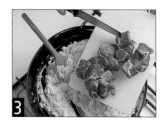

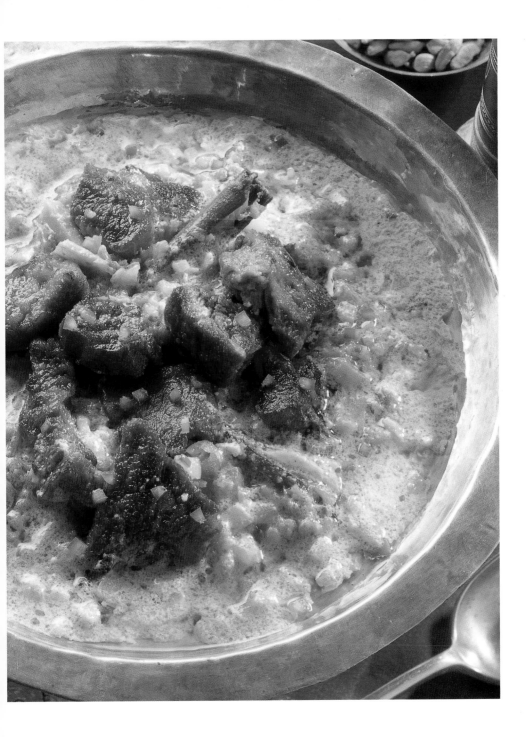

citrus osso bucco

serves six

1–2 tbsp plain flour

salt and pepper

6 meaty slices veal

1 kg/2 lb 4 oz fresh tomatoes, peeled, deseeded and diced, or 800 g/1 lb 12 oz canned chopped tomatoes

1–2 tbsp olive oil

250 g/9 oz onions, very finely chopped

250 g/9 oz carrots, finely diced

225 ml/8 fl oz dry white wine

225 ml/8 fl oz veal stock

6 large fresh basil leaves, torn

1 large garlic clove, very finely chopped

finely grated rind of 1 large lemon

finely grated rind of 1 orange

2 tbsp finely chopped fresh flat-leaved parsley

1 Put the flour in a polythene bag and season to taste with salt and pepper. Add the veal, a few pieces at a time, and shake until well coated. Remove from the bag and shake off the excess flour.

2 If using canned tomatoes, put them in a nylon sieve and leave to drain.

3 Heat 1 tablespoon of the oil in a large, flameproof casserole. Add the veal and fry for 10 minutes on each side until well browned. Remove from the casserole.

4 Add 1–2 teaspoons more oil to the casserole if necessary. Add the onions and cook, stirring, for 5 minutes, or until soft. Stir in the carrots and cook until softened.

5 Add the tomatoes, wine, stock and basil and return the osso bucco to the casserole. Bring to the boil, then reduce the heat, cover and simmer for 1 hour. Check that the meat is tender with the tip of a knife. If not, continue cooking for 10 minutes and test again.

6 When the meat is tender, sprinkle with the garlic and lemon and orange rinds. Cover and cook over a low heat for a further 10 minutes.

7 Taste and adjust the seasoning if necessary. Sprinkle with the parsley and serve immediately.

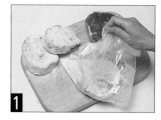

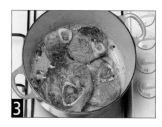

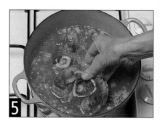

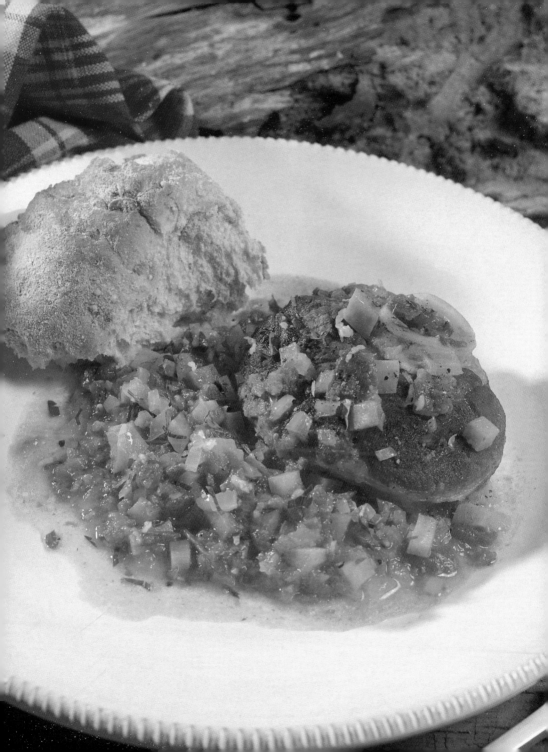

chilli con carne

serves four

750 g/1 lb 10 oz lean braising or
   stewing steak

2 tbsp vegetable oil

1 large onion, sliced

2–4 garlic cloves, crushed

1 tbsp plain flour

425 ml/15 fl oz tomato juice

400 g/14 oz canned tomatoes

1–2 tbsp sweet chilli sauce

1 tsp ground cumin

salt and pepper

425 g/15 oz canned red kidney
   beans, drained

½ teaspoon dried oregano

1–2 tbsp chopped fresh parsley

chopped fresh herbs, to garnish

boiled rice and tortillas, to serve

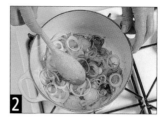

1 Preheat the oven to 160°C/325°F/
Gas Mark 3. Cut the beef into
2-cm/¾-inch cubes. Heat the oil in a
flameproof casserole. Fry the beef until
browned. Remove from the casserole.

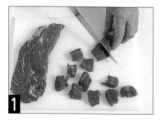

2 Add the onion and garlic to the
casserole and cook until lightly
browned. Stir in the flour and cook for
1–2 minutes. Stir in the tomato juice
and tomatoes and bring to the boil.
Return the beef to the casserole and
add the chilli sauce, cumin and salt
and pepper to taste. Cover and cook
in the oven for 1½ hours, or until
almost tender.

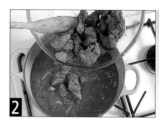

3 Stir in the beans, oregano and
parsley and adjust the seasoning
to taste. Cover the casserole and return
to the oven for 45 minutes. Sprinkle
with herbs and serve with boiled rice
and tortillas.

COOK'S TIP

Because chilli con carne requires
quite a lengthy cooking time, it is
worth preparing double the
quantity you need and freezing
half of it to serve another time.

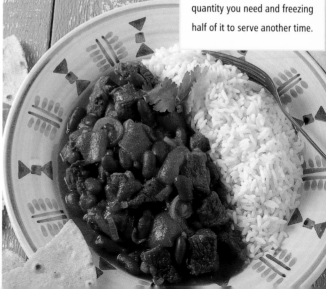

polenta with rabbit stew

butter, for greasing

300 g/10½ oz polenta or cornmeal

1 tbsp coarse sea salt

1.2 litres/2 pints water

4 tbsp olive oil

2 kg/4 lb 8 oz rabbit joints

3 garlic cloves, peeled

3 shallots, sliced

150 ml/5 fl oz red wine

1 carrot, sliced

1 celery stick, sliced

2 bay leaves

1 fresh rosemary sprig

3 tomatoes, peeled and diced

85 g/3 oz stoned black olives

300 ml/10 fl oz water

salt and pepper

2 Meanwhile, heat the oil in a large saucepan and add the rabbit pieces, garlic and shallots. Fry for 10 minutes, or until browned.

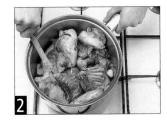

3 Stir in the wine and cook for a further 5 minutes.

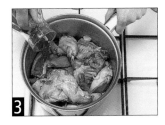

4 Add the carrot, celery, bay leaves, rosemary, tomatoes, olives and water. Cover the pan and simmer for 45 minutes, or until the rabbit is tender. Season to taste with salt and pepper. To serve, spoon or cut a portion of polenta and place on each serving plate. Top with a ladleful of rabbit stew. Serve immediately.

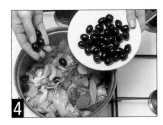

1 Preheat the oven to 190°C/375°F/ Gas Mark 5. Grease a large, ovenproof dish with a little butter. Mix the polenta, salt and water together in a large saucepan, whisking well to prevent lumps from forming. Bring to the boil and boil for 10 minutes, stirring vigorously and constantly. Turn the polenta into the prepared dish and bake in the oven for 40 minutes.

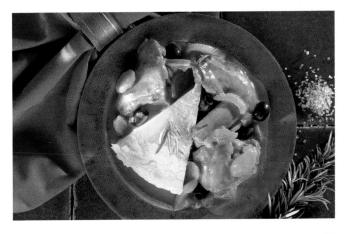

maltese rabbit with fennel

serves four

5 tbsp olive oil

2 large fennel bulbs, sliced

2 carrots, diced

1 large garlic clove, crushed

1 tbsp fennel seeds

about 4 tbsp plain flour

salt and pepper

2 wild rabbits, jointed

225 ml/8 fl oz dry white wine

225 ml/8 fl oz water

1 bouquet garni of 2 fresh
    flat-leaved parsley sprigs,
    1 fresh rosemary sprig and
    1 bay leaf, tied in a 7.5-cm/
    3-inch piece of celery

thick, crusty bread, to serve

TO GARNISH

finely chopped fresh flat-leaved
    parsley or coriander

fresh rosemary sprigs

1 Heat 3 tablespoons of the oil in a large, flameproof casserole over a medium heat. Add the fennel and carrots and cook, stirring occasionally, for 5 minutes. Stir in the garlic and fennel seeds and cook for a further 2 minutes, or until the fennel is tender. Remove the fennel and carrots from the casserole with a slotted spoon and set aside.

2 Put the flour in a polythene bag and season to taste with salt and pepper. Add 2 rabbit pieces and shake to lightly coat, then shake off any excess flour. Continue until all the pieces of rabbit are coated, adding more flour if necessary.

3 Add the remaining oil to the casserole. Fry the rabbit pieces for 5 minutes on each side, or until golden brown, working in batches. Remove the rabbit from the casserole as it is cooked.

4 Pour in the wine and bring to the boil, stirring to scrape up all the sediment from the bottom. Return the rabbit pieces, fennel and carrots to the casserole and pour in the water. Add the bouquet garni and season to taste with salt and pepper.

5 Bring to the boil, then reduce the heat, cover and simmer for 1¼ hours, or until the rabbit is tender.

6 Discard the bouquet garni. Garnish with herbs and serve straight from the casserole with lots of bread to mop up the juices.

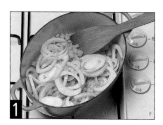

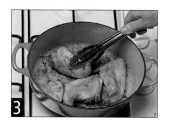

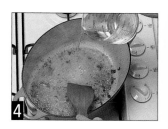

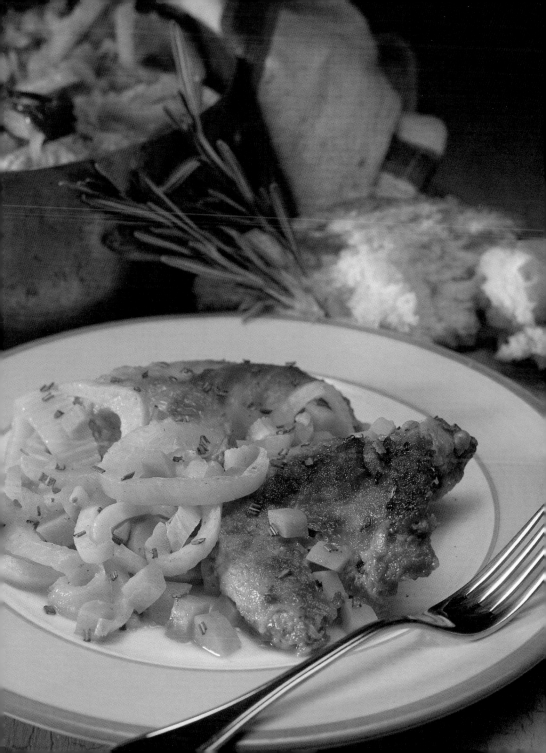

country pork with onions

2 large pork hand and spring

2 large garlic cloves, sliced

3 tbsp olive oil

2 carrots, finely chopped

2 celery sticks, finely chopped

1 large onion, finely chopped

2 fresh thyme sprigs, broken
   into pieces

2 fresh rosemary sprigs, broken
   into pieces

1 large bay leaf

225 ml/8 fl oz dry white wine

225 ml/8 fl oz water

pepper

20 pickling onions

roughly chopped fresh flat-leaved
   parsley, to garnish

1 Preheat the oven to 160°C/325°F/ Gas Mark 3. Using the tip of a sharp knife, make slits all over the pork and insert the garlic slices.

2 Heat 1 tablespoon of the oil in a flameproof casserole over a medium heat. Add the carrots, celery and onion. Cook, stirring occasionally, for 10 minutes, or until softened.

3 Place the pork on top of the vegetables. Sprinkle the thyme and rosemary over the meat. Add the bay leaf, wine and water and season to taste with pepper.

4 Bring to the boil, then remove the casserole from the heat. Cover tightly and cook in the oven for 3½ hours, or until the meat is very tender.

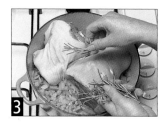

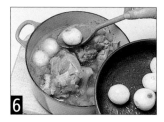

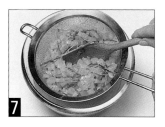

5 Meanwhile, put the onions in a heatproof bowl, pour over boiling water to cover and set aside for 1 minute. Drain, then slip off all the skins. Heat the remaining oil in a large, heavy-based frying pan. Add the onions, partially cover and cook over a low heat for 15 minutes, shaking the pan occasionally, until the onions are just beginning to turn golden.

6 When the pork is tender, add the onions to the casserole and return to the oven for a further 15 minutes. Remove the pork and onions from the casserole and keep warm.

7 Using a large, metal spoon, skim off as much fat as possible from the surface of the cooking liquid. Strain the cooking liquid into a bowl, pressing down lightly to extract the flavour; reserve the strained vegetables. Adjust the seasoning.

8 Cut the pork from the bones, if wished, then arrange on a serving platter with the onions and strained vegetables. Spoon the sauce over and garnish with parsley.

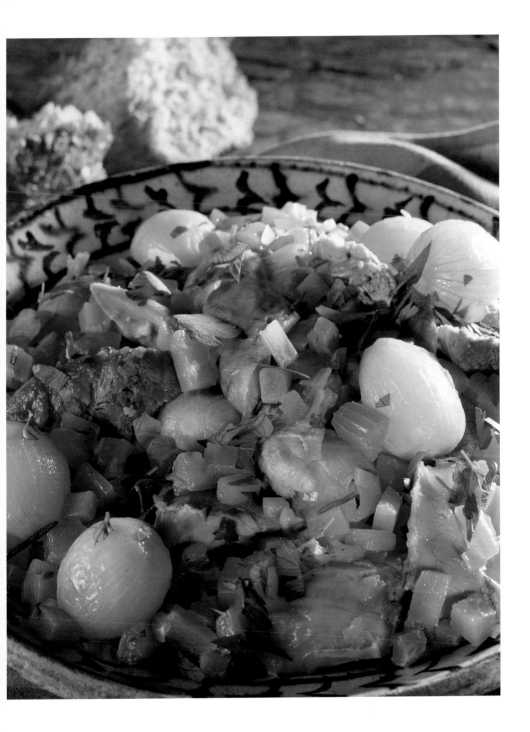

sliced beef with yogurt

serves four

450 g/1 lb lean beef slices, cut into
2.5-cm/1-inch slices

5 tbsp natural yogurt

1 tsp finely chopped fresh
root ginger

1 tsp crushed garlic

1 tsp chilli powder

pinch of ground turmeric

2 tsp garam masala

1 tsp salt

2 green cardamoms

1 tsp black cumin seeds

55 g/2 oz ground almonds

1 tbsp desiccated coconut

1 tbsp poppy seeds

1 tbsp sesame seeds

300 ml/10 fl oz vegetable oil

2 onions, finely chopped

300 ml/10 fl oz water

2 fresh green chillies

few fresh coriander leaves, chopped

1 Place the beef in a large bowl. Combine with the yogurt, ginger, garlic, chilli powder, turmeric, garam masala, salt, cardamoms and cumin seeds and set aside until required.

2 Dry-fry the almonds, coconut and poppy and sesame seeds in a heavy-based frying pan until golden, shaking the pan occasionally.

3 Transfer the spice mixture to a food processor and process until finely ground. (Add 1 tablespoon of water to blend, if necessary.) Add the ground spice mixture to the meat mixture and combine.

4 Heat a little of the oil in a large frying pan, add the onions and cook until golden brown. Remove the onions from the pan. Heat the remaining oil and stir-fry the beef mixture for 5 minutes, then return the onions to the pan and stir-fry for a further 5–7 minutes. Add the water, cover and simmer over a low heat, stirring occasionally, for 25–30 minutes. Add the chillies and coriander and serve hot.

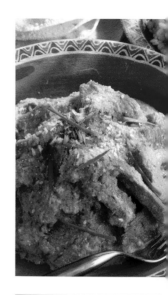

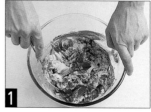

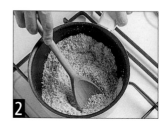

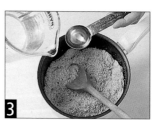

potato, beef & peanut pot

serves four

1 tbsp vegetable oil

5 tbsp butter

450 g/1 lb lean steak, cut into
    thin strips

1 onion, halved and sliced

2 garlic cloves, crushed

600 g/1 lb 5 oz waxy
    potatoes, cubed

½ tsp paprika

4 tbsp crunchy peanut butter

600 ml/1 pint beef stock

4 tbsp unsalted peanuts

2 tsp light soy sauce

55 g/2 oz sugar snap peas

1 red pepper, deseeded and cut
    into strips

few sprigs of fresh parsley, to
    garnish (optional)

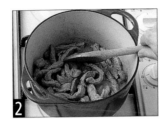

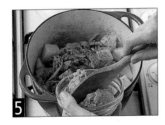

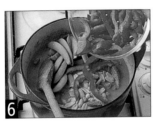

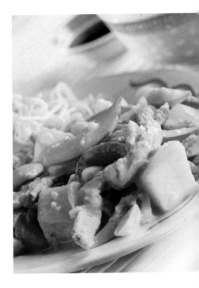

1 Heat the oil and butter in a flameproof casserole.

2 Add the steak strips and fry them gently, stirring and turning the meat, for 3–4 minutes, or until sealed on all sides.

3 Add the onion and garlic to the meat and cook gently for a further 2 minutes, stirring constantly.

4 Add the potato cubes and cook for 3–4 minutes, or until beginning to brown.

5 Stir in the paprika and peanut butter, then gradually stir in the stock. Bring the mixture to the boil, stirring frequently.

6 Add the peanuts, soy sauce, sugar snap peas and pepper.

7 Cover the casserole and cook over a low heat for 45 minutes, or until the beef is cooked right through. Garnish the dish with parsley sprigs, if wished, and serve immediately.

pork stroganoff

serves four

350 g/12 oz lean pork fillet

1 tbsp vegetable oil

1 onion, chopped

2 garlic cloves, crushed

25 g/1 oz plain flour

2 tbsp tomato purée

425 ml/15 fl oz chicken or
vegetable stock

125 g/4½ oz button
mushrooms, sliced

1 large green pepper, deseeded
and diced

salt and pepper

½ tsp ground nutmeg, plus extra
to garnish

4 tbsp low-fat natural yogurt, plus
extra to serve

freshly boiled white rice, to serve

1 Trim away any excess fat
and membrane from the pork,
then cut the meat into slices 1 cm/
½ inch thick.

2 Heat the oil in a large saucepan
over a medium heat, add the
pork, onion and garlic and cook for
4–5 minutes, or until lightly browned.

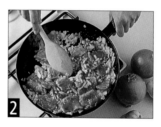

3 Stir in the flour and tomato purée,
then pour in the stock and stir to
mix thoroughly.

COOK'S TIP

You can buy ready-made stock
from leading supermarkets.
Although more expensive, it is
more nutritious than using stock
cubes, which can be high in salt
and artificial flavourings.

4 Add the mushrooms, green
pepper, salt and pepper to taste
and nutmeg. Bring to the boil, then
cover and simmer for 20 minutes, or
until the pork is cooked through.

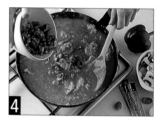

5 Remove the saucepan from the
heat, cool slightly and stir in the
yogurt. Serve the pork and sauce on a
bed of rice, topped with an extra
spoonful of yogurt and garnished with
a dusting of nutmeg.

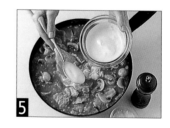

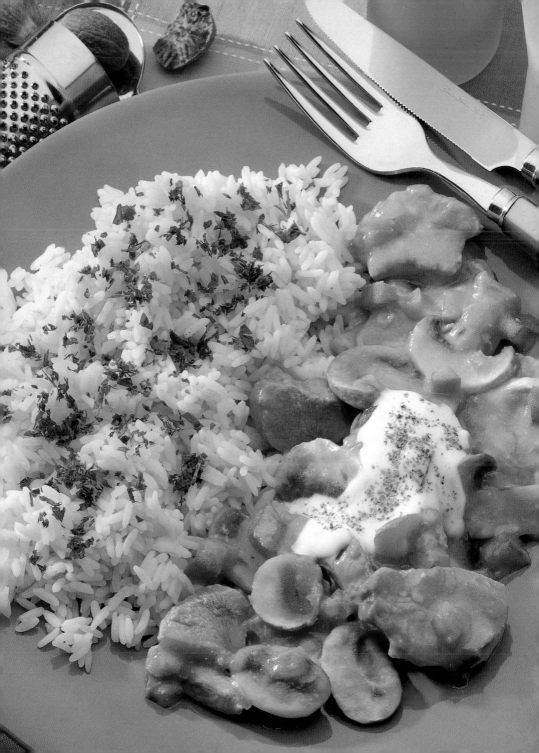

italian sausage & bean casserole

serves four

1 green pepper

8 Italian sausages

1 tbsp olive oil

1 large onion, chopped

2 garlic cloves, chopped

225 g/8 oz fresh tomatoes, peeled
and chopped, or 400 g/14 oz
canned tomatoes, chopped

2 tbsp sun-dried tomato purée

400 g/14 oz canned cannellini
beans, drained

mashed potatoes or rice, to serve

COOK'S TIP

Italian sausages are coarse in texture and have quite a strong flavour. They can be found in specialist sausage shops, Italian delicatessens and some larger supermarkets. Game sausages can be used instead in this recipe.

1 Deseed the pepper and cut it into thin strips.

2 Prick the Italian sausages all over with a fork. Cook under a preheated hot grill, turning occasionally, for 10–12 minutes, or until brown all over. Cut into chunks, set aside and keep warm.

3 Heat the oil in a large frying pan. Add the onion, garlic and pepper and cook, stirring occasionally, for 4 minutes, or until softened.

4 Add the tomatoes to the frying pan and leave the mixture to simmer, stirring occasionally, for 5 minutes, or until slightly reduced and thickened.

5 Stir the sun-dried tomato purée, beans and sausages into the mixture and cook for 4–5 minutes, or until piping hot. Add 4–5 tablespoons of water if the mixture becomes too dry during cooking.

6 Transfer the casserole to warmed serving plates and serve with mashed potatoes or cooked rice.

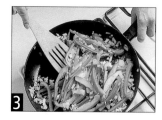

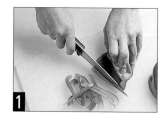

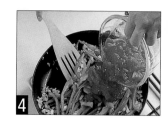

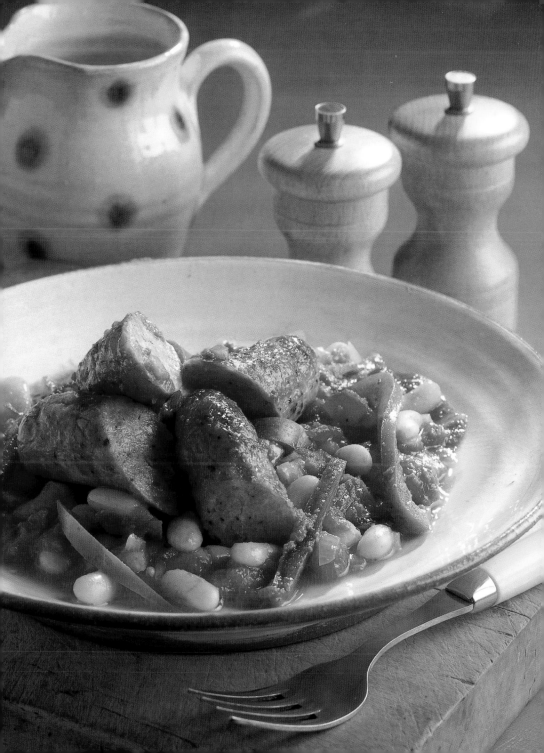

tomatoes cooked with meat & yogurt

serves two–four

1 tsp garam masala

1 tsp finely chopped fresh
   root ginger

1 garlic clove, crushed

2 black cardamoms

1 tsp chilli powder

½ tsp black cumin seeds

2 x 2.5-cm/1-inch cinnamon sticks

1 tsp salt

150 ml/5 fl oz natural yogurt

500 g/1 lb 2 oz lean lamb, cubed

150 ml/5 fl oz oil

2 onions, sliced

600 ml/1 pint water

2 large, firm tomatoes, quartered

2 tbsp lemon juice

2 fresh green chillies, chopped,
   to garnish

1 In a large mixing bowl, mix together the garam masala, ginger, garlic, cardamoms, chilli powder, cumin seeds, cinnamon sticks, salt and the yogurt until well combined.

2 Add the lamb to the yogurt and spice mixture and mix well to coat the meat. Set aside. Heat the oil in a large frying pan, then add the onions and fry until golden brown.

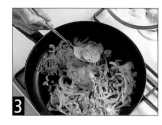

3 Add the lamb to the pan and stir-fry for 5 minutes. Reduce the heat and add the water, then cover the pan and simmer for 1 hour, stirring occasionally.

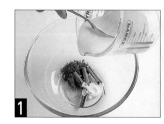

4 Add the tomatoes to the curry and sprinkle with the lemon juice. Leave the curry to simmer for a further 7–10 minutes.

5 Garnish the curry with the green chillies, and serve hot.

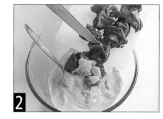

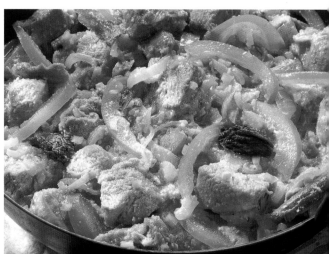

beef korma with almonds

1 Heat the oil in a frying pan, add the onions and stir-fry until golden brown. Remove half the onions from the pan and set aside.

2 Add the meat to the remaining onions in the pan and stir-fry for 5 minutes. Remove the pan from the heat.

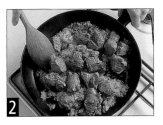

3 Combine the garam masala, ground coriander, ginger, garlic, salt and yogurt in a large bowl. Gradually add the meat to the spice mixture and mix to coat well. Return the meat mixture to the pan. Cook, stirring constantly, for 5–7 minutes, or until the mixture is golden.

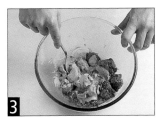

4 Add the cloves, cardamoms and peppercorns, then add the water, and reduce the heat. Cover the pan and simmer for 45–60 minutes. If necessary, add another 300 ml/10 fl oz of water and cook for a further 10–15 minutes, stirring occasionally.

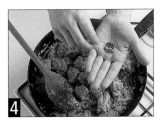

5 Just before serving, garnish with the reserved onions, almonds, chillies and the coriander leaves. Serve with chapatis.

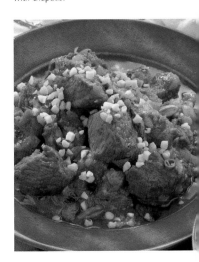

traditional provençal daube

700 g/1 lb 9 oz boneless lean
   stewing beef, such as leg,
   cut into 5-cm/2-inch pieces

400 ml/14 fl oz full-bodied dry
   red wine

2 tbsp olive oil

4 large garlic cloves, crushed

4 shallots, thinly sliced

250 g/9 oz unsmoked lardons

5–6 tbsp plain flour

salt and pepper

250 g/9 oz large chestnut
   mushrooms, sliced

400 g/14 oz canned
   chopped tomatoes

1 large bouquet garni of 1 bay leaf,
   2 dried thyme sprigs and 2 fresh
   parsley sprigs, tied in a 7.5-cm/
   3-inch piece of celery

5-cm/2-inch strip of dried
   orange rind

450 ml/16 fl oz beef stock

50 g/1¾ oz canned anchovy fillets
   in oil

2 tbsp capers in brine, rinsed
   and drained

2 tbsp red wine vinegar

2 tbsp finely chopped fresh parsley

1 Place the beef, wine, oil, half
   the garlic and shallots in a non-
metallic bowl. Cover and refrigerate for
at least 4 hours, stirring occasionally.

2 Meanwhile, place the lardons in
   a saucepan of water and bring to
the boil. Simmer for 10 minutes. Drain.

3 Place 4 tablespoons of the flour in
   a bowl and stir in 2 tablespoons
water to make a thick paste. Cover
with clingfilm and set aside.

4 Preheat the oven to 160°C/325°F/
   Gas Mark 3. Strain the beef,
reserving the marinade. Pat dry and
toss in the remaining flour, seasoned.

5 Arrange a layer of lardons,
   mushrooms and tomatoes, then
beef in a large, flameproof casserole.
Layer the remaining ingredients and
tuck in the bouquet garni and rind.

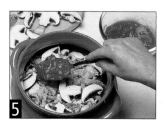

6 Pour in the stock and reserved
   marinade. Spread the flour paste
around the rim of the casserole. Press
on the lid to make a tight seal (make
more paste if necessary).

7 Cook in the preheated oven for
   2½ hours. Meanwhile, drain the
anchovies, then mash with the capers
and remaining garlic in a mortar using
a pestle.

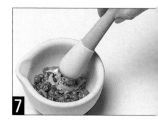

8 Remove the casserole from the
   oven, break the seal and stir in
the mashed anchovies, vinegar and
parsley. Re-cover and cook for a further
1–1½ hours, or until the meat is tender.
Taste and adjust the seasoning and
serve immediately.

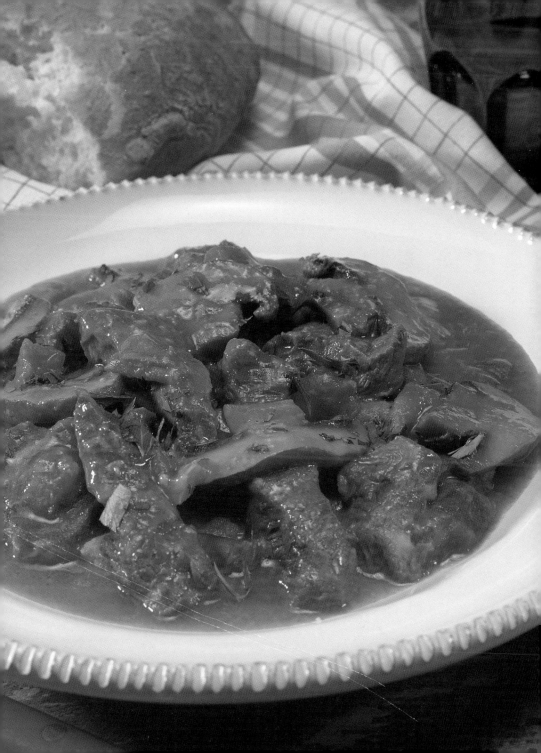

hot spicy lamb in sauce

serves six–eight

175 ml/6 fl oz oil

1 kg/2 lb 4 oz lean leg of lamb, cut
   into large pieces

1 tbsp garam masala

5 onions, chopped

150 ml/5 fl oz natural yogurt

2 tbsp tomato purée

2 tsp finely chopped fresh
   root ginger

2 garlic cloves, crushed

1½ tsp salt

2 tsp chilli powder

1 tbsp ground coriander

2 tsp ground nutmeg

850 ml/1½ pints water

1 tbsp ground fennel seeds

1 tbsp paprika

1 tbsp bhoonay chanay or
   gram flour

3 bay leaves

1 tbsp plain flour

2 tbsp warm water

2–3 fresh green chillies, chopped

2 tbsp chopped fresh coriander, plus
   extra to garnish

thin slivers of fresh root ginger,
   to garnish

naan bread, to serve

1 Heat the oil in a frying pan and add the meat and half the garam masala. Stir-fry the mixture for 7–10 minutes, or until the meat is well coated. Using a slotted spoon, remove the meat and set aside.

2 Add the onions to the pan and fry until golden brown. Return the meat to the pan, reduce the heat and leave to simmer, stirring occasionally.

3 In a bowl, mix together the yogurt, tomato purée, ginger, garlic, salt, chilli powder, ground coriander, nutmeg and the remaining garam masala. Pour the mixture over the meat and stir-fry, mixing the spices well into the meat, for 5–7 minutes.

4 Stir in half the water, then add the fennel seeds, paprika and bhoonay chanay or gram flour. Add the remaining water and the bay leaves, then reduce the heat, cover and cook for 1 hour, stirring occasionally.

5 Mix the flour with the warm water and pour the mixture over the curry. Sprinkle with the chillies and the fresh coriander and cook until the meat is tender and the sauce thickens. Garnish with fresh coriander and ginger and serve with naan bread.

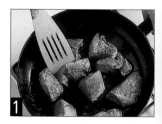

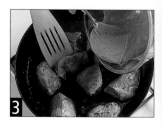

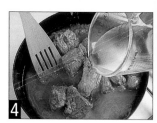

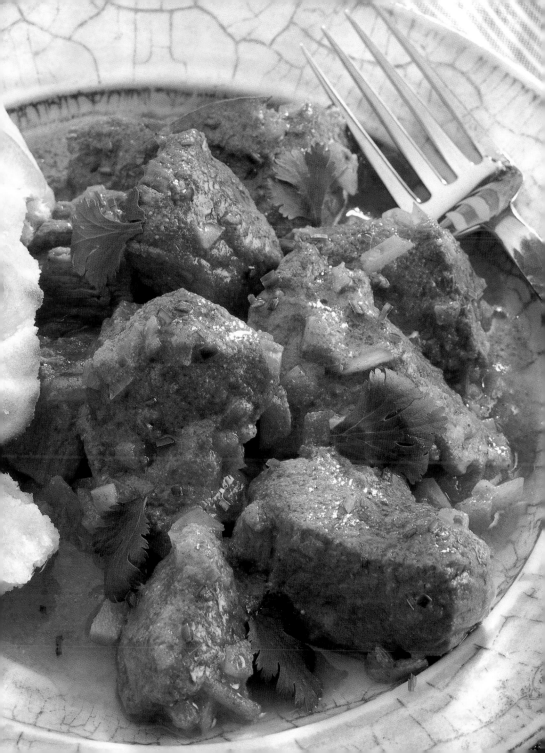

spicy pork with prunes

1 pork joint, such as leg or shoulder, weighing 1.5 kg/3 lb 5 oz

juice of 2–3 limes

10 garlic cloves, chopped

3–4 tbsp mild chilli powder

4 tbsp vegetable oil

salt

2 onions, chopped

500 ml/18 fl oz chicken stock

25 small tart tomatoes, roughly chopped

25 prunes, stoned

1–2 tsp sugar

pinch of ground cinnamon

pinch of ground allspice

pinch of ground cumin

warmed corn tortillas, to serve

1 In a non-metallic dish, combine the pork with the lime juice, garlic, chilli powder, half the oil and salt to taste. Cover and leave to marinate in the refrigerator overnight.

2 Preheat the oven to 180°C/350°F/ Gas Mark 4. Remove the pork from the marinade. Wipe the pork dry with kitchen paper and reserve the marinade. Heat the remaining oil in a flameproof casserole and brown the pork evenly until just golden. Add the onions, the reserved marinade and stock. Cover and cook in the oven for 2–3 hours, or until the pork is tender.

3 Remove from the oven. Spoon off the fat from the surface of the cooking liquid and add the tomatoes. Cook for a further 20 minutes, or until the tomatoes are tender. Mash the tomatoes into a coarse purée. Add the prunes and sugar, then adjust the seasoning, adding cinnamon, allspice and cumin to taste, as well as extra chilli powder, if wished.

4 Increase the oven temperature to 200°C/400°F/Gas Mark 6 and return the meat and sauce to the oven for a further 20–30 minutes, or until the meat has browned on top and the juices have thickened.

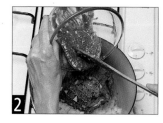

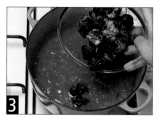

5 Remove the meat from the casserole and set aside for a few minutes. Carefully carve it into thin slices and spoon the sauce over the top. Serve with warmed corn tortillas.

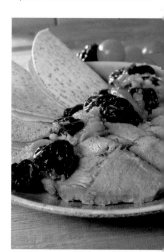

basque pork & beans

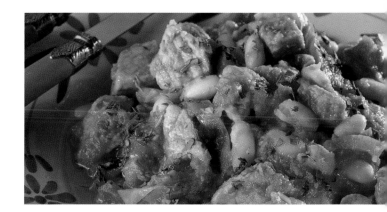

serves four–six

200 g/7 oz dried cannellini beans,
  soaked in cold water overnight

olive oil, for frying

600 g/1 lb 5 oz boneless leg of
  pork, cut into 5-cm/2-inch chunks

1 large onion, sliced

3 large garlic cloves, crushed

400 g/14 oz canned
  chopped tomatoes

2 green peppers, deseeded
  and sliced

finely grated rind of 1 large orange

salt and pepper

finely chopped fresh parsley,
  to garnish

1 Preheat the oven to 180°C/350°F/
Gas Mark 4. Drain the beans and
put in a large saucepan with fresh
water to cover. Bring to the boil and
boil rapidly for 10 minutes. Reduce the
heat and simmer for 20 minutes. Drain.

2 Add enough oil to cover the base
of a frying pan in a very thin
layer. Heat the oil over a medium heat,
add a few pieces of the pork and fry on
all sides until brown. Remove from the
pan and set aside. Repeat with the
remaining pork.

3 Add 1 tablespoon of oil to the
frying pan, if necessary, then add
the onion and cook for 3 minutes. Stir
in the garlic and cook for a further
2 minutes. Return the pork to the pan.

4 Add the tomatoes and bring to
the boil. Reduce the heat and stir
in the pepper slices, orange rind and
the drained beans. Season to taste
with salt and pepper.

5 Transfer to a casserole. Cover the
casserole and cook in the oven for
45 minutes, or until the beans and
pork are tender. Sprinkle with chopped
parsley and serve immediately straight
from the casserole.

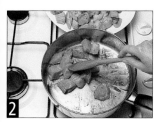

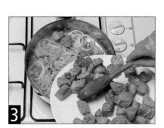

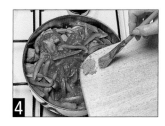

savoury hotpot

serves four

8 middle neck lean lamb chops,
   neck of lamb or any lean
   stewing lamb
salt and pepper
1–2 garlic cloves, crushed
2 lamb's kidneys (optional)
1 large onion, thinly sliced
1 leek, sliced
2–3 carrots, sliced
1 tsp chopped fresh tarragon or
   sage, or ½ tsp dried tarragon
   or sage
1 kg/2 lb 4 oz potatoes, thinly sliced
300 ml/10 fl oz stock
2 tbsp margarine, melted, or 1 tbsp
   vegetable oil
chopped fresh parsley, to garnish

1 Preheat the oven to 180°C/350°F/ Gas Mark 4. Trim any excess fat from the lamb, season well with salt and pepper and arrange in a large, ovenproof casserole. Sprinkle with the crushed garlic.

2 If using kidneys, remove the skin, halve and cut out the cores. Chop into pieces and sprinkle over the lamb.

3 Place the vegetables over the lamb, allowing the pieces to slip in between the meat, then sprinkle with the herbs.

4 Arrange the potato slices on top of the meat and vegetables, in an overlapping pattern.

5 Bring the stock to the boil, season to taste with salt and pepper, then pour over the casserole.

6 Brush the potatoes with the melted margarine or vegetable oil, cover with greased foil or a lid and cook in the oven for 1½ hours.

7 Remove the foil or lid from the casserole, increase the temperature to 220°C/425°F/ Gas Mark 7 and return the casserole to the oven for 30 minutes, or until the potatoes are browned.

8 Garnish the hotpot with parsley and serve immediately.

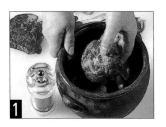

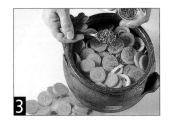

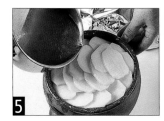

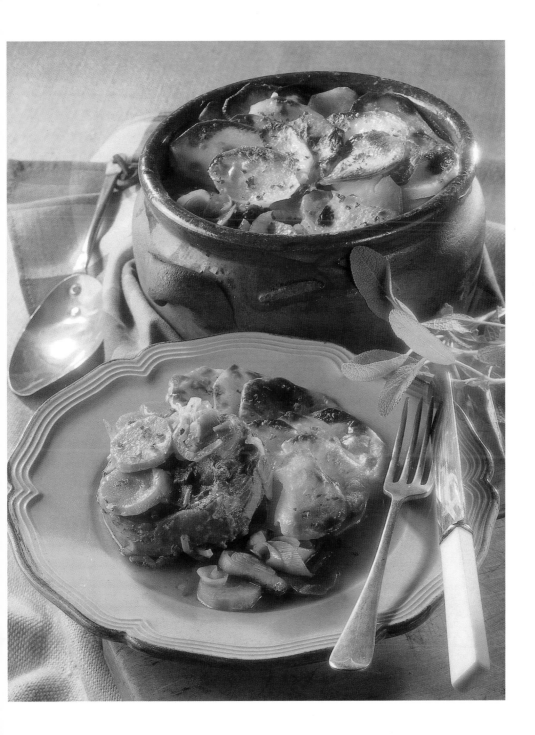

lamb with onions & dried mango powder

serves four

4 onions

300 ml/10 fl oz oil

1 tsp finely chopped fresh
   root ginger

1 garlic clove, crushed

1 tsp chilli powder

pinch of ground turmeric

1 tsp salt

3 fresh green chillies, chopped

450 g/1 lb lean lamb, cubed

600 ml/1 pint water

1½ tsp aamchoor (dried
   mango powder)

1 small bunch fresh
   coriander, chopped

boiled rice, to serve

1 Using a sharp knife, finely chop 3 of the onions.

2 Heat half the oil in a frying pan, add the onions and fry until golden brown. Reduce the heat and add the ginger, garlic, chilli powder, turmeric and salt. Stir-fry the mixture for 5 minutes, then add 2 of the chopped chillies.

3 Add the lamb to the frying pan and stir-fry the mixture for a further 7 minutes.

COOK'S TIP

Aamchoor is made from dried mangoes. It has a sour taste and can be bought in jars.

4 Add the water to the pan, cover and cook over a low heat, stirring occasionally, for 35–45 minutes, or until the lamb is tender.

5 Meanwhile, slice the remaining onion. Heat the remaining oil in a frying pan and fry the onion until golden. Set aside.

6 Once the lamb is tender, add the aamchoor, the remaining chilli and the chopped coriander and stir-fry for 3–5 minutes.

7 Transfer the curry to a serving dish and pour the fried onion slices and oil down the centre. Serve hot, with rice.

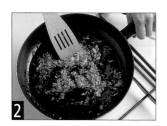

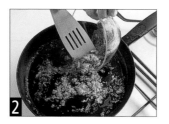

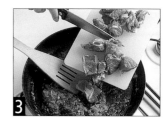

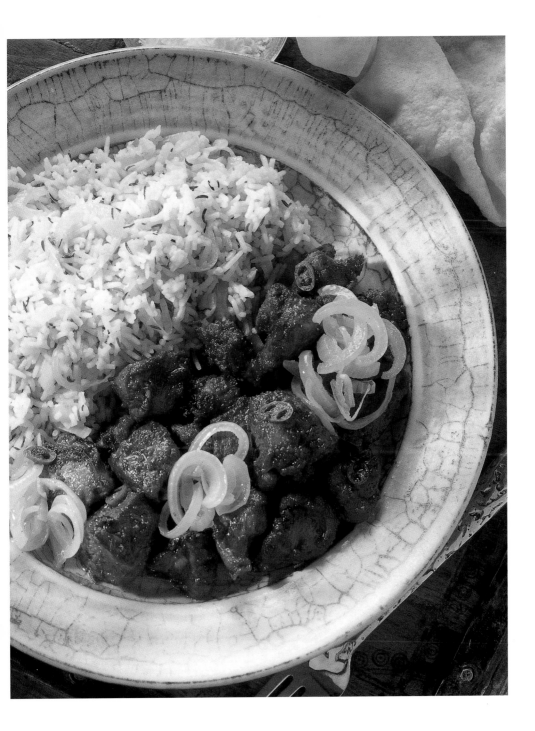

red pork curry

900 g/2 lb boneless pork
    shoulder, sliced

700 ml/1¼ pints coconut milk

2 fresh red chillies, deseeded
    and sliced

2 tbsp Thai fish sauce

2 tsp soft dark brown sugar

1 red pepper, deseeded and sliced

6 kaffir lime leaves, shredded

½ bunch fresh mint
    leaves, shredded

½ bunch fresh Thai basil leaves or
    ordinary basil, shredded

Thai fragrant rice, to serve

RED CURRY PASTE

1 tbsp coriander seeds

2 tsp cumin seeds

2 tsp black or white peppercorns

1 tsp salt

5–8 dried hot red chillies

3–4 shallots, chopped

6–8 garlic cloves

5-cm/2-inch piece fresh root ginger,
    roughly chopped

2 kaffir lime leaves

1 tbsp ground chilli powder

1 tbsp shrimp paste

2 lemon grass stalks, thinly sliced

1 To make the red curry paste, grind the coriander and cumin seeds, peppercorns and salt to a fine powder in a mortar with a pestle. Add the dried chillies, 1 at a time according to taste, until ground.

2 Put the shallots, garlic, ginger, lime leaves, chilli powder and shrimp paste in a food processor. Process for 1 minute. Add the ground spices and process again. Adding water, a few drops at a time, continue to process until a thick paste forms. Scrape into a bowl and stir in the lemon grass.

3 Put about half the red curry paste in a large, deep, heavy-based frying pan with the pork. Cook over a medium heat, stirring gently, for 2–3 minutes, or until the pork is evenly coated and begins to brown.

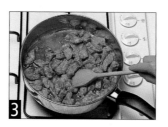

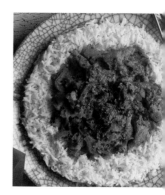

4 Stir in the coconut milk and bring to the boil. Cook, stirring frequently, for 10 minutes. Reduce the heat, stir in the fresh chillies, fish sauce and sugar and simmer for 20 minutes. Add the pepper and simmer for a further 10 minutes.

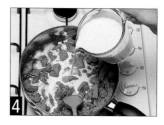

5 Chop the lime leaves and add to the curry with half the mint and basil. Transfer to a serving dish, sprinkle with the remaining mint and basil and serve with the rice.

lamb biryani

serves six

150 ml/5 fl oz milk

1 tsp saffron threads

5 tbsp pure or vegetable ghee

3 onions, sliced

1 kg/2 lb 4 oz lean lamb, cubed

7 tbsp natural yogurt

1½ tsp finely chopped fresh
    root ginger

1–2 garlic cloves, crushed

2 tsp garam masala

2 tsp salt

¼ tsp ground turmeric

600 ml/1 pint water

450 g/1 lb basmati rice

2 tsp black cumin seeds

3 green cardamoms

4 tbsp lemon juice

2 fresh green chillies

¼ bunch fresh coriander, chopped

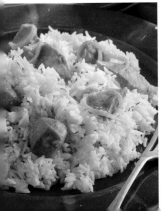

1 Boil the milk in a saucepan with the saffron and set aside. Heat the ghee in a large saucepan and fry the onions until golden. Remove half the onions and ghee from the saucepan and set aside in a bowl.

2 Combine the meat, yogurt, ginger, garlic, garam masala, half the salt and turmeric in a large bowl and mix well.

3 Return the saucepan with the ghee and onions to the heat. Add the meat mixture, stir for 3 minutes, then add the water. Cook over a low heat for 45 minutes, stirring occasionally. Check to see whether the meat is tender; if not, add 150 ml/ 5 fl oz water and cook for a further 15 minutes. Once all the water has evaporated, stir-fry for 2 minutes and set aside.

4 Meanwhile, place the rice in a saucepan. Add the cumin seeds, cardamoms, remaining salt and enough water for cooking, and cook over a medium heat until the rice is half cooked. Drain. Remove half of the rice and place in a bowl.

5 Spoon the meat mixture on top of the rice in the saucepan. Add half each of the saffron milk, lemon juice, chillies and coriander. Then add the reserved onions and ghee, and the remaining rice, saffron milk, lemon juice, chillies and coriander. Cook, covered, over a low heat for 15–20 minutes, or until the rice is cooked. Stir well and serve hot.

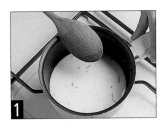

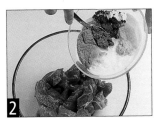

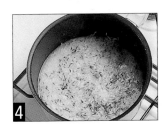

roman pan-fried lamb

serves four

1 tbsp oil

1 tbsp butter

600 g/1 lb 5 oz lamb, shoulder
   or leg, cut into 2.5-cm/
   1-inch chunks

4 garlic cloves, peeled

3 fresh thyme sprigs, stalks removed

6 canned anchovy fillets

150 ml/5 fl oz red wine

150 ml/5 fl oz lamb stock

1 tsp sugar

50 g/1¾ oz black olives, stoned
   and halved

2 tbsp chopped fresh parsley,
   to garnish

mashed potatoes, to serve

COOK'S TIP

Rome is the capital of both Italy and the region of Lazio and thus has become a focal point for specialities from all over Italy. Food from this region tends to be fairly simple and quick to prepare, with plenty of herbs and seasonings giving really robust flavours.

1 Heat the oil and butter in a large frying pan. Add the lamb and cook for 4–5 minutes, stirring, until the meat is browned all over.

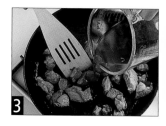

2 Using a pestle and mortar, grind together the garlic, thyme and anchovies to make a smooth paste.

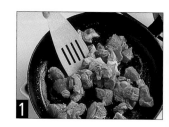

3 Add the wine and stock to the frying pan, then stir in the garlic and anchovy paste together with the sugar.

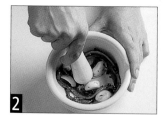

4 Bring the mixture to the boil, then reduce the heat, cover and leave to simmer for 30–40 minutes, or until the lamb is tender. For the last 10 minutes of the cooking time, remove the lid to allow the sauce to reduce slightly.

5 Stir the olives into the sauce and mix to combine.

6 Transfer the lamb and the sauce to a serving bowl and garnish with parsley. Serve with creamy mashed potatoes.

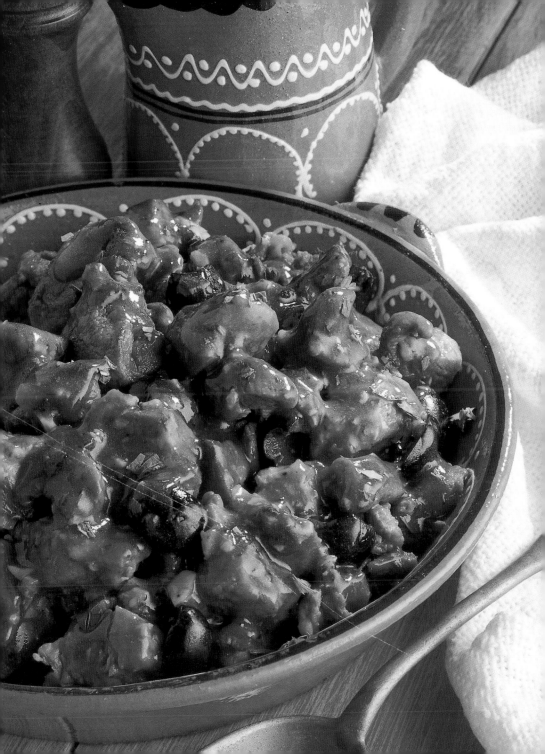

lamb curry in a thick sauce

1 kg/2 lb 4 oz lean lamb

100 ml/3½ fl oz natural yogurt

75 g/2¾ oz almonds

2 tsp garam masala

2 tsp finely chopped fresh
 root ginger

2 garlic cloves, crushed

1½ tsp chilli powder

1½ tsp salt

300 ml/10 fl oz oil

3 onions, finely chopped

4 green cardamoms

2 bay leaves

3 fresh green chillies, chopped

2 tbsp lemon juice

400 g/14 oz canned tomatoes

300 ml/10 fl oz water

1 small bunch fresh
 coriander, chopped

boiled rice, to serve

1 Using a very sharp knife, cut the lamb into small, even-sized pieces.

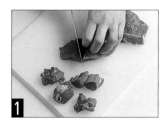

2 In a large mixing bowl, combine the yogurt, almonds, garam masala, ginger, garlic, chilli powder and salt, stirring to mix well.

3 Heat the oil in a large saucepan and fry the onions with the cardamoms and the bay leaves until golden brown, stirring constantly.

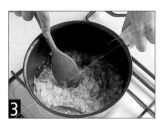

4 Add the meat and the yogurt mixture to the saucepan and stir-fry for 3–5 minutes.

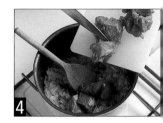

5 Add 2 of the chillies, the lemon juice and tomatoes to the mixture in the saucepan and stir-fry for a further 5 minutes.

6 Add the water to the saucepan, cover and leave to simmer over a low heat for 35–40 minutes.

7 Add the remaining chilli and the coriander and stir until the sauce has thickened. (Remove the lid and increase the heat if the sauce is too watery.)

8 Transfer the curry to warmed serving plates and serve hot with boiled rice.

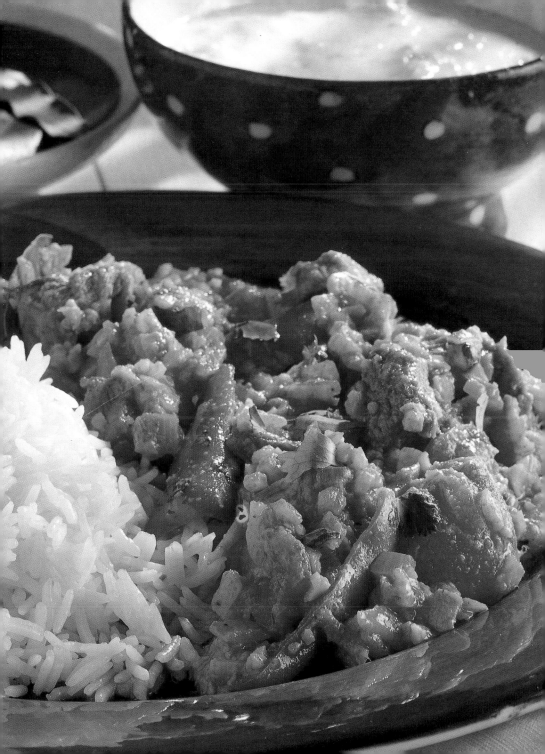

simmered medley

serves six–eight

900 g/2 lb boneless pork

2 bay leaves

1 onion, chopped

8 garlic cloves, finely chopped

2 tbsp chopped fresh coriander

1 carrot, thinly sliced

2 celery sticks, diced

2 chicken stock cubes

½ chicken, cut into portions

4–5 ripe tomatoes, diced

½ tsp mild chilli powder

grated rind of ¼ orange

¼ tsp ground cumin

juice of 3 oranges

1 courgette, cut into
   bite-sized pieces

¼ cabbage, thinly sliced
   and blanched

1 apple, cut into bite-sized pieces

about 10 prunes, stoned

¼ tsp ground cinnamon

pinch of ground ginger

2 hard chorizo sausages, about
   350 g/12 oz in total, cut into
   bite-sized pieces

salt and pepper

rice, tortillas and salsa, to serve

1 Combine the pork, bay leaves, onion, garlic, coriander, carrot and celery in a large saucepan and fill with cold water. Bring to the boil, skimming off the scum on the surface. Reduce the heat and simmer gently for 1 hour.

2 Add the stock cubes to the saucepan with the chicken, tomatoes, chilli powder, orange rind and cumin. Cook for a further 45 minutes, or until the chicken is tender. Spoon off the fat that forms on the top.

3 Add the orange juice, courgette, cabbage, apple, prunes, cinnamon, ginger and chorizo. Simmer for a further 20 minutes, or until the courgette is soft and tender and the chorizo is completely cooked through.

4 Season the stew to taste with salt and pepper. Serve immediately with rice, tortillas and salsa.

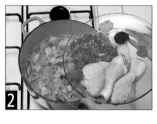

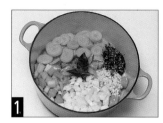

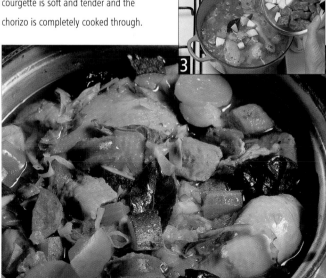

fruity lamb casserole

serves four

450 g/1 lb lean lamb, trimmed and
    cut into 2.5-cm/1-inch cubes

1 tsp ground cinnamon

1 tsp ground coriander

1 tsp ground cumin

2 tsp olive oil

1 red onion, finely chopped

1 garlic clove, crushed

400 g/14 oz canned
    chopped tomatoes

2 tbsp tomato purée

salt and pepper

125 g/4½ oz no-soak dried apricots

1 tsp caster sugar

300 ml/10 fl oz vegetable stock

1 small bunch fresh coriander,
    to garnish

rice, couscous or bulgar wheat,
    to serve

1 Preheat the oven to 180°C/
350°F/Gas Mark 4. Place the
meat in a mixing bowl and add the
cinnamon, coriander, cumin and oil.
Mix thoroughly so that the lamb is
well coated in the spices.

2 Heat a non-stick frying pan for a
few seconds until it is hot, then
add the spiced lamb. Reduce the heat
and cook for 4–5 minutes, stirring,
until browned all over. Using a slotted
spoon, remove the lamb and transfer
to a large, ovenproof casserole.

3 Add the onion, garlic, tomatoes
and tomato purée to the frying
pan and cook, stirring occasionally, for
5 minutes. Season to taste with salt
and pepper. Stir in the apricots, sugar
and stock and bring to the boil.

4 Spoon the sauce over the lamb
and mix well. Cover and cook in
the oven for 1 hour, removing the lid of
the casserole for the last 10 minutes.

5 Roughly chop the coriander and
sprinkle over the casserole to
garnish. Serve with rice, couscous or
bulgar wheat.

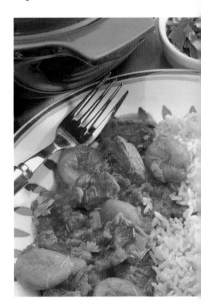

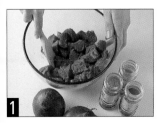

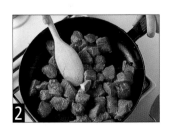

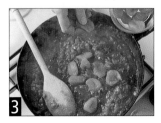

lean lamb cooked in spinach

serves two–four

300 ml/10 fl oz oil

2 onions, sliced

¼ bunch fresh coriander, chopped,
plus extra to garnish

3 fresh green chillies, chopped

1½ tsp finely chopped fresh
root ginger

1–2 garlic cloves, crushed

1 tsp chilli powder

½ tsp ground turmeric

450 g/1 lb lean lamb, cubed

1 tsp salt

1 kg/2 lb 4 oz fresh spinach,
chopped, or 425 g/15 oz
canned spinach

700 ml/1¼ pints water

fresh root ginger, shredded,
to garnish

1 Heat the oil in a frying pan over a medium heat, add the onions and fry until they turn a pale golden colour.

2 Add the coriander and 2 of the chillies to the pan and stir-fry for 3–5 minutes.

3 Reduce the heat and add the ginger, garlic, chilli powder and turmeric to the mixture in the pan, stirring to mix.

4 Add the lamb to the pan and stir-fry for a further 5 minutes. Add the salt and spinach and cook, stirring occasionally, for a further 3–5 minutes.

5 Add the water, stirring, cover the pan and cook over a low heat for 45 minutes. Remove the lid and check the meat; if it is not tender, turn the meat over, increase the heat and cook, uncovered, until the surplus water has been absorbed. Stir-fry the mixture for a further 5–7 minutes.

6 Transfer the lamb and spinach mixture to a serving dish and garnish with shredded ginger, coriander and the remaining chopped chilli. Serve hot.

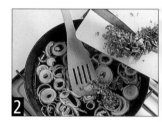

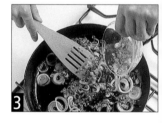

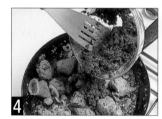

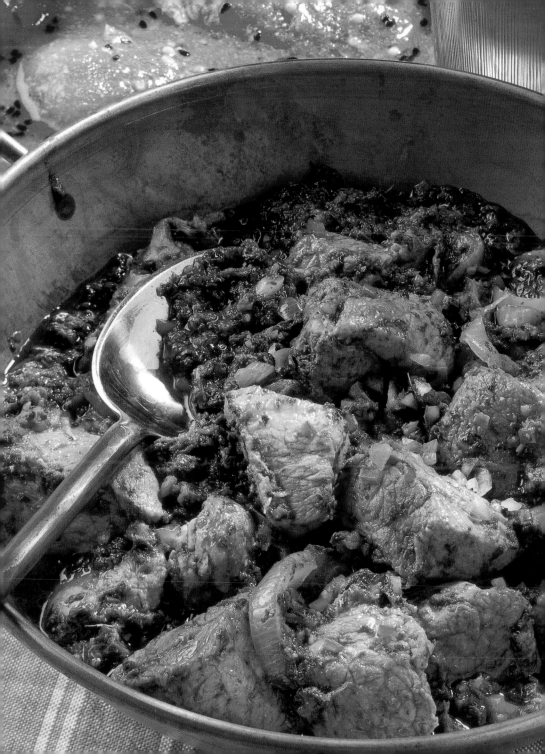

potatoes cooked with meat & yogurt

serves six

3 potatoes

300 ml/10 fl oz oil

3 onions, sliced

1 kg/2 lb 4 oz leg of lamb, cubed

2 tsp garam masala

1½ tsp finely chopped fresh
   root ginger

1–2 garlic cloves, crushed

1 tsp chilli powder

3 black peppercorns

3 green cardamoms

1 tsp black cumin seeds

2 cinnamon sticks

1 tsp paprika

1½ tsp salt

150 ml/5 fl oz natural yogurt

600 ml/1 pint water

TO GARNISH

2 fresh green chillies, chopped

fresh coriander, chopped

1 Peel and cut each potato into 6 pieces.

2 Heat the oil in a saucepan and fry the sliced onions until golden brown. Remove the onions and set aside until required.

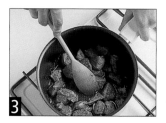

3 Add the meat and half the garam masala to the saucepan and stir-fry for 5–7 minutes over a low heat.

4 Return the cooked onions to the saucepan and remove from the heat.

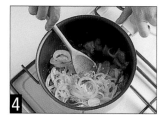

5 In a small bowl, mix together the remaining garam masala and the ginger, garlic, chilli powder, peppercorns, cardamoms, cumin seeds, cinnamon sticks, paprika and salt. Add the yogurt and mix well.

6 Return the saucepan to the heat, gradually add the spice and yogurt mixture to the meat and onions and stir-fry for 7–10 minutes. Add the water, reduce the heat and cook, covered, for 40 minutes, stirring occasionally.

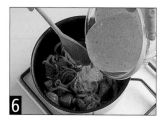

7 Add the potatoes to the saucepan and cook, covered, for a further 15 minutes, gently stirring the mixture occasionally. Garnish with chillies and coriander and serve at once.

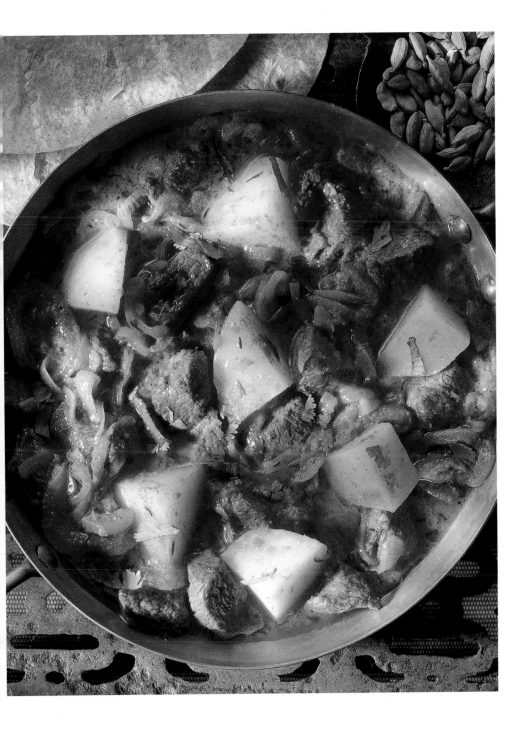

azerbaijani lamb pilaf

serves four–six

2–3 tbsp vegetable oil

650 g/1 lb 7 oz boneless lamb
shoulder, cut into 2.5-cm/
1-inch cubes

2 onions, roughly chopped

1 tsp ground cumin

200 g/7 oz arborio, long-grain or
basmati rice

1 tbsp tomato purée

1 tsp saffron threads

100 ml/3½ fl oz pomegranate juice
(see Cook's Tip)

850 ml/1½ pints lamb or
chicken stock, or water

115 g/4 oz no-soak dried apricots or
prunes, halved

2 tbsp raisins

salt and pepper

TO SERVE

2 tbsp chopped fresh mint

2 tbsp chopped fresh watercress

1 Heat the oil in a large, flameproof casserole or wide pan over a high heat. Add the lamb, in batches, and cook, stirring and turning frequently, for 7 minutes, or until lightly browned.

2 Add the onions, reduce the heat to medium–high and cook for 2 minutes, or until beginning to soften. Add the cumin and rice and cook, stirring to coat, for 2 minutes, or until the rice is translucent. Stir in the tomato purée and the saffron threads.

3 Add the pomegranate juice and stock and bring to the boil, stirring. Stir in the apricots and raisins. Reduce the heat to low, cover and simmer for 20–25 minutes, or until the lamb and rice are tender and the liquid is absorbed.

4 To serve, season to taste with salt and pepper, sprinkle the chopped mint and watercress over the pilaf and serve from the casserole.

COOK'S TIP
Pomegranate juice is available from Middle Eastern grocery stores. If you cannot find it, substitute unsweetened grape or apple juice.

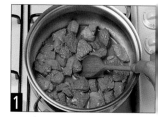

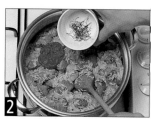

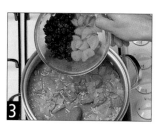

red lamb curry

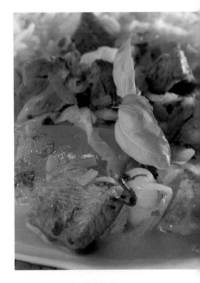

serves four

500 g/1 lb 2 oz boneless lean leg
  of lamb

2 tbsp vegetable oil

1 large onion, sliced

2 garlic cloves, crushed

2 tbsp red curry paste

150 ml/5 fl oz coconut milk

1 tbsp soft light brown sugar

1 large red pepper, deseeded and
  thickly sliced

125 ml/4 fl oz lamb or beef stock

1 tbsp Thai fish sauce

2 tbsp lime juice

225 g/8 oz canned water
  chestnuts, drained

2 tbsp chopped fresh coriander

2 tbsp chopped fresh basil, plus
  extra leaves to garnish

salt and pepper

boiled jasmine rice, to serve

1 Trim the meat and cut it into 3-cm/1¼-inch cubes. Heat the oil in a large frying pan or preheated wok over a high heat and stir-fry the onion and garlic for 2–3 minutes, or until softened. Add the meat and stir-fry until lightly browned.

2 Stir in the curry paste and cook for a few seconds, then add the coconut milk and sugar and bring to the boil. Reduce the heat and simmer for 15 minutes, stirring occasionally.

3 Stir in the pepper, stock, fish sauce and lime juice. Cover and simmer for a further 15 minutes, or until the meat is tender.

4 Add the water chestnuts, coriander and basil and adjust the seasoning to taste. Serve, garnished with basil leaves, with jasmine rice.

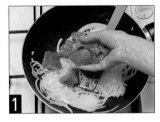

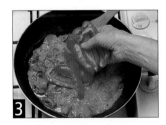

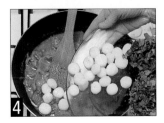

COOK'S TIP

This curry can also be made
with other lean meats.
Try replacing the lamb with
trimmed duck breasts or pieces
of lean braising beef.

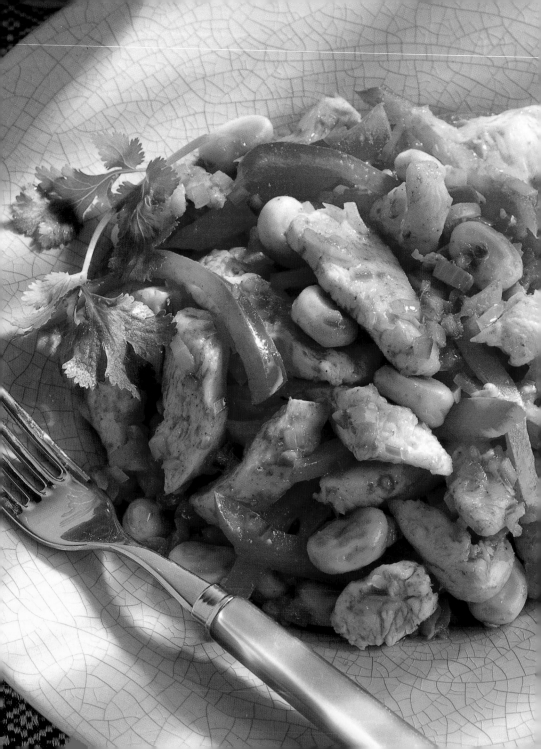

Chicken

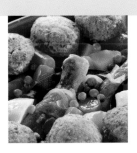

Chicken is the perfect choice for one-pot cooking as there are so many different cuts, from inexpensive thighs to delicate breast meat, as well as the whole bird. In addition, as it is often rather bland in flavour, it benefits from being combined with vegetables, fruit, herbs and aromatics. Almost everyone loves chicken and the recipes in this chapter reflect its universal popularity, with dishes from Mexico, India, Thailand, Spain and Italy, among other countries, and the Middle East. It is a versatile meat and can be cooked in any number of ways, from casseroles to stir-fries and from risottos to curries. There are recipes for all occasions and every time of year, from Sunday lunch with the family to an alfresco dinner party. Hot and spicy, rich and creamy, filling and flavoursome, subtle and delicate – there is a one-pot chicken dish that is sure to please.

chicken & chickpea soup

serves four

25 g/1 oz butter

3 spring onions, chopped

2 garlic cloves, crushed

1 fresh marjoram sprig,
 finely chopped

350 g/12 oz skinless, boneless
 chicken breasts, diced

1.2 litres/2 pints chicken stock

350 g/12 oz canned
 chickpeas, drained

1 bouquet garni

salt and pepper

1 red pepper, deseeded and diced

1 green pepper, deseeded and diced

115 g/4 oz small dried pasta
 shapes, such as elbow macaroni

croûtons, to serve

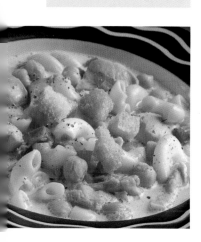

1 Melt the butter in a large saucepan over a medium heat. Add the spring onions, garlic, marjoram and chicken and cook, stirring frequently, for 5 minutes.

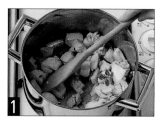

2 Add the stock, chickpeas and bouquet garni and season to taste with salt and pepper.

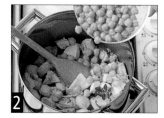

3 Bring the soup to the boil, then reduce the heat and simmer for 2 hours.

4 Add the peppers and pasta to the saucepan, then simmer the soup for a further 20 minutes.

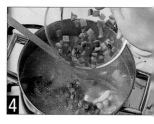

5 To serve, ladle the soup into individual serving bowls and serve immediately, garnished with croûtons.

COOK'S TIP

If you prefer, you can use dried chickpeas. Cover with cold water and set aside to soak for 5–8 hours. Drain and add the beans to the soup, according to the recipe, and allow an additional 30 minutes–1 hour cooking time.

lemon & chicken soup

serves four

4 tbsp butter

8 shallots, thinly sliced

2 carrots, thinly sliced

2 celery sticks, thinly sliced

225 g/8 oz skinless, boneless
   chicken breasts, finely chopped

3 lemons

1.2 litres/2 pints chicken stock

225 g/8 oz dried spaghetti, broken
   into small pieces

salt and pepper

150 ml/5 fl oz double cream

TO GARNISH

fresh parsley sprigs

2 lemon slices, halved

COOK'S TIP

You can prepare this soup in advance up to the end of Step 3, so that all you need do before serving is heat it through very gently before adding the pasta and the finishing touches.

1 Melt the butter in a large saucepan. Add the shallots, carrots, celery and chicken and cook over a low heat, stirring occasionally, for 8 minutes.

2 Thinly pare the lemons and blanch the lemon rind in boiling water for 3 minutes. Squeeze the juice from the lemons.

3 Add the lemon rind and juice to the saucepan, together with the stock. Bring the soup slowly to the boil over a low heat and simmer for 40 minutes, stirring occasionally.

4 Add the spaghetti to the saucepan and cook for 15 minutes. Season to taste with salt and pepper and add the cream. Heat through, but do not allow the soup to boil or it will curdle.

5 Pour the soup into individual bowls, garnish with parsley and half slices of lemon and serve immediately.

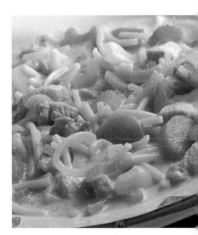

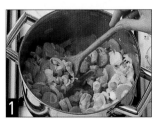

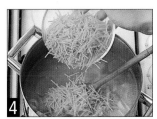

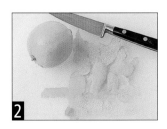

chicken & asparagus soup

serves four

225 g/8 oz asparagus

850 ml/1½ pints chicken stock

150 ml/5 fl oz dry white wine

1 sprig each of fresh parsley, dill
and tarragon

1 garlic clove

55 g/2 oz dried vermicelli
rice noodles

350 g/12 oz lean cooked chicken,
finely shredded

salt and pepper

1 small leek, to garnish

COOK'S TIP

Rice noodles contain no fat and
are an ideal substitute for
egg noodles.

1 Wash the asparagus and trim away the woody ends. Cut each spear into pieces 4 cm/1½ inches long.

2 Pour the chicken stock and wine into a large saucepan and bring to the boil.

3 Wash the herbs and tie them together with clean string. Peel the garlic clove and add to the saucepan with the herbs, asparagus and noodles. Cover and simmer for 5 minutes.

4 Stir in the chicken and season well with salt and pepper. Simmer gently for a further 3–4 minutes, or until heated through.

5 Trim the leek, slice it down the centre and wash under cold running water to remove any dirt. Shake dry and finely shred.

6 Remove the herbs and garlic from the saucepan and discard. Ladle the soup into warmed bowls, sprinkle with shredded leek and serve.

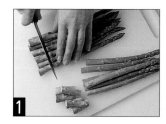

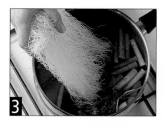

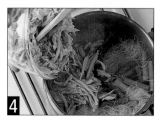

VARIATION

You can use any of your favourite
herbs in this recipe, but choose
those with a subtle flavour so
that they do not overpower the
asparagus. Small, tender
asparagus spears give the best
results and flavour.

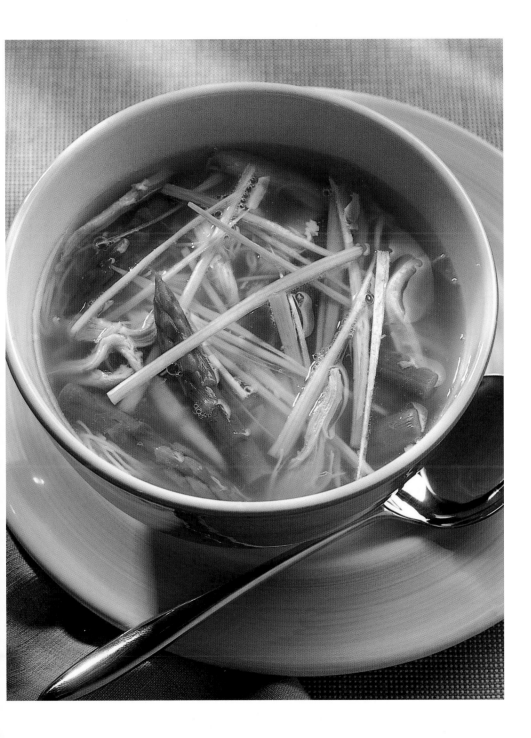

chicken, avocado & chipotle soup

serves four

1.5 litres/2¾ pints chicken stock

2–3 garlic cloves, finely chopped

1–2 dried chipotle chillies,
    reconstituted and cut into very
    thin strips (see Cook's Tip)

1 avocado

lime or lemon juice, for tossing

3–5 spring onions, thinly sliced

350–400 g/12–14 oz cooked
    chicken breast meat, shredded

2 tbsp chopped fresh coriander

TO SERVE

1 lime, cut into wedges

handful of tortilla chips (optional)

COOK'S TIP

Chipotle chillies are smoked and dried jalapeño chillies, available canned or dried from specialist shops. Use chipotles canned in adobo marinade (drained) for this recipe, if possible. Dried chipotles need to be reconstituted before using – place in a heatproof bowl, pour over boiling water and leave for 1–2 hours, or until softened.

1 Place the stock in a large, heavy-based saucepan with the garlic and chillies and bring to the boil.

2 Meanwhile, cut the avocado in half around the stone. Twist apart, then remove the stone with a knife. Carefully peel off the skin, dice the flesh and toss in lime or lemon juice to prevent discoloration.

3 Arrange the spring onions, chicken, avocado and coriander in the base of 4 soup bowls or in a large serving bowl.

4 Ladle hot stock over and serve with lime wedges and a handful of tortilla chips, if wished.

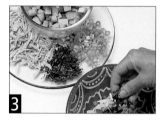

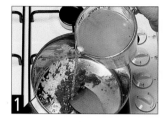

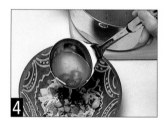

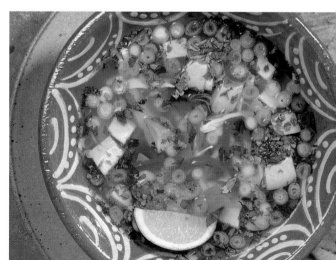

chicken, noodle & corn soup

serves four

450 g/1 lb skinless, boneless
    chicken breasts, cut into strips

1.2 litres/2 pints chicken stock

150 ml/5 fl oz double cream

salt and pepper

100 g/3½ oz dried vermicelli

1 tbsp cornflour

3 tbsp milk

175 g/6 oz sweetcorn kernels

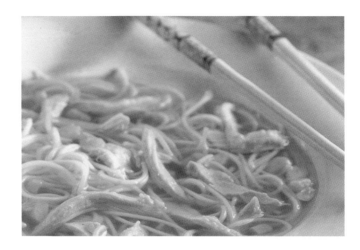

1 Put the chicken, stock and cream into a large saucepan and bring to the boil over a low heat. Reduce the heat slightly and simmer for 20 minutes. Season the soup to taste with salt and pepper.

2 Meanwhile, cook the vermicelli in lightly salted boiling water for 10–12 minutes, or until just tender. Drain the pasta and keep warm.

3 In a small bowl, mix together the cornflour and milk to make a smooth paste. Stir the cornflour into the soup until thickened.

4 Add the sweetcorn and vermicelli to the saucepan and heat through.

5 Transfer the soup to warmed individual soup bowls and serve.

VARIATION

For crab and sweetcorn soup, substitute 450 g/1 lb cooked crabmeat for the chicken breasts. Flake the crabmeat well before adding it to the saucepan and reduce the cooking time by 10 minutes.

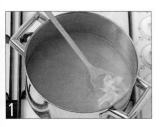

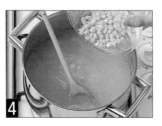

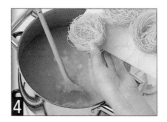

chicken, corn & bean soup

serves six

1½ tbsp butter

1 large onion, finely chopped

1 garlic clove, finely chopped

3 tbsp plain flour

600 ml/1 pint water

1 litre/1¾ pints chicken stock

1 carrot, quartered and thinly sliced

175 g/6 oz French beans, trimmed
    and cut into short pieces

400 g/14 oz canned butter beans,
    rinsed and drained

350 g/12 oz cooked or frozen
    sweetcorn kernels

225 g/8 oz cooked chicken meat

salt and pepper

VARIATION

Replace the canned butter beans
with 300 g/10½ oz cooked fresh
broad beans, peeled if wished.
You could also substitute
sliced runner beans for
the French beans.

---

1 Melt the butter in a large saucepan over a medium–low heat. Add the onion and garlic and cook, stirring frequently, for 3–4 minutes, or until just softened.

2 Stir in the flour and cook for a further 2 minutes, stirring occasionally.

3 Gradually pour in the water, stirring constantly and scraping the bottom of the saucepan to mix in the flour. Bring to the boil, stirring frequently, and cook for 2 minutes. Add the stock and stir until smooth.

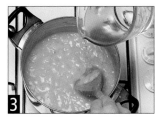

4 Add the carrot, green beans, butter beans, sweetcorn and chicken. Season to taste with salt and pepper. Return to the boil, then reduce the heat to medium–low, cover and simmer for 35 minutes, or until the vegetables are tender.

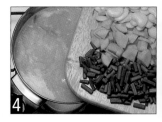

5 Taste the soup and adjust the seasoning, adding salt, if needed, and plenty of pepper.

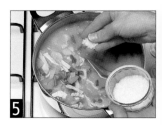

6 Ladle the soup into warmed bowls and serve.

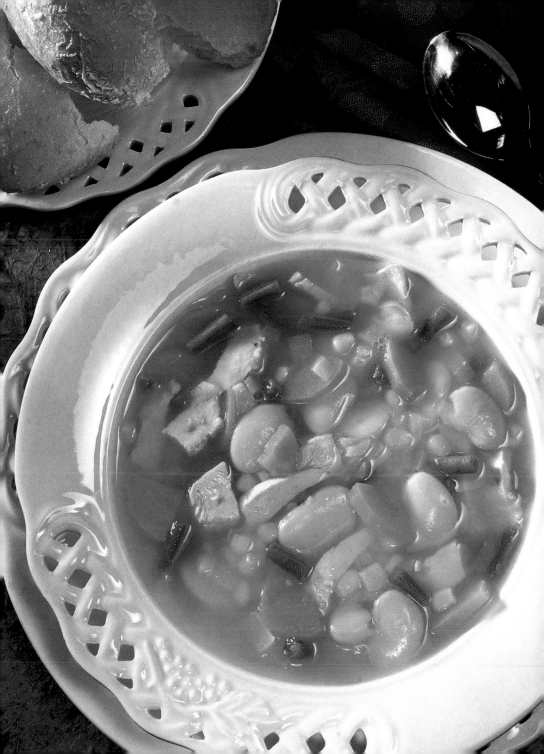

chicken jalfrezi

serves four

1 tsp mustard oil

3 tbsp vegetable oil

1 large onion, finely chopped

3 garlic cloves, crushed

1 tbsp tomato purée

2 tomatoes, peeled and chopped

1 tsp ground turmeric

½ tsp cumin seeds, ground

½ tsp coriander seeds, ground

½ tsp chilli powder

½ tsp garam masala

1 tsp red wine vinegar

1 small red pepper, deseeded
    and chopped

115 g/4 oz frozen broad beans

450 g/1 lb cooked chicken breasts,
    cut into bite-sized pieces

salt

fresh coriander sprigs, to garnish

1 Heat the mustard oil in a large frying pan set over a high heat for 1 minute, or until it begins to smoke. Add the vegetable oil, then reduce the heat, add the onion and garlic and fry until golden.

2 Add the tomato purée, tomatoes, turmeric, cumin, coriander, chilli powder, garam masala and vinegar to the pan. Stir the mixture until fragrant.

3 Add the pepper and beans and stir for 2 minutes, or until the pepper is softened. Stir in the chicken and season to taste with salt. Leave to simmer gently for 6–8 minutes, or until the chicken is heated through and the beans are tender.

4 Serve the chicken, garnished with coriander sprigs.

COOK'S TIP

This dish is an ideal way of making use of leftover cooked poultry or game birds – turkey, duck or quail. Any variety of beans works well, or substitute root vegetables, courgettes, potatoes or broccoli. Leafy vegetables will not be so successful.

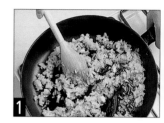

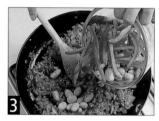

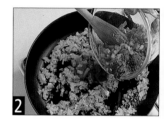

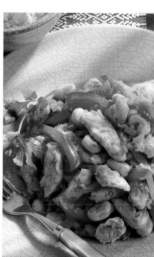

spiced chicken casserole

serves four–six

3 tbsp olive oil

900 g/2 lb chicken, sliced

10 shallots

3 carrots, chopped

55 g/2 oz chestnuts, sliced

55 g/2 oz flaked almonds, toasted

1 tsp freshly grated nutmeg

3 tsp ground cinnamon

300 ml/10 fl oz white wine

300 ml/10 fl oz chicken stock

175 ml/6 fl oz white wine vinegar

1 tbsp chopped fresh tarragon

1 tbsp chopped fresh parsley

1 tbsp chopped fresh thyme

grated rind of 1 orange

1 tbsp dark muscovado sugar

salt and pepper

125 g/4½ oz seedless black
    grapes, halved

fresh herbs, to garnish

freshly cooked wild rice, to serve

COOK'S TIP

This casserole would also be
delicious served with thick slices
of crusty wholemeal bread to
soak up the sauce.

1 Heat the oil in a large, heavy-based saucepan. Add the chicken, shallots and carrots and fry for 6 minutes, or until browned.

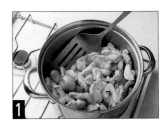

2 Add the remaining ingredients, except the grapes, and simmer over a low heat for 2 hours, or until the meat is very tender. Stir occasionally.

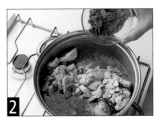

3 Add the grapes just before serving. Transfer to individual plates, garnish with fresh herbs and serve with freshly cooked wild rice.

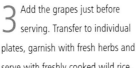

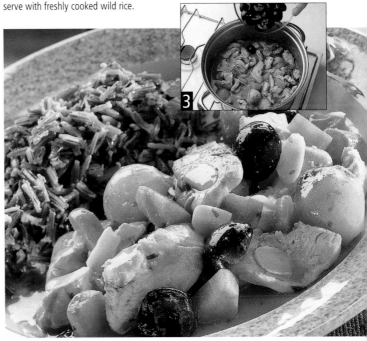

chicken & noodle one-pot

serves four

1 tbsp sunflower oil

1 onion, sliced

1 garlic clove, crushed

2.5-cm/1-inch piece fresh root
ginger, grated

1 bunch spring onions,
diagonally sliced

500 g/1 lb 2 oz skinless, boneless
chicken breasts, cut into
bite-sized pieces

2 tbsp mild curry paste

450 ml/16 fl oz coconut milk

300 ml/10 fl oz chicken stock

salt and pepper

250 g/9 oz dried Chinese
egg noodles

2 tsp lime juice

fresh basil sprigs, to garnish

COOK'S TIP

If you enjoy hot flavours,
substitute the mild curry paste in
the above recipe with hot curry
paste (found in most
supermarkets) but reduce the
quantity to 1 tablespoon.

1 Heat the oil in a preheated wok
or large, heavy-based frying pan.

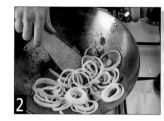

2 Add the onion, garlic, ginger
and spring onions and stir-fry
over a medium heat for 2 minutes,
or until softened.

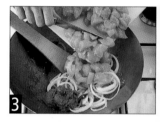

3 Add the chicken and curry paste
and stir-fry for 4 minutes, or until
the vegetables and chicken are golden
brown. Stir in the coconut milk, stock
and salt and pepper to taste and
mix well.

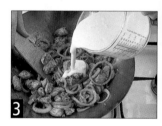

4 Bring to the boil, break the
noodles into large pieces, if
necessary, and add to the wok. Cover
and simmer, stirring occasionally, for
6–8 minutes, or until the noodles are
just tender.

5 Add the lime juice and adjust the
seasoning if necessary.

6 Serve the Chicken and Noodle
One-pot immediately in warmed
deep soup bowls, garnished with
basil sprigs.

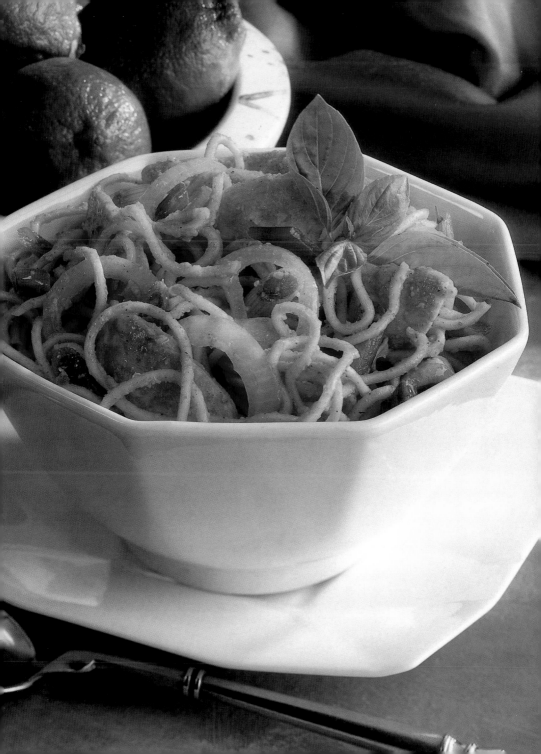

tom's toad in the hole

serves four–six

125 g/4½ oz plain flour

pinch of salt

1 egg, beaten

200 ml/7 fl oz milk

85 ml/3 fl oz water

2 tbsp beef dripping

250 g/9 oz skinless, boneless
chicken breasts

250 g/9 oz Cumberland sausage

VARIATION

Use skinless, boneless chicken
legs instead of chicken breast in
the recipe. Cut up as directed.
Instead of Cumberland sausage,
use your favourite variety
of sausage.

1 Mix the flour and salt in a bowl, then make a well in the centre and add the beaten egg.

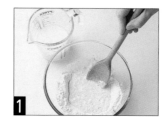

2 Add half the milk and, using a wooden spoon, work in the flour slowly.

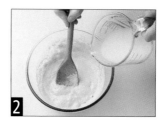

3 Beat the mixture until smooth, then gradually add the remaining milk and water.

4 Beat again until the mixture is smooth. Leave the mixture to stand for at least 1 hour.

5 Preheat the oven to 220°C/425°F/ Gas Mark 7. Add the dripping to individual baking tins or to 1 large baking tin. Cut up the chicken and sausage so that you get a generous piece in each individual tin or several scattered around the large tin.

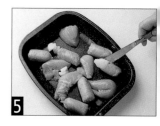

6 Heat in the oven for 5 minutes, or until very hot. Remove the tins from the oven and pour in the batter.

7 Return to the oven to cook for 35 minutes, or until risen and golden brown. Do not open the oven door for at least 30 minutes. Serve hot.

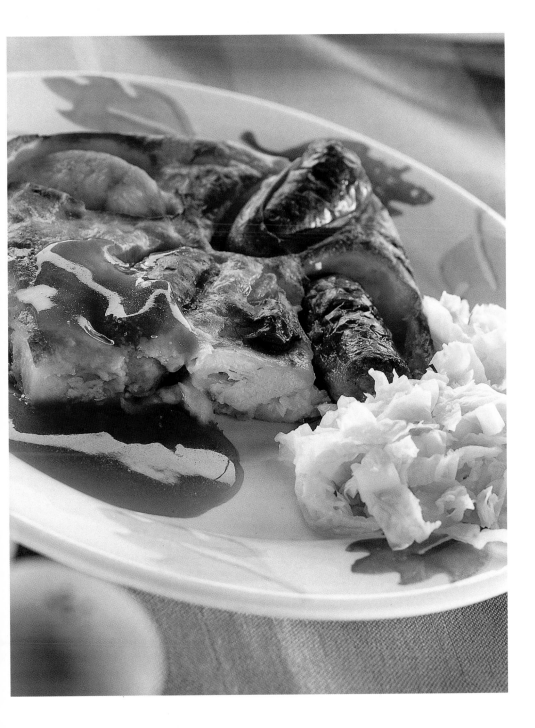

chicken pepperonata

serves four

8 chicken thighs

2 tbsp wholemeal flour

2 tbsp olive oil

1 small onion, thinly sliced

1 garlic clove, crushed

1 each large red, yellow and
    green pepper, deseeded and
    thinly sliced

400 g/14 oz canned
    chopped tomatoes

1 tbsp chopped fresh oregano,
    plus extra to garnish

salt and pepper

crusty wholemeal bread, to serve

COOK'S TIP

If you do not have fresh oregano,
use canned tomatoes with herbs
already added. For extra flavour,
halve the peppers and grill under
a preheated grill until the skins
are charred. Leave to cool, then
remove the skins and seeds. Slice
the peppers thinly and use
in the recipe.

1 Remove the skin from the chicken thighs and toss in the flour.

2 Heat the oil in a wide frying pan. Add the chicken and fry quickly until sealed and lightly browned, then remove from the frying pan. Add the onion to the frying pan and gently fry until soft. Add the garlic, peppers, tomatoes and oregano, then bring to the boil, stirring constantly.

3 Arrange the chicken over the vegetable mixture, season well with salt and pepper, then cover the frying pan tightly and simmer for 20–25 minutes, or until the chicken is tender and the juices run clear when a skewer is inserted into the thickest part of the meat.

4 Taste and adjust the seasoning, if necessary. Garnish with oregano and serve with slices of crusty wholemeal bread.

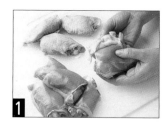

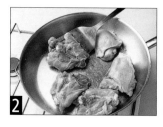

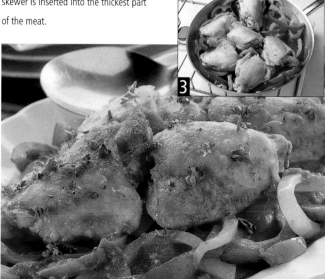

karahi chicken

serves four

2 tbsp ghee or oil

3 garlic cloves, crushed

1 onion, finely chopped

2 tbsp garam masala

1 tsp coriander seeds, ground

½ tsp dried mint

1 bay leaf

750 g/1 lb 10 oz skinless, boneless
  chicken, diced

200 ml/7 fl oz chicken stock

1 tbsp chopped fresh coriander

salt

warmed naan bread or chapatis,
  to serve

1 Heat the ghee in a karahi, wok or a large, heavy-based frying pan. Add the garlic and onion and stir-fry for 4 minutes, or until the onion is golden.

2 Stir in the garam masala, ground coriander, mint and bay leaf.

3 Add the chicken and cook over a high heat, stirring occasionally, for 5 minutes. Add the stock, reduce the heat and simmer for 10 minutes, or until the sauce has thickened, the chicken is tender and the juices run clear when a skewer is inserted into the thickest part of the meat.

4 Stir in the chopped fresh coriander, season to taste with salt and mix well. Serve immediately with warmed naan bread or chapatis.

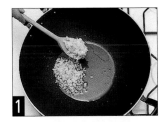

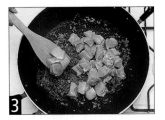

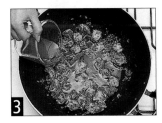

> **COOK'S TIP**
> It is important always to heat a karahi or wok before you add the oil to help maintain the high temperature.

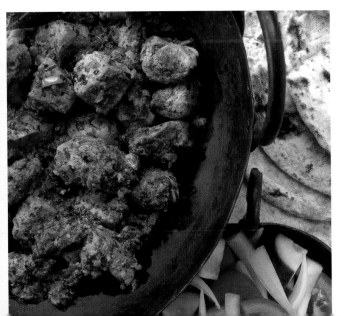

chicken tikka

serves six

1 tsp finely chopped fresh
   root ginger

1 garlic clove, crushed

½ tsp ground coriander

½ tsp ground cumin

1 tsp chilli powder

3 tbsp natural yogurt

1 tsp salt

2 tbsp lemon juice

few drops of red food colouring
   (optional)

1 tbsp tomato purée

1.5 kg/3 lb 5 oz skinless, boneless
   chicken breasts

1 onion, sliced

3 tbsp oil

1 lemon, cut into wedges,
   to garnish

lettuce leaves, to serve

1 Blend together the ginger, garlic, coriander, cumin and chilli powder in a large mixing bowl.

2 Add the yogurt, salt, lemon juice, red food colouring, if using, and the tomato purée to the spice mixture.

3 Using a sharp knife, cut the chicken into pieces. Add the chicken to the spice mixture and toss to coat well. Cover and marinate in the refrigerator for at least 3 hours, preferably overnight.

4 Preheat the grill. Arrange the onion in the base of a flameproof dish. Carefully drizzle half the oil over the onion.

5 Arrange the marinated chicken pieces on top of the onions and cook under the hot grill, turning once and basting with the remaining oil, for 25–30 minutes.

6 Serve on a bed of lettuce, garnished with lemon wedges.

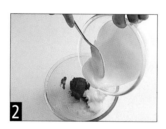

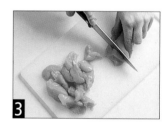

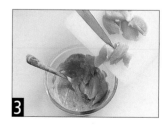

COOK'S TIP

Serve the Chicken Tikka with warmed naan bread, cucumber raita and an Indian chutney, such as mango.

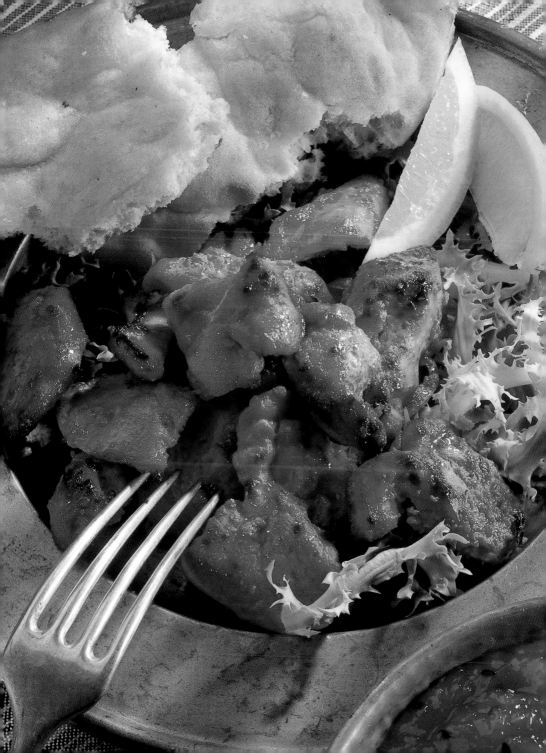

fricassée of chicken in lime sauce

serves four

1 large chicken, cut into
small portions
55 g/2 oz flour, seasoned
2 tbsp sunflower oil
500 g/1 lb 2 oz baby onions or
shallots, sliced
1 each green and red pepper,
deseeded and thinly sliced
150 ml/5 fl oz chicken stock
grated rind and juice of 2 limes
2 fresh chillies, chopped
2 tbsp oyster sauce
1 tsp Worcestershire sauce
salt and pepper

VARIATION

Try this casserole with a cheese
scone topping. About 30 minutes
before the end of cooking time,
simply top with rounds cut from
cheese scone dough.

1 Preheat the oven to 190°C/375°F/
Gas Mark 5. Coat the chicken
pieces in the seasoned flour. Heat the
oil in a large frying pan, add the
chicken and cook for 4 minutes, or
until browned all over.

2 Using a slotted spoon, transfer
the chicken to a large, deep
casserole and sprinkle with the sliced
onions. Keep warm until required.

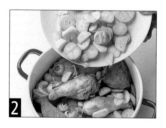

3 Slowly fry the peppers in the
juices remaining in the frying pan.
Add the stock, lime rind and juice and
cook for a further 5 minutes.

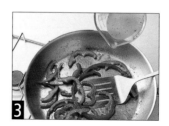

4 Add the chillies, oyster sauce and
Worcestershire sauce. Season to
taste with salt and pepper.

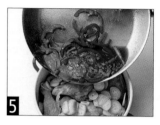

5 Pour the peppers and juices over
the chicken and onions.

6 Cover the casserole with a lid
or foil.

7 Cook in the centre of the oven for
1½ hours, or until the chicken is
very tender, then serve.

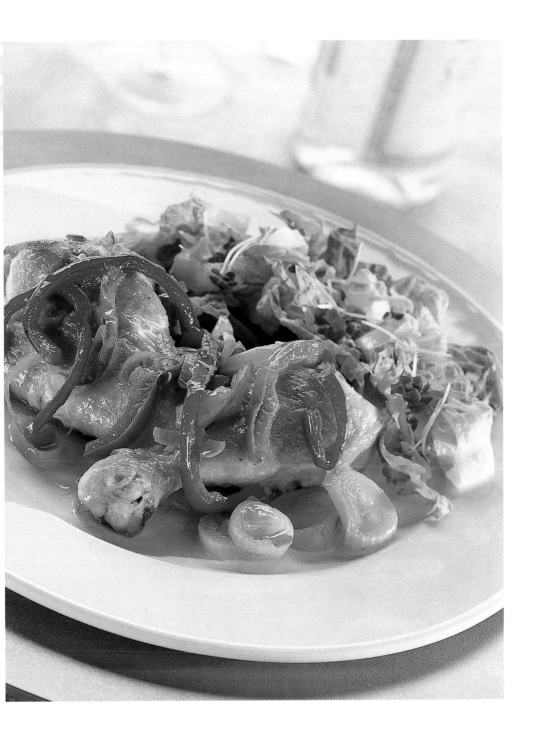

springtime chicken cobbler

serves four

1 tbsp oil

8 skinless chicken drumsticks

1 small onion, sliced

350 g/12 oz baby carrots

2 baby turnips

125 g/4½ oz fresh or frozen peas

1 tsp cornflour

300 ml/10 fl oz chicken stock

2 bay leaves

salt and pepper

COBBLER TOPPING

250 g/9 oz wholemeal plain flour,
   plus extra for dusting

2 tsp baking powder

25 g/1 oz sunflower soft margarine

2 tsp dry mustard

55 g/2 oz Cheddar cheese, grated

2–3 tbsp skimmed milk, plus extra
   for brushing

sesame seeds, for sprinkling

1 Preheat the oven to 200°C/400°F/
Gas Mark 6. Heat the oil in a large
flameproof casserole. Add the chicken
and fry, turning frequently, until golden
brown. Drain well and remove. Add
the onion to the casserole and sauté
for 2–3 minutes, or until softened.

2 Cut the carrots and turnips
into equal-sized pieces. Add to
the casserole with the onion, peas
and chicken.

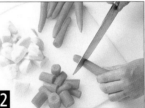

3 Blend the cornflour with a little of
the stock in a small saucepan,
then stir in the remainder and heat
gently, stirring, until boiling. Pour into
the casserole and add the bay leaves
and salt and pepper to taste. Cover the
casserole and bake in the oven for
50–60 minutes, or until the chicken is
tender and the juices run clear when a
skewer is inserted into the thickest part
of the meat.

4 For the topping, sift the flour and
baking powder into a large bowl,
then mix in the margarine with a fork.
Stir in the mustard, cheese and enough
milk to form a fairly soft dough. Roll
out on a lightly floured work surface.
Cut out 16 rounds with a 4-cm/1½-inch
cutter. Uncover the casserole and
arrange the rounds on top. Brush with
milk and sprinkle with sesame seeds.
Bake for a further 20 minutes, or until
the topping is golden and firm.

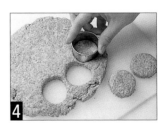

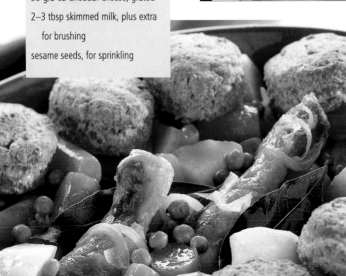

chicken basquaise

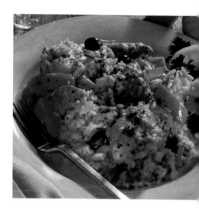

serves four–five

1 chicken, weighing 1.3 kg/3 lb,
    cut into 8 pieces

flour, for coating

salt and pepper

3 tbsp olive oil

1 Spanish onion, thickly sliced

2 red, green or yellow peppers,
    deseeded and cut lengthways
    into thick strips

2 garlic cloves

150 g/5 oz chorizo sausage,
    skinned and cut into 1-cm/
    ½-inch pieces

1 tbsp tomato purée

200 g/7 oz long-grain white rice

450 ml/16 fl oz chicken stock

1 tsp crushed dried chillies

½ tsp dried thyme

115 g/4 oz Bayonne or other air-
    dried ham, diced

12 dry-cured black olives

2 tbsp chopped fresh
    flat-leaved parsley

1 Pat the chicken pieces dry with kitchen paper. Put 2 tablespoons of flour in a polythene bag, season well with salt and pepper and add the chicken pieces. Seal the bag and shake to coat the chicken.

2 Heat 2 tablespoons of the oil in a large, flameproof casserole over a medium–high heat. Add the chicken and cook, turning frequently, for 15 minutes, or until well browned all over. Transfer to a plate.

3 Heat the remaining oil in the casserole and add the onion and peppers. Reduce the heat to medium and stir-fry until beginning to colour and soften. Add the garlic, chorizo and tomato purée and cook, stirring constantly, for about 3 minutes. Add the rice and cook, stirring to coat, for 2 minutes, or until the rice is translucent.

4 Add the stock, crushed chillies and thyme, season to taste with salt and pepper and stir well. Bring to the boil. Return the chicken to the casserole, pressing it gently into the rice. Cover and cook over a very low heat for 45 minutes, or until the chicken is cooked through and the rice is tender.

5 Gently stir the ham, black olives and half the parsley into the rice mixture. Re-cover and heat through for a further 5 minutes. Sprinkle with the remaining parsley and serve immediately.

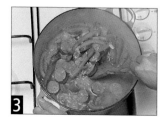

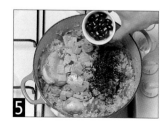

chicken & onions

serves four

300 ml/10 fl oz oil

4 onions, finely chopped

1½ tsp finely chopped fresh
    root ginger

1½ tsp garam masala

1 garlic clove, crushed

1 tsp chilli powder

1 tsp ground coriander

3 green cardamoms

3 peppercorns

3 tbsp tomato purée

8 chicken thighs, skinned

300 ml/10 fl oz water

2 tbsp lemon juice

1 fresh green chilli, finely chopped

¼ bunch fresh coriander
    leaves, chopped

1 fresh green chilli, cut into strips,
    to garnish

1 Heat the oil in a large frying pan. Add the onions and fry, stirring occasionally, until golden brown.

2 Reduce the heat and add the ginger, garam masala, garlic, chilli powder, ground coriander, cardamoms and the peppercorns, stirring to mix.

3 Add the tomato purée to the mixture in the frying pan and stir-fry for 5–7 minutes.

4 Add the chicken thighs to the frying pan and toss to coat with the spice mixture.

COOK'S TIP
This curry definitely improves if it is made in advance and then reheated before serving. This develops and deepens the flavours.

5 Pour the water into the frying pan, cover and leave to simmer for 20–25 minutes.

6 Add the lemon juice, chopped chilli and coriander to the mixture, and stir to combine.

7 Transfer the chicken and onions to serving plates, garnish with chilli strips and serve hot.

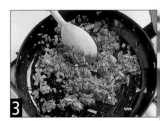

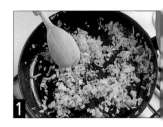

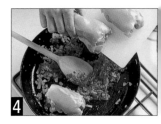

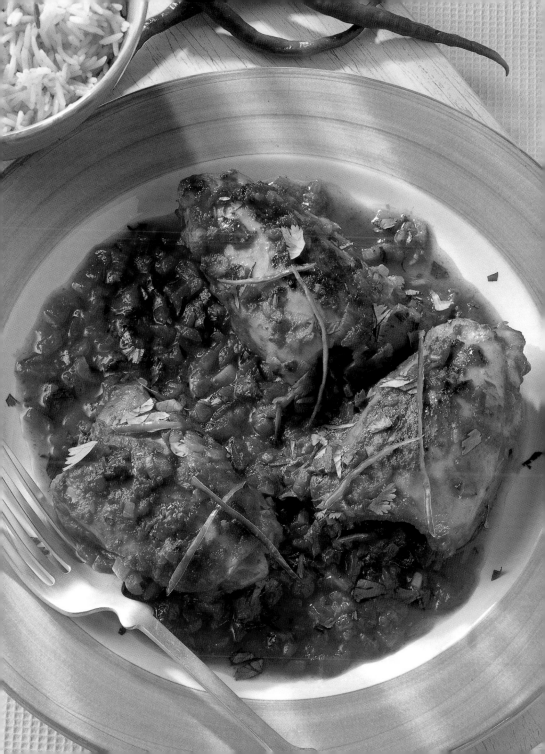

chicken bourguignonne

serves four–six

4 tbsp sunflower oil

900 g/2 lb skinless chicken, diced

250 g/9 oz button mushrooms

125 g/4½ oz rindless smoked
   bacon, diced

16 shallots

2 garlic cloves, crushed

1 tbsp plain flour

150 ml/5 fl oz white Burgundy wine

150 ml/5 fl oz chicken stock

1 bouquet garni (1 bay leaf,
   1 fresh thyme sprig, 1 celery
   stick, 1 fresh parsley sprig and
   1 fresh sage sprig, tied
   together with string)

salt and pepper

TO SERVE

croûtons

selection of cooked vegetables

1 Preheat the oven to 150°C/300°F/ Gas Mark 2. Heat the oil in a flameproof casserole. Add the chicken and cook until browned all over. Remove from the casserole with a slotted spoon and reserve.

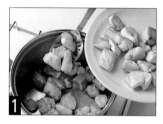

2 Add the mushrooms, bacon, shallots and garlic to the casserole and cook for 4 minutes.

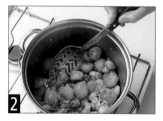

3 Return the chicken to the casserole and sprinkle with flour. Cook for a further 2 minutes, stirring. Add the wine and stock and bring to the boil, stirring constantly. Add the bouquet garni and season well with salt and pepper.

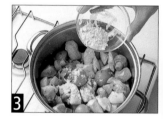

4 Cover the casserole and bake in the centre of the oven for 1½ hours. Remove and discard the bouquet garni.

5 Serve garnished with croûtons and accompanied by a selection of lightly cooked vegetables.

COOK'S TIP

A good quality red wine can be used instead of the white wine, to produce a rich, glossy red sauce.

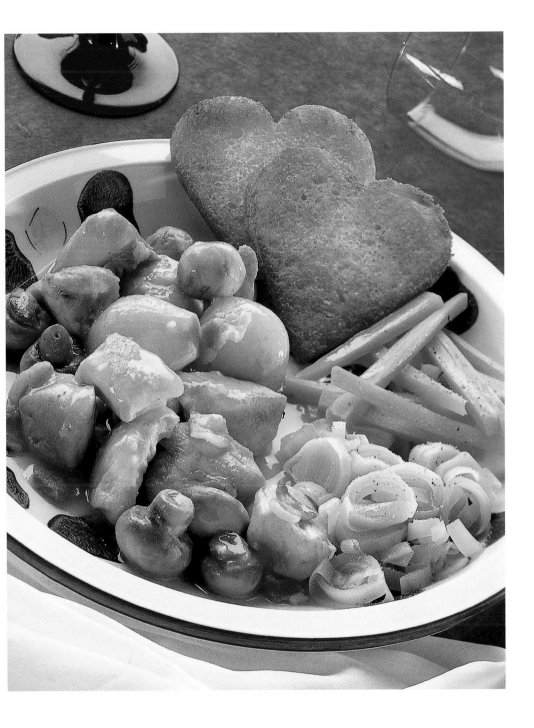

rustic chicken & orange pot

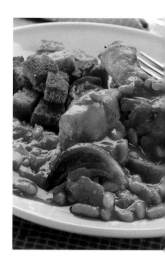

serves four

8 chicken drumsticks, skinned

1 tbsp wholemeal flour

2 tbsp olive oil

2 red onions

1 garlic clove, crushed

1 tsp fennel seeds

1 bay leaf

finely grated rind and juice of
   1 small orange

400 g/14 oz canned
   chopped tomatoes

400 g/14 oz canned cannellini or
   flageolet beans, drained

salt and pepper

TOPPING

3 thick slices wholemeal bread

2 tsp olive oil

1 Preheat the oven to 190°C/375°F/ Gas Mark 5. Toss the chicken drumsticks in the flour to coat evenly. Heat half the oil in a large, flameproof casserole. Add the chicken and fry over a fairly high heat, turning frequently, until golden brown. Transfer to a plate and keep warm until required.

2 Slice the onions into thin wedges. Heat the remaining oil in the casserole and cook the onions until lightly browned. Stir in the garlic.

3 Add the fennel seeds, bay leaf, orange rind and juice, tomatoes and cannellini beans and season to taste with salt and pepper. Add the chicken.

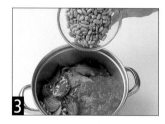

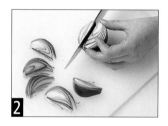

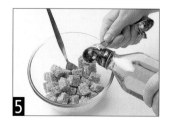

4 Cover tightly and cook in the oven for 30–35 minutes, or until the chicken is tender and the juices run clear when a skewer is inserted into the thickest part of the meat.

5 Cut the bread into small dice and toss in the oil. Remove the lid from the casserole and top with the bread cubes. Bake for a further 15–20 minutes, or until the bread is golden and crisp. Serve hot.

COOK'S TIP

Choose beans that are canned in water with no added sugar or salt. Drain and rinse well before use.

chicken & chilli bean pot

serves four

2 tbsp plain flour

1 tsp chilli powder

salt and pepper

8 chicken thighs or 4 chicken legs

3 tbsp vegetable oil

2 garlic cloves, crushed

1 large onion, chopped

1 green or red pepper, deseeded
  and chopped

300 ml/10 fl oz chicken stock

350 g/12 oz tomatoes, chopped

400 g/14 oz canned red kidney
  beans, rinsed and drained

2 tbsp tomato purée

COOK'S TIP

For extra flavour, use sun-dried
tomato paste instead of
tomato purée.

1 Combine the flour and chilli powder in a shallow dish and add salt and pepper to taste. Rinse the chicken, but do not dry. Dip the chicken into the seasoned flour, turning to coat it on all sides.

2 Heat the oil in a large, deep frying pan or flameproof casserole and add the chicken. Cook over a high heat, turning the pieces frequently, for 3–4 minutes, or until browned all over.

3 Lift the chicken out of the pan with a slotted spoon and drain thoroughly on kitchen paper.

4 Add the garlic, onion and pepper to the pan and cook over a medium heat, stirring occasionally, for 2–3 minutes, or until softened.

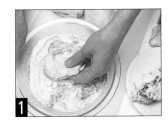

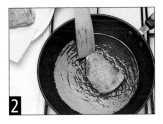

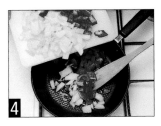

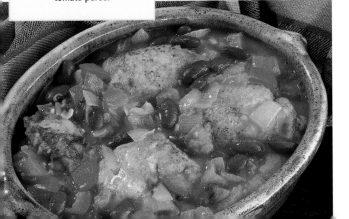

5 Add the stock, tomatoes, beans and tomato purée, stirring well. Bring to the boil, then return the chicken to the pan. Reduce the heat, cover and simmer for 30 minutes, or until the chicken is tender and the juices run clear when a skewer is inserted into the thickest part of the meat. Taste and adjust the seasoning, if necessary, and serve.

chicken korma

serves eight

1½ tsp finely chopped fresh
    root ginger

1–2 garlic cloves, crushed

2 tsp garam masala

1 tsp chilli powder

1 tsp salt

1 tsp black cumin seeds

3 green cardamoms, husks removed
    and seeds crushed

1 tsp ground coriander

1 tsp ground almonds

150 ml/5 fl oz natural yogurt

8 skinless, boneless chicken breasts

300 ml/10 fl oz oil

2 onions, sliced

150 ml/5 fl oz water

¼ bunch fresh coriander, chopped

2 fresh green chillies, chopped

boiled rice, to serve

1 In a bowl, mix the ginger, garlic, garam masala, chilli powder, salt, cumin seeds, cardamoms, ground coriander and ground almonds with the yogurt.

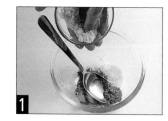

2 Spoon the yogurt and spice mixture over the chicken breasts and set aside to marinate.

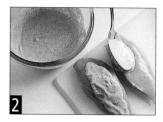

3 Heat the oil in a large frying pan. Add the onions to the pan and fry until golden brown.

4 Add the chicken breasts to the pan, stir-frying for 5–7 minutes.

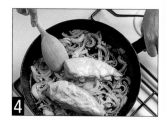

5 Add the water, cover and leave to simmer for 20–25 minutes.

VARIATION

Chicken portions may be used instead of breasts, if preferred, and should be cooked for 10 minutes longer.

6 Add the fresh coriander and chillies. Cook, stirring occasionally, for a further 10 minutes, or until the chicken is tender and the juices run clear when a skewer is inserted into the thickest part of the meat.

7 Transfer to a serving plate and serve with boiled rice.

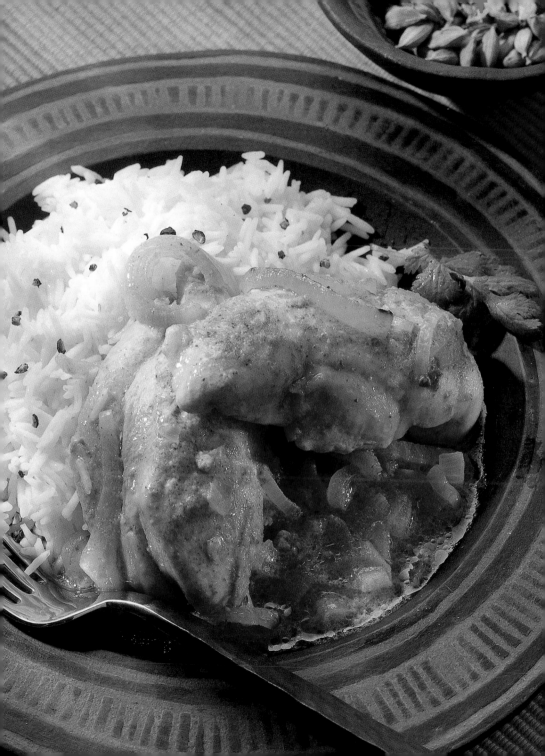

hungarian chicken goulash

900 g/2 lb chicken, diced

55 g/2 oz flour, seasoned with 1 tsp
    paprika, salt and pepper

2 tbsp olive oil

25 g/1 oz butter

1 onion, sliced

24 shallots

1 each red and green pepper,
    deseeded and chopped

1 tbsp paprika

1 tsp fresh rosemary, crushed

4 tbsp tomato purée

300 ml/10 fl oz chicken stock

150 ml/5 fl oz claret

400 g/14 oz canned
    chopped tomatoes

TO GARNISH

150 ml/5 fl oz soured cream

1 tbsp chopped fresh parsley

TO SERVE

crusty bread

crisp salad

1 Preheat the oven to 160°C/325°F/
  Gas Mark 3. Toss the diced
chicken in the seasoned flour until it
is coated all over.

2 Heat the oil and butter in a
  flameproof casserole. Add the
onion, shallots and peppers and fry for
3 minutes.

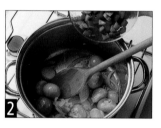

3 Add the chicken and cook for a
  further 4 minutes.

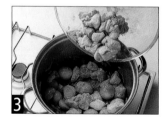

4 Sprinkle with the paprika and
  crushed rosemary.

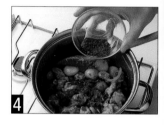

5 Add the tomato purée, stock,
  wine and tomatoes, cover and
cook the casserole in the centre of the
oven for 1½ hours, or until the chicken
is very tender.

6 Remove the casserole from the
  oven, leave it to stand for
4 minutes, then garnish with the
soured cream and parsley.

7 Serve with chunks of bread and a
  crisp salad.

VARIATION

Serve the goulash with buttered
ribbon noodles instead of bread.
For an authentic touch, try
a Hungarian red wine instead
of the claret.

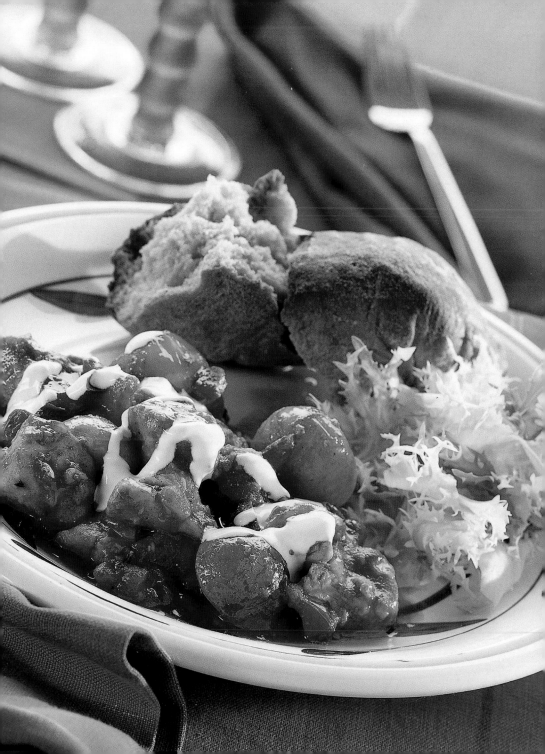

chicken risotto à la milanese

serves four

125 g/4½ oz butter

900 g/2 lb skinless, boneless
chicken breasts, thinly sliced

1 large onion, chopped

500 g/1 lb 2 oz arborio rice

600 ml/1 pint chicken stock

150 ml/5 fl oz white wine

1 tsp crumbled saffron threads

salt and pepper

fresh flat-leaved parsley sprigs,
to garnish

55 g/2 oz freshly grated Parmesan
cheese, to serve

VARIATION

The possibilities for risotto are
endless – try adding the
following at the end of the
cooking time: cashew nuts and
sweetcorn kernels, lightly
sautéed courgettes and
basil or artichokes and
oyster mushrooms.

1 Heat 55 g/2 oz of the butter in a deep frying pan. Add the chicken and onion and fry until golden brown. Add the rice, stir well and cook gently for 5 minutes.

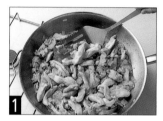

2 Heat the stock in a separate saucepan until boiling, then gradually add to the rice a ladleful at a time. Reserve the last ladleful of stock. Add the wine, saffron and salt and pepper to taste and mix well. Simmer gently for 20 minutes, stirring occasionally and adding extra stock if the risotto becomes too dry.

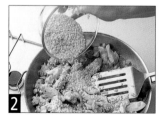

3 Remove the frying pan from the heat and leave to stand for a few minutes. Just before serving, add the reserved stock and simmer for a further 10 minutes. Transfer the risotto to 4 large serving plates and garnish with the parsley. Serve with the grated Parmesan cheese and remaining butter.

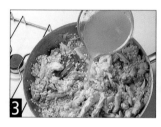

COOK'S TIP

A risotto should have moist but
separate grains. Stock should be
added a little at a time and only
when the previous addition has
been completely absorbed.

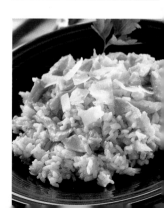

chicken & potato casserole

serves four

2 tbsp vegetable oil

4 chicken portions, about 225 g/
    8 oz each

2 leeks, sliced

1 garlic clove, crushed

4 tbsp plain flour

850 ml/1½ pints chicken stock

300 ml/10 fl oz dry white wine

salt and pepper

125 g/4½ oz baby carrots, halved
    lengthways

125 g/4½ oz baby corn cobs, halved
    lengthways

450 g/1 lb small new potatoes

1 fresh or dried bouquet garni

150 ml/5 fl oz double cream

boiled rice, to serve

VARIATION

Use turkey fillets instead of the
chicken, if preferred, and vary
the vegetables according to
those you have to hand.

1 Preheat the oven to 180°C/
350°F/Gas Mark 4. Heat the oil
in a large frying pan and cook the
chicken, turning, for 10 minutes, or
until browned. Transfer to a casserole
using a slotted spoon.

2 Add the leeks and garlic and cook
for 2–3 minutes, stirring. Stir in
the flour, cook for another minute then
remove from the heat. Stir in stock,
wine and salt and pepper to taste.

3 Return the pan to the heat and
bring to the boil. Stir in the
vegetables and bouquet garni. Transfer
the mixture to the casserole.

4 Cover the casserole and cook in
the oven for 1 hour.

5 Remove the casserole from the
oven and stir in the cream. Return
to the oven, uncovered, and cook for
15 minutes. Remove and discard the
bouquet garni, taste and adjust the
seasoning and serve with rice.

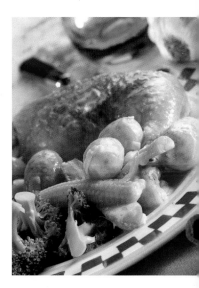

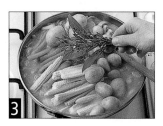

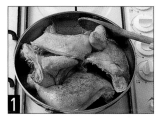

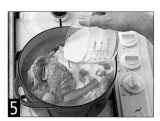

braised chicken with rosemary dumplings

serves four

4 chicken quarters

2 tbsp sunflower oil

2 leeks

250 g/9 oz carrots, chopped

250 g/9 oz parsnips, chopped

2 small turnips, chopped

600 ml/1 pint chicken stock

3 tbsp Worcestershire sauce

2 fresh rosemary sprigs

salt and pepper

ROSEMARY DUMPLINGS

200 g/7 oz self-raising flour

100 g/3½ oz shredded suet

1 tbsp chopped fresh
   rosemary leaves

salt and pepper

about 2–3 tbsp cold water

1 Remove the skin from the chicken, if you prefer. Heat the oil in a large, flameproof casserole or heavy-based saucepan. Add the chicken and fry until golden. Using a slotted spoon, remove the chicken from the casserole. Drain off the excess fat.

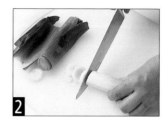

2 Slice the leeks and add to the casserole together with the carrots, parsnips and turnips. Cook for 5 minutes, or until the vegetables are lightly coloured. Return the chicken to the casserole.

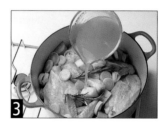

3 Add the stock, Worcestershire sauce and rosemary, season to taste with salt and pepper, then bring to the boil.

4 Reduce the heat, cover and simmer gently for 50 minutes, or until the chicken is tender and the juices run clear when a skewer is inserted into the thickest part of the meat.

5 To make the dumplings, mix the flour, suet, rosemary and salt and pepper to taste together in a large bowl. Stir in just enough water to form a firm dough.

6 Form into 8 small balls between the palms of your hands and place on top of the chicken and vegetables. Cover and simmer for a further 10–12 minutes, or until the dumplings are well risen. Serve immediately with the casserole.

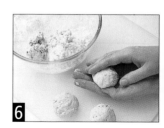

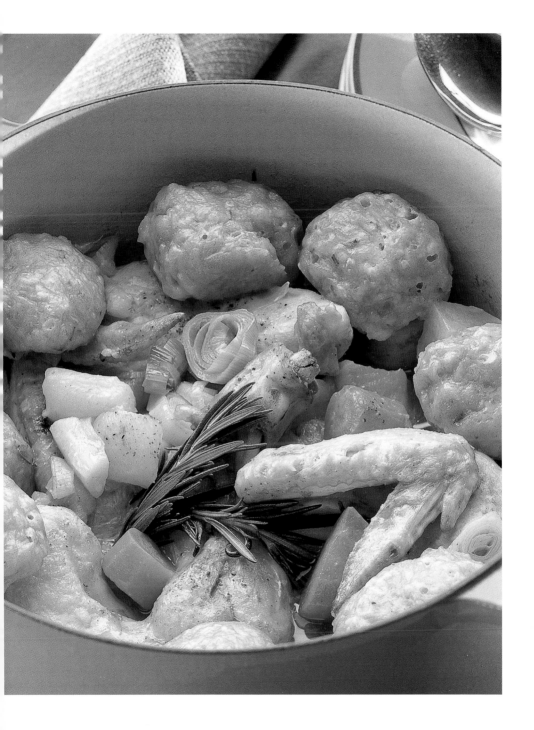

garlic chicken casserole

serves four

4 tbsp sunflower oil

900 g/2 lb chicken, chopped

250 g/9 oz mushrooms, sliced

16 shallots

6 garlic cloves, crushed

1 tbsp plain flour

250 ml/9 fl oz white wine

250 ml/9 fl oz chicken stock

1 bouquet garni (1 bay leaf, 1 fresh
thyme sprig, 1 celery stick, 1 fresh
parsley sprig and 1 fresh sage
sprig, tied together with string)

salt and pepper

400 g/14 oz canned borlotti beans

freshly cooked pattypan squash, to
serve

1 Preheat the oven to 150°C/
300°F/Gas Mark 2. Heat the oil
in a large, flameproof casserole. Add
the chicken and fry until browned all
over. Remove the chicken from the
casserole with a slotted spoon and
reserve until required.

2 Add the mushrooms, shallots and
garlic to the casserole and cook
for 4 minutes.

3 Return the chicken to the
casserole and sprinkle with the
flour, then cook for a further 2 minutes.

4 Add the wine and stock, stir until
boiling, then add the bouquet
garni. Season well with salt and
pepper to taste.

5 Drain the borlotti beans and
rinse thoroughly, then add to
the casserole.

6 Cover and place in the centre of
the oven for 2 hours. Remove and
discard the bouquet garni and serve
the casserole with pattypan squash.

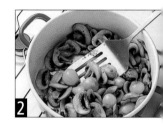

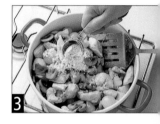

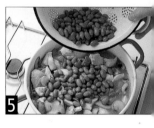

COOK'S TIP

Mushrooms are ideal in a low-fat
diet because they are high in
flavour and contain no fat.
Experiment with the wealth of
varieties that are now available
from supermarkets. Serve the
casserole with brown rice to
make this filling dish go
even further.

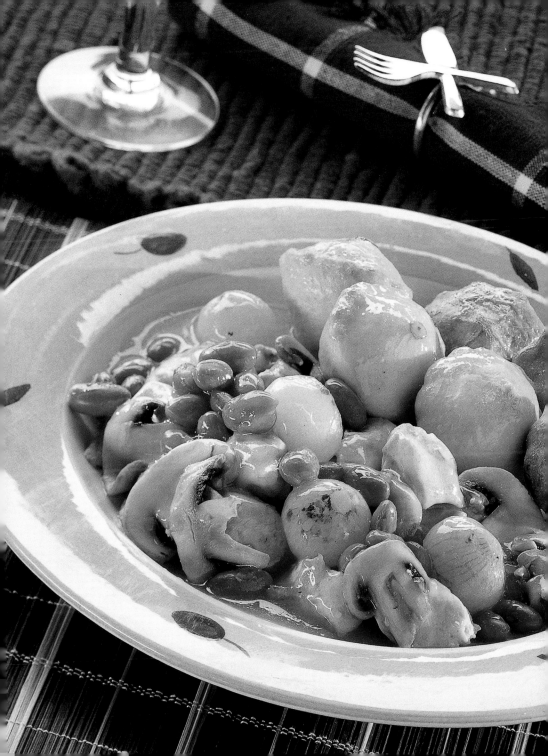

green chicken curry

serves four

6 skinless, boneless chicken thighs

400 ml/14 fl oz coconut milk

2 garlic cloves, crushed

2 tbsp Thai fish sauce

2 tbsp Thai green curry paste

12 baby aubergines

3 fresh green chillies, finely chopped

3 fresh kaffir lime leaves, shredded,
   plus extra to garnish (optional)

salt and pepper

4 tbsp chopped fresh coriander

freshly cooked rice, to serve

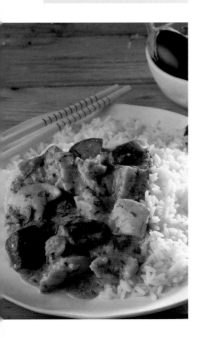

1 Cut the chicken into bite-sized pieces. Pour the coconut milk into a preheated wok or large frying pan over a high heat and bring to the boil.

2 Add the chicken, garlic and fish sauce to the wok and return to the boil. Reduce the heat and simmer gently for 30 minutes, or until the chicken is just tender.

3 Remove the chicken from the wok with a slotted spoon. Keep warm.

4 Stir the curry paste into the wok, add the aubergines, chillies and lime leaves and simmer for 5 minutes.

COOK'S TIP

Baby aubergines, or 'pea aubergines' as they are called in Thailand, are traditionally used in this curry, but they are not always available. If you can't find them in a Thai food shop, use chopped ordinary aubergine, or substitute a few green peas.

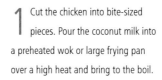

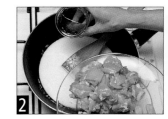

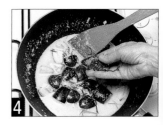

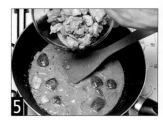

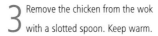

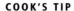

5 Return the chicken to the wok and bring to the boil. Season to taste with salt and pepper, then stir in the coriander. Transfer to warmed serving plates, garnish with lime leaves, if using, and serve with freshly cooked rice.

sage chicken & rice

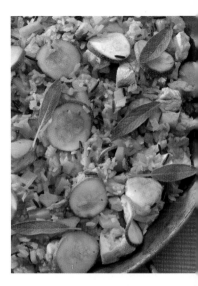

serves four

1 large onion, chopped

1 garlic clove, crushed

2 celery sticks, sliced

2 carrots, diced

2 fresh sage sprigs, plus extra
   to garnish

300 ml/10 fl oz chicken stock

350 g/12 oz skinless, boneless
   chicken breasts

225 g/8 oz mixed brown and
   wild rice

400 g/14 oz canned
   chopped tomatoes

dash of Tabasco sauce

salt and pepper

2 courgettes, thinly sliced

100 g/3½ oz lean ham, diced

TO SERVE

salad leaves

crusty bread

COOK'S TIP

If you do not have fresh sage,
use 1 teaspoon of dried sage
in Step 1.

1 Place the onion, garlic, celery, carrots and sage in a large saucepan and pour in the stock. Bring to the boil, then reduce the heat, cover the saucepan and simmer for 5 minutes.

2 Cut the chicken into 2.5-cm/ 1-inch cubes and stir into the saucepan. Cover and cook for a further 5 minutes.

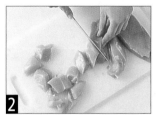

3 Stir in the rice and tomatoes, add Tabasco sauce to taste and season well with salt and pepper. Bring to the boil, then reduce the heat and simmer, covered, for 25 minutes.

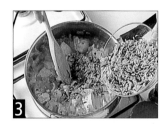

4 Stir in the sliced courgettes and diced ham and cook, uncovered and stirring occasionally, for a further 10 minutes, or until the rice is just tender.

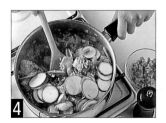

5 Remove and discard the sage. Garnish with a few sage leaves and serve with salad leaves and slices of crusty bread.

buttered chicken

serves four–six

100 g/3½ oz unsalted butter

1 tbsp oil

2 onions, finely chopped

1 tsp finely chopped fresh
   root ginger

2 tsp garam masala

2 tsp ground coriander

1 tsp chilli powder

1 tsp black cumin seeds

1 garlic clove, crushed

1 tsp salt

3 green cardamoms

3 black peppercorns

150 ml/5 fl oz natural yogurt

2 tbsp tomato purée

8 chicken pieces, skinned

150 ml/5 fl oz water

2 bay leaves

150 ml/5 fl oz single cream

TO GARNISH

chopped fresh coriander

2 fresh green chillies, chopped

1 Heat the butter and oil in a large frying pan over a medium heat. Add the onions and fry, stirring frequently, until golden brown. Reduce the heat.

2 Place the ginger in a bowl. Add the garam masala, ground coriander, chilli powder, cumin seeds, garlic, salt, cardamoms and peppercorns and blend. Add the yogurt and tomato purée and stir to combine.

3 Add the chicken pieces to the yogurt and spice mixture and mix to coat well.

4 Add the chicken to the onions in the frying pan and stir-fry vigorously, making semi-circular movements, for 5–7 minutes.

5 Add the water and the bay leaves and leave to simmer for 30 minutes, stirring occasionally.

6 Add the cream and cook for a further 10–15 minutes.

7 Garnish with fresh coriander and chillies and serve hot.

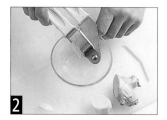

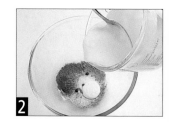

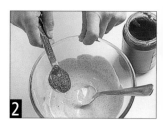

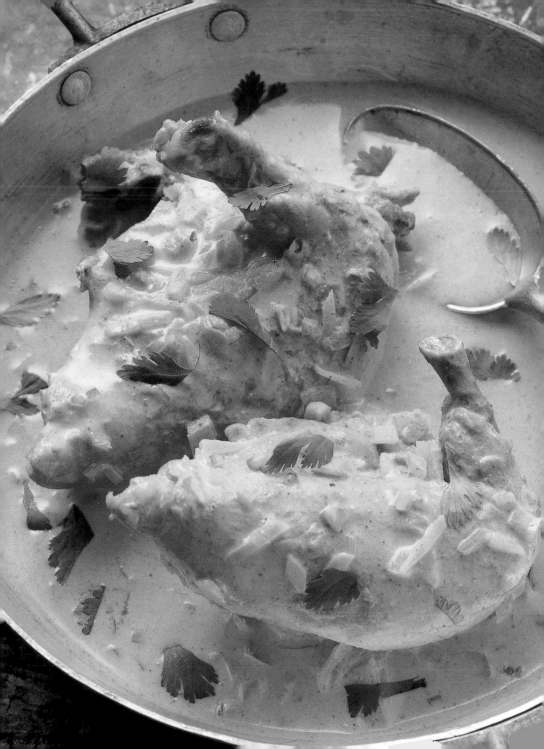

brittany chicken casserole

serves six

500 g/1 lb 2 oz dried beans, such
    as flageolets, soaked overnight
    and drained

25 g/1 oz butter

2 tbsp olive oil

3 rindless bacon rashers, chopped

900 g/2 lb chicken pieces

1 tbsp plain flour

300 ml/10 fl oz cider

150 ml/5 fl oz chicken stock

salt and pepper

14 shallots

2 tbsp clear honey, warmed

225 g/8 oz cooked beetroot,
    chopped

1 Preheat the oven to 160°C/325°F/
Gas Mark 3. Cook the beans in
boiling water for 25 minutes, then
drain thoroughly.

2 Heat the butter and oil in a large,
flameproof casserole. Add the
bacon and chicken and cook for
5 minutes.

3 Sprinkle with the flour, then add
the cider and stock, stirring
constantly to avoid lumps forming.
Season to taste with salt and pepper
and bring to the boil.

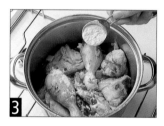

4 Add the drained beans, then
cover the casserole tightly
and bake in the centre of the oven
for 2 hours, or until the chicken is
very tender.

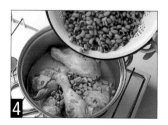

5 About 15 minutes before the
end of the cooking time, uncover
the casserole.

6 Gently cook the shallots and
honey together in a frying pan for
5 minutes, turning the shallots
frequently until golden.

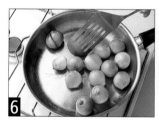

7 Add the shallots and beetroot to
the casserole and return to the
oven for the last 15 minutes of the
cooking time.

COOK'S TIP

To save time, use canned
flageolet beans instead of dried.
Rinse and drain before adding
to the chicken.

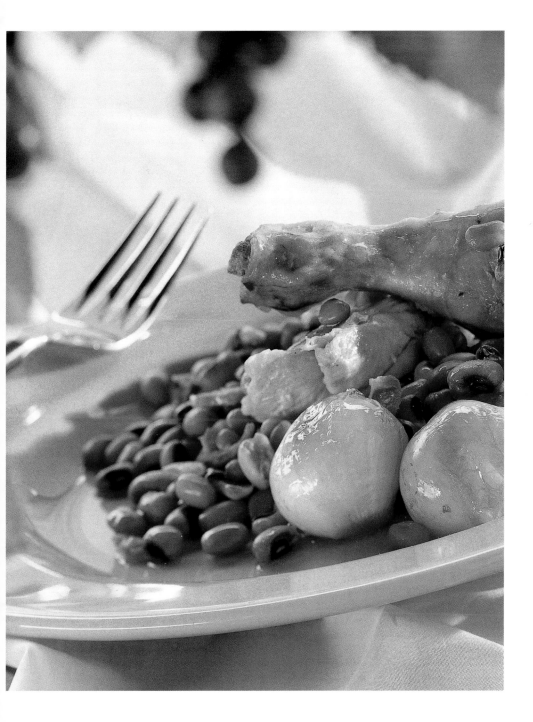

chicken & plum casserole

serves four

2 rindless lean back bacon
rashers, chopped

1 tbsp sunflower oil

450 g/1 lb skinless, boneless
chicken thighs, cut into 4 equal-
sized strips

1 garlic clove, crushed

175 g/6 oz shallots, halved

225 g/8 oz plums, halved or
quartered (if large) and stoned

1 tbsp light muscovado sugar

150 ml/5 fl oz dry sherry

2 tbsp plum sauce

450 ml/16 fl oz chicken stock

2 tsp cornflour, mixed with 4 tsp
cold water

2 tbsp chopped fresh parsley,
to garnish

crusty bread, to serve

VARIATION

Chunks of lean turkey or pork
would also go well with this
combination of flavours.
The cooking time will
remain the same.

1 In a large, non-stick frying pan, dry-fry the bacon for 2–3 minutes until the juices run out. Remove the bacon from the pan with a slotted spoon, set aside and keep warm.

2 In the same frying pan, heat the oil and fry the chicken with the garlic and shallots for 4–5 minutes, stirring occasionally, until well browned all over.

3 Return the bacon to the pan and stir in the plums, sugar, sherry, plum sauce and stock. Bring to the boil, then reduce the heat and simmer for 20 minutes, or until the plums have softened and the chicken is cooked through.

4 Add the cornflour mixture to the pan and cook, stirring, for a further 2–3 minutes, or until thickened.

5 Spoon the casserole on to warmed serving plates and garnish with chopped parsley. Serve with chunks of bread to mop up the fruity gravy.

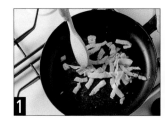

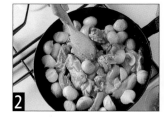

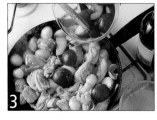

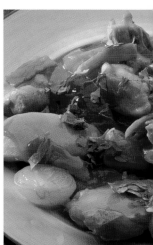

golden chicken risotto

serves four

2 tbsp sunflower oil

1 tbsp butter

1 leek, thinly sliced

1 large yellow pepper, deseeded
   and diced

3 skinless, boneless chicken
   breasts, diced

350 g/12 oz arborio rice

few saffron threads

salt and pepper

1.5 litres/2¾ pints chicken
   stock, simmering

200 g/7 oz canned
   sweetcorn kernels

55 g/2 oz toasted unsalted peanuts

55 g/2 oz freshly grated
   Parmesan cheese

COOK'S TIP

Risottos can be frozen, before
adding the Parmesan cheese, for
up to 1 month, but remember to
reheat this risotto thoroughly as
it contains chicken.

1 Heat the oil and butter in a large,
heavy-based saucepan. Add the
leek and pepper and fry for 1 minute,
then stir in the chicken and cook,
stirring constantly, until golden brown.

2 Stir in the rice and cook for
2–3 minutes.

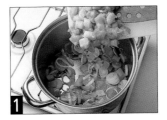

3 Stir in the saffron threads and add
salt and pepper to taste. Add the
stock, a ladleful at a time, then cover
and cook over a low heat, stirring
occasionally, for 20 minutes, or until
the rice is tender and most of the liquid
is absorbed. Do not let the risotto dry
out – add more stock if necessary.

4 Stir in the sweetcorn, peanuts and
Parmesan cheese, then taste and
adjust the seasoning if necessary. Serve
the risotto hot.

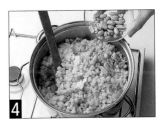

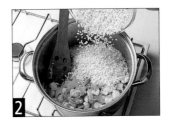

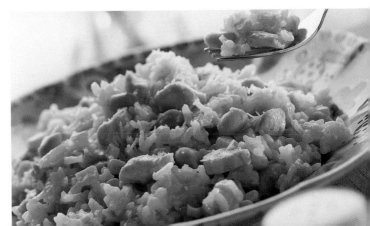

tandoori-style chicken

serves four

8 chicken drumsticks, skinned

150 ml/5 fl oz natural yogurt

1½ tsp finely chopped fresh
  root ginger

1–2 garlic cloves, crushed

1 tsp chilli powder

2 tsp ground cumin

2 tsp ground coriander

1 tsp salt

½ tsp red food colouring

1 tbsp tamarind paste

150 ml/5 fl oz water

150 ml/5 fl oz oil

lettuce leaves, to serve

TO GARNISH

onion rings

sliced tomatoes

lemon wedges

1 Make 2–3 slashes in each chicken drumstick.

2 Place the yogurt in a bowl. Add the ginger, garlic, chilli powder, cumin, coriander, salt and red food colouring and blend together until the mixture is well combined.

3 Add the chicken to the yogurt and spice mixture and mix to coat well. Cover and leave the chicken to marinate in the refrigerator for at least 3 hours.

4 In a separate bowl, mix the tamarind paste with the water and fold into the yogurt and spice mixture. Toss the drumsticks in the mixture, cover and marinate in the refrigerator for a further 3 hours.

5 Preheat the grill to medium–hot. Transfer the drumsticks to a flameproof dish and brush with a little of the oil. Cook, turning the drumsticks occasionally and basting with the remaining oil, for 30–35 minutes, or until tender and the juices run clear when a skewer is inserted into the thickest part of the meat.

6 Arrange the chicken on a bed of lettuce, garnish with onion rings, tomato slices and lemon wedges and serve immediately.

COOK'S TIP

Serve these succulent chicken pieces with warmed naan bread and a raita.

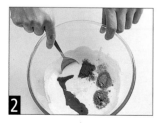

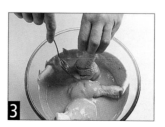

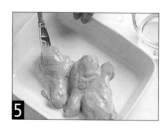

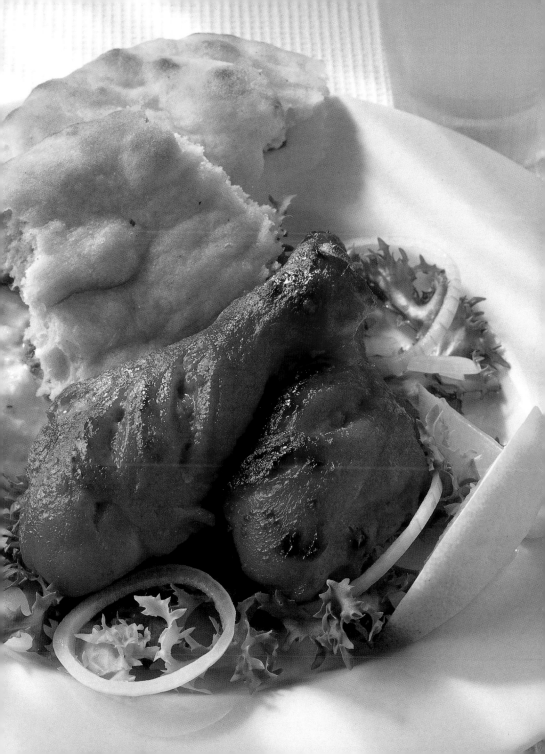

chicken madeira 'french-style'

serves eight

25 g/1 oz butter

20 shallots

250 g/9 oz carrots, sliced

250 g/9 oz rindless bacon, chopped

250 g/9 oz button mushrooms

1 chicken, weighing 1.5 kg/
    3 lb 5 oz

425 ml/15 fl oz white wine

25 g/1 oz plain flour, seasoned

425ml/15 fl oz chicken stock

salt and pepper

1 bouquet garni sachet

150 ml/5 fl oz Madeira wine

mashed potatoes, to serve

COOK'S TIP

You can add any combination of herbs to this recipe – chervil is a popular herb in French cuisine, but add it at the end of cooking so that its delicate flavour is not lost. Other herbs that work well with chicken are parsley and tarragon.

1 Heat the butter in a large, flameproof casserole. Add the shallots, carrots, bacon and mushrooms and fry for 3 minutes, stirring frequently. Transfer to a plate and reserve.

2 Add the chicken to the casserole and cook until browned all over. Add the reserved vegetables and bacon to the casserole.

3 Add the white wine and cook until reduced.

4 Sprinkle with the seasoned flour, stirring to avoid lumps forming.

5 Add the stock, salt and pepper to taste and the bouquet garni. Cover and simmer for 2 hours, or until the chicken is tender and the juices run clear when a skewer is inserted into the thickest part of the meat. About 30 minutes before the end of the cooking time, add the Madeira wine and continue cooking, uncovered.

6 Just before serving, remove and discard the bouquet garni. Carve the chicken and serve with mashed potatoes.

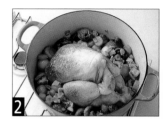

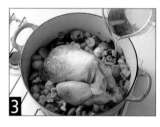

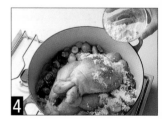

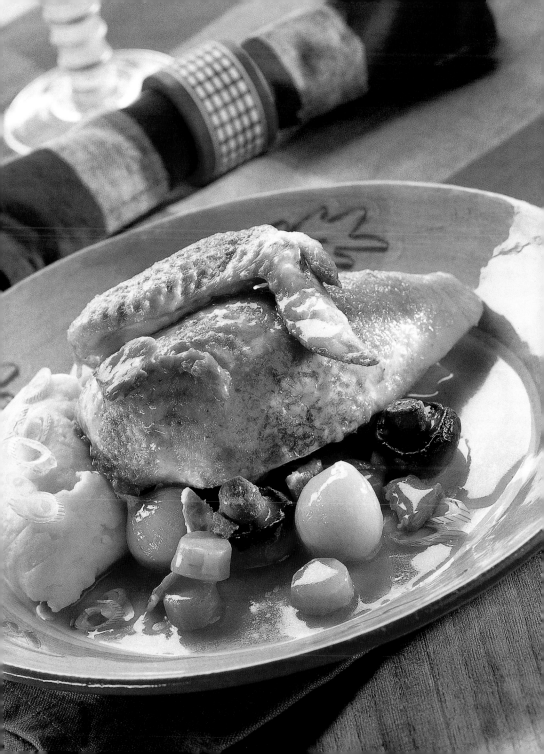

country chicken hotpot

serves four

4 chicken quarters

6 potatoes

salt and pepper

2 fresh thyme sprigs

2 fresh rosemary sprigs

2 bay leaves

200 g/7 oz rindless smoked streaky
    bacon, diced

1 large onion, finely chopped

200 g/7 oz sliced carrots

150 ml/5 fl oz stout

25 g/1 oz melted butter

COOK'S TIP

Serve the hotpot with Rosemary
Dumplings (see page 108) for a
truly hearty meal.

1 Preheat the oven to 150°C/300°F/
Gas Mark 2. Remove the skin
from the chicken quarters, if wished.
Cut the potatoes into 5-mm/¼-inch
thick slices.

2 Arrange a layer of potato slices in
the bottom of a wide casserole.
Season to taste with salt and pepper,
then add the thyme, sprigs of rosemary
and bay leaves.

3 Top with the chicken quarters,
then sprinkle with the bacon,
onion and carrots. Season well
with salt and pepper. Arrange the
remaining potato slices over the top,
overlapping slightly.

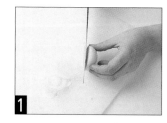

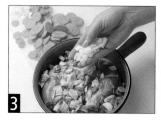

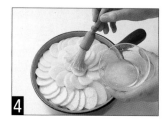

4 Pour over the stout, brush the
potatoes with the melted butter
and cover with a lid.

5 Bake in the oven for 2 hours,
uncovering for the last
30 minutes to allow the potatoes
to brown. Serve hot.

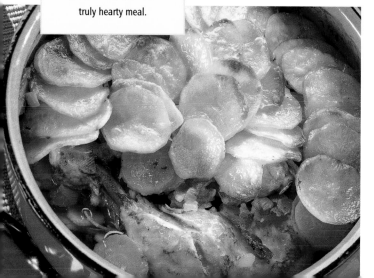

country chicken bake

serves four

2 tbsp sunflower oil

4 chicken quarters

16 small whole onions

3 celery sticks, sliced

400 g/14 oz canned red kidney
    beans, rinsed and drained

4 tomatoes, quartered

200 ml/7 fl oz dry cider or
    chicken stock

4 tbsp chopped fresh parsley

salt and pepper

1 tsp paprika

55 g/2 oz butter

12 slices French bread

COOK'S TIP

Add a crushed garlic clove to the
parsley butter for extra flavour.

1 Preheat the oven to 200°C/400°F/
Gas Mark 6. Heat the oil in a
large, flameproof casserole. Add the
chicken quarters, 2 at a time, and fry
until golden. Using a slotted spoon,
remove the chicken from the casserole
and reserve until required.

2 Add the onions and fry, turning
occasionally, until golden brown.
Add the celery and cook for
2–3 minutes. Return the chicken to
the casserole, then stir in the beans,
tomatoes, cider or stock and half the
parsley. Season to taste with salt and
pepper and sprinkle with the paprika.

3 Cover and cook in the oven for
20–25 minutes, or until the
chicken is tender and the juices run
clear when a skewer is inserted into
the thickest part of the meat.

4 Mix the remaining parsley and
butter together, then spread
evenly over the French bread. Uncover
the casserole, arrange the bread slices
overlapping on top and bake for a
further 10–12 minutes, or until golden
and crisp.

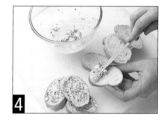

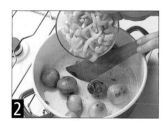

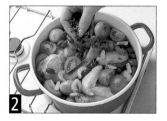

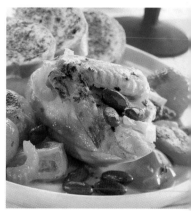

spicy roast chicken

serves four

50 g/1¾ oz ground almonds

50 g/1¾ oz desiccated coconut

150 ml/5 fl oz oil

1 onion, finely chopped

1 tsp chopped fresh root ginger

1 garlic clove, crushed

1 tsp chilli powder

1¼ tsp garam masala

1 tsp salt

150 ml/5 fl oz natural yogurt

4 chicken quarters, skinned

green salad, to serve

TO GARNISH

chopped fresh coriander

1 lemon, cut into wedges

1 Preheat the oven to 160°C/325°F/ Gas Mark 3. In a heavy-based saucepan, dry-fry the almonds and coconut, then set aside.

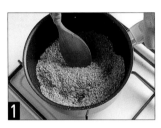

2 Heat the oil in a frying pan and fry the onion, stirring, until golden brown.

3 Place the ginger, garlic, chilli powder, garam masala and salt in a bowl and mix in the yogurt. Add the almonds and coconut and mix well.

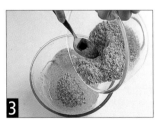

4 Add the onions to the spice mixture, blend and set aside.

5 Arrange the chicken quarters in the base of an ovenproof dish. Spoon the yogurt and spice mixture over the chicken.

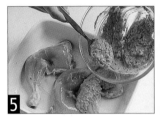

6 Cook in the oven for 35–45 minutes, or until the chicken is tender and the juices run clear when a skewer is inserted into the thickest part of the meat. Garnish with coriander and lemon wedges and serve with a green salad.

COOK'S TIP

If you want a spicier dish, add more chilli powder and garam masala.

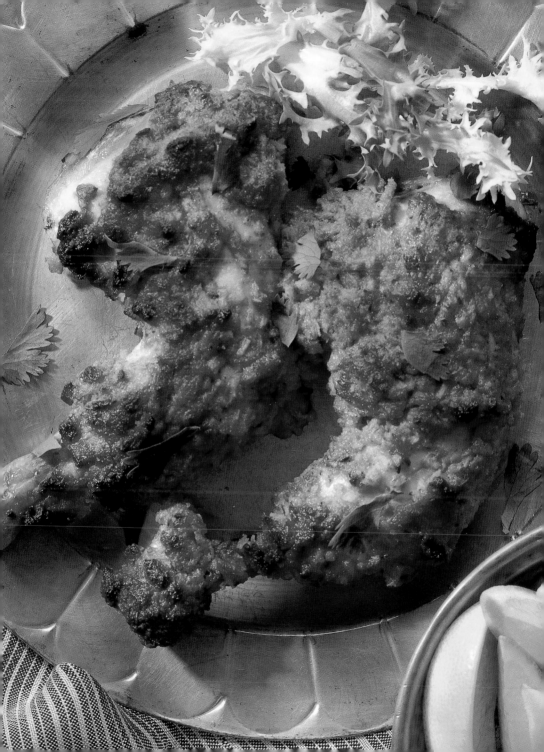

chicken with baby onions & green peas

serves four

250 g/9 oz pork fat

salt and pepper

55 g/2 oz butter

16 small onions or shallots

1 kg/2 lb 4 oz boneless
    chicken pieces

25 g/1 oz plain flour

600 ml/1 pint chicken stock

1 bouquet garni sachet

500 g/1 lb 2 oz shelled fresh peas

COOK'S TIP

If you want to cut down on the fat, use lean bacon, cut into small cubes, rather than pork fat.

1 Preheat the oven to 200°C/400°F/ Gas Mark 6. Cut the pork fat into small cubes. Bring a saucepan of lightly salted water to the boil. Add the pork fat cubes and simmer for 3 minutes. Drain and dry on kitchen paper.

2 Melt the butter in a large frying pan. Add the pork fat and onions or shallots and fry gently for 3 minutes, or until lightly browned.

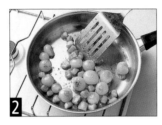

3 Remove the pork fat and onions from the frying pan and reserve until required. Add the chicken pieces to the frying pan and cook until browned all over. Transfer the chicken pieces to a large, flameproof casserole.

4 Add the flour to the frying pan and cook, stirring, until it begins to brown. Slowly blend in the stock.

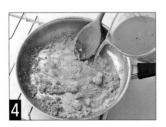

5 Pour the sauce over the chicken and add the bouquet garni. Cover the casserole and cook in the oven for 35 minutes, or until the chicken is tender and the juices run clear when a skewer is inserted into the thickest part of the meat.

6 Remove and discard the bouquet garni about 10 minutes before the end of the cooking time and stir in the peas and reserved pork fat and onions. Taste and adjust the seasoning, if necessary. Return to the oven.

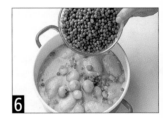

7 To serve, place the chicken pieces on a large platter, surrounded by the pork, peas and onions.

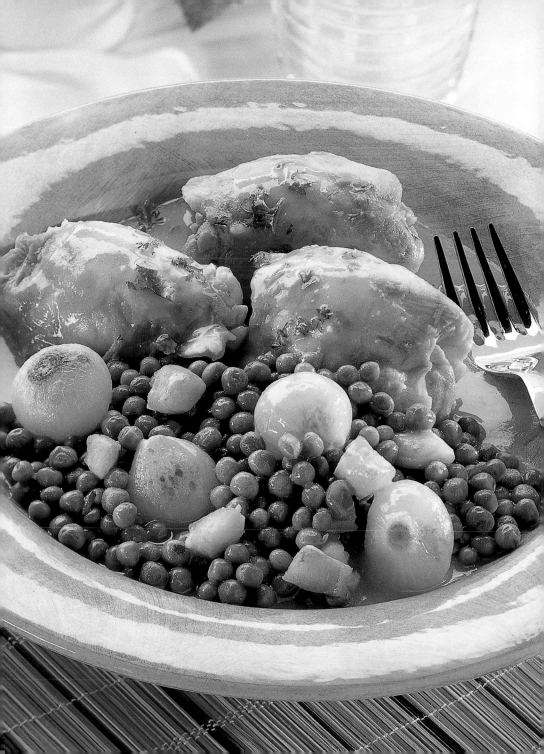

jamaican hotpot

serves four

2 tsp sunflower oil

4 chicken drumsticks

4 chicken thighs

1 onion

750 g/1 lb 10 oz piece pumpkin
    or squash

1 green pepper

2.5-cm/1-inch piece fresh root
    ginger, finely chopped

400 g/14 oz canned
    chopped tomatoes

300 ml/10 fl oz chicken stock

55 g/2 oz split red lentils, washed

garlic salt and cayenne pepper

350 g/12 oz canned sweetcorn
    kernels, drained

crusty bread, to serve

VARIATION

If you can't find fresh root ginger,
add 1 teaspoon of ground
allspice for a fragrant aroma.
If squash or pumpkin is not
available, swede makes a very
good substitute.

---

1 Preheat the oven to 190°C/375°F/
Gas Mark 5. Heat the oil in a
large, flameproof casserole. Add the
chicken joints and fry until golden
brown, turning frequently.

2 Using a sharp knife, slice the
onion, then peel and dice the
pumpkin and deseed and slice the
green pepper.

3 Drain any excess fat from the
casserole and add the onion,
pumpkin and pepper. Gently fry for a
few minutes until lightly browned. Add
the ginger, tomatoes, stock and lentils.
Season lightly with garlic salt and
cayenne pepper.

4 Cover the casserole and cook in
the oven for 1 hour, or until the
vegetables and chicken are tender and
the chicken juices run clear when a
skewer is inserted into the thickest part
of the meat.

5 Add the drained sweetcorn and
cook for a further 5 minutes. Taste
and adjust the seasoning, if necessary,
then serve with crusty bread.

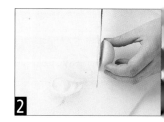
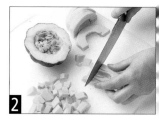
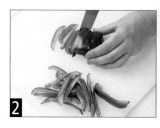
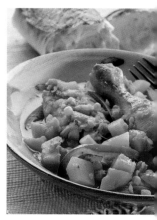

rich mediterranean chicken casserole

serves four

8 boneless chicken thighs

2 tbsp olive oil

1 red onion, sliced

2 garlic cloves, crushed

1 large red pepper, deseeded and
   thickly sliced

thinly pared rind and juice of
   1 small orange

125 ml/4 fl oz chicken stock

400 g/14 oz canned
   chopped tomatoes

25 g/1 oz sun-dried tomatoes,
   thinly sliced

1 tbsp chopped fresh thyme

50 g/1¾ oz stoned black olives

salt and pepper

fresh crusty bread, to serve

TO GARNISH

orange rind

fresh thyme sprigs

COOK'S TIP

Sun-dried tomatoes have a dense
texture and concentrated taste,
and add intense flavour to
slow-cooking casseroles.

---

1 Dry-fry the chicken in a large, heavy-based or non-stick frying pan over a fairly high heat, turning occasionally, until golden brown. Using a slotted spoon, drain off any excess fat from the chicken and transfer to a large, flameproof casserole.

2 Heat the oil in the frying pan. Add the onion, garlic and pepper and fry over a medium heat for 3–4 minutes. Transfer to the casserole.

3 Add the orange rind and juice, stock, canned tomatoes and sun-dried tomatoes and stir to mix.

4 Bring to the boil, then cover the casserole and simmer very gently over a low heat for 1 hour, stirring occasionally, until the chicken is tender. Add the chopped thyme and black olives, then season to taste with salt and pepper.

5 Sprinkle orange rind and thyme sprigs over the casserole to garnish, and serve with crusty bread.

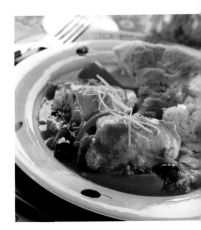

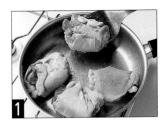

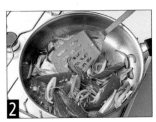

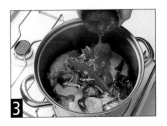

131

pot roast orange & sesame chicken

serves four

2 tbsp sunflower oil

1 chicken, weighing 1.5 kg/
   3 lb 5 oz

2 large oranges

2 small onions, quartered

500 g/1 lb 2 oz small whole carrots
   or thin carrots, cut into 5-cm/
   2-inch lengths

salt and pepper

150 ml/5 fl oz orange juice

2 tbsp brandy

2 tbsp sesame seeds

1 tbsp cornflour

1 tbsp water

VARIATION

Use lemons instead of oranges
for a sharper citrus flavour and
place a fresh thyme sprig in the
chicken cavity with the lemon
half as they are a good
flavour combination.

---

1 Preheat the oven to 190°C/375°F/ Gas Mark 5. Heat the oil in a large, deep, flameproof casserole. Add the chicken and fry, turning occasionally, until evenly browned. Remove the chicken.

2 Cut 1 orange in half and place 1 half inside the chicken cavity. Put the chicken back in the casserole and arrange the onions and carrots around it.

3 Season well with salt and pepper and pour over the orange juice.

4 Cut the remaining oranges into thin wedges and tuck around the chicken in the casserole, among the vegetables.

5 Cover and cook in the oven for 1½ hours, or until the vegetables and chicken are tender and the chicken juices run clear when a skewer is inserted into the thickest part of the meat. Uncover and sprinkle with the brandy and sesame seeds, then return to the oven for 10 minutes.

6 To serve, transfer the chicken to a large platter. Place the vegetables around the chicken. Skim any excess fat from the juices in the casserole. Blend the cornflour with the water, then stir into the juices and bring to the boil, stirring constantly. Season to taste with salt and pepper, then serve the sauce with the chicken.

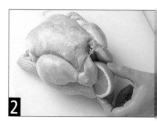

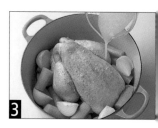

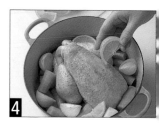

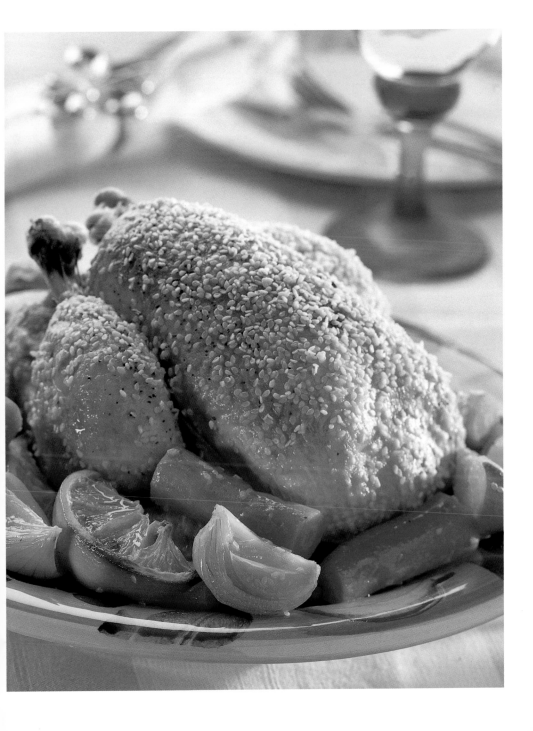

caribbean chicken

COOK'S TIP

When buying mangoes, bear in mind that the skin of ripe mangoes varies in colour from green to pinky-red and the flesh from pale yellow to bright orange. Choose mangoes that yield to gentle pressure.

1 Using a sharp knife, slash the chicken drumsticks at intervals, then place them in a large, non-metallic bowl.

2 Grate the rind from the limes and reserve until required.

3 Squeeze the juice from the limes and sprinkle over the chicken with the cayenne pepper. Cover and leave to marinate in the refrigerator for at least 2 hours, or preferably overnight.

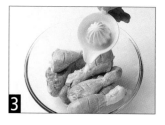

4 Peel the mangoes. Cut lengthways either side of the central stone. Discard the stone and slice the flesh.

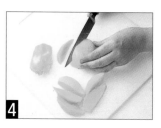

5 Drain the chicken drumsticks using a slotted spoon and reserve the marinade. Heat the oil in a wide, heavy-based frying pan. Add the chicken drumsticks and sauté, turning frequently, until golden. Stir in the marinade, reserved lime rind, mango slices and the sugar.

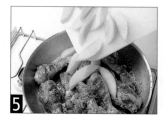

6 Cover the frying pan and simmer gently, stirring occasionally, for 15 minutes, or until the chicken is tender and the juices run clear when a skewer is inserted into the thickest part of the meat. Sprinkle with grated coconut, if using, and garnish with lime wedges and coriander sprigs.

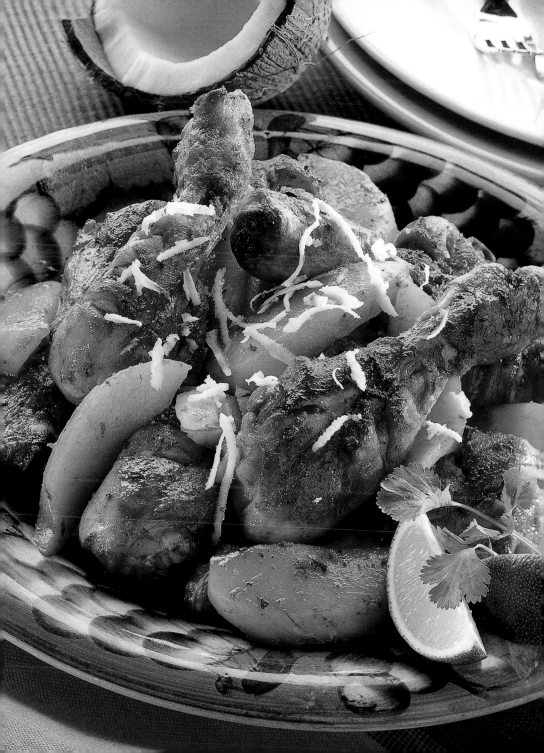

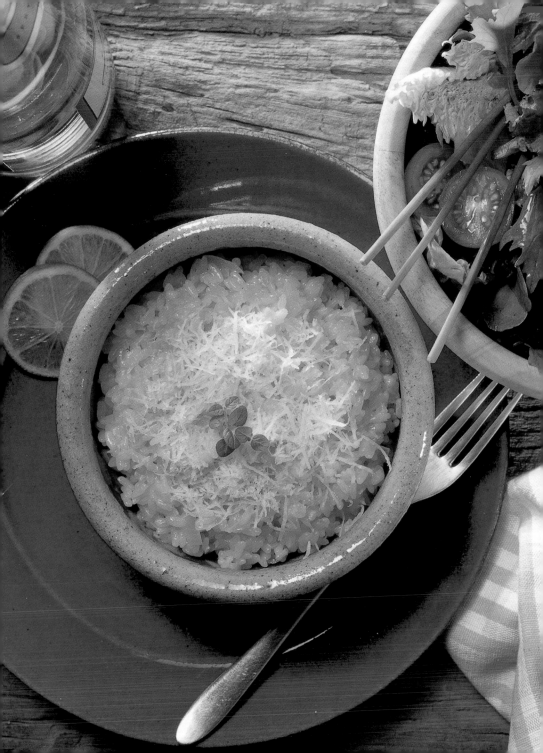

Vegetables

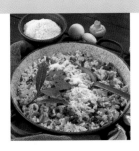

Nutritionists tell us that we should eat more vegetables, but it isn't always easy to persuade the family to eat up their greens, especially if they are sitting in an unappetizing heap on the side of the plate. This chapter provides the answer with a spectacular collection of mouthwatering vegetable dishes – soups, bakes, risottos, casseroles and curries. Beans, peas, lentils, broccoli, cauliflower, mushrooms, peppers, onions, courgettes, tomatoes, even the humble potato, all take a starring role and are combined with each other for a melt-in-the-mouth medley or with other ingredients, such as pasta, to satisfy even the hungriest appetite. A vegetarian main course is an easy way to ring the changes in the weekly menu. From Mushroom and Cheese Risotto (see page 171) to Coconut Vegetable Curry (see page 191), vegetables have never looked – or tasted – so good.

roasted mediterranean vegetable soup

serves six

2–3 tbsp olive oil

700 g/1 lb 9 oz ripe tomatoes,
   peeled, cored and halved

3 large yellow peppers, halved
   and deseeded

3 courgettes, halved lengthways

1 small aubergine, halved
   lengthways

4 garlic cloves, halved

2 onions, cut into eighths

salt and pepper

pinch of dried thyme

1 litre/1¾ pints vegetable stock

125 ml/4 fl oz single cream

shredded fresh basil leaves,
   to garnish

1 Preheat the oven to 190°C/375°F/
Gas Mark 5. Brush a large,
shallow baking dish with oil. Laying
cut-side down, arrange the tomatoes,
peppers, courgettes and aubergine in
1 layer (use 2 dishes if necessary). Tuck
the garlic and onions into the gaps and
drizzle the vegetables with the
remaining oil. Season lightly with salt
and pepper and sprinkle with thyme.

2 Bake the vegetables in the oven,
uncovered, for 30–35 minutes,
or until soft and browned around the
edges. Leave to cool, then scrape out
the aubergine flesh and remove the
skin from the peppers.

3 Working in batches, put the
aubergine and pepper flesh,
together with the courgettes, into a
food processor and chop to the
consistency of salsa or pickle; do not
purée. Alternatively, place in a bowl
and chop with a knife.

4 Combine the stock with the
chopped vegetable mixture in a
saucepan and simmer over a medium
heat for 20–30 minutes, or until all the
vegetables are tender and the flavours
have completely blended.

5 Stir in the cream and heat the
soup through over a low heat
for 5 minutes, stirring occasionally.
Taste and adjust the seasoning,
if necessary. Ladle the soup into
warmed bowls and garnish with basil,
then serve.

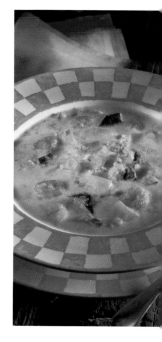

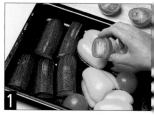

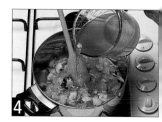

tuscan bean & vegetable soup

serves four

1 onion, chopped

1 garlic clove, finely chopped

2 celery sticks, sliced

1 large carrot, diced

400 g/14 oz canned
    chopped tomatoes

150 ml/5 fl oz Italian dry red wine

1.2 litres/2 pints vegetable stock

1 tsp dried oregano

425 g/15 oz canned mixed beans
    and pulses

2 courgettes, diced

1 tbsp tomato purée

salt and pepper

TO SERVE

Pesto (see page 141) or soured cream

crusty bread

COOK'S TIP

Use a jar of good quality pesto
from the supermarket as the
garnish if you are too busy to
make your own.

1 Place the onion, garlic, celery and carrot in a large saucepan. Stir in the chopped tomatoes, wine, vegetable stock and oregano.

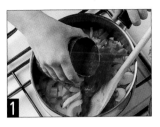

2 Bring to the boil, then reduce the heat, cover and leave to simmer for 15 minutes. Stir the beans and pulses into the mixture with the courgettes, and cook, uncovered, for a further 5 minutes.

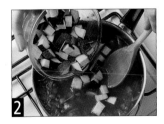

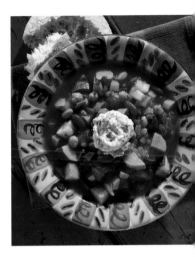

3 Add the tomato purée to the mixture and season to taste with salt and pepper. Heat through, stirring occasionally, for a further 2–3 minutes, but be careful not to allow the mixture to boil again.

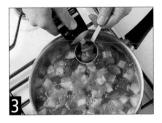

4 Ladle the soup into warmed bowls and serve with a spoonful of Pesto on each portion, accompanied by chunks of crusty bread.

tuscan onion soup

serves four

50 g/1¾ oz pancetta, diced

1 tbsp olive oil

4 large onions, thinly sliced
     into rings

3 garlic cloves, chopped

850 ml/1½ pints hot chicken or
     ham stock

4 slices ciabatta or other
     Italian bread

50 g/1¾ oz butter

75 g/2¾ oz Gruyère or Cheddar
     cheese, coarsely grated

salt and pepper

COOK'S TIP

Pancetta is available from most
delicatessens and some large
supermarkets, but you can use
unsmoked bacon instead.

1 Dry-fry the pancetta in a large saucepan for 3–4 minutes, or until it begins to brown. Remove the pancetta from the saucepan and set aside until required.

2 Add the oil to the saucepan and cook the onions and garlic over a high heat for 4 minutes. Reduce the heat, cover and cook for 15 minutes, or until the onions and garlic are lightly caramelized.

3 Add the stock to the saucepan and bring to the boil, then reduce the heat and leave the mixture to simmer, covered, for 10 minutes.

4 Preheat the grill. Toast the ciabatta under the hot grill for 2–3 minutes on each side, or until golden. Spread the toast with the butter and top each slice with grated cheese. Cut into bite-sized pieces.

5 Add the reserved pancetta to the soup and season to taste with salt and pepper. Pour into 4 soup bowls and top with the toasted bread.

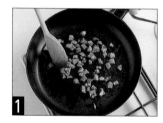

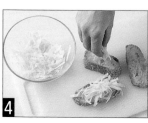

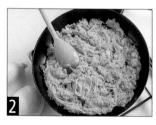

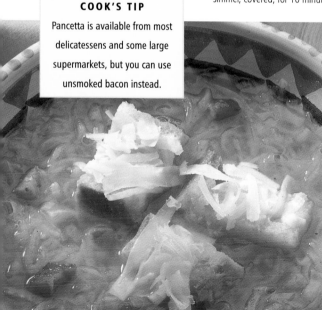

green vegetable soup with basil pesto

serves six

1 tbsp olive oil

1 onion, finely chopped

1 large leek, split and thinly sliced

1 celery stick, thinly sliced

1 carrot, quartered and thinly sliced

1 garlic clove, finely chopped

1.4 litres/2½ pints water

1 potato, diced

1 parsnip, finely diced

1 small kohlrabi or turnip, diced

150 g/5½ oz French beans, cut into
    small pieces

150 g/5½ oz fresh or frozen peas

2 small courgettes, quartered
    and sliced

400 g/14 oz canned flageolet
    beans, rinsed and drained

salt and pepper

100 g/3½ oz fresh spinach leaves,
    finely shredded

PESTO

1 large garlic clove, very
    finely chopped

15 g/½ oz fresh basil leaves

4 tbsp extra virgin olive oil

85 g/3 oz freshly grated
    Parmesan cheese

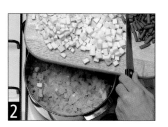

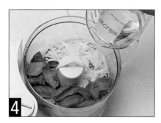

1 Heat the oil in a large saucepan. Cook the onion and leek over a low heat, stirring occasionally, for 5 minutes. Add the celery, carrot and garlic, cover and cook for a further 5 minutes.

2 Add the water, potato, parsnip, kohlrabi or turnip and French beans. Bring to the boil, then reduce the heat, cover and simmer for 5 minutes.

3 Add the peas, courgettes and flageolet beans and season to taste with salt and pepper. Cover and simmer for 25 minutes, or until all the vegetables are tender.

4 Meanwhile, make the pesto. Put all the ingredients in a food processor and process until smooth, scraping down the sides as necessary. Alternatively, pound together using a pestle and mortar.

5 Add the spinach to the soup and simmer for 5 minutes. Stir in a spoonful of the pesto. Ladle the soup into bowls and hand round the remaining pesto separately.

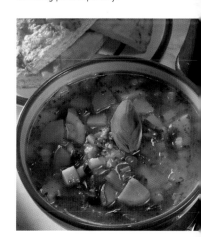

vegetable soup with cannellini beans

serves four

1 small aubergine

2 large tomatoes

1 potato, peeled

1 carrot, peeled

1 leek

400 g/14 oz canned
cannellini beans

850 ml/1½ pints hot vegetable or
chicken stock

2 tsp dried basil

15 g/½ oz dried porcini mushrooms,
soaked for 10 minutes in enough
warm water to cover

50 g/1¾ oz dried vermicelli

3 tbsp Pesto (see page 141 or use
shop-bought)

freshly grated Parmesan cheese,
to serve (optional)

1 Slice the aubergine into rings
about 1 cm/½ inch thick, then cut
each ring into 4.

2 Cut the tomatoes and potato into
small dice. Cut the carrot into
sticks about 2.5 cm/1 inch long and
slice the leek into rings.

3 Place the beans and their liquid in
a large saucepan. Add the
aubergine, tomatoes, potato, carrot
and leek, stirring to mix.

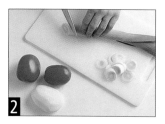

COOK'S TIP

Porcini are a wild mushroom
grown in southern Italy. When
dried and rehydrated they have a
very intense flavour, so although
they are expensive to buy, only a
small amount is required to add
flavour to soups or risottos.

4 Add the stock to the saucepan
and bring to the boil. Reduce the
heat and simmer for 15 minutes.

5 Add the basil, the mushrooms
and their soaking liquid and the
vermicelli and simmer for 5 minutes, or
until all the vegetables are tender.

6 Remove the saucepan from the
heat and stir in the Pesto. Serve
the soup with grated Parmesan cheese,
if wished.

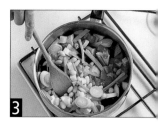

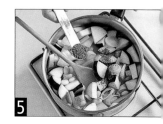

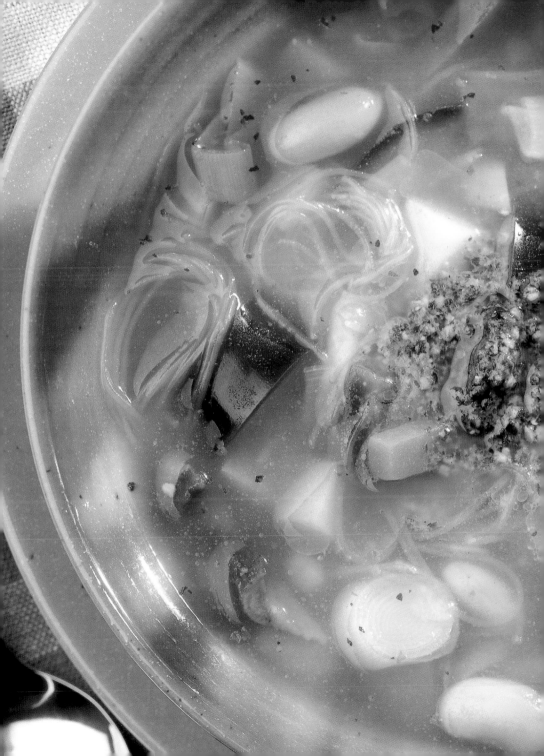

brown lentil soup with pasta

serves four

4 streaky bacon rashers, cut into
  small squares

1 onion, chopped

2 garlic cloves, crushed

2 celery sticks, chopped

50 g/1¾ oz dried farfalline or
  spaghetti broken into
  small pieces

400 g/14 oz canned brown
  lentils, drained

1.2 litres/2 pints hot ham or
  vegetable stock

2 tbsp chopped fresh mint

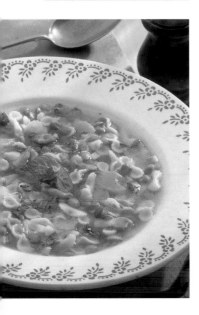

1 Place the bacon in a large frying pan with the onion, garlic and celery. Dry-fry for 4–5 minutes, stirring, until the onion is tender and the bacon is just beginning to brown.

2 Add the pasta pieces to the pan and cook, stirring, for 1 minute to coat the pasta in the oil.

COOK'S TIP

If you prefer to use dried lentils, add the stock before the pasta and cook for 1–1¼ hours, or until the lentils are tender. Add the pasta and cook for a further 12–15 minutes.

VARIATION

Any type of pasta can be used in this recipe – try fusilli, conchiglie or rigatoni, if you prefer.

3 Add the lentils and the stock and bring to the boil. Reduce the heat and leave to simmer for 12–15 minutes, or until the pasta is tender.

4 Remove the pan from the heat and stir in the mint.

5 Transfer the soup to warmed soup bowls and serve immediately.

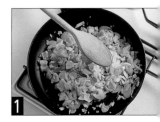
1

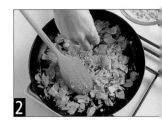
2

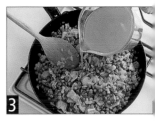
3

lentil, pasta & vegetable soup

serves four

1 tbsp olive oil

1 onion, chopped

4 garlic cloves, finely chopped

350 g/12 oz carrots, sliced

1 celery stick, sliced

225 g/8 oz split red lentils, washed

600 ml/1 pint vegetable stock

700 ml/1¼ pints boiling water

salt and pepper

150 g/5½ oz dried pasta

150 ml/5 fl oz natural low-fat
    fromage frais, plus extra to serve

2 tbsp chopped fresh parsley,
    to garnish

1 Heat the oil in a large saucepan over a medium heat and fry the onion, garlic, carrots and celery, stirring gently, for 5 minutes, or until beginning to soften.

2 Add the lentils, stock and water. Season well with salt and pepper, stir and return to the boil. Reduce the heat and simmer, uncovered, for 15 minutes, or until the lentils are completely tender. Allow to cool for 10 minutes.

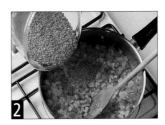

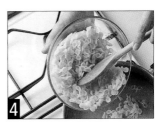

COOK'S TIP

Avoid boiling the soup once the fromage frais has been added or it will separate and become watery, spoiling the appearance of the soup.

3 Meanwhile, bring a separate saucepan of water to the boil and cook the pasta according to the packet instructions. Drain well and set aside.

4 Transfer the soup to a food processor or blender and process until smooth. Return to a clean saucepan and add the pasta. Return to a simmer and heat for 2–3 minutes, or until piping hot. Remove from the heat and stir in the fromage frais. Taste and adjust the seasoning if necessary.

5 Serve, garnished with pepper and parsley, with extra fromage frais, if wished.

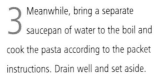

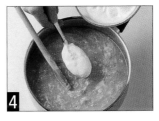

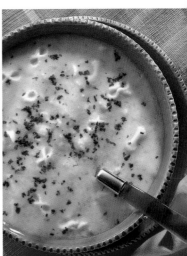

haricot bean & pasta soup

serves four

250 g/9 oz haricot beans, soaked
    for 3 hours in cold water
    and drained

4 tbsp olive oil

2 large onions, sliced

3 garlic cloves, chopped

400 g/14 oz canned
    chopped tomatoes

1 tsp dried oregano

1 tsp tomato purée

850 ml/1½ pints water

100 g/3½ oz dried fusilli or
    conchigliette

salt and pepper

115 g/4 oz sun-dried tomatoes,
    drained and thinly sliced

1 tbsp chopped fresh coriander or
    flat-leaved parsley

2 tbsp Parmesan cheese shavings,
    to serve

1 Put the beans in a large saucepan, add sufficient cold water to cover and bring to the boil. Boil rapidly over a high heat for 15 minutes. Drain the beans and keep warm until required.

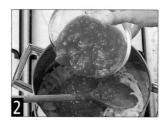

2 Heat the oil in a large saucepan over a medium heat and fry the onions for 2–3 minutes, or until they are just beginning to change colour. Stir in the garlic and cook for 1 minute. Stir in the canned tomatoes, oregano and tomato purée.

3 Add the water and the beans to the saucepan. Bring to the boil, then reduce the heat, cover and simmer for 45 minutes, or until the beans are tender.

COOK'S TIP

If preferred, place the beans in a saucepan of cold water and bring to the boil. Remove from the heat and leave the beans to cool in the water. Drain and rinse the beans before using.

4 Add the pasta to the saucepan and season to taste with salt and pepper. Stir in the sun-dried tomatoes and return to the boil. Reduce the heat, partially cover and simmer for 10 minutes, or until the pasta is tender but still firm to the bite.

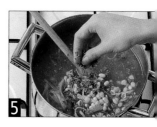

5 Stir the coriander or parsley into the soup. Ladle into warmed bowls, sprinkle over the Parmesan cheese and serve immediately.

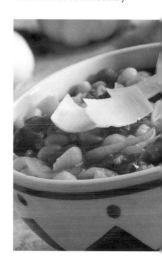

pea & egg noodle soup

serves four

3 rindless smoked bacon
   rashers, diced

1 large onion, chopped

1 tbsp butter

450 g/1 lb dried peas, soaked
   in cold water for 2 hours
   and drained

2.3 litres/4 pints chicken stock

salt and pepper

225 g/8 oz dried egg noodles

150 ml/5 fl oz double cream

chopped fresh parsley, to garnish

Parmesan cheese croûtons (see
   Cook's Tip, to serve)

1 Put the bacon, onion and butter into a large saucepan and cook over a low heat for 6 minutes.

2 Add the peas and the stock to the saucepan and bring to the boil. Season lightly with salt and pepper. Reduce the heat, cover and simmer for 1½ hours.

3 Add the egg noodles to the saucepan and simmer for a further 15 minutes.

4 Pour in the cream and blend thoroughly. Transfer to a warmed tureen and garnish with parsley. Top with the croûtons and serve.

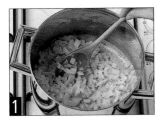

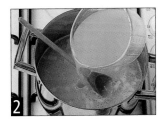

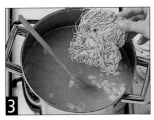

COOK'S TIP

To make Parmesan cheese croûtons, cut a French stick into slices. Coat lightly with olive oil and sprinkle with Parmesan. Grill for about 30 seconds.

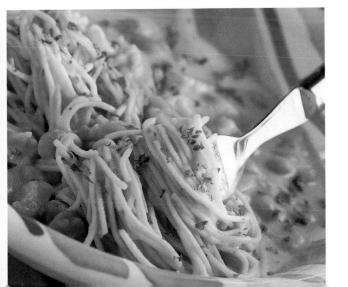

potato, apple & rocket soup

serves four

4 tbsp butter

900 g/2 lb waxy potatoes, diced

1 red onion, quartered

1 tbsp lemon juice

1 litre/1¾ pints chicken stock

450 g/1 lb dessert apples, peeled
and diced

pinch of ground allspice

50 g/1¾ oz rocket leaves, plus
extra to garnish

salt and pepper

warmed crusty bread, to serve

TO GARNISH

slices of red apple

chopped spring onions

COOK'S TIP

If rocket is unavailable, use baby
spinach leaves instead for a
similar flavour.

1 Melt the butter in a large
saucepan and add the potatoes
and onion. Sauté gently for 5 minutes,
stirring constantly.

2 Add the lemon juice, chicken
stock, apples and allspice and stir
to combine.

3 Bring to the boil, then reduce the
heat to a simmer, cover and cook
for 15 minutes.

4 Add the rocket to the soup and
cook for a further 10 minutes, or
until the potatoes are cooked through.

5 Transfer half the soup to a food
processor or blender. Process for
1 minute. Stir the purée into the soup
in the saucepan and heat through.

6 Season to taste with salt and
pepper. Ladle into warmed soup
bowls and garnish with the rocket,
apple slices and spring onions. Serve
at once with warmed crusty bread.

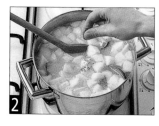

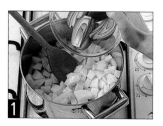

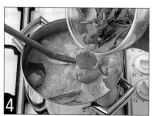

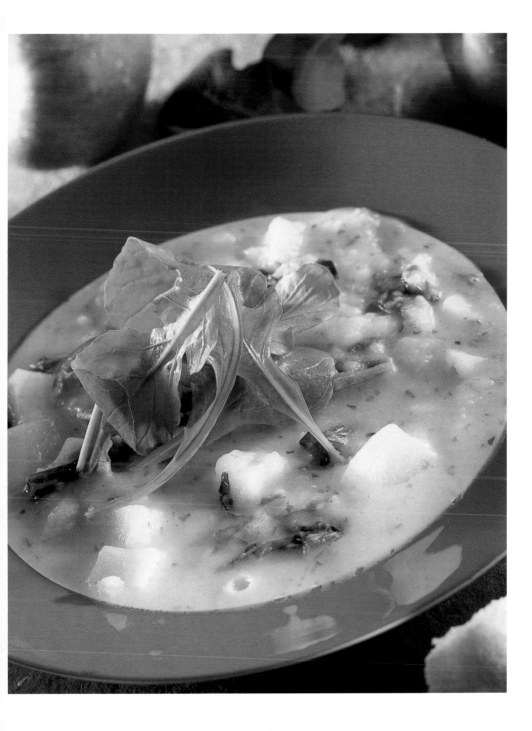

sweet potato & onion soup

serves four

2 tbsp vegetable oil

900 g/2 lb sweet potatoes, diced

1 carrot, diced

2 onions, sliced

2 garlic cloves, crushed

600 ml/1 pint vegetable stock

300 ml/10 fl oz unsweetened
   orange juice

225 ml/8 fl oz low-fat natural yogurt

2 tbsp chopped fresh coriander

salt and pepper

TO GARNISH

fresh coriander sprigs

strips of orange rind

1 Heat the oil in a large, heavy-based saucepan and add the sweet potatoes, carrot, onions and garlic. Sauté the vegetables over a low heat, stirring constantly, for 5 minutes, or until softened.

2 Pour in the stock and orange juice and bring to the boil.

3 Reduce the heat, cover the soup and simmer for 20 minutes, or until the sweet potatoes and carrot are tender.

4 Transfer the mixture to a food processor or blender in batches and process for 1 minute until smooth. Return the purée to the rinsed-out saucepan.

COOK'S TIP

This soup can be chilled before serving, if preferred. If chilling, stir the yogurt into the dish just before serving. Serve in chilled bowls.

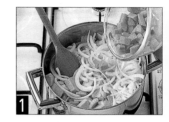

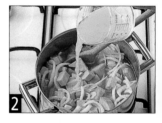

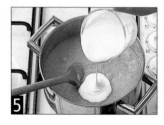

5 Stir in the yogurt and chopped coriander and season to taste with salt and pepper.

6 Serve in warmed soup bowls and garnish with coriander sprigs and orange rind.

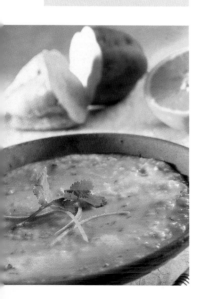

sweetcorn, potato & cheese soup

serves four

25 g/1 oz butter

2 shallots, finely chopped

225 g/8 oz potatoes, diced

4 tbsp plain flour

2 tbsp dry white wine

300 ml/10 fl oz milk

325 g/11½ oz canned sweetcorn
kernels, drained

85 g/3 oz Gruyère, Emmenthal or
Cheddar cheese, grated

8–10 fresh sage leaves, chopped

425 ml/15 fl oz double cream

fresh sage sprigs, to garnish

CROUTONS

2–3 slices day-old white bread

2 tbsp olive oil

1 To make the croûtons, cut the crusts off the bread slices, then cut the remaining bread into 5-mm/ ¼-inch squares. Heat the oil in a heavy-based frying pan and add the bread cubes. Cook, tossing and stirring constantly, until evenly coloured. Drain the croûtons thoroughly on kitchen paper and reserve.

2 Melt the butter in a large, heavy-based saucepan. Add the shallots and cook over a low heat, stirring occasionally, for 5 minutes, or until softened. Add the potatoes and cook, stirring, for 2 minutes.

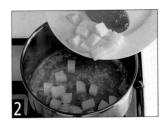

3 Sprinkle in the flour and cook, stirring, for 1 minute. Remove the saucepan from the heat and stir in the wine, then gradually stir in the milk. Return the saucepan to the heat and bring to the boil, stirring constantly, then reduce the heat and simmer.

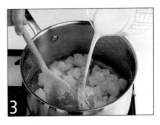

4 Stir in the sweetcorn, cheese, sage and cream and heat through gently until the cheese has just melted. Ladle the soup into warmed bowls, scatter over the croûtons and garnish with sage sprigs. Serve immediately.

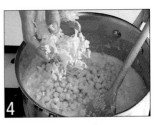

COOK'S TIP

When you are cooking croûtons, make sure that the oil is very hot before adding the bread cubes, otherwise the cubes may turn out soggy rather than crisp.

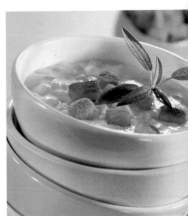

broccoli soup with cream cheese

serves four

400 g/14 oz broccoli
    (from 1 large head)
2 tsp butter
1 tsp oil
1 onion, finely chopped
1 leek, thinly sliced
1 small carrot, finely chopped
3 tbsp long-grain rice
850 ml/1½ pints water
1 bay leaf
salt and pepper
freshly grated nutmeg
4 tbsp double cream
100 g/3½ oz soft cheese
croûtons (see Cook's Tip,
    page 151), to serve

1 Divide the broccoli into small florets and cut off the stems. Peel the large stems and then chop all the stems into small pieces.

2 Heat the butter and oil in a large saucepan over a medium heat and add the onion, leek and carrot. Cook the vegetables for 3–4 minutes, stirring frequently, until the onion is softened.

3 Add the broccoli stems, rice, water, bay leaf and a pinch of salt. Bring just to the boil, then reduce the heat to low. Cover the soup and simmer for 15 minutes. Add the broccoli florets and cook, covered, for a further 15–20 minutes, or until the rice and vegetables are tender. Remove and discard the bay leaf.

4 Season the soup with nutmeg, pepper and, if needed, more salt. Stir in the cream and soft cheese. Simmer over a low heat for a few minutes until heated through, stirring occasionally. Adjust the seasoning if necessary. Ladle into warmed bowls and serve sprinkled with the croûtons.

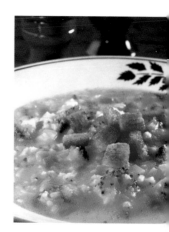

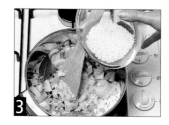

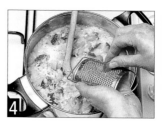

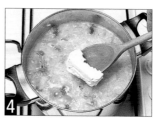

spicy courgette soup with rice & lime

serves four

2 tbsp vegetable oil

4 garlic cloves, thinly sliced

1–2 tbsp mild red chilli powder

¼–½ tsp ground cumin

1.5 litres/2¾ pints chicken,
vegetable or beef stock

2 courgettes, cut into
bite-sized chunks

4 tbsp long-grain rice

salt and pepper

fresh oregano sprigs, to garnish

lime wedges, to serve

COOK'S TIP

Choose courgettes that are firm
to the touch and have shiny skin.
They should not be too large.

1 Heat the oil in a heavy-based saucepan. Add the garlic and cook for 2 minutes, or until softened and just beginning to change colour. Add the chilli powder and cumin and cook over a medium–low heat for 1 minute.

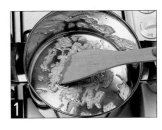

2 Stir in the stock, courgettes and rice, then cook over a medium–high heat for 10 minutes, or until the courgettes are just tender and the rice is cooked through. Season the soup to taste with salt and pepper.

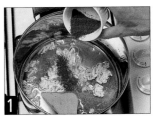

3 Ladle into soup bowls, garnish with oregano sprigs and serve with lime wedges.

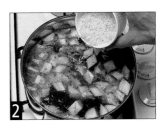

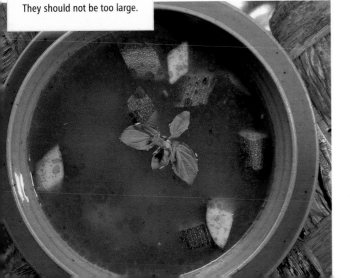

VARIATION

Instead of rice, use rice-shaped
pasta, such as orzo or semone
de melone, or very thin pasta
known as fideo. Use yellow
summer squash instead of the
courgettes and add cooked
pinto beans in place of the rice.
Diced tomatoes also make
a tasty addition.

calabrian mushroom soup

2 tbsp olive oil

1 onion, chopped

450 g/1 lb mixed mushrooms, such
as cep, oyster and button

300 ml/10 fl oz milk

850 ml/1½ pints hot vegetable stock

salt and pepper

8 slices rustic bread or French stick

3 tbsp butter, melted

2 garlic cloves, crushed

75 g/2¾ oz Gruyère cheese,
finely grated

COOK'S TIP

Mushrooms absorb liquid, which
can lessen the flavour and affect
cooking properties. Wipe them
with a damp cloth rather than
rinsing them in water.

---

1 Heat the oil in a large frying pan
and cook the onion for 3–4
minutes, or until softened and golden.

2 Wipe each mushroom with
a damp cloth and cut any
large mushrooms into smaller,
bite-sized pieces.

3 Add the mushrooms to the pan,
stirring quickly to coat in the oil.

4 Add the milk to the pan and bring
to the boil. Reduce the heat,
cover and leave to simmer for
5 minutes. Gradually stir in the hot
stock and salt and pepper to taste.

5 Preheat the grill to medium. Toast
the bread under the hot grill on
both sides until golden.

VARIATION

Supermarkets stock a wide
variety of wild mushrooms. If you
prefer, use a combination of
cultivated and wild mushrooms.

---

6 Mix the butter and garlic together
and spoon generously over
the toast.

7 Place the toast in the bottom of
a large tureen or divide it among
4 individual serving bowls and pour
over the hot soup. Top with the grated
cheese and serve at once.

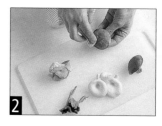

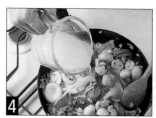

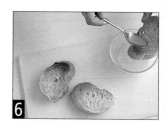

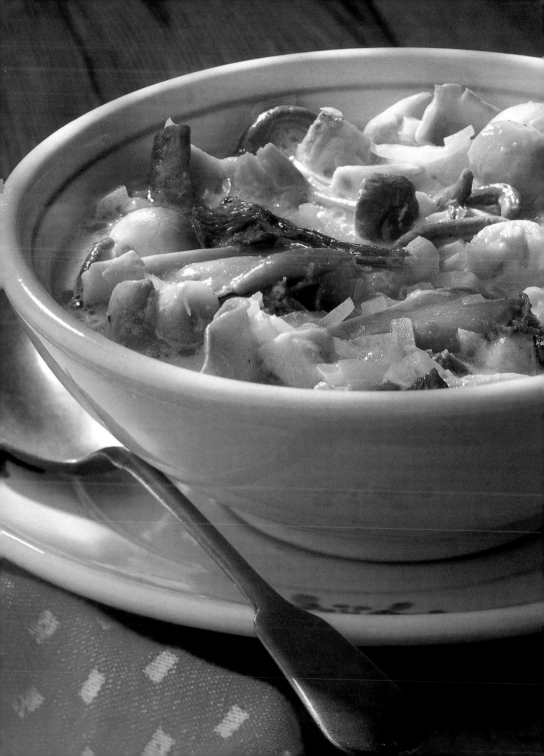

cheese & vegetable chowder

serves four

25 g/1 oz butter

1 large onion, finely chopped

1 large leek, split lengthways and
   thinly sliced

1–2 garlic cloves, crushed

55 g/2 oz plain flour

1.2 litres/2 pints vegetable stock

3 carrots, finely diced

2 celery sticks, finely diced

1 turnip, finely diced

1 large potato, finely diced

3–4 fresh thyme sprigs or
   ⅛ tsp dried thyme

1 bay leaf

350 ml/12 fl oz single cream

300 g/10½ oz mature Cheddar
   cheese, grated

salt and pepper

chopped fresh parsley, to garnish

1 Melt the butter in a large, heavy-based saucepan over a medium–low heat. Add the onion, leek and garlic. Cover and cook, stirring frequently, for 5 minutes, or until the vegetables are beginning to soften.

2 Stir in the flour and cook for 2 minutes. Add a little of the stock and stir, scraping the bottom of the saucepan to mix in the flour. Bring to the boil, stirring frequently, and slowly stir in the remaining stock.

3 Add the carrots, celery, turnip, potato, thyme and bay leaf. Reduce the heat, cover and simmer, stirring occasionally, for 35 minutes, or until the vegetables are tender. Remove the bay leaf and thyme sprigs and discard.

4 Stir in the cream and simmer over a very low heat for 5 minutes.

5 Add the cheese a handful at a time, stirring constantly for 1 minute after each addition to make sure it is completely melted. Taste the soup and adjust the seasoning, adding salt if needed and pepper to taste.

6 Ladle the soup into bowls, sprinkle with parsley and serve.

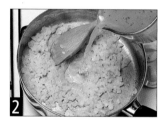

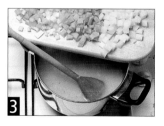

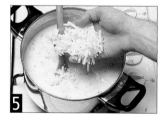

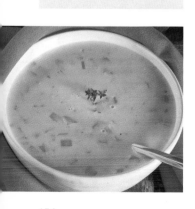

mexican vegetable soup with tortilla chips

serves four–six

2 tbsp vegetable or virgin olive oil

1 onion, finely chopped

4 garlic cloves, finely chopped

¼– ½ tsp ground cumin

2–3 tsp mild chilli powder, such as
    ancho or New Mexico

1 carrot, sliced

1 waxy potato, diced

350 g/12 oz diced fresh or
    canned tomatoes

1 courgette, diced

¼ small cabbage, shredded

1 litre/1¾ pints vegetable or chicken
    stock or water

sweetcorn kernels cut from
    1 corn-on-the-cob or canned

about 10 green or runner beans, cut
    into bite-sized lengths

salt and pepper

TO SERVE

4–6 tbsp chopped fresh coriander

salsa of your choice or chopped
    fresh chilli, to taste

tortilla chips

1 Heat the oil in a heavy-based sauté pan or saucepan. Add the onion and garlic and cook for a few minutes until softened, then sprinkle in the cumin and chilli powder. Stir in the carrot, potato, tomatoes, courgette and cabbage and cook for 2 minutes, stirring the mixture occasionally.

2 Pour in the stock or water. Cover and cook over a medium heat for 20 minutes, or until the vegetables are tender.

3 Add extra stock or water if necessary, then stir in the sweetcorn and beans and cook for a further 5–10 minutes, or until the beans are tender. Season to taste with salt and pepper, bearing in mind that the tortilla chips may be salty.

4 Ladle the soup into soup bowls and sprinkle each portion with chopped coriander. Top with a little salsa or chilli, then add a handful of tortilla chips.

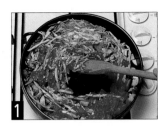

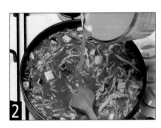

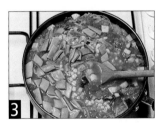

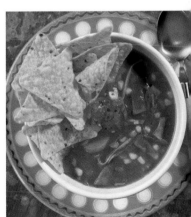

mexican tomato rice

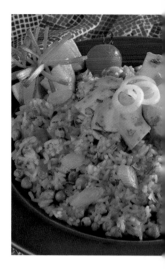

serves six–eight

400 g/14 oz long-grain rice

1 large onion, chopped

2–3 garlic cloves, crushed

350 g/12 oz canned Italian
    plum tomatoes

3–4 tbsp olive oil

1 litre/1¾ pints chicken stock

1 tbsp tomato purée

1 habanero or other hot chilli

salt and pepper

175 g/6 oz frozen peas, thawed

4 tbsp chopped fresh coriander,
    plus extra to serve

TO SERVE

1 large avocado, peeled, stoned,
    sliced and sprinkled with
    lime juice

lime wedges

4 spring onions, chopped

1 In a bowl, cover the rice with hot water and set aside to stand for 15 minutes. Drain, then rinse under cold running water and drain again.

2 Place the onion and garlic in a food processor and process until a smooth purée forms. Scrape the purée into a small bowl and set aside. Put the tomatoes in the food processor and process until smooth, then press through a nylon sieve into another bowl, pushing through any solids with the back of a wooden spoon.

3 Heat the oil in a flameproof casserole over a medium heat. Add the rice and cook, stirring frequently, for 4 minutes until golden and translucent. Add the onion purée and cook, stirring frequently, for a further 2 minutes. Add the stock, processed tomatoes and tomato purée and bring to the boil.

4 Using a pin or long needle, carefully pierce the chilli in 2–3 places. Add to the rice, season to taste with salt and pepper and reduce the heat to low. Cover and simmer for 25 minutes, or until the rice is tender and the liquid is just absorbed. Discard the chilli, stir in the peas and coriander and cook for a further 5 minutes to heat through.

5 To serve, gently fork the rice mixture into a warmed large, shallow serving bowl. Arrange the avocado slices and lime wedges on top. Sprinkle over the spring onions and some chopped coriander and serve immediately.

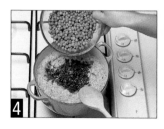

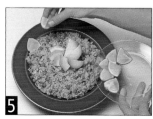

baked tomato rice

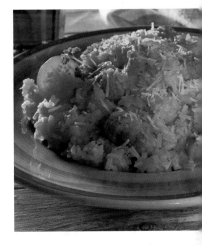

2 tbsp vegetable oil

1 onion, roughly chopped

1 red pepper, deseeded
   and chopped

2 garlic cloves, finely chopped

½ tsp dried thyme

300 g/10½ oz long-grain rice

1 litre/1¾ pints chicken or
   vegetable stock

225 g/8 oz canned
   chopped tomatoes

1 bay leaf

2 tbsp shredded fresh basil

175 g/6 oz mature Cheddar
   cheese, grated

2 tbsp snipped fresh chives

4 herbed pork sausages, cooked
   and cut into 1-cm/½-inch pieces

2–3 tbsp freshly grated
   Parmesan cheese

1 Preheat the oven to 180°C/
350°F/Gas Mark 4. Heat the oil
in a large, flameproof casserole over
a medium heat. Add the onion and
pepper and cook, stirring frequently,
for 5 minutes, or until soft and lightly
coloured. Stir in the garlic and thyme
and cook for a further minute.

2 Add the rice and cook, stirring
frequently, for 2 minutes, or until
the rice is well coated and translucent.
Stir in the stock, tomatoes and bay leaf.
Bring to the boil, then simmer rapidly
for 5 minutes, or until the stock is
almost completely absorbed.

3 Stir in the basil, Cheddar cheese,
chives and sausages and bake,
covered, in the oven for 25 minutes.

4 Sprinkle with the Parmesan
cheese and return to the oven,
uncovered, for 5 minutes, or until the
top is golden. Serve hot.

COOK'S TIP

For a vegetarian version, replace
the pork sausages with 400 g/
14 oz canned drained butter
beans, kidney beans or
sweetcorn kernels. Alternatively,
try a mixture of sautéed
mushrooms and courgettes.

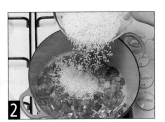

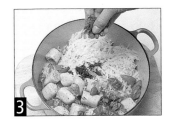

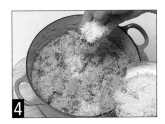

milanese sun-dried tomato risotto

serves four

1 tbsp olive oil

2 tbsp butter

1 large onion, finely chopped

350 g/12 oz arborio rice

about 15 saffron threads

150 ml/5 fl oz white wine

850 ml/1½ pints hot vegetable or
chicken stock

8 sun-dried tomatoes, cut into strips

100 g/3½ oz frozen peas, thawed

50 g/1¾ oz Parma ham, shredded

75 g/2¾ oz freshly grated Parmesan
cheese, plus extra for sprinkling

1 Heat the oil and butter in a large frying pan. Add the chopped onion and cook for 4–5 minutes, or until softened.

2 Add the rice and saffron to the frying pan, stirring well to coat the rice in the oil, and cook for 1 minute.

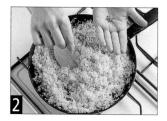

3 Add the wine and stock slowly to the rice mixture in the pan, a ladleful at a time, stirring and making sure that all the liquid is absorbed before adding the next ladleful of liquid.

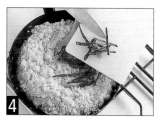

4 About halfway through adding the stock, stir in the tomatoes.

5 When all the wine and stock is incorporated, the rice should be cooked. Test by tasting a grain – if it is still crunchy, add a little more stock and continue cooking. It should take at least 15 minutes to cook.

6 Stir in the peas, Parma ham and Parmesan cheese. Cook, stirring, for 2–3 minutes, or until hot. Serve with extra Parmesan for sprinkling.

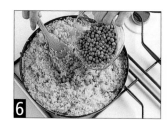

COOK'S TIP
Italian rice is a round, short-grained variety with a nutty flavour, which is essential for a good risotto. Arborio is the very best kind to use.

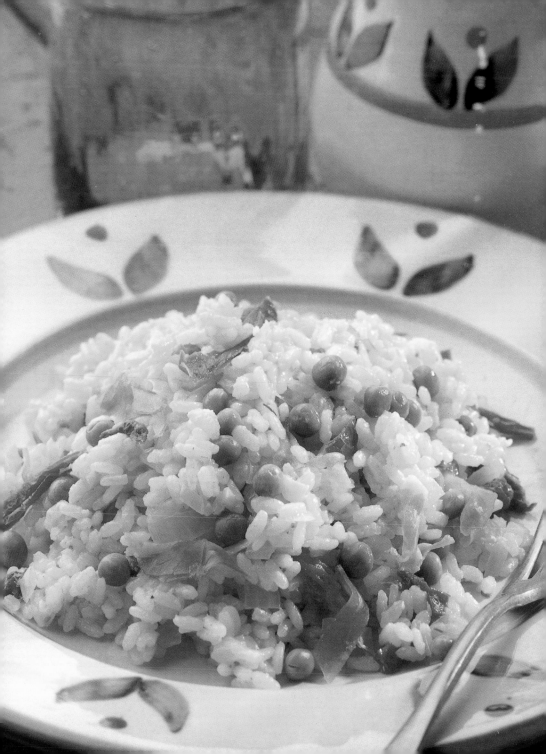

easy cheese risotto

serves four

4–6 tbsp unsalted butter

1 onion, finely chopped

300 g/10½ oz arborio or
  carnaroli rice

125 ml/4 fl oz dry white vermouth
  or white wine

1.2 litres/2 pints chicken or
  vegetable stock, simmering

85 g/3 oz freshly grated Parmesan
  cheese, plus extra for sprinkling

salt and pepper

1 Heat about 2 tablespoons of the butter in a large, heavy-based saucepan over a medium heat. Add the onion and cook for 2 minutes, or until just beginning to soften. Add the rice and cook, stirring, for 2 minutes, or until translucent and well coated with the butter.

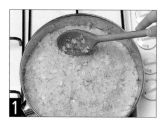

2 Pour in the vermouth; it will bubble and steam rapidly and evaporate almost immediately. Add a ladleful (about 225 ml/8 fl oz) of the simmering stock and cook, stirring constantly, until the stock is completely absorbed.

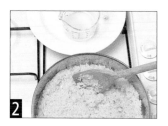

3 Continue adding the stock, about half a ladleful at a time, allowing each addition to be absorbed before adding the next – never allow the rice to cook dry. This should take 20–25 minutes. The risotto should have a creamy consistency and the rice should be tender but still firm to the bite.

4 Switch off the heat and stir in the remaining butter and Parmesan cheese. Season to taste with salt and pepper. Cover, leave to stand for 1 minute, then serve with extra Parmesan for sprinkling.

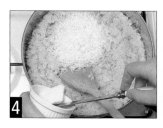

COOK'S TIP

If you prefer not to use butter, soften the onion in 2 tablespoons of olive oil and stir in about 2 tablespoons of extra virgin olive oil with the Parmesan at the end.

minted green risotto

serves six

2 tbsp unsalted butter

450 g/1 lb fresh shelled peas or
thawed frozen peas

1 kg/2 lb 4 oz young spinach leaves

1 bunch of fresh mint, leaves
stripped from stalks

2 tbsp chopped fresh basil

2 tbsp chopped fresh oregano

pinch of freshly grated nutmeg

4 tbsp mascarpone cheese

2 tbsp vegetable oil

1 onion, finely chopped

4 celery sticks, including leaves,
finely chopped

2 garlic cloves, finely chopped

½ tsp dried thyme

300 g/10½ oz arborio or
carnaroli rice

50 ml/2 fl oz dry white vermouth

1 litre/1¾ pints chicken or vegetable
stock, simmering

85 g/3 oz freshly grated
Parmesan cheese

spring onion tassels, to garnish

1 Heat half the butter in a deep frying pan over a medium–high heat. Add the peas, spinach, herbs and nutmeg. Cook, stirring, for 3 minutes, or until the spinach is wilted.

2 Transfer to a food processor and process for 15 seconds. Add the mascarpone and process again for 1 minute. Set aside.

3 Heat the oil and remaining butter in a large, heavy-based saucepan over a medium heat. Add the onion, celery, garlic and thyme and cook for 2 minutes, or until softened. Add the rice and cook, stirring, for 2 minutes, or until translucent and well coated.

4 Pour in the vermouth; it will bubble and steam rapidly. When it is almost absorbed, add a ladleful (about 225 ml/8 fl oz) of the simmering stock. Cook, stirring constantly, until the stock is completely absorbed.

5 Continue adding the stock, about half a ladleful at a time, allowing each addition to be absorbed before adding the next. This should take 20–25 minutes. The risotto should have a creamy consistency and the rice should be tender but still firm to the bite. Stir in the spinach-cream mixture and the Parmesan cheese. Serve the risotto immediately, garnished with spring onion tassels.

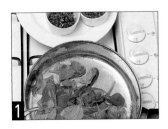

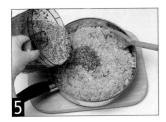

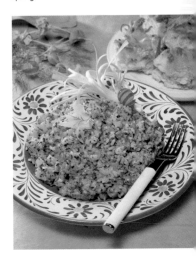

wild mushroom risotto

serves six

55 g/2 oz dried porcini or
morel mushrooms
about 500 g/1 lb 2 oz mixed fresh
wild mushrooms, such as porcini,
girolles, horse mushrooms and
chanterelles, halved if large
4 tbsp olive oil
3–4 garlic cloves, finely chopped
4 tbsp unsalted butter
1 onion, finely chopped
350 g/12 oz arborio or carnaroli rice
50 ml/2 fl oz dry white vermouth
1.2 litres/2 pints chicken
stock, simmering
salt and pepper
115 g/4 oz freshly grated
Parmesan cheese
4 tbsp chopped fresh
flat-leaved parsley
6 fresh parsley sprigs, to garnish
crusty bread, to serve

1 Place the dried mushrooms in a heatproof bowl and pour over enough boiling water to cover. Leave to soak for 30 minutes, then carefully lift out and pat dry. Strain the soaking liquid through a sieve lined with kitchen paper and reserve.

2 Trim the wild mushrooms and gently brush clean.

3 Heat 3 tablespoons of the oil in a frying pan over a low heat. Add the fresh mushrooms and fry for 1–2 minutes. Add the garlic and soaked mushrooms and cook, stirring frequently, for 2 minutes. Transfer to a plate and reserve.

4 Heat the remaining oil and half the butter in a large saucepan over a low heat. Add the onion and cook, stirring occasionally, for 2 minutes, or until softened. Add the rice and cook, stirring, for 2 minutes, or until translucent and well coated. Add the vermouth. When almost absorbed, add a ladleful (about 225 ml/8 fl oz) of the stock. Cook, stirring, until the stock is completely absorbed.

5 Continue adding the stock, about half a ladleful at a time, allowing each addition to be absorbed before adding the next. This should take 20–25 minutes. The risotto should have a creamy consistency and the rice should be tender but still firm to the bite.

6 Add half the reserved mushroom soaking liquid to the risotto and stir in the mushrooms. Season to taste with salt and pepper and add more mushroom liquid, if necessary. Remove from the heat and stir in the remaining butter, the Parmesan cheese and chopped parsley. Transfer to 6 warmed serving dishes, garnish with parsley sprigs and serve with crusty bread.

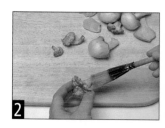

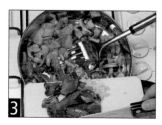

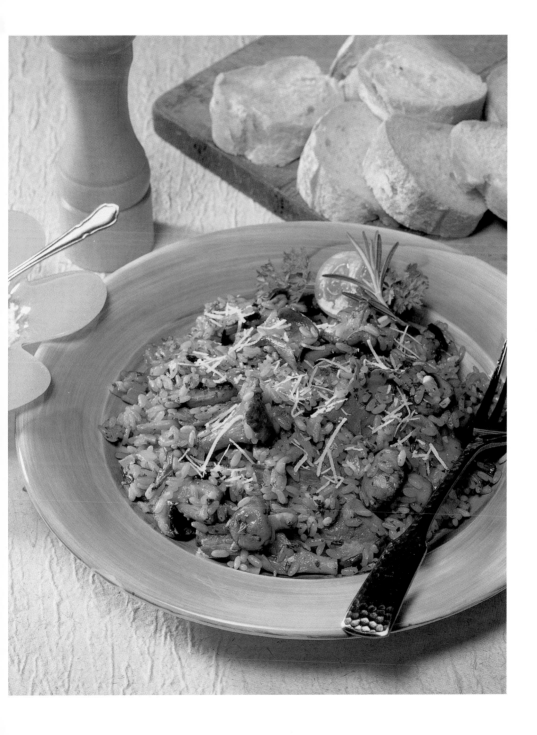

hot pink risotto

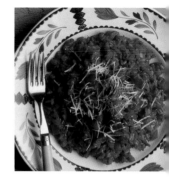

serves four–six

175 g/6 oz dried sour cherries or
  dried cranberries

225 ml/8 fl oz fruity red wine, such
  as Valpolicella

3 tbsp olive oil

1 large red onion, finely chopped

2 celery sticks, finely chopped

½ tsp dried thyme

1 garlic clove, finely chopped

350 g/12 oz arborio or carnaroli rice

1.2 litres/2 pints chicken or
  vegetable stock, simmering

4 cooked fresh beetroot (not
  pickled), diced

2 tbsp chopped fresh dill

2 tbsp snipped fresh chives

salt and pepper

55 g/2 oz freshly grated Parmesan
  cheese, to serve (optional)

1 Put the dried cherries in a saucepan with the wine and bring to the boil. Reduce the heat and simmer for 2–3 minutes, or until slightly reduced. Remove from the heat and set aside.

2 Heat the oil in a large, heavy-based saucepan over a medium heat. Add the onion, celery and thyme and cook, stirring occasionally, for 2 minutes, or until just beginning to soften. Add the garlic and rice and cook, stirring, for 2 minutes, or until the rice is translucent and well coated.

3 Add a ladleful (about 225 ml/ 8 fl oz) of the simmering stock; it will bubble and steam rapidly. Cook, stirring constantly, until the stock is completely absorbed.

4 Continue adding the stock, about half a ladleful at a time, allowing each addition to be absorbed before adding the next. This should take 20–25 minutes. The risotto should have a creamy consistency and the rice should be tender but still firm to the bite. Halfway through the cooking time, remove the cherries or cranberries from the wine with a slotted spoon and add to the risotto with the beetroot and half the wine. Continue adding the stock and remaining wine.

5 Stir in the dill and chives and season to taste with salt and pepper. Serve with Parmesan cheese, if wished.

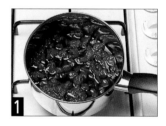

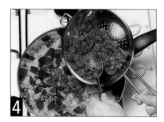

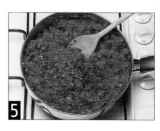

rocket & tomato risotto

serves four–six

2 tbsp olive oil

2 tbsp unsalted butter

1 large onion, finely chopped

2 garlic cloves, finely chopped

350 g/12 oz arborio rice

125 ml/4 fl oz dry white vermouth

1.5 litres/2¾ pints chicken or
    vegetable stock, simmering

6 vine-ripened or Italian
    plum tomatoes, deseeded
    and chopped

125 g/4½ oz wild rocket

handful of fresh basil leaves

115 g/4 oz freshly grated
    Parmesan cheese

225 g/8 oz fresh Italian buffalo
    mozzarella, coarsely grated
    or diced

salt and pepper

1 Heat the oil and half the butter in a large frying pan. Add the onion and cook for 2 minutes, or until just beginning to soften. Stir in the garlic and rice and cook, stirring, for 2 minutes, or until the rice is translucent and well coated.

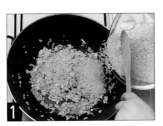

2 Pour in the vermouth; it will bubble and steam rapidly and evaporate almost immediately. Add a ladleful (about 225 ml/8 fl oz) of the stock and cook, stirring, until absorbed.

3 Continue adding the stock, about half a ladleful at a time, allowing each addition to be absorbed before adding the next. Just before the rice is tender, stir in the tomatoes and rocket. Shred the basil leaves and immediately stir into the risotto. Continue to cook, adding more stock, until the risotto is creamy and the rice is tender but still firm to the bite.

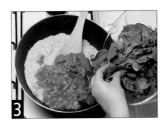

4 Remove from the heat and stir in the remaining butter and cheeses. Season to taste with salt and pepper. Cover and leave to stand for 1 minute. Serve immediately, before the mozzarella melts completely.

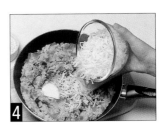

roasted pumpkin risotto

serves six

4 tbsp olive oil

4 tbsp unsalted butter, cut into
  small pieces

450 g/1 lb pumpkin flesh, cut into
  1-cm/½-inch dice

¾ tsp dried sage

2 garlic cloves, finely chopped

salt and pepper

2 tbsp lemon juice

2 large shallots, finely chopped

350 g/12 oz arborio or carnaroli rice

50 ml/2 fl oz dry white vermouth

1.2 litres/2 pints chicken
  stock, simmering

60 g/2¼ oz freshly grated
  Parmesan cheese

300 g/10½ oz dolcelatte cheese, cut
  into small pieces

celery leaves, to garnish

1 Preheat the oven to
200°C/400°F/Gas Mark 6. Put half
the oil and about 1 tablespoon of the
butter in a roasting tin and heat in
the oven.

2 Add the pumpkin to the tin and
sprinkle with the sage, half the
garlic and salt and pepper to taste.
Toss together and roast for 10 minutes,
or until just softened and beginning to
caramelize. Transfer to a plate.

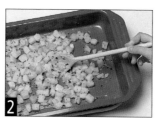

3 Roughly mash about half the
cooked pumpkin with the lemon
juice and reserve with the remaining
diced pumpkin.

4 Heat the remaining oil and
1 tablespoon of the remaining
butter in a large, heavy-based
saucepan over a medium heat. Stir in
the shallots and remaining garlic and
cook for 1 minute. Add the rice and
cook, stirring, for 2 minutes, or until
translucent and well coated.

5 Pour in the vermouth; it will
bubble and steam rapidly and
evaporate almost immediately. Add a
ladleful (about 225 ml/8 fl oz) of the
simmering stock and cook, stirring
constantly, until absorbed.

6 Continue adding the stock, about
half a ladleful at a time, allowing
each addition be absorbed before
adding the next. This should take
20–25 minutes. The finished risotto
should have a creamy consistency and
the rice should be tender but still firm
to the bite.

7 Stir the pumpkin into the risotto
with the remaining butter and the
Parmesan cheese. Remove from the
heat and fold in the dolcelatte. Serve
once, garnished with celery leaves.

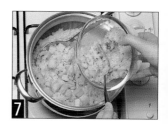

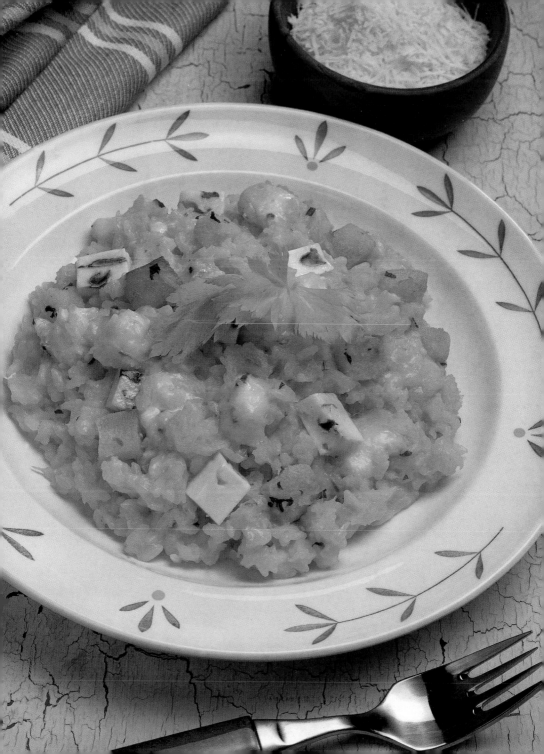

orange-scented risotto

serves four

2 tbsp pine kernels

4 tbsp unsalted butter

2 shallots, finely chopped

1 leek, finely shredded

400 g/14 oz arborio or carnaroli rice

2 tbsp orange-flavoured liqueur or
    dry white vermouth

1.5 litres/2¾ pints chicken or
    vegetable stock, simmering

grated rind of 1 orange

juice of 2 oranges, strained

3 tbsp snipped fresh chives

salt and pepper

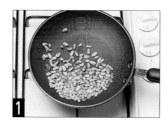

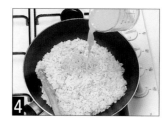

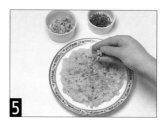

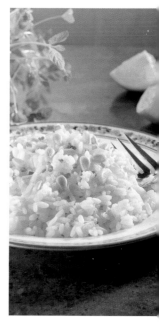

1 Toast the pine kernels in a frying pan over a medium heat, stirring and shaking frequently, for 3 minutes, or until golden brown. Set aside.

2 Heat half the butter in a large, heavy-based pan over a medium heat. Add the shallots and leek and cook for 2 minutes, or until beginning to soften. Add the rice and cook, stirring, for 2 minutes, or until translucent and well coated.

3 Pour in the liqueur or vermouth; it will bubble and steam rapidly and evaporate almost immediately. Add a ladleful (about 225 ml/8 fl oz) of the stock and cook, stirring, until absorbed. Continue adding the stock, about half a ladleful at a time, allowing each addition to be absorbed before adding the next — never allow the rice to cook dry.

4 After about 15 minutes, add the orange rind and juice and continue to cook, adding more stock, until the rice is tender but still firm to the bite. The risotto should have a creamy consistency.

5 Remove from the heat and stir in the remaining butter and 2 tablespoons of the chives. Season to taste with salt and pepper. Spoon into warmed serving dishes and sprinkle with the toasted pine kernels and the remaining chives.

mushroom & cheese risotto

serves four

2 tbsp olive or vegetable oil

225 g/8 oz arborio rice

2 garlic cloves, crushed

1 onion, chopped

2 celery sticks, chopped

1 red or green pepper, deseeded
and chopped

225 g/8 oz mushrooms, sliced

1 tbsp chopped fresh oregano or
1 tsp dried oregano

1 litre/1¾ pints vegetable stock

55 g /2 oz sun-dried tomatoes in
olive oil, drained and chopped
(optional)

salt and pepper

55 g/2 oz finely grated Parmesan
cheese

TO GARNISH

fresh flat-leaved parsley sprigs

fresh bay leaves

1 Heat the oil in a wok or large
frying pan. Add the rice and cook,
stirring constantly, for 5 minutes.

2 Add the garlic, onion, celery and
pepper and cook, stirring
constantly, for 5 minutes. Add the
mushrooms and cook for 3–4 minutes.

3 Stir in the oregano and stock.
Heat until just boiling, then
reduce the heat, cover and simmer for
20 minutes, or until the rice is tender
and creamy.

4 Add the sun-dried tomatoes,
if using, and season to taste
with salt and pepper. Stir in half the
Parmesan cheese. Top with the
remaining Parmesan, garnish with
the parsley sprigs and bay leaves
and serve immediately.

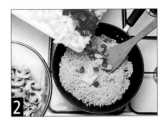

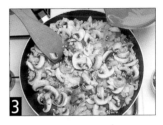

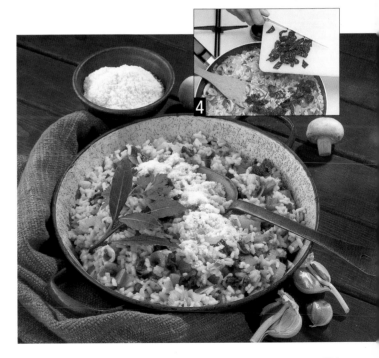

171

vegetable jambalaya

serves four

75 g/2¾ oz brown rice

2 tbsp olive oil

2 garlic cloves, crushed

1 red onion, cut into 8 wedges

1 aubergine, diced

1 green pepper, deseeded and diced

50 g/1¾ oz baby corn cobs,
      halved lengthways

50 g/1¾ oz frozen peas

100 g/3½ oz small broccoli florets

150 ml/5 fl oz vegetable stock

225 g/8 oz canned
      chopped tomatoes

1 tbsp tomato purée

1 tsp Creole seasoning

½ tsp dried chilli flakes

salt and pepper

1 Cook the rice in a large saucepan of boiling water for 20 minutes, or until cooked through. Drain and reserve until required.

2 Heat the oil in a heavy-based frying pan. Add the garlic and onion and cook, stirring constantly, for 2–3 minutes.

3 Add the aubergine, pepper, baby corn cobs, peas and broccoli to the frying pan and cook, stirring occasionally, for 2–3 minutes.

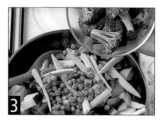

COOK'S TIP
Use a mixture of rice,
such as wild or red rice,
for colour and texture.

4 Stir in the stock, tomatoes, tomato purée, Creole seasoning and chilli flakes. Season to taste with salt and pepper and cook over a low heat for 15–20 minutes, or until the vegetables are tender.

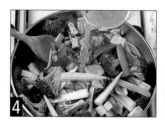

5 Add the rice to the vegetable mixture and heat through, gently stirring, for 3–4 minutes, or until piping hot. Transfer to warmed serving dishes and serve immediately.

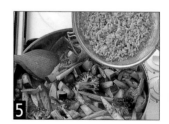

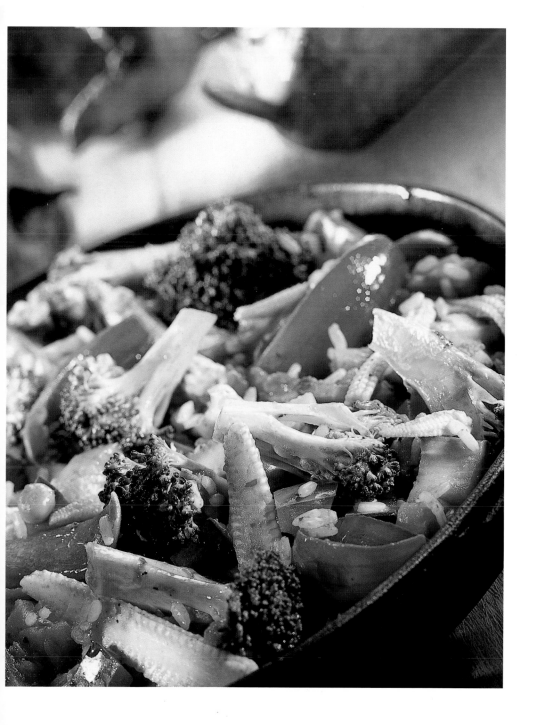

fried rice with spicy beans

serves four

3 tbsp sunflower oil

1 onion, finely chopped

225 g/8 oz long-grain rice

1 green pepper, deseeded and diced

1 tsp chilli powder

600 ml/1 pint boiling water

100 g/3½ oz canned sweetcorn
   kernels, drained

225 g/8 oz canned red kidney
   beans, rinsed and drained

2 tbsp chopped fresh coriander, plus
   extra to garnish (optional)

1 Heat a large wok over a medium heat. Add the oil and heat.

2 Add the onion and stir-fry for 2 minutes, or until softened.

3 Reduce the heat, add the rice, pepper and chilli powder and stir-fry for 1 minute.

4 Pour in the boiling water. Return to the boil, then reduce the heat and simmer for 15 minutes.

5 Stir in the sweetcorn, beans and coriander and heat through, stirring occasionally.

6 Transfer to a warmed serving bowl and serve hot, sprinkled with extra coriander, if wished.

COOK'S TIP

For perfect fried rice, the raw rice should ideally be soaked in a bowl of water for a short time before cooking to remove excess starch. Short-grain Oriental rice can be substituted for the long-grain rice.

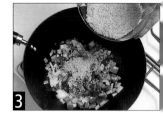

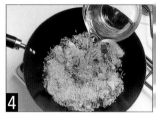

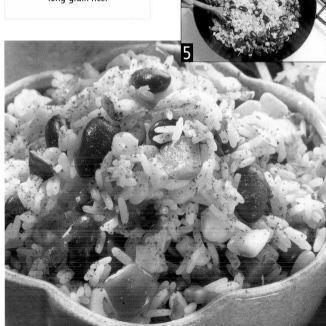

cashew nut paella

serves four

2 tbsp olive oil

1 tbsp butter

1 red onion, chopped

150 g/5½ oz arborio rice

1 tsp ground turmeric

1 tsp ground cumin

½ tsp chilli powder

3 garlic cloves, crushed

1 fresh green chilli, sliced

1 green pepper, deseeded and diced

1 red pepper, deseeded and diced

75 g/2¾ oz baby corn cobs,
   halved lengthways

2 tbsp stoned black olives

1 large tomato, deseeded and diced

450 ml/16 fl oz vegetable stock

75 g/2¾ oz unsalted cashew nuts

25 g/1 oz frozen peas

salt and pepper

2 tbsp chopped fresh parsley

pinch of cayenne pepper

fresh herbs, to garnish

1 Heat the oil and butter in a large frying pan or paella pan until the butter has melted.

2 Add the chopped onion and sauté for 2–3 minutes, stirring constantly, until softened.

3 Stir in the rice, turmeric, cumin, chilli powder, garlic, chilli, peppers, baby corn cobs, olives and tomato and cook over a medium heat for 1–2 minutes, stirring occasionally.

4 Pour in the stock and bring the mixture to the boil. Reduce the heat and cook for 20 minutes, stirring frequently.

5 Add the cashew nuts and peas and cook for a further 5 minutes, stirring occasionally. Season to taste with salt and pepper and sprinkle with parsley and cayenne pepper. Transfer to warmed serving plates, garnish with fresh herbs and serve immediately.

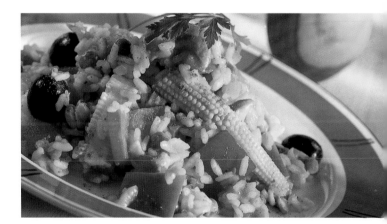

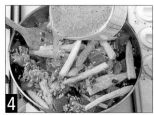
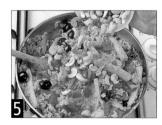

brown rice, vegetable & herb gratin

serves four

100 g/3½ oz brown rice

salt and pepper

2 tbsp butter or margarine,
     plus extra for greasing

1 red onion, chopped

2 garlic cloves, crushed

1 carrot, cut into matchsticks

1 courgette, sliced

75 g/2¾ oz baby sweetcorn,
     halved lengthways

2 tbsp sunflower seeds

3 tbsp chopped fresh mixed herbs

100 g/3½ oz grated
     mozzarella cheese

2 tbsp fresh wholemeal
     breadcrumbs

VARIATION

Use an alternative rice, such as
basmati, and flavour the dish
with curry spices, if you prefer.

1 Preheat the oven to 180°C/
350°F/Gas Mark 4. Lightly grease
an 850-ml/1½-pint ovenproof dish.

2 Cook the rice in a large saucepan
of lightly salted boiling water for
20 minutes. Drain well.

3 Heat the butter in a frying pan.
Add the onion and cook, stirring
constantly, for 2 minutes, or until
softened.

4 Add the garlic, carrot, courgette
and baby corn cobs and cook for
a further 5 minutes, stirring.

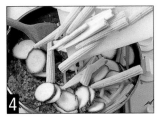

5 Mix the rice with the sunflower
seeds and mixed herbs in a bowl
and stir into the frying pan.

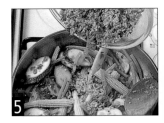

6 Stir in half the cheese and season
to taste with salt and pepper.

7 Spoon the mixture into the
prepared dish and top with the
breadcrumbs and remaining cheese.
Cook in the oven for 25–30 minutes,
or until the cheese begins to turn
golden. Serve immediately.

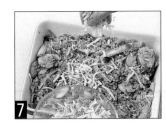

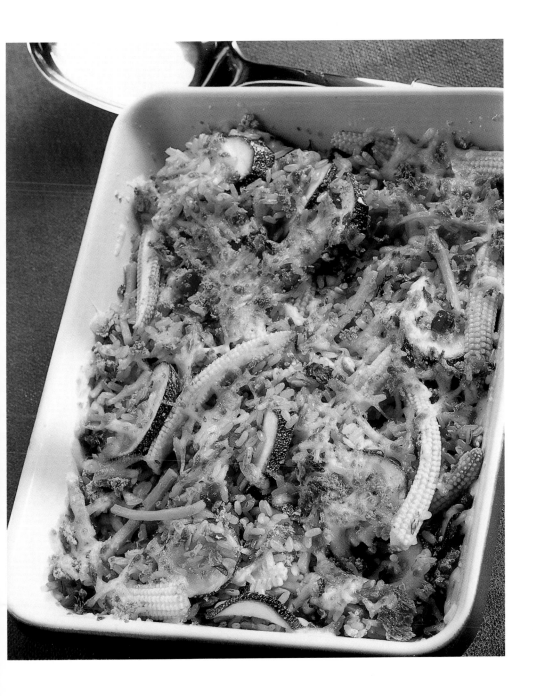

vegetable chilli

serves four

1 aubergine, peeled (optional) and
cut into 2.5-cm/1-inch slices

1 tbsp olive oil, plus extra
for brushing

1 large red or yellow onion,
finely chopped

2 red or yellow peppers, deseeded
and finely chopped

3–4 garlic cloves, finely chopped
or crushed

800 g/1 lb 12 oz canned
chopped tomatoes

1 tbsp mild chilli powder

½ tsp ground cumin

½ tsp dried oregano

salt and pepper

2 small courgettes, quartered
lengthways and sliced

400 g/14 oz canned kidney beans,
rinsed and drained

450 ml/16 fl oz water

1 tbsp tomato purée

TO GARNISH

6 spring onions, finely chopped

115 g/4 oz grated Cheddar cheese

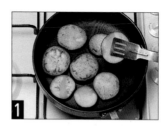

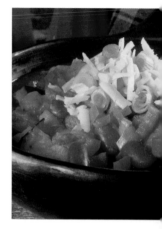

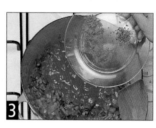

1 Brush the aubergine slices on one side with oil. Heat half the oil in a large, heavy-based frying pan over a medium–high heat. Add the aubergine slices, oiled-side up, and cook for 5–6 minutes, or until browned underneath. Turn over and brown the other side. Remove and cut into bite-sized pieces.

2 Heat the remaining oil in a large saucepan over a medium heat. Add the onion and peppers and cook, stirring occasionally, for 3–4 minutes, or until the onion is just softened but not browned. Add the garlic and cook for a further 2–3 minutes, or until the onion is just beginning to colour.

3 Add the tomatoes, chilli powder, cumin and oregano. Season to taste with salt and pepper. Bring just to the boil, then reduce the heat, cover and simmer gently for 15 minutes.

4 Add the courgettes, aubergine pieces and beans. Stir in the water and the tomato purée. Return to the boil, then reduce the heat, cover and simmer for 45 minutes, or until the vegetables are tender. Taste the chilli and adjust the seasoning if necessary. If you prefer a hotter dish, stir in a little more chilli powder.

5 Ladle into warmed bowls, top with spring onions and cheese and serve.

spicy fragrant black bean chilli

serves four

400 g/14 oz dried black beans

2 tbsp olive oil

1 onion, chopped

5 garlic cloves, roughly chopped

½–1 tsp ground cumin

½–1 tsp mild red chilli powder

1 red pepper, deseeded and diced

1 carrot, diced

400 g/14 oz fresh tomatoes, diced,
    or chopped canned

1 bunch fresh coriander,
    roughly chopped

salt and pepper

COOK'S TIP

You can use canned beans, if
wished – drain and use
225 ml/8 fl oz water in place of
the reserved bean cooking liquid.

1 Soak the beans overnight, then drain. Place in a saucepan, cover with water and bring to the boil. Boil for 10 minutes, then reduce the heat and simmer for 1½ hours, or until tender. Drain well, reserving 225 ml/ 8 fl oz of the cooking liquid.

2 Heat the oil in a frying pan. Add the onion and garlic and cook for 2 minutes until the onion is softened.

3 Stir in the cumin and chilli powder and cook for a few seconds. Add the pepper, carrot and tomatoes. Cook over a medium heat for 5 minutes.

4 Add half the coriander and the beans and their reserved liquid. Season to taste with salt and pepper. Simmer for 30–45 minutes, or until very flavourful and thickened.

5 Stir in the remaining coriander, adjust the seasoning and serve immediately.

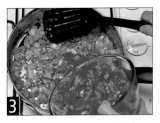

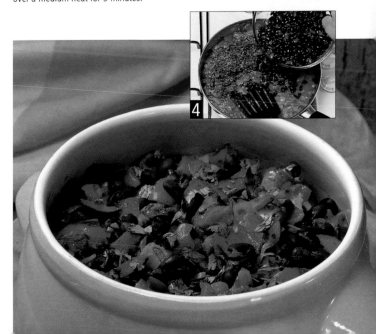

brown rice with fruit & nuts

serves four–six

4 tbsp vegetable ghee or oil

1 large onion, chopped

2 garlic cloves, crushed

2.5-cm/1-inch piece fresh
     root ginger, finely chopped

1 tsp chilli powder

1 tsp cumin seeds

1 tbsp mild or medium curry
     powder or paste

280 g/10 oz brown rice

850 ml/1½ pints boiling
     vegetable stock

400 g/14 oz canned
     chopped tomatoes

salt and pepper

175 g/6 oz no-soak dried apricots or
     peaches, cut into slivers

1 red pepper, deseeded and diced

85 g/3 oz frozen peas

1–2 small, slightly green bananas

55–85 g/2–3oz toasted mixed nuts

1 Heat the ghee in a large frying
pan over a medium heat, add
the onion and fry for 3 minutes.

2 Stir in the garlic, ginger, chilli
powder, cumin seeds, curry
powder and rice. Cook gently for
2 minutes, stirring constantly, until
the rice is coated in the spiced oil.

3 Pour in the boiling stock, stirring
to mix. Add the tomatoes and
season to taste with salt and pepper.
Bring the mixture to the boil, then
reduce the heat, cover and simmer
gently for 40 minutes, or until the rice
is almost cooked and most of the liquid
is absorbed.

4 Add the apricots or peaches,
pepper and peas, cover and cook
for a further 10 minutes.

5 Remove the pan from the heat
and leave to stand, covered, for
5 minutes.

6 Peel and slice the bananas.
Uncover the rice mixture and toss
with a fork to mix. Add the toasted
nuts and sliced banana and toss lightly.

7 Transfer the brown rice, fruit and
nuts to a warmed serving dish
and serve hot.

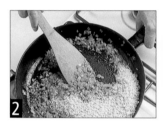

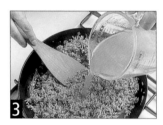

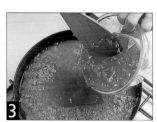

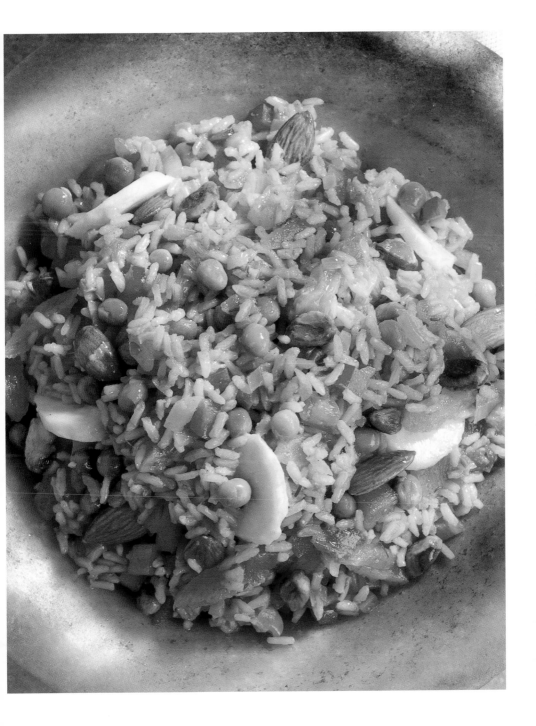

asian-style millet pilau

serves four

300 g/10½ oz millet grains

1 tbsp vegetable oil

1 bunch spring onions, chopped

1 garlic clove, crushed

1 tsp grated fresh root ginger

1 orange pepper, deseeded
   and diced

600 ml/1 pint water

1 orange

salt and pepper

115 g/4 oz chopped stoned dates

2 tsp sesame oil

115 g/4 oz roasted cashew nuts

2 tbsp pumpkin seeds

Oriental salad vegetables, to serve

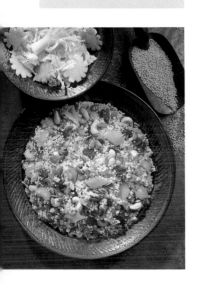

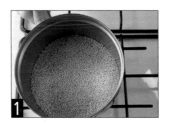

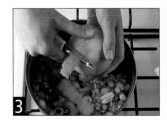

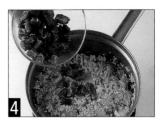

1 Place the millet in a large saucepan and toast over a medium heat, shaking the pan occasionally, for 4–5 minutes, or until the grains begin to crack and pop.

2 Heat the vegetable oil in a separate saucepan. Add the spring onions, garlic, ginger and pepper and cook over a medium heat, stirring frequently, for 2–3 minutes, or until just softened but not browned. Add the millet and pour in the water.

3 Using a vegetable peeler, pare the rind from the orange and add to the saucepan. Squeeze the juice from the orange into the saucepan. Season to taste with salt and pepper.

4 Bring to the boil, then reduce the heat, cover and cook gently for 20 minutes, or until all the liquid has been absorbed. Remove the saucepan from the heat, stir in the dates and sesame oil and set aside. Leave to stand for 10 minutes.

5 Remove and discard the orange rind and stir in the nuts. Pile into a warmed serving dish, sprinkle with pumpkin seeds and serve immediately with Oriental salad vegetables.

vegetable curry

serves four

225 g/8 oz turnips or swede

1 aubergine

350 g/12 oz new potatoes

225 g/8 oz cauliflower

225 g/8 oz button mushrooms

1 large onion

225 g/8 oz carrots

6 tbsp vegetable ghee or oil

2 garlic cloves, crushed

5-cm/2-inch piece fresh root ginger,
    finely chopped

1–2 fresh green chillies, deseeded
    and chopped

1 tbsp paprika

2 tsp ground coriander

1 tbsp mild or medium curry
    powder or paste

450 ml/16 fl oz vegetable stock

400 g/14 oz canned
    chopped tomatoes

salt

1 green pepper, deseeded
    and sliced

1 tbsp cornflour

150 ml/5 fl oz coconut milk

2–3 tbsp ground almonds

fresh coriander sprigs, to garnish

1 Cut the turnips or swede, aubergine and potatoes into 1-cm/½-inch cubes. Divide the cauliflower into small florets. Leave the mushrooms whole, or thickly slice if preferred. Slice the onion and carrots.

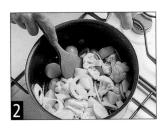

2 Heat the ghee or oil in a large saucepan over a medium heat, add the onion, carrots, turnips or swede, potato and cauliflower and cook for 3 minutes, stirring frequently. Add the garlic, ginger, chillies, paprika, ground coriander and curry powder or paste and cook for 1 minute, stirring.

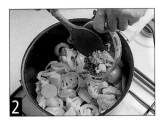

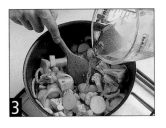

3 Add the stock, tomatoes, aubergine and mushrooms and season to taste with salt. Cover and simmer gently, stirring occasionally, for 30 minutes, or until tender. Add the pepper, cover and cook for a further 5 minutes.

4 Blend the cornflour with the coconut milk and stir into the mixture. Add the almonds and simmer for 2 minutes, stirring constantly. Taste and adjust the seasoning if necessary. Transfer to serving plates and serve hot, garnished with coriander sprigs.

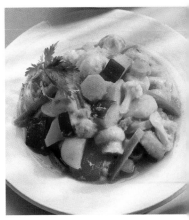

green bean & potato curry

serves four

300 ml/10 fl oz oil

1 tsp cumin seeds

1 tsp mixed mustard and
   onion seeds

4 dried red chillies

3 tomatoes, sliced

1 tsp salt

1 tsp finely chopped fresh
   root ginger

1 garlic clove, crushed

1 tsp chilli powder

200 g/7 oz green beans, sliced

2 potatoes, peeled and diced

300 ml/10 fl oz water

TO GARNISH

chopped fresh coriander

2 fresh green chillies, finely chopped

COOK'S TIP

Mustard seeds are often fried in
oil or ghee (a cooking fat similar
to clarified butter) to bring out
their flavour before being
combined with other ingredients.

1 Heat the oil in a large, heavy-
based saucepan.

2 Add the cumin, mustard and
onion seeds and dried chillies
to the saucepan, stirring well.

3 Add the tomatoes to the
saucepan and stir-fry the mixture
for 3–5 minutes.

4 Mix together the salt, ginger,
garlic and chilli powder and
spoon into the saucepan. Blend the
whole mixture together.

5 Add the beans and potatoes to
the saucepan and stir-fry for
5 minutes.

6 Add the water, then reduce
the heat and simmer for
10–15 minutes, stirring occasionally.

7 Garnish the curry with coriander
and fresh chillies and serve hot.

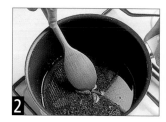

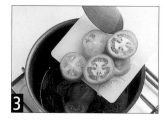

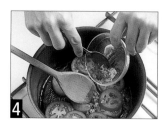

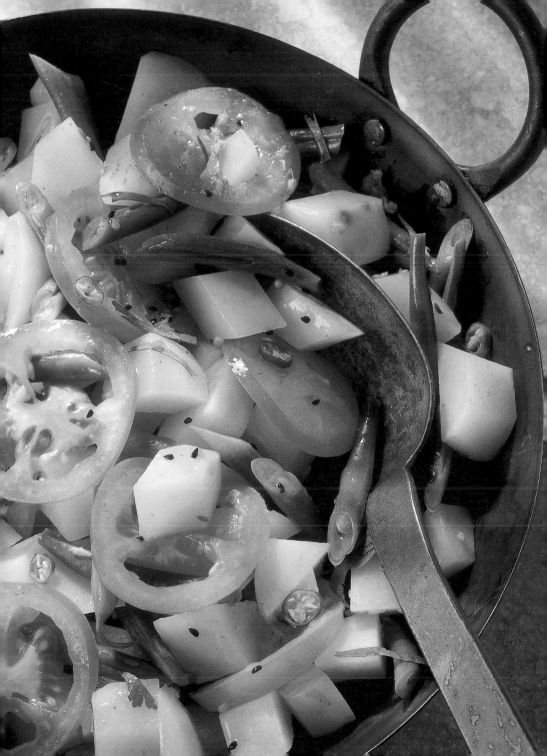

red curry with cashews

serves four

250 ml/9 fl oz coconut milk

1 kaffir lime leaf

¼ tsp light soy sauce

4 baby corn cobs,
    halved lengthways

115 g/4 oz broccoli florets

115 g/4 oz French beans, cut
    into pieces

4 tbsp unsalted cashew nuts

15 fresh basil leaves

1 tbsp chopped fresh coriander

1 tbsp chopped roasted peanuts,
    to garnish

RED CURRY PASTE

7 fresh red chillies, deseeded
    and blanched

2 tsp cumin seeds

2 tsp coriander seeds

2.5-cm/1-inch piece fresh root
    ginger or galangal, chopped

½ lemon grass stalk, chopped

1 tsp salt

grated rind of 1 lime

4 garlic cloves, chopped

3 shallots, chopped

2 kaffir lime leaves, shredded

1 tbsp vegetable oil

1 To make the curry paste, grind all the ingredients in a large mortar with a pestle or in a spice grinder. Alternatively, process briefly in a food processor. (The quantity of red curry paste is more than is required for this recipe. Store for up to 3 weeks in a sealed jar in the refrigerator.)

2 Heat a wok or large, heavy-based frying pan over a high heat, add 3 tablespoons of the red curry paste and stir until it gives off its aroma. Reduce the heat to medium.

3 Add the coconut milk, lime leaf, soy sauce, baby corn cobs, broccoli, beans and cashew nuts. Bring to the boil, then reduce the heat and simmer for 10 minutes, or until the vegetables are cooked but still crunchy.

4 Remove and discard the lime leaf and stir in the basil leaves and coriander. Transfer to a warmed serving dish, garnish with peanuts and serve.

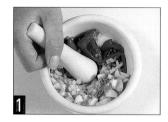
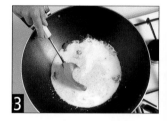
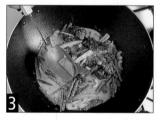
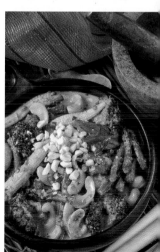

potato & spinach yellow curry

serves four

2 garlic cloves, finely chopped

3-cm/1¼-inch piece fresh root ginger
   or galangal, finely chopped

1 lemon grass stalk,
   finely chopped

1 tsp coriander seeds

3 tbsp vegetable oil

2 tsp Thai red curry paste

½ tsp ground turmeric

200 ml/7 fl oz coconut milk

250 g/9 oz potatoes, cut into
   2-cm/¾-inch cubes

100 ml/3½ fl oz vegetable stock

200 g/7 oz young spinach leaves

1 small onion, thinly sliced
   into rings

COOK'S TIP

Choose a firm, waxy potato for
this dish, one that will keep its
shape during cooking, in
preference to a floury variety,
which will break up easily
once cooked.

1 Place the garlic, galangal, lemon grass and coriander seeds in a mortar and, using a pestle, pound to a smooth paste.

2 Heat 2 tablespoons of the oil in a frying pan or preheated wok. Stir in the garlic paste mixture and stir-fry for 30 seconds. Stir in the curry paste and turmeric, then add the coconut milk and bring to the boil.

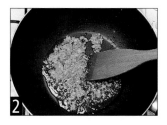

3 Add the potatoes and stock. Return to the boil, then reduce the heat and simmer, uncovered, for 10–12 minutes, or until the potatoes are almost tender.

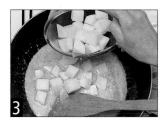

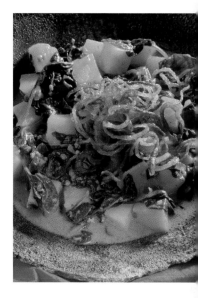

4 Stir in the spinach and simmer until the leaves are wilted.

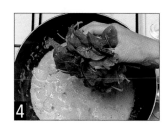

5 Meanwhile, heat the remaining oil in a separate frying pan. Add the onion and fry until crisp and golden brown.

6 Place the fried onions on top of the curry just before serving.

vegetable biryani

serves four

1 large potato, cubed

100 g/3½ oz baby carrots

50 g/1¾ oz okra, thickly sliced

2 celery sticks, sliced

75 g/2¾ oz baby button
  mushrooms, halved

1 aubergine, halved and sliced

300 ml/10 fl oz natural yogurt

1 tbsp grated fresh root ginger

2 large onions, grated

4 garlic cloves, crushed

1 tsp ground turmeric

1 tbsp curry powder

2 tbsp butter

2 onions, sliced

225 g/8 oz basmati rice

fresh coriander leaves, to garnish

1 Cook the potato cubes, carrots and okra in a saucepan of lightly salted boiling water for 7–8 minutes. Drain well and place in a large bowl. Add the celery, mushrooms and aubergine and mix together.

2 Mix the yogurt, ginger, grated onions, garlic, turmeric and curry powder together in a separate bowl and spoon over the vegetables. Cover and leave to marinate in the refrigerator for at least 2 hours.

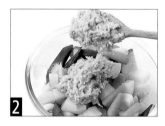

3 Preheat the oven to 190°C/375°F/Gas Mark 5. Heat the butter in a frying pan. Add the sliced onions and cook for 5–6 minutes, or until golden. Remove a few onions from the frying pan and reserve for the garnish.

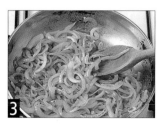

4 Add the vegetables to the onions and cook for 10 minutes.

5 Meanwhile, cook the rice in a saucepan of boiling water for 7 minutes. Drain well and set on one side.

6 Place half the rice in a 2-litre/3½-pint flameproof casserole. Spoon the vegetables on top and cover with the remaining rice. Cover and cook in the oven for 20–25 minutes, or until the rice is tender.

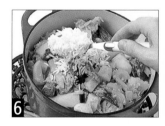

7 Spoon the biryani on to a warmed serving plate, garnish with the reserved onions and coriander leaves and serve immediately.

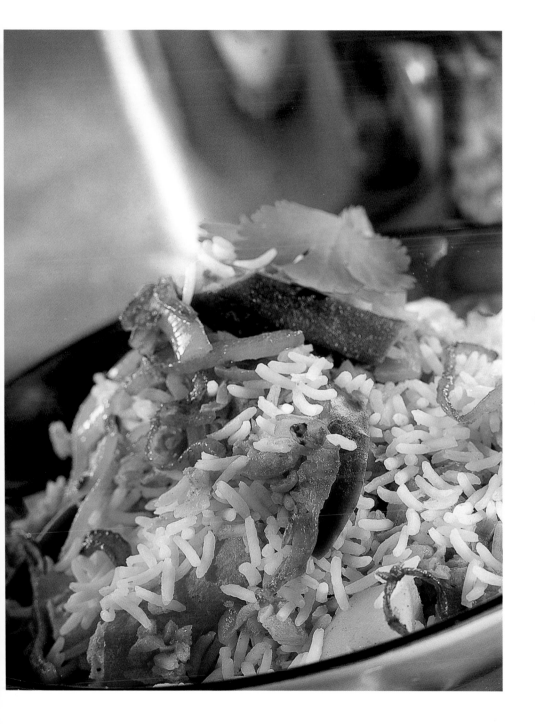

spiced cashew nut curry

serves four

250 g/9 oz unsalted cashew nuts

1 tsp coriander seeds

1 tsp cumin seeds

2 green cardamoms, crushed

1 tbsp sunflower oil

1 onion, thinly sliced

1 garlic clove, crushed

1 small fresh green chilli, deseeded
  and chopped

1 cinnamon stick

½ tsp ground turmeric

4 tbsp coconut cream

300 ml/10 fl oz hot vegetable stock

3 kaffir lime leaves, finely shredded

boiled jasmine rice, to serve

COOK'S TIP

All spices give the best flavour
when freshly crushed, but if you
prefer, you can use ground spices
instead of crushing them yourself
in a mortar with a pestle.

1 Soak the cashew nuts in cold water overnight. Drain thoroughly. Crush the coriander and cumin seeds and cardamoms with a pestle in a mortar.

2 Heat the oil in a frying pan and stir-fry the onion and garlic for 2–3 minutes, or until softened but not browned. Add the chilli, crushed spices, cinnamon stick and turmeric and stir-fry for a further minute.

3 Add the coconut cream and the hot stock to the pan. Bring to the boil, then add the cashew nuts and lime leaves.

4 Cover the pan, reduce the heat and simmer for 20 minutes. Serve hot, accompanied by jasmine rice.

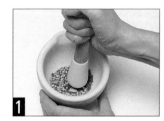

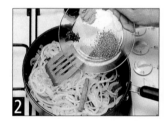

coconut vegetable curry

serves four

1 large aubergine, cut into
    2.5-cm/1-inch cubes

salt and pepper

2 tbsp vegetable oil

2 garlic cloves, crushed

1 fresh green chilli, deseeded and
    finely chopped

1 tsp grated fresh root ginger

1 onion, finely chopped

2 tsp garam masala

8 green cardamoms

1 tsp ground turmeric

1 tbsp tomato purée

700 ml/1¼ pints vegetable stock

1 tbsp lemon juice

225 g/8 oz potatoes, diced

250 g/9 oz small cauliflower florets

225 g/8 oz okra

225 g/8 oz frozen peas

150 ml/5 fl oz coconut milk

flaked coconut, to garnish

naan bread, to serve

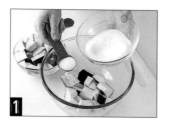

1 Layer the aubergine in a bowl, sprinkling with salt as you go. Set aside for 30 minutes. Rinse well under cold running water. Drain and pat dry. Set aside.

2 Heat the oil in a large saucepan over a medium heat and cook the garlic, chilli, ginger, onion and spices for 4–5 minutes.

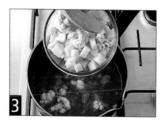

3 Stir in the tomato purée, stock, lemon juice, potatoes and cauliflower and mix well. Bring to the boil, then reduce the heat, cover and simmer for 15 minutes.

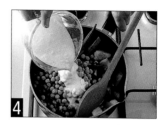

4 Stir in the aubergine, okra, peas and coconut milk and season to taste with salt and pepper. Simmer, uncovered, for a further 10 minutes, or until tender. Discard the cardamoms. Pile the curry on to a warmed serving platter, garnish with flaked coconut and serve with naan bread.

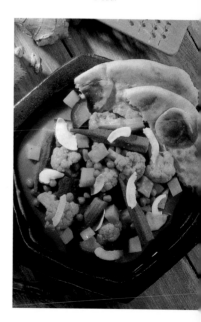

mixed vegetable balti

serves four

225 g/8 oz split yellow peas

3 tbsp vegetable oil

1 tsp onion seeds

2 onions, sliced

115 g/4 oz courgettes, sliced

115 g/4 oz potatoes, cut into
    1-cm/½-inch cubes

115 g/4 oz carrots, sliced

1 small aubergine, sliced

225 g/8 oz tomatoes, chopped

300 ml/10 fl oz water

3 garlic cloves, chopped

1 tsp ground cumin

1 tsp ground coriander

1 tsp salt

2 fresh green chillies, sliced

½ tsp garam masala

2 tbsp chopped fresh coriander

1 Put the split peas in a saucepan and cover with lightly salted water. Bring to the boil, then reduce the heat and simmer for 30 minutes. Drain the peas and keep warm.

2 Heat the oil in a karahi or preheated wok, add the onion seeds and fry until they start popping.

3 Add the onions and stir-fry over a medium heat until golden brown.

4 Add the courgettes, potatoes, carrots and aubergine to the pan. Stir-fry for 2 minutes.

5 Stir in the tomatoes, water, garlic, cumin, ground coriander, salt, chillies, garam masala and the reserved split peas.

6 Bring to the boil, then reduce the heat and simmer for 15 minutes, or until all the vegetables are tender.

7 Stir the fresh coriander into the vegetables. Transfer to a warmed serving dish and serve immediately.

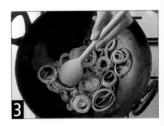

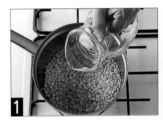

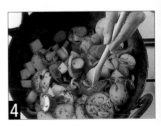

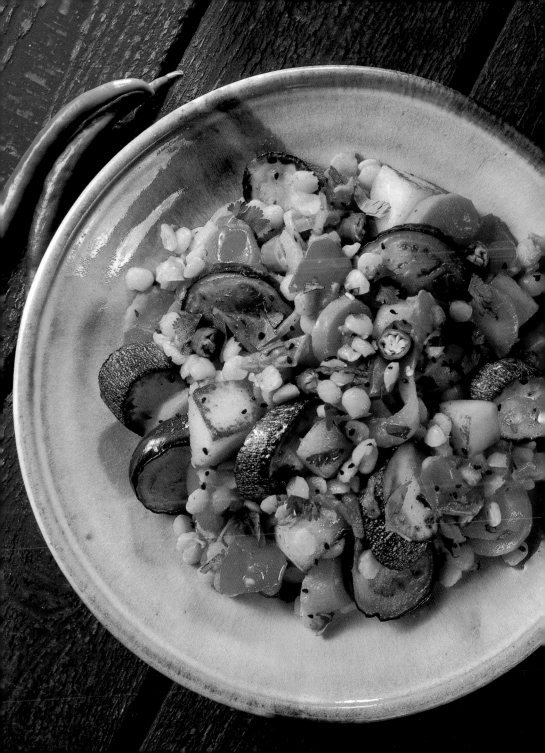

mexican pickles

serves six

3 tbsp vegetable oil

1 onion, thinly sliced

5 garlic cloves, cut into slivers

3 carrots, thinly sliced

2 fresh green chillies, such as
   jalapeño or serrano, deseeded
   and cut into strips

1 small cauliflower, broken
   into florets or cut into
   bite-sized chunks

½ red pepper, deseeded and diced
   or cut into strips

1 celery stick, cut into
   bite-sized pieces

½ tsp oregano leaves

1 bay leaf

¼ tsp ground cumin

5 tbsp cider vinegar

salt and pepper

1 Heat the oil in a heavy-based frying pan and add the onion, garlic, carrots, chillies, cauliflower, pepper and celery. Cook over a low heat, stirring occasionally, for 3–4 minutes, or until just softened but not browned.

2 Add the oregano, bay leaf, cumin and vinegar and season to taste with salt and pepper. Add just enough water to cover the vegetables. Cook for a further 5–10 minutes, or just long enough for the vegetables to be tender but still firm to the bite.

3 Adjust the seasoning, adding more vinegar if needed. Set aside to cool and serve as a relish or with buttered tortillas Mexican-style. The Mexican pickles will keep for up to 2 weeks, if stored in a sealed container in the refrigerator.

COOK'S TIP
Wear rubber gloves when slicing and deseeding fresh chillies and do not touch your eyes during preparation.

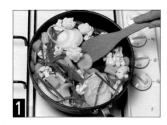

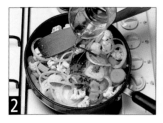

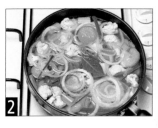

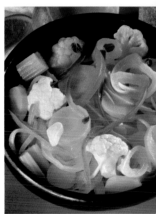

spicy black-eyed beans

serves four

350 g/12 oz black-eyed beans,
    soaked overnight in cold water

1 tbsp vegetable oil

2 onions, chopped

1 tbsp clear honey

2 tbsp treacle

4 tbsp dark soy sauce

1 tsp dry mustard powder

4 tbsp tomato purée

450 ml/16 fl oz vegetable stock

1 bay leaf

1 sprig each of fresh rosemary,
    thyme and sage

1 small orange

pepper

1 tbsp cornflour

2 red peppers, deseeded and diced

2 tbsp chopped fresh parsley,
    to garnish

crusty bread, to serve

1 Preheat the oven to 150°C/300°F/ Gas Mark 2. Rinse the beans and place in a saucepan. Cover with water, bring to the boil and boil rapidly for 10 minutes. Drain and place in an ovenproof casserole.

2 Meanwhile, heat the oil in a frying pan and fry the onions for 5 minutes. Stir in the honey, treacle, soy sauce, mustard and tomato purée. Pour in the stock, bring to the boil and pour over the beans.

3 Tie the bay leaf and herbs together with a clean piece of string and add to the casserole. Using a vegetable peeler, pare 3 pieces of orange rind and mix into the beans, along with plenty of pepper. Cover and bake in the oven for 1 hour.

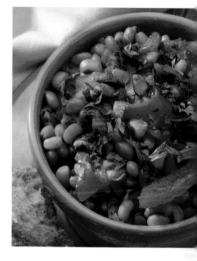

4 Extract the juice from the orange and blend with the cornflour to form a paste. Stir into the beans with the peppers. Cover and cook for a further 1 hour, or until the sauce is rich and thick and the beans are tender. Discard the herbs and orange rind.

5 Garnish with chopped parsley and serve with crusty bread.

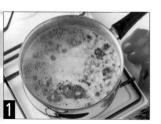

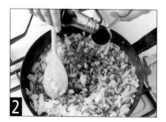

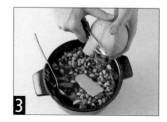

195

spanish tortilla

1 kg/2 lb 4 oz waxy potatoes, thinly sliced

4 tbsp vegetable oil

1 onion, sliced

2 garlic cloves, crushed

1 green pepper, deseeded and diced

2 tomatoes, deseeded and chopped

25 g/1 oz canned sweetcorn kernels, drained

6 large eggs, beaten

2 tbsp chopped fresh parsley

salt and pepper

crisp salad, to serve

COOK'S TIP

Ensure that the handle of your pan is heatproof before placing it under the grill and be sure to use an oven glove when removing it because it will be very hot.

1 Parboil the potatoes in a saucepan of lightly salted boiling water for 5 minutes. Drain well.

2 Heat the oil in a large frying pan, add the potatoes and onion and sauté over a low heat, stirring constantly, for 5 minutes, or until the potatoes have browned.

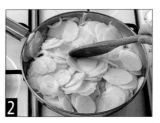

3 Add the garlic, pepper, tomatoes and sweetcorn, mixing well.

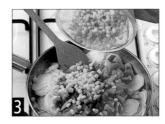

4 Pour in the eggs and add the parsley. Season to taste with salt and pepper. Cook for 10–12 minutes, or until the underside is cooked.

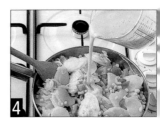

5 Preheat the grill to medium. Remove the frying pan from the heat and continue to cook the tortilla under the hot grill for 5–7 minutes, or until the tortilla is set and the top is golden brown.

6 Cut the tortilla into wedges or cubes, depending on your preference, and transfer to serving dishes. Serve hot, warm or cold with a crisp salad.

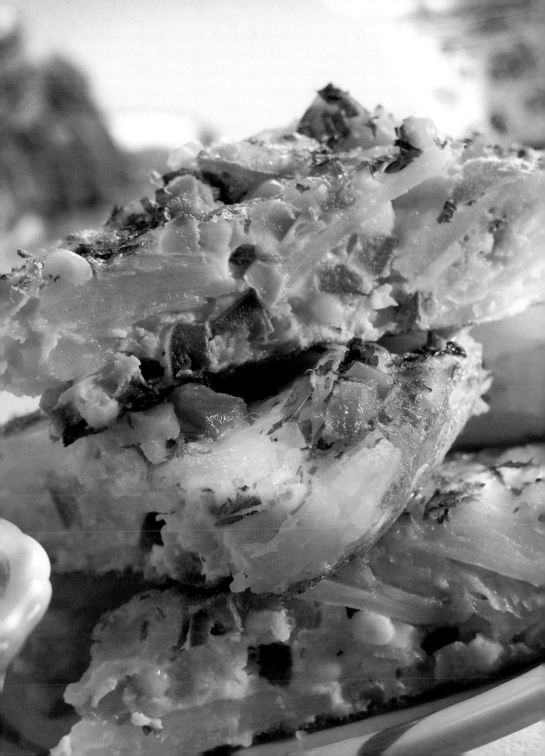

winter vegetable cobbler

serves four

1 tbsp olive oil

1 garlic clove, crushed

8 small onions, halved

2 celery sticks, sliced

225 g/8 oz swede, chopped

2 carrots, sliced

½ small cauliflower, broken
   into florets

225 g/8 oz mushrooms, sliced

400 g/14 oz canned
   chopped tomatoes

55 g/2 oz split red lentils, washed

2 tbsp cornflour

3–4 tbsp water

300 ml/10 fl oz vegetable stock

2 tsp Tabasco sauce

2 tsp chopped fresh oregano, plus
   extra sprigs to garnish

COBBLER TOPPING

225 g/8 oz self-raising flour,
   plus extra for dusting

pinch of salt

4 tbsp butter

115 g/4 oz grated mature
   Cheddar cheese

2 tsp chopped fresh oregano

1 egg, lightly beaten

150 ml/5 fl oz milk

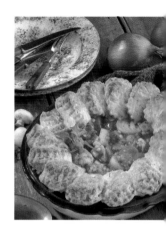

1. Preheat the oven to 180°C/350°F/Gas Mark 4. Heat the oil in a frying pan and cook the garlic and onions for 5 minutes. Add the celery, swede, carrots and cauliflower and cook for 2–3 minutes. Add the mushrooms, tomatoes and lentils. Blend the cornflour with the water and stir into the pan with the stock, Tabasco sauce and oregano.

2. Transfer to an ovenproof dish, cover and bake in the oven for 20 minutes.

3. To make the topping, sift the flour with the salt into a bowl. Rub in the butter, then stir in most of the cheese and the oregano. Beat the egg with the milk and add enough to the dry ingredients to make a soft dough. Knead, roll out on a lightly floured surface to 1 cm/½ inch thick and cut into 5-cm/2-inch rounds.

4. Remove the dish from the oven and increase the temperature to 200°C/400°F/Gas Mark 6. Arrange the scones around the edge of the dish, brush with the remaining egg and milk and sprinkle with the reserved cheese. Bake for a further 10–12 minutes. Garnish with oregano and serve.

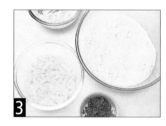

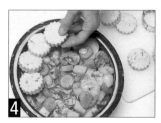

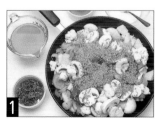

spicy potato & lemon casserole

serves four

100 ml/3½ fl oz olive oil

2 red onions, cut into 8 wedges

3 garlic cloves, crushed

2 tsp ground cumin

2 tsp ground coriander

pinch of cayenne pepper

1 carrot, thickly sliced

2 small turnips, quartered

1 courgette, sliced

450 g/1 lb potatoes, thickly sliced

rind and juice of 2 large lemons

300 ml/10 fl oz vegetable stock

salt and pepper

2 tbsp chopped fresh coriander

COOK'S TIP

A selection of spices and herbs is important for adding variety to your cooking – add to your range each time you try a new recipe.

Check the vegetables while cooking, because they may begin to stick to the casserole. Add a little more boiling water or stock if necessary.

1 Heat the oil in a flameproof casserole.

2 Add the onion wedges and sauté for 3 minutes, stirring.

3 Add the garlic and cook for 30 seconds. Mix in the spices and cook for 1 minute, stirring constantly.

4 Add the carrot, turnips, courgette and potatoes and stir to coat in the oil.

5 Add the lemon rind and juice, stock and salt and pepper to taste, cover and cook over a medium heat for 20–30 minutes, stirring occasionally.

6 Remove the lid, sprinkle in the coriander and stir well. Serve immediately.

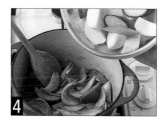

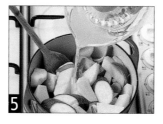

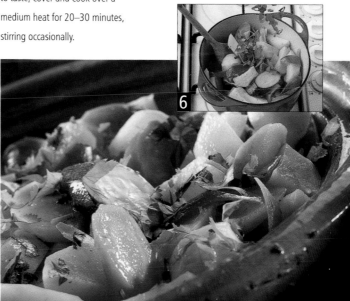

pasta & bean casserole

serves four

225 g/8 oz dried haricot beans,
soaked overnight and drained

225 g/8 oz dried penne, or other
short pasta shapes

6 tbsp olive oil

850 ml/1½ pints vegetable stock

2 large onions, sliced

2 garlic cloves, chopped

2 bay leaves

1 tsp dried oregano

1 tsp dried thyme

5 tbsp red wine

2 tbsp tomato purée

2 celery sticks, sliced

1 fennel bulb, sliced

115 g/4 oz mushrooms, sliced

225 g/8 oz tomatoes, sliced

salt and pepper

1 tsp dark muscovado sugar

55 g/2 oz dry white breadcrumbs

TO SERVE

salad leaves

crusty bread

1 Preheat the oven to 180°C/350°F/ Gas Mark 4. Put the beans in a large saucepan, add water to cover and bring to the boil. Boil rapidly for 20 minutes, then drain and set aside.

2 Cook the pasta for 3 minutes only in a large saucepan of lightly salted boiling water, adding 1 tablespoon of the oil. Drain in a colander and set aside.

3 Put the beans in a large, flameproof casserole, pour in the stock and stir in the remaining oil, the onions, garlic, bay leaves, herbs, wine and tomato purée.

4 Bring to the boil, cover the casserole and cook in the oven for 2 hours.

5 Remove the casserole from the oven, add the reserved pasta, the celery, fennel, mushrooms and tomatoes and season to taste with salt and pepper.

6 Stir in the sugar and sprinkle the breadcrumbs on top. Cover the casserole again, return to the oven and cook for a further 1 hour. Serve straight from the casserole with salad leaves and crusty bread.

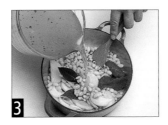

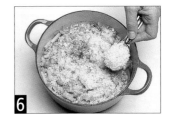

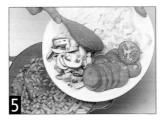

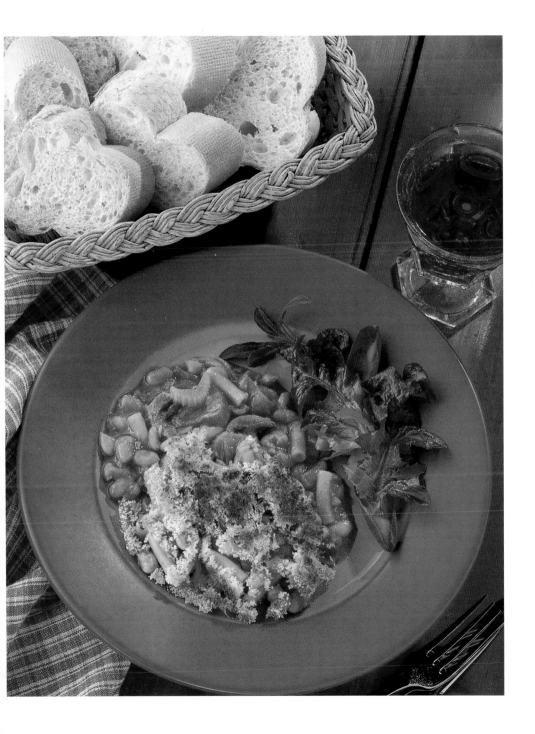

lentil & rice casserole

serves four

225 g/8 oz split red lentils, washed

50 g/1¾ oz long-grain rice

1 litre/1¾ pints vegetable stock

150 ml/5 fl oz dry white wine

1 leek, cut into chunks

3 garlic cloves, crushed

400 g/14 oz canned

    chopped tomatoes

1 tsp ground cumin

1 tsp chilli powder

1 tsp garam masala

1 red pepper, deseeded and sliced

100 g/3½ oz small broccoli florets

8 baby corn cobs,

    halved lengthways

50 g/1¾ oz French beans, halved

1 tbsp shredded fresh basil, plus

    extra sprigs to garnish

salt and pepper

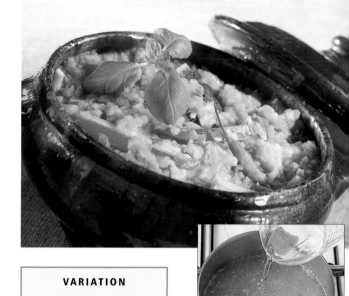

VARIATION

You can vary the rice in this recipe – use brown or wild rice, if you prefer.

1 Place the lentils, rice, stock and wine in a flameproof casserole over a low heat and cook for 20 minutes, stirring occasionally.

2 Add the leek, garlic, tomatoes, cumin, chilli powder, garam masala, pepper, broccoli, baby corn cobs and beans.

3 Bring the mixture to the boil, then reduce the heat, cover and simmer for a further 10–15 minutes, or until the vegetables are tender.

4 Add the shredded basil and season to taste with salt and pepper.

5 Garnish with basil sprigs and serve immediately.

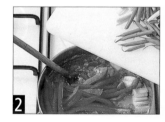

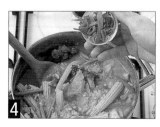

chickpea & vegetable casserole

serves four

1 tbsp olive oil

1 red onion, halved and sliced

3 garlic cloves, crushed

225 g/8 oz spinach leaves

1 fennel bulb, cut into eighths

1 red pepper, deseeded and diced

1 tbsp plain flour

450 ml/16 fl oz vegetable stock

85 ml/3 fl oz dry white wine

400 g/14 oz canned
 chickpeas, drained

1 bay leaf

1 tsp ground coriander

½ tsp paprika

salt and pepper

fennel fronds, to garnish

1 Heat the oil in a large, flameproof casserole. Add the onion and garlic and sauté for 1 minute, stirring. Add the spinach and cook for 4 minutes, or until wilted.

2 Add the fennel and pepper and cook for 2 minutes, stirring.

3 Stir in the flour and cook for 1 minute.

4 Add the stock, wine, chickpeas, bay leaf, coriander and paprika, cover and cook for 30 minutes. Season to taste with salt and pepper, garnish with fennel fronds and serve immediately.

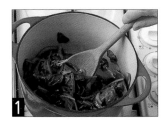

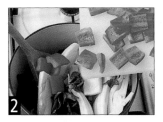

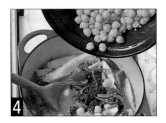

COOK'S TIP
Use other canned pulses or mixed beans instead of the chickpeas, if you prefer.

VARIATION
Replace the coriander with nutmeg, if you prefer, as it works particularly well with spinach.

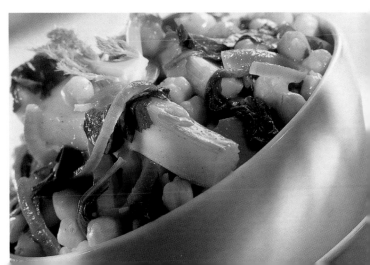

vegetable hotpot

serves four

2 large potatoes, thinly sliced

2 tbsp vegetable oil

1 red onion, halved and sliced

1 leek, sliced

2 garlic cloves, crushed

1 carrot, cut into chunks

100 g/3½ oz broccoli florets

100 g/3½ oz cauliflower florets

2 small turnips, quartered

1 tbsp plain flour

700 ml/1¼ pints vegetable stock

150 ml/5 fl oz dry cider

1 dessert apple, sliced

2 tbsp chopped fresh sage

pinch of cayenne pepper

salt and pepper

50 g/1¾ oz Cheddar cheese, grated

1 Preheat the oven to 190°C/375°F/Gas Mark 5. Cook the potato slices in a saucepan of boiling water for 10 minutes. Drain thoroughly and reserve until required.

2 Heat the oil in a flameproof casserole. Add the onion, leek and garlic and sauté for 2–3 minutes. Add the remaining vegetables and cook for a further 3–4 minutes, stirring.

3 Stir in the flour and cook for 1 minute. Gradually add the stock and cider and bring the mixture to the boil. Add the apple, sage and cayenne pepper and season well with salt and pepper. Remove the casserole from the heat. Transfer the vegetables to an ovenproof dish.

COOK'S TIP

If the potato begins to brown too quickly, cover with foil for the last 10 minutes of the cooking time to prevent the top burning.

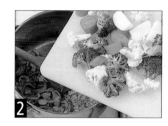

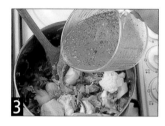

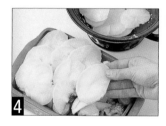

4 Arrange the potato slices on top of the vegetable mixture to cover.

5 Sprinkle the cheese on top of the potato slices and cook in the oven for 30–35 minutes, or until the potato is golden brown and beginning to crisp slightly around the edges. Serve immediately.

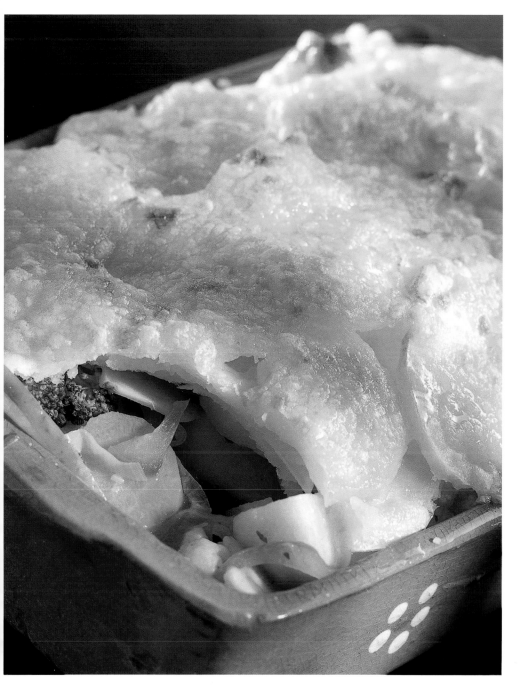

sweet & sour aubergines

serves four

2 large aubergines

salt and pepper

6 tbsp olive oil

4 garlic cloves, crushed

1 onion, cut into 8 wedges

4 large tomatoes, deseeded
and chopped

3 tbsp chopped fresh mint

150 ml/5 fl oz vegetable stock

4 tsp brown sugar

2 tbsp red wine vinegar

1 tsp dried chilli flakes

fresh mint sprigs, to garnish

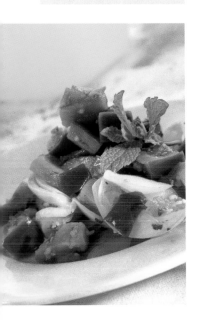

1 Using a sharp knife, cut the aubergines into cubes. Place them in a colander, sprinkle with salt and leave to stand for 30 minutes. Rinse thoroughly under cold running water and drain well. This process removes all the bitter juices from the aubergines. Pat dry with kitchen paper.

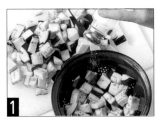

2 Heat the oil in a large frying pan. Add the aubergine and sauté, stirring constantly, for 1–2 minutes.

3 Stir in the garlic and onion and cook for a further 2–3 minutes.

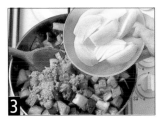

4 Stir in the tomatoes, mint and stock, cover and cook for 15–20 minutes, or until the vegetables are tender.

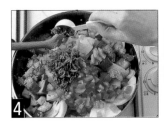

5 Stir in the sugar, vinegar and chilli flakes, season to taste with salt and pepper and cook for 2–3 minutes. Transfer the aubergines to warmed serving plates, garnish with mint sprigs and serve.

COOK'S TIP

Mint is a popular herb in Middle Eastern cooking. It is a useful herb to grow yourself as it can be added to a variety of dishes, particularly salads and vegetable dishes. It can be grown easily in a garden or window box.

cauliflower bake

serves four

450 g/1 lb cauliflower, broken
   into florets

2 large potatoes, cubed

100 g/3½ oz cherry tomatoes

SAUCE

25 g/1 oz butter or margarine

1 leek, sliced

1 garlic clove, crushed

25 g/1 oz plain flour

300 ml/10 fl oz milk

75 g/2¾ oz mixed grated cheese,
   such as Cheddar, Parmesan
   and Gruyère

½ tsp paprika

2 tbsp chopped fresh flat-leaved
   parsley, plus extra to garnish

salt and pepper

1 Preheat the oven to 180°C/
350°F/Gas Mark 4. Cook the
cauliflower in a saucepan of boiling
water for 10 minutes. Drain well and
reserve. Meanwhile, cook the potatoes
in a separate saucepan of boiling water
for 10 minutes, drain and reserve.

2 To make the sauce, melt the
butter or margarine in a
saucepan. Add the leek and garlic and
sauté for 1 minute. Add the flour and
cook for 1 minute. Remove the
saucepan from the heat and gradually
stir in the milk, 50 g/1¾ oz of the
cheese, the paprika and parsley. Return
the saucepan to the heat. Bring to the
boil, stirring. Season to taste with salt
and pepper.

3 Spoon the cauliflower into a
deep, ovenproof dish. Add the
tomatoes and top with the potatoes.
Pour the sauce over the potatoes and
sprinkle over the remaining cheese.

4 Cook in the oven for 20 minutes,
or until the vegetables are cooked
through and the cheese is golden
brown and bubbling. Garnish with
parsley and serve immediately.

VARIATION

This dish could be made with
broccoli instead of the
cauliflower as an alternative.

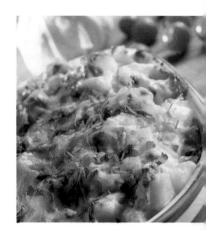

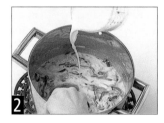

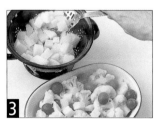

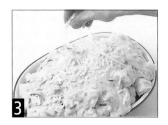

cheese & potato layer bake

450 g/1 lb potatoes

salt and pepper

1 leek, sliced

3 garlic cloves, crushed

50 g/1¾ oz Cheddar cheese, grated

50 g/1¾ oz mozzarella cheese, grated

25 g/1 oz freshly grated Parmesan cheese

2 tbsp chopped fresh flat-leaved parsley, plus extra to garnish

150 ml/5 fl oz single cream

150 ml/5 fl oz milk

1 Preheat the oven to 160°C/ 325°F/Gas Mark 3. Cook the potatoes in a saucepan of lightly salted boiling water for 10 minutes. Drain well.

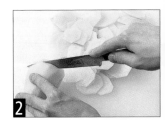

2 Cut the potatoes into thin slices. Arrange a layer of potatoes in the base of an ovenproof dish. Layer with a little of the leek, garlic, cheeses and chopped parsley and season well with salt and pepper.

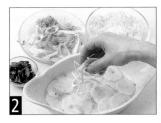

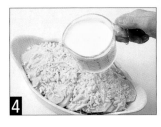

3 Repeat the layers until all of the ingredients have been used, finishing with a layer of cheese on top.

4 Mix the cream and milk together, season to taste with salt and pepper and pour the mixture over the potato layers.

5 Cook in the oven for 1–1¼ hours, or until the cheese is golden brown and bubbling and the potatoes are cooked through.

6 Garnish with chopped parsley and serve immediately.

COOK'S TIP

This tasty bake is perfect for serving as an accompaniment to a whole range of main dishes featured in the book that can be cooked in the oven at the same time, such as a meat or poultry casserole or a gently baked fish dish.

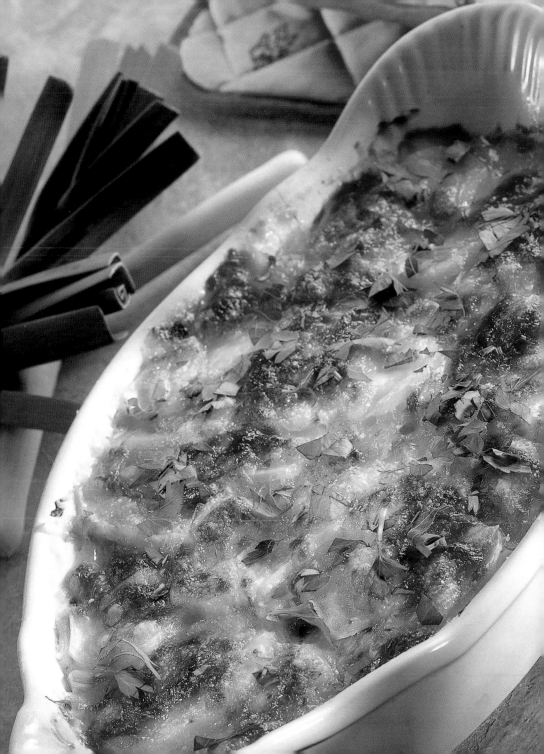

vegetable toad in the hole

serves four

BATTER

100 g/3½ oz plain flour

pinch of salt

2 eggs, beaten

200 ml/7 fl oz milk

2 tbsp wholegrain mustard

2 tbsp vegetable oil

FILLING

75 g/2¾ oz baby carrots,
    halved lengthways

50 g/1¾ oz French beans

2 tbsp butter

2 garlic cloves, crushed

1 onion, cut into 8 wedges

50 g/1¾ oz canned sweetcorn
    kernels, drained

2 tomatoes, deseeded and cut
    into chunks

1 tsp wholegrain mustard

1 tbsp chopped fresh mixed herbs

salt and pepper

COOK'S TIP

It is important that the oil is hot
before adding the batter so that
the batter begins to cook and
rise immediately.

1 Preheat the oven to 200°C/
400°F/Gas Mark 6. To make
the batter, sift the flour and the salt
into a large bowl. Make a well in the
centre and beat in the eggs and milk
to form a batter. Stir in the mustard
and leave the batter to stand until
required.

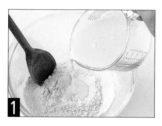

2 Pour the oil into a shallow
ovenproof dish and heat in the
oven for 10 minutes.

3 To make the filling, cook the
carrots and beans in a saucepan
of boiling water for 7 minutes, or until
tender. Drain well. Melt the butter in a
frying pan. Add the garlic and onion
and sauté for 2 minutes, stirring.

4 Add the sweetcorn, tomatoes,
mustard and herbs. Season well
with salt and pepper and add the
carrots and beans.

5 Remove the dish from the oven
and pour in the batter. Spoon the
vegetables into the centre, return to
the oven and cook for 30–35 minutes,
or until the batter has risen and set.
Serve immediately.

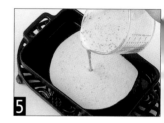

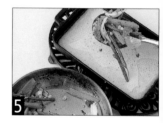

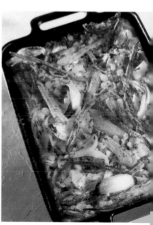

cauliflower & broccoli with herb sauce

serves four

2 baby cauliflowers

225 g/8 oz broccoli

salt and pepper

SAUCE

8 tbsp olive oil

4 tbsp butter

2 tsp grated fresh root ginger

rind and juice of 2 lemons

5 tbsp chopped fresh coriander

5 tbsp grated Cheddar cheese

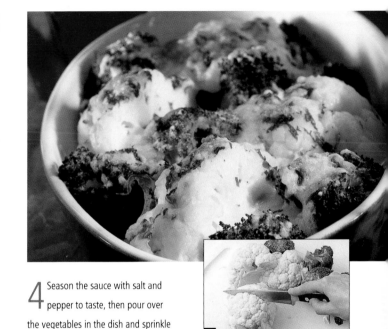

1 Preheat the grill to medium. Using a sharp knife, cut the cauliflowers in half and the broccoli into very large florets.

2 Cook the cauliflower and broccoli in a saucepan of lightly salted boiling water for 10 minutes. Drain well, transfer to a shallow flameproof dish and keep warm until required.

3 To make the sauce, place the oil and butter in a frying pan and heat gently until the butter melts. Add the ginger, lemon rind and juice and coriander and simmer for 2–3 minutes, stirring occasionally.

4 Season the sauce with salt and pepper to taste, then pour over the vegetables in the dish and sprinkle the cheese on top.

5 Cook under the hot grill for 2–3 minutes, or until the cheese is bubbling and golden. Leave to cool for 1–2 minutes, then serve.

VARIATION

Lime or orange could be used instead of the lemon for a fruity and refreshing sauce.

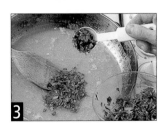

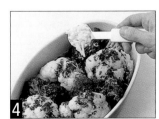

211

green tagliatelle with garlic

serves four

2 tbsp walnut oil

1 bunch spring onions, sliced

2 garlic cloves, thinly sliced

225 g/8 oz sliced mushrooms

salt and pepper

450 g/1 lb fresh green and
white tagliatelle

225 g/8 oz frozen spinach,
thawed and drained

115 g/4 oz full-fat soft cheese with
garlic and herbs

4 tbsp single cream

55 g/2 oz unsalted pistachio
nuts, chopped

2 tbsp shredded fresh basil

fresh basil sprigs, to garnish

Italian bread, to serve

1 Heat the oil in a large frying pan. Add the spring onions and garlic and cook for 1 minute, or until just softened.

2 Add the mushrooms to the pan and stir well. Cover and cook over a low heat for about 5 minutes, or until just softened but not browned.

3 Meanwhile, bring a large saucepan of lightly salted water to the boil. Add the tagliatelle, return to the boil and cook for 3–5 minutes, or until tender but still firm to the bite. Drain the tagliatelle thoroughly and return to the saucepan.

4 Add the spinach to the frying pan and heat through for 1–2 minutes. Add the cheese to the pan and heat until slightly melted. Stir in the cream and cook, without allowing the mixture to come to the boil, until warmed through.

5 Pour the sauce over the pasta, season to taste with salt and pepper the mix well. Heat through gently, stirring constantly, for 2–3 minutes.

6 Transfer the pasta to a warmed serving dish and sprinkle with the pistachio nuts and shredded basil. Garnish with basil sprigs and serve immediately with focaccia, ciabatta or other Italian bread of your choice.

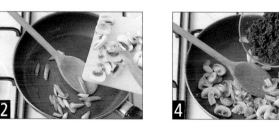

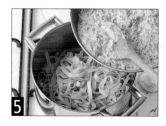

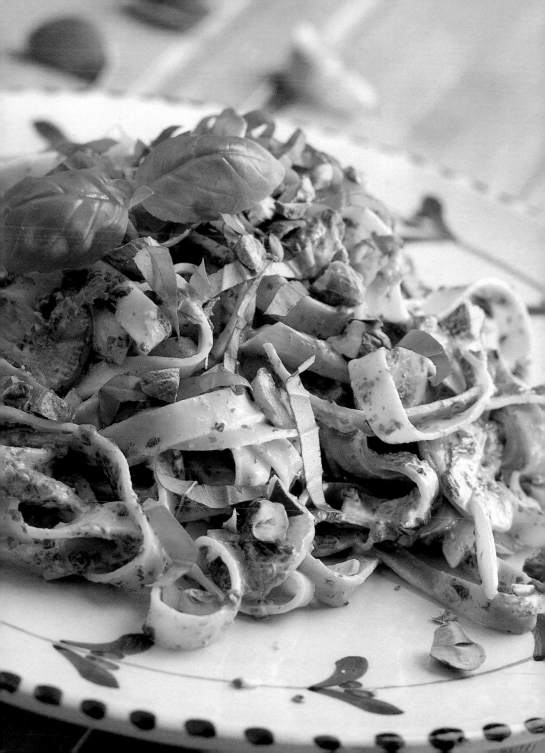

baked cheese & tomato macaroni

serves four

225 g/8 oz dried elbow macaroni

salt and pepper

175 g/6 oz Cheddar cheese,
  grated

100 g/3½ oz freshly grated
  Parmesan cheese

1 tbsp butter or margarine,
  plus extra for greasing

4 tbsp fresh white breadcrumbs

1 tbsp chopped fresh basil

TOMATO SAUCE

1 tbsp olive oil

1 shallot, finely chopped

2 garlic cloves, crushed

450 g/1 lb canned
  chopped tomatoes

1 tbsp chopped fresh basil

salt and pepper

COOK'S TIP

Use other dried pasta shapes,
such as penne, if you have them
to hand, instead of the macaroni.

1 Preheat the oven to 190°C/
375°F/Gas Mark 5. To make
the tomato sauce, heat the oil in a
saucepan. Add the shallot and garlic
and sauté for 1 minute. Add the
tomatoes, basil and salt and pepper
to taste and cook over a medium heat,
stirring, for 10 minutes.

2 Meanwhile, cook the macaroni in
a large saucepan of lightly salted
boiling water for 8 minutes, or until
just undercooked. Drain.

3 Mix both of the cheeses together
in a bowl.

4 Grease a deep, ovenproof dish.
Spoon a third of the tomato sauce
into the base of the dish, top with a
third of the macaroni and then a third
of the cheeses. Season to taste with
salt and pepper. Repeat the layers
twice more.

5 Mix the breadcrumbs and basil
together and sprinkle over the
top. Dot with the butter or margarine
and cook in the oven for 25 minutes,
or until golden brown and bubbling.
Serve immediately.

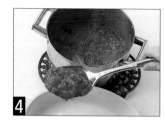

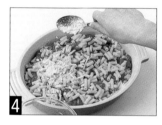

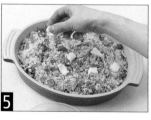

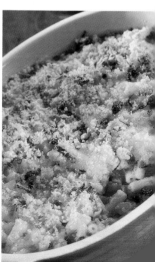

vegetable lasagne

serves four

1 aubergine, sliced

salt and pepper

3 tbsp olive oil

2 garlic cloves, crushed

1 red onion, halved and sliced

1 green pepper, deseeded and diced

1 red pepper, deseeded and diced

1 yellow pepper, deseeded
  and diced

225 g/8 oz mushrooms, sliced

2 celery sticks, sliced

1 courgette, diced

½ tsp chilli powder

½ tsp ground cumin

2 tomatoes, chopped

300 ml/10 fl oz passata

2 tbsp chopped fresh basil

8 no pre-cook lasagne verde sheets

CHEESE SAUCE

2 tbsp butter or margarine

1 tbsp flour

150 ml/5 fl oz vegetable stock

300 ml/10 fl oz milk

75 g/2¾ oz Cheddar cheese,
  grated

1 tsp Dijon mustard

1 tbsp chopped fresh basil

1 egg, beaten

1 Preheat the oven to 180°C/
350°F/Gas Mark 4. Place the
aubergine slices in a colander, sprinkle
with salt and leave to stand for
20 minutes. Rinse under cold running
water, drain and reserve.

2 Heat the oil in a large frying pan.
Add the garlic and onion and
sauté for 1–2 minutes. Add the
peppers, mushrooms, celery and
courgette and cook for 3–4 minutes,
stirring. Stir in the spices and cook for
1 minute.

3 Mix the tomatoes, passata and
basil together, then season well
with salt and pepper.

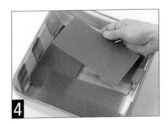

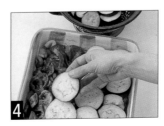

4 To make the sauce, melt the
butter or margarine in a
saucepan. Add the flour and cook for
1 minute. Remove the saucepan from
the heat and stir in the stock and milk.
Return to the heat and add half the
cheese and mustard. Boil, stirring, until
thickened. Stir in the basil and season
to taste with salt and pepper. Remove
the saucepan from the heat and stir in
the egg. Place half the lasagne sheets
in an ovenproof dish. Top with half the
vegetables, then half the tomato
sauce. Cover with half the aubergines.
Repeat and spoon the cheese sauce on
top. Sprinkle with the remaining
cheese and cook in the oven for
40 minutes. Serve immediately.

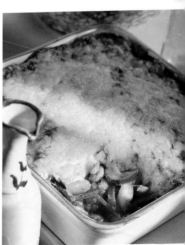

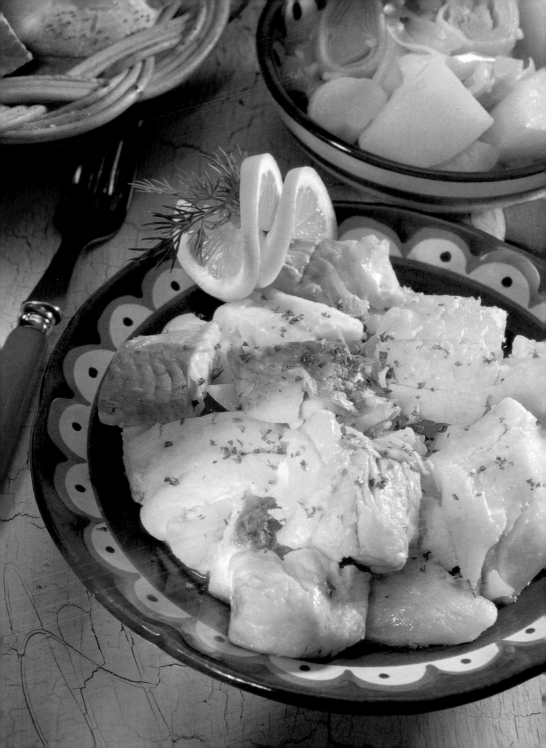

Fish

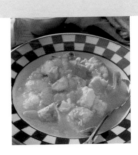

The range of seafood available these days is immense, but sometimes it is difficult to know how to cook unfamiliar fish. The answer might be to put it in a pot and make a fabulous stew. Creole Jambalaya (see page 232), Spanish Fish Stew (see page 250) or Bouillabaisse (see page 236) are as different as their countries of origin, equally delicious and incredibly easy to make. Another answer might be to stir it with rice to make an elegant Prawn and Asparagus Risotto (see page 231) or to combine it with chilli and other spices in a one-pot Goan Fish Curry (see page 234). Then, again, there are soups and chowders, bakes and pasta dishes — and not an unhealthy chip in sight. There are recipes for inexpensive family meals and dishes for sophisticated entertaining featuring seafood of all kinds, from cod to crab and from sardines to squid — even a lobster one-pot.

cullen skink

serves four

225 g/8 oz undyed smoked
   haddock fillet

2 tbsp butter

1 onion, finely chopped

600 ml/1 pint milk

350 g/12 oz potatoes, diced

350 g/12 oz cod, boned, skinned
   and cubed

150 ml/5 fl oz double cream

2 tbsp chopped fresh parsley

salt and pepper

lemon juice, to taste

TO GARNISH

lemon slices

fresh parsley sprigs

1 Put the haddock fillet in a large frying pan and cover with boiling water. Leave for 10 minutes. Drain, reserving 300 ml/10 fl oz of the soaking water. Flake the fish, taking care to remove all the bones.

2 Heat the butter in a large saucepan over a low heat. Add the onion and cook for 10 minutes, or until softened. Add the milk and bring to a gentle simmer before adding the potatoes. Cook for 10 minutes.

3 Add the reserved haddock and cod. Simmer for a further 10 minutes, or until the cod is tender.

COOK'S TIP
Look for Finnan haddock, if you can find it. Do not use yellow-dyed haddock fillet, which is often actually whiting and not haddock at all.

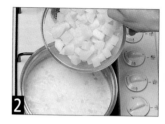

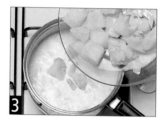

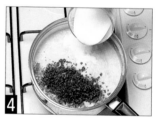

4 Remove about one-third of the fish and potatoes, transfer to a food processor and blend until smooth. Alternatively, push through a sieve into a bowl. Return to the saucepan with the cream, parsley and salt and pepper to taste. Add lemon juice, if wished. Add a little of the reserved soaking water if the soup seems too thick. Reheat gently and serve, garnished with lemon slices and parsley sprigs.

mediterranean fish soup

serves four

1 tbsp olive oil

1 large onion, chopped

2 garlic cloves, finely chopped

450 ml/16 fl oz fish stock

150 ml/5 fl oz dry white wine

1 bay leaf

1 sprig each of fresh thyme,
rosemary and oregano

450 g/1 lb firm white fish fillets,
such as cod, monkfish or halibut,
skinned and cut into
2.5-cm/1-inch cubes

450 g/1 lb live mussels, scrubbed
and debearded

400 g/14 oz canned
chopped tomatoes

225 g/8 oz cooked peeled prawns,
thawed if frozen

salt and pepper

fresh thyme sprigs, to garnish

TO SERVE

lemon wedges

4 slices toasted French bread,
rubbed with a cut garlic clove

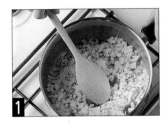

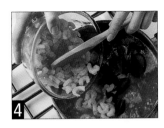

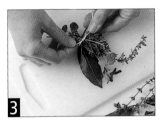

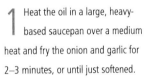

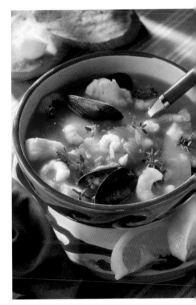

1 Heat the oil in a large, heavy-based saucepan over a medium heat and fry the onion and garlic for 2–3 minutes, or until just softened.

2 Pour in the stock and wine and bring to the boil.

3 Tie the bay leaf and herbs together with a clean piece of string and add to the saucepan with the fish and mussels. Stir, cover and simmer for 5 minutes.

4 Stir in the tomatoes and prawns and cook for a further 3–4 minutes, or until piping hot and the fish is cooked through.

5 Discard the herbs and any mussels that have not opened. Season to taste with salt and pepper, then ladle into warmed soup bowls.

6 Garnish with thyme sprigs and serve with lemon wedges and toasted bread rubbed with garlic.

219

mexican fish & roasted tomato soup

serves four

5 ripe tomatoes

5 garlic cloves, unpeeled

500 g/1 lb 2 oz red snapper,
    cut into chunks

1 litre/1¾ pints fish stock or water
    mixed with 1–2 fish stock cubes

2–3 tbsp olive oil

1 onion, chopped

2 fresh green chillies, such as
    serrano, deseeded and
    thinly sliced

lime wedges, to serve

1 Heat a dry, heavy-based frying pan over a high heat. Add the tomatoes and garlic and cook until the skins are blackened and the flesh is tender. Alternatively, cook under a preheated hot grill, or place the tomatoes and garlic in a roasting tin and bake in a preheated oven at 190°C/375°F/Gas Mark 5 for 40 minutes.

2 Leave the tomatoes and garlic to cool, then remove the skins and roughly chop, combining them with any juices from the frying or grill pan or roasting tin. Set aside.

3 Poach the fish in the stock in a deep frying pan or saucepan over a medium heat until it is just opaque and slightly firm. Remove from the heat and set aside.

4 Heat the oil in a separate deep frying pan or saucepan. Add the onion and cook for 5 minutes, or until softened. Strain in the cooking liquid from the fish, then stir in the tomatoes and garlic.

5 Bring to the boil, then reduce the heat and simmer for 5 minutes to combine the flavours. Add the chillies.

6 Divide chunks of the poached fish between soup bowls and ladle over the hot soup. Serve with lime wedges for squeezing over the top.

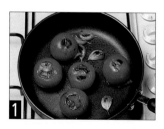

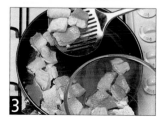

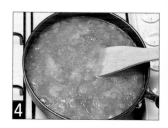

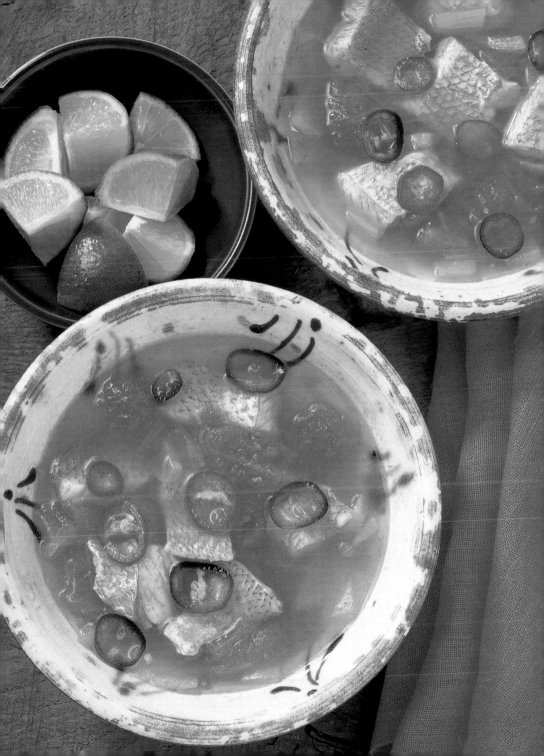

thai fish soup

serves four

450 ml/16 fl oz light chicken stock

2 kaffir lime leaves, chopped

5-cm/2-inch piece fresh lemon grass, chopped

3 tbsp lemon juice

3 tbsp Thai fish sauce

2 small hot fresh green chillies, deseeded and finely chopped

½ tsp sugar

8 small shiitake mushrooms, halved

450 g/1 lb raw prawns, peeled if necessary and deveined

spring onions, to garnish

TOM YAM SAUCE

4 tbsp vegetable oil

5 garlic cloves, finely chopped

1 large shallot, finely chopped

2 large hot dried red chillies, chopped

1 tbsp dried shrimps (optional)

1 tbsp Thai fish sauce

2 tsp sugar

1 First make the tom yam sauce. Heat the oil in a small saucepan. Cook the garlic briefly until just brown, remove with a slotted spoon and set aside. Cook the shallot in the oil until brown and crisp and remove with a slotted spoon. Add the dried chillies and fry until they darken. Remove and drain on kitchen paper, reserving the oil for later use.

2 In a small food processor or spice grinder, grind the dried shrimps, if using, then add the reserved chillies, garlic and shallot. Grind to a smooth paste. Return the paste to the original saucepan over a low heat. Mix in the fish sauce and sugar, then remove from the heat.

> **COOK'S TIP**
>
> Ready-made tom yam sauce in jars can be bought from some Oriental supermarkets.

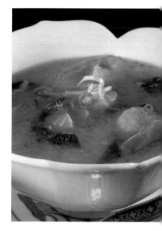

3 Heat the stock and 2 tablespoons of the sauce in a large saucepan. Add the lime leaves, lemon grass, lemon juice, fish sauce, fresh chillies and sugar. Simmer for 2 minutes.

4 Add the mushrooms and prawns and cook for a further 2–3 minutes, or until the prawns are cooked. Ladle the soup into warmed bowls and serve immediately, garnished with spring onions.

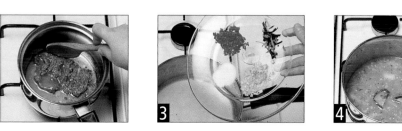

chinese crab & sweetcorn soup

serves four

1 tbsp vegetable oil

1 small onion, finely chopped

1 garlic clove, finely chopped

1 tsp grated fresh root ginger

1 small fresh red chilli, deseeded
and finely chopped

2 tbsp dry sherry or Chinese
rice wine

225 g/8 oz fresh white crabmeat

325 g/11½ oz canned sweetcorn
kernels, drained

600 ml/1 pint light chicken stock

1 tbsp light soy sauce

2 tbsp chopped fresh coriander

2 eggs, beaten

salt and pepper

chilli 'flowers', to garnish (optional)

2 Heat the oil in a large saucepan and add the onion. Cook gently for 5 minutes until softened. Add the garlic, ginger and chilli and cook gently for a further minute.

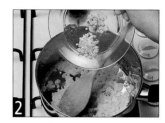

3 Add the sherry and bubble until reduced by half. Add the crabmeat, sweetcorn, stock and soy sauce. Bring to the boil, then simmer for 5 minutes. Stir in the coriander and salt and pepper to taste.

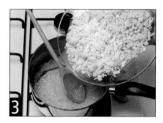

4 Remove from the heat and pour in the eggs. Wait for a few seconds, then stir well to break the eggs into ribbons. Serve the soup immediately, garnished with the chilli 'flowers', if using.

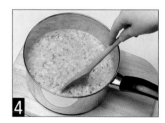

1 To make chilli 'flowers', hold the stem of each chilli with your fingertips and use a small sharp, pointed knife to cut a slit from near the stem end to the tip. Turn a quarter turn and make another cut. Repeat to make a total of 4 cuts, then scrape out the seeds. Cut each 'petal' again, in half or into quarters, to make 8–16 petals. Place the chilli in iced water.

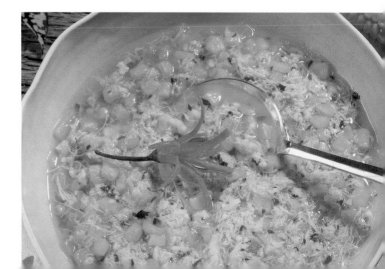

seafood stew

serves four–six

225 g/8 oz live clams

700 g/1 lb 9 oz mixed fish, such as
sea bass, skate, red snapper, rock
fish and any Mediterranean fish
you can find

12–18 raw tiger prawns

about 3 tbsp olive oil

1 large onion, finely chopped

2 garlic cloves, very finely chopped

2 tomatoes, halved, deseeded
and chopped

700 ml/1¼ pints good quality,
ready-made chilled fish stock

1 tbsp tomato purée

1 tsp fresh thyme leaves

pinch of saffron threads

pinch of sugar

salt and pepper

finely chopped fresh parsley,
to garnish

1 Soak the clams in a bowl of lightly salted cold water for 30 minutes. Rinse them under cold running water and lightly scrub to remove any sand from the shells. Discard any broken clams or open clams that do not shut when firmly tapped with the back of a knife, as these will be unsafe to eat.

2 Prepare the fish as necessary, removing any skin and bones, then cut into bite-sized chunks.

3 To prepare the prawns, break off the heads. Peel off the shells, leaving the tails intact, if wished. Using a small knife, make a slit along the back of each and remove the thin black vein. Set all the seafood aside.

4 Heat the oil in a large saucepan. Add the onion and cook for 5 minutes, stirring. Add the garlic and cook for a further 2 minutes, or until the onion is softened but not brown.

5 Add the tomatoes, stock, tomato purée, thyme, saffron and sugar, then bring to the boil, stirring to dissolve the tomato purée. Reduce the heat, cover and simmer for 15 minutes. Season to taste with salt and pepper.

6 Add the seafood and simmer until the clams open and the fish flakes easily. Discard any clams that do not open. Garnish with parsley and serve immediately.

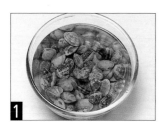

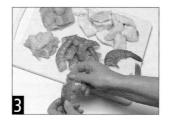

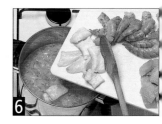

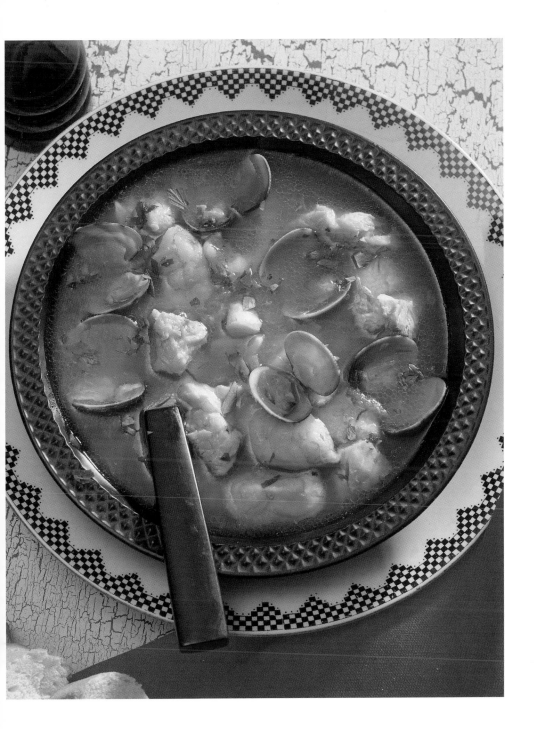

prawns in green bean sauce

serves four

2 tbsp vegetable oil

3 onions, chopped

5 garlic cloves, chopped

5–7 ripe tomatoes, diced

175–225 g/6–8 oz green beans,
  cut into 5-cm/2-inch pieces
  and blanched for 1 minute

¼ tsp ground cumin

pinch of ground allspice

pinch of ground cinnamon

½–1 canned chipotle chilli in
  adobo marinade, with some of
  the marinade

450 ml/l6 fl oz fish stock or water
  mixed with 1 fish stock cube

450 g/1 lb raw prawns, peeled
  and deveined

fresh coriander sprigs, to garnish

1 lime, cut into wedges,
  to serve (optional)

VARIATION

If you can find them, use bottled
nopales (edible cactus), cut into
strips, to add an exotic touch
to the dish.

1 Heat the oil in a large, deep frying pan. Add the onions and garlic and cook over a low heat for 5–10 minutes, or until softened. Add the tomatoes and cook for a further 2 minutes.

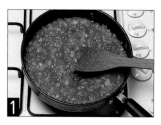

2 Add the beans, cumin, allspice, cinnamon, the chilli and marinade and stock. Bring to the boil, then reduce the heat and simmer for a few minutes to combine the flavours.

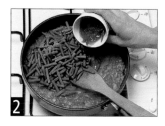

3 Add the prawns and cook for 1–2 minutes only, then remove the frying pan from the heat and leave the prawns to steep in the hot liquid to finish cooking. They are cooked when they have turned a bright pink colour.

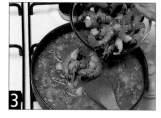

4 Serve the prawns immediately, garnished with the coriander sprigs and accompanied by the lime wedges, if wished.

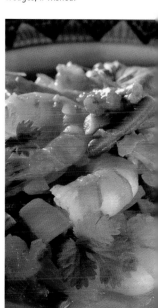

squid simmered with tomatoes & olives

serves four

3 tbsp virgin olive oil

900 g/2 lb cleaned squid, cut into
  rings and tentacles

salt and pepper

1 onion, chopped

3 garlic cloves, chopped

400 g/14 oz canned chopped
  tomatoes

½–1 fresh mild–medium green
  chilli, deseeded and chopped

1 tbsp finely chopped fresh parsley

¼ tsp chopped fresh thyme

¼ tsp chopped fresh oregano

¼ tsp chopped fresh marjoram

large pinch of ground cinnamon

large pinch of ground allspice

large pinch of sugar

15–20 pimento-stuffed green
  olives, sliced

1 tbsp capers

1 tbsp chopped fresh coriander,
  to garnish

1 Heat the oil in a deep, heavy-based frying pan. Add the squid and lightly cook until it turns opaque. Season to taste with salt and pepper and remove from the frying pan with a slotted spoon. Set aside in a bowl.

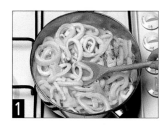

2 Add the onion and garlic to the remaining oil in the frying pan and cook for 5 minutes, or until softened. Stir in the tomatoes, chilli, herbs, cinnamon, allspice, sugar and olives. Cover and cook over a medium–low heat for 5–10 minutes, or until the mixture thickens slightly. Uncover the frying pan and cook for a further 5 minutes to concentrate the flavours.

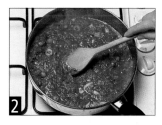

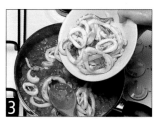

3 Stir in the reserved squid and any of the juices that have gathered in the bowl. Add the capers to the mixture and heat through.

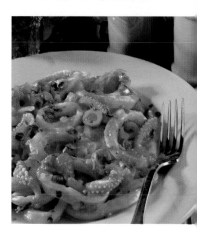

4 Taste and adjust the seasoning, then serve immediately, garnished with coriander.

mussels marinara

2 kg/4 lb 8 oz live mussels

4 tbsp olive oil

4–6 large garlic cloves, halved

800 g/1 lb 12 oz canned
    chopped tomatoes

300 ml/10 fl oz dry white wine

2 tbsp finely chopped fresh
    flat-leaved parsley, plus extra
    to garnish

1 tbsp finely chopped fresh oregano

salt and pepper

French bread, to serve

1 Soak the mussels in a bowl of lightly salted cold water for 30 minutes. Rinse them under cold running water and lightly scrub to remove any sand from the shells. Using a small, sharp knife, remove the 'beards' from the shells.

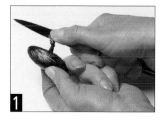

2 Discard any broken mussels or open mussels that do not shut when firmly tapped with the back of a knife. This indicates they are dead and could cause food poisoning if eaten. Rinse the mussels again, then set aside in a colander.

3 Heat the oil in a large saucepan or pot over a medium–high heat. Add the garlic and cook, stirring, for 3 minutes. Using a slotted spoon, remove the garlic from the saucepan.

4 Add the tomatoes and their juice, the wine, parsley and oregano and bring to the boil, stirring. Reduce the heat, cover and simmer for 5 minutes to allow the flavours to blend.

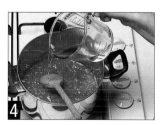

5 Add the mussels, cover the pan and simmer for 5–8 minutes, shaking the pan regularly, until the mussels open. Using a slotted spoon, transfer the mussels to serving bowls, discarding any that remain closed.

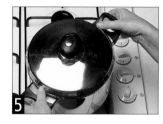

6 Season the sauce to taste with salt and pepper. Ladle the sauce over the mussels, sprinkle with extra chopped parsley and serve immediately with plenty of fresh French bread to mop up the delicious juices.

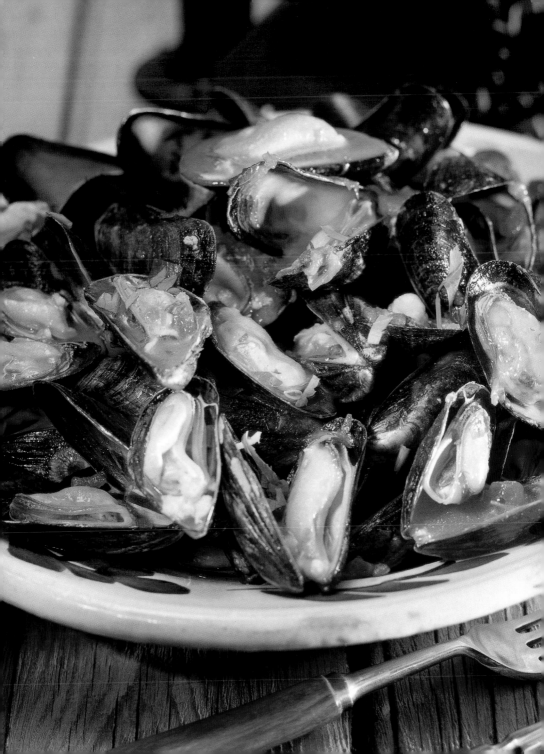

seafood rice

4 tbsp olive oil

16 large raw prawns, peeled

225 g/8 oz cleaned squid, sliced

2 green peppers, deseeded and cut into strips

1 large onion, finely chopped

4 garlic cloves, finely chopped

2 bay leaves

1 tsp saffron threads

½ tsp crushed dried chillies

400 g/14 oz arborio or Valencia rice

225 ml/8 fl oz dry white wine

850 ml/1½ pints fish or chicken stock

salt and pepper

12–16 live clams, scrubbed

12–16 large live mussels, scrubbed and debearded

2 tbsp chopped fresh flat-leaved parsley

RED PEPPER SAUCE

2–3 tbsp olive oil

2 onions, finely chopped

4–6 garlic cloves, finely chopped

4–6 Italian roasted red peppers in olive oil

400 g/14 oz canned chopped tomatoes

1–1½ tsp hot paprika

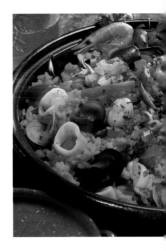

1 To make the red pepper sauce, heat the oil in a frying pan over a medium heat. Add the onions and cook for 6–8 minutes, or until golden. Add the garlic and cook for 1 minute. Add the remaining ingredients and simmer, stirring occasionally, for 10 minutes. Process in a food processor until smooth. Set aside and keep warm.

2 Heat half the oil in a wide frying pan over a high heat. Add the prawns and stir-fry for 2 minutes, or until pink. Transfer to a plate. Add the squid and stir-fry for 2 minutes, or until just firm. Set aside with the prawns.

3 Heat the remaining oil in the pan. Add the peppers and onion and stir-fry for 6 minutes, or until just tender. Stir in the garlic, bay leaves, saffron and chillies and cook for 30 seconds. Add the rice and cook, stirring, until thoroughly coated.

4 Add the wine and stir until absorbed. Add the stock and salt and pepper to taste. Bring to the boil. Reduce the heat, cover and simmer for 20 minutes, or until the rice is just tender and the liquid almost absorbed.

5 Add the clams and mussels, re-cover and cook for 10 minutes, or until the shells open. Discard any that remain closed. Stir in the prawns and squid. Re-cover and heat through gently. Sprinkle with the chopped parsley and serve immediately with the red pepper sauce.

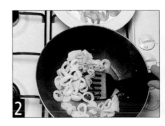

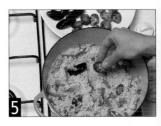

prawn & asparagus risotto

serves four

1.2 litres/2 pints vegetable stock

350 g/12 oz asparagus, cut
into 5-cm/2-inch lengths

2 tbsp olive oil

1 onion, finely chopped

1 garlic clove, finely chopped

350 g/12 oz arborio rice

450 g/1 lb raw tiger prawns, peeled
and deveined

2 tbsp olive paste or tapenade

2 tbsp chopped fresh basil

salt and pepper

Parmesan cheese shavings,
to garnish

1 Bring the stock to the boil in
a large saucepan. Add the
asparagus and cook for 3 minutes, or
until just tender. Strain, reserving the
stock, and refresh under cold running
water. Drain and set aside.

COOK'S TIP

Use a vegetable peeler to make
shavings quickly and easily from
a piece of Parmesan cheese
for the garnish.

2 Heat the oil in a large, heavy-
based frying pan. Add the onion
and cook over a low heat, stirring
occasionally, for 5 minutes, or until
softened. Add the garlic and cook
for a further 30 seconds. Add the
rice and cook, stirring constantly, for
1–2 minutes, or until coated with the
oil and slightly translucent.

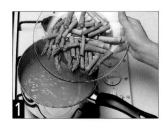

3 Keep the stock on a low heat.
Increase the heat under the
frying pan to medium and begin
adding the stock, a ladleful at a time,
stirring well between additions.
Continue until almost all the stock
has been absorbed. This should take
20–25 minutes.

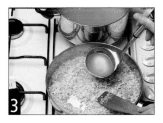

4 Add the prawns and asparagus
with the last ladleful of stock and
cook for a further 5 minutes, or until
the prawns and rice are tender and the
stock has been absorbed. Remove from
the heat.

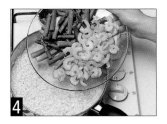

5 Stir in the olive paste, basil and
salt and pepper to taste. Set aside
for 1 minute. Garnish with Parmesan
and serve.

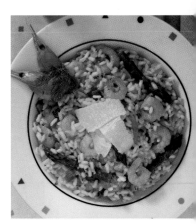

creole jambalaya

serves six–eight

2 tbsp vegetable oil

85 g/3 oz smoked ham, cut into
  bite-sized pieces

85 g/3 oz andouille or other smoked
  pork sausage, cut into chunks

2 large onions, finely chopped

3–4 celery sticks, finely chopped

2 green peppers, deseeded
  and diced

2 garlic cloves, finely chopped

225 g/8 oz skinless, boneless
  chicken breasts or thighs, cut
  into pieces

4 tomatoes, peeled and chopped

175 ml/6 fl oz passata

450 ml/16 fl oz fish stock

400 g/14 oz long-grain rice

4 spring onions, thickly sliced

250 g/9 oz raw prawns, peeled

250 g/9 oz cooked white crabmeat

12 oysters, shelled, with their liquor

SEASONING MIX

2 dried bay leaves

1 tsp salt

1½–2 tsp cayenne pepper

1½ tsp dried oregano

1 tsp ground white pepper

1 tsp black pepper

1 To make the seasoning mix, combine all the ingredients in a bowl until well mixed.

2 Heat the oil in a flameproof casserole over a medium heat. Add the ham and sausage and cook for 8 minutes, stirring frequently, until golden. Using a slotted spoon, transfer to a large plate.

3 Add the onions, celery and peppers to the casserole and cook for 4 minutes, or until just softened. Stir in the chopped garlic, then remove and set aside.

4 Add the chicken to the casserole and cook for 3–4 minutes, or until beginning to colour. Stir in the seasoning mix to coat. Return the ham, sausage and vegetables to the casserole and stir to combine. Add the tomatoes and passata, then pour in the stock. Bring to the boil.

5 Stir in the rice, then reduce the heat, cover and simmer for 12 minutes. Stir in the spring onions and prawns, cover and cook for 4 minutes.

6 Gently stir in the crabmeat and oysters with their liquor. Cook until the rice is just tender. Remove from the heat and leave to stand, covered, for about 3 minutes before serving.

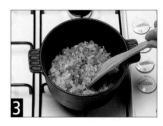

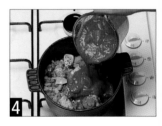

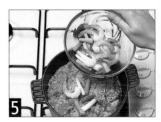

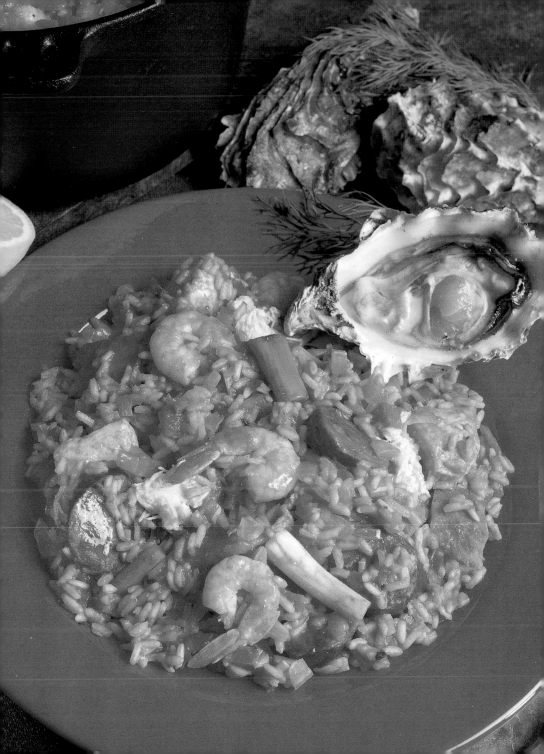

goan fish curry

serves four

750 g/1 lb 10 oz monkfish fillet,
cut into chunks

1 tbsp cider vinegar

1 tsp salt

1 tsp ground turmeric

3 tbsp vegetable oil

2 garlic cloves, crushed

1 small onion, finely chopped

2 tsp ground coriander

1 tsp cayenne pepper

2 tsp paprika

2 tbsp tamarind pulp plus 2 tbsp
boiling water (see Step 4)

85 g/3 oz creamed coconut,
cut into pieces

300 ml/10 fl oz warm water

plain boiled rice, to serve

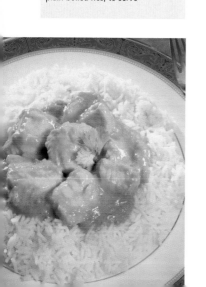

1 Put the fish on a plate and drizzle the vinegar over it. Combine half the salt and half the turmeric and sprinkle evenly over the fish. Cover and set aside for 20 minutes.

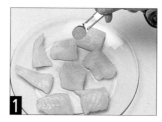

2 Heat the oil in a heavy-based frying pan and add the garlic. Brown slightly, then add the onion and cook, stirring occasionally, for 3–4 minutes, or until softened but not browned. Add the coriander and stir-fry for 1 minute.

3 Mix the remaining turmeric, cayenne pepper and paprika with about 2 tablespoons of water to make a paste. Add to the pan and cook over a low heat for 1–2 minutes.

COOK'S TIP

Tamarind, usually sold in blocks of dried pulp, imparts a sour yet slightly sweet flavour to curries.

4 In a heatproof bowl, stir the tamarind and boiling water together. When thickened and the pulp has separated from the seeds, rub through a sieve. Discard the seeds.

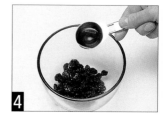

5 Add the coconut cream, warm water and tamarind paste to the pan and stir until the coconut has dissolved. Add the fish and any juices on the plate and simmer gently for 4–5 minutes, or until the sauce has thickened and the fish is just tender. Serve on a bed of plain boiled rice.

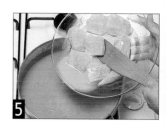

thai green fish curry

serves four

2 tbsp vegetable oil

1 garlic clove, chopped

1 small aubergine, diced

125 ml/4 fl oz coconut cream

2 tbsp Thai fish sauce

1 tsp sugar

225 g/8 oz firm white fish, cut into
    pieces, such as cod, haddock
    or halibut

125 ml/4 fl oz fish stock

2 kaffir lime leaves, finely shredded

about 15 leaves fresh Thai basil or
    ordinary basil

plain boiled rice or noodles, to serve

GREEN CURRY PASTE

5 fresh green chillies, deseeded
    and chopped

2 tsp chopped lemon grass stalks

1 large shallot, chopped

2 garlic cloves, chopped

1 tsp grated fresh root ginger
    or galangal

2 sprigs of fresh coriander, chopped

½ tsp ground coriander

¼ tsp ground cumin

1 kaffir lime leaf, finely chopped

½ tsp salt

1 To make the curry paste, put all the ingredients into a food processor or spice grinder and blend to a smooth paste, adding a little water if necessary. Alternatively, pound together all the ingredients, using a pestle and mortar, until smooth. Set the curry paste aside.

2 Heat the oil in a frying pan or wok until almost smoking. Add the garlic and fry until golden. Add the curry paste and stir-fry for a few seconds. Add the aubergine and stir-fry for 4–5 minutes, or until softened.

3 Add the coconut cream. Bring to the boil and stir until the cream thickens and curdles slightly. Add the fish sauce and sugar and stir into the curry mixture.

4 Add the fish pieces and stock. Simmer, stirring occasionally, for 3–4 minutes, or until the fish is just tender. Add the lime leaves and basil, then cook for a further minute.

5 Transfer to a warmed serving dish and serve with plain boiled rice or noodles.

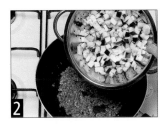

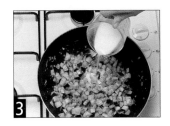

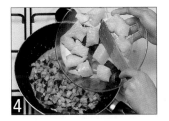

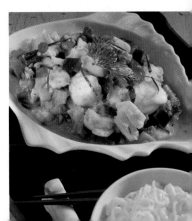

bouillabaisse

5 tbsp olive oil

2 large onions, finely chopped

1 leek, finely chopped

4 garlic cloves, crushed

½ small fennel bulb, finely chopped

5 ripe tomatoes, peeled
  and chopped

1 fresh thyme sprig

2 strips orange rind

salt and pepper

1.7 litres/3 pints hot fish stock

2 kg/4 lb 8 oz mixed seafood,
  such as John Dory, sea bass,
  bream, red mullet, cod and
  skate, roughly chopped;
  soft-shell crabs, raw prawns
  and langoustines, left whole

12–18 thick slices French bread

RED PEPPER & SAFFRON SAUCE

1 red pepper, deseeded
  and quartered

150 ml/5 fl oz light olive oil

1 egg yolk

large pinch of saffron threads

pinch of dried chilli flakes

lemon juice, to taste

salt and pepper

1 To make the sauce, brush the pepper pieces with a little of the oil and cook under a preheated hot grill for 5–6 minutes on each side, or until charred and tender. Remove from the heat and place in a polythene bag until cool enough to handle. Peel the skins away.

2 Place the pepper pieces in a food processor with the egg yolk, saffron, chilli flakes, lemon juice and salt and pepper to taste and process until smooth. Begin adding the remaining oil, drop by drop, until the mixture begins to thicken. Continue adding the oil in a steady stream until it is all incorporated and the mixture is thick. Add a little hot water if too thick.

3 In a large saucepan, heat the oil, add the onions, leek, garlic and fennel and cook for 10–15 minutes, or until softened and beginning to colour. Add the tomatoes, thyme, orange rind and salt and pepper to taste and cook for a further 5 minutes, or until the tomatoes have collapsed.

4 Add the stock and bring to the boil. Reduce the heat and simmer gently for 10 minutes, or until all the vegetables are tender. Add the seafood and return to the boil, then reduce the heat and simmer gently for 10 minutes, or until all the seafood is tender.

5 When the soup is ready, toast the bread on both sides. Using a slotted spoon, divide the fish between serving plates. Add some of the soup to moisten and serve with the bread. Hand round the sauce to accompany. Serve the remaining soup separately.

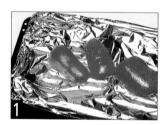

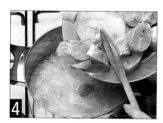

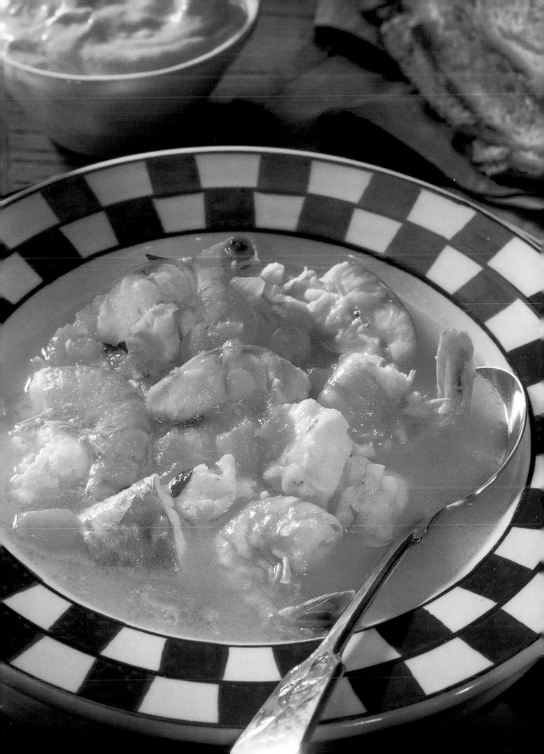

cotriade

serves four

large pinch of saffron threads

600 ml/1 pint hot fish stock

1 tbsp olive oil

2 tbsp butter

1 onion, sliced

2 garlic cloves, chopped

1 leek, sliced

1 small fennel bulb, thinly sliced

450 g/1 lb potatoes, cut into chunks

150 ml/5 fl oz dry white wine

1 tbsp fresh thyme leaves

2 bay leaves

4 ripe tomatoes, peeled
and chopped

900 g/2 lb mixed fish fillets, such as
haddock, hake, mackerel, red or
grey mullet, roughly chopped

2 tbsp chopped fresh parsley

salt and pepper

crusty bread, to serve

COOK'S TIP

Once the fish and vegetables
have been cooked, you could
process the soup in a food
processor or blender and sieve
it to give a smooth fish soup.

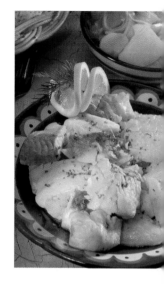

1 Using a pestle and mortar, crush the saffron and add to the stock. Stir the mixture and set aside to infuse for at least 10 minutes.

2 Heat the oil and butter together in a large, heavy-based saucepan. Add the onion and cook over a low heat, stirring occasionally, for 4–5 minutes, or until softened. Add the garlic, leek, fennel and potatoes. Cover and cook for a further 10–15 minutes, or until the vegetables are softened.

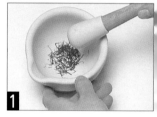

3 Add the wine and simmer rapidly for 3–4 minutes, or until reduced by about half. Add the thyme, bay leaves and tomatoes and stir well. Add the saffron-infused stock. Bring to the boil, then reduce the heat, cover and simmer gently for 15 minutes, or until all the vegetables are tender.

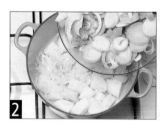

4 Add the fish and return to the boil. Reduce the heat and simmer for a further 3–4 minutes, or until all the fish is tender. Add the parsley and salt and pepper to taste. Using a slotted spoon, transfer the fish and vegetables to a warmed serving dish. Serve with plenty of crusty bread.

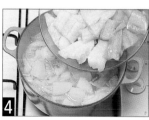

prawns with tomatoes

3 onions

1 green pepper

1 tsp finely chopped fresh
   root ginger

1 garlic clove, crushed

1 tsp salt

1 tsp chilli powder

2 tbsp lemon juice

350 g/12 oz frozen cooked
   peeled prawns

3 tbsp oil

400 g/14 oz canned tomatoes

chopped fresh coriander, to garnish

boiled rice and green salad, to serve

COOK'S TIP

Fresh root ginger looks rather
like a knobbly potato. The
skin should be peeled, then
the flesh either grated, finely
chopped or sliced. Ginger is
also available ground: this can
be used as a substitute for fresh
root ginger, but the flavour of
the fresh root is far superior.

---

1 Using a sharp knife, slice the onions and deseed and slice the green pepper.

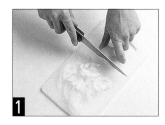

2 Place the ginger, garlic, salt and chilli powder in a small bowl and mix to combine. Add the lemon juice and mix to form a paste.

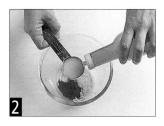

3 Place the prawns in a bowl of cold water and set aside to thaw. Drain thoroughly.

4 Heat the oil in a medium-sized frying pan. Add the onions and fry until golden brown.

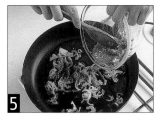

5 Add the spice paste to the onions, reduce the heat to low and cook, stirring and mixing well, for 3 minutes.

6 Add the tomatoes and their juice and the pepper, and cook for 5–7 minutes, stirring occasionally.

7 Add the prawns to the frying pan and cook for 10 minutes, stirring occasionally. Garnish with coriander and serve hot with plain boiled rice and a crisp green salad.

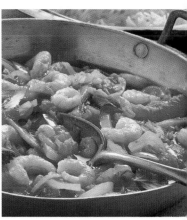

prawn & tuna pasta bake

serves four

225 g/8 oz tricolour pasta shapes

1 tbsp vegetable oil

1 bunch spring onions, chopped

175 g/6 oz button mushrooms,
   sliced

400 g/14 oz canned tuna in brine,
   drained and flaked

175 g/6 oz cooked peeled prawns,
   thawed if frozen

2 tbsp cornflour

425 ml/15 fl oz skimmed milk

salt and pepper

4 tomatoes, thinly sliced

25 g/1 oz fresh breadcrumbs

25 g/1 oz Cheddar cheese,
   grated

TO SERVE

wholemeal bread

fresh salad

1 Preheat the oven to 190°C/
375°F/Gas Mark 5. Bring a large
saucepan of water to the boil and
cook the pasta according to the packet
instructions. Drain well.

2 Meanwhile, heat the oil in a
frying pan and fry all but
a handful of the spring onions and
all of the mushrooms, stirring,
for 4–5 minutes, or until softened.

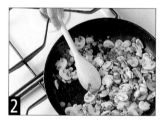

3 Place the cooked pasta in a bowl
and mix in the spring onions and
mushrooms, tuna and prawns. Set
aside until required.

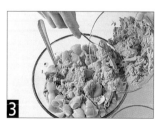

4 Blend the cornflour with a little of
the milk to make a paste. Pour
the remaining milk into a saucepan
and stir in the paste. Heat, stirring,
until the sauce begins to thicken.
Season well with salt and pepper.

5 Pour the sauce over the
pasta mixture and stir until
well combined. Transfer to an
ovenproof gratin dish and place on
a baking sheet.

6 Arrange the tomato slices over
the pasta and sprinkle with the
breadcrumbs and cheese. Bake in the
oven for 25–30 minutes, or until
golden. Serve, sprinkled with the
reserved spring onions and
accompanied by bread and salad.

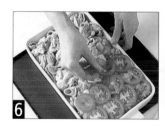

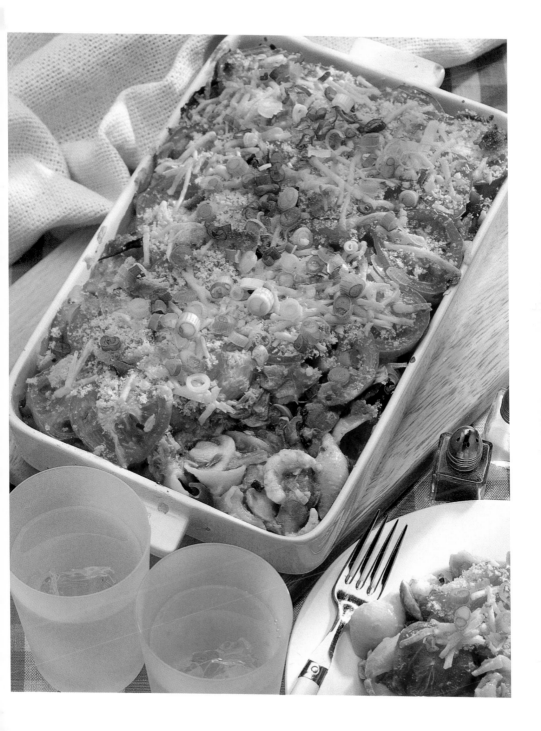

seafood lasagne

serves four

50 g/1¾ oz butter, plus extra
  for greasing
40 g/1½ oz flour
1 tsp mustard powder
600 ml/1 pint milk
2 tbsp olive oil
1 onion, chopped
2 garlic cloves, finely chopped
1 tbsp fresh thyme leaves
450 g/1 lb mixed mushrooms, sliced
150 ml/5 fl oz white wine
400 g/14 oz canned
  chopped tomatoes
salt and pepper
450 g/1 lb mixed skinless white fish
  fillets, cubed
225 g/8 oz shelled scallops, prepared
4–6 sheets fresh lasagne
225 g/8 oz mozzarella cheese,
  drained and chopped

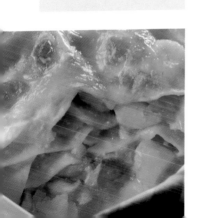

1 Preheat the oven to 200°C/400°F/
Gas Mark 6. Melt the butter in a
saucepan. Add the flour and mustard
powder and stir until smooth. Cook
gently for 2 minutes without colouring.
Gradually add the milk, whisking until
smooth. Bring to the boil, then reduce
the heat and simmer for 2 minutes.
Remove from the heat and set aside.
Cover the surface of the sauce with
clingfilm to prevent a skin forming.

2 Heat the oil in a frying pan over a
medium heat and add the onion,
garlic and thyme. Cook for 5 minutes,
or until softened. Add the mushrooms
and cook for a further 5 minutes, or
until softened. Stir in the wine and boil
rapidly until nearly evaporated. Stir in
the tomatoes. Bring to the boil, then
reduce the heat and simmer, covered,
for 15 minutes. Season to taste with
salt and pepper and set aside.

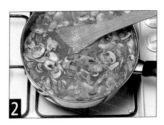

3 Lightly grease a lasagne dish.
Spoon half the tomato sauce over
the base of the dish and top with half
the fish and scallops.

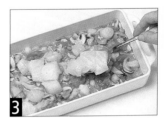

4 Layer half the lasagne over the
fish, pour over half the white
sauce and add half the mozzarella.
Repeat these layers, finishing with the
white sauce and mozzarella.

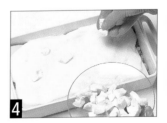

5 Bake the lasagne in the oven
for 35–40 minutes, or until
bubbling and golden and the fish is
cooked through. Remove from the
oven and leave to stand on a heat-
resistant surface or mat for 10 minutes
before serving.

seafood spaghetti

serves four

2 tsp olive oil

1 small red onion, finely chopped

1 tbsp lemon juice

1 garlic clove, crushed

2 celery sticks, finely chopped

150 ml/5 fl oz fish stock

150 ml/5 fl oz dry white wine

small bunch fresh tarragon

450 g/1 lb live mussels, scrubbed
and debearded

225 g/8 oz raw prawns, peeled
and deveined

225 g/8 oz baby squid, cleaned and
cut into rings

8 small cooked crab claws, cracked

225 g/8 oz dried spaghetti

salt and pepper

2 tbsp chopped fresh tarragon,
to garnish

COOK'S TIP

Crab claws contain lean
crabmeat. Ask your fishmonger
to crack the claws for you,
leaving the pincers intact,
because the shell is very tough.

1 Heat the oil in a large saucepan and fry the onion with the lemon juice, garlic and celery for 3–4 minutes, or until just softened.

2 Pour in the stock and wine. Bring to the boil and add the tarragon and mussels. Reduce the heat, cover and simmer for 5 minutes. Add the prawns, squid and crab claws to the pan, mix together and cook for 3–4 minutes, or until the mussels have opened, the prawns are pink and the squid is opaque. Discard the tarragon and any mussels that have not opened.

3 Meanwhile, cook the spaghetti in a saucepan of boiling water according to the packet instructions. Drain well.

4 Add the spaghetti to the shellfish mixture and toss together. Season to taste with salt and pepper.

5 Transfer to warmed serving plates and spoon over the cooking juices. Serve garnished with tarragon.

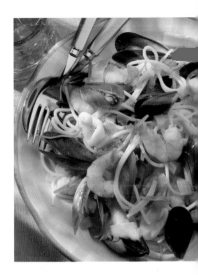

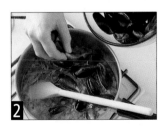

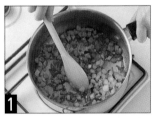

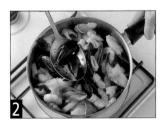

sardinian red mullet

serves four

50 g/1¾ oz sultanas

150 ml/5 fl oz red wine

2 tbsp olive oil

2 onions, sliced

1 courgette, cut into 5-cm/
 2-inch sticks

2 oranges

2 tsp coriander seeds,
 lightly crushed

4 red mullet, boned and filleted

50 g/1¾ oz canned anchovy
 fillets, drained

2 tbsp chopped fresh oregano

COOK'S TIP

Red mullet is usually available all
year round – frozen, if not fresh
– from your fishmonger or
supermarket. If you cannot get
hold of it, try using tilapia.
This dish can also be served
warm, if you prefer.

1 Place the sultanas in a bowl. Pour over the wine and leave to soak for 10 minutes.

2 Heat the oil in a large frying pan. Add the onions and sauté for 2 minutes.

3 Add the courgette to the pan and fry for a further 3 minutes, or until just tender.

4 Using a zester, pare long, thin strips of rind from one of the oranges. Using a sharp knife, remove the skin from both of the oranges, then segment the oranges by slicing between the lines of pith.

5 Add the orange rind to the frying pan. Add the wine, sultanas, coriander seeds, red mullet and anchovies to the pan and leave to simmer for 10–15 minutes, or until the fish is cooked through.

6 Stir in the oregano and orange segments, set aside and leave to cool. Place the mixture in a large bowl and leave to chill, covered, in the refrigerator for at least 2 hours so that the flavours mingle. Transfer to serving plates and serve immediately.

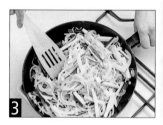

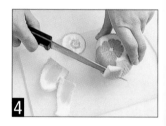

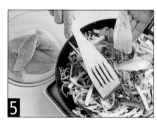

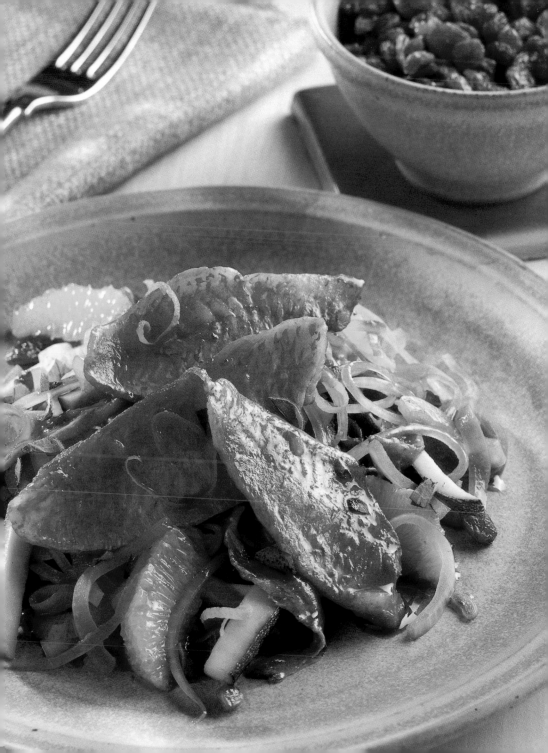

fideua

serves six

3 tbsp olive oil

1 large onion, chopped

2 garlic cloves, finely chopped

pinch of saffron threads, crushed

½ tsp paprika

3 tomatoes, peeled, deseeded
    and chopped

350 g/12 oz dried egg vermicelli,
    broken into 5-cm/2-inch lengths

150 ml/5 fl oz white wine

300 ml/10 fl oz fish stock

12 large raw prawns

18 live mussels, scrubbed
    and debearded

350 g/12 oz cleaned squid, cut
    into rings

18 large live clams, scrubbed

2 tbsp chopped fresh parsley

salt and pepper

lemon wedges, to serve

1 Heat the oil in a large frying pan or paella pan. Add the onion and cook over a low heat for 5 minutes, or until softened. Add the garlic and cook for a further 30 seconds. Add the saffron and paprika and stir well. Add the tomatoes and cook for a further 2–3 minutes until they have collapsed.

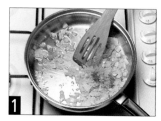

VARIATION
Try using langoustines, prawns and monkfish for a change.

2 Add the vermicelli and stir well. Add the wine to the pan and boil rapidly until it has been absorbed.

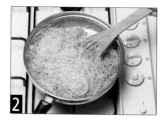

3 Add the stock, prawns, mussels, squid and clams. Stir and return to a low simmer for 10 minutes, or until the prawns and squid are cooked through and the mussels and clams have opened. Discard any that remain shut. The stock should be almost completely absorbed.

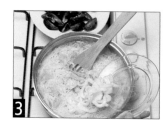

4 Add the parsley and season to taste with salt and pepper. Serve immediately in warmed bowls, with lemon wedges.

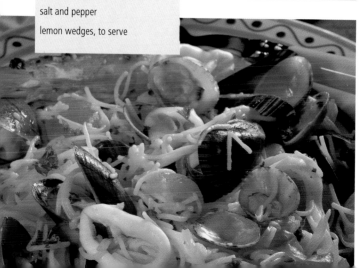

moroccan fish tagine

serves four

2 tbsp olive oil

1 large onion, finely chopped

pinch of saffron threads

½ tsp ground cinnamon

1 tsp ground coriander

½ tsp ground cumin

½ tsp ground turmeric

200 g/7 oz canned
    chopped tomatoes

300 ml/10 fl oz fish stock

4 small red mullet, cleaned, boned
    and heads and tails removed

55 g/2 oz stoned green olives

1 tbsp chopped preserved lemon

3 tbsp chopped fresh coriander

salt and pepper

couscous, to serve

COOK'S TIP

To preserve lemons, take enough
to fill a preserving jar. Quarter
them lengthways without cutting
right through. Pack with 55 g/
2 oz sea salt per lemon. Add the
juice of 1 more lemon and cover
with water. Leave for 1 month.

1 Heat the oil in a large saucepan
or flameproof casserole over a
low heat. Add the onion and cook,
stirring occasionally, for 10 minutes,
or until softened but not coloured.
Add the saffron, cinnamon, ground
coriander, cumin and turmeric and cook
for a further 30 seconds, stirring.

2 Add the tomatoes and stock and
stir well. Bring to the boil, then
reduce the heat, cover and simmer
for 15 minutes. Uncover and allow
the sauce to simmer for a further
20–35 minutes, or until thickened.

3 Cut each red mullet in half, then
add the pieces to the pan,
pushing them into the sauce. Simmer
for a further 5–6 minutes, or until the
fish is just cooked.

4 Carefully stir in the olives,
preserved lemon and the fresh
coriander. Season to taste with salt and
pepper and serve with couscous.

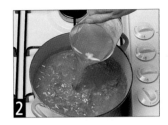

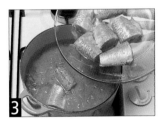

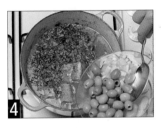

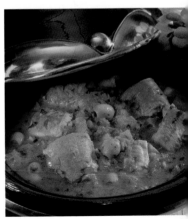

celery & salt cod casserole

serves four

250 g/9 oz salt cod,
  soaked overnight
1 tbsp oil
4 shallots, finely chopped
2 garlic cloves, chopped
3 celery sticks, chopped
400 g/14 oz canned
  tomatoes, chopped
150 ml/5 fl oz fish stock
50 g/1¾ oz pine kernels
2 tbsp roughly chopped
  fresh tarragon
2 tbsp capers
crusty bread or mashed potatoes,
  to serve

COOK'S TIP

Salt cod is a useful ingredient to keep in the storecupboard and, once soaked, can be used in the same way as any other fish. It does, however, have a stronger flavour than normal, and it is, of course, slightly salty. It can be found in fishmongers, larger supermarkets and delicatessens.

1 Drain the salt cod, rinse it under plenty of cold running water and drain again thoroughly. Remove and discard any skin and bones. Pat the fish dry with kitchen paper and then cut it into chunks.

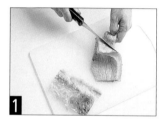

2 Heat the oil in a large frying pan. Add the shallots and garlic and cook for 2–3 minutes. Add the celery and cook for a further 2 minutes, then add the tomatoes and stock.

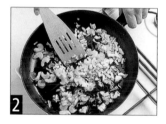

3 Bring the mixture to the boil, then reduce the heat and simmer for 5 minutes.

4 Add the fish and cook for 10 minutes, or until tender.

5 Meanwhile, preheat the grill. Place the pine kernels on a baking tray. Place under the hot grill and toast for 2–3 minutes, or until golden.

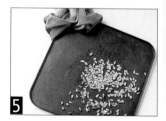

6 Stir the tarragon, capers and pine kernels into the fish casserole and heat gently to warm through.

7 Transfer to serving plates and serve with fresh crusty bread or mashed potatoes.

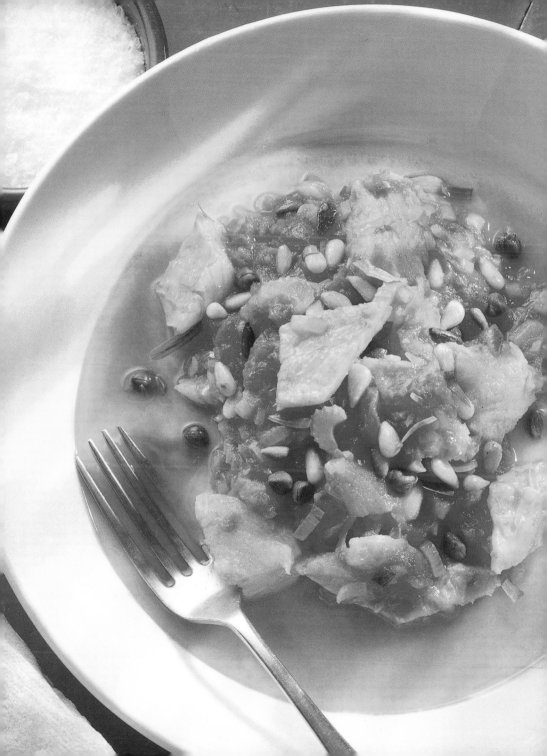

spanish fish stew

serves four

5 tbsp olive oil

2 large onions, finely chopped

2 tomatoes, peeled, deseeded and diced

2 slices white bread, crusts removed

4 almonds, toasted

3 garlic cloves, roughly chopped

350 g/12 oz cooked lobster

200 g/7 oz cleaned squid

200 g/7 oz monkfish fillet

200 g/7 oz cod fillet, skinned

salt and pepper

1 tbsp plain flour

6 large raw prawns

6 langoustines

18 live mussels, scrubbed and debearded

8 large live clams, scrubbed

1 tbsp chopped fresh parsley

125 ml/4 fl oz brandy

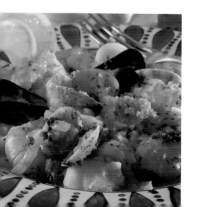

1 Heat 3 tablespoons of the oil in a frying pan over a medium heat and cook the onions for 10–15 minutes, or until lightly golden. Add the tomatoes and cook until they have collapsed. Set aside.

2 Heat 1 tablespoon of the remaining oil in a frying pan and fry the bread until crisp. Break into pieces and put into a mortar with the almonds and 2 garlic cloves. Pound to a fine paste with a pestle. Alternatively, process in a food processor.

3 Split the lobster lengthways. Remove and discard the intestinal vein, the stomach sac and the spongy gills. Crack the claws and remove the meat. Take out the flesh from the tail and chop into large chunks. Slice the squid into rings.

4 Season the monkfish, cod and lobster to taste with salt and pepper and dust with flour. Heat a little of the remaining oil in a flameproof casserole and separately brown the monkfish, cod, lobster, squid, prawns and langoustines. Then return all the fish to the casserole.

5 Add the mussels and clams and the remaining garlic and parsley. Set the casserole over a low heat. Pour over the brandy and ignite. When the flames have died down, add the tomato mixture and just enough water to cover. Bring to the boil, then simmer for 3–4 minutes, or until the mussels and clams have opened. Stir in the bread mixture and season. Simmer for a further few minutes, then serve.

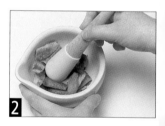

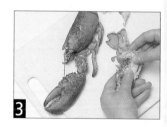

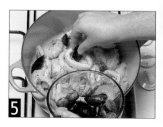

cuttlefish in their own ink

serves four

450 g/1 lb small cuttlefish, with
  their ink sacs

4 tbsp olive oil

1 small onion, finely chopped

2 garlic cloves, finely chopped

1 tsp paprika

175 g/6 oz ripe tomatoes, peeled,
  deseeded and chopped

150 ml/5 fl oz red wine

150 ml/5 fl oz fish stock

salt and pepper

225 g/8 oz instant polenta

3 tbsp chopped fresh
  flat-leaved parsley

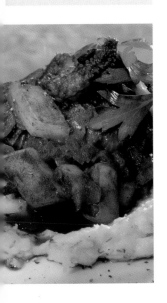

1 Cut off the cuttlefish tentacles in front of the eyes and remove the beak from the centre of the tentacles. Cut the head from the body and discard. Cut open the body section along the dark-coloured back. Remove the cuttle bone and the entrails, reserving the ink sac. Skin the body. Chop the flesh roughly and set aside. Split open the ink sac and dilute the ink in a little water. Set aside.

2 Heat the oil in a large saucepan over a medium heat, add the onion and cook for 8–10 minutes, or until softened and golden. Add the garlic and cook for a further 30 seconds. Add the cuttlefish and cook for a further 5 minutes, or until beginning to brown. Add the paprika and stir for 30 seconds before adding the tomatoes. Cook for 2–3 minutes, or until collapsed.

3 Add the wine, stock and diluted ink and stir well. Bring to the boil, then simmer gently, uncovered, for 25 minutes, or until the cuttlefish is tender and the sauce has thickened. Season to taste with salt and pepper.

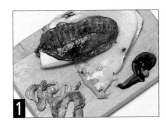

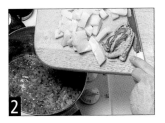

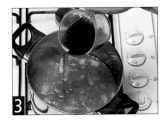

4 Meanwhile, cook the polenta according to the packet instructions. When cooked, remove from the heat and stir in the parsley and salt and pepper to taste.

5 Divide the polenta between plates and top with the cuttlefish and its sauce.

luxury fish pie

serves four

85 g/3 oz butter

3 shallots, finely chopped

115 g/4 oz button
  mushrooms, halved

2 tbsp dry white wine

900 g/2 lb live mussels, scrubbed
  and debearded

600 ml/1 pint fish stock

300 g/10½ oz monkfish fillet, cubed

300 g/10½ oz skinless
  cod fillet, cubed

300 g/10½ oz skinless lemon sole
  fillet, cubed

115 g/4 oz raw tiger prawns,
  peeled and deveined

25 g/1 oz plain flour

50 ml/2 fl oz double cream

salt and pepper

fresh parsley sprigs, to garnish

POTATO TOPPING

1.5 kg/3 lb 5 oz floury potatoes,
  cut into chunks

50 g/1¾ oz butter

2 egg yolks

125 ml/4 fl oz milk

pinch of freshly grated nutmeg

salt and pepper

1 Preheat the oven to 200°C/400°F/Gas Mark 6. For the filling, melt 25 g/1 oz of the butter in a frying pan, add the shallots and cook for 5 minutes, or until softened. Add the mushrooms and cook over a high heat for 2 minutes. Add the wine and simmer until the liquid has evaporated. Transfer to a 1.5-litre/2¾-pint shallow ovenproof dish and set aside.

2 Put the mussels into a large saucepan with just the water clinging to their shells and cook, covered, over a high heat for 3–4 minutes, or until all the mussels have opened. Discard any that remain closed. Drain, reserving the cooking liquid. When cool enough to handle, remove the mussels from their shells and add to the mushrooms.

3 Bring the stock to the boil in a large saucepan and add the monkfish. Poach gently for 2 minutes before adding the cod, sole and prawns. Poach for a further 2 minutes. Remove the seafood with a slotted spoon and add to the mussels and mushrooms.

4 Melt the remaining butter in a saucepan and add the flour. Stir until smooth and cook for 2 minutes without colouring. Gradually stir in the hot stock and mussel cooking liquid until smooth and thickened. Add the cream and simmer gently for 15 minutes, stirring. Season to taste with salt and pepper and pour over the seafood.

5 Meanwhile, make the topping. Boil the potatoes in plenty of salted water for 15–20 minutes, or until tender. Drain well and mash with the butter, egg yolks, milk, nutmeg and salt and pepper to taste. Pipe or spread over the seafood and roughen the surface of the topping with a fork.

6 Bake in the oven for 30 minutes until golden and bubbling. Serve straight from the oven, piping hot, garnished with parsley sprigs.

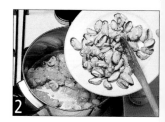

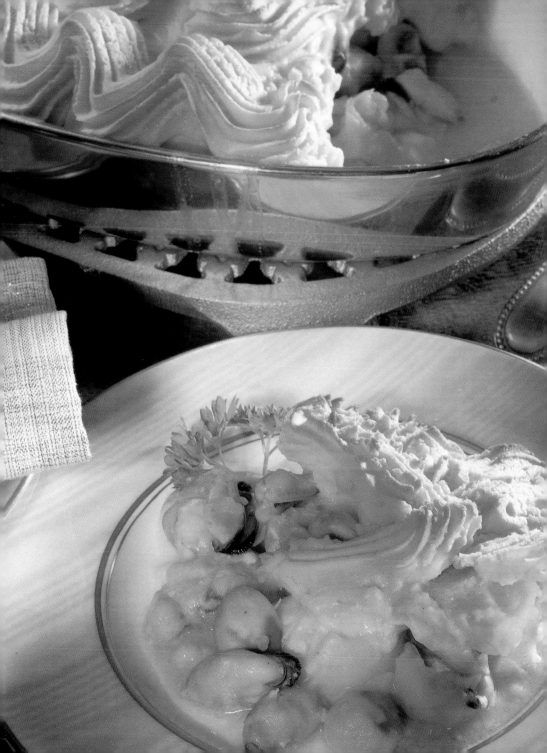